D1170792

NUTRITIONAL ONCOLOGY

Second Edition

EDITOR-IN-CHIEF

David Heber
Center for Human Nutrition
University of California, Los Angeles
Los Angeles, California

SENIOR EDITORS

George L. Blackburn
Beth Israel Deaconess Medical Center
Harvard Medical Center
Boston, Massachusetts

Vay Liang W. Go
David Geffen School of Medicine
University of California, Los Angeles
Los Angeles, California

John Milner
Nutritional Science Research Group
National Cancer Institute
Rockville, Maryland

NUTRITIONAL ONCOLOGY

Second Edition

Editor-in-Chief

David Heber
Center for Human Nutrition
University of California, Los Angeles
Los Angeles, California

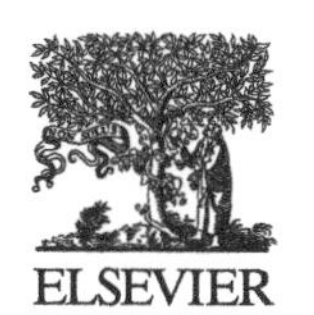

AMSTERDAM • BOSTON • HEIDELBERG • LONDON • NEW YORK • OXFORD
PARIS • SAN DIEGO • SAN FRANCISCO • SINGAPORE • SYDNEY • TOKYO
Academic Press is an imprint of Elsevier

Academic Press is an imprint of Elsevier
30 Corporate Drive, Suite 400, Burlington, MA 01803, USA
525 B Street, Suite 1900, San Diego, California 92101-4495, USA
84 Theobald's Road, London WC1X 8RR, UK

This book is printed on acid-free paper. 

Copyright © 2006, Elsevier Inc. All rights reserved.

No part of this publication may be reproduced or transmitted in any form or by any means, electronic or mechanical, including photocopy, recording, or any information storage and retrieval system, without permission in writing from the publisher.

Permissions may be sought directly from Elsevier's Science & Technology Rights Department in Oxford, UK: phone: (+44) 1865 843830, fax: (+44) 1865 853333, E-mail: permissions@elsevier.com. You may also complete your request on-line via the Elsevier homepage (http://elsevier.com), by selecting "Support & Contact" then "Copyright and Permission" and then "Obtaining Permissions."

Library of Congress Cataloging-in-Publication Data

Nutritional oncology / David L. Heber . . . [et al.].—2nd ed.
p. cm.
Includes bibliographical references and index.
ISBN 0-12-088393-7 (alk. paper)
1. Cancer–Nutritional aspects. 2. Cancer–diet therapy. I. Heber, David.
RC258.45.N886 2006
616.99′40654—dc22 2005059095

British Library Cataloging-in-Publication Data
A catalogue record for this book is available from the British Library.

ISBN 13: 978-0-12-088393-6
ISBN 10: 0-12-088393-7

For information on all Academic Press publications visit our Web site at www.books.elsevier.com

Transferred to Digital Printing in 2011

Working together to grow
libraries in developing countries

www.elsevier.com | www.bookaid.org | www.sabre.org

ELSEVIER BOOK AID International Sabre Foundation

Contents

III. Biological Approaches to Investigating Nutrition and Cancer

13. Endocrine and Paracrine Factors in Carcinogenesis 283

DAVID HEBER AND PINCHAS COHEN

14. Oxidation and Antioxidation in Cancer 297

PAUL DAVIS, DAVID HEBER, AND LESTER PACKER

15. Thiols in Cancer 307

JASON M. HANSEN AND DEAN P. JONES

16. Principles of Tumor Immunology 321

BENJAMIN BONAVIDA

17. Animal Models in Nutritional Oncology Research 333

JIN-RONG ZHOU

IV. Gene–Nutrient Interaction and Cancer Prevention

18. The Challenge of Nutrition in Cancer Prevention 349

PETER GREENWALD AND JOHN MILNER

19. Dietary Assessment 367

CATHERINE L. CARPENTER

20. Prostate Cancer 377

HOWARD PARNES, ASHRAFUL HOQUE, DEMETRIUS ALBANES, PHILIP TAYLOR, AND SCOTT LIPPMAN

21. Breast Cancer 393

DAVID HEBER AND GEORGE BLACKBURN

22. Skin Cancer 405

HOMER S. BLACK

23. Colon Cancer 423

LEO TREYZON, GORDON OHNING, AND DAVID HEBER

24. Gastric Cancer 437

NAI-CHIEH YUKO YOU AND ZUO-FENG ZHANG

25. Pancreatic Cancer 449

DIANE M. HARRIS, MANISH C. CHAMPANERIA, AND VAY LIANG W. GO

26. Bladder Cancer 475

ALLAN J. PANTUCK, RON LIEBERMAN, KELLY KAWAOKA, OLEG SHVARTS, AND DONALD LAMM

27. Differentiation Induction in Leukemia and Lymphoma 491

SVEN DE VOS AND H. PHILLIP KOEFFLER

V. Bioactive Food Components and Botanical Approaches to Cancer

28. Dietary Supplements in Cancer Prevention and Therapy 507

MARY FRANCES PICCIANO, BARBARA E. COHEN, AND PAUL R. THOMAS

29. Dietary Fiber and Carbohydrates 521

MARÍA ELENA MARTÍNEZ AND ELIZABETH T. JACOBS

30. Dietary Lipids 531

HUSEYIN AKTAS, MICHAEL CHOREV, AND J.A. HALPERIN

31. Calcium and Vitamin D 545

JOELLEN WELSH

32. Soy Isoflavones 559

STEPHEN BARNES, JEEVAN PRASAIN, TRACY D'ALESSANDRO, CHAO-CHENG WANG, HUANG-GE ZHANG, AND HELEN KIM

33. Selenium and Cancer Prevention 573

CLEMENT IP, JAMES MARSHALL, YOUNG-MEE PARK, HAITAO ZHANG, YAN DONG, YUE WU, AND ALLEN C. GAO

48. Dietary Interventions 779

LALITA KHAODHIAR AND GEORGE L. BLACKBURN

49. Future Directions in Cancer and Nutrition Research: Gene–Nutrient Interactions, Networks, and the Xenobiotic Hypothesis 807

DAVID HEBER, JOHN MILNER, GEORGE BLACKBURN, AND VAY LIANG W. GO

Contributing Authors

Huseyin Aktas, Brigham and Women's Hospital, Harvard Medical School, Boston, Massachusetts 02115

Demetrius Albanes, Division of Cancer Epidemiology and Genetics, National Cancer Institute, Bethesda, Maryland 20892

Leonard Augenlicht, Department of Oncology, Montefiore Medical Center, Albert Einstein Cancer Center, Bronx, New York 10467

Elisa V. Bandera, The Cancer Institute of New Jersey, Robert Wood Johnson Medical School, New Brunswick, New Jersey 08901

Stephen Barnes, Department of Pharmacology and Toxicology, University of Alabama at Birmingham, Birmingham, Alabama 35294

J. Carl Barrett, Center for Cancer Research, National Cancer Institute, Bethesda, Maryland 20892

Leslie Bernstein, Keck School of Medicine, University of Southern California, Los Angeles, California 90089

Radha M. Bheemreddy, Department of Food Science and Human Nutrition, University of Illinois, Urbana, Illinois 61801

Homer S. Black, Department of Dermatology, Baylor College of Medicine, Houston, Texas 77042

George L. Blackburn, Beth Israel Deaconess Medical Center, Harvard Medical Center, Boston, Massachusetts 02115

Benjamin Bonavida, Department of Microbiology, Immunology, and Molecular Genetics, University of California, Los Angeles, Los Angeles, California 90095

Laszlo G. Boros, Harbor UCLA Medical Center, University of California, Los Angeles, Los Angeles, California 90095

Susan Bowerman, Center for Human Nutrition, University of California, Los Angeles, Los Angeles, California 90095

Eve Callahan, Vanderbilt University Medical Center, Nashville, Tennessee 37232

Catherine L. Carpenter, Center for Human Nutrition, University of California, Los Angeles, Los Angeles, California 90095

David Cella, Institute for Health Services Research and Policy Studies, Northwestern University, Chicago, Illinois 60611

Manish C. Champaneria, Department of Medicine, David Geffen School of Medicine, University of California, Los Angeles, Los Angeles, California 90095

Michael Chorev, Brigham and Women's Hospital, Harvard Medical School, Boston, Massachusetts 02115

Judith Christman, Department of Oncology, Montefiore Medical Center, Albert Einstein Cancer Center, Bronx, New York 10467

Barbara E. Cohen, Division of Cancer Control and Population Sciences, National Cancer Institute, Bethesda, Maryland 20892

Pinchas Cohen, Mattel Children's Hospital, University of California, Los Angeles, Los Angeles, California 90095

Tracy D'Alessandro, Department of Pharmacology and Toxicology, University of Alabama at Birmingham, Birmingham, Alabama 35294

Paul Davis, Department of Nutrition, University of California, Davis, Davis, California 95616

Sven de Vos, Department of Hematology and Oncology, University of California, Los Angeles, Los Angeles, California 90095

Yan Dong, Department of Cancer Prevention and Population Sciences, Roswell Park Cancer Institute, Buffalo, New York 14263

Johanna Dwyer, Tufts University School of Medicine, New England Medical Center, Boston, Massachusetts 02111

Robert M. Elashoff, Department of Biomathematics, University of California, Los Angeles School of Medicine, Los Angeles, California 90095

Karam El-Bayoumy, Penn State Cancer Institute, Pennsylvania State University, Hershey, Pennsylvania 17033

Charles E. Elson, Department of Nutritional Sciences, University of Wisconsin, Madison, Wisconsin 53706

Michele R. Forman, MD Anderson Cancer Center, University of Texas, Houston, Texas 77030

Allen C. Gao, Departments of Medicine and Pharmacology & Therapeutics, Roswell Park Cancer Institute, Buffalo, New York 14263

Jeanine Genkinger, Department of Nutrition, Harvard School of Public Health, Boston, Massachusetts 02115

Ellen Giarelli, University of Pennsylvania School of Nursing, Philadelphia, Pennsylvania 19104

Edward Giovannucci, Department of Nutrition and Epidemiology, Harvard School of Public Health, Boston, Massachusetts 02115

Vay Liang W. Go, David Geffen School of Medicine, University of California, Los Angeles, Los Angeles, California 90095

Peter Greenwald, Division of Cancer Prevention, National Cancer Institute, Bethesda, Maryland 20892

Sandra Guilmeau, Department of Oncology, Montefiore Medical Center, Albert Einstein Cancer Center, Bronx, New York 10467

J.A. Halperin, Laboratory of Membrane Transport, Harvard Medical School, Boston, Massachusetts 02115

Jason M. Hansen, Department of Medicine, Emory University, Atlanta, Georgia 30322

Diane M. Harris, Center for Human Nutrition, University of California, Los Angeles, Los Angeles, California 90095

David Heber, Center for Human Nutrition, University of California, Los Angeles, Los Angeles, California 90095

Barbara Heerdt, Department of Medicine, Montefiore Medical Center, Albert Einstein Cancer Center, Bronx, New York 10467

Dietrich Hoffmann, Division of Cancer Etiology and Prevention, American Health Foundation, Valhalla, New York 10595

Ashraful Hoque, MD Anderson Cancer Center, University of Texas, Houston, Texas 77030

Stephen D. Hursting, Department of Human Ecology, College of Natural Sciences, University of Texas, Austin, Texas 78712

Clement Ip, Department of Cancer Chemoprevention, Roswell Park Cancer Institute, Buffalo, New York 14263

Elizabeth T. Jacobs, Arizona Cancer Center, University of Arizona, Tucson, Arizona 85724

Linda A. Jacobs, University of Pennsylvania Cancer Center, Philadelphia, Pennsylvania 19104

Elizabeth H. Jeffery, Department of Food Science and Human Nutrition, University of Illinois, Urbana, Illinois 61801

Gordon L. Jensen, Vanderbilt Center for Human Nutrition, Vanderbilt University, Nashville, Tennessee 37212

Dean P. Jones, Division of Pulmonary, Allergy, and Critical Care, Department of Medicine, Emory University, Atlanta, Georgia 30322

Kelly Kawaoka, John A. Burns School of Medicine, University of Hawaii at Manoa, Honolulu, Hawaii 96813

Lalita Khaodhiar, Beth Israel Deaconess Medical Center, Harvard Medical School, Boston, Massachusetts, 02115

Helen Kim, Department of Pharmacology and Toxicology, University of Alabama at Birmingham, Birmingham, Alabama 35294

Lidija Klampfer, Montefiore Medical Center, Albert Einstein Cancer Center, Bronx, New York 10467

David M. Klurfeld, Agricultural Research Service, United States Department of Agriculture, Beltsville, Maryland 20705

H. Phillip Koeffler, Jonsson Comprehensive Cancer Center, University of California, Los Angeles, Los Angeles, California 90095

Lawrence H. Kushi, Division of Research, Kaiser Permanente, Oakland, California 94611

Joshua D. Lambert, Department of Chemical Biology, Rutgers University, Piscataway, New Jersey 08854

Donald Lamm, BCG Oncology, Phoenix, Arizona 85032

Janelle M. Landau, Department of Chemical Biology, Rutgers University, Piscataway, New Jersey 08854

Wai-Nang Paul Lee, University of California, Los Angeles School of Medicine, Los Angeles, California 90095

Ron Lieberman, Division of Cancer Prevention, National Cancer Institute, Bethesda, Maryland 20892

Scott Lippman, MD Anderson Cancer Center, University of Texas, Houston, Texas 77030

Somdat Mahabir, Center for Cancer Research, National Cancer Institute, Bethesda, Maryland 20892

Sandra Maier, Montefiore Medical Center, Albert Einstein Cancer Center, Bronx, New York 10467

John Mariadason, Department of Oncology, Montefiore Medical Center, Albert Einstein Cancer Center, Bronx, New York 10467

James Marshall, Department of Cancer Prevention and Population Sciences, Roswell Park Cancer Institute, Buffalo, New York 14263

María Elena Martínez, Arizona Cancer Center, University of Arizona, Tucson, Arizona 85724

Marjorie McCullough, Department of Epidemiology and Surveillance Research, American Cancer Society, Atlanta, Georgia 30329

Anne McTiernan, Fred Hutchinson Cancer Research Center, University of Washington, Seattle, Washington 98109

John Milner, Nutritional Science Research Group, National Cancer Institute, Rockville, Maryland 20852

Huanbiao Mo, Department of Nutrition and Food Sciences, Texas Women's University, Denton, Texas 76204

Joshua E. Muscat, Penn State Cancer Institute, Pennsylvania State University, Hershey, Pennsylvania 17033

Nomeli P. Nunez, Department of Human Ecology, College of Natural Sciences, University of Texas, Austin, Texas 78712

Gordon Ohning, Department of Digestive Diseases and Gastroenterology, UCLA Medical Center, Los Angeles, California 90095

Lester Packer, School of Pharmacy, Molecular Pharmacology, and Toxicology, University of Southern California, Los Angeles, California, 90089

Allan J. Pantuck, Department of Urology, University of California, Los Angeles School of Medicine, Los Angeles, California 90095

Young-Mee Park, Department of Cell Stress Biology, Roswell Park Cancer Institute, Buffalo, New York 14263

Howard Parnes, National Cancer Institute, National Institutes of Health, Bethesda, Maryland 20892

Susan N. Perkins, Division of Cancer Prevention, National Cancer Institute, Bethesda, Maryland 20892

Mary Frances Picciano, Office of Dietary Supplements, National Institutes of Health, Bethesda, Maryland 20892

Jeevan Prasain, Department of Pharmacology and Toxicology, University of Alabama at Birmingham, Birmingham, Alabama 35294

Ramune Reliene, Department of Pathology, University of California, Los Angeles, Los Angeles, California 90089

Connie J. Rogers, Laboratory of Tumor Immunology and Biology, National Cancer Institute, Bethesda, Maryland 20892

Robert H. Schiestl, Department of Pathology, University of California, Los Angeles, Los Angeles, California 90089

Navindra P. Seeram, Center for Human Nutrition, University of California, Los Angeles, Los Angeles, California 90095

Oleg Shvarts, UCLA Medical Center, University of California, Los Angeles, Los Angeles, California 90095

Heidi J. Silver, Vanderbilt Center for Human Nutrition, Vanderbilt University, Nashville, Tennessee 37232

Helena Smartt, Montefiore Medical Center, Albert Einstein Cancer Center, Bronx, New York 10467

Stephanie A. Smith-Warner, Department of Nutrition, Harvard School of Public Health, Boston, Massachusetts 02115

Philip Taylor, Center for Cancer Research, National Cancer Institute, Bethesda, Maryland 20892

N. Simon Tchekmedyian, UCLA School of Medicine, University of California, Los Angeles, Los Angeles, California 90095

Paul R. Thomas, Office of Dietary Supplements, National Institutes of Health, Bethesda, Maryland 20892

Leo Treyzon, Center for Human Nutrition, University of California, Los Angeles, Los Angeles, California 90095

Anna Velcich, Department of Medicine, Montefiore Medical Center, Albert Einstein Cancer Center, Bronx, New York 10467

Chao-Cheng Wang, Department of Pharmacology and Toxicology, University of Alabama at Birmingham, Birmingham, Alabama 35294

JoEllen Welsh, Department of Biological Sciences, University of Notre Dame, South Bend, Indiana 46556

Yue Wu, Department of Cancer Chemoprevention, Roswell Park Cancer Institute, Buffalo, New York 14263

Chung S. Yang, Department of Chemical Biology, Rutgers University, Piscataway, New Jersey 08854

Wancai Yang, Montefiore Medical Center, Albert Einstein Cancer Center, Bronx, New York 10467

Nai-chieh Yuko You, Department of Epidemiology, School of Public Health, University of California, Los Angeles, Los Angeles, California 90095

Haitao Zhang, Department of Cancer Prevention and Population Sciences, Roswell Park Cancer Institute, Buffalo, New York 14263

Huang-Ge Zhang, Department of Medicine, University of Alabama at Birmingham, Birmingham, Alabama 35294

Zuo-Feng Zhang, University of California, Los Angeles School of Public Health, Los Angeles, California 90095

Jin-Rong Zhou, Beth Israel Deaconess Medical Center, Harvard Medical School, Boston, Massachusetts 02115

Preface

Nutritional oncology is an interdisciplinary field that bridges two areas of metabolic homeostasis—nutrition and cancer. Increasingly there are critical links being found between normal metabolic control, normal inflammation, normal genetic and epigenetic homeostasis, DNA repair, and the abnormal processes leading to the multistep process of carcinogenesis. The sequencing of the human genome and the rapidly expanding areas of molecular epidemiology, molecular endocrinology, and cellular signaling have provided new pathways for the study of the abnormal regulatory steps involved in initiating and maintaining carcinogenesis and the steps involved in the progression to metastatic spread.

From these insights it is clear that there are many genetic predispositions that can interact with a Western dietary pattern in experimental models and in human populations to lead to common forms of cancer. The Western dietary pattern does not exist in isolation but is found nested within a sedentary lifestyle and an excess of dietary fats, starches, and refined carbohydrates often combined with excess use of tobacco and alcohol. In the past few decades, the ability to modify environmental factors through nutritional counseling and exercise instruction has been refined, but the ability to modify the behavior of populations through public health measures and dietary guidelines remains a major challenge.

Medical oncologists, nurses, and dietitians will have an increasing opportunity to enhance their care of patients with cancer and those at risk by using the principles and information in this text. Basic scientists moving from a focus on molecular biology, genetics, and metabolism will have an opportunity to integrate basic science with questions important in clinical medicine. In these ways, the field of nutritional oncology aims to modify the environmental factors influencing the genetic changes and their expression at every stage of carcinogenesis, from the initiation of the cancer cell to its metastatic spread to other areas of the body.

This text is divided into the following sections: First, the biology of nutrition and cancer including fundamentals of human nutrition, nutrigenomics and nutrigenetics, genetics and epigenetics, metabolic networks, and energy balance in cancer are described. Second, the evidence from the nutritional epidemiology of cancer is explored, including fruit and vegetable consumption, whole grains, obesity, tobacco-related cancers, alcohol, and environmental toxins. Third, biological approaches to investigating cancer are described, including endocrine and paracrine factors, oxidants and antioxidants, thiols, tumor immunology, and animal models of cancer. Fourth, gene–nutrient interaction in cancer is explored, including an overview of the challenges facing the field, methodological issues in dietary assessment, and the evidence for specific cancers, including prostate cancer, breast cancer, skin cancer, colon cancer, gastric cancer, pancreatic cancer, bladder cancer, leukemia, and lymphoma. Fifth, bioactive food components are examined in detail, including dietary supplements, fiber and carbohydrates, dietary lipids, calcium and vitamin D, soy isoflavones, selenium, glucosinolates, green tea, garlic, berries, and isoprenoids. The sixth section deals with the nutritional assessment and support of the patient with cancer, including cancer anorexia and cachexia, weight management of the breast cancer survivor, nutritional support of the adult patient with cancer, endocrine effects of cancer and ectopic hormone syndromes, counseling the cancer survivor, and nutritional support in quality of life. Finally, the seventh section tackles the problem of implementing nutrition in guidelines and clinical practice, including an analysis of modern statistical methods, evidence-based practice management in prevention and treatment, dietary guidelines in cancer prevention, dietary interventions for cancer prevention, and the future of nutritional oncology with a detailed analysis of the prospects for personalized medicine based on gene–nutrient interaction.

We and our contributors have attempted to provide a comprehensive summary of the field of nutritional oncology from basic principles to the growing edge of research. We would like to thank Susan Bowerman, M.S., R.D., for her excellent editorial assistance and contributions to the organization of the writing efforts of so many authors, and Ms. Tari Paschall and her colleagues at Academic Press for their patience and support of this important publication.

David Heber, M.D., Ph.D. (Los Angeles, California)
George L. Blackburn, M.D., Ph.D. (Boston, Massachusetts)
Vay Liang W. Go, M.D. (Los Angeles, California)
John Milner, Ph.D. (Rockville, Maryland)

Introduction: The Principles of Nutritional Oncology

DAVID HEBER, GEORGE L. BLACKBURN, VAY LIANG W. GO, AND JOHN MILNER

WHAT IS NUTRITIONAL ONCOLOGY?

Nutritional oncology is an interdisciplinary field in which cancers are investigated as both systemic and local diseases originating by changes in the genome and progressing through a multistep process that may be modified by nutritional factors. These points of nutritional preemption are fundamental for the prevention of cancer, the quality of life of cancer patients, and the reduction in cancer recurrence.

Traditional medical oncology in the middle part of the last century sought to kill cancer cells with radiation, surgery, and chemotherapy drugs through a disruption in normal cellular processes, with the premise that the cancer cell is more susceptible to these approaches than the normal tissues, and thus provided a window of therapeutic efficacy. Although this approach succeeded in producing significant cures in childhood leukemia, testicular carcinoma, and Hodgkin's lymphomas, it has brought with it morbidity in patients being treated for more common forms of cancer (Albers et al., 2004; Bonadonna et al., 2005; Redaelli et al., 2005). Empowering the patient and being aware of the multitude of factors affecting quality of life often necessitates that physicians and other health care providers become involved with nutritional issues in cancer patients undergoing treatment. Finally, nutrition has a role to play, not simply in the primary prevention of cancer, but also in the prevention of cancer recurrence, which is of utmost importance in determining survival.

Medical oncology in the postgenomic era has sought to identify targeted treatments that act at a single and/or process-specific site. There has been some success with this approach, as exemplified by the discovery of the overexpression of the Her-2/neu oncogene, which occurs in ~30% of all breast cancer patients (Finn and Slamon, 2003). This observation led to the development of targeted antibody-based therapies that bind to the receptor for this ligand and concentrate chemotherapies on receptor-bearing cells. Although this approach has resulted in some modest improvements in survival in patients with advanced breast cancer, it has minimally affected overall breast cancer morbidity or mortality statistically. On the other hand, the discovery of prostate-specific antigen (PSA) has led to a reduction in prostate cancer mortality largely through the employment of surgery and radiation at an earlier stage in the disease (Anscher, 2005). Just as both targeted therapy and early biomarkers have an important place in the war on cancers, so does nutritional oncology, in which nutritional factors become an important focal point for research and practice.

The very idea that nutrition could affect a serious condition such as cancer was viewed to be both ridiculous and irrelevant by many oncologists 2 decades ago, and this attitude unfortunately persists today among many cancer clinicians and biologists. Increased exposure of medical students and other health professionals to the preventive and therapeutic potential of modern nutrition may ultimately result in an improved appreciation of the proper role of nutrition by those caring for cancer patients. The important role of nutrition in cancer is supported by many signal achievements in nutritional sciences over the last few decades as the result of the advances in human genetics applied to population studies; basic science studies in animals; cellular and molecular discoveries, which demonstrate the effects of nutrients on gene expression (Nowell et al., 2004); and even some limited intervention studies in humans demonstrating the effects of nutritional interventions on the incidence of precancerous precursors such as colon polyps (Wallace et al., 2004). These advances have established the role of nutrition at many levels in the multistep process of carcinogenesis and set the stage for advances in this rapidly expanding interdisciplinary field. Integrating information from various sources, including population studies, basic science studies, and human intervention trials, is critical for scientists in nutritional oncology to develop testable hypotheses that can be used for personalized nutrition approaches for cancer prevention and therapy. These studies are able to examine changes in dietary patterns, physical activity, prevention and treatment of obesity, and the use of plant-derived bioactive substances (not as drugs but as supplements) to modify the natural history of cancer in such a way as to prevent its onset or reduce the risk of cancer recurrence following primary therapy with surgery, radiation, or chemotherapy. The National Institutes of Health has developed interdisciplinary study sections for the first time, which are devoted to the review of scientific applications dealing with diet and the chemoprevention of cancer.

Nutritional oncology is an integrative medical specialty that embraces the best of orthodox and alternative approaches in combination while recognizing the value of proven therapies for cancer. This second edition will revisit and focus on the achievements in nutrition and cancer in relation to the basic mechanism and clinical applicability of the results from human nutrition, intervention, and clinical studies, as well as the evidence provided by the epidemiological case–control and cohort studies as reviewed by experts of their respective field. Through the influence of these scientific achievements on clinical practice, it is hoped that nutrition will soon be integrated into the routine care of the cancer patient in two situations. First, in the diagnosed cancer patient, nutritional support may help to minimize side effects of treatment and improve responses to therapy. Second, in the growing population of cancer survivors, nutrition may help to prevent cancer recurrence through the modulation of hormonal and inflammatory factors that promote angiogenesis and change the invasive and metastatic potential of tumors. However, despite the potential of nutrition, it is not a substitute for definitive therapies of proven curative or preventive benefit. Nutrition can be used as an adjunct but should not be used to delay or avoid appropriate diagnosis and treatment of common forms of cancer.

HISTORY AND FUTURE OF NUTRITIONAL ONCOLOGY

In the early 1920s, prior to the development of chemotherapy, Shields Warren (1932) surmised that cancer killed its victims by depleting the tumor cell's nutrients. This insight led several generations of researchers to investigate the effects of tumors on host metabolism. Nobel laureates, including Warburg and the Coris, discovered much about carbohydrate metabolism while in search of the metabolic aberrations induced by cancer.

Decades later, Waterhouse and others confirmed that there were clear abnormalities of carbohydrate metabolism in the cancer patient (Terepka and Waterhouse, 1956; Holroyde et al., 1975). Protein was also lost from the host and the "nitrogen trap" hypothesis was developed by Fenninger and Midler (1954) in the 1950s to explain the net transfer of protein from tumor to host. In the 1980s, investigations by a number of laboratories, using radioactive and stable isotope tracers of glucose, fatty acids, and amino acids, quantitatively identified increased glucose production, proteolysis, and lipolysis in cancer patients in the 1970s and 1980s (Heber et al., 1986).

The discovery that tumor necrosis factor and other cytokines may account for these metabolic changes in the 1980s and 1990s led ultimately to the concept that the nutritional changes were part of an immune response of the host to the tumor (Shaw and Wolfe, 1987; Lang et al., 1992). Cytokines were shown to exert central nervous system (CNS) effects, which explained in part the anorexia associated with cancer in many patients. Furthermore, cytokines were demonstrated to stimulate tumor growth under certain circumstances.

More recently, investigators have found that the Warburg hypothesis is supported by observations of early changes in the metabolic pathways operative in cancer cells, including an increased rate of aerobic glycolysis and a truncated Krebs cycle mediated by the C-myc oncogene and the hypoxia-inducible factor, Hif-1, which induce the expression of specific glycolytic enzymes (Shaw and Wolfe, 1987). Studies of colonies of cancer cells growing as small spheres have indicated that cancer cell metabolism is also affected by oxygenation (Rempel et al., 1996; Younes et al., 1996). Tumor angiogenesis is relatively inefficient so that the interior of tumor masses carry out anaerobic metabolism, while a 150-micron outer shell carries out enhanced aerobic metabolism. There is a decreasing gradient of oxygen toward the anaerobic core and a decreasing gradient of glucose while lactate increases. All of these metabolic changes based on the induction of specific genes are related to the need of the cancer cell to proliferate and avoid apoptosis.

These stunning discoveries, together with an enhanced understanding of the biology of carcinogenesis, have led to the concept that cancer is a chronic disease of the genome. It begins with genetic changes during tumor cell initiation and progressively moves from tumor growth to tissue invasion to metastasis with many opportunities for nutritional modulation. Many food substances traditionally characterized as nutrients or micronutrients affect DNA replication and cellular differentiation.

Studies of populations based on global prospects (World Cancer Research Fund, 1997) indicate that differences in diet and lifestyle have pronounced effects on tumor incidence, prevalence, and natural history. The promise of nutritional oncology is that it will augment traditional therapies to prolong and improve the life of cancer patients. Clearly, the principles of evidence-based medicine must be developed, demonstrating that these interventions are worthwhile. Healthful changes in diet and lifestyle have benefits for other chronic diseases, including heart disease. Cancer patients often welcome the opportunity to become involved in a meaningful way in their own care. The existing evidence of the impact of nutritional medicine on the quality of life of cancer patients cannot be overestimated.

Since the first edition of this text in 1999, the idea that there is a single gene pathway or single drug cure for cancer has given way to the general view that dietary/environmental factors have an impact on the progression of genetic and cellular changes in common forms of cancer. This broad concept can now be investigated within a basic and clinical research context for specific types of cancer. This book attempts to cover the available knowledge in this new field of nutritional oncology and has been written by invited experts.

GENE–NUTRIENT INTERACTION IN CANCER

Unlike genetic diseases, such as sickle cell disease, cancer is not usually the result of a single mutation and most forms of cancer are unlikely to respond to a single agent targeting a single gene or gene product (Kaiser, 2005). Several genes must be defective before a normal cell will become an invasive cancer cell. Advances in genomics and molecular biology have revealed that alterations in three types of genes are responsible for carcinogenesis, including oncogenes, tumor suppressor genes, and stability genes. Mutations in the oncogenes and tumor suppressor genes increase tumor cell number by stimulating cell proliferation, inhibiting cell death or apoptosis, or providing increased nutrients by stimulating angiogenesis. Stability genes are DNA repair genes that induce the expression of enzymes that carry out multistep processes that repair both spontaneous and mutagen-induced alterations in DNA (Scherer et al., 2005). Mutations in these genes can occur in the germline, resulting in a familial predisposition to cancer or in somatic cells leading to sporadic cancers.

Although inherited cancers are much less common than acquired cancers, germline mutations in DNA repair genes have been shown to confer an increased lifetime risk of cancer. Since only one allele is typically abnormal at birth in the BRCA1 in breast cancer patients, the second mutation must trigger the cancer (Kotsopoulos et al., 2005). Undeniably, lifestyle and diet can influence the onset of even these less common inherited cancers, as demonstrated for the BRCA1 mutation and breast cancer (Kotsopoulos et al., 2005). Although the BRCA1 mutations confer a 90% lifetime risk of breast cancer, the age at onset of breast cancer in a group of such women was shown to be delayed in those who were more physically active during adolescence (King et al., 2003). In addition, studies show that the effects of obesity on breast cancer in postmenopausal women are more easily demonstrated in those with a family history of breast cancer (Carpenter et al., 2003). Therefore, genes and nutrients are not in competition with each other, so a strong genetic predisposition would not necessarily mask or marginalize the response to diet and lifestyle. Rather, there is a gene–nutrient interaction so that genetic predisposition uncovers the influence of nutritional factors.

This model of gene–nutrient interaction can be extended to the most prevalent human cancers, including breast cancer, prostate cancer, ovarian cancer, head and neck cancer, pancreatic cancer, and uterine cancer, among others. In these various cancers, the biochemical, pathological, and genetic markers are under active investigation for the discovery, development, and delivery of appropriate nutrition strategies for prevention or therapy.

Each cancer differs in its natural history, in the factors promoting progression, and in the specific surrogate endpoint biomarkers that may be useful for its study. The emergence of nanotechnology and systems biology—and their application to cancer research—promises to provide a more detailed picture that will ultimately benefit the field of nutritional oncology to a greater extent than classical pharmacological fields looking for a single target, as opposed to multiple effects occurring simultaneously.

AGING AND CANCER

With aging, the risks of many common forms of cancer increase as the amount of oxidant stress in cells increases (Wallace, 2005). The generation of oxygen radicals from aging mitochondria and the DNA damage that follows may mediate age-related changes in cancer incidence. Targeted antioxidation continues to be studied, but many phytochemicals have effects beyond this characteristic. Overnutrition and obesity increase oxidant stress and inflammation, while caloric restriction increases lifespan in sedentary experimental animals and delays the onset of age-associated diseases, including atherosclerosis, diabetes, and cancer. Caloric restriction is recognized to affect the levels of insulin, insulin-like growth factor 1 (IGF-1), and SIRT1, the mammalian analogue of Sir2 protein discovered in the budding yeast *Saccharomyces cerevisiae*. Aging is associated with increased rates of stress-induced apoptosis, and SIRT1 promotes cell survival by inhibiting stress-induced cellular apoptosis. In addition to caloric restriction, small molecules called *STACs* can stimulate SIRT1; the most potent of these recently discovered is resveratrol, a stilbene phytochemical found in grapes and wine (Wood et al., 2004).

Although known as an antioxidant, these effects of resveratrol are independent of its actions as an antioxidant. The case of resveratrol is not an isolated one, as other phytochemicals, including lycopene from tomatoes and other flavonoids such as quercetin (found in fruits and vegetables), can stimulate DNA repair and demonstrate evidence of inhibiting carcinogenesis in various experimental model systems (Heber, 2004).

In the first edition of this text in 1999, we originated the concept of the "Xenobiotic Hypothesis of Cancer," in which the interactions beyond oxidation of phytochemicals trigger protective responses in cells, inhibiting the development of cancer. Research conducted since 1999 has demonstrated that two nuclear receptors function in this metabolic cascade to regulate detoxification and elimination. The constitutive androstane receptor (CAR) mediates the response to a narrow range of phenobarbital-like inducers. In contrast, the human steroid xenobiotic receptor (SXR) responds to many prescription drugs, environmental contaminants, steroids, and toxic bile acids (Xie et al., 2000). Consistent with their role as xenobiotic sensors, both receptors are expressed primarily in the liver and in the small intestine. The CYP 3A enzyme is responsible for metabolizing and clearing >60% of clinically prescribed drugs, and its induction plays a pivotal role in the clearance of hepatotoxic bile salts. CYP 3A gene expression is induced by a large variety of xenobiotic compounds through SXR activation. Two xenobiotic transporters, ABCB1 (or MDR1) and ABCC2 (or MRP2), are also upregulated in hepatocytes and intestinal cells by SXR activators, including a number of phytochemicals. Taken together, the xenobiotic activation of CAR and SXR induces a positive feed-forward loop that aids in clearance of foreign chemicals, including those from plant-based foods, and this process thereby resets the xenosensors for another round of signaling.

Mammalian cells can mirror some events in the plant world, and plant cells contain many homologous genes and gene products. Humans evolved in a plant-based environment where restricted water and light or increased heat is known to lead to increased production of protective colorful phytochemicals that inhibit oxidation. Modern diets in developed countries are typically deficient in these compounds, as fruit, vegetable, and whole grain intakes have declined from those typical in traditional diets. The loss of these substances may lead to a reduction in the activity of cancer-preventive xenobiotic defense mechanisms as outlined earlier.

In summary, massive evidence has accumulated since 1999 that indicates that cancer is the result of a genetic–environmental interaction where nutrition likely has a critical role. A strong association of common forms of cancer with diet and lifestyle suggests that primary prevention of cancer may be possible, and large clinical trials are examining this possibility. It is now appreciated that the process of cancer progression and metastasis may also be modifiable through nutritional intervention. Enhanced understanding of the biology of angiogenesis, tumor invasion of surrounding stroma, stromal–epithelial cell interactions, and factors modifying metastatic spread create new opportunities to modify the natural history of human cancers.

OBESITY AND CANCER

Obesity is the most common nutritional disorder in the United States today, resulting from an imbalance in energy expenditure and intake superimposed on a genetic predisposition to accumulate excess body fat. Obesity has been clearly associated with many forms of cancer, as documented in a number of epidemiological studies (McTiernan, 2005). In common with other chronic diseases, including cancer, it is rare for obesity to be the expression of a pure genetic or medical disorder. In most cases, obesity results from a combination of physiological, psychological, and environmental factors. The endocrine system, which is critically involved in many common forms of cancer, has also been shown to translate environmental influences into excess adiposity.

Fat cells have been found to synthesize and secrete numerous peptides called *adipocytokines,* including leptin and vascular endothelial growth factor (VEGF), which promote angiogenesis, and interleukins, which in turn promote inflammation and oxidation. Obesity is an independent risk factor for heart disease and this increased risk is associated with increased levels of systemic markers of inflammation, including C-reactive protein (CRP), that promote inflammation in the heart (Rose et al., 2004). The possibility that such inflammation and oxidation could promote the development of common forms of cancer is being investigated for a number of common forms of cancer.

Many classic hormones involved in obesity also play a role in the initiation and promotion of cancer at cellular, paracrine, and systemic levels. For example, reproductive hormones are critically involved in both obesity and cancer. In patients with primary anorexia nervosa and malnutrition, reproductive hormone secretion is reduced, resulting in both infertility and a reduced risk of breast cancer. At the same time, women who are very athletic during adolescence have a markedly reduced lifetime risk of breast cancer, as do women who have a later onset of puberty. On the other hand, excess secretion of reproductive hormones (e.g., estrogens) has been observed in overweight and obese women and implicated in the etiology of breast cancer and other reproductive tract cancers (Stephenson and Rose, 2003; Rose et al., 2004).

It is well established that age at menarche, age at menopause, parity, and age at first full-term pregnancy are important determinants of breast cancer risk. Asian women living a traditional lifestyle have lower estrogen levels both before and after menopause, and these lower levels of estrogen have been considered important markers of the differences in breast cancer incidence observed in international epidemiological studies. Increased daily alcohol intake has been associated with increased risk of breast cancer and increased levels of endogenous estrogens in premenopausal women. A number of aspects of dietary intake, physical activity, and body composition affect endogenous estrogen levels.

Increased estrogen production in women with excess fat compared to lean women is probably due to increased peripheral conversion of androstenedione to estrone by fat tissue. Obesity has been associated repeatedly with more advanced breast cancer at the time of diagnosis, higher rates of recurrence, and shorter survival times, even after controlling for tumor size and stage of disease at diagnosis.

There is emerging evidence that insulin and insulin-related hormones, such as IGF-1, may stimulate breast tumor growth. Upper body obesity and a family history of diabetes mellitus increase the risk of developing postmenopausal breast cancer. Therefore, overnutrition, through its stimulation of peptide and steroid hormones, may stimulate tumor growth and progression.

Although there is less known about the influence of nutrition on prostatic cancer, ovarian cancer, uterine cancer, head and neck cancer, and pancreatic cancer, many hypotheses developed using the models of colon cancer and breast cancer are under study.

MICRONUTRIENTS, FIBER, AND CANCER

One of the natural results of eating a modern diet is that along with excess calories and fat comes a deficiency of dietary fiber and the many micronutrients and phytochemicals found in fruits and vegetables (Heber and Bowerman, 2001). It has been estimated that only 10% of the U.S. population eats the five servings per day of fruits and vegetables recommended by the National Cancer Institute. Antioxidants such as vitamin E, vitamin C, and carotenoids are found in fruits and vegetables. In fact, the bright colors of most fruits and vegetables are indicators of their content of antioxidants, where alternating double bonds result in light absorption in the visible spectrum and bright colors. It has been postulated that these antioxidants were developed to protect plants from oxidation by the oxygen produced through photosynthesis. In fact, the concentration of antioxidants can be increased by raising plants under stressful conditions, such as reduced light or water.

Other, less visible phytonutrients, such as organosulfurs in garlic, isoflavones in soy beans, and limonene and geraniol derived from citrus fruit skins, have been reported to have anticancer effects. In some cases, it has been proposed that an accident of nature has resulted in the anticancer activity of substances originally evolved to protect plants from pathogens. Ancient humans ate a variety of fruits, vegetables, cereals, and grains. Although there are 50,000–100,000 edible plant species on earth, modern humans obtain >60% of all plant-derived proteins from a handful of plant species, such as corn, wheat, rice, and soy. Our genetic makeup was designed to complement a high intake of fruits, vegetables, cereals, and grains. The role played by micronutrients in controlling oxidant damage to DNA, mutagenesis, and carcinogenesis may be a significant factor in accounting for the protective effects of these foods observed in cancer epidemiology studies.

NUTRITIONAL ONCOLOGY: THE NEED FOR CONSENSUS

Skeptics demand clinical trial evidence that increasing fruit and vegetable intake reduces cancer risk, and some early evidence from intervention trials is emerging to support this view. However, it is our view that such beneficial maneuvers as improving dietary patterns with more fruits and vegetables and combating obesity with increased physical activity and dietary modification are reasonable at our current state of knowledge and should not wait for the ultimate evidence from definitive clinical trials.

While the research is being accumulated to support the use of nutritional interventions for the reduction of morbidity and mortality, cancer patients continue to demand consensus-based recommendations from their physicians to improve their quality of life and their sense of control over their lives.

This book attempts not only to provide the theoretical and research basis for nutritional oncology, but also to offer the medical oncologist and other members of multidisciplinary groups treating cancer patients practical information on nutrition assessment and nutritional regimens, including micronutrient and phytochemical supplementation. The editors hope that this volume will stimulate increased research, education, and patient application of the principles of nutritional oncology.

References

Albers, P., Weissbach, L., Krege, S., Kliesch, S., Hartmann, M., Heidenreich, A., Walz, P., Kuczyk, M., and Fimmers, R.; the German Testicular Cancer Study Group. 2004. Prediction of necrosis after chemotherapy of advanced germ cell tumors: results of a prospective multicenter trial of the German Testicular Cancer Study Group. *J Urol* **171**: 1835–1838.

Anscher, M.S. 2005. PSA kinetics and risk of death from prostate cancer: in search of the Holy Grail of surrogate end points. *JAMA* **27**: 493–494.

Bonadonna, G., Viviani, S., Bonfante, V., Gianni, A.M., and Valagussa, P. 2005. Survival in Hodgkin's disease patients—report of 25 years of experience at the Milan Cancer Institute. *Eur J Cancer* **41**: 998–1006.

Carpenter, C.L., Paganini-Hill, A., Ross, R.K., and Bernstein, L. 2003. Effect of family history, obesity and exercise on breast cancer risk among postmenopausal women. *Int J Cancer* **206**: 96–102.

Fenninger, L.D., and Midler, G.B. 1954. Energy and nitrogen metabolism in cancer. *Adv Cancer Res* **2**: 229–253.

Finn, R.S., and Slamon, D.J. 2003. Cancer monoclonal antibody therapy for breast cancer: herceptin. *Chemother Biol Response Modif* **21**: 223–233.

Heber, D. 2004. Phytochemicals beyond antioxidation. *J Nutr* **134**: 3175S–3176S.

Heber, D., and Bowerman, S. 2001. Applying science to changing dietary patterns. *J Nutr* **131**: 3078S–3081S.

Heber, D., Byerley, L.O., Chi, J., Grosvenor, M., Bergman, R.N., Coleman, M., and Chlebowski, R.T. 1986. Pathophysiology of malnutrition in the adult cancer patient. *Cancer* **58**: 1867–1873.

Holroyde, C.P., Gabuzda, T., Putnam, R., Paul, P., and Reichard, G. 1975. Carbohydrate metabolism in cancer cachexia. *Cancer Res* **35**: 3710–3714.

Kaiser, J. 2005. Genomics. Tackling the cancer genome. *Science* **309**: 693.

King, M.C., Marks, J.H., and Mandell, J.B.; New York Breast Cancer Study Group. 2003. Breast and ovarian cancer risks due to inherited mutations in BRCA1 and BRCA2. *Science* **302**: 643–646.

Kotsopoulos, J., Lubinski, J., Lynch, H.T., Neuhausen, S.L., Ghadirian, P., Isaacs, C., Weber, B., Kim-Sing, C., Foulkes, W.D., Gershoni-Baruch, R., Ainsworth, P., Friedman, E., Daly, M., Garber, J.E., Karlan, B., Olopade, O.I., Tung, N., Saal, H.M., Eisen, A., Osborne, M., Olsson, H., Gilchrist, D., Sun, P., and Narod, S.A. 2005. Age at menarche and the risk of breast cancer in BRCA1 and BRCA2 mutation carriers. *Cancer Causes Control* **16**: 667–674.

Lang, C.H., Dobrescu, C., and Bagby, G.J. 1992. Tumor necrosis factor impairs insulin action on peripheral glucose disposal and hepatic glucose output. *Endocrinology* **130**: 43–52.

McTiernan, A. 2005. Obesity and cancer: the risks, science, and potential management strategies. *Oncology* **19**: 871–881.

Nowell, S.A., Ahn, J., and Ambrosone, C.B. 2004. Gene–nutrient interactions in cancer etiology. *Nutr Rev* **62**: 427–438.

Redaelli, A., Laskin, B.L., Stephens, J.M., Botteman, M.F., and Pashos, C.L. 2005. A systematic literature review of the clinical and epidemiological burden of acute lymphoblastic leukaemia (ALL). *Eur J Cancer Care* **14**: 53–62.

Rempel, A. et al. 1996. Glucose catabolism in cancer cells: amplification of the gene encoding type II hexokinase. *Cancer Res* **56**: 2468–2471.

Rose, D.P., Komninou, D., and Stephenson, G.D. 2004. Obesity, adipocytokines, and insulin resistance in breast cancer. *Obes Rev* **5**: 153–165.

Scherer, S.J., Avdievich, E., and Edelmann, W. 2005. Functional consequences of DNA mismatch repair missense mutations in murine models and their impact on cancer predisposition. *Biochem Soc Trans* **33**: 689–693.

Schulman, J.A., and Karney, B.R. 2003. Gender and attitudes toward nutrition in prospective physicians. *Am J Health Behav* **27**: 623–632.

Shaw, J.H.F., and Wolfe, R.R. 1987. Fatty acid and glycerol kinetics in septic patients and in patients with gastrointestinal cancer. The response to glucose infusion and parenteral feeding. *Ann Surg* **205**: 368–376.

Stephenson, G.D., and Rose, D.P. 2003. Breast cancer and obesity: an update. *Nutr Cancer* **45**: 1–16.

Terepka, A.R., and Waterhouse, C. 1956. Metabolic observations during force feeding of patients with cancer. *Am J Med* **20**: 225–238.

Wallace, D.C. 2005. A mitochondrial paradigm of metabolic and degenerative diseases, aging, and cancer: a dawn for evolutionary medicine. *Annu Rev Genet* **39**: 359–407.

Wallace, K., Baron, J.A., Cole, B.F., Sandler, R.S., Karagas, M.R., Beach, M.A., Haile, R.W., Burke, C.A., Pearson, L.H., Mandel, J.S., Rothstein, R., and Snover, D.C. 2004. Effect of calcium supplementation on the risk of large bowel polyps. *J Natl Cancer Inst* **96**: 921–925.

Warren, S. 1932. The immediate causes of death in cancer. *Am J Med Sci* **184**: 610–615.

Wood, J.G., Rogina, B., Lavu, S., Howitz, K., Helfand, S.L., Tatar, M., and Sinclair, D. 2004. Sirtuin activators mimic caloric restriction and delay ageing in metazoans. *Nature* **430**: 686–689.

World Cancer Research Fund. 1997. "Food, Nutrition and the Prevention of Cancer: A Global Perspective World Cancer Research Fund/American Institute for Cancer Research." BANTA Book Group, Menasha, WI.

Xie, W., Barwick, J.L., Simon, C.M., Pierce, A.M., Safe, S., Blumberg, B., Guzelian, P.S., and Evans, R.M. 2000. Reciprocal activation of xenobiotic response genes by nuclear receptors SXR/PXR and CAR. *Genes Dev* **14**: 3014–3023.

Younes, M. et al. 1996. Wide expression of the human erythrocyte glucose transporter Glut1 in human cancers. *Cancer Res* **56**: 1164–1167.

CHAPTER

1

Fundamentals of Human Nutrition

DAVID HEBER and SUSAN BOWERMAN

INTRODUCTION

There is accumulating evidence that foods, or their component bioactive substances (Kris-Etherton et al., 2004), offer benefits beyond basic nutrition. Macronutrients alone do not provide complete information about food intake. The types and sources of fats, proteins, and carbohydrates influence dietary patterns, which are composites of the component foods. Dietary patterns characterized as *Western* or *prudent* have been linked to the risk of common forms of cancer (Milner, 2002). Obesity, associated with Western diet patterns, has also been associated with an increased risk of common forms of cancer (Calle and Thun, 2004).

A significant body of evidence suggests that increased consumption of fruits and vegetables along with a reduced intake of fats, especially animal fats, may be related to a reduced risk of cancer (Steinmetz and Potter, 1996; Fung et al., 2003). These effects have been attributed to changes in the pattern of dietary fats, phytochemicals from fruits and vegetables, fiber, and other elements in the diet.

To date, there is no evidence that increasing the amount of fruits and vegetables without making other changes in the diet will have an impact on body fat or body weight (Tohill et al., 2004). However, ongoing research is investigating the impact of specific dietary patterns and physical activity on energetics and obesity. The contribution of specific macronutrients to satiety, especially the impact of increased dietary protein intake together with high-volume/low-caloric density fruits and vegetables, may provide an additional key to controlling energy intake. To understand the rationale for the aforementioned proposed impacts of dietary patterns on cancer prevention and risk, it is necessary to go beyond the classic understanding of food elements in terms of macronutrients.

Diets are made up of numerous foods in varied proportions that are prepared in many ways but ultimately contribute energy to the body to support basic cellular energy needs. How that energy is provided as foods, which are made up of the basic macronutrients—protein, carbohydrate, and fat—plays a major role in determining the impact of dietary patterns on the risk of cancer. Within each category of macronutrient, there are marked differences in how different food sources are digested, absorbed, and metabolized. It is critical both for epidemiological investigations of the role of nutrition in the etiology of cancer and for efforts at modifying dietary behaviors in intervention trials to understand the impact of the specific food sources of these macronutrients.

CLASSIFICATION OF FOOD AND DIETARY QUALITY

Foods can be grouped according to their content of macronutrients combined with their traditional use in an ethnic or societal geographic cuisine. Food groupings such as the basic four food groups [(1) Fruits and Vegetables, (2) Grains and Cereals, (3) Dairy, and (4) Meat, Beans, Nuts, and Cheese] classify foods of very different composition together such as red meat and ocean-caught fish or muffins and whole-grain bread. However, considerations of chemical structure, digestibility, metabolism, and functionality contribute to what is called the *quality of the diet* overall, as well as of individual macronutrients.

Copyright © 2006, Elsevier Inc.
All rights of reproduction in any form reserved.

The quality of dietary macronutrients, such as the ratio of n-3 fatty acids to n-6 fatty acids or of whole grains to refined grains complicates the basic considerations of the effects of diet on cancer incidence and efforts to organize dietary interventions designed to reduce cancer risk. An additional and important consideration is the presence of thousands of phytochemicals in fruits, vegetables, and whole grains, leading to their designation in some cases as "functional foods." The term *functional food* indicates the presence of bioactive substances that affect physiology or cellular and molecular biology.

The term *quality* implies that a value judgment is being leveled against a particular food. Although there is a hierarchical ranking of fats, carbohydrates, and proteins common to the disease prevention literature, the mechanisms underlying the differences among foods that provide protein, fat, and carbohydrate to the diet are simply analyzed in light of fundamental principles of nutrition. Taken together, these aspects of foods contribute to the assessment of the quality of the diet. The lowest quality foods are called *junk foods* because they are high in energy density but low in nutrient density (e.g., French fries). It has been said that there are no junk foods but simply "junk diets." Obviously, if one combines enough junk foods, it leads to a junk diet.

ENERGETICS AND OBESITY

Because humans are well-adapted to starvation and poorly adapted to excess energy intake, the balance of energy taken in as food and energy expenditure through metabolism and exercise has been emphasized as a major factor in cancer etiology (McCullough and Giovannucci, 2004). Evidence that obesity contributes to many common forms of cancer has also accumulated. Among species, animals with a smaller surface area such as mice burn more energy at rest per unit body mass than large mammals such as elephants. Children have higher metabolic rates than adults per unit body mass. Within the same species, there can be significant variations in metabolic rates. For example, the sedentary and overfed laboratory rat has a higher metabolic rate than the desert rat that is better adapted to starvation (Kalman et al., 1993). Energy efficiency may vary as well among humans. There is evidence that the post-obese adult may have a lower metabolism than a never-obese individual of the same size. However, the impact of excess energy is modulated by the location of excess body fat and its effects on hormones and inflammatory cytokines. Therefore, although energy balance is critical, it is not sufficient for an understanding of the effects of nutrition on cancer.

Because obesity results from an imbalance of energy intake and expenditure, certain dietary factors have been identified as contributing to obesity. These include hidden processed fats in foods, added refined sugars in foods, and a high glycemic load (GL) diet rich in refined carbohydrates. Therefore, the quality of the diet in terms of nutrient density can contribute to the tendency of a dietary pattern to promote the development of obesity in genetically susceptible individuals. Low-energy-density foods include all fruits and vegetables, generally because of their high water content. High-energy-density foods include red meats, fats, cheeses, pastries, cookies, cakes, ice cream, snack chips, some fruit juices, and refined grains.

PROTEIN

Roles of Protein

Proteins are involved in the growth, repair, and replacement of tissue and serve numerous functions in the body both as enzymes, antibodies, hormones, and regulators of fluid and acid–base balance and as integral parts of most body structures including skin, muscle, and bone. Within each cell, there is a continuous process of synthesis and breakdown of proteins in the body, referred to as *protein turnover*. The rate of protein turnover affects organ protein mass, body size, and ultimately the body's protein and amino acid requirements (Matthews, 1999; Fuller, 2000). The amino acids are the basic units in protein metabolism, and all have the same basic structure with a central carbon atom with a hydrogen, an amino group, and an acid group attached to it. Attached to the fourth site on the carbon atom is a distinct side chain, which defines the amino acid. Cells link these amino acids in an infinite variety to create proteins that become metabolically essential compounds. There are 21 amino acids in human proteins, and 12 of these are synthesized by the body and are, therefore, known as *nonessential amino acids*. The nine remaining amino acids (histidine, isoleucine, leucine, lysine, methionine, phenylalanine, threonine, tryptophan, and valine) are either not made by the body or not made in sufficient quantities to meet needs and are, thus, termed *essential amino acids*.

The proper balance and sufficient intake of essential amino acids, along with an adequate amount of nitrogen for the production of nonessential amino acids, is required for proper protein nutriture (Berdanier, 2000).

Protein Quality

To manufacture proteins, cells require all the needed amino acids simultaneously with adequate nitrogen-containing amino groups for the manufacturing of the nonessential amino acids. The amino acid composition of a food can vary widely and determines the nutritional quality of the dietary protein. Foods that contain essential amino acids at levels that facilitate tissue growth and repair are known as *complete proteins* and are supplied in the diet from animal sources and soy protein.

There are several ways of measuring protein quality. Most commonly, the term *biological value* is used, which is a measure of the efficiency of a given protein in supporting the body's needs. Complete proteins have a high biological value, which is an expression of the amount of nitrogen absorbed relative to the amount of nitrogen retained by the body. All protein sources are compared with egg white, which provides the most complete protein and has the highest biological value of 100, indicating that 100% of the nitrogen absorbed is retained.

A low concentration of one or more essential amino acids in a food lowers its biological value. With the exception of soy, most plant proteins are deficient in one or more essential amino acids and are, therefore, regarded as incomplete. However, the biological value of incomplete proteins can be improved by combining two proteins that are complementary so that those essential amino acids lacking or deficient in one protein are provided by the other when they are combined. In this way, the two complementary proteins together provide all the essential amino acids in ratios ideal for human protein utilization (Lappe, 1971; Kreutler and Czajka-Narins, 1987; Matthews, 1999). For example, the combination of corn (limited in lysine) with beans (limited in methionine) results in a high-quality protein food combination. Thus, the requirement for adequate essential amino acids can be met in a vegetarian diet by mixing foods of complementary amino acid composition (Lappe, 1971; Committee on Diet and Health, 1989; Berdanier, 2000).

Protein Requirements

The U.S. food supply can provide an average of 102 g of protein per person per day (Nationwide Food Consumption Survey, 1984). Actual daily protein consumption ranges from 88 to 92 g for men and from 63 to 66 g for women (McDowell et al., 1994). Animal products provide ~75% of the essential amino acids in the food supply, followed by dairy products, cereal products, eggs, legumes, fruits, and vegetables (McDowell et al., 1994). The recommended daily allowance (RDA) for protein of high biological value for adults, based on body weight, is ~0.8 g/kg (National Research Council, 1989) or 0.36 g/lb. However, the RDA is set to meet the needs of a defined population group as a whole rather than indicating individual requirements. In a report concerning dietary reference intakes (DRIs), the acceptable macronutrient distribution range (AMDR) was set at 10–35% of total calories from protein. The AMDR is defined as the acceptable range of intakes for protein associated with reduced risk of chronic disease while providing intakes of essential nutrients (Barr et al., 2003). This range was largely set so that the intake of other macronutrients in the diet would be in an acceptable range.

There are many conditions in which extra protein is needed, including periods of growth, pregnancy, lactation, intense strength and endurance training and other forms of physical activity, and possibly in the elderly (Campbell et al., 1994). Additionally, there is research into the role of protein in the regulation of long-term energy balance, maintenance of body weight, and satiety (see the section "Role in Satiety," later in this chapter).

Optimum Protein Intake

Given the variation in the needs for protein throughout the life cycle, there is an individual optimal intake that exists based on lean body mass and activity levels. However, optimal intakes are difficult to determine based on the existing science base in nutrition. In 1977, Garza et al. studied a small number of healthy volunteers and found that 0.8 g/kg/day resulted in positive nitrogen balance. Subsequent studies in endurance athletes found that >1 g/kg/day was required for positive nitrogen balance (Tarnopolsky, 2004), and studies in weightlifters indicated that >2 g/kg/day was needed to achieve positive nitrogen balance (Tarnopolsky et al., 1992). Therefore, although the DRI, which is the same as the RDA, is set at 56 g/day for men consistent with the 1977 study, the allowable range of macronutrient intake is broad (10–35% of total calories), enabling some individual adjustment for optimal intakes both to control hunger and to provide support to lean tissues.

Role in Satiety

In comparison with carbohydrate or fat, protein provides a stronger signal to the brain to satisfy hunger. Although the mechanism of action is unknown, it has been suggested that either single amino acids or small peptides enter the brain to elicit their effects, and several amino acids, including tryptophan, phenylalanine, and tyrosine, have been theorized to affect the hunger control mechanisms once they cross the blood–brain barrier. Small differences in the rates at which proteins release their amino acids into the bloodstream may also affect satiety. In subjects consuming high-protein meals compared with high-carbohydrate meals fed *ad libitum*, a voluntary reduction in energy consumption has been observed.

Researchers in the Netherlands (Westerterp-Plantenga et al., 1999) have studied the effects of protein on hunger perceptions by studying two groups of subjects in a whole-body energy chamber under controlled conditions for >24 hours. Subjects were fed isocaloric diets, which were either high protein/high carbohydrate (protein/carbohydrate/fat, percentage of calories 30/60/10) or high fat (protein/carbohydrate/fat, percentage of calories 10/30/60). Significantly more satiety was reported by subjects on the high-protein/high-carbohydrate diet. At the same time, hunger, appetite, desire to eat, and estimated quantity of food eaten were significantly lower in this group, with less hunger both during and after the high-protein meals. The level of protein in the diet may also have an impact on maintenance of body weight after weight loss. After following a very low energy diet for 4 weeks, subjects who consumed a 20% higher intake of protein than controls (15% vs 18% of energy) showed a 50% lower body weight regain, only consisting of fat-free mass, with increased satiety and decreased energy efficiency during a 3-month maintenance period (Westerterp-Plantenga et al., 2004).

Similar studies have reported improved weight loss and fat loss in subjects consuming a high-protein diet versus a control diet (25% vs 12% energy from protein) *ad libitum*, because of a reduction in daily calorie intake of ~16% (Skov et al., 1999) and improved utilization of body fat with maintenance of lean body mass in subjects consuming 32% of energy from protein compared with controls who consumed 15% of calories as protein (Layman et al., 2003). A similar study comparing diets with 15% versus 30% of calories from protein found that although weight loss in the two groups was similar over the 6-week trial, diet satisfaction was significantly greater in those consuming the higher protein diet (Johnston et al., 2004).

A meta-analysis of studies (Eisenstein et al., 2002) concluded that, on average, high-protein diets were associated with a 9% decrease in total calorie intake. Although the role of protein in affecting overall calorie intake and regulating body weight in comparison to fat and carbohydrate needs further investigation, the evidence is strong that protein affects hunger signaling mechanisms in the brain, induces thermogenesis, and contributes to the building and maintenance of lean body mass.

QUALITY OF LIPIDS, FATS, AND FATTY ACIDS

Fats are a subset of the lipid family, which includes triglycerides (fats and oils), phospholipids, and sterols. Fats play an extremely important role in energy balance by enabling efficient storage of calories in adipose tissue. It is possible for the mythical 70-kg man to carry 130,000 calories in 13.5 kg of fat tissue compared with 54,000 calories stored as protein in an equivalent weight of lean tissue. This efficient storage is accomplished both by largely excluding water from adipose tissues and by storing energy in the chemical bonds of very long chain fatty acids. The typical fatty acids found in digested and stored fat range between 16 and 22 carbons in length.

Triglycerides are the chief form of fat in the diet and the major storage form of fat in the body and are composed of a molecule of glycerol with three fatty acids attached. The principal dietary sources of fat are meats, dairy products, poultry, fish, nuts, and vegetable oils, as well as fats used in processed foods. Vegetables and fruits contain only small amounts of fat, so vegetable oils are only sources of fat due to processing of vegetables. The most commonly used oils and fats for salad oil, cooking oils, shortenings, and margarines in the United States include soybean, corn, cottonseed, palm, peanut, olive, canola (low erucic acid rapeseed oil), safflower, sunflower, coconut, palm kernel, tallow, and lard. These oils contain varying compositions of fatty acids, which have particular physiological properties. The fats stored in tissues reflect to a certain extent the fats in the diet. Humans synthesize saturated fats (e.g., palmitic acid) from carbohydrates, but the polyunsaturated essential fats (linoleic and linolenic acids) must be taken in from the diet and the balance of these fats and the metabolic products of these fats reflect short-term and long-term dietary intake. There is a statistically significant but poor correlation between adipose tissue fatty acid profiles and dietary fatty acid intake as measured on a food frequency questionnaire (London et al., 1991). Red blood cell membranes change their composition in about 3 weeks. However, it is clearly possible to change the amount of fatty acids in tissues (Bagga et al., 1997), and total quantitative fatty acids can be altered by dietary intervention. The quality of fats in the diet is defined as that ratio of fatty acids that can be measured in plasma and tissues.

FATTY ACID STRUCTURE AND CLASSIFICATION

Fatty acids are organic compounds composed of a carbon chain with hydrogens attached at one end and an acid group at the other. Most naturally occurring fatty acids have an even number of carbons in their chain, up to 24 carbons in length, with 18-carbon chains the most abundant fatty acids in the food supply. Saturated fatty acids are completely saturated with hydrogens.

Those fatty acids lacking two hydrogen atoms and containing one double bond are monounsaturated fatty acids, and polyunsaturated fatty acids contain two or more double bonds in the carbon chain. The degree of saturation influences the texture of fats so that, in general, polyunsaturated vegetable oils are liquid at room temperature and the more saturated fats, most of which are animal fats, are solid. Some vegetable oils such as palm and coconut oils are highly saturated, and liquid oils can be hydrogenated in the presence of a nickel catalyst to produce a firmer fat.

The nomenclature of fatty acids is based on location of the double bonds: an omega-3 fatty acid has its first double bond three carbons from the methyl end of the carbon chain. Similarly, an omega-6 fatty acid has its double bond six carbons from the methyl end. Fatty acids are also denoted by the length of the carbon chain and the number of double

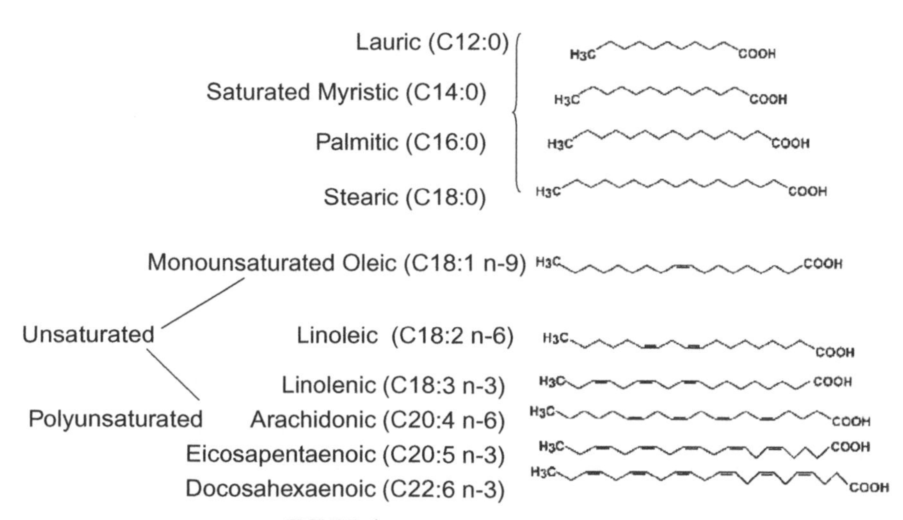

FIGURE 1 Fatty acids in dietary fats.

bonds they contain, such that linoleic acid is an 18:2 fatty acid, which contains 18 carbons and two double bonds. The human body requires fatty acids and can manufacture all but two essential fatty acids: linoleic acid and linolenic acid (18:3) (Figure 1).

Omega-3 fatty acids possess anti-inflammatory, antiarrhythmic, and antithrombotic properties and have been shown to reduce the risk for sudden death caused by cardiac arrhythmias and decrease mortality from all causes in patients with coronary heart disease. Conversely, the omega-6 fatty acids, obtained in the diet primarily from vegetable oils such as corn, safflower, sunflower, and cottonseed, are proinflammatory and prothrombotic. Fish and fish oils are the richest sources of the omega-3 fatty acids eicosapentaenoic acid (EPA) and docosahexaenoic acid (DHA) and are also present in algae. Green leafy vegetables, nuts, seeds, and soybeans contain the omega-3 fatty acid alpha-linolenic acid (AHA). The increased consumption in the United States of omega-6 fats from vegetable oils and grain-fed animals has led to a drastic increase in the ratio of omega-6 to omega-3 fatty acids in the diet from an estimated 1:1 in early human diets to a ratio exceeding 10:1 today (Simopoulos, 2001).

Fatty Acids as Cellular Signals

Increasing evidence from animal and *in vitro* studies indicates that omega-3 fatty acids, especially the long-chain polyunsaturated fatty acids EPA and DHA, present in fatty fish and fish oils inhibit carcinogenesis (Karmali et al., 1984; Lindner, 1991; Rose et al., 1991; Tsai et al., 1998; Boudreau et al., 2001; Narayanan et al., 2001). Several molecular mechanisms have been proposed for the influences on the process, including suppression of arachidonic acid–derived eicosanoid biosynthesis (Okuyama et al., 1996; Rose and Connolly, 1999), and influences on transcription factor activity, gene expression, and signal transduction pathways (Bartsch et al., 1999).

The peroxisome proliferator–activated nuclear receptors (PPARs; α, δ, γ) are activated by polyunsaturated fatty acids, eicosanoids, and various synthetic ligands (Willson et al., 2000). Consistent with their distinct expression patterns, gene-knockout experiments have revealed that each PPAR subtype performs a specific function in fatty acid homeostasis.

More than a decade ago, PPARα was found to respond to hypolipidemic drugs, such as fibrates. Subsequently, it was discovered that fatty acids serve as their natural ligands. Together with the analyses of PPARα-null mice, these studies established PPARα as a global regulator of fatty acid catabolism. PPARα target genes function together to coordinate the complex metabolic changes necessary to conserve energy during fasting and feeding. In the fatty acid metabolic cascade, PPARα activation upregulates the transcription of liver fatty acid–binding protein, which buffers intracellular fatty acids and delivers PPARα ligands to the nucleus (Wolfrum et al., 2001). In addition, expression of two members of the adrenoleukodystrophy subfamily of ABC transporters, ABCD2 and ABCD3, is similarly upregulated to promote transport of fatty acids into peroxisomes (Fourcade et al., 2001) where catabolic enzymes promote beta-oxidation. The hepatocyte CYP4A enzymes complete the metabolic cascade by catalyzing gamma-oxidation, the final catabolic step in the clearance of PPARα ligands (Lee et al., 1995).

PPARγ was identified initially as a key regulator of adipogenesis, but it also plays an important role in cellular differentiation, insulin sensitization, atherosclerosis, and cancer (Rosen and Spiegelman, 2001). Ligands for PPARγ include fatty acids and other arachidonic acid metabolites, antidiabetic drugs (e.g., thiazolidinediones), and triterpenoids. In contrast to PPARα, PPARγ promotes fat storage by increasing adipocyte differentiation and transcription of a number of important lipogenic proteins. Ligand homeostasis is regulated by governing expression of the adipocyte fatty acid–binding protein (A-FABP/aP2) and CYP4B1(Way et al., 2001). In macrophages, PPARγ induces the lipid transporter ABCA1 through an indirect mechanism involving the LXR pathway, which in turn promotes cellular efflux of phospholipids and cholesterol into high-density lipoproteins (Chawla et al., 2001; Chinetti et al., 2001).

QUALITY OF CARBOHYDRATES

As with proteins and fats, one can consider the quality of carbohydrates based on the source of the carbohydrates (fruits, vegetables, or whole grains vs refined grains and simple sugars) and their digestibility (soluble vs insoluble fiber). A quantitative approach to the analysis of dietary carbohydrate has been developed based on glycemic index (GI) and GL, as discussed in the following section.

Sugars and Starches

Simple carbohydrates are present in foods as monosaccharides or disaccharides and are naturally present in such foods as fruit and milk. Glucose, fructose, and galactose are the most common monosaccharides in the human diet and combine to form the disaccharides sucrose (glucose + fructose), lactose (glucose + galactose), and maltose (glucose + glucose). Oligosaccharides are short chains of 3–10 sugar molecules, and the most common ones, raffinose and stachyose, are found in beans, peas, and lentils. Polysaccharides are starches that contain >10 sugar molecules, found in wheat, rice, corn, oats, legumes, and tubers. Starches form long chains that are either straight (amylose) or branched (amylopectin). Amylose and amylopectin occur in a ratio of about 1:4 in plant foods.

Although there are several dietary factors that contribute to obesity, a dietary pattern that is rich in sugars and starches is considered a risk factor for obesity, whereas a high intake of nonstarch polysaccharides in the form of dietary fiber is considered protective (Swinburn et al., 2004). The typical Western diet is high in refined starches and sugars, which are digested and absorbed rapidly, resulting in a high GL and increased demand for insulin secretion. This in turn promotes postprandial carbohydrate oxidation at the expense of fat oxidation. Both acute (Ludwig et al., 1999; Febbraio et al., 2000) and short-term studies (Howe et al., 1996; Agus et al., 2000) indicate that a dietary pattern that produces a high glycemic response affects appetite and promotes body fat storage.

However, diets based on high-fiber foods that produce a low glycemic response can enhance weight control because they promote satiety, minimize postprandial insulin secretion, and maintain insulin sensitivity (Brand-Miller et al., 2002). This is supported by several intervention studies in humans in which energy-restricted diets based on low-GI foods produced greater weight loss than equivalent diets based on high-GI foods. Long-term studies in animal models have also shown that diets based on high-GI starches promote weight gain, visceral adiposity, and higher concentrations of lipogenic enzymes than isoenergetic diets with a low-GI, which are macronutrient controlled.

Soluble and Insoluble Fiber

Insoluble dietary fibers such as cellulose and lignins are not digested in the intestine and pass in the stool intact. These fibers trap water, increase fecal weight, and accelerate transit time in the gastrointestinal tract, thus promoting regularity. Soluble carbohydrates such as pectin, gums, and β-glucans are digested by bacteria in the colon. These fibers delay glucose absorption and are able to bind bile acids in the gastrointestinal tract, thus reducing serum cholesterol levels. Ancient humans ate a great deal of fiber, estimated at >50 g/day, whereas modern humans consume on average 10–15 g/day.

Epidemiological evidence suggests that the risk of colorectal and breast cancers may be decreased by increasing the intake of foods high in fiber such as vegetables, fruits, cereals, and whole grains (Hill, 1998; Jacobs et al., 1998; Martínez et al., 1999), but the findings have not been entirely consistent. Based on 25 years of follow-up data for men in the Seven Countries Study, a 10-g/day increase in fiber intake was associated with a 33% lower 25-year colorectal cancer mortality risk (Jansen et al., 1999). However, 16 years of follow-up data from the Nurses' Health Study showed no association between dietary fiber intake and colorectal cancer risk in women (Fuchs et al., 1999). In the prospective Cancer Study II Nutrition Cohort, higher intakes of plant foods or fiber were not related to lower risk of colon cancer, but it was concluded that very low intakes of plant foods may increase risk (McCullough et al., 2003).

Diets high in fiber have been hypothesized to protect against breast cancer, perhaps because of inhibition of the intestinal reabsorption of estrogens normally excreted in the bile (Goldin et al., 1982). In a meta-analysis of 10 case–control studies, a statistically significant reduction in breast cancer risk with a 20-g/day increase in dietary fiber was observed (Howe et al., 1990), yet prospective studies have been unevenly supportive. In a Canadian prospective study including 519 cases (Rohan et al., 1993), a marginally significant inverse association between dietary fiber and breast cancer risk was seen. In a subsample of >11,000 postmenopausal women in the Malmo Diet and Cancer cohort, high fiber intakes were associated with a lower risk of postmenopausal breast cancer for the highest quintile of fiber intake compared with the lowest quintile, and the combination of high fiber and low fat intakes had the lowest risk (Mattisson et al., 2004). In other prospective cohorts, however, with 344 and 650 cases, no suggestion of a protective effect was found (Graham et al., 1992; Verhoeven et al., 1997). In the Nurses' Health Study, the association between total dietary fiber intake and subsequent breast cancer incidence (1439 cases) was very close to null (Willett et al., 1992).

The evaluation of the role of dietary fiber in cancer prevention is complicated by the varying composition of fiber from different food sources, variations in fiber measurement techniques and dietary assessment, and the possible effects of other substances in high-fiber foods, such as micronutrients and phytochemicals. There are potentially numerous antimutagenic compounds in fruits, vegetables, and whole grains, and fibers may provide one of the simplest mechanisms in their ability to reduce mutagen uptake (Ferguson et al., 2004).

Glycemic Index and Glycemic Load

Conventional approaches to weight loss have focused on decreasing dietary fat because of its high-calorie density. However, the relationship between dietary fat and obesity has been brought into question for several reasons. Low-fat diets have been shown to produce only modest weight loss, and prospective epidemiological studies have not been able to consistently correlate dietary fat intake with weight. Despite a decrease in fat consumption as a percentage of total calories and widespread availability of low-fat and fat-free foods, obesity prevalence in the United States has risen dramatically since the 1970s (Putnam and Allshouse, 1999). At the same time, carbohydrate consumption has increased, and most of this increase has been in the form of refined starches and concentrated sweets with a high GI and/or GL.

In 1981, Jenkins et al. introduced the GI as a system for classifying carbohydrate-containing foods based on their effect on postprandial glycemia. The glycemic response to the ingestion of 50 g of available carbohydrate from the test food is compared with the response from the ingestion of 50 g of the reference food (glucose or white bread), and the GI is expressed as the area under the glucose response curve for the test food divided by the area under the curve for the standard, multiplied by 100. However, the amount of carbohydrate in 50 g of a given food will vary depending on the food, and this observation led to the introduction of the concept of GL. This is an expression of the GI of the food, multiplied by the carbohydrate content of the food, and takes into account the differences in carbohydrate content among foods (Liu, 1998). Foods with a high index but relatively low total carbohydrate content, such as carrots, have a low GL. In general, fruits, nonstarchy vegetables, nuts, and legumes have a low GI (Table 1).

The intake of high-GI/GL meals induces a sequence of hormonal changes, including an increased ratio of insulin to glucagon, which limit the availability of metabolic fuels in the postprandial period and promote nutrient storage (Ludwig, 2002) and would be expected to stimulate hunger and promote food intake. Short-term feeding studies have demonstrated less satiety and greater voluntary food intake after consumption of high-GI meals as compared with

TABLE 1 Glycemic Index and Glycemic Load (GL) Values for Foods

Low GI (<55) and low GL (<16) foods; lowest calorie (≤110 calories/serving)

	GI	GL	Serving size	Calories	Fiber (g)
Most vegetables	<20	<5	1 cup, cooked	40	
Apple	40	6	1 average	75	4
Banana	52	12	1 average	90	3
Cherries	22	3	15 cherries	85	3
Grapefruit	25	5	1 average fruit	75	2
Kiwi	53	6	1 average fruit	45	3
Mango	51	14	1 small fruit	110	3
Orange	48	5	1 average fruit	65	3
Peach	42	7	1 average fruit	70	2
Plums	39	5	2 medium fruits	70	2
Strawberries	40	1	1 cup	50	4
Tomato juice	38	4	1 cup	40	1

High GI (>55) but low GL (<16) foods; all low calorie (≤110)

	GI	GL	Serving size	Calories	Fiber (g)
Apricots	57	6	4 medium	70	4
Orange juice	57	15	1 cup	110	0
Papaya	60	9	1 cup cubes	55	3
Pineapple	59	7	1 cup cubes	75	2
Pumpkin	75	3	1 cup, mashed	85	7
Shredded wheat	75	15	1 cup mini squares	110	5
Toasted oats	74	15	1 cup	110	2
Watermelon	72	7	1 cup cubes	50	1

Low GI (<55) and low GL (<16) foods; moderate calories (110–135 calories/serving)

	GI	GL	Serving size	Calories	Fiber (g)
Apple juice	40	12	1 cup	135	0
Grapefruit juice	48	9	1 cup	115	0
Pear	33	10	1 medium	125	2
Peas	48	3	1 cup	135	9
Pineapple juice	46	15	1 cup	130	0
Whole-grain bread	51	14	1 slice	80–120	2–5

(*continued*)

TABLE 1 *(Continued)*

Low GI (<55) and low GL (<16) foods; higher calorie (160–300 calories/serving)					
	GI	GL	Serving size	Calories	Fiber (g)
Barley	25	11	1 cup, cooked	190	8
Black beans	20	8	1 cup, cooked	235	15
Garbanzo beans	28	13	1 cup, cooked	285	12
Grapes	46	13	40 grapes	160	2
Kidney beans	23	10	1 cup, cooked	210	9
Lentils	29	7	1 cup, cooked	230	15
Soybeans	18	1	1 cup, cooked	300	8
Yam	37	13	1 cup, cooked	160	6
Low GI (<55) and low GL (<16) foods; high fat and high calorie					
	GI	GL	Serving size	Calories	Fiber (g)
Cashews	22	4	1/2 cup	395	2
Premium ice cream	38	10	1 cup	360	0
Low-fat ice cream	37–50	13	1 cup	220	0
Peanuts	14	1	1/2 cup	330	6
Potato chips	54	15	2 ounces	345	3
Whole milk	27	3	1 cup	150	0
Vanilla pudding	44	16	1 cup	250	0
Fruit yogurt	31	9	1 cup	200+	2
Soy yogurt	50	13	1 cup	200+	2
High GI (≥55) and high GL (≥16)					
	GI	GL	Serving size	Calories	Fiber (g)
Baked potato	85	34	1 small	220	3
Cola	63	33	16-ounce bottle	200	0
Corn	60	20	1 ear, 1 cup kernels	130	4
Corn chips	63	21	2 ounces	350	3
Corn flakes	92	24	1 cup	100	1
Cranberry juice	68	24	1 cup	145	1
Cream of wheat	74	22	1 cup, cooked	130	0
Croissant	67	17	1 average	275	1
French fries	75	25	1 large order	515	1
Macaroni and cheese	64	46	1 cup	285	2
Oatmeal	75	17	1 cup, cooked	140	4
High GI (>55) and high GL (>16)					
	GI	GL	Serving size	Calories	Fiber (g)
Pizza	60	20	1 large slice	300	2
Pretzels	83	33	1 ounce	115	1
Raisin bran	61	29	1 cup	185	8
Raisins	66	42	1/2 cup	250	3
Soda crackers	74	18	12 crackers	155	1
Waffles	76	18	1 average	150	0
White bread	73	20	2 small slices	160	1
White rice	64	23	1 cup, cooked	210	1

low-GI meals (Ludwig et al., 1999), for example, the demonstration of prolonged satiety after consumption of a low-GI bean puree versus a high-GI potato puree (Leathwood and Pollett, 1998).

Weight loss on a low-calorie, reduced-fat diet may be enhanced if the diet also has a low GI (Slabber et al., 1994) and even when energy intake is not restricted, low-GI and/or low-GL diets have been shown to produce greater weight loss than conventional low-fat diets (Ebbeling et al., 2003). Additionally, subjects consuming a low-GI diet *ad libitum* have been reported to experience a spontaneous 25% reduction in energy intake, with significant reductions in body weight and waist and hip circumference when compared with controls (Dumesnil et al., 2001).

Other data suggest that low-GI/GL diets may confer protection against certain forms of cancer, cardiovascular disease and the metabolic syndrome, and type 2 diabetes. In the Women's Health Study, a high-GL dietary pattern was associated with an increased risk for colon cancer (Higginbotham et al., 2004), and data from the Iowa Women's Study indicate that a higher GL pattern may be a risk factor for endometrial cancer incidence in nondiabetic women (Folsom et al., 2003). In a study of 244 healthy women, a strong and statistically significant positive association was found between dietary GL and plasma C-reactive protein, a plasma marker for chronic inflammation associated with an increased risk for heart disease (Liu et al., 2002). In large prospective epidemiological studies, both the GI and the GL of the overall diet have been associated with a greater risk of type 2 diabetes in both men and women (Salmeron et al., 1997a,b).

FUNCTIONAL FOODS

Soy Protein

Soy protein is the highest quality protein found in the plant kingdom, and it is eaten by two thirds of the world's population. Interest in soy proteins and cancer prevention arose from the observation that naturally occurring chemicals within soy protein called *soy isoflavones* were able to inhibit the growth of both estrogen-receptor–positive and estrogen-receptor–negative breast cancer cells *in vitro* (Peterson and Barnes 1996).

Soy protein naturally contains isoflavones, primarily genistein and daidzein, which are called *phytoestrogens*. They are usually found in foods linked to sugars called *glycosides*, and these phytoestrogens act like very weak estrogens or antiestrogens similar to raloxifene. When primates have a surgical menopause induced and are given estradiol alone or estradiol in combination with soy isoflavones, the isoflavones antagonize the actions of estradiol in the breast and the uterus but demonstrate estrogen-like beneficial activities in the bone, on serum lipids, and in the brain. These observations are explained by the existence of two estrogen receptors called *alpha* and *beta*. Soy isoflavones bind with very low affinity (1/50,000 to 1/100,000 the affinity of estradiol) to the alpha-estradiol receptor but bind equally well to the beta-estradiol receptor (Clarkson et al., 2001).

In 1994, Messina et al. reviewed 26 studies showing the effects of soy or soy isoflavones on eight cancer sites in animals. Most of the studies (17 of 26, or 65%) showed that soy may have protective effects. None of the studies indicated that soy increased tumor development. In addition, the studies of populations eating soy protein indicated that they had a lower incidence of breast cancer and other common cancers compared with populations such as the U.S. population in which soy foods were rarely eaten (Yamamoto et al., 2003). These studies provided only supportive evidence for a positive role of soy foods, because the diets of the populations eating more soy protein were also richer in fruits, vegetables, and whole cereals and grains in comparison with the U.S. diet.

Soy protein isoflavones have been shown to influence not only sex hormone metabolism and biological activity but also intracellular enzymes, protein synthesis, growth factor action, and malignant cell proliferation, differentiation, and angiogenesis, providing strong evidence that these substances may have a protective role in cancer (Kim et al., 2002).

Soy food intake has also been shown to have beneficial effects on cardiovascular disease, although data directly linking soy food intake to clinical outcomes of cardiovascular disease have been sparse. A study among the participants of the Shanghai Women's Health Study, a population-based prospective cohort study of ~75,000 Chinese women, documented a dose–response relationship between soy food intake and risk of coronary heart disease, providing direct evidence that soy food consumption may reduce the risk of coronary heart disease in women (Zhang et al., 2003).

Phytochemical-Rich Fruits, Vegetables, and Grains

Because fruits and vegetables are high in water and fiber, incorporating them into the diet can reduce energy density, promote satiety, and decrease energy intake while providing phytonutrients. Few interventions have specifically addressed fruit and vegetable consumption and weight loss, but evidence suggests that the recommendation to increase these foods while decreasing total energy intake is an effective strategy for weight management. Obesity, although often considered synonymous with overnutrition, is more accurately depicted as overnutrition of calories but undernutrition of many essential vitamins, minerals, and phytonutrients. This increased incidence of obesity has been associated with an increased incidence of heart disease, breast cancer, prostate cancer, and colon cancer by comparison with populations eating a dietary pattern consisting of less meat and more fruits, vegetables, cereals, and whole grains. The intake of 400–600 g/day of fruits and vegetables is associated with a reduced incidence of many common forms of cancer, heart disease, and many chronic diseases of aging (Willett, 1994, 1995; Temple, 2000).

The common forms of cancer, including breast, colon, and prostate cancer, are the result of genetic–environmental interactions. Most cancers have genetic changes at the somatic cell level, which lead to unregulated growth through activation of oncogenes or inactivation of tumor suppressor genes. Reactive oxygen radicals are thought to damage biological structures and molecules, including lipids, protein, and DNA, and there is evidence that antioxidants can prevent this damage.

Fruits and vegetables provide thousands of phytochemicals to the human diet, and many of these are absorbed into the body. Although these are commonly antioxidants, based on their ability to trap singlet oxygen, they have been demonstrated scientifically to have many functions beyond antioxidation. These phytochemicals can interact with the host to confer a preventive benefit by regulating enzymes important in metabolizing xenobiotics and carcinogens, by modulating nuclear receptors and cellular signaling of proliferation and apoptosis, and by acting indirectly through antioxidant actions that reduce proliferation and protect DNA from damage (Blot et al., 1993).

Phytochemicals found in fruits and vegetables demonstrate synergistic and additive interactions through their effects on gene expression, antioxidation, and cytokine action. Fruits and vegetables are 10-fold to 20-fold less calorie dense than grains, provide increased amounts of dietary fiber compared with refined grains, and provide a balance of omega-3 and omega-6 fatty acids and a rich supply of micronutrients.

Several studies have sought to characterize dietary patterns and relate these patterns to body weight and other nutritional parameters. A prospective study of 737 non-overweight women in the Framingham Offspring/Spouse cohort explored the relationship between dietary patterns and the development of overweight over a 12-year period. Participants were grouped into one of five dietary patterns at baseline, which included a heart-healthy pattern (low fat, nutritionally varied), light eating (lower calories, but proportionately more fat and fewer micronutrients), a wine and moderate-eating pattern, a high-fat pattern, and an empty-calorie pattern (rich in sweets and fat and low in fruits and vegetables). Women in the heart-healthy cluster consumed more servings of vegetables and fruits than women in each of the other four clusters. Over the 12-year period, 214 cases of overweight developed in this cohort. Compared with women in the heart-healthy group, women in the empty-calorie group were at a significantly higher risk for developing overweight (relative risk [RR] 1.4, 95% confidence [CI]) (Quatromoni et al., 2002).

In another analysis of dietary patterns among 179 older rural adults, those in the high-nutrient-dense cluster (higher intake of dark green/yellow vegetables, citrus/melons/berries, and other fruits and vegetables) had lower energy intakes and lower waist circumferences than those in the low-nutrient-dense cluster (higher intake of breads, sweets, desserts, processed meats, eggs, fats, and oil). Those with a low-nutrient-dense pattern were twice as likely to be obese (Ledikewe et al., 2004). Similar observations were reported using data from the Canadian Community Health Survey from 2000 to 2001. The frequency of eating fruits and vegetables was positively related to being physically active and not being overweight (Perez, 2002).

In a controlled clinical trial, families with obese parents and nonobese children were randomized into either a comprehensive behavioral weight management program that featured encouragement to increase fruit and vegetable consumption or to decrease intake of high-fat, high-sugar foods. Over a 1-year period, parents in the increased fruit and vegetable group showed significantly greater decreases in percentage of overweight than in the group attempting to reduce fat and sugar intake (Epstein et al., 2001).

Current National Cancer Institute dietary recommendations emphasize increasing the daily consumption of fruits and vegetables from diverse sources such as citrus fruits, cruciferous vegetables, and green and yellow vegetables (Steinmetz and Potter, 1991). The concept of selecting foods by color was extended in a book for the public to seven different groups based on their content of a primary phytochemical family for which there is evidence of cancer prevention potential (Heber and Bowerman, 2001).

BUILDING DIETS FOR INTERVENTIONAL STUDIES

An improved understanding of the important dietary factors that affect the impact of foods on cellular function is useful when designing diets for clinical trials. So-called "global interventions" attempt to incorporate all that is healthy in a single multifactorial intervention. In the past, these "global" interventions have been criticized for not providing the key functional foods that might be important in cancer prevention (Schatzkin and Lanza, 2002). Instead, they relied on general concepts such as servings of fruits and vegetables or replacing fat with refined carbohydrate. As our scientific understanding of the key physiological roles of the dietary macronutrients has expanded, we are now able to more accurately predict the effects of particular foods on the dietary pattern, energy intake, and physiology. Although additional research is needed, it can now be better focused than the nutrition research studies of 20 years ago.

CONCLUSION

Traditional therapeutic diets provide suggested servings of foods in groups because it is impractical to calculate specific food values for every diet plan that is individually administered. For example, exchange diets are based on the idea that all human diets can be simplified into protein, carbohydrate, or fat exchanges. So a serving of iceberg lettuce and a serving of spinach are equivalent, as would be a serving of grain-fed prime rib and a serving of ocean-caught tuna.

Ultimately, this simplification leads to the idea that food is simply an energy source for the body and that there are certain minimum requirements for avoiding deficiency and promoting health. To some extent, according to these notions, a calorie is a calorie. The body can interconvert from one source to another and this is a key part of our adaptation to starvation. However, there is no genetic pressure for eating a healthful diet that avoids the chronic diseases of aging including cancer because these arise after the age of reproduction has passed. Therefore, the preventive properties of the diet are dissociated from its provision of nutritional energy or calories alone.

As our society is solving the problem of malnutrition throughout the world, we are left with chronic diseases of aging related to too many calories relative to physical activity and poor quality diets with too few servings of fruits, vegetables, and whole grains and too many servings of high-fat, high-sugar processed foods lacking naturally occurring vitamins, minerals, and the thousands of secondary plant substances called *phytonutrients* or *phytochemicals*.

The premise is simple: Diet is a major etiologic factor in chronic disease, responsible for up to one third of most types of cancer. Dietary chemicals change the expression of one's genes and even the genome itself. Genetic variation may explain why two people can eat exactly the same diet and respond very differently. Nutritional genomics emphasizes the interactions at a cellular and molecular level studied through systems biology.

References

Agus, M.S.D., Swain, J.F., Larson, C.L., Eckert, E.A., and Ludwig, D.S. 2000. Dietary composition and physiologic adaptations to energy restriction. *Am J Clin Nutr* **271**: 901–907.

Bagga, D., Capone, S., Wang, H.-J., Heber, D., Lill, M., Chap, L., and Glaspy, J.A. 1997. Dietary modulation of omega-3/omega-6 polyunsaturated fatty acid ratios in patients with breast cancer. *J Natl Cancer Inst* **89**: 1123–1131.

Barr, S.I., Murphy, S.P., Agurs-Collins, T.D., and Poos, M.I. 2003. Planning diets for individuals using the dietary reference intakes. *Nutr Rev* **61**: 352–360.

Bartsch, H., Nair, J., and Owen, R.W. 1999. Dietary polyunsaturated fatty acids and cancers of the breast and colorectum: emerging evidence for their role as risk modifiers. *Carcinogenesis* **20**: 2209–2218.

Berdanier, C. 2000. Proteins. *In* "Advanced Nutrition: Macronutrients," 2nd edition, pp. 130–196. CRC Press, Boca Raton, FL.

Blot, W.J., Li, J.-Y., Taylor, P.R., Guo, W., Dawsey, S., Wang, G.-Q., Yang, C.S., Zheng, S.-F., Gail, M., Li, G.-Y., Yu, Y., Liu, B.-Q., Tangrea, J., Sun, Y.-H., Liu, F., Fraumeni, J.F., Zhang, Y.-H., and Li, B.. 1993. Nutrition intervention trials in Linxiang, China: supplementation with specific vitamin/mineral combinations, cancer incidence, and disease-specific mortality in the general population. *J Nat Cancer Inst* **85**: 1483–1492.

Boudreau, M.D., Sohn, K.H., Rhee, S.H., Lee, S.W., Hunt, J.D., and Hwang, D.H. 2001. Suppression of tumor cell growth both in nude mice and in culture by n-3 polyunsaturated fatty acids: mediation through cyclooxygenase-independent pathways. *Cancer Res* **61**: 1386–1391.

Brand-Miller, J.C., Holt, S.H., Pawlak, D.B., and McMillan, J. 2002. Glycemic index and obesity. *Am J Clin Nutr* **76**: 281S-285S.

Calle, E.E., and Thun, M.J. 2004. Obesity and cancer. *Oncogene* **23**: 6365–6378.

Campbell, W.W., Crim, M.C., Dallal, G.E., Young, V.R., and Evans, W.J. 1994. Increased protein requirements in elderly people: new data and retrospective reassessments. *Am J Clin Nutr* **60**: 501–509.

Chawla, A., Boisvert, W.A., Lee, C.H., Laffitte, B.A., Barak, Y., Joseph, S.B., Liao, D., Nagy, L., Edwards, P.A., Curtiss, L.K., Evans, R.M., and Tontonoz, P. 2001. A PPAR gamma-LXR-ABCA1 pathway in macrophages is involved in cholesterol efflux and atherogenesis. *Mol Cell* **7**: 161–171.

Chinetti, G., Lestavel, S., Bocher, V., Remaley, A.T., Neve, B., Torra, I.P., Teissier, E., Minnich, A., Jaye, M., Duverger, N., Brewer, H.B., Fruchart, J.C., Clavey, V., and Staels, B. 2001. PPAR-alpha and PPAR-gamma activators induce cholesterol removal from human macrophage foam cells through stimulation of the ABCA1 pathway. *Nat Med* **7**: 53–58.

Clarkson, T.B., Anthony, M.S., and Morgan, T.M. 2001. Inhibition of post-menopausal atherosclerosis progression: a comparison of the effects of conjugated equine estrogens and soy phytoestrogens. *J Clin Endocrinol Metab* **86**: 41–47.

Committee on Diet and Health. 1989. Diet and health: protein. *In* "Diet and Health: Implications for Reducing Chronic Disease Risk," pp. 259–271. National Research Council, Food and Nutrition Board, Washington, DC.

Dumesnil, J.G., Turgeon, J., Tremblay, A., Poirier, P., Gilbert, M., Gagnon, L., St-Pierre, S., Garneau, C., Lemieux, I., Pascot, A., Bergeron, J., and Despres, J.P. 2001. Effect of a low-glycaemic index–low-fat–high-protein diet on the atherogenic metabolic risk profile of abdominally obese men. *Br J Nutr* **86**: 557–568.

Ebbeling, C.B., Leidig, M.M., Sinclair, K.B., Hangen, J.P., and Ludwig, D.S. 2003. A reduced-glycemic load diet in the treatment of adolescent obesity. *Arch Pediatr Adolesc Med* **157**: 773–779.

Eisenstein, J., Roberts, S.B., Dallal, G., and Saltzman, E. 2002. High protein weight loss diets: are they safe and do they work? A review of experimental and epidemiologic data. *Nutr Rev* **60**: 189–200.

Epstein, L.H., Gordy, C.C., Raynor, H.A., Beddome, M., Kilanowski, C.K., and Paluch, R. 2001. Increasing fruit and vegetable intake and decreasing fat and sugar intake in families at risk for childhood obesity. *Obes Res* **9**: 171–178.

Febbraio, M.A., Keenan, J., Angus, D.J., Campbell, S.E., and Garnham, A.P. 2000. Pre-exercise carbohydrate ingestion, glucose kinetics, and muscle glycogen use: effect of the glycemic index. *J Appl Physiol* **89**: 1845–1851.

Ferguson, L.R., Philpott, M., and Karunasinghe, N. 2004. Dietary cancer and prevention using antimutagens. *Toxicology* **20**: 147–159.

Folsom, A.R., Demissie, Z., and Harnack, L. 2003. Glycemic index, glycemic load and incidence of endometrial cancer: the Iowa Women's Health Study. *Nutr Cancer* **46**: 119–124.

Fourcade, S., Savary, S., Albet, S., Gauthe, D., Gondcaille, C., Pineau, T., Bellenger, J., Bentejac, M., Holzinger, A., Berger, J., and Bugaut, M. 2001. Fibrate induction of the adrenoleukodystrophy-related gene (ABCD2): promoter analysis and role of the peroxisome proliferator-activated receptor PPARalpha. *Eur J Biochem.* **268**: 3490–3500.

Fuchs, C.S., Giovannucci, E.L., Colditz, G.A., Hunter, D.J., Stampfer, M.J., Rosner, B., Speizer, F.E., and Willett, W.C. 1999. Dietary fiber and the risk of colorectal cancer and adenoma in women. *N Engl J Med* **340**: 169–176.

Fuller, M. 2000. Proteins and amino acid requirements. *In* "Biochemical and Physiological Aspects of Human Nutrition" (M. Stipanuk, Ed.), pp. 287–304. WB Saunders, Philadelphia.

Fung, T., Hu, F.B., Fuchs, C., Giovannucci, E., Hunter, D.J., Stampfer, M.J., Colditz, G.A., and Willett, W.C. 2003. Major dietary patterns and the risk of colorectal cancer in women. *Arch Int Med* **163**: 309–314.

Garza, C., Scrimshaw, N.S., and Young, V.R. 1977. Human protein requirements: a long-term metabolic nitrogen balance study in young men to evaluate the 1973 FAO/WHO safe level of egg protein intake. *J Nutr* **107**: 335–352.

Goldin, B.R., Adlercreutz, H., Gorbach, S.L., Warram, J.H., Dwyer, J.T., Swenson, L., and Woods, M.N. 1982. Estrogen excretion patterns and plasma levels in vegetarian and omnivorous women. *N Engl J Med* **307**: 1542–1547.

Graham, S., Zielezny, M., Marshall, J., Priore, R., Freudenheim, J., Brasure, J., Haughey, B., Nasca, P., and Zdeb, M. 1992. Diet in the epidemiology of postmenopausal breast cancer in the New York State cohort. *Am J Epidemiol* **136**: 1327–1337.

Heber, D., and Bowerman, S. 2001. "What Color is Your Diet?" Harper Collins, New York.

Hill, M.J. 1998. Cereals, cereal fibre and colorectal cancer risk: a review of the epidemiological literature. *Eur J Cancer Prev* **7**: S5–S10.

Higginbotham, S., Zhang, Z.F., Lee, I.M., Cook, N.R., Giovannucci, E., Buring, J.E., and Liu, S. 2004. Dietary glycemic load and risk of colorectal cancer in the Women's Health Study. *J Natl Canc Inst* **96**: 229–233.

Howe, G.R., Hirohata, T., Hislop, T.G., Iscovich, J.M., Yuan, J.M., Katsouyanni, K., Lubin, F., Marubini, E., Modan, B., Rohan, T., Toniolo P., and Shunzhang Y. 1990. Dietary factors and risk of breast cancer: combined analysis of 12 case-control studies. *J Natl Cancer Inst* **82**: 561–569.

Howe, J.C., Rumpler, W.V., and Behall, K.M. 1996. Dietary starch composition and level of energy intake alter nutrient oxidation in "carbohydrate-sensitive" men. *J Nutr* **126**: 2120–2129.

Jacobs, D.R., Marquart, L., Slavin, J., and Kushi, L.H. 1998. Whole-grain intake and cancer: an expanded review and meta-analysis. *Nutr Cancer* **30**: 85–96.

Jansen, M.C., Bueno-de-Mesquita, H.B., Buzina, R., Fidanza, F., Menotti, A., Blackburn, H., Nissinen, A.M., Kok, F.J., and Kromhout, D; the Seven Countries Study Research Group. 1999. Dietary fiber and plant foods in relation to colorectal cancer mortality: the Seven Countries Study. *Int J Cancer* **81**: 174–179.

Jenkins, D.J., Wolever, T.M., Taylor, R.H., Barker, H., Fielden, H., Baldwin, J.M., and Bowling, A.C., Newman, H.C., Jenkins, A.L., and Goff, D.V. 1981. Glycemic index of foods: a physiological basis for carbohydrate exchange. *Am J Clin Nutr* **34**: 362–366.

Johnston, C.S., Tjonn, S.L., and Swan, P.D. 2004. High-protein, low-fat diets are effective for weight loss and favorably alter biomarkers in healthy adults. *J Nutr* **134**: 586–591.

Kalman, R., Adler, J.H., Lazarovici, G., Bar-On, H., and Ziv, E. 1993. The efficiency of sand rat metabolism is responsible for development of obesity and diabetes. *J Basic Clin Physiol Pharmacol* **4**: 57–68.

Karmali, R.A., Marsh, J., and Fuchs, C. 1984. Effect of omega-3 fatty acids on growth of a rat mammary tumor. *J Natl Cancer Inst* **73**: 457–461.

Kim, M.H., Gutierrez, A.M., and Goldfarb, R.H. 2002. Different mechanisms of soy isoflavones in cell cycle regulation and inhibition of invasion. *Anticancer Res.* **22**: 3811–3817.

Kreutler, P., and Czajka-Narins, D. 1987. Protein. *In* "Nutrition in Perspective," pp. 121–162. Prentice Hall, Upper Saddle River, NJ.

Kris-Etherton, P.M., Lefevre, M., Beecher, G.R., Gross, M.D., Keen, C.L., and Etherton, T.D. 2004. Bioactive compounds in nutrition and health-research methodologies for establishing biological function: the antioxidant and anti-inflammatory effects of flavonoids on atherosclerosis. *Ann Rev Nutr* **24**: 511–538.

Lappe, F.M. 1971. "Diet for a Small Planet." Ballantine Books, New York.

Layman, D.K., Boileau, R.A., Erickson, D.J., Painter, J.E., Shiue, H., Sather, C., and Christou, D.D. 2003. Reduced ratio of dietary carbohydrate to protein improves body composition and blood lipid profiles during weight loss in adult women. *J Nutr* **133**: 411–417.

Leathwood, P., and Pollett, P. 1988. Effects of slow release carbohydrates in the form of bean flakes on the evolution of hunger and satiety in man. *Appetite* **10**: 1–11.

Ledikewe, J.H., Smiciklas-Wright, H., Mitchell, D.C., Miller, C.K., and Jensen, G.L. 2004. Dietary patterns of rural older adults are associated with weight and nutritional status. *J Am Geriatr Soc* **52**: 589–595.

Lee, S.S., Pineau, T., Drago, J., Lee, E.J., Owens, J.W., Kroetz, D.L., Fernandez-Salguero, P.M., Westphal, H., and Gonzalez, F.J. 1995. Targeted disruption of the alpha isoform of the peroxisome proliferator-activated receptor gene in mice results in abolishment of the pleiotropic effects of peroxisome proliferators. *Mol Cell Biol* **15**: 3012–3022.

Lindner, M.A. 1991. A fish oil diet inhibits colon cancer in mice. *Nutr Cancer* **15**: 1–11.

Liu, S. 1998. "Dietary Glycemic Load, Carbohydrate and Whole Grain Intakes in Relation to Risk of Coronary Heart Disease." Harvard University, Boston, MA.

Liu, S., Manson, J.E., Buring, J.E., Stampfer, M.J., Willett, W.C., and Ridker, P.M. 2002. Relation between a diet with a high glycemic load and plasma concentrations of high-sensitivity C-reactive protein in middle-aged women. *Am J Clin Nutr* **75**: 492–498.

London, S.J., Sacks, F.M., Caesar, J., Stampfer, M.J., Siguel, E., and Willett, W.C. 1991. Fatty acid composition of subcutaneous adipose tissue and diet in postmenopausal US women. *Am J Clin Nutr* **54**: 340–345.

Ludwig, D.S. 2002. The glycemic index: physiological mechanisms relating to obesity, diabetes, and cardiovascular disease. *JAMA* **287**: 2414–2423.

Ludwig, D.S., Majzoub, J.A., Al-Zahrani, A., Dallal, G.E., Blanco, I., and Roberts, S.B. 1999. High glycemic index foods, overeating, and obesity. *Pediatrics* **103**: E26.

Martínez, M.E., Marshall, J.R., and Alberts, D.S. 1999. Dietary fiber, carbohydrates, and cancer. *In* "Nutritional Oncology" (D. Heber, G.L. Blackburn, and V.L.W. Go, Eds.), pp. 185–194. Academic Press, San Diego.

Matthews, D. 1999. Proteins and amino acids. *In* "Modern Nutrition in Health and Disease" (M. Shils, J. Olson, MD. M. Shike, and A.C. Ross, Eds.), 9th edition, pp. 11–48. Williams & Wilkins, Baltimore.

Mattisson, I., Wirfalt, E., Johansson, U., Gullberg, B., Olsson, H., and Berglund, G. 2004. Intakes of plant foods, fibre and fat and risk of breast cancer—a prospective study in the Malmo Diet and Cancer cohort. *Br J Cancer* **90**: 122–127.

McCullough, M.L., and Giovannucci, E.L. 2004. Diet and cancer prevention. *Oncogene* **23**: 6349–6364.

McCullough, M.L., Robertson, A.S., Chao, A., Jacobs, E.J., Stampfer, M.J., Jacobs, D.R., Diver, W.R., Calle, E.E., and Thun, M.J. 2003. A prospective study of whole grains, fruits, vegetables and colon cancer risk. *Cancer Causes Control* **14**: 959–970.

McDowell, M., Briefel, R., Alaimo, K., Bischof, A.M., Caughman, C.R., Carroll, M.D., Loria, C.M., and Johnson, C.L. 1994. Energy and macronutrient intakes of persons ages 2 months and over in the United States: Third National Health and Nutrition Examination Survey, Phase 1, 1988–91. US Government Printing Office, Vital and Health Statistics, Washington, DC.

Messina, M.J., Persky, V., Setchell, K.D., and Barnes, S. 1994. Soy intake and cancer risk: a review of the in vitro and in vivo data. *Nutr Cancer* **21**: 113–131.

Milner, J. 2002. Strategies for cancer prevention: the role of diet. *Br J Nutr* **87**: S265–S272.

Narayanan, B.A., Narayanan, N.K., and Reddy, B.S. 2001. Docosahexaenoic acid regulated genes and transcription factors inducing apoptosis in human colon cancer cells. *Int J Oncol* **19**: 1255–1262.

National Research Council, Food and Nutrition Board. 1989. "Recommended Dietary Allowances," 10th edition. National Academy Press, Washington, DC.

Nationwide Food Consumption Survey. 1984. Nutrient intakes: individuals in 48 states, year 1977–78. US Dept. of Agriculture, Consumer Nutrition Division, HNIS, Hyattsville, MD. Report No. I-2.

Okuyama, H., Kobayashi, T., and Watanbe, S. 1996. Dietary fatty acids—the n-6/n-3 balance and chronic elderly diseases. Excess linoleic acid and relative n-3 deficiency syndrome seen in Japan. *Prog Lipid Res* **35**: 409–457.

Perez, C.E. 2002. Fruit and vegetable consumption. *Health Rep* **13**: 23–31.

Peterson, G., and Barnes, S. 1996. Genistein inhibits both estrogen and growth factor-stimulated proliferation of human breast cancer cells. *Cell Growth Differ* **7**: 1345–1351.

Putnam, J.J., and Allshouse, J.A. 1999. "Food Consumption, Prices, and Expenditures, 1970–97." US Department of Agriculture, Washington, DC.

Quatromoni, P.A., Copenhafer, D.L., D'Agostino, R.B., and Millen, B.E. 2002. Dietary patterns predict the development of overweight in women: The Framingham Nutrition Studies. *J Am Diet Assoc* **102**: 1240–1246.

Rohan, T.E., Howe, G.R., Friedenreich, C.M., Jain, M., and Miller, A.B. 1993. Dietary fiber, vitamins A, C, and E, and risk of breast cancer: a cohort study. *Cancer Causes Control* **4**: 29–37.

Rose, D.P., and Connolly, J.M. 1999. Omega-3 fatty acids as cancer chemopreventive agents. *Pharmacol Ther* **83**: 217–244.

Rose, D.P., Connolly, J.M., and Meschter, C.L. 1991. Effect of dietary fat on human breast cancer growth and lung metastasis in nude mice. *J Natl Cancer Inst* **83**: 1491–1495.

Rosen, E.D., and Spiegelman, B.M. 2001. PPARgamma: a nuclear regulator of metabolism, differentiation, and cell growth. *J Biol Chem* **276**: 37731–37734.

Salmeron, J., Ascherio, A., Rimm, E.B., Colditz, G.A., Spiegelman, D., Jenkins, D.J., Stampfer, M.J., Wing, A.L., and Willett, W.C. 1997a. Dietary fiber, glycemic load, and risk of NIDDM in men. *Diabetes Care* **20**: 545–550.

Salmeron, J., Manson, J.E., Stampfer, M.J., Colditz, G.A., Wing, A.L., and Willett, W.C. 1997b. Dietary fiber, glycemic load, and risk of non-insulin-dependent diabetes mellitus in women. *JAMA* **277**: 472–477.

Schatzkin, A., and Lanza, E.; the Polyp Prevention Trial Study Group. 2002. Polyps and vegetables (and fat, fibre): the polyp prevention trial. *IARC Sci Publ* **156**: 463–466.

Simopoulos, A.P. 2001. N-3 fatty acids and human health: defining strategies for public policy. *Lipids* **36**: S83–S89.

Skov, A.R., Toubro, S., Ronn, B., Holm, L., and Astrup, A. 1999. Randomized trial on protein vs carbohydrate in ad libitum fat reduced diet for the treatment of obesity. *Int J Obes Related Metab Disord* **23**: 528–536.

Slabber, M., Barnard, H.C., Kuyl, J.M., Dannhauser, A., and Schall, R. 1994. Effects of a low-insulin-response, energy-restricted diet on weight loss and plasma insulin concentrations in hyperinsulinemic obese females. *Am J Clin Nutr* **60**: 48–53.

Steinmetz, K.A., and Potter, J.D. 1991. Vegetables, fruits, and cancer. I. Epidemiology. *Cancer Causes Control* **2**: 325–337.

Steinmetz, K.A., and Potter, J.D. 1996. Vegetables, fruits and cancer prevention: a review. *J Am Diet Assoc* **10**: 1027–1039.

Swinburn, B.A., Caterson, I., Seidell, J.C., and James, W.P. 2004. Diet, nutrition and the prevention of excess weight gain and obesity. *Public Health Nutr* **7**: 123–146.

Tarnopolsky, M. 2004. Protein requirements for endurance athletes. *Nutrition* **20**: 662–668.

Tarnopolsky, M.A., Atkinson, S.A., MacDougall, J.D., Chesley, A., Phillips, S., and Schwarcz, H.P. 1992. Evaluation of protein requirements for trained strength athletes. *J Appl Physiol.* **73**: 1986–1995.

Temple, N.J. 2000. Antioxidants and disease: more questions than answers. *Nutr Res* **20**: 449–559.

Tohill, B.C., Seymour, J., Serdula, M., Kettel-Khan, L., and Rolls, B.J. 2004. What epidemiologic studies tell us about the relationship between fruit and vegetable consumption and body weight. *Nutr Rev* **62**: 365–374.

Tsai, W.S., Nagawa, H., Kaizaki, S., Tsuruo, T., and Muto, T. 1998. Inhibitory effects of n–3 polyunsaturated fatty acids on sigmoid colon cancer transformants. *J Gastroenterol* **33**: 206–212.

Verhoeven, D.T., Assen, N., Goldbohm, R.A., Dorant, E., van 't Veer, P., Sturmans, F., Hermus, R.J., and van den Brandt, P.A. 1997. Vitamins C and E, retinol, beta-carotene and dietary fiber in relation to breast cancer risk: a prospective cohort study. *Br J Cancer* **75**, 149–155.

Way, J.M., Harrington, W.W., Brown, K.K., Gottschalk, W.K., Sundseth, S.S., Mansfield, T.A., Ramachandran, R.K., Willson, T.M., and Kliewer, S.A. 2001. Comprehensive messenger ribonucleic acid profiling reveals that peroxisome proliferator-activated receptor gamma activation has coordinate effects on gene expression in multiple insulin-sensitive tissues. *Endocrinology* **142**: 1269–1277.

Westerterp-Plantega, M.S., Rolland, V., Wilson, S.A.J., and Westerterp, K.R. 1999. Satiety related to 24 h diet-induced thermogenesis during high protein/carbohydrate vs. high fat diets measured in a respiration chamber. *Eur J Clin Nutr* **53**: 495–502.

Westerterp-Plantenga, M.S., Lejeune, M.P., Nihs, I., van Ooijen, M., and Kovacs, E.M. 2004. High protein intake sustains weight maintenance after body weight loss in humans. *Int J Obes Relat Metab Disord* **28**: 57–64.

Willett, W.C. 1994. Diet and health: what should we eat? *Science* **254**: 532–537.

Willett, W.C. 1995. Diet, nutrition and avoidable cancer. *Environ Health Perspect* **103**: 165–171.

Willett, W.C., Hunter, D.J., Stampfer, M.J., Colditz, G., Manson, J.E., Spiegelman, D., Rosner, B., Hennekens, C.H., and Speizer, F.E. 1992. Dietary fat and fiber in relation to risk of breast cancer: an 8-year follow-up. *JAMA* **268**: 2037–2044.

Willson, T.M., Brown, P.J., Sternbach, D.D., and Henke, B.R. 2000. The PPARs: from orphan receptors to drug discovery. *J Med Chem* **43**: 527–550.

Wolfrum, C., Borrmann, C.M., Borchers, T., and Spener, F. 2001. Fatty acids and hypolipidemic drugs regulate peroxisome proliferator-activated receptors alpha- and gamma-mediated gene expression via liver fatty acid binding protein: a signaling path to the nucleus. *Proc Natl Acad Sci USA* **98**: 2323.

World Cancer Research Fund. 1997. "Food, Nutrition and the Prevention of Cancer: A Global Perspective." American Institute for Cancer Research, Washington, DC.

Yamamoto, S., Sobue, T., Kobayashi, M., Sasaki, S., and Tsugane, S.S. 2003. Soy, isoflavones, and breast cancer risk in Japan. Japan Public Health Center–Based Prospective Study on Cancer Cardiovascular Diseases Group. Cancer Information and Epidemiology Division, National Cancer Center Research Institute, Tokyo, Japan. *J Natl Cancer Inst* **95**: 906–913.

Zhang, X., Shu, X.O., Gao, Y.T., Yang, G., Li, Q., Li, H., Jin, F., and Zheng, W. 2003. Soy food consumption is associated with a lower risk of coronary heart disease in Chinese women. *J Nutr* **133**: 2874–2878.

CHAPTER

2

Nutrigenomics and Nutrigenetics

JOHN MILNER

INTRODUCTION

The human genome encodes >30,000 genes and is responsible for >100,000 functionally distinct proteins, which can initiate a host of cellular metabolomic events. Understanding nutrigenomics and how foods and their components interact with the genome at many levels is undeniably fundamental to the identification of those individuals who will benefit most or be placed at risk by nutrition intervention strategies. The identification of individual differences in response to the same food components is the province of the field of nutrigenetics. Evidence is beginning to surface that genetic patterns can influence the response to foods and their components. Likewise, a number of bioactive food components can influence epigenomic, transcriptomic, proteomic, and metabolomic homeostasis. Characterizing the multitude of possible interactions between dietary habits and the "omics" is a daunting task but promises to shed key information about how best to utilize tailored or preemptive dietary intervention approaches for cancer prevention and therapy. As with any new approach, these technologies should be viewed with cautious optimism. It is prudent for nutritionists and other health care professionals to recognize the merits and limitations of genomic technologies and to only allow this type of information to be utilized within a bioethical framework.

Nutrigenomics is best described as the scientific study of the dynamic, yet regulated, manner in which bioactive food components interact with specific genes at multiple levels and vice versa. It is logical that as new information emerges within nutrigenomics, it will provide more specific information about the health consequences of changing eating behaviors at the level of the individual. The overall concept of nutrigenomics builds on the assumptions that (1) dietary patterns or specific dietary components can influence cancer risk by modifying multiple cellular processes involved with the onset, incidence, progression, or severity of these diseases, (2) bioactive food components can influence the human genome directly or indirectly and thereby influence the expression of genes and gene products, and (3) the health consequences of a diet are dependent on the balance of health and disease states and on nutrigenetics (i.e., an individual's genetic background) (Davis and Milner, 2004; Kaput and Rodriguez, 2004; Trujillo et al., 2005). The study of nutrigenomics and its associated changes in proteomics and metabolomics events (often referred to as the "omics") should provide critical clues about molecular targets for bioactive food components and ultimately provide decisive information that can be used for a personalized or preemptive approach to nutrition that is based on predictive data about the likelihood that an individual will respond to a specific intervention.

A host of dietary components likely influence genetic and epigenetic events and thereby influence cancer risk and tumor behavior. Both essential and nonessential nutrients have been found to modify multiple processes associated with cancer. Table 1 provides a list of some of the dietary components with potential anticancer properties. This protection may arise from one or more changes in several cellular mechanisms, including those associated with carcinogen metabolism, hormonal homeostasis, cell signaling regulation, cell cycle controls, cell death, or apoptosis, and angiogenesis (Davis and Milner, 2004). More frequently than not, these bioactive food components modify several processes, and the determination of which is most important is an area of active scientific investigation. The quantity and

Copyright © 2006, Elsevier Inc.
All rights of reproduction in any form reserved.

duration of exposure to these bioactive components are generally the most important factors determining the degree and possibly the direction in which processes are modified. At least some evidence suggests detrimental consequences of consuming too little or too much of some essential nutrients on overall health (Combs, 2005; Miller et al., 2005). Whether this is true or not for nonessential nutrients remains an area of intense investigation. Thus, the intended use or the desired biological response must be considered when evaluating the health consequences associated with a change in the intake of a food or its active component(s). It is plausible that a change in a combination of processes determines the ultimate phenotypic response. Understanding which processes are altered and their interrelationships to the final outcome, as depicted in Figure 1, is fundamental to understanding the dynamic relationship between diet and cancer (Trujillo et al., 2005). Although advances have been made in understanding this interrelationship, the identification of those who will or will not benefit from dietary change remains an area of considerable controversy for the scientific community, as well as a source of bewilderment and frustration for the general public. The genetic revolution and the associated "omics" should provide valuable insights for explaining the inconsistencies in the nutrition and cancer literature.

TABLE 1 Types of Food Components That Have Been Reported to Influence Genetic and Epigenetic Events

Nutrient group	Example
Phytochemicals	Carotenoids, flavonoids, indoles, isothiocyanates, allyl sulfur
Zoochemicals	Conjugated linoleic acid, omega-3 fatty acids, small molecular weight peptides
Fungochemicals	β-glucans, lentinan, schizophyllan, and other compounds found in mushrooms
Bacteriochemicals	Equol, butyrate, and other compounds formed by gastrointestinal tract flora fermentation

The majority of genes appear to have small sequence differences or polymorphisms that occur at about every 1500 base pairs (Livingston et al., 2004). Genetic changes arising as a result of single point mutations (single nucleotide polymorphisms [SNPs]), rearrangements, or copy number involving either deletions or additions can likely influence the response to various dietary components. Some of these polymorphisms may influence the functionality of a protein and how it interacts with substrates or with other proteins. Almost 6 years ago, several gene polymorphisms were iden-

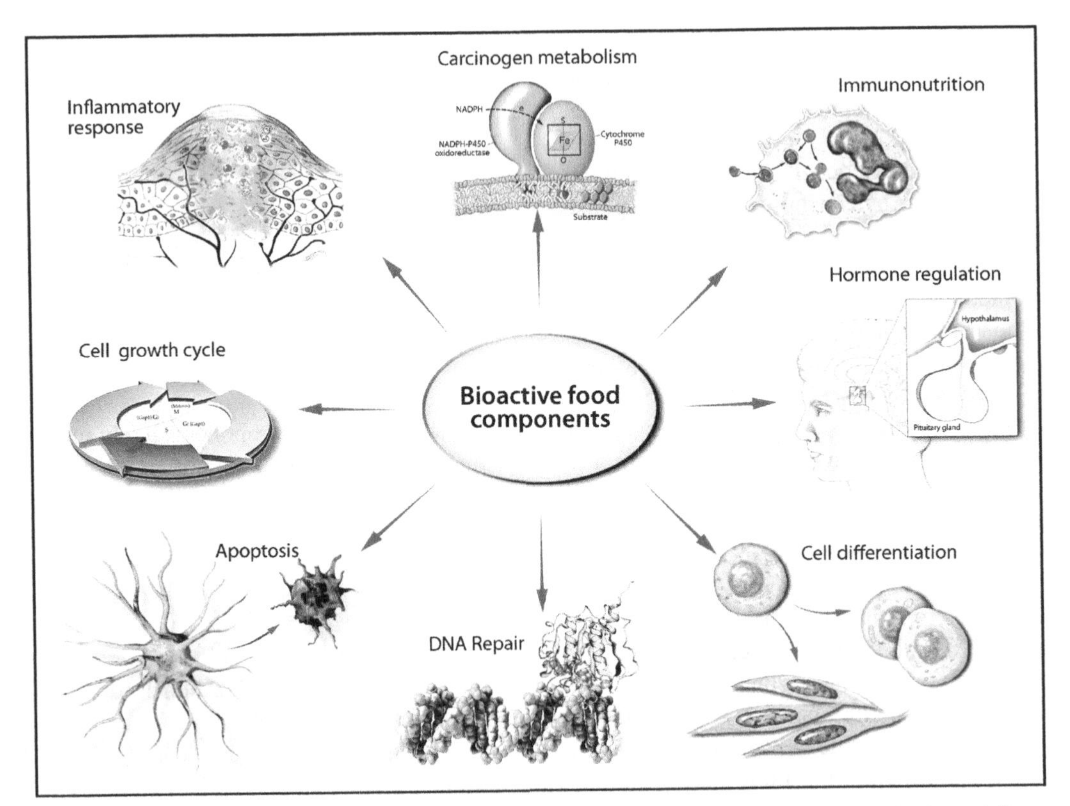

FIGURE 1 Bioactive food components can influence genetic and epigenetic events associated with a host of disease processes. (Modified from Trujillo et al., 2005.)

tified as part of a screening tool to predict disease risk, including the HFE gene for hereditary hemochromatosis and the E4 allele of the APOE gene for cholesterol hemostasis and Alzheimer's disease (Motulsky, 1999). Although these and other SNPs may help explain some health-related conditions, the cancer process appears to be far more complex and, therefore, more dependent on a combination of genetic events and a host of environmental factors. Nevertheless, mounting evidence points to SNPs as important factors in the variation in response to foods and their components. The catalogued SNPs, which are approaching 9 million, suggest the frequency may reach 10–20-fold higher than current estimates and add to the confusion that exists about personalized approaches to health promotion (Wang et al., 2005). Undeniably, SNPs are the most common form of DNA sequence variation and, therefore, can serve as a useful polymorphic marker for investigating genes and responses. However, care must be taken with the interpretation of SNP information because not all directly influence the quality or quantity of the gene product(s). As more information unfolds about the links between SNPs, dietary components, and phenotypes, it should become easier to predict those who might benefit most from dietary change. The simultaneous examination of multiple SNPs may offer special advantages in defining the biological response to food components or drugs because multiple genes are likely involved in determining physiological processes and their ultimate influence of a person's phenotype.

Studies indicate substantial genetic variation among different ethnic groups and that the evaluation of the haplotypes (combination of polymorphisms that are inherited together) can assist in developing a better predictive model for phenotypes than simply relying on individual polymorphisms. Although potentially many haplotypes can occur in a chromosome region, studies suggest their frequency may be far more limited. For example, although many SNPs in the human growth hormone secretagogue receptor (GHSR, or ghrelin receptor) are important in the regulation of food intake and energy homeostasis, Baessler et al. (2005) found a linkage to exist for obesity within the general population for the five SNPs and the two most common haplotypes.

P-glycoprotein (PGP), which is encoded by the *MDR1* gene (*ABCB1*), is a well-characterized adenosine triphosphate (ATP)–binding cassette (ABC) transporter. Its expression is known to vary widely among individuals and is generally overexpressed in multidrug-resistant cancers. Multiple *MDR1* polymorphisms are known to occur in various allelic combinations. The frequencies of variant *MDR1* alleles differ, depending on racial background, and may account for sensitivity to some drugs and possibly dietary components. The C3435T polymorphism (exon 26) has a frequency of 73–84% in individuals of African origin and frequencies of 34–59% in individuals of European and Asian origin (Kim et al., 2001). Grouping these polymorphisms into haplotypes may assist with the prediction of the functional consequences of *MDR1* polymorphisms and their responsiveness to agents, including dietary components.

The grouping of SNPs does not always clarify relationships. Activation of intracellular mitogenic signal transduction pathways driven by the ErbB family of receptor tyrosine kinases has been implicated in various cancers. Among these, the tumorigenic roles of the epidermal growth factor receptor (EGFR) and HER-2 have been most extensively studied. Han et al. (2005) found that individual SNPs, including I655V, and the *HER-2* haplotypes were not associated with increased risk of breast cancer development in Korean women. Regardless, the development of common patterns, or haplotypes, of human genetic variation, as is currently under way across populations in Africa, Asia, and the United States via the International HapMap Consortium, will be an invaluable resource for scientists searching for genes related to health and disease (Crawford and Nickerson, 2005).

NUTRIGENETIC RESPONSE

The study of gene–nutrient interactions is an expanding area of science and one that is becoming increasingly present in the scientific and public press. Discrepancies in the literature may arise from failing to recognize interindividual genetic differences in the response to foods or their components. One of the best examples reflecting how a false conclusion may arise comes from studies with colon cancer animal models. In studies by Yang et al. (2001), a decreased survival of mice was observed when mice were fed a Western-style diet (high in fat and phosphate and low in calcium and vitamin D) compared with an ideal semipurified diet. However, the response was dependent on the frequency of mutated alleles in the p21 tumor suppressor gene. When this allelic variance was not considered, differences between diets were virtually impossible to detect. Wide variation in the response to a food component may occur not only because of genetic determinations of absorption and metabolism but also because of fluctuations in the molecular site of action.

The angiotensinogen gene, which sets the tone for amount of angiotensinogen protein and thus vascular tone and sodium retention, appears to be influenced by several dietary components. A common polymorphism in the angiotensinogen gene encodes threonine (T) instead of methionine (M) at codon 235. Individuals with the angiotensinogen TT genotype appear to have a decrease in blood pressure (BP) when provided a diet with increased amounts (2.7–3.0 g/100 kcal of either insoluble or soluble fiber) of insoluble fiber compared with when increased amounts of soluble fiber are provided. In contrast, BP in individuals with a TM or MM genotype is not influenced by the type of fiber consumed (Hegele et al., 1997). These insights clarify why variations in BP responses to fiber supplementation have been observed in the literature. An association was also reported between angiotensinogen polymorphism (G6A) such that net systolic and diastolic BP response to the Dietary Approaches to Stop Hypertension (DASH) diet was greatest in individuals with the AA genotype (−6.93/−3.68 mm Hg) and least in those with the GG genotype (−2.80/0.20 mm Hg) (Svetkey et al., 2001). Again, some of the reported discrepancies in the response of BP to dietary modification may reflect the populations examined and their genetic variations.

Considerable evidence also points to the ability of dietary selenium to reduce the incidence of chemically induced cancer when provided at above required amounts within physiologically relevant ranges (Kim and Milner, 2001; Combs, 2005). A reduction in the incidence of liver, colon, prostate, and lung cancer has been reported with increasing dietary selenium exposure in humans (Clark et al., 1996). Nevertheless, it is clear from these studies that not all individuals responded equally to exaggerated intake, possibly reflecting genetic differences in the absorption, metabolism, or site of action for this trace element. Polymorphisms in glutathione peroxidase (GPx), a known selenium-dependent enzyme, at codon 198, which causes a substitution of leucine for proline, is associated with an increased risk of lung cancer (Hu and Diamond, 2003). Likewise, in a study nested within the α-Tocopherol, β-Carotene Cancer Prevention Study cohort, individuals with one copy of the allele for leucine (proline/leucine) were at 80% greater risk for lung cancer, and individuals with two copies of the allele for leucine (leucine/leucine) were at 130% greater risk compared with those with the proline genotype (proline/proline) (Ratnasinghe et al., 2000). Similar findings were reported for breast, head and neck, bladder, and skin cancer (Hu et al., 2004; Ichimura et al., 2004). It is conceivable that these relationships reflect cellular differences in the utilization or metabolism of selenium because the activity of GPx was not reported to differ. Support for this belief comes from differences in the ability of selenium to induce GPx activity in breast cancer cells transfected with the leucine or proline coding allele (Hu et al., 2004). Such data provide evidence that it is possible to use information about specific polymorphisms to gain insights into which individuals may need/require increased or decreased amounts of specific nutrients, as has been suggested by Ames et al. (2003). The utility of such information for health benefits comes from the ability of high doses of B vitamins to remedy or ameliorate 50 genetic neurological diseases in humans in which the binding affinity of coenzymes for critically important enzymatic binding sites is reduced, so a higher dose of B vitamin overcomes the effects of the reduced binding affinity normalizing enzymatic activity (Ames et al., 2002).

Shifts in diet may also be needed to help counteract or offset conditions caused by various environmental factors. A study investigating the effect of caffeine on bone loss in elderly women found a positive association with a vitamin D receptor (VDR) (tt genotype) when intakes were > 300 mg/day, compared with those with the TT genotype (Rapuri et al., 2001). Because regular caffeine ingestion is such a common habit in our society, strategies other than recommending abstention from caffeine may be needed. Although it remains to be determined whether increasing the amount of calcium or vitamin D will influence the bone loss occurring in these individuals, this area deserves further consideration because evidence exists that the *FokI* polymorphism of the VDR can influence bone mineral accretion during pubertal growth through an effect on calcium absorption (Abrams et al., 2005).

Many of the effects of vitamin D are likely mediated through changes in the VDR. Several polymorphisms, including *FokI*, *Bsm I*, and *poly-A*, may influence the response to various dietary components and influence risk. The *FokI* VDR polymorphism, with the FF genotype, may be particularly important in determining the effect of dietary calcium on colon cancer risk. Although dietary calcium or fat did not influence colon cancer risk in individuals with an FF genotype, a decreased dietary calcium intake was accompanied by increased colon cancer risk with the f allele. Individuals with the ff genotype exhibited about a 2.5-fold increased colon cancer risk when low calcium was consumed compared with adequate intakes (Wong et al., 2003). Furthermore, high levels of dietary calcium and vitamin D reduced the risk of rectal cancer and provided support for a weak protective effect for the SS (*poly-A*) and BB (*Bsm I*) VDR genotypes (Slattery et al., 2004). Overall, the risk associated with VDR genotypes likely depends not only on the level of dietary calcium and vitamin D consumed but also on the tumor site (Slattery et al., 2004).

Increased intake of some dietary components may lead to depressed health. Unquestionably, high energy intake resulting in obesity is a major public health concern and is associated with several chronic diseases including cancer (Calle et al., 2003). Imbalances in the homeostatic controls between genes and diet may explain the increased morbidity and mortality linked with obesity. It has been estimated that ~90,000 deaths/year from cancer might be avoided if the adult population could maintain a body mass index (BMI) of <25 throughout life (Calle et al., 2003). However, unraveling the relationships among factors influencing obesity, such as amount and type of fat consumed and genetic interactions, will likely be an extremely daunting task. For example, the nuclear receptor peroxisome proliferator-activated receptor-γ (PPARγ) is known to be involved in regulating insulin resistance and BP. In individuals with a Pro12Ala PPARγ polymorphism, the intake of a low polyunsaturated-to-saturated fat ratio is associated with an increased BMI and fasting insulin concentrations in those with multiple copies of the alanine allele. However, in the Pro carriers, increasing the dietary ratio of polyunsaturated (P) to saturated (S) fats to high amounts creates the opposite response (Luan et al., 2001). These data suggest that the dietary P:S ratio should not be set universally across all individuals and that some will likely benefit from a lower ratio, while others will benefit from a higher ratio. The interaction between type of dietary fat and PPARγ genotype illustrates the complexity found in examining gene–nutrient interactions and that blanket recommendations for intakes are likely to lead to unwanted results in subpopulations. As more information surfaces about diet–gene interaction, we should be in a better position to explain the large heterogeneity in findings that has plagued clinical nutrition.

NUTRITIONAL EPIGENETICS

Epigenetic events represent another controlling site for bioactive food components because they are critical for establishing which genes are and are not expressed. Results from numerous investigations provide evidence that tissue-specific differences in vertebrate DNA methylation help maintain patterns of gene expression or are involved in fine-tuning or establishing expression patterns. Various regulatory proteins including DNA methyltransferases, methylcytosine guanine dinucleotide binding proteins, histone-modifying enzymes, chromatin remodeling factors, and their multimolecular complexes are involved in the overall epigenetic process (Ross, 2003; Davis and Milner, 2004; Gallou-Kabani and Junien, 2005). Therefore, vertebrate DNA methylation is responsible for more than simply silencing transposable elements and foreign DNA sequences, as has been suggested. DNA hypomethylation is a nearly universal finding in cancer. These patterns are accompanied by site-specific hypermethylation sites. Hypermethylation of CpG-rich promoters of tumor suppressor genes in cancer has a critical role in downregulating expression of genes and, thus, participates in the cancer process. Nevertheless, evidence exists that creating DNA demethylation increases the formation of certain types of cancers in animal models, and paradoxically, DNA hypermethylation can cause carcinogenesis in other models. Therefore, factors that modify methylation patterns must be used with caution about their overall health consequences. Regardless, chronic administration of methionine- and choline-deficient diets results in global hypomethylation of hepatic DNA and leads to spontaneous liver tumor formation in rats (Poirier, 1986). Actually, several dietary factors may influence the supply of methyl groups and thereby influence the availability of S-adenosylmethionine (SAM) and therefore influence DNA methylation patterns (Ross, 2003). Evidence also exists that dietary factors may modify the utilization of methyl groups by processes including shifts in DNA methyltransferase (Dnmt) activity. A third plausible mechanism may relate to shifts in DNA demethylation activity caused by food components, although this process is not well understood. Finally, DNA methylation patterns may influence the response to bioactive food components and thereby account for differences in response in normal and neoplastic cells (Figure 2).

A series of studies have identified food components ranging from B vitamins to zinc as modifiers of that DNA methylation (Table 2). The physiological relevance of epigenomic events in changing the neonate comes from studies with an Agouti mouse model. Providing supplemental choline, betaine, folic acid, vitamin B12, methionine, and zinc to the maternal diet was found to increase DNA methylation in the Agouti heterozygote mouse and to increase the proportion of offspring with brown compared with the yellow hair color characteristic of Agouti protein expression. This phenotypic change has been found to coincide with a lower susceptibility to obesity, diabetes, and cancer (Cooney, 1993; Cooney et al., 2002). Although the agouti gene does not exist in humans, these types of studies suggest that in principal maternal exposure to some dietary factors may influence lifelong health of the offspring, as has been suggested by others (Brakefield et al., 2005; Hunter, 2005).

Global loss of monoacetylation and trimethylation of histone H4 is also a common occurrence in human tumors (Fraga et al., 2005). Histones are the proteins that form a scaffold around which a cell's DNA is wrapped (Figure 2). Histone deacetylases (HDACs) are a family of 11 enzymes that remove an acetyl group from histones, which allows histones to bind DNA and inhibit gene transcription. Several studies suggest that butyrate, sulforaphane, resveratrol, and diallyl disulfide are dietary modifiers of HDAC (Druesne et al., 2004; Klampfer et al., 2004; Myzak et al., 2004; Galfi et al., 2005). Although much more research is needed to determine how these food components modify histones and ultimately gene expression, the emerging data are very tantalizing. It is certainly conceivable that prolonged exposure to one or more of these may influence the onset and severity of a number of disease conditions, including cancer.

TRANSCRIPTOMICS AND MICROARRAY TECHNOLOGIES

The examination of modifications in DNA and histones is insufficient to provide a clear picture of the impact of diet on a person's phenotype (van Ommen and Stierum, 2002; Davis and Milner, 2004; Kaput and Rodriguez, 2004). The development of microarray technology has given scientists the opportunity to evaluate a number of potential sites of action of food components and begin to explore interactions with various cellular processes and among dietary

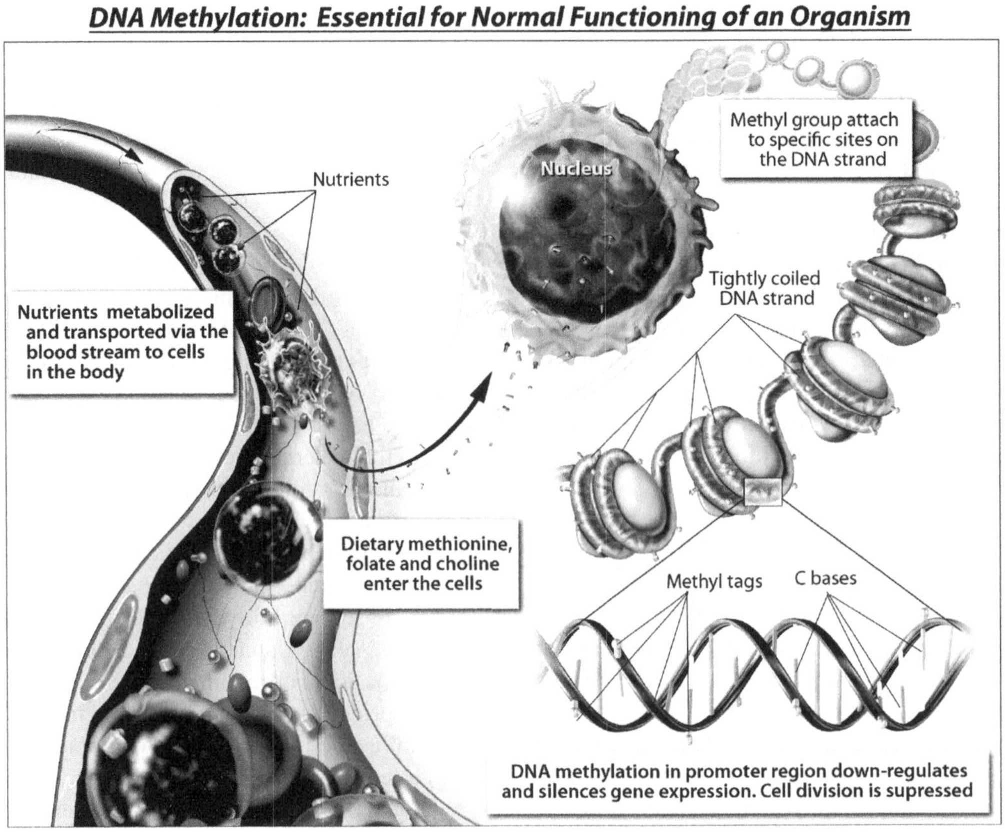

FIGURE 2 Dietary factors and the regulation of DNA methylation. (Modified from Trujillo et al., 2005.)

TABLE 2 Some Dietary Factors Known to Modify DNA Methylation

Arsenic	Betaine
Choline	Equol
Fiber	Folate
Genistein	Methionine
Selenium	Polyphenols
Vitamin A	Vitamin B6
Vitamin B12	Zinc

components. The ability to undertake genome-wide expression patterns permits the simultaneous evaluation of tens of thousands of genes and of their relative expression between normal cells and cancerous cells, as well as the response to an array of dietary components. Evidence is already mounting that the rate of transcription of genes (transcriptomics) can be modified by food components and, thus, represents another intriguing site for influencing an individual's phenotype with foods (Figure 3). Food components within both the essential and the nonessential domain have been reported to influence gene expression patterns (Dong et al., 2003; Herzog et al., 2005; Lu et al., 2005). These components significantly modify gene transcription (both increase and decrease) and lead to a number of biological changes in metabolism, cell growth, apoptosis, and differentiation. With time, this information should assist with the discovery of biomarkers that can be used to evaluate the progression or lack thereof in the cancer process. Likewise, this molecular approach should assist in developing an individualized approach that builds on nutritional preemption.

To prevent transcriptomics from becoming purely descriptive, greater attention is needed on how food components regulate the expression of specific genes. Mounting evidence suggests that messenger RNA (mRNA) abundance may provide little information on protein activity and cannot be a substitute for detailed functional and ecological analyses of candidate genes (Feder and Walser, 2005). Various mouse models, particularly knockouts, may be particularly useful in identifying specific sites of action of specific food components. For example, knockout mice have already assisted in identifying the nuclear factor E2 p45-related factor 2 (Nrf2) and the Kelch domain-containing partner Keap1 as the complex that is influenced by dietary sulforaphane, an active component within broccoli (Thimmu-

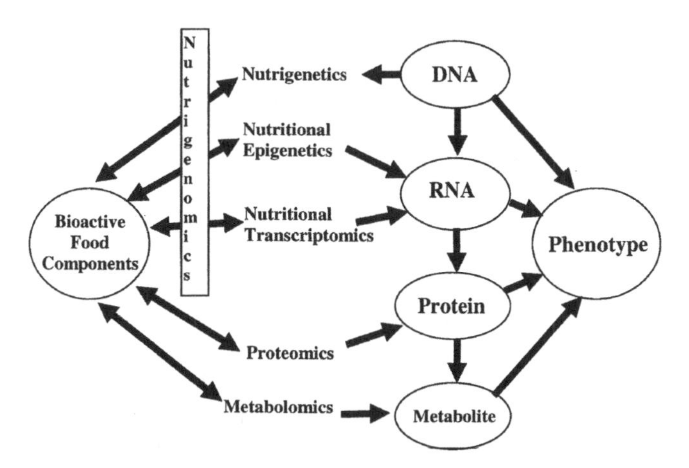

FIGURE 3 Using the "omics" of nutrition to identify how dietary factors contribute to establishing a phenotype. (From Trujillo et al., 2005.)

lappa et al., 2002). Available evidence clearly demonstrates that a comparison of wild type and Nrf2-deficient mice fed sulforaphane helps identify novel downstream events that are influenced by this food component and, thus, clues about those who will likely respond maximally to a diet enriched with cruciferous vegetables, including broccoli. Similar studies with peroxisome proliferator-activated receptor-α (PPARα)–null mice also assisted in the identification of regulatory sites of lipid metabolism that can be influenced by the diet (Pan et al., 2000).

Because microarray technologies provide only a single time event, overinterpretation is a concern. It has long been recognized that adaptive processes occur after the ingestion of foods or components in a number of metabolic pathways (Millward and Jackson, 2004). Thus, the quantity and duration of exposure are critical dimensions to consider when evaluating microarray information. Molecular studies have already revealed that specific events in cell cycle progression that are modified by energy restriction can rather quickly be reversed by refeeding (Jiang et al., 2003). Again, the ability of the body to adapt can determine the frequency by which interventions will be needed to bring about a desired effect.

Another challenge with microarray analysis is how to analyze the massive amounts of data that are generated. Because of the number of genes whose expression can be modified by dietary components, a hierarchical cluster analysis is often used, which may minimize the significance of a particular gene in explaining the overall response. Although most studies use a 50% change in gene expression patterns as a determinant of statistical significance, a shift in mRNA expression at much lower values may be as physiologically relevant, if not more so. As advances in bioinformatics occur, the importance of changes in mRNA expression should help with predicting disease risk and identify those who would benefit from dietary change and those who might be placed at risk because of an intervention (Liu-Stratton et al., 2004).

RNA interference technologies, which can be employed to retard the expression of a particular gene, offer exciting opportunities for defining the site of action of bioactive food components. Through the use of interfering RNAs, investigators systematically disrupted expression of all of the genes in the worm model system *Caenorhabditis elegans* in order to determine which gene inactivation decreased body fat and which increased fat storage (Ashrafi et al., 2003). This approach allowed for the identification of a core set of fat regulatory genes and pathway-specific fat regulators (Ashrafi et al., 2003). Likewise, this technology has been used to identify sites of action of isothiocyanate compounds that arise from broccoli and other related foods (Singh et al., 2005). As transcriptomic information becomes available, it may be possible to identify targets for prevention or treatment of a variety of unhealthy conditions with foods or their components.

BEYOND NUTRIGENOMICS

Dietary components may also influence the translation of RNA to proteins and influence post-translational modification, and both of these can affect protein activity. Just as the genome is the entire set of genes, the proteome is the set of proteins produced by a species. However, unlike the genome, the proteome is dynamic and varies according to the cell type and the functional state of the cell. Although the genomic response to bioactive food components may have limited influence, it could have marked effects on the proteome. One of the frontiers in nutrition and disease prevention research is the development of pioneering technologies for proteomic analysis. Proteomics can be used to identify abnormal protein structures and show how shape affects biology and response to diet. It allows one to determine whether and how bioactive food components influence three-dimensional proteins. Studies with an animal model have shown that dietary fish oil, conjugated linoleic acid (CLA), or elaidic acid can influence lipoprotein metabolism and insulin levels, as indicated by changes in proteomics (deRoos et al., 2005). Fish oil supplementation lowered plasma and liver cholesterol and triglycerides, plasma free fatty acids, and glucose, but increased plasma insulin. Providing CLA was found to reduce plasma cholesterol but increase plasma and liver triglycerides, plasma β-hydroxybutyrate, and insulin. Elaidic acid depressed plasma and liver cholesterol. Overall, the proteomic technique used identified 65 cytosolic and 8 membrane proteins that were modified by dietary components, many of which were related to lipid and glucose metabolism and to oxidative stress. The merging of proteomics and physiological measurements will likely provide key insights into the mechanisms by which dietary components can regulate several metabolic processes, including lipid metabolism, and how these changes bring about a change in phenotype.

As with transcriptomics, proteomic analysis provides a point-in-time snapshot in relation to dietary interventions. Thus, to truly evaluate the impact of diet, there needs to be multiple exposures and varying durations to allow for appropriate predictions about who might respond to a diet.

One of the newest "omics" in nutrition is metabolomics, which refers to the dose and temporal changes in cellular small molecular weight compounds in response to dietary treatments. Unfortunately, few nutrition studies have embraced this newest "omics." One study that did use a metabolomic approach found that plasma profiles of healthy premenopausal women before and after consumption of 60 g of soy provided some clues about changes in energetics (Solanky et al., 2003). Despite the presence of substantial intersubject variability, the metabolomic analysis revealed that soy intervention changed the plasma lipoprotein, amino acid, and carbohydrate profiles, suggesting soy-induced alterations in fat, protein, and carbohydrate metabolism. It is possible that this approach can be expanded to allow for the identification of individuals, based on their metabolic abilities, who would benefit from various foods and/or food patterns. As information in this area surfaces, professionals will be provided with an additional tool for making personalized or preemptive nutritional recommendations.

As with transcriptomics and proteomics, the metabolomic response will also depend on the quantity and timing of exposure to a specific bioactive food component or a blend of components. Timing has already surfaced as a crucial factor in determining whether genistein, the primary isoflavone in soy, is protective against cancer in a rodent model and possibly in humans. In a rat chemical carcinogenesis model, limiting the exposure of dietary genistein to the prenatal or adult periods of life does not predispose or protect against mammary cancer. In contrast, exposure of dietary genistein during the prepubertal and prepubertal plus adult periods protects against chemically induced mammary cancer in this model (Lamartiniere et al., 2002). Epidemiological evidence in humans also suggests an inverse relationship between soy food intake by adolescent girls (13–15 years) and breast cancer incidence later in life but not when introduced in later life (Shu et al., 2001). The mechanisms of these temporal effects may arise from changes in the degree of mammary gland differentiation (Lamartiniere et al., 2002). Such data begin to suggest that more attention is needed to determine the impact of dietary components on fetal and nonfetal stem cells. Because stem cells have the remarkable propensity to develop into many cell types and theoretically divide without limit, they may be particularly sensitive to shifts in the supply of food components. The mounting evidence that a variety of food components can alter differentiation (Zangani et al., 1999; Harris and Go, 2004; Duan, 2005) suggests that the next big issue for nutritionists may be how these cells are influenced by dietary components and how any diet-induced changes influence subsequent health.

CONCLUSIONS

Undeniably an exciting future exists for nutrition as the understanding of the role of the "omics" is unraveled as a determinant of the response in an individual to a food, a blend of foods, or to individual components. This information holds promise to assist with the understanding of the role that environmental and behavioral factors can have on influencing phenotype and ultimately health and wellness. It is likely that health strategies that include a personalized approach to nutrition that builds on recognized targets for bioactive food components or a "nutrition preemption" approach are lofty but realistic goals within the very near future, possibly within the next 5 years. The use of such an approach should allow for prevention measures to block or suppress the initiation, promotion, and progression of pathways that lead to a lethal phenotype including cancer.

Although we must never lose the public health messages that are used for health promotion, it is clear that overly simplistic messages are not appropriate for all individuals. Although unprecedented opportunities exist for the expanded use of foods and bioactive food components to achieve genetic potential, increase productivity, and decrease risk of disease, the science to make such decisions has not reached a level of confidence to achieve personalized nutrition recommendations. The success of nutritional preemption approaches will depend on the ability to identify and validate nutrigenetic, nutritional epigenetic, proteomic, and metabolomic biomarkers to determine cause, effect, and susceptibility to disease. It is essential that health professionals communicate effectively with consumers so that they understand the personal and public health significance of the "omic" approaches to defining dietary needs and that the information obtained is handled within a responsible bioethical framework.

References

Abrams, S.A., Griffin, I.J., Hawthorne, K.M., Chen, Z., Gunn, S.K., Wilde, M., Darlington, G., Shypailo, R.J., and Ellis, K.J. 2005. Vitamin D receptor Fok1 polymorphisms affect calcium absorption, kinetics, and bone mineralization rates during puberty. *J Bone Miner Res* **20**: 945–953.

Ames, B.N., Elson-Schwab, I., and Silver, E.A. 2002. High-dose vitamins stimulate variant enzymes with decreased coenzyme-binding affinity (increased K_m): relevance to genetic disease and polymorphisms. *Am J Clin Nutr* **75**: 616–658.

Ashrafi, K., Chang, F.Y., Watts, J.L., Fraser, A.G., Kamath, R.S., Ahringer, J., and Ruvkun, G. 2003. Genome-wide RNAi analysis of *Caenorhabditis elegans* fat regulatory genes. *Nature* **421**: 268–272.

Ames, B.N. 2003. The metabolic tune-up: metabolic harmony and disease prevention. *J Nutr* **133**: 1544S–1548S.

Baessler, A., Hasinoff, M.J., Fischer, M., Reinhard, W., Sonnenberg, G.E., Olivier, M., Erdmann, J., Schunkert, H., Doering, A., Jacob, H.J., Comuzzie, A.G., Kissebah, A.H., and Kwitek, A.E. 2005. Genetic linkage and association of the growth hormone secretagogue receptor (ghrelin receptor) gene in human obesity. *Diabetes* **54**: 259–267.

Brakefield, P.M., Gems, D., Cowen, T., Christensen, K., Grubeck-Loebenstein, B., Keller, L., Oeppen, J., Rodriguez-Pena, A., Stazi, M.A., Tatar, M., and Westendorp, R.G. 2005. What are the effects of maternal and pre-adult environments on ageing in humans, and are there lessons from animal models? *Mech Ageing Dev* **126**: 431–438.

Calle, E.E., Rodriguez, C., Walker-Thurmond, K., and Thun, M.J. 2003. Overweight, obesity, and mortality from cancer in a prospectively studied cohort of U.S. adults. *N Engl J Med* **348**: 1625–1638.

Clark, L.C., Combs, G.F., Jr., Turnbull, B.W., Slate, E.H., Chalker, D.K., Chow, J., Davis, L.S., Glover, R.A., Graham, G.F., Gross, E.G., Krongrad, A., Lesher, J.L., Jr., Park, H.K., Sanders, B.B., Jr., Smith, C.L., and Taylor, J.R. 1996. Effects of selenium supplementation for cancer prevention in patients with carcinoma of the skin. A randomized controlled trial. Nutritional Prevention of Cancer Study Group. *JAMA* **276**: 1957–1963.

Combs, G.F., Jr. 2005. Current evidence and research needs to support a health claim for selenium and cancer prevention. *J Nutr* **135**: 343–347.

Cooney, C.A. 1993. Are somatic cells inherently deficient in methylation metabolism? A proposed mechanism for DNA methylation loss, senescence and aging. *Growth Dev Aging* **57**: 261–273.

Cooney, C.A., Dave, A.A., and Wolff, G.L. 2002. Maternal methyl supplements in mice affect epigenetic variation and DNA methylation of offspring. *J Nutr* **132**: 2393S–2400S.

Crawford, D.C., and Nickerson, D.A. 2005. Definition and clinical importance of haplotypes. *Annu Rev Med* **56**: 303–320.

Davis, C.D., and Milner, J. 2004. Frontiers in nutrigenomics, proteomics, metabolomics and cancer prevention. *Mutat Res* **551**: 51–64.

de Roos, B., Duivenvoorden, I., Rucklidge, G., Reid, M., Ross, K., Lamers, R.J., Voshol, P.J., Havekes, L.M., and Teusink, B. 2005. Response of apolipoprotein E*3-Leiden transgenic mice to dietary fatty acids: combining liver proteomics with physiological data. *FASEB J* **19**: 813–815.

Dong, Y., Zhang, H., Hawthorn, L., Ganther, H.E., and Ip, C. 2003. Delineation of the molecular basis for selenium-induced growth arrest in human prostate cancer cells by oligonucleotide array. *Cancer Res* **63**: 52–59.

Druesne, N., Pagniez, A., Mayeur, C., Thomas, M., Cherbuy, C., Duee, P.H., Martel, P., and Chaumontet, C. 2004. Diallyl disulfide (DADS) increases histone acetylation and p21(waf1/cip1) expression in human colon tumor cell lines. *Carcinogenesis* **25**: 1227–1236.

Duan, R.D. 2005. Anticancer compounds and sphingolipid metabolism in the colon. *In Vivo* **19**: 293–300.

Feder, M.E., and Walser, J.C. 2005. The biological limitations of transcriptomics in elucidating stress and stress responses. *J Evol Biol* **18**: 901–910.

Fraga, M.F., Ballestar, E., Villar-Garea, A., Boix-Chornet, M., Espada, J., Schotta, G., Bonaldi, T., Haydon, C., Ropero, S., Petrie, K., Iyer, N.G., Perez-Rosado, A., Calvo, E., Lopez, J.A., Cano, A., Calasanz, M.J., Colomer, D., Piris, M.A., Ahn, N., Imhof, A., Caldas, C., Jenuwein, T., and Esteller, M. 2005. Loss of acetylation at Lys16 and trimethylation at Lys20 of histone H4 is a common hallmark of human cancer. *Nat Genet* **37**: 391–400.

Galfi, P., Jakus, J., Molnar, T., Neogrady, S., and Csordas, A. 2005. Divergent effects of resveratrol, a polyphenolic phytostilbene, on free radical levels and type of cell death induced by the histone deacetylase inhibitors butyrate and trichostatin A. *J Steroid Biochem Mol Biol* **94**: 39–47.

Gallou-Kabani, C., and Junien, C. 2005. Nutritional epigenomics of metabolic syndrome: new perspective against the epidemic. *Diabetes* **54**: 1899–1906.

Han, W., Kang, D., Lee, J.E., Park, I.A., Choi, J.Y., Lee, K.M., Bae, J.Y., Kim, S., Shin, E.S., Lee, J.E., Shin, H.J., Kim, S.W., Kim, S.W., and Noh, D.Y. 2005. A haplotype analysis of HER-2 gene polymorphisms: association with breast cancer risk, HER-2 protein expression in the tumor, and disease recurrence in Korea. *Clin Cancer Res* **11**: 4775–4778.

Harris, D.M., and Go, V.L. 2004. Vitamin D and colon carcinogenesis. *J Nutr* **134**: 3463S–3471S.

Hegele, R.A., Jugenberg, M., Connelly, P.W., and Jenkins, D.J.A. 1997. Evidence for gene-diet interaction in the response of blood pressure to dietary fibre. *Nutr Res* **17**: 1229–1238.

Herzog, A., Siler, U., Spitzer, V., Seifert, N., Denelavas, A., Hunziker, P.B., Hunziker, W., Goralczyk, R., and Wertz, K. 2005. Lycopene reduced gene expression of steroid targets and inflammatory markers in normal rat prostate. *FASEB J* **19**: 272–274.

Hu, Y.J., and Diamond, A.M. 2003. Role of glutathione peroxidase 1 in breast cancer: loss of heterozygosity and allelic differences in the response to selenium. *Cancer Res* **63**: 3347–3351.

Hu, Y.J., Dolan, M.E., Bae, R., Yee, H., Roy, M., Glickman, R., Kiremidjian-Schumacher, L., and Diamond, A.M. 2004. Allelic loss at the GPx-1 locus in cancer of the head and neck. *Biol Trace Elem Res* **101**: 97–106.

Hunter, D.J. 2005. Gene-environment interactions in human diseases. *Nat Rev Genet* **6**: 287–298.

Ichimura, Y., Habuchi, T., Tsuchiya, N., Wang, L., Oyama, C., Sato, K., Nishiyama, H., Ogawa, O., and Kato, T. 2004. Increased risk of bladder cancer associated with a glutathione peroxidase 1 codon 198 variant. *J Urol* **172**: 728–732.

Jiang, W., Zhu, Z., and Thompson, H.J. 2003. Effect of energy restriction on cell cycle machinery in 1-methyl-1-nitrosourea–induced mammary carcinomas in rats. *Cancer Res* **63**: 1228–1234.

Kaput, J., and Rodriguez, R.L. 2004. Nutritional genomics: the next frontier in the postgenomic era. *Physiol Genom* **16**: 166–177.

Kim, R.B., Leake, B.F., Choo, E.F., Dresser, G.K., Kubba, S.V., Schwarz, U.I., Taylor, A., Xie, H.G., McKinsey, J., Zhou, S., Lan, L.B., Schuetz, J.D., Schuetz, E.G., and Wilkinson, G.R. 2001. Identification of functionally variant MDR1 alleles among European Americans and African Americans. *Clin Pharmacol Ther* **70**: 189–199.

Kim, Y.S., and Milner, J. 2001. Molecular targets for selenium in cancer prevention. *Nutr Cancer* **40**: 50–54.

Klampfer, L., Huang, J., Swaby, L.A., and Augenlicht, L. 2004. Requirement of histone deacetylase activity for signaling by STAT1. *J Biol Chem* **279**: 30358–30368.

Lamartiniere, C.A., Cotroneo, M.S., Fritz, W.A., Wang, J., Mentor-Marcel, R., and Elgavish, A. 2002. Genistein chemoprevention: timing and mechanisms of action in murine mammary and prostate. *J Nutr* **132**: 552S–558S.

Liu-Stratton, Y., Roy, S., and Sen, C.K. 2004. DNA microarray technology in nutraceutical and food safety. *Toxicol Lett* **150**: 29–42.

Livingston, R.J., von Niederhausern, A., Jegga, A.G., Crawford, D.C., Carlson, C.S., Rieder, M.J., Gowrisankar, S., Aronow, B.J., Weiss, R.B., and Nickerson, D.A. 2004. Pattern of sequence variation across 213 environmental response genes. *Genome Res* **14**: 1821–1831.

Lu, Q.Y., Arteaga, J.R., Zhang, Q., Huerta, S., Go, V.L., and Heber, D. 2005. Inhibition of prostate cancer cell growth by an avocado extract: role of lipid-soluble bioactive substances. *J Nutr Biochem* **16**: 23–30.

Luan, J., Browne, P.O., Harding, A.H., Halsall, D.J., O'Rahilly, S., Chatterjee, V.K., and Wareham, N.J. 2001. Evidence for gene-nutrient interaction at the PPARgamma locus. *Diabetes* **50**: 686–689.

Miller, E.R., 3rd, Pastor-Barriuso, R., Dalal, D., Riemersma, R.A., Appel, L.J., and Guallar, E. 2005. Meta-analysis: high-dosage vitamin E supplementation may increase all-cause mortality. *Ann Intern Med* **142**: 37–46.

Millward, D.J., and Jackson, A.A. 2004. Protein/energy ratios of current diets in developed and developing countries compared with a safe protein/energy ratio: implications for recommended protein and amino acid intakes. *Public Health Nutr* **7**: 387–405.

Motulsky, A.G. 1999. If I had a gene test, what would I have and who would I tell? *Lancet* **354**: SI35–SI37.

Myzak, M.C., Karplus, P.A., Chung, F.L., and Dashwood, R.H. 2004. A novel mechanism of chemoprotection by sulforaphane: inhibition of histone deacetylase. *Cancer Res* **64**: 5767–5774.

Pan, D.A., Mater, M.K., Thelen, A.P., Peters, J.M., Gonzalez, F.J., and Jump, D.B. 2000. Evidence against the peroxisome proliferator-activated receptor alpha (PPARalpha) as the mediator for polyunsaturated fatty acid suppression of hepatic L-pyruvate kinase gene transcription. *J Lipid Res* **41**: 742–751.

Poirier, L.A. 1986. The role of methionine in carcinogenesis in vivo. *Adv Exp Med Biol* **206**: 269–282.

Rapuri, P.B., Gallagher, J.C., Kinyamu, H.K., and Ryschon, K.L. 2001. Caffeine intake increases the rate of bone loss in elderly women and interacts with vitamin D receptor genotypes. *Am J Clin Nutr* **74**: 694–700.

Ratnasinghe, D., Tangrea, J.A., Andersen, M.R., Barrett, M.J., Virtamo, J., Taylor, P.R., and Albanes, D. 2000. Glutathione peroxidase codon 198 polymorphism variant increases lung cancer risk. *Cancer Res* **60**: 6381–6383.

Ross, S.A. 2003. Diet and DNA methylation interactions in cancer prevention. *Ann NY Acad Sci* **983**: 197–207.

Shu, X.O., Jin, F., Dai, Q., Wen, W., Potter, J.D., Kushi, L.H., Ruan, Z., Gao, Y.T., and Zheng, W. 2001. Soyfood intake during adolescence and subsequent risk of breast cancer among Chinese women. *Cancer Epidemiol Biomarkers Prev* **10**: 483–488.

Singh, S.V., Srivastava, S.K., Choi, S., Lew, K.L., Antosiewicz, J., Xiao, D., Zeng, Y., Watkins, S.C., Johnson, C.S., Trump, D.L., Lee, Y.J., Xiao, H., and Herman-Antisiewicz, A. 2005. Sulforaphane-induced cell death in human prostate cancer cells is initiated by reactive oxygen species. *J Biol Chem* **280**: 19911–19924.

Slattery, M.L., Neuhausen, S.L., Hoffman, M., Caan, B., Curtin, K., Ma, K.N., and Samowitz, W. 2004. Dietary calcium, vitamin D, VDR genotypes and colorectal cancer. *Int J Cancer* **111**: 750–756.

Solanky, K.S., Bailey, N.J., Beckwith-Hall, B.M., Davis, A., Bingham, S., Holmes, E., Nicholson, J.K., and Cassidy, A. 2003. Application of biofluid 1H nuclear magnetic resonance–based metabolomic techniques for the analysis of the biochemical effects of dietary isoflavones on human plasma profile. *Anal Biochem* **323**: 197–204.

Svetkey, L.P., Moore, T.J., Simons-Morton, D.G., Appel, L.J., Bray, G.A., Sacks, F.M., Ard, J.D., Mortensen, R.M., Mitchell, S.R., Conlin, P.R., and Kesari, M. 2001. DASH collaborative research group. Angiotensinogen genotype and blood pressure response in the Dietary Approaches to Stop Hypertension (DASH) study. *J Hypertens* **19**: 1949–1956.

Thimmulappa, R.K., Mai, K.H., Srisuma, S., Kensler, T.W., Yamamoto, M., and Biswal, S. 2002. Identification of Nrf2-regulated genes induced by the chemopreventive agent sulforaphane by oligonucleotide microarray. *Cancer Res* **62**: 5196–5203

Trujillo, E., Davis, C., and Milner, J. 2005. Nutrigenomics, proteomics, metabolomics and you. *J Am Diet Assoc* (accepted).

van Ommen, B., and Stierum, R. 2002. Nutrigenomics: exploiting systems biology in the nutrition and health arena. *Curr Opin Biotechnol* **13**: 517–521.

Wang, X., Tomso, D.J., Liu, X., and Bell, D.A. 2005. Single nucleotide polymorphism in transcriptional regulatory regions and expression of environmentally responsive genes. *Toxicol Appl Pharmacol* Jul 4.

Wong, H.L., Seow, A., Arakawa, K., Lee, H.P., Yu, M.C., and Ingles, S.A. 2003. Vitamin D receptor start codon polymorphism and colorectal cancer risk: effect modification by dietary calcium and fat in Singapore Chinese. *Carcinogenesis* **24**: 1091–1095.

Yang, W.C., Mathew, J., Velcich, A., Edelmann, W., Kucherlapati, R., Lipkin, M., Yang, K., and Augenlicht, L.H. 2001. Targeted inactivation of the $p21^{WAF1/cip1}$ gene enhances Apc-initiated tumor formation and the tumor-promoting activity of a Western-style high-risk diet by altering cell maturation in the intestinal mucosa. *Cancer Res* **61**: 565–569.

Zangani, D., Darcy, K.M., Shoemaker, S., and Ip, M.M. 1999. Adipocyte-epithelial interactions regulate the *in vitro* development of normal mammary epithelial cells. *Exp Cell Res* **247**: 399–409.

CHAPTER

3

Genetics and Epigenetics in Cancer Biology

ANNA VELCICH, LIDIJA KLAMPFER, JOHN MARIADASON, HELENA SMARTT, SANDRA GUILMEAU, SANDRA MAIER, WANCAI YANG, JUDITH CHRISTMAN, BARBARA HEERDT, AND LEONARD AUGENLICHT

In this chapter, we consider the role of genetic and epigenetic factors and the pathways of which they are a part in the development of intestinal cancer. This is one of the most prevalent of the solid tumors and is the tumor site for which the greatest insight has been obtained regarding the underlying cell and molecular biology of its etiology, pathogenesis, and response to therapy. We consider the complexity of the pathways that have been linked to development of this tumor. We review the literature and our own data on some of the most interesting pathways involved in the establishment and maintenance of homeostasis in the intestinal mucosa, and the perturbations in these pathways, especially those involved in intestinal cell lineage–specific differentiation, which are linked to tumorigenesis. Finally, we consider the role of the mitochondria, both in the regulation of critical aspects of intestinal cell maturation and in the potential integration of growth and apoptotic pathways. We discuss the role of mitochondrial function and the mitochondrial membrane potential, as well as the influence of both short-chain fatty acids and polyunsaturated fatty acids on the mitochondria, which may be fundamental in determining probability of tumor development.

INTRODUCTION

In this chapter, we explore the relationship among the maintenance and utilization of information encoded in the genome in developing and maintaining the functions and homeostasis of the intestinal mucosa, perturbations that take place that drive tumor development in this tissue, and, in relation to the theme of this volume, the potential modulation of these processes by nutrients.

We have chosen to focus on the intestinal mucosa for a number of reasons: First, the colon is a site of neoplastic disease that has a major impact on human health; second, among the solid tumors, colonic cancer remains the one best understood on the molecular and genetic level; third, it is easy to demonstrate that dietary factors play a major role in both homeostasis of the intestinal mucosa and in risk for and development of tumors.

As to this latter point, there is a wealth of epidemiological and experimental data, some of which is considered in other chapters, that demonstrate the major impact that diet has on intestinal tumor development. Some of the most definitive evidence regarding human colon cancer is the striking alteration in incidence in migrant populations. For example, historically there has been a marked difference in incidence of intestinal cancer in the U.S. white population compared with the indigenous Japanese, with colon cancer the predominant form in the United States and gastric cancer predominant in Japan. However, upon migration to the Hawaiian islands, the first generation Japanese (Issei) show a dramatic shift in this pattern of site-specific disease to that of the Western society, and by the second generation (Nisei), the relative incidence at the two sites is very similar to that seen in the United States (American Institute for Cancer Research, 1997). This is far too short a period to invoke a significant shift in the genetics of the population as an explanation of the altered site-specific tumor incidence. An equally dramatic example of the major importance of diet and its interaction with the genetics of colon cancer comes from one of the genetically highest risk groups for colon cancer: hereditary nonpolyposis colon cancer (HNPCC). In such families, there are inherited defects in DNA mismatch repair that permit mutations in genes important in tissue

Copyright © 2006, Elsevier Inc.
All rights of reproduction in any form reserved.

homeostasis to accumulate, which then cause early and frequent development of tumors. However, even here diet plays a major role: An original HNPCC kindred recognized by Warthin in 1913 in defining hereditary intestinal cancer, Family G, had a high incidence of gastric cancer, then the most common sporadic gastrointestinal cancer in the United States (Warthin, 1913). By 1971, when this kindred was reinvestigated by Lynch and Krush in defining HNPCC, the incidence of gastric cancer in both the kindred and the general population had decreased, but in both cases the incidence of colon cancer had increased. Thus, high risk for cancer was established by the genetics of the family, but environmental factors (i.e., diet) were the major determinant of the site of tumor formation.

Complexity of Tumorigenesis

Every technological development that has permitted more sensitive and comprehensive investigation of the initiation and progression of cancer has revealed greater complexity in these processes. High-throughput methods for screening of altered expression of nearly the entire genome at the messenger RNA (mRNA) level in dozens to hundreds of tumor specimens have documented a complexity and heterogeneity of alterations between normal and tumor tissue, and among tumor tissues, that is enormous. This is likely to grow greater as improvements are made in defining quantitative levels of RNA expression, in validating methods for comparison of the proteins expressed and their post-translational modifications, and in developing and widely using methods for detailed structural comparisons of genomes. For example, Sebat et al. (2004) documented that not only are there myriad single nucleotide polymorphisms (SNPs) present throughout the genome of populations, but small deletions and insertions differ among individuals as well. To compound the problem further, although we review pathways that have been particularly well dissected and the functional interactions among pathways fundamental to transformation, there is as yet no real insight into how quantitative and qualitative alterations among gene products interact within pathways or in coordination of pathways, and there are no extensive studies in transformation regarding intracellular localization of such gene products that may also be essential for dictating functional interactions of importance.

Thus, despite the extensive knowledge gained over the past decade, there is every reason to suspect that the complexity of molecular and biochemical alteration that characterizes the transformed state is far from understood. This issue can be framed as a question: Is the transformed cell an example of biological and regulatory chaos, or is much of this background "noise," and is there a more limited subset of fundamental principles that determine the several characteristics of transformation that are relevant to what we understand, and believe important, regarding its biological and clinical phenotypes? Regarding this, Hanahan and Weinberg (2000) have discussed the fundamental attributes that must be acquired by a cell for it to be malignant. These are as follows:

1. Loss of response to growth regulatory signals and establishment of independence from growth factors
2. Limitless replicative potential
3. Ability to avoid apoptosis
4. Ability to recruit a blood supply for the tumor to nourish itself
5. Ability to invade and metastasize

This provides a useful outline for the discussion of the molecular mechanisms that produce a colon tumor. We focus on the first three, as they are more germane to tumor initiation and its relatively early expansion, rather than progression. And to this, we add another:

- Inability to undergo proper lineage specific differentiation, leading to imbalances in the tissue that are fundamental to tumor development

As we will discuss, accumulating evidence regarding the molecular events in colon tumor formation point to altered differentiation as a key to tumor formation. This might have been expected; loss of growth control may be a necessary element in tumor formation (i.e., numbers 1 and 2, above), but by itself might produce only hyperplasia and hyperplastic growths, which, in the colon, do not have significant malignant potential. Instead, the characteristic early growth that leads to colon cancer is the adenomatous polyp, a lesion whose pathology is defined by its alteration of a differentiated phenotype of the intestinal mucosa—that is, intestinal gland formation.

FUNDAMENTAL CELL BIOLOGY OF MALIGNANT TRANSFORMATION IN THE COLON

Linkage between Cell Proliferation and Differentiation

In the basic histology of the intestinal tract, epithelial cells divide in the lower half to two thirds of the crypt and migrate up to the top of the crypt in the large intestine and up along the villi of the small intestine, until they are sloughed into the lumen and extruded (Lipkin et al., 1983). Along this journey, they undergo differentiation along several lineages and may or may not undergo apoptosis before extrusion. This is an important issue, as there are many reports in the literature indicating rather extensive apoptosis of epithelial cells in the intestinal mucosa, with equally impressive alterations in apoptosis following carcinogenic insult or chemopreventive treatment. However, histologically, apoptotic cells are rare in the intestinal mucosa, and careful analysis by TUNEL staining confirms that at most a small percentage of the cells undergo frank apoptosis. Modulations in these apoptotic rates, especially if they occur focally, may indeed be very important. But reports of very high frequency of, and very large changes in, apoptotic rate should be accepted with caution. Moreover, it is quite frequently stated that for tumor development, cells must develop methods to avoid apoptosis. However, this is not true. In colon tumors, rates of apoptosis are higher than in the normal mucosa. Considering that it takes hundreds of cell generations to create a tumor of clinical significance (Shibata et al., 1996), this must be true, because a simple exponential expansion (i.e., 2^n, where $n > 200$) would form a growth of impossible size. Moreover, apoptosis can be induced in colon tumor cell lines by a variety of stimuli (Hague et al., 1993; Heerdt et al., 1994, 1996, 1997, 1998, 2003), and hence apoptotic pathways are not permanently abrogated in tumors, but modulated in relationship to proliferation.

In general, intestinal tumor development in rodents and humans under either carcinogenic or genetic influence is associated with increased proliferation and, most important, an expansion of the proliferative compartment in the crypt. In simple terms, cells continue to synthesize DNA and divide as they migrate up along the crypt–villus axis. In addition, at a gross level, gland structure is altered. There is a reduction in mucin–secreting, or goblet, cells early, in preneoplastic lesions termed *aberrant crypt foci* (Pretlow et al., 1999). Further, in both benign and malignant tumors, glandular structure and mucin secretion are generally reduced. The extent of these changes yields the histological classification of the tumor, from well differentiated (i.e., many glands and mucin secretion) to moderately well differentiated to poorly differentiated, with most of the tumors falling in the middle category. Pathologically, benign tumors are classified principally in terms of the orderly appearance of their crypt and villi, with increasing disorder characterizing more advanced growths with higher malignant potential.

This fundamental organization, and its disruption in tumors, has guided biochemical and molecular analyses of tumors. This is especially true of the continued proliferation as cells migrate up the crypt. As pointed out previously, lack of response to growth regulatory signals is considered an essential characteristic of tumorigenesis. However, while it is indeed impossible for a tumor to form without loss of growth control and therefore accumulation of cells, such tumors, if only hyperplastic, do not have significant malignant potential in the intestine. The potential for malignancy arises only when overall structure of the mucosa is disorganized and glandular structure, in particular, is altered. Thus, it is probably not wise to try to disconnect the altered proliferation with altered differentiation, consistent with the fact that these processes are fundamentally linked (Zhu and Skoultchi, 2001). Moreover, in the intestine, molecular analysis of the Wnt signaling pathway, the pathway that leads to development of almost all human colon cancer, has now been shown to act in regulating both proliferation and differentiation.

Basic Control of Proliferation/Differentiation in the Intestinal Mucosa

The basics of cell cycle regulation are well understood in the colon and other tissues. Mammalian cell division occurs via progression through the G_1, S, and G_2 and finally, mitotic phases of the cell cycle, with G_1 ("gap1") separating mitosis from DNA synthesis (S) and G_2 ("gap2) separating DNA synthesis from mitosis. Progression through G_1 is mitogen driven until cells reach the "restriction point," beyond which cells are irreversibly committed to DNA synthesis. It is important to note that this G_1 phase exhibits the greatest cell/tissue type specificity of the phases of the cell cycle, with different interactions of growth regulatory factors regulating progression through G_1 in different cell types (Massague, 2004).

In order to ensure proper timing of cell cycle events and the fidelity of DNA synthesis, the cell must proceed through the G_1/S checkpoint. If at this point DNA damage is detected, the cell cycle is halted until DNA repair is complete; if damage is too extensive, the cell undergoes programmed cell death (apoptosis). The G_2 phase, between the S and M phases, also contains a checkpoint (G_2/M), which ensures correct segregation of duplicated chromosomes to the daughter cells. When cells cease proliferation, either as a result of antimitogenic stimulation or in the absence of proper mitogenic signaling, they exit the cycle and enter a state of quiescence known as G_0 (reviewed in Malumbres and Barbacid, 2001; Carnero, 2002).

Progression through the cell cycle is regulated by the cyclin-dependent kinases (CDKs) and their regulatory binding partners, the cyclins. CDK activity is regulated at many levels including phosphorylation and dephosphorylation, cyclin expression levels, and the activity of CDK inhibitors (CKIs) (reviewed in Sherr and Roberts, 1999; Sherr, 2000; Carnero, 2002). Individual cyclins are expressed during specific phases of the cell cycle, regulated via their rate of synthesis and proteasome-mediated degradation. For example, D-type cyclins are induced in early G_1 in response to growth factor stimulation (reviewed in Sherr and Roberts, 1999; Sherr, 2000) and are thought to be involved in passage through the restriction point, beyond which the cell is irreversibly committed to DNA synthesis. The most important target for cyclin D/CDK4 activity is Rb, which binds to and inhibits transcriptional activation by the E2F family of transcription factors. Following phosphorylation of Rb, E2F proteins are released and induce the expression of proteins involved in cell cycle progression (e.g., cyclin E, cyclin A, and CDK1) and DNA synthesis (e.g., thymidylate synthase). The G_2/M checkpoint controlling chromosome segregation is regulated by CDK1 bound to cyclins B or A. G_2/M arrest can be induced by, for example, the p53-inducible proteins 14-3-3 and GADD45 (reviewed in Sherr, 2000). 14-3-3 proteins prevent the phosphatase Cdc25 from removing inhibitory phosphate groups from CDK1/cyclin B, and GADD45 dissociates CDK1 from cyclin B1 (reviewed in Taylor and Stark, 2001).

CKIs belong to two families: the inhibitors of CDK4 (INK4) family ($p16^{INK4a}$, $p15^{INK4b}$, $p18^{INK4c}$, and $p19^{INK4d}$), which inhibit CDK4 and CDK6, and the Cip/Kip family (including $p21^{cip1/waf1}$, $p27^{kip1}$, and $p57^{kip2}$), which share a broader range of inhibition (reviewed in Carnero, 2002). By binding and inhibiting activity of CDK/cyclin complexes, CKIs can control cell cycle progression. For example, induction of p21 protein is a critical part of the p53 response to DNA damage: p21 inhibits cyclin D and E complexes, promoting G_1 arrest (Arellano and Moreno, 1997).

Most of our knowledge concerning the role of cell cycle regulatory proteins in intestinal epithelial cells comes from *in vitro* studies using colorectal cancer cell lines. For example, Caco-2 colon cancer cells undergo differentiation during *in vitro* culture after reaching confluency and this process has been used to model maturation of intestinal epithelial cells as they progress toward the intestinal lumen (Mariadason et al., 2000a, 2001, 2002). During this process, the levels of cyclin D1, cyclin E, CDK2, and CDK4 are decreased while p21 and p27 levels are increased (Evers et al., 1996), concomitant with a reduction in CDK2- and CDK4-kinase activities (Ding et al., 1998). Deschênes et al. (2001) suggested that in post-confluent Caco-2 cells, p21 was involved in the induction of growth arrest, p57 in the maintenance of growth arrest, p27 in the induction of differentiation. In the absence of p27, p57 was markedly induced and appeared to compensate for cell cycle, but not differentiation effects, of p27, highlighting the partially redundant overlapping roles of the Cip/Kip protein family in intestinal epithelial cells (Deschenes et al., 2001). Indeed, crypt–villus architecture is largely unaffected in mice lacking p21 or p27, and p21 knockout mice are relatively normal (Deng et al., 1995), again emphasizing the functional redundancy of CKI proteins (see later discussion).

Relatively little is known about how cell cycle regulatory networks contribute to intestinal epithelial homeostasis *in vivo*. We have reported that among changes in gene expression that characterize cells as they migrate up from the crypt *in vivo* or undergo cell cycle arrest and differentiation *in vitro*, there is a downregulation across the entire network of cell cycle molecules that has been described (Mariadason et al., 2005). For example, levels of cyclin D1, cyclin A2, CDK2, and CDK4 mRNA in epithelial cells decrease toward the crypt lumen, while levels of p21 mRNA increase (Mariadason et al., 2005). The widespread alterations in these functionally related genes are consistent with the predominant characteristic in the intestinal crypt of exit of cells from the cell cycle. However, this result is not consistent with the idea that there is one or a small number of rate-limiting components that regulate cell cycle progression. Thus, either this is further evidence for considerable redundancy in regulation within the network or there are aspects of cell cycle regulation or its interaction with other pathways that we do not understand. In this regard, it will be of considerable interest to determine the CDK–cyclin–CKI complexes formed and their activity in different regions of the crypt–villus axis to gain a clearer picture of how cell cycle regulatory proteins contribute to intestinal epithelial homeostasis. We have begun this effort, and preliminary data suggest that the CDKs are more significantly downregulated than the cyclins during the maturation of intestinal cells *in vivo*, but with considerable heterogeneity even within these classes of molecules (Smartt, unpublished observation).

However, despite the apparent redundancy in cell cycle regulation, considerable evidence suggests deregulation of the G_1 cyclin–CDK–CKI network in colorectal neoplasia, supporting an important role in intestinal epithelial homeostasis. For example, mice lacking p21 or p27 show an increased susceptibility to cancer development in the intestine initiated by a mutation in the Apc gene (Yang et al., 2000, 2003; Philipp-Staheli et al., 2002), with genetic inactivation of p27 sufficient by itself to cause intestinal tumor formation (Yang et al., 2003). Importantly, this is strictly linked to the diet the animals are fed: In p27 knockout mice, intestinal tumors only form in mice fed a defined AIN76A diet and are increased in animals fed a Western-style diet, high in fat and phosphate, low in calcium and vitamin D (Yang, unpublished observations). No tumors form when the same genotypes are maintained on a chow diet. Straightforward explanations for this are that the chow diet contains cancer-inhibiting phytochemicals or that the defined diet, being designed to promote maximal growth of the mice, is a tumor-promoting diet. Nevertheless, the fact that p27 can initiate tumors when inactivated, but that inactivation of p21 requires mutation in the Apc tumor initiator, is consistent with the fact that there is much better evidence for an impact of reduced p27 expression in colon tumors on patient prognosis (reviewed in Yang et al., 2003).

From a mechanistic point of view, it is important that the role of p27 in colorectal cancer may not be directly linked to its role as a regulator of the cell cycle. Ectopic overexpression of p27 in HT29 colon carcinoma cells increased their sensitivity to butyrate-induced differentiation (i.e., expression of alkaline phosphatase [Yamamoto et al., 1999]). Again, in contrast, overexpression of p21 instead decreased sensitivity to butyrate induction of differentiation (Yamamoto et al., 1999). Moreover, Quaroni et al. (2000) also showed that when introduced with an adenoviral vector into a fetal human intestinal cell line, p27 was much more effective than p21 in inducing expression of differentiation markers (e.g., DPPIV, aminopeptidase). Finally, antisense inhibition of p27 expression in differentiating Caco-2 cells repressed villin, sucrase-isomaltase, and alkaline phosphatase expression (Deschenes et al., 2001). In these studies, the effects of altered p27 expression on differentiation were divorced from effects on cell cycling, with the conclusion that "intestinal cell differentiation apparently requires a function of $p27^{Kip1}$ other than that which leads to inhibition of CDKs" (Deschenes et al., 2001). A similar conclusion, that p27 is involved in colonic cell differentiation, was reached by Weinstein's group based on the association of high p27 expression with well-differentiated and moderately differentiated human colorectal tumors, but low levels in poorly differentiated tumors (Ciaparrone et al., 1998). This was echoed by Palmqvist et al. (1999): that the lack of correlation of p27 levels with human tumor cell proliferation "support the view that p27 not merely controls cell cycle progression, but might be associated with other mechanisms responsible for aggressive tumor behavior in colorectal cancer."

In addition to members of the Cip/Kip CKI family, the p16 protein has also been implicated in colorectal maturation and neoplasia. Methylation of the INK4a/Arf locus (which encodes both p16 and Arf proteins) is a common event in colorectal cancer (e.g., see Burri et al., 2001), and ApcMin mice null for the INK4a/Arf locus show increased colonic tumor size and vascularity, suggesting that INK4a/Arf inhibit colon tumor progression (although the relative contributions of p16 and Arf are not yet determined). Furthermore, overexpression of positive cell cycle regulators has also been observed in colorectal neoplasia: For example, cyclin D1 and CDK4 show increased expression in adenomas from both ApcMin mice and human familial adenomatous polyposis (FAP) patients (Zhang et al., 1997), and the targeted inactivation of cyclin D1 reduces tumor formation in mice that is initiated by mutations in Apc (Hulit et al., 2004). Taken together, the evidence supports a crucial role for cyclin-CDK-CKI networks in regulation of intestinal homeostasis and neoplasia, although there is much still to learn about the precise mechanisms involved.

GENE EXPRESSION PROFILING

The complexity of cell phenotypes and functions that characterize the normal colonic mucosa suggested to us that factors that modulate homeostasis, such as oncogenic insults or nutrients, would have complex effects. This was reinforced by findings from hybridization kinetic experiments that suggested that ~10% of expressed genes, or ~1000 loci, might be altered in inducing differentiation or transformation of a variety of cell types (e.g., Hastie, 1976, and discussion in Augenlicht et al., 1992, 1999a). Therefore, in the early 1980s, we began development of methods to analyze the profiles of change in gene expression. Initially, this involved semiquantitative analysis of each of 400 cloned sequences in defined arrays (Augenlicht et al., 1982) but was expanded to 4000 sequences with computerized scanning and image analysis for quantification (Augenlicht et al., 1987). Although these methods were crude by modern standards, they did generate profiles of gene expression, including attempts at clustering of the results, to show that the colonic mucosa at genetic risk for development of colon tumors exhibited a distinct pattern of gene expression compared with the low-risk intestinal mucosa. Moreover, all of the potential uses of gene expression profiling in detection of risk or relative drug sensitivity and in characterization of pathways of cell differentiation were envisioned in this early work (Augenlicht and Kobrin, 1982; Augenlicht et al., 1987, 1992, 1999, 2000; Augenlicht, 1988, 1989, 1997).

A number of groups have applied microarray analysis of gene expression to questions of colon tumor development, demonstrating, for example, that tumor gene expression profiles are distinct from those of normal tissue (Alon et al., 1999; Notterman et al., 2001; Selaru et al., 2002; Zou et al., 2002; Bertucci et al., 2003) and distinguishing tumor subtypes (Selaru et al., 2002). We have used expression profiling approaches to predict sensitivity to chemotherapeutic drugs (Mariadason et al., 2003) and have discovered that constitutive Ras signaling downregulates the interferon response through inhibition of STAT activation (Klampfer et al., 2003). We have also interrogated the complex profiles of expression that characterize lineage-specific differentiation (Mariadason et al., 2002; Velcich et al., 2005), the maturation of cells as they migrate along the crypt–villus axis (Mariadason et al., 2005), and the response of colonic carcinoma cells to chemopreventive agents (Mariadason et al., 2000b).

Such studies of course identify particular sequences that may play an important role in the biological change under investigation and can be pursued for their mechanistic implications. However, in looking at the kinetics of change in gene expression, we noted that in the lineage-specific differentiation of cells in culture or in their response to physiological inducers, such as the SCFA butyrate, there was a monotonic increase in the number of genes altered in expression as a function of time. This progressive increase in the number of genes altered in expression is the hallmark of a defined program that is triggered by the initial stimulus, with each set of changes triggering an expanded set of alterations at the next stage. Thus, from this simple observation, it is straightforward to predict that a large number of signaling pathways and attendant transcriptional regulatory factors would play a role in responding to physiological signals that maintain intestinal homeostasis. This complex network would also then offer multiple targets for disruption of homeostasis in tumor formation. We have, in fact, demonstrated that in response to the short-chain fatty acid butyrate, a physiological regulator of maturation, colon cells do recruit an array of signaling molecules, which expand as a function of time (Mariadason et al., 2000b).

In the next section, we catalogue the data that imply important roles of some of these pathways and factors, with full recognition that such a list is far from comprehensive. Moreover, we have clearly shown that alteration of phenotype, such as arrest of cells in the G_1 phase of the cell cycle, can be achieved by many combinations of events (Mariadason et al., 2000b). Finally, although we discuss some pathways and interactions, the complexity of this network defies simple diagramming. Therefore, in the last section of this chapter, we address the potential that mitochondrial functions have a profound role in integrating the many different signals that are generated from extrinsic and intrinsic signals to determine whether a cell ultimately divides or dies.

SIGNALING PATHWAYS AND TRANSCRIPTIONAL FACTORS IN INTESTINAL CELL MATURATION, TISSUE HOMEOSTASIS, AND TUMORIGENESIS

Wnt Signaling—The Initiator of Tumor Formation—and Its Role in Regulation of c-*myc*

It is clear that loss of APC (adenomatous polyposis coli) function, either by gene mutation or deletion, initiates colonic tumor formation in the human and principally small intestinal tumor formation in the mouse (reviewed and discussed in Kinzler and Vogelstein, 1996). There is strong evidence that it is the role of Apc in β-catenin-Tcf signaling—also known as *Wnt signaling*—that is the key to its transforming ability. However, it must be kept in mind that the Apc gene encodes a protein with multiple functional domains (Van Es et al., 2001), and it has been pointed out that Apc and β-catenin mutations, both of which can initiate intestinal tumor formation in rodents and humans, are not functionally equivalent and that other functions of Apc, such as regulation of cell adhesion, motility, and migration under control of the Apc protein, are necessary for tumorigenesis (Fodde, 2004).

As regards β-catenin–Tcf signaling, Apc protein, in combination with glycogen synthase kinase (GSK) 3β and axin regulates the level of free cytoplasmic β-catenin by binding to and targeting β-catenin for degradation by ubiquitination-dependent proteolysis (Rubinfeld et al., 1993, 1996; Behrens et al., 1996; Ikeda et al., 1998; Sakanaka et al., 1998). Absent or mutant Apc fails to accomplish this targeting, and hence cytoplasmic β-catenin levels accumulate (Korinek et al., 1997; Morin et al., 1997; Rubinfeld et al., 1997). These increased levels lead to an increase in the active transcription complex β-catenin–Tcf, which modulates the expression of important target sequences, such as upregulation of c-*myc* and cyclin D1 (He et al., 1998; Shtutman et al., 1999; Tetsu and McCormick, 1999).

Evidence that loss of regulation of β-catenin is a key event in transformation includes a number of observations: Some human colon tumors have only β-catenin mutations that prevent degradation of β-catenin, in the absence of Apc mutations (Ilyas et al., 1997; Morin et al., 1997). Moreover, rat colon tumors induced by the carcinogen AOM (azoxymethane [Takahashi et al., 1998]) or by heterocyclic amines (putative human colon carcinogens [Dashwood et al., 1998]) frequently exhibit mutant β-catenin, not Apc, mutations. In the AOM model, β-catenin also exhibits mutation and altered subcellular distribution (Takahashi et al., 1998), and overexpression of β-catenin can be found in focal lesions of such AOM-treated rats, which are claimed to be distinct from AOM-induced aberrant crypt foci (ACF) (Yamada et al., 2000), but which may be a subset of dysplastic ACF (Pretlow and Bird, 2000). It is these "β-catenin" lesions that show progressively abnormal histopathology associated with tumor development (Yamada et al., 2001). Regarding the human, ACF with increasing pathology (i.e., dysplasia) show increased levels of β-catenin (Hao et al., 2001). Finally, the β-catenin binding domain of Apc has been reported to be sufficient for tumor suppression (Shih et al., 2000) and stabilized β-catenin has been shown to immortalize colonic epithelial cells (Wagenaar et al., 2001).

The Apc protein, the product of the Apc tumor suppressor gene, is expressed on the basolateral surface of colonic epithelial cells *in situ*, with expression increasing as cells migrate up the crypt toward the lumen (Smith et al., 1993), consequently downregulating β-catenin. This topological distribution of the protein implies that its expression is associated with cell maturation. Indeed, the role of β-catenin in regulating expression of c-*myc* and cyclin D1 strongly suggests that the loss of Apc function deregulates these genes and leads to increased cell proliferation in the mucosa, as discussed earlier. It has also been suggested that Apc participates in regulation of apoptosis (Morin et al., 1996). However, Groden et al. (1995) showed that colon carcinoma cell lines respond to reexpression of wild-type Apc in diverse ways, exhibiting altered morphology and growth in agar, which is also dependent on the expressed form of Apc (Santoro and Groden, 1997). Further, we demonstrated that decreasing β-catenin–Tcf activity in Caco-2 cells by three different means (introduction of wild-type Apc, elevated expression of E-cadherin, and use of a dominant-negative Tcf-4) all caused premature elevation of the promoter activity of genes that encode proteins whose expression defines colonic cell differentiation (Mariadason et al., 2001).

These data suggest that in addition to regulating cell proliferation, a primary role of Apc and β-catenin signaling in normal colonic homeostasis may involve colonic cell differentiation rather than apoptosis. Consistent with this is that in a Tcf-4 knockout mouse (functionally equivalent to reduced β-catenin–Tcf signaling due to expression of wild-type Apc), loss of the stem cell population in the small intestine leads to lethality, but this is due to premature differentiation of the stem cells, rather than apoptotic cell death (Korinet et al., 1998). It has been confirmed that Wnt signaling through β-catenin–Tcf activity is responsible for maintaining intestinal epithelial cells in a progenitor or stem cell–like phenotype, with reduction as cells migrate up the crypt leading to activation of genes involved in colonic cell differentiation (Van de Wetering et al., 2002). This linkage of Wnt signaling to colonic cell differentiation would explain several other observations: that Apc is expressed in almost all colonic epithelial cells as they progress up the crypt, but that only about 1–2% of the cells undergo apoptosis (Augenlicht et al., 1999), indicating that Apc expression may be more tightly linked to differentiation pathways than to apoptotic pathways and that suppression of β-catenin–Tcf by a dominant-negative Tcf-4 restores epithelial cell polarity to a colorectal cancer cell line (Naishiro et al., 2001), a phenotype specifically linked to colon cell differentiation (Augeron and Laboisse, 1984; Mariadason et al., 2001).

In summary, Apc mutation alters β-catenin–Tcf signaling, disrupting mucosal homeostasis leading to tumor formation, and this is likely due to its critical role in proliferation and differentiation pathways, with possibly modest effects on apoptosis. There are a large number of targets of Wnt signaling that may be linked to development of colon tumors, but c-*myc* stands out as one that is particularly important. We have shown that c-*myc* expression decreases as cells mature along their migration toward the lumen, and that this is reciprocal with expression of Max and Mad, two antagonists of c-*myc* function (Mariadason et al., 2005). Moreover, a high percentage of the >1000 sequences we detected as regulated during this *in vivo* maturation are documented c-*myc* target genes (Mariadason et al., 2005). Therefore, downregulation of c-*myc* as cells migrate along the crypt–villus axis appears to play a role in normal colon cell maturation, consistent with reports that c-*myc* is often overexpressed in human colon tumors (Erisman et al., 1985, 1998; Sikora et al., 1987; Finely et al., 1989). In this regard, it has been shown that inactivation (i.e., downregulation) of c-*myc* in hepatocellular carcinoma permits pluripotent cell differentiation, consistent with the concept that it is the important role that c-*myc* plays in differentiation that is fundamental to loss of homeostasis and tumor formation (Shachaf et al., 2004). Further, although β-catenin expression and activation, as indicated by its nuclear localization, are elevated in mouse tumors initiated by inactivation of Apc, this is not true of tumors initiated by targeted inactivation of the major intestinal mucin gene, Muc2 (Velcich et al., 2002). However, in both the Apc and the Muc2 mouse models, c-*myc* is overexpressed in the tumors (Velcich et al., 2002). This suggests that although the mechanisms of tumorigenesis may differ in the two mouse models, in each the pathways converge on c-*myc* overexpression, demonstrating the importance of this locus in both intestinal cell homeostasis and aberrations that lead to tumor formation. Finally, the c-*myc* protein binds to a transcription factor termed *Miz*, which binds to and positively regulates p21WAF1/Cip1 expression, a cell cycle regulatory molecule necessary for both cell cycle arrest and differentiation of colonic epithelial cells that are necessary to maintain intestinal homeostasis and prevent tumor formation. In the presence of elevated β-catenin–Tcf signaling in the proliferative compartment of the intestinal crypt or in intestinal tumors, high c-*myc* expression sequesters Miz, preventing p21 expression. However, when Wnt signaling is driven down as cells undergo normal maturation, myc levels fall and Miz becomes free to induce p21 (Korinek et al., 1998). Thus, the exit of cells from the proliferative compartment and their differentiation along different lineages is temporally, architecturally, and functionally linked to c-*myc* levels along the crypt–villus axis.

At first, the regulation of c-*myc* by Wnt signaling appears to be straightforward: The c-*myc* promoter harbors Tcf-binding sites, providing a means for positive regulation of the locus by elevated β-catenin–Tcf levels. However, we have already pointed out that increased c-*myc* levels in Muc2 tumors are not linked to altered β-catenin signaling. Moreover, the c-*myc* gene is also amplified at a low level in ~30% of human colon tumors (Heerdt et al., 1991), and this amplification, which elevates c-*myc* expression to levels higher than those due to defective β-catenin–Tcf signaling alone, sensitizes the colon cells both *in vitro* and *in vivo* to 5FU (Heerdt, 1991; Augenlicht, 1997; Arango, 2001) and camptothecin (Arango et al., 2002) and is therefore an important marker of prognosis.

We have also investigated two instances of nutritional factors that impinge in complex ways on regulating c-*myc* levels. First, we assumed that the short-chain fatty acid butyrate, which is a physiological inducer of cell maturation in the intestinal tract (Heerdt et al., 1994; Augenlicht et al., 1999b; Mariadason et al., 2000a), would downregulate β-catenin–Tcf signaling, which would mimic what happens to the pathway during cell maturation *in vivo*. However, we found the opposite: that β-catenin–Tcf complex formation and signaling activity were stimulated by butyrate (Bordonaro et al., 1999). This was inconsistent with the many reports that c-*myc* steady state levels were downregulated by butyrate (reviewed in Wilson et al., 2002). We therefore postulated (Bordonaro et al., 1999), based on work reported (Heruth et al., 1993), that butyrate would circumvent the increased β-catenin–Tcf signaling and consequent increased initiation of c-*myc* transcription by a block to transcript elongation and demonstrated this using a novel method of imaging of transcription of the c-*myc* locus (Wilson et al., 2002). We also showed that this block to c-*myc* transcription is actively recruited by 1,25-dihydroxyvitamin D3 (Wilson et al., 2002). Interestingly, we showed that the pharmacological induction of cell cycle arrest by the nonsteroidal anti-inflammatory drug sulindac did not recruit this transcriptional block to c-*myc*, causing steady state levels of c-*myc* to rise during the cell cycle arrest. We have argued that because colonic epithelial cells have evolved in an environment where they utilize SCFAs and vitamin D, they have evolved mechanisms, including the block to c-*myc* transcription, to correctly coordinate events triggered by their interactions with these molecules, but that this is not true of pharmacological agents they have not encountered, such as sulindac (Mariadason et al., 2000b; Wilson et al., 2002). Thus, abnormal situations, such as elevated c-*myc* levels in the presence of cell cycle arrest, which has been shown to trigger apoptosis, can result (Evan et al., 1992; Arango et al., 2001) and hence account for the toxicological side effects of such drugs.

Because even transient inhibition of c-*myc* expression can cause tumor regression (Jain et al., 2002), likely by permitting cell differentiation (Shachaf et al., 2004), it is important that we have shown that nutritional agents can circumvent the increase in c-*myc* transcriptional initiation in colon tumor cells. It also becomes important to understand the mechanism involved, and there are thus far two insights. Trichostatin A (TSA), like butyrate, an inhibitor of histone deacetylase activity (Sealy and Chalkley, 1978; Yoshida et al., 1990; and see below), also increased β-catenin–Tcf signaling (Bordonaro et al., 1999), resulting in increased initiation of c-*myc* transcription (Wilson et al., 2002). However, like butyrate, TSA also recruited the transcriptional block (Wilson et al., 2002), though with different kinetics reflecting the more rapid metabolism and transient effects of TSA (Wilson et al., 2002). Consistent with the integration of the effects on transcription and the downstream block in response to TSA, c-*myc* mRNA steady state levels initially fell and then rose as the effects of TSA on the block were reversed (Wilson et al., 2002). Thus, protein acetylation may play a role in this transcriptional block, although it is not clear from these data whether this is a direct effect on acetylation of molecules at the site of block (e.g., histones, transcription factors) or an upstream effect of acetylation on regulating the expression of such factors (see later discussion). Finally, in HL60 promyelocytic leukemia cell differentiation induced by 1,25-dihydroxyvitamin D3, transcriptional blockage of c-*myc* at the exon 1/intron 1 boundary involves the elevated expression and binding of the homeobox gene product HOXB4 (Pan, 1999; Pan, 2001; Pan, 1996). Preliminary data show induction of HOXB4 in colonic cells treated with either butyrate or 1,2-dihydroxyvitamin D3 (Wilson, unpublished observations). Other factors, such as RFX1, which have been reported to possibly interact with HOXB4 in leukemia cell differentiation at the site of the block (Chen et al., 2000), may also be involved, in addition to post-translational modification (e.g., phosphorylation, acetylation) of HOXB4 or other associated factors.

There are many additional questions raised by these observations, such as the extent to which this mechanism of transcriptional block is utilized *in vivo* as cells normally migrate up the crypt. We have also found that an attenuation of transcription of another Wnt target gene, cyclin D1, is induced by butyrate in a similar fashion and may generate stable short transcripts that could serve as effectors of the butyrate induced reprogramming of the cells (Maier, unpublished observations).

Ras Signaling

Ras proteins are small guanosine triphosphatases (GTPases) that regulate cell growth, differentiation, and apoptosis. There are three isoforms of Ras: H-Ras, N-Ras, and K-Ras. Ras is activated by guanine nucleotide exchange factors (GEFs) that release guanosine diphosphate (GDP) and allow GTP binding. Active GTP-bound Ras interacts with several different effector proteins, such as Raf kinases, PI3K, RalGEFs, and NORE/MST1. GTPase-activating proteins (GAPs) terminate Ras signaling; however, oncogenic forms of Ras are resistant to GAPs and thus remain constitutively activated (reviewed in Rebollo and Martinez, 1999; Shields et al., 2000). Localization of Ras to the plasma membrane is essential for its normal biological function; however, recent data established that Ras can signal from internal membranes as well, such as the endoplasmic reticulum and the Golgi (Bivona and Philips, 2003).

Whereas transient activation of Ras is critical for the response to several growth factors, oncogenic forms of Ras are locked in their active state and thereby constitutively transduce signals for transformation, angiogenesis, invasion, and metastasis in the absence of extracellular stimuli. Point mutations that activate the K-Ras protooncogene are present in up to 50% of sporadic colorectal tumors (Kinzler and Vogelstein, 1996). The majority of the k-ras mutations are gain-of-function mutations at codon 12 and 13, and activated k-ras has been shown to synergize with Apc (D'Abaco et al., 1996) and p53 mutations (Sevignani et al., 1998) in the transformation of intestinal epithelial cells. In addition, targeted expression of oncogenic Ras under control of the villin promoter has been shown to be sufficient to cause spontaneous intestinal tumors, apparently in the absence of Apc mutations (Janssen et al., 2002).

Transmission of proliferative signals by Ras is mediated by the Ras kinase and its downstream effector, ERK1/ERK2.

In normal intestinal epithelium, active MAPK is restricted to the nuclei of cells in the proliferative compartment of the intestinal crypt. The importance of the ERK pathways in tumorigenesis is further underscored by the fact that BRAF mutations, which also result in the activation of the ERK pathway, are found in colorectal tumors that do not carry a Ras mutation (Rajagopalan et al., 2002). BRAF mutations arise primarily in mismatch repair (MMR)–deficient tumors, whereas the incidence of K-Ras mutations is higher in MMR-proficient cancers.

The role of Ras in apoptosis is more complex than its role in proliferation. Ras proteins have been shown either to promote or to inhibit apoptosis (Ohmori et al., 1997; Chang et al., 1998; Nalca et al., 1999; Brooks et al., 2001), depending on the cell type and the nature of the apoptotic stimuli. The antiapoptotic activity of Ras is mediated by the interaction of Ras with the catalytic subunit of the PI3K, which leads to the activation of AKT/PKB, a pro-survival kinase and subsequently to phosphorylation and inactivation of Bad, an antiapoptotic Bcl-2 family member (Datta et al., 1997). We demonstrated that activation of k-ras sensitizes epithelial cells to apoptosis induced by inhibitors of HDAC activity, including butyrate, the short-chain fatty acid that sustains homeostasis of colonic epithelium *in vivo* (Klampfer et al., 2004). This observation is significant because to some extent it explains the "butyrate paradox"—an observation that butyrate selectively induces apoptosis in transformed cells (Gibson et al., 1992). Similarly, we demonstrated that oncogenic mutations of Ras promote apoptosis in response to 5FU and camptothecin, two commonly used chemotherapeutic agents in the treatment of colorectal cancer (Klampfer, unpublished observations).

To identify new effectors of Ras signaling in colon cancer, we used the HCT116 cell line, which harbors an activating mutation in codon 13 of the k-ras protooncogene, and two isogenic clones derived from the HCT116 cell, Hkh2 and Hke-3, both with a targeted inactivation of the mutant k-ras allele (Shirasawa et al., 1993). Disruption of the mutant k-ras allele in HCT116 cells has been shown to result in decreased proliferation, reduced capacity for anchorage independent growth, and reduced tumorigenicity *in vivo* (Shirasawa et al., 1993). Using cDNA microarray analysis, we demonstrated that gelsolin, an actin-binding protein with a potent antiapoptotic activity, is highly downregulated by Ras signaling (Klampfer et al., 2004). Subsequently, we found that Ras inhibits gelsolin expression at the transcriptional level, underlying a frequent downregulation of gelsolin in primary colorectal tumors and colon cancer cell lines (Bertucci et al., 2004). Finally, we showed that silencing of gelsolin expression through siRNA, like Ras mutations, sensitizes cells to butyrate-induced apoptosis, demonstrating that Ras promotes apoptosis, at least in part, through downregulation of gelsolin expression (Klampfer et al., 2004).

Activation of Ras interacts with several other signaling pathways. For example, Ras has been shown to activate Notch signaling (Weijzen et al., 2002) and nuclear factor-κB (NF-κB) signaling (Kim et al., 2002; Millan 12 et al., 2003), two pathways discussed later in this chapter. In contrast, Ras has been shown to negatively regulate signaling by TGF-β (Kretzschmar et al., 1999), an important negative regulator of cell growth, also discussed later. As a result, epithelial cells harboring oncogenic ras often show loss of antimitogenic response to TGF-β. Oncogenic Ras has been shown to inhibit TGF-β–induced SMAD-dependent transcription through phosphorylation of the MAP kinase site in the linker region of SMAD2 and SMAD3 (Kretzschmar et al., 1999). We demonstrated that mutant Ras interferes with signaling by yet another negative regulator of cellular growth, interferon-γ (IFN-γ) (Klampfer et al., 2003). Activated ras inhibited STAT-dependent transcriptional activation in response to IFN-γ and colon cancer cells harboring mutant Ras had reduced expression of STAT1-dependent genes. One of many genes that requires STAT1 for its expression is p21, its central role in normal mucosal homeostasis and transformation having already been discussed. STAT1-deficient colon cancer cells failed to upregulate p21 in response to butyrate and sulindac. Because p21 has been shown to protect colon cancer cells from butyrate-induced apoptosis (Mahyar-Roemer and Roemer, 2001), it was important that cells with silenced STAT1 expression failed to arrest in response to butyrate but underwent accelerated apoptosis (Klampfer, unpublished observations).

TGF-β/BMP Signaling

The TGF-β family comprises a number of members, including TGF betas, bone morphogenetic protein (BMP), and activins, cytokines with antiproliferative and proapoptotic activity. These proteins play an important role in development, wound healing, angiogenesis, proliferation, and cell differentiation. In normal epithelium, TGF-β expression is regulated along the crypt villus axis, suggesting that it regulates growth arrest as cells migrate from the crypt to the villus. Activation of inhibitors of CDKs, such as p15, p21, p57, and p27, inhibition of phosphorylation of Rb, and inhibition of c-Myc underlie the growth inhibitory activity of TGF-β (reviewed in Siegel and Massague, 2003). Whereas the members of the TGF-β family are potent growth suppressors of many different normal cells (via induction of cell cycle arrest and apoptosis), many cancers are resistant to TGF-β, in particular gastric cancers and colon cancers. Mutations of p53, amplification of cyclin D1, and overexpression of mutant Ras have been shown to attenuate the responsiveness to TGF-β. In addition, frequent mutational inactivation of proteins required for signaling by TGF-β has been described in human cancers.

The biological activity of TGF-β is mediated by its binding to its receptor, comprising two subunits, RI and RII. Sporadic colon cancers often carry somatic mutations that inactivate RII (Markowitz et al., 1995). In particular, these mutations occur in tumors with microsatellite instability, a hallmark of defective DNA mismatch repair, which is characteristic of patients with the genetic syndrome hereditary nonpolyposis colon cancer (HNPCC). Most common are mutations affecting a 10-base pair polyadenine repeat (BAT-RII) present in the TGFRII coding region, which generate truncated and inactivating forms of the receptor (Markowitz et al., 1995). The TGF-β RII mutations occur at a relatively late stage of sporadic colorectal tumorigenesis and appear to coincide with the transition of adenomas to malignant carcinoma (Grady et al., 1998). Transfection of HCT116 cells with RII not only restored the responsiveness of cells to TGF-β but also reduced their tumorigenicity both *in vitro* and *in vivo*, demonstrating that RII functions as a tumor suppressor gene (Wang et al., 1995). Mutations of RI are less frequent; however, individuals homozygous for an attenuated allele, TGFRI (6A), appear to be at higher risk for developing colon cancer (Pasche et al., 1999, 2004). From the point of view of nutritional factors, it is important that the RII receptor can also be silenced by methylation of the gene, an epigenetic alteration that can be modulated by diet (see later discussion).

Intracellular messengers of TGF signaling beta are SMAD proteins. The receptor regulated SMADs, which include SMAD1, SMAD2, SMAD3, and SMAD5, associate with SMAD4 and translocate to the nucleus to regulate the expression of target genes. TGF-β signaling is negatively regulated by SMAD6 and SMAD7, inhibitory SMADs (reviewed in Siegel and Massague, 2003). Mutations of SMAD4, originally named DPC4 (deleted in colon and pancreatic carcinoma locus 4), have been identified in 10% of all colon cancers and 30% of metastatic colon cancers (Schutte et al., 1996). Germline mutations of SMAD4 have been found in a subset of patients with Peutz–Jaeger syndrome (JPS), and allelic loss of SMAD4 has been observed in polyps that develop in human JPS (Howe et al., 2001). SMAD4 heterozygous mice develop gastric and duodenal polyps, resembling the JPS and SMAD4 heterozygosity, and SMAD4 inactivation strongly promotes development of adenomas in $Apc^{\Delta716}$ mice (Takaku et al., 1998). In addition, SMAD3-deficient mice have been shown to develop colorectal cancer (Zhu et al., 1998), although this observation has yet to be confirmed.

BMP receptors activate SMAD1, SMAD5, and SMAD8. Villus epithelial cells express phosphorylated SMAD1, SMAD5, and SMAD8, indicating active BMP signaling predominantly in differentiated cells (Haramis et al., 2004). Mutations in the gene encoding BMP receptor type 1A have been found in some patients with JPS who are wild type for SMAD4 (Howe et al., 2001), implying a role for BMP signaling in JPS. Indeed, transgenic expression of the BMP inhibitor noggin results in JPS, with crypts appearing *de novo* throughout the epithelium (Haramis et al., 2004). Adenomatous changes develop in these mice at a later stage, recapitulating the human syndrome. Similarly, conditional inactivation of BMP R1 results in an expansion of the stem cells, leading to intestinal polyposis, resembling human JPS (He et al., 2004).

Thus, it appears that BMP signaling, through suppression of Wnt/β-catenin signaling (He et al., 2004) controls intestinal stem cell self-renewal and thereby prevents crypt fission and the subsequent increase in crypt number.

NF-κB

We have discussed the necessity for the intestinal epithelium to balance proliferation with cell loss in order to maintain homeostasis of the tissue. This cell loss may be passive (i.e., due to mechanical force from neighboring cells or by the luminal contents) or by apoptosis. A major cell survival (i.e., antiapoptotic) pathway that functions in concert with regulation of proliferation is that governed by the NF-κB transcription factor family.

NF-κB was identified by Sen and Baltimore as a nuclear factor binding to the intronic kappa light-chain enhancer element in B cells (Sen and Baltimore, 1986). The term is now used to refer to a family of transcription factors binding a common DNA sequence motif, the κB site. Although NF-κB is constitutively nuclear in mature B cells, in most other resting cell types, it is sequestered in the cytoplasm but can be induced to undergo nuclear translocation by a variety of stimuli (May and Ghosh, 1997). NF-κB exists as homodimers or heterodimers of members of the Rel protein family, of which there are five mammalian members: p50, p52, p65(RelA), RelB, and c-Rel. The most commonly detected NF-κB dimer is p50/p65 (Karin et al., 2002), although many other dimer combinations have been demonstrated *in vivo*. NF-κB nuclear localization, and hence activity, is regulated via binding to members of the IκB protein family; this masks the DNA-binding domain of NF-κB and prevents interaction with the target κB sequences (reviewed in Whiteside et al., 1997a,b). NF-κB is activated by release from IκB-mediated inhibition via phosphorylation followed by ubiquitination (and subsequent degradation) of the IκB protein: In the majority of cases, the IκB kinase complex (IKK) appears to be responsible (Ghosh and Karin, 2002).

NF-κB is activated by >150 distinct upstream stimuli, including a large number of viruses, bacteria, and their products, as well as several inflammatory cytokines (Pahl, 1999). As a result of this and the large number of NF-κB target genes from the immune system (e.g., cytokines, chemokines, immunoreceptors, proteins involved in antigen presentation, cell adhesion molecules, and acute phase proteins), NF-κB has been considered a central mediator of the immune response. However, NF-κB is also activated by hormones, growth factors, mitogens, and other physiological mediators, as well as therapeutic drugs and a range of stress stimuli, and therefore regulates many genes with functions outside the immune system, for example, in growth control and, most notably, in the regulation of apoptosis (reviewed in Pahl, 1999). A number of NF-κB regulated antiapoptotic genes have been identified, including cIAP-1, cIAP-2, XIAP, c-FLIP, and the antiapoptotic Bcl-2 family members Bfl/A1 and Bcl-X_L. Indeed, although most NF-κB knockout mice are viable, p65 knockout mice die at approximately embryonic day 15 due to extensive liver apoptosis (Beg et al., 1995), underscoring the importance of NF-κB in apoptosis. Roles for NF-κB in proliferation and inhibition of differentiation have also been suggested, with NF-κB induction of cyclin D1 implicated in both, although this is not as well established as its role in cell survival (Guttridge et al., 1999; Cao et al., 2001).

Given the multiple roles of NF-κB in growth control, it is not surprising that it has been implicated in intestinal epithelial homeostasis. Active NF-κB dimers (p50/p50 and p50/p65) are detected at the base of the normal mouse colonic crypt while p50/p50 dimers are detected, at lower levels, toward the intestinal lumen. The decreasing levels of active NF-κB toward the intestinal lumen suggest potential pro-proliferative and/or anti-apoptotic roles of NF-κB in the crypt. Nfkb1 knockout mice (which lack p50-containing dimers) showed a significant increase in crypt length and an extended proliferative zone at the base (Inan et al., 2000). This may result from the loss of an inhibitory effect of NF-κB on proliferation rather than an effect on apoptosis, which showed no change. The inhibitory effect of NF-κB on proliferation was suggested to result from suppression by p50/p50 dimers of expression of the potentially growth-enhancing genes TNF-α and NGF, which were both upregulated in the knockout animals. Indeed, dimers of p50 (which, unlike p65, does not contain a transactivation domain) were shown to act as stimulus-specific repressors of p50/p65-regulated genes in a colorectal cell line (Tong et al., 2004). Therefore, p50/p50 dimers may provide a restraining influence on growth-promoting p50/p65 dimers in the crypt base, with the net effect tending toward growth suppression.

In agreement with the apparent role of NF-κB in intestinal homeostasis, a role for NF-κB in initiation of tumors in a mouse model of colitis-associated cancer was suggested, via inhibition of apoptosis in epithelial cells in areas of chronic inflammation (Greten et al., 2004). Constitutive NF-κB activity has also been observed in colon carcinoma cell lines (Dejardin et al., 1999) and there is evidence suggesting that NF-κB activity is increased in human colorectal tumors (Evertsson and Sun, 2002; Maihofner et al., 2003; Yu et al., 2003). The potential role of NF-κB in early stages of colorectal cancer neoplasia is supported by the observation that various agents with chemopreventive activity for intestinal cells (e.g., aspirin and sulindac, curcumin from tumeric, and the SCFA butyrate) all inhibit NF-κB (Inan et al., 2000; Bharti and Aggarwal, 2002). Therefore, modulation of NF-κB by nutritional factors may be a useful tool in reduction of colon cancer risk.

By protecting against apoptosis, NF-κB has the potential to influence intestinal neoplasia at multiple stages of tumor development and in response to therapeutic agents. Constitutive NF-κB activity in colorectal tumor cells could contribute to resistance to standard cancer therapies. Moreover, a number of anticancer agents induce NF-κB activity, which may contribute to inducible chemoresistance. For example, the efficacy of the therapeutic agent CPT-11 in colorectal tumor xenograft models is enhanced by inhibition of NF-κB by either adenoviral expression of mutant IκBa or by the use of NF-κB proteasome inhibitors (Cusack et al., 2000).

In addition to the important roles of NF-κB in growth control, putative roles for NF-κB in metastasis and angiogenesis have recently been suggested. For example, NF-κB has been shown to regulate the expression of cell adhesion molecules ICAM-1 and VCAM-1, matrix metalloproteinase (MMP)-9 and vascular endothelial growth factor (VEGF) (Aggarwal, 2004).

Notch Signaling

Notch genes were first recognized in 1917 by Thomas Hunt Morgan in a strain of *Drosophila* with notches at the end of their wing blades due to haploinsufficiency of what he termed the "Notch" gene. It has been known for decades as a key in cell fate determination (Greenwal, 1998; Artavanis-Tsakonas et al., 1999). The four mammalian Notch genes encode single-pass transmembrane receptors that participate in communication between contiguous cells. They are activated by cell-membrane-associated ligands belonging to Jagged (also known as Serrate) and Delta-like families.

Mature Notch molecules are derived from proteolytic processing of precursors in the Golgi (Blaumueller et al., 1997) that are cleaved by a furin-like protease (Logeat et al., 1998) into heterodimers comprising an extracellular subunit (NEC) noncovalently associated with a transmembrane subunit (NTM) (Rand et al., 2000). NEC contains multiple EGF-like repeats, which are involved in ligand binding, while NTM includes an extracellular domain, containing three "Lin-Notch" repeats, a transmembrane domain and an intracellular domain. This in turn includes a "RAM23" domain, which participates in the binding of the transcription factor CSL, six ankyrin repeats, a polyglutamine region, and a PEST region, which is important for ubiquitination and hence proteolytic degradation (Greenwald, 1998; Artavanis-Tsakonas et al., 1999). The NEC–NTM interaction is Ca^{2+}-dependent, and its dissociation upon binding to ligand triggers receptor activation. Notch heterodimer dissociation causes a two-step proteolytic cleavage; first, the extracellular portion of NTM is clipped by TNF-α–converting enzyme (TACE), a metalloprotease of the disintegrin and metalloprotease (ADAM) family (Brou et al., 2000; Mumm et al., 2000). This makes NTM susceptible to an additional cleavage in the transmembrane domain by a presenilin-1–dependent gamma-secretase activity (DeStrooper et al., 1999; Struhl and Greenwald, 1999; Ye et al., 1999; Huppert et al., 2000; Okochi et al., 2002). This last cleavage releases the intracellular region of NTM (ICN) from the plasma membrane into the cytosol (Schroeter et al., 2002). The generation and stability of ICN is regulated by several E3 ubiquitin ligases, which influence the intensity and duration of Notch signals (Lai, 2002).

CSL-Dependent Notch Signaling

Once released from its membrane anchor, ICN translocates to the nucleus where it subsequently activates the expression of downstream target genes (Fryer et al., 2002) by binding to a highly conserved transcription factor, CSL (also known as *CBF1*, *Suppressor of Hairless*, or *Lag-1*) (Fortini and Artavanis-Tsakonas, 1994; Jarriault et al., 1995; Christensen et al., 1996). The quaternary complex formed by ICN, CSL, DNA-binding protein (Bray and Furriols, 2001), and transcriptional coactivators of the mastermind-like (MAML1) family (Petcherski and Kimble, 2000; Wu et al., 2000) associates with specific regulatory DNA containing CSL-binding sequences (Nam et al., 2003) and recruits additional factors (such as p300 and PCAF) with histone acetylase activity (Wallberg et al., 2002). In the absence of ICN, CSL can recruit repressor complexes to the cis-regulatory region of the CSL-Notch target genes. Therefore, activation of Notch triggers a switch from repression to activation at specific loci.

Notch and Intestinal Cell Fate Determination

The expression and the distribution of Notch receptors and their ligands in the gastrointestinal tract have been described in rodents (Jensen et al., 2000; Schroder and Gossler, 2002; Sander and Powell, 2004). The role of Notch signaling in the intestinal epithelium might be to mediate cell–cell interactions through which a cell that is beginning to differentiate prevents its neighbors from differentiating in the same way at the same time (Jensen et al., 2000; Skipper and Lewis, 2000). This phenomenon is called "lateral inhibition."

Among many other target genes, the expression of the HES (hairy enhancer of split) basic helix-loop-helix (bHLH) transcriptional repressor family is regulated upon Notch activation. In particular, ICN stimulates the expression of Hes1 (Jarriault et al., 1995), which in turn represses the activity of other bHLH transcription factors, including MATH1 (Zheng et al., 2000; Yang et al., 2001).

Both HES and MATH1 bHLH transcription factors have been considered central in gastrointestinal tract cell fate lineage determination, as shown in mice with targeted inactivations of either Hes1 or Math1. In fact, in the duodenum of Hes1$^{-/-}$ mice, there is a striking increase in a number of different enteroendocrine subtypes (CCK/gastrin, serotonin, somatostatin, proglucagon, and GIP-producing cells), as well as goblet cells, concomitant with fewer intestinal enterocytes (Jensen et al., 2000). These data suggest that Notch signaling controls allocation of cells to a secretory fate in the gut. However, because no clustering of secretory cell types was observed in the absence of Hes1 from the intestine, Hes1 function is probably not limited to a lateral inhibitory mechanism between neighboring cells; it may serve as a "prepattern" gene (Jensen et al., 2000).

Hes1 was localized in non-proliferating epithelial cells or confined to the crypts in the duodenum of embryo or adult mice, respectively, suggesting that Hes1 is involved in securing a secondary fate in prospective enterocytes or in controlling a choice between differentiation and proliferation (Jensen et al., 2000).

Math1 is also a key factor for the development of secretory cell lineages in the mouse intestine because its targeted inactivation eliminates the development of goblet, Paneth, and enteroendocrine cells (Yang et al., 2001). Moreover, these mice show no increase in the programmed death of cells at the tip of the villi. Thus, Math1 expression is necessary for cells to make the first secretory lineage-specifying choice. Without Math1, cells remain in the progenitor stem cell pool and can only become enterocytes (189). Math1 is expressed in goblet cells, enteroendocrine cells, and Paneth cells in the gut (Yang et al., 2001) but does not co-localize with all Ki67-expressing cells (Leow et al., 2004), suggesting that Math1 expression is essential only for cells that have just exited the cell cycle.

This intestinal secretory cell fate inhibition by Notch receptors has been confirmed *in vivo*. Thus, in rats, injection for 5 days with gamma-secretase inhibitors that inhibit Notch processing caused a goblet cell metaplasia and an upregulation of secretory cell type markers (somatostatin, mucin, CCK, gastrin) expression (Milano et al., 2004).

Finally, deregulation of the Notch signaling pathway might result in altered equilibria between different gut cell lineages, with cell differentiation, proliferation, and apoptosis being perturbed.

Links between Notch and Colorectal Cancer

As discussed, deregulation of the colonic mucosal homeostatic environment is one of the earliest signs of tumorigenesis. This process normally involves expansion of the proliferative crypt compartment accompanied by a delay or inhibition in cellular differentiation and apoptosis (Augenlicht et al., 1999a). Goblet cells represent one of the major populations of differentiated cells in the colonic mucosa, and loss of goblet cell differentiation and disruption of gland structure of the epithelium have a critical effect on colon cancer development (Velcich et al., 2002). As we have discussed, the loss of the goblet cell phenotype characterizes preneoplastic aberrant crypt foci (Pretlow et al., 1999) and is sufficient in mice with a targeted inactivation of the Muc2 gene to cause intestinal tumor formation (Velcich et al., 2002). If Notch inhibits secretory cell fate determination in the gut, it may, therefore, induce preneoplastic or neoplastic lesions in the intestinal tract. A significant literature has discussed the potential role of Notch as both an oncogene and a tumor suppressor gene (Nickoloff et al., 2003; Radke and Raj, 2003). However, the direct role of Notch receptors in colon tumorigenesis remains unknown.

In colon cancer samples, Notch overexpression has been reported, and downregulation of Hath1, the human orthologue of Math1, has been documented in colon adenocarcinomas and colon cancer cell lines (Leow et al., 2004), confirming that Notch signaling might be upregulated in colon cancer. The same authors show that overexpression of Hath1 in the colon cancer cell line HT29 can inhibit cell proliferation; induce a goblet cell differentiation marker (Muc2); suppress anchorage-independent growth in a soft agar colony formation assay; and more significantly, inhibit growth of HT29 cells as xenografts (Leow et al., 2004). As the loss of proper cell cycle regulation is fundamental to lack of proper cell differentiation and subsequent transformation (discussed earlier), it is important that Hath1 positively regulates p27 but negatively regulates cyclin D1 in HT29 cells. The downregulation of cyclin D1 could contribute to the decrease in cell proliferation, and the upregulation of p27 could potentially facilitate cell cycle exit and, as discussed earlier, differentiation, consequently allowing Hath1 to induce differentiation of colon cancer cells (Leow et al., 2004).

In conclusion, Notch upregulation that activates Hes1 and represses Math1/Hath1 expression might reduce expression of goblet cell differentiation as revealed by the altered expression of the marker, Muc2, which then contributes to the progression of neoplastic growth. However, development of the secretory cell lineage involves complex changes in gene expression (Velcich et al., 2005). Moreover, in mice with a targeted inactivation of Muc2 that develop tumors, as well as in mice with a targeted inactivation of p27 that also develop tumors, ITF, another marker of the lineage and component of mucus, continues to be expressed as it is in the normal mucosa. Therefore, although recognizable goblet cells (e.g., those cells synthesizing, storing and secreting mucin) are decreased in tumor formation, key questions are the extent to which the development of secretory cell lineages are perturbed at the molecular level; what other loci, besides Muc2, are altered, either by altered Notch signaling or by other mechanisms; and which alterations are necessary and sufficient for transformation?

Cdx1 and Cdx2

Among transcription factors that have been identified as important regulators of intestinal epithelial differentiation, the caudal-related genes Cdx1 and Cdx2 stand out as the only intestine-specific transcription factors (James and Kazenwadel, 1991). Cdx proteins are homeobox transcription factors that exert important roles in the determination of the anterior-posterior patterning of the embryo during development, similar to the *Drosophila* caudal (cad) gene from which their names are derived. Loss-of-function and gain-of-function experiments have demonstrated that cdx genes can function as intermediates for signaling molecules like retinoic acids, wint3a, and FGFs by activating the Hox genes involved in patterning (reviewed in Lohnes, 2003).

Cdx1 has been reported to show increased expression along the anterior-posterior axis and to be restricted mainly to the crypt of the small and large intestine in association with the proliferative compartment (Subramanian et al., 1998). However, their role in regulating intestinal epithelial cell proliferation and their involvement in colorectal cancer are not fully elucidated. Regarding the normal mucosa, consistent with Cdx1 localization in the proliferative compartment, *in vivo*, Cdx1 was shown to be a target of β-catenin/Tcf4 activity (Lickert et al., 2000), while *in vitro*, extrinsic expression of Cdx1 in intestinal cell lines induced proliferation (Lorentz et al., 1999; Soubeyran et al., 1999) concomitant with upregulating PCNA (Oh et al., 2002) and repression of p21 (Moucadel et al., 2001). However, overexpression of Cdx1 in confluent cultures of intestinal epithelial cells induced cell differentiation (Lynch et al., 2000, 2003), and Guo et al. (2004) reported that in several colon cancer cell lines, Cdx1 could reduce cell proliferation by blocking β-catenin/Tcf4 transcriptional activity.

The role of Cdx1 in colorectal cancer is likewise controversial: It is not clear whether it acts as an oncogene or tumor suppressor gene. Early reports described a lack of expression of Cdx1 in the majority of human colon carcinoma (Silberg et al., 1997; Vider et al., 1997; Mallo et al., 1998) in line with the hypothesis that Cdx1 could function as a tumor suppressor gene. However, it is noteworthy that cdx1 null mice did not manifest increased risk of tumor development (Subramanian et al., 1998). A 2003 study by Domon-Dell et al., described a more complex pattern of Cdx1 expression during tumor progression. The majority of early polyps analyzed were characterized by elevated levels of Cdx1 expression compared with the adjacent mucosa, in agreement with the fact that Cdx1 was a target of oncogenic pathways most frequently activated in colon cancer (Apc/β-catenin, and mutant Ras). In contrast, the majority of later stage invasive adenocarcinomas were characterized by a reduction of Cdx1 expression, as previously reported. This decreased expression was associated with a high frequency of genomic rearrangement involving the cdx1 locus on chromosome 5q, where Apc is also located, and most commonly linked to allelic imbalance at the Apc locus (Domon-Dell et al., 2003). It is possible that additional mechanisms, such as hypermethylation of its promoter, may also contribute to the decreased level of cdx1 expression in carcinoma (Suh et al., 2002).

In vivo, Cdx2 was shown to be expressed both in the crypt and in the villus compartment in the distal small intestine and proximal colon. Cdx2 has been directly linked to the transcriptional regulation of several genes expressed in enterocytes (Traber and Silberg, 1996) and modulation of cell growth in normal and tumor cells (Suh and Traber, 1996; Mallo et al., 1998). In contrast to cdx1 upregulation, cdx2 is repressed by Wnt signaling and can be induced by Apc (daCosta et al., 1999). This negative regulation is partly mediated by Sox9, a transcription factor of the high mobility group family, the expression of which in the intestinal crypt is dependent on Wnt signaling (Blachet et al., 2004). Therefore, Wnt, through Sox9, maintains cells in a proliferating and undifferentiated state, which has also been termed a *progenitor cell state* (van de Wetering et al., 2002) in the crypt.

An additional level of regulation of Cdx2 is by post-translational modification. Cdx2 can be phosphorylated at ser60, in the activation domain, via the mitogen-activated protein kinase pathway, and in this form has minimal transcriptional activity. *In vivo*, this phosphorylated form of Cdx2 is present mainly in the proliferative compartment of the intestinal epithelium, while the active nonphosphorylated form predominates in the nonproliferating differentiating compartment, coinciding with the expression of genes that are known targets of Cdx2 (Rings et al., 2001). Thus, Cdx2 expression in the crypt is counteracted by a tight regulation of its activity as a transcriptional regulator along the crypt–luminal axis.

To integrate the modulation of gene expression along the spatial-temporal axes, Cdx2 works in conjunction with additional transcription factors, many of which are not intestine restricted. One of the best studied targets of Cdx2 activity is the sucrase isomaltase (SI) gene, which shows an anterior-posterior gradient of expression culminating in the jejunum and absent in the colon. There is also a vertical gradient along the crypt–villus axis characterized by absence of SI expression in the crypt and maximal expression in the lower two thirds of the villi. This pattern of expression is achieved by the contribution of at least two additional transcription factors: HNF1a (hepatocyte nuclear factor) and GATA4 (see later) that cooperate with Cdx2 to impart the spatial-temporal regulation of SI. In fact, Cdx2 expression is not temporally or spatially regulated, but that of HNF1a and GATA4 are and closely reflect the expression of the SI gene (Boudreau et al., 2002).

As mentioned earlier, extrinsic expression of Cdx2 decreases cell proliferation and induces differentiation. Therefore, one question is whether Cdx2 can be considered an integrator of cell proliferation and differentiation. One of the targets of Cdx2 is the p21/Cip1 gene, which has been described as a molecular switch defining the boundary between the proliferative and differentiated compartments along the vertical axes (discussed earlier). In addition, Cdx2 has been shown to regulate the expression of Kruppel-like factor 4 (KLF4), a Zn-finger protein specifically expressed in non-proliferating cells of intestinal and skin cells (Dang et al., 2001). Interestingly, KLF4 has been shown to affect goblet cell maturation without affecting the maturation of other cell lineages (Katz et al., 2002). Goblet cells constitute the major secretory cell lineage of the intestinal mucosa. They synthesize and secrete mucin, which in the intestine is predominantly composed of Muc2. Whether KLF4 directly regulates the Muc2 gene is not known. However, Muc2 was shown to be directly regulated by Cdx2 (Yamamoto et al., 2003), which most likely acts in concert with other members of the Zn^{2+} finger transcription factors, such as Sp1/Sp3 (Aslam et al., 2001), to dictate intestinal specific regulation.

In summary, Cdx2 seems to be a component of the regulatory circuit whose orchestration is required to control epithelial cell proliferation and differentiation. Given this role in cell proliferation and differentiation, it is not surprising that Cdx2 has been shown to have a role in tumorigenesis. $Cdx2^{+/-}$ mice develop either hamartomas or polyps containing heterotopic gastric and small intestinal tissue consistent with the described role in cell proliferation, differentiation, and posterior patterning (Chawengsaksophak et al., 1997; Beck et al., 1999; Tamai, 1999). $Cdx2^{+/-}$ mice were found to be more sensitive to AOM-induced carcinogenesis, suggesting that reduced expression facilitates tumor progression (Bonhomme et al., 2003). Furthermore, Cdx2 becomes highly expressed in intestinal metaplasia of the stomach, one of the most common precursor conditions associated with gastric carcinoma (reviewed in Yuasa, 2003). Cdx2 ectopic expression in the stomach induces intestinal metaplasia in transgenic mice, demonstrating a direct role of cdx2 in the process (Silberg et al., 2002). Expression of Cdx2 is decreased in colorectal cancer compared with normal adjacent mucosa (Ee et al., 1995; Mallo et al., 1997; Silberg et al., 2000; Suh et al., 2002), and the reduction is inversely correlated with the level of differentiation of the tumors (Hinoi et al., 2001). Somatic mutations of cdx2 are infrequent and associated with mismatch repair deficient tumors (Wicking et al., 1998; Woodford-Richens et al., 2001). Further analysis identified lack of expression with absence or severely reduced levels of cdx2 transcripts (Hinoi et al., 2003), suggesting a transcriptional repression of the gene. Upon investigation of the possible mechanisms, it was shown that repression of cdx2 transcription was not due to epigenetic mechanisms like hypermethylation or deacetylation of histones associated with key regulatory elements (Hinoi et al., 2003). Thus, it was suggested that specific repressors may mediate the silencing of cdx2 in tumors, similar to the repression of E-cadherin by SNAIL in breast tumors (Fujita et al., 2003). Interestingly, starting from the observation that in PTEN$^{+/-}$ mice, there was a reduction of Cdx2, Kim et al. (2002) reported that Cdx2 transcriptional regulation may be mediated by the PTEN and the PI3K pathway through a modulation of the NF-κB transcription factor (Kim et al., 2002). Reduction of PTEN would cause a shift from p50 homodimers, which activate cdx2 transcription, to p50/p65 heterodimers that act as repressor, as previously discussed.

These are unusual findings given the current view that p50 is generally a repressor and p65 an activator, and they imply that PTEN/PI3K/AKT may play a role in regulating intestinal cell maturation. A link between Cdx2 and the PI3K/AKT pathway was also revealed by Aoki et al. (2003), which showed the existence of a close relationship between Cdx2 and mTor, a downstream target of PI3K/AKT pathway. Introduction of cdx2 mutation into the Apc$^{\Delta716}$ mouse model caused a shift in tumor development from the small intestine to the colon, where most of human tumors occur. Polyps were characterized by higher frequency of LOH at the Apc locus and chromosomal instability due to activation of the mTor pathway and translational deregulation of cell cycle regulatory proteins (Aoki et al., 2003).

Gata Transcription Factors

Gata factors are Zn-finger transcription factors that can be divided into two classes depending on the pattern of expression and structural characteristics. Gata-4, Gata-5, and Gata-6 are expressed in meso- and endodermal-derived tissues (Molkentin et al., 2000). Their role in regulating intestinal gene expression has been phylogenetically maintained from *C. elegans* to mammals (Britton et al., 1998). In the adult, Gata-4 and Gata-5 are expressed in the villi and not in the crypts of the intestine, while Gata-6 seems to be expressed preferentially in the crypt area of the small intestine, suggesting that Gata-4 and Gata-5 are associated with differentiation and Gata-6 is linked to proliferation (Gao et al., 1998). No expression is detected in the colon.

The different pattern of expression of the Gata factors along the anterior-posterior axis was shown to play a role in the regulation of intestinal-specific genes. As mentioned previously, Gata-4 cooperates with Cdx2 and HNF1 to regulate sucrase-isomaltose (SI) expression (Boudreau et al., 2002). Similar mechanisms have been described to regulate other intestine-specific genes such as FABPi, claudin, lactase-phlorizin hydrolase, and mMuc2 (Gao et al., 1998; Yamamoto et al., 2003; Escaffit et al., 2004; van der Sluis et al., 2004; van Wering et al., 2004). Thus, as described earlier, intestine-specific gene expression is regulated by the interactions of tissue-restricted transcription factors that are coexpressed in the intestine with other nonintestinal-specific factors, which, however, may have a distinct spatial pattern of expression and in the end determine the expression of the target genes.

Modulation of GATA activity in cancer has not been fully investigated. However, it has been reported that in HT29 cells, the SCFA butyrate increased expression of Gata-4 and Gata-5, and in parallel decreased Gata-6 levels (Gao et al., 1998). In agreement, Gata-4 and Gata-5 were shown to be epigenetically silenced in several colon and gastric tumors (Akiyama et al., 2003).

AP-1

As discussed earlier, one class of Ras effectors is represented by the RAF/MAP/ERK kinases. The importance of Ras/Raf signaling in colon cancer is underlined by the fact that 10–15% of tumors that do not have activated K-Ras have activated RAF (BRAF) (Davies et al., 2002; Yuen et al., 2002) and that its inhibition blocks tumor growth in mice (Sebot-Leopold et al., 1999; Sebot-Leopold and Herrera, 2004). The activator protein-1 (AP-1) family of transcription factors is a secondary transcription target of activated ERK. The AP-1 family consists of homodimers or heterodimers of members of the Fos, Jun, activating transcription factor (ATF), and musculoaponeurotic fibrosarcoma (MAF) protein families. Dimer formation occurs through the interaction of the leucin-zipper domain, and the DNA-binding site specificity is dictated by the subunit composition. Binding of AP-1 is rapidly induced in response to several stimuli implicated in cell proliferation, differentiation, and tumorigenesis. The specificity of the responses is dictated by the composition of the dimers, by the cell type, and by interactions with other factors. In general, cFos, FosB, and cJun have strong transforming activities *in vitro* and can cooperate with Ras. These members are characterized by an efficient transactivation domain. Other members, like FRA1 and 2, that have weak transactivation domains either cannot transform efficiently or completely lack transforming activity (JunD and JunB). Further, some members of the Jun family (JunB and JunD) can work as tumor suppressor genes (reviewed in Eferl and Wagner, 2003).

Although there are a large number of reports regarding the role of different members of AP-1 in tumorigenesis, relatively little is known of the role of AP-1 in intestinal tumorigenesis, and whether AP-1 cooperates with activated K-Ras in tumor development. In colorectal cancer cell lines with mutant K-Ras, the predominant AP-1 form induced via the MAPK/ERK pathway is composed of cJun and Fra1 dimers that, in the presence of high level of ERK activity, function to provide survival signals to tumor cells (Vial and Marshall, 2003).

AP-1 has been shown to induce COX2 transcription in intestinal cells in response to gastrin. Transcriptional induction of cyclooxygenase 2 (COX2) occurs through stimulation of AP-1 expression and binding to the COX2 promoter upon Ca^{2+} release, and activation of the MAP kinase pathway (Guo et al., 2001, 2002). This, in addition to alteration of COX2 mRNA stability (Sheng et al., 2001), could be an important mechanism of COX2 deregulation in colon cancer, which is known to play a pivotal role in tumorigenesis (Gupta et al., 2001). In fact, *in vivo*, aberrant expression of gastrin-releasing peptide (GRP) and its receptor GRP receptor (GRP-R) has been identified in premalignant adenomatous polyps and colorectal cancers (Preston et al., 1996; Carroll et al., 1999).

The effects of increased levels of COX2 can be further amplified in a feedback loop involving AP1. Prostaglandin E_2 (PGE_2), a product of COX2 enzymatic activity, was shown to activate EGFR *in vitro* and *in vivo* to cause an increase in Fos levels and the induction of mitogenic signals (Pai et al., 2002).

Finally, AP-1 could also be involved in tumor progression, as it becomes activated in response to hypoxia, which promotes angiogenesis; further, many of the genes that are implicated in the development of metastasis, such as uPAR matrylisin 1 and 3, can be positively regulated by AP-1 (Eferl and Wagner, 2003).

Although AP-1 activity can be regulated at different levels (i.e., transcriptionally, post-transcriptionally, and by dimer composition), it has been reported that dietary components can also modulate AP-1 activity. Curcumin, a natural product of tumeric that is in clinical trials as a chemopreventive agent, was shown to inhibit AP-1 binding and NF-κB activation (Hanazawa et al., 1993).

Peroxisome Proliferator-Activated Receptors (PPARs)

PPARα, PPARβ/δ (henceforth referred to as PPARδ), and PPARγ are ligand-dependent transcription factors belonging to the nuclear-hormone receptor family. PPARs function as heterodimers, RXR being their obligatory partner. Upon activation by fatty acids and their derivatives, PPARs modulate the expression of genes involved in glucose and lipid metabolism. In fact, thiazolidinediones, agonists of PPARγ, are used to control type II diabetes.

These receptors are either expressed ubiquitously or restricted to a subset of tissues (reviewed in Michalik et al., 2004). PPARγ and PPARδ are expressed in the intestinal tract, and while an antiproliferative role and inducer of differentiation has been associated with activation of PPARγ, less clear is the role of PPARδ in the normal intestine, although in skin keratinocytes this receptor has been shown to promote keratinocyte survival.

The role of PPARγ and PPARδ in colorectal tumorigenesis is controversial (Gupta and Dubois, 2002). *In vitro*, PPARγ agonists were shown to be antiproliferative and promote cell differentiation. Xenotransplants of cell lines derived from human tumors showed decreased growth upon treatment with PPARγ ligands (Sarraf et al., 1998). Approximately 10% of primary tumors showed mutational inactivation of PPARγ (Sarraf et al., 1999). These data imply that PPARγ has antitumorigenic activity. Mechanistically, these effects could be linked to the ability of PPARγ to downregulate genes, such as cyclin D1, involved in cell proliferation (Wang et al., 2001), as well as induction of genes involved in differentiation or with tumor-suppressive function (keratin 20 and PTEN) (Gupta et al., 2001; Patel et al., 2001). It was, therefore, surprising that when the agonist was tested in the ApcMin mouse, it promoted, rather than repressed, tumor development (Lefebvre et al., 1998; Saez et al., 1998). Along these lines, it was proposed that the link between a high-fat diet and increased risk of tumor development is due to the activation of PPARγ by fat (Wasan et al., 1997).

A partial reconciliation of these controversial results was provided by Girnun et al. (2002), who showed that the outcome of PPARγ activity is a function of the genetic status of the colon. In the AOM model, $PPAR\gamma^{+/-}$ mice (the null mouse is not viable) developed early and more tumors than the wild-type (wt) animals. Molecularly, reduced PPARγ expression resulted in increased β-catenin levels in the flat mucosa. However, double heterozygous $PPAR\gamma^{+/-}/Apc^{1638}$ mice displayed the same tumor phenotype as the Apc^{1638} mouse (Girnun et al., 2002). These results suggest that in very early stages, PPARγ agonists may be chemopreventive, while activation of PPARγ after Apc mutation may have no effect or even a deleterious effect (Lefebvre et al., 1998; Saez et al., 1998).

The role of PPARδ in cancer has been primarily studied in colon cancer. Originally it was shown that PPARδ was a target of the deregulated Apc–β-catenin pathway (Allgayer et al., 1999; He et al., 1999; Shao et al., 2002) as well as mutant K-Ras (He et al., 1999; Shao et al., 2002), and that it was expressed at high levels in tumors. In agreement with a tumor-promoting activity, xenotransplants of a colon carcinoma cell line null for PPARδ were less tumorigenic than the wild-type counterpart (Park et al., 2001). It has been proposed that PPARδ transcriptional activity is induced indirectly by PGE_2, a metabolite of the COX2 pathway, via PI3K/AKT activity (Gupta et al., 2004). However, these data are challenged by other results showing that deletion of PPARδ was dispensable for tumor formation in the ApcMin mouse model (Barak et al., 2002), and that it even increased the number of tumors in the colon of compound knockout mice (Harman et al., 2004). The latter work further suggests that PPARδ may have a specific protective role in the colon. However, activation of PPARδ with a specific agonist showed increased tumorigenicity in the small intestine of ApcMin+/− mice (Gupta et al., 2004). Even more compelling are data showing that in ApcMin mice treated with PGE_2, a possible activator of PPARδ, there was a dramatic increase in colonic polyp formation and such an effect was abolished in ApcMin mice homozygous for PPARδ deletion (Wang et al., 2004). Although these data do not form a clear picture of the possible role of PPARδ in colon tumorigenesis, the evidence that it can promote tumorigenesis is sufficient to warrant caution when considering use of PPARδ agonists in the treatment of patients with hyperlipidemic states.

EPIGENETIC MECHANISMS OF ALTERED GENE EXPRESSION

As alluded to for several of the pathways discussed, epigenetic mechanisms involving both *cis*- and *trans*-acting regulatory factors that control transcription of specific gene loci are important in cell maturation and transformation, and intestinal cells are no exception. Two mechanisms stand out as having drawn particular interest: histone and other nuclear protein acetylation, and DNA methylation. Further, histones can also undergo other modifications, including methylation and to a lesser extent phosphorylation, ubiquitination, sumoylation, and ribosylation of key amino acid residues within either the N-terminal tail or the globular core, which can have profound effects on gene transcription by regulating access of transcription factors to DNA. Histone acetylation is typically associated with increased transcription, whereas depending on the specific residue modified, histone methylation can either promote or inhibit transcription (Peterson and Laniel, 2004). These and other observations have led to the proposal for the existence of a "histone code" in which specific combinations of histone modifications lead to the recruitment of effector molecules (Strahl and Allis, 2000).

Histone Acetylation

With regards to histone acetylation, net acetylation is determined by the interaction of histone acetyltransferases (HATs) and histone deacetylases (HDACs), which generally act as transcriptional co-activators and co-repressors, respectively. HATS and HDACs can also modulate acetylation of a number of nonhistone proteins, including transcription factors such as p53 (Gu and Roeder, 1997), TFIIEβ and TFIIF (Imhof et al., 1997), Gata-1 (Boyes et al., 1998), Tcf (Waltzer and Bienz, 1998), HMG-1 (Munshi et al., 1998), c-*myb* (Tomita et al., 2000), and E2F1 (Martinez-Balbas et al., 2000), which can regulate transcription by altering their DNA binding affinity. Many of these have already been discussed for their roles in normal and abnormal cell maturation. In conjunction, therefore, HDACs and HATs comprise a major epigenetic mechanism by which cells can be reprogrammed by extrinsic or intrinsic signals.

Eighteen mammalian HDACs have been identified and fall into three classes based on their homology to a prototypical HDAC found in yeast. Class I HDACs (HDACs 1, 2, 3, and 8) show homology to yeast Rpd3; class II HDACs (HDACs 4, 5, 6, 7, 9, and 10) have high homology to Had-1 (Fischle et al., 2001); and class III HDACs (SIRT1 through SIRT7) are homologous to yeast Sir2 (Marks et al., 2001). HDAC11 has been identified (Gao et al., 2002) but has not yet been assigned to a specific class. Class I and II HDACs share some homology, particularly at the catalytic deacetylase domain, but class I HDACs are smaller (40–70 kDa) compared with class II (120–150 kDa) (Bertos et al., 2001) and class I (with the exception of HDAC3) are predominantly nuclear in localization, whereas class II HDACs shuttle between the nucleus and the cytoplasm under regulation by 14-3-3 proteins, as a major mechanism of regulation of their activity (Grozinger and Schrieber, 2000). Class III shares little homology with classes I and II.

The different HDAC family members are recruited to particular loci by different sequence-specific transcription factors, where they then alter chromatin conformation and repress transcription. For example, HDAC1 and HDAC2 interact with the Rb family of pocket proteins and E2Fs to repress E2F target gene expression (Rayman et al., 2002), and HDAC4 interacts with MEF2 to repress muscle-specific genes (Miska et al., 1999). In the latter case, muscle cell differentiation is dependent on 14-3-3 protein-mediated shuttling of HDAC4 out of the nucleus and into the cytoplasm (McKinsey et al., 2000; Miska et al., 2001).

Based on studies in yeast demonstrating that different HDACs regulate distinct cellular processes (i.e., cell cycle progression and carbohydrate utilization) (Bernstein et al., 2000; Robyr et al., 2002), it is likely that different HDACs regulate distinct but overlapping functions in mammalian cells. Butyrate, already discussed as a physiological regulator of colon cell maturation, is a potent inhibitor of HDAC activity (Sealy and Chalkley, 1978; Breneman et al., 1996; Cuisset et al., 1998). Importantly, many, but not all, of butyrate's effects on induction of cell maturation (i.e., cell cycle arrest and apoptosis) are mimicked by trichostatin A (TSA) and other HDAC inhibitors (Archer et al., 1997; Bordonaro et al., 1999; Mariadason et al., 2000b; Wu et al., 2001), suggesting that inhibition of HDAC activity is essential to these components of the butyrate response. Inhibition of HDAC activity by butyrate appears to be by direct interaction of the SCFA with the protein (Emiliani et al., 1998; Wang et al., 1999), although this has not been demonstrated. This inhibition of HDAC activity by SCFAs is structure dependent, with the straight-chain four-carbon structure of butyrate being the most efficient inhibitor (McBain et al., 1997; Mariadason et al., 2001). Consistent with this activity of butyrate, we have shown that butyrate treatment of colon cells results in altered expression of a large number of genes, and the differences in kinetics of altered histone acetylation by butyrate and TSA allowed us to identify a subset of these sequences that were likely regulated in expression by altered levels of histone acetylation (Mariadason et al., 2000b).

Whether cell cycle progression, differentiation, and apoptosis are regulated by similar or distinct HDAC family members is not known. Butyrate and TSA inhibit the activity of most class I and II HDACs, although HDAC6 and HDAC10 are relatively less sensitive to butyrate (Guardiola and Yao, 2002). The effect of butyrate on class III HDACs is unknown, but all are resistant to TSA (Marks et al., 2001), suggesting that at least class III HDACs likely do not play an important role. In Caco-2 cell differentiation along the absorptive cell lineage, we have observed a decrease in HDAC activity concomitant with downregulation of HDAC2 and HDAC4, but not HDAC1, HDAC5, and HDAC8 (Mariadason, unpublished observation).

The link between inhibition of HDAC activity and induction of colon cell maturation *in vitro* suggests that HDACs have a physiological role in these processes. Indeed, we have demonstrated that expression of HDAC2 and HDAC3 and to a lesser extent HDAC1 decreases as cells migrate upwards along the crypt–villus axis in mouse small intestine (Mariadason and Wilson, unpublished observation). Further emphasizing the importance of these molecules in colon cell maturation and transformation, we and others have observed an upregulation of class I HDACs, HDAC1, HDAC2, and HDAC3 in colon cancers (Zhu et al., 2004; Wilson et al., manuscript in preparation).

One mechanism by which these enzymes mediate their effects is through repression of expression of the CDKi, p21WAF1, already discussed as a fundamental element in colonic cell maturation and transformation. Upregulation of p21WAF1 is critical for the coordination of the complete butyrate response, as demonstrated by the failure of p21-deficient cells to undergo cell cycle arrest following butyrate treatment, and the link of the early induction of p21 to the mitochondrial membrane potential (see later). The overexpression of HDAC1 (Choi and Mason, 2000) or HDAC3 or HDAC4 (Mariadason, unpublished observation) abrogates the response of the p21 promoter to butyrate, indicating that at least these three HDACs are important for butyrate induction of p21, and hyperacetylation of histones within the p21 promoter has been reported (Richon et al., 2000).

The precise mechanism, however, by which HDAC inhibitors (HDACi) induce growth inhibition and apoptosis in tumor cells is likely to be complex. For example, HDACi repress expression of key growth-inducing genes including c-*myc* and cyclin D1, while inducing expression of others, including INK4D and GADD45. HDACi are also potent inducers of apoptosis and, depending on the cell type, can mediate this effect through either the intrinsic pathway (mitochondrial) or death receptor pathway (TRAIL and Fas signaling) (Insinga et al., 2005; Nebbioso et al., 2005). HDACi have also been shown to upregulate several proapoptotic genes, including Bax (Bandyopadhyay et al., 2004) and Apaf1, and to induce cleavage of Bid while repressing the expression of the antiapoptotic gene Bcl-2 (Johnstone, 2002).

Finally, as a result of work such as that cited, several HDACi, including phenylbutyrate, valproic acid, TSA, SAHA, pyroxamide, depsipeptide, MS-275, and Cl-994, are in phase I and II clinical trials as either single agents or in combination with existing agents for treatment of solid tumors and hematological malignancies, and promising data have been reported (Marks et al., 2001).

DNA Methylation

CpG islands are stretches of DNA that are usually about 1 kb long that are rich in CpG and GpC dinucleotides (Bird, 1986). The cytosine residues of such sequences can be methylated at the 5′ position by methylases, and such groups removed by demethylases. The CpG sites in these gene-associated regions are rarely methylated in normal cells with the exception of CpG islands of genes on the inactivated X chromosome and CpG islands associated with imprinted genes (Barlow, 1995). Although it was reported that tumors in general exhibit hypomethylation of loci (Feinberg and Vogelstein, 1983; Feinberg et al., 1988), abnormal hypermethylation of CpG islands occurs during aging and during tumor development (Wilson and Jones, 1983; Issa et al., 1996; Baylin et al., 1998; Issa, 2004). Hypermethylation of genes early in tumor formation appears to involve loci in which promoter hypermethylation normally appears as a function of aging. In the colon, the genes with the highest incidence of promoter hypermethylation in tumors fall into this category, and the age-related curves for the increase in hypermethylation and risk for colon cancer are remarkably similar (Toyota et al., 1999; Toyota and Issa, 1999). The mechanism by which hypermethylation of selected CpG islands occurs in tumor cells undergoing an overall decrease in level of cytosine methylation remains to be resolved. Some of the hypermethylated genes appear to be "bystanders" that are not expressed in either the normal tissue or the tumor arising from it but are methylated in the tumor (Silverman et al., 1989). Similarly, some CpG island methylation has no effect on gene activity because it occurs in islands that are not associated with the regulatory regions of genes (Jones, 1999; Nguyen et al., 2001).

There is evidence supporting links of both hypomethylation and hypermethylation of DNA to tumor formation. For example, deficiency of folate, a nutrient that contributes to the methyl donor pool, causes hypomethylation and increased tumor risk in both rodents and humans (Choi and Mason, 2000; Mason and Choi, 2000; Song et al., 2000;

Choi et al., 2002). In contrast, in mice that inherit a mutant Apc allele that causes tumor formation, pharmacological or genetic induction of hypomethylation decreases tumor formation (Laird et al., 1995). Resolution of such apparently conflicting data may come from application of new methods that permit interrogation of CpG methylation status at hundreds to thousands of loci throughout the genome, especially when linked to levels of expression of those loci under different conditions (Costello et al., 2000; Yan et al., 2002).

Over the past 10 years, it has been well documented that loss of tumor suppressor gene function can occur both through mutation and through gene silencing linked to methylation of CpG island promoters (Reviewed in Baylin et al., 1998). An examination of > 600 primary tumor samples from 15 tumor types showed that CpG island promoters of three or more genes from a panel of 12 known tumor suppressor genes were hypermethylated in 5–10% of the samples. At least one CpG island was methylated in ≥80% of samples for each tumor type (Esteller et al., 2001). Using methods that allow genome-wide screening of CpG islands, it has been estimated that, on average, ~1% of CpG island DNA from tumor tissues is abnormally methylated (Costello et al., 2000; Yan et al., 2001, 2002). These studies also provide evidence for tumor-specific patterns of CpG island methylation, with the percentage of CpG island methylation in individual tumors varying from 0–10% of the ~45,000 CpG islands in the human genome (Costello et al., 2000).

There has been interest in studies of the role of methylation at specific loci linked to colon cell maturation and neoplasia. For example, methylation of genes involved in DNA mismatch repair has been demonstrated to result in inactivation and subsequent elevation of tumor formation (Herman et al., 1998). Further, although methylation of the p21 locus at canonical CpG islands is not altered in colon tumors (Kondo and Issa, 2004), we have found that methylation of a CpG "cluster" upstream of the mouse p21 locus likely plays a role in regulation of the gene, and that methylation of cytosine residues in this cluster is sufficient to inhibit induction of the p21 gene by sulindac and to abrogate the tumor-inhibiting effect of this drug (Yang et al., 2001, 2005). There is also evidence of silencing of the p53 tumor suppressor gene as a result of methylation of CpG sites in its "non-CpG island" promoter and of hypermethylation of these sites in human hepatomas (Pogribny et al., 2000, 2002).

MITOCHONDRIA: A MECHANISM OF REGULATION AND INTEGRATION

Establishment and maintenance of the hierarchy of organization that defines living organisms is the antithesis of the entropic drive toward disorganization and is, therefore, strictly dependent on the ability of the organism to efficiently accumulate and manage energy. It is, therefore, no surprise that nutrients are essential components in development, in tissue homeostasis, and in the aberrations that lead to tumor formation. In higher eukaryotes, the physical sites of the most efficient capture and transfer of energy are mitochondria and chloroplasts. These may be considered, therefore, the ultimate achievement of evolution and are at the core of the existence of life as we know it. It is interesting to consider that the mitochondria have also been recruited by evolutionary forces to control cell death (i.e., apoptosis) as well, making them the fundamental arbiters of life and death of the cell and, ultimately, the survival of multicellular organisms. Moreover, discoveries have linked pathways of intermediate metabolism involved in energy capture as important components and regulators of the mitochondrial linked events of cell death and survival (Heerdt et al., 1994, 1996, 2003; Augenlicht and Heerdt, 2001; Danial et al., 2003). This may explain why nutritional factors and their metabolism play major roles in tissue homeostasis and can have major positive and negative impacts on the developmental biology of the organism and on tumor development.

As is well known, differences in metabolism between tumor and normal cells identified > 5 decades ago suggested a role for mitochondria in the tumorigenic process (Warburg, 1956a,b). Consistent with such a role, most tumors exhibit decreased mitochondrial gene expression (Faure Vigny, 1996), mutations and deletions in the mitochondrial genome, alterations in mitochondrial enzymatic activity, and elevations in the mitochondrial membrane potential ($\Delta\psi m$) (Sun et al., 1981; Summerhayes et al., 1982; Davis et al., 1985; Chen, 1988; Wong and Chen, 1988; Modica-Napolitano et al., 1989; Chen and Rivers, 1990). Moreover, by demonstrating depressed expression of mitochondrial genes in the normal appearing colonic mucosa from two high-risk populations (Augenlicht et al., 1987; Heerdt and Augenlicht, 1990), we identified alterations in mitochondrial function as an early event in the transformation of colonic epithelial cells.

As will be reviewed, over the past 15 years, we have dissected how mitochondrial function, particularly the maintenance of the mitochondrial membrane potential, is linked to the role of the short-chain fatty acid butyrate as a physiological regulator of cell maturation for the colonic mucosa. This led to the postulate that through interaction of signaling molecules with the mitochondrial membrane, the mitochondria plays a fundamental role as an integrator of signals for proliferation and apoptosis, determining which of these pathways colonic cells ultimately take (Augenlicht and Heerdt, 2001). We also reported that isogenic cells exhibit different growth properties and response to butyrate based on stable differences in their intrinsic $\Delta\psi m$, and that indeed, this alters the nature, but not the extent, of Bax interaction with the mitochondrial membrane (Heerdt et al., 2003). Further, in unpublished work, we have now found that there is a distribution of mitochondrial membrane potential among colonic tumor cells cloned from a tumor cell line. For each cloned subline, there is a characteristic $\Delta\psi m$ that is stable over many generations, with higher $\Delta\psi m$ linked to properties that favor a metastatic phenotype (Heerdt, unpublished observations). Moreover, as reviewed later, this may be linked to the phospholipid composition of the mitochondrial membrane, therefore establishing a mechanism by which altered dietary intake of polyunsaturated long-chain fatty acids (PUFAs), a determinant of membrane composition and hence function, directly influences tumor development and progression. Our overall hypothesis, therefore, is that a common element in these multiple effects of dietary PUFAs is the ability of n-3 and n-6 PUFAs to determine the function and composition of cellular membranes (Larsson et al., 2004), including those of the mitochondria (Malis et al., 1990; Watkins et al., 1998; Kontogiannea et al., 2000; Chapkin et al., 2002; Hong et al., 2002; Siddiqui et al., 2004; Wu et al., 2004). This, in turn, alters the extent and/or nature of the interaction of the mitochondrial membrane with factors that regulate growth and apoptosis, therefore determining the response of the cell to butyrate and other modulators of colonic cell maturation.

SCFAs can affect mitochondrial activity and have an impact on the probability of colonic tumor formation and progression. The four-carbon atom, unbranched short-chain fatty acid (SCFA) butyric acid is a natural product found in many fruits, vegetables, and milk fat and is generated during the fermentation of fiber by intestinal bacteria. These dietary sources establish butyric acid in the colonic contents at levels of > 20 mM, with total SCFA content of > 200 mM (Roediger, 1980; Cummings, 1983). It has been demonstrated that these SCFAs play a critical role in colonic epithelial cell maturation pathways *in vivo* (Glotzer et al., 1981; Roediger, 1988; Harig et al., 1989; Augenlicht et al., 1999a). This is likely through their role as the principal energy source of colonic epithelial cells (Roediger, 1980, 1982), where they enter the mitochondria, perhaps through porin (Schulz, 1985), and undergo β-oxidation.

Despite the mitochondrial abnormalities that characterize colonic carcinoma cells, we have shown that sodium butyrate significantly increases mitochondrial gene expression and mitochondrial enzymatic activity without altering expression of nuclear genes encoding proteins destined for mitochondrial import. Furthermore, inefficiently oxidized derivatives of butyrate are ineffective in modulating mitochondrial function, again suggesting that the effects of butyrate are linked to its β-oxidation (Heerdt and Augenlicht, 1990, 1991). In mice, the homozygous deletion of the gene for short-chain acyl dehydrogenase, an initial enzyme of mitochondrial SCFA oxidation, abrogates apoptosis in the colonic mucosa, which is further evidence for the necessity of β-oxidation of butyrate in triggering an apoptotic pathway in the mucosa (Augenlicht et al., 1999a).

A critical component in many apoptotic pathways is disruption of the $\Delta\psi m$ and the consequent release of factors from the mitochondria (Hennet et al., 1993, 1998, 2000; Decaudin et al., 1997; Ferri and Kroemer, 2001). We have shown that an intact $\Delta\psi m$ is required not only for butyrate-induced apoptosis but also for its initiation of growth arrest of colonic epithelial cells (Heerdt et al., 1994, 1996, 1997, 1998, 2000). Moreover, there is a link between the intrinsic level of the $\Delta\psi m$ of a cell and the extent to which butyrate induces cell cycle arrest and apoptosis (Heerdt et al., 2003), making it likely that the $\Delta\psi m$ plays a critical role in integrating proliferation and apoptotic pathways (Heerdt et al., 1997, 1998) and as a consequence impacting the probability of colonic tumor formation and progression (Augenlicht and Heerdt, 2001). As will be reviewed later, there is ample evidence suggesting that another major determinant of the $\Delta\psi m$ is dietary intake of PUFAs, thereby linking diet directly to this biochemical function at the heart of probability of tumor development.

Dietary Polyunsaturated Fatty Acids, Mitochondrial Function, and the Modulation of Butyrate Induction of Cell Maturation

Extensive epidemiological evidence has demonstrated an inverse relationship between the risk of colon tumorigenesis and fish consumption, particularly fatty cold-water fish, which are rich in the n-3 PUFAs eicosapentaenoic acid (EPA; C20: 5n-3), and docosahexaenoic acid (DHA; D22: 6n-3) (Fernandez et al., 1999; Larsson et al., 2004). Clinical studies have shown that dietary n-3 PUFAs decrease intestinal proliferation in healthy subjects (Bartram et al., 1993) and in those at risk for colon cancer (Anti et al., 1992, 1994) and inhibit the promotion and progression of colonic carcinogenesis in model systems (Paulsen et al., 1997; Chang et al., 1998).

n-3 fatty acid–mediated protection against colonic tumorigenesis has been linked to inhibition of proliferation (Ramos and Colquhoun, 2003), promotion of differentiation (Chang et al., 1997), decreased expression of Bcl-2 (Chang et al., 1997; Hong et al., 2003), increased production of ROS, and induction of apoptosis (Hong et al., 2002). In contrast, high consumption of dietary n-6 PUFAs, such as linoleic acid (LA; C18: 2n-6), found in corn, safflower, and sunflower seed oils, is linked to inhibition of apoptosis and the promotion and progression of colonic tumors (Nelson et al., 1988; Iigo et al., 1997; Meterissian et al., 2000; Rao et al., 2001).

n-3, but not n-6, PUFAs enhance the effects of butyrate on colonic epithelial cells. The combination of n-3 fatty acids and dietary fiber significantly decreased the formation of aberrant crypt foci induced in rats by AOM (Coleman et al., 2002). *In vitro*, butyrate-mediated production of ROS, lipid peroxidation, Δψm dissipation, cytochrome *c* release, caspase-3 and caspase-9 activation, PARP cleavage, and apoptosis were enhanced by n-3 PUFAs, while expression of antiapoptotic Mcl-1 protein was decreased (Hong et al., 2002; Hofmanova et al., 2004; Sanders et al., 2004). This link of the effects of butyrate to n-3 fatty acids may be a key mechanism by which dietary PUFAs modulate tumor formation.

Approximately 80% of the lipids in mammalian mitochondrial membranes are phospholipids, with phosphatidylcholine (PC), phosphatidylethanolamine (PE), and diphosphatidylglycerol (cardiolipin [CL]) accounting for ~45%, 35%, and 20%, respectively, of total mitochondrial phospholipids. However, CL is unique in that it is exclusively found in the mitochondria, where its synthesis is completed in the inner mitochondrial membrane (Gennis, 1989).

As a specific lipid component of the mitochondrial inner membrane, CL is integrated into the quaternary structure and is essential for the activity of many of the mitochondrial enzyme complexes involved in electron transport (Fry and Green, 1980, 1981; Hoch, 1992; Jiang et al., 2000; Haines and Dencher, 2002). It is also involved in the retention of cytochrome *c* in the intermembranous space and its release during apoptosis (Ott et al., 2002; Poot et al., 2002; Hardy et al., 2003), the function of the adenine nucleotide translocase (Schlame et al., 1991; Ostrander et al., 2001), and the mitochondrial import and activation of nuclear-encoded peptides (Hoch, 1992).

Although the fatty acyl groups of CL in mammalian tissues are almost exclusively 18-carbon fatty acids, the majority of which are LA (18:2n-6) (Schlame et al., 1993), CL has the most diet-responsive and changeable fatty acid composition among phospholipids (Watkins et al., 1998). There is extensive evidence that the fatty acyl chain composition and saturation index of CL can be modified both *in vitro* and *in vivo* by n-3 and n-6 fatty acids (Robblee and Clandinin, 1984; Malis et al., 1990; Groden et al., 1991; Yamaoka-Koseki et al., 1991; Berger et al., 1992; Watkins et al., 1998; Gaposchkin et al., 2000; Chapkin et al., 2002; Hong et al., 2002; Ramos and Colquhoun, 2003; Valianpour et al., 2003). Compared with n-6 fatty acids, n-3 fatty acids decrease the amount of LA and increase the quantity of EPA and DHA that are incorporated into colonic epithelial cell mitochondrial phospholipids (Malis et al., 1990; Chapkin et al., 2002; Hong et al., 2002). n-3 fatty acids also increase mitochondrial phospholipid unsaturation (Watkins et al., 1998; Hong et al., 2002), which is associated with decreased Δψm, elevated production of ROS, and increased cytochrome *c* release (Watkins et al., 1998; Chapkin et al., 2002; Piccotti et al., 2004). Moreover, n-3 fatty acids inhibit migration and decrease metastasis of colonic carcinoma cells (Iigo et al., 1997; Iwamoto et al., 1998; Gaposchkin et al., 2000; Kontogiannea et al., 2000; Ramos and Colquhoun, 2003) while n-6 PUFAs are linked to increased metastatic potential (Nelson et al., 1988; Iigo et al., 1997).

Thus, dietary PUFAs, one of the clearest dietary influences on risk for colon cancer, may alter risk through their modulation of composition and function of the mitochondrial membrane, which in turn, through complex interactions with SCFA metabolism and interaction with the binding and function of multiple effectors of signaling pathways that trigger growth or apoptosis, influence the probability of tumor formation.

References

Aggarwal, B. 2004. Nuclear factor-kappaB: the enemy within. *Cancer Cell* **6**: 203–208.

Akiyama, Y., Watkins, N., Suzuki, H., Jair, K.W., van Engeland, M., Esteller, M., Sakai, H., Ren, C.-Y., Yuasa, Y., Herman, J.G., and Baylin, S.B. 2003. GATA-4 and GATA-5 transcription factor genes and potential downstream antitumor target genes are epigenetically silenced in colorectal and gastric cancer. *Mol Cell Biol* **23**: 8429–8439.

Allgayer, H., Wang, H., Shirasawa, S., Sasazuki, T., and Boyd, D. 1999. Targeted disruption of the K-ras oncogene in an invasive colon cancer cell line down-regulates urokinase receptor expression and plasminogen-dependent proteolysis. *Br J Cancer* **80**: 1884–1891.

Alon, U., Barkai, N., Notterman, D.A., Gish, K., Ybarra, S., Mack, D., and Levine, A.J. 1999. Broad patterns of gene expression revealed by clustering analysis of tumor and normal colon tissues probed by oligonucleotide arrays. *Proc Natl Acad Sci USA* **96**: 6745–6750.

American Institute of Cancer Research. 1997. Colon, rectum. *In* "Food, Nutrition and the Prevention of Cancer" (J. Potter, Ed.), pp. 216–225. American Institute for Cancer Research, Washington, DC.

Anti, M., Marra, G., Armelao, F., Bartoli, G.M., Ficarelli, R., Percesepe, A., De Vitis, I., Maria, G., Sofo, L., Rapaccini, G.L., and et al. 1992. Effect of omega-3 fatty acids on rectal mucosal cell proliferation in subjects at risk for colon cancer. *Gastroenterology* **103**: 883–891.

Anti, M., Armelao, F., Marra, G., Percesepe, A., Bartoli, G.M., Palozza, P., Parrella, P., Canetta, C., Gentiloni, N., De Vitis, I., and et al. 1994. Effects of different doses of fish oil on rectal cell proliferation in patients with sporadic colonic adenomas. *Gastroenterology* **107**: 1709–1718.

Aoki, K., Tamai, Y., Horiike, S., Oshima, M., and Taketo, M. 2003. Colonic polyposis caused by mTOR-mediated chromosomal instability in Apc+/Delta716 Cdx2+/– compound mutant mice. *Nat Genet* **35**: 323–330.

Arango, D., Corner, G.A., Wadler, S., Catalano, P.J., and Augenlicht, L.H. 2001. c-*myc*/p53 interaction determines sensitivity of human colon carcinoma cells to 5-fluorouracil *in vitro* and *in vivo*. *Cancer Res* **61**: 4910–4915.

Arango, D., Mariadason, J., Wilson, C.L., Yang, W., Corner, G., Nicholas, C., Aranes, M.J., and Augenicht, L.H. 2002. c-Myc overexpression senstises colon cancer cells to camptothecin-induced apoptosis. *Br J Cancer* **89**: 1757–1765.

Archer, S.Y., Meng, S., and Hodin, R.A. 1997. Molecular mechanisms underlying the effects of sodium butyrate on intestinal epithelia: the role of histone hyperacetylation. *Gastroenterology* **112**: A345.

Archer, S.Y., Meng, S., Shei, A., and Hodin, R.A. 1998. p21(WAF1) is required for butyrate-mediated growth inhibition of human colon cancer cells. *Proc Natl Acad Sci USA* **95**: 6791–6796.

Arellano, M., and Moreno, S. 1997. Regulation of CDK/cyclin complexes during the cell cycle. *Int J Biochem Cell Biol* **29**: 559–573.

Artavanis-Tsakonas, S., Rand, M.D., and Lake, R.J. 1999. Notch signaling: cell fate control and signal integration in development. *Science* **284**: 770–776.

Aslam, F., Palumbo, L., Augenlicht, L.H., and Velcich, A. 2001. The Sp family of transcription factors in the regulation of the human and mouse MUC2 gene promoters. *Cancer Res* **61**: 570–576.

Augenlicht, L.H., and Kobrin, D. 1982. Cloning and screening of sequences expressed in a mouse colon tumor. *Cancer Res* **42**: 1088–1093.

Augenlicht, L.H., Augeron, C., Yander, G., and Laboisse, C. 1987. Overexpression of ras in mucus-secreting human colon carcinoma cells of low tumorigenicity. *Cancer Res* **47**: 3763–3765.

Augenlicht, L.H. 1988. Gene expression in human colonic biopsies. *In* "Basic and Clinical Perspectives of Colorectal Polyps and Cancer" (G. Steele, R. Burt, S.J. Winawer, and J.P. Karr, Eds.), Vol. 279, pp. 195–202. Alan R. Liss, New York.

Augenlicht, L.H. 1989. Gene structure and expression in colon cancer. *In* "Cell and Molecular Biology of Colon Cancer" (L.H. Augenlicht, Ed.), 1st edition, pp. 165–186. CRC Press, Boca Raton, FL.

Augenlicht, L.H., Corner, G., Molinas, S., and Heerdt, B.G. 1992. Genetic biomarkers. *In* "Cancer Chemoprevention" (L. Wattenberg, M. Lipkin, C.W. Boone, and G.J. Kelloff, Eds.), pp. 559–569. CRC Press, Boca Raton, FL.

Augenlicht, L.H. 1997. Chemoprevention: intermediate markers. *In* "Encyclopedia of Cancer" (J.R. Bertino, Ed.), 1st edition, Vol. 1, pp. 309–318. Academic Press, San Diego.

Augenlicht, L., Velcich, A., Mariadason, J., Bordonaro, M., and Heerdt, B. 1999a. Colonic cell proliferation, differentiation, and apoptosis. *Adv Exp Med Biol* **470**: 15–22.

Augenlicht, L.H., Anthony, G.M., Chruch, T.L., Edelmann, W., Kucherlapati, R., Yang, K.Y., Lipkin, M., and Heerdt, B.G. 1999b. Short chain fatty acid metabolism, apoptosis and Apc initiated tumorigenesis in the mouse gastrointestinal mucosa. *Cancer Res* **59**: 6005–6009.

Augenlicht, L.H., Corner, G., Houston, M., Laboisse, C., Mariadason, J., and Velcich, A. 2000. Microarray analysis of colonic epithelial cell maturation pathways triggered by butryate, sulindac, trichostatin A and curcumin and relationship to pathways of lineage specific differentiation. *Proc Am Assoc Cancer Res.*

Augenlicht, L.H., and Heerdt, B.G. 2001. Mitochondria:integrators in tumorigenesis? *Nat Genet* **28**: 104–105.

Augeron, C., and Laboisse, C.L. 1984. Emergence of permanently differentiated cell clones in a human colonic cancer cell line in culture after treatment with sodium butyrate. *Cancer Res* **44**: 3961–3969.

Bandyopadhyay, D., Mishra, A., and Medrano, E.E. 2004. Overexpression of histone deacetylase 1 confers resistance to sodium butyrate-mediated apoptosis in melanoma cells through a p53-mediated pathway. *Cancer Res* **64**: 7706–7710.

Barak, Y., Liao, D., He, W., Ong, E.S., Nelson, M.C., Olefsky, J.M., Boland, R., and Evans, R.M. 2002. Effects of peroxisome proliferator-activated receptor delta on placentation, adiposity, and colorectal cancer. *PNAS* **99**: 303–308.

Barlow, D.P. 1995. Gametic imprinting in mammals. *Science* **270**: 1610–1613.

Bartram, H.P., Gostner, A., Scheppach, W., Reddy, B.S., Rao, C.V., Dusel, G., Richter, F., Richter, A., and Kasper, H. 1993. Effects of fish oil on rectal cell proliferation, mucosal fatty acids, and prostaglandin E2 release in healthy subjects. *Gastroenterology* **105**: 1317–1322.

Baylin, S., Herman, J., Graff, P., Vertino, and Issa, J.-P. 1998. Alterations in DNA methylation: a fundamental aspect of neoplasia. *Adv Cancer Res* **72**: 141–196.

Beck, F., Chawengsaksophak, K., Waring, P., Playford, R., and Furness, J.B. 1999. Reprogramming of intestinal differentiation and intercalary regeneration in Cdx2 mutant mice. *Proc Natl Acad Sci USA* **96**: 7318–7323.

Beg, A., Sha, W., Bronson, R., Ghosh, S., and Baltimore, D. 1995. Embryonic lethality and liver degeneration in mice lacking the RelA component of NF-κB. *Nature* **376**: 167–170.

Behrens, J., von Kries, J., Kuhl, M., Bruhn, L., Wedlich, D., Grosschedl, R., and Birchmeier, W. 1996. Functional interaction of β-catenin with the transcription factor LEF-1. *Nature* **382**: 638–642.

Berger, A., Gershwin, M.E., and German, J.B. 1992. Effects of various dietary fats on cardiolipin acyl composition during ontogeny of mice. *Lipids* **27**: 605–612.

Bernstein, B., Tong, J., and Schreiber, S. 2000. Genomewide studies ofhistone deacetylase function in yeast. *Proc Natl Acad Sci USA* **97**: 13708–13713.

Bertos, N., Wang, A., and Yang, X. 2001. Class II histone deacetylases: structure, function and regulation. *Biochem Cell Biol* **79**: 243–252.

Bertucci, F., Salas, S., Eysteries, S., Nasser, V., Finetti, P., Ginestier, C., Charafe-Jauffret, E., Loriod, B., Bachelart, L., Montfort, J., Victorero, G., Viret, F., Ollendorff, V., Fert, V., Giovaninni, M., Delpero, J.R., Nguyen, C., Viens, P., Monges, G., Birnbaum, D., and Houlgatte, R. 2004. Gene expression profiling of colon cancer by DNA microarrays and correlation with histoclinical parameters. *Oncogene* **23**: 1377–1391.

Bharti, A., and Aggarwal, B. 2002. Nuclear factor-kappa B and cancer: its role in prevention and therapy. *Biochem Pharmacol* **64**: 883–888.

Bird, A. 1986. CpG-rich islands and the function of DNA methylation. *Nature* **321**: 209–213.

Bivona, T.G., and Philips, M.R. 2003. Ras pathway signaling on endomembranes. *Curr Opin Cell Biol* **15**: 136–142.

Blache, P., van de Wetering, M., Duluc, I., Domon, C., Berta, P., Freund, J.N., Clevers, H., and Jay, P. 2004. SOX9 is an intestine crypt transcription factor, is regulated by the Wnt pathway, and represses the CDX2 and MUC2 genes. *J Cell Biol* **166**: 37–47.

Blaumueller, C.M., Qi, H., Zagouras, P., and Artavanis-Tsakonas, S. 1997. Intracellular cleavage of Notch leads to a heterodimeric receptor on the plasma membrane. *Cell* **90**: 281–291.

Bonhomme, C., Duluc, I., Martin, E., Chawengsaksophak, K., Chenard, M.P., Kedinger, M., Beck, F., Freund, J.N., and Domon-Dell, C. 2003. The Cdx2 homeobox gene has a tumour suppressor function in the distal colon in addition to a homeotic role during gut development. *Gut* **52**: 1465–1471.

Bordonaro, M., Mariadason, J.M., Aslam, F., Heerdt, B.G., and Augenlicht, L.H. 1999. Butyrate induced cell cycle arrest and apoptotic cascade in colonic carcinoma cells: modulation of the β-catenin-Tcf pathway, and concordance with effects of sulindac and trichostatin, but not curcumin. *Cell Growth Differ* **10**: 713–720.

Boudreau, F., Rings, E.H., van Wering, H.M., Kim, R. K., Swain, G.P., Krasinski, S.D., Moffett, J., Grand, R.J., Suh, E.R., and Traber, P.G. 2002. Hepatocyte nuclear factor-1alpha, GATA-4, and caudal related homeodomain protein Cdx2 interact functionally to modulate intestinal gene transcription. Implication for the developmental regulation of the sucrase-isomaltase gene. *J Biol Chem* **277**: 31909–31917.

Boyes, J., Byfield, P., Nakatani, Y., and Ogryzko, V. 1998. Regulation of activity of the transcription factor GATA-1 by acetylation. *Nature* **396**: 594–598.

Bray, S., and Furriols, M. 2001. Notch pathway: making sense of suppressor of hairless. *Curr Biol* **11**: R217–R221.

Breneman, J., Yau, P., Swiger, R., Teplitz, R., Smith, H., Tucker, J., and Bradbury, E. 1996. Activity banding of human chromosomes as shown by histone acetylation. *Chromosoma* **105**: 41–49.

Britton, C., McKerrow, J.H., and Johnstone, I.L. 1998. Regulation of the *Caenorhabditis elegans* gut cysteine protease gene cpr-1: requirement for GATA motifs. *J Mol Biol* **283**: 15–27.

Brooks, D.G., James, R.M., Patek, C.E., Williamson, J., and Arends, M.J. 2001. Mutant K-ras enhances apoptosis in embryonic stem cells in combination with DNA damage and is associated with increased levels of p19(ARF). *Oncogene* **20**: 2144–2152.

Brou, C., Logeat, F., Gupta, N., Bessia, C., LeBail, O., Doedens, J.R., Cumano, A., Roux, P., Black, R.A., and Israel, A. 2000. A novel proteolytic cleavage involved in Notch signaling: the role of the disintegrin-metalloprotease TACE. *Mol Cell* **5**: 207–216.

Burri, N., Shaw, P., Bouzourene, H., Sordat, I., Sordat, B., Gillet, M., Schorderet, D., Bosman, F., and Chaubert, P. 2001. Methylation silencing and mutations of the p14ARF and p16INK4a genes in colon cancer. *Lab Invest* **81**: 217–229.

Cao, Y., Bonizzi, G., Seagroves, T., Greten, F., Johnson, R., Schmidt, E., and Karin, M. 2001. IKK provides an essential link between RANK signalling and cyclin D1 expression during mammary gland development. *Cell* **107**: 763–775.

Carnero, A. 2002. Targeting the cell cycle for cancer therapy. *Br J Cancer* **87**: 129–133.

Carroll, R.E., Matkowskyj, K.A., Chakrabarti, S., McDonald, T.J., and Benya, R.V. 1999. Aberrant expression of gastrin-releasing peptide and its receptor by well-differentiated colon cancers in humans. *Am J Physiol Gastrointest Liver Physiol* **276**: G655–G665.

Chang, M.Y., Jan, M.S., Won, S.J., and Liu, H.S. 1998. Ha-rasVal12 oncogene increases susceptibility of NIH/3T3 cells to lovastatin. *Biochem Biophys Res Commun* **248**: 62–68.

Chang, W.-C.L., Chapkin, R.S., and Lupton, J.R. 1997. Predictive value of proliferation, differentiation, and apoptosis as intermdiate markers for colon tumorigenesis. *Carcinogenesis* **18**: 721–730.

Chapkin, R.S., Hong, M.Y., Fan, Y.Y., Davidson, L.A., Sanders, L.M., Henderson, C.E., Barhoumi, R., Burghardt, R.C., Turner, N.D., and Lupton, J.R. 2002. Dietary n-3 PUFA alter colonocyte mitochondrial membrane composition and function. *Lipids* **37**: 193–199.

Chawengsaksophak, K., James, R., Hammond, V., Kontgen, F., and Beck, F. 1997. Homeosis and intestinal tumours in Cdx2 mutant mice. *Nature* **386**: 84–87.

Chen, L.B. 1988. Mitochondrial membrane potential in living cells. *Annu Rev Cell Biol* **4**: 155–181.

Chen, L.B., and Rivers, E.N. 1990. Mitochondria in cancer cells. *In* "Genes and Cancer" (D. Carney and K. Sikora, Eds.), pp. 127–135. John Wiley & Sons, New York, NY.

Chen, L., Smith, L., Johnson, M.R., Wang, K., Diasio, R.B., and Smith, J.B. 2000. Activation of protein kinase C induces nuclear translocation of RFX1 and down-regulates c-myc via an intron 1 X box in undifferentiated leukemia HL-60 cells. *J Biol Chem* **275**: 32227–32333.

Choi, S.W., and Mason, J.B. 2000. Folate and carcinogenesis: an integrated scheme. *J Nutr* **130**: 129–132.

Choi, S.W., and Mason, J.B. 2002. Folate status: effects on pathways of colorectal carcinogenesis. *J Nutr* **132**: 2413S–2418S.

Christensen, S., Kodoyianni, V., Bosenberg, M., Friedman, L., and Kimble, J. 1996. lag-1, a gene required for lin-12 and glp-1 signaling in *Caenorhabditis elegans*, is homologous to human CBF1 and *Drosophila* Su(H). *Development* **122**: 1373–1383.

Ciaparrone, M., Yamamoto, H., Yao, Y., Sgambato, A., Cattoretti, G., Tomita, N., Monden, T., Rotterdam, H., and Weinstein, I.B. 1998. Localization and expression of p27Kip1 in multistage colorectal carcinogenesis. *Cancer Res* **58**: 114–122.

Coleman, L.J., Landstrom, E.K., Royle, P.J., Bird, A.R., and McIntosh, G.H. 2002. A diet containing alpha-cellulose and fish oil reduces aberrant crypt foci formation and modulates other possible markers for colon cancer risk in azoxymethane-treated rats. *J Nutr* **132**: 2312–2318.

Costello, J.F., Fruhwald, M.C., Smiraglia, D.J., Rush, L.J., Robertson, G.P., Gao, X., Wright, F.A., Feramisco, J.D., Peltomaki, P., Lang, J.C., Schuller, D.E., Yu, L., Bloomfield, C.D., Caligiuri, M.A., Yates, A., Nishikawa, R., Su Huang, H., Petrelli, N.J., Zhang, X., O'Dorisio, M.S., Held, W.A., Cavenee, W.K., and Plass, C. 2000. Aberrant CpG-island methylation has non-random and tumour-type–specific patterns. *Nat Genet* **24**: 132–138.

Cuisset, L., Tichonicky, L., and Delpech, M. 1998. A protein phosphatase is involved in the inhibition of histone deacetylation by sodium butyrate. *Biochem Biophys Res Commun* **246**: 760–764.

Cummings, J.H. 1983. Fermentation in the human large intestine: evidence and implications for health. *Lancet* **1**: 1206–1209.

Cusack, J.J., Liu, R., and Baldwin, A.J. 2000. Inducible chemoresistance to 7-ethyl-10-[4-(1-piperidino)-1-piperidino]-carbonyloxycamptothecin (CPT-11) in colorectal cancer cells and a xenograft model is overcome by inhibition of nuclear factor-κB activation. *Cancer Res* **60**: 2323–2330.

da Costa, L., He, T., Yu, J., Sparks, A., Morin, P., Polyak, K., Laken, S., Vogelstein, B., and KW, K. 1999. CDX2 is mutated in a colorectal cancer with normal APC/beta-catenin signaling. *Oncogene* **18**: 5010–5014.

D'Abaco, G.M., Whitehead, R.H., and Burgess, A.W. 1996. Synergy between Apc min and an activated ras mutation is sufficient to induce colon carcinomas. *Mol Cell Biol* **16**: 884–891.

Dang, D., Mahatan, C., Dang, L., Agboola, I., and Yang, V. 2001. Expression of the gut-enriched Kruppel-like factor (Kruppel-like factor 4) gene in the human colon cancer cell line RKO is dependent on CDX2. *Oncogene* **20**: 4884–4890.

Danial, N.N., Gramm, C.F., Scorrano, L., Zhang, C.Y., Krauss, S., Ranger, A.M., Datta, S.R., Greenberg, M.E., Licklider, L.J., Lowell, B.B., Gygi, S.P., and Korsmeyer, S.J. 2003. BAD and glucokinase reside in a mitochondrial complex that integrates glycolysis and apoptosis. *Nature* **424**: 952–956.

Dashwood, R.H., Suzui, M., Nakagama, H., Sugimura, T., and Nagao, M. 1998. High frequency of β-catenin (Ctnnb1) mutations in the colon tumors induced by two heterocyclic amines in the F344 rat. *Cancer Res* **58**: 1127–1129.

Datta, S.R., Dudek, H., Tao, X., Masters, S., Fu, H., Gotoh, Y., and Greenberg, M.E. 1997. Akt phosphorylation of BAD couples survival signals to the cell-intrinsic death machinery. *Cell* **91**: 231–241.

Davies, H., Bignell, G.R., Cox, C., Stephens, P., Edkins, S., Clegg, S., Teague, J., Woffendin, H., Garnett, M.J., Bottomley, W., Davis, N., Dicks, E., Ewing, R., Floyd, Y., Gray, K., Hall, S., Hawes, R., Hughes, J., Kosmidou, V., Menzies, A., Mould, C., Parker, A., Stevens, C., Watt, S., Hooper, S., Wilson, R., Jayatilake, H., Gusterson, B.A., Cooper, C., Shipley, J., Hargrave, D., Pritchard-Jones, K., Maitland, N., Chenevix-Trench, G., Riggins, G.J., Bigner, D.D., Palmieri, G., Cossu, A., Flanagan, A., Nicholson, A., Ho, J.W., Leung, S.Y., Yuen, S.T., Weber, B.L., Seigler, H.F., Darrow, T.L., Paterson, H., Marais, R., Marshall, C.J., Wooster, R., Stratton, M.R., and Futreal, P.A. 2002. Mutations of the BRAF gene in human cancer. *Nature* **417**: 949–954.

Davis, S., Weiss, M.J., Wong, J.R., Lampidis, T.J., and Chen, L.B. 1985. Mitochondrial and plasma membrane potentials cause unusual accumulation and retention of rhodamine 123 by human breast adenocarcinoma–derived MCF-7 cells. *J Biol Chem* **260**: 13844–13850.

Decaudin, D., Geley, S., Hirsch, T., Castedo, M., Marchetti, P., Macho, A., Kofler, R., and Kroemer, G. 1997. Bcl-2 and Bcl-XL antagonize the mitochondrial dysfunction preceding nuclear apoptosis induced by chemotherapeutic agents. *Cancer Res* **57**: 62–67.

Dejardin, E., Deregowsk, I.V., Chapelier, M., Jacobs, N., Gielen, J., Merville, M.-J., and Bours, V. 1999. Regulation of NF-κB activity by IκB-regulated proteins in adenocarcinoma cells. *Oncogene* **18**: 2567–2577.

Deng, C., Zhang, P., Harper, J.W., Elledge, S.J., and Leder, P. 1995. Mice lacking p21 cip1/waf1 undergo normal development, but are defective in G1 checkpoint control. *Cell* **82**: 675–684.

Deschenes, C., Vezina, A., Beaulieu, J., and Rivard, N. 2001. Role of p27(Kip1) in human intestinal cell differentiation. *Gastroenterology* **120**: 423–438.

De Strooper, B., Annaert, W., Cupers, P., Saftig, P., Craessaerts, K., Mumm, J.S., Schroeter, E.H., Schrijvers, V., Wolfe, M.S., Ray, W.J., Goate, A., and Kopan, R. 1999. A presenilin-1–dependent gamma-secretase–like protease mediates release of Notch intracellular domain. *Nature* **398**: 518–522.

Ding, Q., Ko, T., and Evers, B. 1998. Caco-2 intestinal cell differentiation is associated with G1 arrest and suppression of CDK2 and CDK4. *Am J Physiol* **275**: C1193–C1200.

Domon-Dell, C., Schneider, A., Moucadel, V., Guerin, E., Guenot, D., Aguillon, S., Duluc, I., Martin, E., Iovanna, J., Launay, J., Duclos, B., Chenard, M., Meyer, C., Oudet, P., Kedinger, M., Gaub, M., and JN, F. 2003. Cdx1 homeobox gene during human colon cancer progression. *Oncogene* **22**: 7913–7921.

Ee, H.C., Erler, T., Bhathal, P.S., Young, G.P., and James, R.J. 1995. Cdx-2 homeodomain protein expression in human and rat colorectal adenoma and carcinoma. *Am J Pathol* **147**: 586–592.

Eferl, R., and Wagner, E. 2003. AP-1: a double-edged sword in tumorigenesis. *Nat Rev Cancer* **3**: 859–868.

Emiliani, S., Fischle, W., Van Lint, C., Al-Abed, Y., and Verdin, E. 1998. Characterization of a human RPD3 ortholog, HDAC3. *Proc Natl Acad Sci USA* **95**: 2795–2800.

Erisman, M.D., Rothberg, P.G., Diehl, R.E., Morse, C.C., Spandorfer, J.M., and Astrin, S.M. 1985. Deregulation of c-myc gene expression in human colon carcinoma is not accompanied by amplification or rearrangement of the gene. *Mol Cell Biol* **5**: 1969–1976.

Erisman, M.D., Litwin, S., Keidan, R.D., Comis, R.L., and Astrin, S.M. 1988. Noncorrelation of the expression of the c-myc oncogene in colorectal carcinoma with recurrence of disease or patient survival. *Cancer Res* **48**: 1350–1355.

Escaffit, F., Boudreau, F., and Beaulieu, J.F. 2005. Differential expression of claudin-2 along the human intestine: Implication of GATA-4 in the maintenance of claudin-2 in differentiating cells. *J Cell Physiol* **203**: 15–26.

Esteller, M., Corn, P., Baylin, S., and Herman, J.G. 2001. A gene hypermethylation profile of human cancer. *Cancer Res* **61**: 3225–3229.

Evan, G.I., Wyllie, A.H., Gilbert, C.S., Littlewood, T.D., Land, H., Brooks, M., Waters, C.M., Penn, L.Z., and Hancock, D.C. 1992. Induction of apoptosis in fibroblasts by c-myc protein. *Cell* **69**: 119–128.

Evers, B., Ko, T., Li, J., and Thompson, E. 1996. Cell cycle protein suppression and p21 induction in differentiating Caco-2 cells. *Am J Physiol* **271**: G722–G727.

Evertsson, S., and Sun, X.-F. 2002. Protein expression of NF-κB in human colorectal adenocarcinoma. *Int J Mol Med* **10**: 547–550.

Faure Vigny, H., Heddi, A., Giraud, S., Chautard, D., and Stepien, G. 1996. Expression of oxidative phosphorylation genes in renal tumors and tumoral cell lines. *Mol Carcinogen* **16**: 165–172.

Feinberg, A.P., and Vogelstein, B. 1983. Hypomethylation distinguishes genes of some human cancers from their normal counterparts. *Nature* **301**: 89–92.

Feinberg, A.P., Gehrke, C.W., Kuo, K.C., and Ehrlich, M. 1988. Reduced genomic 5-methylcytosine content in human colonic neoplasia. *Cancer Res* **48**: 1159–1161.

Fernandez, E., Chatenoud, L., La Vecchia, C., Negri, E., and Franceschi, S. 1999. Fish consumption and cancer risk. *Am J Clin Nutr* **70**: 85–90.

Ferri, K., and Kroemer, G. 2001. Mitochondria: the suicide organelles. *Bioessays* **23**: 111–115.

Finely, G.G., Schulz, N.T., Hill, S.A., Geiser, J.R., Pipas, J.M., and Meisler, A.I. 1989. Expression of the myc gene family in different stages of human colorectal cancer. *Oncogene* **4**: 963–971.

Fischle, W., Kiermer, V., Dequiedt, F., and Verdin, E. 2001. The emerging role of class II histone deacetylases. *Biochem Cell Biol* **79**: 337–348.

Fodde, R. 2003. The multiple functions of tumour suppressors: its all in APC. *Nat Cell Biol* **5**: 190–192.

Fortini, M.E., and Artavanis-Tsakonas, S. 1994. The suppressor of hairless protein participates in notch receptor signaling. *Cell* **79**: 273–282.

Fry, M., and Green, D.E. 1980. Cardiolipin requirement by cytochrome oxidase and the catalytic role of phospholipid. *Biochem Biophys Res Commun* **93**: 1238–1246.

Fry, M., and Green, D.E. 1981. Cardiolipin requirement for electron transfer in complex I and III of the mitochondrial respiratory chain. *J Biol Chem* **256**: 1874–1880.

Fryer, C.J., Lamar, E., Turbachova, I., Kintner, C., and Jones, K.A. 2002. Mastermind mediates chromatin-specific transcription and turnover of the Notch enhancer complex. *Genes Dev* **16**: 1397–1411.

Fujita, N., Jaye, D., Kajita, M., Geigerman, C., Moreno, C., and Wade, P. 2003. MTA3, a Mi-2/NuRD complex subunit, regulates an invasive growth pathway in breast cancer. *Cell* **113**: 207–219.

Gao, L., Cueto, M., Asselbergs, F., and Atadja, P. 2002. Cloning and functional characterization ofHDAC11, a novel member of the human histone deacetylase family. *J Biol Chem* **277**.

Gao, X., Sedgwick, T., Shi, Y.-B., and Evans, T. 1998. Distinct functions are implicated for the GATA-4, -5, and -6 transcription factors in the regulation of intestine epithelial cell differentiation. *Mol Cell Biol* **18**: 2901–2911.

Gaposchkin, D.P., Zoeller, R.A., and Broitman, S.A. 2000. Incorporation of polyunsaturated fatty acids into CT-26, a transplantable murine colonic adenocarcinoma. *Lipids* **35**: 181–186.

Gennis, R.B. 1989. "Biomembranes: Molecular Structure and Function." Springer-Verlag, New York.

Ghosh, S., and Karin, M. 2002. Missing pieces in the NF-κB puzzle. *Cell* **109**: S81–S96.

Gibson, P.R., Moeller, I., Kagelari, O., Folino, M., and Young, G.P. 1992. Contrasting effects of butyrate on the expression of phenotypic markers of differentiation in neoplastic and non-neoplastic colonic epithelial cells *in vitro*. *J Gastroenterol Hepatol* **7**: 165–172.

Girnun, G.D., Smith, W.M., Drori, S., Sarraf, P., Mueller, E., Eng, C., Nambiar, P., Rosenberg, D.W., Bronson, R.T., Edelmann, W., Kucherlapati, R., Gonzalez, F.J., and Spiegelman, B.M. 2002. APC-dependent suppression of colon carcinogenesis by PPARgamma *PNAS* **99**: 13771–13776.

Glotzer, D.J., Glick, M.E., and Goldman, H. 1981. Proctitis and colitis following diversion of the fecal stream. *Gastroenterology* **80**: 438–441.

Grady, W.M., Rajput, A., Myeroff, L., Liiu, D.F., Kwon, K., Willis, J., and Markowitz, S. 1998. Mutation of the type II transforming growth factor-beta receptor is coincident with the transformation of human colon adenomas to malignant carcinomas. *Cancer Res* **58**: 3101–3104.

Greenwald, I. 1998. LIN-12/Notch signaling: lessons from worms and flies. *Genes Dev* **12**: 1751–1762.

Greten, F., Eckmann, L., Greten, T., Park, J., Li, Z., Egan, L., Kagnoff, M., and Karin, M. 2004. IKKbeta links inflammation and tumorigenesis in a mouse model of colitis-associated cancer. *Cell* **118**: 285–296.

Groden, J., Thliveris, A., Samowitz, W., Carlson, M., Gelbert, L., Albertson, H., Joslyn, G., Stevens, J., Spiro, L., Robertson, M., Sargeant, L., Krapcho, K., Wolff, E., Burt, R., Hughes, J.P., Warrington, J., McPherson, J., Wasmuth, J., Le Paslier, D., Abderrahim, H., Cohen, D., Leppert, M., and White, R. 1991. Identification and characterization of the familial adenomatous polyposis coli gene. *Cell* **66**: 589–600.

Groden, J., Joslyn, G., Samowitz, W., Jones, D., Bhattacharyya, N., Spirio, L., Thliveris, A., Robertson, M., Egan, S., Meuth, M., and White, R. 1995. Response of colon cancer cell lines to the introduction of APC, a colon-specific tumor suppressor gene. *Cancer Res* **55**: 1531–1539.

Grozinger, C., and Schrieber, S. 2000. Regulation of histone deacetylase 4 and 5 and transcriptional activity by 14-3-3–dependent cellular localization. *Proc Natl Acad Sci USA* **97**: 7835–7840.

Gu, W., and Roeder, R. 1997. Activation of p53 sequence-specific DNA binding by acetylation of the p53 C-terminal domain. *Cell* **90**: 595–606.

Guardiola, A., and Yao, T. 2002. Molecular cloning and characterization of a novel histone deacetylase HDAC10. *J Biol Chem* **277**: 3350–3356.

Guo, R., Suh, E., and Lynch, J. 2004. The role of cdx proteins in intestinal development and cancer. *Cancer Biol Ther* **3**: 592–601.

Guo, Y.-S., Hellmich, M.R., Wen, X.D., and Townsend, C.M., Jr. 2001. Activator protein-1 transcription factor mediates bombesin-stimulated cyclooxygenase-2 expression in intestinal epithelial cells. *J Biol Chem* **276**: 22941–22947.

Guo, Y.-S., Cheng, J.-Z., Jin, G.-F., Gutkind, J.S., Hellmich, M.R., and Townsend, C.M., Jr. 2002. Gastrin stimulates cyclooxygenase-2 expression in intestinal epithelial cells through multiple signaling pathways. Evidence for involvement of erk5 kinase and transactivation of the epidermal growth factor receptor. *J Biol Chem* **277**: 48755–48763.

Gupta, R.A., Brockman, J.A., Sarraf, P., Willson, T.M., and DuBois, R.N. 2001. Target genes of peroxisome proliferator–activated receptor gamma in colorectal cancer cells. *J Biol Chem* **276**: 29681–29687.

Gupta, R.A., and Dubois, R.N. 2002. Controversy: PPARgamma as a target for treatment of colorectal cancer. *Am J Physiol Gastrointest Liver Physiol* **283**: G266–269.

Gupta, R.A., Wang, D., Katkuri, S., Wang, H., Dey, S.K., and DuBois, R.N. 2004. Activation of nuclear hormone receptor peroxisome proliferator–activated receptor-[delta] accelerates intestinal adenoma growth. *Nature Med* **10**: 245–247.

Guttridge, D., Albanese, C., Reuther, J., Pestell, R., and Baldwin, A.J. 1999. NF-κB controls cell growth and differentiation through transcriptional regulation of cyclin D1. *Mol Cell Biol* **19**: 5785–5799.

Hague, A., Manning, A.M., Hanlon, K.A., Huschtscha, L.I., Hart, D., and Paraskeva, C. 1993. Sodium butyrate induces apoptosis in human colonic tumor cell lines in a p53-independent pathway: implications for the possible role of dietary fibre in the prevention of large-bowel cancer. *Int J Cancer* **55**: 498–505.

Haines, T.H., and Dencher, N.A. 2002. Cardiolipin: a proton trap for oxidative phosphorylation. *FEBS Lett* **528**: 35–39.

Hanahan, D., and Weinberg, R. 2000. The Hallmarks of Cancer. *Cell* **100**: 57–70.

Hanazawa, S., Takeshita, A., Amano, S., Semba, T., Nirazuka, T., Katoh, H., and Kitano, S. 1993. Tumor necrosis factor-alpha induces expression of monocyte chemoattractant JE via fos and jun genes in clonal osteoblastic MC3T3-E1 cells. *J Biol Chem* **268**: 9526–9532.

Hao, X.P., Pretlow, T.G., Rao, J.S., and Pretlow, T.P. 2001. β-catenin expression is altered in human colonic aberrant crypt foci. *Cancer Res* **61**: 8085–8088.

Haramis, A.P., Begthel, H., van den Born, M., van Es, J., Jonkheer, S., Offerhaus, G.J., and Clevers, H. 2004. De novo crypt formation and juvenile polyposis on BMP inhibition in mouse intestine. *Science* **303**: 1684–1686.

Hardy, S., El-Assaad, W., Przybytkowski, E., Joly, E., Prentki, M., and Langelier, Y. 2003. Saturated fatty acid-induced apoptosis in MDA-MB-231 breast cancer cells. A role for cardiolipin. *J Biol Chem* **278**: 31861–31870.

Harig, J.M., Soergel, K.H., Komorowski, R.A., and Wood, C.M. 1989. Treatment of diversion colitis with short-chain-fatty acid irrigation. *N Engl J Med* **320**: 23–28.

Harman, F., Nicol, C., Marin, H., Ward, J., Gonzalez, F., and Peters, J. 2004. Peroxisome proliferator-activated receptor-delta attenuates colon carcinogenesis. *Nat Med* **10**: 481–483.

Hastie, N.D., and Bishop, J.O. 1976. The expression of three abundance classes of messenger RNA in mouse tissues. *Cell* **9**: 761–774.

He, T.-C., Sparks, A.B., Rago, C., Hermeking, H., Zawel, L., da Costa, L.T., Morin, P.J., Vogelstein, B., and Kinzler, K.W. 1998. Identification of c-MYC as a target of the APC pathway. *Science* **281**: 1509–1512.

He, T., Chan, T., Vogelstein, B., and Kinzler, K. 1999. PPARdelta is an APC-regulated target of nonsteroidal anti-inflammatory drugs. *Cell* **99**: 335–345.

He, X.C., Zhang, J., Tong, W.G., Tawfik, O., Ross, J., Scoville, D.H., Tian, Q., Zeng, X., He, X., Wiedemann, L.M., Mishina, Y., and Li, L. 2004. BMP signaling inhibits intestinal stem cell self-renewal through suppression of Wnt-beta-catenin signaling. *Nat Genet* **36**: 1117–1121.

Heerdt, B.G., and Augenlicht, L.H. 1990. Changes in the number of mitochondrial genomes during human development. *Exp Cell Res* **186**: 54–59.

Heerdt, B.G., and Augenlicht, L.H. 1991. Effects of fatty acids on expression of genes encoding subunits of cytochrome c oxidase and cytochrome *c* oxidase activity in HT29 human colonic adenocarcinoma cells. *J Biol Chem* **266**: 19120–19126.

Heerdt, B.G., Molinas, S., Deitch, D., and Augenlicht, L.H. 1991. Aggressive subtypes of human colorectal tumors frequently exhibit amplification of the c-myc gene. *Oncogene* **6**: 125–129.

Heerdt, B.G., Houston, M.A., and Augenlicht, L.H. 1994. Potentiation by specific short-chain fatty acids of differentiation and apoptosis in human colonic carcinoma cell lines. *Cancer Res* **54**: 3288–3294.

Heerdt, B.G., Houston, M.A., Rediske, J.J., and Augenlicht, L.H. 1996. Steady state levels of messenger RNA species characterize a predominant pathway culminating in apoptosis and shedding of HT29 human colonic carcinoma cells. *Cell Growth Differ* **7**: 101–106.

Heerdt, B.G., Houston, M.A., and Augenlicht, L.H. 1997. Short chain fatty acid–initiated cell cycle arrest and apoptosis of colonic epithelial cells is linked to mitochondrial function. *Cell Growth Differ* **8**: 523–532.

Heerdt, B.G., Houston, M.A., Anthony, G.M., and Augenlicht, L.H. 1998. Mitochondrial membrane potential in the coordination of p53-independent proliferation and apoptosis pathways in human colonic carcinoma cells. *Cancer Res* **58**: 2869–2875.

Heerdt, B.G., Houston, M.A., Mariadason, J.M., and Augenlicht, L.H. 2000. Dissociation of staurosporine-induced apoptosis from G2-M arrest in SW620 human colonic carcinoma cells: initiation of an apoptotic cascade is associated with elevation of the mitochondrial membrane potential. *Cancer Res* **60**: 6704–6713.

Heerdt, B., Houston, M.A., Wilson, A.J., Augenlicht, L.H. 2003. The intrinsic mitochondrial membrane potential is associated with steady state mitochondrial activity and the extent to which colonic epithelial cells undergo butyrate mediated growth arrest and apoptosis. *Cancer Res* **63**: 6311–6319.

Hennet, T., Bertoni, G., Richter, C., and Peterhans, E. 1993. Expression of BCL-2 protein enhances the survival of mouse fibrosarcoid cells in tumor necrosis factor–mediated cytotoxicity. *Cancer Res* **53**: 1456–1460.

Herman, J.G., Umar, A., Polyak, K., Graff, J.R., Ahuja, N., Issa, J.P., Markowitz, S., Willson, J.K., Hamilton, S.R., Kinzler, K.W., Kane, M.F., Kolodner, R.D., Vogelstein, B., Kunkel, T.A., Baylin, S.B. 1998. Incidence and functional consequences of hMLH1 promoter hypermethylation in colorectal carcinoma. *Proc Natl Acad Sci USA* **95**: 6870–6875.

Heruth, D.P., Zirnstein, G.W., Bradley, J.F., and Rothberg, P.G. 1993. Sodium butyrate causes an increase in the block to transcriptional elongation in the c-myc gene in SW837 rectal carcinoma cells. *J Biol Chem* **268**: 20466–20472.

Hinoi, T., Tani, M., Lucas, P.C., Caca, K., Dunn, R.L., Macri, E., Loda, M., Appelman, H.D., Cho, K.R., and Fearon, E.R. 2001. Loss of CDX2 expression and microsatellite instability are prominent features of large cell minimally differentiated carcinomas of the colon. *Am J Pathol* **159**: 2239–2248.

Hinoi, T., Loda, M., and Fearon, E.R. 2003. Silencing of CDX2 expression in colon cancer via a dominant repression pathway. *J Biol Chem* **278**: 44608–44616.

Hoch, F.L. 1992. Cardiolipins and biomembrane function. *Biochim Biophys Acta* **1113**: 71–133.

Hofmanova, J., Vaculova, A., Lojek, A., and Kozubik, A. 2004. Interaction of polyunsaturated fatty acids and sodium butyrate during apoptosis in HT-29 human colon adenocarcinoma cells. *Eur J Nutr* 1–12.

Hong, M.Y., Chapkin, R.S., Barhoumi, R., Burghardt, R.C., Turner, N.D., Henderson, C.E., Sanders, L.M., Fan, Y.Y., Davidson, L.A., Murphy, M.E., Spinka, C.M., Carroll, R.J., and Lupton, J.R. 2002. Fish oil increases mitochondrial phospholipid unsaturation, upregulating reactive oxygen species and apoptosis in rat colonocytes. *Carcinogenesis* **23**: 1919–1925.

Hong, M.Y., Chapkin, R.S., Davidson, L.A., Turner, N.D., Morris, J.S., Carroll, R.J., and Lupton, J.R. 2003. Fish oil enhances targeted apoptosis during colon tumor initiation in part by downregulating Bcl-2. *Nutr Cancer* **46**: 44–51.

Howe, J.R., Bair, J.L., Sayed, M.G., Anderson, M.E., Mitros, F.A., Petersen, G.M., Velculescu, V.E., Traverso, G., and Vogelstein, B. 2001. Germline mutations of the gene encoding bone morphogenetic protein receptor 1A in juvenile polyposis. *Nat Genet* **28**: 184–187.

Hulit, J., Wang, C., Li, Z., Albanese, C., Rao, M., Di Vizio, D., Shah, S., Byers, S.W., Mahmood, R., Augenlicht, L.H., Russell, R., and Pestell, R.G. 2004. Cyclin D1 genetic heterozygosity regulates colonic epithelial cell differentiation and tumor number in ApcMin mice. *Mol Cell Biol* **24**: 7598–7611.

Huppert, S.S., Le, A., Schroeter, E.H., Mumm, J.S., Saxena, M.T., Milner, L.A., and Kopan, R. 2000. Embryonic lethality in mice homozygous for a processing-deficient allele of Notch1. *Nature* **405**: 966–970.

Iigo, M., Nakagawa, T., Ishikawa, C., Iwahori, Y., Asamoto, M., Yazawa, K., Araki, E., and Tsuda, H. 1997. Inhibitory effects of docosahexaenoic acid on colon carcinoma 26 metastasis to the lung. *Br J Cancer* **75**: 650–655.

Ikeda, S., Kishida, S., Yamamoto, H., Murai, H., and Koyama, S. 1998. Axin, a negative regulator of the Wnt signalling pathway, forms a complex with GSK-3B and β-catenin and promotes GSK-3B–dependent phosphorylation of β-catenin. *EMBO J* **17**: 1371–1384.

Ilyas, M., Tomlinson, I., Rowan, A., Pignatelli, M., and Bodmer, W. 1997. β-catenin mutations in cell lines established from human colorectal cancers. *Proc Natl Acad Sci USA* **94**: 10330–10334.

Imhof, A., Yang, X., Ogryzko, V., Nakatani, Y., Wolffe, A., and Ge, H. 1997. Acetylation of general transcription factors by histone acetyltransferases. *Curr Biol* **7**: 689–692.

Inan, M., Tolmacheva, V., Wang, Q.-S., Rosenberg, D., and Giardina, C. 2000. Transcription factor NF-κB participates in regulation of epithelial cell turnover in the colon. *Am J Physiol* **279**: G1282–G1291.

Insinga, A., Monestiroli, S., Ronzoni, S., Gelmetti, V., Marchesi, F., Viale, A., Altucci, L., Nervi, C., Minucci, S., and Pelicci, P.G. 2005. Inhibitors of histone deacetylases induce tumor-selective apoptosis through activation of the death receptor pathway. *Nat Med* **11**: 71–76.

Issa, J.P., Vertino, P., Boehm, C., Newsham, I., and Baylin, S. 1996. Switch from monoallelic to biallelic human IGF2 promoter methylation during aging and carcinogenesis. *Proc Natl Acad Sci USA* **93**: 11757–11762.

Issa, J.P. 2004. CpG island methylator phenotype in cancer. *Nat Rev Cancer* **4**: 988–993.

Iwamoto, S., Senzaki, H., Kiyozuka, Y., Ogura, E., Takada, H., Hioki, K., and Tsubura, A. 1998. Effects of fatty acids on liver metastasis of ACL-15 rat colon cancer cells. *Nutr Cancer* **31**: 143–150.

Jain, M., Arvanitis, C., Chu, K., Dewey, W., Leonhardt, E., Trinh, M., Sundberg, C.D., Bishop, J.M., and Felsher, D.W. 2002. Sustained loss of a neoplastic phenotype by brief inactivation of MYC. *Science* **297**: 102–104.

James, R., and Kazenwadel, J. 1991. Homeobox gene expression in the intestinal epithelium of adult mice. *J Biol Chem* **266**: 3246–3251.

Janssen, K.P., el-Marjou, F., Pinto, D., Sastre, X., Rouillard, D., Fouquet, C., Soussi, T., Louvard, D., and Robine, S. 2002. Targeted expression of oncogenic K-ras in intestinal epithelium causes spontaneous tumorigenesis in mice. *Gastroenterology* **123**: 492–504.

Jarriault, S., Brou, C., Logeat, F., Schroeter, E.H., Kopan, R., and Israel, A. 1995. Signalling downstream of activated mammalian Notch. *Nature* **377**: 355–358.

Jensen, J., Pedersen, E.E., Galante, P., Hald, J., Heller, R.S., Ishibashi, M., Kageyama, R., Guillemot, F., Serup, P., and Madsen, O.D. 2000. Control of endodermal endocrine development by Hes-1. *Nat Genet* **24**: 36–44.

Jiang, F., Ryan, M.T., Schlame, M., Zhao, M., Gu, Z., Klingenberg, M., Pfanner, N., and Greenberg, M.L. 2000. Absence of cardiolipin in the crd1 null mutant results in decreased mitochondrial membrane potential and reduced mitochondrial function. *J Biol Chem* **275**: 22387–22394.

Johnstone, R.W. 2002. Histone-deacetylase inhibitors: novel drugs for the treatment of cancer. *Nat Rev Drug Discov* **1**: 287–299.

Jones, P. 1999. The DNA methylation paradox. *Trends Genet* **15**: 34–37.

Karin, M., Cao, Y., Greten, F., and Li, Z.-W. 2002. NF-κB in cancer: from innocent bystander to major culprit. *Nature Rev Cancer* **2**: 301–310.

Katz, J.P., Perreault, N., Goldstein, B.G., Lee, C.S., Labosky, P.A., Yang, V.W., and Kaestner, K.H. 2002. The zinc-finger transcription factor Klf4 is required for terminal differentiation of goblet cells in the colon. *Development* **129**: 2619–2628.

Kim, B.Y., Gaynor, R.B., Song, K., Dritschilo, A., and Jung, M. 2002. Constitutive activation of NF-kappaB in Ki-ras–transformed prostate epithelial cells. *Oncogene* **21**: 4490–4497.

Kim, S., Domon-Dell, C., Wang, Q., Chung, D., Di Cristofano, A., Pandolfi, P., Freund, J., and Evers, B. 2002. PTEN and TNF-alpha regulation of the intestinal-specific Cdx-2 homeobox gene through a PI3K, PKB/Akt, and NF-kappaB–dependent pathway. *Gastroenterology* **123**: 1163–1178.

Kinzler, K.W., and Vogelstein, B. 1996. Lessons from hereditary colorectal cancer. *Cell* **87**: 159–170.

Klampfer, L., Huang, J., Corner, G., Mariadason, J., Arango, D., Sasazuki, T., Shirasawa, S., and Augenlicht, L. 2003. Oncogenic Ki-ras inhibits the expression of interferon-responsive genes through inhibition of STAT1 and STAT2 expression. *J Biol Chem* **278**: 46278–46287.

Klampfer, L., Huang, J., Sasazuki, T., Shirasawa, S., and Augenlicht, L. 2004. Oncogenic Ras promotes butyrate-induced apoptosis through inhibition of gelsolin expression. *J Biol Chem* **279**: 36680–36688.

Kondo, Y., and Issa, J.P. 2004. Epigenetic changes in colorectal cancer. *Cancer Metastasis Rev* **23**: 29–39.

Kontogiannea, M., Gupta, A., Ntanios, F., Graham, T., Jones, P., and Meterissian, S. 2000. Omega-3 fatty acids decrease endothelial adhesion of human colorectal carcinoma cells. *J Surg Res* **92**: 201–205.

Korinek, V., Barker, N., Morin, P.J., van Wichen, D., de Weger, R., Kinzler, K.W., Vogelstein, B., and Clevers, H. 1997. Constitutive transcriptional activation by a β-catenin-Tcf complex in APC–/– colon carcinoma. *Science* **275**: 1784–1787.

Korinek, V., Barker, N., Moerer, P., van Donselaar, E., Huls, G., Peters, P.J., and Clevers, H. 1998. Depletion of epithelial stem-cell compartments in the small intestine of mice lacking Tcf-4. *Nat Genet* **19**: 379–383.

Kretzschmar, M., Doody, J., Timokhina, I., and Massague, J. 1999. A mechanism of repression of TGFbeta/ Smad signaling by oncogenic Ras. *Genes Dev* **13**: 804–816.

Lai, E.C. 2002. Protein degradation: four E3s for the notch pathway. *Curr Biol* **12**: R74–R78.

Laird, P.W., Jackson-Grusby, L., Fazell, A., Dickinson, S.L., Jung, W.E., Li, E., Weinberg, R.A., and Jaenisch, R. 1995. Suppression of intestinal neoplasia by DNA hypomethylation. *Cell* **81**: 197–205.

Larsson, S.C., Kumlin, M., Ingelman-Sundberg, M., and Wolk, A. 2004. Dietary long-chain n-3 fatty acids for the prevention of cancer: a review of potential mechanisms. *Am J Clin Nutr* **79**: 935–945.

Lefebvre, A.-M., Chen, I., Desreumaux, P., Najib, J., Fruchart, J.-C., Geboes, K., Briggs, M., Heyman, R., and Auwerx, J. 1998. Activation of the peroxisome proliferator-activated receptor gamma promotes the development of colon tumors in C57BL/6J-ApcMin/+mice. *Nat Med* **4**: 1053–1057.

Leow, C.C., Romero, M.S., Ross, S., Polakis, P., and Gao, W.Q. 2004. Hath1, down-regulated in colon adenocarcinomas, inhibits proliferation and tumorigenesis of colon cancer cells. *Cancer Res* **64**: 6050–6057.

Lickert, H., Domon, C., Huls, G., Wehrle, C., Duluc, I., Clevers, H., Meyer, B., Freund, J., and Kemler, R. 2000. Wnt/(beta)-catenin signaling regulates the expression of the homeobox gene Cdx1 in embryonic intestine. *Development* **127**: 3805–3813.

Lipkin, M., Blattner, W.E., Fraumeni, J.F., Lynch, H.T., Deschner, E., and Winawer, S. 1983. Tritiated thymidine (0p,0h)labeling distribution as a marker for hereditary predisposition to colon cancer. *Cancer Res* **43**: 1899–1904.

Logeat, F., Bessia, C., Brou, C., LeBail, O., Jarriault, S., Seidah, N.G., and Israel, A. 1998. The Notch1 receptor is cleaved constitutively by a furin-like convertase. *Proc Natl Acad Sci USA* **95**: 8108–8112.

Lohnes, D. 2003. The Cdx1 homeodomain protein: an integrator of posterior signaling in the mouse. *Bioessays* **10**: 971–980.

Lorentz, O., Cadoret, A., Duluc, I., Capeau, J., Gespach, C., Cherqui, G., and Freund, J.N. 1999. Downregulation of the colon tumour-suppressor homeobox gene Cdx-2 by oncogenic ras. *Oncogene* **18**: 87–92.

Lynch, H.T., and Krush, A.J. 1971. Cancer family G revisited: 1895–1970. *Cancer* **27**: 1505–1511.

Lynch, J., Suh, E.R., Silberg, D.G., Rulyak, S., Blanchard, N., and Traber, P.G. 2000. The caudal-related homeodomain protein Cdx1 inhibits proliferation of intestinal epithelial cells by down-regulation of D-type cyclins. *J Biol Chem* **275**: 4499–4506.

Lynch, J., Keller, M., Guo, R.J., Yang, D., and Traber, P. 2003. Cdx1 inhibits the proliferation of human colon cancer cells by reducing cyclin D1 gene expression. *Oncogene* **22**: 6395–6407.

Mahyar-Roemer, M., and Roemer, K. 2001. p21 Waf1/Cip1 can protect human colon carcinoma cells against p53-dependent and p53-independent apoptosis induced by natural chemopreventive and therapeutic agents. *Oncogene* **20**: 3387–3398.

Maihofner, C., Charalambous, M., Bhambra, U., Lightfoot, T., Geisslinger, G., and Gooderham, N. 2003. Expression of cyclooxygenase-2 parallels expression of interleukin-1beta, interleukin-6 and NF-kappaB in human colorectal cancer. *Carcinogenesis* **24**: 665–671.

Malis, C.D., Weber, P.C., Leaf, A., and Bonventre, J.V. 1990. Incorporation of marine lipids into mitochondrial membranes increases susceptibility to damage by calcium and reactive oxygen species: evidence for enhanced activation of phospholipase A2 in mitochondria enriched with n-3 fatty acids. *Proc Natl Acad Sci USA* **87**: 8845–8849.

Mallo, G.V., Rechreche, H., Frigerio, J.M., Rocha, D., Zweibaum, A., Lacasa, M., Jordan, B.R., Dusetti, N.J., Dagorn, J.C., and Iovanna, J.L. 1997. Molecular cloning, sequencing and expression of the mRNA encoding human Cdx1 and Cdx2 homeobox. Down-regulation of Cdx1 and Cdx2 mRNA expression during colorectal carcinogenesis. *Int J Cancer* **74**: 35–44.

Mallo, G.V., Soubeyran, P., Lissitzky, J.-C., Andre, F., Farnarier, C., Marvaldi, J., Dagorn, J.-C., and Iovanna, J.L. 1998. Expression of the Cdx1 and Cdx2 homeotic genes leads to reduced malignancy in colon cancer–derived cells. *J Biol Chem* **273**: 14030–14036.

Malumbres, M., and Barbacid, M. 2001. To cycle or not to cycle: a critical decision in cancer. *Nat Rev Cancer* **1**: 222–231.

Mariadason, J.M., Rickard, K.L., Barkla, D.H., Augenlicht, L.H., and Gibson, P.R. 2000a. Divergent phenotypic patterns and commitment to apoptosis of Caco-2 cells during spontaneous and butyrate-induced differentiation. *J Cell Physiol* **183**: 347–354.

Mariadason, J.M., Corner, G.A., and Augenlicht, L.H. 2000b. Genetic reprogramming in pathways of colonic cell maturation induced by short chain fatty acids: comparison with trichostatin A, sulidac, and curcumin and implications for chemoprevention of colon cancer. *Cancer Res* **60**: 4561–4572.

Mariadason, J.M., Bordonaro, M., Aslam, F., Shi, L., Kuraguchi, M., Velcich, A., and Augenlicht, L.H. 2001. Down-regulation of β-catenin-TCF signaling is linked to colonic epithelial cell differentiation. *Cancer Res* **61**: 3465–3471.

Mariadason, J.M., Arango, D., Corner, G.A., Aranes, M.J., Hotchkiss, K.A., Yang, W.C., and Augenlicht, L.H. 2002. A gene expression profile that defines colon cell maturation *in vitro*. *Cancer Res* **62**: 4791–4804.

Mariadason, J.M., Arango, D., Shi, Q., Wilson, A.J., Corner, G.A., Nicholas, C., Aranes, M.J., Lesser, M., Schwartz, E.L., and Augenlicht, L.H. 2003. Gene expression profiling-based prediction of response of colon carcinoma cells to chemotherapeutic agents. *Cancer Res* **63**: 8791–8812.

Mariadason, J., Nicholas, C., L'Italien, K., Zhuang, M., Smartt, H., Heerdt, B., Yang, W., Corner, G., Wilson, A., Klampfer, L., Arango, D., and Augenlicht, L. 2005. Gene expression profiling of intestinal epithelial cell maturation along the crypt-villus axis. *Gastroenterology* **128**: 1081–1088.

Markowitz, S., Wang, J., Myeroff, L., Parsons, R., Sun, L., Lutterbaugh, J., Fan, R.S., Zborowska, E., Kinzler, K.W., Vogelstein, B., Brattain, M., and Willson, J.K.V. 1995. Inactivation of the type II TGF-B receptor in colon cancer cells with microsatellite instability. *Science* **268**: 1336–1338.

Marks, P., Rifkind, R., Richon, V., Breslow, R., Miller, T., and Kelley, W. 2001. Histone deacetylases and cancer: causes and therapies. *Nat Rev Cancer* **1**: 194–202.

Martinez-Balbas, M., Bauer, U., Nielsen, S., Brehm, A., and Kouzarides, T. 2000. Regulation of E2F1 actrivity by acetylation. *EMBO J* **19**: 662–671.

Mason, J.B., and Choi, S.W. 2000. Folate and carcinogenesis: developing a unifying hypothesis. *Adv Enzyme Regul* **40**: 127–141.

Massague, J. 2004. G1 cell-cycle control and cancer. *Nature* **432**: 298–306.

May, M., and Ghosh, S. 1997. Rel/NF-κB and IκB proteins: an overview. *Semin Cancer Biol* **8**: 63–73.

McBain, J., Eastman, A., Nobel, C., and Mueller, G. 1997. Apoptotic cell death in adenocarcinoma cell lines induced by butyrate and other histone deacetylase inhibitors. *Biochem Pharmacol* **53**: 1357–1368.

McKinsey, T., Zhang, C., Lu, J., and Olsen, E. 2000. Signal-dependent nuclear export of a histone deacetylase regulates muscle differentiation. *Nature* **408**: 106–111.

Meterissian, S., Kontogiannea, M., Murty, H., and Gupta, A. 2000. Omega-6 fatty acids can inhibit Fas-mediated apoptosis in a human colorectal carcinoma cell line: a potential mechanism for escape from immune surveillance. *Int J Surg Invest* **2**: 253–257.

Michalik, L., Desvergne, B., and Wahli, W. 2004. Peroxisome-proliferator-activated receptors and cancers: complex stories. *Nat Rev Cancer* **4**: 61–70.

Milano, J., McKay, J., Dagenais, C., Foster-Brown, L., Pognan, F., Gadient, R., Jacobs, R.T., Zacco, A., Greenberg, B., and Ciaccio, P.J. 2004. Modulation of notch processing by gamma-secretase inhibitors causes intestinal goblet cell metaplasia and induction of genes known to specify gut secretory lineage differentiation. *Toxicol Sci* **82**: 341–358.

Millan, O., Ballester, A., Castrillo, A., Oliva, J.L., Traves, P.G., Rojas, J.M., and Bosca, L. 2003. H-Ras–specific activation of NF-kappaB protects NIH 3T3 cells against stimulus-dependent apoptosis. *Oncogene* **22**: 477–483.

Miska, E., Karlsson, C., Langley, E., Nielsen, S., Pines, J., and Kouzarides, T. 1999. HDAC4 deacetylase associaes with and represses the MEF2 transcription factor. *EMBO J* **18**: 5099–5107.

Miska, E., Langley, E., Wolf, D., Karlsson, C., Pines, J., and Kouzarides, T. 2001. Differential localization fo HDAC4 orchestrates muscle differentiation. *Nucleic Acids Res* **29**: 3439–3447.

Modica-Napolitano, J.S., Steele, G.D., and Chen, L.B. 1989. Aberrant mitochondria in two human colon carcinoma cell lines. *Cancer Res* **49**: 3369–3373.

Molkentin, J.D. 2000. The zinc finger–containing transcription factors GATA-4, -5, and -6. Ubiquitously expressed regulators of tissue-specific gene expression. *J Biol Chem* **275**: 38949–38952.

Morin, P.J., Vogelstein, B., and Kinzler, K.W. 1996. Apoptosis and APC in colorectal tumorigenesis. *Proc Natl Acad Sci USA* **93**: 7950–7954.

Morin, P.J., Sparks, A.B., Korinek, V., Barker, N., Clevers, H., Vogelstein, B., and Kinzler, K.W. 1997. Activation of β-catenin-Tcf signaling in colon cancer by mutations in β-catenin or APC. *Science* **275**: 1787–1790.

Moucadel, V., Soubeyran, P., Vasseur, S., Dusetti, N.J., Dagorn, J.C., and Iovanna, J.L. 2001. Cdx1 promotes cellular growth of epithelial intestinal cells through induction of the secretory protein PAP I. *Eur J Cell Biol* **80**: 156–163.

Mumm, J.S., Schroeter, E.H., Saxena, M.T., Griesemer, A., Tian, X., Pan, D.J., Ray, W.J., and Kopan, R.A. 2000. Ligand-induced extracellular cleavage regulates gamma-secretase-like proteolytic activation of Notch1. *Mol Cell* **5**: 197–206.

Munshi, N., Merika, M., Yie, J., Senger, K., Chen, G., and Thanos, D. 1998. Acetylation of HMGI(Y) by CBP turns off IFN beta expression by disrupting teh enhancesome. *Mol Cell* **2**: 457–467.

Naishiro, Y., Yamada, T., Takaoka, A.S., Hayashi, R., Hasegawa, F., Imai, K., and Hirohashi, S. 2001. Restoration of epithelial cell polarity in a colorectal cancer cell line by suppression of β-catenin/T-cell factor 4–mediated gene transactivation. *Cancer Res* **61**: 2751–2758.

Nalca, A., Qiu, S.G., El-Guendy, N., Krishnan, S., and Rangnekar, V.M. 1999. Oncogenic Ras sensitizes cells to apoptosis by Par-4. *J Biol Chem* **274**: 29976–29983.

Nam, Y., Weng, A.P., Aster, J.C., and Blacklow, S.C. 2003. Structural requirements for assembly of the CSL intracellular Notch1 Mastermind-like 1 transcriptional activation complex. *J Biol Chem* **278**: 21232–21239.

Nebbioso, A., Clarke, N., Voltz, E., Germain, E., Ambrosino, C., Bontempo, P., Alvarez, R., Schiavone, E., Ferrara, F., Bresciani, F., Weisz, A., de Lera, A., Gronemeyer, H., and Altucci, L. 2005. Tumor-selective action of HDAC inhibitors involves TRAIL induction in acute myeloid leukemia cells. *Nat Med* **11**: 77–84.

Nelson, R.L., Tanure, J.C., Andrianopoulos, G., Souza, G., and Lands, W.E. 1988. A comparison of dietary fish oil and corn oil in experimental colorectal carcinogenesis. *Nutr Cancer* **11**: 215–220.

Nguyen, C., Liang, G., Nguyen, T., Tsao-Wei, D., Groshen, S., Lubbert, M., Zhou, J., Benedict, W.F., and Jones, P. 2001. Susceptibility of nonpromoter CpG islands to de novo methylation in normal and neoplastic cells. *J Natl Cancer Instit* **93**: 1465–1472.

Nickoloff, B., Osborne, B.A., and Miele, L. 2003. Notch signaling as a therapeutic target in cancer: a new approach to the development of cell fate modifying agents. *Oncogene* **22**: 6596–6608.

Notterman, D.A., Alon, U., Sierk, A.J., and Levine, A.J. 2001. Transcriptional gene expression profiles of colorectal adenoma, adenocarcinoma, and normal tissue examined by oligonucleotide arrays. *Cancer Res* **61**: 3124–3130.

Oh, E.J., Park, J.H., Cho, M., Lee, W.J., Choi, Y.H., and Yoo, M.A. 2002. The caudal-related homeodomain protein CDX1 activates proliferating cell nuclear antigen expression in hepatocellular and colorectal carcinoma cells. *Int J Oncol* **20**: 23–29.

Ohmori, M., Shirasawa, S., Furuse, M., Okumura, K., and Sasazuki, T. 1997. Activated Ki-ras enhances sensitivity of ceramide-induced apoptosis without c-Jun NH2-terminal kinase/stress-activated protein kinase or extracellular signal-regulated kinase activation in human colon cancer cells. *Cancer Res* **57**: 4714–4717.

Okochi, M., Steiner, H., Fukumori, A., Tanii, H., Tomita, T., Tanaka, T., Iwatsubo, T., Kudo, T., Takeda, M., and Haass, C. 2002. Presenilins mediate a dual intramembranous gamma-secretase cleavage of Notch-1. *EMBO J* **21**: 5408–5416.

Ostrander, D.B., Sparagna, G.C., Amoscato, A.A., McMillin, J.B., and Dowhan, W. 2001. Decreased cardiolipin synthesis corresponds with cytochrome *c* release in palmitate-induced cardiomyocyte apoptosis. *J Biol Chem* **276**: 38061–38067.

Ott, M., Robertson, J.D., Gogvadze, V., Zhivotovsky, B., and Orrenius, S. 2002. Cytochrome *c* release from mitochondria proceeds by a two-step process. *Proc Natl Acad Sci USA* **99**: 1259–1263.

Pahl, H. 1999. Activators and target genes of Rel/NF-κB transcription factors. *Oncogene* **18**: 6853–6866.

Pai, R., Soreghan, B., Szabo, I., Pavelka, M., Baatar, D., and Tarnawski, A. 2002. Prostaglandine E_2 transactivates EGF receptor: a novel mechanism for promoting colon cancer growth and gastrointestinal hyperthrophy. *Nat Med* **8**: 289–293.

Palmqvist, R., Stenling, R., Oberg, A., and Landberg, G. 1999. Prognostic significance of p27Kip1 expression in colorectal cancer: a clinico-pathological characterization. *J Pathol* **188**: 18–23.

Park, B.H., Vogelstein, B., and Kinzler, K.W. 2001. Genetic disruption of PPARdelta decreases the tumorigenicity of human colon cancer cells. *Proc Natl Acad Sci USA* **98**: 2598–2603.

Pasche, B., Kolachana, P., Nafa, K., Satagopan, J., Chen, Y.G., Lo, R.S., Brener, D., Yang, D., Kirstein, L., Oddoux, C., Ostrer, H., Vineis, P., Varesco, L., Jhanwar, S., Luzzatto, L., Massague, J., and Offit, K. 1999. TbetaR-I(6A) is a candidate tumor susceptibility allele. *Cancer Res* **59**: 5678–5682.

Pasche, B., Kaklamani, V., Hou, N., Young, T., Rademaker, A., Peterlongo, P., Ellis, N., Offit, K., Caldes, T., Reiss, M., and Zheng, T. 2004. TGFBR1*6A and cancer: a meta-analysis of 12 case–control studies. *J Clin Oncol* **22**: 756–758.

Patel, L., Pass, I., Coxon, P., Downes, C., Smith, S., and Macphee, C. 2001. Tumor suppressor and anti-inflammatory actions of PPARgamma agonists are mediated via upregulation of PTEN. *Curr Biol* **11**: 764–768.

Paulsen, J.E., Elvsaas, I.K., Steffensen, I.L., and Alexander, J. 1997. A fish oil derived concentrate enriched in eicosapentaenoic and docosahexaenoic acid as ethyl ester suppresses the formation and growth of intestinal polyps in the Min mouse. *Carcinogenesis* 18: 1905–1910.

Petcherski, A.G., and Kimble, J. 2000. LAG-3 is a putative transcriptional activator in the C. elegans Notch pathway. *Nature* **405**: 364–368.

Peterson, C.L., and Laniel, M. 2004. Histones and histone modifications. *Curr Biol* **14**: R546–R551.

Philipp-Staheli, J., Kim, K.-H., Payne, S.R., Gurley, K.E., Liggitt, D., Longton, G., and Kemp, C.J. 2002. Pathway-specific tumor suppression: reduction of p27 accelerates gastrointestinal tumorigenesis in Apc mutant mice, but not in Smad3 mutant mice. *Cancer Cell* **1**: 355–368.

Piccotti, L., Buratta, M., Giannini, S., Gresele, P., Roberti, R., and Corazzi, L. 2004. Binding and release of cytochrome *c* in brain mitochondria is influenced by membrane potential and hydrophobic interactions with cardiolipin. *J Membr Biol* **198**: 43–53.

Pogribny, I.P., Pogribna, M., Christman, J.K., and James, S.J. 2000. Single-site methylation within the p53 promoter region reduces gene expression in a reporter gene construct: possible *in vivo* relevance during tumorigenesis. *Cancer Res* **60**: 588–594.

Pogribny, I.P., and James, S.J. 2002. Reduction of p53 gene expression in human primary hepatocellular carcinoma is associated with promoter region methylation without coding region mutation. *Cancer Lett* **176**: 169–174.

Poot, M., Hosier, S., and Swisshelm, K. 2002. Distinct patterns of mitochondrial changes precede induction of apoptosis by all-trans-retinoic acid and N-(4-hydroxyphenyl)retinamide in MCF7 breast cancer cells. *Exp Cell Res* **279**: 128–140.

Preston, S., Miller, G., and Primrose, J. 1996. Bombesin-like peptides and cancer. *Crit Rev Oncol Hematol* **23**: 225–238.

Pretlow, T.P., Siddiki, B., Augenlicht, L.H., Pretlow, T.G., and Kim, Y.S. 1999. Aberrant crypt foci (ACF)—earliest recognized players or innocent bystanders in colon carcinogenesis. *In* "Colorectal Cancer: Molecular Mechanisms, Premalignant State, and Its Prevention" (W. Schmiegel, Ed.). Kluwer Academic Publishers, Lancaster, England.

Pretlow, T.P., and Bird, R.P. 2001. Correspondence re: Y. Yamada et al., Frequent β-catenin gene mutations and accumulations of the protein in the putative preneoplastic lesions lacking macroscopic aberrant crypt foci appearance, in rat colon carcinogenesis. *Cancer Res* **60**: 3323–3327, 2000 and sequential analysis of morphological and biological properties of β-catenin–accumulated crypts, provable premalignant lesions independent of aberrant crypt foci in rat colon carcinogenesis. *Cancer Res* **61**: 1874–1878.

Quaroni, A., Tian, J.Q., Seth, P., and Ap Rhys, C. 2000. p27(Kip1) is an inducer of intestinal epithelial cell differentiation. *Am J Physiol Cell Physiol* **279**: C1045–1057.

Radke, F., and Raj, K. 2003. The role of Notch in tumorigenesis: oncogene or tumour suppressor? *Nat Rev Cancer* **3**: 756–767.

Rajagopalan, H., Bardelli, A., Lengauer, C., Kinzler, K.W., Vogelstein, B., and Velculescu, V.E. 2002. Tumorigenesis: RAF/RAS oncogenes and mismatch-repair status. *Nature* **418**: 934.

Ramos, K.L., and Colquhoun, A. 2003. Protective role of glucose-6-phosphate dehydrogenase activity in the metabolic response of C6 rat glioma cells to polyunsaturated fatty acid exposure. *Glia* **43**: 149–166.

Rand, M.D., Grimm, L.M., Artavanis-Tsakonas, S., Patriub, V., Blacklow, S.C., Sklar, J., and Aster, J.C. 2000. Calcium depletion dissociates and activates heterodimeric notch receptors. *Mol Cell Biol* **20**: 1825–1835.

Rao, C.V., Hirose, Y., Indranie, C., and Reddy, B.S. 2001. Modulation of experimental colon tumorigenesis by types and amounts of dietary fatty acids. *Cancer Res* **61**: 1927–1933.

Rayman, J., Takahasi, Y., Indjeian, V., Dannenberg, J., Catchpole, S., Watson, R., te Riele, H., and Dynlacht, B. 2002. E2F mediates cell cycle-dependent transcriptional repression *in vivo* by recruitment of an HCAC1, mSin3B corepressor complex. *Genes Dev* **16**: 933–947.

Rebollo, A., and Martinez, A.C. 1999. Ras proteins: recent advances and new functions. *Blood* **94**: 2971–2980.

Richon, V., Sandhoff, T., Rifkind, R., and Marks, P. 2000. Histone deacetylase inhibitor selectively induces p21WAF1 expression and gene-associated histone acetylation. *Proc Natl Acad Sci USA* **97**: 10014–10019.

Rings, E., Boudreau, F., Taylor, J., Moffett, J., Suh, E., and Traber, P. 2001. Phosphorylation of the serine 60 residue within the Cdx2 activation domain mediates its transactivation capacity. *Gastroenterology* **121**: 1437–1450.

Robblee, N.M., and Clandinin, M.T. 1984. Effect of dietary fat level and polyunsaturated fatty acid content on the phospholipid composition of rat cardiac mitochondrial membranes and mitochondrial ATPase activity. *J Nutr* **114**: 263–269.

Robyr, D., Suka, Y., Xenarios, I., Kurdistani, S., Wang, A., Suka, N., and Gurunstein, J. 2002. Microarray deacetylation maps determine genome-wide functions for yeast histone deacetylases. *Cell* **109**: 437–446.

Roediger, W.E. 1980. Role of anaerobic bacteria in the metabolic welfare of the colonic mucosa in man. *Gut* **21**: 793–798.

Roediger, W.E.W. 1982. Utilization of metabolic fuels by the colonic mucosa. *Gastroenterology* **83**: 424–429.

Roediger, W.E.W. 1988. Bacterial short-chain fatty acids and mucosal diseases of the colon. *Br J Surg* **75**: 346–348.

Rubinfeld, B., Souza, B., Albert, I., Muller, O., Chamberlain, S.H., Masiarz, F.R., Munemitsu, S., and Polakis, P. 1993. Association of the APC gene product with β-catenin. *Science* **262**: 1731–1734.

Rubinfeld, B., Albert, I., Porfiri, E., Fiol, C., Munemitsu, S., and Polakis, P. 1996. Binding of GSK3b to the APC-β–catenin complex and regulation of complex assembly. *Science* **272**: 1023–1026.

Rubinfeld, B., Albert, I., Porfiri, E., Munemitsu, S., and Polakis, P. 1997. Loss of β-catenin regualtion by the APC tumor suppressor protein correlates with loss of structure due to common somatic mutations of the gene. *Cancer Res* **57**: 4624–4630.

Saez, E., Tontonoz, P., Nelson, M.C., Alvarez, J.G.A., U, T.M., Baird, S.M., Thomazy, V.A., and Evans, R.M. 1998. Activators of the nuclear receptor PPARγ enhance colon polyp formation. *Nature Med* **4**: 1058–1061.

Sakanaka, C., Weiss, J., and Williams, L. 1998. Bridging of β-catenin and glycogen sythase kinase-3B by axin and inhibition of β-catenin–mediated transcription. *Proc Natl Acad Sci USA* **95**: 3020–3023.

Sander, G.R., and Powell, B.C. 2004. Expression of notch receptors and ligands in the adult gut. *J Histochem Cytochem* **52**: 509–516.

Sanders, L.M., Henderson, C.E., Hong, M.Y., Barhoumi, R., Burghardt, R.C., Wang, N., Spinka, C.M., Carroll, R.J., Turner, N.D., Chapkin, R.S., and Lupton, J.R. 2004. An increase in reactive oxygen species by dietary fish oil coupled with the attenuation of antioxidant defenses by dietary pectin enhances rat colonocyte apoptosis. J Nutr **134**: 3233–3238.

Santoro, I.M., and Groden, J. 1997. Alternative splicing of the APC gene and its association with terminal differentiation. *Cancer Res* **57**: 488–494.

Sarraf, P., Mueller, E., Jones, D., King, F.J., DeAngelo, D.J., Partridge, J.B., Holden, S.A., Chen, L.B., Singer, S., Fletcher, C., and Spiegelman, B.M. 1998. Differentiation and reversal of malignant changes in colon cancer through PPARgamma. *Nat Med* **4**: 1046–1052.

Sarraf, P., Muelle, E., Smith, W., Wright, H., Kum, J., Aaltonen, L., de la Chapelle, A., Spiegelman, B., and Eng, C. 1999. Loss-of-function mutations in PPAR gamma associated with human colon cancer. *Mol Cell* **3**: 799–804.

Schlame, M., Beyer, K., Hayer-Hartl, M., and Klingenberg, M. 1991. Molecular species of cardiolipin in relation to other mitochondrial phospholipids. Is there an acyl specificity of the interaction between cardiolipin and the ADP/ATP carrier? *Eur J Biochem* **199**: 459–466.

Schlame, M., Brody, S., and Hostetler, K.Y. 1993. Mitochondrial cardiolipin in diverse eukaryotes. Comparison of biosynthetic reactions and molecular acyl species. *Eur J Biochem* **212**: 727–735.

Schroder, N., and Gossler, A. 2002. Expression of Notch pathway components in fetal and adult mouse small intestine. *Gene Expr Patterns* **2**: 247–250.

Schroeter, E.H., Kisslinger, J.A., and Kopan, R. 1998. Notch-1 signalling requires ligand-induced proteolytic release of intracellular domain. *Nature* **393**: 382–386.

Schulz, H. 1985. Oxidation of fatty acids. *In* "Biochemistry of Lipids and Membranes" (D.E. Vance and J.E. Vance, Eds.), pp. 116–142. Benjamin/Cummings Publishing Co., Reading, MA.

Schutte, M., Hruban, R.H., Hedrick, L., Cho, K.R., Nadasdy, G.M., Weinstein, C.L., Bova, G.S., Isaacs, W.B., Cairns, P., Nawroz, H., Sidransky, D., Casero, R.A., Jr., Meltzer, P.S., Hahn, S.A., and Kern, S.E. 1996. DPC4 gene in various tumor types. *Cancer Res* 56: 2527–2530.

Sealy, L., and Chalkley, R. 1978. The effect of sodium butyrate on histone modification. *Cell* **14**: 115–121.

Sebat, J., Lakshmi, B., Troge, J., Alexander, J., Young, J., Lundin, P., Maner, S., Massa, H., Walker, M., Chi, M., Navin, N., Lucito, R., Healy, J., Hicks, J., Ye, K., Reiner, A., Gilliam, T.C., Trask, B., Patterson, N., Zetterberg, A., and Wigler, M. 2004. Large-scale copy number polymorphism in the human genome. *Science* **305**: 525–528.

Sebolt-Leopold, J.S., Dudley, D.T., Herrera, R., Van Becelaere, K., Wiland, A., Gowan, R.C., Tecle, H., Barrett, S.D., Bridges, A., Przybranowski, S., Leopold, W.R., and Saltiel, A.R. 1999. Blockade of the MAP kinase pathway suppresses growth of colon tumors *in vivo*. *Nat Med* **5**: 810–816.

Sebolt-Leopold, J.S., and Herrera, R. 2004. Targeting the mitogen-activated protein kinase cascade to treat cancer. *Nat Rev Cancer* **4**: 937–947.

Selaru, F.M., Xu, Y., Yin, J., Zou, T., Liu, T.C., Mori, Y., Abraham, J.M., Sato, F., Wang, S., Twigg, C., Olaru, A., Shustova, V., Leytin, A., Hytiroglou, P., Shibata, D., Harpaz, N., and Meltzer, S.J. 2002. Artificial neural networks distinguish among subtypes of neoplastic colorectal lesions. *Gastroenterology* **122**: 606–613.

Sen, R., and Baltimore, D. 1986. Multiple nuclear factors interact with the immunoglobulin enhancer sequences. *Cell* **46**: 705–716.

Sevignani, C., Wlodarski, P., Kirillova, J., Mercer, W.E., Danielson, K.G., Iozzo, R.V., and Calabretta, B. 1998. Tumorigenic conversion of p53-deficient colon epithelial cells by an activated Ki-ras gene. *J Clin Invest* **101**: 1572–1580.

Shachaf, C.M., Kopelman, A.M., Arvanitis, C., Karlsson, A., Beer, S., Mandl, S., Bachmann, M.H., Borowsky, A.D., Ruebner, B., Cardiff, R.D., Yang, Q., Bishop, J.M., Contag, C.H., and Felsher, D.W. 2004. MYC inactivation uncovers pluripotent differentiation and tumour dormancy in hepatocellular cancer. *Nature* **431**: 1112–1117.

Shao, J., Sheng, H., and DuBois, R.N. 2002. Peroxisome proliferator-activated receptors modulate K-Ras–mediated transformation of intestinal epithelial cells. *Cancer Res* **62**: 3282–3288.

Sheng, H., Shao, J., and DuBois, R.N. 2001. K-Ras–mediated increase in cyclooxygenase 2 mRNA stability involves activation of the protein kinase B. *Cancer Res* **61**: 2670–2675.

Sherr, C.J., and Roberts, J.M. 1999. CDK inhibitors: positive and negative regulators of G1-phase progression. *Genes Dev* **13**: 1501–1512.

Sherr, C.J. 2000. The Pezcoller lecture: cancer cell cycles revisited. *Cancer Res* **60**: 3689–3695.

Shibata, D., Navidi, W., Salovaara, R., Li, Z.-H., and Aaltonen, L.A. 1996. Somatic microsatellite mutations as molecular tumor clocks. *Nat Med* **2**: 676–681.

Shields, J.M., Pruitt, K., McFall, A., Shaub, A., and Der, C.J. 2000. Understanding Ras: "it ain't over 'til it's over.'" *Trends Cell Biol* **10**: 147–154.

Shih, I.M., Yu, J., He, T.C., Vogelstein, B., and Kinzler, K.W. 2000. The beta-catenin binding domain of adenomatous polyposis coli is sufficient for tumor suppression. *Cancer Res* **60**: 1671–1676.

Shirasawa, S., Furuse, M., Yokoyama, N., and Sasazuki, T. 1993. Altered growth of human colon cancer cell lines disrupted at activated Ki-ras. *Science* **260**: 85–88.

Shtutman, M., Zhurinsky, J., Simcha, I., Albanese, C., D'Amico, M., Pestell, R., and Ben-Ze'ev, A. 1999. The cyclin D1 gene is a target of the β-catenin/LEF-1 pathway. *Proc Natl Acad Sci USA* **96**: 5522–5527.

Siddiqui, R.A., Shaikh, S.R., Sech, L.A., Yount, H.R., Stillwell, W., and Zaloga, G.P. 2004. Omega 3-fatty acids: health benefits and cellular mechanisms of action. *Mini Rev Med Chem* **4**: 859–871.

Siegel, P.M., and Massague, J. 2003. Cytostatic and apoptotic actions of TGF-beta in homeostasis and cancer. *Nat Rev Cancer* **3**: 807–821.

Sikora, A., Chan, S., Evan, G., Gabra, H., Markham, N., Stewart, J., and Watson, J. 1987. c-myc oncogene expression in colorectal cancer. *Cancer* **59**: 1289–1295.

Silberg, D., Furth, E., Taylor, J., Schuck, T., Chiou, T., and Traber, P. 1997. CDX1 protein expression in normal, metaplastic, and neoplastic human alimentary tract epithelium. *Gastroenterology* **113**: 478–486.

Silberg, D., Swain, G., Suh, E., and Traber, P. 2000. Cdx1 and cdx2 expression during intestinal development. *Gastroenterology* **119**: 961–971.

Silberg, D., Sullivan, J., Kang, E., Swain, G., Moffett, J., Sund, N., Sackett, S., and KH, K. 2002. Cdx2 ectopic expression induces gastric intestinal metaplasia in transgenic mice. *Gastroenterology* **122**: 689–696.

Silverman, A., Park, J., Hamilton, S., Gazdar, A., Luk, G.D., and Baylin, S. 1989. Abnormal methylation of the calcitonin gene in human colonic neoplasms. *Cancer Res* **49**: 3468–3473.

Skipper, M., and Lewis, J. 2000. Getting to the guts of enteroendocrine differentiation. *Nat Genet* **24**: 3–4.

Smith, K.J., Johnson, K.A., Bryan, T.M., Hill, D.E., Markowitz, S., Willson, J.K.V., Paraskeva, C., Petersen, G.M., Hamilton, S.R., Vogelstein, B., and Kinzler, K.W. 1993. The APC gene product in normal and tumor cells. *Proc Natl Acad Sci USA* **90**: 2846–2850.

Song, J., Medline, A., Mason, J.B., Gallinger, S., and Kim, Y.I. 2000. Effects of dietary folate on intestinal tumorigenesis in the ApcMin mouse. *Cancer Res* **60**: 5434–5440.

Soubeyran, P., Andre, F., Lissitzky, J.C., Mallo, G.V., Moucadel, V., Roccabianca, M., Rechreche, H., Marvaldi, J., Dikic, I., Dagorn, J.C., and Iovanna, J.L. 1999. Cdx1 promotes differentiation in a rat intestinal epithelial cell line. *Gastroenterology* **117**: 1326–1338.

Strahl, B.D., and Allis, C.D. 2000. The language of covalent histone modifications. *Nature* **403**: 41–45.

Struhl, G., and Greenwald, I. 1999. Presenilin is required for activity and nuclear access of Notch in *Drosophila*. *Nature* **398**: 522–525.

Subramanian, V., Meyer, B., and Evans, G.S. 1998. The murine Cdx1 gene product localises to the proliferative compartment in the developing and regenerating intestinal epithelium. *Differentiation* **64**: 11–18.

Suh, E., and Traber, P.G. 1996. An intestine-specific homeobox gene regulates proliferation and differentiation. *Mol Cell Biol* **16**: 619–625.

Suh, E.R., Ha, C.S., Rankin, E.B., Toyota, M., and Traber, P.G. 2002. DNA methylation down-regulates CDX1 gene expression in colorectal cancer cell lines. *J Biol Chem* **277**: 35795–35800.

Summerhayes, I.C., Lampidis, T.J., Bernal, S.D., Nadakavukaren, J.J., Nadakaukaren, K.K., Shepherd, E.L., and Chen, L.B. 1982. Unusual retention fo rhodamine 123 by mitochondria in muscle and carcinoma cells. *Proc Natl Acad Sci USA* **79**: 5292–5296.

Sun, A.S., Sepkowitz, B.A., and Geller, S.A. 1981. A study of some mitochondrial and peroxisomal enzymes in human colonic adenocarcinoma. *Lab Invest* **44**: 13–17.

Takahashi, M., Fukuda, K., Sugimura, T., and Wakabayashi, K. 1998. β-catenin is frequently mutated and demonstrates altered cellular location in azoxymethane-induced rat colon tumors. *Cancer Res* **58**: 42–46.

Takaku, K., Oshima, M., Miyoshi, H., Matsui, M., Seldin, M.F., and Taketo, M.M. 1998. Intestinal tumorigenesis in compound mutant mice of both Dpc4(Smad4) and Apc genes. *Cell* **92**: 645–656.

Tamai, Y., Nakajima, R., Ishikawa, T.-O., Takaku, K., Seldin, M.F., and Taketo, M.M. 1999. Colonic hamartoma development by anomalous duplication in Cdx2 knockout mice. *Cancer Res* **59**: 2965–2970.

Taylor, W., and Stark, G. 2001. Regulation of the G2/M transition by p53. *Oncogene* **20**: 1803–1815.

Tetsu, O., and McCormick, F. 1999. β-catenin regulates expression of cyclin D1 in colon carcinoma cells. *Nature* **398**: 422–426.

Tomita, A., Towatari, M., Tsuzuki, S., Hayakawa, F., Kosugi, H., Tamai, K., Miyazaki, T., Kinoshita, T., and Saito, H. 2000. c-Myb acetylation at the carboxyl-terminal conserved domain by transcriptional coactivator p300. *Oncogene* **19**: 444–451.

Tong, X., Yin, L., Washington, R., Rosenberg, D., and Giardina, C. 2004. The p50-p50 NF-kappaB complex as a stimulus-specific repressor of gene activation. *Mol Cell Biochem* **265**: 171–183.

Toyota, M., and Issa, J.-P. 1999. CpG island methylator phenotypes in aging and cancer. *Semin Cancer Biol* **9**.

Toyota, M., Ahuja, N., Ohe-Toyota, M., Herman, J.G., Baylin, S., and Issa, J.-P. 1999. CpG island methylator phenotype in colorectal cancer. *Proc Natl Acad Sci USA* **96**: 8661–8686.

Traber, P.G., and Silberg, D.G. 1996. Intestine-specific gene transcription. *Annu Rev Physiol* **58**: 275–297.

Valianpour, F., Wanders, R.J., Overmars, H., Vaz, F.M., Barth, P.G., and van Gennip, A.H. 2003. Linoleic acid supplementation of Barth syndrome fibroblasts restores cardiolipin levels: implications for treatment. *J Lipid Res* **44**: 560–566.

van de Wetering, M., Sancho, E., Verweij, C., de Lau, W., Oving, I., Hurlstone, A., van der Horn, K., Batle, E., Coudreuse, D., Haramis, A.-P., Tjon-Pon-Fong, M., Moerer, P., van den Born, M., Soete, G., Pals, S., Eilers, M., Medema, R., and Clevers, H. 2002. The β-catenin/TCF-4 complex imposes a crypt progenitor phenotype on coloretal cancer cells. *Cell* **111**: 241–250.

van Den Brink, G.R., de Santa Barbara, P., and Roberts, D.J. 2001. Development. Epithelial cell differentiation—a Mather of choice. *Science* **294**: 2115–2116.

van der Sluis, M., Melis, M., Jonckheere, N., Ducourouble, M., Buller, H., Renes, I., Einerhand, A., and Van Seuningen, I. 2004. The murine Muc2 mucin gene is transcriptionally regulated by the zinc-finger GATA-4 transcription factor in intestinal cells. *Biochem Biophys Res Commun* **325**: 952–960.

van Es, J.H., Giles, R.H., and Clevers, H.C. 2001. The many faces of the tumor suppressor gene APC. *Exp Cell Res* **264**: 126–134.

van Wering, H.M., Bosse, T., Musters, A., de Jong, E., de Jong, N., Hogen Esch, C.E., Boudreau, F., Swain, G.P., Dowling, L.N., Montgomery, R.K., Grand, R.J., and Krasinski, S.D. 2004. Complex regulation of the lactase-phlorizin hydrolase promoter by GATA-4. *Am J Physiol Gastrointest Liver Physiol* **287**: G899–G909.

Velcich, A., Corner, G., Paul, D., Laboisse, C., and Augenlicht, L. 2005. Quantitative rather than qualitative differences in gene expression predominate in intestinal cell maturation along distinct lineages. *Exp Cell Res* **304**: 28–39.

Vial, E., and Marshall, C.J. 2003. Elevated ERK-MAP kinase activity protects the FOS family member FRA-1 against proteasomal degradation in colon carcinoma cells. *J Cell Sci* **116**: 4957–4963.

Vider, B., Zimber, A., Hirsch, D., Estlein, D., Chastre, E., Prevot, S., Gespach, C., Yaniv, A., and A, G. 1997. Human colorectal carcinogenesis is associated with deregulation of homeobox gene expression. *Biochem Biophys Res Commun* **232**: 742–748.

Wagenaar, R.A., Crawford, H.C., and Matrisian, L.M. 2001. Stabilized β-catenin immortalizes colonic epithelial cells. *Cancer Res* **61**: 2097–2104.

Wallberg, A.E., Pedersen, K., Lendahl, U., and Roeder, R.G. 2002. p300 and PCAF act cooperatively to mediate transcriptional activation from chromatin templates by notch intracellular domains *in vitro*. *Mol Cell Biol* **22**: 7812–7819.

Waltzer, L., and Bienz, M. 1998. *Drosophila* CBP represses the transcription factor TCF to antagonize Wingless signalling. *Nature* **395**: 521–525.

Wang, A., Bertos, N., Vezmar, M., Pelletier, N., Crosato, M., Heng, H., Th'ng, J., Han, J., and Yang, X. 1999. HDAC4, a human histone deacetylase related to yeast HDA1, is a transcriptional co-repressor. *Mol Cell Biol* **19**: 7816–7827.

Wang, A., Kruhlak, M., Wu, J., Bertos, N., Vezmar, M., Posner, B., Bazett-Jones, D., and Yang, X. 2000. Regulation of histone deacetylase 4 by binding of 14-3-3 proteins. *Mol Cell Biol* **20**: 6904–6912.

Wang, C., Fu, M., D'Amico, M., Albanese, C., Zhou, J.-N., Brownlee, M., Lisanti, M.P., Chatterjee, V.K.K., Lazar, M.A., and Pestell, R.G. 2001. Inhibition of cellular proliferation through IκB kinase–independent and peroxisome proliferator-activated receptor-γ–dependent repression of cyclin D1. *Mol Cell Biol* **21**: 3057–3070.

Wang, D., Wang, H., Shi, Q., Katkuri, S., Walhi, W., Desvergne, B., Das, S.K., Dey, S.K., and DuBois, R.N. 2004. Prostaglandin E2 promotes colorectal adenoma growth via transactivation of the nuclear peroxisome proliferator-activated receptor-δ. *Cancer Cell* **6**: 285–295.

Wang, J., Sun, L., Myeroff, L., Wang, X., Gentry, L.E., Yang, J., Liang, J., Zborowska, E., Markowitz, S., Willson, J.K.V., and Brattain, M.G. 1995. Demonstration that mutation of the type II transforming growth factor beta receptor inactivates its tumor suppressor activity in replication error-positive colon carcinoma cells. *J Biol Chem* **270**: 22044–22049.

Warburg, O. 1956a. On respiratory impairment in cancer cells. *Science* 124: 269–270.

Warburg, O. 1956b. On the origin of cancer cells. *Science* **123**: 309–314.

Warthin, A.S. 1913. Heredity with reference to carcinoma. *Arch Intern Med* **12**: 546–555.

Wasan, H.S., Novelli, M., Bee, J., and Bodmer, W.F. 1997. Dietary fat influences on polyp phenotype in multiple intestinal neoplasia mice. *Proc Natl Acad Sci USA* **94**: 3308–3313.

Watkins, S.M., Carter, L.C., and German, J.B. 1998. Docosahexaenoic acid accumulates in cardiolipin and enhances HT-29 cell oxidant production. *J Lipid Res* **39**: 1583–1588.

Weijzen, S., Rizzo, P., Braid, M., Vaishnav, R., Jonkheer, S.M., Zlobin, A., Osborne, B.A., Gottipati, S., Aster, J.C., Hahn, W.C., Rudolf, M., Siziopikou, K., Kast, W.M., and Miele, L. 2002. Activation of Notch-1 signaling maintains the neoplastic phenotype in human Ras-transformed cells. *Nat Med* **8**: 979–986.

Whiteside, S., Epinat, J.-C., Rice, N., and A, I. 1997a. I kappa B epsilon, a novel member of the IκB family, controls RelA and cRel NF-κB activity. *EMBO J* **16**: 1413–1426.

Whiteside, S., and Israël, A. 1997b. IκB proteins: structure, function and regulation. *Semin Cancer Biol* **8**: 75–82.

Wicking, C., Simms, L., Evans, T., Walsh, M., Chawengsaksophak, K., Beck, F., Chenevix-Trench, G., Young, J., Jass, J., Leggett, B., and Wainwright, B. 1998. CDX2, a human homologue of *Drosophila* caudal, is mutated in both alleles in a replication error positive colorectal cancer. *Oncogene* **17**: 657–659.

Wilson, A.J., Velcich, A., Arango, D., Kurland, A.R., Shenoy, S.M., Pezo, R.C., Levsky, J.M., Singer, R.H., and Augenlicht, L.H. 2002. Novel detection and differential utilization of a c-myc transcriptional block in colon cancer chemoprevention. *Cancer Res* **62**: 6006–6010.

Wilson, V.L., and Jones, P.A. 1983. DNA methylation decreases in aging but not in immortal cells. *Science* **220**: 1055–1057.

Wong, J.R., and Chen, L.B. 1988. Recent advances in the study of mitochondria in living cells. *Adv Cell Biol* **2**: 263–290.

Woodford-Richens, K.L., Rowan, A.J., Gorman, P., Halford, S., Bicknell, D.C., Wasan, H.S., Roylance, R.R., Bodmer, W.F., and Tomlinson, I.P.M. 2001. SMAD4 mutations in colorectal cancer probably occur before chromosomal instability, but after divergence of the microsatellite instability pathway. *PNAS* **98**: 9719–9723.

Wu, B., Iwakiri, R., Ootani, A., Tsunada, S., Fujise, T., Sakata, Y., Sakata, H., Toda, S., and Fujimoto, K. 2004. Dietary corn oil promotes colon cancer by inhibiting mitochondria-dependent apoptosis in azoxymethane-treated rats. *Exp Biol Med (Maywood)* **229**: 1017–1025.

Wu, J., Archer, S.Y., Hinnebusch, B., Meng, S., and Hodin, R.A. 2001. Transient versus prolonged histone hyperacetylation: effects on colon cancer cell growth, differentiation and apoptosis. *Am J Physiol* **280**: G482–490.

Wu, L., Aster, J.C., Blacklow, S.C., Lake, R., Artavanis-Tsakonas, S., and Griffin, J.D. 2000. MAML1, a human homologue of *Drosophila* mastermind, is a transcriptional co-activator for NOTCH receptors. *Nat Genet* **26**: 484–489.

Yamada, Y., Yoshimi, N., Hirose, Y., Kawabata, K., Matsunaga, K., Shimizu, M., Hara, A., and Mori, H. 2000. Frequent β-catenin gene mutations and accumulations of the protein in the putative preneoplastic lesions lacking macroscopic aberrant crypt foci appearance, in rat colon carcinogenesis. *Cancer Res* **60**: 3323–3327.

Yamada, Y., Yoshimi, N., Hirose, Y., Matsunaga, K., Katayama, M., Sakata, K., Shimizu, M., Kuno, T., and Mori, H. 2001. Sequential analysis of morphological and biological properties of β-catenin–accumulated crypts, provable premalignant lesions independent of aberrant crypt foci in rat colon carcinogenesis. *Cancer Res* **61**: 1874–1878.

Yamaoka-Koseki, S., Urade, R., and Kito, M. 1991. Cardiolipins from rats fed different dietary lipids affect bovine heart cytochrome c oxidase activity. *J Nutr* **121**: 956–958.

Yamamoto, H., Soh, J.-W., Shirin, H., Xing, W-Q., Lim, J.TE., Yao, Y., Slosberg, E., Tomita, N., Schieren, I., and Weinstein, I.B. 1999. Comparative effects of overexpression of p27Kip1 and p21Cip1/Waf1 on growth and differentiation in human colon carcinoma cells. *Oncogene* **18**: 103–115.

Yamamoto, H., Bai, Y., and Yuasa, Y. 2003. Homeodomain protein CDX2 regulates goblet-specific MUC2 gene expression. *Biochem Biophys Res Commun* **300**: 813–818.

Yan, P.S., Chen, C.M., Shi, H., Rahmatpanah, F., Wei, S.H., Caldwell, C.W., and Huang, T.H. 2001. Dissecting complex epigenetic alterations in breast cancer using CpG island microarrays. *Cancer Res* **61**: 8375–8380.

Yan, P.S., Chen, C.M., Shi, H., Rahmatpanah, F., Wei, S.H., and Huang, T.H. 2002. Applications of CpG island microarrays for high-throughput analysis of DNA methylation. *J Nutr* **132**: 2430S–2434S.

Yang, Q., Bermingham, N.A., Finegold, M.J., and Zoghbi, H.Y. 2001. Requirement of Math1 for secretory cell lineage commitment in the mouse intestine. *Science* **294**: 2155–2158.

Yang, W., Bancroft, L., Nicholas, C., Lozonschi, I., Augenlicht, L.H. 2003. Targeted inactivation of p27kip1 is sufficient for large and small intestinal tumorigenesis in the mouse, which can be augmented by a Western-style high-risk diet. *Cancer Res* **63**: 4990–4996.

Yang, W., Bancroft, L., and Augenlicht, L. 2005. Methylation in the p21WAF1/cip1 promoter of Apc+/–,p21+/– mice and lack of response to sulindac. *Oncogene* **24**: 2104–2109.

Yang, W.C., Mathew, J., Edelmann, W., Kucherlapati, R., Lipkin, M., Yang, K., and Augenlicht, L.H. 2000. Enhancement of intestinal tumorigenesis in Apc1638 mice by elimination of p21waf1. *Proc Am Assoc Cancer Res*.

Yang, W.C., Velcich, A., Mariadason, J., Nicholas, C., Corner, G., Houston, M., Edelmann, W., Kucherlapati, R., Holt, P., and Augenlicht, L.H. 2001. p21WAF1/cip1 is an important determinant of intestinal cell response to sulindac *in vitro* and *in vivo*. *Cancer Res* **61**: 6297–6302.

Ye, Y., Lukinova, N., and Fortini, M.E. 1999. Neurogenic phenotypes and altered Notch processing in *Drosophila* presenilin mutants. *Nature* **398**: 525–529.

Yoshida, M., Kijima, M., Akita, M., and Beppu, T. 1990. Potent and specific inhibition of mammalian histone deacetylase both *in vivo* and *in vitro* by trichostatin. *J Biol Chem* **265**: 17174–17179.

Yu, H., Yu, L., Yang, Y., Luo, H., Yu, J., Meier, J., Schrader, H., Bastian, A., Schmidt, W., and Schmitz, F. 2003. Increased expression of RelA/nuclear factor-kappa B protein correlates with colorectal tumorigenesis. *Oncology* **65**: 37–45.

Yuasa, Y. 2003. Control of gut differentiation and intestinal-type gastric carcinogenesis. *Nat Rev Cancer* **3**: 592–600.

Yuen, S.T., Davies, H., Chan, T.L., Ho, J.W., Bignell, G.R., Cox, C., Stephens, P., Edkins, S., Tsui, W.W., Chan, A.S., Futreal, P.A., Stratton, M.R., Wooster, R., and Leung, S.Y. 2002. Similarity of the phenotypic patterns associated with BRAF and KRAS mutations in colorectal neoplasia. *Cancer Res* **62**: 6451–6455.

Zhang, T., Nanney, L., Luongo, C., Lamps, L., Heppner, K., DuBois, R., and Beauchamp, R. 1997. Concurrent overexpression of cyclin D1 and cyclin-dependent kinase 4 (Cdk4) in intestinal adenomas from multiple intestinal neoplasia (Min) mice and human familial adenomatous polyposis patients. *Cancer Res* **57**: 169–175.

Zheng, J., Shou, J., Guillemot, F., Kageyama, R., and Gao, W. 2000. Hes1 is a negative regulator of inner ear hair cell differentiation. *Development* **127**: 4551–4560.

Zhu, L., and Skoultchi, A.I. 2001. Coordinating cell proliferation and differentiation. *Curr Opin Genet Dev* **10**: 91–97.

Zhu, P., Martin, E., Mengwasser, J., Schlag, P., Janssen, K.P., and Gottlicher, M. 1998. Induction of HDAC2 expression upon loss of APC in colorectal tumorigenesis. *Cancer Cell* **5**: 455–463, 2004.

Zhu, Y., Richardson, J.A., Parada, L.F., and Graff, J.M. Smad3 mutant mice develop metastatic colorectal cancer. *Cell* **94**: 703–714.

Zou, T.T., Selaru, F.M., Xu, Y., Shustova, V., Yin, J., Mori, Y., Shibata, D., Sato, F., Wang, S., Olaru, A., Deacu, E., Liu, T.C., Abraham, J.M., and Meltzer, S.J. 2002. Application of cDNA microarrays to generate a molecular taxonomy capable of distinguishing between colon cancer and normal colon. *Oncogene* **21**: 4855–4862.

CHAPTER

4

Metabolic Networks in Cancer Cells

LASZLO G. BOROS AND WAI-NANG PAUL LEE

Like other living cells, tumor cells possess the potential for proliferation, differentiation, growth cycle arrest, and apoptosis. There is a specific metabolic phenotype associated with each of these functions. Tumor cells lock themselves into the proliferative state by employing a metabolic network that is dominated by nonoxidative anabolic reactions and macromolecule synthesis. Therefore, their transformation and growth are associated with the activation of intermediary metabolic enzymes that facilitate glucose carbon utilization for nucleic acid synthesis. The metabolic network possesses many control points composed of metabolic enzymes with high control properties on metabolic reactions that sustain malignant cell proliferation and tumor growth.

INTRODUCTION

Decades of intensive research have identified many possible mechanisms for the transformation of normal regulated cells to those with unregulated proliferation characteristic of cancer cells. The cause for development of common human malignancies is multifactorial, which includes tumor-inducing genes, environmental factors, and signal transduction pathways. In the constraint-based model of cell proliferation, these factors constitute genomic, metabolic, and environmental constraints (Figure 1).

The current understanding of malignant cell behavior places heavy emphasis on genetic regulation of human cell functions. Human cancer is thought to arise from a dysregulation of gene expression resulting from the presence of growth-promoting oncogenes or the absence of tumor suppressor genes. Genetic alterations in cancer reported to date include frequent mutations of the K-ras, p53, p16, and Smad4 genes and are reported to be associated with accelerated disease progression and poor prognosis (Sakai et al., 2000; Yatsuoka et al., 2000; Comin et al., 2001; Boros et al., 2002a; Cascante et al., 2002). Genetic abnormalities influencing cellular responses to hormonal growth regulators and their signaling pathways have been reported in connection with all major tumor types (Issa, 2000; Jung and Messing, 2000; Largaespada, 2000; Martin and Weber, 2000; Ozen and Pathak, 2000; Szabo et al., 2000). However, it is well established through molecular genetic studies that in response to environmental changes, nutrition, lifestyle, and age, there is great variation in the expression of human genes, resulting in variability of the phenotypes. Thus, possible mechanisms for the development of common human malignancies include tumor-inducing genes, growth-modulating signal transduction pathways, and nutritional and environmental factors.

The diverse mechanisms of tumor induction have in common their resultant influence on metabolism (altering the respective metabolic constraints), thus altering normal potential for differentiation, cell cycle arrest, and apoptosis. Figure 2 illustrates the transition of cells from one phenotype to another as changes in metabolic solution spaces under proliferation or differentiation signals (constraints). The metabolic network consisting of all functional metabolic pathways gives rise to the "general solution space," which represents all possible metabolic phenotypes (solutions) for the given metabolic network. Environmental and signaling constraints further narrow the space for possible phenotypes of proliferation, differentiation, and apoptosis.

Many potential growth-modulating factors have been identified and characterized through their signal transduc-

Copyright © 2006, Elsevier Inc.
All rights of reproduction in any form reserved.

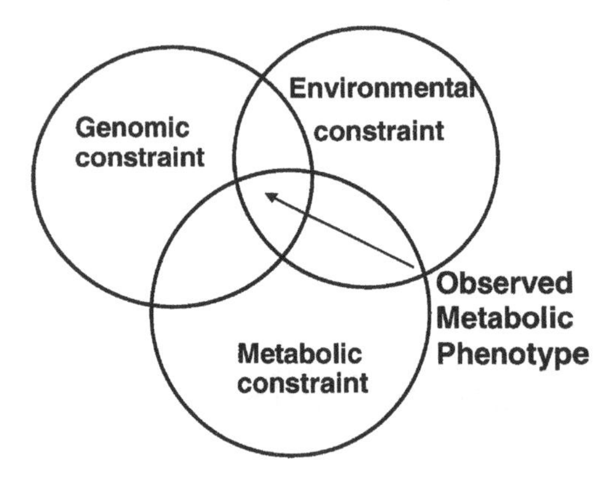

FIGURE 1 Constraint-based model of cell proliferation.

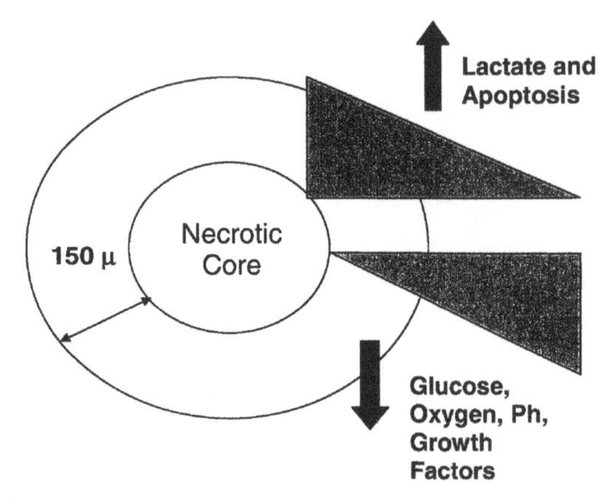

FIGURE 3 Metabolism of tumors is affected by oxygen tension caused by poor blood flow, so lactate *increases*, whereas glucose, oxygen, and pH level *decrease* inside a 150-μ thick well-oxygenated shell.

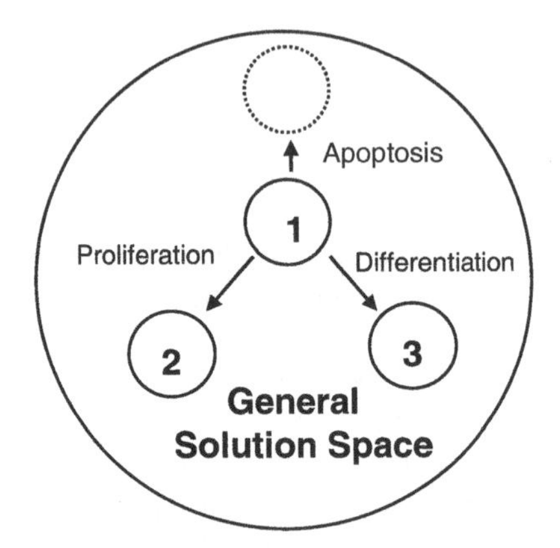

FIGURE 2 Transition of cells from one phenotype to another with changes in metabolic solution spaces under proliferation or differentiation signals (constraints).

tion pathways. These belong to two major signal types: one that acts on intracellular receptors and influences gene expression and the other that acts on cell surface receptors and influences multiple enzyme activities by protein phosphorylation.

Metabolic Alterations in Tumor Tissues

Normal tissues depend on diffusion of oxygen from blood vessels and demonstrate an oxygen gradient across a distance of 400 μ from a blood supply. On the other hand, human tumors and tumor xenografts are hypoxic, and cells adjacent to capillaries have a mean oxygen concentration of 2%. Cells located 200 μ from the nearest capillary have a mean oxygen concentration of only 0.2% (Helmlinger et al., 1997) (Figure 3).

This restrictive environment selects for cells that are adapted to chronic hypoxia. In normal cells, a critical response to hypoxia is the induction of the hypoxia-inducible transcription factor HIF-1 (Wang et al., 1995). Interestingly, HIF-1β is also known as the aryl hydrocarbon receptor nuclear translocator (ARNT) (Wang et al., 1995). HIF-1 binds to the DNA sequence 5′-RCGTG-3′ and increases the expression of genes that encode glycolytic enzymes, including aldolase A, enolase 1, lactate dehydrogenase A (LDH-A), phosphofructokinase L, phosphoglycerate kinase 1, and pyruvate kinase M, as well as the vascular endothelial growth factor (VEGF) gene, which mediates tumor angiogenesis (Firth et al., 1995; Semenza et al., 1996; Carmeliet et al., 1998; Iyer et al., 1998; Ryan et al., 1998).

Changes in glucose concentration can also activate many glycolytic enzyme genes through the carbohydrate-response element (ChoRE; 5′-CACGTG-3′), which matches the consensus binding-site sequences for MYC and HIF-1 (Towle, 1995; Grandori and Eisenman, 1997). Studies of transgenic mice have demonstrated that HIF-1 regulates glycolytic enzyme gene expression via changes in the concentration of cellular oxygen and glucose, respectively (Iyer et al., 1998; Ryan et al., 1998; Vallet et al., 1998). Activation of the HIF-1 pathway may mediate the adaptive responses to hypoxia and hypoglycemia in cancer cells. The activation of oncogenes or loss of tumor suppressors by somatic mutation in tumor cells can also lead directly to nonphysiological alterations of cellular metabolism and provide a selective advantage in hostile metabolic environments. The epigenetic changes and those secondary to metabolic signaling may both mediate the ultimate changes observed in tumor cells when they provide a selective growth advantage.

Elegant studies by Warburg (1930) >70 years ago demonstrate that the vast majority of human and animal tumors display a high rate of glycolysis under aerobic conditions. Prior to World War II and the discovery of DNA, this phenomenon, called *Warburg effect*, was thought to be causally related to cancer. Although Warburg's basic proposal that defective oxidative metabolism was the cause of increased glycolysis via futile cycling was not supported, his original observation has been confirmed repeatedly (Gatenby, 1995).

Magnetic resonance spectroscopy (MRS) and positron emission tomography (PET) studies with 2-[^{18}F]fluoro-2-deoxy-glucose have consistently demonstrated that different clinical tumors show about an order of magnitude more glucose uptake *in vivo* than normal tissue (Gatenby, 1995). Furthermore, glucose uptake correlates with tumor aggressiveness and prognosis, and the expression of the glucose transporter GLUT1 is also increased in cancer cells (Younes et al., 1996).

Increases in glucose transport and type II hexokinase activity in cancer cells cause the increased flux of glucose through the cancer cells (Rempel et al., 1996). Type II hexokinase plays a role in initiation and maintenance of high rates of glucose catabolism in rapidly growing tumors. The enzyme converts glucose to glucose-6-phosphate, the initial phosphorylated intermediate of the glycolytic pathway.

The gene that encodes type II hexokinase has been shown to be amplified fivefold in a hepatoma cell line (Rempel et al., 1996). Its promoter contains a potential glucose-response element and putative p53-responsive elements, and type II hexokinase expression is markedly decreased in HIF-1α–deficient embryonic stem (ES) cells (Iyer et al., 1998). A mutated p53 allele stimulates transcription of the type II hexokinase promoter, which suggests that mutant p53 plays a role in tumor metabolism (Mathupala et al., 1997).

The ability of HIF-1α to interact with and stabilize p53 protein suggests that p53 plays a direct role as a transcription factor in response to hypoxia, although p53 protein is induced by near anoxic conditions (<0.02% oxygen) (An et al., 1998) and HIF-1α expression increases exponentially when oxygen levels fall to <5%. Additional studies are required to elucidate the details of the functional interactions between p53 and HIF-1α. Glucose usage in mutant Chinese hamster ovary (CHO) cells that lack LDH-A (Yamagata et al., 1998), an enzyme that is not considered to be rate limiting for glycolysis, is drastically diminished, compared with that in parental cells. This indicates that alternative pathways of energy metabolism, such as the use of glutamine, exist in cancer cells.

Cells transformed by the oncogenes v-SRC or activated H-RAS exhibit increased rates of aerobic glycolysis. Although cells that express v-SRC display increased expression of HIF-1 and its targets VEGF and enolase 1 (Jiang et al., 1997), in SRC-deficient cells hypoxia-inducible expression of either VEGF or the gene that encodes GLUT1 does not differ from that in wild-type cells (Gleadle and Ratcliffe, 1997).

The oncogene H-RAS stimulates transcription of the gene that encodes VEGF via an intact HIF-1–binding site (Mazure et al., 1996). The *MYC* gene is frequently activated in human cancers. Lewis et al. (1997) identified genes that are differentially expressed in *MYC*-transformed Rat1a fibroblasts. The gene that encodes LDH-A is an MYC target (Lewis et al., 1997), and its expression is frequently increased in human cancers (Shim et al., 1997). LDH-A has been used as a marker of neoplastic transformation and is induced by hypoxia through the activity of HIF-1 (Firth et al., 1995; Semenza et al., 1996).

During normal mitogenesis, *MYC* expression transiently increases in the G_1 phase, which might account for activation of glycolysis and an eightfold increase in LDH-A levels as primary lymphocytes enter into the S phase (Greiner et al., 1994). Studies of transgenic animals that overexpress *MYC* in the liver provide additional evidence for the *in vivo* induction of glycolysis by MYC (Valera et al., 1995). These animals have increased glycolytic enzyme activity in liver and overproduce lactic acid (Valera et al., 1995). Stably transfected rodent fibroblasts that overexpress LDH-A alone and those transformed by *MYC* overproduce lactate; this suggests that overexpression of LDH-A is sufficient to induce the Warburg effect (Gatenby, 1995). From a teleological point of view, anaerobic glycolysis might protect DNA from damage by oxygen radicals that are produced by oxidative phosphorylation (Brand and Hermfisse, 1997), and this may explain the origin of some of the observed metabolic changes because oxidation of DNA can be lethal to the cell.

LDH-A overexpression is required for *MYC*-mediated transformation: Decreasing the expression levels of the former reduces the soft agar clonogenicity of *MYC*-transformed fibroblasts, *MYC*-transformed human lymphoblastoid cells, and Burkitt's lymphoma cells. Likewise, CHO cells that lack LDH-A display a decreased soft agar clonogenicity induced by activated RAS; they form small colonies *in vitro,* and *in vivo* they form tumors that, compared with parental cell populations, have a large proportion of necrotic or apoptotic cells (Yamagata et al., 1998).

Tumor angiogenesis is stimulated by hypoxia and hypoglycemia, which induce expression of VEGF among other angiogenic factors (Hanahan and Folkman, 1996). VEGF recruits new microvessels, which allow delivery of nutrients and expansion of the tumor mass. Prior to microvessel recruitment, a small tumor can remain dormant. This dormancy state is a consequence of the fact that the apoptosis rate equals that of mitosis. As new blood vessels are recruited, the rate of tumor apoptosis decreases, the rate of mitosis increases, and the tumor rapidly grows. Hypoxia remains a strong selective force, however, because new microvessels are limited and disorganized and oxygen-consumption rates tend to exceed the supply rate.

Although tumor cells adapt to the hypoxic and acidic microenvironment, spheroid clusters of avascular tumor cells invariably display a core of necrotic or apoptotic cells that separate from the 150-μ-thick shell of live cells (Sutherland, 1988). Many factors contribute to cell death under these conditions. A major consequence of an elevated rate of glycolysis in tumor cells is that glucose carbons are converted primarily to lactate and are, therefore, no longer the major carbon source for aerobic respiration. In tumor cells that are able to consume limited amounts of oxygen, glutamine is the major oxidizable substrate that enters an abnormal truncated Krebs cycle. Reactive oxygen intermediates that arise from oxidative metabolism of glutamine in L929 fibrosarcoma cells appear to be required for tumor necrosis factor-α (TNF-α)–mediated apoptosis (Goossens et al., 1996). Depletion of glutamine, but not of glucose, from the culture medium desensitizes the L929 cells to TNF-α cytotoxicity.

Like the gradient of oxygen tension (which diminishes toward the center of a tumor mass), the concentration of glucose also tapers drastically, which contributes to the triggering of cell death in the tumor core (Sutherland, 1988). Glucose deprivation is a particularly potent inducer of apoptosis in transformed cells that depend on glucose as a major source of energy. Glucose deprivation or treatment with 2-deoxyglucose, a glycolytic inhibitor, caused nontransformed cells to arrest in the G_1 phase, whereas *MYC*-transformed fibroblasts or lymphoblastoid cells underwent extensive apoptosis, which was blocked by elevated BCL-2 expression (Shim et al., 1998).

HIF-1 modulates gene expression in tumors and induces both angiogenesis and tumor growth (Maxwell et al., 1997). Hypoxia induces the expression of certain genes, such as VEGF and phosphoglycerokinase 1, through HIF-1α, whereas the effects of glucose deprivation on gene expression might be HIF-1 independent (Carmeliet et al., 1998; Iyer et al., 1998; Ryan et al., 1998). Intriguingly, HIF-1α appears to influence the extent of apoptosis in tumors derived from ES cells injected into immunocompromised nude mice (Carmeliet et al., 1998).

Molecular studies of cancer have revealed that in addition to the contributions of oncogenes and tumor suppressor genes to the growth and apoptotic phenotypes of cancer cells, some of these genes directly affect cellular energy metabolism. The products of these genes alter the expression of transcription factors that regulate genes that encode metabolic enzymes and angiogenic factors. Because hypoxia is a key selective pressure on the progression of cancer cells, physiological and nonphysiological (oncogenic) activation of HIF-1 and perhaps other transcription factors might play a central role in promoting the survival of cancer cells in adverse tumor microenvironments. Rekindling interest in the classical biochemical pathways and their intersections with newly discovered signal transduction pathways will provide novel molecular insights into the alterations in metabolic profile that have long been known to occur in cancers. The frequency and severity of tumor hypoxia and its association with malignant progression suggest that therapeutic strategies designed to prevent metabolic adaptation would be particularly efficacious.

Experimental evidence suggests that a number of growth-modulating signals have significant influence on substrate redistribution in cells. For example, transforming growth factor (TGF-β), which uses the tyrosine kinase signaling pathways through the cell surface TGF-β receptor family, promotes invasive transformation of various human cells (Hogo et al., 1999). In response to this growth factor, the human lung epithelial carcinoma cells accumulate glucose carbons in nucleic acid ribose in a dose-dependent manner. Concomitant metabolic changes in response to TGF-β treatment include decreased glucose oxidation in the pentose and TCA cycles, indicating invasive cell transformation accompanied by nonoxidative metabolic changes and increased glucose utilization toward anabolic metabolic reactions of nucleotides (Boros et al., 2000). This increase in the nonoxidative metabolism of glucose in the pentose cycle provides one explanation at the molecular level for the principal metabolic disturbance observed in human tumors: increased glucose uptake with increased glucose utilization for nucleic acid synthesis and decreased glucose oxidation. These metabolic changes also explain how tumor cells are capable of dividing rapidly in the hypoxic environment. On the other hand, growth-modulating agents can exert opposite effects on substrate redistribution depending on their effects on the cell signaling pathway. Genistein, the natural tumor growth-regulating agent found in soybean, has marked tyrosine kinase–(El-Zarruk and van den Berg, 1999) and protein kinase (PK)–(Waltron and Rozengurt, 2000) inhibiting properties resulting in cell cycle arrest (Lian et al., 1998) and limited angiogenesis (Zhou et al., 1999) in several tumor models. Evidence indicates that genistein decreases glucose uptake and glucose carbon incorporation into nucleic acid ribose in MIA pancreatic adenocarcinoma cells (Boros et al., 2001a). After treating tumor cells with growth-promoting or growth-inhibiting agents, opposite changes in glucose carbon deposition into nucleic acid ribose, lactate, glutamate, and fatty acids indicate that glucose carbon redistribution among major metabolic pathways plays a critical role in the cell proliferation and differentiation process.

The degree of oxygenation of tumor cells also affects metabolism. As one moves into the core of a colony of cells growing in agar, there is a progressive increase in lactate and a decrease in oxygenation with a concomitant increase in anaerobic metabolism. Because tumor angiogenesis results in disorganized blood flow, tumor tissues are often poorly vascularized *in vivo*, making aerobic and anaerobic coexist to varying degrees.

METABOLIC HYPOTHESIS OF TUMOR GROWTH

It is clear from previous work on pancreatic, lung, and bone marrow precursor cells that invasive transformation is associated with characteristic metabolic changes. Cell-transforming agents, such as TGF-β and organophosphate pesticides, induce a severe imbalance in glucose carbon redistribution among precursors toward the synthesis of proliferation-related structural and regulatory macromolecules. This phenotype is characterized by increased glucose utilization, specifically for nucleic acid synthesis through the nonoxidative branch of the pentose cycle, with a concomitant decrease in glucose oxidation and the synthesis of glutamate, palmitate, and stearate directly from glucose. On the other hand, agents such as genistein, STI-571 (Boros et al., 2001b), and the fermented wheat germ extract Avemar, which inhibit tumor growth, alter glucose utilization from a pattern typical of the proliferative phenotype to one of differentiated or apoptotic cells. Such evidence suggests the general metabolic hypothesis that cellular functions *in vitro* and physiological functions *in vivo* are both regulated by metabolic changes, and such regulations can be understood in terms of systems biology of the metabolic network. Specific application of the hypothesis to tumor growth (Boros et al., 2002b) implies the following:

1. Cell transformation and tumor growth are associated with the activation of metabolic enzymes that increase glucose carbon utilization toward nucleic acid synthesis, while lipid and amino acid synthesis pathway enzymes are activated during tumor growth inhibition.
2. The phosphorylation, allosteric, and transcriptional regulation of intermediary metabolic enzymes and their substrates together mediate and sustain cell transformation from one condition to another.

Tumor cells, just as other living cells, possess the potential for proliferation, differentiation, and cell cycle arrest or apoptosis (Figure 2). Associated with each of these conditions is a specific distribution of substrates between macromolecule synthesis pathways according to the metabolic needs of the given phenotype. These phenotypes are characterized by different needs for the production of energy and substrates necessary for the cells to function under different physiological and pathophysiological conditions. The effects of abnormal physiological and genetic factors that transform tumor cells from one functional state to another are mediated by metabolic phenotype changes aimed toward supplying the dividing cell with an optimal source of carbons at the expense of cell differentiation and host integrity. On the other hand, factors that control cell growth through differentiation or apoptosis have a very different pattern of substrate redistribution.

Figure 4 illustrates the relationship between extrinsic tumor growth influencing factors and metabolic enzymes that are targets of growth-regulating signals. Tumor growth modulating factors in the form of peptide hormones, which bind to cell surface receptors, oncogenes, and mutated tumor suppressor gene products, environmental pollutants, xenobiotics, and the processes associated with cellular aging can all activate specific signal transduction pathways, which result in activity changes of metabolic enzymes through either protein phosphorylation or gene regulation. Superimposed on this background, glucose, intracellular glucose metabolites and various nutrients directly affect cell functions because they provide the substrates for various intracellular synthetic reactions and energy production, and they are key allosteric regulators of metabolic enzymes.

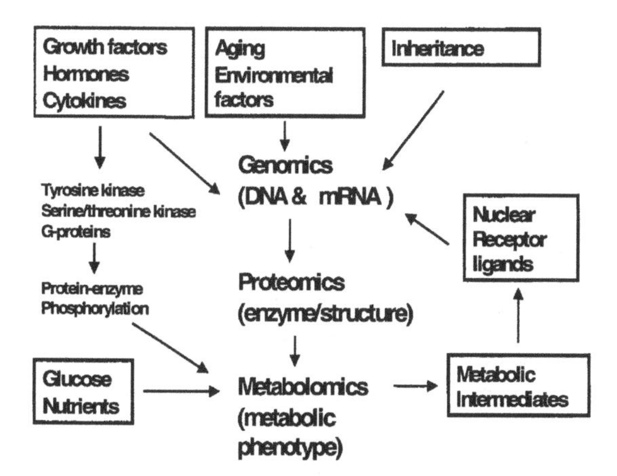

FIGURE 4 Relationship between extrinsic tumor growth influence factors and metabolic enzymes.

The metabolic characteristics of four distinctive phenotypes, namely proliferation, differentiation, cell cycle arrest, and apoptosis, which have been described in tumor cells in response to tumor growth modulating treatments, are summarized (Table 1). Table 1 lists a number of agents (column 4) and their mechanism (column 3) that ultimately results in changes in biological states (column 1) and their associated metabolic phenotypes (column 2). As indicated in the second row of the table, H441 and K562 cells are sensitive to activation of tyrosine kinases/PKs, which subsequently affect substrate flux through the pentose cycle providing metabolic support for cell proliferation. As shown in Table 1 as well, apoptosis can be induced by metabolic inhibitor 2-DOG or by the cytokine TNF-α through actions on the glycolytic, pentose, and TCA cycle metabolic pathways. It is clear from these examples that signaling pathways influence both gene expression and metabolic pathways culminating in the cellular phenotypes of either differentiation or proliferation. Tumor cells adapt to high rates of glucose utilization and macromolecule synthesis and become highly dependent on the availability of glucose carbons. Via a feedback mechanism, the production of intermediary metabolites also regulates gene expression through intracellular nuclear receptors. The proposed constraint-based model we have proposed is based on the direct determination of substrate flow through various metabolic pathways that control the proliferation and differentiation processes under the

TABLE 1 Metabolic Phenotypes of Tumor Cells and Their Biological Characteristics

Biological phenotype and dominant cell cycle	**Metabolic phenotype**	**Metabolic pathway and *enzyme***	**Cell type: induction method; signaling pathway**	**References**
Proliferating: S-phase cycle dominance	Distribution and continuous flow of glucose carbons through the nonoxidative steps of the PC for *de novo* DNA and RNA synthesis	Nonoxidative PC—*transketolase*	H441 lung adenocarcinoma, K562 myeloid blasts; TGF-β or isofenphos pesticide; tyrosine/protein kinases	Boros et al., 1997
Differentiating: "G_0-G_1" phase cycle dominance	Shift of glucose carbons to direct oxidation through G6PD and recycling of ribose carbons back into glycolysis; increased lipid and amino acid synthesis from the carbons of glucose	Oxidative pentose cycle—*G6PD* Glycolysis—*pyruvate kinase*	MIA pancreatic adenocarcinoma; Genistein, Avemar, STI571; Tyrosine/protein kinase inhibitors	Boren et al., 2001; Wang et al., 1995
Cell cycle arrest: "G_0-G_1" or "G_2-M" phase cycle dominance	Limited carbon flow through both the oxidative and the nonoxidative branches of the PC—limited RNA/DNA synthesis, limited NADPH production	Nonoxidative pentose cycle—*transketolase* Oxidative pentose cycle—*G6PD*	MIA pancreatic adenocc, *Ehrlich*'s ascites carcinoma in mice; oxythiamine, DHEAS; no signal transducer pathways are needed	Boros et al., 1997; Rais et al., 1999
Apoptotic: "G_0" cycle arrest	Limited glucose availability or direct inhibition of glycolytic, PC or TCA cycle enzymes	Glycolysis, PC and TCA cycle	Fibroblasts, lymphoblasts, lung carcinoma; DOG or TNF-α; no signal transducer pathways are needed	Shim et al., 1998; Osthus et al., 2000

PC, pentose cycle; DOG, 2-deoxy-d-glucose; TCA, tricarboxylic acid; TNF, tumor necrosis factor.

influence of various signaling regulatory events and nutritional constraints.

In support of our constraint-based model (Figures 1 and 2) are the strong interactions between newly discovered signal transduction pathways and fundamental metabolic pathways, such as the glycolytic and the pentose cycle pathways. Glucose deprivation can induce apoptosis even when other nutrients are plentiful (Shim et al., 1998; Spitz, et al., 2000). The c-myc oncogene directly regulates glucose transporter 1 and glycolytic gene expression in several tumor cells (Osthus et al., 2000). The constraint-based model has as its key metabolic regulatory elements (1) the flow of information from the exterior of cells using specific signal transduction pathways and (2) the flow of substrates necessary to sustain these signaling events. These two elements also determine the optimum activation of metabolic enzymes, which are the key regulatory checkpoints of carbon redistribution between major metabolic pathways.

Metabolic enzymes control substrate flow according to the physiological needs of a given cell as determined by its metabolic phenotype. The direct and indirect interactions between signal transduction pathways, substrates, and their intracellular target enzymes allow a fine regulatory mechanism, which together control cell events such as cell cycle progression, transformation, proliferation, hormone or enzyme secretion, differentiation, apoptosis, and growth. Accordingly, multiple genetic alterations and signaling pathways that cause tumor development directly constrain the "general solution space of metabolism" affecting glycolysis (Kunz-Schughart et al., 2000), the cellular response to hypoxia (Boros et al., 2000), and the ability of tumor cells to recruit new blood vessels (Oku et al., 1998).

Metabolic Control Analysis

If the metabolic model of tumor growth is correct, it will predict that proliferation or differentiation signals will have a strong influence on substrate utilization and redistribution in pancreatic cancer cells exposed to these signals. Conversely, inhibitors of the key metabolic pathways will have a significant impact on the cellular phenotype expression of tumor cells. *How can these effects be quantified and analyzed?* During the past 2 decades, two main theoretical frameworks have been developed for studying the genetic, enzymatic, and substrate level control mechanisms in metabolic networks. They are the Biochemical Systems Theory (BST) developed by Savageau (for reviews, see Savageau, 1976; Voit, 2000) and the Metabolic Control Analysis (MCA) (see as a review, Fell, 1997; Cornish-Bowden and Cardenas, 2000). Although these two theories share many elements, MCA has become the major method used in the study of metabolic control properties of cells because the

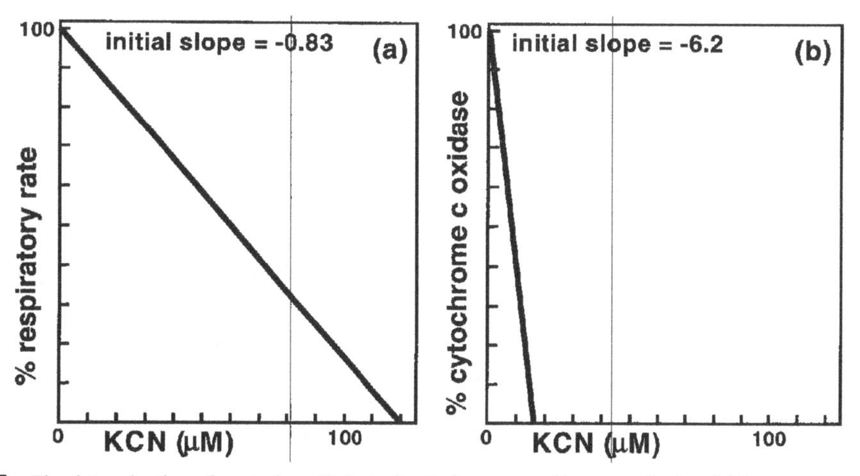

FIGURE 5 The determination of control coefficient of cytochrome *c* oxidase on mitochondrial oxygen consumption.

language used in this method is more accessible for nonmathematicians.

In MCA, the control exerted by each and every enzyme in a metabolic network over substrate flux or any other systemic parameter (i.e., metabolite concentration, hormone secretion, or cell proliferation) can be quantitatively described as a control coefficient. *Control coefficients of enzymatic steps* are defined as the fractional change in the systemic property over the fractional change in enzyme activity exposed using specific enzyme inhibitors. An enzymatic step is considered to have the highest control coefficient when fractional change of enzyme activity is equal to the fractional change of the system parameter. This is illustrated in Figure 5, where the determination of control coefficient of cytochrome *c* oxidase on mitochondrial oxygen consumption is plotted according to the method of Rossignol et al. (2000). In this case, the control coefficient is low. Therefore, in this example, altering the levels of the oxidase has relatively little effect on oxygen consumption of the mitochondrial oxygen generation system. In metabolic networks where the individual enzyme–substrate kinetics are known, MCA can be used to derive the individual control coefficients that predict response of the system to perturbations (Fell, 1997), as, for instance, changes in substrate availability or "genetic" perturbation of the network. On the other hand, in poorly defined systems where enzyme–substrate kinetics are unknown, control coefficients can be determined experimentally by varying the parameter of interest and measuring the changes in the relevant substrate flux. For example, when determining the control coefficient of a metabolic enzyme (enzyme A) on tumor cell proliferation, one would administer the specific inhibitor of enzyme A to cultures of tumor cells and subsequently measure the parallel decrease in enzyme A activity and cell proliferation. The slope of the log–log plot of tumor cell proliferation versus enzyme activity gives the control coefficient of

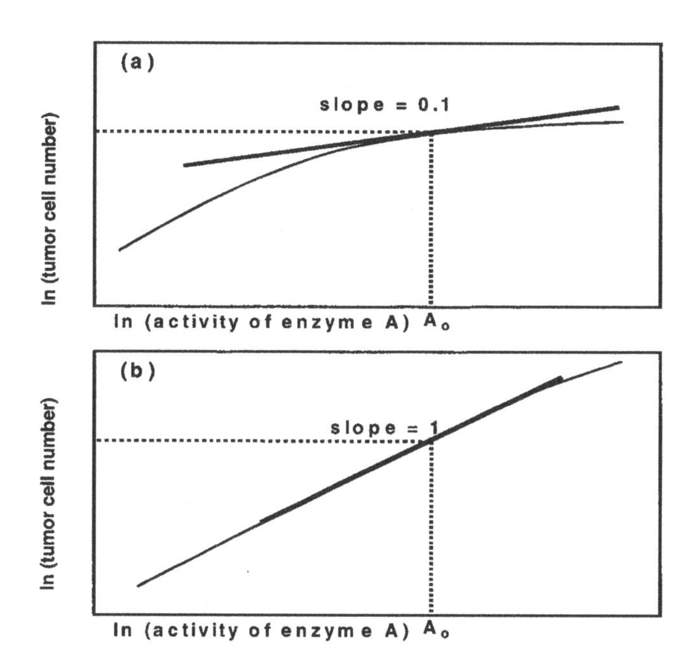

FIGURE 6 Dependence of tumor cell proliferation on activity of a hypothetical enzyme (enzyme A) with low control coefficient (a) and with high control coefficient (b).

enzyme A on cell proliferation (C_A). Where the activity decreases in the same relative amount as cell proliferation, the control coefficient value is unity (or 1). We assume that the enzyme inhibitor we used in this example is a specific inhibitor of enzyme A and does not affect other enzymes in tumor cells.

Figure 6 shows the double log plots of the dependence of tumor cell proliferation on activity of a hypothetical enzyme A having a low (Figure 6a) and high (Figure 6b) control coefficient. An enzyme is considered to have a high control coefficient when changes in its activity are reflected totally in changes of tumor cell proliferation. The control coefficient value for the enzyme is unity. Conversely, an enzyme is considered to have a low control coefficient when changes in its activity have small or negligible effect on the tumor cell proliferation. Thus, by means of control coefficients, MCA provides an easily understandable quantitative description of how metabolic enzymes or transport proteins control biological functions in complex mammalian cells.

The ordering of control coefficients of the various enzymatic steps in a metabolic pathway as co-responders gives us the initial assessment of where to interfere within a metabolic network to alter cell proliferation. By either direct enzyme inhibitors or genetic manipulations of these steps, one hopes to achieve the desired values of metabolic substrate flux that affect systemic parameters such as cell proliferation or cell cycle progression in studies of cancer cells. Despite that the application of MCA in biotechnology is yet a young field, some promising examples have captured the attention of metabolic engineers, drug developers, and basic scientists (for reviews, see Fell, 1997; Cornish-Bowden and Cardenas, 2000).

APPLYING METABOLIC CONTROL ANALYSIS

Cell signaling and metabolic pathways constitute a metabolic network and can be subjected to MCA. The control exerted by hormone signals or enzymes over substrate flux or any other systemic parameter can be calculated and described as their respective control coefficients. Our metabolic hypothesis of tumor growth predicts that cell proliferation or differentiation signals have high control coefficients over characteristics of glucose metabolic pathways. Conversely, inhibitors of these glucose metabolic pathways have a significant impact on the cellular phenotype expression of pancreatic cancer cells. The long-term objective of these studies is to apply MCA to determine the metabolic sensitivity of the proliferation and differentiation signals in pancreatic cancer. Additionally, the measured substrate fluxes and their respective control coefficients can be used as an experimentally determined constraint set for modeling purposes.

The application of MCA complements current approaches to identifying specific targets of proliferative disease pathways. Differential expression of genes between diseased and healthy tissues is commonly used to identify specific disease pathways. Such an approach ignores the obvious fact that the robust metabolic network of feedback loops and cellular regulatory mechanisms has evolved to maintain homeostasis and to withstand various genetic and environmental insults. The linkage of multiple interacting disease pathways through such a metabolic network has made it almost impossible to identify critical pathways or therapeutic targets using information from gene expression analysis alone. On the other hand, MCA approaches the problem by examining the contribution of individual components within a metabolic network, providing a theoretical framework for describing the metabolic outcomes of complex interactions of genes, signaling pathways, and enzymes. An attractive feature of MCA is that it does not require all system components to be characterized a priori (Fell, 1997; Voit, 2000). Moreover, control coefficients can be estimated for different components of the network, including environmental factors pertinent to the network. The control coefficients give us a first approximation of which proteins or pathways may exert more control on the system properties to be modified. Targeting the steps with higher control coefficients on relevant system properties such as cell proliferation can be a good strategy to understand disease processes in systems biology.

METABOLIC PROFILING OF CELL PROLIFERATION AND DIFFERENTIATION

Metabolic profiling is an experimental tool that can be used to determine substrate flux and metabolic control coefficients characteristic of specific metabolic phenotypes. A mammalian cell's genetic program directs the cell's response to specific regulatory ligands, resulting in a distinctive phenotype at any given point during the cell's life cycle (see Figures 1 and 2). This phenotype is expressed as a possible solution space in the constraint-based model in the context of the microenvironment, particularly substrate availability, which determines enzyme activities and substrate utilization/redistribution within and among major metabolic pathways (Sachs, 1980; Yamaji et al., 1994; Lee et al., 1995; Hieter and Bogusky, 1997; Moley and Mueckler, 2000). Alterations in substrate flow in response to hormonal, environmental, or carcinogenic stimuli reflect changes in metabolic enzyme activities and metabolic constraints. These changes occur either through protein phosphorylation/glycosylation or through metabolic enzyme gene expression regulation by transcription factors.

The metabolic profile of a given cell represents the integrated end-point of many growth-modifying signaling events against the background of the cell's genetic and metabolic makeup. Metabolic profiling is the simultaneous assessment of substrate flux within and among major metabolic pathways of macromolecule synthesis and energy production under various physiological conditions, growth phases, and substrate environments. Metabolic profiling greatly assists the study of disease processes by revealing metabolic adaptive changes that occur as a consequence of gene expression and changes in microenvironment. It provides the database for constraint-based modeling and is, therefore, complementary to the constraint-based modeling.

Over the past 5 years, stable isotope techniques have been developed in our laboratory for the metabolic characterization of various mammalian cells *in vitro* (Lee et al., 1995; Boros et al., 1997, 2001a, c). With the use of mass spectrometry and glucose molecules labeled with stable (nonradiating) isotope (^{13}C), the distribution of labeled carbons in various intermediates during *de novo* macromolecule synthesis in cancer cells can be traced. Metabolic profiling is designed to uncover detailed substrate flow modifications in response to pathological processes and in response to new antitumor therapies.

One of the more useful isotopes for applying metabolic profiling is [1,2-$^{13}C_2$]glucose. Changes in the pattern of distribution of ^{13}C carbons from [1,2-$^{13}C_2$]glucose in intracellular metabolic intermediates simultaneously provides a measure of carbon flow toward the pentose cycle, glycolysis, direct glucose oxidation, TCA cycle, and fatty acid synthesis. Metabolic profiling provides measurement of specific flux changes in lactate, glutamate, nucleic acid ribose, palmitate, and CO_2 during oncogenesis and antiproliferative treatments. Thus, it can indicate major changes in glucose utilization for macromolecular synthesis in cancer cells. The stable isotope–based metabolic profiling technique, as introduced in this proposal, utilizes ^{13}C-labeled glucose carbons not only as they accumulate in cells but also by their destinies as they react through specific metabolic steps. The specificity of this tracer technology to follow metabolic reactions makes it possible to study cellular metabolism in the absence or presence of physiological and pathological modulators of cancer cell function.

RELATIVE ROLES OF GENOMICS, PROTEOMICS, AND METABOLOMICS IN CANCER RESEARCH

Genomics, proteomics, and metabolomics are three research approaches in the new field of bioinformatics (Table 2). The study of the expression of genes and the effect of mutations on their expression in many organisms forms the basis of functional genomics (for reviews, see Hieter and Bogusky, 1997; Eisenberg et al., 2000). The functional state of an organism is defined by the outcome of the expression of a large array of genes (Schuster et al., 1999). Emphasis has shifted to understanding cellular function in terms of the expression of the various coded proteins—so-called proteomics. In the field of proteomics, expression of protein is scanned by the use of matrix-assisted laser desorption–time-of-flight (MALDI-TOF) mass spectrometry and structural information determined by tandem mass spectrometry analysis. The cellular function of an organism is defined in terms of the expression of structural and enzyme proteins, as well as their post-translational modification. However, even as new information on DNA, messenger RNA (mRNA), and proteins is collated, such information presents a static picture of the cell and cannot account for the interactions between metabolic substrates and signaling pathways. The fact that signaling events lead to related metabolic reactions, which in turn modify other metabolic functions or gene expression, makes it impossible to understand biological systems merely in terms of a set of components in the genome, transcriptome, or proteome. It is extremely difficult to separate signaling events from their related metabolic reactions and to define the precise boundaries of individual gene action in a biological system of complex regulatory mechanisms (Westerhoff et al., 1990; Dang and Semenza, 1999).

TABLE 2 Comparison of Research Methods Used in Different Fields of Bioinformatics

Research field	Research techniques	Target molecules	Analytical method	Specific information provided
Functional genomics	PCR, microarray, sequencing	DNA, RNA	Pattern recognition	Genetic abnormalities, expression of genes, gene sequences (static and qualitative)
Proteomics	LC/MS/MS, MALDI-TOF	Peptides and proteins	Structure-function relationship	Composition and structure of structural and enzyme proteins (static and qualitative)
Metabolomics	Stable isotope tracers	Carbohydrates, amino acids, lipids, all intermediates of metabolism	Substrate distribution, rate of synthesis, substrate flux ratios (results of the interaction among substrates, genomics, and proteomics)	Substrate flux through metabolic pathways, identification and contribution of substrates to macromolecule synthesis (quantitative and dynamic)

Source: Sakai et al., 2000.
LC/MS, liquid chromatography/mass spectrometry; MALDI-TOF, matrix-assisted laser desorption–time-of-flight mass spectrometry.

The behavior of metabolic networks in mammalian cells, as demonstrated by the individual substrate distribution, the flow of substrates, and the relative fluxes among the various metabolic interconversion, is the culmination of regulatory processes at many levels, including the availability of substrates, expression of enzymes and regulatory proteins, and the transcription of genes into mRNA based on sequence information of genomic components of the DNA. The complex behavior of metabolic network is determined by interactions among building components that determine its ultimate biological behavior such as proliferation or differentiation.

The quantitative study of the relationship among the individual substrate distributions, the flow of substrates, and the relative fluxes among the various metabolic interconversions constitutes the field of metabolomics. Metabolic profiling or metabolic phenotyping consists of the measurements of the individual substrate distribution, the flow of substrates, and the relative fluxes among the various metabolic interconversion. The comparison among genomics, proteomics, and metabolomics is provided in Table 2. It is sufficient to point out that there are major differences in the nature of the information. Genomics and proteomics yield information regarding the presence or absence (binary array) of a genetic expression in the form of RNA and protein. However, the quantitative relationship of this gene expression with the clinical and metabolic behavior cannot be predicted based on such information. The information of metabolomics differs from the others in that it provides quantitative and dynamic measures of the behavior of the metabolic network.

The complementary nature of genetic and metabolic information in cancer research can be illustrated by the story of Gleevec in the treatment of chronic myelogenous leukemia (CML). The expression of a constitutively active tyrosine kinase signaling protein construct by realignment of the breakpoint cluster region and Ableson leukemia virus protooncogene sequences (Bcr/Abl) is the basis of oncogenic transformation of myeloid cells in chronic myeloid leukemia (CML). It is believed that this construct stimulates glucose transport in multipotent hematopoietic cells stimulating the uncontrolled proliferation of these cells. The inhibition of this constitutively active Bcr/Abl tyrosine kinase by the anticancer drug STI571 (Gleevec) has been shown to lead to remission of the CML. The success of the treatment could not have been predicted from the genetic information of the Bcr/Abl gene. Using metabolic profiling techniques, we showed that Gleevec inhibits glucose utilization toward nucleic acid synthesis and leukemia cell proliferation. At doses comparable to those used in the treatment of myelogenous leukemia, STI571 suppresses hexokinase and glucose-6-phosphate dehydrogenase (G6PDH) activities in K562 myeloid leukemia cells. The metabolic profile correlates positively with the response of K562 myeloid leukemia cells and directly suggests that Gleevec is a potential therapeutic agent (Boros et al., 2001).

FUTURE DIRECTIONS

The use of metabolic phenotyping to classify tumor type is novel. The information derived from this analysis can be used to design a chemopreventive approach protocol or the result of complex changes in dietary patterns. The use of MCA to investigate the metabolic sensitivity of proliferation and differentiation signals provides a basic understanding of the interaction between signaling constraints and metabolic constraints in determining cell proliferation and differentiation. Such technology for the study of complex biological system can be extended to investigate the properties of other important proliferating cells such as germ cell lines and stem cell lines. The system biology approach using constraint-based modeling can also be applied to investigate the mechanism of nutrient action. The metabolic constraints imposed by nutrients such as vitamins, minerals, and phytochemicals are represented by the respective metabolomes, which can be used to predict potential nutrient–nutrient interactions and unexpected nutrient effects. It is evident that the novelty, power, and specificity of the stable isotope–based metabolic profiling technology in revealing metabolic pathway substrate flow modifications in health and disease will greatly assist the research community interest in studying physiology and nutritional factors involved in the development of chronic disease processes including cancer.

References

An, W.G., et al. 1998. Stabilization of wild-type p53 by hypoxia-inducible factor 1alpha. *Nature* **392**: 405–408.

Boren, J., Cascante, M., Marin, S., Comin-Anduix, B., Centelles, J.J., Lim, S., Bassilian, S., Ahmed, S., Lee, W.N., and Boros, L.G. 2001. Gleevec (STI571) influences metabolic enzyme activities and glucose carbon flow toward nucleic acid and fatty acid synthesis in myeloid tumor cells. *J Biol Chem* **276**: 37747–37753.

Boros, L.G., Puigjaner, J., Cascante, M., Lee, W.N., Brandes, J.L., Bassilian, S., Yusuf, F.I., Williams, R.D., Muscarella, P., Melvin, W.S., and Schirmer, W.J. 1997. Oxythiamine and dehydroepiandrosterone inhibit the nonoxidative synthesis of ribose and tumor cell proliferation. *Cancer Res* **57**: 4242–4248.

Boros, L.G., Torday, J.S., Lim, S., Bassilian, S., Cascante, M., and Lee, W.N. 2000. Transforming growth factor beta2 promotes glucose carbon incorporation into nucleic acid ribose through the nonoxidative pentose cycle in lung epithelial carcinoma cells. *Cancer Res* **60**: 1183–1185.

Boros, L.G., Bassilian, S., Lim, S., and Lee, W.N.P. 2001a. Genistein inhibits non-oxidative ribose synthesis in MIA pancreatic adenocarcinoma cells: a new mechanism of controlling tumor growth. *Pancreas* **22**: 1–7.

Boros, L.G., Lapis, K., Szende, B., Tömösközi-Farkas, R., Balogh, A., Boren, J., Silvia Marin, S., Cascante, M., Lee, W.N.P., and Hidvégi, M. 2001b. Wheat germ extract decreases glucose uptake and RNA ribose formation in MIA pancreatic adenocarcinoma cells. *Pancreas* **23**: 141–147.

Boros, L.G., Cascante, M.S., and Lee, W.N.P. 2002a. Metabolic profiling of cell growth and death in cancer: applications in drug discovery. *Drug Discov Today* **7**: 364–372.

Boros, L.G., Lee, W.N.P., and Go, V.L.W. 2002b. A metabolic hypothesis of cell growth and death in pancreatic cancer. *Pancreas* **24**: 26–33.

Brand, K.A., and Hermfisse, U. 1997. Aerobic glycolysis by proliferating cells: a protective strategy against reactive oxygen species. *FASEB J* **11**: 388–395.

Carmeliet, P. et al. 1998. Role of HIF-1alpha in hypoxia-mediated apoptosis, cell proliferation and tumour angiogenesis. *Nature* **394**: 485–490.

Cascante, M., Boros, L.G., Comin, B., Atauri, P., Centelles, J.J., and Lee, W.N.P. 2002. Metabolic Control Analysis: a rational approach for new drug development. *Nat Biotechnol* **20**: 243–249.

Comín, B., Boren, J., Martinez, S., Moro, C., Centelles, J.J., Trebukhina, R., Petushok, N., Lee, W.N.P., Boros, L.G., and Cascante, M. 2001. The effect of thiamine supplementation on tumor proliferation: A Metabolic Control Analysis study. *Eur J Biochem* **268**: 4177–4182.

Cornish-Bowden, A., and Cárdenas, M.L. 2000. "Technological and Medical Implications of Metabolic Control Analysis." Kluwer Academic Publishers, Dordrecht.

Dang, C.V., and Semenza, G.L. 1999. Oncogenic alterations of metabolism. *Trends Biochem Sci* **24**: 68–72.

Eisenberg, D., Marcotte, E.M., Xenarios, I., and Yates, T.O. 2000. Protein function in the post-genomic era. *Nature* **405**: 823–826.

El-Zarruk, A.A., and van den Berg, H.W. 1999. The anti-proliferative effects of tyrosine kinase inhibitors towards tamoxifen-sensitive and tamoxifen-resistant human breast cancer cell lines in relation to the expression of epidermal growth factor receptors (EGF-R) and the inhibition of EGF-R tyrosine kinase. *Cancer Lett* **142**: 185–193.

Fell, D. 1997. "Understanding the Control of Metabolism." Portland Press, London.

Firth, J.D., Ebert, B.L., and Ratcliffe, P.J. 1995. Hypoxic regulation of lactate dehydrogenase A. Interaction between hypoxia-inducible factor 1 and cAMP response elements. *J Biol Chem* **270**: 21021–21027.

Gatenby, R.A. 1995. The potential role of transformation-induced metabolic changes in tumor-host interaction. *Cancer Res* **55**: 4151–4156.

Gleadle, J.M., and Ratcliffe, P.J. 1997. Induction of hypoxia-inducible factor-1, erythropoietin, vascular endothelial growth factor, and glucose transporter-1 by hypoxia: evidence against a regulatory role for Src kinase. *Blood* **89**: 503–509.

Goossens, V., Grooten, J., and Fiers, W. 1996. The oxidative metabolism of glutamine. A modulator of reactive oxygen intermediate-mediated cytotoxicity of tumor necrosis factor in L929 fibrosarcoma cells. *J Biol Chem* **271**: 192–196.

Grandori, C., and Eisenman, R.N. 1997. Myc target genes. *Trends Biochem Sci* **22**: 177–181.

Greiner, E.F., Guppy, M., and Brand, K. 1994. Glucose is essential for proliferation and the glycolytic enzyme induction that provokes a transition to glycolytic energy production. *J Biol Chem* **269**: 31484–31490.

Hanahan, D., and Folkman, J. 1996. Patterns and emerging mechanisms of the angiogenic switch during tumorigenesis. *Cell* **86**: 353–364.

Helmlinger, G., Yuan, F., Dellian, M., and Jain, R.K. 1997. Interstitial pH and pO2 gradients in solid tumors in vivo: high-resolution measurements reveal a lack of correlation. *Nat Med* **3**: 177–182.

Hieter, P., and Bogusky, M. 1997. Functional genomics: it's all how you read it. *Science* **278**: 601–602.

Hojo, M., Morimoto, T., Maluccio, M., Asano, T., Morimoto, K., Lagman, M., Shimbo, T., and Suthanthiran, M. 1999. Cyclosporine induces cancer progression by a cell-autonomous mechanism. *Nature* **397**: 530–534.

Issa, J.P. 2000. The epigenetics of colorectal cancer. *Ann NY Acad Sci* **910**: 140–153.

Iyer, N.V., et al. 1998. Cellular and developmental control of O2 homeostasis by hypoxia inducible factor 1 alpha. *Genes Dev* **12**: 149–162.

Jiang, B.H., Agani, F., Passaniti, A., and Semenza, G.L. 1997. V-SRC induces expression of hypoxia-inducible factor 1 (HIF-1) and transcription of genes encoding vascular endothelial growth factor and enolase 1: involvement of HIF-1 in tumor progression. *Cancer Res* **57**: 5328–5335.

Jung, I., and Messing, E. 2000. Molecular mechanisms and pathways in bladder cancer development and progression. Cancer Control **7**: 325–334.

Kunz-Schughart, L.A., Doetsch, J., Mueller-Klieser, W., and Groebe, K. 2000. Proliferative activity and tumorigenic conversion: impact on cellular metabolism in 3-D culture. *Am J Physiol Cell Physiol* **278**: C765–C780.

Largaespada, D.A. 2000. Genetic heterogeneity in acute myeloid leukemia: maximizing information flow from MuLV mutagenesis studies. *Leukemia* **14**: 1174–1184.

Lee, W.N., Byerley, L.O., Bassilian, S., Ajie, H.O., Clark, I., Edmond, J., and Bergner, E.A. 1995. Isotopomer study of lipogenesis in human hepatoma cells in culture: contribution of carbon and hydrogen atoms from glucose. *Anal Biochem* **226**: 100–112.

Lewis, B.C., et al. 1997. Identification of putative c-Myc–responsive genes: characterization of rcl, a novel growth-related gene. *Mol Cell Biol* **17**: 4967–4978.

Lian, F., Bhuiyan, M., Li, Y.W., Wall, N., Kraut, M., and Sarkar, F.H. 1998. Genistein-induced G_2-M arrest, p21WAF1 upregulation, and apoptosis in a non-small-cell lung cancer cell line. *Nutr Cancer* **31**: 184–191.

Martin, A.M., and Weber, B.L. 2000. Genetic and hormonal risk factors in breast cancer. *J Natl Cancer Inst* **92**: 1126–1135.

Mathupala, S.P., Heese, C., and Pedersen, P.L. 1997. Glucose catabolism in cancer cells. The type II hexokinase promoter contains functionally active response elements for the tumor suppressor p53. *J Biol Chem* **272**: 22776–22780.

Maxwell, P.H., et al. 1997. Hypoxia-inducible factor-1 modulates gene expression in solid tumors and influences both angiogenesis and tumor growth. *Proc Natl Acad Sci USA* **94**: 8104–8109.

Mazure, N.M., et al. 1996. Oncogenic transformation and hypoxia synergistically act to modulate vascular endothelial growth factor expression. *Cancer Res.* **56**: 3436–3440.

Moley, K.H., and Mueckler, M.M. Glucose transport and *apoptosis*. (2000) *Apoptosis* **5**: 99–105.

Oku, T., Tjuvajev, J.G., Miyagawa, T., Sasajima, T., Joshi, A., Joshi, R., Finn, R., Claffey, K.P., and Blasberg, R.G. 1998. Tumor growth modulation by sense and antisense vascular endothelial growth factor gene expression: effects on angiogenesis, vascular permeability, blood volume, blood flow, fluorodeoxyglucose uptake, and proliferation of human melanoma intracerebral xenografts. *Cancer Res* **58**: 4185–4192.

Osthus, R.C., Shim, H., Kim, S., Li, Q., Reddy, R., Mukherjee, M., Xu, Y., Wonsey, D., Lee, L.A., and Dang, C.V. 2000. Deregulation of glucose transporter 1 and glycolytic gene expression by c-Myc. *J Biol Chem* **275**: 21797–21800.

Ozen, M., and Pathak, S. 2000. Genetic alterations in human prostate cancer: a review of current literature. *Anticancer Res* **20**: 1905–1912.

Rais, B., Comin, B., Puigjaner, J., Brandes, J.L., Creppy, E., Saboureau, D., Ennamany, R., Lee, W.N., Boros, L.G., and Cascante, M. 1999. Oxythiamine and dehydroepiandrosterone induce a G_1 phase cycle arrest in Ehrlich's tumor cells through inhibition of the pentose cycle. *FEBS Lett* **456**: 113–118.

Rempel, A., et al. 1996. Glucose catabolism in cancer cells: amplification of the gene encoding type II hexokinase. *Cancer Res* **56**: 2468–2471.

Rossignol, R., Letellier, T., Malgrat, M., Rocher, C., and Mazat, J.P. 2000. Tissue variation in the control of oxidative phosphorylation: implication for mitochondrial diseases. *Biochem J* **347**: 45–53.

Ryan, H.E., Lo, J., and Johnson, R.S. 1998. HIF-1 alpha is required for solid tumor formation and embryonic vascularization. *EMBO J* **17**: 3005–3015.

Sachs, L. 1980. Constitutive uncoupling of the controls for growth and differentiation in myeloid leukemia and the development of cancer. *J Natl Cancer Inst* **65**: 675–679.

Sakai, Y., Yanagisawa, A., Shimada, M., Hidaka, E., Seki, M., Tada, Y., Harada, T., Saisho, H., Kato, Y. 2000. K-ras gene mutations and loss of heterozygosity at the p53 gene locus relative to histological characteristics of mucin-producing tumors of the pancreas. *Hum Pathol* **31**: 795–803.

Savageau, M. 1976. "Biochemical System Analysis. A Study of Function and Design in Molecular Biology." Addison-Wesley, Reading, MA.

Schuster, S., Dandekar, T., and Fell, D.A. 1999. Detection of elementary flux modes in biochemical networks: a promising tool for pathway analysis and metabolic engineering. *Trends Biotechnol* **17**: 53–60.

Semenza, G.L., et al. 1996. Hypoxia response elements in the aldolase A, enolase 1, and lactate dehydrogenase A gene promoters contain essential binding sites for hypoxia-inducible factor 1. *J Biol Chem* **271**: 32529–32537.

Shim, H., et al. 1997. c-Myc transactivation of LDH-A: implications for tumor metabolism and growth. *Proc Natl Acad Sci USA* **24**: 6658–6663.

Shim, H., Chun, Y.S., Lewis, B.C., and Dang, C.V. 1998. A unique glucose-dependent apoptotic pathway induced by c-Myc. *Proc Natl Acad Sci USA* **95**: 1511–1516.

Spitz, D.R., Sim, J.E., Ridnour, L.A., Galoforo, S.S., and Lee, Y.J. 2000. Glucose deprivation-induced oxidative stress in human tumor cells. A fundamental defect in metabolism? *Ann NY Acad Sci* **899**: 349–362.

Sutherland, R.M. 1988. Cell and environment interactions in tumor microregions: The multicell spheroid model. *Science* **240**: 177–184.

Szabo, C., Masiello, A., Ryan, J.F., and Brody, L.C. 2000. The Breast Cancer Information Core: Database design, structure, and scope. *Hum Mutat* **16**: 23–131.

Takeda, K., Matsuno, S., and Horii, A. 2000. Association of poor prognosis with loss of 12q, 17p, and 18q, and concordant loss of 6q/17p and 12q/18q in human pancreatic ductal adenocarcinoma. *Am J Gastroenterol* **95**: 2080–2085.

Towle, H.C. 1995. Metabolic regulation of gene transcription in mammals. *J Biol Chem* **270**: 23235–23238.

Valera, A., et al. 1995. Evidence from transgenic mice that myc regulates hepatic glycolysis. *FASEB J* **9**: 1067–1078.

Vallet, V.S., et al. 1998. Differential roles of upstream stimulatory factors 1 and 2 in the transcriptional response of liver genes to glucose. *J Biol Chem* **273**: 20175–20179.

Voit, E.O. 2000. "Computational Analysis of Biochemical Systems." Cambridge University Press, Cambridge.

Waltron, R.T., and Rozengurt, E. 2000. Oxidative stress induces protein kinase D activation in intact cells involvement of Src and dependence on protein kinase C. *J Biol Chem* **275**: 17114–17121.

Wang, G.L., Jiang, B.-H., Rue, E.A., and Semenza, G.L. 1995. Hypoxia-inducible factor 1 is a basic-helix-loop-helix-PAS heterodimer regulated by cellular O_2 tension. *Proc Natl Acad Sci* **9**: 5510–5514.

Warburg, O. 1930. "The Metabolism of Tumours." Constable.

Westerhoff, H.V., Koster, J.G., Van Workum, M., and Rudd, K.E. 1990. On the control of gene expression. *In* "Control of Metabolic Processes" (A. Cornish-Bowden, Ed.), pp. 399–412. Plenum, New York.

Yamagata, M., Hasuda, K., Stamato, T., and Tannock, I.F. 1998. The contribution of lactic acid to acidification of tumours: studies of variant cells lacking lactate dehydrogenase. *Br J Cancer* **77**: 1726–1731.

Yamaji, Y., Shiotani, T., Nakamura, H., Hata, Y., Hashimoto, Y., Nagai, M., Fujita, J., and Takahara, J. 1994. Reciprocal alterations of enzymic phenotype of purine and pyrimidine metabolism in induced differentiation of leukemia cells. *Adv Exp Med Biol* **370**: 747–751.

Yatsuoka, T., Sunamura, M., Gurukawa, T., Fukushige, S., Yokoyama, T., Inoue, H., Shibuya, K., Takeda, K., Matsuno, S., and Horii, A. 2000. Association of poor prognosis with loss of 12q 17p, and 18q, and concordant loss of 6q/17p and 12q/18q in human pancreatic ductal adenocarcinoma. *Am J Gastroenterol* **95**: 2080–2085.

Younes, M., et al. 1996. Wide expression of the human erythrocyte glucose transporter Glut1 in human cancers. *Cancer Res* **56**: 1164–1167.

Zhou, J.R., Gugger, E.T., Tanaka, T., Guo, Y., Blackburn, G.L., and Clinton, S.K. 1999. Soybean phytochemicals inhibit the growth of transplantable human prostate carcinoma and tumor angiogenesis in mice. *J Nutr* **129**: 1628–1635.

C H A P T E R

5

Energy Balance and Cancer

STEPHEN D. HURSTING, CONNIE J. ROGERS, SOMDAT MAHABIR, NOMELI P. NUNEZ, J. CARL BARRETT, SUSAN N. PERKINS, AND MICHELE R. FORMAN

INTRODUCTION

The term "energy balance" refers to the integrated effects of diet, physical activity, and genetics on growth and body weight over an individual's lifetime, including the mechanistic pathways through which physical activity and diet exert their effects. Scientists are increasingly aware of the importance of understanding the effects of energy balance on the development and progression of cancer and in cancer patients' quality of life during and after treatment (U.S. Department of Health and Human Services [U.S. DHHS], 2004). Indeed, a 2003 Institute of Medicine (IOM) report on cancer prevention and control assigns top priority to the development of a national strategy to prevent obesity and sedentary behavior (Curry et al., 2003). The prevalence of overweight and obesity has increased dramatically in the past 2 decades in the United States (Hedley et al., 2004). Among adults 20 years or older in 1999–2002, 65.7% were overweight (body mass index [BMI] = 25.0–29.9), 30.6% were obese (BMI ≥ 30.0), and 5.1% were extremely obese (BMI > 40). On average, this translates to an average gain of > 20 pounds in both men and women between the early 1960s and 2002, while during the same time period mean height increased by ~1 in. (Ogden et al., 2004). Over the same years, mean BMI increased ~3 BMI units in both men and women as well (Ogden et al., 2004). Although this trend has appeared across all ethnic groups and genders, it has occurred disproportionately in members of specific ethnic groups, particularly African Americans, Hispanic whites, and American Indians. Of particular concern is that these same trends have also appeared in children, with ethnic group disparities similar to those in adults (Hedley et al., 2004).

The level of physical activity of U.S. citizens at work and during daily living has been decreasing for decades. Less than 40% of American adults get regular exercise, and some 25% get no activity at all. Similar, maybe even more severe, problems exist for our children, where half of American youths do not engage in vigorous physical activity on a regular basis (U.S. DHHS, 1996). Studies have found that physical activity declines steadily and steeply after childhood. In addition to these ominous trends, daily enrollment in physical activity classes in high school has also steadily declined over the past 2 decades (U.S. DHHS, 1996). Reversing these trends is essential, because physical activity plays a direct role in health and well-being, and inactivity is a major factor in the obesity epidemic that is affecting our population.

Obesity in adults is associated with increased mortality from cancers of the colon, breast (in postmenopausal women), endometrium, kidney (renal cell), esophagus (adenocarcinoma), gastric cardia, pancreas, prostate, gallbladder, and liver in a cohort of men and women aged 57 years in 1982, known as the American Cancer Society (ACS) study (Calle et al., 2003). Estimates from the ACS study, the largest prospective analysis of the weight–cancer relationship, suggest 14% of all cancer deaths in men to 20% of all cancer deaths in women from a range of cancer types are attributed to overweight and obesity (Calle et al., 2003). In addition, a study based on the National Health and Nutrition Surveys (NHANES) I, II, and III, as well as the NHANES 1999–2002, identified those in both the leanest and the highest level of BMI at increased risk of all cause mortality (Flegal et al., 2005). If one examines the NHANES data and the ACS data by birth cohort, the findings are quite similar, indicating the importance of events across the life

Copyright © 2006, Elsevier Inc.
All rights of reproduction in any form reserved.

course and their influence on energy balance and mortality.

An International Agency for Research on Cancer (IARC) Working Group on the Evaluation of Weight Control and Physical Activity (2003) concluded that the avoidance of weight gain reduces the risk of developing cancers of the colon, breast (in postmenopausal women), endometrium, kidney, and esophagus based on epidemiological studies of overweight and/or obese compared with leaner individuals. The IARC Working Group Report also concluded that there is consistent epidemiological evidence for a protective effect of physical activity for some cancers. However, the report stated that the relationship between energy balance and cancer is poorly understood. Furthermore, obesity prevention and treatment regimens are difficult, and research on cancer risk in people who have lost weight is extremely limited (Ogden et al., 2003; Calle et al., 2004). In addition, surprisingly little is known about the mechanisms through which caloric restriction or physical activity (the major lifestyle-based strategies for reducing/maintaining weight) exert their anticancer effects (Rundle et al., 2005).

PHYSICAL ACTIVITY AND ENERGY BALANCE

The positive health benefits from physical activity and high fitness are clear (U.S. DHHS, 1996). The Healthy People 2000 goals described in that U.S. DHHS report recognized the importance of physical activity for the nation's health. There is a growing body of evidence that physical inactivity and low physical fitness are associated with increased risk of several cancers, and the underlying physiological changes associated with the healthful effects of exercise are beginning to be characterized. The evidence for an inverse relationship between physical inactivity is conclusive for colon cancer and quite strong for cancers of the breast (although menopausal status does influence this effect, as reported by Friedenreich, 2004), endometrial, ovarian, prostate, and testicular cancers (IARC, 2003). Work since the IARC report was published is further clarifying the exercise–breast cancer link. A meta-analysis of physical activity in adolescence and young adult years had an overall summary risk estimator of 0.81 for those in the highest compared with those in the lowest category of physical activity in observational epidemiological studies, thereby suggesting a protective effect of physical activity on breast cancer risk (Lagerros et al., 2004). This protection due to physical exercise in youth did not vary by study design (cohort vs case–control) or by menopausal status of the women. A report by Holmes et al. (2005) also suggests that increased physical activity after breast cancer diagnosis may decrease risk of death from the disease in breast cancer patients.

One of the issues in the analysis of physical activity and cancer risk is illustrated in an earlier review of the association with ovarian cancer (Bertone et al., 2001). Older birth cohorts of women might not have experienced a protective effect of physical activity in adult years on ovarian cancer because their birth cohort did not have the variation in and intensity of sports or regular exercise to the extent of more recent birth cohorts of women (Bertone et al., 2001). Few studies on other cancers are available, but serious work in this area has been undertaken.

EXERCISE AND ENERGY BALANCE IN CARCINOGENESIS

Studies of the effects of exercise on carcinogenesis have used a variety of animal models including chemically induced tumors, transplantable tumors, spontaneous tumor models, and transgenic and induced-mutant mice, in addition to experimental metastasis models (Hoffman-Goetz, 2003). Many of the studies have identified some form of protective effect of either voluntary or involuntary exercise on carcinogenesis, although other studies have been less consistent (reviewed in Shephard and Futcher, 1997; Woods, 1998). Colon cancer has been the best-studied type of cancer using exercise regimens in animal models, and a consistent inverse association has been observed. To the detriment of the field, the number of animal studies has not increased dramatically, and perhaps more importantly, few studies have used the newer genetically altered models of cancer or have focused on potential mechanisms that might explain the exercise effects. Mechanisms most commonly cited as potential mediators include enhanced antioxidant defense, reductions in body fat, decreases in reproductive hormones, enhanced immunity, or a change in insulin resistance and the insulin-like growth factor-1 (IGF-1) pathway, including its related binding proteins (IARC, 2002). There are also site-specific mechanisms for various cancers such as a decreased colonic transit time in relation to colon cancer. Many of the mechanisms that have received more attention in humans (estrogen, IGF-1) have not received much focus in exercised animal models and vice versa (e.g., immunity and inflammation in animal models). Some of the more intriguing proposed mechanisms are examined in the following sections.

Calorie Restriction and Cancer

The best-studied perturbation of energy balance in experimental cancer systems is on the energy-intake side of the equation, specifically involving obesity prevention through calorie restriction (CR). CR is the only established intervention that extends mean and maximal lifespan in mammals (Weindruch and Walford, 1988; Roth et al., 2001). The antiaging effects of CR have been observed in diverse organisms, including protozoa, yeast (*Saccharomyces cerevisiae*), nematode (*Caenorhabditis elegans*), several insect species including fruit fly (*Drosophila melanogaster*), mouse (including transgenic and knockout models of cancer susceptibility), rat, hamster, guinea pig, dog, cow, and preliminarily in several nonhuman primate species (Pinney et al., 1972; Weindruch and Walford, 1988; Defossez et al., 2001; Roth et al., 2001; Kealy et al., 2002). Thus, the mechanisms underlying the survival extension in response to CR, imposed using various dietary compositions, feeding strategies, and levels of restriction, appear to be evolutionarily conserved. This suggests that a better understanding of these mechanisms will reveal important clues about the biology of aging, as well as preventive strategies for diseases of aging, including cancer.

CR inhibits a variety of spontaneous neoplasias in experimental cancer model systems (Hursting and Kari, 1998), including tumors arising in several genetically altered mouse models, such as p53-deficient mice, APC^{min} mice, and *Wnt-1* transgenic mice (Hursting et al., 2005). CR also suppresses the carcinogenic action of several classes of chemicals in rodents, including polycyclic aromatic hydrocarbons, for example, benzo(a)pyrene (Tannenbaum, 1940, 1942) and DMBA (Andreous and Morgan, 1981; Boissonneault et al., 1986); alkylating and methylating agents, for example, diethylnitrosamine (Lagopoulous and Stadler, 1987); and aromatic amines, such as *p*-cresidine (Dunn et al., 1997). In addition, CR inhibits several forms of radiation-induced cancers (Gross and Dreyfuss, 1984, 1990). Thus, the inhibitory action of CR on carcinogenesis is effective in several species for a variety of tumor types and for both spontaneous tumors and chemically induced neoplasias. In our view, the central goals of contemporary CR research are to apply its findings to human health concerns and to understand the biological mechanisms of CR's effects.

Observational studies suggest that CR has beneficial effects on longevity in humans. These studies include natural experiments, such as a study of Spanish nursing home residents, suggesting that reduced caloric intake reduces morbidity and mortality (Roth et al., 1999). Moreover, physiological changes analogous to those observed in CR rodents and monkeys, including high-density lipoprotein (HDL) cholesterol increases, are reported in Muslims who fast during the daylight hours of the holy month of Ramadan (Temizhan et al., 2000). In addition, inhabitants of Okinawa, Japan, who are known to consume fewer calories than residents of the main Japanese islands, display lower death rates from cancer and vascular diseases (Kagawa, 1978). The relationship between reduced calories and reduced mortality in Okinawa, relative to the rest of Japan, could be confounded by other factors such as genetic differences or other dietary differences, but these observations are intriguing. Data from certain historical events, such as the Dutch famine during World War II, are also suggestive of decreased mortality from cancer and other age-related diseases following extended reductions in calorie intake, although such observations are difficult to interpret because of confounding factors such as malnutrition (van Noord and Kaaks, 1991).

Another category of studies in humans includes more controlled demonstrations of the antiaging effects of CR, such as occurred with Biosphere 2 and the ongoing Netherlands Toxicology and Nutrition Institute study. Biosphere 2, which took place in a closed ecosystem in Arizona from 1991 to 1993, involved four men and four women who experienced, on average, a 30% restriction in calorie intake relative to their usual intake. Although this sample was too small and uncontrolled to allow clear conclusions, many of the physiological parameters associated with the anticancer effects of CR in rodents and nonhuman primates were observed in these subjects (Walford et al., 1992). The TNO study was more controlled, with 8 *ad libitum* (AL) control subjects and 16 subjects on a 20% CR regimen. As in Biosphere 2, the TNO study subjects on the CR regimen, relative to the controls, displayed positive effects, including decreased fat mass and lowered blood pressure (Velthuis et al., 1994).

In the past decade, four longevity studies involving long-term CR versus AL feeding have been initiated in several nonhuman primate species (Roth et al., 1999; Lane et al., 2001). It remains to be seen whether the extension of lifespan and/or reduction in tumor development demonstrated consistently in rodents will be replicated in nonhuman primates. However, preliminary reports on chronic disease-associated markers and initial tumor incidence and mortality data suggest that monkeys on CR regimens are less likely to develop diabetes, cardiovascular disease, obesity, autoimmune diseases, and cancer than their AL-fed counterparts (Roth et al., 1999; Lane et al., 2001).

Selected Potential Mechanisms

Because perturbations in energy balance act broadly with respect to species, mode of induction, and type of tumor effected, and because CR, obesity, and physical activity each influences the levels of a number of hormones and growth factors (Weindruch and Walford, 1988), several investigators (including us) have suggested that globally active circulating factors may be the key mediators of the energy balance and cancer link (reviewed in Weindruch and Walford, 1988; Hursting et al., 2003). A number of inherited endocrinological disorders may contribute to obesity, although the prevalence of even the most common syndromes is very low. Several central nervous system factors, including neuropeptide Y, proopiomelanocortin, 5-hydroxytryptamine, noradrenaline, dopamine, and corticotrophin-releasing factor, have been shown to play a role in the regulation of normal body weight in rodents (Schwartz et al., 2000; Altman, 2002; Bray, 2004). These neurochemicals interact with the receptors on specific neurons in the arcuate nucleus (ARC) in the hypothalamus (Altman, 2002). The ARC has neurotransmitters and modulators that play a critical role in receiving and transmitting signals that regulate energy intake (Schwartz et al., 2000; Zigman and Elmquist, 2003; Seely et al., 2004). However, the roles of these factors in humans (particularly with respect to cancer risk) are unclear, primarily because of the tremendous technical challenges involved in measuring these neurochemicals. Numerous other hormones are involved in body weight regulation as satiety signals or as regulators of energy metabolism, such as gherelin, cholecystokinin, glucagon, glucagon-like peptide-1, adiponectin, resistin, and bombesin (deGraaf et al., 2004), although the relationships between these factors and cancer have not been well characterized. Finally, several other hormones serve as intermediate and long-term communicators of nutritional state throughout the biosystem and have been implicated in both energy balance and carcinogenesis. These hormones include IGF-1, as well as insulin, leptin, and several factors associated with inflammation and oxidative stress, and are the focus of the following mechanistic discussion.

Potential Role of IGF-1 in Cancer

The possible involvement of IGF-1 in cancer was first suspected when *in vitro* studies consistently showed that IGF-1 enhances the growth of various cancer cell lines. These include prostate, bladder, breast, lung, colon, stomach, esophagus, liver, pancreas, kidney, thyroid, brain, ovarian, cervical, and endometrial cancer cell lines (Macauley, 1992; LeRoith et al., 1995; Fenton et al., 2005; Singh et al., 1996). There is now abundant epidemiological evidence, reviewed elsewhere in this book, supporting the hypothesis that IGF-1 is involved in several types of human cancer. IGF-1 acts directly on cells via the IGF-1 receptor (IGF-1R), which is overexpressed in many tumors, or indirectly through its action with other cancer-related molecules. For example, IGF-1 and the p53 tumor suppressor appear to function together in a regulatory network. The p53 gene regulates the expression of IGF-binding protein-3 (IGFBP-3) (Buckbinder et al., 1996), and IGF-1–induced mitogenesis is associated with phosphorylation and translocation of the p53 protein from the nucleus to the cytoplasm (Takahashi and Suzuki, 1993).

Findings in diverse species, including yeast (*S. cerevisiae*), nematode (*C. elegans*), fruit fly (*D. melanogaster*), and mouse (*Mus* spp.), suggest that IGF-1 is part of an evolutionarily conserved neurosecretory pathway that regulates animal aging in response to food availability (Gems and Partridge, 2001). For example, increased longevity is observed in *Drosophila* Chico mutants and *InR* mutants that display altered insulin/IGF-1 signaling (Clancy et al., 2001; Tatar et al., 2001). In *C. elegans*, mutants in the *daf* (dauer formation) gene, which is part of an IGF-like signal transduction pathway, demonstrate increased change to stresses such as crowding, starvation, and thermal, as well as increased lifespan (Murakami and Johnson, 1996, 1998; Barsyte et al., 2001).

A markedly increased average and maximal lifespan is also observed in several strains of mutant or genetically modified mice that suffer defects in the production of growth hormone or IGF-1 or in responsiveness to growth hormone (and hence express significantly lower levels of circulating IGF-1). The "little" mouse, with its defective response to hypothalamic growth hormone–releasing hormone, lives 20–25% longer than wild-type mice (Flurkey et al., 2001). Laron mice, with a disruption in the growth hormone receptor/binding protein gene, have higher circulating levels of growth hormone than wild-type mice but much lower serum IGF-1 levels, and they live 38–55% longer than wild-type mice (Coschigano et al., 2000). Mice with primary deficiencies in growth hormone, prolactin, and thyrotropin, caused by failure of the pituitary to differentiate during fetal development, live still longer, 40–64% longer than wild-type mice. These latter examples include the Snell and Jackson dwarf mice, which have a point mutation in the homeotic transcription factor, *Pit1* (Flurkey et al., 2002), and the Ames dwarf mouse, which fails to express Pit1 because of an inactivating point mutation in the *Prop1* transcription factor (Brown-Borg et al., 1996). As seen with CR, these mutations appear to reduce the onset and/or rate of aging and age-associated cancers, resulting in an extended lifespan (Anisimov, 2001). In addition, mice displaying an ~75% reduction of circulating IGF-1 levels, due to a liver-specific knockout of IGF-1, show reduced tumor development and growth (Yakar et al., 2005). In contrast, tissue-specific overexpression of IGF-1 via the keratin 5 promoter increases spontaneous tumor development and susceptibility to carcinogens (DiGiovanni et al., 2000).

IGF-1, Growth, and Cell Cycle Regulation

The complex process of growth involves the coordination of environmental signals (including nutritional cues) with programmed neuroendocrine responses that determine body size and composition. IGF-1 is a central component of a complex network of molecules that includes growth hormone, IGF-2, insulin, six (at least) IGFBPs that regulate IGF-1 ligand activity, leptin, adrenal steroid hormones, and several cell surface receptors. IGF-1 (a 70–amino acid polypeptide growth factor that shares ~50% homology with insulin) and pituitary-derived growth hormone are key regulators of an endocrine, paracrine, and autocrine signaling network that controls long bone growth and energy metabolism (LeRoith et al., 2001). The circulating level of IGF-1 is mainly determined by hepatic synthesis, which is regulated by growth hormone and influenced by nutrient intake, particularly intake of energy and protein (Hursting et al.,

1993). Regulation of IGF-1 in extrahepatic tissues is more complex, involving growth hormone, other hormones and growth factors, and IGFBPs, which determine the systemic half-life and local availability of IGF-1 (LeRoith et al., 2001).

IGF-1 also regulates mitogenic and antiapoptotic signaling in many types of normal and cancer cells. IGF-1 has been identified as a cell cycle progression factor based on its ability in many normal and cancer cell types to stimulate progression through the cell cycle from G_1 to S phase, purportedly by activating the phosphatidylinositol-3 kinase/Akt signal transduction pathway and modulating cyclin-dependent kinases. *In vivo*, IGF-1 may also be required for efficiently traversing the later stages of the cell cycle (LeRoith et al., 2001).

IGF-1 and Apoptosis

IGF-1 can suppress apoptosis in various cell types, and cells overexpressing the IGF-1 receptor (IGF-1R) show decreased apoptosis (Resnicoff et al., 1995; Dunn et al., 1998). In addition, apoptosis is induced by reducing the cellular levels of IGF-1R using antisense oligonucleotides or by expression of a dominant-negative IGF-1R (D'Ambrosio et al., 1996). IGF-1 in many cell types stimulates phosphorylation of phosphatidylinositol-3 kinase, resulting in active phospholipid phosphatases that activate Akt (LeRoith et al., 2001). Activated Akt can suppress apoptosis by inhibiting the activation of interleukin-1β–converting enzyme (ICE)–like proteases. Other pathways may also play a role in IGF-1–dependent suppression of apoptosis. The apparently ubiquitous suppression of apoptosis by IGF-1 suggests that it is part of an important regulatory mechanism for maintaining tissue homeostasis that is usurped during the neoplastic process. It is primarily these effects on proliferation and apoptosis that make IGF-1 a plausible target for therapeutic and preventive strategies against cancer.

IGF-1 as a Mediator of the Anticancer Effects of CR

There is mounting evidence that IGF-1 mediates at least some of the anticancer effects of CR through its role in an evolutionarily conserved regulatory pathway that is responsive to energy availability (Gems and Partridge, 2001). In various mouse and rat models, we and others have shown that serum IGF-1 levels are consistently decreased in proportion to the severity of the CR regimen imposed (reviewed in Hursting et al., 2005). For example, we reported that a CR regimen (25% reduction in calorie intake) reduces serum IGF-1, decreases *in situ* leukemia cell proliferation, and inhibits spontaneous and transplanted mononuclear cell leukemia in F344 rats (Hursting et al., 1993) and p53-deficient mice (Hursting et al., 1994). Furthermore, restoration of serum IGF-1 concentrations to control levels in CR-treated rats by infusion via miniature osmotic pumps restores *in situ* leukemia cell proliferation rates to near control levels (Hursting et al., 1993). We also demonstrated that a moderate CR regimen (20% reduction in calorie intake) decreases serum IGF-1, increases the ratio of apoptotic versus proliferating preneoplastic urothelial cells, and suppresses *p*-cresidine–induced bladder carcinogenesis in p53-deficient mice (Dunn et al., 1997). Restoration of serum IGF-1 concentrations (again with miniature osmotic pumps) to control levels in *p*-cresidine–treated CR mice reversed the effects of CR on urothelial cell proliferation, apoptosis, and bladder tumor development (Dunn et al., 1997). Taken together, these studies suggest that IGF-1 mediates at least some of the antiproliferative, proapoptotic, and anticancer effects of CR. This conclusion does not exclude other mediators, which may be regulated by IGF-1 or function independently of IGF-1. In fact, our studies of CR in K5-IGF-1 transgenic mice, which constitutively overexpress IGF-1, and in liver-specific IGF-1–deficient mice, which have only 25% of normal circulating IGF-1 levels, suggest that IGF-1 accounts for some but certainly not all of the effects of CR (Hursting et al., unpublished observations).

Physical Activity and IGF-1 Levels in Men and Women

Because physical activity induces changes in body fat, especially intraabdominal fat, with changes in insulin and insulin sensitivity, as well as the IGF axis (McTiernan, 1998), several physical activity intervention projects have been conducted in women aged 30–50 years (Schmitz et al., 2002) and in postmenopausal women (McTiernan et al., 2004). Interestingly, none of these intervention studies demonstrated a difference in preintervention and postintervention IGF-1 levels even though the intensity of physical activity and duration of the intervention varied by study. Because IGF-1 concentrations in humans decline from late adolescence on and serum levels of IGF-1 are related to age, perhaps the inability to detect differences in IGF-1 levels from exercise may relate to the limited range in age and large interindividual variation in IGF-1 levels in adults (O'Connor et al., 1998). However, using age-matched, inbred mice, which have only modest interindividual variation in IGF-1 levels, we have not observed differences in circulating IGF-1 levels in response to various levels of treadmill (Colbert et al., 2003) or voluntary wheel running (Colbert et al., unpublished observations). These findings are consistent with little or no long-term effects of exercise on circulating IGF-1 levels, as suggested by the human studies. However, we are seeing exercise effects on IGFBPs, so levels of bioavailable IGF-1 may be altered by physical activity.

Another issue described by Rundle et al. (2005) is that there are no available biomarkers of exposure to or biologically effective doses of physical activity on cancer risk or biomarkers of intermediate effects from physical activity training by level and duration.

Other Possible Mechanisms Underlying the Energy Balance and Cancer Association

Insulin: Chronic hyperinsulinemia and insulin resistance increase risk of cancer at several sites (Calle and Kaaks, 2004), although it is unclear whether the tumor-enhancing effects of insulin are due to direct effects via the insulin receptor on preneoplastic cells or alternatively due to indirect effects via stimulation of IGF-1, estrogens, or other hormones. There is certainly important crosstalk between these hormonal pathways that is only now beginning to be understood, and it is clear that high circulating levels of insulin promote the hepatic synthesis of IGF-1 and decrease the production of IGFBP-1, thus increasing the biologic activity of IGF-1 (Calle and Kaaks, 2004). Furthermore, both insulin and IGF-1 act *in vitro* as growth factors to promote cancer cell proliferation and decrease apoptosis (Yakar et al., 2005). Insulin resistance, a state of reduced response of tissues to the physiological actions of insulin, results in a compensatory rise in plasma insulin levels and is affected by both adiposity and physical activity. Intraabdominal obesity is associated with insulin resistance (Abate, 1996), although physical activity improves insulin sensitivity (Grimm et al., 1999). A growing body of epidemiological evidence suggests that type II diabetes, which is usually characterized by hyperinsulinemia and insulin resistance for long periods, is associated with increased risks of endometrial, colon, pancreas, kidney, and postmenopausal breast cancers (Calle and Kaaks, 2004).

Leptin is a 16-kDa peptide hormone secreted from adipocytes that is involved with appetite control and energy metabolism through hypothalamic influence. In the nonobese state, rising leptin levels result in decreased appetite and increased energy metabolism through a series of neuroendocrine changes. The obese state is associated with high circulating leptin levels (Lohnquist et al., 1997; Montague et al., 1997; Woods et al., 1998; Zhang and Leibel, 1998), suggesting that the obese may be leptin resistant. This resistance appears to explain much of the inability of exogenous leptin administration to prevent weight gain. The mechanisms underlying this apparent leptin insensitivity in the obese are not fully understood, although they may be due to defects in leptin signal transduction and/or transport across the blood–brain barrier, resulting in a higher "setpoint" of body weight (Wilding et al., 1997). The limited number of studies are suggestive of an association between circulating leptin levels and cancer risk, with the most consistent findings thus far for colon (Stattin et al., 2004) and prostate cancer (particularly progression of prostate cancer, as suggested by Chang et al. [2001] and Saglam et al. [2003]). *In vitro*, leptin stimulates proliferation of multiple types of preneoplastic and neoplastic cells (but not "normal" cells, as reported by Fenton et al., 2005) and in animal models appears to promote angiogenesis and tumor invasion (Bouloumie et al., 1998).

The primary physiological role of leptin may be regulating energy homeostasis by providing a signal to the central nervous system regarding the size of fat stores, and circulating leptin levels correlate strongly with adipose tissue levels in animals and humans (Ostlund, 1996). Findings reviewed by Rajala and Scherer (2003) also suggest that leptin exerts its metabolic effects, at least in part, by activating 5′-AMP–activated protein kinase (AMPK) in muscle and liver, thus decreasing several anabolic pathways (including glucose-regulated transcription and fatty acid and triglyceride synthesis) and increasing several ATP-producing catabolic pathways (including glucose transport, glycolysis, and mitochondrial biogenesis). In addition, there is significant crosstalk among the leptin pathway, which involves the Jak/Stat family of transcription factors, the insulin/IGF-1/Akt pathway, and AMPK. Furthermore, leptin plays a role in regulating the hypothalamus–pituitary–adrenal axis and, thus, influences IGF-1 synthesis (Rajala and Scherer, 2003). Finally, leptin functions as an inflammatory cytokine and appears to influence immune function (Loffreda et al., 1998). In fact, the immunosuppression associated with acute starvation is reversed by leptin administration (Rajala and Scherer, 2003). Thus, though not well studied, leptin is certainly positioned as a central player in the energy balance and cancer association.

Sex steroid hormones, including estrogens, androgens, and progesterone, also reportedly play a role in the relationship between energy balance and certain types of cancer. Adipose tissue is the main site of estrogen synthesis in men and postmenopausal (or otherwise ovarian hormone–deficient) women, through the ability of aromatase (an enzyme present in adipose tissue) to convert androgenic precursors produced in the adrenals and gonads to estrogens (Calle and Kaaks, 2004). In addition, adipose tissue is the second major source of IGF-1 (liver is the primary source). The increased insulin and bioactive IGF-1 levels that typically accompany increased adiposity can provide feedback to reduce sex hormone binding globulin, resulting in an increased fraction of bioavailable estradiol in men and women (Calle and Kaaks, 2004). This can also result in higher bioavailable testosterone in women, and extreme obesity can lead to polycystic ovary disease, which manifests as hyperandrogenism, chronic anovulation, and progesterone deficiency. The epidemiological literature clearly suggests that the increased bioavailability of sex steroids that accompanies increased adiposity is strongly associated with risk of endometrial and postmenopausal breast cancers (Endogenous Hormones and Breast Cancer Collaborative Group, 2002; Kaaks et al., 2002) and may impact colon and other cancers as well.

The estrogen and androgen receptors, through which the sex steroids exert most of their proliferative and pro-cancer effects, are part of a nuclear receptor superfamily. A review by Ronald Evans (2005) suggests that this family of nuclear receptors has exquisitely evolved to acquire, absorb, distribute, store, and use energy. Examples include (1) dietary and endogenous fats that involve the lipid-sensing peroxisome proliferator-activated receptors (PPARs), which are emerging as key regulators of lipid and glucose homeostasis (Evans et al., 2004); (2) sugar mobilization involving the glucocorticoid receptor; (3) cholesterol through the liver X receptor; and (4) maintenance of metabolic rate through the thyroid hormone receptor. Evans et al. (2004) suggest that these "fuel management–related" receptors interact with gonadal steroid receptors (estrogen, androgen, progesterone receptors) to link nutritional status and fertility. Inflammation, which is the third key component regulated by the nuclear receptor superfamily, is also linked to energy balance through these same pathways that coordinately manage energy and inflammation. For example, the glucocorticoid receptor pathway is capable of mobilizing massive amounts of energy and suppressing inflammation, and the retinoic acid receptors, liver X receptors, PPARα and PPARγ, and the vitamin D receptor can also protect against inflammation, which can have an impact on cancer risk.

Inflammation: The association between chronic inflammation and cancer is widely accepted (reviewed by Coussens and Werb, 2002). The effect of exercise on inflammatory processes has been better characterized than the effects of obesity, CR, or other energy balance perturbations. However, obesity is clearly associated with increased inflammation, and we and others have shown that CR decreases certain inflammatory markers.

The cytokine response to exercise (reviewed by Petersen and Pedersen, 2005) does not involve an increase in the proinflammatory cytokines, tumor necrosis factor-α (TNF-α) and interleukin-1β (IL-1β) but is initiated by IL-6 and then is followed by an increase in the anti-inflammatory mediators, IL-1ra, sTNF-R, and IL-10 (Ostrowski et al., 1999, 2000). Circulating levels of IL-6 have been shown to significantly increase (up to 100-fold) with exercise and decline in the postexercise period, with the relative increase in IL-6 in relation to exercise intensity, duration, and endurance capacity (Pedersen and Hoffman-Goetz, 2000; Pedersen et al., 2001; Suzuki et al., 2002; Febbraio et al., 2004). Interestingly, the main source of the exercise-induced increase in IL-6 is skeletal muscle (Penkowa et al., 2003; Steensberg et al., 2003; Hiscock et al., 2004) rather than monocytes (Ullum et al., 1994; Moldoveannu et al., 2000; Starkie et al., 2001).

This exercise-induced increase in IL-6 is intriguing for several reasons. First, several studies have shown that IL-6 can inhibit the production of the proinflammatory cytokines, TNF-α, and IL-1β. IL-6 has been shown to inhibit lipopolysaccharide (LPS)-induced TNF-α production *in vitro* (Schindler et al., 1990). In both IL-6 knockout mice (Mizuhara et al., 1994) and mice treated with anti-IL-6 antibodies (Matthys et al., 1995), the circulating levels of TNF-α are significantly increased following either bacterial or an injury stimulus. Furthermore, the administration of recombinant human IL-6 to healthy volunteers inhibited the endotoxin-induced increase in TNF-α (Starkie et al., 2003). Second, IL-6 has also been shown to stimulate the production of anti-inflammatory mediators, such as IL-1ra, sTNF-R, and IL-10 (Steensberg et al., 2003). Combined, these data suggest that exercise increases systemic IL-6 and that this exercise-induced increase in IL-6 may result in a reduction of chronic inflammation by reducing proinflammatory mediators and elevating anti-inflammatory mediators. However, additional studies are needed to determine whether regular moderate exercise can significantly reduce systemic inflammation and subsequently affect tumor development.

Oxidative stress: Reactive oxygen species (ROS), involved in the inflammatory response, are important in a variety of normal processes within the body, including energy metabolism, direction of the immune response against pathogens, apoptotic regulation, intracellular signaling, and control of vascular permeability. However, the accumulation of ROS as byproducts of normal energy metabolism and in response to inflammatory conditions or ROS-generating environmental exposures (e.g., to particulates in tobacco smoke) has been associated with the pathogenesis of cancer and nonneoplastic age-related pathologies in rodents, nonhuman primates, and humans (Ames et al., 1993; Marnet et al., 2000). ROS can act as both initiators and promoters of tumors by damaging critical cellular macromolecules, such as DNA, proteins, and lipids, and by acting as cell-signaling molecules, in the manner of nitric oxide (Marnet et al., 2000; Hursting et al., 2005). There are few studies that have examined ROS-related damage or relevant antioxidant enzymes in the context of exercise in a cancer model, although exercise has been shown to effect oxidative stress (Ji, 1999; Fehrenbach et al., 2001; Radak et al., 2001). A 10-week treadmill training program in rats led to increased levels of superoxide dismutase (SOD) and catalase (CAT) in the lung, whereas UDP-glucuronosyl transferase was upregulated in both liver and lung (Duncan et al., 1997). Radak et al. (2004) also reported a decrease in ROS production in the liver following 8 weeks of treadmill training in Fischer 344 rats. Thus, evidence is accumulating that chronic exercise training promotes beneficial effects in many animal antioxidant systems (Radak et al., 2001).

One study has examined wheel running in a tumor-bearing rat model, and its effects on coenzymes Q_9 and Q_{10} in skeletal muscle, as exercise in this same model had been found to delay cancer-induced cachexia, which interestingly is mediated by the inflammatory cytokine TNF-α (Daneryd et al., 1995). Both enzymes appeared to be upregulated in anterior tibialis muscle and Q_9 also in the soleus.

CR is known to decrease oxidative stress and inflammation (Sohal and Weindruch, 1996), and the CR-induced reduction in IGF-1 levels may play a role in these effects. Evidence from diverse species suggests a link among defects in the IGF-1 pathway, increased tolerance to oxidative and other stresses, and extended lifespan. For example, *Daf* gene mutants in *C. elegans*, described earlier because of their defect in IGF-like signaling and extended lifespan, also demonstrate increased tolerance to several types of stress (Murakami and Johnson, 1998). In *Drosophila, InR* mutants mimic *C. elegans Daf-2* mutants (e.g., altered IGF-like signaling, increased lifespan, and tolerance to stress), whereas overexpression of antioxidant proteins, including superoxide dismutase, catalase, and glutathione reductase, also extends lifespan and increases resistance to oxidative stress (Tatar et al., 2001). Furthermore, CR in *S. cerevisiae* increases *Sir2* activity, which extends lifespan and increases genomic stability and stress resistance (Defossez et al., 2001). Mice in which the p66 splice variant of the *shc* protooncogene has been ablated by gene targeting appear not only to be resistant to oxidative stress but also to live 30% longer than wild-type mice (Migliaccio, 1999). Finally, Ames dwarf mice, which are growth-hormone/IGF-1 deficient because of a mutation in *Prop*1, exhibit an upregulation of antioxidative defenses and a significant extension of lifespan relative to wild-type siblings (Brown-Borg et al., 2002).

CR may exert some of its antitumor effects by decreasing ROS production and enhancing antioxidant defenses. CR decreases the rate of accumulation of oxidized DNA and protein that accompanies aging in rodents (Youngman et al., 1992). In addition, a number of intracellular antioxidant defense systems, including SOD, CAT, and glutathione peroxidase, which decline with age, are reportedly maintained or even enhanced by CR (Weindruch and Walford, 1988). CR also reduces nitric oxide production in peritoneal macrophages in p53-deficient and wild-type mice (Mei et al., 1998). Thus, evidence is mounting that CR may decrease oxidative stress by decreasing oxidant production and enhancing antioxidant capacity, although the exact mechanisms involved have yet to be fully established. The reduction in IGF-1 in response to CR may again play a role because cultured hepatocytes treated with IGF-1 demonstrate decreased activity and expression of CAT, glutathione peroxidase, and manganese SOD and, thus, have a decreased ability to counter oxidative stress (Brown-Borg et al., 2002).

FUTURE RESEARCH DIRECTIONS AND CONCLUSIONS

Although the associations between overweight/obesity and several cancers are becoming well defined, the causal relationships between energy balance and cancer risk are not well established. For example, key unanswered questions include the following: (1) Does reversal of obesity through diet, exercise, or pharmacological regimens decrease cancer risk or impact existing cancers? (2) Are there important differences between antiobesity regimens (calorie restriction, exercise, drugs) in terms of anticancer effects, or is weight reduction/maintenance the key irrespective of the means? (3) Which, if any, of the hormonal changes (i.e., IGF-1, insulin, leptin, and sex steroids) or biosystem changes (i.e., weight, adiposity, insulin resistance, inflammation, hypoxia, and alterations in energy metabolism) accompanying energy imbalance are causally linked to carcinogenesis? (4) What is the impact of different energy balance states and their associated effects on physiology (i.e., lean vs obese; insulin resistant vs insulin sensitive; high vs low postmenopausal estrogen levels) on the response to cancer prevention or cancer therapy regimens? As illustrated in Figure 1, progress in this area will require a multidisciplinary approach, and these and other key questions will only be answered through well-designed studies in both animals and humans that incorporate molecular, genetic, and metabolic/nutritional tools and expertise.

As discussed in this chapter, the components of several interacting pathways associated with aging and carcinogenesis are altered by perturbations in energy balance, such as physical activity and CR. One approach to deciphering the complex network of mediators underlying the energy

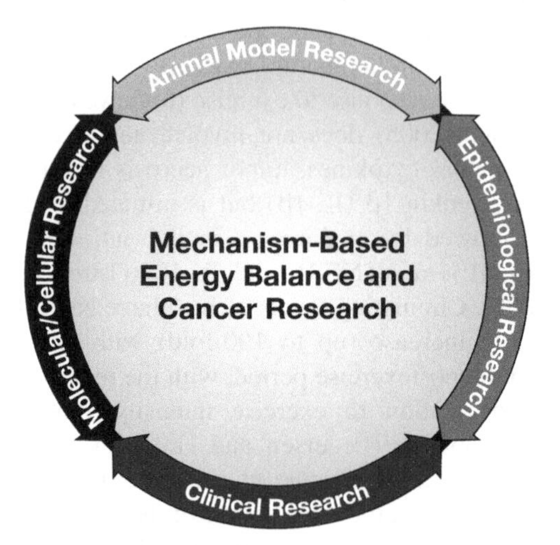

FIGURE 1 The transdisciplinary nature of mechanism-based energy balance and cancer prevention research. Progress in the translation of mechanism-based findings in energy balance and carcinogenesis to cancer prevention strategies in humans requires the integration of observational epidemiological and clinical findings, the development and use of relevant animal models that can model the key events of both energy balance and carcinogenesis, the characterization of basic mechanisms at the molecular, cellular, and metabolic level, and the ultimate application of these findings to the clinic and community.

TABLE 1 Selected Microarray Studies of Gene Expression in Mice in Response to Aging and Calorie Restriction (CR)

Reference	Tissue: model	Age of "aged" animals	Age, proportional to maximal longevity[a]	No. of genes measured	No. of genes significantly altered by aging	Percentage of genes changed by aging	Percent ameliorated by CR[b,c]
Lee et al., 1999	Gastrocnemius muscle: male C57BL/6 mice	30 months	~0.95	6,347	113	1.8	29% completely 34% partially
Lee et al., 2000	Brain: male C57BL/6 mice	30 months	~0.95	6,347	110	1.7	30% completely 75% partially
Cao et al., 2001	Liver: female C3B10RF1 mice	27 months	~0.75	~5,300	46	0.7	59% completely
Prolla, 2002	Brain: male C57BL/6 mice	30 months	~0.95	6,347	114 (neocortex) 108 (cerebellum)	~1 (neocortex and cerebellum similar)	30% completely or partially; similar patterns in neocortex and cerebellum
Tsuchiya et al., 2004	Liver: female Ames homozygous (Dwarf) vs heterozygous (normal) littermates	6 months	~0.19	12,252	212 (Dwarf vs normal); 77 (CR only)	—	77 genes independently affected by CR; 212 independently altered by dwarfism; 95 additively affected by CR and Dwarfism (including several in IGF-1 pathway)
Dhabi et al., 2004	Liver: male B6C3F1 mice, with CR begun at 7 months of age	34 months	~0.98	12,422	—	—	6% (123) genes changed in response to CR begun at seven months vs *ad lib* throughout life
Higami et al., 2004	Adipose: male C57BL/6 mice	11 months	~0.33	~11,200	—	—	5.5% (345) of total *lib*genes expressed in adipose from controls altered by long-term (9-month) CR

[a]Maximal longevity data obtained from Weindruch and Walford, 1988.

[b]*Ameliorated* = either a change occurred in aged AL-fed animals but not in aged CR-fed animals, or changes occurred in both groups but in opposite directions.

[c]CR also induced multiple gene alterations different from those occurring with age.

[d]Investigated gene expression changes in response to aging over time: 7, 18, 23, 28, 42, and 47 days.

balance and cancer link is to incorporate genomic and proteomic (and very soon metabolomic) analyses into these studies. Weindruch; Prolla and colleagues; and Spindler, Dhabi, and colleagues were among the first to use microarray technology to investigate the antiaging effects of CR, and a selection of these studies is summarized in Table 1. For example, Weindruch's and Prolla's initial experiments involved the comparison of global gene expression patterns in muscle (Lee et al., 1999) and brain (Lee et al., 2000) of young (3-month-old) AL-fed mice, aged (30-month-old) AL-fed mice, and aged CR-fed mice. Their findings linked aging with a gene expression pattern indicative of decreased metabolism and biosynthesis in muscle, increased inflammatory response in brain, and an increased stress response in both tissues (Weindruch, et al., 2002). CR either completely or partially attenuated many of these changes (Table 1). A similar reversal of age-related gene expression changes was evident in a comparative whole-genome transcript profiling of AL-fed and CR-fed aged *D. melanogaster* (Pletcher et al., 2002). Microarray analysis of gene expression in livers of both short- and long-term CR mice indicates that CR also reverses many of the gene expression changes associated with aging in the livers of C3B10RF1 female mice (Cao et al., 2001), and the reversal of these age-related gene expression patterns by CR is rapid (Dhabi et al., 2004). AL-fed aged, relative to AL-fed young, rhesus monkeys demonstrated significant upregulation in skeletal muscle of transcripts involved in inflammation and oxidative stress, as well as downregulation of genes involved in mitochondrial electron transport, consistent with the age-related gene expression changes observed in mice. In addition, adult-onset CR in rhesus monkeys decreased the expression of skeletal muscle genes involved in mitochondrial bioenergetics and upregulated several cytoskeletal-related genes, but it did not reverse the age-related changes in gene expression (Kayo et al., 2001). A review by Han and Hickey (2005) of the nearly 25 reports of microarray analyses in various organisms (mostly mice) that included some aspect of CR in their study suggests that no specific genes were altered across all the studies, possibly because of differences in microarray platform, species, strain and tissue differences, and other study differences. However, several functional categories of genes universally emerge as responsive to CR, including energy metabolism, stress responses (such as heat shock and oxidative), immune/inflammation pathways, and transcriptional regulation.

To our knowledge, no studies using microarray or proteomic approaches to directly investigate the anticancer effects of CR have been published. Because carcinogenesis is a multistage process, the temporal design of such experiments requires careful consideration. Although many tissues share similarities in the classes of genes altered by CR, as discussed previously, relevant gene expression patterns will change throughout the carcinogenesis process and will vary from tissue to tissue. The challenge is to recognize those causal pathways and their upstream regulators that can serve as targets for cancer prevention. This process will involve validating microarray findings, tying gene expression findings to protein expression findings, and testing hypotheses about perturbations in causal pathways both *in vitro* and *in vivo*. Comparisons of energy balance perturbations in normal versus preneoplastic versus tumor tissue across a time course may also provide important insights and facilitate the identification of the most relevant pathways in the midst of a large number of individual gene expression changes.

A better understanding of the physiological interactions between IGF-1 and other pathways involved in processes associated with energy balance and carcinogenesis (including new pathways that emerge from genomic and proteomic studies) will be very important in the translation of mechanism-based studies to disease prevention. Examples discussed in this chapter include important interactions among IGF-1, insulin, and other factors involved in glucose metabolism and insulin sensitivity, estrogens and other hormones linking energy balance and reproductive processes, as well as leptin and several other hormones and cytokines that bridge energy balance and inflammation. Although much of the excitement and attention centers on cytokines such as IL-6, TNF-α, monocyte chemoattractant protein-1, and several others, some of the classic hormones, like the adrenal steroids (which are not discussed in detail here) also likely play a role. Glucocorticoids such as corticosterone are known to affect the cell cycle, induce apoptosis, and reduce inflammation in a variety of cells and tissues and are an integral component of glucose metabolism and mobilization. Several laboratories have shown that CR increases plasma levels and urinary excretion of corticosterone and its metabolites in rodents (Birt et al., 1999; Berrigan et al., 2002; Mai et al., 2003). Therefore, the increase in corticosterone levels with CR could interact with alterations in IGF-1 signaling to significantly contribute to the antiaging and anticancer effects of CR. There is also a host of emerging energy balance–related factors, including adiponectin, resistin, gherelin, glucagon-like peptide-1, C-reactive protein, and several others. Many of these are produced in adipose tissue or in the gut, and at least some will likely turn out to play an important role in energy balance and carcinogenesis. Little will be gained by addressing these factors individually; the central goal has to be deciphering how these pathways interact to link energy balance and the carcinogenesis process.

The insights from basic and applied research concerning the benefits of CR, exercise, and other antiobesity interventions on healthy aging and cancer prevention require translation into medical interventions and public health recommendations. Unfortunately, the direct translation of CR to humans may never be broadly accepted because major dietary and lifestyle changes, such as a 20–40% decrease in calorie intake, are very difficult for most people (McGuire et al., 1999). Exercise regimens may have broader appeal, although again not everyone can successfully make this change in lifestyle. New approaches to translation are, therefore, needed to fulfill the promise of the health benefits of CR and exercise. In this section, we propose areas relevant to translation that merit further basic and applied research.

As described earlier, the IGF-1 pathway has emerged as a potential key mediator of CR's anticancer and antiaging effects. Agents or interventions that reduce IGF-1 without requiring drastic dietary changes may provide an effective physiological or pharmacological mimetic of those effects, which could be readily adopted by a large proportion of the population, particularly those at high risk for cancer or other chronic diseases associated with high IGF-1 levels. Small-molecule inhibitors of IGF-1 (Vogt et al., 1998) or IGF/IGFBP (Chen et al., 2001), as well as antisense IGF-1 inhibitor approaches (Scotlandi et al., 2002) and anti-IGF-1 antibody therapies (Granerus and Engstrom, 2001), are under development.

It is important to note that any interventions involving IGF-1 modulation must be viewed cautiously. IGF-1 levels decrease with age, and increased IGF-1, directly or indirectly through growth hormone supplementation, in aged rodents and humans has been associated with decreased muscle wasting and improved mobility (Rudman et al., 1990). IGF-1 also plays a key role in bone mineralization

(Rosen and Donahue, 1998), and studies in rodents have pointed out that CR and other interventions associated with decreased IGF-1 levels reduce bone mineral density (Ferguson et al., 1999). Such findings have prompted proposals that growth hormone supplementation to elevate IGF-1 levels in the elderly would increase bone density and muscle tone (Rudman, 1990). However, three studies have found that higher bone mineral density is associated with increased risk of breast cancer in postmenopausal women (Cauley et al., 1996; Zhang et al., 1997; Buist et al., 2001), consistent with the evidence discussed earlier that links higher IGF-1 levels with higher cancer risk. Taken together, these findings suggest that lowering IGF-1 levels pharmacologically or through lifestyle changes would involve tradeoffs, having positive effects on cancer risk and some aspects of aging but also negative effects such as increased risk of fracture through osteoporosis and decreased muscle tone. Therefore, interventions targeting IGF-1 should proceed with caution. Combination approaches, such as diet or pharmacological modulation of IGF-1 combined with an exercise regimen, may increase the effectiveness of the IGF modulation while protecting the bones and improving muscle tone and insulin sensitivity. In addition, progress in the characterization of the molecular mediators underlying both the desired and the undesired effects of reduced IGF-1 levels will greatly facilitate the translation of CR research into safe and effective interventions.

Another strategy for developing pharmacological mimetics of CR is to identify agents that can emulate the modulation of energy metabolism and glucoregulation observed with CR. 2-Deoxyglucose (2DG), a glucose analogue, is the first proposed candidate compound of this type. 2DG is a strong competitor of the enzyme phosphohexose isomerase, which converts glucose 6 phosphate to fructose 6-phosphate. Administration of 2DG greatly reduces the metabolism of glucose. Low-dose regimens (0.3–0.4% of diet) of 2DG had no effect on food intake or body weight but did result in several physiological/metabolic changes observed with CR, such as reduced insulin levels, reduced body temperature, and lower rates of tumor development (Zhu et al., 2005). IGF-1 levels were not reported. These preliminary findings suggest that metabolic mimetics of CR may provide a promising approach. Again, successful translation of this aspect of CR-related research will require attention to the entire biosystem to maximize the benefits while minimizing adverse effects.

In conclusion, this chapter, and much of our own research, focuses on the molecular and hormonal mechanisms linking energy balance and cancer. In the postgenomic era, we have access to powerful new research tools that can further elucidate the pathogenesis of human carcinogenesis and the mechanisms underlying effective anticancer interventions such as CR and physical activity. There is tremendous optimism surrounding the application of these new tools in cancer research, including energy balance–related studies as discussed previously, to hopefully result in the development of important new targets and strategies for both treatment and prevention of human cancer. However, we think a transdisciplinary approach that integrates molecular/cellular/biochemical tools and information with diet and other lifestyle variables in future basic, epidemiological, and clinical studies (as illustrated in Figure 1) is essential to the successful translation of the cancer-preventing effects of energy balance–related interventions such as CR and physical activity into human disease prevention strategies.

References

Abate, N. 1996. Insulin resistance and obesity. The role of fat distribution pattern. *Diabetes Care* **19**: 292–294.

Altman, J. 2002. Weight in the balance. *Neuroendocrinology* **76**: 131–136.

Ames, B.N., Shigenaga, M.K., and Hagen, T.M. 1993. Oxidants, antioxidants, and the degenerative diseases of aging. *Proc Natl Acad Sci USA* **90**: 7915–7922.

Andreous, K.K., and Morgan, P.R. 1981. Effect of dietary restriction on induced hamster cheek pouch carcinogenesis. *Arch Oral Biol* **26**: 525–531.

Anisimov, V.N. 2001. Mutant and genetically modified mice as models for studying the relationship between aging and carcinogenesis. *Mech Ageing Dev* **122**: 1221–1255.

Barsyte, D., Lovejoy, D.A., and Lithgow, G.J. 2001. Longevity and heavy metal resistance in *daf-2* and *age-1* long-lived mutants of *Caenorhabditis elegans. FASEB J* **15**: 627–634.

Berrigan, D., Perkins, S., Haines, D., and Hursting, S. 2002. Adult-onset calorie restriction and fasting delay spontaneous tumorigenesis in p53-deficient mice. *Carcinogenesis* **23**: 817–822.

Bertone, E.R., Willett, W.C., Rosner, B.A., Hunter, D.J., Fuchs, C.S., Speizer, F.E., Colditz, G.A., and Hankinson, S.E. 2001. Prospective study of recreational physical activity and ovarian cancer. *J Natl Cancer Inst* **93**: 942–948.

Birt, D.F., Yaktine, A., and Duysen, E. 1999. Glucocorticoid mediation of dietary energy restriction inhibition of mouse skin carcinogenesis. *J Nutr* **129**: 571S–574S.

Boissonneault, G.A., Elson, C.E., and Pariza, M.W. 1986. Net energy effects of dietary fat on chemically induced mammary carcinogenesis in F344 rats. *J Natl Cancer Inst* **76**: 335–338.

Bouloumie, A., Drexler, H.C., and Lafontan, M. 1998. Leptin, the product of Ob gene, promotes angiogenesis. *Circ Res* **83**: 1059–1066.

Bray, G. 2004. Obesity is a chronic, relapsing neurochemical disease. *Int J Obesity* **28**: 34–38.

Brown-Borg, H.M., Borg, K.E., Meliska, C.J., and Bartke, A. 1996. Dwarf mice and the ageing process. *Nature* **384**: 33.

Brown-Borg, H.M., Rakoczy, S.G., Romanick, M.A., and Kennedy, M.A. 2002. Effects of growth hormone and insulin-like growth factor-1 on hepatocyte antioxidative enzymes. *Exp Biol Med* **227**: 94–104.

Buckbinder, L., Talbott, R., Velasco-Miguel, S., et al. 1995. Induction of the growth inhibitor IGF–binding protein 3 by p53. *Nature* **377**: 646–649.

Buist, D.S., LaCroix, A.Z., and Barlow, W.E. 2001. Bone mineral density and endogenous hormones and risk of breast cancer in postmenopausal women (United States). *Cancer Causes Control* **12**: 213–222.

Calle, E., and Kaaks, R. 2004. Overweight, obesity and cancer: epidemiological evidence and proposed mechanisms. *Nat Rev* **4**: 579–591.

Calle, E., Rodriguez, C., Walker-Thurmond, K., and Thun, M. 2003. Overweight, obesity, and mortality from cancer in a prospectively studied cohort of U.S. adults. *N Engl J Med* **348**: 1625–1638.

Cao, S.X., Dhahbi, J.M., Mote, P.L., and Spindler, S.R. 2001. Genomic profiling of short- and long-term caloric restriction effects in the liver of aging mice. *Proc Natl Acad Sci USA* **98**: 10630–10635.

Cauley, J.A., Lucas, F.L., Kuller, L.H., Vogt, M.T., Browner, W.S., and Cummings, S.R. 1996. Bone mineral density and risk of breast cancer in older women: the study of osteoporotic fractures. Study of Osteoporotic Fractures Research Group. *JAMA* **276**: 1404–1408.

Chang, S., Hursting, S.D., Contois, J.H., Strom, S.S., Yamamura, Y., Babaian, R.J., Troncoso, P., Scardino, P.S., Wheeler, T.M., Amos, C.I., and Spitz, M.R. 2001. Leptin and prostate cancer. *Prostate* **46**: 62–67.

Chen, C., Zhu, Y.F., Liu, X.J., Lu, Z.X., Xie, Q., and Ling, N. 2001. Discovery of a series of nonpeptide small molecules that inhibit the binding of insulin-like growth factor (IGF) to IGF-binding proteins. *J Med Chem* **44**: 4001–4010.

Clancy, D.J., Gems, D., Harshman, L.G., Oldham, S., Stocker, H., Hafen, E., Leevers, S.J., and Partridge, L. 2001. Extension of life-span by loss of CHICO, a *Drosophila* insulin receptor substrate protein. *Science* **292**: 104–106.

Colbert, L.H., Mai, V., Perkins, S.N., Berrigan, D., Lavigne, J.A., Wimbrow, H.H., Alvord, W.G., Haines, D.C., Srinivas, P., and Hursting, S.D. 2003. Exercise and intestinal polyp development in APC^{Min} mice. *Med Sci Sports Exerc* **35**: 1662–1669.

Coschigano, K.T., Clemmons, D., Bellush, L.L., and Kopchick, J.J. 2000. Assessment of growth parameters and life span of GHR/BP gene–disrupted mice. *Endocrinology* **141**: 2608–2613.

Coussens, L.M., and Werb, Z. 2002. Inflammation and cancer. *Nature* **420**: 860–867.

Curry, S.J., Byers, T., and Hewitt, M.E. 2003. "Fulfilling the Potential of Cancer Prevention and Early Detection." National Academies Press, Washington, DC.

D'Ambrosio, C., Ferber, A., Resnicoff, M., and Baserga, R. 1996. A soluble insulin-like growth factor I receptor that induces apoptosis of tumor cells *in vivo* and inhibits tumorigenesis. *Cancer Res* **56**: 4013–4020.

Daneryd, P., Åberg, F., Dallner, G., Ernster, L., Scherstén, T., and Soussi, B. 1995. Coenzymes Q9 and Q10 in skeletal and cardiac muscle in tumour-bearing exercising rats. *Eur J Cancer* **31A**: 760–765.

Defossez, P.A., Lin, S.J., and McNabb, D.S. 2001. Sound silencing: the Sir2 protein and cellular senescence. *Bioessays* **23**: 327–232.

deGraaf, C., Blom, W., Smeets, P., Stafleu, A., and Hendriks, H. 2004. Biomarkers of satiation and satiety. *Am J Clin Nutr* **79**: 946–961.

Dhabi, J.M., Kim, H., Mote, P.L., Beaver, R.J., and Spindler, S.R. 2004. Temporal link between the phenotypic and genomic responses to caloric restriction. *Proc Natl Acad Sci USA* **101**: 5524–5529.

DiGiovanni, J., Bol, D.K., Wilker, E., Beltran, L., Carbajal, S., Moats, S., Ramirez, A., Jorcano, J., and Kiguchi, K. 2000. Constitutive expression of insulin-like growth factor-1 in epidermal basal cells of transgenic mice leads to spontaneous tumor promotion. *Cancer Res* **60**: 1561–1570.

Duncan, K., Harris, S., and Ardies, C. 1997. Running exercise may reduce risk for lung and liver cancer by inducing activity of antioxidant and phase II enzymes. *Cancer Lett* **116**: 151–158.

Dunn, S.E., Ehrlich, M., Sharp, N.J., Reiss, K., Solomom, G., Hawkins, R., Baserga, R., and Barrett, J.C. 1998. A dominant negative mutant of the insulin-like growth factor-I receptor inhibits the adhesion, invasion, and metastasis of breast cancer. *Cancer Res* **58**: 3353–3361.

Dunn, S.E., Kari, F.W., French, J., Leininger, J.R., Travlos, G., Wilson, R., and Barrett, J.C. 1997. Dietary restriction reduces insulin-like growth factor I levels, which modulates apoptosis, cell proliferation, and tumor progression in p53-deficient mice. *Cancer Res* **57**: 4667–4672.

Endogenous Hormones and Breast Cancer Collaborative Group. 2002. Endogenous sex hormones and breast cancer in postmenopausal women: reanalysis of nine prospective studies. *J Natl Cancer Inst* **94**: 606–616.

Evans, R., Barish, G., and Wang, Y.-X. 2004. PPARs and the complex journey to obesity. *Nat Med* **10**: 1–7.

Evans, R.M. 2005. The nuclear receptor superfamily: a rosetta stone for physiology. *Mol Endocrinol* **19**: 1429–1438.

Febbraio, M.A., Hiscock, N., Sacchetti, M., Fischer, C.P., and Pedersen, B.K. 2004. Interleukin-6 is a novel factor mediating glucose homeostasis during skeletal muscle contraction. *Diabetes* **53**: 1643–1648.

Fehrenbach, E., Northoff, H. 2001. Free radicals, exercise, apoptosis, and heat shock proteins. *Exerc Immunol Rev* **7**: 66–89.

Fenton, J.L., Hord, N.G., Lavigne, J.L., Perkins, S.N., and Hursting, S.D. 2005. Leptin, insulin-like growth factor-1 and insulin-like growth factor-2 are mitogens in ApcMin/+ but not Apc+/+ colonic epithelial cell lines. *Cancer Epidemiol Biomarkers Prev* **14**: 1646–1652.

Ferguson, V.L., Greenberg, A.R., Bateman, T.A., et al. 1999. The effects of age and dietary restriction without nutritional supplementation on whole bone structural properties in C57BL/6J mice. *Biomed Sci Instrum* **35**: 85–91.

Flegal, K.M., Graubard, B.L., Williamson, D.F., and Gail, M.H. 2005. Excess deaths associated with underweight, overweight and obesity. *JAMA* **293**: 1861–1867.

Flurkey, K., Papaconstantinou, J., and Harrison, D.E. 2002. The Snell dwarf mutation *Pit1*^{dw} can increase life span in mice. *Mech Ageing Dev* **123**: 121–130.

Flurkey, K., Papaconstantinou, J., Miller, R.A., Harrison, D.E. 2001. Lifespan extension and delayed immune and collagen aging in mutant mice with defects in growth hormone production. *Proc Natl Acad Sci USA* **98**: 6736–6741.

Friedenreich, C. 2004. Physical activity and breast cancer risk: the effect of menopausal status. *Exerc Sports Sci Rev* **32**: 180–184.

Gems, D., and Partridge, L. 2001. Insulin/IGF signalling and ageing: seeing the bigger picture. *Curr Opin Genet Dev* **11**: 287–292.

Granerus, M., and Engstrom, W. 2001. Effects of insulin-like growth factor–binding protein 2 and an IGF-type I receptor–blocking antibody on apoptosis in human teratocarcinoma cells *in vitro*. *Cell Biol Int* **25**: 825–828.

Grimm, J. 1999. Interaction of physical activity and diet: implications for insulin-glucose dynamics. *Public Health Nutr* **2**: 363–368.

Gross, L., and Dreyfuss, Y. 1984. Reduction in the incidence of radiation-induced tumors in rats after restriction of food intake. *Proc Natl Acad Sci USA* **81**: 7596–7598.

Gross, L., and Dreyfuss, Y. 1990. Prevention of spontaneous and radiation-induced tumors in rats by reduction of food intake. *Proc Natl Acad Sci USA* **87**: 6795–6797.

Han, S., and Hickey, M. 2005. Microarray evaluation of dietary restriction. *J Nutr* **135**: 1343–1346.

Hedley, A., Ogden, C., Johnson, C., Carroll, M., Curtin, L., and Flegal, K. 2004. Prevalence of overweight and obesity among US children, adolescents, and adults, 1999–2002. *JAMA* **291**: 2847–2850.

Higami, Y., Pugh, T.D., Page, G.P., Allison, D.B., Prolla, T.A., and Weindruch, R. 2004. Adipose tissue energy metabolism: altered gene expression profile of mice subjected to long-term calorie restriction. *FASEB J* **18**: 415–417.

Hiscock, N., Chan, M.H., Bisucci, T., Darby, I.A., and Febbraio, M.A. 2004. Skeletal myocytes are a source of interleukin-6 mRNA expression and protein release during contraction: evidence of fiber type specificity. *FASEB J* **18**: 992–994.

Hoffman-Goetz, L. 2003. Physical activity and cancer prevention: animal-tumor models. *Med Sci Sports Exerc* **35**: 1828–1833.

Holmes, M.D., Chen, W.Y., Feskanich, D., Kroenke, C.H., and Colditz, G.A. 2005. Physical activity and survival after breast cancer diagnosis. *JAMA* **29**: 32479–3286.

Hursting, S.D., and Kari, F.W. 1999. The anti-carcinogenic effects of dietary restriction: mechanisms and future directions. *Mutat Res* **443**: 235–249.

Hursting, S.D., Nunez, N.N., Patel, A.C., Perkins, S.N., Lubet, R.A., and Barrett, J.C. 2005. The utility of genetically altered mouse models for nutrition and cancer prevention research. *Mut Res* **576**: 80–92.

Hursting, S.D., Switzer, B.R., French, J.E., and Kari, F.W. 1993. The growth hormone: insulin-like growth factor 1 axis is a mediator of diet restriction–induced inhibition of mononuclear cell leukemia in Fischer rats. *Cancer Res* **53**: 2750–2757.

Hursting, S., Lavigne, J., Berrigan, D., Perkins, S., and Barrett, J. 2003. Calorie restriction, aging, and cancer prevention: mechanisms of action and applicability to humans. *Annu Rev Med* **54**: 131–152.

Hursting, S., Perkins, S., and Phang, J. 1994. Calorie restriction delays spontaneous tumorigenesis in p53-knockout transgenic mice. *Proc Natl Acad Sci USA* **91**: 7036–7040.

"IARC Handbooks of Cancer Prevention, " Vol 6, 2002, "Weight Control and Physical Activity." IARC Press, Lyon, France.

Ji, L. 1999. Antioxidants and oxidative stress in exercise. *Proc Soc Exp Biol Med* **222**: 283–292.

Kaaks, R., Lukanova, A., and Kurzer, M.S. 2002. Obesity, endogenous hormones and endometrial cancer risk: a synthetic review. *Cancer Epidemiol Biomarkers Prev* **11**: 1531–1543.

Kagawa, Y. 1978. Impact of Westernization on the nutrition of Japanese: changes in physique, cancer, longevity and centenarians. *Prev Med* **7**: 205–217.

Kayo, T., Allison, D.B., Weindruch, R., and Prolla, T.A. 2001. Influences of aging and caloric restriction on the transcriptional profile of skeletal muscle from Rhesus monkeys. *Proc Natl Acad Sci USA* **98**: 5093–5098.

Kealy, R.D., Lawler, D.E., Ballam, J.M., et al. 2002. Effects of diet restriction on life span and age-related changes in dogs. *J Am Vet Med Assoc* **220**: 1315–1320.

Lagerros, Y.T., Hsieh, S.F., and Hsieh, C.C. 2004. Physical activity in adolescence and young adulthood and breast cancer risk: a quantitative review. *Eur J Cancer Prev* **13**: 5–12.

Lagopoulos, L., and Stalder, R. 1987. The influence of food intake on the development of diethylnitrosamine-induced liver tumours in mice. *Carcinogenesis* **8**: 33–37.

Lane, M.A., Black, A., Handy, A., Tilmont, E.M., Ingram, D.K., and Roth, G.S. 2001. Caloric restriction in primates. *Ann NY Acad Sci* **928**: 287–295.

Lee, C.K., Klopp, R.G., Weindruch, R., and Prolla, T.A. 1999. Gene expression profile of aging and its retardation by caloric restriction. *Science* **285**: 1390–1393.

Lee, C.K., Weindruch, R., and Prolla, T.A. 2000. Gene-expression profile of the ageing brain in mice. *Nat Genet* **25**: 294–297.

LeRoith, D., Baserga, R., Helman, L., and Roberts, C.T., Jr. 1995. Insulin-like growth factors and cancer. *Ann Intern Med* **122**: 54–59.

LeRoith, D., Bondy, C., Yakar, S., et al. 2001. The somatomedin hypothesis: 2001. *Endocr Rev* **22**: 53–74.

Loffreda, S., Yang, S.Q., Lin, H.Z., et al. 1998. Leptin regulates proinflammatory immune responses. *FASEB J* **12**: 57–65.

Lonnqvist, F., Wennlung, A., and Arner, P. 1997. Relationship between circulating leptin and peripheral fat distribution in obese subjects. *Int J Obes Relat Metab Disord* **21**: 255–260.

Macaulay, V.M. 1992. Insulin-like growth factors and cancer. *Br J Cancer* **65**: 311–320.

Mai, V., Colbert, L., Berrigan, D., Perkins, S., Pfeiffer, R., Lavigne, J., Lanza, E., Haines, D., Schatzkin, A., and Hursting, S. 2003. Calorie restriction and diet composition modulate spontaneous intestinal tumorigenesis in Apc-min mice through different mechanisms. *Cancer Res* **63**: 1752–1755.

Marnett, L. 2000. Oxyradicals and DNA damage. *Carcinogenesis* **21**: 361–370.

Matthys, P., Mitera, T., Heremans, H., Van Damme, J., and Billiau, A. 1995. Anti-gamma interferon and anti-interleukin-6 antibodies affect staphylococcal enterotoxin B–induced weight loss, hypoglycemia, and cytokine release in D-galactosamine–sensitized and unsensitized mice. *Infect Immun* **63**: 1158–1164.

McGuire, M.T., Wing, R.R., Klem, M.L., and Hill, J.O. 1999. Behavioral strategies of individuals who have maintained long-term weight losses. *Obes Res* **7**: 334–341.

McTiernan, A., Tworoger, S.S., Ulrich, C.M., Yasui, Y., Irwin, M.L., Rajan, K.B., Sorensen, B., Rudolph, R.E., Bowen, D., Stanczyk, F.Z., Potter, J.D., and Schwartz, R.S. 2004. Effects of moderate intensity exercise intervention on estrogen metabolism in postmenopausal women. *Cancer Res* **64**: 2923–2928.

McTiernan, A., Ulrich, C., Slate, S., and Potter, J. Physical activity and cancer etiology: associations and mechanisms. 1998. *Cancer Causes Control* **9**: 487–509.

Mei, J.J., Hursting, S.D., Perkins, S.N., and Phang, J.M. 1998. p53-independent inhibition of nitric oxide generation by cancer preventive interventions in *ex vivo* mouse peritoneal macrophages. *Cancer Lett.* **129**: 191–197.

Migliaccio, E., Giorgio, M., Mele, S., Pelicci, G., Reboldi, P., Pandolfi, P.P., Lanfrancone, L., and Pelicci, P.G. 1999. The p66^{shc} adaptor protein controls oxidative stress response and life span in mammals. *Nature* **402**: 309–313.

Mizuhara, H., O'Neill, E., Seki, N., Ogawa, T., Kusunoki, C., Otsuka, K., Satoh, S., Niwa, M., Senoh, H., and Fujiwara, H. 1994. T cell activation-associated hepatic injury: mediation by tumor necrosis factors and protection by interleukin 6. *J Exp Med* **179**: 1529–1537.

Moldoveanu, A.I., Shephard, R.J., and Shek, P.N. 2000. Exercise elevates plasma levels but not gene expression of IL-1beta, IL-6, and TNF-alpha in blood mononuclear cells. *J Appl Physiol* **89**: 1499–1504.

Montague, C.T., Prins, J.B., Sanders, L., Digby, J.E., and O'Rahilly, S. 1997. Depot- and sex-specific differences in human leptin mRNA expression: implications for the control of regional fat distribution. *Diabetes* **46**: 342–347.

Murakami, S., and Johnson, T.E. 1996. A genetic pathway conferring life extension and resistance to UV stress in *Caenorhabditis elegans*. *Genetics* **143**: 1207–1218.

Murakami, S., and Johnson, T.E. 1998. Life extension and stress resistance in *Caenorhabditis elegans* modulated by the tkr-1 gene. *Curr Biol* **8**: 1091–1094.

O'Connor, K.G., Tobin, J.D., Harman, S.M., Plato, C.C., Roy, T.A., Sherman, S.S., and Blackman, M.R. 1998. Serum levels of insulin-like growth factor-I are related to age and not to body composition in healthy women and men. *J Gerontol A Biol Sci Med Sci* **53**: M176–M182.

Ogden, C.L., Carroll, M.D., and Flegal, K.M. 2003. Epidemiologic trends in overweight and obesity. *Endocrinol Metab Clin North Am* **32**: 741–760.

Ogden, C. 2004. Advance Data from Vital Health Statistics. Centers for Disease Control and Prevention. October.

Ostlund, R.E., Yang, J.W., Klein, S., and Gingerich, R. 1996. Relation between plasma leptin concentration and body fat, gender, diet, age, and metabolic covariates. *J Clin Endocrin Metab* **81**: 3909–3913.

Ostrowski, K., Rohde, T., Asp, S., Schjerling, P., and Pedersen, B.K. 1999. Pro- and anti-inflammatory cytokine balance in strenuous exercise in humans. *J Physiol* **515**(Pt 1): 287–291.

Ostrowski, K., Schjerling, P., and Pedersen, B.K. 2000. Physical activity and plasma interleukin-6 in humans—effect of intensity of exercise. *Eur J Appl Physiol* **83**: 512–515.

Pedersen, B.K., and Hoffman-Goetz, L. 2000. Exercise and the immune system: regulation, integration, and adaptation. *Physiol Rev* **80**: 1055–1081.

Pedersen, B.K., Steensberg, A., and Schjerling, P. 2001. Muscle-derived interleukin-6: possible biological effects. *J Physiol* **536**(Pt 2): 29–37.

Penkowa, M., Keller, C., Keller, P., Jauffred, S., and Pedersen, B.K. 2003. Immunohistochemical detection of interleukin-6 in human skeletal muscle fibers following exercise. *FASEB J* **17**: 2166–2168.

Petersen, A.M., and Pedersen, B.K. 2005. The anti-inflammatory effect of exercise. *J Appl Physiol* **98**: 1154–1162.

Pinney, D.O., Stephens, D.F., and Pope, L.S. 1972. Lifetime effects of winter supplemental feed level and age at first parturition on range beef cows. *J Animal Sci* **34**: 1067–1074.

Pletcher, S.D., Macdonald, S.J., Marguerie, R., et al. 2002. Genome-wide transcript profiles in aging and calorically restricted *Drosophila melanogaster*. *Curr Biol* **12**: 712–723.

Prolla, T.A. 2002. DNA microarray analysis of the aging brain. *Chem Senses* **27**: 299–306.

Radák, Z., Chung, H., Naito, H., Takahashi, R., Jung, K., Kim, H.-J., and Goto, S. 2004. Age-associated increases in oxidative stress and nuclear transcription factor κβ_activation are attenuated in rat liver by regular exercise. *FASEB J* **18**: 749–750.

Radak, Z., Taylor, A., Ohno, H., and Goto, S. 2001. Adaptation to exercise-induced oxidative stress: from muscle to brain. *Exercise Immunol Rev* **7**: 90–107.

Rajala, M., and Scherer, P. 2003. Minireview: the adipocyte—at the crossroads of energy homeostasis, inflammation, and atherosclerosis. *Endocrinology* **144**: 3765–3773.

Renehan, A.G., Zwahlen, M., Minder, C., O'Dwyer, S.T., Shalet, S.M., and Egger, M. 2004. Insulin-like growth factor (IGF)-1, IGF binding protein-3, and cancer risk: systematic review and meta-regression analysis. *Lancet* **363**: 1346–1353.

Resnicoff, M., Abraham, D., Yutanawiboonchai, W.H.L., Kajstura, J., Rubin, R., Zoltick, P., and Baserga, R. 1995. The insulin-like growth factor I receptor protects tumor cells from apoptosis *in vivo*. *Cancer Res* **55**: 2463–2469.

Rosen, C.J., and Donahue, L.R. 1998. Insulin-like growth factors and bone: the osteoporosis connection revisited. *Proc Soc Exp Biol Med* **219**: 1–7.

Roth, G.S., Ingram, D.K., and Lane, M.A. 1999. Calorie restriction in primates: will it work and how will we know? *J Am Geriatr Soc* **47**: 896–903.

Roth, G.S., Ingram, D.K., and Lane, M.A. 2001. Caloric restriction in primates and relevance to humans. *Ann NY Acad Sci* **928**: 305–315.

Rudman, D., Feller, A.G., Nagraj, H.S., Gergans, G.A., Lalitha, P.Y., Goldberg, A.F., Schlenker, R.A., Cohn, L., Rudman, I.W., and Mattson, D.E. 1990. Effects of human growth hormone in men over 60 years old. *N Engl J Med* **323**: 1–6.

Rundle, A. Molecular epidemiology of physical activity and cancer. 2005. *Cancer Epidemiol Biomarkers Prev* **14**: 227–236.

Saglam, K., Aydur, E., Yilmaz, M., and Goktas, S. 2003. Leptin influences cellular differentiation and progression in prostate cancer. *J Urol* **169**: 1308–1311.

Schindler, R., Mancilla, J., Endres, S., Ghorbani, R., Clark, S.C., and Dinarello, C.A. 1990. Correlations and interactions in the production of interleukin-6 (IL-6), IL-1, and tumor necrosis factor (TNF) in human blood mononuclear cells: IL-6 suppresses IL-1 and TNF. *Blood* **75**: 40–47.

Schmitz, K.H., Ahmed, R.L., and Yee, D. 2002. Effects of a 9-month strength training intervention on insulin, insulin-like growth factor (IGF)-I, IGF-binding protein (IGFBP)-1, and IGFBP-3 in 30–50 year old women. *Cancer Epidemiol Biomarkers Prev* **11**: 1597–1604.

Schwartz, M., Woods, S., Porte, D., Jr., Seely, R., and Baskin, D. 2000. Central nervous system control of food intake. *Nature* **404**: 661–671.

Scotlandi, K., Maini, C., Manara, M.C., Benini, S., Serra, M., Cerisano, V., Strammiello, R., Baldini, N., Lollini, P.L., Nanni, P., Nicoletti, G., and Picci, P. 2002. Effectiveness of insulin-like growth factor I receptor antisense strategy against Ewing's sarcoma cells. *Cancer Gene Ther* **9**: 296–307.

Seeley, R., Drazen, D., and Clegg, D. 2004. The critical role of the melanocortin system in the control of energy balance. *Annu Rev Nutr* **24**: 133–149.

Shephard, R.J., and Futcher, R. 1997. Physical activity and cancer: how may protection be maximized? *Crit Rev Oncogenesis* **8**: 219–272.

Singh, P., Dai, B., Yallampalli, U., Lu, X., and Schroy, P.C. 1996. Proliferation and differentiation of a human colon cancer cell line (CaCo2) is associated with significant changes in the expression and secretion of insulin-like growth factor (IGF) IGF-II and IGF binding protein-4: role of IGF-II. *Endocrinology* **137**: 1764–1774.

Sohal, R.S., and Weindruch, R. 1996. Oxidative stress, caloric restriction, and aging. *Science* **273**: 59–63.

Starkie, R., Ostrowski, S.R., Jauffred, S., Febbraio, M., and Pedersen, B.K. 2003. Exercise and IL-6 infusion inhibit endotoxin-induced TNF-alpha production in humans. *FASEB J* **17**: 884–886.

Starkie, R.L., Rolland, J., Angus, D.J., Anderson, M.J., and Febbraio, M.A. 2001. Circulating monocytes are not the source of elevations in plasma IL-6 and TNF-alpha levels after prolonged running. *Am J Physiol Cell Physiol* **280**: C769–C774.

Stattin, P., Lukanova, A., Biessy, C., Soderberg, S., Palmquist, R., Kaaks, R., Olsson, T., and Jellum, E. 2004. Obesity and colon cancer: does leptin provide a link? *Int J Cancer* **109**: 149–152.

Steensberg, A., Fischer, C.P., Keller, C., Moller, K., and Pedersen, B.K. 2003. IL-6 enhances plasma IL-1ra, IL-10, and cortisol in humans. *Am J Physiol Endocrinol Metab* **285**: E433–E437.

Suzuki, K., Nakaji, S., Yamada, M., Totsuka, M., Sato, K., and Sugawara, K. 2002. Systemic inflammatory response to exhaustive exercise. Cytokine kinetics. *Exercise Immunol Rev* **8**: 6–48.

Takahashi, K., and Suzuki, K. 1993. Association of insulin-like growth-factor-I–induced DNA synthesis with phosphorylation and nuclear exclusion of p53 in human breast cancer MCF-7 cells. *Int J Cancer* **55**: 453–458.

Tannenbaum, A. 1940. The initiation and growth of tumors. Introduction. I. Effects of underfeeding. *Am J Cancer* **38**: 335–350.

Tannenbaum, A. 1942. The genesis and growth of tumors. II. Effects of caloric restriction per se. *Cancer Res* **2**: 460–464.

Tatar, M., Kopelman, A., Epstein, D., Tu, M.P., Yin, C.M., and Garofalo, R.S. 2001. A mutant *Drosophila* insulin receptor homolog that extends life-span and impairs neuroendocrine function. *Science* **292**: 107–110.

Temizhan, A., Tandogan, I., Donderici, O., and Demirbas, B. 2000. The effects of Ramadan fasting on blood lipid levels. *Am J Med* **109**: 341–342.

Tsuchiya, T., Dhabi, J.M., Cui, X., Mote, P.L., Bartke, A., and Spindler, S.R. 2004. Additive regulation of hepatic gene regulation by dwarfism and caloric restriction. *Physiol Genomics* **17**: 307–315.

Ullum, H., Haahr, P.M., Diamant, M., Palmo, J., Halkjaer-Kristensen, J., and Pedersen, B.K. 1994. Bicycle exercise enhances plasma IL-6 but does not change IL-1 alpha, IL-1 beta, IL-6, or TNF-alpha pre-mRNA in BMNC. *J Appl Physiol* **77**: 93–97.

US Department of Health and Human Services. 1996. Physical Activity and Health: A Report of the US Surgeon General. US Dept of Health and Human Services, Centers for Disease Control and Prevention, Atlanta, GA.

U.S. Department of Health and Human Services. 2004. National Institutes of Health. Strategic Plan for NIH Obesity Research. A Report of the NIH Obesity Research Task Force. NIH Publication No. 04-5493.

van Noord, P.A., and Kaaks, R. 1991. The effect of wartime conditions and the 1944–45 "Dutch famine" on recalled menarcheal age in participants of the DOM breast cancer screening project. *Ann Hum Biol* **18**: 57–70.

Velthuis, T., Wierik, E.J., van den Berg, H., Schaafsma, G., et al. 1994. Energy restriction, a useful intervention to retard human ageing? Results of a feasibility study. *Eur J Clin Nutr* **48**: 138–148.

Vogt, A., Rice, R.L., Settineri, C.E., et al. 1998. Disruption of insulin-like growth factor-1 signaling and down-regulation of cdc2 by SCααδ9, a novel small molecule antisignaling agent identified in a targeted array library. *J Pharmacol Exp Ther* **287**: 806–813.

Walford, R.L., Harris, S.B., and Gunion, M.W. 1992. The calorically restricted low-fat nutrient-dense diet in Biosphere 2 significantly lowers blood glucose, total leukocyte count, cholesterol, and blood pressure in humans. *Proc Natl Acad Sci USA* **89**: 11533–11537.

Weindruch, R., Kayo, T., Lee, C.K., and Prolla, T.A. 2002. Gene expression profiling of aging using DNA microarrays. *Mech Ageing Dev* **123**: 177–193.

Weindruch, R., and Walford, R.L. 1988. "The Retardation of Aging and Disease by Dietary Restriction." Charles C. Thomas, Springfield, IL.

Wilding, J., Widdowson, P., and Williams, G. 1997. Obesity: neurobiology. *Br Med Bull* **53**: 286–306.

Woods, J. 1998. Exercise and resistance to neoplasia. *Can J Physiol Pharmacol* **76**: 581–588.

Woods, S., Seeley, R.J., Porte, D., and Schwartz, M.W. 1998. Signals that regulate food intake and energy homeostasis. *Science* **280**: 1378–1382.

Yakar, S., LeRoith, D., and Brodt, P. 2005. The role of the growth hormone/insulin-like growth factor axis in tumor growth and progression: Lessons from animal models. *Cytokine Growth Factor Rev* **16**: 407–420.

Youngman, L.D., Park, J.Y., and Ames, B.N. 1992. Protein oxidation associated with aging is reduced by dietary restriction of protein or calories. *Proc Natl Acad Sci USA* **89**: 9112–9116.

Yu, H., and Rohan, T. 2000. Role of the insulin-like growth factor family in cancer development and progression. *J Natl Cancer Inst* **92**: 1472–1489.

Zhang, Y., and Leibel, R. 1998. Molecular physiology of leptin and its receptor. *Growth Genet Hormones* **14**: 17–35.

Zhang, Y., Kiel, D.P., Kreger, B.E., Cupples, L.A., Ellison, R.C., Dorgan, J.F., Schatzkin, A., Levy, D., and Felson, D.T. 1997. Bone mass and the risk of breast cancer among postmenopausal women. *N Engl J Med* **336**: 611–617.

Zhu, Z., Jiang, W., McGinley, J.N., and Thompson, H.J. 2005. 2-Deoxyglucose as an energy restriction mimetic agent: effects on mammary carcinogenesis and on mammary tumor cell growth *in vitro*. *Cancer Res* **65**: 7023–7030.

Zigman, J., and Elmquist, J. 2003. Minireview: from anorexia to obesity—the yin and yang of body weight control. *Endocrinology* **144**: 3749–3756.

C H A P T E R

6

Nutritional Epidemiology

MARJORIE MCCULLOUGH AND EDWARD GIOVANNUCCI

INTRODUCTION

Nutritional epidemiology examines dietary or nutritional factors in relation to disease occurrence in populations. Findings from nutritional epidemiology often contribute toward the evidence used in guiding dietary recommendations for prevention of cancer and other diseases (Byers, 1999). Epidemiological methods have been used to study the relationship between diet and disease for centuries, originally to identify nutritional deficiencies and target foods to ameliorate them (Cervantes-Laurean et al., 1999; Jacob, 1999). A classic example is scurvy, a condition observed among sailors of the sixteenth to the eighteenth century manifested by bleeding gums, swollen and inflamed joints, and eventual death. The observation that vegetables and fruits could cure scurvy led Lind to compare the efficacy of various types of these foods. He discovered that lemons and oranges had the most sudden influence on course of the disease. The molecular structure of vitamin C, the nutritional component responsible for the positive effect, was not discovered until centuries later in 1933 (Jacob, 1999). In contrast to studies of nutritional deficiency syndromes, modern nutritional epidemiology focuses on the etiology of chronic diseases such as cardiovascular disease and cancer, the two leading causes of death today (National Center for Health Statistics, 2003). Similar to the early studies of nutrition deficiency, associations between dietary factors and chronic disease may be observed long before a specific etiologic factor can be identified (Jacob, 1999). However, the path from observing to curing disease is more complicated for chronic diseases than deficiency diseases, because chronic disease etiology is multifactorial and diseases take many years to develop or manifest.

Evidence from a variety of study designs is required to establish a definitive relationship between diet and disease. Basic biochemistry and physiology, cell culture experiments, laboratory animal studies, and human metabolic studies provide pertinent mechanistic data to implicate a role for a specific dietary factor in carcinogenesis. However, these studies cannot prove that a particular dietary factor will cause or prevent a cancer in humans. Proof can only be established in human studies, preferably through randomized intervention trials. However, such trials are not always feasible. One challenge is the high cost of long-term studies, given that cancer takes years to develop. In addition, it is ethically implausible to test the relationship between a potentially harmful exposure and cancer in humans. For these reasons, the bulk of the available evidence for a particular diet–cancer relationship is garnered from observational nutritional epidemiological studies. This chapter provides an overview of the nutritional epidemiology of cancer, with particular emphasis on study design, dietary assessment, and analysis, as well as interpretation of findings.

STUDY DESIGNS

Epidemiologists use a variety of population-based approaches to study the relationship between diet and cancer (Table 1). The two major classifications are observational and intervention studies. Most studies are observational, in which cancer rates are observed among individuals or groups with variable levels of dietary exposure. Observational studies can be further categorized into ecologic and analytical epidemiology studies. Ecologic studies, including

Copyright © 2006, Elsevier Inc.
All rights of reproduction in any form reserved.

TABLE 1 Study Designs in Nutritional Epidemiology

Study design	Population	Exposure assessment	Outcome assessment	Advantages	Special Considerations
Observational					
Ecologic:					
Correlational	Country or region	Population-based, e.g., food balance sheets	Population rates of cancer incidence or death	Examine wide range of exposure; population dietary estimates may be more stable than individual diets	Potential for uncontrolled confounding, e.g., unmeasured or uncontrolled aspects of lifestyle related to diet and risk of cancer; potential for biased food estimates because of wastage
Migrant study	Immigrants	Variety of diet assessment tools measured cross-sectionally or over time	Cancer rates in immigrants to new country or region	Examine individuals or ethnic group in transition	Other lifestyle factors are likely to change from country to country and over time in both immigrant and time-trend studies
Time-trend study	Same population, measured over time (usually as cross-sections of the population)	Population-based methods or varied	Rates of cancer within a population over time	Differences in rates less likely to be influenced by genetics; similar covariates	Changes in screening procedures may influence rates
Analytical					
Case–control:	Cases with cancer (or proxies) vs control	Food frequency questionnaire (FFQ) or other; validate FFQ with daily records or recall or other method	Verified cancer outcome, identified in clinic or hospital	Used for rare cancers; low cost; can tailor exposure assessment to the study	Recall bias or misinformation from proxies difficult to avoid
Hospital-based controls			Controls admitted to the same hospital for other disease(s)		Dietary factor must be unrelated to the other control disease
Population-based controls			Controls sampled from the population from which the cases arose		Volunteers may be more health conscious; keep participation rates high to avoid this bias
Prospective cohort	Identify population and follow over time	FFQ, multiple daily records or recalls or biomarkers; method should be validated	Cancer incidence or mortality	Recall bias avoided	Potential for confounding; repeat exposure assessments ideal
Nested case–control	Cases and controls within a larger study, e.g., prospective cohort	FFQ, multiple daily records or recalls or biomarker (collected before disease development)	Cancer incidence	Saves money for data analysis, e.g., biomarker or genetic analysis, or more detailed analysis of diet	Choose controls of same age, alive at time of case diagnosis
Intervention study	Randomize participants to treatment	FFQ or daily measures if required to assess baseline diet and changes over time; otherwise, exposure is assigned	Development of cancer or intermediate endpoint	Randomization avoids confounding	Long time required to study cancer; questionable utility of intermediate outcomes; expensive; test limited number of doses; compliance may be difficult; subject may not be blinded to status

correlational, migrant, and time-trend studies, are based on population rates of cancer and population estimates of dietary intake, whereas analytical epidemiology studies are based on individual disease outcomes and individual estimates of dietary intake. In contrast to observational studies, intervention studies randomize individuals to a particular exposure and then follow participants for disease outcome.

Observational Studies

Ecologic Studies

Correlational studies: Correlational studies compare population disease rates with population-based estimates of dietary exposure, most often across countries or regions. Dietary intake on a population basis can be estimated from food disappearance data, which are calculated from governmental food balance sheets as the sum of food produced and imported, and excluding food that is exported, fed to animals, or unavailable for human consumption. Correlation coefficients range from 0, signifying no correlation of per capita dietary intake with cancer rates, to −1.0 or +1.0, signifying a perfect inverse or positive correlation, respectively. Ecologic investigations of diet and cancer in the mid to late 1900s generated several hypotheses for a role of diet in cancer. In a classic ecologic analysis, Armstrong and Doll (1975) noted, among other findings, a positive correlation between estimated meat intake (disappearance) and colon cancer incidence rates of 0.85 for men and 0.89 for women across 23 countries.

Migrant studies: Migrant populations provide the opportunity to study environmental risk factors and their interaction with genetic susceptibility. Rates of some cancers vary by up to 100-fold by geographical location (International Agency for Research on Cancer, 2002), and migrating populations have been observed to acquire disease rates of the host country. For example, rates of colorectal cancer in Japan have traditionally been among the lowest in the world, but among Japanese immigrants to Hawaii, these rates have surpassed that of Caucasians. That this phenomenon occurred within one generation further supports an environmental role in carcinogenesis (Le Marchand, 1999). Comparative studies in Hawaii and Japan suggest the discrepancy in disease rates may be attributed to the consumption of Western foods by the Japanese immigrants (Stemmermann et al., 1979). One hypothesis is that certain genotypes for carcinogen metabolism common among Japanese may increase risk among individuals who consume well-done red meat (Le Marchand, 1999).

Time-trend studies: These studies examine disease patterns over time within defined populations and geographic locations. From 1963 to 1992, rates of colon cancer in Japan increased fivefold (International Agency for Research on Cancer, 2002). The reasons are unclear, but hypotheses include rapid changes in diet. Ecologic studies typically cannot precisely identify causal factors for changing cancer rates, but they provide compelling evidence for an important role of environmental factors in carcinogenesis. Diagnostic techniques and screening practices may change over time and differ across populations and partially explain sudden changes in disease rates (Potosky et al., 1990).

Interpretation of Results from Ecologic Studies

Ecologic studies have unquestionably provided important hypotheses regarding diet and lifestyle patterns with cancer risk. Their major strength is that contrasts in dietary intake may be substantial. For example, sodium excretion (a highly correlated marker for sodium consumption) across 32 countries varies from 0.2 to 242.0 mEq/day (Intersalt Cooperative Research Group, 1988). Within populations, ranges are narrower, for example 150–170 mEq sodium/day among hypertensive adults in the United States (Intersalt Cooperative Research Group, 1988; Anonymous, 1992). An additional advantage of ecologic studies is that the average diet of individuals within a country is more stable than an individual's diet, which may fluctuate more dramatically.

The primary disadvantage of ecologic studies is that potential determinants of disease other than those under consideration may also vary markedly among populations and regions with extreme incidences of disease. When populations differ by variables other than the main exposure being studied, these other variables could in part explain the exposure–disease relation. For example, smoking, alcohol consumption, physical activity, genetic factors, solar radiation (proxy for vitamin D production and status), selenium intake (based on soil content), and reproductive patterns vary widely across populations. To further illustrate this point, consider an ecologic study of fat intake and cancer among adults in rural 1980s China and current United States. Dietary fat consumption is low among the Chinese and high in U.S. populations. However, the diet–cancer relation may be confounded by differences in physical activity, where physical activity among the Chinese agrarian population exceeds that of most U.S. adults. Even if physical activity were measured perfectly, statistical control for the confounding effects of physical activity may not be feasible if substantial overlap of physical activity level does not exist across both populations. In addition, international comparisons can also be problematic if heterogeneous subgroups living within the same country are considered to represent one entity.

Another limitation is the use of food disappearance data in most ecologic studies, which do not account for discarded food and selective avoidance of fat or meat. Higher disappearance of food and nutrients such as meat, fat, and calories for the United States compared with most countries may relate in part to a greater amount of wasted food, which correlates with socioeconomic factors. Disappearance data suggest an increase in per capita food availability of fat over time (Enns et al., 1997), whereas evidence based on actual dietary intake from a compilation of 171 studies suggests per capita dietary fat intake has decreased in the United States since 1950 (Stephen and Wald, 1990). Thus, analyses could provide spurious or even opposite conclusions, depending on which data source is used.

Analytical Epidemiology Studies

In analytical epidemiology, information on diet and disease occurrence is collected on an individual basis, and risk or rates of disease among individuals with a particular exposure are compared with those with no or low levels of exposure. The most common analytical epidemiology studies are case-control, prospective cohort, and nested case-control studies, although additional designs exist (Rothman and Greenland, 1998).

Case-Control Studies

In case-control studies, individuals who have been diagnosed with cancer (or family members, if the individual has already deceased) are interviewed with respect to past diet and other risk factors and compared with individuals without cancer, usually matched on age and other pertinent factors. These are often termed *retrospective studies* because information about diet is collected after cancer has occurred. Because diet before diagnosis is of interest, reference is usually made to a time before diagnosis. For example, if vegetable intake were hypothesized to lower risk of the disease, one would expect that cases had a lower previous intake of vegetables than control subjects. Statistical models would then control for age and other known risk factors for cancer that are also related to fruit and vegetable intakes to determine whether the observation may have been due to another related risk factor. Results from case-control studies are usually presented as "odds ratios" or the odds of developing disease given a certain dietary exposure, compared with the odds of developing disease with no or very low levels of that dietary factor (Hennekens and Buring, 1987).

Data for case-control studies can be collected more rapidly compared with other study designs (described later in this chapter) because there are typically fewer participants and no follow-up is necessary. Dietary questionnaires can be tailored to the specific research question; for example, a study of phytoestrogen intake and breast cancer would include major food sources of phytoestrogens in the questionnaires (Pillow et al., 1999). For relatively rare cancers, case-control studies may be the only feasible option because other designs require cancer cases to accumulate over time.

Two major drawbacks of case-control studies include recall bias and selection bias. Recall bias occurs because dietary information is obtained after the diagnosis and individuals aware of their disease status may systematically overreport or underreport consumption of a food relative to controls. Cases may be more conscious than disease-free controls about past diet, especially if they are aware of a potential diet–disease hypothesis. To test whether this potential problem influenced epidemiological studies of fat and breast cancer, Giovannucci et al. (1993) mailed dietary questionnaires to nurses in a prospective cohort who recently developed breast cancer. More recent self-reports of past diet were compared with information that the same nurses completed before knowledge of cancer diagnosis. Positive associations were observed between total and saturated fat and breast cancer risk when using diet reports completed after diagnosis but not with earlier prediagnostic diet reports. In this case, the relation between fat and breast cancer was overestimated using the case-control approach. Study interviewers not blinded to a participant's disease status could also contribute to recall bias by inadvertent prompting.

The second major concern, selection bias, pertains to the appropriate selection of a control group for the case-control study. Conceptually, controls should be selected from individuals who, had they developed the cancer, would have been identified as a case in that study. Case-control studies can be categorized as "population based," in which the comparison group is identified from the population from which the cases arise, and "hospital based," in which the comparison group is identified from other patients hospitalized at the institutions where the cases were diagnosed. In hospital-based case-control studies, an important assumption is that the exposure under study is unrelated to the condition of the control group. For example, when studying dietary fat and cancer, one should avoid designating patients with gallstones or heart disease as controls. Because diet may affect many diseases, it is often difficult to identify hospitalized patients with conditions that are definitely unrelated to the aspect of diet under investigation. Investigators may choose different sets of controls hospitalized for several diverse conditions; the consistency of results comparing different sets of controls supports the absence of selection bias. In population-based case-control studies, population lists may be used to randomly select a control group from individuals of a particular geographic region. Selection bias may occur in population-based approaches because diet is typically associated with the level of general health consciousness, and the diets of volunteers may differ substantially from those of nonvolunteers (Maclure and Hankinson, 1990). To minimize selection bias, it is essential for case-control studies to have high participation response rates. This may be a challenge for studies in large cities, where participation rates are often low (Hartge et al., 1984). In general, there is a greater likelihood that validity is compromised in studies with lower participation rates. Acceptable ranges for response rates have yet to be established.

Several features of study design can minimize the influence of potential biases. In case-control studies, the collection of information from cases and controls should occur concurrently and in similar settings. Ideally the study interviewer should be unaware of the case status of the interviewee and of the specific study hypotheses. It is critical that response rates be maximized and similar among cases and controls.

Prospective Cohort Study

The second major type of analytical epidemiology study design is the prospective cohort study. Conceptually, prospective cohort studies are more appealing than case-control studies because dietary exposures are measured before the development of disease, thus avoiding recall bias. Typically tens of thousands of individuals are enrolled. Participants complete questionnaires on diet, lifestyle factors, and medical history and are then followed over many years until adequate cases of cancer(s) develop. Follow-up questionnaires may be mailed periodically to inquire about new disease diagnosis and update exposure information. The rate of disease development over time among individuals with different dietary exposures is then compared using Cox proportional hazards modeling (Cox, 1972) or other longitudinal statistical methods while adjusting for potential confounders. For example, after adjusting for age, smoking, and other risk factors, the rate of developing a new colon cancer in individuals whose diet is relatively high in processed meat is compared with the rate of those who consume relatively low amounts of processed meat. The results are usually expressed as a "hazard rate" or "relative risk," which reflects the rate of disease occurrence in one group divided by the rate of disease occurrence in a specified comparison or "reference" group. A relative risk of 2.0 would imply, for example, that individuals with high consumption of processed meat had twice the incidence of disease as the reference group of individuals with low consumption of processed meat. Repeated assessments of diet may also be obtained over time for several purposes. First, new hypothesized exposures such as heterocyclic amines, phytoestrogens, and acrylamide can be added to questionnaires during follow-up. Second, multiple assessments of diet reduce measurement error and provide the opportunity to study major diet change in relation to disease risk. Finally, multiple assessments of exposure may help identify potentially important exposure periods.

Prospective cohort studies avoid most potential sources of methodological bias associated with case-control studies because information is collected from individuals before disease onset. However, as in case-control studies, high follow-up response rates in cohort studies are also important, as losses to follow-up that vary by level of dietary factors can result in distorted associations. Also, examining study results that exclude the early follow-up period (e.g., first 2 years) is desirable, as they could be influenced by underlying undiagnosed disease at the beginning of the study, known as "reverse causality." For example, a prediagnostic cancer-induced weight loss would distort the results between body mass and risk of cancer in the short term. Although biases are largely minimized in prospective cohort studies, unmeasured or inadequate control for confounding remains a concern for both case-control and prospective studies and is reviewed in detail later.

Approximately 60 prospective cancer cohort studies with > 10,000 participants each exist worldwide. Most have extensive data on dietary intake, although many have just begun publishing findings. Over the past decade, several prospective cohort studies have reported weaker or null associations between diet and cancer compared with those reported previously from case-control studies. For example, findings from prospective studies of fruit, vegetables, and gastrointestinal cancers are generally weaker than those of case-control studies (International Agency for Research on Cancer, 2003). One potential explanation is that the relationships were overestimated in case-control studies if individuals with cancer systematically recalled their prediagnosis diet erroneously, either because they had a preconception about how diet might influence disease or their current diet changed because of cancer. If this is the primary explanation, it suggests fruit and vegetable consumption is not as strongly associated with gastrointestinal cancers as previously thought. Other methodological issues such as limited ranges of exposure or dietary assessment (discussed later) are unlikely to explain these discrepancies because both study designs are equally susceptible to these limitations. Finally, more potential confounders have been extensively measured and controlled for in prospective studies, suggesting that some associations in case-control studies were confounded. Two large consortium projects may help resolve these questions: the Pooling Project of Diet and Cancer Cohorts (Smith-Warner et al., In press) is a collaborative effort of researchers from 16 cohorts in six countries and includes more than one million study participants. The European Prospective Investigation of Cancer (EPIC) (Riboli and Kaaks, 1997) is a multicenter cohort study of ~500,000 participants representing 22 European centers. These studies enable epidemiologists to evaluate wider ranges of dietary intake and have greater statistical power to examine differences in diet effects among subsets of the participants.

Nested Case-Control Study

The nested case-control study includes individuals with and without cancer typically sampled from an existing study population such as a prospective cohort. Cases are individuals who develop a cancer during the follow-up; controls are individuals from the same cohort who were cancer free at the time of diagnosis of the case and usually matched on age, time period of case diagnosis, and other factors. This design has been popular when biological markers of exposure or disease status are analyzed, to help save on analytical costs and to preserve finite biological resources collected on an entire cohort. A critical advantage of the nested case-control design over the standard case-control design is that the exposure is measured before disease development. This advantage may be especially pertinent in studies of biological markers of dietary exposure, which may change in response to underlying disease.

Special Considerations in Observational Studies

As discussed, bias and confounding represent two important potential problems that should be addressed in observational studies. *Bias* refers to a distortion in the way data were collected that may produce spurious results. *Confounding* is a distinct concept that may occur when another factor that is related to risk of disease is correlated with the factor of interest. Generally, bias must be avoided or minimized, whereas confounding represents a characteristic of the specific population that cannot be avoided but must be dealt with statistically or in the study design stage.

The major inherent limitation of both ecologic and analytical observational studies is that the exposure, diet, is not randomized. Confounding, from the Latin word "cunfundere," to mix together, results when the apparent effect of one exposure on risk is brought about by the association with other factors that can influence the outcome (Last, 1983). There are a few key concepts about confounding. First, for a factor to be a confounder, it must be a causal risk factor for the specific disease and be correlated with the exposure of interest. Second, if a study excludes individuals affected by the confounder, then that factor is no longer considered a confounder. For example, smoking would not be considered a confounder if the study excludes tobacco users. Third, the same factor can be a confounder in one population but not another, depending on how it correlates with the factor of interest. In Western populations individuals with healthier diets tend to smoke less, exercise more, weigh less, and take more vitamin supplements, so all of these would be considered potential confounders. In populations where these factors are not all interrelated, these unrelated factors would not be confounders. Overall, confounding is an especially important issue in nutritional epidemiology because dietary factors are often highly correlated. For example, saturated fat and total fat are positively associated, and dietary fiber and total fat intake are inversely associated.

In analytical studies several strategies are used to minimize the influence of confounding. In the study design, cases and controls can be matched and individuals restricted on a potential confounder. In dietary-based studies, confounding is usually dealt with by statistical analysis. An "adjusted relative risk" is a weighted, pooled average of the relative risk across different categories or levels of the confounder. By controlling for smoking, the adjusted relative risk will represent some average of the relative risks between diet and cancer among nonsmokers, past smokers, and current smokers. The ability to control for a confounder statistically is maximized when detailed data are available. "Residual confounding," or incomplete control for confounding, occurs when information on a confounding factor is measured crudely. For example, if "ever" versus "never" smoking were the only assessment of smoking status, this categorization would fail to distinguish duration of smoking among current and past smokers. Because comprehensive knowledge of disease risk factors is rare, the possibility for uncontrolled confounding persists. The goal of the epidemiologist is to assess the plausibility of uncontrolled confounding based on available information. For a factor to be an important confounder, it must have a strong relationship both with the disease endpoint and with the dietary factor of interest.

If research findings vary by category of another variable, results within each stratum should be presented. For example, a dietary factor may influence cancer risk in men but not women or in smokers but not nonsmokers. When associations are different across subgroups, this is referred to as "effect modification" or "interaction."

In addition to concerns for selection and recall bias outlined in the section Case-Control Studies, earlier in this chapter, differential detection rates of cancer by exposure status can distort study results from both case-control and cohort studies. For example, this could arise if dietary intake were related to the likelihood that an individual undergoes a cancer screening test. An implicit assumption in cancer epidemiology is that given the aggressive nature of cancer, individuals with disease would eventually be diagnosed regardless of exposure status. This assumption is reasonable for lung cancer but not for prevalent prostate cancer in the United States because screening by the prostate-specific antigen (PSA) test detects many innocuous cancers (Platz et al., 2004). In addition, individuals who follow breast and colorectal screening recommendations may have healthier lifestyles. Studies should, therefore, examine medical and screening background by diet status when possible. The validity of the relative risk estimate does not require that every cancer be detected but that detection rates are equal across levels of dietary intake.

Randomized Intervention Trials

Randomized intervention studies in humans are often considered the gold standard in epidemiological study design because random assignment of treatment naturally controls for important confounders. Dietary exposures can be clearly defined and comparisons among groups maximized, making this the most definitive test of a diet–cancer hypothesis. Because cancer may take decades to develop, intervention studies measuring cancer outcomes can be cost prohibitive. Intervention studies of diet and cancer prevention, therefore, often utilize surrogate cancer endpoints, such as adenomatous polyp recurrence or other intermediate markers of carcinogenesis, including neoplastic changes or molecular markers (Bostick, 1997; Schatzkin and Gail, 2002). Whether diet influences cancer initiation or progression similarly is not often feasible to study because once a cancer or intermediate risk factor such as a polyp is detected, it is typically removed. Individuals with a history of cancer have also been enrolled in intervention studies, for example, to determine whether high fruit and vegetable/low-fat diets influence breast cancer recurrence or survival (Pierce et al., 2002; Winters et al., 2004).

Both dietary supplements and food-based interventions have been tested. Supplementation trials that investigate the biological effects associated with nutrients individually or in combination with others are easier and less costly to conduct than interventions involving foods or whole diet patterns. An additional advantage of providing supplements is that observed effects can be attributed to the specific nutrient(s) under study, because unlike in dietary interventions, nutrient composition of the diet does not change. Furthermore, nutrients can be formulated into pills, which can be counted at follow-up visits to assess compliance.

A major limitation of supplement interventions is that the ideal dose and form of interventional supplement are not always known. For example, observational studies that suggested diets high in β-carotene (average U.S. intake < 5 mg/day [Institute of Medicine, 2000]) were associated with lower risk of lung cancer inspired intervention trials to study lung cancer risk. However, two trials using 20–30 mg of β-carotene supplements reported increased risk of lung cancer in smokers (Institute of Medicine, 1997), whereas in a third trial, 50 mg every other day did not influence risk of malignant neoplasms (Hennekens et al., 1996). These trials led many to believe that β-carotene causes cancer or the hasty conclusion made by the press and public: "Diet is unrelated to cancer risk." It remains possible that different levels of β-carotene intake reduce the risk of lung cancer, suggesting a nonlinear association, but it is also possible that the earlier studies attributed benefits of foods high in β-carotene to β-carotene alone (Marshall, 1999). Unfortunately, testing various doses and sources of β-carotene is costly. In contrast to β-carotene, intervention trials of 1200 mg and 2000 mg elemental calcium daily (slightly higher than normal intake levels [Institute of Medicine, 1997]) found consistent modest reductions in recurrence of colorectal adenomas (Baron et al., 1999; Bonithon-Kopp et al., 2000); however, whether lower doses have the same effect is still unknown. Underlying interactions may also obscure the full effect of a particular intervention. For example, the inverse association with calcium in one colorectal adenoma trial (Baron et al., 1999) was most notable among individuals with adequate serum 25(OH) vitamin D levels (a measure of vitamin D status) (Grau et al., 2003). Follow-up studies are evaluating the effect of calcium and vitamin D on polyp recurrence using a 2 × 2 factorial design (Bostick, personal communication). Another consideration for supplementation trials is whether individuals change their diet during the intervention. A trial of fiber supplementation and colorectal polyp recurrence documented that all participants increased their micronutrient intake and decreased their fat intake; however, few differences in the diets of intervention and control groups were significant (Jacobs et al., 2004).

Dietary intervention studies involving changes in food intakes or dietary patterns more closely reflect realistic differences in nutrient intake levels. However, this approach is more labor intensive for both investigators and participants and more costly than supplementation trials, especially when all food is provided to participants. Compliance with dietary regimens in free-living populations is a major concern with food-based intervention trials but has been feasible, as documented by biomarkers, anthropometrics, and self-reports (Bingham, 1987; Windhauser et al., 1999). For dietary intervention studies in which participants are taught how to follow a research diet on their own, studies also suggest that with regular support, participants can learn and sustain major dietary changes (Lanza et al., 2001; Pierce et al., 2004; Rock et al., 2004). Nevertheless, the differences in intervention and control diets may narrow as the study progresses if diet in the control group improves, motivation in the intervention group wanes, or some combination thereof. Although providing food may better test a hypothesis, especially when major dietary differences are required, the diet instruction method addresses long-term feasibility; thus, both approaches are valuable.

Advantages and Limitations

The major theoretical advantage of randomized intervention studies over observational studies is they naturally control for known and unknown confounders. Additional practical advantages include the ability to test specific doses, durations, and endpoints. Because these studies usually involve several in-person clinic visits, anthropometric measures and other relevant biological parameters can easily be assessed. Despite the superior design of intervention studies, however, theoretical, ethical, and scientific limitations exist. First, null findings may simply reflect that the outcome measure or the duration, dose, or form of diet under investigation was not appropriate to test the research question. Second, how definitive a marker the surrogate endpoint is for cancer development has direct bearing on whether the relationship between a dietary factor and surrogate endpoint mirrors the relationship between the dietary factor and cancer itself (Schatzkin and Gail, 2002). Third, for intervention studies of dietary factors, it is difficult to blind participants to the intervention unless micronutrients are formulated into pills. Fourth, these studies take years to evaluate one or two doses of a potential chemopreventive agent. Fifth, whether nutrients supplied in pill form have the same biological effect as those found in food is unclear because food sources contain numerous other dietary factors that may act additively or synergistically to influence carcinogenesis. Pills may also contain doses that exceed amounts found in the diet or forms that do not occur naturally in the diet. Dietary fiber interventions in the form of a high-fiber diet (Schatzkin et al., 2000) or cereal fiber supplements (Alberts et al., 2000) yielded null results for colorectal adenoma recurrence (Alberts et al., 2000; Schatzkin et al., 2000), but the fiber supplement ispaghula husk was associated with increased polyp recurrence (Bonithon-Kopp et al., 2000). Although "fiber" was tested in each trial, the source, form, and vehicle for fiber varied in each study. Sixth, for ethical reasons intervention trials cannot evaluate dietary factors hypothesized to increase cancer risk. Many dietary factors that have hypothesized benefits for various cancers also have potential benefits for other chronic diseases, particularly cardiovascular disease. If a benefit is established for cardiovascular disease, it may be unethical to seek consent for randomization that would lead to long-term deprivation of a factor among those randomized to the placebo group. Seventh, an important scientific limitation relates to generalizability of findings from intervention studies. Populations are heterogeneous with regard to both physiological and lifestyle risk factors, and results in one population may not correspond to those of others. Furthermore, individuals who volunteer to participate in trials may often be quite different from the general population, restricting generalizability of results. For all of these reasons, knowledge of cancer risk in humans is usually based on observational studies and the totality of evidence from several study designs.

SPECIAL ISSUES IN NUTRITIONAL EPIDEMIOLOGY

A number of specific issues in nutritional epidemiology may critically influence the quality of a particular study. These include issues regarding the nature of diet and its measurement, statistical analysis, and the induction period required to observe a diet–cancer association. Although not all concepts reviewed in the following section are unique to nutritional epidemiology, each is important to consider when interpreting the quality of epidemiological studies of diet and cancer.

Nutrients, Foods, and Diet Patterns

Nutritional epidemiology research examines individual nutrients, foods, or diet patterns. Human diets are complex, and foods contain a wide range of vitamins, minerals, phytochemicals, estrogenic compounds, chemical and natural pesticides, microbial toxins, and chemicals formed during cooking. A single dietary component is typically the focus when it is supported by a hypothesis and is measurable from the questionnaire and its corresponding nutrient database. Nutrients are usually spread out among many different food sources, and a biological association may be overlooked if that factor is not measured across all dietary sources. Because some nutrients are highly intercorrelated because of shared food sources, known as "collinearity," it is often difficult to attribute an association to a single factor. Usually one of the first steps in nutrition analyses is to examine the correlational structure of various nutrients of interest in the study population. Supplements generally contain much higher nutrient levels than foods; thus, supplement users are usually in the highest of several nutrient intake categories. One approach to evaluate potential confounding or effect modification by supplements is to stratify the results by supplement use patterns. Finally, foods may also be the focus of study when the exact component responsible for a particular health effect is not known (e.g., tomatoes) or when evaluating the effects of adherence to a specific recommendation (e.g., "reduce meat intake").

Researchers have also begun to assess dietary patterns in epidemiology because individuals eat foods in various combinations, and manipulation of a single nutrient (e.g., fiber) usually affects several dietary exposures. Further, many components in a total diet may have additive or interactive effects on health. Diet patterns can be tested in nutritional epidemiology using a variety of approaches (Kant, 1996; Hu, 2002), including empirically based methods such as principal component or factor analysis, the diet-score method reflecting a hypothetically protective diet or dietary guidance (McCullough et al., 2002), or some combination of both (Schulze et al., 2003). The diet-patterns approach characterizes foods that are consumed together (as in factor and cluster analysis) or foods that have hypothesized additive or interactive beneficial effects when consumed together (a priori diet scores). Dietary patterns offer one way to test the effects of dietary combinations on disease prevention, but the specific mechanisms for any observed associations in studies of diet patterns are less transparent.

Another issue is that nutrients, food, and diet-pattern studies differ among populations. For example, a study of vegetable consumption and stomach cancer in the United States may not be comparable to a similar study in China because the vegetables consumed and preparation methods differ (not to mention differences in proportion of gastric cancer subtypes by country). That studies of empirically derived food patterns have not always been replicated across countries (Slattery et al., 1998; Terry et al., 2001) is not surprising given differences in tradition and food availability.

Ranges of Intake

The range of dietary intake should be considered when interpreting study results. For example, the range of fat intake within many Western populations studied is somewhat limited, ranging from ~30–40% of total energy. These studies can be informative across this range, but evidence from populations with a different dietary pattern is required to assess any influence at lower levels of intake. Studies that span multiple populations can usually address wider ranges of exposure (Riboli and Kaaks, 1997; Smith-Warner et al., In press), although confounding and dietary differences should still be considered. Consistency of a finding across populations offers support for a given hypothesis.

Energy Adjustment

Because many nutrients are correlated with energy intake, study results can be seriously confounded by other dietary factors that track with higher calorie consumption if not controlled for energy. Generally, changes in nutrient composition of the diet are more relevant than changes in absolute intake. For example, by controlling for energy, a statistical model for the association of fat with disease would be interpreted as the effect of increasing fat intake while reducing calories from protein and/or carbohydrates. This is relevant because most people do not simply add more fat or other sources of calories to the diet (unless they are on a path to weight gain); they usually make substitutions. In the case where energy consumption is also a risk factor for the disease under study, energy may be an independent confounder. Control for energy also reduces measurement error due to overreporting or underreporting total food intake. Several methods are available to control for energy (Willett and Stampfer, 1986; Willett, 1998).

Measurement Error

The measurement of many exposures in epidemiology is subject to error, and epidemiologists try to minimize and correct for them when possible. Random or nonsystematic measurement error in dietary studies tends to obscure or weaken any true association with disease. For example, if high intake of a factor has a true relative risk of 2.5 with a specific cancer, error in measurement may attenuate the relative risk to, say, 1.8. Thus, when a significant positive or inverse association is observed in a study, random error in dietary measurement alone cannot account for this, and the true relationship is probably stronger. When an association with a dietary factor exists, potential for bias and confounding should be the major consideration. For a null association, it would be important to evaluate whether the degree of error in dietary measurement was so large that it could have obscured a true relationship entirely. Specific statistical techniques have been formulated to quantify the influence of measurement error on relative risks, including the correction of relative risks for measurement error using data from a validation study (Rosner et al., 1990; Spiegelman et al., 2001). Specific concerns have arisen regarding correction for measurement error if the validation study used a comparison method with errors that correlated with the primary method under study (Kipnis et al., 2003). Validation studies should ideally use methods with independent error structures including biomarkers when feasible.

Measurement error in several dietary factors and nondietary covariates may produce spurious and erroneous findings (Marshall et al., 1999). It would theoretically be ideal to validate and correct for measurement errors in the assessment of the main exposure and all other confounders. Unfortunately, this is not practical for most studies. Further, not all confounders (e.g., physical activity) have a readily available standard of comparison. It was shown that proper adjustment for energy may partly ameliorate these problems in nutritional analyses (Michels et al., 2004).

Relevant Exposure Periods

The long induction period between exposure and cancer diagnosis for most cancers may influence dietary measurement. A typical assessment of diet for an epidemiological study spans a year. Individuals' diets tend to track over time, but the extent varies across populations and is difficult to assess directly. In response, some cohort studies have repeated assessments of diet. For example, diet has been assessed seven times over 22 years in the Nurses' Health Study of women (in 1980, 1984, 1986, 1990, 1994, 1998, and 2002) and five times over 16 years in the male Health Professionals Follow-up Study (in 1986, 1990, 1994, 1998, and 2002). Repeated measures provide powerful data to evaluate long-term dietary patterns on cancer risk and enable epidemiologists to examine specific temporal relationships, including latency periods and the effect of changes in diet on disease risk. Repeated measures also reduce measurement error over the long term.

GENE–DIET INTERACTIONS

Nutritional factors may influence cancer risk differently according to genotype, haplotype, or molecular characteristic of the tumor. Genetic studies additionally provide a greater understanding of the biological role of certain nutrients in carcinogenesis. Past inconsistencies in nutritional epidemiology literature may be explained in part by differences in the distribution of polymorphisms for important cancer-related genes across studies. Ultimately, genetic studies may lead to improved understanding of biological processes and offer potential for targeted interventions for prevention or treatment of cancer. However, cancer genes involve complex pathways with multiple potentially important allelic variants (Vogelstein and Kinzler, 2004). Statistical methods used to test the relationship between multiple genetic polymorphisms, either within a metabolic pathway or between pathways, need further development (Hoh et al., 2001; Kooperberg et al., 2001; Devlin et al., 2003; Ritchie et al., 2003).

INTERPRETATION OF EPIDEMIOLOGICAL STUDIES

Because epidemiological studies are correlative in nature, statistical associations do not necessarily represent cause-and-effect relationships. When interpreting results from individual studies, the potential for bias and confounding should always be considered, as should the appropriateness of dietary assessment methods, ranges of intake, potential for measurement error, and control for energy and latency period. Ultimately, epidemiologists are interested in whether observed associations represent a true causal relationship and whether modifying the specific dietary factor influences the frequency of disease.

Hill (1965) summarized several criteria to establish causality, including the strength of association, the consistency of a finding in various studies and populations, the presence of a dose–response gradient, the appropriate temporal relationship, the biological plausibility, and the coherence of existing data. Though helpful, none can be considered requirements and satisfaction of these cannot be considered proof of a causal relationship. As discussed previously, the greater the magnitude of an association, the less likely the association is due to bias or confounding. The dose–response gradient may be useful, but linear dose–response relationships could also be generated by bias and confounding. Further, nonlinear causal associations in nutrition are certainly plausible. An understanding of underlying mechanisms may enhance the plausibility of a finding but is not required for assessing a diet–disease relationship. For example, obesity is strongly associated with death from many cancers (Calle et al., 2003), although the exact reason for these associations is not clearly understood.

One of the most important criterion to consider in observational studies is consistency of results across studies. For epidemiologists, "replication" of findings has a somewhat different connotation than for the experimental scientist. In the laboratory, it is important to replicate findings by creating the circumstances of the experiment as closely as possible. If results cannot be replicated, the question of validity of the initial experiment may be raised. By the nature of epidemiology, settings can never be replicated precisely, so one typically cannot expect identical results across different studies. Results may vary for methodological and biological reasons.

Because findings from epidemiological studies contribute to dietary recommendations for chronic disease reduction (Byers, 1999), several important criteria have been outlined for reviewing the literature in relation to dietary guidance (Freudenheim, 1999; Potischman and Weed, 1999). Evaluation of dietary behaviors that are likely to reduce chronic disease risk requires the consideration of all available epidemiological studies and other evidence bearing on the association. To draw conclusions from a single or even a few epidemiological studies is not desirable; hopefully, numerous well-designed studies possess relevant information. The World Cancer Research Fund and the American Institute for Cancer Research are conducting systematic literature reviews on the epidemiology of dietary factors and several cancers to update their earlier review (World Cancer Research Fund, 1997); this is due out in 2006.

SUMMARY

Many types of studies contribute to our understanding of the association between dietary factors and various cancers. Epidemiological data contribute an important part of the total evidence. Data from epidemiological studies must be carefully evaluated using various criteria to determine whether a relationship is likely to be causal, and if so, what factors may modify the relationship. Although randomized trials may eventually provide definitive answers to some of these questions, our knowledge of many of these relationships will depend largely on data from observational studies. Advancements in epidemiological methods, assessment of dietary exposures, and gene–diet interaction studies will improve our ability to identify important dietary factors in the etiology of cancer. Findings can then be applied to reduce the risk of cancer development and recurrence.

References

Alberts, D.S., Martinez, M.E., Roe, D.J., Guillen-Rodriguez, J.M., Marshall, J.R., van Leeuwen, J.B., Reid, M.E., Ritenbaugh, C., Vargas, P.A., Bhattacharyya, A.B., Earnest, D.L., and Sampliner, R.E. 2000. Lack of effect of a high-fiber cereal supplement on the recurrence of colorectal adenomas. Phoenix Colon Cancer Prevention Physicians' Network. *N Engl J Med* **342**: 1156–1162.

Anonymous. 1992. The effects of nonpharmacologic interventions on blood pressure of persons with high normal levels. Results of the Trials of Hypertension Prevention, Phase I. *JAMA* **267**: 1213–1220.

Armstrong, B., and Doll, R. 1975. Environmental factors and cancer incidence and mortality in different countries, with special reference to dietary practices. *Int J Cancer* **15**: 617–631.

Baron, J.A., Beach, M., Mandel, J.S., van Stolk, R.U., Haile, R.W., Sandler, R.S., Rothstein, R., Summers, R.W., Snover, D.C., Beck, G.J., Bond, J.H., and Greenberg, E.R. 1999. Calcium supplements for the prevention of colorectal adenomas. The Calcium Polyp Prevention Study Group. *N Engl J Med* **340**: 101–107.

Bingham, S.A. 1987. The dietary assessment of individuals: methods, accuracy, new techniques and recommendations. *Nutr Abstr Rev* **57**: 705–743.

Bonithon-Kopp, C., Kronborg, O., Giacosa, A., Rath, U., and Faivre, J. 2000. Calcium and fibre supplementation in prevention of colorectal adenoma recurrence: a randomized intervention trial. *Lancet* **356**: 1300–1306.

Bostick, R.M. 1997. Human studies of calcium supplementation and colorectal epithelial cell proliferation. *Cancer Epidemiol Biomarkers Prev* **6**: 971–980.

Byers, T. 1999. The role of epidemiology in developing nutritional recommendations: past, present, and future. *Am J Clin Nutr* **69**: 1304S–1308S.

Calle, E.E., Rodriguez, C., Walker-Thurmond, K., and Thun, M.J. 2003. Overweight, obesity, and mortality from cancer in a prospectively studied cohort of U.S. adults. *N Engl J Med* **348**: 1625–1638.

Cervantes-Laurean, D., McElvaney, N.G., and Moss, J. 1999. Niacin. *In* "Modern Nutrition in Health and Disease" (M.E. Shils, J.A. Olson, M. Shike, and A.C. Ross, Eds.). Lippincott, Williams & Wilkins, Philadelphia.

Cox, D.R. 1972. Regression models and life-tables. *J R Stat Soc B* **34**: 187–220.

Devlin, B., Roeder, K., and Wasserman, L. 2003. Analysis of multilocus models of association. *Genet Epidemiol* **25**: 36–47.

Enns, C.W., Goldman, J.D., and Cook, A. 1997. Trends in food and nutrient intakes by adults: NFCS 1977–78, CSFII 1989–91, and CSFII 1994–95. *Fam Econ Nutr Rev* **10**: 2–15.

Freudenheim, J.L. 1999. Study design and hypothesis testing: issues in the evaluation of evidence from research in nutritional epidemiology. *Am J Clin Nutr* **69**: 1315S–1321S.

Giovannucci, E., Stampfer, M.J., Colditz, G.A., Manson, J.E., Rosner, B.A., Longnecker, M., Speizer, F.E., and Willett, W.C. 1993. A comparison of prospective and retrospective assessments of diet in the study of breast cancer. *Am J Epidemiol* **137**: 502–511.

Grau, M.V., Baron, J.A., Sandler, R.S., Haile, R.W., Beach, M.L., Church, T.R., and Heber, D. 2003. Vitamin D, calcium supplementation, and colorectal adenomas: results of a randomized trial. *J Natl Cancer Inst* **95**: 1765–1771.

Hartge, P., Brinton, L.A., Rosenthal, J.F.A., Cahill, J.I., Hoover, R.N., and Waksberg, J. 1984. Random digit dialing in selecting a population-based control group. *Am J Epidemiol* **120**: 825–833.

Hennekens, C.H., and Buring, J.E. 1987. "Epidemiology in Medicine." Little, Brown and Co., Boston.

Hennekens, C.H., Buring, J.E., Manson, J.E., Stampfer, M., Rosner, B., Cook, N.R., Belanger, C., LaMotte, F., Gaziano, J.M., Ridker, P.M., Willett, W., and Peto, R. 1996. Lack of effect of long-term supplementation with beta carotene on the incidence of malignant neoplasms and cardiovascular disease. *N Engl J Med* **334**: 1145–1149.

Hill, A.B. 1965. The environment and disease: association or causation? *Proc R Soc Med* **58**: 295–300.

Hoh, J., Wille, A., and Ott, J. 2001. Trimming, weighting, and grouping SNPs in human case–control association studies. *Genome Res* **11**: 2115–2119.

Hu, F.B. 2002. Dietary pattern analysis: a new direction in nutritional epidemiology. *Curr Opin Lipidol* **13**: 3–9.

Institute of Medicine. 1997. "Dietary Reference Intakes for Calcium, Phosphorus, Magnesium, Vitamin D and Fluoride." National Academy Press, Washington, DC.

Institute of Medicine. 2000. "Dietary Reference Intakes for Vitamin C, Vitamin E, Selenium and Carotenoids." National Academy Press, Washington, DC.

International Agency for Research on Cancer. 2002. "Cancer Incidence in Five Continents." IARC Scientific Publications, Lyon, France.

International Agency for Research on Cancer. 2003. Fruits and vegetables. *In* "IARC Handbook of Cancer Prevention." IARC Press, Lyon, France.

Intersalt Cooperative Research Group. 1988. Intersalt: an international study of electrolyte excretion and blood pressure. Results for 24 hour urinary sodium and potassium excretion. *BMJ* **297**: 319–328.

Jacob, R.A. 1999. Vitamin C. *In* "Modern Nutrition in Health and Diseases" (M.E. Shils, J.A. Olson, M. Shike, and A.C. Ross, Eds.), pp. 467–483. Lippincott, Williams & Wilkins, Philadelphia.

Jacobs, E.T., Giuliano, A.R., Roe, D.J., Guillen-Rodriguez, J.M., Hartz, V.L., Whitsacre, R.C., Albers, D.S., and Martinez, M.E. 2004. Dietary change in an intervention trial of wheat bran fiber and colorectal adenoma recurrence. *Ann Epidemiol* **14**: 280–286.

Kant, A.K. 1996. Indexes of overall diet quality: a review. *J Am Diet Assoc* **96**: 785–791.

Kipnis, V., Subar, A.F., Midthune, D., Freedman, L.S., Ballard-Barbash, R., Troiano, R.P., Bingham, S., Schoeller, D.A., Schatzkin, A., and Carroll, R.J. 2003. Structure of dietary measurement error: results of the OPEN biomarker study. *Am J Epidemiol* **158**: 14–21.

Kooperberg, C., Ruczinski, I., LeBlanc, M.L., and Hsu, L. 2001. Sequence analysis using logic regression. *Genet Epidemiol* **21**: S626–S631.

Lanza, E., Schatzkin, A., Daston, C., Corle, D., Freedman, L., Ballard-Barbash, R., Caan, B., Lance, P., Marshall, J., Iber, F., Shike, M., Weissfeld, J., Slattery, M., Paskett, E., Mateski, D., and Albert, P. 2001. Implementation of a 4-y, high-fiber, high-fruit-and-vegetable, low-fat dietary intervention: results of dietary changes in the Polyp Prevention Trial. PPT Study Group. *Am J Clin Nutr* **74**: 387–401.

Last, J.M. 1983. "A Dictionary of Epidemiology." Oxford University Press, Oxford.

Le Marchand, L. 1999. Combined influence of genetic and dietary factors on colorectal cancer incidence in Japanese Americans. *J Natl Cancer Inst Monogr* **26**: 101–105.

Maclure, M., and Hankinson, S. 1990. Analysis of selection bias in a case–control study of renal adenocarcinoma. *Epidemiology* **1**: 441–447.

Marshall, J.R. 1999. Beta-carotene: a miss for epidemiology. *J Natl Cancer Inst* **91**: 2068–2069.

Marshall, J.R., Hastrup, J.L., and Ross, J.S. 1999. Mismeasurement and the resonance of strong confounders: correlated errors. *Am J Epidemiol* **150**: 88–96.

McCullough, M.L., Feskanich, D., Stampfer, M.J., Giovannucci, E.L., Rimm, E.B., Hu, F.B., Spiegelman, D., Hunter, D.J., Colditz, G.A., and Willett, W.C. 2002. Diet quality and major chronic disease risk in men and women: moving toward improved dietary guidance. *Am J Clin Nutr* **76**: 1261–1271.

Michels, K.B., Bingham, S.A., Luben, R., Welch, A.A., and Day, N.E. 2004. The effect of correlated measurement error in multivariate models of diet. *Am J Epidemiol* **160**: 59–67.

National Center for Health Statistics. 2003. "National Vital Statistics Reports," Vol 52. Centers for Disease Control and Prevention, Atlanta, GA.

Pierce, J.P., Faerber, S., Wright, F.A., Rock, C.L., Newman, V., Flatt, S.W., Kealey, S., Jones, V.E., Caan, B.J., Gold, E.B., Haan, M., Hollenbach, K.A., Jones, L., Marshall, J.R., Ritenbaugh, C., Stefanick, M.L., Thomson, C., Wasserman, L., Natarajan, L., Thomas, R.G., and Gilpin, E.A. 2002. A randomized trial of the effect of a plant-based dietary pattern on additional breast cancer events and survival: the Women's Healthy Eating and Living (WHEL) Study. *Control Clin Trials* **23**: 728–756.

Pierce, J.P., Newman, V.A., Flatt, S.W., Faerber, S., Rock, C.L., Natarajan, L., Caan, B.J., Gold, E.B., Hollenbach, K.A., Wasserman, L., Jones, L., Ritenbaugh, C., Stefanick, M.L., Thomson, C.A., and Kealey, S. 2004. Telephone counseling intervention increases intakes of micronutrient- and phytochemical-rich vegetables, fruit and fiber in breast cancer survivors. Women's Healthy Eating and Living (WHEL) Study Group. *J Nutr* **134**: 452–458.

Pillow, P.C., Duphorne, C.M., Chang, S., Contois, J.H., Strom, S.S., Spitz, M.R., and Hursting, S.D. 1999. Development of a database for assessing dietary phytoestrogen intake. *Nutr Cancer* **33**: 3–19.

Platz, E.A., De Marzo, A.M., and Giovannucci, E. 2004. Prostate cancer association studies: pitfalls and solutions to cancer misclassification in the PSA era. *J Cell Biochem* **91**: 553–571.

Potischman, N., and Weed, D.L. 1999. Causal criteria in nutritional epidemiology. *Am J Clin Nutr* **69**: 1309S–1314S.

Potosky, A.L., Kessler, L., Gridley, G., Brown, C.C., and Horm, J.W. 1990. Rise in prostatic cancer incidence associated with increased use of transurethral resection. *J Natl Cancer Inst* **82**: 1624–1628.

Riboli, E., and Kaaks, R. 1997. The EPIC project: rationale and study design. *Int J Epidemiol* **26**: S6–S14.

Reproducibility and validity of a expanded self-administered semiquantitative food frequency questionnaire among male health professionals. *Am J Epidemiol* **135**: 1114–1126.

Ritchie, M.D., Hahn, L.W., and Moore, J.H. 2003. Power of multifactor dimensionality reduction for detecting gene–gene interactions in the presence of genotyping error, missing data, phenocopy, and genetic heterogeneity. *Genet Epidemiol* **24**: 150–157.

Rock, C.L., Flatt, S.W., Thomson, C.A., Stefanick, M.L., Newman, V.A., Jones, L., Natarajan, L., Pierce, J.P., Chang, R.J., and Witztum, J.L. 2004. Plasma triacylglycerol and HDL cholesterol concentrations confirm self-reported changes in carbohydrate and fat intakes in women in a diet intervention trial. Women's Healthy Eating and Living (WHEL) Study Group. *J Nutr* **134**: 342–347.

Rosner, B., Spiegelman, D., and Willett, W.C. 1990. Correction of logistic regression relative risk estimates and confidence intervals for measurement error: the case of multiple covariates measured with error. *Am J Epidemiol* **132**: 734–745.

Rothman, K.J., and Greenland, S. 1998. "Modern Epidemiology." Lippincott–Raven Publishers, Philadelphia.

Schatzkin, A., and Gail, M. 2002. The promise and peril of surrogate end points in cancer research. *Nat Rev Cancer* **2**: 19–27.

Schatzkin, A., Lanza, E., Corle, D., Lance, P., Iber, F., Caan, B., Shike, M., Weissfeld, J., Burt, R., Cooper, M.R., Kikendall, J.W., and Cahill, J. 2000. Lack of effect of a low-fat, high-fiber diet on the recurrence of colorectal adenomas. Polyp Prevention Trial Study Group. *N Engl J Med* **342**: 1149–1155.

Schulze, M.B., Hoffmann, K., Kroke, A., and Boeing, H. 2003. Risk of hypertension among women in the EPIC-Potsdam Study: comparison of relative risk estimates for exploratory and hypothesis oriented dietary patterns. *Am J Epidemiol* **158**: 365–373.

Slattery, M.L., Boucher, K.M., Caan, B.J., Potter, J.D., and Ma, K.N. 1998. Eating patterns and risk of colon cancer. *Am J Epidemiol* **148**: 4–16.

Smith-Warner, S.A., Spiegelman, D., Ritz, J., Albanes, D., Beeson, L., Bernstein, L., Berrino, F., van den Brandt, P., Buring, J.E., Cho, E., Colditz, A., Folsom, A., Freudenheim, J., Giovannucci, E., Goldbohm, R., Graham, S., Harnack, L., Horn-Ross, P.L., Krogh, V., Leitzmann, M.F., McCullough, M.L., Miller, A., Rodriguez, C., Rohan, T., Schatzkin, A., Shore, R.E., Virtanen, M., Willett, W.C., Wolk, A., Zeleniuch-Jacquotte, A., Zhang, S.M., and Hunter, D.J. In press. Methods for pooling results of epidemiologic studies: the pooling project of prospective studies of diet and cancer, *Am J Epidemiol.*

Spiegelman, D., Carroll, R.J., and Kipnis, V. 2001. Efficient regression calibration for logistic regression in main study/internal validation study designs with an imperfect reference instrument. *Stat Med* **20**: 139–160.

Stemmermann, G.N., Mandel, M., and Mower, H.F. 1979. Colon cancer: its precursors and companions in Hawaii Japanese. *Natl Cancer Inst Monogr* **53**: 175–179.

Stephen, A.M., and Wald, N.J. 1990. Trends in individual consumption of dietary fat in the United States, 1920–1984. *Am J Clin Nutr* **52**: 457–469.

Terry, P., Hu, F.B., Hansen, H., and Wolk, A. 2001. Prospective study of major dietary patterns and colorectal cancer risk in women. *Am J Epidemiol* **154**: 1143–1149.

Vogelstein, B., and Kinzler, K.W. 2004. Cancer genes and the pathways they control. *Nat Med* **10**: 789–799.

Willett, W.C. 1998. "Nutritional Epidemiology," 2nd edition. Oxford University Press, New York.

Willett, W.C., and Stampfer, M.J. 1986. Total energy intake: implications for epidemiologic analyses. *Am J Epidemiol* **124**: 17–27.

Windhauser, M.M., Evans, M.A., McCullough, M.L., Swain, J.F., Lin, P.H., Hoben, K.P., Plaisted, C.S., Karanja, N.M., and Vollmer, W.M. 1999. Dietary adherence in the Dietary Approaches to Stop Hypertension trial. DASH Collaborative Research Group. *J Am Diet Assoc* **99**: S76–S83.

Winters, B.L., Mitchell, D.C., Smiciklas-Wright, H., Grosvenor, M.B., Liu, W., and Blackburn, G.L. 2004. Dietary patterns in women treated for breast cancer who successfully reduce fat intake: the Women's Intervention Nutrition Study (WINS). *J Am Diet Assoc* **104**: 551–559.

World Cancer Research Fund. 1997. "Food, Nutrition, and the Prevention of Cancer: A Global Perspective." American Institute for Cancer Research, Washington, DC.

C H A P T E R

7

Fruit and Vegetable Consumption and Cancer

STEPHANIE A. SMITH-WARNER, JEANINE GENKINGER, AND EDWARD GIOVANNUCCI

The association between fruit and vegetable consumption and cancer risk has been reported in hundreds of epidemiological studies (Block et al., 1992; Steinmetz and Potter, 1996; World Cancer Research Fund et al., 1997; The Working Group on Diet and Cancer of the Committee on Medical Aspects of Food and Nutrition Policy, 1998; International Agency for Research on Cancer [IARC], 2003). These studies have been conducted in numerous countries with diverse diets, have evaluated many types of cancer, and have used different dietary assessment methods to assess fruit and vegetable intake. Various aspects of fruit and vegetable consumption have been examined. Studies have evaluated broad subgroups such as total fruits and total vegetables, finer categorization of these groups such as botanically defined groups or groups based on phytochemical content, and individual fruits and vegetables.

It has been hypothesized that the wide variety of nutrients and bioactive compounds in fruits and vegetables can inhibit carcinogenesis during the initiation, promotion, and progression stages. The nutrients and bioactive compounds present in fruits and vegetables have been shown to inhibit the deactivation of procarcinogens, induce detoxification pathways, affect the cell cycle by regulating cell cycle progression, influence cell-to-cell communication, quench free radicals, stimulate the immune system, modulate hormone metabolism, and dilute and bind carcinogens, all of which should help to prevent the development of cancer (Table 1). For example, sulforaphanes and isothiocyanates, present in cruciferous vegetables, induce phase I and phase II enzymes to detoxify and eliminate carcinogens (Dragsted et al., 1993; Fahey et al., 1997; Verhoeven et al., 1997a; Belanger, 1998; Crowell, 1999; Hecht, 1999a; van Poppel et al., 1999; Sato and Miyata, 2000; Greenwald et al., 2001; Lamm and Riggs, 2001; IARC, 2003), regulate cell cycle progression (Bianchini and Vainio, 2001; Greenwald et al., 2001; Pinto et al., 2001), and induce apoptosis (Crowell, 1999; Greenwald et al., 2001; Pinto et al., 2001). The vitamin C found in many fruits and vegetables and organosulfur compounds found in onions, leeks, and garlic may additionally stimulate the immune system (Sato and Miyata, 2000; Venket Rao and Agarwal, 2000; Greenwald et al., 2001; Lee et al., 2003a; Pinto et al., 2001). By promoting the proliferation of lymphocytes, stimulating macrophage phagocytosis, and enhancing the activity of natural killer cells, these nutrients may protect cells against microbes, bacteria, and viral and fungal agents (Head, 1998; Lamm and Riggs, 2001; Lee et al., 2003a). Fruits and vegetables are also rich sources of antioxidants (Cao et al., 1996; Wang et al., 1996), which help to quench exogenous and endogenous free radicals. If the free radicals remain in an oxidative state, they may cause oxidative damage to nucleotides, proteins, and cell membranes and result in the initiation of carcinogenesis. Because randomized clinical trials of β-carotene, vitamin C, and vitamin E have shown no or questionable benefits on cancer outcomes (Hennekens et al., 1996; Lee et al., 1999; Malila et al., 1999; Bjelakovic et al., 2004) and in some cases, a rise in cancer outcomes (The Alpha-Tocopherol and Beta Carotene Cancer Prevention Study Group, 1994; Omenn et al., 1996a), synergism of the variety of phytochemicals present in fruits and vegetables may be more important than consuming high doses of a single nutrient or phytochemical, because of complementary and overlapping mechanisms of action (La Vecchia and Tavani, 1998; Lampe, 1999).

Copyright © 2006, Elsevier Inc.
All rights of reproduction in any form reserved.

TABLE 1

Potential anticarcinogenic mechanisms	Examples of phytochemicals	Examples of food sources
• **Enzyme induction of phase I enzymes** ◦ **Inhibits carcinogen uptake and formation** (Ariyoshi et al., 1975; Austin et al., 1988; Belanger, 1998; Crowell, 1999; Crowell et al., 1992; Dragsted et al., 1993; Greenwald et al., 2001; Hecht, 1999b; IARC, 2003; Lamm and Riggs, 2001; Maltzman et al., 1991; van Poppel et al., 1999; Verhoeven et al., 1997a) ◦ **P450, CYP 2B1, CYP 2C, epoxide hydratase**	**Carotenoids**	Yellow-orange vegetables
	Organosulfur compounds Allyl sulfides (allicin) Allyl disulfides	Liliaceas (e.g., chives, garlic, leeks, onions)
	Sulforaphanes **Glucosinolates** Indoles Isothiocyanates	Cruciferous (e.g., broccoli, cabbage, cauliflower, greens)
	Terpenes/D-limonene Carveol Carvone Geranoil	Citrus fruits, cherries, lemons, oranges, grapefruit, spearmint, tomatoes
• **Inhibition of phase I enzymes** ◦ P450 (Bianchini and Vainio, 2003; Gusman et al., 2001)	**Resveratrol**	Vitaceae (e.g., grapes, currants)
• **Enzyme induction of phase II enzymes** ◦ **Inactivates carcinogens** (Crowell, 1999; Dragsted et al., 1993; Fahey et al., 1997; Greenwald et al., 2001; Hecht, 1999b; IARC, 2003; Kris-Etherton et al., 2002; Pinto et al., 2001; Sato and Miyata, 2000; Shapiro et al., 2001; Talalay and Fahey, 2001; van Poppel et al., 1999)	**Carotenoids**	Yellow-orange vegetables
	Flavonoids/Flavonols Quercetin Kaempferol Myricetin Isorhamnetin	Apple, blueberry, broccoli, brussels sprout, grape (red), lemon, onion, orange, pear (red/green), pepper (green/red), strawberry
	Organosulfur compounds Allyl sulfides (allicin) Allyl disulfides	Liliaceae (e.g., chives, garlic, leeks, onions)
◦ **GST, Quinine reductase** (Jang et al., 1997), **UDP-glucuronyl transferase** (Belanger, 1998; Crowell, 1999; Elegbede et al., 1993)	**Resveratrol**	Vitaceae (e.g., grapes, currants)
	Sulforaphanes **Glucosinolates** Indoles Isothiocyanates	Cruciferous (e.g., broccoli, cabbage, cauliflower, greens)
	Terpenes/D-limonene Carveol Carvone Geranoil	Citrus fruits, cherries, lemons, oranges, grapefruit, spearmint, tomatoes
May affect cell cycle/DNA through one or more of the following mechanisms • **May regulate cell cycle progression** (Pinto et al., 2001; Bianchini and Vainio, 2001; Greenwald et al., 2001) ◦ Inhibition of tumor cell prolifeation (Belanger, 1998; Crowell, 1999; Morse and Stoner, 1993) ◦ Induction of tumor cell differentiation (Belanger, 1998; Crowell, 1999; Greenwald et al., 2001; Haag and Gould, 1994; Haag et al., 1992; Morse and Stoner, 1993) ◦ Growth control (Agarwal and Rao, 2000; Sengupta and Das, 1999) ◦ Induce cell cycle arrest (Greenwald et al., 2001) ▪ Ability to block G_2/M phase (Knowles and Milner, 2001) ◦ Induce apoptosis (Crowell, 1999; Greenwald et al., 2001; Mills et al., 1995; Morse and Stoner, 1993; Pinto et al., 2001)	**Sulforaphanes** **Glucosinolates** Indoles Isothiocyantes	Cruciferous (e.g., broccoli, cabbage, cauliflower, greens)
	Organosulfur compounds Allyl sulfides (allicin) Allyl disulfides	Liliaceae (e.g., chives, garlic, leeks, onions)
	Vitamin E	Avocado; apples; blackberries; bananas; broccoli; dark, green, leafy vegetables; kiwifruit; spinach
	Beta-Carotene	Yellow-orange fruits and vegetables
	Lycopene	Grapefruit (red/pink), guava, tomato, watermelon
	Beta-cryptoxanthin	Apple, avocado, broccoli, cantaloupe, corn, grapefruit, kiwi, mango, orange, peach, pepper (red), plum, spinach, tomato, winter squash
• **Role in DNA metabolism** (Choi and Mason, 2000; Krishnaswamy and Madhavan Nair, 2001; Terry et al., 2001c) (Pinto et al., 2001)	**Folate**	Citrus fruits, dark green leafy vegetables
• **Increasing growth factor receptors** (Belanger, 1998)	**D-limonene**	Cherries, lemons, oranges, grapefruit, peppermint, grasses, tomatoes

TABLE 1 (*Continued*)

Potential anticarcinogenic mechanisms	Examples of phytochemicals	Examples of food sources
• **Inhibits platelet aggregation and adhesion** (Kris-Etherton et al., 2002) • **DNA/lipoproteins** ◦ Shields sensitive structures such as DNA (Dragsted et al., 1993; Kris-Etherton et al., 2002) ◦ Inhibits LDL oxidation ◦ Reduced DNA adduct formation (Bianchini and Vainio, 2001; Verhoeven et al., 1997a) ◦ Maintains DNA integrity and repair (Choi and Mason, 2000; Dragsted et al., 1993; Kris-Etherton et al., 2002; La Vecchia and Tavani, 1998; Schorah, 1999; Terry et al., 2001c) • **May enhance cell to cell communication** (Greenwald et al., 2001; Paiva and Russell, 1999) ◦ Upregulate gap junction communication (Sengupta and Das, 1999) • **Metabolic pathways regulations** (Agarwal and Rao, 2000; Venket Rao, 2000) ◦ May modulate enzyme activities (Bianchini and Vainio, 2001) • **Provitamin A activity** (Paiva and Russell, 1999; Agarwal and Rao, 2000; Venket Rao and Agarwal, 2000)	**Flavonoids/flavonols** Quercetin Kaempferol Myricetin Isorhamnetin	Apple, blueberry, broccoli, Brussels sprout, grape (red), lemon, onion, orange, pear (red/green), pepper (green/red), strawberry
• **Stimulate immune system** (Agarwal and Rao, 2000; Greenwald et al., 2001; Lee et al., 2003a; Pinto et al., 2001; Sato and Miyata, 2000; Venket Rao and Agarwal, 2000) ◦ Regulate nuclear factors and inflammation (Pinto et al., 2001) ◦ Antibacterial effect, particularly with *H. pylori* (Fleischauer and Arab, 2001; Sato and Miyata, 2000) ◦ Antimicrobial (Sato and Miyata, 2000) ◦ Antifungal (Sato and Miyata, 2000) ◦ Stimulates proliferation of lymphocytes and macrophage phagocytosis, interleukin-2, tumor necrosis factor-α and interferon-γ (Lamm and Riggs, 2001) ◦ Stimulates release of enhanced natural killer cell and lymphokine-activated killer cell activity (Lamm and Riggs, 2001)	**Organosulfur compounds** Allyl sulfides (allicin) Allyl disulfides	Liliaceae (e.g., chives, garlic, leeks, onions)
	Vitamin C	Rutaceae (citrus fruits) Cruciferous vegetables (broccoli, Brussels sprouts, cabbage) Solanaceae (tomato, peppers, potatoes)
	Vitamin E	Avocado; apples; blackberries; bananas; broccoli; dark, green, leafy vegetables; kiwifruit; spinach
	Beta-carotene	Yellow-orange fruits and vegetables
	Lycopene	Grapefruit (red/pink), guava, tomato, watermelon
• **Antioxidant properties** (Bianchini and Vainio, 2003; Greenwald et al., 2001; Gusman et al., 2001; Jang et al., 1997; Kris-Etherton et al., 2002; Lee et al., 2003a; Paiva and Russell, 1999) ◦ Quenches exogenous and endogenous oxidants (free radicals, ROS/RNS/RCS) in aqueous solutions, blood, membranes, and within cells (Evans and Halliwell, 2001; IARC, 2003; Schorah, 1999) ▪ Nitrosamines (Dragsted et al., 1993; Lee et al., 2003a) lipid carbon-centered hydroperoxyl, lipid peroxyl radicals ▪ O_2^-, H_2O_2, singlet oxygen, hypochlorite (Evans and Halliwell, 2001), nitrogen dioxide, thiyl, sulphonyl radical (Kris-Etherton et al., 2002)	**Resveratrol** **Vitamin C** **Vitamin E** **β-Carotene** **Lycopene**	Vitaceae (red grapes) Rutaceae (citrus fruits) Cruciferous vegetables (broccoli, Brussels sprouts, cabbage) Avocado; apples; blackberries; bananas; broccoli; dark, green, leafy vegetables; kiwifruit; spinach Apricot, broccoli, Brussels, sprouts, cantaloupe, grapefruit (red/pink), mustard greens, peach, pepper (red), romaine, spinach, sweet potato, tomato, turnip greens, winter squash Grapefruit (red/pink), guava, tomato, watermelon

(*continues*)

TABLE 1 *(Continued)*

Potential anticarcinogenic mechanisms	Examples of phytochemicals	Examples of food sources
▪ Singlet oxygen and radical (Agarwal and Rao, 2000; Dragsted et al., 1993; Giovannucci, 1999; Nishino et al., 2000; Paiva and Russell, 1999; Pool-Zobel et al., 1997; Sengupta and Das, 1999; Venket Rao and Agarwal, 2000) ▪ Alkoxyl and peroxyl radicals (Greenwald et al., 2001; Paiva and Russell, 1999) ▪ Ultraviolet light and cigarette smoke (Kris-Etherton et al., 2002) ▪ Activated mutagens and carcinogens (Dragsted et al., 1993; Kris-Etherton et al., 2002) ◦ May inhibit free radical generating reactions (carbon-centered radicals) (Kris-Etherton et al., 2002; Paiva and Russell, 1999) ◦ Can regenerate other antioxidants such as vitamin E (Evans and Halliwell, 2001) ◦ May chelate prooxidant metal ions (Kris-Etherton et al., 2002) ◦ Protects lipids, DNA, lipoproteins (Agarwal and Rao, 2000; Kris-Etherton et al., 2002; Sengupta and Das, 1999)	**Flavonoids/flavonols** Quercetin Kaempferol Myricetin Isorhamnetin	Apple, blueberry, broccoli, Brussels sprout, cherry, cranberry, grape (red), grapefruit, lemon, orange, onion, pear (red/green), pepper (green/red), plum, raspberry, strawberry, tangerine
• **Increase fecal bulk** (Greenwald et al., 2001; IARC, 2003; La Vecchia, 2001) ◦ Decrease concentration of bile acid and other carcinogens (Havas, 1997) • **Dilution and binding of carcinogens** (IARC, 2003) ◦ Secondary bile acids and hydrophobic carcinogens (Havas, 1997) ◦ Binding of steroid hormones • **Increase transit time** ◦ Decrease time that colon is exposed to carcinogens (Havas, 1997) • **Produce short-chain fatty acids, which may affect pH** • **Increase availability of butyrate** (Greenwald et al., 2001; IARC, 2003; La Vecchia, 2001) ◦ Promotes growth arrest ◦ Promotes differentiation ◦ Promotes apoptosis • May affect enterohepatic circulation of estrogens and the actions of fiber associated phytoestrogens (Rose, 1990; Rose et al., 1991)	**Fiber**	Apple, apricot, asparagus, bamboo shoots, bananas, bean sprout, beets, blueberries, broccoli, Brussels sprouts, cabbage, cantaloupe, carrots, cauliflower, celery, cherries, corn, cucumber, grapefruit, grapes, green beans, mushrooms, nectarine, onion, orange, pear, pepper (green), pineapple, plum, potato, pumpkin, radish, squash, strawberry, sweet potato, tangerine, tomatoes, turnip greens, watermelon (Marlett, 1992)

PUBLISHED REVIEWS

Several panels have reviewed the results from observational studies on fruit and vegetable consumption and specific cancer sites. In 1997, a panel sponsored by the World Cancer Research Fund and American Institute of Cancer Research reviewed 14 ecologic, 37 cohort, and 196 case-control studies that had examined the relationship between fruits and vegetables and cancer risk (World Cancer Research Fund et al., 1997). The most extensively studied cancers were stomach, colon and rectum, esophagus, mouth, oral cavity, and pharynx. Of the case-control studies, 78% reported a statistically significant inverse association between a specific cancer site and intake of at least one fruit and/or vegetable item or group. The panel determined that the evidence for a protective relationship for fruits and vegetables was convincing for cancers of the mouth and pharynx, esophagus, lung, and stomach; probable for cancers of the larynx, pancreas, breast, and bladder; and possible for cancers of the cervix, ovary, endometrium, and thyroid.

Associations were examined separately for vegetable consumption in 74 case-control and cohort studies. In these studies, 80% showed an inverse association for at least one vegetable group or item and 12% found positive associations. Among the specific vegetable subgroups that were reviewed, an inverse association was most consistently observed for raw vegetables. For the 56 case-control and cohort studies that examined associations for fruit intake alone, the corresponding numbers were 64% and 9%, respectively. Null findings were more common for fruit compared with vegetable intakes (27% vs 8%, respectively). For vegetables, the evidence was determined to be convincing for cancers of the colon and rectum and possible for cancers of the liver, prostate, and kidney. No consensus statement was made regarding fruit consumption alone. Moreover, the evidence did not suggest that fruits and vegetables increased the risk of any of the cancer sites evaluated (World Cancer Research Fund et al., 1997).

The conclusions from a 1998 review of epidemiological and experimental studies on fruits and vegetables and cancer risk by the Working Group on Diet and Cancer of the Committee on Medical Aspects (COMA) of Food and Nutrition Policy made more conservative conclusions than the World Cancer Research Fund and American Institute for Cancer Research panel, even though the two panels reviewed essentially the same studies (The Working Group on Diet and Cancer of the Committee on Medical Aspects of Food and Nutrition Policy, 1998). The COMA Working Group concluded that (1) there is moderate evidence that higher intakes of fruits and vegetables would reduce the risk of gastric cancer, (2) there is moderate evidence that higher intakes of vegetables would reduce the risk of colorectal cancer, and (3) there is weak evidence that higher intakes of fruits and vegetables would reduce the risk of breast cancer. Based on the lack of data showing that fruits and vegetables increase the risk of cancer and the suggestion of a graded decrease in risk with increasing fruit and vegetable consumption, the panel concluded that the "overall picture, therefore, is consistent [with] and supports the hypothesis that the consumption of fruits and vegetables protects against the development of some cancers," although the evidence is insufficient to define an optimal level of fruit and vegetable consumption to reduce cancer risk.

A meta-analysis summarized the association between total fruit and total vegetable intakes and the risk of several cancers (Riboli and Norat, 2003) (Table 2). To reduce the heterogeneity in the exposures examined across studies, the authors limited their meta-analysis to only categories representing total fruit and total vegetable intake. The study-specific relative risks were extracted from each publication and then reexpressed based on an increase in 100 g/day of intake. For fruit, statistically significant decreases in risk were observed among case-control studies for cancers of the mouth and pharynx, larynx, esophagus, stomach, colon and rectum, colon, bladder, and lung; a nonsignificant inverse association was observed only for breast cancer. Vegetable consumption was associated with a statistically significant decrease in the risk of cancers of the esophagus, stomach, colon and rectum, bladder, and lung. The magnitude of the association for vegetables generally was stronger than that for fruits only for colorectal and breast cancers. Associations among cohort studies generally were weaker than those observed among case-control studies, with statistically significant decreases in risk being observed only for cancers of the colon (for vegetables only), rectum (for fruit only), bladder (for fruit only), and lung (for fruit only). There was significant heterogeneity in the study-specific results for most cancer sites overall and when case-control studies and cohort studies were examined separately. However, for some cancer sites (i.e., esophagus and stomach), the heterogeneity occurred because the magnitude of the inverse association differed across studies, not because of the directionality of the association.

In 2003, a working group sponsored by the IARC reviewed the results on total fruit consumption and total vegetable consumption and the risk of specific cancers (IARC, 2003). Although both positive and inverse associations were observed for the risk of specific cancers with fruit and vegetable consumption, the mean of the study-specific relative risks suggested that higher compared with lower intakes of total fruit intake and total vegetable intake were each associated with a lower risk of most cancers. In general, the results from cohort studies were weaker than those observed in case-control studies. The working group concluded that the evidence indicated that higher fruit consumption probably reduces the risk of esophageal, stomach, and lung cancer and that higher vegetable consumption probably reduces the risk of esophageal and colorectal cancer. For several cancer sites, no conclusion was made because the data were too limited or the results were inconclusive.

INDIVIDUAL CANCER SITES

In this chapter, the results for lung, breast, colorectal, stomach, and prostate cancers are summarized in more detail. We chose these five sites because they represent the five most common incident cancers in the world (Ferlay et al., 2004). The discussion follows the progression from broad to specific fruit and vegetable exposures to examine whether specific combinations of fruits and vegetables are more strongly associated with cancer risk compared with overall measures of fruit and vegetable consumption. For each cancer site, associations are summarized for total fruits, citrus fruits, total vegetables, cruciferous vegetables, and green vegetables.

TABLE 2 Summary of Meta-Analysis of Case-Control and Cohort Studies Examining Fruit and Vegetable Consumption and Cancer Risk (Adapted from Riboli and Norat, 2003)

		Fruit			Vegetables		
Cancer site	**Study design**	**n**	**RR (95% CI)**	***p* for heterogeneity**	**n**	**RR (95% CI)**	***p* for heterogeneity**
Oral and pharynx	All	9	0.53 (0.37–0.76)		7	0.84 (0.67–1.07)	
	Case-control	9	0.53 (0.37–0.76)		7	0.84 (0.67–1.07)	
	Cohort	0			0		
Larynx	All	5	0.73 (0.64–0.84)		4	0.92 (0.83–1.02)	
	Case-control	5	0.73 (0.64–0.84)		4	0.92 (0.83–1.02)	
	Cohort	0			0		
Esophagus	All	13	0.72 (0.62–0.83)	<.01	13	0.89 (0.82–0.97)	.002
	Case-control	12	0.72 (0.62–0.83)		12	0.89 (0.82–0.97)	
	Cohort						
Gastric	All	31	0.74 (0.69–0.81)	<.01	22	0.81 (0.75–0.87)	<.01
	Case-control	24	0.69 (0.62–0.77)	<.01	17	0.78 (0.71–0.86)	<.01
	Cohort	7	0.89 (0.73–1.09)	<.01	5	0.89 (0.75–1.05)	<.01
Colorectal	All	31	0.94 (0.90–0.98)	<.01	46	0.91 (0.86–0.97)	<.01
	Case-control	15	0.93 (0.87–0.99)	.003	29	0.87 (0.80–0.95)	<.01
	Cohort	16	0.96 (0.90–1.01)	.001	17	0.96 (0.90–1.05)	.13
Colon	All	19	0.94 (0.89–1.00)	<.01	27	0.91 (0.83–1.00)	<.01
	Case-control	10	0.90 (0.82–0.99)	.002	17	0.90 (0.78–1.03)	<.01
	Cohort	9	0.97 (0.91–1.04)	.003	11	0.91 (0.86–0.96)	.59
Rectum	All				9	0.95 (0.80–1.11)	.01
	Case-control				4	0.75 (0.51–1.08)	<.01
	Cohort	5	0.88 (0.81–0.96)	.30	5	1.06 (0.90–1.25)	.32
Bladder	All	8	0.81 (0.73–0.91)	.007	6	0.91 (0.82–1.00)	.12
	Case-control	5	0.82 (0.70–0.94)	.004	4	0.90 (0.78–1.03)	.06
	Cohort	3	0.80 (0.65–0.99)	.13	2	0.92 (0.75–1.14)	.24
Breast	All	18	0.99 (0.98–1.00)	.88	20	0.96 (0.94–0.98)	.89
	Case-control	8	0.92 (0.84–1.01)	<.01	10	0.86 (0.78–0.94)	<.01
	Cohort	10	0.99 (0.98–1.00)	.99	10	1.00 (0.97–1.02)	.99
Lung	All	35	0.85 (0.78–0.92)	<.01	25	0.89 (0.82–0.93)	.003
	Case-control	22	0.83 (0.74–0.94)	<.01	14	0.85 (0.77–0.92)	.006
	Cohort	13	0.86 (0.78–0.94)	<.01	11	0.92 (0.84–1.07)	.14

Lung Cancer

Lung cancer is the most common cancer in the world (Ferlay et al., 2004). Although cigarette smoking is the primary cause of lung cancer, with relative risks exceeding 10–15 for comparisons of current smokers with nonsmokers (Chyou et al., 1992; Szabo and Mulshine, 1993; Ernster, 1994), other factors, such as diet, have been hypothesized to influence lung cancer risk. This hypothesis is based, in part, on the observation that ~15–20% of lung cancer cases are not attributed to smoking (Chyou et al., 1992; Ernster, 1994; Parkin et al., 1994).

Fruits and vegetables have been the most extensively evaluated dietary variables in relation to lung cancer risk with > 50 case-control (MacLennan et al., 1977; Mettlin et al., 1979; Pisani et al., 1986; Ziegler et al., 1986; Bond et al., 1987; Fontham et al., 1988; Koo, 1988; Le Marchand et al., 1989, 2000; Mettlin, 1989; Pierce et al., 1989; Sakai, 1989; Jain et al., 1990; Kalandidi et al., 1990; Wu-Williams et al., 1990a; Harris et al., 1991; Candelora et al., 1992; Forman et al., 1992; Swanson et al., 1992; Alavanja et al., 1993, 2001; Dorgan et al., 1993; Gao et al., 1993; Mayne et al., 1994; Sankaranarayanan et al., 1994; Suzuki et al., 1994; Lei et al., 1996; Xu et al., 1996; Agudo et al., 1997; Hu et al., 1997; Ko et al., 1997; Pawlega et al., 1997; Pillow et al., 1997; Nyberg et al., 1998; Brennan et al., 2000; Darby et al., 2001; Takezaki et al., 2001; Axelsson and Rylander, 2002; De Stefani et al., 2002b; Kreuzer et al., 2002; Marchard et al., 2002; Pisa and Barbone, 2002; Rachtan, 2002a; Ruano-Ravina et al., 2002; Seow et al., 2002; Chan-Yeung et al., 2003; Wright et al., 2003; Zatloukal et al., 2003) and 20 cohort (Kvale et al., 1983; Long-de and Hammond, 1985; Hirayama, 1990; Fraser et al., 1991; Chow et al., 1992; Shibata et al., 1992; Steinmetz et al., 1993; Ocke et al., 1997;

Yong et al., 1997; Knekt et al., 1999; Breslow et al., 2000; Feskanich et al., 2000; Voorrips et al., 2000b; Ozasa et al., 2001; Appleby et al., 2002; Holick et al., 2002; Neuhouser et al., 2003; Sauvaget et al., 2003; Liu et al., 2004; Miller et al., 2004) studies reporting associations (Table 3). The studies have evaluated data from the 1940s through 2001. For the cohort studies, follow-up times have ranged from 3 (Steinmetz et al., 1993) to 40 years (Bond et al., 1987). Most studies have evaluated associations with incident lung cancer; however, some case-control (Bond et al., 1987; Lei et al., 1996) and cohort (Hirayama, 1979; Long-de and Hammond, 1985; Chow et al., 1992; Breslow et al., 2000; Ozasa et al., 2001; Appleby et al., 2002; Sauvaget et al., 2003) studies have evaluated fatal lung cancer. About half of the case-control studies used hospital controls.

An important confounder in examining diet and lung cancer associations is smoking habits because smoking is strongly associated with lung cancer risk (Chyou et al., 1992; Szabo and Mulshine, 1993; Ernster, 1994) and smokers eat fewer fruits and vegetables compared with never smokers (Subar et al., 1990; Nuttens et al., 1992; Agudo and Pera, 1999; Smith-Warner et al., 2003). In some studies, the difference in intakes between never and current smokers is more pronounced for fruit consumption than for vegetable consumption (Agudo and Pera, 1999; Smith-Warner et al., 2003). Although most, but not all (Hirayama, 1979; Mettlin et al., 1979; Long-de and Hammond, 1985; Pisani et al., 1986; Swanson et al., 1992; Lei et al., 1996; Le Marchand et al., 2000), studies have adjusted for smoking habits, a variety of parameterizations have been used to model smoking habits including smoking status only, pack-years of smoking, the number of years smoked, or the amount smoked; thus, the degree of residual confounding by other unmeasured smoking habits and environmental tobacco smoke may differ across studies and impact the strength of the associations observed. Among cohort studies, changes in smoking habits during follow-up are rarely measured, which may confound the observed results. Several studies have been conducted among never smokers only (Kalandidi et al., 1990; Candelora et al., 1992; Nyberg et al., 1998) or among never and former smokers (Koo, 1988; Alavanja et al., 1993; Mayne et al., 1994; Ko et al., 1997; Brennan et al., 2000; Kreuzer et al., 2002) to reduce the possibility of residual confounding by smoking.

In summarizing the results for total fruit consumption, the categories of total fruits, all fruits, fresh fruits, and fruits and berries were considered. More than 35 case-control (Ziegler et al., 1986; Fontham et al., 1988; Koo, 1988; Le Marchand et al., 1989; Pierce et al., 1989; Jain et al., 1990; Kalandidi et al., 1990; Wu-Williams et al., 1990a; Candelora et al., 1992; Forman et al., 1992; Swanson et al., 1992; Alavanja et al., 1993, 2001; Gao et al., 1993; Mayne et al., 1994; Suzuki et al., 1994; Lei et al., 1996; Xu et al., 1996; Agudo et al., 1997; Hu et al., 1997; Ko et al., 1997; Pawlega et al., 1997; Pillow et al., 1997; Nyberg et al., 1998; Brennan et al., 2000; Takezaki et al., 2001; Axelsson and Rylander, 2002; De Stefani et al., 2002b; Kreuzer et al., 2002; Marchand et al., 2002; Rachtan, 2002a; Ruano-Ravina et al., 2002; Seow et al., 2002; Chan-Yeung et al., 2003; Wright et al., 2003) and 15 cohort studies (Kvale et al., 1983; Long-de and Hammond, 1985; Fraser et al., 1991; Chow et al., 1992; Shibata et al., 1992; Steinmetz et al., 1993; Ocke et al., 1997; Knekt et al., 1999; Breslow et al., 2000; Feskanich et al., 2000; Voorrips et al., 2000b; Appleby et al., 2002; Holick et al., 2002; Neuhouser et al., 2003; Sauvaget et al., 2003; Liu et al., 2004; Miller et al., 2004) have reported on associations for fruit consumption and lung cancer risk. An inverse association has been observed in most, but not all, studies. The majority of studies have reported at least a 20% reduction in risk with higher fruit consumption, and several studies have found that lung cancer risk was reduced by at least half with higher compared with lower fruit consumption. For most of the latter studies, the association was statistically significant. However, in some studies, the significant association was limited to a specific population subgroup (e.g., men [Mayne et al., 1994; Lei et al., 1996; Takezaki et al., 2001; Appleby et al., 2002], women [Axelsson and Rylander, 2002], nonsmokers [Seow et al., 2002], or the placebo group in a randomized clinical trial [Neuhouser et al., 2003]). Only two case-control and no cohort studies have reported a statistically significant elevation in lung cancer risk for higher compared with lower fruit consumption (Wu-Williams et al., 1990a; Ruano-Ravina et al., 2002).

Relatively few studies have examined citrus fruits as a separate category in relation to the risk of lung cancer (Fraser et al., 1991; Candelora et al., 1992; Alavanja et al., 1993; Agudo et al., 1997; Nyberg et al., 1998; Feskanich et al., 2000; Voorrips et al., 2000b; Marchand et al., 2002; Pisa and Barbone, 2002; Neuhouser et al., 2003; Wright et al., 2003; Zatloukal et al., 2003). The results for citrus fruit consumption generally have not been statistically significant, although statistically significant positive (Alavanja et al., 1993) and inverse (Feskanich et al., 2000; Voorrips et al., 2000b) associations have also been reported.

More than 30 case-control (MacLennan et al., 1977; Ziegler et al., 1986; Mayne et al., 1994; Fontham et al., 1988; Nyberg et al., 1998; Le Marchand et al., 1989; Pierce et al., 1989; Jain et al., 1990; Kalandidi et al., 1990; Candelora et al., 1992; Forman et al., 1992; Alavanja et al., 1993; Gao et al., 1993; Lei et al., 1996; Sankaranarayanan et al., 1994; Agudo et al., 1997; Hu et al., 1997; Ko et al., 1997; Pawlega et al., 1997; Pillow et al., 1997; Brennan et al., 2000; Darby et al., 2001; Takezaki et al., 2001; Axelsson and Rylander, 2002; De Stefani et al., 2002b; Kreuzer et al., 2002; Marchand et al., 2002; Rachtan, 2002a; Seow et al., 2002; Wright et al., 2003; Zatloukal et al., 2003) and 10 cohort (Breslow et al., 2000; Chow et al., 1992;

TABLE 3 Summary of Case-Control and Cohort Studies of Fruit and Vegetable Consumption and Lung Cancer Risk[a]

Author, year, country	Study dates	Study population	Comparison	Odds ratio/relative risk (95% CI), unless otherwise noted	
				Total fruit	Citrus fruit
Case-control studies					
MacLennan et al., 1977, Singapore	1972–1973	233 cases, 300 hospital controls	Low vs high[b]		
Pisani et al., 1986, Italy	1979–1981	417 cases, 849 hospital controls	0 vs ≥7		
Ziegler et al., 1986, USA	1980–1981	763 cases (465 current, 13 nonsmokers), 900 population controls	Lowest vs highest quartile	1.0, p for trend = 0.35	
Fontham et al., 1988, USA	1979–1982	1253 cases, 1274 hospital controls	Highest vs lowest tertile	0.67 (0.52–0.86), p for trend = 0.002	
Koo, 1988, China	1981–1983	88 cases, 137 population controls	Lowest vs highest tertile[b]	Fresh: 2.39 (1.09–5.23), [0.42, 0.19–0.92], p for trend = 0.002	
Le Marchand et al., 1989, USA	1983–1985	332 cases (230 men, 102 women), 865 population controls (597 men, 268 women)	Lowest vs highest quartile[b]	No association	
Pierce et al., 1989, Australia	1984–1985	71 cases, 71 hospital controls	High vs low	Fresh: 0.99 (0.45–2.17), p for trend = 0.98	
Jain et al., 1990, Canada	1981–1985	839 cases, 772 population controls	Highest vs lowest quartile	1.10, p for trend = 0.76	
Kalandidi et al., 1990, Greece	1987–1989	91 cases, 120 hospital controls	Highest vs lowest quartile	0.33 (0.13–0.86), p for trend = 0.02	
Wu-Williams et al., 1990, China	1985–1987	965 cases, 959 population controls	>132 vs <19 times/year	Fresh: 1.5 (1.2–2.0)	
Harris et al., 1991, UK	1979–1981	96 cases, 97 hospital controls			
Candelora et al., 1992, USA	Initiated in 1987	124 cases, 263 population controls	Highest vs lowest quartile	0.6 (0.3–1.1), p for trend = 0.04	0.6 (0.3–1.1), p for trend = 0.20
Forman et al., 1992, China	1985–1986	183 cases, 183 occupational controls	Lowest vs highest quartile[b]	0.91 (0.48–1.74), [1.10, 0.57–2.08]	
Swanson et al., 1992, China	1984–1988	428 cases, 1011 population controls	Highest vs lowest quartile	Fresh: 0.94, p for trend = 0.31	
Alavanja et al., 1993, USA	1986–1991	429 cases, 1021 population controls	Highest vs lowest quintile	1.14, p for trend = 0.99	1.68, p for trend = 0.03
Dorgan et al., 1993, USA	1980–1983	1951 cases, 1238 population controls	Lowest vs highest tertile[b]		
Gao et al., 1993, Japan	1988–1991	282 cases, 282 outpatient controls	Every day vs almost none and sometimes	0.45 (0.30–0.67)	

Odds ratio/relative risk (95% CI), unless otherwise noted				
Total vegetables	Cruciferous vegetables	Green vegetables	Matching and adjustment factors	Miscellaneous
2.23 (1.49–3.33), [0.45, 0.30–0.67]			Age, sex, dialect, smoking, socioeconomic status	
		Green leafy: 1.9 [0.53]	Age, sex, and study area	Also stratified by cell type and smoking status
All: 1.4 (1.0–2.0) [0.71, 0.5–1.0], p for trend = 0.01; current: 1.8, [0.56], p for trend = 0.004; nonsmokers: 0.3 [3.33], p for trend = 0.20		Dark green: 1.5 [0.67], p for trend = 0.02	Age, race, residence, smoking	Men only. Also stratified by smoking and cell type
0.80 (0.62–1.04), p for trend = 0.09			Race, sex, age, pack-years of cigarette use, family income, ethnic group, and respondent status	Also stratified by cell type
	1.04 [0.96], p for trend = 0.36	Fresh leafy green: 2.06 [0.49], p for trend = 0.24	Age, number of live births and schooling	Female nonsmokers only. Also stratified by cell type
Women: 7.0 [0.14], p for trend < 0.001; men: 2.7 [0.37], p for trend < 0.001	Women: 4.7 [0.21], p for trend < 0.001]; men: 2.2 [0.45], p for trend = 0.001,	Dark green, women: 3.9 [0.26], p for trend = 0.001; men: 2.0 [0.5], p for trend = 0.003	Age, ethnicity, smoking status, pack-years of cigarette smoking, and cholesterol intake (men only)	Also stratified by smoking and cell type
1.69 (0.75–3.78), p for trend = 0.19	1.58 (0.71–3.50), p for trend = 0.25		Age and smoking	Men only
0.60 (0.40–0.88), p for trend = 0.01			Age, residence, and cumulative cigarette smoking	
1.09 (0.44–2.68), p for trend = 0.86			Age, years of schooling, interviewer, and total energy intake	Female never smokers only
			Age, education, personal smoking, and study area	Women only
		Green: 1.09, p for trend = 0.35	Age and cigarette smoking 1 year before diagnosis	Men only. Reported one-sided p values
0.2 (0.1–0.5), p for trend = 0.0003		Green and yellow: 0.4 (0.2–0.7), p for trend = 0.0001	Age, education, and total calories	Female never smokers only
1.68 (0.85–3.29), [0.60, 0.30–1.18]		Dark green leafy: 0.82 (0.41–1.61) [1.22, 0.62–2.44]; yellow and light green: 2.39 (1.15–4.96) [0.42, 0.20–0.87]	Age, total tobacco intake, height, number of meals at home per day, per capita income, education, and 2 measures of occupational exposure to radon and arsenic	Men only
		Dark green leafy: 0.41, p for trend < 0.01; light green: 0.35, p for trend < 0.01	Age, respondent type, study site, education, and income	Men only. Also stratified by cell type and smoking status
0.99, p for trend = 0.89	0.73, p for trend = 0.36	Yellow and green leafy: 0.81, p for trend = 0.44	Age, smoking history, previous lung disease, interview type, and total calories per day	Female nonsmokers only. Also stratified by cell type
		Yellow/green: 1.37 (1.12–1.69) [0.73, 0.59–0.89]	Age, race, sex, education, occupation, residence, smoking, passive smoking, and study phase	Also stratified by cell type and smoking
Raw: 0.64 (0.43–0.97)		Green: 0.44 (0.26–0.73)	Age, time of first visit to hospital, and smoking status	Men only. Also stratified by cell type and smoking

(*continues*)

TABLE 3 *(Continued)*

Author, year, country	Study dates	Study population	Comparison	Odds ratio/relative risk (95% CI), unless otherwise noted	
				Total fruit	Citrus fruit
Mayne et al., 1994, USA	1982–1985	413 cases (212 male, 201 female), 413 population controls	Highest vs lowest quartile	Fresh: 0.44, p < 0.05, *p* for trend < 0.01; women: 0.58, *p* for trend < 0.10; men: 0.65, *p* for trend ns	
Sankaranarayanan et al., 1994, India	1990	281 cases, 1207 hospital visitor control	Highest vs lowest quartile		
Suzuki et al., 1994, Brazil	1991–1992	123 cases, 123 hospital controls	Daily vs <1/wk	1.2 (0.4–3.1), *p* for trend = 0.57	
Lei et al., 1996, China	1986	792 deceased cases (563 males, 229 females), 792 deceased hospital controls	Not regularly vs regularly[b]	Women: NS diff; men: 1.36 (1.04–1.78) [0.74, 0.56–0.96]	
Xu et al., 1996, China	1987–1993	610 cases, 959 controls from same work site	≥55 vs 0 jing/yr	0.6 (0.5–0.9)	
Agudo et al., 1997, Spain	1989–1992	103 cases (80 never smokers), 206 hospital controls	Highest vs lowest tertile	Fresh: 1.20 (0.56–2.56), *p* for trend = 0.66	1.43 (0.66–3.13), *p* for trend = 0.37
Hu et al., 1997, China	1985–1987	227 cases, 227 hospital controls	Highest vs lowest quartile	0.7 (0.4–1.2), *p* for trend = 0.10	
Ko et al., 1997, Taiwan	1992–1993	105 cases, 105 outpatient controls	Daily vs 0–6/wk	1.0 (0.5–1.7)	
Pawlega et al., 1997, Poland	1992–1994	176 cases, 341 population controls	<1/wk vs >1/wk[b] for fruit, <3/wk vs >3/wk[b] for vegetables and green vegetables	2.4 (1.3–4.4) [0.42, 0.23–0.77], *p* for trend < 0.05	
Pillow et al., 1997, USA		137 cases, 187 population controls	Increment = g/1000 kcal	0.56 (0.31–0.99), *p* for trend = 0.05	
Nyberg et al., 1998, Sweden	1989–1995	124 cases, 235 population controls	Highest vs lowest tertile for fruit and vegetable analyses; daily or almost daily vs ≤ 1/wk for citrus fruit and green leafy vegetables, >1/wk vs <1/wk for cruciferous vegetables	0.67 (0.33–1.36), *p* for trend ns	1.52 (0.82–2.81), *p* for trend = 0.21
Brennan et al., 2000, Europe	1988–1994	506 cases, 1045 hospital and population controls (depended on center)	Highest vs lowest tertile	1.0 (0.6–1.5), *p* for trend = 0.81	

Odds ratio/relative risk (95% CI), unless otherwise noted			Matching and adjustment factors	Miscellaneous
Total vegetables	Cruciferous vegetables	Green vegetables		
Women: 0.47, $p < 0.05$, p for trend < 0.025; men: 0.55 (ns), p for trend ns		All cooked greens and salad greens (except lettuce): 0.42, $p < 0.05$, p for trend < 0.01	Age, sex, residence, prior cigarette use, religion, education, body mass index, and income	Nonsmokers only. Also stratified by smoking history and cell type
0.32 (0.13–0.78)			Age, education, religion, and smoking	Men only
		Green: 2.0 (0.7–5.8), p for trend = 0.21	Age, sex, race, income, and tobacco consumption	
Men: 3.75 (1.75–8.00) [0.27, 0.13–0.57]			Age, sex	
			Age, sex, smoking, income, education, tea consumption, pulmonary disease, and family history of lung cancer	
0.65 (0.32–1.31), p for trend = 0.23	0.54 (0.26–1.13), p for trend = 0.13	Leafy green: 0.61 (0.30–1.22), p for trend = 0.19; dark green: 0.58 (0.29–1.15), p for trend = 0.11	Age, residence, hospital, smoking status, and total pack-years smoked	Women only. Also presented results for never smokers and adenocarcinomas
Fresh: 0.8 (0.4–1.3), p for trend = 0.65			Age, sex, residence, cigarettes per day, duration of smoking, and family income	Also stratified by smoking status
0.4 (0.2–0.8)			Age, socioeconomic status, residence, and education	Female nonsmokers only
Boiled: 4.6 (2.3–9.2) [0.22, 0.11–0.43], p for trend < 0.05		Green: 1.1 (0.5–2.7) [0.91, 0.37–2.0], p for trend < 0.05	Age, education, place of permanent residence, pack-years of smoking, and years of occupational exposure	Men only
1.49 (0.84–2.63), p for trend = 0.17			Pack-years smoked, calories consumed, age, sex, and ethnicity	Also stratified by ethnicity (African-American and Mexican American)
0.57 (0.29–1.13), p for trend = 0.35	1.06 (0.58–1.92), p for trend = 0.33	Green leafy: 1.09 (0.59–2.00), p for trend = 0.38	Gender, age, catchment area, occasional smoking, degree of urban residence, years of exposure to risk occupations, ever-exposure status, years since last exposure and hour-years of exposure to environmental tobacco smoke, carrot consumption (for fruit, citrus fruit and cruciferous vegetable analyses), and other fruit consumption (for citrus fruit, vegetable, cruciferous vegetables and green leafy vegetables analyses)	Never smokers only. Also stratified by cell type
Fresh: 0.7 (0.5–1.0), p for trend = 0.09	1.1 (0.7–1.6), p for trend = 0.76		Age, sex, and center	Nonsmokers only (<400 cigarettes in lifetime). Also stratified by cell type. No heterogeneity by age, sex, residence

(*continues*)

TABLE 3 *(Continued)*

Author, year, country	Study dates	Study population	Comparison	Odds ratio/relative risk (95% CI), unless otherwise noted	
				Total fruit	**Citrus fruit**
Alavanja et al., 2001, USA	1993–1996	360 cases, 574 population controls	Highest vs lowest quintile	1.4 (0.7–2.5)	
Darby et al., 2001, England	1988–1993	982 cases, 1486 population controls	Highest vs lowest quartile for vegetables; highest quartile vs quartile 3 for green vegetables		
Takezaki et al., 2001, Japan	1988–1997	1045 cases (240 women, 367 men), 4153 hospital controls (1189 women, 2964 men)	Highest vs lowest quartile	Men, adenocarcinomas: 0.98 (0.61–1.58), p for trend = 0.38; small and squamous: 0.61 (0.40–0.95), p for trend = 0.007; women, adenocarcinomas: 0.68 (0.27–1.70), p for trend = 0.54; small and squamous: 0.49 (0.11–2.13), p for trend = 0.67	
Axelsson and Rylander, 2002, Sweden	1989–1994	536 cases, 916 population controls	Highest vs lowest quartile	Women: 0.5 (0.2–1.0), p for trend = 0.05; men: 0.8 (0.5–1.2), p for trend = 0.19	
De Stefani et al., 2002, Uruguay	1988–2000	1032 cases, 1030 hospital controls	Highest vs lowest quartile	0.84 (0.62–1.13), p for trend = 0.14	
Kreuzer et al., 2002, Germany	1991–1996	234 cases, 535 population controls	Daily vs ≤weekly	0.66 (0.37–1.19), p for trend = 0.94	
Marchand et al., 2002, New Caledonia	1993–1995	134 cases (25 women, 109 men), 295 (68 women, 227 men)	Highest vs lowest tertile	Men: 0.7 (0.4–1.5), p for trend = 0.09	Men: 0.8 (0.4–1.7), p for trend = 0.09
Pisa and Barbone, 2002, Italy	1996	111 cases, 247 population controls	≥7 vs ≤1/wk		1.3 (0.6–3.0)
Rachtan, 2002, Poland	1991–1997	242 cases, 352 controls who were healthy relatives of other hospital patients	Every day	0.49 (0.32–0.74), p for trend = 0.0008	
Ruano-Ravina et al., 2002, Spain	1992–1994	157 cases, 236 population controls	≥1/day vs <1/wk	2.16 (1.02–4.58)	

Odds ratio/relative risk (95% CI), unless otherwise noted				
Total vegetables	**Cruciferous vegetables**	**Green vegetables**	**Matching and adjustment factors**	**Miscellaneous**
		Yellow-green: 0.4 (0.2–0.7), *p* for trend = 0.018	Age, education, pack-years of smoking, smoking history, yellow-green vegetables (for fruit analyses), fruit (for yellow-green vegetable analyses), previous lung disease, alcohol consumption, body mass index, saturated fat, cholesterol, and nutrient density calories	Women only
0.90 (0.69–1.17), *p* for trend = 0.75		Green: 1.38 (1.11–1.70), *p* for trend = 0.40	Age, sex, smoking	
Raw, men, adenocarcinomas: 1.01 (0.62–1.65), *p* for trend = 0.66; small and squamous: 0.80 (0.51–1.25), *p* for trend = 0.004; women, adenocarcinomas: 0.84 (0.45–1.55), *p* for trend = 0.90; small and squamous: 1.01 (0.28–3.58), *p* for trend = 0.90		Green, men, adenocarcinomas: 0.77 (0.51–1.15), *p* for trend = 0.04; small and squamous: 0.49 (0.32–0.74), *p* for trend = 0.002; women, adenocarcinomas: 0.64 (0.35–1.15), *p* for trend = 0.23; small and squamous: 1.37 (0.46–4.09), *p* for trend = 0.31	Age, season and year of visit, occupation, prior lung diseases, smoking, passive smoking from husband (females), consumption of green vegetables and meat	
Women: 0.8 (0.4–1.5), *p* for trend = 0.23; men: 0.4 (0.2–0.6), *p* for trend < 0.001			Age, marital status, smoking duration, number of cig/day, milk consumption, fruit intake (for vegetable analyses) and vegetable intake (for fruit analyses)	Update of Axelsson et al., 1996. Also stratified by number of cigarettes/day and by cell type
0.72 (0.54–0.97), *p* for trend = 0.008			Age, sex, residence, urban/rural status, education, year of diagnosis, smoking status, years since quitting, intensity of smoking, age at start, and energy intake	Update of De Stefani, et al. 1999 and 2002. Also stratified by cell type and smoking
Fresh: 0.45 (0.25–0.82), *p* for trend = 0.03			Age and region	Female nonsmokers only
Men: 1.4 (0.7–2.9), *p* for trend = 0.72		Men, green: 0.8 (0.4–1.5), *p* for trend = 0.40; dark green: 0.5 (0.2–1.2), *p* for trend = 0.12	Age, ethnicity, and smoking (pack-years)	Did geometric mean analysis for women; no significant associations with any food among women (not shown)
		Green salad: 0.7 (0.3–1.6)	Year of birth, sex, and dose of smoking	
Vegetables except carrots and spinach: 0.23 (0.13–0.41), *p* for trend < 0.0001			Age and pack-years	Women only Update of Rachtan, 1997; same population as Rachtan, 2002
		Green leafy: 0.63 (0.24–1.63)	Age, gender, and smoking habit (in packs smoked over a lifetime)	

(*continues*)

TABLE 3 *(Continued)*

Author, year, country	Study dates	Study population	Comparison	Odds ratio/relative risk (95% CI), unless otherwise noted	
				Total fruit	Citrus fruit
Seow et al., 2002, Singapore	1996–1998	303 cases (176 never smokers, 127 smokers) and 765 hospital controls (663 never smokers, 102 smokers)	Highest vs lowest tertile	Smokers: 0.63 (0.28–1.44), *p* for trend = 0.4; nonsmokers: 0.60 (0.39–0.93), *p* for trend = 0.03	
Chan-Yeung et al., 2003, Hong Kong	1999–2001	331 cases, 331 hospital controls	30+ vs <15 portions/mo for fruit, 65+ vs <45 portions/mo for green vegetables	Women: 1.25 (0.65–2.44); men: 0.65 (0.36–1.16)	
Wright et al., 2003, USA	1993–1994	587 cases, 624 population controls	Increment = difference in interquartile range	No association	No association
Zatloukal et al., 2003, Czechoslovakia	1998–2002	366 cases (145 adenocarcinoma, 221 squamous + small + large cell), 1624 controls who were relatives/friends of other patients	Daily vs never/no for citrus fruit, daily vs ≤weekly for vegetables		Adenocarcinoma: 1.14 (0.63–2.03), *p* for trend = 0.13; Squamous + small + large:1.07 (0.63–1.82), *p* for trend = 0.81
Cohort studies					
Kvale et al., 1983, Norway	1964–1978	168 cases, cohort of 13,785	≥50 vs <20	Fruits and berries: 1.10, p = 0.9	
Long-de et al., 1985, USA	1959–1970	671 fatal cases, cohort of 136,281	0–2 vs 5–7 d/wk[b]	1.75 [0.57]	
Hirayama, 1990, Japan	1965–1982	1917 fatal cases, cohort of 265,118	Daily vs <daily		
Fraser et al., 1991, USA	1977–1982	61 cases, cohort of 34,198	≥2/day vs <3/wk for fruit; ≥3/wk vs <3/wk for citrus fruit; ≥7 vs <3/wk for cooked green vegetables and green salads	0.26 (0.10–0.70), *p* for trend = 0.006	Fresh: 0.64 (0.35–1.17)
Chow et al., 1992, USA	1966–1986	219 fatal cases, cohort of 17,633	>90 vs <31/mo for fruit; >160 vs <46/mo for vegetables; >8 vs <2/mo for cruciferous vegetables	0.7 (0.4–1.3)	
Shibata et al., 1992, USA	1981–1989	164 cases (94 male, 70 female), cohort of 13,981	Highest vs lowest tertile	Women: 0.68 (0.37–1.24); men: 0.99 (0.59–1.66)	
Steinmetz et al., 1993, USA	1986–1989	138 cases, cohort of 35,115 (analyzed as a nested case-control study with 2814 controls)	Highest vs lowest quartile	0.75 (0.44–1.23), *p* for trend = 0.08	
Ocke et al., 1997, Netherlands	1971–1990	54 cases, cohort of 561	Lowest 2 tertiles vs highest tertile[b]	Average intake: 1.39 (0.80–2.41) [0.72, 0.41–1.25]	
Knekt et al., 1999, Finland	1967–1991	138 cases, cohort of 4545	Highest vs lowest tertile	0.58 (0.37–0.93), *p* for trend = 0.013	
Breslow, et al., 2000, USA	1987–1995	158 fatal cases, cohort of 20,004	Highest vs lowest quartile	0.9 (0.5–1.6), *p* for trend < 0.489	

Odds ratio/relative risk (95% CI), unless otherwise noted			Matching and adjustment factors	Miscellaneous
Total vegetables	Cruciferous vegetables	Green vegetables		
Smokers: 0.48 (0.23–1.00), p for trend = 0.04; nonsmokers: 0.78 (0.51–1.20), p for trend = 0.3	Smokers: 0.46 (0.22–0.96), p for trend = 0.06; nonsmokers: 0.89 (0.59–1.35), p for trend = 0.6		Age, date of admission, place of birth, and first degree relative with history of cancer. For smokers, adjusted for duration and intensity.	Women only. Also stratified by cell type
		Green, women: 1.74 (0.86–3.52); men: 2.23 (1.28–3.89)	Age, education, smoking, place of birth (for men), family history of lung cancer (for men)	Similar results observed for nonsmoking men
Total: 0.67 (0.55–0.82), p for trend < 0.0001; total: 0.45 (0.30–0.69) for highest vs lowest quintile, p for trend = 0.0007; raw: 0.74 (0.62–0.88), p for trend = 0.0007		Dark green and deep yellow vegetables: 0.84 (0.75–0.94), p for trend = 0.002	Age, total calorie intake, pack-years of smoking, and education	Women only. Also stratified by smoking status and cell type
Adenocarcinoma: 0.93 (0.54–1.59), p for trend = 0.79; Squamous + small + large: 0.69 (0.44–1.08), p for trend = 0.11			Age, residence, education, and pack-years of smoking	Women only. Update of Kubik et al., 2001, Kubik et al., 2002
0.74, p = 0.37			Age, cigarette smoking, region, and urban/rural residence	Men only. Also stratified by cell type
		Green salad: 1.30 [0.77]	Age	Also stratified by smoking status
		Green-yellow: 0.85 (0.79–0.93)	Age, sex	90% confidence interval
		Cooked green: 1.09 (0.41–2.87), p for trend = 0.50; green salads: 0.65 (0.29–1.47), p for trend = 0.52	Age, sex, and smoking history	Also stratified by smoking status and cell type
1.2 (0.6–2.3)	0.8 (0.5–1.4)		Age, smoking status, and industry/occupation	Men only
Women: 0.58 (0.32–1.05); men: 1.37 (0.74–2.25)		Dark green, women: 0.64 (0.35–1.18); men: 1.16 (0.71–1.91)	Age and smoking	
0.50 (0.29–0.87), p for trend = 0.01		Green leafy: 0.45 (0.26–0.79), p for trend = 0.0003	Age, energy intake, and pack-years of smoking	Women only. Also stratified by smoking status and cell type
Average intake: 1.19 (0.68–2.06) [0.84, 0.48–1.47]			Age, pack-years of cigarettes, and energy intake	Men only. Used average intake from 1960, 1965 and 1970 interviews
0.83 (0.54–1.26), p for trend = 0.20			Age and smoking status	Men only. Update of Knekt et al., 1991 and 1997
0.9 (0.5–1.5), p for trend < 0.786			Age, sex, smoking duration, packs/day smoked	Excluded individuals who died within 1 year of baseline

(continues)

TABLE 3 (*Continued*)

Author, year, country	Study dates	Study population	Comparison	Odds ratio/relative risk (95% CI), unless otherwise noted	
				Total fruit	Citrus fruit
Feskanich et al., 2000, USA	Women: 1984–1996; men: 1986–1996	Women: 519 cases, cohort of 77,283; men: 274 cases, cohort of 47,778	Highest vs lowest quintile	All: 0.94 (0.59–1.49); women: 0.76 (0.56–1.02); men: 1.22 (0.80–1.87)	Women: 0.72 (0.54–0.97); men: 1.12 (0.77–1.61)
Voorrips et al., 2000, Netherlands	1986–1992	1074 cases for the fruit analyses, 1010 cases for vegetable analyses, cohort of 120,852 (analyzed as a case–cohort with a subcohort of 3123 for the fruit analyses and 2953 for the vegetable analyses)	Highest vs lowest quintile except for raw leafy vegetables, which used highest vs lowest tertile	0.8 (0.6–1.1), p for trend < 0.0001	0.7 (0.5–0.9), p for trend < 0.0001
Ozasa et al., 2001, Japan	1988–1997	572 fatal cases (126 women, 446 men), cohort of 98,248 (55,308 women, 42,940 men)	Almost every day vs ≤1–2/wk		
Appleby et al., 2002, UK	1973–1997	81 fatal cases, cohort of 10,771	Daily vs <daily	All: 0.53 (0.33–0.85); women: 0.62 (0.28–1.38); men: 0.47 (0.27–0.84)	
Holick et al., 2002, Finland	1985–1998	1644 cases, cohort of 27,084	Highest vs lowest quintile	0.87 (0.74–1.02), p for trend = 0.01	
Neuhouser et al., 2003, USA	1989–2001	740 cases (326 placebo, 414 intervention), cohort of 14,120 (7048 placebo, 7072 intervention)	Highest vs lowest quintile	Intervention: 0.79 (0.57–1.11), p for trend = 0.13; placebo: 0.56 (0.39–0.81), p for trend = 0.003	Intervention: 0.84 (0.58–1.21), p for trend = 0.22; placebo: 0.72 (0.46–1.10), p for trend = 0.15
Sauvaget et al., 2003, Japan	1980–1998	563 fatal cases, cohort of 38,540	Highest vs lowest tertile	0.80 (0.65–0.98), p for trend = 0.03	
Liu et al., 2004, Japan	1990–1999 for cohort I; 1993–1999 for cohort II	428 cases (177 cohort I, 251 cohort II), cohort of 93,338 (42,224 cohort I, 51,114 cohort II)	Highest vs lowest tertile	Cohort I: 1.40 (0.92–2.13); cohort II: 1.01 (0.72–1.41); both: 1.16 (0.84–1.58)	
Miller et al., 2004, Europe	1992–2002	860 cases, cohort of 478,021	Highest vs lowest quintile	Total fruits: 0.60 (0.46–0.78), p for trend = 0.01; fruits: 0.56 (0.43–0.73), p for trend = 0.01	

Odds ratio/relative risk (95% CI), unless otherwise noted			Matching and adjustment factors	Miscellaneous
Total vegetables	**Cruciferous vegetables**	**Green vegetables**		
All: 0.82 (0.54–1.25); women: 0.68 (0.51–0.90); men 1.04 (0.69–1.57)	Women: 0.74 (0.55–0.99); men: 1.11 (0.76–1.64)	Green leafy, women: 0.90 (0.68–1.20); men: 0.99 (0.65–1.49)	Age, follow–up cycle, smoking status, years since quitting among past smokers, cigarettes smoked/day among current smokers, age at start of smoking, total energy intake, and availability of diet data after baseline measure	Update of Speizer, et al., 1999. Also stratified by smoking status and cell type
Vegetables: 0.7 (0.5–1.00), *p* for trend = 0.001; cooked: 0.8 (0.6–1.1), *p* for trend = 0.01; raw: 0.7 (0.6–1.0), *p* for trend = 0.04	Brassicas: 0.7 (0.5–1.0), *p* for trend = 0.009	Leafy cooked: 0.7 (0.5–1.0), *p* for trend = 0.04; leafy raw: 0.9 (0.7–1.1), *p* for trend = 0.06	Age, sex, family history of lung cancer, education, current smoker, years of smoking, number of cigarettes/day	Men only
		Green leafy, women: 1.19 (0.75–1.90), *p* for trend = 0.45; men: 0.76 (0.59–0.98), *p* for trend = 0.04	Age, parents' history of lung cancer, smoking status, smoking pack-years for current smokers, and time since quitting smoking	Also stratified by smoking status
			Age at recruitment, sex, and smoking	Update of Key et al., 1996. Also stratified by smoking status
0.75 (0.63–0.88), *p* for trend < 0.0001			Age, years smoked, cigarettes per day, intervention (alpha-tocopherol and beta-carotene supplement), supplement use (beta-carotene, vitamin A), energy intake, cholesterol, and fat	Male current smokers only
Intervention: 0.81 (0.65–1.21), *p* for trend = 0.46; placebo: 0.82 (0.59–1.14), *p* for trend = 0.39	Intervention: 0.91 (0.65–1.28), *p* for trend = 0.36; placebo: 0.68 (0.45–1.04), *p* for trend = 0.01		Sex, age, smoking status, total pack-years of smoking, asbestos exposure, race/ethnicity, enrollment center, total fruits (for citrus fruits), and total vegetables (for cruciferous vegetables)	Men only. Heavy smokers and asbestos-exposed workers Also stratified by cell type
		Green-yellow: 0.95 (0.76–1.19), *p* for trend = 0.68	Sex, age, radiation dose, city, body mass index, smoking status, alcohol habits, and education	Also stratified by smoking
Cohort I: 1.11 (0.77–1.61); cohort II: 0.97 (0.71–1.33); both: 1.03 (0.81–1.30)			Age, gender, areas, sports, frequency of alcohol intake, body mass index, vitamin supplement use, salted fish and meat, pickled vegetables, smoking status, smoking duration, and number of cigarettes per day	
1.00 (0.76–1.30), *p* for trend = 0.85	1.21 (0.92–1.60), *p* for trend = 0.25	Leafy: 0.89 (0.66–1.19), *p* for trend = 0.30	Smoking, weight, height, sex, and center	Also stratified by smoking

(*continues*)

TABLE 3 (*Continued*)

Author, year, country	Study dates	Study population	Comparison	Odds ratio/relative risk (95% CI), unless otherwise noted	
				Total fruit	Citrus fruit
Pooled analyses					
Jansen et al., 2001, Europe	Around 1970–1995	149 fatal cases, 1578	Highest vs lowest tertile	0.69 (0.46–1.02), *p* for trend = 0.05	
Smith-Warner, et al., 2003, USA, Canada, Europe	1976–1996	3206 cases 430,281	Highest vs lowest quintile for fruits and vegetables; ≥1/2 serving/day vs <1 serving/wk for green leafy vegetables	All: 0.77 (0.67–0.87), *p* for trend < 0.001; women: 0.83 (0.70–1.00), *p* for trend = 0.07; men: 0.70 (0.57–0.87), *p* for trend = 0.003	

[a]The following studies have examined the association between fruit and vegetable consumption and lung cancer risk but did not report associations for the groups included in the table: Mettlin et al., 1979; Bond et al., 1987; Mettlin et al., 1989; Saka et al., 1989; Le Marchand et al., 2000; Yong et al., 1997.

[b]The inverse of the relative risk was calculated to represent a comparison of high vs low intake and is included in brackets after the published estimate.

Feskanich et al., 2000; Holick et al., 2002; Knekt et al., 1999; Kvale et al., 1983; Liu et al., 2004; Miller et al., 2004; Neuhouser et al., 2003; Ocke et al., 1997; Shibata et al., 1992; Steinmetz et al., 1993; V oorrips et al., 2000b) studies have examined the association between vegetable consumption and lung cancer risk. Overall, vegetable consumption has been inversely associated with the risk of lung cancer. Many studies have found statistically significant reductions in the risk of lung cancer by at least 50% with higher compared with lower vegetable consumption. In some studies, the reduction in risk was limited to a particular subgroup (such as men [Axelsson and Rylander, 2002], women [Mayne et al., 1994], or smokers [Seow et al., 2002]). Very few studies have suggested that higher vegetable intakes increase the risk of lung cancer, and none of these results has been statistically significant (Pierce et al., 1989; Chow et al., 1992; Shibata et al., 1992; Pillow et al., 1997; Marchand et al., 2002).

Associations with cruciferous vegetables have been examined rarely in relation to the risk of lung cancer (Koo, 1988; Le Marchand et al., 1989; Pierce et al., 1989; Chow et al., 1992; Alavanja et al., 1993; Agudo et al., 1997; Nyberg et al., 1998; Brennan et al., 2000; Feskanich et al., 2000; Voorrips et al., 2000b; Seow et al., 2002; Neuhouser et al., 2003; Miller et al., 2004). Although statistically significant reductions in the risk of lung cancer of at least 25% have been observed for high compared with low cruciferous vegetable consumption in some studies (Le Marchand et al., 1989; Feskanich et al., 2000; Voorrips et al., 2000b; Seow et al., 2002; Neuhouser et al., 2003), most studies have reported nonsignificant associations.

Green vegetable consumption has been examined in numerous studies using various definitions including dark green vegetables, dark green leafy vegetables, green leafy vegetables, green vegetables, green and yellow vegetables, yellow and green leafy vegetables, and all cooked greens and salad greens (except lettuce). For the case-control studies, an inverse association has been observed in most (Ziegler et al., 1986; Pisani et al., 1986; Koo, 1988; Le Marchand et al., 1989; Candelora et al., 1992; Forman et al., 1992; Swanson et al., 1992; Alavanja et al., 1993, 2001; Dorgan et al., 1993; Gao et al., 1993; Mayne et al., 1994; Agudo et al., 1997; Pawlega et al., 1997; Takezaki et al., 2001; Marchand et al., 2002; Pisa and Barbone, 2002; Ruano-Ravina et al., 2002; Wright et al., 2003), but not all (Darby et al., 2001; Harris et al., 1991; Forman et al., 1992; Suzuki et al., 1994; Nyberg et al., 1998; Takezaki et al., 2001; Chan-Yeung et al., 2003) studies. Typically, a 40–60% reduction in lung cancer risk has been observed for the uppermost compared with the lowermost quantile of green vegetable intake. The association has been less consistent among cohort studies (Long-de and Hammond, 1985; Fraser et al., 1991; Shibata et al., 1992; Steinmetz et al., 1993; Terry et al., 1998; Feskanich et al., 2000; Voorrips et al., 2000b; Ozasa et al., 2001; Sauvaget et al., 2003; Miller et al., 2004). In only four cohort studies (Hirayama, 1990; Steinmetz et

Odds ratio/relative risk (95% CI), unless otherwise noted				
Total vegetables	**Cruciferous vegetables**	**Green vegetables**	**Matching and adjustment factors**	**Miscellaneous**
0.90 (0.61–1.33), *p* for trend = 0.59			Age, number of cigarettes smoked at baseline, country/cohort, energy intake, vegetable intake (for fruit analyses), and fruit intake (for vegetable analyses)	Male smokers only. Also stratified by smoking status
All: 0.88 (0.78–1.00), *p* for trend = 0.12; women: 0.93 (0.78–1.12), *p* for trend = 0.59; men: 0.83 (0.69–1.00), *p* for trend = 0.08		Green leafy: 0.93 (0.81–1.07), *p* for trend = 0.07	Age, education, body mass index, alcohol intake, energy intake, smoking status, smoking duration for past smokers, smoking duration for current smokers, amount smoked for current smokers	Also stratified by smoking and cell type

al., 1993; Voorrips et al., 2000b; Ozasa et al., 2001) has a statistically significant association been observed; the magnitude of the association ranged from a 15 to 55% decrease in risk comparing high versus low intakes of green vegetables.

Associations between carrot consumption and lung cancer risk have been reported in several studies (Kvale et al., 1983; Bond et al., 1987; Fontham et al., 1988; Koo, 1988; Le Marchand et al., 1989; Mettlin, 1989; Pierce et al., 1989; Pisani et al., 1986; Harris et al., 1991; Candelora et al., 1992; Chow et al., 1992; Steinmetz et al., 1993; Sankaranarayanan et al., 1994; Pawlega et al., 1997; Nyberg et al., 1998; Knekt et al., 1999; Brennan et al., 2000; Feskanich et al., 2000; Voorrips et al., 2000b; Takezaki et al., 2001; Darby et al., 2001; Ozasa et al., 2001; Kreuzer et al., 2002; Marchand et al., 2002; Pisa and Barbone, 2002; Rachtan, 2002a; Ruano-Ravina et al., 2002; Chan-Yeung et al., 2003; Wright et al., 2003). Although most of the associations have not been statistically significant, the relative risks consistently have been in the protective direction for comparisons of high versus low intakes. In the Lutheran Brotherhood Cohort Study, a nonsignificant inverse association was observed for carrot consumption; however, the relative risk was not provided (Chow et al., 1992). Only four studies have reported positive associations (Pierce et al., 1989; Ozasa et al., 2001; Takezaki et al., 2001; Chan-Yeung et al., 2003) with the association being statistically significant in only two studies (Takezaki et al., 2001; Chan-Yeung et al., 2003), which reported at least a 50% higher risk of lung cancer among individuals eating the most compared to the least amount of carrots.

Several studies have examined whether the association between fruit and vegetable consumption and lung cancer risk is modified by smoking status (Pisani et al., 1986; Ziegler et al., 1986; Le Marchand et al., 1989; Fraser et al., 1991; Swanson et al., 1992; Dorgan et al., 1993; Gao et al., 1993; Steinmetz et al., 1993; Hu et al., 1997; Yong et al., 1997; Brennan et al., 2000; Feskanich et al., 2000; Voorrips et al., 2000b; Ozasa et al., 2001; Appleby et al., 2002; Axelsson and Rylander, 2002; De Stefani et al., 2002b; Sauvaget et al., 2003; Wright et al., 2003; Liu et al., 2004; Miller et al., 2004); many of these studies had limited power to examine never smokers or nonsmokers because they included < 100 cases among never smokers or nonsmokers. For fruit intake, results by smoking status have been inconsistent (Fraser et al., 1991; Gao et al., 1993; Steinmetz et al., 1993; Hu et al., 1997; Yong et al., 1997; Feskanich et al., 2000; De Stefani et al., 2002b; Voorrips et al., 2000b; Sauvaget et al., 2003; Liu et al., 2004; Miller et al., 2004). For vegetables, a stronger inverse association frequently has been observed for vegetable consumption among current smokers compared with smokers (Ziegler et al., 1986; Le Marchand et al., 1989; Gao et al., 1993; Steinmetz et al., 1993; Feskanich et al., 2000; Voorrips et al., 2000b; De Stefani et al., 2002b; Wright et al., 2003; Miller et al., 2004), although a number of studies have found opposite (Hu et al., 1997; Le Marchand et al., 1989;

Feskanich et al., 2000) or equivalent (Axelsson and Rylander, 2002; Liu et al., 2004) findings between never and current smokers.

Pooled Analyses

Two pooled analyses have examined the association between fruit and vegetable consumption and the risk of lung cancer (Jansen et al., 2001; Smith-Warner et al., 2003). In the first pooled analysis, data from 1578 male smokers who participated in 16 population samples from the Seven Countries Study were followed for 25 years. During this time 149 lung cancer deaths occurred. About a 30% decrease in the risk of lung cancer death was observed for individuals in the highest versus lowest tertile of fruit intake, but no association was observed for vegetable consumption (Jansen et al., 2001). The second pooled analysis included eight prospective cohort studies (many of which are included separately in Table 3) in which 3206 incident lung cancer cases were diagnosed among 430,281 women and men followed for up to a maximum of 6–16 years across studies (Smith-Warner et al., 2003). For comparisons of the highest versus lowest quintile of intake, the pooled multivariate relative risks were 0.77 (95% confidence interval [CI] = 0.67–0.87) for total fruits and 0.88 (95% CI = 0.78–1.00) for total vegetables. Individuals with elevated risk were limited to the lowest quintile of intake. Green leafy vegetable and carrot intakes were not associated with the risk of lung cancer. Associations for fruits, vegetables, and total fruits and vegetables did not differ by smoking status or by cell type.

Summary

Although the most important risk factor for lung cancer is smoking, fruit and vegetable intakes have been consistently associated with a lower risk of lung cancer, with similar associations being observed for fruits and for vegetables. Inverse associations have been consistently observed for green vegetables and carrots, but not for cruciferous vegetables and citrus fruit. Although it was hypothesized that the β-carotene in fruits and vegetables was the agent responsible for the protective associations observed, randomized clinical trials of β-carotene have shown an increase in lung cancer incidence rates (the Alpha-Tocopherol and Beta Carotene Cancer Prevention Study Group, 1994; Omenn et al., 1996b) or similar rates (Hennekens et al., 1996; Lee et al., 1999) in those receiving β-carotene supplements compared with placebo albeit at nonphysiologic intakes. In addition, studies that have examined the association between intakes of specific carotenoids and the risk of lung cancer have not consistently shown an inverse association for β-carotene. Associations for α-carotene, β-cryptoxanthin, lutein/zeaxanthin, and lycopene also have been inconsistent across studies (Candelora et al., 1992; Le Marchand et al., 1993; Ziegler et al., 1996; Garcia-Closas et al., 1998; Knekt et al., 1999; Wright et al., 2003; Mannisto et al., 2004). Thus, intake of a specific carotenoid alone is unlikely to account for the observed benefit of a high fruit and vegetable diet on lung cancer risk. Instead the combination of various carotenoids or other unidentified phytochemicals, which are common in a variety of fruits and vegetables, may be important for decreasing lung cancer risk. Alternatively, residual confounding in observational studies because of imperfect classification and measurement of factors such as smoking may have led to an overestimation of the strength of the association between fruit and vegetable consumption and lung cancer risk (Stram et al., 2002).

Breast Cancer

Although breast cancer is the leading cause of cancer incidence and mortality in women worldwide, there is considerable international variation in breast cancer rates across countries (Ferlay et al., 2004). The highest rates tend to be in North America, Europe, and Oceania; the lowest rates tend to be in Asia and Africa (Ferlay et al., 2004). In addition, migrant studies have suggested that lifestyle factors may contribute to the differences in incidence rates among countries (McMichael and Giles, 1988; Kelsey and Horn-Ross, 1993). Endogenous hormones have been found to influence breast cancer risk. Elevations in breast cancer risk have been found for a younger age at menarche, older age at first birth, lower parity, and older age at menopause (Henderson et al., 1991; Bernstein and Ross, 1993; Zografos et al., 2004). Opposite associations have been observed for body mass index (BMI) in premenopausal compared with postmenopausal women. In premenopausal women, BMI has been inversely associated with risk, whereas in postmenopausal women a positive association has been observed (van den Brandt et al., 2000; Carmichael and Bates, 2004; Lahmann et al., 2004). Dietary factors typically have not been strongly associated with breast cancer risk (Holmes and Willett, 2004). Studies that combined data from multiple studies have shown that breast cancer risk increased linearly with increasing alcohol consumption (Smith-Warner et al., 1998; Hamajima et al., 2002). Associations with dietary fat have been inconsistent. Fat intake generally has not been associated with breast cancer risk in cohort studies (Boyd et al., 1993; Smith-Warner et al., 2001a), although more recent studies have shown positive associations with saturated fat (Boyd et al., 2003). Case-control and ecologic studies have been more supportive of a positive association between fat intake and breast cancer risk (Boyd et al., 2003).

At least 50 case-control (Graham et al., 1982; Zemla, 1984; Katsouyanni et al., 1986; Hislop et al., 1986; Iscovich et al., 1989; Toniolo et al., 1989; Young, 1989; Ingram et al., 1991; Richardson et al., 1991; Zaridze et al., 1991; Pawlega, 1992; Levi et al., 1993; Holmberg et al., 1994; Landa et al.,

1994; Qi et al., 1994; Franceschi et al., 1995; Yuan et al., 1995; Byrne et al., 1996; Freudenheim et al., 1996; Challier et al., 1998; Thorand et al., 1998; Potischman et al., 1999; Ronco et al., 1999; Tavani et al., 1999; Terry et al., 2001d; Amaral et al., 2002; Dos Santos Silva et al., 2002; Hermann et al., 2002; Adzersen et al., 2003; Hirose et al., 2003; Malin et al., 2003; Shannon et al., 2003; Frazier et al., 2004) and cohort (Hirayama, 1990; Shibata et al., 1992; Rohan et al., 1993; Jarvinen et al., 1997; Verhoeven et al., 1997b; Zhang et al., 1999; Appleby et al., 2002; Maynard et al., 2003; Sauvaget et al., 2003; Mattisson et al., 2004) studies have reported on associations between fruit and vegetable intake and breast cancer risk in women (Table 4). Studies have been conducted over the past 40 years in North and South America, Australia, Asia, and Europe. Although most studies have examined associations with breast cancer incidence, some studies have examined associations with mortality (Appleby et al., 2002; Maynard et al., 2003). Most case-control studies have measured dietary intake during the 1–5 years prior to diagnosis, although some studies have assessed dietary intakes during childhood (Hislop et al., 1986), adolescence (Hislop et al., 1986; Potischman et al., 1999; Frazier et al., 2004), and young adulthood (Hislop et al., 1986). Cohort studies generally have measured recent diet at baseline. Associations with total fruit consumption and breast cancer risk have been measured in at least 18 case-control studies (Katsouyanni et al., 1986; Toniolo et al., 1989; Ingram et al., 1991; Zaridze et al., 1991; Levi et al., 1993; Holmberg et al., 1994; Landa et al., 1994; Qi et al., 1994; Freudenheim et al., 1996; Thorand et al., 1998; Potischman et al., 1999; Ronco et al., 1999; Terry et al., 2001d; Dos Santos Silva et al., 2002; Hermann et al., 2002; Adzersen et al., 2003; Hirose et al., 2003; Malin et al., 2003; Shannon et al., 2003) and eight cohort studies (Shibata et al., 1992; Rohan et al., 1993; Jarvinen et al., 1997; Verhoeven et al., 1997b; Zhang et al., 1999; Appleby et al., 2002; Maynard et al., 2003; Sauvaget et al., 2003; Mattisson et al., 2004). Among case-control studies, the association between fruit consumption and breast cancer risk appears to be relatively weak; with most relative risks ranging between 0.8 and 1.1 or being nonsignificant, suggesting that fruit consumption is not associated with the risk of breast cancer. A statistically significant lower risk of breast cancer of at least 30% has been observed for women in the highest versus lowest category of fruit consumption in a few case-control studies. Only two case-control studies have found at least a 25% increase in breast cancer risk with elevated fruit consumption (Zaridze et al., 1991; Holmberg et al., 1994). In one of these studies (Holmberg et al., 1994), breast cancer risk was increased by 70% (odds ratio [OR] = 1.7, 95% CI 1.0–3.0) in women older than 50 years but was not associated with the risk of breast cancer in women 50 years or younger (OR = 0.7, 95% CI 0.3–2.1). The test for effect modification by age group was not statistically significant. The same type of pattern was observed in the other case-control study showing a positive association (Zaridze et al., 1991). Breast cancer risk was elevated (but the increase was not statistically significant) among postmenopausal women for comparisons of women who had increased versus decreased their fruit consumption in the past 10 years. However, a nonsignificant inverse association was observed for premenopausal women (Zaridze et al., 1991). Among cohort studies, no statistically significant associations have been observed for fruit intake (Shibata et al., 1992; Rohan et al., 1993; Jarvinen et al., 1997; Verhoeven et al., 1997b; Zhang et al., 1999; Appleby et al., 2002; Maynard et al., 2003; Sauvaget et al., 2003; Mattisson et al., 2004), even though the risk of breast cancer was reduced by ~20% in half the studies. None of the studies has reported that the association between fruit consumption and breast cancer risk was significantly modified by menopausal status (Rohan et al., 1993; Franceschi et al., 1995; Trichopoulou et al., 1995; Ronco et al., 1999).

Reporting of associations with citrus fruits has been limited (Iscovich et al., 1989; Richardson et al., 1991; Levi et al., 1993; Franceschi et al., 1995; Hermann et al., 2002; Malin et al., 2003; Shannon et al., 2003). Both decreases (Iscovich et al., 1989; Malin et al., 2003) and increases (Richardson et al., 1991; Hermann et al., 2002) of at least 30% in the risk of breast cancer have been observed in case-control studies. However, in one of the studies showing a positive association, the association for citrus fruits was attenuated and nonsignificant after further adjustment for other dietary factors (Richardson et al., 1991). No association with citrus fruits has been reported in other case-control studies (Levi et al., 1993; Franceschi et al., 1995; Shannon et al., 2003). No cohort studies were identified that have reported on citrus fruit consumption and breast cancer risk.

For total vegetable consumption and the risk of breast cancer, at least 22 case-control (Zemla, 1984; Katsouyanni et al., 1986; Toniolo et al., 1989; Richardson et al., 1991; Ingram et al., 1991; Zaridze et al., 1991; Pawlega, 1992; Landa et al., 1994; Qi et al., 1994; Freudenheim et al., 1996; Braga et al., 1997; Thorand et al., 1998; Potischman et al., 1999; Tavani et al., 1999; Amaral et al., 2002; Dos Santos Silva et al., 2002; Hermann et al., 2002; Adzersen et al., 2003; Hirose et al., 2003; Malin et al., 2003; Shannon et al., 2003; Frazier et al., 2004) and 6 cohort (Shibata et al., 1992; Rohan et al., 1993; Jarvinen et al., 1997; Verhoeven et al., 1997b; Zhang et al., 1999; Maynard et al., 2003; Mattisson et al., 2004) studies were identified. The evidence that vegetables are inversely associated with breast cancer risk is more consistent than that observed for fruit consumption. Most case-control studies, but not all, have found that the risk of breast cancer is lower among women who eat more vegetables. Of the case-control studies with statistically significant associations, the risk of breast cancer was generally 40–60% lower among women with the highest versus lowest intakes of total

TABLE 4 Summary of Case-Control and Cohort Studies of Fruit and Vegetable Consumption and Breast Cancer Risk[a]

Author, year, country	Study dates	Study population	Comparison	Odds ratio/relative risk (95% CI), unless otherwise noted	
				Total fruit	Citrus fruit
Case-control studies					
Graham et al., 1982, USA	1958–1965	2024 cases, 1463 hospital controls	≤3 vs ≥20/mo[b]		
Zemla, 1984, Poland	1979–1981	328 cases (214 Native Upper Silesians, 114 migrants), 585 hospital visitor controls (405 Native Upper Silesians, 180 migrants)	Rather regular vs none		
Katsouyanni et al., 1986, Greece	1983–1984	120 cases, 120 hospital controls	Highest vs lowest quintile	χ for trend = −1.74, $p < 0.10$	
Iscovich et al., 1989, Argentina	1984–1985	150 cases, 150 hospital controls, 150 neighborhood controls	Highest vs lowest quartile		hospital controls: 0.75, Z for trend = −0.63, ns; vs neighborhood controls: 0.58, $p < 0.05$
Toniolo et al., 1989, Italy	1983–1984	250 cases (70 premenopausal, 180 postmenopausal), 499 population controls (128 premenopausal, 371 postmenopausal)	Highest vs lowest quartile	1.1, χ^2 for trend = 0.29, ns	
Young, 1989, USA	1981–1982	277 cases, 372 population controls	8 vs 0/mo		
Ingram et al., 1991, Australia	1985–1987	99 cases, 209 population controls	High vs low	0.9 (0.5–1.6)	
Richardson et al., 1991, France	1983–1987	409 cases, 515 hospital controls	≥525 vs <300 g/wk		1.4 (1.0–2.0), p for trend = 0.061
Zaridze et al., 1991, Russia	1987–1989	139 cases (58 premenopausal, 81 postmenopausal), 139 hospital controls (54 premenopausal, 85 postmenopausal)	Decreased vs increased intake in past 10 years[b]	Premenopausal: 1.22 (0.19–7.64) [0.82, 0.13–5.26]; Postmenopausal: 0.55 (0.14–2.15) [1.82, 0.46–7.14]	
Pawlega, 1992, Poland	1987	127 cases (33 < 50 years, 94 ≥ 50 years), 250 population controls (61 < 50 years, 189 ≥ 50 years)	>3 vs <1/wk		

Odds ratio/relative risk (95% CI), unless otherwise noted				
Total vegetables	Cruciferous vegetables	Green vegetables	Matching and adjustment factors	Miscellaneous
	1.00, p for trend > 0.05		Age	No association among women > 55 years or among women < 55 years
Raw, Upper Silesians: 0.73, $\chi^2 = 2.49$, ns; migrants: 1.57, $\chi^2 = 1.81$, ns			Age	
0.09 (0.03–0.30)			Age, interviewer, years of schooling. For the vegetable analyses additional adjustment was made for parity, age at first birth, marital status, menopausal status, age at menopause, age at menarche, and place of residence.	No interaction with age, years of schooling, menopausal status
		Green leafy vegetables, vs hospital controls: 0.32, $p < 0.05$; vs neighborhood controls: 0.15, $p < 0.05$; All green vegetables, vs hospital controls: 0.52, $p < 0.05$; vs neighborhood controls: 0.40, $p < 0.05$	Age, age at birth of first child, husband's occupation, and body mass index	
1.2, $\chi^2 = 0.32$, ns			Age, energy intake	
	18–35 years: 0.66 (0.42–1.02); > 35 years: 0.64 (0.41–1.00)		Age, alcohol consumption	
1.4 (0.8–2.4)		Leafy and orange/red vegetables: 1.0 (0.6–1.7)	Age, residence	
Nonsignificant difference in mean intake between cases (1092 g/wk) vs controls (1064 g/wk)			Age, menopausal status, alcohol consumption, family history of breast cancer, past history of benign breast disease, age at menopause, age at menarche, parity, age at first full-term pregnancy, education	RR was attenuated and nonsignificant when further adjusted for meat, processed pork meat, high-fat cheese, margarine, olive oil, fruits rich in beta-carotene, desserts and chocolate, nuts
Premenopausal: 3.23 (0.27–39.07) [0.31, 0.02–3.70]; Postmenopausal:1.45 (0.22–9.72) [0.69, 0.10–4.54]			Age, neighborhood, age at menarche, age at first birth (premenopausal only), education (postmenopausal only)	
Boiled, >50 years: 0.4 (0.2–0.8), p for trend = 0.01			Age, residence, education, social class, marital status, number of persons in household, years of smoking, body mass index, drinking of vodka 20 years earlier	Data on boiled vegetables among women < 50 years were not accepted because of low reproducibility

(continues)

TABLE 4 (*Continued*)

Author, year, country	Study dates	Study population	Comparison	Odds ratio/relative risk (95% CI), unless otherwise noted	
				Total fruit	Citrus fruit
Levi et al., 1993, Switzerland	1990–1992	107 cases, 318 hospital controls	Highest vs lowest tertile	Fresh: 0.8, χ^2 for trend = 0.9, ns	1.1, χ^2 for trend = 0.7, ns
Holmberg et al., 1994, Sweden	1987–1990	265 cases (55 ≤ 50 years, 210 > 50 years), 432 screening controls	Highest vs lowest quartile	All: 1.4 (0.9–2.3); ≤50 years: 0.7 (0.3–2.1); >50 years: 1.7 (1.0–3.0)	
Landa et al., 1994, Spain	1987–1988	100 cases, 100 hospital controls	Lowest vs highest tertile[b]	Fresh: 3.83 [0.26] (p < 0.05)	
Qi et al., 1994, China	1986–1987	244 cases, 244 hospital controls	≥600 vs <400 g	No association	
Franceschi et al., 1995, Braga et al., 1997, Italy	1991–1994	2569 cases, 2588 hospital controls	Highest vs lowest quintile for total population, increment = difference in upper cutpoint of highest quartile — lowest quartile for analyses of premenopausal and postmenopausal women separately		1.06 (0.89–1.28), χ^2 for trend = 0.10, ns
Yuan et al., 1995, China	1984–1985	534 cases, 534 community controls (Shanghai)	Mean intake for cases vs controls		
Yuan et al., 1995, China	1985–	300 cases, 300 community controls (Tianjin)	Mean for cases vs controls		
Freudenheim et al., 1996, USA	1986–1991	297 premenopausal cases, 311 population controls	Highest vs lowest quartile	0.67 (0.42–1.09), p for trend = 0.05	
Challier et al., 1998, France	1986–1989	345 cases, 345 controls undergoing a preventive exam	>3 vs <2/mo		
Thorand et al., 1998, Germany	1991–1992	43 cases, 106 population controls	Increment = difference in 75th and 25th percentile	0.82 (0.51–1.32)	
Potischman et al., 1999, USA	1990–1992	568 cases with *in situ* or invasive localized disease (did not report chemotherapy treatment), 1451 population controls	Highest vs lowest quartile	Fruit and fruit juice: 1.08 (0.8–1.4); fruit: 1.02 (0.8–1.4)	

Odds ratio/relative risk (95% CI), unless otherwise noted				
Total vegetables	Cruciferous vegetables	Green vegetables	Matching and adjustment factors	Miscellaneous
	0.6, p for trend < 0.05	Green vegetables: 0.4, p for trend < 0.05	Age	
			Age, country of residence, month of mammography	Effect modification by age-group nonsignificant
Vegetables: 1.92 [0.52] (p < 0.05), raw: 3.1 [0.32] (p < 0.01)			Age	
0.26 (0.14–0.47)			Age, length of stay in Tianjin, date of diagnosis, age at menarche, age at menopause, age at first birth	
Raw, all: 0.73 (0.60–0.88), p for trend < 0.01; premenopausal: 0.73 (0.6–0.9), p < 0.01; postmenopausal: 0.92 (0.8–1.0), $\chi^2 = 1.46$, ns; cooked vegetables: 0.96 (0.79–1.16), χ^2 for trend = 0.34, ns			Age, study center, education, parity, energy intake, alcohol intake (for total population), age at first birth (for premenopausal and postmenopausal groups)	No significant interaction by study center, age-group, menopausal status, education, parity, and body mass index
		Medium/dark green vegetables: 164.4 vs 189.1 g/day (p = 0.0001); light-green vegetables. 1.0 vs 0.7 g/day (p = 0.21)	Age	
		Medium/dark green vegetables: 19.4 vs 20.0 g/day (p = 0.37); light-green vegetables. 87.8 vs 93.5 g/day (p = 0.04)		
0.46 (0.28–0.74), p for trend < 0.001			Age, residence, education, age at first birth, age at menarche, first-degree relative with breast cancer, previous benign breast disease, body mass index, energy intake	Premenopausal women only
	1.45 (1.03–2.06), p for trend = 0.03		Age, socioeconomic status, parity, weight, corporeal surface, energy intake	
Total (excluding potatoes): 0.86 (0.51–1.46); total (including potatoes): 0.88 (0.53–1.46)			Age, body mass index, exogenous hormone use, age at menarche, nulliparity, smoking status, socioeconomic status, energy intake	Postmenopausal women only
0.86 (0.6–1.1)	0.95 (0.7–1.3)		Age at diagnosis, study site, ethnicity, education, age at first birth, alcohol intake, years of oral contraceptive use, smoking status	Results were similar when limited to the 353 cases with localized disease or to those who were interviewed within 3 months of diagnosis 0.78 (0.5–1.2) for >2/wk vs 0

(*continues*)

TABLE 4 *(Continued)*

Author, year, country	Study dates	Study population	Comparison	Odds ratio/relative risk (95% CI), unless otherwise noted	
				Total fruit	Citrus fruit
Ronco et al., 1999, Uruguay	1994–1997	400 cases, 405 hospital controls	Highest vs lowest quartile	0.57 (0.36–0.89), p for trend = 0.05	
Tavani et al., 1999, Italy	1983–1994	579 cases, 668 hospital controls	>8 servings/wk		
Terry et al., 2001, Sweden	1993–1995	2832 cases, 2650 population controls	Highest vs lowest quartile	0.96 (0.79–1.17), p = 0.81	
Amaral et al., 2002, Portugal	1993–1996	127 cases, 158 hospital controls	Highest vs lowest quartile		
Dos Santos Silva et al., 2002, UK	1995–1999	240 cases, 477 population controls	Highest vs lowest quartile	0.89 (0.50–1.57), p for trend = 0.45	
Hermann et al., 2002, Germany	1992–1995	355 cases, 838 population controls	Highest vs lowest quartile among consumers	1.13 (0.77–1.66), p for trend = 0.374	1.53 (1.04–2.25)
Adzersen et al., 2003, Germany	1998–1999	310 cases, 353 hospital controls	Highest vs lowest quartile	0.84 (0.51–1.39), p for trend = 0.19	

Total vegetables	Cruciferous vegetables	Green vegetables	Matching and adjustment factors	Miscellaneous
Odds ratio/relative risk (95% CI), unless otherwise noted				
		Green leafy vegetables: 0.36 (0.23–0.55)	Age, residence, urban/rural status, family history of breast cancer in a first-degree relative, body mass index, age at menarche, parity, menopausal status, energy intake	
Raw: 0.57 (0.33–0.98)			Study, center, year of recruitment, age, education, body mass index, family history of breast cancer, parity, age at first birth	Subset of women < 40 years from studies by Franceschi et al. 1995; and Negri et al. 1991
	0.76 (0.62–0.93)		Age, height, body mass index, current smoking, socioeconomic status, alcohol intake, consumption of high-fiber grains and cereals, fatty fish consumption, multivitamin use, parity, hormone replacement therapy, history of benign breast disease, family history of breast cancer, type of menopause, age at menopause, age at menarche, age at first birth	Postmenopausal women only
0.34 (0.15–0.76)			Age, education, height, age at first birth, length of exposure to endogenous estrogens, family history of breast cancer; nonremoval of visible fat in meat and total energy	Postmenopausal women only
Vegetables dishes: 0.48 (0.27–0.85), *p* for trend = 0.005			Age, general practitioner, energy intake, age at menarche, age at first birth, parous, parity, breast-feeding, family history of breast cancer, menopausal status, time since menopause, education	Population: women of South Asian ethnicity who had migrated to England
Total: 0.64 (0.43–0.96), *p* for trend = 0.034; raw: 0.89 (0.61–1.30), *p* for trend = 0.268; cooked: 0.77 (0.52–1.15), *p* for trend = 0.219			Age, study region, education, duration of breast-feeding, family history of breast cancer, number of births, body mass index, energy intake, alcohol consumption, and nonconsumers of each specific food group	Also stratified by menopausal status
Total: 0.62 (0.38–1.02), *p* for trend = 0.04; raw: 0.51 (0.31–0.84), *p* for trend = 0.09; cooked: 1.26 (0.77–2.06), *p* for trend = 0.90			Age, total energy without alcohol intake, age at menarche, age at first birth, age at menopause, mother/sister with breast cancer, current smoking, history of benign breast disease and/or operation, body mass index, consumption of alcohol, current or within past year hormone replacement therapy	

(*continues*)

TABLE 4 *(Continued)*

Author, year, country	Study dates	Study population	Comparison	Odds ratio/relative risk (95% CI), unless otherwise noted	
				Total fruit	Citrus fruit
Frazier et al., 2003, USA	1980–1986	843 cases, 8430 controls			
Hirose et al., 2003, Japan	1989–2000	2385 cases (1336 premenopausal, 1049 postmenopausal), 19,013 hospital controls (12,003 premenopausal, 7010 postmenopausal)	Highest vs lowest quartile	Premenopausal: 0.87 (0.65–1.16), p for trend = 0.14; postmenopausal: 0.61 (0.41–0.91), p for trend = 0.02	
Malin et al., 2003, China	1996–1998	1459 cases (852 premenopausal, 421 postmenopausal), 1556 population controls (859 premenopausal, 447 postmenopausal)	Highest vs lowest quintile	All: 1.01 (0.80–1.28), p for trend = 0.89	All: 0.68 (0.54–0.86), p for trend = 0.002, premenopausal: 0.65 (0.48–0.88), p for trend < 0.001; postmenopausal: 0.78 (0.53–1.16), p for trend = 0.23
Shannon et al., 2003, USA	1988–1990	441 cases, 370 population controls	Highest vs lowest quartile for fruit, citrus fruit, vegetables, cruciferous vegetables; highest vs lowest tertile for dark green vegetables	0.72 (0.48–1.08), p for trend = 0.16	1.16 (0.77–1.74), p for trend = 0.77
Cohort studies					
Hirayama et al., 1990, Japan	1965–1982	243 fatal cases (241 women, 2 men), cohort of 265,118 (142,857 women, 122,261 men)			
Shibata et al., 1992, USA	1981–1989	219 cases, cohort of 11,580 (~2/3 are women)	Highest vs lowest tertile	0.82 (0.60–1.12)	
Rohan et al., 1993, Canada	1982–1987	519 cases, cohort of 56,837 (analyzed as nested case-control study with 1182 controls)	Highest vs lowest quintile	0.81 (0.57–1.14), p for trend = 0.174	
Järvinen et al., 1997, Finland	1966–1991	88 cases, cohort of 4697		Fruits and berries: no association	
Verhoeven et al., 1997, Netherlands	1986–1990	607 cases, cohort of 62,573 (analyzed as a case-cohort study with a subcohort of 1598)	Highest vs lowest quintile	0.76 (0.54–1.08), p for trend = 0.10	

Odds ratio/relative risk (95% CI), unless otherwise noted				
Total vegetables	Cruciferous vegetables	Green vegetables	Matching and adjustment factors	Miscellaneous
No association			Age at diagnosis, age at menarche, menopausal status, family history, benign breast disease, adult height, parity/age at first birth, postmenopausal hormone use, body mass index at age 18, alcohol intake in 1980, 1980 vitamin A intake excluding supplements in 1980	Nested case-control study within Nurses' Health Study. Similar relative risks for premenopausal and postmenopausal breast cancer
Raw, premenopausal: 1.28 (0.87–1.89), *p* for trend = 0.74; postmenopausal: 1.17 (0.84–1.62), *p* for trend = 0.91		Green leafy vegetables: 0.89 (0.71–1.11), *p* for trend < 0.05	Age, visit year, family history, age at menarche, parity and age at first full-term pregnancy, age at menopause (for analyses of postmenopausal women), body mass index (for analyses of postmenopausal women)	Update of Hirose, 1995
1.05 (0.81–1.40), *p* for trend = 0.81	1.10 (0.87–1.40), *p* for trend = 0.21	Dark green vegetables: 1.02 (0.82–1.28), *p* for trend = 0.83	Age, education, family history of breast cancer, history of breast fibroadenoma, waist-to-hip ratio, menarche age, ever had live birth, age at first birth, total energy	Also stratified by menopausal status
0.86 (0.56–1.31), *p* for trend = 0.35	0.91 (0.61–1.38), *p* for trend = 0.69	Dark green vegetables: 1.04 (0.73–1.46), *p* for trend = 0.63	Age, energy intake, number of pregnancies, education	
		Green-yellow vegetables: 1.04 (0.81–1.33)		
0.96 (0.69–1.34)		Dark green vegetables. 0.91 (0.66–1.25)	Age, smoking	
0.86 (0.61–1.23), *p* for trend = 0.752			Age, age at menarche, surgical menopause, age at first live birth, education, family history of breast cancer, history of benign breast disease, and other contributors to total food intake	Update of Simard, 1990. No statistically significant difference by menopausal status
No association			Age, body mass index, parity, region, occupation, smoking	
0.94 (0.67–1.31), *p* for trend = 0.30			Age, energy intake, alcohol intake, history of benign breast disease, maternal breast cancer, breast cancer in sister(s), age at menarche, age at menopause, age at first birth, parity	Postmenopausal women only

(*continues*)

TABLE 4 *(Continued)*

Author, year, country	Study dates	Study population	Comparison	Odds ratio/relative risk (95% CI), unless otherwise noted	
				Total fruit	**Citrus fruit**
Appleby et al., 1996, UK	1973–1997	90 fatal cases, cohort of 6416	Daily vs <daily	Fresh fruit: 0.77 (0.46–1.27)	
Zhang et al., 1999, USA	1980–1994	2697 cases (784 premenopausal, 1913 postmenopausal), cohort of 83,234	>5.0 vs <2 servings/day for fruits and vegetables; >1 vs <0.25 servings/day for cruciferous vegetables	Premenopausal: 0.74 (0.45–1.24), *p* for trend = 0.13; postmenopausal: 0.84 (0.64–1.09), *p* for trend = 0.10; current hormone replacement therapy users: 0.57 (0.33–1.00)	
Maynard et al., 2003, UK	1937–2000	118 cases (82 incident, 36 fatal), cohort of 1959	Highest vs lowest quartile	Incidence: 1.08 (0.52–2.25); *p* for trend = 0.61; mortality: 1.25 (0.40–3.92), *p* for trend = 0.73	
Sauvaget et al., 2003, Japan	1980–1998	76 fatal cases, cohort of 23,667	Highest vs lowest tertile	0.91 (0.48–1.72), *p* for trend = 0.71	
Mattisson et al., 2004, Sweden	1991–2001	342 cases, cohort of 11,726	Continuous	Total fruits and berries: no association	
Pooled analyses					
Smith-Warner et al., 2001a,b	Follow-up times:1976–1994	7377 cases from 8 cohort studies with total baseline population of 351,825 women	Highest vs lowest quartile for fruits and vegetables for total population. Increment = 100 g/day for citrus fruit, cruciferous, vegetables, and green leafy vegetables and for all results presented separately for premenopausal and postmenopausal women.	All: 0.93 (0.86–1.00), *p* for trend = 0.08; premenopausal: 0.98 (0.94–1.02); postmenopausal: 0.99 (0.98–1.01); fruits, all: 0.93 (0.84–1.02), *p* for trend = 0.08; premenopausal: 0.95 (0.90–1.00); postmenopausal: 1.00 (0.97–1.02)	Rutaceae, all: 0.99 (0.97–1.01)

[a]The following studies have examined the association between fruit and vegetable consumption and breast cancer risk but did not report associations for the groups included in the table: Nislop et al. 1986; Yuan et al., 1995; Byrne et al., 1996.

[b]The inverse of the relative risk was calculated to represent a comparison of high vs low intake and is included in brackets after the published estimate.

vegetables (Katsouyanni et al., 1986; Pawlega, 1992; Landa et al., 1994; Qi et al., 1994; Franceschi et al., 1995; Freudenheim et al., 1996; Tavani et al., 1999; Amaral et al., 2002; Dos Santos Silva et al., 2002; Hermann et al., 2002; Adzersen et al., 2003). The risk of breast cancer was also lower (but the estimates were not statistically significant) among women who had increased versus decreased their vegetable consumption during the past 10 years (Zaridze et al., 1991). In all of the case-control studies that showed at least a 20% increase in risk with higher vegetable consumption, the association was not statistically significant. Among cohort studies (Hirayama, 1990; Shibata et al., 1992; Rohan et al., 1993;

Odds ratio/relative risk (95% CI), unless otherwise noted				
Total vegetables	Cruciferous vegetables	Green vegetables	Matching and adjustment factors	Miscellaneous
			Age and smoking	
Premenopausal: 0.64 (0.43–0.95), *p* for trend = 0.10; postmenopausal: 1.02 (0.85–1.24), *p* for trend = 0.61; postmenopausal, current hormone replacement therapy users: 0.87 (0.63–1.20)	Premenopausal: 0.83 (0.52–1.32), *p* for trend = 0.19; postmenopausal: 0.98 (0.77–1.25), *p* for trend = 0.83		Age, length of follow-up, energy intake, parity, age at first birth, age at menarche, history of breast cancer in mother or sister, history of benign breast disease, alcohol intake, body mass index at age 18, weight change from age 18, height	Update of Hunter, 1993. Also stratified by family history and alcohol intake
Incidence: 1.43 (0.70–2.92), *p* for trend = 0.59; mortality: 0.86 (0.30–2.47), *p* for trend = 0.35			Age, energy intake, food expenditure, Townsend score, season	
		Green-yellow vegetables: 1.28 (0.64–2.54), *p* for trend = 0.53	Age, radiation dose, city, body mass index, smoking status, alcohol habits, education	Atomic bomb survivors only
No association			Diet interviewer, season of diet interview, method version, age, change of dietary habits, total energy, current hormone use, age at first child, height, waist, leisure time physical activity, age at menarche, educational	Postmenopausal women only
All: 0.96 (0.89–1.04), *p* for trend = 0.54; premenopausal: 0.99 (0.93–1.06); postmenopausal: 1.00 (0.97–1.02)	All: 0.96 (0.87–1.06)	All, green leafy vegetables: 0.99 (0.92–1.06)	Age, at menarche, interaction between parity and age at birth of first child, oral contraceptive use, history of benign breast disease, menopausal status at follow-up, postmenopausal hormone use, family history of breast cancer, smoking status, education, body mass index, body mass index, menopausal status interaction, height, alcohol intake, and energy intake.	Study-specific RRs were calculated using the primary data and then were combined using the random effects model

Jarvinen et al., 1997; Verhoeven et al., 1997b; Zhang et al., 1999; Maynard et al., 2003; Mattisson et al., 2004), a statistically significant inverse association with total vegetable consumption was observed only in the Nurses' Health Study when the analysis was limited to premenopausal breast cancer (Zhang et al., 1999).

Relatively few studies have examined whether the association between vegetable consumption and breast cancer risk is modified by menopausal status. Among those studies that have evaluated associations separately by menopausal status (Katsouyanni et al., 1986; Rohan et al., 1993; Freudenheim et al., 1996; Hirose et al., 1995; Trichopoulou et al., 1995; Braga et al., 1997; Ronco et al., 1999; Tavani et al., 1999) or age-group (Katsouyanni et al., 1986; Holmberg et al., 1994; Braga et al., 1997), most have found that the associations did not differ between groups. However, some case-control studies have suggested that higher vegetable consumption is associated with a reduced risk of premenopausal, but not postmenopausal, breast cancer (Freudenheim et al., 1996; Braga et al., 1997; Tavani et al., 1999). In the Nurses' Health Study, the risk of premenopausal breast cancer was reduced by ~35% comparing intakes of more than five versus less than 2 servings of vegetables per day (relative risk [RR] = 0.64, 95% CI 0.43–0.95) (Zhang et al., 1999). Although vegetable consumption was not associated with the risk of postmenopausal breast cancer overall, there was a suggestion of an inverse association among postmenopausal women who were current users of hormone replacement therapy.

For cruciferous vegetables, many studies have found no relation with the risk of breast cancer (Graham et al., 1982; Potischman et al., 1999; Malin et al., 2003; Shannon et al., 2003), although some case-control studies have shown at least a 24–40% reduction in the risk of breast cancer with high compared with low intake (Young, 1989; Levi et al., 1993; Terry et al., 2001d). Only a case-control study that used a recalled 6-day food diary covering the period before diagnosis to estimate dietary intakes has suggested that eating cruciferous vegetables may increase the risk of breast cancer. In that study, eating at least three versus ≤ 2 servings of cruciferous vegetables a month was associated with a 45% higher risk of breast cancer (RR = 1.45, 95% CI 1.03–2.06) (Challier et al., 1998). Cruciferous vegetable consumption was not associated with breast cancer risk in the Nurses' Health Study (Zhang et al., 1999).

Similar types of green vegetables have been examined in relation to the risk of breast cancer, as were evaluated for lung cancer. Collectively, these groups are referred to as *green vegetables*. Green vegetable consumption has been associated with a reduced risk of breast cancer in some (Iscovich et al., 1989; Levi et al., 1993; Ronco et al., 1999; Hirose et al., 2003) but not all (Hirayama, 1990; Ingram et al., 1991; Malin et al., 2003; Sauvaget et al., 2003; Shannon et al., 2003) studies evaluating this exposure. Relative risks for breast cancer comparing high versus low green vegetable consumption have ranged from 0.3 (Iscovich et al., 1989) to 0.91 (Shibata et al., 1992). Further, in a case-control study of Chinese women residing in Shanghai, mean daily consumption of medium/dark green vegetables was significantly higher in controls compared with breast cancer cases (Yuan et al., 1995).

Pooled Analyses

In a pooled analysis of eight prospective cohort studies including 7377 breast cancer cases, intakes of total fruits and vegetables, total fruit, citrus fruit, total vegetables, cruciferous vegetables, and green leafy vegetables were not associated with the risk of breast cancer (Smith-Warner et al., 2001b). The associations for total fruit and vegetable, total fruit, and total vegetable consumption were not modified by menopausal status.

Summary

The evidence that fruits and vegetables may protect against breast cancer is weak. Total fruits and vegetables, fruits, and vegetables generally have not been significantly associated with the risk of breast cancer. Moreover, the majority of relative risks for these three exposure categories have been between 0.8 and 1.2, which suggests that these broad categories of fruit and vegetable consumption are not strongly related to the risk of developing breast cancer in either a protective or harmful direction. Because of the limited data available on associations for other fruit and vegetable groups, it is unclear whether stronger associations may exist for more specific fruit and vegetable exposures.

Colon Cancer

Colon cancers were rare before the twentieth century, but now the incidence is high among economically developed areas, particularly in North America and northern Europe (Potter et al., 1993; Giovannucci and Willett, 1994). However, rates of this malignancy remain relatively low in Asia and Africa. Environmental factors, particularly dietary patterns, account for most of this marked variation in rates (Doll and Peto, 1981). The current epidemiological evidence indicates that physical inactivity (Lee et al., 1991) or excess energy intake relative to requirements increases the risk of colon cancer (Lee and Paffenbarger, 1992). Also, intake of red meat appears to increase risk, but protein-rich sources other than red meat probably do not elevate risk and may even reduce the occurrence of this cancer (Willett et al., 1990). Alcohol intake may increase risk of cancers of the colon and rectum, although the evidence is not entirely consistent (Cho et al., 2004; Kune and Vitetta, 1992). The influence of alcohol may be particularly strong when combined with a diet low in methionine, folate, and vitamin B6, suggesting that the effect of alcohol may be through antagonism of one-carbon metabolism (Stover, 2004). Cigarette smoking at an early age may also enhance the risk of this cancer (Giovannucci et al., 1994). Because the etiology of colon cancer may differ from that of rectal cancer (Potter, 1996; Wei et al., 2004), only the studies on colon cancer are summarized here.

More than 38 case-control studies (Wynder et al., 1969; Wynder and Shigematsu, 1967; Bjelke, 1974; Modan et al., 1975; Phillips, 1975; Graham et al., 1978, 1988; Miller et al., 1983; Pickle et al., 1984; Tajima and Tominaga, 1985; Kune et al., 1987; Vlajinac et al., 1987; Slattery et al., 1988;

Tuyns et al., 1988; Young and Wolf, 1988; Lee et al., 1989; Peters et al., 1989; Benito et al., 1990; Hu et al., 1991; Negri et al., 1991; Bidoli et al., 1992; Iscovich et al., 1992; Peters et al., 1992; Steinmetz and Potter, 1993; Inoue et al., 1995; Kampman et al., 1995; Kotake et al., 1995; Shannon et al., 1996; Slattery et al., 1997; Franceschi et al., 1998; Boutron-Ruault et al., 1999; Levi et al., 1999; Murata et al., 1999; Deneo-Pellegrini et al., 2002; Chiu et al., 2003; Sauvaget et al., 2003; Yeh et al., 2003; Satia-Abouta et al., 2004) and 12 cohort studies (Phillips and Snowdon, 1985; Heilbrun et al., 1989; Hirayama, 1990; Shibata et al., 1992; Thun et al., 1992; Deneo-Pellegrini et al., 1996; Sellers et al., 1998; Singh and Fraser, 1998; Hsing et al., 1998a; Michels et al., 2000; Voorrips et al., 2000a; Terry et al., 2001a; McCullough et al., 2003) have examined the association between fruit and vegetable consumption and cancer risk (Table 5). Studies have been conducted since the 1950s in multiple countries throughout the world. For fruit intake, most case-control studies have found nonsignificant associations (Wynder and Shigematsu, 1967; Phillips, 1975; Pickle et al., 1984; Slattery et al., 1988; Tuyns et al., 1988; Bidoli et al., 1992; Iscovich et al., 1992; Peters et al., 1992; Steinmetz and Potter, 1993; Inoue et al., 1995; Kampman et al., 1995; Kotake et al., 1995; Deneo-Pellegrini et al., 1996, 2002; Slattery et al., 1997; Franceschi et al., 1998; Murata et al., 1999; Satia-Abouta et al., 2004), with most of the associations being close to the null or not reported. However, a few studies have shown a significant reduction in the risk of colon cancer with higher compared with lower fruit consumption, but in most cases, the association was limited to particular subgroups. In one case-control study, the risk of colon cancer was not associated with fresh fruit intake but was 50% higher in participants in the highest versus lowest quartile of stewed and canned fruit intake (Tuyns et al., 1988). Cohort studies are even less supportive of the association between fruit consumption and colon cancer risk (Shibata et al., 1992; Sellers et al., 1998; Singh and Fraser, 1998; Michels et al., 2000; Voorrips et al., 2000a; Terry et al., 2001a; McCullough et al., 2003). Although several cohort studies have reported about a 25% reduction in the risk of colon cancer with higher compared with lower fruit intake, in only one study was the association statistically significant, but this association was observed only in women and no association was evident in men (Shibata et al., 1992). In addition, other studies have shown at least a 50% higher risk of colon cancer with high compared with low fruit consumption (Hsing et al., 1998a).

Citrus fruit consumption has not been associated with colon cancer risk in most studies that have examined this group (Wynder et al., 1969; Miller et al., 1983; Tuyns et al., 1988; Young and Wolf, 1988; Bidoli et al., 1992; Slattery et al., 1997; Franceschi et al., 1998; Levi et al., 1999; Michels et al., 2000; Voorrips et al., 2000a; Deneo-Pellegrini et al., 2002; McCullough et al., 2003; Satia-Abouta et al., 2004).

Vegetable consumption has been evaluated in > 20 case-control studies (Bjelke, 1974; Graham et al., 1978; Miller et al., 1983; Pickle et al., 1984; Slattery et al., 1988; Tuyns et al., 1988; Lee et al., 1989; Hu et al., 1991; Bidoli et al., 1992; Iscovich et al., 1992; Steinmetz and Potter, 1993; Inoue et al., 1995; Kampman et al., 1995; Kotake et al., 1995; Deneo-Pellegrini et al., 1996; Shannon et al., 1996; Slattery et al., 1997; Franceschi et al., 1998; Levi et al., 1999; Deneo-Pellegrini et al., 2002; Chiu et al., 2003; Satia-Abouta et al., 2004). Several studies have shown that the risk of colon cancer is at least 50% lower among individuals with the highest versus lowest vegetable intakes. Other studies have shown statistically significant but more modest reductions in risk, although many studies have found weak or nonsignificant positive or inverse associations. In contrast to the inverse association observed in most case-control studies, none of the cohort studies (Colditz et al., 1985; Shibata et al., 1992; Hsing et al., 1998a; Sellers et al., 1998; Thun et al., 1992; Levi et al., 1999; Michels et al., 2000; Voorrips et al., 2000a; Terry et al., 2001a; McCullough et al., 2003) has found a significant reduction in the risk of colon cancer with higher vegetable intake. A cohort study of > 35,000 postmenopausal women found no association among women without a family history of colon cancer; however, a twofold increased risk of colon cancer was observed among women with a family history of colon cancer in the highest compared with the lowest tertile of vegetable intake (Sellers et al., 1998).

Associations with cruciferous vegetables have been reported in many case-control studies (Miller et al., 1983; Pickle et al., 1984; Kune et al., 1987; Graham et al., 1988; Young and Wolf, 1988; Lee et al., 1989; West et al., 1989; Benito et al., 1990; Bidoli et al., 1992; Peters et al., 1992; Steinmetz and Potter, 1993; Slattery et al., 1997; Franceschi et al., 1998; Deneo-Pellegrini et al., 2002; Chiu et al., 2003). Although several case-control studies have shown reductions in the risk of colon cancer of at least 40% for the highest compared with the lowest cruciferous vegetable intakes, many other studies have shown that cruciferous vegetable intake was not associated with the risk of colon cancer. The evidence from cohort studies (Heilbrun et al., 1989; Hsing et al., 1998a; Sellers et al., 1998; Michels et al., 2000; Voorrips et al., 2000a; McCullough et al., 2003) is less suggestive of an inverse association compared with that from case-control studies with a statistically significant inverse association being observed in only one cohort study (Voorrips et al., 2000a). However, in this study, the inverse association was statistically significant only in the women; the association was weaker and nonsignificant in the men.

The association between green vegetables and colon cancer risk has been inconsistent in case-control studies (Wynder and Shigematsu, 1967; Phillips, 1975; Pickle et al., 1984; Hu et al., 1991; Negri et al., 1991; Iscovich et al., 1992; Steinmetz and Potter, 1993; Inoue et al., 1995; Slattery et al.,

TABLE 5 Summary of Case-Control and Cohort Studies of Fruit and Vegetable Consumption and Colon Cancer Risk[a]

Author, year, country	Study dates	Study population	Comparison	Odds ratio/relative risk (95% CI), unless otherwise noted	
				Total fruit	Citrus fruit
Case-control studies					
Wynder and Shigematsu, 1967, USA		468 (204 women, 264 men) cases, 409 hospital controls		No association	
Wynder et al., 1969, Japan		69 (31 women, 38 men) cases, 307 hospital controls			Women: lower intake in controls; men: lower intake in controls
Bjelke, 1974, Norway		162 cases, 1394 hospital controls			
Bjelke, 1974, USA		259 cases, 1657 hospital controls			
Phillips, 1975, USA	1969–1973	41 cases, 106 hospital controls and population controls	Highest vs lowest tertile	Fresh: 2.0 (ns)	
Graham et al., 1978, USA	1959–1965	256 cases, 783 hospital controls	0–20 vs >61 times/mo[b] for total vegetables; 0–10 vs >21 times/mo[b] for raw vegetables		
Miller et al., 1983, Canada	1976–1978	348 (177 women, 171 men) cases, 542 neighborhood controls, 535 hospital controls	Highest vs lowest tertile		Women: 0.9 (ns), *p* for trend = 0.24; men: 1.3 (ns), *p* for trend = 0.06
Pickle et al., 1984, USA	1970–1977	58 (32 women, 26 men) cases, 178 hospital controls	High vs low	1.12 (ns)	
Kune et al., 1987, Australia	1980–1981	392 (190 women, 202 men) cases, 727 community controls	High vs low		
Graham et al., 1988, USA	1975–1984	428 cases, 428 neighborhood controls			
Slattery et al., 1988, West et al., 1989, USA	1979–1983	231 (119 women, 112 men) cases, 391 population controls	Highest vs lowest quartile	Women: 0.6 (0.3–1.3); men: 0.3 (0.1–0.6)	
Tuyns et al., 1988, Belgium	1978–1982	453 cases, 2851 population controls	Highest vs lowest quartile for fruits and vegetables; highest vs lowest tertile for citrus fruit	Fresh: 0.91 (p = 0.11), *p* for trend = 0.19; stewed and canned: 1.50 (*p* = 0.0016), *p* for trend = 0.0013	1.08 (p = 0.77), *p* for trend = 0.55
Young and Wolf, 1988, USA	1981–1982	353 cases, 618 population controls	Highest vs lowest quartile		No association
Lee et al., 1989, Singapore	1985–1987	132 cases, 425 hospital controls	Highest vs lowest tertile		
Benito et al., 1990, Spain	1984–1988	144 (72 women, 72 men) cases, 295 population controls, 203 hospital controls	Highest vs lowest quartile		

Odds ratio/relative risk (95% CI), unless otherwise noted				
Total vegetables	**Cruciferous vegetables**	**Green vegetables**	**Matching and adjustment factors**	**Miscellaneous**
		Green and yellow vegetables: no association		
			Age	
Lower intake in cases				
Lower intake in cases				
		Green leafy vegetables: 0.5 (ns)	Age, sex, race	
Total: 2.12 [0.47] (p = 0.02); raw: 1.76 [0.57] (p = 0.002)			Age	Men only
Women: 0.7 (ns), p for trend = 0.06; men: 0.8 (ns), p for trend = 0.19	Women: 0.7 ($p < 0.05$), p for trend = 0.05; men: 0.9 (ns), p for trend = 0.35		Age, saturated fat (for cruciferous vegetable analysis)	
1.77 (ns)	0.78 (ns)	1.21 (ns)	Age, race, sex, hospital, year of hospitalization, residence, Bohemian ancestry and Moravian ancestry	Also stratified by Bohemian ancestry
	All: 0.52, women: 0.43, men: 0.58		Age, sex	
	No association		Age, sex, education	
Women: 0.3 (0.1–0.9); men: 0.6 (0.3–1.3)	Women: 0.9 (0.4–1.8); men: 0.3 (0.1–0.8)		Age, body mass index, religion (for fruit, vegetable analyses), crude fiber (for cruciferous vegetable analyses), energy intake	Also stratified by tumor site
Raw: 0.37 ($p < 0.0001$), p for trend <0.0001; cooked: 0.71 (p = 0.41), p for trend = 0.0094			Age, sex, province	
	Diet under age 18: 0.57 (0.39–0.83); diet between 18–35 yr: 0.53 (0.36–0.77); diet older than age 35: 0.59 (0.41–0.85)		Age, sex, age^{x} sex	
0.79 (0.48–1.28), p for trend = ns	0.47 (0.27–0.81), p for trend < 0.01		Age, sex, dialect group, occupation	Significant interaction with age and sex for cruciferous vegetables
	vs population controls: 0.48, p for trend < 0.01; vs hospital controls: 0.43, p for trend < 0.01		Age, sex, weight 10 years prior to the interview, education, physical activity on the job, number of meals per day, cereals, potatoes, meat, dairy products, eggs	Also stratified by tumor site

(*continues*)

TABLE 5 *(Continued)*

Author, year, country	Study dates	Study population	Comparison	Odds ratio/relative risk (95% CI), unless otherwise noted	
				Total fruit	Citrus fruit
Hu et al., 1991, China	1985–1988	111 cases, 111 hospital controls	<75.5 vs >193 kg/year for vegetables in 1985[b]; <95 vs >345 kg/year for vegetables in 1966[b]; <28.5 vs >57 kg/year for green vegetables in 1985[b]; <48.5 vs >151 kg/year for green vegetables in 1966[b]		
Negri et al., 1991, Italy	1983–1990	673 cases, 6147 hospital controls	Highest vs lowest tertile	0.6 (0.5–0.7)	
Bidoli et al., 1992, Italy	1986–1990	123 cases, 699 hospital controls	Highest vs lowest tertile	Fresh: 1.0 (ns), χ^2 for trend = 0.00	0.9 (ns), χ^2 for trend = 0.17
Iscovich et al., 1992, Argentina	1985–1987	110 (48 women, 62 men) cases, 220 neighborhood controls	Highest vs lowest quartile	No association	
Peters et al., 1992, USA	1983–1986	746 (327 women, 419 men) cases, 746 neighborhood controls	Increment = 10 servings/mo	1.00 (0.97–1.03)	
Steinmetz and Potter, 1993, Australia	1979–1980	220 (99 women, 121 men) cases, 438 (197 women, 241 men) population controls	Highest vs lowest quartile	Total, women: 0.90 (0.38–2.11); men: 1.74 (0.88–3.46); raw, women: 0.80 (0.34–1.89); men: 1.16 (0.59–2.29)	
Kampman et al., 1995, Netherlands	1989–1993	232 cases, 259 population controls	Highest vs lowest quartile	All: 0.82 (0.84–1.41), *p* for trend = 0.37; women: 0.54 (0.23–1.23), *p* for trend = 0.13; men: 1.00 (0.49–2.03), *p* for trend = 0.88	
Inoue et al., 1995, Japan	1988–1992	231 (42 women proximal, 50 men proximal, 61 women distal, 75 men distal) cases, 31,782 (23,161 women, 8621 men) hospital controls	High vs low	Women, proximal: 1.3 (0.7–2.4); women, distal: 0.4 (0.3–0.8); men, proximal: 1.0 (0.6–1.9); men, distal: 1.4 (0.9–2.3)	
Kotake et al., 1995, Japan	1992–1994	187 cases, 213 screening controls, 150 hospital controls	Daily vs <1–2 week	0.8 (0.27–2.41)	
Deneo-Pellegrini et al., 1996, Uruguay	1992–1994	160 (61 women, 99 men) cases, 287 (107 women, 180 men) hospital controls	Highest vs lowest quartile	0.46 (0.25–0.82), *p* for trend = 0.005	
Shannon et al., 1996, USA	1985–1989	424 (186 women, 238 men) cases, 414 (190 women, 224 men) population controls	Highest vs lowest quartile	Women: 0.44 (0.24–0.82), *p* for trend = 0.007; men: 0.77 (0.44–1.36), *p* for trend = 0.21	
Slattery et al., 1997, USA	1991–1994	1993 (894 women, 1099 men) cases, 2410 controls from the Kaiser Permanente Medical Care Program	Highest vs lowest quintile for fruits and vegetables; >3 vs 0/wk for citrus fruit; >5.5 vs 0 servings/wk for cruciferous vegetables; >5 vs 1 servings/wk for salad greens	Women: 1.0 (0.7–1.4), *p* for trend = 0.54; men: 1.1 (0.8–1.4), *p* for trend = 0.74	Women: 0.8 (0.6–1.0) 1.0 (0.9–1.1)

Odds ratio/relative risk (95% CI), unless otherwise noted				
Total vegetables	Cruciferous vegetables	Green vegetables	Matching and adjustment factors	Miscellaneous
Fresh, diet in 1985: 5.50 (1.65–18.29) [0.18, 0.05–0.61]; fresh, diet in 1966: 8.80 (2.09–37.02) [0.11, 0.03–0.48]		Green vegetables, diet in 1985: 8.85 (2.65–29.61) [0.11, 0.03–0.38] green vegetables, diet in 1966: 6.48 (1.51–27.88) [0.15, 0.04–0.66]	Age, sex, residential area	
		0.5 (0.4–0.6)	Age, area of residence, education, smoking, sex, plus vegetable and fruit consumption	Update of LaVecchia, et al., 1988, which includes citrus fruits
0.7 (ns), χ^2 for trend = 1.02	0.6 (ns), χ^2 for trend = 2.11		Age, sex, social status	
0.12 (0.04–0.34), *p* for trend < 0.001		Green leafy: 0.24 (0.12–0.49), *p* for trend <0.001	Age, sex, residency	
	1.00 (0.99–1.01)		Age, sex, neighborhood, fat, protein, carbohydrates, alcohol, calcium, family history, weight, physical activity, pregnancy history (women)	
Total, women: 1.11 (0.50–2.45); men: 1.29 (0.67–2.51) raw, women: 1.34 (0.67–2.72), men: 1.27 (0.62–2.60)	Women: 1.12 (0.51–2.46); men: 1.10 (0.57–2.14)	Green leafy, women: 1.02 (0.47–2.21); men: 0.82 (0.45–1.52)	Age, protein intake, Quetelet's index, alcohol intake, occupation (men), age at first live birth (women)	Also stratified by tumor site
0.40 (0.23–0.69), *p* for trend = 0.0004			Age, gender, urbanization level, energy intake, alcohol consumption, cholecystectomy, family history of colon cancer	Also stratified by sex
Fresh, women, proximal: 0.9 (0.5–1.6); women, distal: 0.8 (0.5–1.4); men, proximal: 1.1 (0.6–1.9); men, distal: 0.9 (0.6–1.5)		Green, women, proximal: 0.8 (0.5–1.6); women, distal: 0.9 (0.6–1.6); men, proximal: 1.4 (0.8–2.4); men, distal: 1.7 (1.0–2.6)	Age	Also stratified by tumor site
1.0 (0.24–4.22)			Age and sex	
0.39 (0.21 - 0.75), *p* for trend = 0.007			Age, sex, residence, education, family history of colon cancer, body mass index, energy intake, alcohol intake	
Women: 0.51 (0.28–0.93), *p* for trend = 0.02; men: 0.78 (0.45–1.35), *p* for trend = 0.46			Age, energy intake	Also stratified by tumor site
Women: 0.7 (0.5–1.0), *p* for trend = 0.04; men: 0.7 (0.5–0.9), *p* for trend < 0.01	Women: 1.0 (0.7–1.8), *p* for trend = 0.68; men: 0.8 (0.6–1.1), *p* for trend = 0.08	Salad greens, women: 0.7 (0.5–1.0), *p* for trend = 0.04; men: 0.8 (0.6–1.1), *p* for trend = 0.02	Age, body mass index, physical activity, use of aspirin/NSAID, presence or absence of a first-degree relative with colorectal cancer, total energy intake and calcium	Also stratified by age-group, family history and tumor site

(*continues*)

TABLE 5 *(Continued)*

Author, year, country	Study dates	Study population	Comparison	Odds ratio/relative risk (95% CI), unless otherwise noted	
				Total fruit	**Citrus fruit**
Franceschi et al., 1998, Italy	1991–1996	1225 cases, 5155 hospital controls	Increment = difference in 80th and 20th percentile	1.0 (0.9–1.0)	
Levi et al., 1999, Switzerland	1992–1997	119 cases, 491 hospital controls	Increment = 1 serving/day increase		0.90 (0.79–1.03)
Murata et al., 1999, Japan	1989–1997	265 (108 women, 157 men) cases, 794 (399 women, 395 men) hospital controls	Increment = 1 unit increase in frequency score	0.94 (0.78–1.13)	
Deneo-Pellegrini et al., 2002, Uruguay	1996–	260 cases, 1452 hospital controls	Highest vs lowest quartile	All: 0.9 (0.8–1.0); women: 0.7 (0.4–1.3); men: 0.7 (0.4–1.2)	All: 0.9 (0.9–1.1); women: 1.3 (0.7–2.3); men: 0.7 (0.4–1.2)
Chiu et al., 2003, China	1990–1993	931 (469 women, 462 men) cases, 1552 (701 women, 851 men) population controls	Highest vs lowest quartile	Women: 0.6 (0.4–0.9), p for trend = 0.02; men: 0.7 (0.5–1.0), p for trend = 0.06	
Satia-Abouta et al., 2004, USA	1996–2000	613 cases (337 Caucasians, 276 African-Americans), 1048 population controls (596 Caucasians, 400 African-Americans)	Highest vs lowest quartile of mean daily intake	Caucasians: 0.8 (0.5–1.2), p for trend = 0.37; African-Americans: 0.7 (0.4–1.1), p for trend = 0.07	Caucasians: 1.0 (0.6–1.5), p for trend = 0.69; African-Americans: 1.0 (0.6–1.6), p for trend = 0.69
Cohort studies					
Heilbrun et al., 1989, USA	1965–1985	102 cases, cohort of 8006 (analyzed as a case-cohort study with a subcohort of 361 men)			
Hirayama, 1990, Japan	1965–1982	552 (304 women, 248 men), cohort of 265,118	Daily vs <daily		
Shibata et al., 1992, USA	1981–1989	202 (105 women, 97 men) cases, cohort of 11,580	Highest vs lowest tertile	Women: 0.50 (0.31–0.80); men: 1.12 (0.69–1.81)	
Thun et al., 1992, USA	1982–1988	1150 (539 women, 611 men) cases, cohort of 764,343 (analyzed as nested case-control study with 5746 controls)	Highest vs lowest quintile		
Sellers et al., 1998, USA	1986–1995	241 cases (61 with a positive family history of colon cancer), cohort of 35,216 (4239 with a positive family history of colon cancer)	Highest vs lowest tertile	No family history of colon cancer: 0.9 (0.6–1.2), p for trend = 0.4; positive family history: 1.4 (0.7–2.8), p for trend = 0.3	

Odds ratio/relative risk (95% CI), unless otherwise noted				
Total vegetables	**Cruciferous vegetables**	**Green vegetables**	**Matching and adjustment factors**	**Miscellaneous**
Raw: 0.7 (0.7–0.8); cooked: 0.7 (0.6–0.8)	Cooked: 0.9 (0.7–1.0)	Spinach and other greens: 0.8 (0.7–0.9)	Age, sex, center, year of interview, education, physical activity, alcohol, energy intake	
Raw: 0.90 (0.76–1.07); cooked: 0.69 (0.54–0.88)			Age, sex, education, smoking, alcohol, body mass index, physical activity, and energy intake	
		0.87 (0.67–1.12)	Age, sex, population density, alcohol intake, smoking, meal time, meal amount, meal speed, meat intake, fish intake, fruit intake (for green vegetable analyses)	
Total, all: 0.9 (0.8–1.1); total, women: 0.9 (0.5–1.5); total, men: 0.8 (0.5–1.3); raw, all: 0.9 (0.8–0.9); raw, women: 0.5 (0.3–0.9); raw, men: 0.8 (0.5–1.4); cooked, all: 1.0 (0.9–1.2); cooked, women: 0.5 (0.3–0.9); cooked, men: 0.8 (0.5–1.4)	All: 1.0 (0.9–1.2); women: 1.5 (0.8–2.8); men: 0.7 (0.4–1.3)	Green leafy, all: 0.9 (0.8–1.0); women: 0.6 (0.3–1.0); men: 0.9 (0.5–1.6)	Age, sex, residence, urban/rural status, education, family history of colon cancer, body mass index, energy and red meat intakes	
Women: 1.0 (0.7–1.5), *p* for trend = 0.5; men: 0.8 (0.5–1.1), *p* for trend = 0.04	Women: 1.2 (0.8–1.7), *p* for trend = 0.3; men: 0.7 (0.5–1.0), *p* for trend = 0.07	Dark green leafy, women: 0.9 (0.6–1.2), *p* for trend = 0.5; men: 0.7 (0.5–1.0), *p* for trend = 0.07	Age, energy intake, education, body mass index, income, and occupational physical activity	
Caucasians: 0.5 (0.3–0.9), *p* for trend = 0.006; African-Americans 0.5 (0.3–0.8), *p* for trend = 0.003		Dark green, deep yellow, Caucasians: 0.6 (0.4–1.0), *p* for trend = 0.09; African-Americans: 0.7 (0.4–1.2), *p* for trend = 0.04	Total energy, age, gender, education, body mass index, smoking history, physical activity, family history of colon cancer, NSAID use, fat, carbohydrates, dietary fiber, Vitamin C, Vitamin E, beta-carotene, calcium, folate, fruits and vegetables	Also did analyses using weekly frequency of consumption
	No significant association	Green vegetables and seaweed: No significant association	Age	Men only
		Green-yellow vegetables: 0.85 (0.73–0.99)	Age, sex	
Women: 0.72 (0.45–1.16); men: 1.39 (0.84–2.30)		Dark green vegetables, women: 1.04 (0.63–1.73); men: 2.28 (1.33–3.91)	Age, smoking	
Women: 0.66; men: 0.80			Age, race	No interaction between fat and vegetable intakes
No family history of colon cancer: 1.1 (0.7–1.6), *p* for trend = 0.8, positive family history = 2.0 (1.0–4.2), *p* for trend = 0.1	No family history of colon cancer: 1.1 (0.8–1.6), *p* for trend = 0.6; positive family history: 1.3 (0.7–2.4), *p* for trend = 0.5	Green leafy: No family history of colon cancer: 1.3 (0.9–1.8), *p* for trend = 0.2; positive family history: 1.3 (0.7–2.5), *p* for trend = 0.4	Age, energy intake, history of rectal/colon polyps	Update of Steinmetz et al., 1994. Women only

(*continues*)

TABLE 5 *(Continued)*

Author, year, country	Study dates	Study population	Comparison	Odds ratio/relative risk (95% CI), unless otherwise noted	
				Total fruit	Citrus fruit
Hsing et al., 1998, USA	1966–1986	120 fatal cases, cohort of 17,633	Highest vs lowest quartile	1.6 (0.9–2.9), *p* for trend = 0.05	
Singh and Fraser, 1998, USA	1976–1982	157 cases, cohort of 32,051	>1/day vs <2/wk	No association	
Michels et al., 2000, USA	Women: 1980–1996; Men: 1986–1996	Women: 569 cases, cohort of 88,764; men: 368 cases, cohort of 47,325	≥5 vs ≤1 servings/day for fruits and vegetables; ≥2 servings/day vs ≤1 servings/wk for citrus fruits; ≥5 vs ≤1 servings/wk for cruciferous vegetables	Women: 0.80; men: 1.35	All: 1.05 (0.80–1.39); women: 0.97; men: 1.19
Voorrips et al., 2000, Netherlands	1986–1992	578 (266 women, 312 men) cases, cohort of 120,852 (62,573 women, 58,279 men) (analyzed as a case–cohort study with a subcohort of 1812 women and 1688 men)	Highest vs lowest quintile for all groups except raw leafy vegetables for which comparison is highest vs lowest tertile	Women: 0.73 (0.48–1.11), *p* for trend = 0.12; men: 1.33 (0.90–1.97), *p* for trend = 0.22	Women: 1.00 (0.66–1.52), *p* for trend = 0.99; men: 1.09 (0.75–1.59), *p* for trend = 0.44
Terry et al., 2001, Sweden	1987–1998	291 cases, cohort of 61,463	Highest vs lowest quartile	0.76 (0.55–1.06), *p* for trend = 0.23	
McCullough et al., 2003, USA	1992–1997	508 cases (210 women, 298 men) cases, cohort of 133,163 (70,554 women, 62,609 men)	Highest vs lowest quintile	Women: 0.74 (0.47–1.16), *p* for trend = 0.47; men: 1.11 (0.76–1.62), *p* for trend = 0.52	Women: 0.71 (0.47–1.07), *p* for trend = 0.40; men: 0.85 (0.58–1.26), *p* for trend = 0.94

[a]The following studies have examined the association between fruit and vegetable consumption and colon cancer risk but did not report associations for the groups included in the table: Tajima and Tominga, 1985; Vlajinac et al., 1987; Peters et al., 1989; Boutron-Rualt et al., 1999; Yeh et al., 2003; Phillips and Snowden, 1985.

[b]The inverse of the relative risk was calculated to represent a comparison of high vs low intake and is included in brackets after the published estimate.

Odds ratio/relative risk (95% CI), unless otherwise noted				
Total vegetables	Cruciferous vegetables	Green vegetables	Matching and adjustment factors	Miscellaneous
1.5 (0.8–2.8), p for trend = 0.3	1.4 (0.9–2.4), p for trend = 0.2		Age, smoking, alcohol intake, energy intake	Men only
		Green vegetables: 0.74 (0.46–1.19), p for trend = 0.10	Age, sex, body mass index, physical activity, parental history of colon cancer, smoking, alcohol consumption, and aspirin use	
All: 1.00 (0.72–1.38); women: 0.96; men: 1.24	All: 0.89 (0.68–1.15); women: 0.94; men: 0.83	Green leafy, all: 1.10 (0.88–1.37); women: 1.02; men: 1.23	Age, family history of colorectal cancer, sigmoidoscopy, height, body mass index, smoking, alcohol intake, physical activity, aspirin use, vitamin supplement intake, energy intake, red meat consumption, menopausal status (among women only) and postmenopausal hormone use (among women only)	Also stratified by supplement use, smoking status, folate intake, body mass index
Total, women: 0.83 (0.54–1.26), p for trend = 0.31; men: 0.85 (0.57–1.27), p for trend = 0.45; raw, women: 1.02 (0.67–1.54), p for trend = 0.53; men: 0.79 (0.54–1.16), p for trend = 0.47; cooked, women: 0.75 (0.49–1.14), p for trend = 0.43; men: 0.94 (0.64–1.39), p for trend = 0.72	Women: 0.51 (0.33–0.80), p for trend = 0.004; men: 0.76 (0.51–1.13), p for trend = 0.11	Leafy vegetables, cooked, women: 0.62 (0.40–0.96), p for trend = 0.06; men: 0.75 (0.50–1.13), p for trend = 0.05; leafy vegetables, raw, women: 0.98 (0.71–1.35), p-trend = 0.85; men: 1.02 (0.75–1.38), p for trend = 0.92	Age, family history of colorectal cancer, and alcohol intake	Also stratified by tumor site
0.90 (0.66–1.24), p for trend = 0.43			Age, red meat consumption, dairy product consumption and energy intake	Also stratified by alcohol consumption, body mass index, and tumor site
Women: 0.91 (0.56–1.48), p for trend = 0.56; men: 0.69 (0.47–1.03), p for trend = 0.10	Women: 0.91 (0.58–1.44), p for trend = 0.55; men: 0.74 (0.51–1.08), p for trend = 0.15		Age, exercise, aspirin, smoking, family history of colorectal cancer, body mass index, energy, education, multivitamin use, total calcium, red meat, hormone replacement therapy use (for women)	

1997; Franceschi et al., 1998; Murata et al., 1999; Deneo-Pellegrini et al., 2002; Chiu et al., 2003; Satia-Abouta et al., 2004). Approximately half of the case-control studies have shown statistically significant inverse associations; the magnitude of the association has varied from odds ratios of 0.11 (Hu et al., 1991) to 0.8 (Slattery et al., 1997; Franceschi et al., 1998). Although most of the other case-control studies have reported nonsignificant inverse associations, a few studies have suggested that green vegetable consumption could possibly increase the risk of colon cancer (Pickle et al., 1984; Inoue et al., 1995). Among cohort studies, nonsignificant or null associations have been commonly observed (Heilbrun et al., 1989; Hsing et al., 1998b; Sellers et al., 1998; Singh and Fraser, 1998; Michels et al., 2000), although in a cohort study of elderly retired men and women, more than a twofold increased risk of colon cancer was observed for men in the highest compared with the lowest tertile of green vegetable consumption (Shibata et al., 1992). Only in the Netherlands Cohort Study, a population-based cohort study of > 120,000 men and women, has a statistically significant inverse association been observed, but the association was limited to cooked leafy vegetable consumption among women only (Voorrips et al., 2000a). A more modest inverse association was observed for fatal colon cancer in a cohort of ~265,000 Japanese men and women (Hirayama, 1990).

Summary

The association between fruit and vegetable consumption and colon cancer risk has been evaluated in many case-control and cohort studies. Although many case-control studies have suggested that total fruit and total vegetable intakes are associated with a lower risk of colon cancer, the results from cohort studies generally have been null. Associations for cruciferous vegetable and green vegetable intakes have been inconsistent, although the case-control studies have been more suggestive of an inverse association than the cohort studies. Although risk factors for proximal and distal colon cancers may differ (Iacopetta, 2002), relatively few studies have examined associations separately for cancers of the proximal colon and distal.

Stomach Cancer

Although stomach cancer incidence rates have been decreasing over the past few decades (Plummer et al., 2004), stomach cancer is still a major cause of cancer incidence and mortality in the world. Overall, stomach cancer is the fourth most common incident cancer and second highest cause of cancer death worldwide, with incidence rates in less developed countries at least 1.5 times higher compared with those in more developed countries (Ferlay et al., 2004).

Case-control and cohort studies over the with 15 years have shown that stomach cancer is positively associated with *Helicobacter pylori* infection, and ~40–70% of stomach cancer may be attributed to its infection (Stewart and Kleihues, 2003). *H. pylori* infection causes gastritis, which may lead to stomach cancer (Asaka et al., 1994; Graham, 2000). Other factors that have been associated with stomach cancer risk are increasing age; male gender; lack of refrigeration of foods; tobacco use; and intakes of salted foods, nitrate products, and red meat (barbecued or well done) (Stewart and Kleihues, 2003; Crew and Neugut, 2004).

At least 47 case-control studies (Higginson, 1966; Correa et al., 1985; Risch et al., 1985; Tajima and Tominaga, 1985; Trichopoulos et al., 1985; Jedrychowski et al., 1986, 1992; La Vecchia et al., 1987b, 1997; Kono et al., 1988; You et al., 1988; Buiatti et al., 1989; Coggon et al., 1989; De Stefani et al., 1990, 2000, 2001; Demirer et al., 1990; Graham et al., 1990; Kato et al., 1990; Lee et al., 1990, 1995, 2003b; Wu-Williams et al., 1990b; Boeing et al., 1991a,b; Gonzalez et al., 1991; Yu and Hsieh, 1991; Hoshiyama and Sasaba, 1992; Memik et al., 1992; Palli et al., 1992; Sanchez-Diez et al., 1992; Tuyns et al., 1992; Hansson et al., 1993; Ramon et al., 1993; Inoue et al., 1994; Comee et al., 1995; Harrison et al., 1997; Munoz et al., 1997, 2001; Ji et al., 1998; Gao et al., 1999; Ward and Lopez-Carrillo, 1999; Ekstrom et al., 2000; Huang et al., 2000; Mathew et al., 2000; Terry et al., 2000, 2001b; Hamada et al., 2002; Kim et al., 2002; Nishimoto et al., 2002; Xibin et al., 2002; Cai et al., 2003; Hara et al., 2003; Ito et al., 2003; Nomura et al., 2003) and sixteen cohort studies (Chyou et al., 1990; Nomura et al., 1990; Kneller et al., 1991; Kato et al., 1992; Guo et al., 1994; Inoue et al., 1996; Botterweck et al., 1998; Galanis et al., 1998; Terry et al., 1998; Jansen et al., 1999; McCullough et al., 2001; Appleby et al., 2002; Kasum et al., 2002; Kobayashi et al., 2002; Ngoan et al., 2002; Sauvaget et al., 2003) have examined the association between fruit and vegetable consumption and stomach cancer risk between 1959 and 2001 (Table 6). All of the case-control studies have evaluated incident stomach cancer, and seven of the cohort studies have examined fatal stomach cancer. Most of the studies have been conducted in Asia, Europe, and North America. Most of the case-control studies and all of the cohort studies were initiated before the knowledge of the role of *H. pylori* in stomach carcinogenesis, so the results in only one case-control study have adjusted for *H. pylori* infection.

More than 50 case-control (Higginson, 1966; Correa et al., 1985; Trichopoulos et al., 1985; Jedrychowski et al., 1986, 1992; La Vecchia et al., 1987b, 1997; You et al., 1988; Coggon et al., 1989; De Stefani et al., 1990, 2000, 2001; Kato et al., 1990; Lee et al., 1990, 2003b; Wu-Williams et al., 1990b; Boeing et al., 1991a,b; Yu and Hsieh, 1991; Hoshiyama and Sasaba, 1992; Memik et al., 1992; Sanchez-Diez et al., 1992; Tuyns et al., 1992; Ramon et al., 1993; Inoue et al., 1994; Comee et al., 1995; Xu et al., 1996; Harrison et al., 1997; Mathew et al., 2000; Munoz et al., 1997, 2001; Ji et al., 1998; Gao et al., 1999; Ward and

Lopez-Carrillo, 1999; Ekstrom et al., 2000; Huang et al., 2000; Terry et al., 2001b; Hamada et al., 2002; Kim et al., 2002; Nishimoto et al., 2002; Xibin et al., 2002; Cai et al., 2003; Ito et al., 2003) and cohort (Chyou et al., 1990; Nomura et al., 1990; Kneller et al., 1991; Kato et al., 1992; Guo et al., 1994; Inoue et al., 1996; Botterweck et al., 1998; Galanis et al., 1998; Jansen et al., 1999; Appleby et al., 2002; Kasum et al., 2002; Kobayashi et al., 2002; Ngoan et al., 2002; Sauvaget et al., 2003) studies have assessed the association between stomach cancer risk and intake of fruits. About half of the case-control studies have shown a statistically significant lower risk of stomach cancer with a higher versus lower intake of fruits; odds ratios ranged between 0.30 and 0.72 across studies. Of the remaining case-control studies, several have shown nonsignificant inverse associations. Of the cohort studies, three studies have shown a statistically significant lower risk of stomach cancer with higher intakes of fruits, and among these studies, the magnitude of the association has varied. Most of the cohort studies have reported nonsignificant inverse associations. However, three studies have suggested that fruit intake increases the risk of stomach cancer. Of these studies, two found statistically significant twofold elevations in the risk of stomach cancer with higher intake of fruits. A nonsignificant 50% elevation in the risk of stomach cancer also was observed in a U.S. cohort study.

More than 15 case-control (Demirer et al., 1990; Boeing et al., 1991a; Gonzalez et al., 1991; Palli et al., 1992; Rose, 1992; Tuyns et al., 1992; Ramon et al., 1993; Comee et al., 1995; Harrison et al., 1997; Ward and Lopez-Carrillo, 1999; Ekstrom et al., 2000; Terry et al., 2000; De Stefani et al., 2001; Kim et al., 2002) and cohort studies (Botterweck et al., 1998; Jansen et al., 1999; McCullough et al., 2001) of stomach cancer have evaluated citrus fruits. All of these studies have reported inverse associations comparing high versus low intakes, although only five studies reported few associations that were statistically significant.

Similar to total fruits, a higher intake of vegetables has been associated with a lower risk of stomach cancer in most case-control studies examining this association. Of the 40 studies conducted (Higginson, 1966; Correa et al., 1985; Risch et al., 1985; Trichopoulos et al., 1985; Jedrychowski et al., 1986, 1992; Kono et al., 1988; You et al., 1988; De Stefani et al., 1990; Graham et al., 1990; Kato et al., 1990, 2002; Boeing et al., 1991a; Gonzalez et al., 1991; Kim et al., 2002; Hoshiyama and Sasaba, 1992; Memik et al., 1992; Palli et al., 1992; Sanchez-Diez et al., 1992; Tuyns et al., 1992; Ramon et al., 1993; Inoue et al., 1994; Comee et al., 1995; Lee et al., 1995, 2003b; Rimm, 1996; Xu et al., 1996; Harrison et al., 1997; La Vecchia et al., 1997; Ji et al., 1998; Gao et al., 1999; Ward and Lopez-Carrillo, 1999; Ekstrom et al., 2000; Huang et al., 2000; Mathew et al., 2000; De Stefani et al., 2001; Munoz et al., 2001; Terry et al., 2001b; Xibin et al., 2002; Cai et al., 2003; Hara et al., 2003; Ito et al., 2003; Nomura et al., 2003), more than half of the studies have reported a statistically significant inverse association; of these studies, about half have reported at least a 50% reduction in stomach cancer risk with higher vegetable consumption. Only three case-control studies have reported weak positive associations and none of these was statistically significant. In the cohort studies, the association between vegetable consumption and stomach cancer risk generally has been weaker and not statistically significant in contrast to the consistent inverse association observed in the case-control studies.

Few studies on stomach cancer have evaluated associations with cruciferous vegetable consumption and stomach cancer risk (Risch et al., 1985; Chyou et al., 1990; Kneller et al., 1991; Harrison et al., 1997; Botterweck et al., 1998; Ji et al., 1998; Ekstrom et al., 2000; De Stefani et al., 2001; Hara et al., 2003; Nomura et al., 2003). Although all of these studies have reported nonsignificant associations, the association was in the protective direction in most of the studies.

Green vegetables that have been examined in relation to stomach cancer risk are green and yellow vegetables, leafy vegetables, dark green vegetables, raw green vegetables, and pale green vegetables. Of the case-control studies (Risch et al., 1985; Kono et al., 1988; Demirer et al., 1990; Kato et al., 1990; Lee et al., 1990; Jedrychowski et al., 1992; Tuyns et al., 1992; Ramon et al., 1993; Ji et al., 1998; Ward and Lopez Carrillo, 1999; Ekstrom et al., 2000; Mathew et al., 2000; De Stefani et al., 2001; Hamada et al., 2002; Nishimoto et al., 2002; Ito et al., 2003; Nomura et al., 2003) conducted, about half have reported a statistically significant inverse association, and several others have reported a nonsignificant inverse association. Most of the cohort studies have reported a nonsignificant lower risk of stomach cancer with higher intakes of green vegetables. The risk estimates reported ranged between 0.05 and 1.54.

Summary

Overall, case-control studies generally have shown that fruit and vegetable consumption is inversely associated with the risk of stomach cancer, although the associations in many studies have not been statistically significant. Among cohort studies, weaker and nonsignificant inverse associations have frequently been observed. Studies examining intakes of citrus fruit, cruciferous vegetables, and green vegetables were each suggestive of an inverse association, although many associations were not statistically significant. Because of the small number of studies that have examined different subtypes of stomach cancer (e.g., cardia, noncardia, antrum, intestinal, diffuse, differentiated, and nondifferentiated), we could not examine whether the results differ among these subtypes. In the future, it will be important to understand whether *H. pylori* modifies the association between fruit and vegetable consumption and stomach cancer.

TABLE 6 Summary of Case-Control and Cohort Studies of Fruit and Vegetable Consumption and Stomach Cancer Risk[a]

Author, year, country	Study dates	Study population	Comparison	Odds ratio/relative risk (95% CI), unless otherwise noted	
				Total fruit	Citrus fruit
Case-control studies					
Higginson et al., 1966, USA	1959-	93 cases, 1020 hospital controls	Daily vs never	Cases = 50% daily, Controls = 59.5% daily; Cases = 5.7% never, Controls = 2.3% never	
Correa et al., 1985, USA	1979–1983	391 cases, 391 hospital controls	Highest vs lowest quartile	White: 0.47 (0.24–0.92), p for trend < 0.005; black: 0.33 (0.16–0.66), p for trend < 0.01	
Risch et al., 1985, Canada	1979–1982	246 cases, 246 population controls	Increment = 100 g/day		
Trichopoulous et al., 1985, Greece	1981–1984	110 cases, 100 hospital controls	Highest vs lowest quartile	No association, $\chi^2 = 0.3$	
Jedrychowski et al., 1986, Poland	1980–1981	110 cases, 110 hospital controls	Less frequently vs daily or almost daily[b]	3.24 (1.56–6.77), [0.31, 0.15–0.64]	
Kono et al., 1988, Japan	1979–1982	139 cases, 2574 hospital controls	Highest vs lowest tertile		
You et al., 1988, China	1984–1986	564 cases, 1131 population controls	>30 g vs <5 g for fruits; >156 g vs <73 g for vegetables	Fresh: 0.6 (0.4–0.8)	
Coggon et al., 1989, United Kingdom	1985–1987	95 cases, 190 population controls	>5 times/wk vs <1 time/wk	0.6 (0.2–1.5)	
Demirer et al., 1990, Turkey	1987–1988	100 cases, 61 hospital and 39 population controls	>1–2 times/wk vs <1–2 times/mo		0.06 (0.03–0.13)
De Stefani et al., 1990, Uruguay	1985–1988	210 cases, 630 hospital controls	≤2 times /wk vs 5–7 times/wk[b]	2.8 (1.8–4.3), [0.36, 0.23–0.56], p for trend < 0.001	
Graham et al., 1990, USA	1975–1985	293 cases, 285 population controls (Male: 186 cases, 181 controls)	Unknown	No association	
Kato et al., 1990, Japan	1985–1989	427 cases, 1247 hospital controls	Daily vs 1–2 times/mo	Women: 0.77 (0.33–1.78); men: 0.83 (0.51–1.33)	
Lee et al., 1990, Taiwan, China	1954–1988	217 cases, 820 hospital controls	6+ vs <1 meals/wk for fruits; 15+ vs <14 meals/wk for green vegetables	Diet before age 20: 0.91, ns; Diet age 20 to 39: 1.09, ns	
Wu-Williams et al., 1990, USA	1975–1982	137 cases, 137 population controls	≤1/wk vs ≥5/wk[bb]	1.5 (0.6–3.5), [0.67, 0.29–1.67]	

Odds ratio/relative risk (95% CI), unless otherwise noted				
Total vegetables	**Cruciferous vegetables**	**Green vegetables**	**Matching and adjustment factors**	**Miscellaneous**
Cooked: Cases = 36.6% >daily, controls = 35.1% >daily; Cases = 6.5% never, Controls = 2.5% never raw: Cases = 11.8% >daily, Controls = 12.9% >daily; Cases = 25.8% never, Controls = 17.9% never				
White: inverse; black: 0.50 (0.25–1.00), p for trend < 0.05			Sex, age, race, respondent status, income, and duration of smoking	
0.84 (0.72–0.96), p for trend = 0.01	0.65 (0.38–1.12), p for trend = 0.11	Pale green: 0.29 (0.07–1.11), p for trend = 0.05	Sex, age, province of residence, total food consumption and ethnicity (for pale green vegetables, also grains, grain products, chocolate, fibrous foods, smoked meats, eggs, and public water supply) (for vegetables, also dietary fiber, nitrite, chocolate, carbohydrate, and duration without refrigeration)	
Inverse trend, < 0.001			Age, sex, and years of schooling	
1.63 (0.67–3.97), [0.61, 0.25–1.49]			Residence and smoking	
Raw vegetables: 0.8, χ^2 trend = 1.74		Green-yellow vegetables: 1.3, χ^2 trend = 0.46	Age and sex, occupational class	
Fresh: 0.4 (0.3–0.6)			Sex, age, and family income	
			Age, sex, length of refrigerator use, dietary variables, and socioeconomic class	
		Raw, yellow and green: 0.05 (0.02–0.10)	Age, sex, and residential area	
2.7 (1.7–4.3), [0.37, 0.23–0.59], p for trend < 0.001			Age, sex, residence, smoking duration, wine ingestion and meat, salted meat, mate, and fruit and vegetable	
Raw: 0.43 (0.23–0.78)			Age, neighborhood, sex, and education	
Raw, women: 0.84 (0.47–1.51); raw, men: 0.59 (0.37–0.93)		Green-yellow vegetables, women: 0.81 (0.61–1.09); men: 0.81 (0.56–1.16)	Adjusted for age and residence	Also stratified by subtype
		Green vegetable diet before age 20: 0.82, ns; Green vegetable diet age 20–39: 0.92, ns	Age, sex, and hospital	Also stratified by subsite
			Sex, year of birth, and race	

(*continues*)

TABLE 6 *(Continued)*

Author, year, country	Study dates	Study population	Comparison	Odds ratio/relative risk (95% CI), unless otherwise noted: Total fruit	Citrus fruit
Boeing et al., 1991, Germany	1985–1988	143 cases, 579 hospital and visitor controls	Highest vs lowest tertile	Fruit: 0.56 (0.35–0.91); domestic: 0.62 (0.39–0.98)	0.42 (0.26–0.69)
Gonzalez et al., 1991, Spain	1987–1989	354 cases, 354 hospital controls	Highest vs lowest quartile		0.99, *p* for trend = 0.89
Yu & Hsieh, 1991, China	1976–1980	84 cases, 2676 population controls	Users vs nonusers	0.5 (0.3–0.8)	
Hoshiyama and Sasaba, 1992, Japan	1984–1990	216 cases, 483 population controls	Highest vs lowest tertile	0.8 (0.5–1.3), *p* for trend = 0.34	
Jedrychowski, 1992, Poland	1986–1990	741 cases, 741 household controls	Highest vs lowest tertile	0.72 (0.56–0.94), *p* for trend = 0.015	
Memik et al., 1992, Turkey	1977–1991	252 cases, 609 controls	5+ times/wk vs 0–1 times/wk	Fresh: nonsignificant	
Palli et al., 1992, Italy	1985–1987	923 cases, 1159 population controls	Highest vs lowest tertile		All other gastric: 0.6 (0.4–0.7); cardia: 0.3 (0.2–0.6)
Sanchez-Diez et al., 1992, Spain	1975–1986	109 cases, 123 population controls	Daily vs nonconsumption	Fresh: 3.26 (1.15–9.24), [0.31, 0.11–0.87]	
Tuyns et al., 1992, Belgium	1979–1982	449 cases, 3524 population controls	Highest vs lowest quartile	Fresh: 0.56, *p* for trend = 0.0001	0.82, *p* for trend = 0.40
Ramon et al., 1993, Spain	1986–1989	117 cases, 234 population controls	Highest vs lowest quartile for fruit, vegetables, and green vegetables; highest vs lowest tertile for citrus fruit	0.85 (0.21–1.11)	0.47 (0.21–0.76)
Inoue et al., 1994, Japan	1988–1991	668 cases, 668 hospital controls	3–4 times or more/wk vs less	All: 0.86 (0.70–1.10); cardia: 0.97 (0.69–1.48); middle: 0.86 (0.64–1.21); antrum: 0.84 (0.62–1.14)	
Cornee et al., 1995, France	1985–1988	92 cases, 128 hospital controls	Highest vs lowest tertile	Fresh: 0.50 (0.25–1.03), *p* for trend = 0.02	0.57 (0.26–1.25), *p* for trend = 0.17

Odds ratio/relative risk (95% CI), unless otherwise noted				
Total vegetables	**Cruciferous vegetables**	**Green vegetables**	**Matching and adjustment factors**	**Miscellaneous**
Vegetables: 0.86 (0.54–1.36); raw: 0.63 (0.39–1.02)			Adjusted for age, sex, and hospital	
Raw: 0.8, *p* for trend = 0.25; cooked: 0.6 (0.3–1.0), *p* for trend = 0.12			Total calories (and other dietary foods for cooked vegetables and other fruits), age, sex, and area of residence	
			Age, sex, family income, family history of stomach cancer, family history of other cancer, history of tuberculosis, blood type, cigarette smoking, alcohol, strong tea, fruit, and milk consumption	
Raw: 0.6 (0.3–1.0), *p* for trend = 0.04			Age and smoking status	
0.60 (0.46–0.78), *p* for trend < 0.001		Green leafy: 0.76 (0.58–1.00), *p* for trend = 0.048	Age, sex, education, occupation of the index person and for residency, source of vegetable and fruits and status of respondent	Update of Boeing et al., 1991
0.6 (0.31–1.23), *p* for trend < 0.05			Age and sex	
Raw, all other gastric: 0.6 (0.3–0.8); raw, cardia: 0.4 (0.2–0.8); cooked, all other gastric: 1.1 (0.9–1.4); cooked, cardia: 1.5 (0.8–2.8)			Age and sex, area, place of residence, migration from the south, socioeconomic status, familial GC history and body mass index, along with dietary or other variables of interest, and log total caloric intake	Update of Buiatti et al., 1989. Only analyzed by subtype
Fresh: 1.42 (0.93–2.43), [0.70, 0.41–1.08]			Age, sex, and municipality of residence	
Cooked: 0.33, *p* for trend < 0.0001; raw: 0.40, *p* for trend < 0.0001		Cooked leafy vegetables: 0.35, *p* for trend = < 0.001	Sex, age, and province	
0.66, ns		Raw, green: 0.56 (0.29–0.84)	Sex, age, and telephone ownership, education, cig/day, rice, cereals, smoked and pickled foods, salt (and citrus fruits, raw green veg, and all fruits)	
All: 0.70 (0.55–0.88); cardia: 0.60 (0.41–0.90); middle: 0.78 (0.56–1.08), antrum: 0.68 (0.50–0.93)			Age, sex, and time of hospital visit	Also stratified by subtype
Total: 0.77 (0.37–1.60), *p* for trend = 0.68; raw: 0.41 (0.19–0.88), *p* for trend = 0.02; cooked: 1.06 (0.53–2.13), *p* for trend = 0.51; raw and cooked: 0.95 (0.46–1.96), *p* for trend = 0.53			Age, sex, occupation, and total energy intake	

(*continues*)

TABLE 6 *(Continued)*

Author, year, country	Study dates	Study population	Comparison	Odds ratio/relative risk (95% CI), unless otherwise noted	
				Total fruit	Citrus fruit
Lee et al., 1995, Korea	1990–1991	213 cases, 213 hospital controls	Highest vs lowest tertile		
Xu et al., 1996, China	1989–1993	293 cases, 959 population controls	55+ jing/year vs 0 jing/year for fruit; 7.4+ jing/wk vs <5.4 jing/wk for vegetables	0.5 (0.4–0.8)	
Harrison et al., 1997, USA	1992–1994	91 cases, 132 hospital controls	Increment = one standard deviation	Intestinal: 0.5 (0.3–0.9), p for trend < 0.05; diffuse: 0.5 (0.2–0.99), p for trend < 0.05; raw, intestinal: 0.6 (0.3–0.99), p for trend < 0.05; raw, diffuse: 0.7 (0.4–1.3)	Citrus fruit + juice, Intestinal: 0.8 (0.5–1.3); Citrus fruit + juice, diffuse: 0.6 (0.2–1.3); Citrus fruit, intestinal: 0.7 (0.4–1.3); Citrus fruit, diffuse: 0.8 (0.4–1.4)
La Vecchia et al., 1997, Italy	1985–1993	746 cases, 2053 hospital controls	≥3 vs <2 times for fruit; >7 vs ≤5 times for vegetables	0.6 (0.5–0.8), p for trend < 0.001	
Ji et al., 1998, China	1988–1989	1124 cases, 1451 population controls	Highest vs lowest quartile	Women: 0.5 (0.3–0.8), p for trend = 0.0006; men: 0.4 (0.3–0.6), p for trend < 0.001	
Gao et al., 1999, China	1995	153 cases, 234 population controls	≥1 vs ≤1 time/mo for fruit, frequently vs almost never for vegetables	0.88 (0.47–1.67)	
Ward and Lopez-Carrillo, 1999, Mexico	1989–1990	220 cases, 752 population controls	≥5 vs <2 times/day for fruit; ≥9 vs <2 times/wk for citrus fruit; ≥6 vs <4 times/day for vegetables; ≥10 vs <5 times/wk for dark green vegetables	All: 1.0 (0.5–2.2), p for trend = 0.67; intestinal: 0.8 (0.3–2.2); diffuse: 1.4 (0.5–3.8)	All: 0.7 (0.3–1.5), p for trend = 0.07; intestinal: 0.9 (0.3–2.7); diffuse: 0.5 (0.2–1.8)
Ekstrom et al., 2000, Sweden	1989–1995	567 cases, 1165 population controls	>1/day vs ≤2/wk for fruit; ≥3–4/wk vs <1/mo for citrus fruit; ≥2/day vs <5/wk for vegetables; ≥2/wk vs never/seldom for green vegetables	Cardia: 0.5 (0.2–1.0), p for trend = 0.03; non-cardia: 0.6 (0.4–0.8), p for trend < 0.01; intestinal: 0.6 (0.4–0.9), p for trend = 0.01; diffuse: 0.5 (0.3–0.9), p for trend = 0.05	Cardia: 0.8 (0.4–2.0), p for trend = 0.26; non-cardia: 0.8 (0.5–1.2), p for trend = 0.04; intestinal: 0.9 (0.6–1.5), p for trend = 0.09; diffuse: 0.6 (0.3–1.1), p for trend = 0.16
Huang et al., 2000, Japan	1988–1995	1111 cases, 26,996 controls	>3 times /wk vs <3 times/ month	Family history: 1.39 (0.69–2.82); No family history: 1.11 (0.74–1.67)	

Odds ratio/relative risk (95% CI), unless otherwise noted				
Total vegetables	Cruciferous vegetables	Green vegetables	Matching and adjustment factors	Miscellaneous
Fresh: 1.2 (0.8–1.9), ns			Age, sex, education, economic status, residence, and mutually adjusted for other dietary factors	
0.5 (0.4–0.8)			Age and sex, birth year, smoking, education, stomach disease, family stomach cancer (and fruit and vegetable and pickled veg)	
Intestinal: 0.8 (0.5–1.3); diffuse: 0.7 (0.4–1.2); raw, intestinal: 0.6 (0.4–1.1); raw, diffuse: 0.6 (0.3–1.2)	Intestinal: 0.8 (0.5–1.5); diffuse: 0.9 (0.5–1.7)		Caloric intake, age, gender, race, education, pack-years of smoking, alcohol drinking, and body mass index	Only analyzed by subtype
0.5 (0.4–0.7), *p* for trend < 0.001			Age, sex, area of residence, education, family history of stomach cancer, total number of servings, body mass index, and total energy intake	Update of La Vecchia, 1987 and Munoz et al., 1997
Women: 0.7 (0.5–1.1), *p* for trend = 0.09; men: 0.4 (0.3–0.5), *p* for trend < 0.001	Women: 0.8 (0.5–1.1), *p* for trend = 0.20; men: 0.8 (0.6–1.1), *p* for trend = 0.07	Yellow and green vegetable, women: 0.7 (0.5–1.1), *p* for trend = 0.08; yellow and green vegetable, men: 0.5 (0.4–0.7), *p* for trend = 0.001	Age and sex, income, education, smoking (males only) and alcohol drinking (males only)	
Raw: 0.07 (0.04–0.13)			Age, sex, and neighborhood	
All: 0.3 (0.1–0.6), *p* for trend = 0.001; intestinal: 0.3 (0.1–0.6); diffuse: 0.3 (0.1–0.7)		All dark green: 1.0 (0.6–1.8), *p* for trend = 0.90; intestinal dark green: 0.9 (0.5–1.9); diffuse dark green: 1.1 (0.5–2.5)	Age, gender, total calories, chili pepper consumption, added salt, history of peptic ulcer, cig smoking and socioeconomic status	Also stratified by subtype
Cardia: 0.5 (0.3–1.1), *p* for trend = 0.05; non-cardia: 0.7 (0.5–1.0), *p* for trend = 0.02; intestinal: 0.6 (0.3–0.9), *p* for trend = 0.02; diffuse: 0.7 (0.4–1.1), *p* for trend = 0.08	Cardia: 0.7 (0.3–1.4), *p* for trend = 0.24; non-cardia: 0.8 (0.6–1.2), *p* for trend = 0.19; intestinal: 0.6 (0.4–1.0), *p* for trend = 0.10; diffuse: 1.0 (0.6–1.6), *p* for trend = 0.52	Dark green, cardia: 0.4 (0.2–0.9), *p* for trend < 0.01; non-cardia: 0.9 (0.6–1.3), *p* for trend = 0.40; intestinal: 0.7 (0.4–1.2), *p* for trend = 0.20; diffuse: 0.9 (0.51–1.6), *p* for trend = 0.71	Age, sex, total caloric intake, tobacco use, body mass index, geographic risk area, number of siblings, SES, number of meals/day, multivitamin supplement, table salt use, and urban environment	Update of Hansson et al., 1993. Also stratified by subtype
Raw, family history: 0.52 (0.27–0.99), *p* for trend < 0.05; raw, no family history: 0.95 (0.64–1.41)			Age at diagnosis, gender, habitual smoking and drinking, and carrots, lettuce, pumpkin, raw vegetables, and picked vegetables	

(*continues*)

TABLE 6 (*Continued*)

Author, year, country	Study dates	Study population	Comparison	Odds ratio/relative risk (95% CI), unless otherwise noted	
				Total fruit	Citrus fruit
Mathew et al., 2000, India	1988–1991	194 cases, 305 hospital visitor controls	>9 vs ≤3 for fruits and vegetables; >2 times/week vs never/occasional for leafy vegetables	0.7 (0.2–3.6), *p* for trend = 0.99	
Terry et al., 2000, Sweden; Terry et al., 2001, Sweden	1994–1997	258 cases, 815 population controls	Highest vs lowest quartile	1.0 (0.6–1.4), *p* for trend = 0.23	0.9 (0.6–1.5), *p* for trend = 0.84
De Stefani et al., 2001, Uruguay	1997–2000	160 cases, 320 hospital controls	Highest vs lowest tertile	0.33 (0.20–0.56), *p* for trend < 0.001	0.51 (0.31–0.85), *p* for trend = 0.01
Munoz et al., 2001, Venezuala	1991–1997	292 cases, 485 population controls	Highest vs lowest quartile	2.27 (1.40–3.70), *p* for trend = 0.001	
Hamada et al., 2002, Brazil	1991–1994	96 cases, 192 hospital controls	Daily vs <3–4 d/wk for fruits; daily vs <1 d/wk for green vegetables	0.4 (0.2–0.9)	
Kim et al., 2002, Korea	1997–1998	136 cases, 136 hospital controls	Highest vs lowest tertile	Total: 0.67 (0.33–1.39), *p* for trend = 0.56	0.66 (0.31–1.41), *p* for trend = 0.27
Nishimoto et al., 2002, Brazil	1991–1994	236 cases, 236 hospital controls	Daily vs 1d/wk	0.6 (0.3–1.2), *p* for trend = 0.08	
Xibin et al., 2002, China	1998–1999	210 cases, 630 hospital controls	Highest vs lowest quartile	1.24, *p* for trend = 0.44	
Cai et al., 2003, China	2000–2001	381 (191 cardia, 190 non-cardia) cases, 222 hospital controls	≥3 times/wk vs <1 times/mo for fruit and pickled vegetables; ≥3 vs <3 times/wk for fresh vegetables	Fresh fruit, cardia: 0.23 (0.11–0.45), *p* for trend < 0.001; non-cardia: 0.29 (0.15–0.56), *p* for trend < 0.001	
Hara et al., 2003, Japan	1998–2002	115 cases, 115 population controls	Highest vs lowest tertile		
Ito et al., 2003, Japan	1988–1998	508 cases, 36,490 controls	Highest vs lowest quartile	0.68 (0.40–1.16), *p* for trend < 0.001	

Odds ratio/relative risk (95% CI), unless otherwise noted				
Total vegetables	Cruciferous vegetables	Green vegetables	Matching and adjustment factors	Miscellaneous
1.1 (0.2–5.0), p for trend = 0.08		Leafy vegetable: 1.2 (0.7–2.0), p for trend = 0.18	Age, sex, religion, residential area, education, income, smoking and alcohol habits	
0.8 (0.6–1.3), p for trend = 0.44			Age, gender, body mass index, total energy, energy adjusted alcohol, total fruit and vegetable intake, cig smoking and use of antacids (gastroesophageal reflux symptoms)	
All: 0.64 (0.38–1.08), p for trend = 0.10; raw: 0.52 (0.31–0.86), p for trend = 0.01; cooked: 0.93 (0.57–1.51), p for trend = 0.81	1.59 (0.88–2.86), p for trend = 0.34	Green leafy: 0.73 (0.46–1.18), p for trend = 0.19	Sex, age, residence and urban/rural status, education, body mass index, and total energy intake	Update of De Stefani et al., 2000
0.35 (0.21–0.59), p for trend < 0.001			Age, sex, SES (also tobacco, alcohol, total calories for starchy veg, vegetable and fruit)	
		0.9 (0.4–1.9)	Age, gender, country of birth (and beef consumption for fruit analysis)	
Total: 0.64 (0.31–1.32), p for trend = 0.02; raw: 0.55 (0.28–1.09), p for trend = 0.16; cooked: 0.98 (0.50–1.90), p for trend = 0.67			Age sex, socioeconomic status, fam history and refrigerator use	
		0.7 (0.4–1.3), p for trend = 0.33	Age and gender, race and education, smoking, and fruit and vegetable intake	
0.27, p for trend < 0.01			Age, income, resident space, refrigerator use, and educational level	
Fresh vegetable, cardia: 0.44 (0.21–0.91), p for trend = 0.03; non-cardia: 0.64 (0.30–1.37), p for trend = 0.25; pickled vegetable, cardia: 1.76 (1.04–2.97), p for trend = 0.03; non-cardia:1.27 (0.77–2.10), p for trend = 0.36			Age, gender, smoking, drinking and family cancer history in the first degree relative	Also stratified by histopathological status and tumor
1.12 (0.61–2.05), p for trend = 0.70	1.11 (0.58–2.13), p for trend = 0.76		Smoking status, alcohol intake, family history of stomach cancer, salt intake, energy intake and Japan, Agricultural Cooperatives membership	Only analyzed by subtype
Raw: 0.50 (0.36–0.71), p for trend < 0.001		0.60 (0.43–0.83), p for trend < 0.001	Age, year, and season of first hospital visit, smoking habit and fam history of gastric cancer	Analyses stratified by differentiated/ nondifferentiated

(*continues*)

TABLE 6 *(Continued)*

Author, year, country	Study dates	Study population	Comparison	Odds ratio/relative risk (95% CI), unless otherwise noted	
				Total fruit	Citrus fruit
Lee S, 2003, J Epidemiol, Korea	1999	69 cases, 199 healthy controls	>5 vs <3/wk for fruit; >7 vs 2/mo for seasoned, raw vegetables; >6/wk vs <4/wk for raw veg	Fruits: 0.3 (0.1–0.7), p for trend < 0.01; fruits or fruit juice: 0.5 (0.2–1.2), p for trend < 0.01	
Nomura et al., 2003, USA	1993–1999	300 cases, 446 population controls	Highest vs lowest tertile		
Cohort studies					
Chyou et al., 1990, Hawaii	1965–1986	111 cases, 8006 (analyzed as a case-cohort study with a subcohort of 361)	≥301 vs 0 g/day for fruits; ≥80 vs 0 g/day for vegetables vs 0 g/day for green vegetables; ≥60 vs 0 g/day for cruciferous vegetables	0.8 (0.4–1.3), p for trend = 0.20	
Nomura, 1990, Cancer Res, Hawaii	1965–1986	150 cases, cohort of 7990	≥5/wk vs ≤1/wk	0.8 (0.5–1.3)	
Kneller et al., 1991, USA	1966–1986	75 fatal cases, cohort of 17,633	Highest vs lowest quartile	1.5 (0.75–2.93), p for trend ns	
Kato et al., 1992, Japan	1985–1991	57 fatal cases, cohort of 9753	Daily vs ≤1–2/wk	1.92 (1.03–3.59), p for trend = 0.04	
Guo et al., 1994, China	1986–1991	539 cases, cohort of ~30,000 (analyzed as a nested case-control study with 2695 population controls)	≥1 vs 0 times/mo for fruits; ≥60 vs ≤30 times/mo for vegetables	Fresh: 0.9 (0.8–1.1)	
Inoue et al., 1996, Japan	1985–1995	69 cases, cohort of 5373	Highest vs lowest tertile	0.55 (0.22–1.35)	
Botterweck et al., 1998, Netherlands	1986–1992	282 cases, cohort of 120,852 (analyzed as a case-cohort study with a subcohort of 3500)	Highest vs lowest quintile for fruit, citrus fruit, vegetables, cruciferous vegetables; prepared leafy vegetables; highest vs lowest tertile for raw leafy vegetables	Total: 0.97 (0.64–1.48), p for trend = 0.51	0.86 (0.57–1.29), p for trend = 0.20
Galanis et al., 1998, USA	1975 (+14.8 yr mean follow-up)	108 cases, cohort of 11,907	7+ vs 0–6 times/wk	All: 0.6 (0.4–0.9); women: 0.7 (0.4–1.4); men: 0.6 (0.3–1.0)	
Terry et al., 1998, Sweden	1967–1992	116 cases, cohort of 11,546 twins	None/very little vs high[b]		

Odds ratio/relative risk (95% CI), unless otherwise noted				
Total vegetables	**Cruciferous vegetables**	**Green vegetables**	**Matching and adjustment factors**	**Miscellaneous**
Seasoned, raw: 0.2 (0.1–0.6), p for trend = 0.01; raw: 0.2 (0.1–0.5), p for trend < 0.01			Age, sex, education, family history of gastric cancer, smoking, drinking, and *H. pylori* infection	
Women: 0.4 (0.2–0.8), p for trend = 0.01; men: 0.4 (0.2–0.6), p for trend < 0.001	Women: 0.6 (0.3–1.1), p for trend = 0.09; men: 0.6 (0.4–1.0), p for trend = 0.07	Dark green, women: 0.4 (0.2–0.8), p for trend = 0.01; dark green, men: 0.3 (0.2–0.6), p for trend < 0.001; light green, women: 0.5 (0.2–1.0), p for trend = 0.02; light green, men: 0.4 (0.3–0.7), p for trend < 0.001	Age, ethnicity, cig smoking status, education, history of gastric ulcer, NSAID use, fam history of gastric cancer, and total calories	
All: 0.7 (0.4–1.1), p for trend = 0.001	0.7 (0.4–1.2), p for trend = 0.07	0.7 (0.4–1.2), p for trend = 0.06	Age and smoking	
			Age	
0.9 (0.48–1.78), p for trend ns	1.3 (0.67–2.68), p for trend ns		Year of birth, current cigarette smoking	
		Green-yellow vegetables: 1.54 (0.77–3.11), p for trend = 0.23	Age and sex	
Fresh: 1.1 (0.8–1.4)			Age, sex, years of smoking and cancer history in first degree relatives	
Raw: 0.67 (0.29–1.57)		Green-yellow vegetables: 0.74 (0.17–3.20)	Gender and age	
Total: 0.86 (0.58–1.26), p for trend = 0.25; prepared: 0.81 (0.56–1.19), p for trend = 0.26; raw: 0.97 (0.64–1.46), p for trend = 0.96	0.93 (0.61–1.43), p for trend = 0.29	Prepared leafy: 0.96 (0.63–1.44), p for trend = 0.98; raw leafy: 0.90 (0.64–1.25), p for trend = 0.76	Age, sex, education, stomach disorders, and family history of stomach cancer (and fruit and vegetable consumption)	
Raw, all: 0.8 (0.5–1.2); raw, women: 0.7 (0.4–1.4); raw, men: 0.9 (0.5–1.5)			Age, years of education, Japanese place of birth and gender (in combined analyses). Men were also adjusted for cigarette smoking and alcohol intake status	
			Alcohol intake, age, gender, smoking status, body mass index at age 25, and childhood socioeconomic status	

(*continues*)

TABLE 6 (*Continued*)

Author, year, country	Study dates	Study population	Comparison	Odds ratio/relative risk (95% CI), unless otherwise noted	
				Total fruit	Citrus fruit
Jansen et al., 1999, Seven Countries	1958–1989	267 fatal cases, cohort of 12,761	Increment = change in intake of 10% of the mean	0.96 (0.91–0.99)	0.95 (0.92–0.98)
McCullough et al., 2001, USA	1982–1996	1349 fatal cases, cohort of 1,184,657	Highest vs lowest tertile		Women: 0.97 (0.78–1.21), *p* for trend = 0.79; men: 0.88 (0.75–1.03), *p* for trend = 0.11
Appleby et al., 2002, United Kingdom	1973–1997	40 fatal cases, cohort of 10,741	Daily vs <daily	All: 0.88 (0.41–1.88); women: 0.52 (0.20–1.34); men: 1.73 (0.49–6.16); nonsmokers: 1.12 (0.43–2.93)	
Kasum et al., 2002, USA	1986–1999	56 cases, cohort of 34,351	Unknown	Inverse, ns	
Kobayashi et al., 2002, Japan	1990–1999	404 cases, cohort of 39,993	Almost daily vs <1/day for fruits and green vegetables; highest vs lowest quintile for vegetables	0.70 (0.48–1.01), *p* for trend = 0.25	
Ngoan et al., 2002, Japan	1986–1998	116 fatal cases, cohort of 13,250	Highest vs lowest tertile	All: 0.9 (0.3–2.1); women: 1.5 (0.6–3.8); men: 1.6 (0.8–3.3)	
Sauvaget et al., 2003, Japan	1980–1998	617 fatal cases, cohort of 38,540	Highest vs lowest tertile	0.80 (0.65–0.98), *p* for trend = 0.03	

[a]The following studies have examined the association between fruit and vegetable consumption and stomach cancer risk but did not report associations for the groups included in the table: Tajima and Tuminaga, 1985.

[b] The inverse of the relative risk was calculated to represent a comparison of high vs low intake and is included in brackets after the published estimate.

Prostate Cancer

Worldwide prostate cancer is the second most common incident cancer and the sixth highest cause of cancer mortality in men (Ferlay et al., 2004). Leading the world in the highest rates are North America, northwest Europe (particularly Scandinavian countries), and the Caribbean, while Asia and South America have some of the lowest rates. In the United States, prostate cancer is the leading cause of cancer and the second highest cause of cancer mortality among men (American Cancer Society, 2005).

One of the most influential advances in prostate cancer prevention has been the widespread use of prostate-specific antigen (PSA), which was introduced between 1988 and 1992 for screening (Platz et al., 2004). Use of the PSA measure has led to a shift in the diagnosis of the prostate cancers being detected, with more prostate cancers being diagnosed at earlier or localized stages (Crawford, 2003; Quaglia et al., 2003; Hugosson et al., 2004). In the Prostate, Lung, Colorectal, and Ovary Cancer trial, in the group receiving screening, only 6% of the prostate cancers were poorly differentiated, whereas 17–25% would have been

Odds ratio/relative risk (95% CI), unless otherwise noted				
Total vegetables	**Cruciferous vegetables**	**Green vegetables**	**Matching and adjustment factors**	**Miscellaneous**
0.96 (0.82–1.11)			Energy and smoking	
Women: 1.25 (0.99–1.58), p for trend = 0.06; men: 0.89 (0.76–1.05), p for trend = 0.17			Age, education, smoking, body mass index, multivitamin and vitamin C use, aspirin use, race and family history	
			Adjusted for age at recruitment, and where applicable, sex and smoking	Update of Key et al., 1996
Inverse, ns			Whole grains, refined grains, alcohol, smoking, age, and energy intake	
0.75 (0.54–1.04), p for trend = 0.17		0.77 (0.40–1.46), p for trend = 0.62	Age, gender, area, educational level, smoking status, body mass index, alcohol intake, use of vitamin A, C, E supplement, total energy intake, highly salted food intake, history of peptic ulcer, and family history of gastric cancer	
		Green and yellow, all: 0.4 (0.2–1.1); green and yellow, women: 1.0 (0.3–3.5); green and yellow, men: 0.9 (0.5–1.8)	Age	
		Green and yellow: 0.91	Sex, age, radiation dose, city, body mass index, smoking status, alcohol habits and education level	Also stratified by smoking status and gender

poorly differentiated in the nonscreened group (de Koning et al., 2002).

Although in the United States the 5-year survival rate in 2004 was 100% for local and regional stages and 98% for all stages, much needs to be learned about the risk factors and preventive measures for prostate cancer. Epidemiological studies have shown that advancing age, African-American race, and family history of prostate cancer are risk factors for prostate cancer (Crawford, 2003). Studies conducted among men of Japanese ancestry have shown that prostate cancer incidence rates are higher among Japanese men who have immigrated to the United States and among men of Japanese ancestry born in the United States compared with Japanese men (Shimizu et al., 1991; Whittemore et al., 1995; Cook et al., 1999). These studies have led to hypotheses that environmental factors, including diet, may influence the risk of prostate cancer. Typically, Asian diets are lower in fat and red meat intake and higher in soy intake than Western diets, and Asian diets have been associated with a lower prostate cancer risk in ecological and migrant studies (Rose et al., 1986; Yu et al., 1991; Tominaga and Kuroishi, 1997). Although a study conducted in the NHANES Epidemiological Follow-up suggested that the red meat–starch pattern was not associated with prostate cancer risk (Tseng et al., 2004), red meat intake has been shown to be positively associated with prostate cancer risk in two case-control studies and four cohort studies (Kolonel, 2001). Other studies have shown that lower intakes of selenium may lead to a higher risk of prostate cancer (Dagnelie et al., 2004; Li et al., 2004). Diets high in dairy products, possibly related to calcium, have been associated with an increased risk of advanced prostate cancer (Giovannucci, 2005).

The relationship between fruit and vegetable consumption and the risk of prostate cancer has been examined in at least 28 case-control (Schuman et al., 1982; Graham et al., 1983; Mishina et al., 1985; Ross et al., 1987; Oishi et al., 1988; Le Marchand et al., 1991; Negri et al., 1991; Talamini et al., 1986, 1992; Walker et al., 1992; Beckett, 1993; Andersson et al., 1995; De Stefani et al., 1995; Whittemore et al., 1995; Ewings and Bowie, 1996; Key et al., 1997; Lee et al., 1998; Deneo-Pellegrini et al., 1999; Hayes et al., 1999; Jain et al., 1999; Sung et al., 1999; Tzonou et al., 1999; Villeneuve et al., 1999; Bosetti et al., 2000, 2004; Cohen et al., 2000; Kolonel et al., 2000; Norrish et al., 2000; Hsing et al., 2002; Sonoda et al., 2004) and 15 cohort studies (Snowdon et al., 1984; Mills et al., 1989; Severson et al., 1989; Hirayama, 1990; Hsing et al., 1990; Shibata et al., 1992; Le Marchand et al., 1994; Giovannucci et al., 1995, 2002, 2003; Gronberg et al., 1996; Rodriguez et al., 1997; Schuurman et al., 1998; Fraser, 1999; Chan et al., 2000; Appleby et al., 2002; Key et al., 2004) (Table 7). Approximately half of the case-control studies used hospital controls; the remainder of the case-control studies used population or neighborhood controls. Most studies were conducted in North America and Europe. The studies were conducted from 1957 until 2002. Approximately half of the case-control studies and almost all of the cohort studies were initiated prior to the PSA era, with only one case-control and one cohort study adjusting for or stratifying by PSA screening. By restricting the analysis to men who were screened by a PSA test, the analysis limited the potential for detection bias in those studies that have included prostate cancer cases diagnosed when PSA screening was prevalent. Furthermore, because PSA screening has shifted the stage distribution of the cases over the past decade to more localized-stage cancers, future analyses should take into account PSA screening to be able to compare similar case populations. This stratification is particularly important if associations with prostate cancer are different for localized versus advanced or metastatic prostate cancer. In addition, four cohort studies focused on fatal prostate cancer (Snowdon et al., 1984; Hsing et al., 1990; Rodriguez et al., 1997; Appleby et al., 2002), which should be less influenced by the increase in PSA screening.

At least 13 case-control (Negri et al., 1991; Talamini et al., 1992; De Stefani et al., 1995; Lee et al., 1998; Deneo-Pellegrini et al., 1999; Hayes et al., 1999; Jain et al., 1999; Tzonou et al., 1999; Sung et al., 1999; Villeneuve et al., 1999; Cohen et al., 2000; Kolonel et al., 2000; Sonoda et al., 2004) and 11 cohort studies (Snowdon et al., 1984; Mills et al., 1989; Severson et al., 1989; Hsing et al., 1990; Shibata et al., 1992; Le Marchand et al., 1994; Giovannucci et al., 1995; Schuurman et al., 1998; Chan et al., 2000; Appleby et al., 2002; Key et al., 2004) have evaluated whether fruit intake is associated with the risk of prostate cancer. Most of the studies have found nonsignificant associations. Only one case-control study has reported a statistically significant lower risk of prostate cancer with higher intake of fruits (OR = OA, 95% CI 0.3–0.8). A statistically significant inverse trend also has been observed in the Adventist Health Study, a cohort study of ~14,000 Seventh Day Adventist men. However, three case-control studies have shown that men who consumed the highest quantity of fruits compared with the lowest quantity had at least a 50% higher risk of prostate cancer. Additionally, in the Netherlands Cohort Study, a population-based study of >58,000 men, a statistically significant positive trend was observed between fruit consumption and prostate cancer risk.

Relatively few studies have examined the association between citrus fruits and prostate cancer (Mills et al., 1989; Whittemore et al., 1995; Key et al., 1997; Schuurman et al., 1998; Jain et al., 1999; Cohen et al., 2000; Bosetti et al., 2004). As observed for total fruits, citrus fruit consumption has not been significantly associated with prostate cancer risk in most studies, although one case–control study found a nonsignificant increase in prostate cancer risk of at least 40%. Statistically significant increases and decreases in prostate cancer risk of ~50% also have been reported. In the Netherlands Cohort Study, a statistically significant positive trend was also observed.

Of the case-control studies (Oishi et al., 1988; Le Marchand et al., 1991; Talamini et al., 1992; De Stefani et al., 1995; Key et al., 1997; Lee et al., 1998; Deneo-Pellegrini et al., 1999; Hayes et al., 1999; Jain et al., 1999; Tzonou et al., 1999; Villeneuve et al., 1999; Bosetti et al., 2000, 2004; Cohen et al., 2000; Kolonel et al., 2000; Sonoda et al., 2004) evaluating associations with vegetable consumption, three studies have shown a statistically significant 25–50% reduction in prostate cancer risk with high compared with low intake, one has shown a significant inverse trend, and one has reported that vegetable consumption was significantly lower in men with prostate cancer compared with a group of population controls. The associations in the remaining studies, including three studies showing an elevation in risk of at least 20% with higher vegetable intake, have not been statistically significant. A nonsignificant association has been reported consistently in cohort studies. The one exception is the Cancer Prevention Study II in which men in the highest compared with the lowest quartile of vegetable intake had a 21% lower risk of fatal prostate cancer.

Cruciferous vegetable consumption has been examined in few studies of prostate cancer (Graham et al., 1983; Hsing et al., 1990; Le Marchand et al., 1991; Lee et al., 1998; Schuurman et al., 1998; Jain et al., 1999; Villeneuve et al., 1999; Cohen et al., 2000; Kolonel et al., 2000; Giovannucci et al., 2003). Nonsignificant, inverse associations have been found in most of the case-control and cohort studies. However, in two case-control studies, a higher intake of cruciferous vegetables has been associated with a 20–45% lower risk of prostate cancer.

Tomatoes have been commonly studied in association with prostate cancer risk. Analyses have examined intakes of total tomatoes, raw tomatoes, cooked tomatoes, tomato sauce, tomato juice, and tomato-based products. Of the 11 case-control and cohort studies conducted (Schuman et al., 1982; Mills et al., 1989; Le Marchand et al., 1991; Giovannucci et al., 1995; Key et al., 1997; Hayes et al., 1999; Jain et al., 1999; Villeneuve et al., 1999; Bosetti et al., 2000; Cohen et al., 2000; Kolonel et al., 2000; Norrish et al., 2000; Sonoda et al., 2004), one reported a statistically significant lower risk of prostate cancer of at least 25% with higher intake of tomatoes. However, in one case-control study, a 90% increase in the risk of prostate cancer also has been observed for cooked tomatoes, in which lycopene is more bioavailable (Gartner et al., 1997).

For the remaining case-control studies showing nonsignificant associations, the odds ratios have varied from 0.71 to 1.55. In contrast, two of the three cohort studies that examined tomato products and prostate cancer risk showed inverse associations between tomato and tomato sauce intake and prostate cancer risk.

Because associations with prostate cancer may differ by stage at diagnosis, limiting analyses to localized cancers separately from advanced and metastatic prostate cancers may provide important insight into different etiologies. For cruciferous vegetable consumption, the Health Professionals Follow-up Study found a stronger inverse association with organ-confined cancers compared with extraprostatic cancers (Giovannucci et al., 2003), and the study by Kolonel et al. (2000) found a stronger inverse association for advanced cases compared with all cases. For tomato product consumption, only one (Hayes et al., 1999) of three (Hayes et al., 1999; Kolonel et al., 2000; Giovannucci et al., 2003) studies has suggested that the association differed by stage with a stronger association observed for advanced prostate cancer.

Summary

Overall, fruits and vegetables have not been found to be strongly associated with the risk of prostate cancer, although consumption of tomato-based products and possibly cruciferous vegetables may lower the risk of prostate cancer. With the increase in the use of PSA screening, it will be important to evaluate the association separately for localized versus advanced cancers, as the risk factors for prostate cancer may vary by stage of disease.

ALL CANCER

Few cohort studies have examined associations with all cancer types combined (Colditz et al., 1985; Hirayama, 1990; Shibata et al., 1992; Hertog et al., 1996; Sahyoun et al., 1996; Appleby et al., 2002; Maynard et al., 2003; Sauvaget et al., 2003; Hung et al., 2004). Most of these studies used mortality data (Colditz et al., 1985; Hirayama, 1986; Hertog et al., 1996; Sahyoun et al., 1996; Appleby et al., 2002; Maynard et al., 2003; Sauvaget et al., 2003); three studies assessed cancer incidence (Shibata et al., 1992; Maynard et al., 2003; Hung et al., 2004). The number of cases varied 300-fold across the studies (range: 42–14, 740).

Fruit intake has been associated with a 12–50% lower risk of cancer in many (Shibata et al., 1992; Hertog et al., 1996; Appleby et al., 2002; Maynard et al., 2003; Sauvaget et al., 2003), but not all (Sahyoun et al., 1996; Hung et al., 2004), studies for comparisons of the highest versus lowest intakes. Citrus fruit consumption has been examined in only two studies (Sahyoun et al., 1996; Hung et al., 2004), and the associations observed were similar to those for total fruit intake in these studies. Total vegetable intake has been examined in fewer studies than total fruits (Shibata et al., 1992; Sahyoun et al., 1996; Maynard et al., 2003; Hung et al., 2004). No association was evident in each study. For green vegetables, no association generally has been reported (Shibata et al., 1992; Hirayama, 1990; Sahyoun et al., 1996; Sauvaget et al., 2003; Hung et al., 2004), although a small cohort study reported a 70% decrease in cancer risk for comparisons of individuals in the highest versus lowest quintile of intake (Colditz et al., 1985). The only other study reporting a statistically significant association found that cancer risk was 5% lower among men and women who ate green leafy vegetables daily versus less than daily (Hirayama, 1990).

METHODOLOGICAL ISSUES

In addition to general methodological issues related to the conduct of epidemiological studies examining diet and cancer associations, several distinct issues arise in summarizing fruit and vegetable and cancer associations. First, the specific fruits and vegetables assessed have varied across studies based on culinary custom and scientific hypotheses. Classification of foods as fruits or vegetables has been based on both culinary usage and botanical definitions, which may result in the inclusion of different items in the fruit and vegetable groups. For example, squash, tomatoes, and peppers

TABLE 7 Summary of Case-Control and Cohort Studies of Fruit and Vegetable Consumption and Prostate Cancer Risk[a]

Author, year, country	Study dates	Study population	Comparison for relative risk	Odds ratio/relative risk (95% CI), unless otherwise noted	
				Total fruit	Citrus fruit
Case-control studies					
Schuman et al., 1982, USA	1976–1979	223 cases, 223 hospital controls, 223 neighborhood controls	<3 vs >14 times/mo[b]		
Graham et al., 1983, USA	1957–1965	262 cases, 259 hospital controls	5 times/mo vs 1 time/mo		
Oishi et al., 1988, Japan	1981–1984	100 cases, 100 controls with benign prostatic hyperplasia (BPH), 100 hospital controls	Highest vs lowest tertile		
Le Marchand et al., 1991, USA	1977–1983	452 cases, 899 population controls	Highest vs lowest quartile		
Negri et al., 1991, Italy	1983–1990	107 cases, 2,522 hospital controls	Highest vs lowest tertile	0.4 (0.3–0.8), p for trend < 0.01	
Talamini et al., 1992, Italy	1986–1990	271 cases, 685 hospital controls	Highest vs lowest tertile	Fresh: 1.41 (0.96–2.07), p for trend = 0.06	
De Stefani et al., 1995, Uruguay	1988–1994	156 cases, 302 hospital controls	≥261 vs ≤96 times/year for fruit; ≥131 vs ≤51 times/year for vegetables	1.7 (1.1–2.8), p for trend = 0.04	
Whittemore et al., 1995, USA	1987–1991	1,655 cases, 1,645 population controls			No consistent association
Key TJ, 1997, UK	1989–1992	328 cases, 328 population controls	≥5/wk vs never for citrus; >1/day vs ≤4/wk for cooked veg; ≥5/wk vs ≤3/mo for raw tomatoes; ≥2/wk vs ≤1/mo for cooked tomatoes		1.45 (0.83–2.52), p for trend = 0.09
Lee et al., 1998, China	1989–1992	133 cases, 265 population controls		No difference in mean intake, $p = 0.89$	
Deneo-Pellegrini H, 1999, Uruguay	1994–1997	175 cases, 233 hospital controls	Highest vs lowest quartile	0.8 (0.4–1.4), p for trend = 0.08	
Hayes et al., 1999, USA	1986–1989	932 cases, 1201 population controls	Highest vs lowest quartile for fruits and vegetables; 5+/wk vs never for all tomato groups	All: 1.1, p for trend = 0.48; black:1.3 p for trend = 0.29; white: 1.0, p for trend = 0.98	

Odds ratio/relative risk (95% CI), unless otherwise noted				
Total vegetables	**Cruciferous vegetables**	**Tomatoes**	**Matching and adjustment factors**	**Miscellaneous**
		vs neighborhood controls: 1.41 [0.71]; vs hospital controls: 1.09 [0.92]	Age	
	1.06, p for trend >0.05		Age	
vs BHP controls: 1.53 (0.78–3.00); vs hospital controls: 0.87 (0.43–1.76)			Age	
<70 yrs: 0.8, p for trend = 0.11; >70 yrs: 1.2, p for trend = 0.58	<70 yrs: 0.8, p for trend = 0.27; >70 yrs: 1.1, p for trend = 0.40	<70 yrs: 0.9, p for trend = 0.35; >70 yrs: 1.1, p for trend = 0.57	Age, ethnicity	Also stratified by age
			Age, residence, education, smoking, green vegetable consumption	
1.39 (0.88–2.17), p for trend = 0.17			Age, residence, education, body mass index	Also stratified by age
1.1 (0.6–1.9), p for trend = 0.71)			Age, residence, education, smoking and beer consumption	
Cooked: 0.71 (0.34,1.48), p for trend = 0.42		Raw: 1.06 (0.55–1.62), p for trend = 0.88; Cooked: 0.92 (0.59–1.42), p for trend = 0.64	Social class	
Lower mean intake in cases, p = 0.04	No difference in mean intake, p = 0.17		Age and residence	
0.6 (0.3–1.1), p for trend = 0.02			Age, residence, urban/rural status, education, family history of prostate cancer, body mass index and energy	
All: 1.0, p for trend = 0.89; black: 1.2, p for trend = 0.30; white: 0.8, p for trend = 0.38		All, raw: 0.8, p for trend = 0.16; Black, raw: 0.8, p for trend = 0.41; White, raw: 0.9, p for trend = 0.23; All, cooked sauce: 1.3, p for trend = 0.71; Black, cooked sauce: 1.3, p for trend = 0.98; White, cooked sauce: 0.9, p for trend = 0.62 All, juice: 1.4, p for trend = 0.20; Black, juice: 1.3, p for trend = 0.36; White, juice: 1.5, p for trend = 0.36	Age, calories, study site, and race (for all analyses)	Analyses also for advanced cancers

(*continues*)

TABLE 7 *(Continued)*

Author, year, country	Study dates	Study population	Comparison for relative risk	Odds ratio/relative risk (95% CI), unless otherwise noted	
				Total fruit	Citrus fruit
Jain et al., 1999, Canada	1990–1992 Ontario; 1989–1993 Quebec; 1989–1991 British Columbia	617 cases, 636 population controls	Highest vs lowest quartile	1.51 (1.14–2.01)	1.48 (1.12–1.96)
Sung et al., 1999, Cancer, Taiwan	1995–1996	90 cases, 180 hospital controls	2–7/wk vs less	1.16 (0.57–2.35)	
Tzonou et al., 1999, Greece; Bosetti et al., 2000, Greece	1994–1997	320 cases, 246 hospital controls	Increment = one quintile for fruit and vegetables; highest vs lowest tertile for tomatoes	0.92 (0.86–1.11), *p* for trend = 0.67	
Villeneuve et al., 1999, Canada	1994–1997	1,623 cases, 1,623 population controls	≥28 vs <7 servings/wk for fruit; ≥28 vs <14 servings/wk for total vegetables; ≥4 vs <1 serving/wk for cruciferous vegetables; ≥7 vs <1 serving/wk for tomatoes	1.5 (1.1–1.9), *p* for trend = 0.03	
Kolonel et al., 2000, USA/ Canada	1989–1991 (African-Americans and Whites) and 1987–1991 (Chinese and Japanese)	1,619 cases, 1,618 population controls	Highest vs lowest quintile	All: 1.01 (0.79–1.28), *p* for trend = 0.48	
Cohen et al., 2000, USA	1993–1996	628 cases, 602 population controls	≥14 vs <3 servings/wk for 5/day fruit; ≥21 vs <7 servings/wk for fruit summation and 5/day vegetables; ≥3 vs <1 servings/wk for citrus fruit and juice, cruciferous vegetables and tomatoes; ≥28 vs <14 servings/wk for vegetables summation	Total fruit, 5/day method: 0.80 (0.53–1.23), *p* for trend = 0.38; Total fruit, summation: 1.07 (0.72, 1.60), *p* for trend = 0.96	Citrus fruit: 0.93 (0.66–1.30), *p* for trend = 0.81 Citrus juice: 1.00 (0.75–1.35), *p* for trend = 0.91

Odds ratio/relative risk (95% CI), unless otherwise noted				
Total vegetables	Cruciferous vegetables	Tomatoes	Matching and adjustment factors	Miscellaneous
0.95 (0.68–1.33)	0.85 (0.64–1.13)	0.64 (0.45–0.91)	Age and log total energy intake, vasectomy, ever smoked, marital status, study area, body mass index, education, ever used multivitamin supplements in 1 year before diagnosis/interview, area of study, and log-converted amounts for grain, fruit, vegetables, total plants, total carotenoids, folic acid, dietary fiber, conjugated linoleic acid, vit E, vit C, retinol, total fat and linoleic acid	
			Age, treatment hospital, and date of admission	
0.97 (0.85–1.10), *p* for trend = 0.64		Raw: 1.55 (1.00–2.52); cooked: 1.91 (1.20–3.04)	Age, height, body mass index, years of schooling, and total energy intake	
1.0 (0.8–1.3), *p* for trend = 0.79	0.9 (0.7–1.1), *p* for trend = 0.57	1.0 (0.7–1.3), *p* for trend = 0.29	Age, province of residence, race, years since quitting smoking, cig pack-years, body mass index, rice and pasta, coffee, grains and cereals, alcohol, fruit and fruit juices, tofu, meat, income and family history of cancer	
All: 0.74 (0.58–0.96), *p* for trend = 0.04	0.78 (0.61–1.00), *p* for trend = 0.02	Tomatoes: 1.07 (0.83–1.38), *p* for trend = 0.85; Cooked: 0.94 (0.58–1.52), *p* for trend = 0.56	Age, education, ethnicity, geographic area, and calories	Analyses also for all cases/normal controls AND advanced cases/ all controls Also stratified by race
Total veg, 5/day method: 0.52 (0.31–0.84), *p* for trend = 0.05; total veg, summation: 0.65 (0.45–0.94), *p* for trend = 0.01	0.54 (0.38–0.76), *p* for trend = 0.01	Raw: 0.93 (0.67–1.30), *p* for trend = 0.76; cooked: 0.73 (0.48–1.10), *p* for trend = 0.68	Fat, energy, race, age, family history of prostate cancer, body mass index, PSA tests in previous 5 years and education	

(*continues*)

TABLE 7 (*Continued*)

Author, year, country	Study dates	Study population	Comparison for relative risk	Odds ratio/relative risk (95% CI), unless otherwise noted	
				Total fruit	Citrus fruit
Norrish et al., 2000, New Zealand	1996–1997	317 cases, 480 population controls	Highest vs lowest quartile		
Bosetti et al., 2004, Italy	1991–2002	1,294 cases, 1,451 hospital controls	Highest vs lowest quintile		0.90 (0.70–1.16), *p* for trend = 0.12
Sonoda et al., 2004, Japan	1996–2002	140 cases, 140 hospital controls	≥239.9 vs ≤78.7 g/day for fruits; ≥300 vs ≤151.7 g/day for vegetables; ≥100 vs ≤28.5 g/day day for tomatoes	0.63 (0.29–1.38), *p* for trend = 0.13	
Cohort studies					
Snowden et al., 1984, USA	1960–1980	99 fatal cases, cohort of 6,763		No association	
Mills et al., 1989, USA	1976–1982	180 cases, cohort of 14,000	≥2 times/day vs <3 times/wk for fruit; ≥5 times/wk vs <1/wk for citrus fruit and tomatoes	0.70 (0.32–1.51), *p* for trend = 0.04	Fresh: 0.53 (0.34–0.86), *p* for trend = 0.008
Severson et al., 1989, USA	1965–1986	174 cases, cohort of 7,999	≥5 vs ≤1/wk	1.57 (0.95–2.61)	
Hsing et al., 1990, USA	1966–1986	149 fatal cases, cohort of 17,633	Highest vs lowest quartile	0.9 (0.6–1.4)	
Shibata et al., 1992, USA	1981–1989	208 cases, cohort of ~4,000	Highest vs lowest tertile	1.04 (0.74–1.46)	
Le Marchand et al., 1994, USA	1975–1989	198 cases, cohort of 20,316	Highest vs lowest quartile	Fresh: 1.0 (0.7–1.6), *p* for trend = 0.99	
Giovannucci et al., 1995, USA	1986–1992	812 (773 non stage A1) cases, cohort of 47,894	>4 vs <1 serving/day for fruit; >5 vs <2 servings/day for vegetables; ≥2/wk vs 0 for tomatoes, tomato juice, and tomato sauce; >10 vs <1.5 servings/wk for tomato-based products	0.84 (0.59–1.84), *p* for trend = 0.21	
Rodriguez et al., 1997, USA	1982–1991	1,748 fatal cases, cohort of 450,279	Highest vs lowest quartile		
Schuurman et al., 1998, Netherlands	1986–1992	610 (veg) and 642 (fruit), 58,279 men (subcohort = 1688)	Highest vs lowest quintile	1.31 (0.96–1.79), *p* for trend = 0.02	1.27 (0.93–1.73), *p* for trend = 0.01

Odds ratio/relative risk (95% CI), unless otherwise noted				
Total vegetables	**Cruciferous vegetables**	**Tomatoes**	**Matching and adjustment factors**	**Miscellaneous**
		Tomato-based foods: 0.82 (0.53–1.26), *p* for trend = 0.30; Raw: 1.01 (0.66–1.53), *p* for trend = 0.93	Age, height, total nonsteroidal anti-inflammatory drugs, and socioeconomic status	
Raw: 0.87 (0.65–1.16), *p* for trend = 0.32; Cooked: 0.74 (0.57–0.95), *p* for trend = 0.01			Age, study center, years of education, social class, body mass index, family history of prostate cancer, and total calorie intake	
0.65 (0.28–1.48), *p* for trend = 0.35		0.86 (0.37–2.01), *p* for trend = 0.87	Matched on age. Adjusted for cigarette smoking and energy intake	
No association			Age	
		0.57 (0.35–0.93), *p* for trend = 0.06	Age	
			Age	
0.7 (0.4–1.2)	1.3 (0.8–2.0)		Age, smoking	
1.04 (0.74–1.46)			Age, smoking	
Raw: 1.1 (0.7–1.7), *p* for trend = 0.69			Age, ethnicity, income	
1.04 (0.81–1.34), *p* for trend = 0.68		Tomatoes: 0.74 (0.58–0.93), *p* for trend = 0.03; tomato juice: 1.15 (0.90–1.49), *p* for trend = 0.67; tomato sauce: 0.66 (0.49–0.90), *p* for trend = 0.001; all tomato-based products: 0.65 (0.44–0.95), *p* for trend = 0.01	Age, energy	Update on advanced cancer in Giovannucci, 1998 and updated in Giovannucci, 2002
1.26 (1.07–1.48) [0.79 (0.68–0.93)]			Age, race, family history of prostate cancer, education, vasectomy, exercise, body mass index, alcohol use, fat meat intake	
Total: 0.80 (0.57–1.12), *p* for trend = 0.51; Prepared: 0.85 (0.61–1.19), *p* for trend = 0.46; Raw: 0.96 (0.69–1.34), *p* for trend = 0.61	Brassicas: 0.82 (0.59–1.12), *p* for trend = 0.06		Age, family history of prostate cancer, socioeconomic status, total fruit consumption (for all vegetable analyses), total vegetable consumption (for all fruit analyses)	Analyses for different grades of disease (well-differentiated, moderately differentiated, poorly or undifferentiated)

(*continues*)

TABLE 7 *(Continued)*

Author, year, country	Study dates	Study population	Comparison for relative risk	Odds ratio/relative risk (95% CI), unless otherwise noted	
				Total fruit	Citrus fruit
Chan et al., 2000, Finland	1985–1993	184 cases, cohort of 27,062	Highest vs lowest quintile	1.3 (0.8–2.2), *p* for trend = 0.13	
Appleby et al., 2002, UK	1973–1997	41 fatal cases, cohort of 4,325	Daily vs <daly	Male: 0.66 (0.34–1.29); Non-smokers 1.18 (0.49–2.85)	
Giovannucci et al., 2003, USA	1986–2000	2,969 cases, cohort of 47,365	>5/wk vs ≤1/wk		
Key et al., 2004, Europe	1993–1999	1,104 cases, cohort of 130,544	Highest vs lowest quintile	All: 1.06 (0.84–1.34), *p* for trend = 0.74; Denmark: 0.98 (0.46–2.09), *p* for trend = 0.43; Germany: 1.03 (0.53–2.01), *p* for trend = 0.99; Spain: 0.62 (0.31–1.22), *p* for trend = 0.53; Sweden: 1.24 (0.85–1.81), *p* for trend = 0.94; UK: 1.45 (0.84–2.50), *p* for tend = 0.66	

[a]The following studies have examined the association between fruit and vegetable consumption and prostate cancer risk but did not report associations for the groups included in the table: Tajima and Tominaga et al., 1985; Mishina et al., 1985, Japan; Talamini et al., 1986, Italy; Ross et al., 1987, USA; Walker et al., 1992, South Africa; Andersson et al., 1995, Sweden; Ewings and Bowie, 1996, UK; Hsing et al., 2002, China; Hirayama et al., 1990, Japan; Grönberg et al., 1996, Sweden.

[b]The inverse of the relative risk was calculated to represent a comparison of high vs low intake and is included in brackets after the published estimate.

are botanical fruits but are generally considered culinary vegetables. In addition, some studies have included potatoes or mature beans in their total vegetables category, and other studies have not. Because potatoes are commonly consumed in some cultures, they may be an important contributor to total vegetable intake if they are included as a vegetable.

Second, fruit and vegetable exposures have been measured differently across studies. Some diet questionnaires have been developed to assess the intake of a specific nutrient (such as β-carotene) such that total fruit and vegetable consumption cannot be assessed. Other questionnaires have been designed to measure total diet; these questionnaires have varied from those including a single question on fruit and vegetable consumption to those including many questions on fruit and vegetables. The number of fruit and vegetable items on the food frequency questionnaire may affect estimated intakes because the number of reported fruit and vegetable servings has been found to increase the number of specific items on the questionnaire (Krebs-Smith et al., 1995), whereas combining multiple foods as a single item tends to underestimate intake (Serdula et al., 1992). Mis-

Odds ratio/relative risk (95% CI), unless otherwise noted				
Total vegetables	**Cruciferous vegetables**	**Tomatoes**	**Matching and adjustment factors**	**Miscellaneous**
0.8 (0.5–1.3), p for trend = 0.84			Supplementation group (alpha-tocopherol, beta-carotene, both, or placebo), education, age, body mass index, energy, and number of years as a smoker	
			Adjusted for age at recruitment, and where applicable, sex and smoking	Update of Key et al., 1996
	0.93 (0.82–1.05), p for trend = 0.30		Body mass index at age 21, body mass index in 1986, height, cigarette pack-years in previous 10 yrs, fam history of prostate cancer, history of diabetes mellitus, vigorous physical activity, and intakes of total calories, red meat, processed meat, fish, alpha-linoleic acid, calcium, and tomato sauce	Analyses by type of prostate cancer (organ-confined, extraprostatic), by age, including only those with PSA, and excluding those who reported increased vegetable intake in past 10 years
All: 1.00 (0.81–1.22), p for trend = 0.74; Denmark: 0.91 (0.44–1.88), p for trend = 0.61; Germany: 1.63 (0.78–3.41), p for trend = 0.27; Spain: 0.85 (0.40–1.79), p for trend = 0.70; Sweden: 1.01 (0.74–1.37), p for trend = 0.97; UK: 0.76 (0.46–1.25), p for trend = 0.62			Height, weight, and energy	

classification in the evaluation of fruit and vegetable subgroups also may occur when multiple foods are included on the same line on a questionnaire, because the quantity of the individual foods consumed is unknown. Some studies have included summary questions about fruit and vegetable intake on their questionnaires to adjust intake estimates derived from the sum of the individual fruit and vegetable questions (Block and Subar, 1992; Krebs-Smith et al., 1995; Subar et al., 1995). The impact of these different ways in measuring and analyzing fruit and vegetable consumption on reported cancer associations is unknown.

SUMMARY

Numerous bioactive compounds present in fruits and vegetables have been hypothesized to act as cancer preventive agents by inhibiting the activation of procarcinogens, enhancing the detoxification of carcinogens, preventing carcinogens from interacting with critical target sites, or impeding the progression of carcinogenesis (Steinmetz and Potter, 1991; Wattenberg, 1992; Lampe, 1999; IARC, 2003). Because fruits and vegetables are heterogeneous in phytochemical content, color, size, and culinary usage

(Wattenberg, 1990; Steinmetz and Potter, 1991; Mangels et al., 1993; Smith et al., 1995), associations may vary among different types of fruits and vegetables. Fruit and vegetable intakes have been categorized on the basis of culinary usage, botanical taxonomy, and phytochemical content. Thus, difficulty arises in summarizing the literature examining the association between fruit and vegetable consumption and cancer risk as a result of the different ways in which fruit and vegetable intakes have been measured, the variety of fruit and vegetable groups evaluated, and the tendency for investigators to report individual foods or groups for which results are statistically significant, leading to publication bias. In 1997, the World Cancer Research Fund review concluded that the epidemiological and experimental evidence that diets rich in fruits and vegetables could reduce the risk of many cancer sites was very strong and estimated that "diets high in vegetables and fruits (more than 400 g/day) could prevent at least 20% of all cancer incidence." However, conclusions regarding the strength of a cancer preventive association have become weaker during the past few years, primarily because of the weak or null results published in several prospective cohort studies. In 2003, the review by the IARC stated that higher fruit and vegetable consumption was associated with a lower risk of various types of cancer. The review concluded that the evidence indicates the higher fruit intake probably lowers the risk of cancers of the esophagus, stomach, and lung, whereas higher vegetable intake probably lowers the risk of cancers of the esophagus and colon and rectum. The preventable fraction for total cancer for low fruit and vegetable intake was estimated to fall into the range of 5–12% (IARC, 2003). The overall data did not suggest that fruits and vegetables increase the risk of any individual cancer site (IARC, 2003). Thus, eating a diet rich in fruits and vegetables may have a modest impact on preventing cancer but is unlikely to increase the risk of developing cancer. Furthermore, fruits and vegetables have been found to lower the risk of cardiovascular disease (Hung et al., 2004; Ness and Powles, 1997), an important contributor to overall morbidity and mortality in the world, leading to the continued recommendation that fruits and vegetables are an important component of a healthy diet.

References

Adzersen, K.H., Jess, P., Freivogel, K.W., Gerhard, I., and Bastert, G. 2003. Raw and cooked vegetables, fruits, selected micronutrients, and breast cancer risk: a case–control study in Germany. *Nutr Cancer* **46**: 131–137.

Agarwal, S., and Rao, A.V. 2000. Tomato lycopene and its role in human health and chronic diseases. *Can Med Assoc* **163**: 739–744.

Agudo, A., Esteve, M.G., Pallares, C., Martinez-Ballarin, I., Fabregat, X., Malats, N., Machengs, I., Badia, A., and Gonzalez, C.A. 1997. Vegetable and fruit intake and the risk of lung cancer in women in Barcelona, Spain. *Eur J Cancer* **33**: 1256–1261.

Agudo, A., and Pera, G. 1999. Vegetable and fruit consumption associated with anthropometric, dietary and lifestyle factors in Spain. EPIC Group of Spain. European Prospective Investigation into Cancer. *Public Health Nutr* **2**: 263–271.

Alavanja, M.C., Field, R.W., Sinha, R., Brus, C.P., Shavers, V.L., Fisher, E.L., Curtain, J., and Lynch, C.F. 2001. Lung cancer risk and red meat consumption among Iowa women. *Lung Cancer* **34**: 37–46.

Alavanja, M.C.R., Brown, C.C., Swanson, C., and Brownson, R.C. 1993. Saturated fat intake and lung cancer risk among nonsmoking women in Missouri. *J Natl Cancer Inst* **85**: 1906–1916.

Amaral, T., de Almeida, M.D., and Barros, H. 2002. Diet and postmenopausal breast cancer in Portugal. *IARC Sci Publ* **156**: 297–299.

American Cancer Society. 2005. "Cancer Facts and Figures 2005." American Cancer Society, Atlanta.

Andersson, S.-O., Baron, J., Wolk, A., Lindgren, C., Bergstrom, R., and Adami, H.-A. 1995. Early life risk factors for prostate cancer: a population-based case–control study in Sweden. *Cancer Epidemiol Biomarkers Prev* **4**: 187–192.

Appleby, P.N., Key, T.J., Burr, M.L., and Thorogood, M. 2002. Mortality and fresh fruit consumption. *IARC Sci Publ* **156**: 131–133.

Ariyoshi, T., Arakaki, M., Ideguchi, K., Ishizuka, Y., and Noda, K. 1975. Studies on the metabolism of d-limonene (p-mentha-l, 8-diene). III. Effects of d-limonene on the lipids and drug-metabolizing enzymes in rat livers. *Xenobiotica* **5**: 33–38.

Asaka, M., Kimura, T., Kato, M., Kudo, M., Miki, K., Ogoshi, K., Kato, T., Tatsuta, M., and Graham, D.Y. 1994. Possible role of *Helicobacter pylori* infection in early gastric cancer development. *Cancer* **73**: 2691–2694.

Austin, C.A., Shephard, E.A., Pike, S.F., Rabin, B.R., and Phillips, I.R. 1988. The effect of terpenoid compounds on cytochrome P-450 levels in rat liver. *Biochem Pharmacol* **37**: 2223–2229.

Axelsson, G., Liljeqvist, T., Andersson, L., Bergman, B., and Rylander, R. 1996. Dietary factors and lung cancer among men in West Sweden. *Int J Epidemiol* **25**: 32–39.

Axelsson, G., and Rylander, R. 2002. Diet as risk for lung cancer: a Swedish case–control study. *Nutr Cancer* **44**: 145–151.

Beckett, W.S. 1993. Epidemiology and etiology of lung cancer. *Clin Chest Med* **14**: 1–15.

Belanger, J.T. 1998. Perillyl alcohol: applications in oncology. *Alt Med Rev* **3**: 448–457.

Benito, E., Obrador, A., Stiggelbout, A., Bosch, F.X., Mulet, M., Munoz, N., and Kaldor, J. 1990. A population-based case–control study of colorectal cancer in Majorca. I. Dietary factors. *Int J Cancer* **45**: 69–76.

Bernstein, L., and Ross, R.K. 1993. Endogenous hormones and breast cancer risk. *Epidemiol Rev* **15**: 48–65.

Bianchini, F., and Vainio, H. 2001. Allium vegetables and organosulfur compounds: do they help prevent cancer? *Env Health Perspect* **109**: 893–902.

Bianchini, F., and Vainio, H. 2003. Wine and resveratrol: mechanisms of cancer prevention? *Eur J Cancer Prevention* **12**: 417–425.

Bidoli, E., Franceschi, S., Talamini, R., Barra, S., and La Vecchia, C. 1992. Food consumption and cancer of the colon and rectum in North-Eastern Italy. *Int J Cancer* **50**: 223–229.

Bjelakovic, G., Nikolova, D., Simonetti, R.G., and Gluud, C. 2004. Antioxidant supplements for prevention of gastrointestinal cancers: a systematic review and meta-analysis. *Lancet* **364**: 1219–1228.

Bjelke, E. 1974. Epidemiologic studies of cancer of the stomach, colon and rectum; with special emphasis on the role of diet. *Scan J Gastroenterol* **31**(Suppl): 1–235.

Block, G., Patterson, B., and Subar, A. 1992. Fruit, vegetables, and cancer prevention: a review of the epidemiological evidence. *Nutr Cancer* **18**: 1–29.

Block, G., and Subar, A.F. 1992. Estimates of nutrient intake from a food frequency questionnaire: the 1987 National Health Interview Survey. *J Am Diet Assoc* **92**: 969–977.

Boeing, H., Frentzel-Beyme, R., Berger, M., Berndt, V., Gores, W., Komer, M., Lohmeier, R., Menarcher, A., Mannl, H.F., Meinhardt, M., and et al. 1991a. Case–control study on stomach cancer in Germany. *Int J Cancer* **47**: 858–864.

Boeing, H., Jedrychowski, W., Wahrendorf, J., Popiela, T., Tobiasz-Adamczyk, B., and Kulig, A. 1991b. Dietary risk factors in intestinal and diffuse types of stomach cancer: a multicenter case–control study in Poland. *Cancer Causes Control* **2**: 227–233.

Bond, G.G., Thompson, F.E., and Cook, R.R. 1987. Dietary vitamin A and lung cancer: results of a case–control study among chemical workers. *Nutr Cancer* **9**: 109–121.

Bosetti, C., Micelotta, S., Dal Maso, L., Talamini, R., Montella, M., Negri, E., Conti, E., Franceschi, S., and La Vecchia, C. 2004. Food groups and risk of prostate cancer in Italy. *Int J Cancer* **110**: 424–428.

Bosetti, C., Tzonou, A., Lagiou, P., Negri, E., Trichopoulos, D., and Hsieh, C.C. 2000. Fraction of prostate cancer incidence attributed to diet in Athens, Greece. *Eur J Cancer Prevention* **9**: 119–123.

Botterweck, A.A., van den Brandt, P.A., and Goldbohm, R.A. 1998. A prospective cohort study on vegetable and fruit consumption and stomach cancer risk in The Netherlands. *Am J Epidemiol* **148**: 842–853.

Boutron-Ruault, M.C., Senesse, P., Faivre, J., Chatelain, N., Belghiti, C., and Meance, S. 1999. Foods as risk factors for colorectal cancer: a case–control study in Burgundy (France). *Eur J Cancer Prevention* **8**: 229–235.

Boyd, N.F., Martin, L.J., Noffel, M., Lockwood, G.A., and Tritchler, D.L. 1993. A meta–analysis of studies of dietary fat and breast cancer risk. *Br J Cancer* **68**: 627–636.

Boyd, N.F., Stone, J., Vogt, K.N., Connelly, B.S., Martin, L.J., and Minkin, S. 2003. Dietary fat and breast cancer risk revisited: a meta-analysis of the published literature. *Br J Cancer* **89**: 1672–1685.

Braga, C., La Vecchia, C., Negri, E., Franceschi, S., and Parpinel, M. 1997. Intake of selected foods and nutrients and breast cancer risk: an age- and menopause-specific analysis. *Nutr Cancer* **28**: 258–263.

Brennan, P., Fortes, C., Butler, J., Agudo, A., Benhamou, S., Darby, S., Gerken, M., Jockel, K.H., Kreuzer, M., Mallone, S., Nyberg, F., Pohlabeln, H., Ferro, G., and Boffetta, P. 2000. A multicenter case–control study of diet and lung cancer among non-smokers. *Cancer Causes Control* **11**: 49–58.

Breslow, R.A., Graubard, B.I., Sinha, R., and Subar, A.F. 2000. Diet and lung cancer mortality: a 1987 National Health Interview Survey cohort study. *Cancer Causes Control* **11**: 419–431.

Buiatti, E., Palli, D., Decarli, A., Amadori, D., Avellini, C., Bianchi, S., Biserni, R., Cipriani, F., Cocco, P., Giacosa, A., and et al . . . 1989. A case–control study of gastric cancer and diet in Italy. *Int J Cancer* **44**: 611–616.

Byrne, C., Ursin, G., and Ziegler, R.G. 1996. A comparison of food habit and food frequency data as predictors of breast cancer in the NHANES I/NHEFS cohort. *J Nutr* **126**: 2757–2764.

Cai, L., Zheng, Z.L., and Zhang, Z.F. 2003. Risk factors for the gastric cardia cancer: a case–control study in Fujian Province. *World J Gastroenterol* **9**: 214–218.

Candelora, E.C., Stockwell, H.G., Armstrong, A.W., and Pinkham, P.A. 1992. Dietary intake and risk of lung cancer in women who never smoked. *Nutr Cancer* **17**: 263–270.

Cao, G., Sofic, E., and Prior, R.L. 1996. Antioxidant capacity of tea and common vegetables. *J Agric Food Chem* **44**: 3426–3431.

Carmichael, A.R., and Bates, T. 2004. Obesity and breast cancer: a review of the literature. *The Breast* **13**: 85–92.

Challier, B., Peramau, J.M., and Viel, J.F. 1998. Garlic, onion and cereal fibre as protective factors for breast cancer: a French case–control study. *Eur J Epidemiol* **14**: 737–747.

Chan, J.M., Pietinen, P., Virtanen, M., Malila, N., Tangrea, J., Albanes, D., and Virtamo, J. 2000. Diet and prostate cancer risk in a cohort of smokers, with a specific focus on calcium and phosphorus (Finland). *Cancer Causes Control* **11**: 859–867.

Chan-Yeung, M., Koo, L.C., Ho, J.C., Tsang, K.W., Chau, W.S., Chiu, S.W., Ip, M.S., and Lam, W.K. 2003. Risk factors associated with lung cancer in Hong Kong. *Lung Cancer* **40**: 131–140.

Chiu, B.C., Ji, B.T., Dai, Q., Gridley, G., McLaughlin, J.K., Gao, Y.T., Fraumeni, J.F., Jr., and Chow, W.H. 2003. Dietary factors and risk of colon cancer in Shanghai, China. *Cancer Epidemiol Biomarkers Prev* **12**: 201–208.

Cho, E., Smith-Warner, S.A., Ritz, J., van den Brandt, P.A., Colditz, G.A., Folsom, A.R., Freudenheim, J.L., Giovannucci, E., Goldbohm, R.A., Graham, S., Holmberg, L., Kim, D.H., Malila, N., Miller, A.B., Pietinen, P., Rohan, T.E., Sellers, T.A., Speizer, F.E., Willett, W.C., Wolk, A., and Hunter, D.J. 2004. Alcohol intake and colorectal cancer: a pooled analysis of 8 cohort studies. *Ann Intern Med* **140**: 603–613.

Choi, S.W., and Mason, J.B. 2000. Folate and carcinogenesis: an integrated scheme. *J Nutr* **130**: 129–132.

Chow, W.-H., Schuman, L.M., McLaughlin, J.K., Bjelke, E., Gridley, G., Wacholder, S., Co Chien, H.T., and Blot, W.J. 1992. A cohort study of tobacco use, diet, occupation, and lung cancer mortality. *Cancer Causes Control* **3**: 247–254.

Chyou, P.H., Nomura, A.M., Hankin, J.H., and Stemmermann, G.N. 1990. A case–cohort study of diet and stomach cancer. *Cancer Res* **50**: 7501–7504.

Chyou, P.-H., Nomura, A.M.Y., and Stemmermann, G.N. 1992. A prospective study of the attributable risk of cancer due to cigarette smoking. *Am J Public Health* **82**: 37–40.

Coggon, D., Barker, D.J., Cole, R.B., and Nelson, M. 1989. Stomach cancer and food storage. *J Natl Cancer Inst* **81**: 1178–1182.

Cohen, J.H., Kristal, A.R., and Stanford, J.L. 2000. Fruit and vegetable intakes and prostate cancer risk. *J Natl Cancer Inst* **92**: 61–68.

Colditz, G.A., Branch, L.G., Lipnick, R.J., Willett, W.C., Rosner, B., Posner, B.M., and Hennekens, C.H. 1985. Increased green and yellow vegetable intake and lowered cancer deaths in an elderly population. *Am J Clin Nutr* **41**: 32–36.

Cook, L.S., Goldoft, M., Schwartz, S.M., and Weiss, N.S. 1999. Incidence of adenocarcinoma of the prostate in Asian immigrants to the United States and their descendants. *J Urol* **161**: 152–155.

Cornee, J., Pobel, D., Riboli, E., Guyader, M., and Hernon, B. 1995. A case–control study of gastric cancer and nutritional factors in Marseille, France. *Eur J Epidemiol* **11**: 55–65.

Correa, P., Fontham, E., Pickle, L.W., Chen, V., Lin, Y.P., and Haenszel, W. 1985. Dietary determinants of gastric cancer in south Louisiana inhabitants. *J Natl Cancer Inst* **75**: 645–654.

Crawford, E.D. 2003. Epidemiology of prostate cancer. *Urology* **62**: 3–12.

Crew, K.D., and Neugut, A.I. 2004. Epidemiology of upper gastrointestinal malignancies. *Semin Oncol* **31**: 450–464.

Crowell, P.L. 1999. Prevention and therapy of cancer by dietary monoterpenes. *J Nutr* **129**: 775S–778S.

Crowell, P.L., Kennan, W.S., Haag, J.D., Ahmad, S., Vedejs, E., and Gould, M.N. 1992. Chemoprevention of mammary carcinogenesis by hydroxylated derivatives of d-limonene. *Carcinogenesis* **13**: 1261–1264.

Dagnelie, P.C., Schuurman, A.G., Goldbohm, R.A., and Van den Brandt, P.A. 2004. Diet, anthropometric measures and prostate cancer risk: a review of prospective cohort and intervention studies. *BJU Int* **93**: 1139–1150.

Darby, S., Whitley, E., Doll, R., Key, T., and Silcocks, P. 2001. Diet, smoking and lung cancer: a case–control study of 1000 cases and 1500 controls in South-West England. *Br J Cancer* **84**: 728–735.

de Koning, H.J., Auvinen, A., Berenguer Sanchez, A., Calais da Silva, F., Ciatto, S., Denis, L., Gohagan, J.K., Hakama, M., Hugosson, J., Kranse, R., Nelen, V., Prorok, P.C., and Schroder, F.H. 2002. Large-scale randomized prostate cancer screening trials: program performances in the European Randomized Screening for Prostate Cancer trial and the Prostate, Lung, Colorectal and Ovary cancer trial. *Int J Cancer* **97**: 237–244.

De Stefani, E., Boffetta, P., Deneo-Pellegrini, H., Mendilaharsu, M., Carzoglio, J.C., Ronco, A., and Olivera, L. 1999. Dietary antioxidants and lung cancer risk: a case–control study in Uruguay. *Nutr Cancer* **34**: 100–110.

De Stefani, E., Boffetta, P., Ronco, A.L., Brennan, P., Deneo-Pellegrini, H., Carzoglio, J.C., and Mendilaharsu, M. 2000. Plant sterols and risk of stomach cancer: a case–control study in Uruguay. *Nutr Cancer* **37**: 140–144.

De Stefani, E., Brennan, P., Boffetta, P., Mendilaharsu, M., Deneo-Pellegrini, H., Ronco, A., Olivera, L., and Kasdorf, H. 2002a. Diet and adenocarcinoma of the lung: a case–control study in Uruguay. *Lung Cancer* **35**: 43–51.

De Stefani, E., Brennan, P., Ronco, A., Fierro, L., Correa, P., Boffetta, P., Deneo-Pellegrini, H., and Barrios, E. 2002b. Food groups and risk of lung cancer in Uruguay. *Lung Cancer* **38**: 1–7.

De Stefani, E., Correa, P., Boffetta, P., Ronco, A., Brennan, P., Deneo-Pellegrini, H., and Mendilaharsu, M. 2001. Plant foods and risk of gastric cancer: a case–control study in Uruguay. *Eur J Cancer Prevention* **10**: 357–364.

De Stefani, E., Correa, P., Fierro, L., Carzoglio, J., Deneo-Pellegrini, H., and Zavala, D. 1990. Alcohol drinking and tobacco smoking in gastric cancer. A case–control study. *Rev Epidemiol Sante Publ* **38**: 297–307.

De Stefani, E., Fierro, L., Barrios, E., and Ronco, A. 1995. Tobacco, alcohol, diet and risk of prostate cancer. *Tumori* **81**: 315–320.

Demirer, T., Icli, F., Uzunalimoglu, O., and Kucuk, O. 1990. Diet and stomach cancer incidence. A case–control study in Turkey. *Cancer* **65**: 2344–2348.

Deneo-Pellegrini, H., Boffetta, P., De Stefani, E., Ronco, A., Brennan, P., and Mendilaharsu, M. 2002. Plant foods and differences between colon and rectal cancers. *Eur J Cancer Prevention* **11**: 369–375.

Deneo-Pellegrini, H., De Stefani, E., and Ronco, A. 1996. Vegetables, fruits, and risk of colorectal cancer: a case–control study from Uruguay. *Nutr Cancer* **25**: 297–303.

Deneo-Pellegrini, H., De Stefani, E., Ronco, A., and Mendilaharsu, M. 1999. Foods, nutrients and prostate cancer: a case–control study in Uruguay. *Br J Cancer* **80**: 5917.

Doll, R., and Peto, R. 1981. The causes of cancer: quantitative estimates of avoidable risks of cancer in the United States today. *J Natl Cancer Inst* **66**: 1191–1308.

Dorgan, J.F., Ziegler, R.G., Schoenberg, J.B., Hartge, P., McAdams, M.J., Falk, R.T., Wilcox, H.B., and Shaw, G.L. 1993. Race and sex differences in associations of vegetables, fruits, and carotenoids with lung cancer risk in New Jersey (United States). *Cancer Causes Control* **4**: 273–281.

Dos Santos Silva, I., Mangtani, P., McCormack, V., Bhakta, D., Sevak, L., and McMichael, A.J. 2002. Lifelong vegetarianism and risk of breast cancer: a population-based case–control study among youth Asian migrant women living in England. *Int J Cancer* **99**: 238–244.

Dragsted, L.O., Strube, M., and Larsen, J.C. 1993. Cancer-protective factors in fruits and vegetables: biochemical and biological background. *Pharmacol Toxicol* **72**(Suppl): 116–135.

Ekstrom, A.M., Serafini, M., Nyren, O., Hansson, L.E., Ye, W., and Wolk, A. 2000. Dietary antioxidant intake and the risk of cardia cancer and noncardia cancer of the intestinal and diffuse types: a population-based case–control study in Sweden. *Int J Cancer* **87**: 133–140.

Elegbede, J.A., Maltzman, T.H., Elson, C.E., and Gould, M.N. 1993. Effects of anti carcinogenic monoterpenes on phase II hepatic metabolizing enzymes. *Carcinogenesis* **14**: 1221–1223.

Ernster, V.L. 1994. The epidemiology of lung cancer in women. *Ann Epidemiol* **4**: 102–110.

Evans, P., and Halliwell, B. 2001. Micronutrients: oxidant/antioxidant status. *Br J Nutr* **85**(Suppl 2): S67–S74.

Ewings, P., and Bowie, C. 1996. A case–control study of cancer of the prostate in Somerset and east Devon. *Br J Cancer* **74**: 661–666.

Fahey, J.W., Zhang, Y., and Talalay, P. 1997. Broccoli sprouts: an exceptionally rich source of inducers of enzymes that protect against chemical carcinogens. *Proc Nat Acad Sci* **94**: 10367–10372.

Ferlay, J., Bray, F., Pisani, P., and Parkin, D.M. 2004. "GLOBOCAN 2002: Cancer Incidence, Mortality and Prevalence Worldwide." IARC Press, Lyon, France.

Feskanich, D., Ziegler, R.G., Michaud, D.S., Giovannucci, E.L., Speizer, F.E., Willett, W.C., and Colditz, G.A. 2000. Prospective study of fruit and vegetable consumption and risk of lung cancer among men and women. *J Natl Cancer Inst* **92**: 1812–1823.

Fleischauer, A.T., and Arab, L. 2001. Garlic and cancer: a critical review of the epidemiologic literature. *J Nutr* **131**: 1032S–1040S.

Fontham, E.T.H., Pickle, L.W., Haenszel, W., Correa, P., Lin, Y., and Falk, R.T. 1988. Dietary vitamins A and C and lung cancer risk in Louisiana. *Cancer* **62**: 2267–2273.

Forman, M.R., Yao, S.X., Graubard, B.I., Qiao, Y.L., McAdams, M., Mao, B.L., and Taylor, P.R. 1992. The effect of dietary intake of fruits and vegetables on the odds ratio of lung cancer among Yunnan tin miners. *Int J Epidemiol* **21**: 437–441.

Franceschi, S., Favero, A., La Vecchia, C., Negri, E., Dal Maso, L., Salvini, S., Decarli, A., and Giacosa, A. 1995. Influence of food groups and food diversity on breast cancer risk in Italy. *Int J Cancer* **63**: 785–789.

Franceschi, S., Parpinel, M., La Vecchia, C., Favero, A., Talamini, R., and Negri, E. 1998. Role of different types of vegetables and fruit in the prevention of cancer of the colon, rectum, and breast. *Epidemiology* **9**: 338–341.

Fraser, G.E. 1999. Associations between diet and cancer, ischemic heart disease, and all-cause mortality in non-Hispanic white California Seventh-day Adventists. *Am J Clin Nutr* **70**: 532S–538S.

Fraser, G.E., Beeson, W.L., and Phillips, R.L. 1991. Diet and lung cancer in California Seventh-day Adventists. *Am J Epidemiol* **133**: 683–693.

Frazier, A.L., Tomeo, C.A., Rockett, H., Willett, W.C., and Colditz, G.A. 2004. Adolescent diet and risk of breast cancer. *Breast Cancer Res.* **5**: R59–64.

Freudenheim, J.L., Marshall, J.R., Vena, J.E., Laughlin, R., Brasure, J.R., Swanson, M.K., Nemoto, T., and Graham, S. 1996. Premenopausal breast cancer risk and intake of vegetables, fruits, and related nutrients. *J Natl Cancer Inst* **88**: 340–348.

Galanis, D.J., Kolonel, L.N., Lee, J., and Nomura, A. 1998. Intakes of selected foods and beverages and the incidence of gastric cancer among the Japanese residents of Hawaii: a prospective study. *Int J Epidemiol* **27**: 173–180.

Gao, C.-M., Tajima, K., Kuroishi, T., Hirose, K., and Inoue, M. 1993. Protective effects of raw vegetables and fruit against lung cancer among smokers and ex-smokers: a case–control study in the Tokai Area of Japan. *Jpn J Cancer Res* **84**: 594–600.

Gao, C.M., Takezaki, T., Ding, J.H., Li, M.S., and Tajima, K. 1999. Protective effect of allium vegetables against both esophageal and stomach cancer: a simultaneous case-referent study of a high-epidemic area in Jiangsu Province, China. *Jpn J Cancer Res* **90**: 614–621.

Garcia-Closas, R., Agudo, A., Gonzalez, C.A., and Riboli, E. 1998. Intake of specific carotenoids and flavonoids and the risk of lung cancer in women in Barcelona, Spain. *Nutr Cancer* **32**: 154–158.

Gartner, C., Stahl, W., and Sies, H. 1997. Lycopene is more bioavailable from tomato paste than from fresh tomatoes. *Am J Clin Nutr* **66**: 116–122.

Giovannucci, E. 1999. Tomatoes, tomato-based products, lycopene, and cancer: review of the epidemiologic literature. *J Natl Cancer Inst* **91**: 317–331.

Giovannucci, E. (2005). The epidemiology of vitamin D and cancer incidence and mortality: a review. *Cancer Causes Control* **16**: 83–95.

Giovannucci, E., Ascherio, A., Rimm, E.B., Stampfer, M.J., Colditz, G.A., and Willett, W.C. 1995. Intake of carotenoids and retinol in relation to risk of prostate cancer. *J Natl Cancer Inst* **87**: 1767–1776.

Giovannucci, E., Rimm, E.B., Liu, Y., Stampfer, M.J., and Willett, W.C. 2002. A prospective study of tomato products, lycopene, and prostate cancer risk. *J Natl Cancer Inst* **94**: 391–398.

Giovannucci, E., Rimm, E.B., Liu, Y., Stampfer, M.J., and Willett, W.C. 2003. A prospective study of cruciferous vegetables and prostate cancer. *Cancer Epidemiol Biomarkers Prev* **12**: 1403–1409.

Giovannucci, E., Rimm, E.B., Stampfer, M.J., Colditz, G.A., Ascherio, A., Kearney, J., and Willett, W.C. 1994. A prospective study of cigarette smoking and risk of colorectal adenoma and colorectal cancer in U.S. men. *J Natl Cancer Inst* **86**: 183–191.

Giovannucci, E., Rimm, E.B., Wolk, A., Ascherio, A., Stampfer, M.J., Colditz, G.A., and Willett, W.C. 1998. Calcium and fructose intake in relation to risk of prostate cancer. *Cancer Res* **58**: 442–447.

Giovannucci, E., and Willett, W.C. 1994. Dietary factors and risk of colon cancer. *Ann Med* **26**: 443–452.

Gonzalez, C.A., Sanz, J.M., Marcos, G., Pita, S., Brullet, E., Saigi, E., Badia, A., and Riboli, E. 1991. Dietary factors and stomach cancer in Spain: a multi-centre case–control study. *Int J Cancer* **49**: 513–519.

Graham, D.Y. 2000. *Helicobacter pylori* infection is the primary cause of gastric cancer. *J Gastroenterol* **35**(Suppl) **12**: 90–97.

Graham, S., Dayal, H., Swanson, M., Mittelman, A., and Wilkinson, G. 1978. Diet in the epidemiology of cancer of the colon and rectum. *J Natl Cancer Inst* **61**: 709–714.

Graham, S., Haughey, B., Marshall, J., Brasure, J., Zielezny, M., Freudenheim, J., West, D., Nolan, J., and Wilkinson, G. 1990. Diet in the epidemiology of gastric cancer. *Nutr Cancer* **13**: 19–34.

Graham, S., Haughey, B., Marshall, J., Priore, R., Byers, T., Rzepka, T., Mettlin, C., and Pontes, J.E. 1983. Diet in the epidemiology of carcinoma of the prostate gland. *J Natl Cancer Inst* **70**: 687–692.

Graham, S., Marshall, J., Haughey, B., Mittelman, A., Swanson, M., Zielezny, M., Byers, T., Wilkinson, G., and West, D. 1988. Dietary epidemiology of cancer of the colon in Western New York. *Am J Epidemiol* **128**: 490–503.

Graham, S., Marshall, J., Mettlin, C., Rzepka, T., Nemoto, T., and Byers, T. 1982. Diet in the epidemiology of breast cancer. *Am J Epidemiol* **116**: 68–75.

Greenwald, P., Clifford, C.K., and Milner, J.A. 2001. Diet and cancer prevention. *Eur J Cancer* **37**: 948–965.

Gronberg, H., Damber, L., and Damber, J.-E. 1996. Total food consumption and body mass index in relation to prostate cancer risk: a case–control study in Sweden with prospectively collected exposure data. *J Urol* **155**: 969–974.

Guo, W., Blot, W.J., Li, J.Y., Taylor, P.R., Liu, B.Q., Wang, W., Wu, Y.P., Zheng, W., Dawsey, S.M., Li, B., and et al. 1994. A nested case–control study of oesophageal and stomach cancers in the Linxian nutrition intervention trial. *Int J Epidemiol* **23**: 444–450.

Gusman, J., Malonne, H., and Atassi, G. 2001. A reappraisal of the potential chemopreventive and chemotherapeutic properties of resveratrol. *Carcinogenesis* **22**: 1111–1117.

Haag, J.D., and Gould, M.N. 1994. Mammary carcinoma regression induced by perillyl alcohol, a hydroxylated analog of limonene. *Cancer Chemother Pharmacol* **34**: 477–483.

Haag, J.D., Lindstrom, M.J., and Gould, M.N. 1992. Limonene-induced regression of mammary carcinomas. *Cancer Res* **52**: 4021–4026.

Hamada, G.S., Kowalski, L.P., Nishimoto, I.N., Rodrigues, J.J., Iriya, K., Sasazuki, S., Hanaoka, T., and Tsugane, S. 2002. Risk factors for stomach cancer in Brazil (II. a case–control study among Japanese Brazilians in Sao Paulo. *Jpn J Clin Oncol* **32**: 284–290.

Hamajima, N., Hirose, K., Tajima, K., Rohan, T., Calle, E.E., Heath, C.W., Jr., Coates, R.J., Liff, J.M., Talamini, R., Chantarakul, N., Koetsawang, S., Rachawat, D., Morabia, A., Schuman, L., Stewart, W., Szklo, M., Bain, C., Schofield, F., Siskind, V., Band, P., Coldman, A.J., Gallagher, R.P., Hislop, T.G., Yang, P., Kolonel, L.M., Nomura, A.M., Hu, J., Johnson, K.C., Mao, Y., De Sanjose, S., Lee, N., Marchbanks, P., Ory, H.W., Peterson, H.B., Wilson, H.G., Wingo, P.A., Ebeling, K., Kunde, D., Nishan, P., Hopper, J.L., Colditz, G., Gajalanski, V., Martin, N., Pardthaisong, T., Silpisomkosol, S., Theetranont, C., Boosiri, B., Chutivongse, S., Jimakom, P., Virutamasen, P., Wongsrichanalai, C., Ewertz, M., Adami, H.O., Bergkvist, L., Magnusson, C., Persson, I., Chang-Claude, J., Paul, C., Skegg, D.C., Spears, G.F., Boyle, P., Evstifeeva, T., Daling, J.R., Hutchinson, W.B., Malone, K., Noonan, E.A., Stanford, J.L., Thomas, D.B., Weiss, N.S., White, E., Andrieu, N., Bremond, A., Clavel, F., Gairard, B., Lansac, J., Piana, L., Renaud, R., Izquierdo, A., Viladiu, P., Cuevas, H.R., Ontiveros, P., Palet, A., Salazar, S.B., Aristizabel, N., Cuadros, A., Tryggvadottir, L., Tulinius, H., Bachelot, A., Le, M.G., Peto, J., Franceschi, S., Lubin, F., Modan, B., Ron, E., Wax, Y., Friedman, G.D., Hiatt, R.A., Levi, F., Bishop, T., Kosmelj, K., et al. 2002. Alcohol, tobacco and breast cancer—collaborative reanalysis of individual data from 53 epidemiological studies, including 58,515 women with breast cancer and 95,067 women without the disease. *Br J Cancer* **87**: 1234–1245.

Hansson, L.E., Nyren, O., Bergstrom, R., Wolk, A., Lindgren, A., Baron, J., and Adami, H.O. 1993. Diet and risk of gastric cancer. A population-based case–control study in Sweden. *Int J Cancer* **55**: 181–189.

Hara, M., Hanaoka, T., Kobayashi, M., Otani, T., Adachi, H.Y., Montani, A., Natsukawa, S., Shaura, K., Koizumi, Y., Kasuga, Y., Matsuzawa, T., Ikekawa, T., Sasaki, S., and Tsugane, S. 2003. Cruciferous vegetables, mushrooms, and gastrointestinal cancer risks in a multicenter, hospital-based case–control study in Japan. *Nutr Cancer* **46**: 138–147.

Harris, R.W.C., Key, T.J.A., Silcocks, P.B., Bull, D., and Wald, N.J. 1991. A case–control study of dietary carotene in men with lung cancer and in men with other epithelial cancers. *Nutr Cancer* **15**: 63–68.

Harrison, L.E., Zhang, Z.F., Karpeh, M.S., Sun, M., and Kurtz, R.C. 1997. The role of dietary factors in the intestinal and diffuse histologic subtypes of gastric adenocarcinoma: a case–control study in the U.S. *Cancer* **80**: 1021–1028.

Havas, S. 1997. Diet and cancer. *Md Med J* **46**: 477–480.

Hayes, R.B., Ziegler, R.G., Gridley, G., Swanson, C., Greenberg, R.S., Swanson, G.M., Schoenberg, J.B., Silverman, D.T., Brown, L.M., Pottern, L.M., Liff, J., Schwartz, A.G., Fraumeni, J.F., Jr., and Hoover, R.N. 1999. Dietary factors and risks for prostate cancer among blacks and whites in the United States. *Cancer Epidemiol Biomarkers Prev* **8**: 25–34.

Head, K.A. 1998. Ascorbic acid in the prevention and treatment of cancer. *Alt Med Rev* **3**: 174–186.

Hecht, S.S. 1999a. Chemoprevention of cancer by isothiocyanates, modifiers of carcinogen metabolism. *J Nutr* **129**: 768S–774S.

Hecht, S.S. 1999b. Chemoprevention of cancer by isothiocyanates, modifiers of carcinogen metabolism. *J Nutr* **129**: 768S–774S.

Heilbrun, L.K., Nomura, A., Hankin, J.H., and Stemmermann, G.N. 1989. Diet and colorectal cancer with special reference to fiber intake. *Int J Cancer* **44**: 1–6.

Henderson, B.E., Ross, R.K., and Pike, M.C. 1991. Toward the primary prevention of cancer. *Science* **254**: 1131–1138.

Hennekens, C.H., Buring, J.E., Manson, J.E., Stampfer, M., Rosner, B., Cook, N.R., Belanger, C., LaMotte, F., Gaziano, J.M., Ridker, P.M., Willett, W., and Peto, R. 1996. Lack of effect of long-term supplementation with beta carotene on the incidence of malignant neoplasms and cardiovascular disease. *N Engl J Med* **334**: 1145–1149.

Hermann, S., Linseisen, J., and Chang-Claude, J. 2002. Nutrition and breast cancer risk by age 50: a population-based case–control study in Germany. *Nutr Cancer* **44**: 23–34.

Hertog, M.G.L., Bueno-de-Mesquita, H.B., Fehily, A.M., Sweetnam, P.M., Elwood, P.C., and Kromhout, D. 1996. Fruit and vegetable consumption and cancer mortality in the Caerphilly Study. *Cancer Epidemiol Biomarkers Prev* **5**: 673–677.

Higginson, J. 1966. Etiological factors in gastrointestinal cancer in man. *J Natl Cancer Inst* **37**: 527–545.

Hirayama, T. 1979. Diet and cancer. *Nutr Cancer* **1**: 67–81.

Hirayama, T. 1986. A large scale cohort study on cancer risks by diet—with special reference to the risk reducing effects of green-yellow vegetable consumption. *In* "Diet, Nutrition, and Cancer" (Y. Hayashi, M. Magao, T. Sugimura, and et al., Eds.), pp. 41–53. Japan Scientific Societies Press, Tokyo.

Hirayama, T. 1990. Life-style and mortality: a large-scale census-based cohort study in Japan. *In* "Contributions to Epidemiology and Biostatistics" (J. Wahrendorf, Ed.), pp. 1–133. Karger, Basel.

Hirose, K., Tajima, K., Hamajima, N., Inoue, M., Takezaki, T., Kuroishi, T., Yoshida, M., and Tokudome, S. 1995. A large-scale, hospital-based case–control study of risk factors of breast cancer according to menopausal status. *Jpn J Cancer Res* **86**: 146–154.

Hirose, K., Takezaki, T., Hamajima, N., Miura, S., and Tajima, K. 2003. Dietary factors protective against breast cancer in Japanese premenopausal and postmenopausal women. *Int J Cancer* **107**: 276–282.

Hislop, T.G., Coldman, A.J., Elwood, J.M., Brauer, G., and Kan, L. 1986. Childhood and recent eating patterns and risk of breast cancer. *Cancer Detect Prev* **9**: 47–58.

Holick, C.N., Michaud, D.S., Stolzenberg-Solomon, R., Mayne, S.T., Pietinen, P., Taylor, P.R., Virtamo, J., and Albanes, D. 2002. Dietary carotenoids, serum β-carotene and retinol and risk of lung cancer in the alpha-tocopherol, beta-carotene cohort study. *Am J Epidemiol* **156**: 536–547.

Holmberg, L., Ohlander, E.M., Byers, T., Zack, M., Wolk, A., Bergstrom, R., Bergkvist, L., Thurfjell, E., Bruce, A., and Adami, H.-O. 1994. Diet and breast cancer risk: results from a population-based, case–control study in Sweden. *Arch Intern Med* **154**: 1805–1811.

Holmes, M.D., and Willett, W.C. 2004. Does diet affect breast cancer risk? *Breast Cancer Res* **6**: 170–178.

Hoshiyama, Y., and Sasaba, T. 1992. A case–control study of single and multiple stomach cancers in Saitama Prefecture, Japan. *Jpn J Cancer Res* **83**: 937–943.

Hsing, A.W., Chokkalingam, A.P., Gao, Y.T., Madigan, M.P., Deng, J., Gridley, G., and Fraumeni, J.F., Jr. 2002. Allium vegetables and risk of prostate cancer: a population based study. *J Natl Cancer Inst* **94**: 1648–1651.

Hsing, A.W., McLaughlin, J.K., Chow, W.H., Schuman, L.M., Co Chien, H.T., Gridley, G., Bjelke, E., Wacholder, S., and Blot, W.J. 1998a. Risk factors for colorectal cancer in a prospective study among U.S. white men. *Int J Cancer* **77**: 549–553.

Hsing, A.W., McLaughlin, J.K., Cocco, P., Co Chien, H.T., and Fraumeni, J.F., Jr. 1998b. Risk factors for male breast cancer (United States). *Cancer Causes Control* **9**: 26975.

Hsing, A.W., McLaughlin, J.K., Schuman, L.M., Bjelke, E., Gridley, G., Wacholder, S., Co Chien, H.T., and Blot, W.J. 1990. Diet, tobacco use, and fatal prostate cancer: results from the Lutheran Brotherhood Cohort Study. *Cancer Res* **50**: 6836–6840.

Hu, J., Johnson, K.C., Mao, Y., Xu, T., Lin, Q., Wang, C., Zhao, F., Wang, G., Chen, Y., and Yang, Y. 1997. A case–control study of diet and lung cancer in Northeast China. *Int J Cancer* **71**: 924–931.

Hu, J., Liu, Y., Yu, Y., Zhao, T., Liu, S., and Wang, Q. 1991. Diet and cancer of the colon and rectum: a case–control study in China. *Int J Epidemiol* **20**: 362–367.

Huang, X.E., Tajima, K., Hamajima, N., Xiang, J., Inoue, M., Hirose, K., Tominaga, S., Takezaki, T., Kuroishi, T., and Tokudome, S. 2000. Comparison of lifestyle and risk factors among Japanese with and without gastric cancer family history. *Int J Cancer* **86**: 421–424.

Hugosson, J., Aus, G., Lilja, H., Lodding, P., and Pihl, C.G. 2004. Results of a randomized, population-based study of biennial screening using serum prostate-specific antigen measurement to detect prostate carcinoma. *Cancer* **100**: 1397–1405.

Hung, H.C., Jiang, R., Joshipura, K.J., Hu, F.B., Hunter, D.J., Smith-Warner, S.A., Colditz, G.A., Rosner, B., Spiegelman, D., and Willett, W.C. 2004. Fruit and vegetable intake and the risk of major chronic disease. *J Natl Cancer Inst* **96**: 1577–1584.

Hunter, D.J., Manson, J.E., Colditz, G.A., Stampfer, M.J., Rosner, B., Hennekens, C.H., Speizer, F.E., and Willett, W.C. 1993. A prospective study of the intake of vitamins C, E, and A and the risk of breast cancer. *N Engl J Med* **329**: 234–240.

Iacopetta, B. 2002. Are there two sides to colorectal cancer? *Int J Cancer* **101**: 403–408.

IARC. 2003. "Fruit and Vegetables: IARC Handbooks of Cancer Prevention." IARC Press, Lyon, France.

Ingram, D.M., Nottage, E., and Roberts, T. 1991. The role of diet in the development of breast cancer: a case–control study of patients with breast cancer, benign epithelial hyperplasia and fibrocystic disease of the breast. *Br J Cancer* **64**: 187–191.

Inoue, M., Tajima, K., Hirose, K., Hamajima, N., Takezaki, T., Hirai, T., Kato, T., and Ohno, Y. 1995. Subsite-specific risk factors for colorectal cancer: a hospital-based case–control study in Japan. *Cancer Causes Control* **6**: 14–22.

Inoue, M., Tajima, K., Hirose, K., Kuroishi, T., Gao, C.M., and Kitoh, T. 1994. Life-style and subsite of gastric cancer—joint effect of smoking and drinking habits. *Int J Cancer* **56**: 494–499.

Inoue, M., Tajima, K., Kobayashi, S., Suzuki, T., Matsuura, A., Nakamura, T., Shirai, M., Nakamura, S., Inuzuka, K., and Tominaga, S. 1996. Protective factor against progression from atrophic gastritis to gastric cancer—data from a cohort study in Japan. *Int J Cancer* **66**: 309–314.

Iscovich, J.M., Iscovich, R.B., Howe, G., Shiboski, S., and Kaldor, J.M. 1989. A case–control study of diet and breast cancer in Argentina. *Int J Cancer* **44**: 770–776.

Iscovich, J.M., L'Abbe, K.A., Castelleto, R., Calzona, A., Bemedo, A., Chopita, N.A., Jmelnitzsky, A.C., and Kaldor, J. 1992. Colon cancer in Argentina. I: Risk from intake of dietary items. *Int J Cancer* **51**: 851–857.

Ito, L.S., Inoue, M., Tajima, K., Yamamura, Y., Kodera, Y., Hirose, K., Takezaki, T., Hamajima, N., Kuroishi, T., and Tominaga, S. 2003. Dietary factors and the risk of gastric cancer among Japanese women: a comparison between the differentiated and nondifferentiated subtypes. *Ann Epidemiol* **13**: 24–31.

Jain, M., Burch, J.D., Howe, G.R., Risch, H.A., and Miller, A.B. 1990. Dietary factors and risk of lung cancer: results from a case–control study, Toronto, 1981–1985. *Int J Cancer* **45**: 287–293.

Jain, M.G., Hislop, G.T., Howe, G.R., and Ghadirian, P. 1999. Plant foods, antioxidants, and prostate cancer risk: findings from case–control studies in Canada. *Nutr Cancer* **34**: 173–184.

Jang, M., Cai, L., Udeani, G.O., Slowing, K.V., Thomas, C.F., Beecher, C.W., Fong, H.H., Farnsworth, N.R., Kinghorn, A.D., Mehta, R.G., Moon, R.C., and Pezzuto, J.M. 1997. Cancer chemopreventive activity of resveratrol, a natural product derived from grapes. *Science* **275**: 218–220.

Jansen, M.C., Bueno-de-Mesquita, H.B., Rasanen, L., Fidanza, F., Menotti, A., Nissinen, A., Feskens, E.J., Kok, F.J., and Kromhout, D. 1999. Consumption of plant foods and stomach cancer mortality in the seven countries study. Is grain consumption a risk factor? Seven Countries Study Research Group. *Nutr Cancer* **34**: 49–55.

Jansen, M.C., Bueno-de-Mesquita, H.B., Rasanen, L., Fidanza, F., Nissinen, A.M., Menotti, A., Kok, F.J., and Kromhout, D. 2001. Cohort analysis of fruit and vegetable consumption and lung cancer mortality in European men. *Int J Cancer* **92**: 913–918.

Jarvinen, R., Knekt, P., Seppanen, R., and Teppo, L. 1997. Diet and breast cancer risk in a cohort of Finnish women. *Cancer Lett* **114**: 251–253.

Jedrychowski, W., Boeing, H., Popiela, T., Wahrendorf, J., Tobiasz-Adamczyk, B., and Kulig, J. 1992. Dietary practices in households as risk factors for stomach cancer: a familial study in Poland. *Eur J Cancer Prevention* **1**: 297–304.

Jedrychowski, W., Wahrendorf, J., Popiela, T., and Rachtan, J. 1986. A case–control study of dietary factors and stomach cancer risk in Poland. *Int J Cancer* **37**: 837–842.

Ji, B.T., Chow, W.H., Yang, G., McLaughlin, J.K., Zheng, W., Shu, X.O., Jin, F., Gao, R.N., Gao, Y.T., and Fraumeni, J.F., Jr. 1998. Dietary habits and stomach cancer in Shanghai, China. *Int J Cancer* **76**: 659–664.

Kalandidi, A., Katsouyanni, K., Voropoulou, N., Bastas, G., Saracci, R., and Trichopoulos, D. 1990. Passive smoking and diet in the etiology of lung cancer among non-smokers. *Cancer Causes Control* **1**: 15–21.

Kampman, E., Verhoeven, D., Sloots, L., and van'tVeer, P. 1995. Vegetable and animal products as determinants of colon cancer risk in Dutch men and women. *Cancer Causes Control* **6**: 225–234.

Kasum, C.M., Jacobs, D.R., Jr., Nicodemus, K., and Folsom, A.R. 2002. Dietary risk factors for upper aerodigestive tract cancers. *Int J Cancer* **99**: 267–272.

Kato, I., Tominaga, S., Ito, Y., Kobayashi, S., Yoshii, Y., Matsuura, A., Kameya, A., and Kano, T. 1990. A comparative case–control analysis of stomach cancer and atrophic gastritis. *Cancer Res* **50**: 6559–6564.

Kato, I., Tominaga, S., and Matsumoto, K. 1992. A prospective study of stomach cancer among a rural Japanese population: a 6-year survey. *Jpn J Cancer Res* **83**: 568–575.

Katsouyanni, K., Trichopoulos, D., Boyle, P., Xirouchaki, E., Trichopoulou, A., Lisseos, B., Vasilaros, S., and MacMahon, B. 1986. Diet and breast cancer: a case–control study in Greece. *Int J Cancer* **38**: 815–820.

Kelsey, J.L., and Horn-Ross, P.L. 1993. Breast cancer: magnitude of the problem and descriptive epidemiology. *Epidemiol Rev* **15**: 7–16.

Key, T.J., Allen, N., Appleby, P., Overvad, K., Tjonneland, A., Miller, A., Boeing, H., Karalis, D., Psaltopoulou, T., Berrino, F., Palli, D., Panico, S., Tumino, R., Vineis, P., Bueno-De-Mesquita, H.B., Kiemeney, L., Peeters, P.H., Martinez, C., Dorronsoro, M., Gonzalez, C.A., Chirlaque, M.D., Quiros, J.R., Ardanaz, E., Berglund, G., Egevad, L., Hallmans, G., Stattin, P., Bingham, S., Day, N., Gann, P., Kaaks, R., Ferrari, P., and Riboli, E. 2004. Fruits and vegetables and prostate cancer: no association among 1104 cases in a prospective study of 130544 men in the European Prospective Investigation into Cancer and Nutrition (EPIC). *Int J Cancer* **109**: 119–124.

Key, T.J., Silcocks, P.B., Davey, G.K., Appleby, P.N., and Bishop, D.T. 1997. A case–control study of diet and prostate cancer. *Br J Cancer* **76**: 678–687.

Key, T.J.A., Thorogood, M., Appleby, P.N., and Burr, M.L. 1996. Dietary habits and mortality in 11,000 vegetarians and health conscious people: results of a 17 year follow up. *BMJ* **313**: 775–779.

Kim, H.J., Chang, W.K., Kim, M.K., Lee, S.S., and Choi, B.Y. 2002. Dietary factors and gastric cancer in Korea: a case–control study. *Int J Cancer* **97**: 531–535.

Knekt, P., Jarvinen, R., Seppanen, R., Heliovaara, M., Teppo, L., Pukkala, E., and Aromaa, A. 1997. Dietary flavonoids and the risk of lung cancer and other malignant neoplasms. *Am J Epidemiol* **146**: 223–230.

Knekt, P., Jarvinen, R., Seppanen, R., Rissanen, A., Aromaa, A., Heinonen, O.P., Albanes, D., Heinonen, M., Pukkala, E., and Teppo, L. 1991. Dietary antioxidants and the risk of lung cancer. *Am J Epidemiol* **134**: 471–479.

Knekt, P., Jarvinen, R., Teppo, L., Aromaa, A., and Seppanen, R. 1999. Role of various carotenoids in lung cancer prevention. *J Natl Cancer Inst* **91**: 182–184.

Kneller, R.W., McLaughlin, J.K., Bjelke, E., Schuman, L.M., Blot, W.J., Wacholder, S., Gridley, G., CoChien, H.T., and Fraumeni, J.F., Jr. 1991. A cohort study of stomach cancer in a high-risk American population. *Cancer* **68**: 672–678.

Knowles, L.M., and Milner, J.A. 2001. Possible mechanism by which allyl sulfides suppress neoplastic cell proliferation. *J Nutr* **131**: 106IS–106S.

Ko, Y.-C., Lee, C.-H., Chen, M.-J., Huang, C.-C., Chang, W.-Y., Lin, H.-J., Wang, H.-Z., and Chang, P.-Y. 1997. Risk factors for primary lung cancer among non-smoking women in Taiwan. *Int J Epidemiol* **26**: 24–31.

Kobayashi, M., Tsubono, Y., Sasazuki, S., Sasaki, S., and Tsugane, S. 2002. Vegetables, fruit and risk of gastric cancer in Japan: a 10-year follow-up of the JPHC Study Cohort I. *Int J Cancer* **102**: 39–44.

Kolonel, L.N. 2001. Fat, meat, and prostate cancer. *Epidemiol Rev* **23**: 72–81.

Kolonel, L.N., Hankin, J.H., Whittemore, A.S., Wu, A.H., Gallagher, R.P., Wilkens, L.R., John, E.M., Howe, G.R., Dreon, D.M., West, D.W., and Paffenbarger, R.S., Jr. 2000. Vegetables, fruits, legumes and prostate cancer: a multiethnic case–control study. *Cancer Epidemiol Biomarkers Prev* **9**: 795–804.

Kono, S., Ikeda, M., Tokudome, S., and Kuratsune, M. 1988. A case–control study of gastric cancer and diet in northern Kyushu, Japan. *Jpn J Cancer Res* **79**: 1067–1074.

Koo, L.C. 1988. Dietary habits and lung cancer risk among Chinese females in Hong Kong who never smoked. *Nutr Cancer* **11**: 155–172.

Kotake, K., Koyama, Y., Nasu, J., Fukutomi, T., and Yamaguchi, N. 1995. Relation of family history of cancer and environmental factors to the risk of colorectal cancer: a case–control study. *Jpn J Clin Oncol* **25**: 195–202.

Krebs-Smith, S.M., Heimendinger, J., Subar, A.F., Patterson, B.H., and Pivonka, E. 1995. Using food frequency questionnaires to estimate fruit and vegetable intake: association between the number of questions and total intakes. *J Nutr Education* **27**: 80–85.

Kreuzer, M., Heinrich, J., Kreienbrock, L., Rosario, A.S., Gerken, M., and Wichmann, H.E. 2002. Risk factors for lung cancer among nonsmoking women. *Int J Cancer* **100**: 706–713.

Kris-Etherton, P.M., Hecker, K.D., Bonanome, A., Coval, S.M., Binkoski, A.E., Hilpert, K.F., Griel, A.E., and Etherton, T.D. 2002. Bioactive compounds in foods: their role in the prevention of cardiovascular disease and cancer. *Am J Med* **113**(Suppl 9B): 71S–88S.

Krishnaswamy, K., and Madhavan Nair, K. 2001. Importance of folate in human nutrition. *Br J Nutr* **85**(Suppl 2): S115–S124.

Kubik, A., Zatloukal, P., Tomasek, L., Kriz, J., PetrliZelka, L., and Plesko, I. 2001. Diet and the risk of lung cancer among women. A hospital-based case–control study. *Neoplasma* **48**: 262–266.

Kubik, A.K., Zatloukal, P., Tomasek, L., and Petruzelka, L. 2002. Lung cancer risk among Czech women: a case–control study. *Prev Med* **34**: 436–444.

Kune, G.A., and Vitetta, L. 1992. Alcohol consumption and the etiology of colorectal cancer: a review of the scientific evidence from 1957 to 1991. *Nutr Cancer* **18**: 97–111.

Kune, S., Kune, G.A., and Watson, L.F. 1987. Case-control study of dietary etiologic factors: the Melbourne Colorectal Cancer Study. *Nutr Cancer* **9**: 21–42.

Kvale, G., Bjelke, E., and Gart, J.J. 1983. Dietary habits and lung cancer risk. *Int J Cancer* **31**: 397–405.

La Vecchia, C. 2001. Diet and human cancer: a review. *Eur J Cancer Prevention* **10**: 177–181.

La Vecchia, C., Decarli, A., Franceschi, S., Gentile, A., Negri, E., and Parazzini, F. 1987a. Dietary factors and the risk of breast cancer. *Nutr Cancer* **10**: 205–214.

La Vecchia, C., Munoz, S.E., Braga, C., Fernandez, E., and Decarli, A. 1997. Diet diversity and gastric cancer. *Int J Cancer* **72**: 255–257.

La Vecchia, C., Negri, E., Decarli, A., D'Avanzo, B., and Franceschi, S. 1987b. A case–control study of diet and gastric cancer in northern Italy. *Int J Cancer* **40**: 484–489.

La Vecchia, C., Negri, E., Decarli, A., D'Avanzo, B., Gallotti, L., Gentile, A., and Franceschi, S. 1988. A case–control study of diet and colo-rectal cancer in Northern Italy. *Int J Cancer* **41**: 492–498.

La Vecchia, C., and Tavani, A. 1998. Fruit and vegetables, and human cancer. *Eur J Cancer Prevention* **7**: 3–8.

Lahmann, P.H., Hoffmann, K., Allen, N., van Gils, C.H., Khaw, K.T., Tehard, B., Berrino, F., Tjonneland, A., Bigaard, J., Olsen, A., Overvad,

K., Clavel-Chapelon, F., Nagel, G., Boeing, H., Trichopoulos, D., Economou, G., Bellos, G., Palli, D., Tumino, R., Panico, S., Sacerdote, C., Krogh, V., Peeters, P.H., Bueno-de-Mesquita, H.B., Lund, E., Ardanaz, E., Amiano, P., Pera, G., Quiros, J.R., Martinez, C., Tormo, M.J., Wirfalt, E., Berglund, G., Hallmans, G., Key, T.J., Reeves, G., Bingham, S., Norat, T., Biessy, C., Kaaks, R., and Riboli, E. 2004. Body size and breast cancer risk: findings from the European Prospective Investigation into Cancer And Nutrition (EPIC). *Int J Cancer* **111**: 762–771.

Lamm, D.L., and Riggs, D.R. 2001. Enhanced immunocompetence by garlic: role in bladder cancer and other malignancies. *J Nutr* **131**: 1067S–1070S.

Lampe, J.W. 1999. Health effects of vegetables and fruit: assessing mechanisms of action in human experimental studies. *Am J Clin Nutr* **70**: 475S–490S.

Landa, M.-C., Frago, N., and Tres, A. 1994. Diet and the risk of breast cancer in Spain. *Eur J Cancer Prevention* **3**: 313–320.

Le Marchand, L., Hankin, J.H., Kolonel, L.N., Beecher, G.R., Wilkens, L.R., and Zhao, L.P. 1993. Intake of specific carotenoids and lung cancer risk. *Cancer Epidemiol Biomarkers Prev* **2**: 183–187.

Le Marchand, L., Hankin, J.H., Kolonel, L.N., and Wilkins, L.R. 1991. Vegetable and fruit consumption in relation to prostate cancer risk in Hawaii: a reevaluation of the effect of dietary beta-carotene. *Am J Epidemiol* **133**: 215–219.

Le Marchand, L., Kolonel, L.N., Wilkens, L.R., Myers, B.C., and Hirohata, T. 1994. Animal fat consumption and prostate cancer: a prospective study in Hawaii. *Epidemiology* **5**: 276–282.

Le Marchand, L., Murphy, S.P., Hankin, J.H., Wilkens, L.R., and Kolonel, L.N. 2000. Intake of flavonoids and lung cancer. *J Natl Cancer Inst* **92**: 154–160.

Le Marchand, L., Yoshizawa, C.N., Kolonel, L.N., Hankin, J.H., and Goodman, M.T. 1989. Vegetable consumption and lung cancer risk: a population-based case–control study in Hawaii. *J Natl Cancer Inst* **81**: 1158–1164.

Lee, H.H., Wu, H.Y., Chuang, Y.C., Chang, A.S., Chao, H.H., Chen, K.Y., Chen, H.K., Lai, G.M., Huang, H.H., and Chen, C.J. 1990. Epidemiologic characteristics and multiple risk factors of stomach cancer in Taiwan. *Anticancer Research* **10**: 875–881.

Lee, H.P., Gourley, L., Duffy, S.W., Esteve, J., Lee, J., and Day, N.E. 1989. Colorectal cancer and diet in an Asian population—A case–control study among Singapore Chinese. *Int J Cancer* **43**: 1007–1016.

Lee, I.-M., Cook, N.R., Manson, J.E., Buring, J.E., and Hennekens, C.H. 1999. β-carotene supplementation and incidence of cancer and cardiovascular disease: the Women's Health Study. *J Natl Cancer Inst* **91**: 2102–2106.

Lee, I.-M., and Paffenbarger, R.S. 1992. Quetelet's index and risk of colon cancer in college alumni. *J Natl Cancer Inst* **84**: 1326–1331.

Lee, I.-M., Paffenbarger, R.S., Jr., and Hsieh, C.-C. 1991. Physical activity and risk of developing colorectal cancer among college alumni. *J Natl Cancer Inst* **83**: 1324–1329.

Lee, J.K., Park, B.J., Yoo, K.Y, and Ahn, Y.O. 1995. Dietary factors and stomach cancer: a case–control study in Korea. *Int J Epidemiol* **24**: 33–41.

Lee, K.W., Lee, H.J., Surh, Y.J., and Lee, C.Y. 2003a. Vitamin C and cancer chemoprevention: reappraisal. *Am J Clin Nutr* **78**: 1074–1078.

Lee, M.M., Wang, R.T., Hsing, A.W., Gu, F.L., Wang, T., and Spitz, M. 1998. Case-control study of diet and prostate cancer in China. *Cancer Causes Control* **9**: 545–552.

Lee, S.A., Kang, D., Shim, K.N., Choe, J.W., Hong, W.S., and Choi, H. 2003a. Effect of diet and *Helicobacter pylori* infection to the risk of early gastric cancer. *J Epidemiol* **13**: 162–168.

Lei, Y.-X., Cai, W.-C., Chen, Y.-Z., and Du, Y.-X. 1996. Some lifestyle factors in human lung cancer: a case–control study of 792 lung cancer cases. *Lung Cancer* **14**(Suppl): S121–S136.

Levi, F., La Vecchia, C., Gulie, C., and Negri, E. 1993. Dietary factors and breast cancer risk in Vaud, Switzerland. *Nutr Cancer* **19**: 327–335.

Levi, F., Pasche, C., La Vecchia, C., Lucchini, F., and Franceschi, S. 1999. Food groups and colorectal cancer risk. *Br J Cancer* **79**: 1283–1287.

Li, H., Stampfer, M.J., Giovannucci, E.L., Morris, J.S., Willett, W.C., Gaziano, J.M., and Ma, J. 2004. A prospective study of plasma selenium levels and prostate cancer risk. *J Natl Cancer Inst* **96**: 696–703.

Liu, Y., Sobue, T., Otani, T., and Tsugane, S. 2004. Vegetables, Fruit Consumption and Risk of Lung Cancer among Middle-Aged Japanese Men and Women: JPHC Study. *Cancer Causes Control* **15**: 349–357.

Long-de, W., and Hammond, E.C. 1985. Lung cancer, fruit, green salad and vitamin pills. *Chin Med J* **98**: 206–210.

MacLennan, R., Da Costa, J., Day, N.E., Law, C.H., Ng, Y.K., and Shanmugaratnam, K. 1977. Risk factors for lung cancer in Singapore Chinese, a population with high female incidence rates. *Int J Cancer* **20**: 854–860.

Malila, N., Virtamo, J., Virtanen, M., Albanes, D., Tangrea, J.A., and Huttunen, J.K. 1999. The effect of alpha-tocopherol and beta-carotene supplementation on colorectal adenomas in middle-aged male smokers. *Cancer Epidemiol Biomarkers Prev* **8**: 489–493.

Malin, A.S., Qi, D., Shu, X.O., Gao, Y.T., Friedmann, J.M., Jin, F., and Zheng, W. 2003. Intake of fruits, vegetables and selected micronutrients in relation to the risk of breast cancer. *Int J Cancer* **105**: 413–418.

Maltzman, T.H., Christou, M., Gould, M.N., and Jefcoate, C.R. 1991. Effects of monoterpenoids on *in vivo* DMBA-DNA adduct formation and on phase I hepatic metabolizing enzymes. *Carcinogenesis* **12**: 2081–2087.

Mangels, A.R., Holden, J.M., Beecher, G.R., Forman, M.R., and Lanza, E. 1993. Carotenoid content of fruits and vegetables: an evaluation of analytic data. *J Am Diet Assoc* **93**: 284–296.

Mannisto, S., Smith-Warner, S.A., Spiegelman, D., Albanes, D., Anderson, K., van den Brandt, P., Cerhan, J., Colditz, G., Feskanich, D., Freudenheim, J.L., Giovannucci, E., Goldbohm, R., Graham, S., Miller, A., Rohan, T., Virtamo, J., Willett, W.C., and Hunter, D.J. 2004. Dietary carotenoids and risk of lung cancer in a pooled analysis of seven cohort studies. *Cancer Epidemiol Biomarkers Prev* **13**: 40–48.

Marchand, J.L., Luce, D., Goldberg, P., Bugel, I., Salomon, C., and Goldberg, M. 2002. Dietary factors and the risk of lung cancer in New Caledonia (South Pacific). *Nutr Cancer* **42**: 18–24.

Marlett, J.A. 1992. Content and composition of dietary fiber in 117 frequently consumed foods. *J Am Diet Assoc* **92**: 175–186.

Mathew, A., Gangadharan, P., Varghese, C., and Nair, M.K. 2000. Diet and stomach cancer: a case–control study in South India. *Eur J Cancer Prevention* **9**: 89–97.

Mattisson, I., Wirfalt, E., Johansson, U., Gullberg, B., Olsson, H., and Berglund, G. 2004. Intakes of plant foods, fibre and fat and risk of breast cancer—a prospective study in the Malmo Diet and Cancer cohort. *Br J Cancer* **90**: 122–127.

Maynard, M., Gunnell, D., Emmett, P., Frankel, S., and Davey Smith, G. 2003. Fruit, vegetables, and antioxidants in childhood and risk of adult cancer: the Boyd Orr cohort. *J Epidemiol Community Health* **57**: 218–225.

Mayne, S.T., Janerich, D.T., Greenwald, P., Chorost, S., Tucci, C., Zaman, M.B., Melamed, M.R., Kiely, M., and McKneally, M.F. 1994. Dietary beta carotene and lung cancer risk in U.S. nonsmokers. *J Natl Cancer Inst* **86**: 33–38.

McCullough, M.L., Robertson, A.S., Chao, A., Jacobs, E.J., Stampfer, M.J., Diver, R., Calle, E.E., and Thun, M.J. 2003. A prospective study of whole grains, fruits, vegetables, and colon cancer risk. *Cancer Causes Control* **14**: 959–970.

McCullough, M.L., Robertson, A.S., Jacobs, E.J., Chao, A., Calle, E.E., and Thun, M.J. 2001. A prospective study of diet and stomach cancer mortality in United States men and women. *Cancer Epidemiol Biomarkers Prev* **10**: 1201–1205.

McMichael, A.J., and Giles, G.G. 1988. Cancer in migrants to Australia: extending the descriptive epidemiological data. *Cancer Res* **48**: 751–756.

Memik, F., Nak, S.G., Gulten, M., and Ozturk, M. 1992. Gastric carcinoma in northwestern Turkey: epidemiologic characteristics. *J Environ Pathol Toxicol Oncol* **11**: 335–338.

Mettlin, C. 1989. Milk drinking, other beverage habits, and lung cancer risk. *Int J Cancer* **43**: 608–612.

Mettlin, C., Graham, S., and Swanson, M. 1979. Vitamin A and lung cancer. *J Natl Cancer Inst* **62**: 1435–1438.

Michels, K.B., Giovannucci, E., Joshipura, K.J., Rosner, B.A., Stampfer, M.J., Fuchs, C.S., Colditz, G.A., Speizer, F.E., and Willett, W.C. 2000. Prospective study of fruit and vegetable consumption and incidence of colon and rectal cancers. *J Natl Cancer Inst* **92**: 1740–1752.

Miller, A.B., Altenburg, H.P., Bueno-de-Mesquita, B., Boshuizen, H.C., Agudo, A., Berrino, F., Gram, I.T., Janson, L., Linseisen, J., Overvad, K., Rasmuson, T., Vineis, P., Lukanova, A., Allen, N., Amiano, P., Barricarte, A., Berglund, G., Boeing, H., Clavel Chapelon, F., Day, N.E., Hallmans, G., Lund, E., Martinez, C., Navarro, C., Palli, D., Panico, S., Peeters, P.H., Quiros, J.R., Tjonneland, A., Turnino, R., Trichopoulou, A., Trichopoulos, D., Slimani, N., and Riboli, E. 2004. Fruits and vegetables and lung cancer: Findings from the European Prospective Investigation into Cancer and Nutrition. *Int J Cancer* **108**: 269–276.

Miller, A.B., Howe, G.R., Jain, M., Craib, K.J.P., and Harrison, L. 1983. Food items and food groups as risk factors in a case–control study of diet and colo-rectal cancer. *Int J Cancer* **32**: 155–161.

Mills, J.J., Chari, R.S., Boyer, I.J., Gould, M.N., and Jirtle, R.L. 1995. Induction of apoptosis in liver tumors by the monoterpene perillyl alcohol. *Cancer Res* **55**: 979–983.

Mills, P.K., Beeson, W.L., Phillips, R.L., and Fraser, G.E. 1989. Cohort study of diet, lifestyle, and prostate cancer in Adventist men. *Cancer* **64**: 598–604.

Mishina, T., Watanabe, H., Araki, H., and Nakao, M. 1985. Epidemiological study of prostatic cancer by matched-pair analysis. *Prostate* **6**: 423–436.

Modan, B., Barell, V., Lubin, F., Modan, M., Greenberg, R.A., and Graham, S. 1975. Low fiber intake as an etiologic factor in cancer of the colon. *J Natl Cancer Inst* **55**: 15–18.

Morse, M.A., and Stoner, G.D. 1993. Cancer chemoprevention: principles and prospects. *Carcinogenesis* **14**: 1737–1746.

Munoz, N., Plummer, M., Vivas, J., Moreno, V., De Sanjose, S., Lopez, G., and Oliver, W. 2001. A case–control study of gastric cancer in Venezuela. *Int J Cancer* **93**: 417–423.

Munoz, S.E., Ferraroni, M., La Vecchia, C., and Decarli, A. 1997. Gastric cancer risk factors in subjects with family history. *Cancer Epidemiol Biomarkers Prev* **6**: 137–140.

Murata, M., Tagawa, M., Watanabe, S., Kimura, H., Takeshita, T., and Morimoto, K. 1999. Genotype difference of aldehyde dehydrogenase 2 gene in alcohol drinkers influences the incidence of Japanese colorectal cancer patients. *Jpn J Cancer Res* **90**: 711–79.

Negri, E., La Vecchia, C., Franceschi, S., D'Avanzo, B., and Parazzini, F. 1991. Vegetable and fruit consumption and cancer risk. *Int J Cancer* **48**: 350–354.

Ness, A.R., and Powles, J.W. 1997. Fruit and vegetables, and cardiovascular disease—a review. *Int J Epidemiol* **26**: 1–13.

Neuhouser, M.L., Patterson, R.E., Thomquist, M.D., Omenn, G.S., King, I.B., and Goodman, G.E. 2003. Fruits and Vegetables are associated with lower lung cancer risk only in the placebo arm of the β-carotene and retinol efficacy trial (CARET). *Cancer Epidemiol Biomarkers Prev* **12**: 350–358.

Ngoan, L.T., Mizoue, T., Fujino, Y., Tokui, N., and Yoshimura, T. 2002. Dietary factors and stomach cancer mortality. *Br J Cancer* **87**: 37–42.

Nishimoto, I.N., Hamada, G.S., Kowalski, L.P., Rodrigues, J.G., Iriya, K., Sasazuki, S., Hanaoka, T., and Tsugane, S. 2002. Risk factors for stomach cancer in Brazil (I. a case–control study among non-Japanese Brazilians in Sao Paulo). *Jpn J Clin Oncol* **32**: 277–283.

Nishino, H., Tokuda, H., Murakoshi, M., Satomi, Y., Masuda, M., Onozuka, M., Yamaguchi, S., Takayasu, J., Tsuruta, J., Okuda, M., Khachik, F., Narisawa, T., Takasuka, N., and Yano, M. 2000. Cancer prevention by natural carotenoids. *Biofactors* **13**: 89–94.

Nomura, A., Grove, J.S., Stemmermann, G.N., and Severson, R.K. 1990. A prospective study of stomach cancer and its relation to diet, cigarettes, and alcohol consumption. *Cancer Res* **50**: 627–631.

Nomura, A.M., Hankin, J.H., Kolonel, L.N., Wilkens, L.R., Goodman, M.T., and Stemmermann, G.N. 2003. Case–control study of diet and other risk factors for gastric cancer in Hawaii (United States). *Cancer Causes Control* **14**: 547–558.

Norrish, A.E., Jackson, R.T., Sharpe, S.J., and Skeaff, C.M. 2000. Prostate cancer and dietary carotenoids. *Am J Epidemiol* **151**: 119–123.

Nuttens, M.C., Romon, M., Ruidavets, J.B., Arveiler, D., Ducimetiere, P., Lecerf, J.M., Richard, J.L., Cambou, J.P., Simon, C., and Salomez, J.L. 1992. Relationship between smoking and diet: the MONICA-France project. *J Intern Med* **231**: 349–356.

Nyberg, F., Agrenius, V., Svartengren, K., Svensson, C., and Pershagen, G. 1998. Dietary factors and risk of lung cancer in never-smokers. *Int J Cancer* **78**: 430–436.

Ocke, M.C., Bueno-de-Mesquita, H.B., Feskens, E.J.M., van Staveren, W.A., and Kromhout, D. 1997. Repeated measurements of vegetables, fruits, β-carotene, and vitamins C and E in relation to lung cancer: The Zutphen Study. *Am J Epidemiol* **145**: 358–365.

Oishi, K., Okada, K., Yoshida, O., Yamabe, H., Ohno, Y., Hayes, R.B., and Schroeder, F.H. 1988. A case–control study of prostatic cancer with reference to dietary habits. *Prostate* **12**: 179–190.

Omenn, G.S., Goodman, G.E., Thomquist, M.D., Balmes, J., Cullen, M.R., Glass, A., Keogh, J.P., Meyskens, F.L., Jr., Valanis, B., Williams, J.H., Jr., Barnhart, S., Cherniack, M.G., Brodkin, C.A., and Hammar, S. 1996a. Risk factors for lung cancer and for intervention effects in CARET, the Beta-Carotene and Retinol Efficacy Trial. *J Natl Cancer Inst* **88**: 1550–1559.

Omenn, G.S., Goodman, G.E., Thomquist, M.D., Balmes, J., Cullen, M.R., Glass, A., Keogh, J.P., Meyskens, F.L., Jr., Valanis, B., Williams, J.H., Jr., Barnhart, S., and Hammar, S. 1996b. Effects of a combination of beta carotene and vitamin A on lung cancer and cardiovascular disease. *N Engl J Med* **334**: 1150–1155.

Ozasa, K., Watanabe, Y., Ito, Y., Suzuki, K., Tamakoshi, A., Seki, N., Nishino, Y., Kondo, T., Wakai, K., Ando, M., and Ohno, Y. 2001. Dietary habits and risk of lung cancer death in a large-scale cohort study (JACC Study) in Japan by sex and smoking habit. *Jpn J Cancer Res* **92**: 1259–1269.

Paiva, S.A., and Russell, R.M. 1999. Beta-carotene and other carotenoids as antioxidants. *J Am Col Nutr* **18**: 426–433.

Palli, D., Bianchi, S., Decarli, A., Cipriani, F., Avellini, C., Cocco, P., Falcini, F., Puntoni, R., Russo, A., Vindigni, C., and et al. 1992. A case–control study of cancers of the gastric cardia in Italy. *Br J Cancer* **65**: 263–266.

Parkin, D.M., Pisani, P., Lopez, A.D., and Masuyer, E. 1994. At least one in seven cases of cancer is caused by smoking. Global estimates for 1985. *Int J Cancer* **59**: 494–504.

Pawlega, J. 1992. Breast cancer and smoking, vodka drinking and dietary habits. *Acta Oncol* **31**: 387–392.

Pawlega, J., Rachtan, J., and Dyba, T. 1997. Evaluation of certain risk factors for lung cancer in Cracow (Poland). *Acta Oncol* **36**: 471–476.

Peters, R.K., Garabrant, D.H., Yu, M.C., and Mack, T.M. 1989. A case–control study of occupational and dietary factors in colorectal cancer in young men by subsite. *Cancer Res* **49**: 5459–5468.

Peters, R.K., Pike, M.C., Garabrandt, D., and Mack, T.M. 1992. Diet and colon cancer in Los Angeles County, California. *Cancer Causes Control* **3**: 457–473.

Phillips, R.L. 1975. Role of life-style and dietary habits in risk of cancer among Seventh-Day Adventists. *Cancer Res* **35**: 3513–3522.

Phillips, R.L., and Snowdon, D.A. 1985. Dietary relationships with fatal colorectal cancer among Seventh-Day Adventists. *J Natl Cancer Inst* **74**: 307–317.

Pickle, L.W., Green, M.H., Ziegler, R.G., Toledo, A., Hoover, R., Lynch, H.T., and Fraumeni, J.F.J. 1984. Colorectal cancer in rural Nebraska. *Cancer Res* **44**: 363–369.

Pierce, R.J., Kune, G.A., Kune, S., Watson, L.F., Field, B., Merenstein, D., Hayes, A., and Irving, L.B. 1989. Dietary and alcohol intake, smoking pattern, occupational risk, and family history in lung cancer patients: results of a case–control study in males. *Nutr Cancer* **12**: 237–248.

Pillow, P.C., Hursting, S.D., Duphorne, C.M., Jiang, H., Honn, S.E., Chang, S., and Spitz, M.R. 1997. Case-control assessment of diet and lung cancer risk in African Americans and Mexican Americans. *Nutr Cancer* **29**: 169–173.

Pinto, J.T., Lapsia, S., Shah, A., Santiago, H., and Kim, G. 2001. Antiproliferative effects of garlic-derived and other allium related compounds. *Adv Exp Med Biol* **492**: 83–106.

Pisa, F.E., and Barbone, F. 2002. Diet and the risk of cancers of the lung, oral cavity and pharynx, and larynx: a population-based case–control study in north-east Italy. *IARC Scientific Publication* **156**: 141–143.

Pisani, P., Berrino, F., Macaluso, M., Pastorino, U., Crosignani, P., and Baldasseroni, A. 1986. Carrots, green vegetables and lung cancer: a case–control study. *Int J Epidemiol* **15**: 463–468.

Platz, E.A., De Marzo, A.M., and Giovannucci, E. 2004. Prostate cancer association studies: pitfalls and solutions to cancer misclassification in the PSA era. *J Cell Biochem* **91**: 553–571.

Plummer, M., Franceschi, S., and Munoz, N. 2004. Epidemiology of gastric cancer. *In* "IARC Scientific Publications No. 157: Mechanisms of Carcinogenesis: Contributions of Molecular Epidemiology" (S. Publ. Ed.), pp. 311–326. IARC Press, Lyon, France.

Pool-Zobel, B.L., Bub, A., Muller, H., Wollowski, I., and Rechkemmer, G. 1997. Consumption of vegetables reduces genetic damage in humans: first results of a human intervention trial with carotenoid-rich foods. *Carcinogenesis* **18**: 1847–1850.

Potischman, N., Swanson, C.A., Coates, R.J., Gammon, M.D., Brogan, D.R., Curtin, J., and Brinton, L.A 1999. Intake of food groups and associated micronutrients in relation to risk of early-stage breast cancer. *Int J Cancer* **82**: 315–321.

Potter, J.D. 1996. Nutrition and colorectal cancer. *Cancer Causes Control* **7**: 127–146.

Potter, J.D., Slattery, M.L., Bostick, R.M., and Gapstur, S.M. 1993. Colon cancer: a review of the epidemiology. *Epidemiol Rev* **15**: 499–545.

Qi, X.-Y., Zhang, A.-Y., Wu, G.-L., and Pang, W.-Z. 1994. The association between breast cancer and diet and other factors. *Asia-Pacific J Publ Health* **7**: 98–104.

Quaglia, A., Vercelli, M., Puppo, A., Casella, C., Artioli, E., Crocetti, E., Falcini, F., Ramazzotti, V., and Tagliabue, G. 2003. Prostate cancer in Italy before and during the "PSA era": survival trend and prognostic determinants. *Eur J Cancer Prevention* **12**: 145–152.

Rachtan, J. 2002a. A case–control study of lung cancer in Polish women. *Neoplasma* **49**: 75–80.

Rachtan, J. 2002b. Dietary habits and lung cancer risk among Polish women. *Acta Oncol* **41**: 389–394.

Rachtan, J., and Sokolowski, A. 1997. Risk factors for lung cancer among women in Poland. *Lung Cancer* **18**: 137–145.

Ramon, J.M., Serra, L., Cerdo, C., and Oromi, J. 1993. Dietary factors and gastric cancer risk. A case–control study in Spain. *Cancer* **71**: 1731–1735.

Riboli, E., and Norat, T. 2003. Epidemiologic evidence of the protective effect of fruit and vegetables on cancer risk. *Am J Clin Nutr* **78**: 559S–569S.

Richardson, S., Gerber, M., and Cenee, S. 1991. The role of fat, animal protein and some vitamin consumption in breast cancer: a case–control study in Southern France. *Int J Cancer* **48**: 1–9.

Rimm, E.B. 1996. Invited commentary—alcohol consumption and coronary heart disease: good habits may be more important than just good wine. *Am J Epidemiol* **143**: 1094–1098.

Risch, H.A., Jain, M., Choi, N.W., Fodor, J.G., Pfeiffer, C.J., Howe, G.R., Harrison, L.W., Craib, K.J., and Miller, A.B. 1985. Dietary factors and the incidence of cancer of the stomach. *Am J Epidemiol* **122**: 947–959.

Rodriguez, C., Tatham, L.M., Thun, M.J., Calle, E.E., and Heath, C.W.J. 1997. Smoking and fatal prostate cancer in a large cohort of adult men. *Am J Epidemiol* **145**: 466–475.

Rohan, T.E., Howe, G.R., Friedenreich, C.M., Jain, M., and Miller, A.B. 1993. Dietary fiber, vitamins A, C, and E, and risk of breast cancer: a cohort study. *Cancer Causes Control* **4**: 29–37.

Ronco, A., De Stefani, E., Boffetta, P., Deneo-Pellegrini, H., Mendilaharsu, M., and Leborgne, F. 1999. Vegetables, fruits, and related nutrients and risk of breast cancer: a case–control study in Uruguay. *Nutr Cancer* **35**: 111–119.

Rose, D.P. 1990. Dietary fiber and breast cancer. *Nutr Cancer* **13**: 1–8.

Rose, D.P. 1992. Dietary fiber, phytoestrogens, and breast cancer. *Nutrition* **8**: 47–51.

Rose, D.P., Boyar, A.P., and Wynder, E.L. 1986. International comparisons of mortality rates for cancer of the breast, ovary, prostate, and colon, and per capita food consumption. *Cancer* **58**: 2363–2371.

Rose, D.P., Goldman, M., Connolly, J.M., and Strong, L.E. 1991. High-fiber diet reduces serum estrogen concentrations in premenopausal women. *Am J Clin Nutr* **54**: 520–525.

Ross, R.K., Shimizu, H., Paganini-Hill, A., Honda, G., and Henderson, B.E. 1987. Case–control studies of prostate cancer in Blacks and Whites in Southern California. *J Natl Cancer Inst* **78**: 869–874.

Ruano-Ravina, A., Figueiras, A., Dosil-Diaz, O., Barreiro-Carracedo, A., and Barros-Dios, J.M. 2002. A population-based case–control study on fruit and vegetable intake and lung cancer: a paradox effect? *Nutr Cancer* **43**: 47–51.

Sahyoun, N.R., Jacques, P.F., and Russell, R.M. 1996. Carotenoids, vitamins C and E, and mortality in an elderly population. *Am J Epidemiol* **144**: 501–511.

Sakai, R. 1989. Epidemiologic survey on lung cancer with respect to cigarette smoking and plant diet. *Jpn J Cancer Res* **80**: 513–520.

Sanchez-Diez, A., Hernandez-Mejia, R., and Cueto-Espinar, A. 1992. Study of the relation between diet and gastric cancer in a rural area of the Province of Leon, Spain. *Eur J Epidemiol* **8**: 233–237.

Sankaranarayanan, R., Varghese, C., Duffy, S.W., Padmakumary, G., Day, N.E., and Nair, M.K. 1994. A case–control study of diet and lung cancer in Kerala, South India. *Int J Cancer* **58**: 644–649.

Satia-Abouta, J., Galanko, J.A., Martin, C.F., Ammerman, A., and Sandler, R.S. 2004. Food groups and colon cancer risk in African-Americans and Caucasians. *Int J Cancer* **109**: 728–736.

Sato, T., and Miyata, G. 2000. The nutraceutical benefit, part iv: garlic. *Nutrition* **16**: 787–788.

Sauvaget, C., Nagano, J., Hayashi, M., Spencer, E., Shimizu, Y., and Allen, N. 2003. Vegetables and fruit intake and cancer mortality in the Hiroshimal Nagasaki Life Span Study. *Br J Cancer* **88**: 689–694.

Schorah, C.J. 1999. Micronutrients, vitamins, and cancer risk. *Vitamins and Hormones* **57**: 123.

Schuman, L.M., Mandel, J.S., Radke, A., Seal, U., and Halberg, F. 1982. Some selected features of the epidemiology of prostatic cancer: Minneapolis-St. Paul, Minnesota case–control study, 1976–1979. *In* "Trends in Cancer Incidence: Causes and Practical Implications" (K. Magnus, Ed.), pp. 345–354. Hemisphere Publishing Corp, Washington, DC.

Schuurman, A.G., Goldbohm, R.A., Dorant, E., and van den Brandt, P.A. 1998. Vegetable and fruit consumption and prostate cancer risk: a cohort study in The Netherlands. *Cancer Epidemiol Biomarkers Prev* **7**: 673–680.

Sellers, T.A., Bazyk, A.E., Bostick, R.M., Kushi, L.H., Olson, J.E., Anderson, K.E., Lazovich, D., and Folsom, A.R. 1998. Diet and risk of colon cancer in a large prospective study of older women: an analysis stratified on family history (Iowa, United States). *Cancer Causes Control* **9**: 357–367.

Sengupta, A., and Das, S. 1999. The anti-carcinogenic role of lycopene, abundantly present in tomato. *Eur J Cancer Prevention* **8**: 325–330.

Seow, A., Poh, W.T., Teh, M., Eng, P., Wang, Y.T., Tan, W.C., Chia, K.S., Yu, M.C., and Lee, H.P. 2002. Diet, reproductive factors and lung cancer risk among Chinese women in Singapore: evidence for a protective effect of soy in nonsmokers. *Int J Cancer* **97**: 365–371.

Serdula, M., Byers, T., Coates, R., Mokdad, A., Simoes, E.J., and Eldridge, L. 1992. Assessing consumption of high-fat foods: the effect of grouping foods into single questions. *Epidemiology* **3**: 503–508.

Severson, R.K., Nomura, A.M.Y., Grove, J.S., and Stemmermann, G.N. 1989. A prospective study of demographics, diet, and prostate cancer among men of Japanese ancestry in Hawaii. *Cancer Res* **49**: 1857–1860.

Shannon, J., Cook, L.S., and Stanford, J.L. 2003. Dietary intake and risk of postmenopausal breast cancer (United States). *Cancer Causes Control* **14**: 19–27.

Shannon, J., White, E., Shattuck, A.L., and Potter, J.D. 1996. Relationship of food groups and water intake to colon cancer risk. *Cancer Epidemiol Biomarkers Prev* **5**: 495–502.

Shapiro, T.A., Fahey, J.W., Wade, K.L., Stephenson, K.K., and Talalay, P. 2001. Chemoprotective glucosinolates and isothiocyanates of broccoli sprouts: metabolism and excretion in humans. *Cancer Epidemiol Biomarkers Prev* **10**: 501–508.

Shibata, A., Paganini-Hill, A., Ross, R.K., and Henderson, B.E. 1992. Intake of vegetables, fruits, beta-carotene, vitamin C and vitamin supplements and cancer incidence among the elderly: a prospective study. *Br J Cancer* **66**: 673–679.

Shimizu, H., Ross, R.K., Bernstein, L., Yatani, R., Henderson, B.E., and Mack, T.M. 1991. Cancers of the prostate and breast among Japanese and white immigrants in Los Angeles County. *Br J Cancer* **63**: 963–966.

Simard, A., Vobecky, J., and Vobecky, J.S. 1990. Nutrition and lifestyle factors in fibrocystic disease and cancer of the breast. *Cancer Detect Prev* **14**: 567–572.

Singh, P.N., and Fraser, G.E. 1998. Dietary risk factors for colon cancer in a low-risk population. *Am J Epidemiol* **148**: 761–774.

Slattery, M.L., Potter, J.D., Coates, A., Ma, K.-N., Berry, T.D., Duncan, D.M., and Caan, B.J. 1997. Plant foods and colon cancer: an assessment of specific foods and their related nutrients (United States). *Cancer Causes Control* **8**: 575–590.

Slattery, M.L., Sorenson, A.W., Mahoney, A.W., French, T.K., Kritchevsky, D., and Street, J.C. 1988. Diet and colon cancer: assessment of risk by fiber type and food source. *J Natl Cancer Inst* **80**: 1474–1480.

Smith, S.A., Campbell, D.R., Elmer, P.J., Martini, M.C., Slavin, J.L., and Potter, J.D. 1995. The University of Minnesota Cancer Prevention Research Unit vegetable and fruit classification scheme (United States). *Cancer Causes Control* **6**: 292–302.

Smith-Warner, S.A., Spiegelman, D., Adami, H.O., Beeson, L., van den Brandt, P., Folsom, A., Fraser, G., Freudneheim, J., Goldbohm, R., Graham, S., Kushi, L., Miller, A., Rohan, T., Speizer, F.E., Toniolo, P., Willett, W.C., Wolk, A., Zeleniuch-Jacquotte, A., and Hunter, D.J. 2001a. Types of dietary fat and breast cancer: a pooled analysis of cohort studies. *Int J Cancer* **92**: 767–774.

Smith-Warner, S.A., Spiegelman, D., Yaun, S.-S., Albanes, D., Beeson, W.L., van den Brandt, P.A., Feskanich, D., Folsom, A.R., Fraser, G.E., Freudenheim, J.L., Giovannucci, E., Goldbohm, R.A., Graham, S., Kushi, L., Miller, A.B., Pietinen, P., Rohan, T., Speizer, F.E., Willett, W.C., and Hunter, D.J. 2003. Fruits, vegetables and lung cancer: a pooled analysis of cohort studies. *Int J Cancer* **107**: 1001–1011.

Smith-Warner, S.A., Spiegelman, D., Yaun, S.-S., Beeson, L., van den Brandt, P., Folsom, A., Fraser, G., Freudneheim, J., Goldbohm, R., Graham, S., Miller, A., Potter, J., Rohan, T., Speizer, F.E., Toniolo, P., Willett, W.C., Wolk, A., Zeleniuch-Jacquotte, A., and Hunter, D.J. 2001b. Intake of fruits and vegetables and risk of breast cancer: a pooled analysis of cohort studies. *JAMA* **285**: 769–776.

Smith-Warner, S.A., Spiegelman, D., Yaun, S.-S., van den Brandt, P.A., Folsom, A.R., Goldbohm, R.A., Graham, S., Holmberg, L., Howe, G.R., Marshall, J.R., Miller, A.B., Potter, J.D., Speizer, F.E., Willett, W.C., Wolk, A., and Hunter, D.J. 1998. Alcohol and breast cancer in women: a pooled analysis of cohort studies. *JAMA* **279**: 535–540.

Snowdon, D.A., Phillips, R.L., and Choi, W. 1984. Diet, obesity, and risk of fatal prostate cancer. *Am J Epidemiol* **120**: 244–250.

Sonoda, T., Nagata, Y., Mori, M., Miyanaga, N., Takashima, N., Okumura, K., Goto, K., Naito, S., Fujimoto, K., Hirao, Y., Takahashi, A., Tsukamoto, T., Fujioka, T., and Akaza, H. 2004. A case–control study of diet and prostate cancer in Japan: possible protective effect of traditional Japanese diet. *Cancer Sci* **95**: 238–242.

Speizer, F.E., Colditz, G.A., Hunter, D.J., Rosner, B., Hennekens, C., Willett, W.C., and Kawachi, I. 1999. Prospective study of smoking, antioxidant intake, and lung cancer in middle-aged women (USA). *Cancer Causes Control* **10**: 475–482.

Steinmetz, K.A., Kushi, L.H., Bostick, R.M., Folsom, A.R., and Potter, J.D. 1994. Vegetables, fruit, and colon cancer in the Iowa Women's Health Study. *Am J Epidemiol* **139**: 1–15.

Steinmetz, K.A., and Potter, J.D. 1991. Vegetables, fruit, and cancer. II. Mechanisms. *Cancer Causes Control* **2**: 427–442.

Steinmetz, K.A., and Potter, J.D. 1993. Food-group consumption and colon cancer in the Adelaide Case-Control Study. I. Vegetables and fruit. *Int J Cancer* **53**: 711–719.

Steinmetz, K.A., and Potter, J.D. 1996. Vegetables, fruit, and cancer prevention: a review. *J Am Diet Assoc* **96**: 1027–1039.

Steinmetz, K.A., Potter, J.D., and Folsom, A.R. 1993. Vegetables, fruit, and lung cancer in the Iowa Women's Health Study. *Cancer Res* **53**: 536–543.

Stewart, B.W., and Kleihues, P. 2003. "World Cancer Report," pp. 1–19. IARC, Lyon, France.

Stover, P.J. 2004. Physiology of folate and vitamin B12 in health and disease. *Nutr Rev* **62**: S3–S13.

Stram, D.O., Huberman, M., and Wu, A.H. 2002. Is residual confounding a reasonable explanation for the apparent protective effects of beta-carotene found in epidemiologic studies of lung cancer in smokers? *Am J Epidemiol* **155**: 622–628.

Subar, A.F., Harlan, L.C., and Mattson, M.E. 1990. Food and nutrient intake differences between smokers and non-smokers in the US. *Am J Public Health* **80**: 1323–1329.

Subar, A.F., Heimendinger, J., Patterson, B.H., Krebs-Smith, S.M., Pivonka, E., and Kessler, R. 1995. Fruit and vegetable intake in the United States: the baseline survey of the Five A Day for Better Health Program. *Am J Health Promotion* **9**: 352–360.

Sung, J.F., Lin, R.S., Pu, Y.S., Chen, Y.C., Chang, H.C., and Lai, M.K. 1999. Risk factors for prostate carcinoma in Taiwan: a case–control study in a Chinese population. *Cancer* **86**: 484–491.

Suzuki, I., Hamada, G.S., Zamboni, M.M., Cordeiro Pde, B., Watanabe, S., and Tsugane, S. 1994. Risk factors for lung cancer in Rio de Janeiro, Brazil: a case–control study. *Lung Cancer* **11**: 179–190.

Swanson, C.A., Mao, B.L., Li, J.Y., Lubin, J.H., Yao, S.X., Wang, J.Z., Cai, S.K., Hou, Y., Luo, Q.S., and Blot, W.J. 1992. Dietary determinants of lung-cancer risk: results from a case–control study in Yunnan Province, China. *Int J Cancer* **50**: 876–880.

Szabo, E., and Mulshine, J. 1993. Epidemiology, prognostic factors, and prevention of lung cancer. *Curr Opin Oncol* **5**: 302–309.

Tajima, K., and Tominaga, S. 1985. Dietary habits and gastro-intestinal cancers. A comparative case–control study of stomach and large intestinal cancers in Nagoya, Japan. *Jpn J Cancer Res* **76**: 705–716.

Takezaki, T., Hirose, K., Inoue, M., Hamajima, N., Yatabe, Y., Mitsudomi, T., Sugiura, T., Kuroishi, T., and Tajima, K. 2001. Dietary factors and lung cancer risk in Japanese: with special reference to fish consumption and adenocarcinomas. *Br J Cancer* **84**: 1199–1206.

Talalay, P., and Fahey, J.W. 2001. Phytochemicals from cruciferous plants protect against cancer by modulating carcinogen metabolism. *J Nutr* **131**: 3027S–3033S.

Talamini, R., Franceschi, S., La Vecchia, C., Serraino, D., Barra, S., and Negri, E. 1992. Diet and prostatic cancer: a case–control study in Northern Italy. *Nutr Cancer* **18**: 277–286.

Talamini, R., La Vecchia, C., Decarli, A., Negri, E., and Franceschi, S. 1986. Nutrition, social factors and prostatic cancer in a Northern Italian population. *Br J Cancer* **53**: 817–821.

Tavani, A., Gallus, S., La Vecchia, C., Negri, E., Montella, M., Dal Maso, L., and Franceschi, S. 1999. Risk factors for breast cancer in women under 40 years. *Eur J Cancer* **35**: 1361–1367.

Terry, P., Giovannucci, E., Michels, K.B., Bergkvist, L., Hansen, H., Holmberg, L., and Wolk, A. 2001a. Fruit, vegetables, dietary fiber, and risk of colorectal cancer. *J Natl Cancer Inst* **93**: 525–533.

Terry, P., Lagergren, J., Hansen, H., Wolk, A., and Nyren, O. 200lb. Fruit and vegetable consumption in the prevention of oesophageal and cardia cancers. *Eur J Cancer Prevention* **10**: 365–369.

Terry, P., Lagergren, J., Wolk, A., and Nyren, O. 2000. Reflux-inducing dietary factors and risk of adenocarcinoma of the esophagus and gastric cardia. *Nutr Cancer* **38**: 186–191.

Terry, P., Nyren, O., and Yuen, J. 1998. Protective effect of fruits and vegetables on stomach cancer in a cohort of Swedish twins. *Int J Cancer* **76**: 35–37.

Terry, P., Terry, J.B., and Wolk, A. 2001c. Fruit and vegetable consumption in the prevention of cancer: an update. *J Intern Med* **250**: 280–290.

Terry, P., Wolk, A., Persson, I., and Magnusson, C. 2001d. Brassica vegetables and breast cancer risk (Letter). *JAMA* **285**: 2975–2977.

The Alpha-Tocopherol, and Beta Carotene Cancer Prevention Study Group. 1994. The effect of vitamin E and beta carotene on the incidence of lung cancer and other cancers in male smokers. *N Engl J Med* **330**: 1029–1035.

The Working Group on Diet and Cancer of the Committee on Medical Aspects of Food and Nutrition Policy. 1998. Nutritional aspects of the development of cancer. Controller of Her Majesty's Stationery Office.

Thorand, B., Kohlmeier, L., Simonsen, N., Croghan, C., and Thamm, M. 1998. Intake of fruits, vegetables, folic acid and related nutrients and risk of breast cancer in postmenopausal women. *Public Health Nutr* **1**: 147–156.

Thun, M.J., Calle, E.E., Namboodiri, M.M., Flanders, W.D., Coates, R.J., Byers, T., Boffetta, P., Garfinkel, L., and Heath, C.W.J. 1992. Risk factors for fatal colon cancer in a large prospective study. *J Natl Cancer Inst* **84**: 1491–1500.

Tominaga, S., and Kuroishi, T. 1997. An ecological study on diet/nutrition and cancer in Japan. *Int J Cancer* **l0**(Suppl): 2–6.

Toniolo, P., Riboli, E., Protta, F., Charrel, M., and Cappa, A.P.M. 1989. Calorie-providing nutrients and risk of breast cancer. *J Natl Cancer Inst* **81**: 278–286.

Trichopoulos, D., Ouranos, G., Day, N.E., Tzonou, A., Manousos, O., Papadimitriou, C., and Trichopoulos, A. 1985. Diet and cancer of the stomach: a case–control study in Greece. *Int J Cancer* **36**: 291–297.

Trichopoulou, A., Katsouyanni, K., Stuver, S., Tzala, L., Gnardellis, C., Rimm, E., and Trichopoulos, D. 1995. Consumption of olive oil and specific food groups in relation to breast cancer risk in Greece. *J Natl Cancer Inst* **87**: 110–116.

Tseng, M., Breslow, R.A., DeVellis, R.F., and Ziegler, R.G. 2004. Dietary patterns and prostate cancer risk in the National Health and Nutrition Examination Survey Epidemiological Follow-up Study cohort. *Cancer Epidemiol Biomarkers Prev* **13**: 71–77.

Tuyns, A.J., Kaaks, R., and Haelterman, M. 1988. Colorectal cancer and the consumption of foods: a case–control study in Belgium. *Nutr Cancer* **11**: 189–204.

Tuyns, A.J., Kaaks, R., Haelterman, M., and Riboli, E. 1992. Diet and gastric cancer. A case–control study in Belgium. *Int J Cancer* **51**: 1–6.

Tzonou, A., Signorello, L.B., Lagiou, P., Wuu, J., Trichopoulos, D., and Trichopoulou, A. 1999. Diet and cancer of the prostate: a case–control study in Greece. *Int J Cancer* **80**: 704–708.

van den Brandt, P.A., Spiegelman, D., Yaun, S.-S., Adami, H.-O., Beeson, L., Folsom, A.R., Fraser, G.E., Goldbohm, R.A., Graham, S., Kushi, L.H., Marshall, J.R., Miller, A.B., Rohan, T., Smith-Warner, S.A., Speizer, F.E., Willett, W.C., Wolk, A., and Hunter, D.J. 2000. Pooled analysis of prospective cohort studies on height, weight and breast cancer risk. *Am J Epidemiol* **152**: 514–527.

van Poppel, G., Verhoeven, D.T., Verhagen, H., and Goldbohm, R.A. 1999. Brassica vegetables and cancer prevention. Epidemiology and mechanisms. *Adv Exp Med Biol* **472**: 159–168.

Venket Rao, A., and Agarwal, S. 2000. Role of antioxidant lycopene in cancer and heart disease. *J Am Col Nutr* **19**: 563–569.

Verhoeven, D.T., Verhagen, H., Goldbohm, R.A., van den Brandt, P.A., and van Poppel, G. 1997a. A review of mechanisms underlying anti carcinogenicity by brassica vegetables. *Chemico-Biol Inter* **103**: 79–129.

Verhoeven, D.T.H., Assen, N., Goldbohm, R.A., Dorant, E., van't Veer, P., Sturmans, F., Hermus, R.J.J., and van den Brandt, P.A. 1997b. Vitamins C and E, retinol, betacarotene and dietary fibre in relation to breast cancer risk: a prospective cohort study. *Br J Cancer* **75**: 149–155.

Villeneuve, P.J., Johnson, K.C., Kreiger, N., and Mao, Y. 1999. Risk factors for prostate cancer: results from the Canadian National Enhanced Cancer Surveillance System. The Canadian Cancer Registries Epidemiology Research Group. *Cancer Causes Control* **10**: 355–367.

Vlajinac, H., Adanja, B., and Jarebinski, M. 1987. Case-control study of the relationship of diet and colon cancer. *Arch Geschwulstforschung* **57**: 493–498.

Voorrips, L.E., Goldbohm, R.A., van Poppel, G., Sturmans, F., Hermus, R.J., and van den Brandt, P.A. 2000a. Vegetable and fruit consumption and risks of colon and rectal cancer in a prospective cohort study: The Netherlands Cohort Study on Diet and Cancer. *Am J Epidemiol* **152**: 1081–1092.

Voorrips, L.E., Goldbohm, R.A., Verhoeven, D.T.H., van Poppel, G.A.F.C., Sturmans, F., Hermus, R.J.J., and van den Brandt, P.A. 2000b. Vegetable and fruit consumption and lung cancer risk in the Netherlands Cohort Study on Diet and Cancer. *Cancer Causes Control* **11**: 101–115.

Walker, A.R.P., Walker, B.F., Tsotetsi, N.G., Sebitso, C., Siwedi, D., and Walker, A.J. 1992. Case-control study of prostate cancer in black patients in Soweto, South Africa. *Br J Cancer* **65**: 438–441.

Wang, H., Cao, G., and Prior, R.L. 1996. Total antioxidant capacity of fruits. *J Agric Food Chem* **44**: 701–705.

Ward, M.H., and Lopez-Carrillo, L. 1999. Dietary factors and the risk of gastric cancer in Mexico City. *Am J Epidemiol* **149**: 925–932.

Wattenberg, L.W. 1990. Inhibition of carcinogenesis by minor anutrient constituents of the diet. *Proc Nutr Soc* **49**: 173–183.

Wattenberg, L.W. 1992. Inhibition of carcinogenesis by minor dietary constituents. *Cancer Res* **52**: 2085S–2091S.

Wei, E.K., Giovannucci, E., Wu, K., Rosner, B., Fuchs, C.S., Willett, W.C., and Colditz, G.A. 2004. Comparison of risk factors for colon and rectal cancer. *Int J Cancer* **108**: 433–442.

West, D.W., Slattery, M.L., Robison, L.M., Schuman, K.L., Ford, M.H., Mahoney, A.W., Lyon, J.L., and Sorensen, A.W. 1989. Dietary intake and colon cancer: sex- and anatomic site-specific associations. *Am J Epidemiol* **130**: 883–894.

Whittemore, A.S., Kolonel, L.N., Wu, A.H., John, E.M., Gallagher, R.P., Howe, G.R., Burch, J.D., Hankin, J., Dreon, D.M., West, D.W., Teh, C.-Z., and Paffenbarger, R.S., Jr. 1995. Prostate cancer in relation to diet, physical activity, and body size in Blacks, Whites, and Asians in the United States and Canada. *J Natl Cancer Inst* **87**: 652–661.

Willett, W.C., Stampfer, M.J., Colditz, G.A., Rosner, B.A., and Speizer, F.A. 1990. Relation of meat, fat, and fiber intake to the risk of colon cancer in a prospective study among women. *N Engl J Med* **323**: 1664–1672.

Word Cancer Research Fund, American Institute for Cancer Research Expert Panel (J.D. Potter and Chair) 1997. "Food, Nutrition and the Prevention of Cancer: A Global Perspective." American Institute for Cancer Research, Washington, DC.

Wright, M.E., Mayne, S.T., Swanson, C.A., Sinha, R., and Alavanja, M.C.R. 2003. Dietary carotenoids, vegetables, and lung cancer risk in women: the Missouri Women's Health Study (United States). *Cancer Causes Control* **14**: 85–96.

Wu-Williams, A.H., Dai, X.D., Blot, W., Xu, Z.Y., Sun, X.W., Xiao, H.P., Stone, B.J., Yu, S.F., Feng, Y.P., Ershow, A.G., Sun, J., Fraumeni, J.F., Jr., and Henderson, B.E. 1990a. Lung cancer among women in north-east China. *Br J Cancer* **62**: 982–987.

Wu-Williams, A.H., Yu, M.C., and Mack, T.M. 1990b. Life-style, work-place, and stomach cancer by subsite in young men of Los Angeles County. *Cancer Res* **50**: 2569–2576.

Wynder, E.L., Kajitani, T., Ishikawa, S., Dodo, H., and Takano, A. 1969. Environmental factors of cancer of the colon and rectum. II. Japanese epidemiological data. *Cancer* **23**: 1210–1220.

Wynder, E.L., and Shigematsu, T. 1967. Environmental factors of cancer of the colon and rectum. *Cancer* **20**: 1520–1561.

Xibin, S., Moller, H., Evans, H.S., Dixing, D., Wenjie, D., and Jianbang, L. 2002. Residential Environment, Diet and Risk of Stomach Cancer: a Case-control Study in Linzhou, China. *Asian Pacific J Cancer Prev* **3**: 167–172.

Xu, Z., Brown, L.M., Pan, G.W., Liu, T.F., Gao, G.S., Stone, B.J., Cao, R.M., Guan, D.X., Sheng, J.H., Yan, Z.S., Dosemeci, M., Fraumeni, J.F., Jr., and Blot, W.J. 1996. Cancer risks among iron and steel workers in Anshan, China, Part II: Case-control studies of lung and stomach cancer. *Am J Industrial Med* **30**: 7–15.

Yeh, C.C., Hsieh, L.L., Tang, R., Chang-Chieh, C.R., and Sung, F.C. 2003. Risk factors for colorectal cancer in Taiwan: a hospital-based case–control study. *J Formos Med Assoc* **102**: 305–312.

Yong, L.-C., Brown, C.C., Schatzkin, A., Dresser, C.M., Slesinski, M.J., Cox, C.S., and Taylor, P.R. 1997. Intake of vitamins E, C, and A and risk of lung cancer: the NHANES I Epidemiologic Followup Study. *Am J Epidemiol* **146**: 231–243.

You, W.C., Blot, W.J., Chang, Y.S., Ershow, A.G., Yang, Z.T., An, Q., Henderson, B., Xu, G.W., Fraumeni, J.F., Jr., and Wang, T.G. 1988. Diet and high risk of stomach cancer in Shandong, China. *Cancer Res* **48**: 3518–3523.

Young, T.B. 1989. A case–control study of breast cancer and alcohol consumption habits. *Cancer* **64**: 552–558.

Young, T.B., and Wolf, D.A. 1988. Case-control study of proximal and distal colon cancer and diet in Wisconsin. *Int J Cancer* **42**: 167–175.

Yu, G.P., and Hsieh, C.C. 1991. Risk factors for stomach cancer: a population-based case–control study in Shanghai. *Cancer Causes Control* **2**: 169–174.

Yu, H., Harris, R.E., Gao, Y.-T., Gao, R., and Wynder, E.L. 1991. Comparative epidemiology of cancers of the colon, rectum, prostate and breast in Shanghai, China versus the United States. *Int J Epidemiol* **20**: 76–81.

Yuan, J.-M., Wang, Q.-S., Ross, R.K., Henderson, B.E., and Yu, M.C. 1995. Diet and breast cancer in Shanghai and Tianjin, China. *Br J Cancer* **71**: 1353–1358.

Zaridze, D., Lifanova, Y., Maximovitch, D., Day, N.E., and DuffY, S.W. 1991. Diet, alcohol consumption and reproductive factors in a case–control study of breast cancer in Moscow. *Int J Cancer* **48**: 493–501.

Zatloukal, P., Kubik, A., Pauk, N., Tomasek, L., and Petruzelka, L. 2003. Adenocarcinoma of the lung among women: risk associated with smoking, prior lung disease, diet and menstrual and pregnancy history. *Lung Cancer* **41**: 283–293.

Zemla, B. 1984. The role of selected dietary elements in breast cancer risk among native and migrant populations in Poland. *Nutr Cancer* **6**: 187–195.

Zhang, S., Hunter, D.J., Forman, M.R., Rosner, B.A., Speizer, F.E., Colditz, G.A., Manson, J.E., Hankinson, S.E., and Willett, W.C. 1999. Dietary carotenoids, and vitamins A, C, and E and risk of breast cancer. *J Natl Cancer Inst* **91**: 547–556.

Ziegler, R.G., Colavito, E.A., Hartge, P., McAdams, M.J., Schoenberg, J.B., Mason, T.J., and Fraumeni, J.F., Jr. 1996. Importance of ex-carotene, β-carotene, and other phytochemicals in the etiology of lung cancer. *J Natl Cancer Inst* **88**: 612–615.

Ziegler, R.G., Mason, T.J., Sternhagen, A., Hoover, R., Schoenberg, J.B., Gridley, G., Virgo, P.W., and Fraumeni, J.F., Jr. 1986. Carotenoid intake, vegetables, and the risk of lung cancer among white men in New Jersey. *Am J Epidemiol* **123**: 1080–1093.

Zografos, G.C., Panou, M., and Panou, N. 2004. Common risk factors of breast and ovarian cancer: recent view. *Int J Gynecol Cancer* **14**: 721–740.

CHAPTER

8

Are Whole Grains Protective Against a Variety of Cancers?

DAVID M. KLURFELD

INTRODUCTION

Whole grains have received increased emphasis in dietary recommendations because they are linked epidemiologically to reduced incidence of a variety of chronic diseases including diabetes, heart disease, and cancer. Their consumption is also linked with less obesity, which is a risk factor for the other conditions. The 2005 revision of the dietary guidelines for Americans suggests that people consume half of their grain servings as whole grain products (U.S. Department of Health and Human Services and U.S. Department of Agriculture, 2005). The rationale for this recommendation is that whole grains contain various phytonutrients such as dietary fiber, vitamins, minerals, lignans, phytoestrogens, phenolic compounds, and phytic acid. Many of these compounds, particularly those without established nutrient functions, have been studied in isolation for protection against several types of cancer, but it is thought that the package of nutrients available from whole grains may be greater than the sum of the individual components. This could happen as a result of synergistic effects of individual phytonutrients on processes leading to tumor development. Both observational epidemiology and intervention studies with laboratory animals or cell lines point toward a protective role of whole grains or their constituent products in the development of several types of cancer. This chapter focuses on the epidemiological studies because the experimental studies are of uncertain relevance to human cancer.

Epidemiological research on whole grain consumption in relation to most chronic diseases has been hampered by the scientific approach of focusing on nutrients contained in foods rather than on the foods eaten. This has led to emphasis on dietary fiber, as well as a few other minor constituents such as phytate or lignans, as putative protective factors against cancer and, in particular, colon cancer. Though an attractive hypothesis, there is still no conclusive evidence that dietary fiber or these other ingredients found in grains protect against development of benign or malignant colon tumors in humans. An unexamined question is whether the whole is greater than the sum of the parts. That is, does consumption of whole grains provide health benefits that are not derived from intake of nutrients such as dietary fiber? This is relevant for multiple reasons. First, dietary fiber is not a single entity and experimental studies in rodents clearly indicate that some sources of fiber protect against colon tumor formation while others actually increase that process. Second, whole grains and products made from them may not be digested at the same rate as more refined products derived from the same grains. This leads to differences in glycemic load and changes in location of absorption in the gastrointestinal tract of nutrients from these foods. Finally, the satiety effect of whole grain consumption may prevent weight gain, which is a risk factor for many types of cancer. However, it is unlikely that epidemiological investigation will elucidate a definitive answer to the question of whether the whole is greater than the sum of the parts of grains. A direct answer is only possible through long-term interventions in humans, which will not be done, or from studies of animals and then the question of relevance to the human situation remains open.

One of the real problems in addressing the relationship of whole grain intake with cancer risk is how whole grains are defined in questionnaires and databases in common use. The definition would be expected to include all components of the kernel or seed: bran, germ, and endosperm; if the grain is processed, the proportion of the three components should

Copyright © 2006, Elsevier Inc.
All rights of reproduction in any form reserved.

be close to that found in the whole grain. However, a definition of that sort is rarely used in epidemiological studies. Large prospective studies use food frequency questionnaires that usually include bran cereals, wheat germ, and any dark breads or crackers as whole grain products. Therefore, determination of actual intake of whole grain products is overestimated by some unknown proportion. One could legitimately conclude that the protective effect of whole grains is, therefore, stronger than suggested by observational studies. However, if whole grain intake is found associated with protection against cancer, the relationship may be due to other ingredients in foods identified as "whole grain," or purported whole grain intake may simply be a marker for a constellation of health habits such as greater fruit and vegetable intake, more exercise, less smoking, and less obesity. In addition, quantitation of intake varies among the different questionnaires used. Some ask about various specific foods made from whole grains, some request number of servings, and some simply ask about preference of whole grain over refined flour products. Because there are no biomarkers of either whole grain or fiber intake, there is no way to validate accuracy of these instruments to estimate intake. The correlation coefficients for nutrients that can be measured suggest that low and high consumers can be distinguished, but the quantitative limitations need to be acknowledged. Dietary fiber intake should correlate to some extent with whole grain intake, so it is surprising that some studies find a disconnect between dietary fiber and whole grain affecting risk of colon cancer. Most studies on whole grains and cancer have looked at various sites within the gastrointestinal tract, but the risk of cancer in numerous organs has been analyzed in relation to whole grain intake.

WHOLE GRAINS AND CANCER

In 1998, Jacobs et al. reviewed the relationship between whole grain consumption and cancer and included a meta-analysis of 40 case-control studies. This is the most comprehensive published review on this subject correlating whole grain intake with cancer risk and should still be considered the definitive work in this area. Cancers included in this analysis were oral, laryngeal, esophageal, gastric, colon, colorectal, rectal, pancreatic, hepatic, breast, endometrial, ovarian, soft tissue sarcoma, Hodgkin's disease, non-Hodgkin's lymphoma, brain, myeloma, bladder, thyroid, and nonmalignant colorectal polyps. Therefore, 20 tumor types plus one precancerous lesion were grouped for analytical purposes. It is possible that whole grain intake may have a protective effect on only one type of cancer or a limited range of cancers, so this approach could be considered the most conservative in regard to establishing a correlation. Or it could reflect differences in a constellation of risk factors that vary with whole grain intake, such as normal body weight, lower fat intake, higher fruit and vegetable intake, less tobacco use, and a variety of other health behaviors not well studied. With regard to grain intake, high versus low intake was defined within each population so that high intake in one group was not comparable in absolute amount to that in other groups. The pooled odds ratio (OR) for these studies was 0.66 (95% confidence interval [CI] = 0.60–0.72). When whole grain intake was examined quantitatively, the reduced ORs were significant when intake was expressed as "never, occasional, or habitual" (OR of 1, 0.82, and 0.59, respectively) or by tertile (OR of 1, 0.81, and 0.62 from lowest to highest intake), but not when expressed more quantitatively as number of servings per day (OR ranging from 0.98 to 0.85). This difference in results of qualitative and quantitative reporting of whole grain intake associated with cancer risk may be real, but it is likely due to the lower number of studies using the latter indicator of intake, therefore reducing the statistical ability to discern a difference. Jacobs et al. (1998) adjusted their analyses for potential confounders including demographics (age, gender, education), body mass index (BMI), lifestyle (physical activity, smoking, alcohol intake), reproductive factors, other dietary factors (fruits, vegetables, energy intake, other foods), nutrients (B vitamins, calcium, retinol, carotene), and history of disease. None of these factors significantly attenuated the protective association of whole grain intake with cancer risk. The researchers pointed out that there were a small number of studies of cancers except those on the aerodigestive tract. They expressed concern about the OR for breast and prostate cancer, which were close to or more than 1. Although it is not likely that additional meta-analyses will change the fundamental conclusions of Jacobs et al. (1998), it is instructive to examine some representative individual studies in greater detail, with an emphasis on studies not included in the previous review.

Another analysis of multiple tumor sites in relation to whole grain intake was conducted by Chatenoud et al. (1998), who reported on 181 oropharyngeal cancers, 242 laryngeal, 316 esophageal, 745 gastric, 828 colonic, 498 rectal, 428 hepatic, 60 gallbladder, 362 pancreatic, 3,412 breast, 750 endometrial, 971 ovarian, 127 prostate, 431 bladder, 190 renal, 208 thyroid, 80 Hodgkin's disease, 200 non-Hodgkin's lymphomas, and 120 multiple myelomas. This resulted in 10,149 cancer cases who were compared with 7,990 hospitalized, noncancer control subjects in Northern Italy. Whole grain intake (mainly from bread) was divided into tertiles and was associated with significantly reduced risk for 13 of 18 tumor locations. Tumors not correlated inversely with whole grain intake were those of pancreas, endometrium, prostate, Hodgkin's disease, and multiple myeloma. In Italy, whole grain intake is associated with high socioeconomic status and generally healthier habits as it is in most countries. Covariates adjusted for in this analysis included age, gender, education, smoking, alcohol intake, and BMI, but these were entered into the regression analysis singly rather than as a combined group. When factored individually, there was little effect of these covariates on the relative risk (RR) reduction associated with the highest whole grain intake. But unmeasured confounding could still have a major effect on the estimated relationship. Nevertheless, whole grain intake could be an indicator of such a healthier lifestyle, rather than having a direct protective effect. One of the limitations of this study is the very low whole grain intake in the area studied. Only about one-quarter of the population consumed whole grains, and the questionnaire used did not seek information on quantity or portion size, so only frequency of use was measured. The authors of this study suggested that those who consumed whole grain products consumed fewer refined grain products, and this may have lessened risk for cancer. Such a relationship has been suggested for stomach and colon cancer but not for most of the tumors studied here.

WHOLE GRAINS AND GASTROINTESTINAL TRACT CANCERS

The greatest number of studies linking whole grain intake with reduced rate of cancer are those examining gastrointestinal tract cancers. Franceschi et al. (1992) studied 102 patients with cancer of the tongue and 104 with cancer of the mouth who were compared with 726 control subjects in Northern Italy in relation to various risk factors. The investigators included all whole grain bread and pasta into a single category and expressed consumption into tertiles of low, intermediate, and high intake, but the amounts were not revealed. Highly significant reductions in trend for OR were seen for both cancer of the tongue (1, 0.6, and 0.1; 95% CI = 0.01–0.8) and cancer of the mouth (1, 0.1, and 0.5; 95% CI = 0.2–1.4). Strong adverse effects of alcohol and tobacco (OR up to 22 and 9, respectively) were identified, and the authors suggested that certain foods showing protection might have a mechanical cleansing effect on the tissues of the oropharyngeal area. These foods included whole grain bread and pasta, green vegetables, carrots, fresh fruits, coffee, tea, milk, and cola beverages. These results also point out the relative strength of association with inducing factors that are well established versus the uncertainty that still remains concerning possible reductions in cancer with consumption of whole grains or other foods. (In most areas of environmental epidemiology, RRs under three tend to be ignored as noise. In diet and disease epidemiology, it is rare to find a RR greater than two. One could argue the effect of diet is weak, but one could also legitimately make the case that because our determination of diet is so imprecise, that finding an RR of two signifies a strong effect.) Multiple adjustment for confounding was not done in this study, as is often the case in observational studies. This is important because individuals who eat the most whole grain foods are also likely to be consumers of large amounts of fruits and vegetables, which showed similar reductions in OR.

Cancers of the upper aerodigestive tract were analyzed by Kasum et al. (2002) for relation to dietary risk factors as part of the Iowa Women's Health Study in which 34,651 postmenopausal women completed a mailed food frequency questionnaire and were followed for 14 years. During this time, 169 women developed one of the cancers studied in this report: oropharyngeal, laryngeal, nasopharyngeal/salivary, esophageal, and salivary. The number of individual tumor types was too small to allow statistical analysis, but as a group of all aerodigestive cancers combined, the highest tertile of whole grain consumption was associated with a significantly lower RR of 0.53 (95% CI = 0.34–0.81). This was approximately the same as that found for the highest intake of yellow/orange vegetables, which had an RR of 0.58 (95% CI = 0.39–0.87) or for dietary fiber intake from whole grains (RR of 0.56, 95% CI = 0.37–0.84), but total grain fiber was not associated with a significant reduction in risk (RR of 0.82, 95% CI = 0.57–1.19). In this analysis, increased intake of refined grains or ethanol did not affect the RR for these tumors. Smoking, older age, and energy intake were all significant risk factors for these tumors.

The risk for oral, esophageal, and laryngeal cancers was studied according to intake of whole and refined grains in Switzerland. Levi et al. (2000) used 156 cases of oral cancer, 101 of esophageal cancer, and 40 of laryngeal cancer who were compared with 349 controls admitted to a hospital for nonneoplastic conditions. Data were collected over an 8-year period at a single hospital, and a food frequency questionnaire was used to estimate dietary intake. ORs for each tumor site were reduced in the highest tertile of consumption of whole grains, although only that for esophagus was statistically significant individually; combining all three sites gave a significant OR of 0.5 (95% CI = 0.3–1). The highest tertile of refined grain intake was associated with statistically significant elevations of risk for all three sites individually, and for the combined analysis, the OR was 5.7 (95% CI = 2.8–11.4). The authors point out that the relatively small number of cases may have precluded their finding statistical significance for the reduced risk of all three types of cancer. They describe relatively high consumption of both refined and whole grain products but only provide estimates of frequency of intake. For whole grains, the range of consumption for the highest tertile was >10 times/wk. It was indicated in the paper that allowance was made for tobacco, ethanol, fruit, vegetable, and total energy intake and that there was no effect on the RR, but the data were not presented.

A case-control study on stomach cancer done in Milan, Italy, compared dietary intake of 206 cases with that of 474 controls who were hospitalized for nondigestive reasons (La

Vecchia et al., 1987). Intake for each food was divided into tertiles of consumption, and most were not related significantly to risk of stomach cancer. However, nine foods were significantly related to risk. These included pasta or rice (as a single food group), polenta, sugar, ham, green vegetables, fresh fruit, citrus fruit, melon, and whole grain bread or pasta. The first four food groups were associated with significantly elevated risk, while the last five food groups were associated with significantly lower risks. The RR for stomach cancer in the highest tertile was 0.34 when adjusted for age and gender; it was 0.4 when also adjusted for education and area of residence. Once all these foods were entered into a single multiple logistic regression analysis, the RR associated with the highest consumption of whole grain bread or pasta was 0.44, but this was no longer statistically significant ($p = 0.11$), indicating some attenuation of the apparent relationship. This result could be interpreted as meaning higher consumption of whole grain foods along with lower consumption of the positive risk factors such as polenta and ham may be required to show a statistically significant protective association.

A prospective study of 61,433 Swedish women who completed a food frequency questionnaire and were followed for a mean of ~15 years found 805 cases of colorectal cancer (Larsson et al., 2005a). The RR for highest quintile of intake of whole grain foods was 0.67 (95% CI = 0.47–0.96) for colon cancer, but the risk for rectal cancer was not significantly affected by whole grain intake. Another analysis by the same group (Larsson et al., 2005b) on the same patients reported that magnesium intake was associated with significantly lower RR in the highest quintile for colon and rectal tumors analyzed together but only for rectal cancer when analyzed separately, suggesting that magnesium intake may mediate some of the protective effect from whole grains. For the highest magnesium intake, the RR was 0.59 (95% CI = 0.4–0.87) for those in the upper quintile. For colon cancer the RR was 0.66 (95% CI = 0.41–1.07), and for rectal cancer, the RR was 0.45 (95% CI = 0.22–0.89). However, since colon cancer was the tumor principally affected in the whole grain analysis and rectal cancer in the magnesium analysis, the data are not complementary. Although it is possible that the smaller numbers preclude finding a significant difference, if there is a cause-and-effect relationship, it simply may not be strong enough to see with the numbers reported here. This uncertainty about cause and effect is a recurring theme with all epidemiological studies of this nature.

A large case-control study conducted in California, Utah, and Minnesota assessed the relationship of individual plant foods with risk of colon cancer in 1993 cases and 2410 controls (Slattery et al., 1997). Whole grain intake was analyzed as quintiles of consumption for men and women separately. In addition, subjects were analyzed by age (younger than 67 years or 67 years or older), and by location of the cancer in the colon (proximal vs distal). For men, there was a statistically significant reduction in OR for the quintile of highest intake (0.8; 95% CI = 0.6–1) but not for women (OR of 1; 95% CI = 0.8–1.4). For men, the lowest and highest quintiles of intake were < 0.5 and > 2.3 servings of whole grain foods per day. In men the effect was restricted to those older than 67 years and was primarily for distal tumors. None of the ORs in women approached statistical significance. In women the quintiles of intake were <0.5 and >1.9 servings per day. The model used here adjusted for age, BMI, physical activity, use of nonsteroidal anti-inflammatory drugs, family history of colon cancer, total energy intake, and calcium. The results of this study call into question the possible protective effect of whole grain intake because this was observed only in men and the difference in consumption between the genders was less than a half a serving per day. There were 894 female cases and 1099 male cases, so it would be difficult to argue that there was a lack of statistical power for the women in this study. This study did not find any consistent relationship of magnesium intake with risk of colon cancer. High intake of refined grains was suggested as being associated with increased risk in men, but none of the analyses for this food group achieved statistical significance, except when grain intake was adjusted for dietary fiber in men. Mixed results were found with analyses of dietary fiber and colon cancer risk. Fiber was analyzed as total dietary fiber, soluble fiber, pectin, and insoluble fiber. Seven of forty comparisons were statistically significant, suggesting a generally weak effect of dietary fiber intake on risk of colon tumors.

The same investigators who conducted the previous study also examined a large population of colon cancer (n = 1308) and rectal cancer (n = 952) patients and controls (n = 1544 and 1205, respectively) from California and Utah (Slattery et al., 2003). This study attempted to identify dietary patterns associated with risk of cancer. Pooled analysis of the two tumor types revealed that a Western diet pattern enhanced risk, while a prudent diet pattern reduced risk. The Western pattern was defined by those foods with high factor loadings in factor analysis and included processed meats, red meat, fast-food meat, eggs, butter, margarine, potatoes, high-fat dairy foods, legumes, refined grains, added sugar, sugar drinks, and sugar desserts; several of these foods loaded into the model only for men. The prudent pattern was characterized by all types of fruits and vegetables, whole grains, fish, and poultry. The effect of the two diet patterns was stronger in subjects who had a family history of first-degree relatives with the same type of cancer. Although this study does not isolate whole grain intake as a potential protective factor, it points out that foods are not eaten in isolation and that individuals who consume the most whole grains generally have a number of dietary characteristics that differentiate their diet from those whose intake of whole grains is low. In addition, a variety of health behaviors that may affect propensity toward development and/or diagnosis of colon or rectal cancer such as sigmoidoscopic screening, cigarette smoking, BMI, and nonsteroidal anti-inflammatory drug use may co-vary with dietary pattern more than with intake of a single food group.

One of the largest prospective cohort studies to address the potential link between whole grain intake and cancer risk is the Cancer Prevention Study II Nutrition Cohort, run by the American Cancer Society in 21 states in the United States. An analysis of >133,000 men and women found 298 cases of colon cancer among men and 210 among women after 4.5 years of follow-up (McCullough et al., 2003) and focused on whole grains, fruit, and vegetables. Those reporting higher intakes of these foods were slightly older, more physically active, more likely to use vitamin and calcium supplements over the long term, and less likely to use tobacco. Quintiles of whole grain servings in both men and women ranged from < 2 to >11/wk, so the range should have been adequate to see a protective effect. Whole grains analyzed separately or a composite score for the three plant food groups showed no significant difference from unity. Multivariate adjustments included age, exercise, aspirin, tobacco use, family history of colorectal cancer, BMI, education, energy intake, multivitamin use, calcium intake, and red meat consumption. This suggests that some of the co-varying factors may mediate the putative protective effect of whole grain intake against colon cancer. Very low consumption of dietary fiber from vegetables in men and from fruits in women was associated with a doubling of the risk, suggesting that a threshold effect with low intakes may increase tumor formation. However, there was no indication of this for whole grain intake.

Another approach at evaluating food group intake in relation to colorectal cancer was done in Switzerland in which 119 cases of colon cancer and 104 cases of rectal cancer were compared with 491 hospital-based controls (Levi et al., 1999). An interviewer-administered food frequency questionnaire was used to assess diet. There were eight questions related to bread and cereal dishes, so it is not clear what proportion of whole grain intake was captured by this dietary instrument. Intake was divided into tertiles and related to risk of the combined 223 cases of colorectal cancer. Highest whole grain intake was associated with an OR of 0.54 (95% CI = 0.34–0.85). In contrast, refined grain intake was associated with a significantly elevated OR of 1.79 (95% CI = 1.12–2.87). However, when refined grains were analyzed in a multiple logistic regression that included meat and vegetable intake along with several other factors, the increased risk was reduced somewhat and no longer statistically significant. The authors calculated population attributable risks from the dietary factors reported here and concluded that low intake of whole grains accounted for 41% of the attributable risk, which was the strongest single factor identified. They suggested that a food pattern of low intake of whole grains, vegetables, fruit, and high red meat implied an attributable risk of 80%. Although this is theoretically possible, in a genetically heterogenous population this degree of risk is likely to be a considerable overestimate.

A relatively small study of 147 case-control pairs from Los Angeles that examined dietary and occupational factors in men younger than the age of 45 years was reported by Peters et al. (1989). One could approach this type of study as indicating those individuals most susceptible to environmental factors because they developed colorectal cancer at a very young age or that the subjects in this study developed tumors at such early ages that this process would not be affected by external factors. Unfortunately, we do not know enough yet to adequately address this dichotomous interpretation. Whole grain preference was associated with an OR of 0.6 (95% CI = 0.4–1.1), which was not statistically significant. This study was likely underpowered to address this dietary question, as there were only 39 cases and 51 controls who preferred whole grain bread to white bread. Cases were divided according to site within the colon (right side, transverse/descending, sigmoid and rectum), and none of these subsites was associated with a significant reduction in risk, which is understandable given the lack of power for the group as a whole. The magnitude of risk reduction is similar in this study to those from previously described analyses that found statistically significant reductions in risk associated with whole grain intake, but in this study the confidence interval included 1, probably as a result of too few subjects. This is another characteristic shared by many of the epidemiologic studies published on this topic. Although there is no specific cutoff for minimum number of subjects (since power calculations are easily affected by choosing slightly different predicted differences in means or standard deviations), studies in which the population is divided into quintiles of intake of whole grains include few individuals in the lowest and highest quintiles, and it is those extremes of intake that have the greatest effect on the eventual determination of statistical significance. This is because intake of most foods is relatively normally distributed, so most individuals will fall into the central three quintiles of consumption. Therefore, the determination of significance is strongly influenced by far less than two fifths of the number of cases (not total population), and the numbers in those two quintiles can be about one tenth of the total number of cases.

Two case-control studies of whole grain bread and pasta intake in northern Italy reflect the natural heterogeneity in findings typical of observational studies. One study done in Milan compared 339 colon cancer and 236 rectal cancer cases with 778 hospitalized controls (La Vecchia et al., 1988). In this study there was no association of whole grain intake with risk of these cancers with the RR for colon cancer in the highest tertile at 0.72 and that for rectal cancer at 0.88. Some of the same investigators conducted a similar study in Pordenone province in northeastern Italy with 123 colon cancer and 125 rectal cancer cases who were compared with 699 hospitalized controls (Bidoli et al., 1992). In this second study, those in the highest tertile of whole grain bread and pasta consumption had an RR of 0.7 ($p = 0.08$) for colon cancer and an RR of 0.3 ($p = 0.002$) for rectal cancer. This second study had less than half the case numbers of the first study yet found a much stronger relationship with whole grain intake. However, none of the foods identified as significantly related to cancer in the colon or rectum in the Milanese population were also found in the residents of Pordenone and vice versa. These studies call into question the repeatability of such studies. Although food frequency questionnaires ask about habitual intake over an extended period of time, often up to 1 year, they are strongly influenced by recent intake. Most food frequency questionnaires have been validated for a limited number of nutrients, rather than foods, by comparison with another measure of dietary intake or a limited number of biomarkers in serum. Just because a questionnaire approximates intake for a limited number of nutrients does not guarantee its accuracy for the entire range of foods.

In a study of rectal cancer and diet, Slattery et al. (2004) compared 952 cases with 1205 population-based controls in California. In this study, men and women were evaluated separately and together. Consumption of whole grain foods was divided into quintiles, with the extremes being less than a half serving daily to more than three per day. The mean number of servings in this sample was about 1.7, so the intake was considerably higher than average for the U.S. population with the mean for cases being 1.64 and that for controls at 1.81; these values were significantly different, although one must wonder if it is possible to discern such small differences with any accuracy given the current state of the art in assessing dietary intake. For men, the OR was 0.67 (95% CI = 0.46–0.98) and for women the OR was a non-significant 0.74 (95% CI = 0.43–1.27); for all subjects the OR was 0.69 (95% CI = 0.51–0.94). This study also found that intakes of fruit, vegetables, and dietary fiber were inversely associated with risk of rectal cancer, while high consumption of refined grain products produced an increased risk.

WHOLE GRAINS AND NONINTESTINAL CANCERS

Non-Hodgkin's lymphoma is a malignancy of lymphocytes that is heterogenous in cell origin with 10 disease types and 20 entities recognized by current classification schemes. Given that limitation, a group of 208 cases was compared with 401 hospitalized controls in northeastern Italy. In this group of cases, there were 11 different histological types of non-Hodgkin's lymphoma with numbers ranging from four to 39 for each histological type (Franceschi et al., 1989). One must question whether the different types have similar etiologies. It is equally reasonable to assume they do and that host reactions modify the response, or that the different histological types do not share causative factors and that exposure to initiators, promoters, and epigenetic factors influence the cellular manifestations. Intake of whole grain pasta and bread was divided into tertiles, and the highest tertile had an RR of 0.53, which was statistically significant. Entering whole grain consumption into multivariate models including age, gender, education, weight, tobacco, and four food groups identified as significant risks in this study (liver, milk, fats in seasonings, methylxanthine-containing beverages) did not attenuate the relationship with the RR in the highest tertile of 0.44.

The same investigators also evaluated dietary risk factors for soft-tissue sarcoma in northeastern Italy by analyzing data from 88 cases of soft-tissue sarcoma in comparison with 610 controls (Serraino et al., 1991). Intake of whole grain bread or pasta showed a significant negative association in the third tertile (OR of 0.4, 95% CI = 0.2–0.9). This was the only seemingly protective dietary factor and high intake of dairy products and vegetable oils were the only apparent positive dietary risk factors. One must question the validity of any of these findings given the small number of cases.

Two studies on whole grain intake and endometrial cancer have been conducted, one in the United States, and one in Italy. The Italian study also included some patients from Switzerland (Levi et al., 1993). This is problematic because 50% of the cases were from Switzerland while 71% of the controls were from there, with the remainders of both groups from two locations in northern Italy. Even though the Swiss canton borders northwestern Italy, there are considerable differences in diet between the two countries; however, the authors examined the results from the Swiss and Italian centers separately and reported they appeared consistent. A total of 274 cases of endometrial cancer were compared with 572 hospitalized controls. The investigators found that whole grain bread or pasta intake was related to a significantly lower OR of 0.43 in the highest tertile. This study found numerous dietary relationships with risk of endometrial cancer. Other factors associated with reduced risk were total vegetables, total fruit, carrots, artichokes, onions, garlic, pears, and melon. Dietary factors associated with increased risk were beef, pork, ham, canned meat, "other" meats, eggs, beans and peas, butter, seed oils, sugar, tea, total added fats, and total energy. The authors used several logistic regression models to control for confounding but pointed out that the only substantial confounding was derived from including total energy intake along with age and study center. The American study on endometrial cancer is from the Iowa Women's Health Study (Kasum et al., 2001). This is a large prospective study in which more than 41,000 women returned a food frequency questionnaire in 1986 and then were followed for 12 years. A total of 382 cases of endometrial cancer were identified from a population of

23,014 eligible participants. Women in the highest quintile of whole grain consumption had an RR of 0.89 (95% CI = 0.61–1.29), which was not statistically significant. Women were then classified whether they had or had not used hormone replacement therapy (HRT). Those women in the highest quintile of whole grain intake who never used HRT had an RR of 0.63 (95% CI = 0.39–1.1); the trend was statistically significant at p = 0.05 even though the confidence interval included 1. Women in the highest quintile of whole grain consumption who had ever used HRT had an RR of 1.54 (95% CI = 0.80–2.98). It is possible that weak estrogenic effects of some components of whole grain foods may manifest protective effects in women not exposed to exogenous hormones, but in those who have used HRT, the weak phytoestrogenic effects may be masked.

Also in the Iowa Women's Health Study, the relationship between whole grain intake and breast cancer risk were assessed (Nicodemus et al., 2001). The follow-up was 9 years, and 977 cases of breast cancer were identified. Regular whole grain intake was a marker for what the authors described as a healthier lifestyle and that included a higher incidence of mammography. There was a statistically significant elevation in risk of breast cancer in the quintile of highest intake of whole grains with an RR of 1.21 (95% CI = 0.96–1.5, p for trend of 0.02). Controlling for screening mammography did not have an effect on the RR, while use of HRT seemed to have varied results. For hormone current users, the RR increased to 1.85 (95% CI = 1.01–3.4, p for trend of 0.05), while former users and never users of HRT showed attenuation of the RR to insignificant values. The authors concluded that the increased RR in women who ate the most whole grains was a function of their increased likelihood of participating in screening mammography. This is a reasonable interpretation but also calls into question how much bias there is, whether recognized or not, in similar diet and cancer studies. Such bias can be in other dietary components that may change in relation to frequency of whole grain food consumption including sporadic inadequate intake of vitamins, or in nondietary factors such as participation in exercise, better medical care, and so forth.

The other study that examined a relationship between breast cancer risk and whole grain intake was a case-control study done in Heidelberg, Germany (Adzersen et al., 2003). Three hundred ten cases of breast cancer were matched to 353 hospitalized controls. Whole grain intake was divided into quartiles with a range of less than 8.9 grams/day to more than 47.1 grams/day. The OR for the highest quartile was 0.57 (95% CI = 0.34–0.95, p of 0.01 for trend). Protective associations were also seen for total vegetables and raw vegetables. Zinc was the individual nutrient to show the strongest significant negative relationship (RR of 0.35, 95% CI = 0.15–0.78), and this could have been the result of the higher zinc content of many whole grain cereals.

The single analysis on prostate cancer and whole grains was from a case-control study done in Canada (Jain et al., 1999). This included 617 cases and 636 population-based controls from three provinces. Consumption of whole grain breakfast cereals was associated with a statically significant elevation in risk in the highest quartile of intake with an OR of 1.41 (95% CI = 1.05–1.88) when analyzed in a multivariate model that adjusted for 22 factors. Whole grain bread intake was not associated with any difference in risk (OR of 0.99, 95% CI = 0.76–1.28), even though the authors claim that was there was an overall decrease in risk in their discussion of the findings, but high intake of refined grain breads showed an OR of 0.65 (95% CI = 0.48–0.88, p for trend of 0.02). Also in this study, there was a negative association with green vegetable intake but a significant positive association with fruit consumption. This study provides an example of potential spurious significant findings when numerous statistical analyses are conducted. Twenty-nine food groups were separately analyzed along with 12 nutrients in both univariate and multivariate models, generating a large number of comparisons that are likely to present a number of false positives. This does not make this study different from other comprehensive attempts to tease out relationships in diet and environment with risk of developing any chronic disease.

CONCLUSIONS

It is possible, even likely, that whole grain consumption protects against development of cancer at a variety of sites. However, it is also important to admit that this is currently an educated guess and given the limitations of observational epidemiology, one must realize that despite numerous investigations into this relationship we cannot say with a high degree of confidence that whole grain intake definitely prevents cancer of any organ in the body. This could be a result of few people consuming enough whole grains over the long term that the protective effects do not show up, or it could simply reflect that other factors overwhelm a protective effect of eating whole grains. This does not make the situation for whole grains different from that for other foods or nutrients tentatively linked to development of cancer as either a positive or negative risk factor. In fact, we refer to risk factors precisely because there is a change in the level of risk but no definitive link of cause and effect. This should not be taken as a reason to avoid whole grain foods, but it is important to admit the current state of the art in this area of science so as not to lose credibility in making future recommendations for diet and prevention of cancer. One must ask if the measures of dietary intake are sophisticated enough to accurately estimate dietary intake, particularly for whole grain foods that are not accurately quantifiable from existing nutrient databases. Is the inability of large, cohort studies to see any protective effect from whole grains caused by their use of semi-quantitative food frequency questionnaires in contrast to case-control studies that were more likely to have used diet histories? Most food frequency questionnaires do not contain specific questions on grain types and cereal brands used, so they probably lack sufficient detail to differentiate whole grain intake from refined grain products.

An interesting analysis of food consumption and total mortality in women was reported by Michels and Wolk (2002), who used data from 59,038 Swedish women. At the time of the analysis, there had been 3710 deaths in almost 10 years of follow-up. A healthy diet was defined as including more fruits, vegetables, whole grain breads, cereals, fish, and low-fat dairy products. Women who were in the highest quintile of consumption of these foods as measured by a composite score had an RR of 0.58 (95% CI = 0.5–0.68); excluding the first 5 years of follow-up had no effect on the RR. Diets that contained more red meat, refined carbohydrates and sugar, and foods high in saturated or trans fats were not associated with higher mortality. This led the authors to conclude that it is more important to increase the number of healthy foods consumed regularly than to decrease other foods. Clearly this recommendation needs to be put into the context of energy balance and increased physical activity would allow greater consumption of foods from either category without adverse effects on body weight.

Plausible mechanism(s) by which whole grain consumption prevents cancer should exist, and many have been proposed. Both dietary fiber and resistant starch are fermented to short chain fatty acids (SCFAs). The SCFAs, butyrate in particular, have been linked with reduced proliferation and increased differentiation of colonic cells. The phenolics, especially ferulic acids, are antioxidants, and these compounds exert a plethora of beneficial effects including improving membrane and DNA stability. Whole grain foods generally have low glycemic index/load, and elevations in these have been related to increased insulin secretion, which is a putative risk factor for several tumor types. The lignans and related compounds have estrogenic effects, induce apoptosis, modulate cell cycle dynamics, alter levels of transcription factors, and collectively function to inhibit growth of tumor cells. One example of this is the recent report that intake of whole grains affects the plasma concentration of enterolactone (Johnsen et al., 2004). In addition, consumption of cabbage, leafy vegetables, and coffee also increased enterolactone levels, although the cumulative effective of these foods was about one third that from intake of whole grains. This study was conducted in Denmark, so it is not unexpected that most of this effect was from ingestion of whole grain rye products, which are particularly rich in the precursor to this phytoestrogen. Some of the chemicals in whole grains may induce cytochrome p450 enzymes that detoxify carcinogens. It is also likely that we have not yet identified all the potentially beneficial chemical constituents of whole grains and should not expect that those in highest concentrations are the most beneficial. Despite all these beneficial effects, we do not know if the relationship between whole grain intake and cancer should be viewed as high consumption of whole grains reducing the risk or low consumption increasing the risk. Slavin (2000) has summarized mechanisms by which whole grain intake could modify the carcinogenic process. She points out that whole grains are concentrated sources of a variety of nutrients already implicated in protection against tumor development such as dietary fiber, resistant starch, antioxidants, and phytoestrogens, as well as resulting in a lower glycemic load. Her review supports the plausibility that whole grain intake could modulate development of cancer.

One important limitation of observational epidemiology is that quite often a single diet analysis is obtained via a semi-quantitative food frequency questionnaire, and subjects are followed for a number of years until a sufficient number develop the cancer of interest to yield a meaningful statistical analysis. Assuming the diet does not change over many years is patently incorrect. Only a few of the major longitudinal studies have employed repeated diet analyses, and those that have indicate the majority of individuals modify their dietary fiber intake enough so that 77% will move two or more quintiles over an 8-year period (Willett et al., 1990). This implies potential for major changes in whole grain intake over time, even though average consumption in the United States is only about one serving per day.

In evaluating the observational data linking whole grain intake with reduced risk of cancer, it is imperative to keep in mind the principals needed before one can discern causation from correlation. These were elegantly stated by Hill (1965) 40 years ago and remain valid today. He pointed out that there were nine criteria that could be fulfilled, and the more of them specifically related to the subject, the more certain one could be. These include strength of association, consistency of the observations, specificity, temporality, biological gradient, plausibility, coherence, experimental evidence, and analogy. These criteria have yet to be fulfilled for any foods and reduced risk of cancer. So, for now, it is mostly an unproven hypothesis that whole grain intake reduces the risk of cancer. Although there is likely to be no downside to increasing consumption of whole grain foods, we simply do not know enough to suggest whether, or by how much, whole grain intake will affect cancer risk.

References

Adzersen, K.-H., Jess, P., Freivogel, K.W., Gerhard, I., and Bastert, G. 2003. Raw and cooked vegetables, fruits, selected micronutrients, and breast cancer risk: a case-control study in Germany. *Nutr Cancer* **46**: 131–137.

Bidoli, E., Franceschi, S., Talamini, R., Barra, S., and La Vecchia, C. 1992. Food consumption and cancer of the colon and rectum in North-eastern Italy, *Int J Cancer* **50**: 223–239.

Chatenoud, L., Tavani, A., La Vecchia, C., Jacobs, D.R., Jr., Negri, E., Levi, F., and Franceschi, S. 1998. Whole grain food intake and cancer risk. *Int J Cancer* **77**: 24–28.

Franceschi, S., Barra, S., La Vecchia, C., Bidoli, E., Negri, E., and Talamini, R. 1992. Risk factors for cancer of the tongue and the mouth. A case-control study from Northern Italy. *Cancer* **70**: 2227–2233.

Franceschi, S., Serraino, D., Carbone, A., Talamini, R., and La Vecchia, C. 1989. Dietary factors and non-Hodgkin's lymphoma: a case-control study in the Northeastern part of Italy. *Nutr Cancer* **12**: 333–341.

Hill, A.B. 1965. The environment and disease: association or causation? *Proc R Soc Med* **58**: 295–300.

Jacobs, D.R., Jr., Marquart, L., Slavin, J., and Kushi, L.H. 1998. Whole-grain intake and cancer: an expanded review and meta-analysis. *Nutr Cancer* **30**: 85–96.

Jain, M.G., Hislop, G.T., Howe, G.R., and Ghadirian, P. 1999. Plant foods, antioxidants, and prostate cancer risk: findings from case-control studies in Canada. *Nutr Cancer* **34**: 173–184.

Johnsen, N.F., Hausner, H., Olsen, A., Tetens, I., Christensen, J., Knudsen, K.E., Overvad, K., and Tjonneland, A. 2004. Intake of whole grains and vegetables determines the plasma enterolactone concentration of Danish women. *J Nutr* **134**: 2691–2697.

Kasum, C.M., Jacobs, D.R. Jr., Nicodemus, K., and Folsom, A.R. 2002. Dietary risk factors for upper aerodigestive tract cancers. *Int J Cancer* **99**: 267–272.

Kasum, C.M., Nicodemus, K., Harnack, L.J., Jacobs, D.R., Jr., and Folsom, A.R. 2001. Whole grain intake and incident endometrial cancer: The Iowa Women's Health Study. *Nutr Cancer* **39**: 180–186.

Larsson, S.C., Giovannucci, E., Bergkvist, L., and Wolk, A. 2005a. Whole grain consumption and risk of colorectal cancer: a population-based cohort of 60,000 women. *Br J Cancer* **92**, 1803–1807.

Larsson, S.C., Bergkvist, L., and Wolk, A. 2005b. Magnesium intake in relation to risk of colorectal cancer in women. *JAMA* **293**: 86–89.

La Vecchia, C., Negri, E., Decarli, A., D'Avanzo B., and Franceschi, S. 1987. A case-control study of diet and gastric cancer in Northern Italy. *Int J Cancer* **40**: 484–489.

La Vecchia, C., Negri, E., Decarli, A., D'Avanzo B., Gallotti, L., Gentile, A., and Franceschi, S. 1988. A case-control study of diet and gastric cancer in Northern Italy. *Int J Cancer* **41**: 492–498.

Levi, F., Franceschi, S., Negri, E., and La Vecchia, C. 1993. Dietary factors and the risk of endometrial cancer. *Cancer* **71**: 3575–3581.

Levi, F., Pasch, C., La Vecchia, C., Lunching, F., and Franceschi, S. 1999. Food groups and colorectal cancer risk. *Br J Cancer* **79**: 1283–1287.

Levi, F., Pasch, C., Lunching, F., Chatenoud, L., Jacobs, D.R., Jr., and La Vecchia, C. 2000. Refined and whole grain cereal and the risk of oral, esophageal and laryngeal cancer. *Eur J Clin Nutr* **54**: 487–489.

McCullough, M.L., Robertson, A.S., Chad, A., Jacobs, L.J., Sampler, L.J., Jacobs, D.R., Diver, W.R., Calls, E.E., and Thun, L.J. 2003. A prospective study of whole grains, fruits, vegetables and colon cancer risk. *Cancer Causes Control* **14**: 959–970.

Michels, K.W., and Wolk, A. 2002. A prospective study of variety of healthy foods and mortality in women. *Int J Epidemiol* **31**: 847–854.

Miller, H.E., Rigelhof, F., Marquart, L., Prakash, A., and Kanter, M. 2000. Antioxidant content of whole grain breakfast cereal, fruits and vegetables. *J Am Coll Nutr* **19**: 312S–319S.

Nicodemus, K.K., Jacobs, D.R., Jr., and Folsom, A.R. 2001. Whole and refined grain intake and risk of incident postmenopausal breast cancer (United States). *Cancer Causes Control* **12**: 917–925.

Peters, R.K., Garabrant, D.H, Yu, M.C., and Mack, T.M. 1989. A case-control study of occupational and dietary factors in colorectal cancer in young men by subsite. *Cancer Res* **49**: 5459–5468.

Serraino, D., Franceschi, S., Talamini, R., Frustaci, S., and La Vecchia, C. 1991. Non-occupational risk factors for adult soft-tissue sarcoma in northern Italy. *Cancer Causes Control* **2**: 157–164.

Slattery, M.L., Curtin, K.P., Edwards, S.L., and Schaffer, D.M. 2004. Plant foods, fiber, and rectal cancer. *Am J Clin Nutr* **79**: 274–281.

Slattery, M.L., Levin, T.R., Ma, K., Goldgar, D., Holubkov, R., and Edwards, S. 2003. Family history and colorectal cancer: predictors of risk. *Cancer Causes Control* **14**: 879–887.

Slattery, M.L., Potter, J.D., Coates, A., Ma, K.N., Berry, T.D., Duncan, D.M., and Caan, B.J. 1997. Plant foods and colon cancer: an assessment of specific foods and their related nutrients (United States). *Cancer Causes Control* **8**: 575–590.

Slavin, J.L. 1994. Epidemiological evidence for the impact of whole grains on health. *Crit Rev Food Sci Nutr* **34**: 427–434.

Slavin, J.L. 2000. Mechanisms for the impact of whole grain foods in cancer risk. *J Am Coll Nutr* **19**: 300S–307S.

U.S. Department of Health and Human Services and U.S. Department of Agriculture. 2005. "Dietary Guidelines for Americans," 6th edition. US Government Printing Office, Washington, DC.

Willett, W.C., Stampfer, M.J., Colditz, G.A., Rosner, B.A., and Speizer, F.E. 1990. Relation of meat, fat, and fiber intake to the risk of colon cancer in a prospective study among women. *N Engl J Med* **323**: 1664–1672.

CHAPTER

9

Obesity and Cancer Risk

CATHERINE L. CARPENTER AND LESLIE BERNSTEIN

INTRODUCTION

Obesity is characterized by excessive amounts of adipose tissue. Adipose tissue primarily serves the function of energy storage but in excess can lead to increased risk of disease. Obesity is an epidemic in both the United States and other developed countries. After remaining stable in the 1960s and 1970s, the prevalence of obesity among U.S. adults increased by ~50% throughout the 1980s and 1990s (Flegal et al., 2002). Almost one-fourth of the U.S. population overall is considered obese (body mass index [BMI], measured as weight in kg divided by height in meters^2, >30), with obesity prevalence among U.S. adults 20 years or older increasing from 19.4% in 1997 to 23.9% in 2002 (U.S. Department of Health and Human Services, 2002). Among older adults (55–64 years), 43% of U.S. women and 33% of U.S. men are obese.

An interrelated epidemic of physical inactivity is also occurring. Surveys of physical activity in the year 2000 indicate that 27% of U.S. adults did no physical activity and another 28% were not regularly active (Mokdad et al., 2001). Children who engage in the least amount of vigorous physical activity or the greatest amount of television viewing tend to be the most overweight (Anderson, 1998).

The obesity epidemic is not just limited to the United States. Almost all countries (high income and low income) are experiencing an obesity epidemic, although the magnitude of this impact varies (World Health Organization [WHO], 2001). In many developing countries undergoing economic transition to increasingly industrialized and mechanized lifestyles, rising levels of obesity often coexist in the same population with chronic undernutrition. In developed countries, the rising prevalence of obesity cuts across all classes, with the highest levels reported among lower socioeconomic groups (WHO, 2001).

The rising obesity epidemic not only affects chronic diseases such as congestive heart failure, atherosclerosis, and diabetes but may cause increased cancer incidence. Obesity raises the risk for several types of cancer, including endometrial, kidney, and colon cancer, esophageal adenocarcinoma, and breast cancer among postmenopausal women. Obesity is also thought to be associated with non-Hodgkin's lymphoma (NHL), pancreatic cancer, and prostate cancer. This chapter describes risk factors for obesity and suggests mechanisms that explain the obesity–cancer association for different types of cancer.

ETIOLOGY OF OBESITY

Obesity is a multifactorial disease that arises from interactions of genes, environmental factors, and behavior (Comuzzie and Allison, 1998). Features of the physical environment affect both energy expenditure and dietary intake. These environmental factors include modern technology and availability of fast, inexpensive, high-fat food, and large portion sizes in the American diet (Hill and Peters, 1998). Moreover, efforts to reduce weight through diet and exercise are often thwarted by personal, social, and environmental barriers. Reasons such as lack of perceived benefit, time availability, motivation, and lack of social support affect the initiation and maintenance of exercise and dietary changes (Sternfeld et al., 1999; Sherwood and Jeffery, 2000; Manson et al., 2004). Access to exercise is often restricted to the middle and upper classes (Parks et al., 2003). Density of fast-food restaurants in lower socioeconomic communi-

Copyright © 2006, Elsevier Inc.
All rights of reproduction in any form reserved.

ties, long commuting distances to work, high crime rates impacting exercise outside the home, and architectural designs for inexpensive housing may function to limit access to exercise and healthy food choices (Hill and Peters, 1998). Furthermore, lack of healthy food in institutions such as schools and businesses weakens efforts to make dietary changes (Manson et al., 2004).

Life expectancy in the United Statues in the twentieth century may be shortened because of the effects of obesity, according to a report in the *New England Journal of Medicine* (Olshansky et al., 2005). The authors reanalyzed life expectancy in the United States and found that the steady rise in life expectancy during the past 2 centuries may be coming to an end because of the effects of obesity on longevity. The most important group affected by obesity is children, among whom the rise in obesity prevalence represents the greatest number of potential years of life lost because of complications from obesity. As obesity onset occurs at younger ages in the current generation of children and young adults, more adverse effects of obesity will occur than those observed in previous generations (Olshansky et al., 2005).

Increases in obesity during the twentieth century have already had a major impact on cancer mortality. Among the morbidly obese participants (BMI > 40) of a prospective study of >900,000 U.S. adults free of cancer in 1992, the death rate from all cancers combined was 52% higher for men and 62% higher for women than the rates found in men and women of normal weight (Calle et al., 2003). BMI was significantly associated with higher rates of death from cancers of the esophagus, colon and rectum, gallbladder, pancreas, kidney, NHL, and multiple myeloma among men and women. Also consistent with an impact of obesity on mortality were results for cancers of the stomach and prostate in men and cancers of the breast, uterus, cervix, and ovary in women (Calle et al., 2003).

Obesity and Hormones

Energy storage for future times of nutritional scarcity is the main biological function of adipose tissue. However, adipose tissue is also the source of hormones and cytokines that serve signaling functions and contribute to inflammation throughout the body. Accumulating evidence suggests that adipose tissue functions as an endocrine organ. Some of the major hormones related to body fat and body fat distribution include estrogen (estrone), insulin, insulin-like growth factors (IGFs), leptin, and sex hormone–binding globulin (SHBG).

Adipose tissue cells are a source of reproductive hormones in both men and women. The androgen androstenedione is converted to estrone by adipocytes (adipose tissue cells) in the presence of aromatase (Tchernof and Despres, 2000). SHBG is a protein that binds estradiol (a conversion product of estrone) and testosterone. Circulating levels of SHBG are lower among obese men and women, resulting in higher circulating levels of free or non–protein-bound estradiol and testosterone, which are considered the biologically active fractions of these hormones and are implicated in risk of breast cancer and prostate cancer, respectively (Tchernof and Despres, 2000).

Obesity is also associated with high levels of insulin, insulin resistance, and non–insulin-dependent diabetes mellitus in men and women (Kaaks, 1996; Hsing et al., 2001, 2003). Insulin resistance, diabetes, and elevated insulin and insulin-related growth factors may increase cancer risk at several sites including prostate cancer among men (Hsing et al., 2001, 2003; Barnard et al., 2002), breast cancer among women (Bruning et al., 1992; Hankinson et al., 1998; Agurs-Collins et al., 2000; Toniolo et al., 2000), and colon cancer among men and women (Ma et al., 1999; Giovannucci et al., 2000; Palmqvist et al., 2003).

The IGFs are proteins that control vital cell functions in multiple tissue sites including the breast, colon, and prostate. Many studies of the IGF system and cancer have focused on IGF-1 and its associated binding protein, IGF-BP3; however, the exact mechanism for explaining the role of IGF-1 in oncogenesis has not yet been determined.

Leptin, a cytokine produced by body fat (adipocytokine), is angiogenic (Sierra-Honigmann et al., 1998) and may enhance the metastatic potential of tumors (Hu et al., 2002). Leptin is increased in association with androgens and insulin (Brzechffa et al., 1996; Ryan and Elahi, 1996; Kennedy et al., 1997; Ambrosius et al., 1998), as well as with abdominal obesity, such that higher leptin levels are more strongly associated with visceral rather than subcutaneous fat (Fruehwald-Schultes et al., 1998). Leptin binds to specific receptors in the hypothalamus and is involved in appetite control and thermogenesis (Fruehwald-Schultes et al., 1998). Women of all ages have higher plasma leptin levels than men (Ryan and Elahi, 1996; Castracane et al., 1998). This may be due to estrogens, androgens, or a variation in body fat distribution, but this has not been definitively established.

Leptin has only been recently implicated as a hormonal factor that may partially account for the association between obesity and cancers of the breast, colon, prostate, and kidney.

Obesity and Inactivity

Obesity does not result from inactivity alone. Instead, obesity arises from an imbalance between energy intake and energy expenditure, where energy intake exceeds energy expenditure (Hill, 2004). According to Hill, one way to prevent obesity in the context of a sedentary lifestyle is to restrict dietary intake. Human physiology, however, has not evolved to support energy restriction, and it is difficult for most people to reduce intake of food over time (Hill, 2004).

Physically active people are less likely to gain weight over the course of their lifetime and as a consequence are more likely to have a low prevalence of obesity (U.S. Department of Health and Human Services, 1996). The Surgeon General's report additionally reviewed the literature on the impact of exercise training on body weight and obesity and has concluded (U.S. Department of Health and Human Services, 1996):

1. "Physical activity generally affects body composition and weight favorably by promoting fat loss while preserving or increasing lean mass.
2. The rate of weight loss is positively related, in a dose–response manner, to the frequency and duration of the physical activity session, as well as to the duration of the physical activity program (e.g., months, years).
3. Although the rate of weight loss resulting from increased physical activity without caloric restriction is slow, the combination of increased physical activity and dieting appears to be more effective for long-term weight regulation than is dieting alone."

Physical activity reduces the risk of breast and colon cancer. These protective effects may operate through obesity-related mechanisms such as weight loss and changes to body composition, through the functional effects of mobility, or through the effect of exercise on hormone and growth factor levels. Most likely the mechanisms for reduction in risk of colon cancer and breast cancer result from combinations of the aforementioned factors.

Obesity, Inflammation, and Metabolism

Adipose tissue, in addition to functioning as an endocrine organ, also serves as a metabolic organ. Adipose tissue, in response to endocrine and metabolic stimuli, increases or decreases release of fatty acids that provide fuel for skeletal muscle and other tissues. Adipose tissue also contributes to the inflammatory response.

Elevated levels of several proinflammatory cytokines, interleukin-6 (IL-6), IL-18, tumor necrosis factor-α (TNF-α), and C-reactive protein (CRP), in addition to leptin and adiponectin, have been associated with excess BMI (Aronson et al., 2004; Trayhurn and Wood, 2004). Weight loss studies consistently demonstrate reductions of leptin and hsCRP in the short and long term, and reduction of TNF-α, cyclooxygenase-2 (COX-2), IL-6, and high-density lipoprotein C (HDL-C) in the long term (Laimer et al., 2002; Esposito et al., 2003; van Dielen et al., 2004).

Serum CRP closely correlates with circulating levels of proinflammatory cytokines and is associated with atherosclerosis, an inflammation of blood vessel walls (Ridker et al., 2000). CRP is produced in the liver and is thought to be a sensitive and particularly stable marker for subclinical inflammation (Ridker, 2001). Serum CRP is also linked to insulin resistance, prediabetes (Haffner, 2003), and fasting insulin (Pradhan et al., 2003).

The obesity phenotype is heterogeneous and can affect cancer risk in multiple ways. Possible consequences of obesity that are thought to be associated with cancer risk include: alterations in hormones and growth factors; metabolic complications; immune system dysregulation; inflammation; inactivity; and changes in adiposity at different ages.

OBESITY AND CANCER RISK OF SPECIFIC SITES

Breast Cancer in Women

Obesity and weight gain during adulthood are associated with increased breast cancer risk among postmenopausal women (Hunter and Willett, 1993; Huang et al., 1997; Endogenous Hormones and Breast Cancer Collaborative Group, 2003). Most studies report relative risks that range from 1.5 to 2, comparing women in the highest BMI category to those in the lowest category or those with the greatest weight gain to those with no weight gain or minimal weight gain (International Agency for Research on Cancer [IARC], 2002). Obesity has the opposite effect on breast cancer risk among younger premenopausal women, with those with high BMI at lower risk than those with low BMI (Ursin et al., 1995; Swanson et al., 1996; Cleary and Maihle, 1997; Stoll, 1998; Coates et al., 1999; Peacock et al., 1999).

Obesity, Hormones, and Breast Cancer

Endogenous estrogens and progesterone, as well as exogenous formulations of these hormones, drive cellular proliferation in the breast and thus are key to the development of breast cancer (Feigelson and Henderson, 2000). Estrone has been shown to be the principal hormone responsible for the association between obesity and breast cancer risk among postmenopausal women (Endogenous Hormones and Breast Cancer Collaborative Group, 2003). The major source of estrone (precursor to estrogen) after menopause is the conversion of androstenedione to estrone by adipose tissue cells (adipocytes) in the presence of aromatase (Endogenous Hormones and Breast Cancer Collaborative Group, 2003). Larger amounts of adipose tissue in obese women increase circulating estrone levels in direct proportion to the amount of adipose tissue (MacDonald et al., 1978). Estrone itself is converted to the more potent estrogen estradiol during this process.

Most epidemiological studies that have evaluated body fat distribution have observed an association between upper body obesity and postmenopausal breast cancer risk, although a few studies have found visceral obesity predictive of breast cancer risk (Cleary and Maihle, 1997). A reduction in circulating SHBG levels may mediate the relationship between upper body obesity and postmenopausal breast cancer risk, although the relationship is probably indirect. Key and Pike (1988b) estimate that doubling the weight of a postmenopausal woman from 54 kg to 108 kg will reduce her SHBG levels by 85% and increase her total and bioavailable estradiol levels by 60%.

Hormone therapy modifies the relationship between obesity and postmenopausal breast cancer risk (Huang et al., 1997; Morimoto et al., 2002). Obesity does not increase breast cancer risk among women who have taken hormone therapy; in the milieu of exogenous estrogen (and progestin), the added impact of obesity-related increases on circulating estrogens is negligible.

Heavy body weight is associated with a 10–30% reduction of breast cancer risk in premenopausal women (Ursin et al., 1995). Among premenopausal women, obesity may increase circulating estrogen levels to the same extent that they are increased among postmenopausal women, but within the milieu of ovarian estrogen production, the additional estrogen due to obesity has little or no impact. Further, younger women who are obese may experience menstrual cycle disturbances, including anovulatory menstrual cycles or secondary amenorrhea, reducing their cumulative exposure to estradiol and progesterone (Key and Pike, 1988b). Some evidence suggests that obesity during adolescence shows the strongest inverse relationship (Stoll, 1998). One explanation for this observation is the induction of insulin resistance, particularly if obesity occurs in adolescence (Stoll, 1998).

Obese postmenopausal women have increased insulin levels, insulin resistance, and IGF-1 levels (Stoll, 2000). IGFs are peptides that serve signaling functions in many tissues, including the breast, and circulate as endocrine factors that regulate tissue growth and fat deposition (Lipworth et al., 1996). IGF-1 serves as a strong stimulator of mitosis in breast cancer cells and may be increased concurrent with diminished SHBG concentrations observed in obese women (Lipworth et al., 1996).

Serum IGF-1 levels are controlled by hormonal, nutritional, and genetic factors. IGF levels are related to IGF-1 gene polymorphisms and are linked to body composition and weight, in age- and gender-specific manners (Jernstrom et al., 2001; Johnston et al., 2003; Rietveld et al., 2003, 2004; Rivadeneira et al., 2003). IGF levels are higher among obese postmenopausal women (Stoll, 2000). Most epidemiological studies have found an association between IGF-1 level and premenopausal breast cancer, but not postmenopausal breast cancer risk (Hankinson et al., 1998; Toniolo et al., 2000). The biological function of IGF-1 suggests an association with both premenopausal and postmenopausal breast cancer; however, risk is only increased among premenopausal women. The IGF pathway in relationship to postmenopausal breast cancer remains speculative. At this stage of understanding, we do not know enough about how IFG-1 changes at menopause.

Leptin has been implicated as a hormonal factor that might partially account for the association between obesity and cancer of the breast. A study of human cell lines, leptin-deficient mice and leptin receptor–deficient mice, suggests that leptin controls proliferation of normal and malignant breast epithelial cells (Hu et al., 2002). The current epidemiological literature on leptin and breast cancer risk is limited. Studies have been small, were not specifically designed for studying a leptin–breast cancer association, and have shown no association between leptin and breast cancer risk (Mantzoros et al., 1999; Stattin et al., 2004b).

Obesity, Inflammation, and Breast Cancer

The inflammation pathway may be important in the multistep process of breast carcinogenesis; however, many questions remain unanswered. In particular, malignant breast tumors have high levels of prostaglandins (Rolland et al., 1980; Brueggemeier et al., 2003), which may promote mitogenesis, cellular adhesion, immune surveillance, and angiogenesis (Brueggemeier et al., 2003). Presence of a high omega-6/omega-3 fatty acid ratio, associated with high levels of prostaglandins, has been found in adipose tissue of obese women with breast cancer (Brueggemeier et al., 2003; London et al., 1993). We have evidence that breast tissue selectively concentrates omega-3 fatty acids by comparison to gluteal fat (Bagga et al., 1997).

Colon Cancer

Evidence is fairly consistent that excess weight is associated with an increased risk of colon cancer (Potter et al., 1993; Caan et al., 1998; Ford, 1999; Murphy et al., 2000; Giovannucci, 2003). The adverse impact of overweight and obesity on colon cancer risk is stronger for the distal than for the proximal colon and stronger among men than among women (IARC, 2002). One possible explanation for this gender difference is that the increase in estrogen exposure that women receive as a result of obesity (through aromatization of androstenedione to estrone in body fat) may counteract somewhat other mechanisms operating to increase risk, in the same way as use of hormone therapy appears to reduce women's risk of colon cancer (Rossouw et al., 2002). Heavier weight earlier in life appears to carry the same risk as recent weight (IARC, 2002), suggesting that immediate weight reduction efforts could affect colon cancer risk.

Obesity, Hormones, and Colon Cancer

The insulin pathway has been suggested as an essential link between obesity and colon cancer (Giovannucci, 1995, 2003). Insulin is an important growth factor of colonic epithelial cells and promotes tumor growth *in vitro* (Watkins et al., 1990; Bjork et al., 1993). Additionally, colon cancer tissue has both insulin and IGF-1 receptors that have higher rates of expression than surrounding normal tissue (Freier et al., 1999). A case-control study nested within the prospective Northern Sweden Health and Disease Cohort found a moderate though nonsignificant association between fasting insulin and colon cancer risk (Palmqvist et al., 2003). Diabetes risk is strongly associated with obesity (Centers for Disease Control and Prevention [CDC], 2004) and diabetes has a modest association with colon cancer risk in case-control studies (Giovannucci, 1995), although results for cohort studies are mixed (Weiderpass et al., 1997; Kim, 1998; Will et al., 1998). Indirect associations have been observed between polymorphisms of insulin-related genes and colon cancer risk (insulin receptor substrate-1 [IRS1], insulin receptor substrate 2 [IRS2], and IGF-1) (Slattery et al., 2004, 2005).

Several case-control studies nested within large prospective cohorts found associations between serum level IGFs and colon cancer risk (Ma et al., 1999; Giovannucci et al., 2000; Kaaks et al., 2000b). In the Physicians' Health Study, plasma IGF-BP3, adjusted for IGF-1, was associated with colon cancer risk among both younger and older men (Ma et al., 1999). Among women in the Nurses' Health Study, an association between IGF-BP3 and risk of intermediate/late-stage colorectal adenoma was observed (Giovannucci et al., 2000). In another case-control study nested within a cohort of women in New York, colorectal cancer risk showed a modest association with the highest quintile of IGF-BP3 adjusting for IGF-1 (Kaaks et al., 2000b). It is possible that the impact of IGF-related factors is independent of BMI, as shown in the analyses of the Physicians' Health Study and the Nurses' Health Study adjusted for BMI; however, biologically, the IGF system is most likely interrelated with obesity and diabetes.

Experimental studies point to a possible role for leptin in development of colon cancer, as the leptin receptor is expressed in human colon cancer cell lines and human colonic tissue (Hardwick et al., 2001). Stimulation with leptin leads to increased cell proliferation, indirectly demonstrating that leptin may be partially responsible for the observed association between obesity and colon cancer risk (Hardwick et al., 2001).

Leptin plays an important role in fat storage and metabolism and is associated with higher insulin levels. Therefore, it may be important in colon cancer etiology. Two epidemiological studies provide some support for the role of leptin in colon cancer development. One study in Norway showed a 2.7-fold increased risk of colon cancer among individuals with leptin concentrations in the highest versus lowest quartile (Stattin et al., 2004a). A second similar study conducted in Sweden found that colon cancer risk increased with increasing leptin levels in men, but not women (Stattin et al., 2003b).

Obesity, Inflammation, and Colon Cancer

Inflammation increases the risk for several gastrointestinal malignancies. Chronic bowel inflammation, also known as inflammatory bowel disease (IBD), (both ulcerative colitis and Crohn's colitis), increases the risk of colorectal cancer (Itzkowitz and Yio, 2004). Suppression of inflammation in the bowel through pharmacological agents such as nonsteroidal anti-inflammatory drugs (NSAIDs), 5-aminosalicylates, and steroids may prevent the development of colorectal cancer (Thun et al., 2002). Moreover, NSAIDs, particularly the highly selective COX-2 inhibitors, restore normal apoptosis in human adenomatous colorectal polyps and inhibit angiogenesis in both cell culture and rodent models (Thun et al., 2002).

Clinical trials have established that aspirin can reduce the risk of sporadic colorectal adenomas, but whether aspirin can prevent development of colorectal cancer remains to be determined. The randomized clinical trial that was primarily conducted to evaluate aspirin in prevention of cardiovascular disease (Physicians' Health Study) found no reduction in invasive or *in situ* colorectal cancer incidence or mortality (Steering Committee of the Physicians' Health Study Research Group, 1989). In randomized prevention trials of colorectal adenomas, moderate to strong protective associations were observed for aspirin and adenoma incidence, recurrence, and adenomas among patients with colorectal cancer (Benamouzig et al., 2003; Sandler et al., 2003; Baron et al., 2005).

Other markers of inflammation, such as CRP, may be related to colon cancer risk. The chronic inflammation caused by obesity contributes to oxidative stress that promotes mutagenic assault and sustained DNA damage resulting in neoplastic transformation of the colonic mucosa (Itzkowitz and Yio, 2004). A paired study of fecal calprotectin, a marker of bowel inflammation, and serum CRP was conducted in south London among 320 healthy men and women (Poullis et al., 2004). Fecal calprotectin was positively associated with increasing age, obesity, and physical inactivity and was inversely associated with fiber intake and vegetable consumption. Further, a significant independent association was found between CRP and fecal calprotectin. When models were adjusted for CRP, the relationship between calprotectin and obesity disappeared, suggesting that CRP mediated the obesity and calprotectin association.

Endometrial Cancer in Women

Endometrial cancer is a hormone-dependent cancer associated with a deficiency in progesterone and an excess of estrogen, and estrogen therapy after menopause is an acknowledged cause of this cancer (Kaaks et al., 2002). Thus, it is not surprising that obesity is associated with greater risk of endometrial cancer, particularly among postmenopausal women (IARC, 2002). Among premenopausal women, the effect appears to be limited to women in the obese category (BMI > 30 kg/m^2), but among postmenopausal women, risk increases linearly with increasing body mass. Heavier postmenopausal women are exposed to excess levels of estrogen, resulting from the aromatization of androstenedione in body fat in the absence of progesterone, which counteracts the proliferative effects of estrogen on endometrial tissue. Findings from a nested case-control analysis of postmenopausal women in three prospective cohorts from New York, Sweden, and Italy showed that prediagnostic levels of circulating estrogens were directly associated with endometrial cancer risk and that SHBG levels were inversely related to risk (Lukanova et al., 2004).

Hormones implicated in energy metabolism are also related to increased endometrial cancer risk. A review of endometrial cancer risk by Kaaks et al. (2002) noted that, in addition to the reproductive hormones, chronic hyperinsulinemia was also a risk factor for endometrial cancer, with both elevated insulin and diabetes increasing endometrial cancer risk. In a Norwegian cohort study, a linear association between fasting glucose and endometrial cancer risk was found, with the association appearing stronger among overweight women (BMI > 25 kg/m^2), and almost absent among normal-weighted women (Furburg and Thune, 2003). A small case-control study of IGF-1, IGF-BP3, insulin, and hormone replacement therapy (HRT) showed that elevated IGF-BP1 levels increased endometrial cancer risk only among users of HRT (Wiederpass et al., 2003). Overall associations among IGF-1, IGF-BP3, and insulin, however, were unrelated to endometrial risk. The study did not measure hormones before endometrial cancer diagnosis, so tumor status may have affected circulating levels among the cases. Another small case-control study conducted in Greece found a strong association between serum leptin and endometrial cancer risk; however, when data were adjusted for BMI, the association disappeared (Petridou et al., 2002), suggesting that obesity and leptin may share a common pathway with respect to endometrial cancer. The study did not, however, measure leptin prior to diagnosis and tumor status may have biased the results.

Adenocarcinoma of the Esophagus

An epidemic of adenocarcinoma of the esophagus, which was extremely rare 30 years ago, has paralleled the epidemic of obesity in developed countries (IARC, 2002). During this 30-year period, rates of esophageal adenocarcinoma have increased >350%. The epidemic has been most apparent among white men whose rates of esophageal adenocarcinoma are three to four greater than those of black men and at least eight times greater than those of white women (Bernstein, 1999). In studies of esophageal adenocarcinoma, obesity has been consistently observed to increase risk of this disease (Chow et al., 1998; Wu et al., 2001; Lagergren et al., 2005). Gastroesophageal reflux symptoms, which are common among obese patients and increase as BMI increases (Nilsson et al., 2003; Wu et al., 2003), are also associated with risk of esophageal adenocarcinoma (Chow et al., 1995; Lagergren et al., 1999; Ye et al., 2001). Thus, one of the mechanisms by which obesity may have an impact on esophageal adenocarcinoma risk is through changes in the esophageal epithelium induced by reflux that leads to Barrett's esophagus, a lesion of columnar cells in the squamous cell–lined esophagus that is a precursor to esophageal adenocarcinoma cancer.

Kidney or Renal Cell Cancer

Previous investigations of the relationship of BMI, a measure of obesity, and renal cancer risk have shown increased risks among obese women, but the results have been less consistent among men. Three cohort studies from the United States and Denmark have reported increased mortality and incidence rates for renal cell cancer (RCC) in obese women and to a lesser degree for obese men (Lew and Garfinkel, 1979; Mellemgaard et al., 1991; Wolk et al., 2001). Similarly, most case-control studies of RCC have observed associations with measures of body size among women, but there is variance with regard to the magnitude of effect and what was observed for men (Wynder et al., 1974; Goodman et al., 1986; Yu et al., 1986; Mellemgaard et al., 1995; Chow et al., 1996). One case-control study found increased risk of renal cell carcinoma associated with overweight and obesity among both men and women (Hu et al., 2003), and a large prospective study of almost 400,000 Swedish men found a strong linear association between increasing percentiles of BMI and risk for RCC (Chow et al., 2000).

Obesity is one component of the metabolic syndrome. It is possible the metabolic syndrome itself is associated with RCC. Other features of the metabolic syndrome include hypertension; decreased insulin sensitivity; increased levels of IGFs; and in women, anovulation and excessive androgen production (Wolk et al., 1996). Renal damage may occur as a result of hypertension and metabolic complications from obesity that could predispose the kidney to the putative effects of carcinogens. Many studies have identified obesity and hypertension as risk factors for RCC (Chow et al., 1996, 2000; Yuan et al., 1998). Although these associations appear statistically independent, biologically, they are interrelated, as obesity increases the risk for hypertension.

CANCER SITES SUSPECTED TO BE ASSOCIATED WITH OBESITY

Several types of cancer such as prostate cancer, pancreatic cancer, and NHL may be associated with obesity; however, the evidence for such relationships is not conclusive.

Obesity and Prostate Cancer in Men

Conversion of the adrenal androgen androstenedione to estrone by adipose tissue in the presence of aromatase occurs in men and women (Pasquali et al., 1991). The exact role of estrogen in prostate cancer development and progression is unclear, but animal and experimental studies suggest that elevated estradiol levels may play an important role in testosterone-induced prostate tumorigenesis. Studies of mice with genetically altered aromatase or estrogen receptor expression have shown that estradiol combined with testosterone regulates proliferation and apoptosis of prostate cells (McPherson et al., 2001; Ho et al., 2004). Leav et al. (1989) demonstrated that testosterone needs to be combined with estrogen for development of proliferative lesions in mouse prostate tissue. On the basis of these experimental data, excess estradiol in obese men may enhance the growth-promoting effect of testosterone on prostate cancer.

Clear evidence exists showing that increasing levels of testosterone and decreasing levels of SHBG are predictive of prostate cancer risk (Gann et al., 1996). Thus, these hormonal factors may mediate any association between obesity and prostate cancer. In particular, larger waist circumference is associated with lower testosterone and SHBG levels and higher estradiol levels (Svartberg et al., 2004).

Insulin and insulin resistance may be related to prostate cancer development (Barnard et al., 2002). Several studies have shown that insulin resistance, diabetes, and elevated insulin/glucose levels are associated with increased prostate cancer risk (Hsing et al., 2001, 2003). Other studies have not observed an association of prostate cancer risk with diabetes (Giovannucci et al., 1998; Weiderpass et al., 2002; Stattin and Kaaks, 2003). Because of conflicting data in the literature, additional studies need to be conducted to determine the impact of insulin resistance or diabetes on prostate cancer development.

Evidence has accumulated linking IGF-1 levels and prostate cancer risk on the basis of prospective studies in which blood samples were collected before disease diagnosis. In the Physicians' Health Study, a strong positive association between plasma IGF-1 and prostate cancer risk was observed (Chan et al., 1998). Men in the highest quartile of IGF-1 level had more than a fourfold greater risk of prostate cancer compared with men in the lowest quartile (Chan et al., 1998). The association remained when adjusted for weight, height, BMI, and other covariates such as estrogen, lycopene, and SHBG. Other studies have found similar associations (Kaaks et al., 2000a). In a Swedish cohort study, an increase in prostate cancer risk was associated with IGF-1 among men who developed a prostate tumor before age 60 years (Stattin et al., 2000).

Leptin also may be associated with prostate cancer risk, although studies have not been consistent. One cohort study found an association between prediagnostic serum leptin concentrations and prostate cancer risk (Stattin et al., 2001), but other studies have not found an association (Hsing et al., 2001; Stattin et al., 2003). Two studies among men with prostate cancer found that serum leptin concentrations were associated with larger, higher-grade, and more advanced tumors (Chang et al., 2001; Saglam et al., 2003).

Emerging epidemiological and experimental evidence suggests that inflammation may play an important role in the development and progression of prostate cancer. A meta-analysis by Dennis et al. (2002) found that a history of prostatitis (inflammation of the prostate) was associated with increased prostate cancer risk. In addition, inflammatory atrophy in prostate tissue is frequently found in close association with prostatic intraepithelial neoplasia, which is known to be precancerous (De Marzo et al., 1999).

Numerous mechanisms have been proposed linking initiation and promotion of prostate cancer with inflammation, including release of cytokines and chemokines, as well as generation of reactive oxygen species (Coussens and Werb, 2002). Few studies have evaluated associations between CRP levels and prostate cancer risk or progression (Platz and Giovannucci, 2004). Elevated serum levels of the cytokine IL-6 have been associated with more advanced stages of prostate cancer, and higher preoperative serum IL-6 levels predict recurrence following radical prostatectomy (Shariat et al., 2004). IL-6 is produced by adipocytes, prostate cancer cells, and immune cells including activated macrophages (Ho et al., 2004).

The COX-2 and the prostaglandin E_2 (PGE_2) inflammation pathway may also play a key role in prostate cancer progression. COX-2 is overexpressed in prostate cancer, and increased expression and levels of COX-2 have been reported in malignant as compared with benign prostate tissue (Tsujii et al., 1997; Gupta et al., 2000; Kirschenbaum et al., 2000). PGE_2, a conversion product of COX-2, affects cell proliferation and tumor cell invasion (Levy, 1997; Nithipatikom et al., 2002). High levels of PGE_2 have been shown to play an important role in controlling growth and metastasis in prostate cancer (Ablin and Shaw, 1986).

Results from a prospective study of healthy men suggest that prostate cancer detection may be influenced by BMI. BMI and prostate-specific antigen (PSA) levels were examined in 2779 men without prostate carcinoma in a study conducted by the San Antonio Center of Biomarkers of Risk (Baillargeon et al., 2005). Mean PSA value decreased in a linear fashion with increasing BMI from 1.01 ng/ml in normal-weighted men to 0.69 ng/ml in obese men, adjusting for race/ethnicity and age. In another study of men consecutively referred for abnormal digital rectal examination (DRE) results or high levels of PSA that was followed up by biopsy, detection rates of cancer were highest among normal-weighted men (Presti et al., 2004). Lower levels of PSA that occur in obese men might mask detection of prostate carcinoma. Moreover, obesity may inhibit accurate

DRE results. That is, if obesity increases the risk of prostate cancer, studies that rely on PSA or DRE results for prostate cancer detection may fail to observe an underlying association.

Obesity and Non-Hodgkin's Lymphoma

The incidence of NHL has rapidly increased among both men and women over the past 30 years. Since the mid-1980s, the acquired immunodeficiency syndrome (AIDS) epidemic has affected NHL incidence rates; however, the marked increase in incidence of NHL preceded the AIDS epidemic by several decades, and the AIDS epidemic has affected female NHL incidence rates minimally (Devesa and Fears, 1992; Groves et al., 2000; Eltom et al., 2002). The incidence of AIDS-related NHL has begun to decrease (Eltom et al., 2002). Thus, any changes in incidence of NHL due to AIDS have been superimposed upon a background of clearly increasing incidence that has been maintained since the 1980s and into the new century.

The dramatic rise in incidence has prompted investigators to consider changes in prevalence of risk factors that might be associated with NHL. Obesity is suspected as a risk factor for NHL because of the dramatic increase in obesity prevalence, but more importantly, obesity is suspected as a risk factor because of inflammation and its corresponding effects on immunity (Marti et al., 2001). A review of clinical and epidemiological data relating obesity to immune function noted that the incidence and severity of specific types of infection are higher in obese persons, and that the antibody response tends to be compromised in obese persons (Marti et al., 2001).

Leptin also is implicated in immune response. Leptin production is increased during infection and inflammation. Leptin appears to modulate helper T-lymphocyte function, through regulation of cell proliferation. Leptin also promotes nitric oxide synthesis and production of proinflammatory cytokines (Otero et al., 2005).

Results for BMI differ between the Iowa Women's Health Study and a case-control study in the San Francisco Bay area. No relationship of obesity to NHL was observed among Iowa women (Cerhan et al., 2002). In contrast, NHL risk increased with increasing BMI among San Francisco women, such that relative to lean women, those who were considered obese (BMI > 30) had a threefold elevated risk (Skibola et al., 2005). In a linkage study of a population-based cohort of hospitalized patients with any discharge diagnosis of obesity and the Swedish Cancer Registry, a significant risk elevation of NHL was noted for women but not men (Chang et al., 2005).

Results from these studies suggest that much work remains in determining whether obesity might be a risk factor for NHL. One of the difficulties in studying risk factors for NHL is that NHL is composed of many different subtypes. The WHO NHL classification system considers morphology, immunophenotype, genotype, normal cell counterpart, and clinical features in grouping tumors into categories thought to be etiologically distinct, and few studies have examined the association of obesity with NHL risk within these categories (Jaffee et al., 2001). Another complication factor is that hormonal exposures among women appear to reduce risk of NHL, providing one possible explanation for the lower incidence of NHL among women (Nelson et al., 2001) Thus, a modest protection from obesity-related increases in circulating estrogen might counteract the adverse effects of inflammation on risk. The impact of male hormones on NHL risk among men is not known.

Obesity and Pancreatic Cancer

Established risk factors for pancreatic cancer are few, and with the exception of tobacco smoking (Michaud, 2004), the causes of pancreatic cancer are still unknown. Obesity, diabetes mellitus, glucose intolerance, high serum glucose, and hyperinsulinemia are some of the suspected risk factors for pancreatic cancer (Michaud, 2004).

Previous case-control studies of obesity and pancreatic cancer have yielded inconclusive results; however, several prospective studies found increased risks for obesity. A meta-analysis of obesity and pancreas cancer risk based on six case-control studies and eight cohort studies estimated that risk of pancreas cancer increased 2% per unit increase of BMI (Berrington de Gonzalez et al., 2003). Although this estimate of the impact of obesity on pancreatic cancer risk was statistically significant, it is of relatively small magnitude and may reflect confounding by other risk factors.

The American Cancer Society cohort was studied in relationship to obesity, recreational activity, and risk of pancreatic cancer (Patel et al., 2005). Results showed an increased risk of pancreatic cancer among obese (BMI > 30) men and women compared wtih normal-sized men and women (BMI < 25). Risk was independently increased among men and women who reported a tendency for central weight gain. No difference in pancreatic cancer risk was noted for high levels of activity among men and women compared to no reported recreational activity. Central adiposity reflects development of insulin resistance and hyperinsulinemia, which may be the underlying mechanism that explains the obesity relationship with pancreatic cancer.

In a prospective cohort study of >1 million Koreans 30–95 years of age, all cancer mortality was positively associated with fasting serum glucose level. By cancer site, the association was strongest for pancreatic cancer (Jee et al., 2005). Because of the co-occurrence of obesity, diabetes, and impaired glucose metabolism, these and other results suggest a possible etiological role for obesity. In one study that combined data from two U.S. cohort studies and evaluated effects from physical activity, height, and BMI, obesity significantly increased the risk of pancreatic cancer, whereas physical activity appeared to decrease the risk, especially among overweight and obese subjects who had a BMI of at least 25 kg/m^2 (Michaud et al., 2001). Among overweight and obese subjects, a low level of physical activity actually increased risk, suggesting a synergism between obesity and inactivity. In a commentary about the study, Gapstur and Gann (2001) suggested that hyperinsulinemia could be the etiological mechanism for pancreatic carcinogenesis. The pathogenic relationship of pancreatic cancer to insulin could, in part, be explained by anatomy: The exocrine cells of the pancreas, which give rise to fatal pancreatic cancers, are exposed to extremely high concentrations of insulin because their blood supply passes through the islet cell region (Gapstur and Gann, 2001).

SUMMARY

Obesity is associated with elevation in risk for several types of cancer, including endometrial, kidney, and colon cancer, as well as esophageal adenocarcinoma, and breast cancer among postmenopausal women. Obesity is thought to be associated with NHL, pancreatic cancer, and prostate cancer. We described risk factors for obesity and discussed suggested mechanisms that explain the obesity–cancer association for different types of cancer.

The pathways that appear to promote elevated cancer risk due to obesity include reproductive hormones; hormones and growth factors involved in energy utilization; lack of exercise; and inflammation. Although obesity is associated with each cancer site uniquely, some common aspects of obesity appear to promote risk in more than one cancer. The rising obesity prevalence may translate into increases in cancer incidence. In particular, increasing numbers of obese children and adolescents may have a dramatic impact on cancer incidence when adulthood is reached.

Acknowledgment

This research is supported by the National Cancer Institute (1 P01 CA 42710), California Breast Cancer Research Program (9PB-0117), and the UCLA Center for Human Nutrition.

References

Ablin, R.J., and Shaw, M.W. 1986. Prostaglandin modulation of prostate tumor growth and metastases. *Anticancer Res* **6**: 327–328.

Agurs-Collins, T., Adams-Campbell, L., Sook, K., and Cullen, K.J. 2000. Insulin-like growth factor-1 and breast cancer risk in postmenopausal African-American women. *Cancer Detect Prev* **24**: 199–206.

Ambrosius, W.T., Compton, J.A., Bowsher, R.R., and Pratt, J.H. 1998. Relation of race, age, and sex hormone differences to serum leptin concentrations in children and adolescents. *Horm Res* **49**: 240–246.

Andersen, R.E., Crespo, C.J., Bartlett, S.J., Cheskin, L.J., and Pratt, M. 1998. Relationship of physical activity and television watching with body weight and level of fatness among children: Results from the Third National Health and Nutrition Examination Survey. *JAMA* **279**: 938–942.

Aronson, D., Bartha, P., Zinder, O., Kerner, A., Markiewicz, W., Avizohar, O. et al. 2004. Obesity is the major determinant of elevated C-reactive protein in subjects with the metabolic syndrome. *Int J Obes Relat Metab Disord* **28**: 674–679.

Bagga, D., Capone, S., Wang, H.J., Heber, D., Lill, M., Chap, L. et al. 1997. Dietary modulation of omega-3/omega-6 polyunsaturated fatty acid ratios in patients with breast cancer. *J Natl Cancer Inst* **89**: 1123–1131.

Baillargeon, J., Pollock, B.H., Kristal, A.R., Bradshaw, P., Hernandez, J., Basler, J. et al. 2005. The association of body mass index and prostate-specific antigen in a population-based study. *Cancer* **103**: 1092–1095.

Barnard, R.J., Aronson, W.J., Tymchuk, C.N., and Ngo, T.H. 2002. Prostate cancer: another aspect of the insulin-resistance syndrome? *Obes Rev* **3**: 303–308.

Baron, J.A., Cole, B.F., Sandler, R.S., Haile, R.W., Ahnen, D., and Brasalier, R. 2005. A randomized trial of aspirin to prevent colorectal adenomas. *N Engl J Med* **348**: 891–899.

Benamouzig, R., Deyra, J., Martin, A., Girard, B., Julian, E., and Piednoir, B. 2003. Daily soluble aspirin and prevention of colorectal adenoma recurrence: one-year results of the APACC trial. *Gastroenterology* **12**: 328–336.

Bernstein, L. 1999. Barrett's esophagus and adenocarcinoma: epidemiology. *In* "American Society of Clinical Oncology Education Book" (M.C. Perry, Ed.), pp. 99–105. ASCO, Alexandria, VA.

Berrington de Gonzalez, A., Sweetland, S., and Spencer, E. 2003. A meta-analysis of obesity and the risk of pancreatic cancer. *Br J Cancer* **89**: 519–523.

Bjork, J., Nilsson, J., Hultcrantz, R., and Johansson, C. 1993. Growth-regulatory effects of sensory neuropeptides, epidermal growth factor, insulin, and somatostatin on the non-transformed intestinal epithelial cell line IEC-6 and the colon cancer cell line HT 29. *Scand J Gastroenterol* **28**: 879–884.

Brueggemeier, R.W., Richards, J.A., and Petrel, T.A. 2003. Aromatase and cyclooxygenases: enzymes in breast cancer. *J Steroid Biochem Mol Biol* **86**: 501–507.

Bruning, P.F., Bonfrer, J.M., Van Noord, P.A., Hart, A.A., de Jong-Bakker, M., and Nooijen, W.J. 1992. Insulin resistance and breast-cancer risk. *Int J Cancer* **52**: 511–516.

Brzechffa, P.R., Jakimiuk, A.J., Agarwal, S.K., Weitsman, S.R., Buyalos, R.P., and Magoffin, D.A. 1996. Serum immunoreactive leptin concentrations in women with polycystic ovary syndrome. *J Clin Endocrinol Metab* **81**: 4166–4169.

Caan, B.J., Coates, A.O., Slattery, M.L., Potter, J.D., Quesenberry, C.P., Jr., and Edwards, S.M. 1998. Body size and the risk of colon cancer in a large case-control study. *Int J Obes Relat Metab Disord* **22**: 178–184.

Calle, E.E., Rodriguez, C., Walker-Thurmond, K., and Thun, M.J. 2003. Overweight, obesity, and mortality from cancer in a prospectively studied cohort of U.S. adults. *N Engl J Med* **348**: 1625–1638.

Castracane, V.D., Kraemer, R.R., Franken, M.A., Kraemer, G.R., and Gimpel, T. 1998. Serum leptin concentration in women: effect of age, obesity, and estrogen administration. *Fertil Steril* **70**: 472–477.

Centers for Disease Control and Prevention. 2004. Prevalence of overweight and obesity among adults with diagnosed diabetes—United States. *MMWR Morb Mortal Wkly Rep* **53**: 1066–1068.

Cerhan, J.R., Janney, C.A., Vachon, C.M., Habermann, T.M., Kay, N.E., Potter, J.D. et al. 2002. Anthropometric characteristics, physical activity, and risk of non-Hodgkin's lymphoma subtypes and B-cell chronic lymphocytic leukemia: a prospective study. *Am J Epidemiol* **156**: 527–535.

Chan, J.M., Stampfer, M.J., Giovannucci, E., Gann, P.H., Ma, J., Wilkinson, P. et al. 1998. Plasma insulin-like growth factor-I and prostate cancer risk: a prospective study. *Science* **279**: 563–566.

Chang, E.T., Hjalgrim, H., Smedby, K.E., Akerman, M., Tani, E., Johnsen, H.E. et al. 2005. Body-mass index and risk of malignant lymphoma in Scandinavian men and women. *J Natl Cancer Inst* **97**: 310–318.

Chang, S., Hursting, S.D., Contois, J.H., Strom, S.S., Yamamura, Y., Babaian, R.J. et al. 2001. Leptin and prostate cancer. *Prostate* **46**: 62–67.

Chow, W.H., Finkle, W.D., and McLaughlin, J.K. 1995. The relation of gastroesophageal reflux disease and its treatment to adenocarcinomas of the esophagus and gastric cardia. *JAMA* **274**: 474–477.

Chow, W.H., McLaughlin, J.K., Mandel, J.S., Wacholder, S., Niwa, S., and Fraumeni, J.F., Jr. 1996. Obesity and risk of renal cell cancer. *Cancer Epidemiol Biomarkers Prev* **5**: 17–21.

Chow, W.H., Blot, W.J., Vaughan, T.L., et al. 1998. Body mass index and risk of adenocarcinomas of the esophagus and gastric cardia. *J Natl Cancer Inst* **1998**: 150–155.

Chow, W.H., Gridley, G., Fraumeni, J.F., Jr., and Jarvholm, B. 2000. Obesity, hypertension, and the risk of kidney cancer in men. *N Engl J Med* **343**: 1305–1311.

Cleary, M.P., and Maihle, N.J. 1997. The role of body mass index in the relative risk of developing premenopausal versus postmenopausal breast cancer. *Proc Soc Exp Biol Med* **216**: 28–43.

Coates, R.J., Uhler, R.J., Hall, H.I., Potischman, N., Brinton, L.A., Ballard-Barbash, R. et al. 1999. Risk of breast cancer in young women in relation to body size and weight gain in adolescence and early adulthood. *Br J Cancer* **81**: 167–174.

Comuzzie, A.G., and Allison, D.B. 1998. The search for human obesity genes. *Science* **280**: 1374–1377.

Coussens, L.M., and Werb, Z. 2002. Inflammation and cancer. *Nature* **420**: 860–867.

De Marzo, A.M., Marchi, V.L., Epstein, J.I., and Nelson, W.G. 1999. Proliferative inflammatory atrophy of the prostate: implications for prostatic carcinogenesis. *Am J Pathol* **155**: 1985–1992.

Dennis, L.K., Lynch, C.F., and Torner, J.C. 2002. Epidemiologic association between prostatitis and prostate cancer. *Urology* **60**: 78–83.

Devesa, S.S., and Fears, T. 1992. Non-Hodgkin's lymphoma time trends: United States and international data. *Cancer Res* **52**: 5432s–5440s.

Eltom, M.A., Jemal, A., Mbulaiteye, S.M., Devesa, S.S., and Biggar, R.J. 2002. Trends in Kaposi's sarcoma and non-Hodgkin's lymphoma incidence in the United States from 1973 through 1998. *J Natl Cancer Inst* **94**: 1204–1210.

Endogenous Hormones and Breast Cancer Collaborative Group. 2003. Body mass index, serum sex hormones, and breast cancer risk in postmenopausal women. *J Natl Cancer Inst* **95**: 1218–1226.

Esposito, K., Pontillo, A., Di, P.C., Giugliano, G., Masella, M., Marfella, R. et al. 2003. Effect of weight loss and lifestyle changes on vascular inflammatory markers in obese women: a randomized trial. *JAMA* **289**: 1799–1804.

Feigelson, H.S., and Henderson, B.E. 2000. Future possibilities in the prevention of breast cancer role of genetic variation in breast cancer prevention. *Breast Cancer Res* **2**: 277–282.

Flegal, K.M., Carroll, M.D., Ogden, C.L., and Johnson, C.L. 2002. Prevalence and trends in obesity among US adults, 1999–2000. *JAMA* **288**: 1723–1727.

Ford, E.S. 1999. Body mass index and colon cancer in a national sample of adult US men and women. *Am J Epidemiol* **150**: 390–398.

Freier, S., Weiss, O., Eran, M., Flyvbjerg, A., Dahan, R., Nephesh, I. et al. 1999. Expression of the insulin-like growth factors and their receptors in adenocarcinoma of the colon. *Gut* **44**: 704–708.

Fruehwald-Schultes, B., Peters, A., Kern, W., Beyer, J., and Pfutzner, A. 1998. Influence of sex differences in subcutaneous fat mass on serum leptin concentrations. *Diabetes Care* **21**: 1204–1205.

Furburg, A.-S., and Thune, I. 2003. Metabolic abnormalities (hypertension, hyperglycemia, and overweight), lifestyle (high energy intake and physical inactivity) and endometrial cancer risk in a Norwegian cohort. *Int J Cancer* **104**: 669–676.

Gann, P.H., Hennekens, C.H., Ma, J., Longcope, C., and Stampfer, M.J. 1996. Prospective study of sex hormone levels and risk of prostate cancer. *J Natl Cancer Inst* **88**: 1118–1126.

Gapstur, S.M., and Gann, P.H. 2001. Is pancreatic cancer a preventable disease? *JAMA* **286**: 967–968.

Giovannucci, E. 1995. Insulin and colon cancer. *Cancer Causes Control* **6**: 164–179.

Giovannucci, E., Rimm, E.B., Stampfer, M.J., Colditz, G.A., and Willett, W.C. 1998. Diabetes mellitus and risk of prostate cancer (United States). *Cancer Causes Control* **9**: 3–9.

Giovannucci, E., Pollak, M.N., Platz, E.A., Willett, W.C., Stampfer, M.J., Majeed, N. et al. 2000. A prospective study of plasma insulin-like growth factor-1 and binding protein-3 and risk of colorectal neoplasia in women. *Cancer Epidemiol Biomarkers Prev* **9**: 345–349.

Giovannucci, E. 2003. Diet, body weight, and colorectal cancer: a summary of the epidemiologic evidence. *J Womens Health (Larchmt)* **12**: 173–182.

Goodman, M.T., Morgenstern, H., and Wynder, E.L. 1986. A case-control study of factors affecting the development of renal cell cancer. *Am J Epidemiol* **124**: 926–941.

Groves, F.D., Linet, M.S., Travis, L.B., and Devesa, S.S. 2000. Non-Hodgkin's lymphoma incidence by histologic subtypes in the United States from 1978 through 1995. National Cancer Institute. Cancer Surveillance Series.

Gupta, S., Srivastava, M., Ahmad, N., Bostwick, D.G., and Mukhtar, H. 2000. Over-expression of cyclooxygenase-2 in human prostate adenocarcinoma. *Prostate* **42**: 73–78.

Haffner, S.M. 2003. Insulin resistance, inflammation, and the prediabetic state. *Am J Cardiol* **92**: 18J–26J.

Hankinson, S.E., Willett, W.C., Colditz, G.A., Hunter, D.J., Michaud, D.S., Deroo, B. et al. 1998. Circulating concentrations of insulin-like growth factor-I and risk of breast cancer. *Lancet* **351**: 1393–1396.

Hardwick, J.C., van den Brink, G.R., Offerhaus, G.J., van Deventer, S.J., and Peppelenbosch, M.P. 2001. Leptin is a growth factor for colonic epithelial cells. *Gastroenterology* **121**: 79–90.

Hill, J. 2004. Physical activity and obesity. *Lancet* **363**: 182.

Hill, J.O., and Peters, J.C. 1998. Environmental contributions to the obesity epidemic. *Science* **280**: 1371–1374.

Ho, E., Boileau, T.W., and Bray, T.M. 2004. Dietary influences on endocrine-inflammatory interactions in prostate cancer development. *Arch Biochem Biophys* **428**: 109–117.

Hsing, A.W., Chua, S. Jr., Gao, Y.T., Gentzschein, E., Chang, L., Deng, J. et al. 2001. Prostate cancer risk and serum levels of insulin and leptin: a population-based study. *J Natl Cancer Inst* **93**: 783–789.

Hsing, A.W., Gao, Y.T., Chua, S., Jr., Deng, J., and Stanczyk, F.Z. 2003. Insulin resistance and prostate cancer risk. *J Natl Cancer Inst* **95**: 67–71.

Hu, X., Juneja, S.C., Maihle, N.J., and Cleary, M.P. 2002. Leptin–a growth factor in normal and malignant breast cells and for normal mammary gland development. *J Natl Cancer Inst* **94**: 1704–1711.

Hu, J., Mao, Y., and White, K. 2003. Overweight and obesity in adults and risk of renal cell carcinoma in Canada. *Soz Praventivmed* **48**: 178–185.

Hu, X., Juneja, S.C., Maihle, N.J., and Cleary, M.P. 2002. Leptin–a growth factor in normal and malignant breast cells and for normal mammary gland development. *J Natl Cancer Inst* **94**: 1704–1711.

Huang, Z., Hankinson, S.E., Colditz, G.A. et al. 1997. Dual effects of weight and weight gain on breast cancer risk. *JAMA* **278**: 1407–1411.

Hunter, D.J., and Willett, W.C. 1993. Diet, body size, and breast cancer. *Epidemiol Rev* **15**: 110–132.

International Agency for Research on Cancer. 2002. "Weight Control and Physical Activity." IARC Press, Lyon, France.

Itzkowitz, S.H., and Yio, X. 2004. Inflammation and cancer, IV. Colorectal cancer in inflammatory bowel disease: the role of inflammation. *Am J Physiol Gastrointest Liver Physiol* **287**: G7–G17.

Jaffee, E.S., Harris, N.L., Stein, H., Vardiman, J.W. et al. 2001. "World Health Organization Classification of Tumors of Haematopoietic and Lymphoid Tissues." IARC Press, Lyon, France.

Jee, S.H., Ohrr, H.S., Suli, J.W., Yun, J.E., and Samet, J.M. 2005. Fasting serum glucose level and cancer risk in Korean men and women. *JAMA* **293**: 194–202.

Jernstrom, H., Deal, C., Wilkin, F., Chu, W., Tao, Y., Majeed, N. et al. 2001. Genetic and nongenetic factors associated with variation of plasma levels of insulin-like growth factor-I and insulin-like growth factor-binding protein-3 in healthy premenopausal women. *Cancer Epidemiol Biomarkers Prev* **10**: 377–384.

Johnston, L.B., Dahlgren, J., Leger, J., Gelander, L., Savage, M.O., Czernichow, P. et al. 2003. Association between insulin-like growth factor I (IGF-I) polymorphisms, circulating IGF-I, and pre- and post-natal growth in two European small for gestational age populations. *J Clin Endocrinol Metab* **88**: 4805–4810.

Kaaks, R. 1996. Nutrition, hormones, and breast cancer: is insulin the missing link? *Cancer Causes Control* **7**: 605–625.

Kaaks, R., Lukanova, A., and Sommersberg, B. 2000a. Plasma androgens, IGF-1, body size, and prostate cancer risk: a synthetic review. *Prostate Cancer Prostatic Dis* **3**: 157–172.

Kaaks, R., Toniolo, P., Akhmedkhanov, A., Lukanova, A., Biessy, C., Dechaud, H. et al. 2000b. Serum C-peptide, insulin-like growth factor (IGF)-I, IGF-binding proteins, and colorectal cancer risk in women. *J Natl Cancer Inst* **92**: 1592–1600.

Kaaks, R., Lukanova, A., and Kurzer, M.S. 2002. Obesity, endogenous hormones and endometrial cancer risk: A synthetic review. *Cancer Epidemiol Biomarkers Prev* **11**: 1531–1543.

Kennedy, A., Gettys, T.W., Watson, P., Wallace, P., Ganaway, E., Pan, Q. et al. 1997. The metabolic significance of leptin in humans: gender-based differences in relationship to adiposity, insulin sensitivity, and energy expenditure. *J Clin Endocrinol Metab* **82**: 1293–1300.

Key, T.J., and Pike, M.C. 1988a. The dose–effect relationship between "unopposed" oestrogens and endometrial mitotic rate: its central role in explaining and predicting endometrial cancer risk. *Br J Cancer* **57**: 205–212.

Key, T.J., and Pike, M.C. 1988b. The role of oestrogens and progestagens in the epidemiology and prevention of breast cancer. *Eur J Cancer Clin Oncol* **24**: 29–43.

Kim, Y.I. 1998. Diet, lifestyle, and colorectal cancer: is hyperinsulinemia the missing link? *Nutr Rev* **56**: 275–279.

Kirschenbaum, A., Klausner, A.P., Lee, R., Unger, P., Yao, S., Liu, X.H. et al. 2000. Expression of cyclooxygenase-1 and cyclooxygenase-2 in the human prostate. *Urology* **56**: 671–676.

Lagergren, J., Bergstrom, R., Lindgren, A., and Nyren, O. 1999. Symptomatic gastroesophageal reflux as a risk factor for esophageal adenocarcinoma. *N Engl J Med* **340**: 825–831.

Lagergren, J., Bergstron, R., Lindgren, A. et al. 2005. Symptomatic gastroesophageal reflux as a risk factor for esophageal adenocarcinoma. *N Engl J Med* **340**: 825–831.

Laimer, M., Ebenbichler, C.F., Kaser, S., Sandhofer, A., Weiss, H., Nehoda, H. et al. 2002. Markers of chronic inflammation and obesity: a prospective study on the reversibility of this association in middle-aged women undergoing weight loss by surgical intervention. *Int J Obes Relat Metab Disord* **26**: 659–662.

Leav, I., Merk, F.B., Kwan, P.W., and Ho, S.M. 1989. Androgen-supported estrogen-enhanced epithelial proliferation in the prostates of intact Noble rats. *Prostate* **15**: 23–40.

Levy, G.N. 1997. Prostaglandin H synthases, nonsteroidal anti-inflammatory drugs, and colon cancer. *FASEB J* **11**: 234–247.

Lew, E.A., and Garfinkel, L. 1979. Variations in mortality by weight among 750,000 men and women. *J Chronic Dis* **32**: 563–576.

Lipworth, L., Adami, H.O., Trichopoulos, D., Carlstrom, K., and Mantzoros, C. 1996. Serum steroid hormone levels, sex hormone-binding globulin, and body mass index in the etiology of postmenopausal breast cancer. *Epidemiology* **7**: 96–100.

London, S.J., Sacks, F.M., Stampfer, M.J., Henderson, I.C., Maclure, M., Tomita, A. et al. 1993. Fatty acid composition of the subcutaneous adipose tissue and risk of proliferative benign breast disease and breast cancer. *J Natl Cancer Inst* **85**: 785–793.

Lukanova, A., Lundin, E., Micheli, A., Arslan, A., Ferrari, P., Rinaldi, S. et al. 2004. Circulating levels of sex steroid hormones and risk of endometrial cancer in postmenopausal women. *Int J Cancer* **108**: 425–432.

Ma, J., Pollak, M.N., Giovannucci, E., Chan, J.M., Tao, Y., Hennekens, C.H. et al. 1999. Prospective study of colorectal cancer risk in men and plasma levels of insulin-like growth factor (IGF)-I and IGF-binding protein-3. *J Natl Cancer Inst* **91**: 620–625.

MacDonald, P.C., Edman, C.D., Hemsell, D.L., Porter, J.C., and Siiteri, P.K. 1978. Effect of obesity on conversion of plasma androstenedione to estrone in postmenopausal women with and without endometrial cancer. *Am J Obstet Gynecol* **130**: 448–455.

Manson, J.E., Skerrett, P.J., Greenland, P., and VanItallie, T.B. 2004. The escalating pandemics of obesity and sedentary lifestyle. A call to action for clinicians. *Arch Intern Med* **164**: 249–258.

Mantzoros, C.S., Bolhke, K., Moschos, S., and Cramer, D.W. 1999. Leptin in relation to carcinoma in situ of the breast: a study of pre-menopausal cases and controls. *Int J Cancer* **80**: 523–526.

Marti, A., Marcos, A., and Martinez, J.A. 2001. Obesity and immune function relationships. *Obes Rev* **2**: 131–140.

McPherson, S.J., Wang, H., Jones, M.E., Pedersen, J., Iismaa, T.P., Wreford, N. et al. 2001. Elevated androgens and prolactin in aromatase-deficient mice cause enlargement, but not malignancy, of the prostate gland. *Endocrinology* **142**: 2458–2467.

Mellemgaard, A., Moller, H., Olsen, J.H., and Jensen, O.M. 1991. Increased risk of renal cell carcinoma among obese women. *J Natl Cancer Inst* **83**: 1581–1582.

Mellemgaard, A., Lindblad, P., Schlehofer, B., Bergstrom, R., Mandel, J.S., McCredie, M. et al. 1995. International renal-cell cancer study. III. Role of weight, height, physical activity, and use of amphetamines. *Int J Cancer* **60**: 350–354.

Michaud, D.S., Giovannucci, E., Willett, W.C., Colditz, G.A., Stampfer, M.J., and Fuchs, C.S. 2001. Physical activity, obesity, height and the risk of pancreatic cancer. *JAMA* **286**: 921–929.

Michaud, D.S. 2004. Epidemiology of pancreatic cancer. *Minerva Chir* **59**: 99–111.

Mokdad, A.H., Bowman, B.A., Ford, E.S. et al. 2001. The continuing epidemics of obesity and diabetes in the United States. *JAMA* **296**: 1195–1200.

Morimoto, L.M., White, E., Chen Z. et al. 2002. Obesity, body size, and risk of postmenopausal breast cancer: the Women's Health Initiative (United States). *Cancer Causes Control* **13**: 741–751.

Murphy, T.K., Calle, E.E., Rodriguez, C., Kahn, H.S., and Thun, M.J. 2000. Body mass index and colon cancer mortality in a large prospective study. *Am J Epidemiol* **152**: 847–854.

Nelson, R.A., Levine, A.M., and Bernstein, L. 2001. Reproductive factors and risk of intermediate- or high-grade B-cell non-Hodgkin's lymphoma in women. *J Clin Oncol* **19**: 1381–1387.

Nilsson, M., Johnsen, R., and Ye, W., Hveem, K., and Langergen J. 2003. Obesity and estrogen as risk factors for gastroesophageal reflux symptoms. *JAMA* **290**: 66–72.

Nithipatikom, K., Isbell, M.A., Lindholm, P.F., Kajdacsy-Balla, A., Kaul, S., and Campell, W.B. 2002. Requirement of cyclooxygenase-2 expression and prostaglandins for human prostate cancer cell invasion. *Clin Exp Metastasis* **19**: 593–601.

Olshansky, S.J., Passaro, D.J., Hershow, R.C., Layden, J., Carnes, B.A., Brody, J. et al. 2005. A potential decline in life expectancy in the United States in the 21st century. *N Engl J Med* **352**: 1138–1145.

Otero, M., Lago, R., Lago, F., Casanueva, F.F., Dieguez, C., and Gomez-Reino, J.J. 2005. Leptin, from fat to inflammation: Old questions and new insights. *FEBS Letters* **579**: 295–301.

Palmqvist, R., Stattin, P., Rinaldi, S., Biessy, C., Stenling, R., Riboli, E. et al. 2003. Plasma insulin, IGF-binding proteins-1 and -2 and risk of colorectal cancer: a prospective study in northern Sweden. *Int J Cancer* **107**: 89–93.

Parks, S.E., Housemann, R.A., and Brownson, R.C. 2003. Differential correlates of physical activity in urban and rural adults of various socioeconomic backgrounds in the United States. *J Epidemiol Community Health* **57**: 29–35.

Pasquali, R., Casimirri, F., Cantobelli, S., Melchionda, N., Morselli Labate, A.M., Fabbri, R. et al. 1991. Effect of obesity and body fat distribution on sex hormones and insulin in men. *Metabolism* **40**: 101–104.

Patel, A.V., Rodriguez, C., Bernstein, L., Chao, A., Thun, M.J., and Calle, E.E. 2005. Obesity, recreational physical activity, and risk of pancreatic cancer in a large US cohort. *Cancer Epidemiol Biomarkers Prev* **14**: 459–466.

Peacock, S.L., White, E., Daling, J.R., Voigt, L.F., and Malone, K.E. 1999. Relation between obesity and breast cancer in young women. *Am J Epidemiol* **149**: 339–346.

Petridou, E., Belechri, M., Dessypris, N., Koukoulomatis, P., Diakomanolis, E., Spanos, E. et al. 2002. Leptin and body mass index in relation to endometrial cancer risk. *Ann Nutr Metab* **46**: 147–181.

Platz, E.A., and Giovannucci, E. 2004. The epidemiology of sex steroid hormones and their signaling and metabolic pathways in the etiology of prostate cancer. *J Steroid Biochem Mol Biol* **92**: 237–253.

Potter, J.D., Slattery, M.L., Bostick, R.M., and Gapstur, S.M. 1993. Colon cancer: a review of the epidemiology. *Epidemiol Rev* **15**: 499–545.

Poullis, A., Foster, R., Shetty, A., Fagerhol, M.K., and Mendall, M.A. 2004. Bowel inflammation as measured by fecal calprotectin: a link between lifestyle factors and colorectal cancer risk. *Cancer Epidemiol Biomarkers Prev* **13**: 279–284.

Pradhan, A.D., Cook, N.R., Buring, J.E., Manson, J.E., and Ridker, P.M. 2003. C-reactive protein is independently associated with fasting insulin in nondiabetic women. *Arterioscler Thromb Vasc Biol* **23**: 650–655.

Presti, J.C., Jr., Lee, U., Brooks, J.D., and Terris, M.K. 2004. Lower body mass index is associated with a higher prostate cancer detection rate and less favorable pathological features in a biopsy population. *J Urol* **171**: 2199–2202.

Ridker, P.M. 2001. High-sensitivity C-reactive protein: potential adjunct for global risk assessment in the primary prevention of cardiovascular disease. *Circulation* **103**: 1813–1818.

Ridker, P.M., Hennekens, C.H., Buring, J.E., and Rifai, N. 2000. C-reactive protein and other markers of inflammation in the prediction of cardiovascular disease in women. *N Engl J Med* **342**: 836–843.

Rietveld, I., Janssen, J.A., Hofman, A., Pols, H.A., van Duijn, C.M., and Lamberts, S.W. 2003. A polymorphism in the IGF-I gene influences the age-related decline in circulating total IGF-I levels. *Eur J Endocrinol* **148**: 171–175.

Rietveld, I., Janssen, J.A., van Rossum, E.F., Houwing-Duistermaat, J.J., Rivadeneira, F., Hofman, A. et al. 2004. A polymorphic CA repeat in the IGF-I gene is associated with gender-specific differences in body height, but has no effect on the secular trend in body height. *Clin Endocrinol (Oxf)* **61**: 195–203.

Rivadeneira, F., Houwing-Duistermaat, J.J., Vaessen, N., Vergeer-Drop, J.M., Hofman, A., Pols, H.A. et al. 2003. Association between an insulin-like growth factor I gene promoter polymorphism and bone mineral density in the elderly: the Rotterdam Study. *J Clin Endocrinol Metab* **88**: 3878–3884.

Rolland, P.H., Martin, P.M., Jacquemier, J., Rolland, A.M., and Toga, M. 1980. Prostaglandin in human breast cancer: Evidence suggesting that an elevated prostaglandin production is a marker of high metastatic potential for neoplastic cells. *J Natl Cancer Inst* **64**: 1061–1070.

Rossouw, J.E., Anderson, G.L., Prentice, R.L., LaCroix, A.Z., Kooperberg, C., Stefanick, M.L. et al. 2002. Risks and benefits of estrogen plus progestin in healthy postmenopausal women: principal results From the Women's Health Initiative randomized controlled trial. *JAMA* **288**: 321–333.

Ryan, A.S., and Elahi, D. 1996. The effects of acute hyperglycemia and hyperinsulinemia on plasma leptin levels: its relationships with body fat, visceral adiposity, and age in women. *J Clin Endocrinol Metab* **81**: 4433–4438.

Saglam, K., Aydur, E., Yilmaz, M., and Goktas, S. 2003. Leptin influences cellular differentiation and progression in prostate cancer. *J Urol* **169**: 1308–1311.

Sandler, R.S., Halabi, S., Baron, J.A., Budinger, S., Paskett, E., Keresztes, R. et al. 2003. A randomized trial of aspirin to prevent colorectal adenomas in patients with previous colorectal cancer. *N Engl J Med* **348**: 883–890.

Shariat, S.F., Kattan, M.W., Traxel, E., Andrews, B., Zhu, K., Wheeler, T.M. et al. 2004. Association of pre- and postoperative plasma levels of transforming growth factor beta(1) and interleukin 6 and its soluble receptor with prostate cancer progression. *Clin Cancer Res* **10**: 1992–1999.

Sherwood, N.E., and Jeffery, R.W. 2000. The behavioral determinants of exercise: implications for physical activity interventions. *Annu Rev Nutr* **20**: 21–44.

Sierra-Honigmann, M.R., Nath, A.K., Murakami, C., Garcia-Cardena, G., Papapetropoulos, A., Sessa, W.C. et al. 1998. Biological action of leptin as an angiogenic factor. *Science* **281**: 1683–1686.

Skibola, C.F., Holly, E.A., Forrest, M.S., Hubbard, A., Bracci, P.M., Skibola, D.R. et al. 2005. Body mass index, leptin and leptin receptor polymorphisms, and non-Hodgkin lymphoma. *Cancer Epidemiol Biomarkers Prev* **13**: 779–786.

Slattery, M.L., Samowitz, W., Hoffman, M., Ma, K.N., Levin, T.R., and Neuhausen, S. 2004. Aspirin, NSAIDs, and colorectal cancer: possible involvement in an insulin-related pathway. *Cancer Epidemiol Biomarkers Prev* **13**: 538–545.

Slattery, M.L., Murtaugh, M., Caan, B., Ma, K.N., Neuhausen, S., and Samowitz, W. 2005. Energy balance, insulin-related genes and risk of colon and rectal cancer. *Int J Cancer* **115**: 148–154.

Stattin, P., Bylund, A., Rinaldi, S., Biessy, C., Dechaud, H., Stenman, U.H. et al. 2000. Plasma insulin-like growth factor-I, insulin-like growth factor-binding proteins, and prostate cancer risk: a prospective study. *J Natl Cancer Inst* **92**: 1910–1917.

Stattin, P., Soderberg, S., Hallmans, G., Bylund, A., Kaaks, R., Stenman, U.H. et al. 2001. Leptin is associated with increased prostate cancer risk: a nested case-referent study. *J Clin Endocrinol Metab* **86**: 1341–1345.

Stattin, P., and Kaaks, R. 2003. Prostate cancer, insulin, and androgen deprivation therapy. *Br J Cancer* **89**: 1814–1815.

Stattin, P., Kaaks, R., Johansson, R., Gislefoss, R., Soderberg, S., Alfthan, H. et al. 2003a. Plasma leptin is not associated with prostate cancer risk. *Cancer Epidemiol Biomarkers Prev* **12**: 474–475.

Stattin, P., Palmqvist, R., Soderberg, S., Biessy, C., Ardnor, B., Hallmans, G. et al. 2003b. Plasma leptin and colorectal cancer risk: a prospective study in Northern Sweden. *Oncol Rep* **10**: 2015–2021.

Stattin, P., Lukanova, A., Biessy, C., Soderberg, S., Palmqvist, R., Kaaks, R. et al. 2004a. Obesity and colon cancer: does leptin provide a link? *Int J Cancer* **109**: 149–152.

Stattin, P., Soderberg, S., Biessy, C., Lenner, P., Hallmans, G., Kaaks, R. et al. 2004b. Plasma leptin and breast cancer risk: a prospective study in northern Sweden. *Breast Cancer Res Treat* **86**: 191–196.

Steering Committee of the Physicians' Health Study Research Group. 1989. Final report on the aspirin component of the ongoing Physicians' Health Study. *N Engl J Med* **321**: 129–135.

Sternfeld, B., Ainsworth, B.E., and Quesenberry, C.P. 1999. Physical activity patterns in a diverse population of women. *Prev Med* **28**: 313–323.

Stoll, B.A. 1998. Teenage obesity in relation to breast cancer risk. *Int J Obes Relat Metab Disord* **22**: 1035–1040.

Stoll, B.A. 2000. Adiposity as a risk determinant for postmenopausal breast cancer. *Int J Obes Relat Metab Disord* **24**: 527–533.

Svartberg, J., von, M.D., Sundsfjord, J., and Jorde, R. 2004. Waist circumference and testosterone levels in community dwelling men. The Tromso study. *Eur J Epidemiol* **19**: 657–663.

Swanson, C.A., Coates, R.J., Schoenberg, J.B., Malone, K.E., Gammon, M.D., Stanford, J.L. et al. 1996. Body size and breast cancer risk among women under age 45 years. *Am J Epidemiol* **143**: 698–706.

Tchernof, A., and Despres, J.P. 2000. Sex steroid hormones, sex hormone-binding globulin, and obesity in men and women. *Horm Metab Res* **32**: 526–536.

Thun, M.J., Henley, S.J., and Patrono, C. 2002. Nonsteroidal anti-inflammatory drugs as anticancer agents: mechanistic, pharmacologic, and clinical issues. *J Natl Cancer Inst* **94**: 252–266.

Toniolo, P., Bruning, P.F., Akhmedkhanov, A., Bonfrer, J.M., Koenig, K.L., Lukanova, A. et al. 2000. Serum insulin-like growth factor-I and breast cancer. *Int J Cancer* **88**: 828–832.

Trayhurn, P., and Wood, I.S. 2004. Adipokines: inflammation and the pleiotropic role of white adipose tissue. *Br J Nutr* **92**: 347–355.

Tsujii, M., Kawano, S., and DuBois, R.N. 1997. Cyclooxygenase-2 expression in human colon cancer cells increases metastatic potential. *Proc Natl Acad Sci USA* **94**: 3336–3340.

U.S. Department of Health and Human Services. 2004. NHANES III, II, I, and NHES I, and preliminary estimates updated in 2002. National Center for Health Statistics. Unpublished Tabulations.

U.S. Department of Health and Human Services. 1996. Physical activity and health. National Center for Chronic Disease Prevention and Health Promotion, Centers for Disease Control and Prevention. A Report of the Surgeon General.

Ursin, G., Longnecker, M.P., Haile, R.W., and Greenland, S. 1995. A meta-analysis of body mass index and risk of premenopausal breast cancer. *Epidemiology* **6**: 137–141.

van Dielen, F.M., Buurman, W.A., Hadfoune, M., Nijhuis, J., and Greve, J.W. 2004. Macrophage inhibitory factor, plasminogen activator inhibitor-1, other acute phase proteins, and inflammatory mediators normalize as a result of weight loss in morbidly obese subjects treated with gastric restrictive surgery. *J Clin Endocrinol Metab* **89**: 4062–4068.

Watkins, L.F., Lewis, L.R., and Levine, A.E. 1990. Characterization of the synergistic effect of insulin and transferrin and the regulation of their receptors on a human colon carcinoma cell line. *Int J Cancer* **45**: 372–375.

Weiderpass, E., Gridley, G., Nyren, O., Ekbom, A., Persson, I., and Adami, H.O. 1997. Diabetes mellitus and risk of large bowel cancer. *J Natl Cancer Inst* **89**: 660–661.

Weiderpass, E., Ye, W., Vainio, H., Kaaks, R., and Adami, H.O. 2002. Reduced risk of prostate cancer among patients with diabetes mellitus. *Int J Cancer* **102**: 258–261.

Wiederpass, E., Brismar, K., Bellocco, R., Vainio, H., and Kaaks, R. 2003. Serum levels of insulin-like growth factor-1, IGF-binding protein 1 and 3, and insulin and endometrial cancer risk. *Br J Cancer* **89**: 1697–1704.

Will, J.C., Galuska, D.A., Vinicor, F., and Calle, E.E. 1998. Colorectal cancer: another complication of diabetes mellitus? *Am J Epidemiol* **147**: 816–825.

Wolk, A., Lindblad, P., and Adami, H.O. 1996. Nutrition and renal cell cancer. *Cancer Causes Control* **7**: 5–18.

Wolk, A., Gridley, G., Svensson, M., Nyren, O., McLaughlin, J.K., Fraumeni, J.F. et al. 2001. A prospective study of obesity and cancer risk (Sweden). *Cancer Causes Control* **12**: 13–21.

World Health Organization. 2001. Obesity: preventing and managing the global epidemic. Report on a WHO consultation. Technical Report Series 894.

Wu, A.H., Tseng, C.-C., and Bernstein, L. 2003. Hiatal hernia, reflux symptoms, body size, and risk of esophageal and gastric adenocarcinoma. *Cancer Causes Control* **98**: 940–948.

Wu, A.H., Wan, P., and Bernstein, L. 2001. A multiethnic population-based study of smoking, alcohol and body size and risk of adenocarcinoma of the stomach and esophagus (United States). *Cancer Causes Control* **8**: 721–732.

Wynder, E.L., Mabuchi, K., and Whitmore, W.F., Jr. 1974. Epidemiology of adenocarcinoma of the kidney. *J Natl Cancer Inst* **53**: 1619–1634.

Ye, W., Chow, W.H., Lagergren, J. et al. 2001. Risk of adenocarcinoma of the esophagus and gastric cardia in patients with gastroesophageal reflux diseases and after antireflux surgery. *Gastroenterology* **121**: 1286–1293.

Yu, M.C., Mack, T.M., Hanisch, R., Cicioni, C., and Henderson, B.E. 1986. Cigarette smoking, obesity, diuretic use, and coffee consumption as risk factors for renal cell carcinoma. *J Natl Cancer Inst* **77**: 351–356.

Yuan, J.M., Castelao, J.E., Gago-Dominguez, M., Ross, R.K., and Yu, M.C. 1998. Hypertension, obesity and their medications in relation to renal cell carcinoma. *Br J Cancer* **77**: 1508–1513.

CHAPTER

10

Nutrition and Tobacco-Related Cancers

KARAM EL-BAYOUMY, JOSHUA E. MUSCAT, AND DIETRICH HOFFMANN

INTRODUCTION

Tobacco use is the leading cause of mortality in the United States, accounting for 478,082 deaths (18.1% of total deaths) in 2002 (Twombly, 2005). Smoking causes 90% of lung cancer cases and up to one third of all cancer deaths. More than 8.6 million Americans suffer from tobacco-induced illnesses, and one in every five deaths in the United States is smoking related according to the Centers for Disease Control and Prevention (CDCP). Cigarette smoking is the single most preventable cause of cancer deaths in America, as it is responsible for cancers of the lung, head and neck, kidney, bladder, and pancreas (Thun et al., 1997). Cigarette smoking has also been implicated as a possible cause of other cancers (Vineis et al., 2004). In fact, while the 1982 Surgeon General's Report concluded that smoking caused lung cancer, in addition to other cancers (The Health Consequences of Smoking, 1982), the most recent edition implied all organs are at risk of developing tobacco-related cancers (The Health Consequences of Smoking, 2004). The role of cigarette smoking in the development of pancreatic cancer was uncertain in 1982, but subsequent studies established a twofold to threefold risk in cigarette smokers (Risch, 2003). The 1982 and 2001 Surgeon General's Reports (Women and Smoking, 2001) concluded that there was insufficient evidence that tobacco use caused cancer of the breast, prostate, colon, and uterine cervix. However, scientists continue to investigate whether cigarette smoking causes cancer of reproductive and other organs (Vineis et al., 2004; The Health Consequences of Smoking, 2004). The role of tobacco use as a risk for cancer has also been investigated in conjunction with high-risk genetic or phenotypic traits, such as advanced age, family history, positive or negative hormone receptor status, and mutations in critical genes. If cigarette smoking increases the risk of breast, prostate, and colon cancer in some smokers, there will be a need to stress, even further, the importance of measures that can postpone or prevent the onset of smoking among youths and will hasten smoking cessation among adults.

Although the risk of cancer from cigarette smoking was shown to be a dose–response effect, reductions in cigarette tar yield and nicotine levels over the past several decades have not effectively reduced the cancer mortality rates from smoking; smokers of low-yield products simply increased smoking intensity and depth of inhalation (Thun and Burns, 2001). Clearly, from a public health standpoint, the only harmless cigarette is the one that is not smoked. Yet, smoking control efforts should include the development of less toxic and carcinogenic cigarettes as long as millions of current and future smokers remain at risk. Although quitting the smoking habit obviously reduces the risk of tobacco-related cancers, dietary and/or chemoprevention might be a plausible alternative for smokers who are unable to quit. Chemopreventive agents, along with dietary modulation, may have the potential to reduce the risk of cancer in former smokers as well, because their risk remains elevated above those who have never smoked, even for many years after cessation (Khuder and Mutgi, 2001). The importance of chemoprevention research and dietary modification is underscored by the fact that in the United States, nearly one half of all cancer deaths can be linked to tobacco and diet (Doll and Peto, 1981; Stein and Colditz, 2004). Emphasis needs to be made, however, that chemoprevention should never be considered a substitute for primary prevention efforts, but a complementary approach.

Copyright © 2006, Elsevier Inc.
All rights of reproduction in any form reserved.

An important goal for the development of cancer prevention strategies is the identification of molecular pathways by which normal cells progress to the first definable stage of cancer. Genomics, proteomics, transcriptomics, and metabolomics are highly useful and complementary approaches to the understanding of mechanisms of cancer development at the molecular level (Davis and Milner, 2004) and can provide novel markers that can be employed for early detection (Desai et al., 2002; Michener et al., 2002; Etzioni et al., 2003; Wagner et al., 2004). Knowledge gathered from the varied disciplines, collectively referred to as an "omics" approach, is requisite to the design of an appropriate strategy for clinical chemoprevention intervention trials. Clearly, the goal is to gain insights into individually tailored cancer prevention and treatment modalities. Today, it seems promising that investigators can apply high-throughput screening techniques to develop new hypotheses and to identify new molecular targets and/or pathways in the multistep tobacco carcinogenesis and chemoprevention processes (El-Bayoumy and Sinha, 2005).

This chapter updates information on tobacco carcinogenesis and the role of tobacco and nutrition in established tobacco-related cancers (details are discussed in the first edition of *Nutritional Oncology*; Hoffmann and El-Bayoumy, 1999). Furthermore, we discuss findings on the relationship of cigarette smoking and cancers of the breast, prostate, colon, and uterine cervix, as well as leukemia and the role of dietary factors in cancer prevention.

TOBACCO CARCINOGENESIS

Likely Causative Agents

In previous reports (Hoffmann and El-Bayoumy, 1999; Hoffmann et al., 2001), we have detailed the chemical composition and toxic and carcinogenic agents in cigarette smoke. Briefly, cigarette smoke is composed of vapor and particulate phases. The vapor phase is arbitrarily defined as that portion of the smoke that passes through a Cambridge glass fiber filter. The particulate phase is the portion that is trapped on the glass fiber filter; the size of particles ranges from 0.1 to $<1\,\mu m$ in diameter. This definition does not fully reflect the conditions prevailing in freshly generated cigarette smoke because some semivolatile agents, such as phenol, appear somewhat in the vapor phase. Some of the substituted phenols, the semi-volatile *N*-nitrosamines, and volatile compounds, such as hydrogen cyanide and low-boiling aldehydes, are partially trapped as aerosol inclusion in the particulate matter. The vapor phase accounts for up to 96% of the weight of the mainstream smoke of a nonfilter cigarette with the following compounds as major constituents: nitrogen ~60%, oxygen ~13%, carbon dioxide 13%, carbon monoxide 3.5%, water 2%, argon 1%, hydrogen 0.1–0.2%, acetone ~1%, nitrogen oxides (NO, NO_2, N_2O) <0.1%, and volatile sulfur compounds likewise <0.1%. Major components of the particulate phase include nicotine (0.2–0.6% of the weight of the total smoke), other *Nicotiana* alkaloids (~0.02%), and compounds specific to *Solanaceae*, namely *n*-hentriacontane ($C_{31}H_{64}$) and solanesol (0.1–0.2%). In addition, the particulate phase contains catechols (~1%), 2- and 4-ring noncarcinogenic polynuclear aromatic hydrocarbons (PAHs) (0.003–0.007% = 3–7 ppm), and the carcinogenic PAH (0.00002–0.00007% = 0.3–0.7 ppm). These relative proportions of smoke components are approximate.

The number of known carcinogens in tobacco smoke increased from 68 in the year 2000 to 81 in 2003. This increase has been attributed to advances in chemical analytical techniques and increased knowledge of genotoxic environmental agents (Smith et al., 2003). These agents include PAHs other than benzo[a]pyrene, aromatic amines, including known human bladder carcinogens, nitrosamines, aldehydes, and several other classes of organic and inorganic compounds. An International Agency for Research on Cancer (IARC) working group concluded that exposure to the tobacco-specific nitrosamines *N'*-nitrosonornicotine (NNN) and 4-(methylnitrosamino)-1-(3-pyridyl)-1-butanone (NNK) is carcinogenic to humans (Cogliano et al., 2004). Table 1 summarizes likely causative agents for tobacco-related cancers.

Biomarkers of Tobacco Carcinogens

For many years, suspected chemical carcinogens were identified primarily from increased cancer rates in occupational settings (Siemiatycki et al., 2004). Beginning in 1976, sensitive methods were developed to measure the uptake and

TABLE 1 Likely Causative Agents for Tobacco-Related Cancers

Cancer type	Agent
Lung, larynx	TSNA (NNK), PAH (B[a]P), benzene, ROS, aldehydes, polonium-210
Oral cavity	TSNA (NNK, NNN), PAH (B[a]P), ROS, alkenals
Esophagus	TSNA (NNN)
Cervix	TSNA (NNK), PAH (B[a]P), human papilloma virus (HPV), ROS
Leukemia	Benzene, nitrosamines, polonium-210, ROS
Pancreas	TSNA (NNK, NNAL)
Bladder	Aromatic amines
Liver	NNK, other nitrosamines, furan
Breast	PAH, aromatic amines, heterocyclic amines
Colon	Heterocyclic amines
Prostate	[ROS?]

Source: From Hoffmann et al., 1991, 2001; Hecht, 1999, 2003.

metabolism of carcinogens. This required an understanding of the metabolic pathways of such carcinogens. We now know that the metabolism of tobacco carcinogens leads to the formation of active electrophiles that can either react with macromolecules, such as DNA, or undergo detoxification reactions. The balance between metabolic activation, detoxification, and DNA repair capacity in a given organ determines the levels of DNA-adduct formation. If these adducts escape repair and persist, they will lead to mutations in critical genes and, consequently, result in the disruption of the normal growth of cells.

There are three types of carcinogen biomarkers: DNA adducts, protein adducts, and urinary metabolites. Literature has thoroughly discussed the accuracy and validity of assays that measure these markers (El-Bayoumy and Hoffmann, 1999; Hecht, 2003). These biomarkers have been widely used in studies aimed at assessing carcinogen exposure and cancer risk. Carcinogen–DNA adducts have been measured by ^{32}P-postlabeling and immunoassays, although neither is precise for specific carcinogens; there are more exact methods for the quantification of DNA adducts. For example, B[*a*]P diol epoxide (BPDE)–DNA adducts were quantified using a high-performance liquid chromatography–mass spectrometry (HPLC-MS) approach. Quantitative analysis of 7-methylguanine, derived from carcinogenic agents such as *N*-nitrosodimethylamine and NNK, was performed by HPLC with ultraviolet (UV) and fluorescence detection (Hecht et al., 1986). HPB–DNA adducts derived from NNK and NNN were analyzed by liquid chromatography with electrospray ionization–MS (LC-ESI-MS) with selected ion monitoring (Wang et al., 2003).

Among protein adducts, the bladder carcinogen 4-aminobiphenyl is known to bind to hemoglobin and serum albumin following metabolic activation (Kadlubar et al., 1988). In a population-based case–control study (Gan et al., 2004), levels of hemoglobin adducts derived from arylamines were associated with bladder cancer risk among nonsmokers. These results emphasize the need for studies aimed at the identification of environmental sources of these compounds. Metabolic activation of NNK and NNN results in the formation of HPB-releasing hemoglobin adducts (Wang et al., 2003). *N*-(2-hydroxyethyl)valine is an established biomarker derived from ethylene oxide (Wu et al., 2004a).

Urinary metabolites reported in the literature include those derived from PAH, for example, 1-hydroxypyrene from pyrene, *r*-1,*t*-2,3*c*-4-tetrahydroxy-1,2,3,4-tetrahydrophenanthrene from phenanthrene, and *t,t*-muconic acid from benzene (Melikian et al., 1999a, b; Hecht et al., 2003). Metabolism of NNK leads to its reduction products (NNAL and NNAL-Gluc), which are excreted in the urine. Of particular significance is the proposal by Hecht et al. (2003) that determining urinary phenanthrene metabolite ratios could be useful for testing the hypothesis that individual differences in PAH metabolism determine cancer risk. Hecht (2003) also proposed that carcinogen–metabolite phenotyping by measuring urinary metabolites could provide a useful determinant for individual susceptibility; clearly, this proposal is based on the results of many studies that have found inconsistencies or merely modest associations of variants of the genes encoding certain enzymes with cancer. Studies that examined carcinogen uptake in smokers are numerous, but limited data are available on carcinogen uptake in smokers who have reduced their smoking levels. Hecht et al. (2004) studied whether reducing the number of cigarettes smoked per day would lead to a corresponding reduction in carcinogen uptake. They found statistically significant reductions in urinary metabolites of NNK as measured by NNAL and NNAL-Gluc. However, the reductions were generally modest and sometimes transient. These results emphasize that some smokers may benefit from reduced smoking; however, most of the effects are modest and probably due to compensation (i.e., more intense puffing and deeper inhalation). Hatsukami et al. (2004) studied smokeless tobacco users who switched to Snus, a smokeless tobacco product from Sweden containing low levels of NNK, as well as cigarette smokers who switched to OMNI cigarettes. Switchers had decreased urinary levels of NNK metabolites, although the greatest reductions were in subjects who had switched to medicinal nicotine. Hatsukami et al. (2004) stated that medicinal nicotine is a safer alternative than modified tobacco products. In another study, Hecht et al. (2005) demonstrated that lung carcinogen and nicotine uptake, as measured by urinary 1-hydroxypyrene, total NNAL, and total cotinine, is the same in smokers of regular, light, and ultralight cigarettes; these results are consistent with epidemiological studies that show no difference in lung cancer risk to smokers of these cigarettes.

Biomarkers of Oxidative Damage

Tobacco smoke is a rich source of free radicals that are thought to play an important role in carcinogenesis and the depletion of blood antioxidant levels (Mayne, 2003). Certain tobacco carcinogens are known to enhance levels of 8-hydroxy-2′-deoxyguanosine (8-OHdG), a marker of DNA oxidative damage (Palozza et al., 2004). 8-OHdG has been detected with single solid-phase extraction and gas chromatography–MS (GC-MS) using selective ion monitoring (Lin et al., 2004). Biomarkers of oxidative damage include oxidation products of DNA, and of lipids and proteins. The use of direct markers, rather than proxy markers of oxidative damage, will potentially lead to a better understanding of the role of oxidative stress in cancer development. Methodologic concerns regarding the accurate measurement and interpretation of studies involving damage to macromolecules include laboratory artifacts, the different affinities for substrates of various reactive oxygen species, and the effectiveness of different biological antioxidants (Mayne,

2003). Levels of 8-OHdG in peripheral lymphocytes and urine are higher in smokers than in nonsmokers, although the findings have been inconsistent (van Zeeland et al., 1999) and a wide degree of interindividual variation has been reported (Pilger et al., 2001). The levels of lipid peroxidation products such as F_2-isoprostanes are also higher in smokers than in nonsmokers (Morrow et al., 1995). Similarly, levels of nitrated proteins that are generated by the uptake of cigarette smoke, are higher in smokers and in lung cancer patients (Pignatelli et al., 2001).

Iron particles in cigarette smoke induce oxidative stress in lung cells. It is possible that the observation in recent decades of both more frequent tumor occurrence and more oxidative damage in the peripheral lung than in the central lung is linked to the use of low-yield cigarettes. Differences in the chemical composition of the smoke of such cigarettes, as well as the modification of inhalation patterns associated with their use, may account for this observation (Brooks et al., 2005).

There are few population-based data on the influence of race, sex, diet, and other factors on levels of these biomarkers (Block et al., 2002). Further, it is uncertain whether such biomarkers of oxidative damage to macromolecules ideally reflect the subtle and chronic changes in human oxidative stress levels. Some concepts in oxidative stress measurement have emphasized the regulation of key cellular activities through pathways that do not involve direct and irreversible damage of macromolecules (Filomeni et al., 2002). Toward this end, there is interest in the glutathiolation of proteins at key cysteine residues, because this is an important redox-sensitive, post-translational signaling mechanism in the regulation of critical cellular functions. Several methods have already been developed to measure glutathione (GSH) and protein glutathiolation (Niwa et al., 2000; Kleinman et al., 2003; Pastore et al., 2003). The results of the selenium trial conducted by Clark et al. (1996) and Duffield-Lillico et al. (2002) led us to conduct a pilot study aimed at understanding the effect of selenium yeast on biomarkers of oxidative damage in healthy subjects. We showed that selenium-enriched yeast enhances blood levels of GSH and reduces blood levels of protein-bound GSH (El-Bayoumy et al., 2002). A small but nonsignificant decrease in urinary 8-OHdG was also observed in this pilot study.

The intraindividual variation in blood levels of protein-bound glutathione (GSSP) is low, so GSSP serves as an attractive biomarker for human studies of post-translational signaling. The sensitivity of blood levels of GSSP as a marker of oxidative stress was demonstrated by comparing its concentrations in cigarette smokers with those in nonsmokers. The mean concentration of blood GSSP (μmol/L) was 32% higher in cigarette smokers and even 43% higher when standardized by hemoglobin concentrations ($p < .01$; Muscat et al., 2004). These differences suggest that substantial oxidative protein modification may occur in cells and tissues; however, this remains to be demonstrated. Several critical proteins involved in carcinogenesis are glutathiolated, including c-Jun (Klatt et al., 1997), spectrin (Sangerman et al., 2001), protein kinase C (Ward et al., 2002), and carbonic anhydrase III (Mallis et al., 2001). The efficacy of specific antioxidants in cancer prevention can be anticipated on the basis of the underlying mechanisms by which oxidative stress affects cellular proliferation, apoptosis, and transcription.

NUTRITION AND TOBACCO-RELATED CANCERS

Lung Cancer

Cigarette smoking causes about 80–90% of all lung cancers. Genetic susceptibility to tobacco carcinogens and lifestyle, including dietary habits, must be important determinants in lung cancer risk because only about 11% of cigarette smokers develop lung cancer (Amos et al., 1999). Inherited factors have been difficult to study because familial aggregation of lung cancer may be due, in part, to shared common environmental risk factors such as cigarette smoking. In one report that accounted for familial smoking status, the relative risk of lung cancer in immediate family members of a lung cancer proband (age 55 years or older) was 1.71 ($p < .01$; Etzel et al., 2003). Several single nucleotide polymorphisms in genes encoding for phase I, phase II, and DNA repair enzymes have been linked to an increased or decreased lung cancer risk (Goode et al., 2002; Kiyohara et al., 2002; Spitz et al., 2003), but the genetic factors that contribute to most of the lung cancers in smokers have, for the most part, not been identified.

Cigarette smoke contains abundant reactive free radicals that cause oxidative damage to DNA, lipids, and proteins (Mayne, 2003). Chronic exposure to free radicals from cigarette smoke is considered an important cause of lung cancer, but this hypothesis has not been demonstrated empirically. Studies of oxidative stress and cancer risk have used proxy measures of antioxidant exposure via fruit and vegetable intake. The rates of nearly all cancers are lower in populations who consume relatively high amounts of fruits and vegetables (Steinmetz et al., 1991). The inverse correlation between carotenoid intake and lung cancer rates was a major reason for conducting the Finnish Alpha-Tocopherol, Beta-Carotene Cancer Prevention (ATBC) Study and the Beta-Carotene and Retinol Efficacy Trial (CARET) (Bendrich, 2004). However, both studies failed to find a protective effect of β-carotene supplement intake on lung cancer incidence. The adverse effects of β-carotene and retinyl palmitate supplements on lung cancer incidence, all-cause mortality in cigarette smokers, as well as in individuals with occupational exposure to asbestos, persisted upon cessation of supplemental administration. Yet, their assessment is no longer statistically significant (Goodman et al.,

2004). Despite the disappointing trial results, subsequent prospective studies ascertained that high fruit consumption confers a protective effect against lung cancer. In the Netherlands Cohort Study, high total consumption of both fruits and vegetables was inversely related to lung cancer risk, particularly in smokers (Voorrips et al., 2000). Similar findings for high fruit intake were reported in a study of a European cohort of Finnish, Italian, and Dutch men (Jansen et al., 2001). In the European Prospective Investigation Into Cancer and Nutrition (EPIC), which surveyed 478,021 individuals, the hazard ratio for lung cancer in the highest quintile of fruit consumption relative to the lowest was 0.60 (95% confidence interval [CI] = 0.46–0.78) (Miller et al., 2004). No association was found with total and specific vegetable consumption.

Hung et al. (2004) analyzed data from >100,000 participants in two large cohort studies, the Nurses' Health Study and the Health Professionals' follow-up study, and found an increase in the beneficial association between total fruit and vegetable intake and the risk of cardiovascular disease, but not with cancer incidence. However, accurate exposure assessment of fruits and vegetables is essential if nutrition and cancer epidemiology studies are to allow unequivocal conclusions. Furthermore, other confounding factors may explain the lack of protective effect of fruits and vegetables on cancer. There has been little success in identifying the specific nutrients that appear to reduce the risk of lung cancer, although the development of nutritional databases has improved the accuracy of these types of studies. Among such studies, a pooled analysis from seven prospective cohorts in North America and Europe found no association between the intake of α-carotene, β-carotene, lutein/zeaxanthin, lycopene, and lung cancer risk (Männistö et al., 2004). A significantly decreased risk was observed for intake of β-cryptoxanthin and citrus fruits that contain high concentrations of it (Smith-Warner et al., 2003). In the CARET trial, the mean levels of almost all micronutrients measured, including zeaxanthin, β-cryptoxanthin, α-carotene, α-tocopherol, retinol, and retinyl palmitate, were lower in prerandomized serum samples from lung cancer cases than in controls (Goodman et al., 2003). Smokers tend to have lower blood levels of many micronutrients and tend to eat fewer fruits and vegetables. However, the correlation between nutrient intake and nutrient levels in blood or tissue is only modest. Cooking method, bioavailability, and laboratory error contribute to the variation in biological measurements, whereas food frequency data may not reflect recent intake of foods (Mayne, 2003). Improved research methods are necessary to verify and validate the correlation between food intake data and blood micronutrient levels.

The U.S. Preventive Services Task Force (USPSTF) concluded that there was insufficient evidence to recommend for or against the use of supplemental vitamins A, C, or E; multivitamins with folic acid; or antioxidant combinations to prevent cancer in healthy individuals (USPSTF, 2003). Actually, the USPSTF recommended against the use of β-carotene alone or in combination with other micronutrients for cancer prevention. Other groups have made similar recommendations (Byers et al., 2002; Bourgeois, 2003).

A protective role of supplemental selenium is supported by numerous epidemiological studies conducted in the United States and abroad, as well as in preclinical investigations (reviewed in El-Bayoumy, 2001). To date, although the use of selenium in human clinical trials is limited, it is known that selenium-enriched yeast inhibits the development of prostate, lung, and colon cancer in one of the most noteworthy randomized placebo-controlled clinical trials in the United States, conducted by the late Larry Clark (Clark et al., 1996; Duffield-Lillico et al., 2002). Participants were subjects with a history of nonmelanoma skin cancer. The treatment group received 200 μg selenium supplements per day for 4.5 years and was followed on average for 6.2 years. In the initial trial, the subsequent incidence of nonmelanoma skin cancer was not significantly different from that in controls, but in a follow-up report, selenium yeast was associated with an increased risk of recurrence of nonmelanoma skin cancer (Duffield-Lillico et al., 2003). However, the results clearly showed a reduction in the incidence of prostate cancer and a reduction in colon and lung cancer incidence that was dependent upon baseline selenium levels. The incidence of breast cancer in this trial was too low to permit any conclusions about a possible effect of selenium.

One area of research on the effects of antioxidants against cancer of the lung and other tobacco-related cancers that has received relatively little attention is the role of GSH. This most abundant intracellular antioxidant is synthesized from cysteine and is considered to play a key role in cancer and aging (Richie, 1992). There is little known about the relationship between GSH intake from foods and GSH blood levels because methods determining GSH concentrations are based largely on plasma levels. New methods that determine GSH concentrations in erythrocytes may shed more light on this relationship (Kleinman and Richie, 1995). Alcoholics suffering from liver cirrhosis or hepatitis have depleted GSH blood levels (Fiorelli et al., 2002; Lee et al., 2004). Tumors increase GSH production and increase GST expression, which is associated with their resistance to chemotherapy. Blood GSH is highly correlated with GST activity in non–small-cell lung cancer and squamous cell carcinoma of the head and neck (Ferruzi et al., 2003).

There are many nonnutritive components in plant foods that inhibit tumor formation in laboratory animals exposed to carcinogens. These include phenols, terpenes, and indoles, among others (Dragsted et al., 1997). For example, a compound that reduces cigarette smoke– or B[*a*]P-induced DNA damage is curcumin, an antioxidant in the Indian spice turmeric (Mukundan et al., 1993; Polasa et al., 2004). Considerable progress has been made in the study of glucosinolates in cruciferous vegetables, including isothiocyanates (ITCs), which inhibit the initiation and promotion of lung tumorigenesis in bioassays with tobacco-specific nitrosamines (Chung, 2001). In Shanghai, China, men who had a high intake of ITCs showed a reduced risk of lung cancer (London et al., 2000). The study examined the correlation between intake frequency of ITC-containing foods and urinary ITC levels; other studies in China examined the same correlation, but with varied genotypes (Seow et al., 1998; Fowke et al., 2003). ITCs induce phase II enzymes; high intake and urinary ITC correlation was strongest for homozygous-null glutathione *S*-transferase GSTT1 and for GSTP1-A/A (Seow et al., 1998).

The role of macronutrients in the development and inhibition of lung cancer still needs further exploration. For many years scientific data pointed to a role of high-fat diet in lung cancer risk, although new evidence from prospective studies has challenged this perspective. Nationally and internationally, there are high correlations between per capita fat intake and lung cancer mortality (Wynder et al., 1987, 1992; Taioli et al., 1991), and increased risks associated with red meat consumption have been reported in case-control studies (Alavanja et al., 2001).

A pooled analysis of eight prospective studies conducted in the United States, Canada, Finland, and the Netherlands found no association between high intake of dietary fat and lung cancer risk (Smith-Warner et al., 2002). The risk was unrelated to both the amount of fat intake and the specific types of fats. The findings from cohort studies that were not included in the pooled data were inconclusive or mixed (Veierod et al., 1997; Breslow et al., 2000). In a separate pooled analysis of five prospective studies that compared lung cancer death rates in vegetarians and nonvegetarians, the smoking-adjusted rate ratio was 0.84 (0.59–1.18; Key et al., 1999). However, in four of the five studies, the lung cancer death rate in vegetarians was lower by ≥30%. The interpretation of these results begs the question whether a pooled analysis is the most appropriate measure for analyzing these data and whether, in some respect, there was bias in the study that found few differences in death rates between groups.

The data from epidemiologic and laboratory animal studies are too conflicting to enable recommendations on lowering fat intake to reduce lung cancer risk. It has been suggested that the range of dietary fat intake in a typical Western diet is too high to measure the effects of low fat intake and cancer risk (Wynder et al., 1993). Although Asian countries such as China and Japan are increasingly adopting Western lifestyles, there are still large differences in nutrient intake. The recent INTERMAP study compared 24-hour dietary recall and urine samples from 17 population samples of middle-aged adults in China, Japan, the United Kingdom, and the United States (Zhou et al., 2003). The mean intake of total fat and saturated fat, assessed as a percentage of calories, was substantially lower in Japan and China (Table 2). Both men and women in the United Kingdom and the United States derive about one third of their calories from fat. This is similar to figures from the eight cohort studies (31.9–43.0%) (Smith-Warner et al., 2002). In Japan and China, the percentage of caloric intake from fat is between 20 and 26%. Future studies are necessary to determine the basis for the discrepancies between the high international correlations of fat intake and lung cancer and the lack of an overall association in Western cohort studies.

The international data on dietary intake suggest that high intake of fish might prevent lung cancer (Table 2), although a nonsignificant inverse correlation was reported between omega-3 fatty acid intake and international lung cancer mortality (Hursting et al., 1990). The findings from case-control studies examining intake of fish or fish oil in relation to lung cancer risk have been suggestive but mixed (Kvale et al., 1983; Veierod et al., 1997; Darby et al., 2001; Ozasa et al., 2001; Marchand et al., 2002; Takezaki et al., 2003).

The results from certain laboratory animal studies support epidemiologic observations indicating that dietary fats play a role in lung cancer. A high-fat diet given to animals exposed to tobacco carcinogens increased lung tumor size and decreased latency of tumor appearance (Hoffmann et al., 1993). Specific mechanisms that may account for the enhancing effect of a high-fat diet could, in part, involve increased cyclooxygenase-2 (COX-2) expression (El-Bayoumy et al., 1999). This appears to be consistent with some epidemiologic observations of reduced lung cancer incidence in users of nonsteroidal anti-inflammatory drugs (Harris et al., 2002, 2005; Muscat et al., 2004). In the A/J mouse model, a Western-style diet consisting of mixed lipids (20% of calories from fat) increased cellular proliferation and tumor size (Patolla et al., 2004). Fish oil fatty acids inhibited human lung carcinoma growth in an animal bioassay (de Bravo et al., 1991).

Cancer of the Head and Neck, Bladder, Pancreas, and Kidney

A major risk factor for these cancers is cigarette smoking. Smokeless tobacco use, a risk factor for head and neck cancer, has declined in U.S. youths (Tomar, 2003), yet 22% of male youths continued to use smokeless tobacco products in 2001, which remains a concern. In a large population-based case-control study, smokeless tobacco and cigar smoking increased the risk of pancreatic cancer (Augustine et al., 1988; Muscat et al., 1992, 1995, 1997; Alguacil and Silverman, 2004).

Numerous studies have established that plant-based nutrients protect against the development of head and neck cancers (Chainani-Wu, 2002). A high intake of green, yellow, and cruciferous vegetables reduces the risk, as does total fruit and citrus fruit intake. Specific nutrients that are

TABLE 2 Daily Intake of Fat in Four Countries: 1997–1999

	Japan		Peoples Republic of China		United Kingdom		United States	
	Mean	SD	Mean	SD	Mean	SD	Mean	SD
Energy (kcal/day)								
Men	2278	428	2347	532	2470	635	2609	694
Women	1798	325	1733	443	1827	419	1876	474
Total fat (%kcal)								
Men	23.7	4.8	20.5	6.2	33.0	6.5	33.3	6.7
Women	26.1	4.9	19.5	6.0	32.5	6.5	32.6	7.1
SFA (%kcal)								
Men	6.1	1.6	5.2	2.0	12.0	3.4	10.8	2.8
Women	7.1	1.8	4.8	2.1	12.2	3.3	10.6	2.9
MFA (%kcal)								
Men	8.6	2.1	8.3	2.8	11.2	2.5	12.4	2.8
Women	6.6	1.4	5.7	2.2	6.1	1.8	6.9	2.2
PFA								
Men	6.2	1.5	5.9	2.2	6.4	1.9	7.0	2.2
Women	5.2	1.3	5.2	2.1	5.4	1.7	6.3	2.0
Omega-3 PFA (%kcal)								
Men	1.3	0.4	0.6	0.4	0.7	0.3	0.7	0.3
Women	1.4	0.4	0.5	0.4	0.7	0.2	0.8	0.3

Source: Modified from Zhou et al., 2003.

thought to be protective include carotene, vitamin C, and vitamin E.

There are relatively few epidemiologic and experimental data on the relationship of fat intake to cancer of the head and neck, bladder, and kidney (Hoffmann and El-Bayoumy, 1999). In particular, there is a paucity of prospective cohort data on these associations. The results of published studies are summarized in Table 3.

TABLE 3 Summary of Findings on Meat and Fish Intake and Risk of Oral, Bladder, Kidney, and Pancreas Cancers

Tumor site	Exposure	Risk	Citation
Pancreas	High red meat intake	↑↔	Howe and Burch, 1996 Michaud et al., 2003 Stolzenberg-Solomon et al., 2002
Bladder	High fat intake High red meat intake Fish	↑ ↔ ?	Steinmaus et al., 2000
Oral/pharynx	High fat/meat intake Unsalted fish Salted/smoked fish	↑ ↓↔ ↑	Levi et al., 1998 De Stefani et al., 1999 Winn et al., 1984 Franceshi et al., 1999 Rajkumar et al., 2003 Rogers et al., 1995 Zheng et al., 1992
Kidney	High fat/meat intake Heterocyclic amines Fish	↑? ↔ ?	Chow et al., 1994 Augustsson et al., 1999

?, limited data; ↑, increased risk; ↓, decreased risk; ↔, null findings.

Breast Cancer

Hormonal and reproductive risk factors for breast cancer include early age at menarche, parity, late age at first birth, age at menopause, and obesity (Muti, 2005). A family history of breast cancer and specifically germline BRCA1- and BRCA2-mutations are also established risk factors. There is growing evidence that physical inactivity increases the risk (Sasco, 2001). A pooled analysis of prospective cohort studies that comprised data on about 83,000 women found that spontaneous and induced abortions were unrelated to subsequent risk of breast cancer (Beral et al., 2004). In a Finnish cohort, breast cancer risk increased in premenopausal women who had used antibiotics to treat urinary tract infections (Knekt et al., 2000). Similarly, an American cohort found a significant dose–response trend with the use of all antibiotic classes and breast cancer mortality (Velicer et al., 2004). These findings are significant in that they establish, for the most part, that breast cancer risk factors cannot be modified or would require cultural changes that are incompatible with modern lifestyles (e.g., giving birth at a younger age). Whether the association with antibiotic use is a consequence of poor immunity or specific clinical indications requires further study.

In a meta-analysis of 53 studies of smoking and breast cancer, smoking was highly correlated with alcohol consumption (Hamajima et al., 2002). When restricted to the 22,255 nondrinking cases and 40,832 nondrinking controls, the relative breast cancer risk for ever smokers versus never smokers was 1.03 (95% CI 0.98–1.07). In current smokers, the relative risk (RR) was 0.99 (95% CI 0.92–1.05). A prospective cohort study, not included in the pooled analyses, also found that cigarette smoking did not increase the risk (Vessey et al., 2003). By contrast, the RR for current smokers in the California Teachers' Study of >116,544 members was 1.32 (95% CI 1.1–1.57; Reynolds et al., 2004). The RR for estrogen receptor–positive women who smoked ≥20 years was 1.37 (95% CI 1.07–1.74) in the Nurses' Health Study II (Al-Delaimy et al., 2004). Lifelong smoking was not a risk factor for estrogen receptor–negative women. A comprehensive review noted that in many studies, breast cancer risk was decreased in smokers, perhaps because of an antiestrogenic effect (Terry and Rohan, 2002). A form of endocrine therapy that has gained acceptance is the use of agents that specifically suppress estrogen biosynthesis by inhibiting the aromatization of androgens to estrogens (Brodie, 1991). Because smoking has a profound effect on estrogen-related processes, Kadohama et al. (1993) examined the ability of tobacco constituents to suppress estrogen production in two human breast cancer cell lines (MDA-MB-231, SK-BR-3). They observed that acyl derivatives of nornicotine and anabasine block estrogen formation and suggest that this observation may explain the decreased estrogen levels in women who smoke. An increased risk was found in some studies for early age at smoking onset or duration of smoking. The increased risk with early age at smoking onset was also shown in a separate meta-analysis (RR = 1.14, CI = 1.06–1.23; Khuder et al., 2001). Cigarette smoking might increase the risk only in women who are highly susceptible to tobacco carcinogens. Smoking increases the risk in women with a familial disposition to breast and ovarian cancer (Couch et al., 2001). Some studies indicate an increased risk for women with certain genetic polymorphisms, although the findings are often limited to subgroups and remain inconsistent between study populations (Garcia-Closas et al., 1999; Zheng et al., 1999; van der Hel et al., 2003a, b).

Several tobacco smoke carcinogens known to induce mammary cancer in laboratory animals (Amin and El-Bayoumy, 2005) should be regarded as potential human risk factors and need to be evaluated more closely. Literature data document that nicotine and its metabolite, cotinine, are present in the breast fluid of nonlactating women who smoke (Petrakis et al., 1978); clearly, tobacco smoke constituents are reaching the human breast (Hecht, 2002). The characteristically high lipid content of the mammary gland makes this organ a reservoir for lipid-soluble, toxic, and carcinogenic agents (Beer and Billingham, 1978; Martin et al., 1996). Mutagenic activity has been detected in nipple aspirates and breast cyst fluid (reviewed in Amin and El-Bayoumy, 2005), and several studies describe the detection of DNA adducts in human mammary tissues. These adducts still remain largely unknown, so future studies should focus on determining their structure. In a case-control study conducted in New York, PAH–DNA adduct levels were higher in blood samples from women with breast cancer than from controls (Gammon et al., 2002). Environmental PAHs from various sources may increase DNA adduct formation in blood. These sources include cigarette smoke, urban and indoor air pollution, and diet. The case-control study by Gammon et al. (2002) showed no dose–response relationship between amount smoked and adduct levels; it suggests that breast tissues, rather than blood, are the appropriate biological matrix to analyze for PAH–DNA adducts and to determine their role in the development of breast cancer (Perera and Rundle, 2003).

The role of diet in the development of breast cancer remains controversial and not well understood (Blackburn et al., 2003). As with lung cancer, ecological studies and case-control studies have shown that high fat intake is associated with breast cancer mortality rates and breast cancer risk, respectively. In pooled prospective cohort studies, diets high in fat, specific types of fat, red meat, and dairy foods were not associated with breast cancer risk (Hunter et al., 1996; Smith-Warner et al., 2001a, b; Missmer et al., 2002). The combined RR for the upper quartile of fat intake (verses lowest quartile) in a separate meta-analysis of cohort and case-control studies was 1.14 (95% CI 1.03–1.25) (Boyd et al., 2003). The risk estimates were similar, though not statistically significant, when the analysis was restricted to case-control or cohort studies only. Because most of these studies were conducted in Western countries, it is possible that the variation in dietary fat intake was too minimal to produce large effects. Another methodological concern is the imprecision of food frequency questionnaires that do not accurately reflect dietary intake (Bingham et al., 2003). There might be critical time periods, such as the reproductive years, when dietary or caloric intake could affect breast cancer risk. There are few data that directly address this issue, but some findings provide intriguing results. For example, a high intake of animal fat increased the risk of subsequent breast cancer in premenopausal women participating in the Nurses' Health Study (Cho et al., 2003). A low caloric intake 20 years before diagnosis was associated with a reduction in breast cancer risk (Caygill et al., 1998). In Swedish women younger than 40 years hospitalized for anorexia nervosa, the incidence of breast cancer was 53% lower than in the general Swedish female population (Michels and Ekbom, 2004). These studies are consistent with laboratory animal studies in which energy restriction reduced spontaneous mammary cancers in mice irrespective of nutrient intake (Dirx et al., 2003; Tannenbaum, 1944).

The effect of fat, at least in the case-control studies of breast cancer, is independent of the dietary source, suggesting that fat and caloric intake might both be factors in breast cancer risk (Macrae, 1993). The possibility exists that early severe caloric restriction prevents breast cancer; however, this is clearly not a lifestyle option. Again, further investigation could show that modest energy restriction may reduce breast cancer risk. Other specific dietary nutrients that may protect against breast cancer include marine fatty acids, but the findings have been conflicting (Terry et al., 2003). Although a diet high in fruits and vegetables is associated with lower risk in some studies, pooled prospective cohort studies found no association with total fruit and vegetable intake (Smith-Warner et al., 2001a, b; Hung et al., 2004). Efforts are under way to identify specific dietary micronutrients that confer a protective effect (Kim, 2002). High serum β-carotene and lycopene levels reportedly have protective effects (Sato et al., 2002), whereas a prospective study using dietary intake data found protective effects only with preformed vitamin A levels in smokers (Cho et al., 2003).

Several agents have been characterized as useful in chemoprevention in preclinical investigations. Efforts continue to develop even more effective agents for cancer prevention (Sporn, 1976; Wattenberg, 1978, 1985; El-Bayoumy, 1994; Kelloff et al., 1994).

Prostate Cancer

In the United States, prostate cancer represents a major clinical and public health challenge. The American Cancer Society (ACS) estimates that in 2005, about 232,090 men will be diagnosed with prostate cancer and an estimated 30,350 will die from it (ACS, 2005). The rates are substantially higher in older persons, African-Americans, and in persons with a family history (Schaid, 2004). The identification of prostate cancer susceptibility genes has become an important focus of research, but the causes of prostate cancer remain poorly understood.

Most prospective cohort studies of smoking and prostate cancer incidence, as well as case-control studies, found no association (Lumey, 1996; Hickey et al., 2001). However, positive associations have been observed in studies of smoking and prostate cancer mortality (Giovannucci et al., 1999), suggesting that smoking affects the aggressiveness of the tumor. In a tumor registry study, current smoking was associated with metastatic spread of prostate cancer (RR = 1.53, $p < 0.01$) (Kobrinsky et al., 2003).

Many investigations have shown that dietary and nutritional factors are associated with the risk of prostate cancer. In particular, dietary antioxidants such as vitamins A, C, and E, as well as minerals like selenium, are candidates for chemoprevention. Lycopene has inhibitory effects, but these appear to be limited to sporadic prostate cancer (Kristal, 2004; Wu et al., 2004b). Other carotenoids such as β-carotene appear to play a minor role in preventing prostate cancer. The protective effect of selenium in Clark's trial (Clark et al., 1996; Duffield-Lillico et al., 2002) provided the basis for further trials around the world, including the SELECT trial in the United States (Klein et al., 2000, 2003), the PRECISE trial in Europe (Rayman, 2000), and the Negative Biopsy Trial in New Zealand (Karunasinghe et al., 2004).

Colon Cancer

Cancer of the colon is one of the leading causes of death in both men and women in Western countries, including the United States, where about 104,950 new cases of colorectal cancer were diagnosed in 2005, with an expected 56,290 related deaths (ACS, 2005). The causes of colon cancer are still not well understood, although in general, most cases are thought to be due to poor diet and sedentary lifestyle (Giovannucci, 2002a, b). For example, physical inactivity is associated with increased risk, even though the mechanisms have not been well elucidated (Quadrilatero and Hoffman-Goetz, 2003).

Cigarette smoking has been increasingly implicated in the risk of colon cancer and adenomatous polyps (Table 4). Some of the most convincing and thorough evidence comes from the ACS's prospective Cancer Prevention Study II, which included 312,332 men and 469,019 women (Chao et al., 2000). With 4432 colorectal cancer deaths in the follow-up period, colorectal cancer mortality rates were highest in current smokers, intermediate in former smokers, and lowest in lifelong nonsmokers. The RR for current versus never smokers was 1.32 (95% CI 1.16–1.49) in men and 1.41 (95% CI 1.26–1.58) in women. The risk in current and former smokers increased with duration of smoking, average number of cigarettes smoked per day, and years since quitting. The authors estimated that ~12% of colorectal cancer deaths in the general U.S. population during 1997 are attributable to smoking. There is now sufficient evidence to recognize smoking as a causal factor in colon carcinoma (Giovannucci, 2001; Colditz and Yaus, 2004).

Several of the aforementioned studies visibly show that smoking cessation reduces the risk of colon cancer when compared with persons who continue to smoke. Because the effects of cigarette smoke appear to be manifested after

TABLE 4 Prospective Studies of Smoking and Colon/Colorectal Cancer

Author/year	Study	Smoking measure	Relative risk; 95% CI
Colangelo et al., 2004	Chicago Heart Association	>20 years	1.87; 1.1–3.2
Sanjoaquin et al., 2004	Oxford Vegetarian Study	Current	1.88; 1.03–3.44
Otani et al., 2003	Japan Public Health Center-based Prospective Study	Current	1.4; 1.1–1.8
Wakai et al., 2003	Japan Collaborative Cohort Study	Current	1.07; 0.72–1.59
Van der Hel et al., 2003b	Diagnostisch Onderzoek Mammacarcinoom Study	Current and Rapid Acetylation Genotype	1.56; 1.03–2.37
Terry et al., 2002	Canadian National Breast Screening Study	Current >40 years	0.93; 0.71–1.24 3.14, 1.33–7.42 (rectal)
Terry et al., 2001	Swedish Twin Registry	Current	0.4–0.7 (colon) 5.3; 1.9–15.0 (rectal)
Chao et al., 2000	Cancer Prevention Study II	Current	1.32; 1.16–1.49 (men) 1.41; 1.26–1.58 (women)
Hsing et al., 1998	Lutheran Brotherhood Insurance Society	Current GE 30 cpd	2.3, 95% CI 0.9–5.7
Knekt et al., 1998	Finnish Cohort	After 11–20 years follow-up	1.57; 1.09–2.24
Dreyer and Olsen 1998	Danish survivors of acute myocardial infarct	Not measured	1.0; 0.9–1.0 (SIR)
Nyren et al., 1996	Swedish construction workers	Current	0.98; 0.82–1.17 (colon) 1.16; 0.94–1.44 (rectum)
Engeland et al., 1996	Migrant Study-Norway	Current	1.2; 0.8–1.6 (men) 1.1; 0.8–1.4 (women)
Heineman et al., 1994	US Veterans, service from 1917–1940	Current	1.2; 1.1–1.4 colon 1.4; 1.2–1.7 rectum
Giovannucci et al., 1994a,b	Health Professionals Follow-up Study	GE 35 years	1.94; 1.13–3.35
Giovannucci et al., 1994a,b	Nurses Health Study	35–39 years and >10 cpd	1.47; 1.07–2.01
Wu et al., 1987	Leisure World Cohort	Current	1.8; 0.6–5.2 (men) 1.4; 0.7–1.0 (women)

decades of smoking, quitting smoking must now be considered a primary prevention strategy that not only reduces the risk of cancer of the lung and head and neck cancers, but also diminishes colorectal cancer risk.

Obesity and a high-fat, high-caloric diet are thought to significantly contribute to the high incidence of colon cancer in Western countries. Epidemiological observations support an important protective role for fruit and vegetable intake. Much more research is necessary to identify the imbalance of specific macronutrients and micronutrients that leads to colon cancer. High fiber intake has long been considered important in reducing risk, but it has not been born out in clinical trials. Strong evidence exists for testing folate, calcium, and vitamin D in randomized trials (Lamprecht and Lipkin, 2003). As described earlier, the randomized trial of selenium by Clark et al. (1996) and Duffield-Lillico et al. (2002) found a reduced incidence of colon cancer, as well as other cancers, after years of follow-up; the protective effect was dependent on the basal levels of selenium prior to the intervention.

Cervical Cancer

Because cigarette smoking is highly correlated with sexual history, the contribution of smoking has been uncertain. In a pooled analysis of 10 case-control studies that was limited to human papilloma virus (HPV)–positive women and positive controls, cigarette smoking was significantly associated with cervical cancer risk (odds ratio [OR] 2.17; 95% CI 1.46–3.22) (Plummer et al., 2003). HPV DNA is found in >90% of cervical tumor specimens, and HPV infection is considered a necessary condition for the development of cervical cancer (Zur Hausen, 1974). However, Vineis et al. (2004) concluded that HPV infection alone cannot explain the association between cervical cancer and smoking.

Cervical tissue is capable of metabolizing TSNA to intermediate forms that damage DNA (Prokopczyk et al., 2001). Cervical specimens from smokers contain detectable levels of tobacco-specific *N*-nitrosamines (Prokopczyk et al., 1997). Evidence from studies conducted in our laboratory, together with evaluating smoking-associated DNA adduct formation, provides additional support for epidemiological observations related to tobacco smoking and cancer of the uterine cervix. Melikian et al. (1999a) detected metabolites derived from B[*a*]P in cervical mucus and a higher level of B[*a*]P–DNA adducts in cervical tissues of smokers than in nonsmokers. These results add significantly to the evidence that smoking is an important cofactor in the etiology of this tumor.

For many decades, the relationship between micronutrients and cervical dysplasia/cancer has been examined in several case-control studies. Protective effects were found for high intake of β-carotene and vitamins C and E (Wassertheil-Smoller et al., 1981; La Vecchia et al., 1984; Slattery et al., 1990; Herrero et al., 1991; Buckley et al., 1992), folate (Goodman et al., 2001), vitamin A, retinol, lycopene (Kanetsky et al., 1998; Shannon et al., 2002), and high serum vitamin C (VanEenwyk et al., 1991), as well as retinol (Nagata et al., 1999; Yeo et al., 2000) and β-carotene (Potischman et al., 1991). However, other studies do not support the effects of these micronutrients (Ziegler et al., 1990).

Leukemia

Cigarette smoking was associated, in some studies, with a modest increase in risk for both forms of leukemia (Brownson et al., 1993), but large-scale population-based studies found no association of leukemia with smoking (Stagnaro et al., 2001). There has been a substantial interest in maternal tobacco smoking during pregnancy and childhood leukemia, but the weight of the evidence shows no association (Boffetta et al., 2000). Parental alcohol consumption and cured meat may be relevant to factors in infant leukemia (Shu, 1997).

The leukemias are a heterogeneous group of acute and chronic forms. Except for benzene, a constituent of cigarette smoke and occupational agent, and high-dose radiation, the environmental causes of adult leukemia remain largely unknown (Zeeb and Blettner, 1998).

Smokers have much higher levels of benzene in their blood than nonsmokers. According to Korte et al. (2000), linear extrapolation from the known effects of high doses of benzene suggests that this agent is responsible for about one third of smoking-induced acute myeloid leukemia. On the basis of literature data, Vineis et al. (2004) concluded that sufficient evidence exists that smoking causes myeloid leukemia, but that there is no association between smoking and the risk of lymphatic leukemia.

There are few data on diet and adult leukemia. There is an international correlation between caloric intake and incidence rates (Hursting et al., 1993) and consistent evidence for an association with obesity (Pan et al., 2004; Samanic et al., 2004). High vegetable intake was protective in a case-control study (Kwiatkowski, 1993) and in a prospective cohort study (Ross et al., 2002). A protective effect was also found with fresh fish consumption (Fritschi et al., 2004).

SUMMARY

The first conclusive studies that linked cigarette smoking to lung cancer (Wynder and Graham, 1950, 1985; Doll and Hill, 1950) were published more than a half a century ago. In addition to target organs for which there is already an established association between cancer and exposure to tobacco carcinogens, epidemiologic studies are now providing new information linking tobacco smoking with breast and colon cancer; some data suggest that tobacco smoking also enhances metastasis of the prostate. Future laboratory studies should focus specifically on the role of nutrition in tobacco-related breast, colon, and prostate cancer. This is important not only for understanding the mechanisms of tobacco carcinogenesis, but also for developing appropriate nutritional intervention strategies for cancer prevention.

Efforts toward clinical chemoprevention of lung cancer remain highly disappointing. Therefore, studies are urgently necessary that focus on both elucidating tobacco carcinogenesis mechanisms and developing appropriate animal model systems that mimic human exposure to the complex mixture of tobacco smoke. Toward this end, Fiala et al. (2005) reported the development of such a model. Male Hartley guinea pigs treated with cigarette smoke by inhalation twice a day for 28 days developed preneoplastic lung lesions, including bronchial hyperplasia, dysplasia, and squamous metaplasia analogous contrast. In contrast, no lung lesions were found in guinea pigs (sham exposed) submitted to identical procedures, but without cigarettes.

The cancer burden and the prevalence of different types of cancer have differed substantially in developed and developing countries, but the reduction in smoking prevalence continues to be the most important prevention measure worldwide. Quitting the tobacco habit is the best strategy for prevention of all tobacco-related cancers. In addition to smoking, factors such as infections, alcohol consumption, exposure to sunlight, occupational, and environmental pollutants, as well as physical inactivity and obesity, are important contributors to cancer (Peto, 2001). The contribution of diet to cancer risk is important, but specific dietary recommendations to avoid cancer are speculative (Peto, 2001). Because it is inevitable that people will continue smoking, the design of the least toxic and carcinogenic cigarettes (Hoffmann et al., 2001), combined with tailored dietary interventions, could have a significant impact on cancer rates. Future studies need to more clearly define the mechanisms of cigarette-induced cancers, the modification of these effects by specific dietary constituents, and the additional impact of individual genotypes. The "omics" approach will assist in the discovery of molecular markers critical in the development of tobacco-related cancers (El-Bayoumy and Sinhu, 2005). Studies combining gene array analyses with proteomic profiling will constitute the most meaningful strategy for elucidating the mechanisms of tobacco carcinogenesis. This will allow for intervention with chemopreventive agents in conjunction with nutritional manipulation and prevent the epidemic of deaths due to tobacco use. Similarly, such efforts will be significant in designing mechanism-based, randomized dietary/chemoprevention trials to combat the cancer epidemic attributable to tobacco smoking.

Acknowledgments

Our studies reported here are supported by the National Cancer Institute, Grant Nos. PO1 CA 70972 and RO1 CA 100924. The authors thank Mrs. Ilse Hoffmann for editing this chapter and Ms. Kathy Cannon and Ms. Suanne Wilson for word processing skills.

References

Alavanja, M.C., Field, R.W., Sinha, R., Brus, C.P., Shavers, V.L., Fisher, E.L., Curtain, J., and Lynch, C.F. 2001. Lung cancer risk and red meat consumption among Iowa women. *Lung Cancer* **34**: 37–46.

Al-Delaimy, W.K., Cho, E., Chen, W.Y., Colditz, G., and Willet, W.C. 2004. A prospective study of smoking and risk of breast cancer in young adult women. *Cancer Epidemiol Biomarkers Prev* **13**: 398–404.

Alguacil, J., and Silverman, D.T. 2004. Smokeless and other noncigarette tobacco use and pancreatic cancer: a case–control study based on direct interviews. *Cancer Epidemiol Biomarkers Prev* **13**: 55–58.

American Cancer Society. 2005. "Cancer Facts and Figures." American Cancer Society, Atlanta, GA.

Amin, S., and El-Bayoumy, K. 2005. Tumorigenicity of polycyclic aromatic hydrocarbons. *In* "The Carcinogenic Effects of Polycyclic Aromatic Hydrocarbons" (A. Luch, Ed.). World Scientific Publishing Co., London.

Amos, C.I., Xu, W., and Spitz, M.R. 1999. Is there a genetic basis for lung cancer susceptibility? *Recent Results Cancer Res* **151**: 3–12.

Augustine, A., Hebert, J.R., Kabat, G.C., Wynder, E.L. 1988. *Cancer Res* **48**: 4405–4408.

Augustsson, K., Skog, K., Jagerstad, M., Dickman, P.W., and Steineck, G. 1999. Dietary heterocyclic amines and cancer of the colon, rectum, bladder, and kidney: a population-based study. *Lancet* **353**: 703–707.

Beer, A.E., and Billingham, R.E. 1978. Adipose tissue, a neglected factor in aetiology of breast cancer? *Lancet* **2**: 296.

Bendich, A. 2004. From 1989 to 2001: what have we learned about the "biological actions of beta-carotene"? *J Nutr* **134**: 225S–230S.

Beral, V., Bull, D., Doll, R., Peto, R., and Reeves, G.; the Collaborative Group on Hormonal Factors in Breast Cancer. 2004. Breast cancer and abortion: collaborative reanalysis of data from 53 epidemiological studies, including 83,000 women with breast cancer from 16 countries. *Lancet* **363**: 1007–1016.

Bingham, S.A., Luben, R., Welch, A., Wareham, N., Khaw, K.T., and Day, N. 2003. Are imprecise methods obscuring a relation between fat and breast cancer? *Lancet* **362**: 212–214.

Blackburn, G.L., Copeland, T., Khaodhiar, L., and Buckley, R.B. 2003. Diet and breast cancer. *J Womens Health (Larchmt)* **12**: 183–192.

Block, G., Dietrich, M., Norkus, E.P., Morrow, J.D., Hudes, M., Caan, B., and Packer, L. 2002. Factors associated with oxidative stress in human populations. *Am J Epidemiol* **156**: 274–285.

Boffetta, P., Tredaniel, J., and Greco, A. 2000. Risk of childhood cancer and adult lung cancer after childhood exposure to passive smoke: a meta-analysis. *Environ Health Perspect* **108**: 73–82.

Bourgeois, C.F. 2003. Antioxidant vitamins and health. *In* "Cardiovascular Disease, Cancer, Cataracts, and Aging," p. 240. HNB Publishing, New York.

Boyd, N.F., Stone, J., Vogt, K.N., Connelly, B.S., Martin, L.J., and Minkin, S. 2003. Dietary fat and breast cancer risk revisited: a meta-analysis of the published literature. *Br J Cancer* **89**: 1672–1685.

Breslow, R.A., Graubard, B.I., Sinha, R., and Subar, A.F. 2000. Diet and lung cancer mortality: a 1987 National Health Interview Survey cohort study. *Cancer Causes Control* **11**: 419–431.

Brodie, A. 1991. Aromatase and its inhibitors—an overview. *J Steroid Biochem Mol Biol* **40**: 255–261.

Brooks, D.R., Austin, J.H., Heelan, R.T., Ginsberg, M.S., Shin, V., Olson, S.H., Muscat, J.E., and Stellman, S.D. 2005. Influence of type of cigarette on peripheral versus central lung cancer. *Cancer Epidemiol Biomarkers Prev* **14**: 576–581.

Brownson, R.C., Novotny, T.E., and Perry, M.C. 1993. Cigarette smoking and adult leukemia. A meta-analysis. *Arch Intern Med* **22**: 469–475.

Bruemmer, B., White, E., Vaughan, T.L., and Cheney, C.L. 1996. Nutrient intake in relation to bladder cancer among middle-aged men and women. *Am J Epidemiol* **144**: 485–495.

Buckley, D.I., McPherson, R.S., North, C.Q., and Becker, T.M. 1992. Dietary micronutrients and cervical dysplasia in southwestern American Indian women. *Nutr Cancer* **17**: 179–185.

Byers, T., Nestle, M., McTiernan, A., Doyle, C., Currie-Williams, A., Gansler, T., Thun, M., and the American Cancer Society. 2001 Nutrition and Physical Activity Guidelines Advisory Committee. 2002. American Cancer Society guidelines on nutrition and physical activity for cancer prevention: reducing the risk of cancer with healthy food choices and physical activity. *CA Cancer J Clin* **52**: 92–119.

Caygill, C.P., Charlett, A., and Hill, M.J. 1998. Relationship between the intake of high-fibre foods and energy and the risk of cancer of the large bowel and breast. *Eur J Cancer Prev* **7**: S11–S17.

Chainani-Wu, N. 2002. Diet and oral, pharyngeal, and esophageal cancer. *Nutr Cancer* **44**: 104–126.

Chao, A., Thun, M.J., Jacobs, E.J., Henley, S.J., Rodriguez, C., and Calle, E.E. 2000. Cigarette smoking and colorectal cancer mortality in the cancer prevention study II. *J Natl Cancer Inst* **92**: 1888–1896.

Cho, E., Spiegelman, D., Hunter, D.J., Chen, W.Y., Stampfer, M.J., Colditz, G.A., and Willett, W.C. 2003. Premenopausal fat intake and risk of breast cancer. *J Natl Cancer Inst* **95**: 1079–1085.

Cho, E., Spiegelman, D., Hunter, D.J., Chen, W.Y., Zhang, S.M., Colditz, G.A., and Willett, W.C. 2003. Premenopausal intakes of vitamins A, C, and E, folate, and carotenoids, and risk of breast cancer. *Cancer Epidemiol Biomarkers Prev* **12**: 713–720.

Chow, W.H., Gridley, G., McLaughlin, J.K., Mandel, J.S., Wacholder, S., Blot, W.J., Niwa, S., and Fraumeni, J.F., Jr. 1994. Protein intake and risk of renal cell cancer. *J Natl Cancer Inst* **86**: 1131–1139.

Chung, F.L. 2001. Chemoprevention of lung cancer by isothiocyanates and their conjugates in A/J mouse. *Exp Lung Res* **27**: 319–330.

Clark, L.C., Combs, G.F.J., Turnbull, B.W., Slate, E.H., Chalker, D.K., Chow, J., Davis, L.S., Glover, R.A., Graham, G.F., Gross, E.G., Krongrad, A., Lesher, J.L., Jr., Park, H.K., Sanders, B.B., Jr., Smith, C.L, and Taylor, J.R. 1996. Effects of selenium supplementation for cancer prevention in patients with carcinoma of the skin. A randomized controlled trial. Nutritional Prevention of Cancer Study Group. *JAMA* **276**: 1957–1963.

Cogliano, V., Straif, K., Baan, R., Grosse, Y., Secretan, B., and El Ghissassi, F. 2004. Smokeless tobacco and tobacco-related nitrosamines. *Lancet Oncol* **5**(12): 708.

Colangelo, L.A., Gapstur, S.M., Gann, P.H., and Dyer, A.R. 2004. Cigarette smoking and colorectal carcinoma mortality in a cohort with long-term follow-up. *Cancer* **100**: 288–293.

Colditz, G.A., and Yaus, K.P. 2004. Smoking causes colon carcinoma. *Cancer* **100**: 223–224.

Couch, F.J., Cerhan, J.R., Vierkant, R.A., Grabrick, D.M., Therneau, T.M., Pankratz, V.S., Hartmann, L.C., Olson, J.E., Vachon, C.M., and Sellers, T.A. 2001. Cigarette smoking increases risk for breast cancer in high-risk breast cancer families. *Cancer Epidemiol Biomarkers Prev* **10**: 327–332.

Darby, S., Whitley, E., Doll, R., Key, T., and Silcocks, P. 2001. Diet, smoking and lung cancer: a case–control study of 1000 cases and 1500 controls in South-West England. *Br J Cancer* **84**: 728–735.

Davis, C.D., and Milner, J. 2004. Frontiers in nutrigenomics, proteomics, metabolomics and cancer prevention. *Mutat Res* **551**(1–2): 51–64.

de Bravo, M.G., de Antueno, R.J., Toledo, J., De Tomas, M.E., Mercuri, O.F., and Quintans, C. 1991. Effects of an eicosapentaenoic and docosahexaenoic acid concentrate on a human lung carcinoma grown in nude mice. *Lipids* **26**: 866–870.

Desai, K.V., Kavanaugh, C.J., Calvo, and Green, J.E. 2002. Chipping away at breast cancer: insights from microarray studies of human and mouse mammary cancer. *Endocr Relat Cancer* **9**: 207–220.

De Stefani, E., Deneo-Pellegrini, H., Mendilaharsu, M., and Ronco, A. 1999. Diet and risk of cancer of the upper aerodigestive tract; I. Foods. *Oral Oncol* **35**: 17–21.

Dirx, M.J., Zeegers, M.P., Dagnelie, P.C., van den Bogaard, T., and van den Brandt, P.A. 2003. Energy restriction and the risk of spontaneous mammary tumors in mice: a meta-analysis. *Int J Cancer* **106**: 766–770.

Doll, R., and Hill, A.B. 1950. Smoking and carcinoma of the lung. Preliminary report. *Br Med J* **ii**: 739–748.

Doll, R., and Peto, R. 1981. The causes of cancer: quantitative estimates of avoidable risks of cancer in the United States today. *J Natl Cancer Inst* **66**: 1191–1308.

Dragsted, L.O., Strube, M., and Leth, T. 1997. Dietary levels of plant phenols and other non-nutritive components: could they prevent cancer? *Eur J Cancer Prev* **6**: 522–528.

Dreyer, L., and Olsen, J.H. 1998. Cancer risk of patients discharged with acute myocardial infarct. *Epidemiology* **9**: 178–183.

Duffield-Lillico, A.J., Reid, M.E., Turnbull, B.W., Combs, G.F., Jr., Slate, E.H., Fischbach, L.A., Marshall, J.R., and Clark, L.C. 2002. Baseline characteristics and the effect of selenium supplementation on cancer incidence in a randomized clinical trial: a summary report of the Nutritional Prevention of Cancer Trial. *Cancer Epidemiol Biomarkers Prev* **11**: 630–639.

Duffield-Lillico, A.J., Slate, E.H., Reid, M.E., Turnbull, B.W., Wilkins, P.A., Combs, G.F., Jr., Park, H.K., Gross, E.G., Graham, G.F., Stratton, M.S., Marshall, J.R., Clark, L.C., and Nutritional Prevention of Cancer Study Group. 2003. Selenium supplementation and secondary prevention of nonmelanoma skin cancer in a randomized trial. *J Natl Cancer Inst* **95**: 1477–1481.

El-Bayoumy, K. 1994. Evaluation of chemopreventive agents against breast cancer and proposed strategies for future clinical intervention trials. *Carcinogenesis* **15**: 2395–2420.

El-Bayoumy, K. 2001. The protective role of selenium on genetic damage and on cancer. *Mutat Res* **475**: 123–139.

El-Bayoumy, K., and Hoffmann, D. 1999. Nutrition and tobacco-related cancer. *In* "Nutritional Oncology" (D. Heber and G. Blackburn, Eds.), pp. 299–324. Academic Press, San Diego, CA.

El-Bayoumy, K., Iatropoulos, M., Amin, S., Hoffmann, D., and Wynder, E.L. 1999. Increased expression of cyclooxygenase-2 in rat lung tumors induced by the tobacco-specific nitrosamine 4-(methylnitrosamino)-4-(3-pyridyl)-1-butanone: the impact of a high-fat diet. *Cancer Res* **59**: 1400–1403.

El-Bayoumy, K., Richie, J.P., Jr., Boyiri, T., Komninou, D., Prokopczyk, B., Trushin, N., Kleinman, W., Cox, J., Pittman, B., and Colosimo, S. 2002. Influence of selenium-enriched yeast supplementation on biomarkers of oxidative damage and hormone status in healthy adult males: a clinical pilot study. *Cancer Epidemiol Biomarkers Prev* **11**: 1459–1465.

El-Bayoumy, K., and Sinha, R. 2005. Molecular chemoprevention by selenium: a genomic approach. *Mutat Res* **591**: 224–236.

Engeland, A., Andersen, A., Haldorsen, T., and Tretli, S. 1996. Smoking habits and risk of cancers other than lung cancer: 28 years' follow-up of 26,000 Norwegian men and women. *Cancer Causes Control* **7**: 497–506.

Etzel, C.J., Amos, C.I., and Spitz, M.R. 2003. Risk for smoking-related cancer among relatives of lung cancer patients. *Cancer Res* **63**: 8531–8535.

Etzioni, R., Urban, N., Ramsey, S., McIntosh, M., Schwartz, S., Reid, B., Radich, J., Anderson, G., Hartwell, L. 2003. The case for early detection. *Nat Rev Cancer* **3**: 243–252.

Ferruzzi, E., Franceschini, R., Cazzolato, G., Geroni, C., Fowst, C., Pastorino, U., Tradati, N., Tursi, J., Dittadi, R., and Gion, M. 2003. Blood glutathione as a surrogate marker of cancer tissue glutathione S-transferase activity in non–small cell lung cancer and squamous cell carcinoma of the head and neck. *Eur J Cancer* **39**: 1019–1029.

Fiala., E.S., Sohn, O.S., Wang, C.X., Seibert, E., Tsurutani, J., Dennis, P.A., El-Bayoumy, K., Sodum, R., Desai, D., Reinhardt, J., and Aliaga, C. 2005. Induction of preneoplastic lung lesions in guinea pigs by cigarette smoke inhalation and their exacerbation by high dietary levels of vitamins C and E. *Carcinogenesis* **26**(3): 605–612.

Filomeni, G., Rotilio, G., and Ciriolo, M.R. 2002. Cell signalling and the glutathione redox system. *Biochem Pharmacol* **64**: 1057–1064.

Fiorelli, G., De Feo, T.M., Duca, L., Tavazzi, D., Nava, I., Fargion, S., and Cappellini, M.D. 2002. Red blood cell antioxidant and iron status in alcoholic and nonalcoholic cirrhosis. *Eur J Clin Invest* **32**(Suppl 1): 21–27.

Fowke, J.H., Shu, X.O., Dai, Q., Shintani, A., Conaway, C.C., Chung, F.L., Cai, Q., Gao, Y.T., and Zheng, W. 2003. Urinary isothiocyanate excretion, brassica consumption, and gene polymorphisms among women living in Shanghai, China. *Cancer Epidemiol Biomarkers Prev* **12**: 1536–1539.

Fritschi, L., Ambrosini, G.L., Kliewer, E.V., Johnson, K.C.; Canadian Cancer Registries Epidemiologic Research Group. 2004. Dietary fish intake and risk of leukaemia, multiple myeloma, and non-Hodgkin lymphoma. *Cancer Epidemiol Biomarkers Prev* **13**: 532–537.

Gammon, M.D., Santella, R.M., Neugut, A.I., Eng, S.M., Teitelbaum, S.L., Paykin, A., Levin, B., Terry, M.B., Young, T.L., Wang, L.W., Wang, Q., Britton, J.A., Wolff, M.S., Stellman, S.D., Hatch, M., Kabat, G.C., Senie, R., Garbowski, G., Maffeo, C., Montalvan, P., Berkowitz, G., Kemeny, M., Citron, M., Schnabel, F., Schuss, A., Hajdu, S., and Vinceguerra, V. 2002. Environmental toxins and breast cancer on Long Island. I. Polycyclic aromatic hydrocarbon DNA adducts. *Cancer Epidemiol Biomarkers Prev* **11**: 677–685.

Gan, J., Skipper, P.L., Gago-Dominguez, M., Arakawa, K., Ross, R.K., Yu, M.C., and Tannenbaum, S.R. 2004. Alkylaniline-hemoglobin adducts and risk of non–smoking-related bladder cancer. *J Natl Cancer Inst* **96**: 1425–1431.

Garcia-Closas, M., Kelsey, K.T., Hankinson, S.E., Spiegelman, D., Springer, K., Willett, W.C., Speizer, F.E., and Hunter, D.J. 1999. Glutathione S-transferase mu and theta polymorphisms and breast cancer susceptibility. *J Natl Cancer Inst* **91**: 1960–1964.

Giovannucci, E. 2001. An updated review of the epidemiological evidence that cigarette smoking increases risk of colorectal cancer. *Cancer Epidemiol Biomarkers Prev* **10**: 725–731.

Giovannucci, E. 2002a. Modifiable risk factors for colon cancer. *Gastroenterol Clin North Am* **31**: 925–943.

Giovannucci, E. 2002b. Epidemiologic studies of folate and colorectal neoplasia: a review. *J Nutr* **132**: 2350S–2355S.

Giovannucci, E., Colditz, G.A., Stampfer, M.J., Hunter, D., Rosner, B.A., Willett, W.C., and Speizer, F.E. 1994a. A prospective study of cigarette smoking and risk of colorectal adenoma and colorectal cancer in U.S. women. *J Natl Cancer Inst* **86**: 192–199.

Giovannucci, E., Rimm, E.B., Ascherio, A., Colditz, G.A., Spiegelman, D., Stampfer, M.J., and Willett, W.C. 1999. Smoking and risk of total and fatal prostate cancer in United States health professionals. *Cancer Epidemiol Biomarkers Prev* **8**: 277–282.

Giovannucci, E., Rimm, E.B., Stampfer, M.J., Colditz, G.A., Ascherio, A., Kearney, J., and Willett, W.C. 1994b. A prospective study of cigarette smoking and risk of colorectal adenoma and colorectal cancer in U.S. men. *J Natl Cancer Inst* **86**: 183–191.

Goode, E.L., Ulrich, C.M., and Potter, J.D. 2002. Polymorphisms in DNA repair genes and associations with cancer risk. *Cancer Epidemiol Biomarkers Prev* **11**: 1513–1530.

Goodman, G.E., Schaffer, S., Omenn, G.S., Chen, C., and King, I. 2003. The association between lung and prostate cancer risk, and serum micronutrients: results and lessons learned from beta-carotene and retinol efficacy trial. *Cancer Epidemiol Biomarkers Prev* **12**: 518–526.

Goodman, G.E., Thornquist, M.D., Balmes, J., Cullen, M.R., Meyskens, F.L., Jr., Omenn, G.S., Valanis, B., and Williams, J.H., Jr. 2004. The Beta-Carotene and Retinol Efficacy Trial: incidence of lung cancer and cardiovascular disease mortality during 6-year follow-up after stopping beta-carotene and retinol supplements. *J Natl Cancer Inst* **96**(23): 1743–1750.

Goodman, M.T., McDuffie, K., Hernandez, B., Wilkens, L.R., Bertram, C.C., Killeen, J., Le Marchand, L., Selhub, J., Murphy, S., and Donlon, T.A. 2001. Association of methylenetetrahydrofolate reductase polymorphism C677T and dietary folate with the risk of cervical dysplasia. *Cancer Epidemiol Biomarkers Prev* **10**: 1275–1280.

Hamajima, N., Hirose, K., Tajima, K., Rohan, T., Calle, E.E., Heath, C.W., Jr., Coates, R.J., Liff, J.M., Talamini, R., Chantarakul, N., Koetsawang, S., Rachawat, D., Morabia, A., Schuman, L., Stewart, W., Szklo, M., Bain, C., Schofield, F., Siskind, V., Band, P., Coldman, A.J., Gallagher, R.P., Hislop, T.G., Yang, P., Kolonel, L.M., Nomura, A.M., Hu, J., Johnson, K.C., Mao Y., De Sanjose, S., Lee, N., Marchbanks, P., Ory, H.W., Peterson, H.B., Wilson, H.G., Wingo, P.A., Ebeling, K., Kunde, D., Nishan, P., Hopper, J.L., Colditz, G., Gajalanski, V., Martin, N., Pardthaisong, T., Silpisornkosol, S., Theetranont, C., Boosiri, B., Chutivongse, S., Jimakorn, P., Virutamasen, P., Wongsrichanalai, C., Ewertz, M., Adami, H.O., Bergkvist, L., Magnusson, C., Persson, I., Chang-Claude, J., Paul, C., Skegg, D.C., Spears, G.F., Boyle, P., Evstifeeva, T., Daling, J.R., Hutchinson, W.B., Malone, K., Noonan, E.A., Stanford, J.L., Thomas, D.B., et. al.; the Collaborative Group on Hormonal Factors in Breast Cancer. 2002. Alcohol, tobacco and breast cancer—collaborative reanalysis of individual data from 53 epidemiological studies, including 58,515 women with breast cancer and 95,067 women without the disease. *Br J Cancer* **87**: 1234–1245.

Harris, R.E., Beebe-Donk, J., and Schuller, H.M. 2002. Chemoprevention of lung cancer by non-steroidal anti-inflammatory drugs among cigarette smokers. *Oncol Rep* **9**: 693–695.

Harris, R.E., Beebe-Donk, J., Doss, H. and Doss, D.B. 2005. Aspirin, ibuprofen, and other non-steroidal anti-inflammatory drugs in cancer prevention: a critical review of non-selective COX-2 blockade. *Oncol Rep* **13**: 559–583.

Hatsukami, D.K., Lemmonds, C., Zhang, Y., Murphy, S.E., Le, C., Carmella, S.G., and Hecht, S.S. 2004. Evaluation of carcinogen exposure in people who used "reduced exposure" tobacco products. *J Natl Cancer Inst* **96**(11): 844–852.

Hecht, S.S. 1999. Tobacco smoke carcinogens and lung cancer. *J Natl Cancer Inst* **91**: 1194–1210.

Hecht, S.S. 2002. Tobacco smoke carcinogens and breast cancer. *Environ Mol Mutagen* **39**: 119–126.

Hecht, S.S. 2003. Tobacco carcinogens, their biomarkers and tobacco-induced cancer (erratum appears in *Nat Rev Cancer* **4**: 84). *Nat Rev Cancer* **3**: 733–744.

Hecht, S.S., Chen, M., Yagi, H., Jerina, D.M., Carmella, S.G. 2003. r-1,t-2,3,c-4-Tetrahydroxy-1,2,3,4-tetrahydrophenanthrene in human urine: a potential biomarker for assessing polycyclic aromatic hydrocarbon metabolic activation. *Cancer Epidemiol Biomarkers Prev* **12**: 1501–1508.

Hecht, S.S., Murphy, S.E., Carmella, S.G., Zimmerman, C.L., Losey, L., Kramarczuk, I., Roe, M.R., Puumala, S.S., Li, S., Le, D., Jensen, J., and Hatsukami, D.K. 2004. Effects of reduced cigarette smoking on the uptake of a tobacco-specific lung carcinogen. *J Natl Cancer Inst* **96**: 107–115.

Hecht, S.S, Murphy, S.E., Carmella, S.G., Li, S., Jensen, J., Le, C., Joseph, A.M. and Hatsukami, D.K. 2005. Similar uptake of lung carcinogens by smokers of regular, light and ultralight cigarettes. *Cancer Epidemiol Biomarkers Prev* **14**: 693–698.

Hecht, S.S., Trushin, N., Castonguay, A., and Rivenson, A. 1986. Comparative tumorigenicity and DNA methylation in F344 rats by 4-(methylnitrosamino)-1-(3-pyridyl)-1-butanone and N-nitrosodimethylamine. *Cancer Res* **46**: 498–502.

Heineman, E.F., Zahm, S.H., McLaughlin, J.K., and Vaught, J.B. 1994. Increased risk of colorectal cancer among smokers: results of a 26-year follow-up of US veterans and a review. *Int J Cancer* **59**: 728–738.

Herrero, R., Potischman, N., Brinton, L.A., Reeves, W.C., Brenes, M.M., Tenorio, F., de Britton, R.C., and Gaitan, E. 1991. A case–control study of nutrient status and invasive cervical cancer. I. Dietary indicators. *Am J Epidemiol* **134**: 1335–1346.

Hickey, K., Do, K.A., and Green, A. 2001. Smoking and prostate cancer. *Epidemiol Rev* **23**: 115–125.

Hoffmann, D., and El-Bayoumy, K. 1999. Nutrition and tobacco-related cancer, Chapter 20, pp. 299–324. [D. Heber, G.L. Blackburn and V.L.W. Go, eds.] Nutritional Oncology. Academic Press: San Diego, CA.

Hoffmann, D., Hoffmann, I., and El-Bayoumy, K. 2001. The less harmful cigarette: a controversial issue. a tribute to Ernst L. *Wynder Chem Res Toxicol* **14**(7): 767–790.

Hoffmann, D., Rivenson, A., Abbi, R., and Wynder, E.L. 1993. A study of tobacco carcinogenesis: effect of the fat content of the diet on the carcinogenic activity of 4-(methylnitrosamino)-1-(3-pyridyl)-1-butanone in F344 rats. *Cancer Res* **53**: 2758–2761.

Hoffmann, D., Rivenson, A., Chung, F.L., and Hecht, S.S. 1991. Nicotine-derived N-nitrosamines (TSNA) and their relevance in tobacco carcinogenesis. *Crit Rev Toxicol* **21**: 305–311.

Howe, G.R., and Burch, J.D. 1996. Nutrition and pancreatic cancer. *Cancer Causes Control* **7**: 69–82.

Hsing, A.W., McLaughlin, J.K., Chow, W.H., Schuman, L.M., Co Chien, H.T, Gridley, G., Bjelke, E., Wacholder, S., and Blot, W.J. 1998. Risk factors for colorectal cancer in a prospective study among U.S. white men. *Int J Cancer* **77**: 549–553.

Hung, H.C., Joshipura, K.J., Jiang, R., Hu, F.B., Hunter, D., Smith-Warner, S.A., Colditz, G.A., Rosner, B., Spiegelman, D., and Willett, W.C. 2004. Fruit and vegetable intake and the risk of major chronic disease. *J Natl Cancer Inst* **96**: 1577–1584.

Hunter, D.J., Spiegelman, D., Adami, H.O., Beeson, L., van den Brandt, P.A., Folsom, A.R., Fraser, G.E., Goldbohm, R.A., Graham, S., Howe, G.R, et al. 1996. Cohort studies of fat intake and the risk of breast cancer—a pooled analysis. *N Engl J Med* **334**: 356–361.

Hursting, S.D., Margolin, B.H., and Switzer, B.R. 1993. Diet and human leukemia: an analysis of international data. *Prev Med* **22**: 409–422.

Hursting, S.D., Thornquist, M., and Henderson, M.M. 1990. Types of dietary fat and the incidence of cancer at five sites. *Prev Med* **19**: 242–253.

International Agency for Research on Cancer. 1972–2000. "IARC Monographs on the Evaluation of Carcinogenic Risks of Chemicals to Humans," Vol. 1–77. IARC: Lyon, France.

Jansen, M.C., Bueno-de-Mesquita, H.B., Rasanen, L., Fidanza, F., Nissinen, A.M., Menotti, A., Kok, F.J., and Kromhout, D. 2001. Cohort analysis of fruit and vegetable consumption and lung cancer mortality in European men. *Int J Cancer* **92**: 913–918.

Kadlubar, F.F., Talaska, G., Lang, N.P., Benson, R.W., and Roberts, D.W. 1988. Assessment of exposure and susceptibility to aromatic amine carcinogens. *IARC Sci Publ* **89**: 166–174.

Kadohama, N., Shintani, K., and Osawa, Y. 1993. Tobacco alkaloid derivatives as inhibitors of breast cancer aromatase. *Cancer Lett* **75**: 175–182.

Kagan, M.R., Cunningham, J.A., and Hoffmann, D. 1999. 53rd Tobacco Science Research Conference, Montreal, Quebec, Canada, Abstr. 41.

Kanetsky, P.A., Gammon, M.D., Mandelblatt, J., Zhang, Z.F., Ramsey, E., Dnistrian, A., Norkus, E.P., and Wright, T.C., Jr. 1998. Dietary intake and blood levels of lycopene: association with cervical dysplasia among non-Hispanic, black women. *Nutr Cancer* **31**: 31–40.

Karunasinghe, N., Ryan, J., Tuckey, J., Masters, J., Jamieson, M., Clarke, L.C., Marshall, J.R., and Ferguson, L.R. 2004. DNA stability and serum selenium levels in a high-risk group for prostate cancer. *Cancer Epidemiol Biomarkers Prev* **13**: 391–397.

Kelloff, G.J., Boone, C.W., Steel, V.E., et al. 1994. Progression in cancer chemoprevention: perspectives on agent selection and short-term clinical intervention trials. *Cancer Res* **54**: 2015s–2024s.

Key, T.J., Fraser, G.E., Thorogood, M., Appleby, P.N., Beral, V., Reeves, G., Burr, M.L., Chang-Claude, J., Frentzel-Beyme, R., Kuzma, J.W., Mann, J., and McPherson, K. 1999. Mortality in vegetarians and non-vegetarians: detailed findings from a collaborative analysis of 5 prospective studies. *Am J Clin Nutr* **70**: 516S–524S.

Khuder, S.A., and Mutgi, A. 2001. Effect of smoking cessation on major histologic types of lung cancer. *Chest* **120**: 1577–1583.

Khuder, S.A., Mutgi, A.B., and Nugent, S. 2001. Smoking and breast cancer: a meta-analysis. *Rev Environ Health* **16**: 253–261.

Kim, D.J. 2002. Report from a symposium on diet and breast cancer. *Cancer Causes Control* **13**: 591–594.

Kiyohara, C., Otsu, A.,. Shirakawa, T., Fukuda, S., and Hopkin, J.M. 2002. Genetic polymorphisms and lung cancer susceptibility: a review. *Lung Cancer* **37**: 241–256.

Klatt, P., Molina, E.P., De Lacoba, M.G., Padilla, C.A., Martinez-Galesteo, E., Barcena, J.A., and Lamas, S. 1997. Redox regulation of c-Jun DNA binding by reversible S-glutathiolation. *FASEB J* **13**: 1481–1490.

Klein, E.A., Thompson, I.M., Lippman, S.M., Goodman, P.J., Albanes, D., Taylor, P.R., and Coltman, C. 2000. SELECT: the Selenium and Vitamin E Cancer Prevention Trial: rationale and design. *Prostate Cancer Prostatic Dis* **3**: 145–151.

Klein, E.A., Thompson, I.M., Lippman, S.M., Goodman, P.J., Albanes, D., Taylor, P.R., and Coltman, C. 2003. SELECT: the selenium and vitamin E cancer prevention trial. *Urol Oncol* **21**: 59–65.

Kleinman, W.A., Komninou, D., Leutzinger, Y., Colosimo, S., Cox, J., Lang, C.A., and Richie, J.P., Jr. 2003. Protein glutathiolation in human blood. *Biochem Pharmacol* **65**: 741–746.

Kleinman, W.A., and Richie, J.P., Jr. 1995. Determination of thiols and disulfides using high-performance liquid chromatography with electrochemical detection. *J Chromatogr B Biomed Appl* **672**: 73–80.

Knekt, P., Adlercreutz, H., Rissanen, H., Aromaa, A., Teppo, L., and Heliovaara, M. 2000. Does antibacterial treatment for urinary tract infection contribute to the risk of breast cancer? *Br J Cancer* **82**: 1107–1110.

Knekt, P., Hakama, M., Jarvinen, R., Pukkala, E., and Heliovaara, M. 1998. Smoking and risk of colorectal cancer. *Br J Cancer* **78**: 136–139.

Kobrinsky, N.L., Klug, M.G., Hokanson, P.J., Sjolander, D.E., and Burd, L. 2003. Impact of smoking on cancer stage at diagnosis. *J Clin Oncol* **21**: 907–913.

Korte, J.E., Hertz-Picciotto, I., Schulz, M.R., Ball, L.M., and Duell, E.J. 2000. The contribution of benzene to smoking-induced leukemia. *Environ Health Perspect* **108**: 333–339.

Kristal, A.R. 2004. Vitamin A, retinoids and carotenoids as chemopreventive agents for prostate cancer. *J Urol* **171**: S54–S58.

Kushi, L.H., Sellers, T.A., Potter, J.D., Nelson, C.L., Munger, R.G., Kaye, S.A., and Folsom, A.R. 1992. Dietary fat and postmenopausal breast cancer. *J Natl Cancer Inst* **84**: 1092–1099.

Kvale, G., Bjelke, E., and Gart, J.J. 1983. Dietary habits and lung cancer risk. *Int J Cancer* **31**: 397–405.

Kwiatkowski, A. 1993. Dietary and other environmental risk factors in acute leukaemias: a case–control study of 119 patients. *Eur J Cancer Prev* **2**: 139–146.

Lamprecht, S.A., and Lipkin, M. 2003. Chemoprevention of colon cancer by calcium, vitamin D and folate: molecular mechanisms. *Nat Rev Cancer* **3**: 601–614.

La Vecchia, C., Franceschi, S., Decarli, A., Gentile, A., Fasoli, M., Pampallona, S., and Tognoni, G. 1984. Dietary vitamin A and the risk of invasive cervical cancer. *Int J Cancer* **34**: 319–322.

La Vecchia, C., Negri, E., Decarli, A., D'Avanzo, B., Liberati, C., and Franceschi, S. 1989. Dietary factors in the risk of bladder cancer. *Nutr Cancer* **12**: 93–101.

Lee, T.D., Sadda, M.R., Mendler, M.H., Bottiglieri, T., Kanel, G., Mato, J.M., and Lu, S.C. 2004. Abnormal hepatic methionine and glutathione metabolism in patients with alcoholic hepatitis. *Alcohol Clin Exp Res* **28**: 173–181.

Levi, F., Pasche, C., La Vecchia, C., Lucchini, F., Franceschi, S., and Monnier, P. 1998. Food groups and risk of oral and pharyngeal cancer. *Int J Cancer* **77**: 705–709.

Lin, H.S., Jenner, A.M., Ong, C.N., Huang, S.H., Whiteman, M., and Halliwell, B. 2004. High-throughput and sensitive methodology for the quantitation of urinary 8-hydroxy-2′-deoxyguanosine: measurement with gas chromatography-mass spectrometry after single solid phase extraction. *Biochem J* **380**: 541–548.

London, S.J., Yuan, J.M., Chung, F.L., Gao, Y.T., Coetzee, G.A., Ross, R.K., and Yu, M.C. 2000. Isothiocyanates, glutathione S-transferase M1 and T1 polymorphisms, and lung-cancer risk: a prospective study of men in Shanghai, China. *Lancet* **356**: 724–729.

Lumey, L.H. 1996. Prostate cancer and smoking: a review of case–control and cohort studies. *Prostate* **29**: 249–260.

Macrae, F.A. 1993. Fat and calories in colon and breast cancer: from animal studies to controlled clinical trials. *Prev Med* **22**: 750–766.

Mallis, R.J., Buss, J.E., and Thomas, J.A. 2001. Oxidative modification of H-ras: S-thiolation and S-nitrosylation of reactive cysteines. *Biochem J* **355**: 145–153.

Männistö, S., Smith-Warner, S.A., Spiegelman, D., Albanes, D., Anderson, K., van den Brandt, P.A., Cerhan, J.R., Colditz, G., Feskanich, D., Freudenheim, J.L., Giovannucci, E., Goldbohm, R.A., Graham, S., Miller, A.B., Rohan, T.E., Virtamo, J., Willett, W.C., and Hunter, D.J. 2004. Dietary carotenoids and risk of lung cancer in a pooled analysis of seven cohort studies. *Cancer Epidemiol Biomarkers Prev* **13**: 40–48.

Marchand, J.L., Luce, D., Goldberg, P., Bugel, I., Salomon, C., and Goldberg, M. 2002. Dietary factors and the risk of lung cancer in New Caledonia (South Pacific). *Nutr Cancer* **42**: 18–24.

Martin, F.L., Carmichael, P.L., Crofton-Sleigh, C., Venitt, S., Phillips, D.H., and Grover, P.L. 1996. Genotoxicity of human mammary lipid. *Cancer Res* **56**: 5342–5346.

Mayne, S.T. 2003. Antioxidant nutrients and chronic disease: use of biomarkers of exposure and oxidative stress status in epidemiologic research. *J Nutr* **133**(Suppl 3): 933S–940S.

Mayo, J.J., Kohlhepp, P., Zhang, D., and Winzerling, J.J. 2004. Effects of sham air and cigarette smoke on A549 lung cells: implications for iron-mediated oxidative damage. *Am J Physiol Lung Cell Mol Physiol* **286**(4): L866–L876.

Melikian, A.A., Meng, M., O'Connor, R., and Hu, P., Thompson S.M. 1999b. Development of liquid chromatography-electrospray ionization-tandem mass spectrometry methods for determination of urinary metabolites of benzene in humans. *Res Rep Health Eff Inst* **87**: 1–36.

Melikian, A.A., Sun, P., Prokopczyk, B., El-Bayoumy, K., Hoffmann, D., Wang, X., and Waggoner, S. 1999a. Identification of benzo[a]pyrene metabolites in cervical mucus and DNA adducts in cervical tissues in humans by gas chromatography-mass spectrometry. *Cancer Lett* **146**: 127–134.

Michaud, D.S., Giovannucci, E., Willett, W.C., Colditz, G.A., and Fuchs, C.S. 2003. Dietary meat, dairy products, fat, and cholesterol and pancreatic cancer risk in a prospective study. *Am J Epidemiol* **157**: 1115–1125.

Michels, K.B., and Ekbom, A. 2004. Caloric restriction and incidence of breast cancer. *JAMA* **291**: 1226–1230.

Michener, C.M., Ardekani, A.M., Petricoin, E.F., Liotta, L.A., and Kohn, E.C. 2002. Genomics and proteomics: application of novel technology to early detection and prevention of cancer. *Cancer Detect Prev* **26**: 249–255.

Miller, A.B., Altenburg, H.P., Bueno-de-Mesquita, B., Boshuizen, H.C., Agudo, A., Berrino, F., Gram, I.T., Janson, L., Linseisen, J., Overvad, K., Rasmuson, T., Vineis, P., Lukanova, A., Allen, N., Amiano, P., Barricarte, A., Berglund, G., Boeing, H., Clavel-Chapelon, F., Day, N.E., Hallmans, G., Lund, E., Martinez, C., Navarro, C., Palli, D., Panico, S., Peeters, P.H., Quiros, J.R., Tjonneland, A., Tumino, R., Trichopoulou, A., Trichopoulos, D., Slimani, N., and Riboli, E. 2004. Fruits and vegetables and lung cancer: Findings from the European Prospective Investigation into Cancer and Nutrition. *Int J Cancer* **108**: 269–276.

Mills, P.K., Beeson, W.L., Phillips, R.L., and Fraser, G.E. 1991. Bladder cancer in a low risk population: results from the Adventist Health Study. *Am J Epidemiol* **133**: 230–239.

Missmer, S.A., Smith-Warner, S.A., Spiegelman, D., Yaun, S.S., Adami, H.O., Beeson, W.L., van den Brandt, P.A., Fraser, G.E., Freudenheim, J.L., Goldbohm, R.A., Graham, S., Kushi, L.H., Miller, A.B., Potter, J.D., Rohan, T.E., Speizer, F.E., Toniolo, P., Willett, W.C., Wolk, A., Zeleniuch-Jacquotte, A., and Hunter, D.J. 2002. Meat and dairy food consumption and breast cancer: a pooled analysis of cohort studies. *Int J Epidemiol* **31**: 78–85.

Morrow, J.D., Frei, B., Longmire, A.W., Gaziano, J.M., Lynch, S.M., Shyr, Y., Strauss, W.E., Oates, J.A., and Roberts, L.J., 2nd. 1995. Increase in circulating products of lipid peroxidation (F2-isoprostanes) in smokers. Smoking as a cause of oxidative damage. *N Engl J Med* **332**: 1198–1203.

Mukundan, M.A., Chacko, M.C., Annapurna, V.V., and Krishnaswamy, K. 1993. Effect of turmeric and curcumin on BP-DNA adducts. *Carcinogenesis* **14**: 493–496.

Muscat, J.E., Hoffmann, D., and Wynder, E.L. 1995. The epidemiology of renal cell carcinoma. A second look. *Cancer* **75**: 2552–2557.

Muscat, J.E., Kleinman, W., Colosimo, S., Muir, A., Lazarus, P., Park, J., and Richie, J.P., Jr. 2004. Enhanced protein glutathiolation and oxidative stress in cigarette smokers. *Free Radic Biol Med* **36**: 464–470.

Muscat, J.E., Stellman, S.D., Hoffmann, D., and Wynder, E.L. 1997. Smoking and pancreatic cancer in men and women. *Cancer Epidemiol Biomarkers Prev* **6**: 15–19.

Muscat, J.E., and Wynder, E.L. 1992. Tobacco, alcohol, asbestos and occupational risk factors for laryngeal cancer. *Cancer* **69**: 2244–2251.

Muti, P. 2005. The role of endogenous hormones in the etiology and prevention of breast cancer: the epidemiologic evidence. *Rev Results Cancer Res* **166**: 245–256.

Nagata, C., Shimizu, H., Higashiiwai, H., Sugahara, N., Morita, N., Komatsu, S., and Hisamichi, S. 1999. Serum retinol level and risk of subsequent cervical cancer in cases with cervical dysplasia. *Cancer Invest* **17**: 253–258.

Niwa, T., Naito, C., Mawjood, A.H., and Imai, K. 2000. Increased glutathionyl hemoglobin in diabetes mellitus and hyperlipidemia demonstrated by liquid chromatography/electrospray ionization-mass spectrometry. *Clin Chem* **46**: 82–88.

Nyren, O., Bergstrom, R., Nystrom, L., Engholm, G., Ekbom, A., Adami, H.O., Knutsson, A., and Stjernberg, N. 1996. Smoking and colorectal cancer: a 20-year follow-up study of Swedish construction workers. *J Natl Cancer Inst* **88**: 1302–1307.

Otani, T., Iwasaki, M., Yamamoto, S., Sobue, T., Hanaoka, T., Inoue, M., Tsugane, S., and Japan Public Health Center–based Prospective Study Group. 2003. Alcohol consumption, smoking, and subsequent risk of colorectal cancer in middle-aged and elderly Japanese men and women: Japan Public Health Center–based prospective study. *Cancer Epidemiol Biomarkers Prev* **12**: 1492–1500.

Ozasa, K., Watanabe, Y., Ito, Y., Suzuki, K., Tamakoshi, A., Seki, N., Nishino, Y., Kondo, T., Wakai, K., Ando, M., and Ohno, Y. 2001. Dietary habits and risk of lung cancer death in a large-scale cohort study (JACC Study) in Japan by sex and smoking habit. *Jpn J Cancer Res* **92**: 259–269.

Palozza, P., Serini, S., DiNicuolo, F., Boninsegna, A., Torsello, A., Maggiano, N., Ranelletti, F.O., Wolf, F.I., Calviello, G., and Cittandini, A. 2004. Beta-Carotene exacerbates DNA oxidative damage and modifies p53-related pathways of cell proliferation and apoptosis in cultured cells exposed to tobacco smoke condensate. *Carcinogenesis* **25**: 1315–1325.

Pan, S.Y., Johnson, K.C., Ugnat, A.M., Wen, S.W., Mao, Y., and Canadian Cancer Registries Epidemiology Research Group. 2004. Association of obesity and cancer risk in Canada. *Am J Epidemiol* **159**: 259–268.

Pastore, A., Francesca Mozzi, A., Tozzi, G., Maria Gaeta, L., Federici, G., Bertini, E., Lo Russo, A., Mannucci, L., and Piemonte, F. 2003. Determination of glutathionyl-hemoglobin in human erythrocytes by cation-exchange high-performance liquid chromatography. *Anal Biochem* **312**: 85–90.

Patolla, J.M., Ragu, J., Swamy, M.V., Herzog, C.R., Desai, D.H., Amin, S., and Rao, C.V. 2004. Enhancement of NNK-induced lung tumorigenesis by Western-style diet. *Proc AACR* **45**: 897–898.

Perera, F., and Rundle, A. 2003. Correspondence re: Gammon et al., Environmental toxins and breast cancer on Long Island. I. Polycyclic aromatic hydrocarbon DNA adducts. **11**: 677–685, 2002. *Cancer Epidemiol Biomarkers Prev* **12**: 75.

Peto, J. 2001. Cancer epidemiology in the last century and the next decade. *Nature* **411**: 390–395.

Petrakis, N.L. 1978. Breast secretory activity in nonlactating women, postpartum breast involution, and the epidemiology of breast cancer. *Natl Cancer Inst Monogr* **47**: 161–164.

Pignatelli, B., Li, C.Q., Boffetta, P., Chen, Q., Ahrens, W., Nyberg, F., Mukeria, A., Bruske-Hohlfeld, I., Fortes, C., Constantinescu, V., Ischiropoulos, H., and Ohshima, H. 2001. Nitrated and oxidized plasma proteins in smokers and lung cancer patients. *Cancer Res* **61**: 778–784.

Pilger, A., Germadnik, D., Riedel, K., Meger-Kossien, I., Scherer, G., and Rudiger, H.W. 2001. Longitudinal study of urinary 8-hydroxy-2′-deoxyguanosine excretion in healthy adults. *Free Radic Res* **35**: 273–280.

Plummer, M., Herrero, R., Franceschi, S., Meijer, C.J., Snijders, P., Bosch, F.X., de Sanjose, S., Munoz, N., and IARC Multi-centre Cervical Cancer Study Group. 2003. Smoking and cervical cancer: pooled analysis of the IARC multi-centric case–control study. *Cancer Causes Control* **14**: 805–814.

Polasa, K., Naidu, A.N., Ravindranath, I., and Krishnaswamy, K. 2004. Inhibition of B(a)P induced strand breaks in presence of curcumin. *Mutat Res* **557**: 203–213.

Potischman, N., Herrero, R., Brinton, L.A., Reeves, W.C., Stacewicz-Sapuntzakis, M., Jones, C.J., Brenes, M.M., Tenorio, F., de Britton, R.C., and Gaitan, E. 1991. A case–control study of nutrient status and invasive cervical cancer. II. Serologic indicators. *Am J Epidemiol* **134**: 1347–1355.

Prokopczyk, B., Cox, J.E., Hoffmann, D., and Waggoner, S.E. 1997. Identification of tobacco-specific carcinogen in the cervical mucus of smokers and nonsmokers. *J Natl Cancer Inst* **18**: 868–873.

Prokopczyk, B., Trushin, N., Leszczynska, J., Waggoner, S.E., and El-Bayoumy, K. 2001. Human cervical tissue metabolizes the tobacco-specific nitrosamine, 4-(methylnitrosamino)-1-(3-pyridyl)-1-butanone, via alpha-hydroxylation and carbonyl reduction pathways. *Carcinogenesis* **22**: 107–114.

Quadrilatero, J., and Hoffman-Goetz, L. 2003. Physical activity and colon cancer. A systematic review of potential mechanisms. *J Sports Med Phys Fitness* **43**: 121–138.

Rajkumar, T., Sridhar, H., Balaram, P., Vaccarella, S., Gajalakshmi, V., Nandakumar, A., Ramdas, K., Jayshree, R., Munoz, N., Herrero, R., Franceschi, S., and Weiderpass, E. 2003. Oral cancer in Southern India: the influence of body size, diet, infections and sexual practices. *Eur J Cancer Prev* **12**: 135–143.

Rayman, M.P. 2000. The importance of selenium to human health. *Lancet* **356**: 233–241.

Reynolds, P., Hurley, S., Goldberg, D.E., Anton-Culver, H., Bernstein, L., Deapen, D., Horn-Ross, P.L., Peel, D., Pinder, R., Ross, R.K., West, D., Wright, W.E., and Ziogas, A. 2004. Active smoking, household passive smoking, and breast cancer: evidence from the California Teachers Study. *J Natl Cancer Inst* **96**: 29–37.

Richie, J.P., Jr. 1992. The role of glutathione in aging and cancer. *Exp Gerontol* **27**: 615–626.

Richie, J.P., Jr., Skowronski, L., Abraham, P., and Leutzinger, Y. 1996. Blood glutathione concentrations in a large-scale human study. *Clin Chem* **42**: 64–70.

Risch, H.A. 2003. Etiology of pancreatic cancer, with a hypothesis concerning the role of N-nitroso compounds and excess gastric acidity. *J Natl Cancer Inst* **95**: 948–960.

Rogers, M.A., Vaughan, T.L., Davis, S., and Thomas, D.B. 1995. Consumption of nitrate, nitrite, and nitrosodimethylamine and the risk of upper aerodigestive tract cancer. *Cancer Epidemiol Biomarkers Prev* **4**: 29–36.

Ross, J.A., Kasum, C.M., Davies, S.M., Jacobs, D.R., Folsom, A.R., and Potter, J.D. 2002. Diet and risk of leukemia in the Iowa Women's Health Study. *Cancer Epidemiol Biomarkers Prev* **11**: 777–781.

Samanic, C., Gridley, G., Chow, W.H., Lubin, J., Hoover, R.N., and Fraumeni, J.F., Jr. 2004. Obesity and cancer risk among white and black United States veterans. *Cancer Causes Control* **15**: 35–43.

Sangerman, J., Kakhniashvili, D., Brown, A., Shartava, A., and Goodman, S.R. 2001. Spectrin ubiquitination and oxidative stress: potential roles in blood and neurological disorders. *Cell Mol Biol Lett* **6**: 607–636.

Sanjoaquin, M.A., Appleby, P.N., Thorogood, M., Mann, J.I., and Key, T.J. 2004. Nutrition, lifestyle and colorectal cancer incidence: a prospective investigation of 10998 vegetarians and non-vegetarians in the United Kingdom. *Br J Cancer* **90**: 118–121.

Sasco, A.J. 2001. Epidemiology of breast cancer: an environmental disease? *APMIS* **109**: 321–332.

Sato, R., Helzlsouer, K.J., Alberg, A.J., Hoffman, S.C., Norkus, E.P., and Comstock, G.W. 2002. Prospective study of carotenoids, tocopherols, and retinoid concentrations and the risk of breast cancer. *Cancer Epidemiol Biomarkers Prev* **11**: 451–457.

Schaid, D.J. 2004. The complex genetic epidemiology of prostate cancer. *Hum Mol Genet* **13**(Suppl 1): R103–R121.

Seow, A., Shi, C.Y, Chung, F.L, Jiao, D., Hankin, J.H., Lee, H.P., Coetzee, G.A., and Yu, M.C. 1998. Urinary total isothiocyanate (ITC) in a population-based sample of middle-aged and older Chinese in Singapore: relationship with dietary total ITC and glutathione S-transferase M1/T1/P1 genotypes. *Cancer Epidemiol Biomarkers Prev* **7**: 775–781.

Shannon, J., Thomas, D.B., Ray, R.M., Kestin, M., Koetsawang, A., Koetsawang, S., Chitnarong, K., Kiviat, N., and Kuypers, J. 2002. Dietary risk factors for invasive and in-situ cervical carcinomas in Bangkok, Thailand. *Cancer Causes Control* **13**: 691–699.

Shu, X.O. 1997. Epidemiology of childhood leukemia. *Curr Opin Hematol* **4**: 227–232.

Siemiatycki, J., Richardson, L., Straif, K., Latreille, B., Lakhani, R., Campbell, S., Rousseau, M.C., and Boffetta, P. 2004. Listing occupational carcinogens. *Environ Health Perspect* **112**: 1447–1459.

Sies, H., Brigelius, R., and Graf, P. 1987. Hormones, glutathione status and protein S-thiolation. Adv. *Enzyme Regul* **26**: 175–189.

Slattery, M.L., Abbott, T.M., Overall, J.C., Jr., Robison, L.M., French, T.K., Jolles, C., Gardner, J.W., and West, D.W. 1990. Dietary vitamins A, C, and E and selenium as risk factors for cervical cancer. *Epidemiology* **1**: 8–15.

Smith, C.J., Perfetti, T.A., Garg, R., and Hansch, C. 2003. IARC carcinogens reported in cigarette mainstream smoke and their calculated log P values. *Food Chem Toxicol* **41**: 807–817.

Smith-Warner, S.A., Ritz, J., Hunter, D.J., Albanes, D., Beeson, W.L., van den Brandt, P.A., Colditz, G., Folsom, A.R., Fraser, G.E., Freudenheim, J.L., Giovannucci, E., Goldbohm, R.A., Graham, S., Kushi, L.H., Miller, A.B., Rohan, T.E., Speizer, F.E., Virtamo, J., and Willett, W.C. 2002. Dietary fat and risk of lung cancer in a pooled analysis of prospective studies. *Cancer Epidemiol Biomarkers Prev* **11**: 987–992.

Smith-Warner, S.A., Spiegelman, D., Adami, H.O., Beeson, W.L., van den Brandt, P.A., Folsom, A.R., Fraser, G.E., Freudenheim, J.L., Goldbohm, R.A., Graham, S., Kushi, L.H., Miller, A.B., Rohan, T.E., Speizer, F.E., Toniolo, P., Willett, W.C., Wolk, A., Zeleniuch-Jacquotte, A., and Hunter, D.J. 2001a. Types of dietary fat and breast cancer: a pooled analysis of cohort studies. *Int J Cancer* **92**: 767–774.

Smith-Warner, S.A., Spiegelman, D., Yaun, S.S., Adami, H.O., Beeson, W.L., van den Brandt, P.A., Folsom, A.R., Fraser, G.E., Freudenheim, J.L., Goldbohm, R.A., Graham, S., Miller, A.B., Potter, J.D., Rohan, T.E., Speizer, F.E., Toniolo, P., Willett, W.C., Wolk, A., Zeleniuch-Jacquotte, A., and Hunter, D.J. 2001b. Intake of fruits and vegetables and risk of breast cancer: a pooled analysis of cohort studies. *JAMA* **285**: 769–776.

Smith-Warner, S.A., Spiegelman, D., Yaun, S.S., Albanes, D., Beeson, W.L., van den Brandt, P.A., Feskanich, D., Folsom, A.R., Fraser, G.E., Freudenheim, J.L., Giovannucci, E., Goldbohm, R.A., Graham, S., Kushi, L.H., Miller, A.B., Pietinen, P., Rohan, T.E., Speizer, F.E., Willett, W.C., and Hunter, D.J. 2003. Fruits, vegetables and lung cancer: a pooled analysis of cohort studies. *Int J Cancer* **107**: 1001–1011.

Spitz, M.R., Wei, Q., Dong, Q., Amos, C.I., and Wu, X. 2003. Genetic susceptibility to lung cancer: the role of DNA damage and repair. *Cancer Epidemiol Biomarkers Prev* **12**: 689–698.

Stagnaro, E., Ramazzotti, V., Crosignani, P., Fontana, A., Masala, G., Miligi, L., Nanni, O., Neri, M., Rodella, S., Costantini, A.S., Tumino, R., Vigano, C., Vindigni, C., and Vineis, P. 2001. Smoking and hematolymphopoietic malignancies. *Cancer Causes Control* **12**: 325–334.

Stein, C.J., and Colditz, G.A. 2004. Modifiable risk factors for cancer. *Br J Cancer* **90**: 299–303.

Steinmaus, C.M., Nunez, S., and Smith, A.H. 2000. Diet and bladder cancer: a meta-analysis of six dietary variables. *Am J Epidemiol* **151**: 693–702.

Steinmetz, K.A., and Potter, J.D. 1991. Vegetables, fruit, and cancer. I. Epidemiology. *Cancer Causes Control* **2**: 325–357.

Stolzenberg-Solomon, R.Z., Pietinen, P., Taylor, P.R., Virtamo, J., and Albanes, D. 2002. Prospective study of diet and pancreatic cancer in male smokers. *Am J Epidemiol* **155**: 783–792.

Taioli, E., Nicolosi, A., and Wynder, E.L. 1991. Possible role of diet as a host factor in the aetiology of tobacco-induced lung cancer: an ecological study in southern and northern Italy. *Int J Epidemiol* **20**: 611–614.

Takezaki, T., Inoue, M., Kataoka, H., Ikeda, S., Yoshida, M., Ohashi, Y., Tajima, K., and Tominaga, S. 2003. Diet and lung cancer risk from a 14-year population-based prospective study in Japan: with special reference to fish consumption. *Nutr Cancer* **45**: 160–167.

Tannenbaum, A. 1944. The importance of differential consideration of the stages of carcinogenesis in the evaluation of cocarcinogenic and anticarcinogenic effects. *Cancer Res* **4**: 678–687.

Terry, P.D., Miller, A.B., and Rohan, T.E. 2002. Prospective cohort study of cigarette smoking and colorectal cancer risk in women. *Int J Cancer* **99**: 480–483.

Terry, P.D., and Rohan, T.E. 2002. Cigarette smoking and the risk of breast cancer in women: a review of the literature. *Cancer Epidemiol Biomarkers Prev* **11**: 953–971.

Terry, P.D., Rohan, T.E., and Wolk, A. 2003. Intakes of fish and marine fatty acids and the risks of cancers of the breast and prostate and of other hormone-related cancers: a review of the epidemiologic evidence. *Am J Clin Nutr* **77**: 532–543.

Terry, P., Ekbom, A., Lichtenstein, P., Feychting, M., and Wolk, A. 2001. Long-term tobacco smoking and colorectal cancer in a prospective cohort study. *Int J Cancer* **91**: 585–587.

The Health Consequences of Smoking: A report of the Surgeon General, May 2004.

The Health Consequences of Smoking. Cancer. A Report of the Surgeon General. 1982. U.S. Department of Health and Human Services. Public Health Services Office of Smoking and Health, Rockville, MD.

Thun, M.J., and Burns, D.M. 2001. Health impact of "reduced yield" cigarettes: a critical assessment of the epidemiological evidence. *Tob Control* **10**(Suppl 1): i4–11.

Thun, M.J., Day-Lailly, C., Myers, D.G., Calle, E.E., Flanders, D., Zhu, B., Namboodiri, M., and Health, C.W., Jr. 1997. Trends in tobacco smoking and mortality from cigarette use in Cancer Prevention Studies I (1959 through 1965) and II (1982 through 1988). *In* "Changes in Cigarette-Related Disease Risks and Their Implication for Prevention and Control: Smoking and Tobacco Control Monograph 8," pp. 305–382. U.S. Dept. of Health and Human Services, Public Health Service, National Institutes of Health, Bethesda, MD.

Tomar, S.L. 2003. Trends and patterns of tobacco use in the United States. *Am J Med Sci* **326**: 208–254.

Twombly, R. 2005. Cancer surpasses heart disease as leading cause of death for all but the very elderly. *J Natl Cancer Inst* **97**: 330–331.

U.S. Preventive Services Task Force. 2003. Routine vitamin supplementation to prevent cancer and cardiovascular disease: recommendations and rationale. *Ann Intern Med* **139**: 51–55.

van der Hel, O.L., Bueno de Mesquita, H.B., Sandkuijl, L., van Noord, P.A., Pearson, P.L., Grobbee, D.E., and Peeters, P.H. 2003b. Rapid N-acetyltransferase 2 imputed phenotype and smoking may increase risk of colorectal cancer in women (Netherlands). *Cancer Causes Control* **14**: 293–298.

van der Hel, O.L., Peeters, P.H., Hein, D.W., Doll, M.A., Grobbee, D.E., Kromhout, D., and Bueno de Mesquita, H.B. 2003a. NAT2 slow acetylation and GSTM1 null genotypes may increase postmenopausal breast cancer risk in long-term smoking women. *Pharmacogenetics* **13**: 399–407.

VanEenwyk, J., Davis, F.G., and Bowen, P.E. 1991. Dietary and serum carotenoids and cervical intraepithelial neoplasia. *Int J Cancer* **48**: 34–38.

van Zeeland, A.A., de Groot, A.J., Hall, J., and Donato, F. 1999. 8-Hydroxydeoxyguanosine in DNA from leukocytes of healthy adults: relationship with cigarette smoking, environmental tobacco smoke, alcohol and coffee consumption. *Mutat Res* **439**: 249–257.

Veierod, M.B., Laake, P., and Thelle, D.S. 1997. Dietary fat intake and risk of lung cancer: a prospective study of 51,452 Norwegian men and women. *Eur J Cancer Prev* **6**: 540–549.

Velicer, C.M., Heckbert, S.R., Lampe, J.W., Potter, J.D., Robertson, C.A., and Taplin S.H. 2004. Antibiotic use in relation to the risk of breast cancer. *JAMA* **291**: 827–835.

Vessey, M., Painter, R., and Yeates, D. 2003. Mortality in relation to oral contraceptive use and cigarette smoking. *Lancet* **362**: 185–191.

Vineis, P., Alavanja, M., Buffler, P., Fontham, E., Franceschi, S., Gao, Y.T., Gupta, P.C., Hackshaw, A., Matos, E., Samet, J., Sitas, F., Smith, J., Stayner, L., Straif, K., Thun, M.J., Wichmann, H.E., Wu, A.H., Zaridze, D., Peto, R., and Doll, R. 2004. Tobacco and cancer: recent epidemiological evidence. *J Natl Cancer Inst* **96**(2): 99–106.

Voorrips, L.E., Goldbohm, R.A., Verhoeven, D.T., van Poppel, G.A., Sturmans, F., Hermus, R.J., and van den Brandt, P.A. 2000. Vegetable and fruit consumption and lung cancer risk in the Netherlands Cohort Study on diet and cancer. *Cancer Causes Control* **11**: 101–115.

Wagner, P.D., Maruvada, P., and Srivastava, S. 2004. Molecular diagnostics: a new frontier in cancer prevention. *Expert Rev Mol Diagn* **4**: 503–511.

Wakai, K., Hayakawa, N., Kojima, M., Tamakoshi, K., Watanabe, Y., Suzuki, K., Hashimoto, S., Tokudome, S., Toyoshima, H., Ito, Y., Tamakoshi, A., and JACC Study Group. 2003. Smoking and colorectal cancer in a non-Western population: a prospective cohort study in Japan. *J Epidemiol* **13**: 323–332.

Wang, M., Cheng, G., Sturla, S.J., Shi, Y., McIntee, E.J., Villalta, P.W., Upadhyaya, P., Hecht, S.S. 2003. Identification of adducts formed by pyridyloxobutylation of deoxyguanosine and DNA by 4-(acetoxymethylnitrosamino)-1-(3-pyridyl)-1-butanone, a chemically activated form of tobacco specific carcinogens. *Chem Res Toxicol* **16**: 616–626.

Ward, N.E., Chu, F., and O'Brian, C.A. 2002. Regulation of protein kinase C isozyme activity by S-glutathiolation. *Methods Enzymol* **353**: 89–100.

Wassertheil-Smoller, S., Romney, S.L., Wylie-Rosett, J., Slagle, S., Miller, G., Lucido, D., Duttagupta, C., and Palan, P.R. 1981. Dietary vitamin C and uterine cervical dysplasia. *Am J Epidemiol* **114**: 714–724.

Wattenberg, L.W. 1978. Inhibition of chemical carcinogenesis. *J Natl Cancer Inst* **60**: 11–18.

Wattenberg, L.W. 1985. Chemoprevention of cancer. *Cancer Res* **45**: 1–8.

Winn, D.M., Ziegler, R.G., Pickle, L.W., Gridley, G., Blot, W.J., and Hoover, R.N. 1984. Diet in the etiology of oral and pharyngeal cancer among women from the southern United States. *Cancer Res* **44**: 1216–1222.

"Women and Smoking. A Report of the Surgeon General." 2001. Rockville, MD: U.S. Department of Health and Human Services. Public Health Services, Office of the Surgeon General, Washington, DC.

Wu, A.H., Paganini-Hill, A., Ross, R.K., and Henderson, B.E. 1987. Alcohol, physical activity and other risk factors for colorectal cancer: a prospective study. *Br J Cancer* **55**: 687–694.

Wu, K., Erdman, J.W., Jr., Schwartz, S.J., Platz, E.A., Leitzmann, M., Clinton, S.K., DeGroff, V., Willett, W.C. and Giovannucci, E. 2004b. Plasma and dietary carotenoids, and the risk of prostate cancer: a nested case–control study. *Cancer Epidemiol Biomarkers Preven* **13**: 260–269.

Wu, K.Y., Chiang, S.Y., Huang, T.H., Tseng, Y.S., Chen, Y.L., Kuo, H.W., and Hsieh, C.L. 2004d. Formation of N-(2-hydroxyethyl)valine in human hemoglobin-effect of lifestyle factors. *Mutat Res* **559**: 73–82.

Wynder, E.L., Cohen, L., and Stellman, S.D. 1993. Breast cancer risk from diet, tobacco, and alcohol. *JAMA* **269**: 1791.

Wynder, E.L., and Graham, E.A. 1985. Landmark article May 27, 1950: Tobacco Smoking as a possible etiologic factor in bronchiogenic carcinoma. A study of six hundred and eighty-four proved cases. *JAMA* **253**: 2986–2994.

Wynder, E.L., Hebert, J.R., and Kabat, G.C. 1987. Association of dietary fat and lung cancer. *J Natl Cancer Inst* **79**: 631–637.

Wynder, E.L., Taioli, E., and Fujita, Y. 1992. Ecologic study of lung cancer risk factors in the U.S. and Japan, with special reference to smoking and diet. *Jpn J Cancer Res* **83**: 418–423.

Yeo, A.S., Schiff, M.A., Montoya, G., Masuk, M., van Asselt-King, L., and Becker, T.M. 2000. Serum micronutrients and cervical dysplasia in Southwestern American Indian women. *Nutr Cancer* **38**: 141–150.

Zeeb, H., and Blettner, M. 1998. Adult leukaemia: what is the role of currently known risk factors? *Radiat Environ Biophys* **36**: 217–228.

Zheng, W., Blot, W.J., Shu, X.O., Diamond, E.L., Gao, Y.T., Ji, B.T., and Fraumeni, J.F., Jr. 1992. Risk factors for oral and pharyngeal cancer in Shanghai, with emphasis on diet. *Cancer Epidemiol Biomarkers Prev* **1**: 441–448.

Zheng, W., Deitz, A.C., Campbell, D.R., Wen, W.Q., Cerhan, J.R., Sellers, T.A., Folsom, A.R., and Hein, D.W. 1999. N-acetyltransferase 1 genetic polymorphism, cigarette smoking, well-done meat intake, and breast cancer risk. *Cancer Epidemiol Biomarkers Prev* **8**: 233–239.

Zheng, W., McLaughlin, J.K., Gridley, G., Bjelke, E., Schuman, L.M., Silverman, D.T., Wacholder, S., Co-Chien, H.T., Blot, W.J., and Fraumeni, J.F., Jr. 1993. A cohort study of smoking, alcohol consumption, and dietary factors for pancreatic cancer (United States). *Cancer Causes Control* **4**: 477–482.

Zhou, B.F., Stamler, J., Dennis, B., Moag-Stahlberg, A., Okuda, N., Robertson, C., Zhao, L., Chan, Q., and Elliott, P., and INTERMAP Research Group. 2003. Nutrient intakes of middle-aged men and women in China, Japan, United Kingdom, and United States in the late 1990s: the INTERMAP study. *J Hum Hypertens* **17**: 623–630.

Ziegler, R.G., Brinton, L.A., Hamman, R.F., Lehman, H.F., Levine, R.S., Mallin, K., Norman, S.A., Rosenthal, J.F., Trumble, A.C., and Hoover, R.N. 1990. Diet and the risk of invasive cervical cancer among white women in the United States. *Am J Epidemiol* **132**: 432–445.

Zur Hausen, H. 1974. Attempts to detect virus specific DNA in human tumors. *Int J Cancer* **13**: 650–656.

CHAPTER

11

Alcohol and Cancer

ELISA V. BANDERA AND LAWRENCE H. KUSHI

INTRODUCTION

Alcohol consumption has been designated a *known human carcinogen* (International Agency on Research for Cancer [IARC], 1988; 10th Report on Carcinogens, 2002), and acetaldehyde, the major metabolite of alcohol, has been classified an *animal carcinogen* (IARC, 1988).

It has been estimated that ~2–3% of all cancers are attributable to alcohol consumption (Longnecker and Tseng, 1999). Several international panels found convincing evidence that alcohol is causally related to cancers of the mouth, larynx, pharynx, liver, and esophagus (Table 1). Alcohol may also increase colorectal and breast cancer risk. For other cancer sites, the association is controversial (lung, ovary, endometrium, prostate). The current evidence does not seem to indicate that cancers of the stomach, pancreas, and bladder are related to alcohol intake.

A number of meta-analyses (Longnecker et al., 1990; Longnecker, 1994; Holman et al., 1996; Corrao et al., 1999; Zeegers et al., 1999; Bagnardi et al., 2001a,b; Ellison et al., 2001; Korte et al., 2002) have been published attempting to summarize and quantify the relationship between alcohol and cancer. These meta-analyses, summarized in Table 2, varied widely in methodology, but in general, confirm the conclusions of the international panels in Table 1.

Given the large body of literature examining alcohol and cancer, we have chosen not to display the evidence for cancer sites that have been already classified as causally related to alcohol (i.e., oral, pharynx, larynx, esophagus, and liver cancers). For these, we summarize the current knowledge, highlighting new findings. For other sites with a less established or in some cases controversial relationship with alcohol (i.e., colorectal, breast, lung, endometrial, ovarian, and prostate cancers), we show the results of selected studies meeting our inclusion criteria described later in this chapter.

ALCOHOL CONSUMPTION: TRENDS AND PREVALENCE

According to a report by the National Institute on Alcohol Abuse and Alcoholism (NIAAA, 2003) reporting trends of alcohol consumption for the period 1977–2000, consumption of spirits and beer has declined (38.7% and 5.4% lower in 2000 than in 1977, respectively), whereas wine consumption has increased (6.9% higher in 2000 than in 1977). Overall, total per capita intake has decreased. In this report estimates of alcohol consumption were based on alcoholic beverage sales data. In 2000, 56% of total ethanol consumption in the United States was from beer, whereas 14.2% was from wine and 29.8% was from spirits.

Another source of national prevalence and trend data on alcohol consumption is the Behavioral Risk Factor Surveillance System (http://www.cdc.gov/brfss/#about_BRFSS), a survey on health risk factors established by the Centers for Disease Control and Prevention (CDC), conducted each year in a random sample of the population 18 years and older residing in each state. According to these data, the prevalence of chronic alcohol drinking, defined as drinking an average of more than two drinks per day for males and more than one drink per day for females, has increased, particularly among females. In 2002, the U.S. prevalence of chronic alcohol drinking was 7.1% for males and 4.5% for females, while binge drinking (having five or more drinks per occasion, one or more times in the past month) was reported by 24.4% of males and 8.1% of females.

Copyright © 2006, Elsevier Inc.
All rights of reproduction in any form reserved.

TABLE 1 Alcohol and Cancer: Judgment Regarding the Overall Scientific Evidence by International Panels

Cancer site	IARC (1988)	WCRF/AICR (1997)	WHO/FAO (2003)
Oral	"Causally related"	Convincing	Convincing
Pharynx	"Causally related"	Convincing	Convincing
Larynx	"Causally related"	Convincing	Convincing
Esophagus	"Causally related"	Convincing	Convincing
Stomach	Inconclusive	Probable (no association)	—
Colon	Inconclusive	Probable	—
Rectum	Inconclusive	Probable	—
Lung	Not causally related	Possible	—
Liver	"Causally related"	Convincing	Convincing
Pancreas	"Unlikely to be causally related"	Probable (no association)	—
Breast	Inconclusive	Probable	Convincing
Endometrium	Insufficient data		—
Ovary	No association		—
Prostate	No association	Possible (no association)	—
Bladder	No association	Convincing (no association)	—

These trends on alcohol consumption are confirmed by data from another national survey conducted by CDC, the National Health Interview Survey (NHIS). Also, according to NHIS 1999–2001 data, 68.6% of men and 56.3% of women are current drinkers. White adults are more likely to be current drinkers and to have had five drinks or more in 1 day in the past year than black and Asian adults (Schoenborn et al., 2004).

ALCOHOLIC BEVERAGES COMPOSITION

Alcoholic beverages are produced by fermentation of high-carbohydrate foods, such as grains (in the case of beer) and grapes (in the case of wine). Distilled spirits are made from the distillation of the ethanol after fermentation. A number of fruits and vegetables can be fermented and then distilled. The type of alcohol drunk by humans is almost exclusively ethanol. The content of alcohol by volume varies by ingredient, processes, and alcoholic beverages, but it is ~4–7% for beer, 10–13% for wine, and 30–50% for spirits (WCRF, 1997). In the United States, a drink of beer (12 oz or 355 ml), wine (5 oz or 148 ml), and liquor (1.5 oz or 44 ml) provide the same amount of alcohol, ~15 g or 0.5 oz (Anonymous, 2000). In addition to ethanol, alcoholic beverages contain contaminants with known or suspected carcinogenic properties, such as nitrosamines, mycotoxins, urethane, asbestos, arsenic compounds, and pesticides (IARC, 1988). There are also anticarcinogenic compounds in alcoholic beverages, including polyphenols and flavonoids, mainly in wine. In particular, there is a growing interest in the beneficial effects of the polyphenol resveratrol, as an anti-inflammatory, antioxidant agent, capable of inhibiting the metabolic activation of carcinogens and cell proliferation and inducing apoptosis (Bianchini and Vainio, 2003). Resveratrol, as a phytoestrogen, can also bind to estrogen receptors (ERs) and exhibit estrogenic and anti-estrogenic activity (Bowers et al., 2000).

ALCOHOL METABOLISM

Alcohol is absorbed in the stomach and small intestine and metabolized mainly in the liver. Three systems in the hepatocyte are capable of metabolizing alcohol: alcohol dehydrogenase (ADH), the microsomal ethanol oxidizing system (MEOS), and catalase (Caballeria, 2003; Quertemont, 2004). Each of these pathways leads to the production of acetaldehyde, which in turn is metabolized to acetate by acetaldehyde dehydrogenase (ALDH). Acetate produced in the liver is metabolized by peripheral tissues to carbon dioxide, fatty acids, and water. Alcohol consumed at moderate levels is mostly metabolized by the ADH system, whereas at higher and chronic levels, the MEOS system (involving mostly CYP 2E1) is activated. The catalase system plays a minor role in metabolizing alcohol.

There is great individual variability in alcohol metabolism mainly because of genetic variations in the main ethanol and acetaldehyde-metabolizing enzymes ADH and ALDH (Quertemont, 2004). These genetic polymorphisms affect both alcohol metabolism and drinking behavior (Bosron and Li, 1986), and there is a growing interest in their role on influencing cancer susceptibility. In general, polymorphisms that favor the production of acetaldehyde or reduce its oxidation to acetate can potentially increase cancer risk. Higher acetaldehyde levels have been found in subjects with the alleles ALDH2*2, ADH2*2, and ADH3*1 (Stickel et al., 2002). New findings in this area are highlighted later in this chapter in the corresponding cancer site section. Other factors can affect alcohol blood levels after alcohol consumption, including gender, race, and food intake (Caballeria, 2003). For example, women are more susceptible to the toxic effects of ethanol due mainly to a lower gastric mucosal ADH activity and different body composition. The main enzyme that metabolizes acetaldehyde, ALDH2, is polymorphic and varies by race. The ADH3*1 allele is present in 40–50% of Caucasians and in ~95% of Japanese (Muto et al., 2002). The ALDH2*2 allele is found only in Orientals, with a prevalence of about 50% (Muto et al., 2002). Subjects with the inactive ALDH2 (ALDH2*2 genotype) experience elevated levels of acetaldehyde after drinking, leading to a series of unpleasant symptoms that have been labeled the "flushing response" (Yokoyama and

TABLE 2 Meta-analyses of Alcohol and Cancer

Author, year	No. of studies included	Subgroup	Drinking level	Pooled OR/RR (95% CL)
Oral cancer				
Bagnardi et al., 2001a	26		25 g/day	1.73 (1.67, 1.78)
			50 g/day	2.77 (2.67, 2.95)
Oral and pharyngeal cancer				
Corrao et al., 1999	8	Males,	25 g/day	2.2 (1.9, 2.5)
		Mediterranean areas	50 g/day	4.2 (3, 5.5)
		Males,	25 g/day	1.9 (1.5, 2.3)
		Other areas	50 g/day	3 (1.9, 4.8)
		Females,	25 g/day	2.3 (1.7, 3)
		Mediterranean areas	50 g/day	4.5 (2.4, 7.7)
		Females, other	25 g/day	1.9 (1.3, 2.8)
		areas	50 g/day	3.2 (1.5, 7.1)
Bagnardi et al., 2001b	26		25 g/day	1.75 (1.7, 1.82)
			50 g/day	2.85 (2.7, 3.04)
Laryngeal cancer				
Corrao et al., 1999	20	Mediterranean areas	25 g/day	1.6 (1.6, 1.7)
			50 g/day	2.7 (2.4, 2.9)
		Other areas	25 g/day	1.2 (1.1, 1.3)
			50 g/day	1.5 (1.2, 1.8)
Bagnardi et al., 2001	20		25 g/day	1.35 (1.31, 1.4)
			50 g/day	1.83 (1.72, 1.95)
Esophageal cancer				
Corrao et al., 1999	14	Mediterranean areas	25 g/day	1.6 (1.5, 1.7)
			50 g/day	2.5 (2.2, 2.8)
		Other areas	25 g/day	1.5 (1.3, 1.7)
			50 g/day	2.2 (1.7, 2.8)
Bagnardi et al., 2001a,b	28		25 g/day	1.51 (1.48, 1.55)
			50 g/day	2.21 (2.11, 2.31)
	18	Males	25 g/day	1.43 (1.38, 1.48)
			50 g/day	1.98 (1.87, 2.11)
	5	Females	25 g/day	1.52 (1.42, 1.63)
			50 g/day	2.24 (1.95, 2.58)
Stomach cancer				
Bagnardi et al., 2001a,b	16		25 g/day	1.07 (1.04, 1.1)
			50 g/day	1.15 (1.09, 1.22)
Colon cancer				
Longnecker, 1990	14		24 g/day	1.1 (1.03, 1.17)
Corrao et al., 1999	16 total	Case-control studies	25 g/day	(1, 1.1)
			50 g/day	1.1 (1, 1.2)
		Cohort studies	25 g/day	1.4 (1.1, 1.7)
			50 g/day	1.9 (1.3, 2.9)
Bagnardi et al., 2001a	17		25 g/day	1.14 (1.07, 1.21)
			50 g/day	1.21 (1.11, 1.32)
Rectal cancer				
Longnecker, 1990	14		24 g/day	1.1 (1.02, 1.18)
Corrao et al., 1999	3	Men	25 g/day	1.1 (1, 1.2)
			50 g/day	1.2 (1.1, 1.5)
		Women	25 g/day	2.3 (1.3, 4)
			50 g/day	5 (1.6, 16.4)
Bagnardi et al., 2001a	16		25 g/day	1.11 (1.03, 1.2)
			50 g/day	1.17 (1.06, 1.3)
Lung cancer				
Bagnardi et al., 2001a,b	6		25 g/day	1.02 (1, 1.04)
			50 g/day	1.04 (1, 1.08)

(*continues*)

TABLE 2 *(Continued)*

Author, year	No. of studies included	Subgroup	Drinking level	Pooled OR/RR (95% CL)
Korte et al., 2002	10	Case-control studies	Highest level of alcohol reported	1.39 (1.06, 1.83)
	8	Cohort studies	Highest level of alcohol reported	1.19 (1.11, 1.29)
Liver cancer				
Corrao et al., 1999	10		25 g/day	1.2 (1.1, 1.3)
			50 g/day	1.4 (1.2, 1.6)
Bagnardi et al., 2001a	19		25 g/day	1.20 (1.13, 1.27)
			50 g/day	1.41 (1.26, 1.56)
	10	Males	25 g/day	1.28 (1.13, 1.45)
			50 g/day	1.51 (1.27, 2.1)
	3	Females	25 g/day	1.97 (1.3, 3)
			50 g/day	3.57 (1.56, 8.21)
Pancreatic cancer				
Bagnardi et al., 2001a,b	17		25 g/day	0.98 (0.9, 1.05)
			50 g/day	1.05 (0.93, 1.18)
Breast cancer				
Longnecker, 1994	38		1 drink/day	1.11 (1.07, 1.16)
			2 drinks/day	1.24 (1.15, 1.34)
			3 drinks/day	1.38 (1.23, 1.55)
Holman et al., 1996	26		<2 drinks/day	1.09 (1.06, 1.12)
			2–4 drinks/day	1.31 (1.24, 1.39)
			>4 drinks/day	1.68 (1.51, 1.87)
Corrao et al., 1999	29	Mediterranean areas	25 g/day	1.4 (1.3, 1.5)
			50 g/day	1.8 (1.6, 2.1)
		Other areas	25 g/day	1.2 (1, 1.4)
			50 g/day	1.5 (1.1, 2)
Bagnardi et al., 2001a,b	49		25 g/day	1.31 (1.27, 1.36)
			50 g/day	1.67 (1.56, 1.78)
Ellison et al., 2001	42		24 g/day	1.21 (1.13, 1.3)
Endometrial cancer				
Bagnardi et al., 2001a,b	6		25 g/day	1.05 (0.88, 1.24)
			50 g/day	1.09 (0.78, 1.54)
Ovarian cancer				
Bagnardi et al., 2001a,b	5		25 g/day	1.11 (1, 1.24)
			50 g/day	1.23 (1.01, 1.54)
Webb et al., 2004	7	Population-based studies	Highest level of alcohol reported	0.72 (0.54–0.97)
	7	Hospital-based studies	Highest level of alcohol reported	1.1 (0.83–1.44)
Prostate cancer				
Bagnardi et al., 2001a,b	11		25 g/day	1.05 (1, 1.08)
			50 g/day	1.09 (1.02, 1.17)
Dennis and Hayes, 2001	15		4 drinks/day	1.21 (1.05, 1.39)
Bladder cancer				
Zeegers et al., 1999	11		Current drinkers vs nondrinker	1.3 (1.1, 1.5)
Bagnardi et al., 2001a,b	11		25 g/day	1.04 (0.99, 1.09)
			50 g/day	1.08 (0.98, 1.89)

Omori, 2003). Because of the unpleasant immediate effects of drinking, these subjects are less likely to drink, but those who do are more susceptible to the effects of alcohol. This has implications for epidemiological research, in that studies evaluating risk associated with ALDH2*1/2*2 genotype should adjust for alcohol intake to avoid an underestimation of the relationship (Yokoyama and Omori, 2003).

CHALLENGES IN STUDYING ALCOHOL AND CANCER

Assessment of Alcohol Intake

Most studies have attempted to characterize current alcohol consumption using quantity–frequency methods or retrospective or prospective diaries. However, the relevant aspect of alcohol consumption is uncertain. Some studies have examined the role of cumulative measures such as lifetime drinking or even drinking patterns. Although alcohol consumption is usually underreported in epidemiological surveys, self-reported alcohol intake has generally been found to have adequate validity and reliability (Feunekes et al., 1999; Del Boca and Darkes, 2003) and to provide enough information for ranking of individuals according to intake to allow the examination of the relationship between alcohol and cancer. However, because these methods may not provide an accurate estimate of the absolute level of intake, their use to issue recommendations for safe drinking has been criticized (Feunekes et al., 1999). A systematic review of the literature on alcohol assessment methods (Feunekes et al., 1999) found that retrospective methods tended to give estimates ~20% lower than quantity-frequency methods and prospective diaries. Furthermore, they found that studies obtaining information about alcoholic beverage type reported estimates ~20% higher. Underreporting due to assessment method and beverage specificity occurred at all levels of drinking but was larger for heavy drinkers. These findings suggest that studies should collect frequency and quantity data on alcoholic beverage type to optimize the estimation of alcohol consumption. More importantly, they imply that the resulting misclassification of alcohol exposure is level dependent and, therefore, may lead to an underestimation of the strength of the association between alcohol and cancer. An additional study (Carlsson et al., 2003) comparing self-reported alcohol intake with biological markers (γ-glutamyltransferase, mean corpuscular volume, and carbohydrate-deficient transferrin) found an increase in the levels of these markers with self-reported consumption. However, the strength of the correlation was inversely proportional to the drinking level. These findings provide support for the use of self-report methods of alcohol consumption assessment in epidemiology. However, the underestimation of heavy drinking using questionnaire data is of concern, particularly as it hampers the ability to detect weak associations between alcohol and certain types of cancer. There currently are no well-established biological markers to monitor alcohol consumption for use in epidemiological research (Nasca, 2001).

International Comparisons

Comparison of results of studies of alcohol and cancer conducted in different countries is very informative, mainly because it allows the examination of the alcohol-cancer link at wider ranges of intake. Also, cultural values may affect the level of underreporting alcohol intake across countries. For instance, studies conducted in Italy and other European countries tend to report much higher levels of intake than those conducted in the United States, particularly among women. However, international comparisons of alcohol studies pose several methodological issues that should be taken into account in the interpretation of results. For example, differences in drink sizes, conversion factors used to estimate ethanol intake, degree of underreporting, drinking patterns, and beverage preference, as well as in production techniques leading to some variability in alcoholic beverage composition, may have explained some of the conflicting results across countries.

Design/Statistical Issues

Studies of alcohol and cancer are confronted by a number of issues. The selection of an appropriate control group in case-control studies is one of them. For example, the selection of hospitalized patients as a control group may not be appropriate, as heavy drinking might be related to the reasons for seeking medical attention and moderate consumption might be associated with a reduced likelihood of a hospital visit.

Confounding is a major issue because alcohol drinking tends to be correlated with other cancer risk factors, such as smoking and dietary intake. Confounding by cigarette smoking is particularly challenging in studies of lung cancer, given the strong relationship of cigarette smoking with this cancer type. Cigarette smoking needs to be carefully assessed and controlled for in the analysis to avoid residual confounding. Diet is another important factor to consider, as drinking affects dietary patterns and diet has been linked to certain cancer sites (WCRF, 1997). Alcohol affects appetite, digestion, absorption, and metabolism of nutrients (Feinman and Lieber, 1999), as well as dietary patterns. Heavy drinkers tend to consume diets high in fat and low in fruits and vegetables (Hebert and Kabat, 1991), whereas moderate drinkers have been found to consume less fat than nondrinkers (Swanson et al., 1993). Alcohol calories (7 kcal/g) are added to the diet, rather than replacing calories derived from foods, resulting in an overall increase in total energy intake (Lands, 1995). However, alcohol consumption has been consistently found to be associated with lower body weight (Lands, 1995), which is not explained by a higher level of physical activity among drinkers (Jones et al., 1982; Gruchow et al., 1985). For these reasons, both total energy intake and body mass index (BMI) should also be considered as potential confounders. Studies should also evaluate possible effect modification by gender, race, menopausal status, genotype, and BMI.

Statistical power has been limited in many studies. Even a large cohort study including thousands may have limited power to examine the relationship between alcohol and cancer if only a few subjects drink at a level likely to have an impact. This has been the case in many studies evaluating the effect on women, where the number of drinkers was small and the reported drinking levels were low. In some studies, for example, the highest level of consumption was less than half a drink per day or even per week. Clearly, these studies can only report on the effect of moderate drinking. Furthermore, at least for some cancers, the relationship with alcohol does not seem to be linear. For example, moderate alcohol drinking does not seem to increase the risk of cancers of the lung, endometrium, ovary, and prostate, whereas heavy drinking might. Former drinkers tend to appear to be at increased cancer risk, perhaps reflecting poor health that led to the cessation of drinking. Therefore, not excluding ex-drinkers from the comparison group may lead to an underestimation of risk among heavy drinkers.

SUMMARY OF THE EPIDEMIOLOGICAL EVIDENCE

Methodology

As previously mentioned, for cancers with an established relationship with alcohol intake (i.e., oral, pharynx, larynx, esophagus, and liver), we summarize the current knowledge, highlighting new findings. For cancers with a less established relationship, we display the results of selected studies. Studies were identified by conducting Medline searches through April 2004, complemented with manual searches of references in other published articles. We selected studies based on the following inclusion criteria: (1) publication language: manuscript written in English, (2) publication type: peer-reviewed articles, (3) study design: population-based case–control and cohort studies, (4) interview type: collecting individual data on alcohol and smoking through direct interview with participants, (5) outcome: cancer incidence, not mortality, (6) alcohol assessment: not using a 24-hour recall, (7) alcohol data: presented in at least three levels of consumption in terms of frequency or quantity, (8) adjustment for covariates: controlling for age and cigarette smoking (for oral, pharynx, larynx, lung, esophagus, stomach, liver, bladder, pancreas, and endometrium), and (9) sample size: including at least 100 cases. For some studies, only analyses with ≥100 cases are shown in the tables. Also, studies using two control groups (e.g., community controls and hospital controls) are included only if separate results are presented for the population controls.

We show in the tables risk estimates corresponding to the highest level of alcohol consumption reported. We also include five relevant covariates for each cancer site and whether the analysis was adjusted for those covariates. Case-control studies that were matched on age were considered to be adjusted for age, even if age was not included in the analysis.

Site-Specific Relationships

Cancers with an Established Relationship with Alcohol Consumption

Head and Neck Cancers

There is convincing evidence that alcohol use is associated with cancers of the mouth, pharynx, and larynx (IARC, 1988; WCRF, 1997; WHO, 2003). There is a strong dose–response relationship between levels of alcohol consumption and the risk of developing these cancer types (Longnecker and Tseng, 1999). Results by beverage type are inconsistent, but some studies have suggested stronger associations for beer and liquor consumption (Longnecker and Tseng, 1999). Alcohol and smoking interact, and their combined effect in head and neck cancers is more than additive (Longnecker and Tseng, 1999). However, an independent effect of alcohol has been demonstrated by studies showing increased risk of head and neck cancers associated with alcohol consumption among nonsmokers (Longnecker and Tseng, 1999).

Japanese studies conducted among alcoholics have consistently found markedly elevated risk of head and neck cancers for those with the inactive variant of ALDH2 (ALDH2*1/2*2 genotype), whereas studies conducted in the general population have not offered consistent results (Yokoyama and Omori, 2003). An association between ADH2*1/2*1 genotype, the less active variant, and head and neck cancers has also been found among alcoholics or moderate/heavy drinkers in studies conducted in Japan (Yokoyama and Omori, 2003). The gene combination ALDH2*1/2*2 and ADH2*1/2*1 has been reported to increase the risk of head and neck cancers in a multiplicative fashion (Yokoyama and Omori, 2003). ADH3*1, the fast metabolizing ADH3 allele, has also been found to be associated with elevated head and neck cancers in studies conducted among French alcoholics (Coutelle et al., 1997) and Puerto Ricans (Harty et al., 1997), but not in another study conducted among French Caucasians (Bouchardy et al., 2000). The role of CYP2E1 genotype has also been evaluated with inconsistent results (Bouchardy et al., 2000).

Cancer of the Esophagus

There is a large body of literature consistently showing an increased risk of esophageal cancer associated with alcohol consumption, and overall, there is convincing evidence that alcohol consumption is an independent risk factor for this type of cancer (IARC, 1988; WCRF, 1997; WHO, 2003). There is a dose–response relationship between consumption level and risk, and the association appears to be stronger for squamous cell carcinomas than for adenocarcinomas (Longnecker and Tseng, 1999). Smoking and alcohol are both independent risk factors, but they also act synergistically in a multiplicative fashion (Nyren and Adami, 2002). The combination of smoking and alcohol also causes head and neck cancers, and esophageal cancer is found in ~1–2% of head and neck cancer patients (Enzinger and Mayer, 2003). Although there have been suggestions that type of alcoholic beverage may be important, results are inconclusive and seem to indicate that total alcohol consumption is the important factor regardless of beverage type (Nyren and Adami, 2002). There has been some interest in evaluating the effect by subsite within the esophagus, but results are inconclusive (Nyren and Adami, 2002).

The notion of a simple dose–response relationship between alcohol and esophageal cancer has been challenged by studies showing important variability in individual susceptibility to alcohol even at light drinking levels (Yokoyama et al., 2002). Studies in Japanese drinkers and Chinese alcoholics have fairly consistently found an elevated risk of squamous cell esophageal cancer for those with inactive forms of ALDH2 encoded by ALDH2*1/2*2 genotype (Yokoyama and Omori, 2003). ADH2 genotype has also been found to be related to esophageal cancer, with those with the less active ADH2*1/2*1 being at increased risk (Yokoyama and Omori, 2003), which does not provide support for the role of acetaldehyde on esophageal carcinogenesis. A multiplicative interaction has also been reported for the gene combination ADH2*1/2*1 and ALDH2*1/2*2, with a substantial elevation in risk of esophageal cancer (odds ratio [OR] = 30, 95% confidence interval [CI]: 13–69) (Yokoyama et al., 2002). Currently, there is little support for a role of ADH3 genotype in esophageal carcinogenesis (Yokoyama et al., 2002). A relationship with CYP2E1 genotype was suggested in a case-control study (Itoga et al., 2002). However, other studies have not confirmed this association (Nyren and Adami, 2002).

Liver Cancer

There is convincing evidence that alcohol consumption increases liver cancer risk (IARC, 1988; WCRF, 1997; WHO, 2003). Chronic alcohol consumption leads to liver cirrhosis, which is a risk factor for hepatocellular carcinoma (Stickel et al., 2002). Chronic hepatitis C virus (HCV) infection interacts with alcohol consumption in producing cirrhosis (Pawlotsky, 2004). Several reviews have been published in this area (Stickel et al., 2002; Jamal and Morgan, 2003; Pawlotsky, 2004). Interactions of alcohol with smoking and hepatitis B virus (HBV) on liver cancer have also been reported (Nasca, 2001). Some studies have suggested that ALDH2 and CYP 2E1 polymorphisms may modify the risk of developing liver cancer (Kato et al., 2003; Munaka et al., 2003). However, earlier studies failed to find a relationship with CYP 2E1 (Lee et al., 1997), ALDH2 (Takeshita et al., 2000), or ADH2 genotypes (Takeshita et al., 2000).

Cancers Probably Caused by Alcohol Consumption

Breast Cancer

The association between alcohol intake with breast cancer has become generally accepted. Two early case-control studies (Williams and Horm, 1977; Rosenberg et al., 1982) created substantial interest in this area and have resulted in a large literature that has examined this association. In a review of this literature through 1997, the WCRF Report noted that "high alcohol intake probably increases the risk of breast cancer" (WCRF, 1997). Several meta-analyses of the literature have been published (Longnecker, 1994; Holman et al., 1996; Corrao et al., 1999; Bagnardi et al., 2001a,b; Ellison et al., 2001), and these uniformly suggest that alcohol intake increases the risk of breast cancer. In an earlier meta-analysis based on 10 cohort and 28 case-control studies (Longnecker, 1994), it was estimated that one drink per day would increase risk by 1.11 (95% confidence limits [CLs]: 1.08, 1.16) in comparison to non-drinkers, whereas three drinks per day would carry a relative risk of 1.38 (95% CL: 1.23, 1.55). One estimate based on 12 cohort and 37 case-control studies reported a pooled relative risk of 1.67 (95% CL: 1.56, 1.78) for an intake of 50 g/day (Bagnardi et al., 2001a). Other meta-analyses generally report risks associated with intakes in these ranges that are comparable to these reports. Based on these and other analyses, it has been estimated that ~4% of breast cancers in developed countries may be attributable to alcohol intake (Hamajima et al., 2002).

Results from population-based case-control and cohort studies that met our inclusion criteria are listed in Table 3. As can be seen, although there is variation in the magnitude of the OR or relative risk comparing extreme intake categories, a substantial preponderance of studies suggest an increased risk with increased intake. Pooled analyses using original data from a number of studies have been conducted in cohort studies (Smith-Warner et al., 1998), case-control studies (Howe et al., 1991), or both (Hamajima et al., 2002). The earliest of these, combining data from six case-control studies,

TABLE 3 Population-Based Case-Control and Cohort Studies Examining Total Alcohol Consumption and Breast Cancer

Author, publication year	Study location	Cases n	Controls/cohort size n	Age range years (mean)	Subgroup	Alcohol variable
Case-control studies						
Webster et al., 1983	USA	1,206	1,256	20–54		Alcohol, g/wk
Harvey et al., 1987	USA	1,524	1,896			Alcohol, g/wk
Adami et al., 1988	NOR, SWE	422	527	<45		Alcohol, g/day
Rohan and McMichael, 1988	Adelaide, AUS	451	451	20–74		Alcohol, g/day
		146	132		Premenopausal	Alcohol, g/day
		281	288		Postmenopausal	Alcohol, g/day
Chu et al., 1989	USA	3,217	2,945	20–54		Alcohol, drinks/wk
		1,535	1,289		Premenopausal	Alcohol, drinks/wk
		577	489		Perimenopausal	Alcohol, drinks/wk
		399	429		Postmenopausal, natural	Alcohol, drinks/wk
		706	738		Postmenopausal, surgical	Alcohol, drinks/wk
Young, 1989	WI, USA	277	372	35–89		Alcoholic drinks/wk, age 18–35 yr
		255	358	35–89		Alcoholic drinks/wk, age >35 yr
Toniolo et al., 1989	Vercelli, ITA	250	499	25–75		Alcohol, g/day
Rosenberg et al., 1990	Toronto, CAN	607	1,214	<70		Alcoholic drinks
Nasca et al., 1990	NY, USA	1,608	1,609	20–79		Alcohol, g/day
Ewertz et al., 1991	DEN	1,486	1,336	<70		
		?	?	<50	<50 yr	Alcohol, g/day
		?	?	60–69	60+ y	Alcohol, g/day
Sneyd et al., 1991	NZL	891	1,864	25–54		Alcohol, drinks/wk
		603	1,432	25–54	Premenopausal	Alcohol, drinks/wk
		115	166	25–54	Postmenopausal (artificial)	Alcohol, drinks/wk
		170	259	25–54	Postmenopausal (natural)	Alcohol, drinks/wk
Martin-Moreno et al., 1993	ESP	762	988	18–75		Alcohol, g/day
		247	356		Premenopausal	Alcohol, g/day
		515	632		Postmenopausal	Alcohol, g/day
Rookus and van Leeuwen, 1994	NED	918	918	<55		Alcohol, glasses/wk
Nasca et al., 1994	NY, USA	790	1,609	20–79	ER+	Alcohol, g/day
		355	1,609	20–79	ER−	Alcohol, g/day
		1,230	1,609	20–79	Ductal carcinoma	Alcohol, g/day
		104	1,609	20–79	Lobular carcinoma	Alcohol, g/day
Freudenheim et al., 1995	Western NY, USA	738	810	40–85		Alcohol 2 yr ago, drinks/mo
		736	807	40–85		Alcohol 10 yr ago, drinks/mo
		735	802	40–85		Alcohol 20 yr ago, drinks/mo
		735	807	40–85		Alcohol at age 16 yr, drinks/mo

Contrast	OR/RR (95% CL)	Covariate adjustment				
		Age	Smoking[a]	BMI/weight	Reproductive factors	Total energy intake
≥300 vs never	1.1 (0.6, 18)	Y	Y *(cont.)*	Y	Y	N
≥183 vs nondrinker	1.66 (1.2, 2.4)	Y	N	N	N	N
15+ vs 0	0.5 (0.2, 1.3)	Y	Y *(cont.)*	N	Y	N
>9.3 vs 0	1.57 (0.99, 2.51)	Y	Y (?)	N	Y	N
>9.3 vs 0	2.33 (0.85, 6.37)	Y	Y (?)	N	Y	N
>9.3 vs 0	1.27 (0.69, 2.33)	Y	Y (?)	N	Y	N
22+ vs <1	1.2 (0.9, 1.6)	Y	Y *(cont.)*	N	Y	N
≥8 vs 0	0.9	Y	Y *(cont.)*	N	Y	N
≥8 vs 0	1.7	Y	Y *(cont.)*	N	Y	N
≥8 vs 0	1	Y	Y *(cont.)*	N	Y	N
≥8 vs 0	1.1	Y	Y *(cont.)*	N	Y	N
10 vs 0 (continuous)	2.12 (1.27, 3.52)	Y	N	Y	N	N
10 vs 0 (continuous)	1.93 (1.25, 2.98)	Y	N	Y	N	N
>40 vs 0	1.6 (0.9, 2.9)	Y	N	Y	N	Y
≥2/day vs <1/mo	1 (0.7, 1.5)	Y	Y (?)	Y	Y	N
≥15 vs none	1.26 (0.98, 1.64)	Y	N	N	Y	N
≥24 vs 0	0.63 (0.34, 1.17)	Y	N	N	Y	N
≥24 vs 0	0.95 (0.44, 2.07)	Y	N	N	Y	N
>14 vs never	1.8 (0.87, 3.8)	Y	Y *(status)*	N	Y	N
≥8 vs <1	1	Y	Y *(status)*	N	Y	N
≥8 vs <1	0.84	Y	Y *(status)*	N	Y	N
≥8 vs <1	0.96	Y	Y *(status)*	N	Y	N
>20.4 vs 0	1.7 (1.3, 2.3)	Y	N	Y	Y	Y
>23 vs 0	1.6 (0.9, 2.8)	Y	N	Y	Y	Y
>18.8 vs 0	1.9 (1.3, 2.8)	Y	N	Y	Y	Y
>10 vs 0	1.2	Y	Y *(status)*	Y	Y	N
≥15 vs 0	1.35 (0.99, 1.85)	Y	N	N	N	N
≥15 vs 0	1.05 (0.7, 1.59)	Y	N	N	N	N
≥15 vs 0	1.32 (1.01, 1.72)	Y	N	N	N	N
≥15 vs 0	1.76 (0.83, 3.71)	Y	N	N	N	N
≥28 vs 0	0.89 (0.62, 1.3)	Y	N	Y	Y	Y
≥28 vs 0	0.91 (0.63, 1.32)	Y	N	Y	Y	Y
≥28 vs 0	0.74 (0.51, 1.07)	Y	N	Y	Y	Y
≥28 vs 0	0.72 (0.22, 2.4)	Y	N	Y	Y	Y

(continues)

TABLE 3 (*Continued*)

Author, publication year	Study location	Cases n	Controls/cohort size n	Age range years (mean)	Subgroup	Alcohol variable
Longnecker et al., 1995a	ME, MA, NH, WI, USA	6,390	8,794	(58.7)		Alcohol, g/day
		6,163	8,480			Lifetime average alcohol, g/day
		1,392	2,504		Premenopausal	Alcohol, g/day
		4,563	5,733		Postmenopausal	Alcohol, g/day
Longnecker et al., 1995b	Los Angeles County, USA	1,431	1,431	55–64		Alcohol, recent, g/day
		1,431	1,431	55–64		Alcohol at age 40 yr
		1,431	1,431	55–64		Alcohol at age 25 yr
		1,431	1,431	55–64		Lifetime average alcohol, g/day
Holmberg et al., 1995	Uppsala and Västmanland counties, SWE	276	452	40–74		Alcohol, g/day
		54	97	40–50	≤50 yr	Alcohol, g/day
		222	355	51–74	>50 y	Alcohol, g/day
Weiss et al., 1996	Atlanta, GA, Puget Sound, WA, and NJ,	228	1,505	20–44	In situ	Alcohol, drinks/wk
	USA	784	1,505	20–44	Local	Alcohol, drinks/wk
		602	1,505	20–44	Regional/distant	Alcohol, drinks/wk
Viladiu et al., 1996	Girona, ESP	330	346	<75		Alcohol, drinks/day
Swanson et al., 1997	Atlanta, GA, Puget Sound, WA and NJ,	1,645	1,497	20–44		Recent alcohol intake, g/day
	USA	220	1,497	20–44	In situ	Recent alcohol intake, g/day
		753	1,497	20–44	Localized	Recent alcohol intake, g/day
		577	1,497	20–44	Regional, distant	Recent alcohol intake, g/day
Bowlin et al., 1997	Long Island, NY, USA	1,413	1,214	20–79		Alcohol, g/day
		281	281	20–79	Premenopausal	Alcohol, g/day
		775	776	20–79	Postmenopausal	Alcohol, g/day
Brinton et al., 1997	Atlanta, GA and NJ, USA	960	1,033	20–54	White	
		?	340	20–39	White, <40 yr	Alcoholic drinks
		?	693	40–54	White, ≥40 yr	Alcoholic drinks
		281	296	20–54	Black	
		?	102	20–39	Black, <40 yr	Alcoholic drinks
		?	194	40–54	Black, ≥40 yr	Alcoholic drinks
Royo-Bordonada et al., 1997	GER, GBR, NED, SUI, ESP	315	364	50–74		Alcohol intake
McCredie et al., 1998	Melbourne and Sydney, AUS	453	408	<40		Alcohol, drinks/wk
Enger et al., 1999	Los Angeles County, USA	205	726	21–40	Premenopausal, ER+/PR+	Alcohol, g/day
		149	726	21–40	Premenopausal, ER–/PR–	Alcohol, g/day
		302	726	21–40	Premenopausal, ER/PR unknown	Alcohol, g/day

Contrast	OR/RR (95% CL)	Covariate adjustment				
		Age	Smoking[a]	BMI/weight	Reproductive factors	Total energy intake
≥46 vs 0	1.96 (1.43, 2.67)	Y	N	Y	Y	N
≥46 vs 0	1.75 (1.16, 2.64)	Y	N	Y	Y	N
≥46 vs 0	1.61 (0.9, 2.86)	Y	N	Y	Y	N
≥46 vs 0	2.28 (1.51, 3.44)	Y	N	Y	Y	N
≥46 vs 0	1.36 (0.79, 2.35) (*p* trend = 0.02)	Y	N	Y	Y	N
≥46 vs 0	1.11 (0.7, 1.77) (*p* trend = 0.03)	Y	N	Y	Y	N
≥46 vs 0	0.99 (0.44, 2.2) (*p* trend = 0.25)	Y	N	Y	Y	N
≥46 vs 0	0.94 (0.46, 1.93) (*p* trend = 0.01)	Y	N	Y	Y	N
≥2 vs never	1.6 (1, 2.4)	Y	N	Y	Y	N
≥2 vs never	0.8 (0.4, 1.4)	Y	N	Y	Y	N
≥2 vs never	1.8 (1.1, 2.9)	Y	N	Y	Y	N
≥14 vs non drinker	0.65 (0.2, 1.8)	Y	N	Y	Y	N
≥14 vs non drinker	1.62 (1, 2.6)	Y	N	Y	Y	N
≥14 vs non drinker	2.52 (1.6, 4.1)	Y	N	Y	Y	N
>15 vs never	1.3 (0.8, 2)	Y	N	N	Y	N
≥14 vs nondrinker	1.73 (1.2, 2.5)	Y	N	N	Y	N
≥14 vs nondrinker	1.17 (0.4, 2.1)	Y	N	N	Y	N
≥14 vs nondrinker	1.53 (1, 2.4)	Y	N	N	Y	N
≥14 vs nondrinker	2.42 (1.6, 3.8)	Y	N	N	Y	N
≥5 vs 0	1.46 (1.13, 1.89)	Y	Y *(cat.)*	N	Y	N
≥5 vs 0	1.54 (0.87, 2.74)	Y	Y *(cat.)*	N	Y	N
≥5 vs 0	1.51 (1.09, 2.08)	Y	Y *(cat.)*	N	Y	N
≥7 vs none	1.1 (0.6, 1.9)	Y	N	N	Y	N
≥7 vs none	1.4 (1, 2)	Y	N	N	Y	N
≥7 vs none	1.9 (0.7, 5.5)	Y	N	N	Y	N
≥7 vs none	1.6 (0.8, 3)	Y	N	N	Y	N
Current (highest tertile) vs never	0.99 (0.48, 2.01)	Y	Y *(cat.)*	Y	Y	N
10+ vs 0	1.2 (0.8, 1.7)	Y	N	Y	Y	N
14+ vs 0	1.1 (0.67, 1.8)	Y	N	N	Y	N
14+ vs 0	1.04 (0.6, 1.81)	Y	N	N	Y	N
14+ vs 0	1.27 (0.83, 1.94)	Y	N	N	Y	N

(*continues*)

TABLE 3 *(Continued)*

Author, publication year	Study location	Cases n	Controls/cohort size n	Age range years (mean)	Subgroup	Alcohol variable
		450	1,091	55–64	Postmenopausal, ER+/PR+	Alcohol, g/day
		159	1,091	55–64	Postmenopausal, ER+/PR−	Alcohol, g/day
		127	1,091	55–64	Postmenopausal, ER−/PR−	Alcohol, g/day
		400	1,091	55–64	Postmenopausal, ER/PR unknown	Alcohol, g/day
Kinney et al., 2000	NC, USA	856	784	20–74		Current alcohol, g/wk
		332	328	20–74	Blacks	Current alcohol, g/wk
		524	456	20–74	Whites	Current alcohol, g/wk
		332	784	20–74	Localized brca	Current alcohol, g/wk
		452	784	20–74	Regional or distant brca	Current alcohol, g/wk
		323	784	20–74	ER−	Current alcohol, g/wk
		457	784	20–74	ER+	Current alcohol, g/wk
Mannisto et al., 2000	Eastern FIN	113	172	25–75	Premenopausal	Current alcohol, g/wk
		188	271	25–75	Postmenopausal	Current alcohol, g/wk
		113	172	25–75	Premenopausal	Total lifetime alcohol intake, g
		188	271	25–75	Postmenopausal	Total lifetime alcohol intake, g
Marcus et al., 2000	NC, USA	860	784	20–74		Alcohol, drinks/wk
Trentham-Dietz et al., 2000	WI, USA	293	3,924	20–74	*In situ*	Alcohol, g/wk
		3,721	3,924	28–74	Invasive	Alcohol, g/wk
Johnson et al., 2000	CAN	802	774	25–54	Premenopausal	Alcohol, drinks/wk
		1,452	1,601	35–74	Postmenopausal	Alcohol, drinks/wk
Kropp et al., 2001	GER	706	1,381	20–50		Current alcohol, g/day
Baumgartner et al., 2002	NM, USA	326	379	30–74	Hispanic	Alcohol, g/wk
		377	451	30–74	Non-Hispanic white	Alcohol, g/wk
		128	379	30–74	Hispanic, ER+/PR+	Alcohol, g/wk
		153	451	30–74	Non-Hispanic white, ER+/PR+	Alcohol, g/wk
Wrensch et al., 2003	Marin County, USA	285	286	(55.4)		Alcoholic drinks, average after age 21 y
		201	201		Age ≥ 50 yr	Alcoholic drinks, average after age 21 y
		84	85		Age < 50 yr	Alcoholic drinks, average after age 21 y

Contrast	OR/RR (95% CL)	Covariate adjustment: Age	Smoking[a]	BMI/weight	Reproductive factors	Total energy intake
14+ vs 0	1.76 (1.14, 2.71)	Y	N	Y	Y	N
14+ vs 0	1.1 (0.53, 2.26)	Y	N	Y	Y	N
14+ vs 0	1.37 (0.68, 2.76)	Y	N	Y	Y	N
14+ vs 0	1.43 (0.9, 2.27)	Y	N	Y	Y	N
≥182 vs nondrinker	1 (0.6, 1.6)	Y	Y *(status)*	Y	Y	N
≥182 vs nondrinker	0.8 (0.3, 1.8)	Y	Y *(status)*	Y	Y	N
≥182 vs nondrinker	1.2 (0.6, 2.3)	Y	Y *(status)*	Y	Y	N
≥91 vs nondrinker	1.4 (0.8, 2.3)	Y	Y *(status)*	Y	Y	N
≥91 vs nondrinker	1.1 (0.7, 1.8)	Y	Y *(status)*	Y	Y	N
≥91 vs nondrinker	1.1 (0.6, 1.7)	Y	Y *(status)*	Y	Y	N
≥91 vs nondrinker	1.3 (0.8, 2)	Y	Y *(status)*	Y	Y	N
>36 vs nondrinker	1 (0.4, 2.2)	Y	Y (?)	Y	Y	N
>29 vs nondrinker	0.8 (0.4, 1.6)	Y	Y (?)	Y	Y	N
>28,657 vs nondrinker	0.9 (0.4, 2.2)	Y	Y (?)	Y	Y	N
>28,028 vs nondrinker	0.6 (0.3, 1.3)	Y	Y (?)	Y	Y	N
≥14 vs none	1.2 (0.8, 1.8)	Y	N	N	N	N
≥183 vs none	2.34 (1.32, 4.16)	Y	N	Y	Y	N
≥183 vs none	1.76 (1.37, 2.25)	Y	N	Y	Y	N
>3.5 vs 0	1.1 (0.8, 1.4)	Y	N	Y	Y	N
>5 vs 0	1.1 (0.9, 1.4)	Y	N	Y	Y	N
≥31 vs 0	1.94 (1.18, 3.2)	Y	N	N	Y	N
≥85 (5–7 drinks) vs nondrinker	1.35 (0.63, 2.93)	Y	Y (?)	Y	Y	Y
≥148 (8+ drinks) vs nondrinker	1.56 (0.85, 2.86)	Y	Y (?)	Y	Y	Y
≥42 (3+ drinks) vs nondrinker	1.78 (0.86, 3.68)	Y	Y (?)	Y	Y	Y
≥148 (8+ drinks) vs nondrinker	2.13 (1.03, 4.43)	Y	Y (?)	Y	Y	Y
≥3/day vs <1/wk	3.6 (1.2, 11.5)	Y	Y *(cat.)*	Y	Y	N
≥3/day vs <1/wk	2.9 (0.8, 10.9)	Y	Y *(cat.)*	Y	Y	N
2/day vs <1/wk	3.6 (0.79, 16.5)	Y	Y *(cat.)*	Y	Y	N

(continues)

TABLE 3 *(Continued)*

Author, publication year	Study location	Cases n	Controls/cohort size n	Age range years (mean)	Subgroup	Alcohol variable
Althius et al., 2003	Atlanta, GA, Puget Sound, WA, and NJ, USA	265	280	20–34	Age < 35 yr	Alcohol, drinks/wk
	Atlanta, GA, Puget Sound, WA, and NJ, USA	1,212	1,031	35–44	Age 35–44 yr	Alcohol, drinks/wk
	Atlanta, GA, USA	270	244	45–54		Alcohol, drinks/wk
Li et al., 2003	Puget Sound, WA, USA	967	998	65–79		Current alcohol, g/day
		651	998	65–79	Ductal carcinoma	Current alcohol, g/day
		195	998	65–79	Lobular carcinoma	Current alcohol, g/day
		789	998	65–79	ER+	Current alcohol, g/day
		106	998	65–79	ER–	Current alcohol, g/day
		648	998	65–79	PR+	Current alcohol, g/day
		244	998	65–79	PR–	Current alcohol, g/day
		642	998	65–79	ER+/PR+	Current alcohol, g/day
		144	998	65–79	ER+/PR–	Current alcohol, g/day
		100	998	65–79	ER–/PR–	Current alcohol, g/day
Freudenheim et al., 2004	New York State, USA	52	494	40–85	P53+	Alcohol 2 yr ago, drinks/mo
		138	494	40–85	P53–	Alcohol 2 yr ago, drinks/mo
Pooled case-control studies						
Howe et al., 1991	AUS, CAN, ITA, GRE, ARG	1,575	1,974			Alcohol, g/day
Hamajima et al., 2002	World	38,675	45,794			Alcohol, g/day
Cohort studies						
Paganini-Hill, 1983[b]	Los Angeles, USA	239	239			Alcohol intake, drinks/day
Hiatt and Bawol, 1984	San Francisco Bay Area, USA	654	3,911	>15		Alcohol, drinks/day
		?	16,662	≥30		Alcohol, drinks/day
		?	?	≥30	White	Alcohol, drinks/day
		?	?	≥30	Black	Alcohol, drinks/day
Schatzkin, 1987	USA	121	7,188	25–74		Alcohol, g/day
Willett et al., 1987	USA	601	89,538	34–59		Alcohol, g/day
		298	49,693		Premenopausal	Alcohol, g/day
		205	26,745		Postmenopausal	Alcohol, g/day
		86	11,911		Hysterectomy	Alcohol, g/day

		Covariate adjustment				
Contrast	OR/RR (95% CL)	Age	Smoking[a]	BMI/weight	Reproductive factors	Total energy intake
14+ vs none	1.71 (0.7, 4)	Y	N	Y	Y	N
14+ vs none	1.95 (1.2, 3.3)	Y	N	Y	Y	N
14+ vs none	4.24 (1.2, 14.6)	Y	N	Y	Y	N
≥30 vs never	1.8 (1.2, 2.9)	Y	N	Y	N	N
≥30 vs never	1.5 (0.9, 2.6)	Y	N	Y	N	N
≥30 vs never	3.3 (1.7, 6.4)	Y	N	Y	N	N
≥30 vs never	1.9 (1.2, 3.1)	Y	N	Y	N	N
≥30 vs never	1.5 (0.5, 4)	Y	N	Y	N	N
≥30 vs never	2 (1.2, 3.2)	Y	N	Y	N	N
≥30 vs never	1.7 (0.9, 3.3)	Y	N	Y	N	N
≥30 vs never	2 (1.2, 3.3)	Y	N	Y	N	N
≥30 vs never	1.8 (0.8, 4)	Y	N	Y	N	N
≥30 vs never	1.5 (0.6, 4.1)	Y	N	Y	N	N
>16 vs 0	1.47 (0.5, 4.32)	Y	Y *(status)*	Y	Y	Y
>16 vs 0	1.08 (0.6, 1.95)	Y	Y *(status)*	Y	Y	Y
≥40 vs 0	1.69 (1.19, 2.4)	Y	N	N	N	N
10 g (continuous)	1.074 (1.052, 1.096)	Y	N	N	N	N
2+ vs never	1.02	Y	N	N	N	N
3+ vs none	1.38	Y	Y (?)	Y	Y	N
3+ vs none	1.49 (1.13, 1.95)	Y	N	N	N	N
3+ vs none	1.46 (1.09, 1.94)	Y	N	N	N	N
3+ vs none	1.08 (0.62, 1.88)	Y	N	N	N	N
≥5 vs 0	2 (1.1, 3.7)	Y	N	Y	Y	N
≥15 vs none	1.6 (1.3, 2)	Y	N	N	Y	N
≥5 vs none	1.5	Y	N	N	N	N
≥5 vs none	1.3	Y	N	N	N	N
≥5 vs none	1.4	Y	N	N	N	N

(continues)

TABLE 3 *(Continued)*

Author, publication year	Study location	Cases n	Controls/cohort size n	Age range years (mean)	Subgroup	Alcohol variable
Hiatt et al., 1988	San Francisco Bay Area, USA	303	58,347			Alcohol, drinks/day
		227	?		White or Hispanic	Alcohol, drinks/day
		76	?		Black	Alcohol, drinks/day
Schatzkin et al., 1989	Framingham, MA, USA	143	2,636	29–62		Alcohol at baseline, g/day
		141		29–62		Most recent alcohol, g/day
Gapstur et al., 1992	Iowa, USA	459	133,074[e]	55–69		Alcohol, g/day
Friedenreich et al., 1993[b]	CAN	519	1,182	40–59		Alcohol, g/day
		235	491		Premenopausal	Alcohol, g/day
		284	691		Postmenopausal	Alcohol, g/day
van den Brandt et al., 1995[c]	NED	422	1,579	55–69		Alcohol, g/day
Zhang et al., 1999b	Framingham, MA, USA	287	4,761	12–62		Alcohol, g/day
		221	2,543	28–62	"original" cohort	Alcohol, g/day
		66	2,218	12–60	"offspring" cohort	Alcohol, g/day
Garland et al., 1999	USA	400	569,657[e]	25–42		Alcohol, g/day
		435	595,210[e]	25–42		Lifetime alcohol intake, g/day
Rohan et al., 2000[a]	CAN	1,336	5,238	40–59		Alcohol, g/day
		598			Premenopausal	Alcohol, g/day
		542			Postmenopausal	Alcohol, g/day
Hines et al., 2000[b]	USA	455	608	43–69		Alcohol, g/day
		99	206	43–69	ADH3 fast genotype	Alcohol, g/day
		235	296	43–69	ADH3 intermediate genotype	Alcohol, g/day
		71	110	43–69	ADH3 slow genotype	Alcohol, g/day
Chen et al., 2002	USA	1,722	44,187	30–55	Postmenopausal only	Alcohol, g/day
Horn-Ross et al., 2002	California, USA	711	111,256	21–103		Alcohol, g/day
Sellers et al., 2002	Iowa, USA	1,191		55–69	ER+	Alcohol, g/day
		225		55–69	ER−	Alcohol, g/day
		459		55–69	ER missing	Alcohol, g/day
		989		55–69	PR+	Alcohol, g/day
		353		55–69	PR−	Alcohol, g/day
		533		55–69	PR missing	Alcohol, g/day
Feigelson et al., 2003	USA	1,303	66,561	40–87		Alcohol, g/day
Tjønneland et al., 2003	Copenhagen and Aarhus, DEN	425	23,778	55–64		Alcohol, g/day
		425	23,778	55–64		Alcohol, g/day
Tjønneland et al., 2004	Copenhagen and Aarhus, DEN	423	23,683	55–64		Alcohol at baseline, g/day
		394	21,901	55–64		Cumulative alcohol, g/day
Horn-Ross et al., 2004	California, USA	1,742	103,460	22–84		
		295	172,715[e]		Premenopausal/ perimenopausal	Alcohol, g/day in past year
		973	195,223[e]		Postmenopausal	Alcohol, g/day in past year

Contrast	OR/RR (95% CL)	Covariate adjustment				
		Age	Smoking[a]	BMI/weight	Reproductive factors	Total energy intake
6+ vs never drinker	3.3 (1.18, 9.28)	Y	Y *(status)*	Y	N	N
6+ vs never drinker	3.55 (1.07, 11.79)	Y	Y *(status)*	Y	N	N
6+ vs never drinker	2.8 (0.35, 22.58)	Y	Y *(status)*	Y	N	N
≥5 vs none	0.6 (0.4, 1)	Y	Y (?)	Y	Y	N
≥5 vs none	0.8 (0.5, 1.2)	Y	N	Y	Y	N
≥15.0 vs 0	1.46 (1.04, 2.04)	Y	N	Y	Y	N
≥30 vs 0	1.22 (0.78, 1.9)	Y	Y *(status)*	N	Y	Y
≥30 vs 0	1.88 (0.96, 3.66)	Y	Y *(status)*	N	Y	Y
≥30 vs 0	0.86 (0.46, 1.59)	Y	Y *(status)*	N	Y	Y
≥30 vs nondrinker	1.72 (0.9, 3.28)	Y	Y *(status)*	Y	Y	Y
≥15 vs nondrinker	0.7 (0.5, 1.1)	Y	Y *(cont.)*	Y	Y	N
≥15 vs nondrinker	0.7 (0.5, 1.1)	Y	Y *(cont.)*	Y	Y	N
≥15 vs nondrinker	1 (0.4, 2.2)	Y	Y *(cont.)*	Y	Y	N
>20 vs none	1.23 (0.68, 2.21)	Y	N	Y	Y	N
≥10 vs none	1.2 (0.68, 2.11)	Y	N	Y	Y	N
>50 vs 0	1.7 (0.97, 2.98)	Y	N	N	Y	Y
10g (continuous)	1.06 (0.97, 1.15)	Y	N	N	Y	Y
10g (continuous)	1.05 (0.98, 1.11)	Y	N	N	Y	Y
≥10 vs none	1.1 (0.7, 1.6)	Y	N	Y	Y	N
≥10 vs none	0.8 (0.4, 1.5)	Y	N	Y	Y	N
≥10 vs none	0.8 (0.4, 1.4)	Y	N	Y	Y	N
≥10 vs none	1.1 (0.5, 2.4)	Y	N	Y	Y	N
≥20 vs none	1.33 (1.12, 1.58)	Y	N	Y	Y	N
≥20 vs nondrinkers	1.5 (1.2, 2)	Y	N	Y	Y	Y
>4 vs 0	1.07 (0.9, 1.26)	Y	Y *(status)*	Y	Y	Y
>4 vs 0	1.64 (1.14, 2.35)	Y	Y *(status)*	Y	Y	Y
>4 vs 0	1.02 (0.79, 1.32)	Y	Y *(status)*	Y	Y	Y
>4 vs 0	1.12 (0.93, 1.34)	Y	Y *(status)*	Y	Y	Y
>4 vs 0	1.28 (0.96, 1.71)	Y	Y *(status)*	Y	Y	Y
>4 vs 0	1 (0.79, 1.28)	Y	Y *(status)*	Y	Y	Y
15+ vs none	1.26 (1.04, 1.53)	Y	N	Y	Y	Y
>60 vs >0 to ≥6	1.35 (0.68, 2.66)	Y	N	Y	Y	N
10g (continuous)	1.1 (1.04, 1.16)	Y	N	Y	Y	N
10g (continuous)	1.1 (1.03, 1.16)	Y	N	Y	Y	N
10g (continuous)	1.02 (0.99, 1.05)	Y	N	Y	Y	N
≥20 vs <5	1.21 (0.76, 1.92)	Y	N	Y	Y	Y
≥20 vs <5	1.32 (1.06, 1.63)	Y	N	Y	Y	Y

(continues)

TABLE 3 (*Continued*)

Author, publication year	Study location	Cases n	Controls/cohort size n	Age range years (mean)	Subgroup	Alcohol variable
Petri et al., 2004	DEN	473	13,074	20+		Alcohol, drinks/wk
		76			Premenopausal	Alcohol, drinks/wk
		396			Postmenopausal	Alcohol, drinks/wk
Pooled cohort studies						
Smith-Warner et al., 1998	CAN, NED, SWE, USA	4,335	322,647	40–93		Alcohol, g/day
	CAN, NED, SWE, USA				Premenopausal	Alcohol, g/day
	CAN, NED, SWE, USA				Postmenopausal	Alcohol, g/day
Hamajima et al., 2002	World	9,693	38,431			Alcohol, g/day

[a]*(status)*: adjusted for smoking status, *(cont.)*: adjusted for cigarette smoking in pack-years or cigarettes/day as a continuous variable, *(cat.)*: Adjusted for cigarette smoking in categories of pack-years or cigarettes per day, (?): adjustment method not specified.

[b]Nested case-control design.

[c]Case-cohort design.

[d]Based on 88 cases with complete covariate information.

[e]Person-years.

both population based and hospital based, reported an increased risk of 1.69 for 40 g/day of alcohol (Howe et al., 1991). Another analysis based on 30 population-based case-control studies combining 38,675 cases and 45,794 controls reported an increased risk of 7.4% for 10 g/day of alcohol, corresponding to a relative risk of about 1.33 for 40 g/day of alcohol; these analyses also suggest that the pooled estimate from hospital-based case-control studies was comparable (7.1% for 10 g/day) to the population-based case-control studies. In comparable analyses, this group reported that for cohort studies, 10 g/day of alcohol increased risk of breast cancer by 5% (Hamajima et al., 2002). Another pooled analysis of cohort studies also noted increased breast cancer risk with increased alcohol intake that was of comparable magnitude (Smith-Warner et al., 1998).

As noted previously, studies that examine alcohol–cancer associations may be limited by a relatively narrow range of intake or a large proportion of nondrinkers. This may be particularly true for studies that focus on women. Thus, the magnitude of the association may be relatively small, as it is for breast cancer, on the order of 1.1–1.5 for one drink per day compared with nondrinkers. As a result, there has been interest in determining whether there may be particular subgroups of the population in which alcohol carries a more substantial risk. There have been studies that have stratified results by menopausal status, family history of breast cancer, BMI, stage of disease, hormone receptor status, and tumor histology, race, educational status, and other factors. Studies have also examined whether various aspects of alcohol use, such as age at onset of drinking, duration of drinking, or drinking habits at different ages, may result in differences in risk of breast cancer.

Among studies that have examined differences in risk of breast cancer due to alcohol by menopausal status or younger compared with older ages, some found that risk may be greater for premenopausal or early onset breast cancers (O'Connell et al., 1987; Rohan and McMichael, 1988; Friedenreich et al., 1993), some found a suggestion that risk was higher among postmenopausal breast cancers (Ewertz, 1991; Martin-Moreno et al., 1993; Holmberg et al., 1995; Longnecker et al., 1995a; Enger et al., 1999), and others found little difference in risk by menopausal status (Willett et al., 1987; Sneyd et al., 1991; Bowlin et al., 1997; Johnson et al., 2000; Mannisto et al., 2000; Rohan et al., 2000a; Wrensch et al., 2003; Horn-Ross et al., 2004). The Pooling Project of cohort studies found elevated risks for postmenopausal breast cancer, but not for premenopausal breast cancer (Smith-Warner et al., 1998). Among studies limited largely to premenopausal breast cancer or younger age-groups, alcohol was associated with increased risk in 7 (Sneyd et al., 1991; Viladiu et al., 1996; Weiss et al., 1996; Brinton et al., 1997; Swanson et al., 1997; Kropp et al., 2001; Althuis et al., 2003) of 11 (Webster et al., 1983; Sneyd et al., 1991; Rookus and van Leeuwen, 1994; Viladiu et al.,

		Covariate adjustment				
Contrast	OR/RR (95% CL)	Age	Smoking[a]	BMI/weight	Reproductive factors	Total energy intake
>27 vs <1	1.19 (0.58, 2.41)	Y	N	N	Y	N
>27 vs <1	3.49 (1.36, 8.99)	Y	N	N	Y	N
>27 vs <1	0.57 (0.18, 1.78)	Y	N	N	Y	N
≥60 vs nondrinkers	1.31 (0.86, 1.98) *p* trend <0.001	Y	Y *(status)*	Y	Y	Y
10g (continuous)	1 (0.87, 1.15)	Y	Y *(status)*	Y	Y	Y
10g (continuous)	1.05 (1.01, 1.1)	Y	Y *(status)*	Y	Y	Y
10g (continuous)	1.05 (1.016, 1.082)	Y	N	N	N	N

1996; Weiss et al., 1996; Brinton et al., 1997; Swanson et al., 1997; McCredie et al., 1998; Garland et al., 1999; Kropp et al., 2001; Althuis et al., 2003) studies, whereas those limited largely to older age-groups observed increased risk in 7 (Gapstur et al., 1992; Longnecker et al., 1995b; van den Brandt et al., 1995; Chen et al., 2002; Sellers et al., 2002; Li, 2003; Tjonneland et al., 2003) of 10 (Paganini-Hill, 1983; Gapstur et al., 1992; Graham et al., 1992; Longnecker et al., 1995b; van den Brandt et al., 1995; Royo-Bordonada et al., 1997; Chen et al., 2002; Sellers et al., 2002; Li, 2003; Tjonneland et al., 2003) studies. In one study that separated perimenopausal women from premenopausal or postmenopausal women, an increased risk of breast cancer due to alcohol was seen only in the perimenopausal group (Chu et al., 1989). In the pooled analysis, risk of breast cancer due to alcohol was slightly lower but similar for premenopausal or early-age-at-onset breast cancers compared with postmenopausal or later-age-at-onset cancers (Hamajima et al., 2002). Overall, there appears to be both mixed evidence that the effect of alcohol on breast cancer risk differs by menopausal status and consistent evidence that alcohol increases the risk of both premenopausal and postmenopausal breast cancers.

Fewer studies have examined whether the association between alcohol and breast cancer risk differs by other characteristics. Regarding BMI, some studies found that the alcohol-breast cancer association was stronger among women with higher body mass (Sneyd et al., 1991; Enger et al., 1999), whereas other studies suggested higher alcohol-related risk of breast cancer among leaner women (Willett et al., 1987; Gapstur et al., 1992; Longnecker et al., 1995b). Others have found little evidence of differences in the effect of alcohol by BMI (Chu et al., 1989; Rosenberg et al., 1990; van den Brandt et al., 1995; Rohan et al., 2000a; Horn-Ross et al., 2004). The Pooling Project of cohort studies found little evidence that BMI modified the alcohol–breast cancer association (Smith-Warner et al., 1998). Interactions with family history of breast cancer are similarly inconsistent, with some studies suggesting increased risk among those with a family history (Webster et al., 1983; Gapstur et al., 1992; van den Brandt et al., 1995); others suggesting an increased risk among those without a family history (Longnecker et al., 1995b); and others (Willett et al., 1987; Chu et al., 1989; Rohan et al., 2000a), including the Pooling Project of cohort studies (Smith-Warner et al., 1998), suggesting no modification by family history. Overall, the large Collaborative Study provided little evidence that family history, BMI, or other factors for which adequate data were available, including parity, age at first birth, breast-feeding, education, use of hormone replacement therapy, or hormonal contraceptive use, had an important effect in modifying the effect of alcohol on breast cancer risk (Hamajima et al., 2002). There was some suggestion in these pooled analyses that the effect may be weaker or null in nonwhite populations or studies conducted in developing countries, but the number of such studies was inadequate to provide much confidence in the pooled estimate of effect for alcohol in these subgroups (Hamajima et al., 2002). The few individual studies (Hiatt and Bawol, 1984; Hiatt et al., 1988; Brinton et al., 1997; Kinney et al., 2000; Baumgartner et al., 2002) that fit our criteria and reported results stratified by race or ethnicity also provided mixed evidence that this was an important effect modifier of the alcohol–breast cancer association, although some suggested the alcohol effect may be stronger among whites than nonwhites (Hiatt and Bawol, 1984; O'Connell et al., 1987).

One of the few factors to demonstrate consistently an interaction with alcohol on breast cancer risk is folate intake. It is well known that alcohol intake may compromise folic acid nutriture, and folic acid itself is involved in methyl-group donor reactions that are important in DNA metabolism (Bailey, 2003). For this reason, it has been of interest to determine whether the effect of alcohol on breast cancer risk may be particularly strong among women with low folate intake. One of the first studies to examine this hypothesis, the Nurses' Health Study (Zhang et al., 1999a), demonstrated such an interaction. Women with low folate intake and high alcohol consumption carried the highest risk of breast cancer, compared with women with higher folate or lower alcohol intake. Similar findings have been observed in other cohort studies (Rohan et al., 2000b; Sellers et al., 2001) and case-control studies (Negri et al., 2000), although one cohort study failed to find an interaction between alcohol and folate intakes and breast cancer risk (Feigelson et al., 2003). Another study examined blood folate levels and its interaction with alcohol intake on breast cancer risk and, consistent with the majority of studies that have examined dietary folate, found that low plasma levels of folate and high alcohol intake carry the highest risk of breast cancer (Zhang et al., 2003).

Several studies have examined whether the alcohol–breast cancer association differs by tumor characteristics. Among studies that have examined associations by hormone receptor status, several suggested higher risks associated with alcohol intake among ER-positive or ER-positive/PR-positive breast cancers (Nasca et al., 1994; Enger et al., 1999; Kinney et al., 2000; Li, 2003), whereas only one suggested that ER-negative tumors may carry a higher risk associated with alcohol (Sellers et al., 2002). There is some suggestion that alcohol-associated risk of hormone receptor–positive breast cancer may be further modified by body mass (Enger et al., 1999) or use of hormone replacement therapy (Gapstur et al., 1995), but few studies have examined these interactions. Nasca et al. (1994) and Li (2003) provide some evidence that the alcohol-associated risk may be somewhat higher for lobular as compared with ductal breast cancers. Weiss et al. (1996) and Swanson et al. (1997) suggest breast cancers diagnosed at more advanced stages may also be more strongly associated with alcohol, although another study that examined this found somewhat higher risks for localized rather than regional or distant breast cancers (Kinney et al., 2000). In a case-only study, Vaeth and Satariano (1998) noted that women diagnosed with regional breast cancer were more likely to consume alcohol frequently compared with those diagnosed with localized breast cancer. In one of the few studies to compare alcohol-associated risks for *in situ* and invasive breast cancers, it was noted that alcohol was associated with increased risk for both breast carcinomas (Trentham-Dietz et al., 2000).

Case-control studies that have examined the alcohol–breast cancer association have focused primarily on recent prediagnosis intake among cases, as well as a comparable time period or current intake among controls. Cohort studies have typically used alcohol intake assessed at a baseline data collection point as their primary measure of exposure, although when follow-up assessments have been available, studies have also examined the effect of using more recent or averaged alcohol intake (e.g., see Schatzkin et al., 1989). A number of studies have examined other aspects of alcohol drinking, including age at which alcohol drinking was first initiated (Nasca et al., 1990; Holmberg et al., 1995; Bowlin et al., 1997; Royo-Bordonada et al., 1997; Swanson et al., 1997; Mannisto et al., 2000; Marcus et al., 2000; Wrensch et al., 2003; Tjonneland et al., 2004), alcohol intake at different ages (Harvey et al., 1987; Young, 1989; Graham et al., 1991; Longnecker et al., 1995a; Swanson et al., 1997; Garland et al., 1999; Kropp et al., 2001; Horn-Ross et al., 2004; Tjonneland et al., 2004), duration of alcohol intake (Nasca et al., 1990; Graham et al., 1992; Holmberg et al., 1995; Longnecker et al., 1995a; Bowlin et al., 1997; Swanson et al., 1997), or average or total lifetime intake (Nasca et al., 1990; Longnecker et al., 1995a,b; Swanson et al., 1997; Garland et al., 1999; Kinney et al., 2000; Mannisto et al., 2000; Tjonneland et al., 2004). In general, exposures that are indicative of greater alcohol intake are associated with greater risk of breast cancer (e.g., longer duration of intake compared with never drinkers), whereas findings related to other nuances of alcohol exposure are inconsistent. For example, some studies suggest later age at onset of alcohol drinking may be associated with increased risk (Wrensch et al., 2003) or the effect of alcohol on breast cancer may be stronger among those who started drinking at a later age (Nasca et al., 1990), others suggest earlier age at onset increases risk (Holmberg et al., 1995; Royo-Bordonada et al., 1997), and others largely show no association with age at onset (Bowlin et al., 1997; Swanson et al., 1997; Mannisto et al., 2000; Marcus et al., 2000; Tjonneland et al., 2004).

There has been growing interest in whether the effect of alcohol on risk of breast cancer is modified by polymorphisms in selected genes that encode for enzymes involved in alcohol metabolism. At least two studies (Freudenheim et al., 1999; Hines et al., 2000) have examined polymorphisms in the ADH3 gene and its effect on the alcohol–breast cancer association. In one of these studies (Freudenheim et al., 1999), alcohol increased risk only among premenopausal women with the ADH31-1 (fast oxidizing) genotype (OR = 3.6, 95% CL: 1.5–8.8). However, no substantive difference in the modest alcohol–breast cancer association according to ADH3 genotype was observed in the other study, in either premenopausal or postmenopausal women (Hines et al., 2000). In a case-only study in Germany, Sturmer et al. (2002) examined whether an RFLP in exon 3 of ADH2 demonstrated an interaction with alcohol intake in breast cancer risk. Cases who consumed larger amounts of alcohol had a lower prevalence of the $\beta1/\beta2$ (more rapid) ADH2 polymorphism. A case-control study in Korea reported on interactions between ALDH2 polymorphisms and alcohol on breast cancer risk (Choi et al., 2003); no interaction was observed. This study also examined alcohol interactions with polymorphisms in CYP 2E1 c2 allele (Choi et al., 2003) and CYP 19 and CYP 1B1 (Lee et al., 2003). Women who carried the CYP 2E1 c2 allele and drank alcohol at least once per month had a relative risk of breast cancer of 1.9 (0.99, 3.83), compared with women who carried the c1/c1 genotype and drank less than one drink per month (Choi et al., 2003). There was no increased risk with either the c2 genotype or more frequent alcohol drinking alone. No association was observed between CYP 1B1 genotypes and breast cancer risk, whereas there appeared to be an interaction between alcohol drinking and CYP19 genotypes on breast cancer risk (Lee et al., 2003). Women who drank at least once per month and had the CYP19 arg/cys or cys/cys genotype had an increased relative risk of 3.3 (1.7, 6.5) compared with women with the CYP19 arg/arg genotype who drank less than once per month (Lee et al., 2003). Unlike CYP 2E1, for which alcohol is a known substrate, CYP19 (aromatase) is thought to be involved primarily in estrogen synthesis from testosterone and androstenedione. Two studies examined the interactions of GSTM1 and GSTT1 polymorphisms and alcohol on breast cancer risk (Park et al., 2000). In one study, presence of both GSTM1 null and GSTT1 null genotypes increased risk of breast cancer overall compared with no null polymorphisms for both GST isoforms, and the increased risk was stronger among ever drinkers than never drinkers (Park et al., 2000). The specific effect of alcohol by GST polymorphisms was not reported, although the crude OR for ever drinkers compared with never drinkers was 3.9 for women with two null genotypes, 1.5 for women with one null, and 1.5 for women with no nulls (Park et al., 2000). In the other study, alcohol was associated with increased breast cancer risk among women with the GSTM1-A genotype, but not among women with GSTM1-B or who were GSTM1 null (Zheng et al., 2003). In contrast, alcohol increased risk among women who were GSTT1 null and not among women with the GRTT1 positive (Zheng et al., 2003). One study examined alcohol intake and p53 mutations (Freudenheim et al., 2004). There was some suggestion that alcohol was associated with increased risk of breast cancer only among women with p53+ mutations. However, this was confined to premenopausal women and was stronger for alcohol intake 20 years ago than alcohol intake 10 years ago; no impact was seen for recent intake.

A number of studies have examined whether the type of alcoholic beverage—beer, wine, or liquor—has differential effects on breast cancer risk. A few studies reported that beer or alcohol intake from beer is associated directly with breast cancer risk (Willett et al., 1987; Ranstam and Olsson, 1995; Kropp et al., 2001), whereas other studies (Webster et al., 1983; Harvey et al., 1987; Adami et al., 1988; Hiatt et al., 1988; Rohan and McMichael, 1988; Chu et al., 1989; Rosenberg et al., 1990; Ewertz, 1991; Graham et al., 1991; Sneyd et al., 1991; Friedenreich et al., 1993; Martin-Moreno et al., 1993; Freudenheim et al., 1995; Longnecker et al., 1995b; van den Brandt et al., 1995; Bowlin et al., 1997; Swanson et al., 1997; Zhang et al., 1999b; Kinney et al., 2000; Rohan et al., 2000a; Horn-Ross et al., 2002; Tjonneland et al., 2003; Petri et al., 2004) did not. Significant increased risks of breast cancer were observed for wine intake in several studies (Willett et al., 1987; Toniolo et al., 1989; Friedenreich et al., 1993; Martin-Moreno et al., 1993; Bowlin et al., 1997; Horn-Ross et al., 2002; Tjonneland et al., 2003), but not in others (Webster et al., 1983; Adami et al., 1988; Hiatt et al., 1988; Rohan and McMichael, 1988; Rosenberg et al., 1990; Ewertz, 1991; Graham et al., 1991; Howe et al., 1991; Sneyd et al., 1991; Freudenheim et al., 1995; Longnecker et al., 1995b; Ranstam and Olsson, 1995; van den Brandt et al., 1995; Swanson et al., 1997; Zhang et al., 1999b; Kinney et al., 2000; Rohan et al., 2000a; Kropp et al., 2001; Petri et al., 2004). For liquor or spirits, significantly increased risks were observed in a few studies (Willett et al., 1987; Rohan and McMichael, 1988; Martin-Moreno et al., 1993; Longnecker et al., 1995b; Bowlin et al., 1997; Horn-Ross et al., 2002; Petri et al., 2004), and not in others (Webster et al., 1983; Adami et al., 1988; Hiatt et al., 1988; Chu et al., 1989; Rosenberg et al., 1990; Ewertz, 1991; Graham et al., 1991; Sneyd et al., 1991; Friedenreich et al., 1993; Freudenheim et al., 1995; Ranstam and Olsson, 1995; van den Brandt et al., 1995; Zhang et al., 1999b; Kinney et al., 2000; Rohan et al., 2000a; Kropp et al., 2001; Tjonneland et al., 2003). Many of the studies that did not report significant increased risks with specific alcoholic beverages nonetheless reported risk estimates higher than 1. In general, it appears that the ability to observe direct associations with specific beverages is in part a reflection of the prevalence of drinking that beverage. A greater proportion of women tend to be wine drinkers rather than beer or liquor drinkers, a probable source of the differences in the qualitative results for these three classes of alcoholic beverages.

Overall, there is little evidence that source of alcohol results in different effects on breast cancer risk.

In addition to the studies that we include in our tables or reference in this text, a substantial number of studies that did not fit our criteria have also been conducted examining the association of alcohol with breast cancer. Selected examples include studies with hospital-based (Rosenberg et al., 1982; Katsouyanni et al., 1994) or clinic-based (Smith et al., 1994) case-control studies, case-control studies that combine hospital and population controls (Iscovich et al., 1989), studies using cancer controls (e.g., Williams and Horm, 1977; Kato et al., 1989) or other unique designs (Haile et al., 1996; Vachon et al., 2001), prospective studies focusing on mortality from breast cancer (Garfinkel et al., 1988; Fuchs et al., 1995; Feigelson et al., 2001), or smaller studies with few cases (van't Veer et al., 1989; Pawlega, 1992; Thorand et al., 1998). Although results from these studies vary, overall, as evidenced by reviews or meta-analyses that may have included such studies (Longnecker, 1994; Holman et al., 1996; Ellison et al., 2001; Hamajima et al., 2002), this additional literature adds to the evidence that alcohol intake is associated with increased risk of breast cancer.

Colorectal Cancer

In 1988, the evidence linking alcohol and colorectal cancer was deemed inconclusive (IARC, 1988). Nine years later, in the WCRF Report (WCRF, 1997) alcohol was found to "possibly increase the risk of cancers of the colon and rectum," with an estimated elevation in risk of 1.5–2 for those consuming >30–50 g of alcohol per day compared with nondrinkers. The strength of the association was suggested to be somewhat weaker in two meta-analyses (Longnecker et al., 1990; Bagnardi et al., 2001b), in which an elevated risk of cancer of the colon and rectum of about 10% was found for those consuming ~24 g/day. For drinkers of 50 g/day, the summary risk estimate was 1.21 (1.11, 1.32) for colon cancer and 1.17 (1.06, 1.30) for rectal cancer (Bagnardi et al., 2001b). A review of the literature from 1957 to 1991 concluded that the relationship between alcohol and colorectal cancer tended to be more frequently found for males than for females, for rectal cancer than for colon cancer, and for beer than for other alcoholic beverages (Kune and Vitetta, 1992). However, the specificity of the alcohol–colorectal link to beer has been challenged (Potter, 1999).

Population-based case-control studies and cohort studies meeting our inclusion criteria are listed in Tables 4A and 4B. Because of the claim that the association may be different for colon cancer and rectal cancer, only studies examining the two sites separately were included in our tables. As shown in Table 4A, most studies have suggested an increased risk of colon cancer associated with alcohol consumption (Potter and McMichael, 1986; Kune et al., 1987; Klatsky et al., 1988; Longnecker, 1990; Peters et al., 1992; Meyer and White, 1993; Newcomb et al., 1993; Giovannucci et al., 1995; Le Marchand et al., 1997; Fuchs et al., 2002; Sharpe et al., 2002; Otani et al., 2003; Shimizu et al., 2003; Cho et al., 2004). However, other studies failed to find an association (Graham et al., 1988; Slattery et al., 1990; Gerhardsson de Verdier et al., 1993; Goldbohm et al., 1994; Harnack et al., 2002; Pedersen et al., 2003). In two of the negative studies (Slattery et al., 1990; Harnack et al., 2002), alcohol consumption was fairly low, which may have affected their ability to detect a relationship. For rectal cancer (Table 4B), studies have also fairly consistently suggested an elevated risk with alcohol intake (Kune et al., 1987; Freudenheim et al., 1990; Longnecker, 1990; Newcomb et al., 1993; Goldbohm et al., 1994; Sharpe et al., 2002; Otani et al., 2003; Pedersen et al., 2003; Cho et al., 2004). In contrast, some studies reported no association (Gerhardsson de Verdier et al., 1993; Hoshiyama et al., 1993; Le Marchand et al., 1997). As previously suggested, a stronger relationship for the rectum than for the colon has been suggested in a few studies (Freudenheim et al., 1990; Longnecker, 1990; Newcomb et al., 1993; Goldbohm et al., 1994; Otani et al., 2003; Pedersen et al., 2003). However, similar estimates were obtained for both sites in meta-analyses of published studies (Longnecker et al., 1990; Bagnardi et al., 2001b) (Table 2). Furthermore, a pooled analysis of eight cohort studies (Cho et al., 2004) reported essentially identical risk estimates for cancers of the colon and rectum.

Whether the relationship is stronger in males than females, as previously suggested, is unclear. As shown in Tables 4A and 4B, studies have generally reported a stronger association in males than females, but this could be due to lower drinking levels among women. Furthermore, there is no conclusive evidence pointing to a stronger effect for beer than other alcoholic beverages, particularly for colon cancer. For rectal cancer, a number of studies have suggested a stronger effect for beer (Kune et al., 1987; Longnecker, 1990; Gerhardsson de Verdier et al., 1993; Newcomb et al., 1993; Freudenheim et al., 2003; Cho et al., 2004). However, in other studies there was an indication of a stronger association for liquor (Goldbohm et al., 1994; Sharpe et al., 2002). It is possible that the association with alcohol appears to be stronger for the alcoholic beverage most commonly consumed in the study population. In the pooled analysis of cohort studies (Cho et al., 2004), which included populations from several countries, there was a 50–60% increase in rectal cancer for drinkers of 15 g/day of beer or wine. However, liquor consumption was unrelated to rectal cancer (Table 4B).

Given the inconsistencies in results, there has been some interest in examining the relationship by anatomical subsite within the colon (Peters et al., 1992; Le Marchand et al., 1997; Sharpe et al., 2002; Cho et al., 2004). However, studies have varied in their classification of tumors and no conclusive pattern has emerged. Nevertheless, the finding of

TABLE 4A Population-Based Case-Control and Cohort Studies Examining Alcohol Consumption and Colon Cancer

Author, publication year	Study location	Cases n	Controls/ cohort size n	Age range years (mean)	Subgroup	Alcohol variable	Contrast	OR/RR (95% CL)	Covariate adjustment				
									Age	Smoking[a]	BMI/ weight	Total energy intake	Physical activity
Total alcohol													
Case-control studies													
Kune et al., 1987	Australia	202	398	20–80+	Males	Recent intake	High vs low quartile	0.96 (not shown, $p > 0.05$)	Y	N	N	N	N
		190	329	20–80+	Females	Recent intake	High vs low quartile	1.41 (not shown, $p > 0.05$)	Y	N	N	N	N
Graham et al., 1988	Western NY, US	428	428					No association					
Longnecker, 1990	Various locations, US	251	992	>31	Males	Consumption 5 years ago	>5 drinks/day vs none	1.8 (1, 3.2)	Y	Y (?)	N	N	N
						Consumption 20 years ago	>5 drinks/day vs none	1.2 (0.6, 1.9)	Y	Y (?)	N	N	N
Slattery et al., 1990	Utah, US	112	185	40–79	Males	Recent intake	>15 g/week vs none	1.1 (0.5, 2.4)	Y	N	Y	Y	N
Peters et al., 1992	California, USA	419	419	45–69	Males	Recent intake	≥100 drinks/mo vs none	1.84 (1.15, 2.96)	Y	N	Y	N	Y
		327	327	45–69	Females	Recent intake	≥100 drinks/mo vs none	1.42 (0.61, 3.32)	Y	N	Y	N	Y
Gerhardsson de Verdier et al., 1993	Sweden	163	236		Males	Recent intake	≥30 vs 0–9.9 g/day	1.2 (0.6, 2.4)	Y	Y (?)	Y	Y	Y
		189	276		Females	Recent intake	≥10 vs 0–9.9 g/day	0.4 (0.2, 1)	Y	Y(?)	Y	Y	Y
Meyer and White, 1993	Washington State, USA	424 men and women	414 men and women	30–62	Males	Recent intake	≥30 g/day vs none	2.58 (not shown)	Y	N	N	N	N
					Females	Recent intake	≥30 g/day vs none	2.46 (not shown)	Y	N	N	N	N
Newcomb et al., 1993	Wisconsin, USA	779	2,315	<75	Females	Recent intake	≥11 drinks/wk vs none	1.35 (0.84, 2.16)	Y	N	Y	N	N
Le Marchand et al., 1997	Hawaii, USA	197	698	<84	Males, right colon	Lifetime intake	>83 drink-years vs none	2 (1.1, 3.6)	Y	Y *(cont.)*	Y	Y	Y

(continues)

TABLE 4A (*Continued*)

Author, publication year	Study location	Cases n	Controls/ cohort size n	Age range years (mean)	Subgroup	Alcohol variable	Contrast	OR/RR (95% CL)	Covariate adjustment: Age	Smoking[a]	BMI/ weight	Total energy intake	Physical activity
		270	698	<84	Males, left colon	Lifetime intake	>83 drink-years vs none	1.3 (0.7, 2.1)	Y	Y *(cont.)*	Y	Y	Y
		164	494	<84	Females, right colon	Lifetime intake	>29 drink-years vs none	1.4 (0.5, 3.9)	Y	Y *(cont.)*	Y	Y	Y
		194	494	<84	Females, left colon	Lifetime intake	>29 drink-years vs none	0.8 (0.4, 1.8)	Y	Y *(cont.)*	Y	Y	Y
Sharpe et al., 2002	Canada	176	500	35–70	Males, proximal colon	Recent intake	Daily drinker of ≥5 drinks/day vs never drank daily	1.6 (0.9, 2.9)	Y	Y (?)	N	N	N
		179	500	35–79	Males, distal colon	Recent intake	Daily drinker of ≥5 drinks/day vs never drank daily	3 (1.6, 5.6)	Y	Y (?)	N	N	N
		176	500	35–70	Males, proximal colon	Lifetime intake	>125 drink-years vs never drank daily	1.5 (0.8, 2.7)	Y	Y (?)	N	N	N
		179	500	35–79	Males, distal colon	Lifetime intake	>125 drink-years vs never drank daily	2.5 (1.3, 4.6)	Y	Y (?)	N	N	N
Cohort studies													
Klatsky et al., 1988	USA (Kaiser Permanente)	173	10,593		Males and females[b]	Recent intake	≥3 drinks/day vs never drinker	1.85 (0.95, 3.61)	Y	Y *(cont.)*	Y	N	N
		111			Females	Recent intake	≥3 drinks/day vs never drinker	2.56 (1.03, 6.4)	Y	Y *(cont.)*	Y	N	N
Goldbohm et al., 1994	The Netherlands	217	3,500	55–69	Males and females[b]	Recent intake	≥30 g/day vs none	1.1 (0.3, 3.6)	Y	Y (?)	Y	Y	N
Giovannucci et al., 1995	USA (Health Professionals Study)	205	47,931	40–75	Males	Recent intake	>2 vs 0–0.25 drinks/day	2.07 (1.29, 3.32)	Y	Y *(cont.)*	Y	Y	Y

Harnack et al., 2002[c]	USA (Iowa Women's Health Study)	598	41,836	55–69	Females	Recent intake	≥20 vs <20 g/day	1.08 (0.72, 1.62)	Y	Y *(cat.)*	Y	Y	N
Pedersen et al., 2003	Denmark	411	29,132	23–95	Males and females[b]	Recent intake	≥41 vs <1 drinks/week	0.8 (0.5, 1.5)	Y	Y *(status)*	Y	N	N
Otani et al., 2003	Japan	299	90,004	40–69	Males	Regular drinking	>300 g/wk vs none	1.9 (1.4, 2.7)	Y	Y *(status)*	Y	N	Y
Shimizu et al., 2003	Japan	105	13,392	>35	Males	Recent intake	>36.7 g/day vs none	2.67 (1.06, 6.76)	Y	Y (?)	Y	N	N
Cho et al., 2004	US (Pooling Project)[d]	3,291	489,979		Males and females	Recent intake	≥45 g/day vs none	1.45 (1.14, 1.83)	Y	Y *(cat.)*	Y	Y	Y
Beer													
Case-control studies													
Longnecker, 1990	Various locations, USA	251	992	>31	Males	Consumption 5 years ago	Continuous (5 drinks/day)	2.3 (1.4, 3.8)	Y	Y (?)	N	N	N
						Consumption 20 years ago	Continuous (5 drinks/day)	1.3 (0.8, 1.9)	Y	Y (?)	N	N	N
Gerhardsson de Verdier et al., 1993	Sweden	163	236		Males	Recent intake	≥10 vs 0–9.9 g/day	1.2 (0.6, 2.5)	Y	Y (?)	Y	Y	Y
		189	276		Females	Recent intake	≥10 vs 0–9.9 g/day	0.9 (0.5, 1.5)	Y	Y (?)	Y	Y	Y
Meyer and White, 1993	Washington State, USA	424 men and women	414 men and women	30–62	Males	Recent intake	≥30 g/day vs none	1.44 (not shown)	Y	N	N	N	N
					Females	Recent intake	≥30 g/day vs none	3.58 (not shown)	Y	N	N	N	N
Sharpe et al., 2002	Canada	176	500	35–70	Males, proximal colon	Recent intake	Daily drinker of ≥5 drinks/day vs never drank daily	2.4 (1.2, 4.6)	Y	Y (?)	N	N	N
		179	500	35–79	Males, distal colon	Recent intake	Daily drinker of ≥5 drinks/day vs never drank daily	2.4 (1.2, 5)	Y	Y (?)	N	N	N
Cohort studies													
Goldbohm et al., 1994	The Netherlands	217	3,500	55–69	Males and females[b]	Recent intake	≥5 g/day vs none	0.9 (0.4, 2.1)	Y	Y (?)	Y	Y	N
Pedersen et al., 2003	Denmark	411	29,132	23–95	Males and females[b]	Recent intake	≥14 vs 0 drinks/week	1.2 (0.8, 1.7)	Y	Y *(status)*	Y	N	N

(continues)

TABLE 4A (*Continued*)

Author, publication year	Study location	Cases n	Controls/ cohort size n	Age range years (mean)	Subgroup	Alcohol variable	Contrast	OR/RR (95% CL)	Covariate adjustment: Age	Smoking[a]	BMI/ weight	Total energy intake	Physical activity
Cho et al., 2004	USA (Pooling Project)[d]	3,291	489,979		Males and females	Recent intake	≥15 g/day vs none	1.38 (1.05, 1.82)	Y	Y *(cat.)*	Y	Y	Y
Wine													
Case-control studies													
Longnecker, 1990	Various locations, USA	251	992	>31	Males	Consumption 5 years ago	Continuous (5 drinks/ day)	1.6 (0.4, 6.3)	Y	Y (?)	N	N	N
						Consumption 20 years ago	Continuous (5 drinks/ day)	0.5 (0.1, 2.2)	Y	Y (?)	N	N	N
Gerhardsson de Verdier et al., 1993	Sweden	163	236		Males	Recent intake	≥10 vs 0–9.9 g/day	1.9 (0.6, 5.8)	Y	Y (?)	Y	Y	Y
		189	276		Females	Recent intake	≥10 vs 0–9.9 g/day	0.6 (0.4, 0.9)	Y	Y (?)	Y	Y	Y
Meyer and White, 1993	Washington State, USA	424 men and women	414 men and women	30–62	Males	Recent intake	≥30 g/day vs none	2.36 (not shown)	Y	N	N	N	N
					Females	Recent intake	≥30 g/day vs none	0.83 (not shown)	Y	N	N	N	N
Sharpe et al., 2002	Canada	176	500	35–70	Males, proximal colon	Recent intake	Daily drinker of ≥5 drinks/day vs never drank daily	0.7 (0.2, 2.4)	Y	Y (?)	N	N	N
		179	500	35–79	Males, distal colon	Recent intake	Daily drinker of ≥5 drinks/day vs never drank daily	1.1 (0.4, 3.6)	Y	Y (?)	N	N	N
Cohort studies													
Goldbohm et al., 1994	The Netherlands	217	3,500	55–69	Males and females[b]	Recent intake	≥5 g/day vs none	1 (0.6, 1.6)	Y	Y (?)	Y	Y	N
Pedersen et al., 2003	Denmark	411	29,132	23–95	Males and females[b]	Recent intake	≥14 vs <1 drinks/wk	0.5 (0.2, 1)	Y	Y *(status)*	Y	N	N
Cho et al., 2004	USA (Pooling Project)[d]	3,291	489,979		Males and females	Recent intake	≥15 g/day vs none	1.33 (1, 1.77)	Y	Y *(cat.)*	Y	Y	Y

Liquor													
Case-control studies													
Potter and McMichael, 1986	Australia	121	241	30–74	Males	Recent intake	Continuous (glass/wk)	1.08 (1.02, 1.15)	Y	N	N	N	N
Longnecker, 1990	Various locations, USA	251	992	>31	Males	Consumption 5 years ago	Continuous (5 drinks/day)	1.1 (0.7, 2)	Y	Y (?)	N	N	N
						Consumption 20 years ago	Continuous (5 drinks/day)	1.3 (0.7, 2.1)	Y	Y (?)	N	N	N
Gerhardsson de Verdier et al., 1993	Sweden	163	236		Males	Recent intake	≥10 vs 0–9.9 g/day	1.1 (0.6, 2)	Y	Y (?)	Y	Y	Y
		189	276		Females	Recent intake	≥10 vs 0–9.9 g/day	0.8 (0.2, 2.8)	Y	Y (?)	Y	Y	Y
Meyer and White, 1993	Washington State, USA	424 men and women	414 men and women	30–62	Males	Recent intake	≥30 g/day vs none	3.08 (not shown)	Y	N	N	N	N
					Females	Recent intake	≥30 g/day vs none	2.87 (not shown)	Y	N	N	N	N
Sharpe et al., 2002	Canada	176	500	35–70	Males, proximal colon	Recent intake	Daily drinker of ≥5 drinks/day vs never drank daily	2 (0.9, 4.7)	Y	Y (?)	N	N	N
		179	500	35–79	Males, distal colon	Recent intake	Daily drinker of ≥5 drinks/day vs never drank daily	1.3 (0.5, 3.3)	Y	Y (?)	N	N	N
Cohort studies													
Goldbohm et al., 1994	The Netherlands	217	3,500	55–69	Males and females[b]	Recent intake	≥7.5 g/day vs none	0.6 (0.3, 1.3)	Y	Y (?)	Y	Y	N
Pedersen et al., 2003	Denmark	411	29,132	23–95	Males and females[b]	Recent intake	≥14 vs <1 drinks/wk	1 (0.5, 1.9)	Y	Y *(status)*	Y	N	N
Cho et al., 2004	USA (Pooling Project)[d]	3,291	489,979		Males and females	Recent intake	≥15 g/day vs none	1.06 (0.86, 1.3)	Y	Y *(cat.)*	Y	Y	Y

[a]*(status)*, adjusted for smoking status; *(cont.)*, adjusted for cigarette smoking in pack-years or cigarettes/day as a continuous variable; *(cat.)*, Adjusted for cigarette smoking in categories of pack-years or cigarettes per day; (?), adjustment method not specified.

[b]Adjusted for gender.

[c]An earlier report from the same study (Iowa Women's Health Study) by Gapstur et al. (1994) with a shorter period of follow-up and fewer cases suggested a weak inverse association between light drinking and distal colon cancer, specific to wine.

[d]Includes the Iowa Women's Health Study, the Health Professionals Follow-up Study, and the Nurses' Health Study.

TABLE 4B Population-Based Case-Control and Cohort Studies Examining Alcohol Consumption and Rectal Cancer

Author, publication year	Study location	Cases n	Controls/ cohort size n	Age range Years (mean)	Subgroup	Alcohol variable	Contrast	OR/RR (95% CL)	Covariate adjustment: Age	Smoking[a]	BMI/ weight	Total energy intake	Physical activity
Total alcohol													
Case-control studies													
Kune et al., 1987	Australia	186	398	20–80+	Males	Recent intake	High vs low quartile	1.54 (not shown, p > 0.05)	Y	N	N	N	N
		137	329	20–80+	Females	Recent intake	High vs low quartile	0.93 (not shown, p > 0.05)	Y	N	N	N	N
Longnecker, 1990	Various locations, USA	393	992	>31	Males	Consumption 5 years ago	>5 drinks/day vs none	1.5 (0.9, 2.5)	Y	Y (?)	N	N	N
						Consumption 20 years ago	>5 drinks/day vs none	1.9 (1.2, 3)	Y	Y (?)	N	N	N
Freudenheim et al., 1990	Western NY, USA	277	277	>40	Males	Lifetime intake	High vs Low quartile	1.8 (1.12, 2.89)	Y	N	N	N	N
		145	145	>40	Females	Lifetime intake	High vs Low tertile	1.88 (0.98, 3.58)	Y	N	N	N	N
Newcomb et al., 1993	Wisconsin, USA	779	2,315	<75	Females	Recent intake	≥11 drinks/wk vs none	1.88 (1.02, 3.45)	Y	N	Y	N	N
Hoshiyama et al., 1993	Japan	102	623	40–69	Males and females[b]	Recent intake	Daily drinking of ≥50 ml/day vs never	0.6 (0.3, 1.3)	Y	N	N	N	N
						Lifetime intake	≥500 liters/ lifetime vs nondrinker	0.9 (0.4, 2.2)	Y	N	N	N	N
Gerhardsson de Verdier et al., 1993	Sweden	107	236		Males	Recent intake	≥30 vs 0–9.9 g/day	1.2 (0.5, 2.7)	Y	Y (?)	Y	Y	Y
		110	276		Females	Recent intake	≥10 vs 0–9.9 g/day	0.9 (0.4, 1.9)	Y	Y (?)	Y	Y	Y
Le Marchand et al., 1997	Hawaii, USA	221	698	<84	Males	Lifetime intake	>83 drink-years vs none	1 (0.6, 1.8)	Y	Y *(cont.)*	Y	Y	Y
		129	494	<84	Females	Lifetime intake	>29 drink-years vs none	1.6 (0.6, 4.5)	Y	Y *(cont.)*	Y	Y	Y

Sharpe et al., 2002[c]	Canada	230	500	35–70	Males	Recent intake	Daily drinker of ≥5 drinks/day vs never drank daily	2 (1.1, 3.6)	Y	Y (?)	N	N	N
						Lifetime intake	>125 drink-years vs never drank daily	2.1 (1.2, 3.7)	Y	Y (?)	N	N	N
Cohort studies													
Goldbohm et al., 1994	The Netherlands	113	3,500	55–69	Males and females[b]	Recent intake	≥30 g/day vs none	2 (0.4, 9.6)	Y	Y (?)	Y	Y	N
Harnack 2002	US (Iowa Women's Health Study)	123	41,836	55–69	Females	Recent intake	≥20 g/day vs <20	0.91 (0.39, 2.1)	Y	Y *(cat.)*	Y	Y	N
Pedersen et al., 2003	Denmark	202	29,132	23–95	Males and females[b]	Recent intake	≥41 vs <1 drinks/wk	2.2 (1, 4.6)	Y	Y *(status)*	Y	N	N
Otani et al., 2003	Japan	148	90,004	40–69	Males	Regular drinking	>300 g/wk vs none	2.4 (1.5, 4)	Y	Y *(status)*	Y	N	Y
Cho et al., 2004	USA (Pooling Project)[d]	3,291	489,979		Males and females	Recent intake	≥45 g/day vs none	1.49 (1.04, 2.12)	Y	Y *(cat.)*	Y	Y	Y
Beer													
Case-control studies													
Longnecker, 1990	Various locations, USA	393	992	>31	Men	Consumption 5 years ago	Continuous (5 drinks/ day)	1.8 (1.2, 2.8)	Y	Y (?)	N	N	N
						Consumption 20 years ago	Continuous (5 drinks/ day)	1.5 (1.1, 2.1)	Y	Y (?)	N	N	N
Freudenheim et al., 1990	Western NY, US	277	277	>40	Males	Lifetime intake	High vs low quartile	1.86 (1.13, 3.06)	Y	N	N	N	N
		145	145	>40	Females	Lifetime intake	High vs low tertile	1.25 (0.69, 2.26)	Y	N	N	N	N
Gerhardsson de Verdier et al., 1993	Sweden	107	236		Males	Recent intake	≥10 vs 0–9.9 g/day	1.4 (0.6, 3.1)	Y	Y (?)	Y	Y	Y
		110	276		Females	Recent intake	≥10 vs 0–9.9 g/day	0.9 (0.5, 1.6)	Y	Y(?)	Y	Y	Y
Sharpe et al., 2002	Canada	230	500	35–70	Males	Recent intake	Daily drinker of ≥5 drinks/day vs never drank daily	1.5 (0.8, 3)	Y	Y (?)	N	N	N
Cohort studies													
Goldbohm et al., 1994	The Netherlands	113	3,500	55–69	Males and females[b]	Recent intake	≥5 g/day vs none	1.7 (0.6, 4.8)	Y	Y (?)	Y	Y	N

(continues)

TABLE 4B (*Continued*)

Author, publication year	Study location	Cases n	Controls/ cohort size n	Age range Years (mean)	Subgroup	Alcohol variable	Contrast	OR/RR (95% CL)	Covariate adjustment: Age	Smoking[a]	BMI/ weight	Total energy intake	Physical activity
Pedersen et al., 2003	Denmark	202	29,132	23–95	Males and females[b]	Recent intake	≥14 vs 0 drinks/wk	1.4 (0.8, 2.4)	Y	Y *(status)*	Y	N	N
Cho et al., 2004	USA (Pooling Project)[d]	3,291	489,979		Males and females	Recent intake	≥15 g/day vs none	1.59 (1.12, 2.25)	Y	Y *(cat.)*	Y	Y	Y
Wine													
Case-control studies													
Longnecker, 1990	Various locations, USA	393	992	>31	Men	Consumption 5 years ago	Continuous (5 drinks/ day)	1.4 (0.4, 5.1)	Y	Y (?)	N	N	N
						Consumption 20 years ago	Continuous (5 drinks/ day)	1.1 (0.4, 3.3)	Y	Y (?)	N	N	N
Freudenheim et al., 1990	Western NY, USA	277	277	>40	Males	Lifetime intake	High vs low quartile	0.87 (0.55, 1.38)	Y	N	N	N	N
		145	145	>40	Females	Lifetime intake	High vs low tertile	0.94 (0.58, 1.67)	Y	N	N	N	N
Gerhardsson de Verdier et al., 1993	Sweden	107	236		Males	Recent intake	≥10 vs 0–9.9 g/day	1 (0.2, 4.2)	Y	Y (?)	Y	Y	Y
		110	276		Females	Recent intake	≥10 vs 0–9.9 g/day	1 (0.6, 1.6)	Y	Y (?)	Y	Y	Y
Cohort studies													
Goldbohm et al., 1994	The Netherlands	113	3,500	55–69	Males and females[b]	Recent intake	≥5 g/day vs none	1.4 (0.4, 9.6)	Y	Y (?)	Y	Y	N
Pedersen et al., 2003	Denmark	202	29,132	23–95	Males and females[b]	Recent intake	≥14 vs 0 drinks/wk	0.9 (0.7, 2.9)	Y	Y *(status)*	Y	N	N
Cho et al., 2004	USA (Pooling Project)[d]	3,291	489,979		Males and females	Recent intake	≥15 g/day vs none	1.55 (1.11, 2.17)	Y	Y *(cat.)*	Y	Y	Y
Liquor													
Case-control studies													
Longnecker, 1990	Various locations, USA	393	992	>31	Men	Consumption 5 years ago	Continuous (5 drinks/ day)	1 (0.6, 1.7)	Y	Y (?)	N	N	N
						Consumption 20 years	Continuous (5 drinks/	0.9 (0.6, 1.5)	Y	Y (?)	N	N	N

						ago	day)						
Freudenheim et al., 1990	Western NY, USA	277	277	>40	Males	Lifetime intake	High vs low quartile	1.23 (0.78, 1.94)	Y	N	N	N	N
		145	145	>40	Females	Lifetime intake	High vs low tertile	1.33 (0.76, 2.35)	Y	N	N	N	N
Gerhardsson de Verdier et al., 1993	Sweden	107	236		Males	Recent intake	≥10 vs 0–9.9 g/day	1.1 (0.5, 2.1)	Y	Y (?)	Y	Y	Y
		110	276		Females	Recent intake	≥10 vs 0–9.9 g/day	0.7 (0.2, 3.7)	Y	Y (?)	Y	Y	Y
Sharpe et al., 2002	Canada	230	500	35–70	Males	Recent intake	Daily drinker of ≥5 drinks/day vs never drank daily	1.9 (0.9, 3.9)	Y	Y (?)	N	N	N
Cohort studies													
Goldbohm et al., 1994	The Netherlands	113	3500	55–69	Males	Recent intake	≥7.5 g/day vs none	2.7 (1, 7.5)	Y	Y (?)	Y	Y	N
Pedersen et al., 2003	Denmark	202	29,132	23–95	Males and females[b]	Recent intake	≥14 vs 0 drinks/wk	1.3 (0.6, 3)	Y	Y *(status)*	Y	N	N
Cho et al., 2004	USA (Pooling Project)[d]	3,291	489,979		Males and females	Recent intake	≥15 g/day vs none	1.1 (0.85, 1.41)	Y	Y *(cat.)*	Y	Y	Y

[a]*(status)*, adjusted for smoking status; *(cont.)*, adjusted for cigarette smoking in pack-years or cigarettes/day as a continuous variable; *(cat.)*, Adjusted for cigarette smoking in categories of pack-years or cigarettes per day; (?), adjustment method not specified.

[b]Adjusted for gender.

[c]Analyses on wine are also presented in the manuscript, but they were based on very few cases and are not included here.

[d]Includes the Iowa Women's Health Study, the Health Professionals Follow-up Study, and the Nurses' Health Study.

a stronger effect for the distal colon than for the proximal colon found in a case-control study (Sharpe et al., 2002) and a pooled analysis of cohort studies (Cho et al., 2004) is intriguing and deserves further exploration. Interestingly, alcohol, and particularly beer, has been found to be more strongly associated with colorectal polyps that overexpress p53 than those that do not, and polyps overexpressing p53 were reported to be more likely to be located in the distal colon and rectum (Terry et al., 2003).

Alcohol consumption has been found to exacerbate the elevation in colorectal cancer risk associated with having a family history of the disease at least in two studies (Le Marchand et al., 1999; Fuchs et al., 2002). Because alcohol is known to act as an antagonist of methyl-group metabolism, there has been some interest in exploring its interaction with folate and methionine intakes. In the Health Professionals Follow-up Study, an increased risk of colon cancer was found for those with high alcohol and low folate and methionine intakes, particularly for carcinomas of the distal colon (Giovannucci et al., 1995). In the pooled analysis of eight prospective studies (Cho et al., 2004), the observed relationship with alcohol was limited to those in the lowest tertile of methionine intake, whereas there was no indication of a folate–alcohol interaction.

Some studies have examined the possible influence of genetic susceptibility to the effect of alcohol on colorectal cancer. For example, an interaction of alcohol with polymorphisms in methylenetetrahydrofolate reductase (MTHFR) and methionine synthase (Ma et al., 1999), two enzymes involved in the generation of *S*-adenosylmethionine, the primary methyl donor for DNA methylation, has been reported. The role of polymorphisms in enzymes involved in alcohol metabolism has also been explored. In a nested case-control study within the Physician's Health Study (Chen et al., 2001), ADH3 polymorphism was unrelated to colorectal cancer, but there was a suggestion of an interaction with alcohol intake. An association and effect modification of the alcohol effect by ALDH2 genotype was reported in two studies conducted in Japan (Murata et al., 1999; Matsuo et al., 2002).

Cancers with a Controversial Association with Alcohol

Lung Cancer

A relationship between lung cancer and alcohol has been suggested in a number of studies (Bandera et al., 2001), but it has generally been attributed to residual confounding by cigarette smoking. Studying this relationship is indeed a challenge given the strong relationship between cigarette smoking and lung cancer and the fact that smoking and drinking behaviors tend to correlate, at least in some cultures. The 1988 IARC Report concluded that alcohol and lung cancer were "not causally related," whereas the 1997 WCRF Report concluded that the association was "possible." A meta-analysis (Bagnardi et al., 2001a) including three case-control studies and three cohort studies found a modest increase in risk of 4% and 8% for approximately four drinks per day and eight drinks per day, respectively. Another more comprehensive meta-analysis (Korte et al., 2002) reported overall pooled smoking-adjusted risk estimates on the basis of highest consumption category in each study of 1.19 (95% CI: 1.11, 1.29) for 11 cohort studies and 1.39 (95% CI: 1.06, 1.83) for 7 case-control studies. This meta-analysis also found that smoking-adjusted risk estimates in hospital-based case-control studies (pooled OR = 1.69, 95% CI: 1.35, 2.12) tended to be of greater magnitude than those reported in population-based case-control studies (pooled OR = 1.09 (95% CI: 0.63, 1.88). This could be explained in part by the fact that two of the hospital-based studies included in these analyses were conducted in Uruguay (De Stefani et al., 1993) and Turkey (Dosemeci et al., 1997) and participants reported much higher levels of intake than in other studies.

Population-based studies evaluating the association between alcohol and lung cancer meeting our inclusion criteria are shown in Table 5. Of the 10 studies identified, 6 (Bandera et al., 1992; Potter et al., 1992; Carpenter et al., 1998; Prescott et al., 1999; Djousse et al., 2002; Freudenheim et al., 2003) reported elevated risk for at least one type of alcohol, whereas there was no evidence of an association in other studies (Mayne et al., 1994; Bandera et al., 1997; Woodson et al., 1999; Hu et al., 2002). For example, one study conducted in California (Carpenter et al., 1998) found a relationship only for liquor, whereas in the other studies conducted in western New York (Bandera et al., 1992; Freudenheim et al., 2003) and Iowa (Potter et al., 1992), the association with alcohol was mostly explained by beer consumption. It is uncertain whether there is a true different effect by each alcohol type or an association tends to be found with the most prevalent alcoholic beverage consumed in that population. As illustrated in Table 5, studies examining the effect by alcoholic beverage type have not offered consistent results, but in general they tend to suggest an increased risk with beer, and perhaps liquor, and a decreased lung cancer risk associated with moderate wine consumption. This is of particular interest because wine drinking has been shown to be unrelated to smoking (Prescott et al., 1999). It also points out the need for evaluating the role of the different alcoholic beverages rather than that of total alcohol.

To avoid the issue of residual confounding by smoking, studies in never smokers could be particularly informative. However, evaluating the relationship among non/never smokers has been difficult given the low incidence of lung cancer and low prevalence of drinking in this population. In general, studies evaluating the relationship among nonsmokers have presented conflicting results (Bandera et al.,

TABLE 5 Population-Based Case-Control and Cohort Studies Examining Alcohol Consumption and Lung Cancer

Author, publication year	Study location	Cases n	Controls/ cohort size n	Age range Years (mean)	Subgroup	Alcohol variable	Contrast	OR/RR (95% CL)	Covariate adjustment				
									Age	Smoking[a]	ETS	Total energy intake	Other dietary factors
Total alcohol													
Case-control studies													
Bandera et al., 1992	Western New York, USA	280	564	35–79	M, heavy smokers	Recent intake	≥22 drinks/ month vs less	1.6 (1, 2.4)	Y	Y *(cont.)*	N	N	Y
Carpenter, 1998	California, USA	261	615	40–84	M and F	Recent intake	≥3 drinks/ day vs 0–3 drinks/mo	1.07 (0.46, 2.47)	Y	Y *(cat.)*	N	N	Y
Hu et al., 2002	Canada	161	483	20– >70	F, never smoker	Recent intake	>1 servings/wk vs none	0.8 (0.5, 1.2)	Y	N	N	N	N
Freudenheim et al., 2003	Western New York, USA	111	1546	35–79	M and F	Recent intake	>2.5 L vs none	1.35 (0.54, 3.41)	Y	Y *(cont.)*	Y	Y	Y
						Lifetime intake	>82 L vs none	1.13 (0.47, 2.72)	Y	Y *(cont.)*	Y	Y	Y
Cohort studies													
Woodson et al., 1999	Finland, ATBC study population	1,059	27,111	50–69	M, smokers	Recent intake	High vs low drinking quartile (>27.7 g/day vs <5.2)	1 (0.8, 1.2)	Y	Y *(cont.)*	N	Y	Y
Prescott et al., 1999	Denmark	480	15,107	>20	M	Recent intake	>41 vs <1 drinks/wk	1.57 (1.06, 2.33)	Y	Y *(cat.)*	N	N	N
		194	13,053	>20	F	Recent intake	>41 vs <1 drinks/wk	0.8 (0.11, 5.79)	Y	Y *(cat.)*	N	N	N
Bandera et al., 1997	New York State, USA	395	27,544	<40– >80	M	Recent intake	>48 drinks/mo vs none	1.15 (0.8, 1.65)	Y	Y *(cont.)*	N	Y	N
		130	20,456	<40– >80	F	Recent intake	High vs low tertile	1.01 (0.64, 1.58)	Y	Y *(cont.)*	N	Y	N
Djousse et al., 2002	Framingham, US	269	8969	28–62	M and F	Recent intake	>24 g/day vs none	1.3 (0.7, 2.4)	Y	Y *(cont.)*	N	N	N
Beer													
Case-control studies													
Bandera et al., 1992	Western New York, USA	280	564	35–79	M	Recent intake	≥113 drinks/mo vs none	1.95 (1, 3.7)	Y	Y *(cont.)*	N	N	Y
Mayne et al., 1994	New York State, USA	413	413	20–80	M and F,[b] nonsmokers	"Usual intake"	High vs low quartiles (cut points not shown)	1.18 (CI not presented, includes one)	Y	Y (cont.)	Y	N	N

(*continues*)

TABLE 5 *(Continued)*

Author, publication year	Study location	Cases n	Controls/ cohort size n	Age range Years (mean)	Subgroup	Alcohol variable	Contrast	OR/RR (95% CL)	Covariate adjustment: Age	Smoking[a]	ETS	Total energy intake	Other dietary factors
Carpenter et al., 1998	California, USA	261	615	40–84	M and F	Recent intake	≥1 drinks/ day vs 0–3 drinks/mo	0.86 (0.44, 1.75)	Y	Y *(cat.)*	N	N	Y
Hu et al., 2002	Canada	161	483	20 to >70	F, never smoker	Recent intake	>0.5 bottles or cans/week vs none	0.5 (0.2, 1.1)	Y	N	N	N	N
Freudenheim et al., 2003	Western New York, USA	111	1,546	35–79	M and F	Recent intake	>1.6 liters vs none	1.67 (0.96, 2.92)	Y	Y *(cont.)*	Y	Y	Y
						Lifetime intake	>62 liters vs none	1.36 (0.82, 2.27)	Y	Y *(cont.)*	Y	Y	Y
Cohort studies													
Woodson et al., 1999	Finland, ATBC study population	1,059	27,111	50–69	M, smokers	Recent intake	High vs low drinking quartile (>11.6 g/day vs <1.6)	0.9 (0.7, 1.1)	Y	Y *(cont.)*	N	Y	Y
Potter et al., 1992[c]	Iowa, US	109	1,900	55–69	W	Recent intake	≥1 drink/ day vs less	2 (1.02, 3.8)	Y	Y *(cat.)*	N	N	N
Prescott et al., 1999	Denmark	480	15,107	>20	M	Recent intake	>13 vs <1 drinks/week	1.36 (1.02, 1.82)	Y	Y *(cat.)*	N	N	N
		194	13,053	>20	F	Recent intake	>13 vs <1 drinks/week	1.49 (0.7, 3.13)	Y	Y *(cat.)*	N	N	N
Wine													
Case-control studies													
Bandera et al., 1992	Western New York,	280	564	35–79	M	Recent intake	≥2 drinks/mo vs none	0.7 (0.5, 1.1)	Y	Y *(cont.)*	N	N	N
Carpenter et al., 1998	California, USA	261	615	40–84	M and F	Recent intake	≥1 drinks/day vs 0–3 drinks/mo	0.79 (0.34, 1.86)	Y	Y *(cat.)*	N	N	Y
Hu et al., 2002	Canada	161	483	20 to >70	F, never smoker	Recent intake	>0.5 glasses/wk vs none	0.7 (0.4, 1.2)	Y	N	N	N	N
Freudenheim et al., 2003	Western New York, USA	111	1,546	35–79	M and F	Recent intake	>1 liter vs none	0.72 (0.4, 1.29)	Y	Y *(cont.)*	Y	Y	Y
						Lifetime intake	>19 liters vs none	0.80 (0.51, 1.25)	Y	Y *(cont.)*	Y	Y	Y

Cohort studies													
Woodson et al., 1999	Finland, ATBC study population	1,059	27,111	50–69	M, smokers	Recent intake	High vs low drinking (>2.1 g/day vs<2)	0.8 (0.6, 1.1)	Y	Y *(cont.)*	N	Y	Y
Prescott et al., 1999	Denmark	480	15,107	>20	M	Recent intake	>13 vs <1 drinks/wk	0.44 (0.22, 0.86)	Y	Y *(cat.)*	N	N	N
		194	13,053	>20	F	Recent intake	>13 vs <1 drinks/wk	0.18 (0.03, 1.33)	Y	Y *(cat.)*	N	N	N
Liquor													
Case-control studies													
Bandera et al., 1992	Western New York, USA	280	564	35–79	M	Recent intake	≥9 drinks/mo vs none	1.1 (0.7, 1.6)	Y	Y *(cont.)*	N	N	N
Carpenter et al., 1998	California, US	261	615	40–84	M and F	Recent intake	≥1 drinks/day vs 0–3 drinks/mo	1.87 (1.02, 3.42)	Y	Y *(cat.)*	N	N	Y
Hu et al., 2002	Canada	161	483	20 to >70	F, never smoker	Recent intake	>0.5 shots/wk vs none	1.1 (0.6, 2.1)	Y	N	N	N	N
Freudenheim et al., 2003	Western New York, USA	111	1,546	35–79	M and F	Recent intake	>1 liter vs none	0.87 (0.51, 1.48)	Y	Y *(cont.)*	Y	Y	Y
						Lifetime intake	>28 liters vs none	0.79 (0.52, 1.2)	Y	Y *(cont.)*	Y	Y	Y
Cohort studies													
Woodson et al., 1999	Finland, ATBC study population	1,059	27,111	50–69	M, smokers	Recent intake	High vs low drinking quartile (>22.8 g/day vs <2.6)	1.1 (0.9, 1.3)	Y	Y *(cont.)*	N	Y	Y
Potter et al., 1992[c]	Iowa, USA	109	1,900	55–69	W	Recent intake	≥1 drink/day vs none	1.1 (0.6, 2.3)	Y	Y *(cat.)*	N	N	N
Prescott et al., 1999	Denmark	480	15,107	>20	M	Recent intake	>13 vs <1 drinks/wk	1.46 (0.99, 2.14)	Y	Y *(cat.)*	N	N	N
		194	13,053	>20	F	Recent intake	>13 vs <1 drinks/wk	0.67 (0.21, 2.18)	Y	Y *(cat.)*	N	N	N

[a] *(status)*, adjusted for smoking status; *(cont.)*, adjusted for cigarette smoking in pack-years or cigarettes/day as a continuous variable; *(cat.)*, adjusted for cigarette smoking in categories of pack-years or cigarettes per day; (?), adjustment method not specified.

[b] Unadjusted by gender.

[c] Nested case-control design.

ETS, environmental tobacco smoke; M, males; F, females.

2001; Korte et al., 2002). The two population-based studies conducted among nonsmokers (Mayne et al., 1994) or never smokers (Hu et al., 2002) did not find an association.

If alcohol has an effect in lung carcinogenesis, current drinking rather than lifetime or past drinking appears to be the relevant period (Bandera et al., 2001). The effect by gender and histological type has been evaluated in a number of studies with inconclusive results (Bandera et al., 2001). The few studies that evaluated the effect of alcohol on lung cancer by levels of vitamin A, carotenoids, or vegetable consumption reported with some consistency a stronger association for the lower category of consumption (Bandera et al., 2001). Because one of the proposed mechanisms of action of alcohol is through direct damaging effects of acetaldehyde on the lung tissue, the role of ADH genotype has received some attention. Yang et al. (2002) found that ADH3*1 genotype was associated with higher pulmonary ADH activity and acetaldehyde–DNA adduct levels in Caucasian lung tissue. In contrast, a case-control study (Freudenheim et al., 2003) did not find elevated risk of lung cancer for those with the ADH31-1 genotype, the variant that has been shown to catalyze alcohol to acetaldehyde more rapidly (Bosron and Li, 1986). Furthermore, there was no indication in this study (Freudenheim et al., 2003) of an interaction of alcohol consumption and ADH genotype on lung cancer risk, but these analyses were based on small numbers.

Endometrial Cancer

The relationship between alcohol and endometrial cancer has been examined in relatively few epidemiological studies. The 1988 IARC Report concluded that there were insufficient data to judge the evidence, and the 1997 WCRF Report did not even mention the possible role of alcohol on endometrial cancer risk. In general, epidemiological studies have not offered much support for the association, although there are some aspects of this potential relationship that warrant further examination (Bandera et al., 2003). Population-based studies examining this relationship (Webster and Weiss, 1989; Gapstur et al., 1993; Swanson et al., 1993; Goodman et al., 1997a,b; Newcomb et al., 1997; Terry et al., 1999; Jain et al., 2000a; Jain et al., 2000b; McCann et al., 2000; Littman et al., 2001; Weiderpass and Baron, 2001), shown in Table 6, have reported risk estimates for total alcohol fluctuating around the null value. However, these studies were confronted with very limited range of alcohol consumption. Hospital-based studies conducted in Italy reporting much higher drinking levels reported an elevated risk (Bandera et al., 2003). A meta-analysis including two cohort studies and four case-control studies reported a 20% increased risk for an alcohol consumption of 100 g/day, whereas for 25 or 50 g/day, there was no association (Bagnardi et al., 2001a). Studies evaluating alcohol type suggested a reduced risk for moderate intake of beer and wine, whereas liquor intake appeared to increase risk. This may be explained by the beneficial effects of antioxidants and phytoestrogens in beer and wine when consumed at moderate levels (Bandera et al., 2003). Overall, it seems that at moderate levels, alcohol consumption does not increase endometrial cancer risk or it may even be beneficial. The role of heavy alcohol consumption is not clear. Furthermore, important aspects of this relationship that have received limited attention and need to be considered in studies are the possible effect modification by menopausal status and use of estrogen replacement therapy.

Ovarian Cancer

Compared with other cancer sites, the relationship between alcohol and ovarian cancer has not been widely investigated. The 1988 IARC Report concluded that there was no association between alcohol and ovarian cancer, whereas the relationship was not even mentioned in the 1997 WCRF/AICR Report (WCRF, 1997). A meta-analysis (Bagnardi et al., 2001b) including five case-control studies computed elevated pooled ORs (95% CIs) of 1.11 (1.0–1.24), 1.23 (1.01–1.54), and 1.53 (1.03–2.32) for 25, 50, and 100 g of alcohol per day, respectively (Table 2). Another meta-analysis including seven population-based studies (Webb et al., 2004) computed a pooled risk estimate of 0.72 (95% CI: 0.54–0.97) for the highest level of consumption reported in each study.

Results from population-based studies examining the relationship between alcohol and ovarian cancer risk are displayed in Table 7. A decreased risk associated with drinking levels of fewer than three drinks per day was suggested by several case-control studies (Gwinn et al., 1986; Godard et al., 1998; Goodman and Tung, 2003; Webb et al., 2004) and in the Iowa Women's Health Study (Kushi et al., 1999). The remaining case-control study suggested an elevated risk for drinkers of more than three drinks per day (Kuper et al., 2000). There was no indication of an association among participants in the Netherlands Cohort Study (Schouten et al., 2004).

Two case-control studies (Goodman and Tung, 2003; Modugno et al., 2003) have suggested that the effect of alcohol on ovarian cancer risk might vary by histology, perhaps explaining in part the inconsistent results. One of these studies (Modugno et al., 2003) reported an elevated risk only for mucinous tumors, with an OR for those consuming more than 24 g/day of ethanol of 1.93 (95 % CI: 1.02, 3.65). In contrast, another study (Goodman and Tung, 2003) found similar risk estimates for mucinous and nonmucinous tumors but reported a strong protective effect for total alcohol only for invasive epithelial ovarian cancer (OR = 0.36; 95% CI: 0.19, 0.70) and an elevated risk for borderline serous tumors associated with the consumption of spirits (OR = 2.66, 95% CI: 1.46, 4.85). However, a large case-control study found an inverse association between

TABLE 6 Population-Based Case–Control and Cohort Studies Examining Alcohol Consumption and Endometrial Cancer

								Covariate adjustment				
Author, publication year	**Study location**	**Cases n**	**Controls/ Cohort size n**	**Age range Years (mean)**	**Alcohol variable**	**Contrast**	**OR/RR (95% CL)**	**Age**	**Smoking[a]**	**BMI/ weight**	**Total energy intake**	**HRT/ERT use**
Total alcohol												
Case-control studies												
Webster and Weiss, 1989	USA	351	2,247	20–54	Recent intake	0 vs ≥150 g/wk	1.83 (1.11, 3.01)	Y	Y *(status)*	N	N	N
Newcomb et al., 1997	Wisconsin, USA	739	2,313	40–79	Recent intake	≥14 vs 0 drinks/wk	1.27 (0.78, 2.07)	Y	Y *(status)*	Y	N	Y
Goodman et al., 1997a	Hawaii, USA	332	511	18–84	Recent intake	>17.8 vs 0 g/day	0.8	Y	N	Y	Y	N
Jain et al., 2000a	Ontario, Canada	391	298		Recent intake	>8.3 vs 0 g/day	0.72 (0.52, 0.99)	Y	Y *(status)*	Y	Y	Y
McCann et al., 2000	Western NY, USA	232	639	40–85	Recent intake	>9 vs ≤0.5 g/day	1 (0.5, 1.8)	Y	Y *(cont.)*	Y	Y	Y
Littman et al., 2001	Washington State, USA	679	944	45–74	Recent intake	≥1 vs 0 drinks/day	0.95 (0.66, 1.4)	Y	Y *(status)*	Y	Y	Y
Weiderpass and Baron, 2001	Sweden	704	2,859	50–74	Recent intake	>4 vs 0 g/day	0.92 (0.7, 1.2)	Y	Y *(status)*	Y	N	Y
Swanson et al., 1993	USA	400	297	20–74	Intake during adulthood	>4 vs 0 drinks/wk	0.72 (0.39, 1.35)	Y	Y *(status)*	Y	N	N
Newcomb et al., 1997	Wisconsin, USA	739	2,313	40–79	Intake as young adult	≥14 vs 0 drinks/wk	1 (0.58, 1.73)	Y	Y *(status)*	Y	N	Y
Cohort studies												
Gapstur et al., 1993	Iowa, USA	167	24,848	55–69	Recent intake	≥4 vs 0 g/day	1 (0.7, 1.6)	Y	N	Y	N	Y
Terry et al., 1999	Sweden	133	11,659		Recent intake	>4 vs 0 drinks/wk	1.3 (0.6, 2.8)	Y	N	Y	N	N
Jain et al., 2000b	Canada	221	56,837	40–59	Recent intake	H vs L quartile	1 (0.67, 1.5)	Y	Y *(status)*	Y	Y	Y
Beer												
Case-control studies												
Goodman et al., 1997b	Hawaii, USA	332	511	18–84	Recent intake	>154 vs 0 g of beer/day	0.54 (0.18, 1.62)	Y	N	Y	Y	Y
Cohort studies												
Gapstur et al., 1993	Iowa, USA	167	24,848	55–69	Recent intake	≥4 vs 0 g/day	0.7 (0.3, 1.6)	Y	N	Y	N	Y

(continues)

TABLE 6 (*Continued*)

Author, publication year	Study location	Cases n	Controls/ Cohort size n	Age range Years (mean)	Alcohol variable	Contrast	OR/RR (95% CL)	Covariate adjustment				
								Age	Smoking[a]	BMI/ weight	Total energy intake	HRT/ERT use
Wine												
Case-control studies												
Goodman et al., 1997a	Hawaii, USA	332	511	18–84	Recent intake	>3.95 vs 0 g of wine/day	0.7	Y	N	Y	Y	N
Cohort studies												
Gapstur et al., 1993	Iowa, USA	167	24,848	55–69	Recent intake	≥4 vs 0 g/day	0.8 (0.4, 1.7)	Y	N	Y	N	Y
Liquor												
Case-control studies												
Goodman et al., 1997a	Hawaii, USA	332	511	18–84	Recent intake	>37 vs 0 g of liquor/day	2.1	Y	N	Y	Y	N
Cohort studies												
Gapstur et al., 1993	Iowa, USA	167	24,848	55–69	Recent intake	≥4 vs 0 g/day	1.4 (0.8, 2.4)	Y	N	Y	N	Y

[a]*(status)*, adjusted for smoking status; *(cont.)*, adjusted for cigarette smoking in pack-years or cigarettes/day as a continuous variable; *(cat.)*, Adjusted for cigarette smoking in categories of pack-years or cigarettes per day; (?), adjustment method not specified.

TABLE 7 Population-Based Case-Control and Cohort Studies Examining Alcohol Consumption and Ovarian Cancer

Author, publication year	Study location	Cases n	Controls/ cohort size n	Age range years (mean)	Subgroup	Alcohol variable	Contrast	OR/RR (95% CL)	Covariate adjustment				
									Age	Smoking[a]	BMI/weight/ WHR	Total energy	OC use
Total alcohol													
Case-control studies													
Gwinn et al., 1986	USA (multicenter)	433	2,915	20–54		Recent intake	≥250 g/wk vs never drank	0.5 (0.2, 0.9)	Y	Y *(?)*	N	N	Y
Godard et al., 1998	Canada	170	170	20–84		Recent intake	≥10 drinks/wk vs none	0.46 (0.13, 1.69)	Y	N	N	N	Y
Kuper et al., 2000	Massachusetts and New Hampshire, USA	549	516	<30–70		Recent intake	>3 drinks/day vs 0	1.35 (0.8, 2.26)	Y	Y *(cont.)*	Y	N	Y
Modugno et al., 2003	Delaware Valley, USA	761	1,352	20–69	Mucinous tumors (n = 112)	Current	≥24 g/day vs never	1.93 (1.02, 3.65)	Y	Y *(status)*	N	N	Y
						Former	≥24 g/day vs never	0.64 (0.22, 1.85)	Y	Y *(status)*	N	N	Y
					Nonmucinous tumors (n = 649)	Current	≥24 g/day vs never	0.88 (0.57, 1.37)	Y	Y *(status)*	N	N	Y
						Former	≥24 g/day vs never	1.29 (0.83, 2)	Y	Y *(status)*	N	N	Y
Goodman and Tung, 2003	Hawaii and Los Angeles, USA	558	607	>18		Current	≥14 drinks/wk vs never	0.84 (0.55, 1.28)	Y	N	N	N	Y
						Drink-years	≥25 vs never	0.88 (0.58, 1.34)	Y	N	N	N	Y
					Invasive tumors (n = 355)	Current	≥14 drinks/wk vs never	0.36 (0.19, 0.7)	Y	N	N	N	Y
						Drink-years	≥25 vs never	0.59 (0.35, 1)	Y	N	N	N	Y
Webb et al., 2004	Australia	696	786	18–79		Recent intake	≥2 drinks/day vs none	0.49 (0.3, 0.81)	Y	Y *(status)*	Y	N	Y
Cohort studies													
Kushi et al., 1999	Iowa, USA	139	29,083	55–69		Recent intake	>10 g/day vs 0	0.49 (0.24, 1.01)	Y	Y *(cont.)*	Y	Y	N
Schouten et al., 2004	The Netherlands	214	62,573	55–69		Recent intake	>15 g/day vs none	0.92 (0.55, 1.54)	Y	Y (status)	Y	Y	Y

(continues)

TABLE 7 *(Continued)*

Author, publication year	Study location	Cases n	Controls/ cohort size n	Age range years (mean)	Subgroup	Alcohol variable	Contrast	OR/RR (95% CL)	Covariate adjustment: Age	Smoking[a]	BMI/weight/ WHR	Total energy	OC use
Beer													
Case-control studies													
Gwinn et al., 1986	USA (multicenter)	433	2,915	20–54		Recent intake	≥150 g/wk vs never drank	0.9 (0.5, 1.8)	Y	Y (?)	N	N	Y
Modugno et al., 2003	Delaware Valley, USA	761	1,352	20–69	Mucinous tumors (n = 112)	Current	≥24 g/day vs never	2.53 (0.86, 7.42)	Y	Y *(status)*	N	N	Y
						Former	≥24 g/day vs never	1.25 (0.4, 3.93)	Y	Y *(status)*	N	N	Y
					Nonmucinous tumors (n = 649)	Current	≥24 g/day vs never	0.92 (0.39, 2.14)	Y	Y *(status)*	N	N	Y
						Former	≥24 g/day vs never	1.24 (0.63, 2.45)	Y	Y *(status)*	N	N	Y
Goodman and Tung, 2003	Hawaii and Los Angeles, US	558	607	>18		Current	≥14 drinks/wk vs never	0.93 (0.53, 1.64)	Y	N	N	N	Y
						Drink-years	≥25 vs never	1.05 (0.62, 1.77)	Y	N	N	N	Y
Webb et al., 2004	Australia	696	786	18–79		Recent intake	≥1 drink/day vs none	1.26 (0.65, 2.46)	Y	Y *(status)*	Y	N	Y
Wine													
Case-control studies													
Gwinn et al., 1986	USA (multicenter)	433	2,915	20–54		Recent intake	≥150 g/wk vs never drank	0.7 (0.3, 1.4)	Y	Y (?)	N	N	Y
Modugno et al., 2003	Delaware Valley, USA	761	1,352	20–69	Mucinous tumors (n = 112)	Current	0–24 g/day vs never	0.59 (0.28, 1.24)	Y	Y *(status)*	N	N	Y
						Former	0–24 g/day vs never	0.71 (0.29, 1.74)	Y	Y *(status)*	N	N	Y
					Nonmucinous tumors (n = 649)	Current	≥24 g/day vs never	0.92 (0.38, 2.23)	Y	Y *(status)*	N	N	Y
						Former	≥24 g/day vs never	0.71 (0.25, 2.04)	Y	Y *(status)*	N	N	Y
Goodman and Tung, 2003	Hawaii and Los Angeles, USA	558	607	>18		Current	≥14 drinks/wk vs never	0.81 (0.52, 1.26)	Y	N	N	N	Y
						Drink-years	≥25 vs never	1.07 (0.71, 1.63)	Y	N	N	N	Y

Webb et al., 2004	Australia	696	786	18–79		Recent intake	≥1 drink/day vs none	0.56 (0.33, 0.93)	Y	Y *(status)*	Y	N	Y
Cohort studies													
Schouten et al., 2004	The Netherlands	214	62,573	55–69		Recent intake	>15 g/day vs none	1 (0.57, 1.75)	Y	Y (status)	Y	Y	Y
Liquor													
Case-control studies													
Gwinn et al., 1986	US (multicenter)	433	2,915	20–54		Recent intake	≥150 g/week vs never drank	0.6 (0.3, 1.1)	Y	Y (?)	N	N	Y
Modugno et al., 2003	Delaware Valley, USA	761	1,352	20–69	Mucinous tumors (n = 112)	Current	≥24 g/day vs never	8.83 (2.89, 27.01)	Y	Y *(status)*	N	N	Y
						Former	≥24 g/day vs never	1.07 (0.3, 3.79)	Y	Y *(status)*	N	N	Y
					Nonmucinous tumors (n = 649)	Current	≥24 g/day vs never	1.53 (0.58, 4)	Y	Y *(status)*	N	N	Y
						Former	≥24 g/day vs never	1.42 (0.79, 2.57)	Y	Y *(status)*	N	N	Y
Goodman and Tung, 2003	Hawaii and Los Angeles, USA	558	607	>18		Current	≥14 drinks/wk vs never	1.07 (0.64, 1.78)	Y	N	N	N	Y
						Drink-years	≥25 vs never	0.69 (0.42, 1.14)	Y	N	N	N	Y
Webb et al., 2004	Australia	696	786	18–79		Recent intake	≥1 drink/day vs none	1.07 (0.59, 1.95)	Y	Y *(status)*	Y	N	Y

[a]*(status)*, adjusted for smoking status; *(cont.)*, adjusted for cigarette smoking in pack-years or cigarettes/day as a continuous variable; *(cat.)*, adjusted for cigarette smoking in categories of pack-years or cigarettes per day; (?), adjustment method not specified.

BMI, body mass index; WHR, waist-to-hip ratio.

alcohol consumption and ovarian cancer, which was of similar magnitude for all histological types (Webb et al., 2004). Although the findings are not conclusive, they suggest that future ovarian cancer studies should examine the effect by histological type. Overall, these results, though inconsistent, tend to indicate that moderate levels of alcohol drinking might be associated with a reduced risk of ovarian cancer. As Table 7 shows, there is no consistent evidence that any particular source of alcohol may be more beneficial or detrimental than another, but in general there is a tendency for studies to show reduced risk for wine consumption and elevated risk estimates for beer and liquor. The high content of antioxidants and resveratrol in wine has been proposed to explain these findings (Webb et al., 2004). If alcohol drinking is related to ovarian cancer, current rather than lifetime drinking seems to be the relevant factor (Goodman and Tung, 2003).

Prostate Cancer

Both the IARC (1988) and WCRF/AICR (1997) Reports concluded that there was no association between alcohol consumption and prostate cancer risk. A review of the literature reported no association with moderate consumption of alcohol (less than three drinks per day), whereas an elevated risk for drinking more than seven drinks per day was suggested (Dennis and Hayes, 2001). Two independent meta-analyses (Dennis, 2000; Bagnardi et al., 2001b) found an ~20% increased risk associated with drinking levels of about four drinks per day (Table 2).

The results of population-based studies examining the role of alcohol on prostate cancer and meeting our inclusion criteria are displayed in Table 8. As shown in the table, results are inconsistent. An increased risk was suggested in several case-control studies (Andersson et al., 1996; Hayes et al., 1996; Breslow et al., 1999; Sharpe and Siemiatycki, 2001) and cohort studies (Breslow et al., 1999; Putnam et al., 2000; Sesso et al., 2001). However, other studies failed to find an association (Hiatt et al., 1994; Le Marchand et al., 1994; Gronberg et al., 1996; Key et al., 1997; Jain et al., 1998; Schuurman et al., 1999; Villeneuve et al., 1999; Ellison, 2000; Albertsen and Gronbaek, 2002). A cohort study (Breslow et al., 1999) reported an inverse association for distant past heavy drinking, but this finding was based on a small number of subjects and has not been confirmed nor evaluated in other investigations to our knowledge. Nevertheless, this aspect of drinking might be important to consider in future studies. The studies evaluating the effect by alcoholic beverage type did not offer consistent results. Unlike other cancer sites, there is no indication that wine, even at moderate levels, may exert a protective effect. The overall evidence does not seem to indicate that recent consumption of alcohol at moderate levels plays a major role in the etiology of prostate cancer.

Cancers Probably Not Associated with Alcohol Consumption

Epidemiological studies have generally not shown an association with cancer of the pancreas (IARC, 1988; WCRF, 1997; Longnecker and Tseng, 1999; Nasca, 2001). However, given the high fatality rate for this cancer, most studies used proxy interviews, perhaps leading to considerable random measurement error. If there is a weak association between alcohol and cancer of the pancreas, the relationship may have been missed because of the resulting misclassification. Heavy alcohol consumption increases the risk of chronic pancreatitis, which in turn is a risk factor for pancreatic cancer (Longnecker and Tseng, 1999).

Alcohol consumption does not appear to increase the risk of stomach and bladder cancers (IARC, 1988; WCRF, 1997).

ALCOHOL DRINKING AND CANCER SURVIVAL

Considering the extensive literature on alcohol and cancer, the relatively small body of literature examining the role of alcohol in cancer survival is surprising. There is a growing interest in this research area, with most research focusing on head and neck and breast cancers.

Alcohol in the Prognosis of Head and Neck Cancers

Head and neck cancer patients are at increased risk of developing second primary esophageal squamous cell carcinomas, and chronic use of alcohol and smoking, in particular acetaldehyde, has been implicated in its etiology (Muto et al., 2002). A case-control study found a strong relationship with heavy alcohol consumption but not with cigarette smoking for second primary esophageal cancer among head and neck cancer patients (Tanabe et al., 2001). Confirming the role of acetaldehyde, a case-control study found an interaction between drinking and the ALDH2-2 genotype (coding for the inactive ALDH2) and a weak interaction with ADH3-1 (coding for the more active ADH3) (Muto et al., 2002) on multiple esophageal dysplasia, a precursor for squamous cell esophageal carcinoma, among head and neck cancer patients.

In addition to esophageal cancer, head and neck cancer patients who drink and smoke have elevated risk of other second tumors in the aerodigestive tract, and an independent role of alcohol has been suggested in a number of studies (Franco et al., 1991; Day et al., 1994; Barbone et al., 1996).

Heavy alcohol drinking has also been associated with decreased survival for head and neck cancer patients. A cohort study found that head and neck cancer patients who drank heavily around the time of diagnosis experienced

TABLE 8 Population-Based Case-Control and Cohort Studies Examining Alcohol Consumption and Prostate Cancer

Author, publication year	Study location	Cases n	Controls/cohort size n	Age range years (mean)	Alcohol variable	Contrast	OR/RR (95% CL)	Covariate adjustment: Age	Smoking[a]	BMI/weight	Total energy intake	Physical activity
Total alcohol												
Case-control studies												
Hayes et al., 1996	USA (Georgia, Michigan, New Jersey)	981	1,315	40–79	"Usual consumption"	≥57 drinks/wk vs never	1.9 (1.3, 2.7)	Y	N	N	N	N
Andersson et al., 1996	Sweden	256	252	<80	Recent intake	>96 g/wk vs none	1.5 (0.8, 2.8)	Y	N	N	N	N
					Years drinking	54–61 years vs none	1.2 (0.7, 2.3)	Y	N	N	N	N
Key et al., 1997	England	328	328	<75	Recent intake	>16.6 g/day vs <3.6 g/day	1.04 (0.71, 1.54)	Y	N	N	N	N
Jain et al., 1998	Canada	617	637	(69.8)	Recent intake	≥30 g/day vs none	0.89 (0.64, 1.25)	Y	N	N	Y	N
Villeneuve et al., 1999	Canada	1,623	1,623	50–74	Recent intake	≥4 drinks/day vs none	1.1 (0.9, 1.6)	Y	Y *(cont.)*	Y	N	N
Sharpe et al., 2001	Canada	399	476	45–70	Lifetime drinking among daily drinkers	>125 drink-years vs never drank weekly	2.1 (1.3, 3.3)	Y	Y *(?)*	N	N	N
Cohort studies												
Le Marchand et al., 1994	Hawaii, USA	198	20,316	>18	Lifetime intake	≥5261 g vs 0	1.1 (0.7, 1.7)	Y	N	N	N	N
Hiatt et al., 1994	California, USA	238	43,432	>30	Recent intake	≥6 drinks/day vs never	1 (0.4, 2.8)	Y	Y *(status)*	N	N	N
Breslow et al., 1999	USA (NHANES cohort I)	252	5,766	25–65+	"Usual intake"	>22 drinks/wk vs none	1.42 (0.84, 2.4)	Y	N	N	N	N
Breslow et al., 1999	USA (NHANES cohort II)	134	3,775	25–65+	"Usual intake"	>22 drinks/wk vs none	0.23 (0.06, 0.95)	Y	N	N	N	N
Schuurman et al., 1999	The Netherlands	680	58,279	55–69	Recent intake	≥30 g/day vs none	1.1 (0.8, 1.6)	Y	N	N	N	N
Putnam et al., 2000	Iowa, USA	101	1,572	40–86	Recent intake	>92 g/wk vs 0	1.5 (0.8, 2.7)	Y	N	N	N	N
Ellison, 2000	Canada	145	3,400	50–84	Recent intake	≥25 ml/day vs none	0.93 (0.55, 1.57)	Y	N	N	N	N
Sesso et al., 2001	Harvard Alumni, US	366	7,612	(66.6)	Recent intake	>3 drinks/day vs almost never	1.33 (0.86, 2.05)	Y	Y *(cat.)*	Y	N	Y
Albertsen and Gronbaek, 2002	Denmark	233	12,989	20–98	Recent intake	>41 drinks/wk vs <1	0.66 (0.29, 1.49)	Y	Y *(status)*	Y	N	Y

(continues)

TABLE 8 *(Continued)*

Author, publication year	Study location	Cases n	Controls/ cohort size n	Age range years (mean)	Alcohol variable	Contrast	OR/RR (95% CL)	Covariate adjustment: Age	Smoking[a]	BMI/ weight	Total energy intake	Physical activity
Beer												
Case-control studies												
Hayes et al., 1996	USA (Georgia, Michigan, New Jersey)	981	1,315	40–79	"Usual consumption"	≥29 drinks/wk vs never	2.1 (1.4, 3.1)	Y	N	N	N	N
Gronberg et al., 1996	Sweden	406	1,218	47–91	Recent intake	Almost daily vs none	0.84 (0.56, 1.24)	Y	N	N	N	N
Jain et al., 1998	Canada	617	637	(69.8)	Recent intake	≥10 g/day vs none	0.68 (0.49, 0.94)	Y	N	N	Y	N
Villeneuve et al., 1999	Canada	1,623	1,623	50–74	Recent intake	≥4 drinks/day v none	0.5 (0.2, 1)	Y	Y *(cont.)*	Y	N	N
Sharpe et al., 2001	Canada	399	476	45–70	Lifetime drinking among daily drinkers	>102 drink-years vs never drank weekly	1.7 (1, 2.9)	Y	Y (?)	N	N	N
Cohort studies												
Breslow et al., 1999	USA (NHANES cohort II)	134	3,775	25–65+	"Usual intake"	15–21 drinks/wk vs none	0.34 (0.12, 0.92)	Y	N	N	N	N
Schuurman et al., 1999	The Netherlands	680	58,279	55–69	Recent intake	≥30 g/day vs none	0.5 (0.2, 1.3)	Y	N	N	N	N
Putnam et al., 2000	Iowa, USA	101	1,572	40–86	Recent intake	>3 cans/week vs none	1.7 (0.9, 3)	Y	N	N	N	N
Sesso et al., 2001	Harvard Alumni, US	366	7,612	(66.6)	Recent intake	>3 drinks/day vs almost never	0.72 (0.18, 2.9)	Y	Y *(cat.)*	Y	N	Y
Albertsen and Gronbaek, 2002	Denmark	233	12,989	20–98	Recent intake	>13 drinks/wk vs none	0.98 (0.63, 1.54)	Y	Y *(status)*	Y	N	Y
Wine												
Case-control studies												
Hayes et al., 1996	USA (Georgia, Michigan, New Jersey)	981	1,315	40–79	"Usual " consumption	>14 drinks/wk vs never	1.4 (0.9, 2.2)	Y	N	N	N	N
Gronberg et al., 1996	Sweden	406	1,218	47–91	Recent intake	Almost daily vs none	1.18 (0.23, 5.44)	Y	N	N	N	N
Jain et al., 1998	Canada	617	637	(69.8)	Recent intake	≥10 g/day vs none	1.12 (0.8, 1.55)	Y	N	N	Y	N
Villeneuve et al., 1999	Canada	1,623	1,623	50–74	Recent intake	≥1 drinks/day vs none	0.9 (0.7, 1.5)	Y	Y *(cont.)*	Y	N	N

Sharpe et al., 2001	Canada	399	476	45–70	Lifetime drinking among daily drinkers	>105 drink-years vs never drank weekly	1 (0.5, 2.1)	Y	Y *(?)*	N	N	N
Cohort studies												
Breslow et al., 1999	USA (NHANES cohort II)	134	3,775	25–65+	"Usual intake"	15–21 drinks/wk vs none	1.22 (0.38, 3.88)	Y	N	N	N	N
Schuurman et al., 1999	The Netherlands	680	58,279	55–69	Recent intake	≥30 g/day vs none	2.3 (1, 5.3)	Y	N	N	N	N
Putnam et al., 2000	Iowa, USA	101	1,572	40–86	Recent intake	>0.9 glasses/week vs none	1.9 (0.9, 3.7)	Y	N	N	N	N
Sesso et al., 2001	Harvard Alumni, USA	366	7,612	(66.6)	Recent intake	>3 drinks/day vs almost never	1.05 (0.49, 2.27)	Y	Y *(cat.)*	Y	N	Y
Albertsen and Gronbaek, 2002	Denmark	233	12,989	20–98	Recent intake	>13 drinks/day vs none	0.92 (0.42, 2.02)	Y	Y *(status)*	Y	N	Y
Liquor												
Case-control studies												
Hayes et al., 1996	USA (Georgia, Michigan, New Jersey)	981	1,315	40–79	"Usual consumption"	≥29 drinks/wk vs never	1.9 (1.4, 2.7)	Y	N	N	N	N
Gronberg et al., 1996	Sweden	406	1,218	47–91	Recent intake	Almost daily vs none	0.78 (0.26, 2.23)	Y	N	N	N	N
Jain et al., 1998	Canada	617	637	(69.8)	Recent intake	≥16 g/day vs none	0.86 (0.63, 1.18)	Y	N	N	Y	N
Villeneuve et al., 1999	Canada	1,623	1,623	50–74	Recent intake	≥4 drinks/day vs none	1.8 (0.9, 3.8)	Y	Y *(cont.)*	Y	N	N
Sharpe et al., 2001	Canada	399	476	45–70	Lifetime drinking among daily drinkers	>68 drink-years vs never drank weekly	1.7 (0.9, 3.1)	Y	Y *(?)*	N	N	N
Cohort studies												
Breslow et al., 1999	USA (NHANES cohort II)	134	3,775	25–65+	"Usual intake"	15–21 drinks/wk vs none	1.01 (0.50, 2.04)	Y	N	N	N	N
Schuurman et al., 1999	The Netherlands	680	58,279	55–69	Recent intake	≥30 g/day vs none	1.1 (0.6, 2)	Y	N	N	N	N
Putnam et al., 2000	Iowa, USA	101	1,572	40–86	Recent intake	>2.5 shots/wk vs none	1.7 (0.9, 3)	Y	N	N	N	N
Sesso et al., 2001	Harvard Alumni, USA	366	7,612	(66.6)	Recent intake	>3 drinks/day vs almost never	1.12 (0.64, 1.94)	Y	Y *(cat.)*	Y	N	Y
Albertsen and Gronbaek, 2002	Denmark	233	12,989	20–98	Recent intake	>13 drinks/week vs none	1.02 (0.52, 2.01)	Y	Y *(status)*	Y	N	Y

[a] *(status)*, adjusted for smoking status; *(cont.)*, adjusted for cigarette smoking in pack-years or cigarettes/day as a continuous variable; *(cat.)*, adjusted for cigarette smoking in categories of pack-years or cigarettes per day; (?), adjustment method not specified.

BMI, body mass index.

decreased survival after controlling for age, site of cancer, histopathological grade, anatomical stage, antineoplastic treatment, and cigarette smoking (Deleyiannis et al., 1996). Alcohol intake was shown to predict laryngeal cancer survival in one study conducted in Argentina (Pradier et al., 1993), but not in another one conducted in Italy (Boffetta et al., 1997).

Alcohol and Breast Cancer Survival

Drinking has been found to be associated with stage of breast cancer at diagnosis, with frequent drinkers in one study (Vaeth and Satariano, 1998) or those drinking ≥14 drinks/wk in another (Weiss et al., 1996) being at increased risk of a regional stage diagnosis. Although these findings could be explained by confounding by other factors affecting survival or detection, such as unhealthy behaviors, access to medical care, or other socioeconomic factors, it is also possible that alcohol affects cancer progression.

The few cohort studies that have examined the effect of alcohol drinking on breast cancer survival have offered conflicting results. Overall, most of these studies had limited power due to a small number of events (recurrences or deaths) and/or drinking range, and some of them failed to control for potentially relevant prognostic factors, such as stage at diagnosis, smoking, and treatment. We identified seven cohort studies examining the role of alcohol on breast cancer survival. Of these studies, four (Rohan et al., 1993; Zhang et al., 1995; Holmes et al., 1999; Saxe et al., 1999) did not find an association between drinking and breast cancer survival (death and/or recurrence), whereas one suggested slightly elevated risk of death, though not statistically significant (Ewertz et al., 1991), and two reported elevated risk (Hebert et al., 1998; McDonald et al., 2002). One of these positive studies (Hebert et al., 1998) reported a 41% increased risk of recurrence and a 58% increased risk of death for each additional beer consumed, after adjusting for stage, estrogen receptor status, age, BMI, other dietary factors, and menopausal status. The other positive study conducted among African American women (McDonald et al., 2002) reported an RR of 2.7 (95% CI: 1.3, 5.8) for regular drinkers, after adjusting for stage, radiotherapy, and smoking. Drinking levels were low in these studies, with the highest quartile of intake shown being one drink per day. The effect of heavy alcohol use on breast cancer prognosis has not been evaluated. Overall, there are insufficient data to conclude that drinking has no effect on cancer survival and there is a clear need for research in this area.

Alcohol in the Prognosis of Other Cancers

A cohort study of Memorial Sloan-Kettering Cancer Center's patients found that among nonsmokers, alcohol drinkers with oral and pancreatic cancers experienced poorer prognosis than nondrinkers (Yu et al., 1997). Alcohol consumption was shown in another study to increase the risk of liver metastasis in colorectal cancer patients (Maeda et al., 1998). A Japanese study reported better bladder cancer survival for alcohol drinkers (Wakai et al., 1993), but to our knowledge, this finding has not been replicated in other studies.

Possible Biological Mechanisms

A number of causal pathways have been proposed by which alcohol drinking may affect cancer risk. These include direct effects of alcohol on specific organs and tissues, particularly in cancers of the aerodigestive tract, as well as indirect effects by, for example, inducing changes in hormonal levels, interfering with metabolism and absorption of dietary factors, or affecting the metabolism of other carcinogens (WCRF, 1997).

Acetaldehyde, the main metabolite of ethanol, is a known carcinogen in experimental animals (IARC, 1988). Elevated DNA adducts of acetaldehyde have been found in peripheral blood cells among alcoholics (Fang and Vaca, 1997). Ethanol has also been shown to generate free radicals and impair DNA repair and immune function (Bandera et al., 2001). Moreover, alcohol drinking can interfere with absorption and/or metabolism of certain dietary factors that have been implicated in cancer etiology, such as retinoids (Wang, 2003) and folate (Bailey, 2003).

Although the literature on hormonal effects of alcohol consumption is not consistent, moderate alcohol use has been associated with higher levels of circulating estrogens in premenopausal and postmenopausal women (Gill, 2000). This may explain, at least in part, the increased breast cancer risk associated with alcohol intake. Changes in insulin resistance and the growth hormone–insuline-like growth factor-1 (GH/IGF1) axis have also been implicated (Stoll, 1999).

Alcohol may also increase cancer risk by acting as a solvent for tobacco or other carcinogens or affecting the metabolism of carcinogens by reducing their detoxification and/or catalyzing the metabolic activation of procarcinogens (Blot, 1999). These mechanisms may explain the interaction between smoking and alcohol on certain cancers.

Besides ethanol, alcoholic beverages contain other substances with carcinogenic (e.g., asbestos filtration products, tannins, *N*-nitroso compounds, urethan, arsenic, and pesticide residues [Blot, 1999]) and anticarcinogenic potential (e.g., polyphenols, particularly resveratrol in wine [Bianchini and Vainio, 2003]).

CONCLUSIONS AND PUBLIC HEALTH IMPLICATIONS

There is convincing evidence that heavy alcohol consumption is strongly related to cancers of the mouth,

TABLE 9 National and International Guidelines Regarding Alcohol and Health

Source	Year	Recommendation
Alcohol and cancer		
World Research Fund/American Institute for Cancer Research (WCRF/AICR)	1997	"Alcohol consumption is not recommended. If consumed at all, limit alcoholic drinks to less than two drinks a day for men and one for women"
National Cancer Institute (NCI)	Current	"Consume alcoholic beverages in moderation, if at all."
American Cancer Society (ACS)	2002	"If you drink alcoholic beverages, limit consumption (no more than two drinks per day for men and one drink for women.)"
World Health Organization (WHO)	2003	"Consumption of alcoholic beverages is not recommended: if consumed do not exceed two units (one glass of beer, wine or spirits) per day."
Alcohol and health		
National Research Council (NRC)	1989	"The committee does not recommend alcohol consumption. For those who drink alcoholic beverages, the committee recommends limiting consumption to the equivalent of less than two cans of beer, two small glasses of wine, or two average cocktails."
United States Department of Agriculture (USDA)	2000	"If you drink alcoholic beverages, do so in moderation. Limit intake to one drink per day for women or two per day for men, and take with meals to slow alcohol absorption."

pharynx, larynx, esophagus, and liver. Alcohol also probably increases the risk of colorectal and breast cancer. For other cancers, such as lung, ovarian, prostate, and endometrial cancers, the relationship remains controversial. Evidence is accumulating that certain populations may be more susceptible to alcohol on the basis of genetic variations on alcohol metabolism. Although the biological mechanisms by which alcohol increases cancer risk are not established, several plausible pathways have been proposed.

Issuing recommendations regarding alcohol intake is difficult given the potential beneficial and detrimental effects for both the general public (Anonymous, 2000) and cancer patients (Brown et al., 2003). National and international guidelines regarding alcohol and health are listed in Table 9. Most scientific panels do not recommend drinking for health or cancer prevention, but for those who elect to drink, moderate consumption is recommended (i.e., less than one drink per day for women and two per day for men). Although moderate wine drinking has been shown to be beneficial for certain cancers, there is insufficient evidence to recommend one alcoholic beverage type over another.

Acknowledgments

We thank Nirupa Ghai, MPH, and Dina Considine, MPH, for their assistance in conducting searches and in acquiring hundreds of manuscripts.

References

10th Report on Carcinogens. 2002. U.S. Department of Health and Human Services, Public Health Service, National Toxicology Program, December 2002.

Adami, H.O., Lund, E., Bergstrom, R., and Meirik, O. 1988. Cigarette smoking, alcohol consumption and risk of breast cancer in young women. *Br J Cancer* **58**: 832–837.

Albertsen, K., and Gronbaek, M. 2002. Does amount or type of alcohol influence the risk of prostate cancer? *Prostate* **52**: 297–304.

Althuis, M.D., Brogan, D.D., Coates, R.J., Daling, J.R., Gammon, M.D., Malone, K.E., Schoenberg, J.B., and Brinton, L.A. 2003. Breast cancers among very young premenopausal women (United States). *Cancer Causes Control* **14**: 151–160.

Andersson, S.O., Baron, J., Bergstrom, R., Lindgren, C., Wolk, A., and Adami, H.O. 1996. Lifestyle factors and prostate cancer risk: a case-control study in Sweden. *Cancer Epidemiol Biomarkers Prev* **5**: 509–513.

Anonymous. 2000. Health risks and benefits of alcohol consumption. *Alcohol Res Health* **24**: 5–11.

Bagnardi, V., Blangiardo, M., La Vecchia, C., and Corrao, G. 2001a. Alcohol consumption and the risk of cancer: a meta-analysis. *Alcohol Res Health* **25**: 263–270.

Bagnardi, V., Blangiardo, M., La Vecchia, C., and Corrao, G. 2001b. A meta-analysis of alcohol drinking and cancer risk. *Br J Cancer* **85**: 1700–1705.

Bailey, L.B. 2003. Folate, methyl-related nutrients, alcohol, and the MTHFR 677C– > T polymorphism affect cancer risk: intake recommendations. *J Nutr* **133**: 3748S–3753S.

Bandera, E.V., Freudenheim, J.L., Graham, S., Marshall, J.R., Haughey, B.P., Swanson, M., Brasure, J., and Wilkinson, G. 1992. Alcohol consumption and lung cancer in white males. *Cancer Causes Control* **3**: 361–369.

Bandera, E.V., Freudenheim, J.L., Marshall, J.R., Zielezny, M., Priore, R.L., Brasure, J., Baptiste, M., and Graham, S. 1997. Diet and alcohol consumption and lung cancer risk in the New York State Cohort (United States). *Cancer Causes Control* **8**: 828–840.

Bandera, E.V., Freudenheim, J.L., and Vena, J.E. 2001. Alcohol consumption and lung cancer: a review of the epidemiologic evidence. *Cancer Epidemiol Biomarkers Prev* **10**: 813–821.

Bandera, E.V., Kushi, L.H., Olson, S.H., Chen, W.Y., and Muti, P. 2003. Alcohol consumption and endometrial cancer: some unresolved issues. *Nutr Cancer* **45**: 24–29.

Barbone, F., Franceschi, S., Talamini, R., Barzan, L., Franchin, G., Favero, A., and Carbone, A. 1996. A follow-up study of determinants of second tumor and metastasis among subjects with cancer of the oral cavity, pharynx, and larynx. *J Clin Epidemiol* **49**: 367–372.

Baumgartner, K.B., Annegers, J.F., McPherson, R.S., Frankowski, R.F., Gilliland, F.D., and Samet, J.M. 2002. Is alcohol intake associated with breast cancer in Hispanic women? The New Mexico Women's Health Study. *Ethn Dis* **12**: 460–469.

Bianchini, F., and Vainio, H. 2003. Wine and resveratrol: mechanisms of cancer prevention? *Eur J Cancer Prev* **12**: 417–425.

Blot, W.J. 1999. Invited commentary: more evidence of increased risks of cancer among alcohol drinkers. *Am J Epidemiol* **150**: 1138–1140; discussion 1141.

Boffetta, P., Merletti, F., Faggiano, F., Migliaretti, G., Ferro, G., Zanetti, R., and Terracini, B. 1997. Prognostic factors and survival of laryngeal cancer patients from Turin, Italy. A population-based study. *Am J Epidemiol* **145**: 1100–1105.

Bosron, W.F., and Li, T.K. 1986. Genetic polymorphism of human liver alcohol and aldehyde dehydrogenases, and their relationship to alcohol metabolism and alcoholism. *Hepatology* **6**: 502–510.

Bouchardy, C., Hirvonen, A., Coutelle, C., Ward, P.J., Dayer, P., and Benhamou, S. 2000. Role of alcohol dehydrogenase 3 and cytochrome P-4502E1 genotypes in susceptibility to cancers of the upper aerodigestive tract. *Int J Cancer* **87**: 734–740.

Bowers, J.L., Tyulmenkov, V.V., Jernigan, S.C., and Klinge, C.M. 2000. Resveratrol acts as a mixed agonist/antagonist for estrogen receptors alpha and beta. *Endocrinology* **141**: 3657–3667.

Bowlin, S.J., Leske, M.C., Varma, A., Nasca, P., Weinstein, A., and Caplan, L. 1997. Breast cancer risk and alcohol consumption: results from a large case-control study. *Int J Epidemiol* **26**: 915–923.

Breslow, R.A., Wideroff, L., Graubard, B.I., Erwin, D., Reichman, M.E., Ziegler, R.G., and Ballard-Barbash, R. 1999. Alcohol and prostate cancer in the NHANES I epidemiologic follow-up study. First National Health and Nutrition Examination Survey of the United States. *Ann Epidemiol* **9**: 254–261.

Brinton, L.A., Benichou, J., Gammon, M.D., Brogan, D.R., Coates, R., and Schoenberg, J.B. 1997. Ethnicity and variation in breast cancer incidence. *Int J Cancer* **73**: 349–355.

Brown, J.K., Byers, T., Doyle, C., Coumeya, K.S., Demark-Wahnefried, W., Kushi, L.H., McTieman, A., Rock, C.L., Aziz, N., Bloch, A.S., Eldridge, B., Hamilton, K., Katzin, C., Koonce, A., Main, J., Mobley, C., Morra, M.E., Pierce, M.S., and Sawyer, K.A. 2003. Nutrition and physical activity during and after cancer treatment: an American Cancer Society guide for informed choices. *CA Cancer J Clin* **53**: 268–291.

Caballeria, J. 2003. Current concepts in alcohol metabolism. *Ann Hepatol* **2**: 60–68.

Carlsson, S., Hammar, N., Hakala, P., Kaprio, J., Marniemi, J., and Ronnemaa, T. 2003. Assessment of alcohol consumption by mailed questionnaire in epidemiological studies: evaluation of misclassification using a dietary history interview and biochemical markers. *Eur J Epidemiol* **18**: 493–501.

Carpenter, C.L., Morgenstern, H., and London, S.J. 1998. Alcoholic beverage consumption and lung cancer risk among residents of Los Angeles County. *J Nutr* **128**: 694–700.

Chen, J., Ma, J., Stampfer, M.J., Hines, L.M., Selhub, J., and Hunter, D.J. 2001. Alcohol dehydrogenase 3 genotype is not predictive for risk of colorectal cancer. *Cancer Epidemiol Biomarkers Prev* **10**: 1303–1304.

Chen, W.Y., Colditz, G.A., Rosner, B., Hankinson, S.E., Hunter, D.J., Manson, J.E., Stampfer, M.J., Willett, W.C., and Speizer, F.E. 2002. Use of postmenopausal hormones, alcohol, and risk for invasive breast cancer. *Ann Intern Med* **137**: 798–804.

Cho, E., Smith-Warner, S.A., Ritz, J., van den Brandt, P.A., Colditz, G.A., Folsom, A.R., Freudenheim, J.L., Giovannucci, E., Goldbohm, R.A., Graham, S., Holmberg, L., Kim, D.H., Malila, N., Miller, A.B., Pietinen, P., Rohan, T.E., Sellers, T.A., Speizer, F.E., Willett, W.C., Wolk, A., and Hunter, D.J. 2004. Alcohol intake and colorectal cancer: a pooled analysis of 8 cohort studies. *Ann Intern Med* **140**: 603–613.

Choi, J.Y., Abel, J., Neuhaus, T., Ko, Y., Harth, V., Hamajima, N., Tajima, K., Yoo, K.Y., Park, S.K., Noh, D.Y., Han, W., Choe, K.J., Ahn, S.H., Kim, S.U., Hirvonen, A., and Kang, D. 2003. Role of alcohol and genetic polymorphisms of CYP2E1 and ALDH2 in breast cancer development. *Pharmacogenetics* **13**: 67–72.

Chu, S.Y., Lee, N.C., Wingo, P.A., and Webster, L.A. 1989. Alcohol consumption and the risk of breast cancer. *Am J Epidemiol* **130**: 867–877.

Corrao, G., Bagnardi, V., Zambon, A., and Arico, S. 1999. Exploring the dose-response relationship between alcohol consumption and the risk of several alcohol-related conditions: a meta-analysis. *Addiction* **94**: 1551–1573.

Coutelle, C., Ward, P.J., Fleury, B., Quattrocchi, P., Chambrin, H., Iron, A., Couzigou, P., and Cassaigne, A. 1997. Laryngeal and oropharyngeal cancer, and alcohol dehydrogenase 3 and glutathione S-transferase M1 polymorphisms. *Hum Genet* **99**: 319–325.

Day, G.L., Blot, W.J., Shore, R.E., McLaughlin, J.K., Austin, D.F., Greenberg, R.S., Liff, J.M., Preston-Martin, S., Sarkar, S., Schoenberg, J.B., and et al. 1994. Second cancers following oral and pharyngeal cancers: role of tobacco and alcohol. *J Natl Cancer Inst* **86**: 131–137.

De Stefani, E., Correa, P., Fierro, L., Fontham, E.T., Chen, V., and Zavala, D. 1993. The effect of alcohol on the risk of lung cancer in Uruguay. *Cancer Epidemiol Biomarkers Prev* **2**: 21–26.

Del Boca, F.K., and Darkes, J. 2003. The validity of self-reports of alcohol consumption: state of the science and challenges for research. *Addiction* **98**(Suppl 2): 1–12.

Deleyiannis, F.W., Thomas, D.B., Vaughan, T.L., and Davis, S. 1996. Alcoholism: independent predictor of survival in patients with head and neck cancer. *J Natl Cancer Inst* **88**: 542–549.

Dennis, L.K. 2000. Meta-analysis for combining relative risks of alcohol consumption and prostate cancer. *Prostate* **42**: 56–66.

Dennis, L.K., and Hayes, R.B. 2001. Alcohol and prostate cancer. *Epidemiol Rev* **23**: 110–114.

Djousse, L., Dorgan, J.F., Zhang, Y., Schatzkin, A., Hood, M., D'Agostino, R.B., Copenhafer, D.L., Kreger, B.E., and Ellison, R.C. 2002. Alcohol consumption and risk of lung cancer: the Framingham Study. *J Natl Cancer Inst* **94**: 1877–1882.

Dosemeci, M., Gokmen, I., Unsal, M., Hayes, R.B., and Blair, A. 1997. Tobacco, alcohol use, and risks of laryngeal and lung cancer by subsite and histologic type in Turkey. *Cancer Causes Control* **8**: 729–737.

Ellison, L.F. 2000. Tea and other beverage consumption and prostate cancer risk: a Canadian retrospective cohort study. *Eur J Cancer Prev* **9**: 125–130.

Ellison, R.C., Zhang, Y., McLennan, C.E., and Rothman, K.J. 2001. Exploring the relation of alcohol consumption to risk of breast cancer. *Am J Epidemiol* **154**: 740–747.

Enger, S.M., Ross, R.K., Paganini-Hill, A., Longnecker, M.P., and Bernstein, L. 1999. Alcohol consumption and breast cancer oestrogen and progesterone receptor status. *Br J Cancer* **79**: 1308–1314.

Enzinger, P.C., and Mayer, R.J. 2003. Esophageal cancer. *N Engl J Med* **349**: 2241–2252.

Ewertz, M. 1991. Alcohol consumption and breast cancer risk in Denmark. *Cancer Causes Control* **2**, 247–252.

Ewertz, M., Gillanders, S., Meyer, L., and Zedeler, K. 1991. Survival of breast cancer patients in relation to factors which affect the risk of developing breast cancer. *Int J Cancer* **49**: 526–530.

Fang, J.L., and Vaca, C.E. 1997. Detection of DNA adducts of acetaldehyde in peripheral white blood cells of alcohol abusers. *Carcinogenesis* **18**: 627–632.

Feigelson, H.S., Calle, E.E., Robertson, A.S., Wingo, P.A., and Thun, M.J. 2001. Alcohol consumption increases the risk of fatal breast cancer (United States). *Cancer Causes Control* **12**: 895–902.

Feigelson, H.S., Jonas, C.R., Robertson, A.S., McCullough, M.L., Thun, M.J., and Calle, E.E. 2003. Alcohol, folate, methionine, and risk of incident breast cancer in the American Cancer Society Cancer Prevention Study II Nutrition Cohort. *Cancer Epidemiol Biomarkers Prev* **12**: 161–164.

Feinman, L., and Lieber, C.S. 1999. Nutrition and diet in alcoholism. *In* "Modern Nutrition in Health and Disease" (M.E. Shils, J.A. Olson, M.

Shike, and A.C. Ross, Eds.), 9th edition, Chapter 94, Lippincott Williams & Wilkins, Books@Ovid.

Feunekes, G.I., van't Veer, P., van Staveren, W.A., and Kok, F.J. 1999. Alcohol intake assessment: the sober facts. *Am J Epidemiol* **150**: 105–112.

Franco, E.L., Kowalski, L.P., and Kanda, J.L. 1991. Risk factors for second cancers of the upper respiratory and digestive systems: a case-control study. *J Clin Epidemiol* **44**: 615–625.

Freudenheim, J.L., Graham, S., Marshall, J.R., Haughey, B.P., and Wilkinson, G. 1990. Lifetime alcohol intake and risk of rectal cancer in western New York. *Nutr Cancer* **13**: 101–109.

Freudenheim, J.L., Marshall, J.R., Graham, S., Laughlin, R., Vena, J.E., Swanson, M., Ambrosone, C., and Nemoto, T. 1995. Lifetime alcohol consumption and risk of breast cancer. *Nutr Cancer* **23**: 1–11.

Freudenheim, J.L., Ambrosone, C.B., Moysich, K.B., Vena, J.E., Graham, S., Marshall, J.R., Muti, P., Laughlin, R., Nemoto, T., Harty, L.C., Crits, G.A., Chan, A.W., and Shields, P.G. 1999. Alcohol dehydrogenase 3 genotype modification of the association of alcohol consumption with breast cancer risk. *Cancer Causes Control* **10**: 369–377.

Freudenheim, J.L., Ram, M., Nie, J., Muti, P., Trevisan, M., Shields, P.G., Bandera, E.V., Campbell, L.A., McCann, S.E., Schunemann, H.J., Carosella, A.M., Vito, D., Russell, M., Nochajski, T.H., and Goldman, R. 2003. Lung cancer in humans is not associated with lifetime total alcohol consumption or with genetic variation in alcohol dehydrogenase 3 (ADH3). *J Nutr* **133**: 3619–3624.

Freudenheim, J.L., Bonner, M., Krishnan, S., Ambrosone, C.B., Graham, S., McCann, S.E., Moysich, K.B., Bowman, E., Nemoto, T., and Shields, P.G. 2004. Diet and alcohol consumption in relation to p53 mutations in breast tumors. *Carcinogenesis* **25**: 931–939.

Friedenreich, C.M., Howe, G.R., Miller, A.B., and Jain, M.G. 1993. A cohort study of alcohol consumption and risk of breast cancer. *Am J Epidemiol* **137**: 512–520.

Fuchs, C.S., Stampfer, M.J., Colditz, G.A., Giovannucci, E.L., Manson, J.E., Kawachi, I., Hunter, D.J., Hankinson, S.E., Hennekens, C.H., and Rosner, B. 1995. Alcohol consumption and mortality among women. *N Engl J Med* **332**: 1245–1250.

Fuchs, C.S., Willett, W.C., Colditz, G.A., Hunter, D.J., Stampfer, M.J., Speizer, F.E., and Giovannucci, E.L. 2002. The influence of folate and multivitamin use on the familial risk of colon cancer in women. *Cancer Epidemiol Biomarkers Prev* **11**: 227–234.

Gapstur, S.M., Potter, J.D., Sellers, T.A., and Folsom, A.R. 1992. Increased risk of breast cancer with alcohol consumption in postmenopausal women. *Am J Epidemiol* **136**: 1221–1231.

Gapstur, S.M., Potter, J.D., Sellers, T.A., Kushi, L.H., and Folsom, A.R. 1993. Alcohol consumption and postmenopausal endometrial cancer: results from the Iowa Women's Health Study. *Cancer Causes Control* **4**: 323–329.

Gapstur, S.M., Potter, J.D., Drinkard, C., and Folsom, A.R. 1995. Synergistic effect between alcohol and estrogen replacement therapy on risk of breast cancer differs by estrogen/progesterone receptor status in the Iowa Women's Health Study. *Cancer Epidemiol Biomarkers Prev* **4**: 313–318.

Garfinkel, L., Boffetta, P., and Stellman, S.D. 1988. Alcohol and breast cancer: a cohort study. *Prev Med* **17**: 686–693.

Garland, M., Hunter, D.J., Colditz, G.A., Spiegelman, D.L., Manson, J.E., Stampfer, M.J., and Willett, W.C. 1999. Alcohol consumption in relation to breast cancer risk in a cohort of United States women 25–42 years of age. *Cancer Epidemiol Biomarkers Prev* **8**: 1017–1021.

Gerhardsson de Verdier, M., Romelsjo, A., and Lundberg, M. 1993. Alcohol and cancer of the colon and rectum. *Eur J Cancer Prev* **2**: 401–408.

Gill, J. 2000. The effects of moderate alcohol consumption on female hormone levels and reproductive function. *Alcohol Alcohol* **35**: 417–423.

Giovannucci, E., Rimm, E.B., Ascherio, A., Stampfer, M.J., Colditz, G.A., and Willett, W.C. 1995. Alcohol, low-methionine–low-folate diets, and risk of colon cancer in men. *J Natl Cancer Inst* **87**: 265–273.

Godard, B., Foulkes, W.D., Provencher, D., Brunet, J.S., Tonin, P.N., Mes-Masson, A.M., Narod, S.A., and Ghadirian, P. 1998. Risk factors for familial and sporadic ovarian cancer among French Canadians: a case-control study. *Am J Obstet Gynecol* **179**: 403–410.

Goldbohm, R.A., Van den Brandt, P.A., Van't Veer, P., Dorant, E., Sturmans, F., and Hermus, R.J. 1994. Prospective study on alcohol consumption and the risk of cancer of the colon and rectum in the Netherlands. *Cancer Causes Control* **5**: 95–104.

Goodman, M.T., Hankin, J.H., Wilkens, L.R., Lyu, L.C., McDuffie, K., Liu, L.Q., and Kolonel, L.N. 1997a. Diet, body size, physical activity, and the risk of endometrial cancer. *Cancer Res* **57**: 5077–5085.

Goodman, M.T., Wilkens, L.R., Hankin, J.H., Lyu, L.C., Wu, A.H., and Kolonel, L.N. 1997b. Association of soy and fiber consumption with the risk of endometrial cancer. *Am J Epidemiol* **146**: 294–306.

Goodman, M.T., and Tung, K.H. 2003. Alcohol consumption and the risk of borderline and invasive ovarian cancer. *Obstet Gynecol* **101**: 1221–1228.

Graham, S., Marshall, J., Haughey, B., Mrttleman, A., Swanson, M., Zielezny, M., Byers, T., Wilkinson, G., and West, D. 1988. Dietary epidemiology of cancer of the colon in western New York. *Am J Epidemiol* **128**: 490–503.

Graham, S., Hellmann, R., Marshall, J., Freudenheim, J., Vena, J., Swanson, M., Zielezny, M., Nemoto, T., Stubbe, N., and Raimondo, T. 1991. Nutritional epidemiology of postmenopausal breast cancer in western New York. *Am J Epidemiol* **134**: 552–566.

Graham, S., Zielezny, M., Marshall, J., Priore, R., Freudenheim, J., Brasure, J., Haughey, B., Nasca, P., and Zdeb, M. 1992. Diet in the epidemiology of postmenopausal breast cancer in the New York State Cohort. *Am J Epidemiol* **136**: 1327–1337.

Gronberg, H., Damber, L., and Damber, J.E. 1996. Total food consumption and body mass index in relation to prostate cancer risk: a case-control study in Sweden with prospectively collected exposure data. *J Urol* **155**: 969–974.

Gruchow, H.W., Sobocinski, K.A., Barboriak, J.J., and Scheller, J.G. 1985. Alcohol consumption, nutrient intake and relative body weight among US adults. *Am J Clin Nutr* **42**: 289–295.

Gwinn, M.L., Webster, L.A., Lee, N.C., Layde, P.M., and Rubin, G.L. 1986. Alcohol consumption and ovarian cancer risk. *Am J Epidemiol* **123**: 759–766.

Haile, R.W., Witte, J.S., Ursin, G., Siemiatycki, J., Bertolli, J., Douglas Thompson, W., and Paganini-Hill, A. 1996. A case-control study of reproductive variables, alcohol, and smoking in premenopausal bilateral breast cancer. *Breast Cancer Res Treat* **37**: 49–56.

Hamajima, N., Hirose, K., Tajima, K., Rohan, T., Calle, E.E., Heath, C.W., Jr., Coates, R.J., Liff, J.M., Talamini, R., Chantarakul, N., Koetsawang, S., Rachawat, D., Morabia, A., Schuman, L., Stewart, W., Szklo, M., Bain, C., Schofield, F., Siskind, V., Band, P., Coldman, A.J., Gallagher, R.P., Hislop, T.G., Yang, P., Kolonel, L.M., Nomura, A.M., Hu, J., Johnson, K.C., Mao, Y., De Sanjose, S., Lee, N., Marchbanks, P., Ory, H.W., Peterson, H.B., Wilson, H.G., Wingo, P.A., Ebeling, K., Kunde, D., Nishan, P., Hopper, J.L., Colditz, G., Gajalanski, V. 2002. Alcohol, tobacco and breast cancer–collaborative reanalysis of individual data from 53 epidemiological studies, including 58,515 women with breast cancer and 95,067 women without the disease. *Br J Cancer* **87**: 1234–1245.

Harnack, L., Jacobs, D.R., Jr., Nicodemus, K., Lazovich, D., Anderson, K., and Folsom, A.R. 2002. Relationship of folate, vitamin B-6, vitamin B-12, and methionine intake to incidence of colorectal cancers. *Nutr Cancer* **43**: 152–158.

Harty, L.C., Caporaso, N.E., Hayes, R.B., Winn, D.M., Bravo-Otero, E., Blot, W.J., Kleinman, D.V., Brown, L.M., Armenian, H.K., Fraumeni, J.F., Jr., and Shields, P.G. 1997. Alcohol dehydrogenase 3 genotype and risk of oral cavity and pharyngeal cancers. *J Natl Cancer Inst* **89**: 1698–1705.

Harvey, E.B., Schairer, C., Brinton, L.A., Hoover, R.N., and Fraumeni, J.F., Jr. 1987. Alcohol consumption and breast cancer. *J Natl Cancer Inst* **78**: 657–661.

Hayes, R.B., Brown, L.M., Schoenberg, J.B., Greenberg, R.S., Silverman, D.T., Schwartz, A.G., Swanson, G.M., Benichou, J., Liff, J.M., Hoover, R.N., and Pottern, L.M. 1996. Alcohol use and prostate cancer risk in US blacks and whites. *Am J Epidemiol* **143**: 692–697.

Hebert, J.R., and Kabat, G.C. 1991. Implications for cancer epidemiology of differences in dietary intake associated with alcohol consumption. *Nutr Cancer* **15**: 107–119.

Hebert, J.R., Hurley, T.G., and Ma, Y. 1998. The effect of dietary exposures on recurrence and mortality in early stage breast cancer. *Breast Cancer Res Treat* **51**: 17–28.

Hiatt, R.A., and Bawol, R.D. 1984. Alcoholic beverage consumption and breast cancer incidence. *Am J Epidemiol* **120**: 676–683.

Hiatt, R.A., Klatsky, A.L., and Armstrong, M.A. 1988. Alcohol consumption and the risk of breast cancer in a prepaid health plan. *Cancer Res* **48**: 2284–2287.

Hiatt, R.A., Armstrong, M.A., Klatsky, A.L., and Sidney, S. 1994. Alcohol consumption, smoking, and other risk factors and prostate cancer in a large health plan cohort in California (United States). *Cancer Causes Control* **5**: 66–72.

Hines, L.M., Hankinson, S.E., Smith-Warner, S.A., Spiegelman, D., Kelsey, K.T., Colditz, G.A., Willett, W.C., and Hunter, D.J. 2000. A prospective study of the effect of alcohol consumption and ADH3 genotype on plasma steroid hormone levels and breast cancer risk. *Cancer Epidemiol Biomarkers Prev* **9**: 1099–1105.

Holman, C.D., English, D.R., Milne, E., and Winter, M.G. 1996. Meta-analysis of alcohol and all-cause mortality: a validation of NHMRC recommendations. *Med J Aust* **164**: 141–145.

Holmberg, L., Baron, J.A., Byers, T., Wolk, A., Ohlander, E.M., Zack, M., and Adami, H.O. 1995. Alcohol intake and breast cancer risk: effect of exposure from 15 years of age. *Cancer Epidemiol Biomarkers Prev* **4**: 843–847.

Holmes, M.D., Stampfer, M.J., Colditz, G.A., Rosner, B., Hunter, D.J., and Willett, W.C. 1999. Dietary factors and the survival of women with breast carcinoma. *Cancer* **86**: 826–835.

Horn-Ross, P.L., Hoggatt, K.J., West, D.W., Krone, M.R., Stewart, S.L., Anton, H., Bernstei, C.L., Deapen, D., Peel, D., Pinder, R., Reynolds, P., Ross, R.K., Wright, W., and Ziogas, A. 2002. Recent diet and breast cancer risk: the California Teachers Study (USA). *Cancer Causes Control* **13**: 407–415.

Horn-Ross, P.L., Canchola, A.J., West, D.W., Stewart, S.L., Bernstein, L., Deapen, D., Pinder, R., Ross, R.K., Anton-Culver, H., Peel, D., Ziogas, A., Reynolds, P., and Wright, W. 2004. Patterns of alcohol consumption and breast cancer risk in the California Teachers Study cohort. *Cancer Epidemiol Biomarkers Prev* **13**: 405–411.

Hoshiyama, Y., Sekine, T., and Sasaba, T. 1993. A case-control study of colorectal cancer and its relation to diet, cigarettes, and alcohol consumption in Saitama Prefecture, Japan. *Tohoku J Exp Med* **171**: 153–165.

Howe, G., Rohan, T., Decarli, A., Iscovich, J., Kaldor, J., Katsouyanni, K., Marubini, E., Miller, A., Riboli, E., Toniolo, P., and et al. 1991. The association between alcohol and breast cancer risk: evidence from the combined analysis of six dietary case-control studies. *Int J Cancer* **47**: 707–710.

Hu, J., Mao, Y., Dryer, D., and White, K. 2002. Risk factors for lung cancer among Canadian women who have never smoked. *Cancer Detect Prev* **26**: 129–138.

IARC. 1988. "Alcohol drinking. IARC Monographs on the Evaluation of Carcinogenic Risks to Humans." International Agency for Research on Cancer, Lyon, France.

Iscovich, J.M., Iscovich, R.B., Howe, G., Shiboski, S., and Kaldor, J.M. 1989. A case-control study of diet and breast cancer in Argentina. *Int J Cancer* **44**: 770–776.

Itoga, S., Nomura, F., Makino, Y., Tomonaga, T., Shimada, H., Ochiai, T., Iizasa, T., Baba, M., Fujisawa, T., and Harada, S. 2002. Tandem repeat polymorphism of the CYP2E1 gene: an association study with esophageal cancer and lung cancer. *Alcohol Clin Exp Res* **26**: 15S–19S.

Jain, M.G., Hislop, G.T., Howe, G.R., Burch, J.D., and Ghadirian, P. 1998. Alcohol and other beverage use and prostate cancer risk among Canadian men. *Int J Cancer* **78**: 707–711.

Jain, M.G., Howe, G.R., and Rohan, T.E. 2000a. Nutritional factors and endometrial cancer in Ontario, Canada. *Cancer Control* **7**: 288–296.

Jain, M.G., Rohan, T.E., Howe, G.R., and Miller, A.B. 2000b. A cohort study of nutritional factors and endometrial cancer. *Eur J Epidemiol* **16**: 899–905.

Jamal, M.M., and Morgan, T.R. 2003. Liver disease in alcohol and hepatitis C. *Best Pract Res Clin Gastroenterol* **17**: 649–662.

Johnson, K.C., Hu, J., and Mao, Y. 2000. Passive and active smoking and breast cancer risk in Canada, 1994–97. The Canadian Cancer Registries Epidemiology Research Group. *Cancer Causes Control* **11**: 211–221.

Jones, B.R., Barrett-Connor, E., Criqui, M.H., and Holdbrook, M.J. 1982. A community study of calorie and nutrient intake in drinkers and non-drinkers of alcohol. *Am J Clin Nutr* **35**: 135–139.

Kato, I., Tominaga, S., and Terao, C. 1989. Alcohol consumption and cancers of hormone-related organs in females. *Jpn J Clin Oncol* **19**: 202–207.

Kato, S., Tajiri, T., Matsukura, N., Matsuda, N., Taniai, N., Mamada, H., Yoshida, H., Kiyam, T., and Naito, Z. 2003. Genetic polymorphisms of aldehyde dehydrogenase 2, cytochrome p450 2E1 for liver cancer risk in HCV antibody-positive japanese patients and the variations of CYP2E1 mRNA expression levels in the liver due to its polymorphism. *Scand J Gastroenterol* **38**: 886–893.

Katsouyanni, K., Trichopoulou, A., Stuver, S., Vassilaros, S., Papadiamantis, Y., Bournas, N., Skarpou, N., Mueller, N., and Trichopoulos, D. 1994. Ethanol and breast cancer: an association that may be both confounded and causal. *Int J Cancer* **58**: 356–361.

Key, T.J., Silcocks, P.B., Davey, G.K., Appleby, P.N., and Bishop, D.T. 1997. A case-control study of diet and prostate cancer. *Br J Cancer* **76**: 678–687.

Kinney, A.Y., Millikan, R.C., Lin, Y.H., Moorman, P.G., and Newman, B. 2000. Alcohol consumption and breast cancer among black and white women in North Carolina (United States). *Cancer Causes Control* **11**: 345–357.

Klatsky, A.L., Armstrong, M.A., Friedman, G.D., and Hiatt, R.A. 1988. The relations of alcoholic beverage use to colon and rectal cancer. *Am J Epidemiol* **128**: 1007–1015.

Korte, J.E., Brennan, P., Henley, S.J., and Boffetta, P. 2002. Dose-specific meta-analysis and sensitivity analysis of the relation between alcohol consumption and lung cancer risk. *Am J Epidemiol* **155**: 496–506.

Kropp, S., Becher, H., Nieters, A., and Chang-Claude, J. 2001. Low-to-moderate alcohol consumption and breast cancer risk by age 50 years among women in Germany. *Am J Epidemiol* **154**: 624–634.

Kune, G.A., and Vitetta, L. 1992. Alcohol consumption and the etiology of colorectal cancer: a review of the scientific evidence from 1957 to 1991. *Nutr Cancer* **18**: 97–111.

Kune, S., Kune, G.A., and Watson, L.F. 1987. Case-control study of alcoholic beverages as etiological factors: the Melbourne Colorectal Cancer Study. *Nutr Cancer* **9**: 43–56.

Kuper, H., Titus-Ernstoff, L., Harlow, B.L., and Cramer, D.W. 2000. Population based study of coffee, alcohol and tobacco use and risk of ovarian cancer. *Int J Cancer* **88**: 313–318.

Kushi, L.H., Mink, P.J., Folsom, A.R., Anderson, K.E., Zheng, W., Lazovich, D., and Sellers, T.A. 1999. Prospective study of diet and ovarian cancer. *Am J Epidemiol* **149**: 21–31.

Lands, W.E. 1995. Alcohol and energy intake. *Am J Clin Nutr* **62**: 1101S–1106S.

Le Marchand, L., Kolonel, L.N., Wilkens, L.R., Myers, B.C., and Hirohata, T. 1994. Animal fat consumption and prostate cancer: a prospective study in Hawaii. *Epidemiology* **5**: 276–282.

Le Marchand, L., Wilkens, L.R., Kolonel, L.N., Hankin, J.H., and Lyu, L.C. 1997. Associations of sedentary lifestyle, obesity, smoking, alcohol use, and diabetes with the risk of colorectal cancer. *Cancer Res* **57**: 4787–4794.

Le Marchand, L., Wilkens, L.R., Hankin, J.H., Kolonel, L.N., and Lyu, L.C. 1999. Independent and joint effects of family history and lifestyle on colorectal cancer risk: implications for prevention. *Cancer Epidemiol Biomarkers Prev* **8**: 45–51.

Lee, H.S., Yoon, J.H., Kamimura, S., Iwata, K., Watanabe, H., and Kim, C.Y. 1997. Lack of association of cytochrome P450 2E1 genetic polymorphisms with the risk of human hepatocellular carcinoma. *Int J Cancer* **71**: 737–740.

Lee, K.M., Abel, J., Ko, Y., Harth, V., Park, W.Y., Seo, J.S., Yoo, K.Y., Choi, J.Y., Shin, A., Ahn, S.H., Noh, D.Y., Hirvonen, A., and Kang, D. 2003. Genetic polymorphisms of cytochrome P450 19 and 1B1, alcohol use, and breast cancer risk in Korean women. *Br J Cancer* **88**: 675–678.

Li, C.I.M., Kathleen; Porter, Peggy; Weiss, Noel; Tang, Mei-Tzu; Daling, Janet. 2003. The Relationship between Alcohol Use and Risk of Breast Cancer by Histology and Hormone Receptor Status among Women 65–79 Years of Age. *Cancer Epidemiol Biomarkers Prev* **12**: 1061–1066.

Littman, A.J., Beresford, S.A., and White, E. 2001. The association of dietary fat and plant foods with endometrial cancer (United States). *Cancer Causes Control* **12**: 691–702.

Longnecker, M.P. 1990. A case-control study of alcoholic beverage consumption in relation to risk of cancer of the right colon and rectum in men. *Cancer Causes Control* **1**: 5–14.

Longnecker, M.P., Orza, M.J., Adams, M.E., Vioque, J., and Chalmers, T.C. 1990. A meta-analysis of alcoholic beverage consumption in relation to risk of colorectal cancer. *Cancer Causes Control* **1**: 59–68.

Longnecker, M.P. 1994. Alcoholic beverage consumption in relation to risk of breast cancer: meta-analysis and review. *Cancer Causes Control* **5**: 73–82.

Longnecker, M.P., Newcomb, P.A., Mittendorf, R., Greenberg, E.R., Clapp, R.W., Bogdan, G.F., Baron, J., MacMahon, B., and Willett, W.C. 1995a. Risk of breast cancer in relation to lifetime alcohol consumption. *J Natl Cancer Inst* **87**: 923–929.

Longnecker, M.P., Paganini-Hill, A., and Ross, R.K. 1995b. Lifetime alcohol consumption and breast cancer risk among postmenopausal women in Los Angeles. *Cancer Epidemiol Biomarkers Prev* **4**: 721–725.

Longnecker, M.P., and Tseng, M. 1999. Alcohol and cancer. *In* "Nutritional Oncology" (D. Heber, G.L. Blackburn, and V.L.W. Go, Eds.), 1st edition, pp. 277–298. Academic Press, San Diego.

Ma, J., Stampfer, M.J., Christensen, B., Giovannucci, E., Hunter, D.J., Chen, J., Willett, W.C., Selhub, J., Hennekens, C.H., Gravel, R., and Rozen, R. 1999. A polymorphism of the methionine synthase gene: association with plasma folate, vitamin B12, homocyst(e)ine, and colorectal cancer risk. *Cancer Epidemiol Biomarkers Prev* **8**: 825–829.

Maeda, M., Nagawa, H., Maeda, T., Koike, H., and Kasai, H. 1998. Alcohol consumption enhances liver metastasis in colorectal carcinoma patients. *Cancer* **83**: 1483–1488.

Mannisto, S., Virtanen, M., Kataja, V., Uusitupa, M., and Pietinen, P. 2000. Lifetime alcohol consumption and breast cancer: a case-control study in Finland. *Public Health Nutr* **3**: 11–18.

Marcus, P.M., Newman, B., Millikan, R.C., Moorman, P.G., Baird, D.D., and Qaqish, B. 2000. The associations of adolescent cigarette smoking, alcoholic beverage consumption, environmental tobacco smoke, and ionizing radiation with subsequent breast cancer risk (United States). *Cancer Causes Control* **11**: 271–278.

Martin-Moreno, J.M., Boyle, P., Gorgojo, L., Willett, W.C., Gonzalez, J., Villar, F., and Maisonneuve, P. 1993. Alcoholic beverage consumption and risk of breast cancer in Spain. *Cancer Causes Control* **4**: 345–353.

Matsuo, K., Hamajima, N., Hirai, T., Kato, T., Koike, K., Inoue, M., Takezaki, T., and Tajima, K. 2002. Aldehyde dehydrogenase 2 (ALDH2) genotype affects rectal cancer susceptibility due to alcohol consumption. *J Epidemiol* **12**: 70–76.

Mayne, S.T., Janerich, D.T., Greenwald, P., Chorost, S., Tucci, C., Zaman, M.B., Melamed, M.R., Kiely, M., and McKneally, M.F. 1994. Dietary beta carotene and lung cancer risk in U.S. nonsmokers. *J Natl Cancer Inst* **86**: 33–38.

McCann, S.E., Freudenheim, J.L., Marshall, J.R., Brasure, J.R., Swanson, M.K., and Graham, S. 2000. Diet in the epidemiology of endometrial cancer in western New York (United States). *Cancer Causes Control* **11**: 965–974.

McCredie, M.R., Dite, G.S., Giles, G.G., and Hopper, J.L. 1998. Breast cancer in Australian women under the age of 40. *Cancer Causes Control* **9**: 189–198.

McDonald, P.A., Williams, R., Dawkins, F., and Adams-Campbell, L.L. 2002. Breast cancer survival in African American women: is alcohol consumption a prognostic indicator? *Cancer Causes Control* **13**: 543–549.

Meyer, F., and White, E. 1993. Alcohol and nutrients in relation to colon cancer in middle-aged adults. *Am J Epidemiol* **138**: 225–236.

Modugno, F., Ness, R.B., and Allen, G.O. 2003. Alcohol consumption and the risk of mucinous and nonmucinous epithelial ovarian cancer. *Obstet Gynecol* **102**: 1336–1343.

Munaka, M., Kohshi, K., Kawamoto, T., Takasawa, S., Nagata, N., Itoh, H., Oda, S., and Katoh, T. 2003. Genetic polymorphisms of tobacco- and alcohol-related metabolizing enzymes and the risk of hepatocellular carcinoma. *J Cancer Res Clin Oncol* **129**: 355–360.

Murata, M., Tagawa, M., Watanabe, S., Kimura, H., Takeshita, T., and Morimoto, K. 1999. Genotype difference of aldehyde dehydrogenase 2 gene in alcohol drinkers influences the incidence of Japanese colorectal cancer patients. *Jpn J Cancer Res* **90**: 711–719.

Muto, M., Nakane, M., Hitomi, Y., Yoshida, S., Sasaki, S., Ohtsu, A., Ebihara, S., and Esumi, H. 2002. Association between aldehyde dehydrogenase gene polymorphisms and the phenomenon of field cancerization in patients with head and neck cancer. *Carcinogenesis* **23**: 1759–1765.

Nasca, P. 2001. Alcohol and cancer. *In* "Fundamentals of Cancer Epidemiology" (P.C. Nasca and H. Pastides, Eds.), pp. 175–205. Aspen Publishers, Inc, Gaithersburg, MD.

Nasca, P.C., Baptiste, M.S., Field, N.A., Metzger, B.B., Black, M., Kwon, C.S., and Jacobson, H. 1990. An epidemiological case-control study of breast cancer and alcohol consumption. *Int J Epidemiol* **19**: 532–538.

Nasca, P.C., Liu, S., Baptiste, M.S., Kwon, C.S., Jacobson, H., and Metzger, B.B. 1994. Alcohol consumption and breast cancer: estrogen receptor status and histology. *Am J Epidemiol* **140**: 980–988.

Negri, E., La Vecchia, C., and Franceschi, S. 2000. Re: dietary folate consumption and breast cancer risk. *J Natl Cancer Inst* **92**: 1270–1271.

Newcomb, P.A., Storer, B.E., and Marcus, P.M. 1993. Cancer of the large bowel in women in relation to alcohol consumption: a case-control study in Wisconsin (United States). *Cancer Causes Control* **4**: 405–411.

Newcomb, P.A., Trentham-Dietz, A., and Storer, B.E. 1997. Alcohol consumption in relation to endometrial cancer risk. *Cancer Epidemiol Biomarkers Prev* **6**: 775–778.

NIAAA. 2003. "Surveillance Report #62. Apparent per capita alcohol consumption: national, state, and regional trends, 1977–2000." U.S. Department of Health and Human Services, Bethesda, MD.

Nyren, O., and Adami, H.-O. 2002. Esophageal cancer. *In* "Textbook of Cancer Epidemiology" (H.-O. Adami, D. Hunter, and D. Trichopoulos, Eds.), pp. 137–161. Oxford University Press, New York.

O'Connell, D.L., Hulka, B.S., Chambless, L.E., Wilkinson, W.E., and Deubner, D.C. 1987. Cigarette smoking, alcohol consumption, and breast cancer risk. *J Natl Cancer Inst* **78**: 229–234.

Otani, T., Iwasaki, M., Yamamoto, S., Sobue, T., Hanaoka, T., Inoue, M., and Tsugane, S. 2003. Alcohol consumption, smoking, and subsequent risk of colorectal cancer in middle-aged and elderly Japanese men and women: Japan Public Health Center-based prospective study. *Cancer Epidemiol Biomarkers Prev* **12**: 1492–1500.

Paganini-Hill, A.R., RK. 1983. Breast cancer and alcohol consumption. *Lancet* 626–627.

Park, S.K., Yoo, K.Y., Lee, S.J., Kim, S.U., Ahn, S.H., Noh, D.Y., Choe, K.J., Strickland, P.T., Hirvonen, A., and Kang, D. 2000. Alcohol consumption, glutathione S-transferase M1 and T1 genetic polymorphisms and breast cancer risk. *Pharmacogenetics* **10**: 301–309.

Pawlega, J. 1992. Breast cancer and smoking, vodka drinking and dietary habits. A case-control study. *Acta Oncol* **31**: 387–392.

Pawlotsky, J.M. 2004. Pathophysiology of hepatitis C virus infection and related liver disease. *Trends Microbiol* **12**: 96–102.

Pedersen, A., Johansen, C., and Gronbaek, M. 2003. Relations between amount and type of alcohol and colon and rectal cancer in a Danish population based cohort study. *Gut* **52**: 861–867.

Peters, R.K., Pike, M.C., Garabrant, D., and Mack, T.M. 1992. Diet and colon cancer in Los Angeles County, California. *Cancer Causes Control* **3**: 457–473.

Petri, A.L., Tjonneland, A., Gamborg, M., Johansen, D., Hoidrup, S., Sorensen, T.I., and Gronbaek, M. 2004. Alcohol intake, type of beverage, and risk of breast cancer in pre- and postmenopausal women. *Alcohol Clin Exp Res* **28**: 1084–1090.

Potter, J.D., and McMichael, A.J. 1986. Diet and cancer of the colon and rectum: a case-control study. *J Natl Cancer Inst* **76**: 557–569.

Potter, J.D., Sellers, T.A., Folsom, A.R., and McGovern, P.G. 1992. Alcohol, beer, and lung cancer in postmenopausal women. The Iowa Women's Health Study. *Ann Epidemiol* **2**: 587–595.

Potter, J.D. 1999. Colorectal cancer: molecules and populations. *J Natl Cancer Inst* **91**: 916–932.

Pradier, R., Gonzalez, A., Matos, E., Loria, D., Adan, R., Saco, P., and Califano, L. 1993. Prognostic factors in laryngeal carcinoma. Experience in 296 male patients. *Cancer* **71**: 2472–2476.

Prescott, E., Gronbaek, M., Becker, U., and Sorensen, T.I. 1999. Alcohol intake and the risk of lung cancer: influence of type of alcoholic beverage. *Am J Epidemiol* **149**: 463–470.

Putnam, S.D., Cerhan, J.R., Parker, A.S., Bianchi, G.D., Wallace, R.B., Cantor, K.P., and Lynch, C.F. 2000. Lifestyle and anthropometric risk factors for prostate cancer in a cohort of Iowa men. *Ann Epidemiol* **10**: 361–369.

Quertemont, E. 2004. Genetic polymorphism in ethanol metabolism: acetaldehyde contribution to alcohol abuse and alcoholism. *Mol Psychiatry* **9**: 570–581.

Ranstam, J., and Olsson, H. 1995. Alcohol, cigarette smoking, and the risk of breast cancer. *Cancer Detect Prev* **19**: 487–493.

Rohan, T.E., and McMichael, A.J. 1988. Alcohol consumption and risk of breast cancer. *Int J Cancer* **41**: 695–699.

Rohan, T.E., Hiller, J.E., and McMichael, A.J. 1993. Dietary factors and survival from breast cancer. *Nutr Cancer* **20**: 167–177.

Rohan, T.E., Jain, M., Howe, G.R., and Miller, A.B. 2000a. Alcohol consumption and risk of breast cancer: a cohort study. *Cancer Causes Control* **11**: 239–247.

Rohan, T.E., Jain, M.G., Howe, G.R., and Miller, A.B. 2000b. Dietary folate consumption and breast cancer risk. *J Natl Cancer Inst* **92**: 266–269.

Rookus, M.A., and van Leeuwen, F.E. 1994. Oral contraceptives and risk of breast cancer in women aged 20–54 years. Netherlands Oral Contraceptives and Breast Cancer Study Group. *Lancet* **344**: 844–851.

Rosenberg, L., Slone, D., Shapiro, S., Kaufman, D.W., Helmrich, S.P., Miettinen, O.S., Stolley, P.D., Levy, M., Rosenshein, N.B., Schottenfeld, D., and Engle, R.L., Jr. 1982. Breast cancer and alcoholic-beverage consumption. *Lancet* **1**: 267–270.

Rosenberg, L., Palmer, J.R., Miller, D.R., Clarke, E.A., and Shapiro, S. 1990. A case-control study of alcoholic beverage consumption and breast cancer. *Am J Epidemiol* **131**: 6–14.

Royo-Bordonada, M.A., Martin-Moreno, J.M., Guallar, E., Gorgojo, L., van't Veer, P., Mendez, M., Huttunen, J.K., Martin, B.C., Kardinaal, A.F., Fernandez-Crehuet, J., Thamm, M., Strain, J.J., Kok, F.J., and Kohlmeier, L. 1997. Alcohol intake and risk of breast cancer: the euramic study. *Neoplasma* **44**: 150–156.

Saxe, G.A., Rock, C.L., Wicha, M.S., and Schottenfeld, D. 1999. Diet and risk for breast cancer recurrence and survival. *Breast Cancer Res Treat* **53**: 241–253.

Schatzkin, A., Carter, C.L., Green, S.B., Kreger, B.E., Splansky, G.L., Anderson, K.M., Helsel, W.E., and Kannel, W.B. 1989. Is alcohol consumption related to breast cancer? Results from the Framingham Heart Study. *J Natl Cancer Inst* **81**: 31–35.

Schoenborn, C.A., Adams, P.F., Barnes, P.M., Vickerie, J.L., and Schiller, J.S. 2004. "Health behaviors of adults: United States: 1999–2001." National Center for Health Statistics. Vital Health Statistics, Hyattsville, MD.

Schouten, L.J., Zeegers, M.P., Goldbohm, R.A., and van den Brandt, P.A. 2004. Alcohol and ovarian cancer risk: results from the Netherlands Cohort Study. *Cancer Causes Control* **15**: 201–209.

Schuurman, A.G., Goldbohm, R.A., and van den Brandt, P.A. 1999. A prospective cohort study on consumption of alcoholic beverages in relation to prostate cancer incidence (The Netherlands). *Cancer Causes Control* **10**: 597–605.

Sellers, T.A., Kushi, L.H., Cerhan, J.R., Vierkant, R.A., Gapstur, S.M., Vachon, C.M., Olson, J.E., Therneau, T.M., and Folsom, A.R. 2001. Dietary folate intake, alcohol, and risk of breast cancer in a prospective study of postmenopausal women. *Epidemiology* **12**: 420–428.

Sellers, T.A., Vierkant, R.A., Cerhan, J.R., Gapstur, S.M., Vachon, C.M., Olson, J.E., Pankratz, V.S., Kushi, L.H., and Folsom, A.R. 2002. Interaction of dietary folate intake, alcohol, and risk of hormone receptor-defined breast cancer in a prospective study of postmenopausal women. *Cancer Epidemiol Biomarkers Prev* **11**: 1104–1107.

Sesso, H.D., Paffenbarger, R.S., Jr., and Lee, I.M. 2001. Alcohol consumption and risk of prostate cancer: The Harvard Alumni Health Study. *Int J Epidemiol* **30**: 749–755.

Sharpe, C.R., and Siemiatycki, J. 2001. Case-control study of alcohol consumption and prostate cancer risk in Montreal, Canada. *Cancer Causes Control* **12**: 589–598.

Sharpe, C.R., Siemiatycki, J., and Rachet, B. 2002. Effects of alcohol consumption on the risk of colorectal cancer among men by anatomical subsite (Canada). *Cancer Causes Control* **13**: 483–491.

Shimizu, N., Nagata, C., Shimizu, H., Kametani, M., Takeyama, N., Ohnuma, T., and Matsushita, S. 2003. Height, weight, and alcohol consumption in relation to the risk of colorectal cancer in Japan: a prospective study. *Br J Cancer* **88**: 1038–1043.

Slattery, M.L., West, D.W., Robison, L.M., French, T.K., Ford, M.H., Schuman, K.L., and Sorenson, A.W. 1990. Tobacco, alcohol, coffee, and caffeine as risk factors for colon cancer in a low-risk population. *Epidemiology* **1**: 141–145.

Smith, S.J., Deacon, J.M., and Chilvers, C.E. 1994. Alcohol, smoking, passive smoking and caffeine in relation to breast cancer risk in young women. UK National Case-Control Study Group. *Br J Cancer* **70**: 112–119.

Smith-Warner, S.A., Spiegelman, D., Yaun, S.S., van den Brandt, P.A., Folsom, A.R., Goldbohm, R.A., Graham, S., Holmberg, L., Howe, G.R., Marshall, J.R., Miller, A.B., Potter, J.D., Speizer, F.E., Willett, W.C., Wolk, A., and Hunter, D.J. 1998. Alcohol and breast cancer in women: a pooled analysis of cohort studies. *JAMA* **279**: 535–540.

Sneyd, M.J., Paul, C., Spears, G.F., and Skegg, D.C. 1991. Alcohol consumption and risk of breast cancer. *Int J Cancer* **48**: 812–815.

Stickel, F., Schuppan, D., Hahn, E.G., and Seitz, H.K. 2002. Cocarcinogenic effects of alcohol in hepatocarcinogenesis. *Gut* **51**: 132–139.

Stoll, B.A. 1999. Alcohol intake and late-stage promotion of breast cancer. *Eur J Cancer* **35**: 1653–1658.

Sturmer, T., Wang-Gohrke, S., Arndt, V., Boeing, H., Kong, X., Kreienberg, R., and Brenner, H. 2002. Interaction between alcohol dehydrogenase

II gene, alcohol consumption, and risk for breast cancer. *Br J Cancer* **87**: 519–523.

Swanson, C.A., Wilbanks, G.D., Twiggs, L.B., Mortel, R., Berman, M.L., Barrett, R.J., and Brinton, L.A. 1993. Moderate alcohol consumption and the risk of endometrial cancer. *Epidemiology* **4**: 530–536.

Swanson, C.A., Coates, R.J., Malone, K.E., Gammon, M.D., Schoenberg, J.B., Brogan, D.J., McAdams, M., Potischman, N., Hoover, R.N., and Brinton, L.A. 1997. Alcohol consumption and breast cancer risk among women under age 45 years. *Epidemiology* **8**: 231–237.

Takeshita, T., Yang, X., Inoue, Y., Sato, S., and Morimoto, K. 2000. Relationship between alcohol drinking, ADH2 and ALDH2 genotypes, and risk for hepatocellular carcinoma in Japanese. *Cancer Lett* **149**: 69–76.

Tanabe, H., Yokota, K., Shibata, N., Satoh, T., Watari, J., and Kohgo, Y. 2001. Alcohol consumption as a major risk factor in the development of early esophageal cancer in patients with head and neck cancer. *Intern Med* **40**: 692–696.

Terry, M.B., Neugut, A.I., Mansukhani, M., Waye, J., Harpaz, N., and Hibshoosh, H. 2003. Tobacco, alcohol, and p53 overexpression in early colorectal neoplasia. *BMC Cancer* **3**: 29.

Terry, P., Baron, J.A., Weiderpass, E., Yuen, J., Lichtenstein, P., and Nyren, O. 1999. Lifestyle and endometrial cancer risk: a cohort study from the Swedish Twin Registry. *Int J Cancer* **82**: 38–42.

Thorand, B., Kohlmeier, L., Simonsen, N., Croghan, C., and Thamm, M. 1998. Intake of fruits, vegetables, folic acid and related nutrients and risk of breast cancer in postmenopausal women. *Public Health Nutr* **1**: 147–156.

Tjonneland, A., Thomsen, B.L., Stripp, C., Christensen, J., Overvad, K., Mellemkaer, L., Gronbaek, M., and Olsen, J.H. 2003. Alcohol intake, drinking patterns and risk of postmenopausal breast cancer in Denmark: a prospective cohort study. *Cancer Causes Control* **14**: 277–284.

Tjonneland, A., Christensen, J., Thomsen, B.L., Olsen, A., Stripp, C., Overvad, K., and Olsen, J.H. 2004. Lifetime alcohol consumption and postmenopausal breast cancer rate in Denmark: a prospective cohort study. *J Nutr* **134**: 173–178.

Toniolo, P., Riboli, E., Protta, F., Charrel, M., and Cappa, A.P. 1989. Breast cancer and alcohol consumption: a case-control study in northern Italy. *Cancer Res* **49**: 5203–5206.

Trentham-Dietz, A., Newcomb, P.A., Storer, B.E., and Remington, P.L. 2000. Risk factors for carcinoma in situ of the breast. *Cancer Epidemiol Biomarkers Prev* **9**: 697–703.

Vachon, C.M., Cerhan, J.R., Vierkant, R.A., and Sellers, T.A. 2001. Investigation of an interaction of alcohol intake and family history on breast cancer risk in the Minnesota Breast Cancer Family Study. *Cancer* **92**: 240–248.

Vaeth, P.A., and Satariano, W.A. 1998. Alcohol consumption and breast cancer stage at diagnosis. *Alcohol Clin Exp Res* **22**: 928–934.

van den Brandt, P.A., Goldbohm, R.A., and van't Veer, P. 1995. Alcohol and breast cancer: results from The Netherlands Cohort Study. *Am J Epidemiol* **141**: 907–915.

van't Veer, P., Kok, F.J., Hermus, R.J., and Sturmans, F. 1989. Alcohol dose, frequency and age at first exposure in relation to the risk of breast cancer. *Int J Epidemiol* **18**: 511–517.

Viladiu, P., Izquierdo, A., de Sanjose, S., and Bosch, F.X. 1996. A breast cancer case-control study in Girona, Spain. Endocrine, familial and lifestyle factors. *Eur J Cancer Prev* **5**: 329–335.

Villeneuve, P.J., Johnson, K.C., Kreiger, N., and Mao, Y. 1999. Risk factors for prostate cancer: results from the Canadian National Enhanced Cancer Surveillance System. The Canadian Cancer Registries Epidemiology Research Group. *Cancer Causes Control* **10**: 355–367.

Wakai, K., Ohno, Y., Obata, K., and Aoki, K. 1993. Prognostic significance of selected lifestyle factors in urinary bladder cancer. *Jpn J Cancer Res* **84**: 1223–1229.

Wang, X.D. 2003. Retinoids and alcohol-related carcinogenesis. *J Nutr* **133**: 287S–290S.

WCRF. 1997. "Food, nutrition and the prevention of cancer: a global perspective." World Cancer Research Fund/American Cancer Institute for Cancer Research, Washington, DC.

Webb, P.M., Purdie, D.M., Bain, C.J., and Green, A.C. 2004. Alcohol, wine, and risk of epithelial ovarian cancer. *Cancer Epidemiol Biomarkers Prev* **13**: 592–599.

Webster, L.A., Layde, P.M., Wingo, P.A., and Ory, H.W. 1983. Alcohol consumption and risk of breast cancer. *Lancet* **2**: 724–726.

Webster, L.A., and Weiss, N.S. 1989. Alcoholic beverage consumption and the risk of endometrial cancer. Cancer and Steroid Hormone Study Group. *Int J Epidemiol* **18**: 786–791.

Weiderpass, E., and Baron, J.A. 2001. Cigarette smoking, alcohol consumption, and endometrial cancer risk: a population-based study in Sweden. *Cancer Causes Control* **12**: 239–247.

Weiss, H.A., Brinton, L.A., Brogan, D., Coates, R.J., Gammon, M.D., Malone, K.E., Schoenberg, J.B., and Swanson, C.A. 1996. Epidemiology of in situ and invasive breast cancer in women aged under 45. *Br J Cancer* **73**: 1298–1305.

Willett, W.C., Stampfer, M.J., Colditz, G.A., Rosner, B.A., Hennekens, C.H., and Speizer, F.E. 1987. Moderate alcohol consumption and the risk of breast cancer. *N Engl J Med* **316**: 1174–1180.

Williams, R.R., and Horm, J.W. 1977. Association of cancer sites with tobacco and alcohol consumption and socioeconomic status of patients: interview study from the Third National Cancer Survey. *J Natl Cancer Inst* **58**: 525–547.

Woodson, K., Albanes, D., Tangrea, J.A., Rautalahti, M., Virtamo, J., and Taylor, P.R. 1999. Association between alcohol and lung cancer in the alpha-tocopherol, beta-carotene cancer prevention study in Finland. *Cancer Causes Control* **10**: 219–226.

World Health Organization. 2003. "Diet, nutrition and the prevention of chronic diseases." World Health Organization, Geneva.

Wrensch, M., Chew, T., Farren, G., Barlow, J., Belli, F., Clarke, C., Erdmann, C.A., Lee, M., Moghadassi, M., Peskin-Mentzer, R., Quesenberry, C.P., Jr., Souders-Mason, V., Spence, L., Suzuki, M., and Gould, M. 2003. Risk factors for breast cancer in a population with high incidence rates. *Breast Cancer Res* **5**: R88–102.

Yang, M., Coles, B.F., Delongchamp, R., Lang, N.P., and Kadlubar, F.F. 2002. Effects of the ADH3, CYP2E1, and GSTP1 genetic polymorphisms on their expressions in Caucasian lung tissue. *Lung Cancer* **38**: 15–21.

Yokoyama, A., Kato, H., Yokoyama, T., Tsujinaka, T., Muto, M., Omori, T., Haneda, T., Kumagai, Y., Igaki, H., Yokoyama, M., Watanabe, H., Fukuda, H., and Yoshimizu, H. 2002. Genetic polymorphisms of alcohol and aldehyde dehydrogenases and glutathione S-transferase M1 and drinking, smoking, and diet in Japanese men with esophageal squamous cell carcinoma. *Carcinogenesis* **23**: 1851–1859.

Yokoyama, A., and Omori, T. 2003. Genetic polymorphisms of alcohol and aldehyde dehydrogenases and risk for esophageal and head and neck cancers. *Jpn J Clin Oncol* **33**: 111–121.

Young, T.B. 1989. A case-control study of breast cancer and alcohol consumption habits. *Cancer* **64**, 552–558.

Yu, G.P., Ostroff, J.S., Zhang, Z.F., Tang, J., and Schantz, S.P. 1997. Smoking history and cancer patient survival: a hospital cancer registry study. *Cancer Detect Prev* **21**: 497–509.

Zeegers, M.P., Tan, F.E., Verhagen, A.P., Weijenberg, M.P., and van den Brandt, P.A. 1999. Elevated risk of cancer of the urinary tract for alcohol drinkers: a meta-analysis. *Cancer Causes Control* **10**: 445–451.

Zhang, S., Folsom, A.R., Sellers, T.A., Kushi, L.H., and Potter, J.D. 1995. Better breast cancer survival for postmenopausal women who are less overweight and eat less fat. The Iowa Women's Health Study. *Cancer* **76**: 275–283.

Zhang, S., Hunter, D.J., Hankinson, S.E., Giovannucci, E.L., Rosner, B.A., Colditz, G.A., Speizer, F.E., and Willett, W.C. 1999a. A prospective study of folate intake and the risk of breast cancer. *JAMA* **281**: 1632–1637.

Zhang, S.M., Willett, W.C., Selhub, J., Hunter, D.J., Giovannucci, E.L., Holmes, M.D., Colditz, G.A., and Hankinson, S.E. 2003. Plasma folate, vitamin B6, vitamin B12, homocysteine, and risk of breast cancer. *J Natl Cancer Inst* **95**: 373–380.

Zhang, Y., Kreger, B.E., Dorgan, J.F., Splansky, G.L., Cupples, L.A., and Ellison, R.C. 1999b. Alcohol consumption and risk of breast cancer: the Framingham Study revisited. *Am J Epidemiol* **149**: 93–101.

Zheng, T., Holford, T.R., Zahm, S.H., Owens, P.H., Boyle, P., Zhang, Y., Zhang, B., Wise, J.P., Sr., Stephenson, L.P., and Ali-Osman, F. 2003. Glutathione S-transferase M1 and T1 genetic polymorphisms, alcohol consumption and breast cancer risk. *Br J Cancer* **88**: 58–62.

CHAPTER

12

Environmental Toxins, Nutrition, and Cancer

RAMUNE RELIENE AND ROBERT H. SCHIESTL

INTRODUCTION

A wide range of environmental toxins have been associated with carcinogenesis of the respiratory system and other organs. Cigarette smoke, particulate matter (PM), and its component diesel exhaust particles (DEPs), as well as arsenic and chromium, are among common environmental toxins that cause a number of adverse health effects predominantly affecting inhabitants of highly populated or industrialized areas. These pollutants have been identified as causative factors for lung cancer, and some are associated with carcinogenesis at other sites. These agents induce oxidative stress and genetic damage, which seem to be the major biological mechanisms responsible for adverse health effects, particularly carcinogenesis. Genetic damage (genotoxicity) includes various aspects of DNA damage ranging from oxidative DNA base lesions and point mutations to chromosomal alterations. Oxidative stress can cause genetic damage. Research data are accumulating that oxidative stress can be alleviated by higher intake of antioxidant vitamins or other antioxidants. In this chapter, we review DNA-damaging effects of cigarette smoke, DEP, arsenic, and chromium and discuss the possible beneficial role of antioxidant dietary supplementation under circumstances of heightened oxidant stress.

TOBACCO SMOKE

Adverse Health Effects of Tobacco Smoke

Cigarette smoking is a major risk factor for lung, oral, and pharyngeal cancer (Bergen and Caporaso, 1999). The other most prevalent smoke-related disorders include chronic obstructive pulmonary disease (COPD) and cardiovascular diseases. Inhalation of environmental tobacco smoke (ETS) by nonsmokers is associated with many of the same deleterious health effects as active smoking (Cal-EPA, 1997; Witschi et al., 1997; Collier and Pritsos, 2003). For example, nonsmokers living with smokers have 20–50% access risk of coronary heart disease and a 1.2–2 times elevated risk of developing lung cancer. The U.S. Environmental Protection Agency (EPA) estimates that annually 38,000 heart disease deaths, 3000 lung cancer deaths, and 12,000 other cancer deaths can be attributed to ETS exposure (Cal-EPA, 1997). ETS is particularly hazardous for the developing fetus or young children.

Environmental Tobacco Smoke Exposure and Children's Health

More than 150 studies have described effects of ETS on respiratory diseases in children (Jinot and Bayard, 1996). Exposure to ETS increases the prevalence of asthma, wheeze, cough, bronchitis, bronchiolitis, pneumonia, and impaired pulmonary function. Other health effects including ear infections, sudden infant death syndrome, behavioral problems, and neurocognitive deficits are also linked to ETS and prenatal maternal smoking (DiFranza et al., 2004). A very comprehensive study on maternal smoking during pregnancy and childhood ETS exposure in almost 6000 children showed an approximate twofold to threefold significantly elevated risk of asthma and wheezing of different subcategories (Gilliland et al., 2001). The study showed that *in utero* exposure to maternal smoking without subsequent postnatal ETS exposure had a more pronounced effect on

Copyright © 2006, Elsevier Inc.
All rights of reproduction in any form reserved.

prevalence of asthma and wheezing than current and previous postnatal ETS exposure. *In utero* exposure was associated with increased prevalence of asthma and wheezing, while current and previous ETS exposure was not linked to higher prevalence of asthma, although it was associated with wheezing. Other studies showed similarly that effects of *in utero* smoke exposure on asthma and wheezing are stronger than effects of postnatal ETS exposure (Ehrlich et al., 1996; Strachan and Cook, 1998; Gold et al., 1999). Asthma is a risk factor for lung cancer even in nonsmokers (Boffett et al., 2002; Santillan et al., 2003), and therefore, asthma provoked by ETS at young age poses a risk of developing lung cancer after several decades. A meta-analysis of 30 studies provides evidence that parental smoking is associated with increased risk of childhood cancers (Boffetta et al., 2000).

Genotoxicity of Tobacco Smoke

It is generally accepted that cancer develops as a result of multiple genetic events, where gene mutations and particularly large genome rearrangements (deletions, translocations, duplications) are a prerequisite in the process of carcinogenesis. Tobacco smoke contains >4700 chemical compounds, and hundreds of them are mutagenic and carcinogenic (Church and Pryor, 1985). Polycyclic aromatic hydrocarbons (PAHs), heterocyclic nitrosamines, redox cycling quinones, reactive oxygen species (ROS), reactive nitrogen species (RNS), and volatile saturated and unsaturated aldehydes are among the reactive ingredients of tobacco smoke. Many of these structurally diverse chemicals have their own mechanism of action. Perhaps the most common mechanism of tobacco smoke constituents involves oxidative damage of macromolecules because free radicals and other oxidants comprise a high fraction of cigarette smoke (Bluhm et al., 1971; Church and Pryor, 1985; Pryor and Stone, 1993). It has been estimated that each puff of cigarette smoke contains $\sim 10^{16}$ oxidant molecules (Church and Pryor, 1985). Oxidative DNA lesions have been found in human smokers and ETS-exposed individuals, indicated by elevated levels of 8-OH deoxyguanosine (8-OHdG), indicating oxidative damage to DNA (Fraga et al., 1996; Howard et al., 1998). Although DNA repair systems evolved to replace damaged DNA bases, 8-OHdG frequently mispairs with an adenosine (A) base (Cheng et al., 1992), causing point mutations (GC $\rightarrow$ TA transversions) and thereby increasing the gene mutation rate (Ames et al., 1993; Cerutti, 1994). Another prevalent DNA lesion induced by cigarette smoke is formation of covalent DNA adducts. DNA adducts have been detected in various organs of lung cancer patients with a history of smoking (Randerath and Randerath, 1993), "healthy" smokers (Tang et al., 2001), placenta of smoking women (Everson et al., 1986; Hansen et al., 1993), and experimental animals exposed to cigarette smoke (Balansky et al., 1996). DNA adducts, if not eliminated in a timely manner, may cause miscoding resulting in gene mutations or cause DNA breaks leading to genome rearrangements. For example, specific deletions in the short arm of chromosomes 3, 9, and 17 appear to be associated with lung tumorigenesis (Hung et al., 1995; Kishimoto et al., 1995; Virmani, 1995).

The fetus and young child are especially vulnerable to toxic effects of environmental pollutants (Perera et al., 1999; Whyatt et al., 2001), and several experimental and human studies suggest that the fetus clears toxicants less efficiently than the adult (Lu et al., 1986; Lu and Wang, 1990; Whyatt et al., 2001). Some cancer-associated genotoxicity markers detected in newborn infants are particularly concerning. A significant difference in the HPRT mutational spectrum was found in *in utero* smoke-exposed newborn infants born to mothers exposed to passive cigarette smoke, where the most notable change was an increase in DNA deletions mediated by V(D)J recombinase, a recombination event associated with childhood hematopoietic malignancies (Finette et al., 1998). The micronucleus assay revealed that the frequency of micronuclei, a marker of chromosomal fragmentation, was significantly higher in children of smoking parents and was slightly higher in children with both parents smoking than those with one parent smoking (Baier et al., 2002). Other genetic alterations, such as sister chromatid exchange, have been found in infants born to smoking mothers (Sardas et al., 1995). Interestingly, an animal study has shown a significant increase in the frequency of DNA deletions in the offspring of pregnant mice exposed for only 4 hours to a cigarette smoke concentration that caused the same concentration of blood nicotine as that found in smokers after smoking one cigarette (Jalili et al., 1998).

Antioxidant Dietary Supplementation against Tobacco Smoke

Oxidative stress has been implicated in the pathogenesis of tobacco-related diseases, such as COPD, lung cancer, and cardiovascular illness. Numerous studies suggest that a fruit- and vegetable-rich diet can reduce the risk of cancer (Block et al., 1992). Smokers are exposed to higher level of oxidants and have lower dietary intake of fruits and vegetables (Traber et al., 2000). It is estimated that vitamin C metabolic turnover of smokers is approximately double that of nonsmokers (Lykkesfeldt et al., 2000). Consequently, plasma levels of major antioxidant vitamins C and E are significantly reduced in smokers, rendering them more susceptible to oxidative damage than nonsmokers (Traber et al., 2000). Besides oxidants derived from cigarette smoke, more oxidants are produced in the organism of a smoker because they have higher numbers of circulating phagocytes primed to produce ROS and RNS as part of the inflammatory immune response against environmental pathogens and xenobiotics (Cross et al., 1999). ETS causes qualitatively similar oxidative stress as active smoking. Passive smokers exhibit intermediate vitamin C concentration in their plasma between smokers and nonsmokers who were not exposed to ETS, despite similar intake of vitamin C (Tribble et al., 1993). Thus, it is expected that higher antioxidant intake would minimize some of the smoke-induced effects, and results of the following studies support that. Dietary supplementation of antioxidant vitamins (vitamin C, vitamin E, β-carotene) reduces oxidative DNA damage and single-strand DNA breaks in smokers (Duthie et al., 1996; Lee et al., 1998). A study on healthy human volunteers exposed to ETS showed that prior ingestion of vitamin C prevented smoke-induced decrease in antioxidant capacity (assessed by the TRAP assay [total peroxyl radical trapping potential of the serum]) and the increase in lipid peroxidation that otherwise were observed after 1.5 hours of passive smoking (Valkonen and Kuusi, 2000). Vitamin C or a combination of vitamin C and E suppressed formation of lipid peroxidation products in chronic smokers (Reilly et al., 1996). Supplementary vitamin E (≥100 IU/day) significantly lowered progression of early preintrusive atherosclerosis compared with non–vitamin E users (Azen et al., 1996). Vitamins C and E seem to ameliorate endothelial dysfunction, an early indicator of atherosclerotic process, in smokers (Traber et al., 2000). An epidemiological study suggested that vitamin E may inhibit lung cancer development by as much as 20% (Woodson et al., 1999). In some studies, however, adverse effects of β-carotene supplements were observed. In human intervention trials, β-carotene supplements actually increased the risk of acquiring lung cancer when administered to heavy smokers of more advanced preclinical stages of carcinogenesis (Greenberg et al., 1996; Omenn et al., 1996). Most of the lung cancers appear in former smokers, and little information is available on the chemosuppression of these tumors. In any case, recommendations on taking antioxidant supplements have to be made with precaution considering compound's action mechanism, dosage, possible side effects, and the stage of disease.

Antismoke Effects of *N*-Acetylcysteine

N-acetylcysteine (NAC) is a thiol antioxidant that is nontoxic at high doses, tasteless, odorless, and well established in clinical practice (Kelly, 1998). NAC, a synthetic precursor of intracellular cysteine and glutathione (GSH), has been used as a mucolytic drug for more than 4 decades. NAC lowers the viscosity of the mucus and thereby alleviates symptoms of bronchitis and other bronchopulmonary diseases. NAC is an efficient antidote against acute acetaminophen (paracetamol) poisoning (Mitchell et al., 1974; Smilkstein et al., 1988). NAC mitigates acetaminophen-induced hepatorenal toxicity because of its ability to block reactive metabolites of acetaminophen and replenish GSH stores that are rapidly depleted by reactive metabolites of xenobiotics. NAC appears to be efficient in inactivating reactive electrophiles and free radical reactions and appears more effective for clinical application than GSH or its precursor cysteine. This is because GSH does not easily cross cell membranes and cysteine is toxic at higher concentrations. Further studies showed that NAC is protective against carcinogenesis-associated end-points (De Flora et al., 1985, 1986, 2001). For example, NAC blocks metabolites of promutagens; inhibits formation of carcinogenic DNA adducts and oxidative DNA damage; and is able to inhibit tumor promotion, progression, and metastases in experimental models.

Substantial research on the effects of NAC on DNA damage following cigarette smoke exposure were carried out in Silvio De Flora's laboratory (De Flora et al., 2001, 2003). Studies showed that dietary NAC administration results in reduction or inhibition of many smoke-induced DNA-damaging effects in experimental animals. This includes decreased levels of DNA adducts in nuclear and mitochondrial DNA, inhibition of oxidative DNA damage, and attenuation of micronucleus formation. All these data indicate that NAC might be protective against smoke-related lung cancer. Unfortunately, this can hardly be tested in animal studies because it has been extremely difficult to induce lung tumors by cigarette smoke in rodent animals (Coggins, 1998). The ability of NAC to modulate smoke-induced biomarkers has been assessed in humans. Oral NAC given at 600–800 mg/day reduced urinary excretion of mutagens in smokers starting on the first day of administration, which was reversed when treatment was withdrawn (De Flora et al., 1996). A battery of biomarkers was examined in healthy smoking volunteers given NAC (2 × 600-mg tablets/day) or placebo in a randomized double-blind phase II chemoprevention trial (Van Schooten et al., 2002). In the placebo group, there was no variation in any of the biomarkers studied, whereas in the NAC group, a significant decrease occurred in some of the markers, including lipophilic DNA adducts and oxidative DNA damage in bronchoalveolar lavage cells. Effect of NAC was studied in a clinical phase III trial in cancer patients. Supplementation with NAC (600 mg/day) and/or retinyl palmitate for 2 years had no beneficial effect on tumor recurrences in the upper or lower airways in the large study composed of almost 2600 patients who have previously been treated for head and neck cancer or lung cancer, and most of them were previous or current smokers (van Zandwijk et al., 2000). Those studies provided some evidence that NAC may possibly reduce cancer risk in healthy human smokers, although it may no longer be effective in cancer patients. Those studies suggest, however, that NAC may be beneficial for ETS-exposed individuals who have not yet developed cancer but suffer from similar health problems as active smokers, albeit to a lesser degree.

PARTICULATE MATTER

PM is airborne sphere-shaped particles forming smog. The particles constitute a carbon core and adsorbed to it organic compounds, low amounts of inorganic compounds (sulphate, nitrate), and metals. The main source of PM is the combustion of fossil fuels (gasoline or diesel) in automobiles and in heavy industries. Some PM comes from natural sources, and secondary particles originate from chemical transformation of the emitted particles in the air. The particles vary in size (categorized as ultrafine, fine, and coarse particles) and composition, although humans are exposed to a complex ambient PM mixture, the concentration of which is high in urban and industrial areas. Exposure to high PM levels has been associated with a variety of adverse health effects, including asthma and pneumonia (Hruba et al., 2001), COPD (Ebelt et al., 2000), heart disease, lung and upper respiratory tract disease, cancer (Dockery et al., 1993; Beeson et al., 1998; Schwela, 2000; Pope et al., 2002), and mortality (Lippmann et al., 2000; Schwartz, 2001). Each 10-$\mu g/m^3$ elevation in fine PM is associated with an increased risk of mortality by 4%, 6%, and 8%, respectively (Pope et al., 2002).

DIESEL EXHAUST PARTICLES

Diesel exhaust (DE) is a complex mixture of gases and particles emitted by combustion engines using diesel oil as a fuel. The diesel engines are used mainly in trucks, buses, locomotives, ships, agricultural, and other off-road equipment. Although diesel fuel is more economic and durable than gasoline fuel, diesel engines emit 30–100 times more PM than gasoline engines (McClellan, 1987). Increased usage of diesel-powered engines has contributed to ambient PM concentrations so that DE particles (DEP) became a significant component of ambient PM, amounting to 20–80% (EPA, 2002). Average DEP concentration in the United States is ~1 $\mu g/m^3$, but it increases dramatically in big cities. For example, DEP concentration is higher than average in the Los Angeles Basin (1.3–3.6 $\mu g/m^3$), and at a bus stop in Manhattan, levels reached 13–47 $\mu g/m^3$ (EPA, 2002). Estimated occupational DEP exposures vary from 2 to 27 $\mu g/m^3$ for truck drivers, 42–155 $\mu g/m^3$ for railway workers, and 150–500 $\mu g/m^3$ for miners (Steenland, 1998).

Both the gaseous phase and particulate component are associated with adverse health effects of DEP. There are several toxic components in the gaseous phase of DE such as aldehydes, benzene, carbon monoxide, nitrogen oxides, sulfur dioxides, PAHs, and nitro-PAHs. The particulate component of DE is composed of >450 different organic compounds including toxic PAHs, quinones and aldehydes, and traces of heavy metals (Barfknecht et al., 1982; Casellas et al., 1995). More than 100 of the chemicals in the particles are carcinogenic and mutagenic. Benzo(a)pyrene, indeno (1,2,3-cd)pyrene, dibenz(a,h)anthracene, benz(a,h)anthracene, benzo(b)fluoranthene, and benzo(k)fluorantene, naphthalene, and chrysene are just a few carcinogenic PAHs that are found in DEP.

Epidemiological studies suggest that exposure to DE is associated with an increased risk (20–50%) of lung cancer in transportation workers, railroad workers, miners, and operators of heavy construction equipment (McClellan, 1987; Garshick et al., 1988; Stayner et al., 1998; Steenland et al., 1998; Larkin et al., 2000; EPA, 2002). The Multiple Air Toxic Exposure Study (MATES II) conducted by the South Coast Air Quality Management District estimates that DEP contributes >71% of the total lifetime cancer risk from ambient particles (Mates(II)Study, 2000). There is also weak evidence linking exposure to DE and bladder cancer. Non-cancer adverse health effects of DE include acute irritation of the eye and nose, respiratory symptoms (cough and phlegm), and allergic reactions (EPA, 2002).

Genotoxic Effects of Diesel Exhaust Particles

The genotoxicity of DE is often expressed in relationship to its particulate component. The lung is the major target organ for PM, and the metabolism of PM is similar to that of other insoluble foreign bodies. The particles are taken up by macrophages followed by inflammatory responses accompanied by the formation of ROS. Research studies show that DEP induces oxidative stress and is mutagenic in bacterial and mammalian cell assays (McClellan, 1987; Schins, 2002). DEP exposure by inhalation or intratracheal instillation induces oxidative DNA damage (Tokiwa et al., 1999; Adachi et al., 2000; Iwai et al., 2000; Risom et al., 2003), DNA adduct formation (Bond et al., 1988; Gallagher et al., 1994), and mutations (Sato et al., 2000) in lung cells. Long-term inhalation exposure causes tumors in the respiratory tract in rodent animals (Mauderly et al., 1987; McClellan, 1987; Schins, 2002). The particle effect, however, is not limited to the lung tissue. Some particle-bound material enters blood circulation and becomes bioavailable. Experimental animal studies show that labeled PAHs were detected in blood, liver, and kidney after inhalation exposure (Sun et al., 1982). Elevated levels of DNA adducts are found in peripheral blood lymphocytes of bus maintenance workers (Hou et al., 1995). The most concerning issue is that the particle genotoxic effect can be transmitted to the next generations. A research study by Somers et al. (2004) showed that airborne particles induced heritable alterations at noncoding repetitive DNA loci in mouse offspring after exposed male mice were mated with unexposed females.

ARSENIC

Chronic exposure of humans to high concentrations of inorganic arsenic is associated with skin lesions, peripheral vascular disease, hypertension, blackfoot disease (vasoocclusive disease, which leads to gangrene of the extremities), and cancer at various sites (Tseng, 1977; International Agency for Research on Cancer [IARC], 1987; EPA, 1988; Engel et al., 1994; Chen et al., 1995; Tondel et al., 1999). An increased mortality from lung cancer has been observed in humans exposed primarily through inhalation. An increased incidence of skin cancer and cancers of other organs (liver, bladder, and kidney) has been found in the general population consuming water contaminated with high arsenic concentration. Arsenic has been used in a variety of industries, including manufacturing of semiconductor, glass, pigments, paints, alloys, pesticide, and herbicide. Arsenic, as an environmental pollutant, arises from burning coal containing high arsenic concentrations, the mining and smelting of metal ores, or improper disposal of industrial byproduct. The major sources of arsenic in drinking water are the presence of arsenic-rich minerals and rocks in aquifers. More than 200 million people in many countries are chronically exposed to arsenic. Intermediate to high levels of arsenic in ground water (2–5000 μg/liter) is found in Asian countries (Taiwan, Thailand, China, India, Mongolia, Vietnam), South America (Chile, Bolivia, Argentina), Bangladesh, Mexico, and the United States (Arizona, California, Nevada). The highest levels of exposure occur in South America, Taiwan, and the Gulf of Bengal. Intermediate levels of arsenic (≤200 μg/liter) are found in some countries in Europe, such as Hungary, Spain, Greece, and Germany. Most of the epidemiological studies have been conduced in areas with high levels of arsenic contamination (typically >200 μg/liter). Even low or intermediate contamination might be a risk factor for bladder cancer. For example, an ecological study showed that exposure to arsenic concentrations at doses 0.1–0.5 and >0.5 μg/liter relative to the doses below 0.1 μg/liter during 2–9 years prior to cancer diagnosis increases the risk of bladder cancer by 1.5-fold and 2.44-fold, respectively (Kurttio et al., 1999).

Action Mechanism of Arsenic Carcinogenicity

Inorganic arsenic in the environment exists as pentavalent inorganic arsenate (AsV) and to a lesser extent as the trivalent arsenite (AsIII). In most mammals, ingested arsenate is readily converted to arsenite, and inorganic arsenic is metabolized to organic forms, namely, first to monomethyl arsonic acid (MMA) and then to dimethylarsinic acid (DMA), and in rats further to trimethylarsine oxide (TMAO) (Aposhian, 1997). Humans exposed to arsenic excrete 10–20% inorganic arsenic, 10–20% MMA, and 60–80% DMA (Vahter and Concha, 2001). The exact action mechanism of arsenic is not known, although at least several mechanisms are postulated on the basis of experimental data (Hughes, 2002; Kitchin and Ahmad, 2003). The most prevalent theories include oxidative stress, chromosomal alterations, tumor promotion, and cocarcinogenesis.

In vitro and *in vivo* studies indicate that arsenic induces oxidative stress. ROS are formed within 5 minutes after arsenite exposure in human–hamster hybrid cells (Liu et al., 2001). Peroxyl radicals of DMA, a major metabolite of ingested inorganic arsenic, are detected *in vitro* (Yamanaka et al., 1990). Oxidative damage is observed in lungs of DMA-exposed mice (Yamanaka et al., 1991; Wanibuchi et al., 2004). Arsenite is a potent clastogenic compound capable of inducing chromosome aberrations (chromatid gaps, breaks, fragmentation, endoreduplication, chromosomal breaks), sister chromatid exchange, micronuclei formation, and large deletions in cultured cells and rodent animals (Tinwell et al., 1991; Jha et al., 1992; Das et al., 1993; RoyChoudhury et al., 1996; Rasmussen and Menzel, 1997; Schiestl et al., 1997; Hei et al., 1998). In contrast, arsenic (inorganic As or its organic metabolites) does not cause point mutations in standard assays.

Research studies using animal models show that arsenic is involved in tumor promotion and initiation. DMA given in drinking water significantly enhances tumor induction in the urinary bladder, kidney, liver, and thyroid gland after multiorgan tumor initiation with organ-specific carcinogens in rats (Wanibuchi et al., 2004). Arsenite is cocarcinogenic with ultraviolet (UV) irradiation (Rossman et al., 2001). Mice exposed to arsenite in drinking water and UV irradiation had a 2.4-fold higher skin tumor rate as mice exposed to UV alone. A 2-year carcinogenicity study showed that DMA itself causes bladder tumors in rats (Wanibuchi et al., 2004). Mutational analysis of the tumors shows that no mutations were present in p53, K-ras, or β-catenin genes, or low levels (10%) were found in the H-ras gene and no microsatellite instability using 18 microsatellite loci. The level of oxidative DNA damage, however, was increased after DMA administration in drinking water for 2 weeks, suggesting that ROS may play a role in the early phases of DMA carcinogenesis.

Fortunately, some arsenic-induced effects can be reduced by antioxidants. Antioxidative enzymes (catalase and superoxide dismutase) reduce arsenite-induced micronuclei formation (Wang and Huang, 1994), and vitamin E reduces cell killing (Lee and Ho, 1994). Free radical scavenger dimethyl sulfoxide lowers ROS concentration to control level (Liu et al., 2001) and the frequency of deletions by about 75% (Hei et al., 1998). Garlic extract given to mice before exposure to arsenite reduces its clastogenic effects (Das et al., 1993; RoyChoudhury et al., 1996). Vitamin C seems not to be beneficial. DMA enhanced iron release from ferritin in the presence of vitamin C, which may lead to higher levels of ROS, because ROS can be formed via cellular iron and other transition metals (Ahmad et al., 2000).

CHROMIUM

Chromium exists predominantly as compounds of trivalent chromium (CrIII) or hexavalent chromium (CrVI) (EPA, 2000; IARC, 1990; Cohen et al., 1993; Costa, 1997; Barceloux, 1999). CrIII is suggested to be an essential micronutrient element, while CrVI is carcinogenic. CrIII is found at higher concentrations in green beans, broccoli, cereals, and some brands of beer and wine. It is claimed that insufficient dietary intake of chromium leads to impaired glucose tolerance, glycosuria, and elevations of serum insulin, cholesterol, and total triglycerides. CrIII dietary supplements are recommended for diabetes patients because of its proposed beneficial effect on glucose metabolism (Anderson et al., 1997; Vincent, 2004). Chromite ore is the major source of CrIII. CrVI occurs rarely in nature in the mineral crocoite ($PbCrO4$). Most CrVI compounds (chromates and Cr trioxide) are produced from chromite ores for commercial applications. CrVI compounds are used in a variety of industries including leather tanning, chrome plating, stainless steel production, chrome pigment manufacturing, and as an antirust agent added to water-cooled machinery. Occupational exposure to CrVI has been associated with respiratory distress, asthma, skin rashes, liver damage, duodenal ulcer formation, and gastritis. The first epidemiological study conducted on chromate production workers in the United States in the 1940s showed that cancer of the respiratory system represented 63% of all deaths from cancer in the exposed group and 21.8% in the general population. Numerous epidemiological studies in different countries confirmed that an increased risk of lung cancer is associated with CrVI exposure and CrVI has been classified as a known human lung carcinogen by the inhalation route of exposure (EPA; IARC, 1990). There is suggestive evidence of an increased incidence of other types of cancer (lymphoma, leukemia, bone, stomach, prostate, genital, bladder, renal cancers) in chrome industry workers (Costa, 1997; Barceloux, 1999). Although CrVI primarily affects individuals in occupational settings, industrial waste contamination and emissions of fossil fuel combustion led to elevated levels of CrVI in the atmosphere, drinking water, and soil. It has been reported that the fourfold increase in childhood leukemia in Woburn, Massachusetts, was attributed to consumption of CrVI-contaminated drinking water at levels two times above the state drinking water standard of 50 ppb (50 μg/liter) (Durant et al., 1995). Epidemiological studies are suggestive that oral exposure to CrVI could lead to increased risk of cancer at various sites, although there is lack of sufficient evidence (Costa, 1997). Experimental studies found that chronic CrVI ingestion via drinking water causes malignant forestomach tumors (Borneff et al., 1968) or enhances susceptibility to UV-induced skin tumors in mice (Davidson et al., 2004). Other rodent studies showed that CrVI exposure via oral route leads to fetal and embryonic toxicity (Kanojia et al., 1998) and teratogenicity (Kanojia et al., 1996).

Mechanism of Chromium Genotoxicity

CrIII is poorly absorbed into the body and does not enter a cell easily, whereas CrVI can be absorbed from gastrointestinal and respiratory tracts or through the skin (Costa, 1997; Barceloux, 1999). Chromium distributes throughout the body and concentrates in the liver and kidney. Absorbed CrVI (highly toxic) is readily taken up into a cell via sulphate and phosphate transporters and is reduced by cellular reducing agents (glutathione, cysteine, ascorbic acid, riboflavin, and others) to CrV, CrIV, and ultimately to relatively inert CrIII. CrVI does not interact with DNA, although its reduced form CrV leads to ROS formation, oxidative DNA damage, and DNA strand breaks. An end product of CrVI metabolism, CrIII, forms DNA adducts, mediates DNA interstrand crosslinks, and protein–DNA crosslinks. The outcome of these DNA–Cr interactions has not been studied in depth. Although available data indicate that CrIII can cause chromosomal aberrations and sister chromatid exchanges, there is little evidence on CrIII-induced point mutations. Thus, chromium induces many different types of genetic lesions. Findings that CrIII (micronutrient element), the end-metabolite of CrVI (classified carcinogen), accumulates in the body (Stearns et al., 1995) and causes DNA damage provokes questions about the safety of CrIII dietary supplements when used in excess dosages or for an extended time. In these supplements, CrIII is bound to its delivery agents (e.g., picolinate) that allow much better CrIII absorption and cell penetration. This is particularly concerning because the lack of toxicity associated with CrIII is commonly attributed to its inability to penetrate the cellular membrane.

Oxidative stress appears to be a major event of CrVI-mediated genotoxicity, suggesting that antioxidant therapy might be protective against CrVI toxicity. Indeed, as an extracellular agent, vitamin C provides some protection (Cohen et al., 1993). The intravenous administration of large doses of vitamin C has been recommended against CrVI-induced acute renal toxicity (Barceloux, 1999). It appears to be effective when administered immediately after chromium poisoning because 1–2 hours after chromium treatment, vitamin C had no effect or increased nephrotoxicity in animal studies. Intracellularly, however, vitamin C and glutathione (GSH) correlates with increased genetic damage (Costa, 1997). For example, increased cellular concentration of vitamin C led to an increased level of CrVI-induced DNA–protein crosslinks, and an increase in GSH was associated with DNA strand breaks and Cr–DNA adducts. Apparently intracellular CrVI reduction acts as bioactivation rather than protection.

CONCLUSIONS

Common environmental pollutants, such as environmental tobacco smoke, PM, DEP, arsenic, and chromium, cause lung cancer, and some are also risk factors for cancer in other organs. The mechanism of carcinogenesis is largely unknown and it might be different for the different agents. Some of the action mechanisms of these agents, however, appear to be common. Namely, they all induce oxidative stress and damage. Additionally and/or as a consequence of oxidative DNA damage, they can cause a wide variety of genetic alterations. Oxidative stress and genetic alterations can act as tumor initiators or promoters. Thus, it seems that maintaining a physiological antioxidant balance may be essential to prevent or reduce genetic damage and possibly the frequency of long-term disease. Under circumstances of elevated oxidant stress, which occurs in individuals exposed to cigarette smoke, PM, or metals, antioxidant balance could potentially be maintained by increasing the intake of dietary antioxidants. Available research data support the notion that dietary antioxidant vitamin intake is beneficial in smokers or ETS-exposed individuals. A thiol antioxidant NAC (a synthetic dietary supplement) seems to be a good candidate to suppress oxidative stress in smokers. For other agents, effects of dietary antioxidant supplementation are yet to be explored.

Acknowledgments

We thank Zhanna Kirpnick of our laboratory for helpful suggestions during the writing of this manuscript. Supported by a research grant from the University of California Toxic Substances Research and Teaching Program (UC TSR&TP) and funds from the UCLA Center for Occupational and Environmental Health to RHS and postgraduate research fellowships of the UC TSR&TP and Philip Morris USA, Inc., to R.R.

References

Ahmad, S., Kitchin, K.T., and Cullen, W.R. 2000. Arsenic species that cause release of iron from ferritin and generation of activated oxygen. *Arch Biochem Biophys* **382**: 195–202.

Ames, B.N., Shigenaga, M.K., and Haen, T.M. 1993. Oxidants, antioxidants, and the degenerative diseases of aging. *Proc Natl Acad Sci USA* **90**: 7915–7922.

Anderson, R.A., Cheng, N., Bryden, N.A., Polansky, M.M., Chi, J., and Feng, J. 1997. Elevated intakes of supplemental chromium improve glucose and insulin variables in individuals with type 2 diabetes. *Diabetes* **46**: 1786–1791.

Aposhian, H.V. 1997. Enzymatic methylation of arsenic species and other new approaches to arsenic toxicity. *Annu Rev Pharmacol Toxicol* **37**: 397–419.

Azen, S.P., Qian, D., Mack, W.J., Sevanian, A., Selzer, R.H., Liu, C.R., Liu, C.H., and Hodis, H.N. 1996. Effect of supplementary antioxidant vitamin intake on carotid arterial wall intima-media thickness in a controlled clinical trial of cholesterol lowering. *Circulation* **94**: 2369–2372.

Baier, G., Stopper, H., Kopp, C., Winkler, U., and Zwirner-Baier, I. 2002. Respiratory diseases and genotoxicity in tobacco smoke exposed children. *Laryngorhinootologie* **81**: 217–225.

Balansky, R., Izzotti, A., Scatolini, L., D'Agostini, F., and De Flora, S. 1996. Induction by carcinogens and chemoprevention by N-acetylcysteine of adducts to mitochondrial DNA in rat organs. *Cancer Res* **56**: 1642–1647.

Barceloux, D.G. 1999. Chromium. *J Toxicol Clin Toxicol* **37**: 173–194.

Barfknecht, T.R., Hites, R.A., Cavaliers, E.L., and Thilly, W.G. 1982. Human cell mutagenicity of polycyclic aromatic hydrocarbon components of diesel emissions. *Dev Toxicol Environ Sci* **10**: 277–294.

Beeson, W.L., Abbey, D.E., and Knutsen, S.F. 1998. Long-term concentrations of ambient air pollutants and incident lung cancer in California adults: results from the AHSMOG study. Adventist Health Study on Smog. *Environ Health Perspect* **106**: 813–823.

Bergen, A.W., and Caporaso, N. 1999. Cigarette smoking. *J Natl Cancer Inst* **91**: 1365–1375.

Block, G., Patterson, B., and Subar, A. 1992. Fruit, vegetables, and cancer prevention: a review of the epidemiological evidence. *Nutr Cancer* **18**: 1–29.

Bluhm, A.L., Weinstein, J., and Sousa, J.A. 1971. Free radicals in tobacco smoke. *Nature* **229**: 500.

Boffett, P., Ye, W., Boman, G., and Nyren. 2002. Lung cancer risk in a population-based cohort of patients hospitalized for asthma in Sweden. *Eur Respir J* **19**: 127–133.

Boffetta, P., Tredaniel, J., and Greco, A. 2000. Risk of childhood cancer and adult lung cancer after childhood exposure to passive smoke: a meta-analysis. *Environ Health Perspect* **108**: 73–82.

Bond, J.A., Wolff, R.K., Harkema, J.R., Mauderly, J.L., Henderson, R.F., Griffith, W.C., and McClellan, R.O. 1988. Distribution of DNA adducts in the respiratory tract of rats exposed to diesel exhaust. *Toxicol Appl Pharmacol* **96**: 336–346.

Borneff, J., Engelhardt, K., Griem, W., Kunte, H., and Reichert, J. 1968. Carcinogens in water and soil. XXII. Experiment with 3,4-benzopyrene and potassium chromate in mice drink. *Arch Hyg Bakteriol* **152**: 45–53.

Cal-EPA. 1997. Health effects of exposure to environmental tobacco smoke, Final Draft. California Environmental Protection Agency.

Casellas, M., Fernandez, P., Bayona, J.M., and Solanas, A.M. 1995. Bioassay-directed chemical analysis of genotoxic components in urban airborne particulate matter from Barcelona (Spain). *Chemosphere* **30**: 725–740.

Cerutti, P.A. 1994. Oxy-radicals and cancer. *Lancet* **344**: 862–863.

Chen, C.J., Hsueh, Y.M., Lai, M.S., Shyu, M.P., Chen, S.Y., Wu, M.M., Kuo, T.L., and Tai, T.Y. 1995. Increased prevalence of hypertension and long-term arsenic exposure. *Hypertension* **25**: 53–60.

Cheng, K.C., Cahill, D.S., Kasai, H., Nishimura, S., and Loeb, L.A. 1992. 8-Hydroxyguanine, an abundant form of oxidative DNA damage, causes G–T and A–C substitutions. *J Biol Chem* **267**: 166–172.

Church, D.F., and Pryor, W.A. 1985. Free-radical chemistry of cigarette smoke and its toxicological implications. *Environ Health Perspect* **64**: 111–126.

Coggins, C.R. 1998. A review of chronic inhalation studies with mainstream cigarette smoke in rats and mice. *Toxicol Pathol* **26**: 307–314; discussion 315.

Cohen, M.D., Kargacin, B., Klein, C.B., and Costa, M. 1993. Mechanisms of chromium carcinogenicity and toxicity. *Crit Rev Toxicol* **23**: 255–281.

Collier, A.C., and Pritsos, C.A. 2003. Environmental tobacco smoke in the workplace: markers of exposure, polymorphic enzymes and implications for disease state. *Chem Biol Interact* **146**: 211–224.

Costa, M. 1997. Toxicity and carcinogenicity of Cr(VI) in animal models and humans. *Crit Rev Toxicol* **27**: 431–442.

Cross, C.E., Traber, M., Eiserich, J., and van der Vliet, A. 1999. Micronutrient antioxidants and smoking. *Br Med Bull* **55**: 691–704.

Das, T., Roychoudhury, A., Sharma, A., and Talukder, G. 1993. Modification of clastogenicity of three known clastogens by garlic extract in mice *in vivo*. *Environ Mol Mutagen* **21**: 383–388.

Davidson, T., Kluz, T., Burns, F., Rossman, T., Zhang, Q., Uddin, A., Nadas, A., and Costa, M. 2004. Exposure to chromium (VI) in the drinking water increases susceptibility to UV-induced skin tumors in hairless mice. *Toxicol Appl Pharmacol* **196**: 431–437.

De Flora, S., Astengo, M., Serra, D., and Bennicelli, C. 1986. Inhibition of urethan-induced lung tumors in mice by dietary *N*-acetylcysteine. *Cancer Lett* **32**: 235–241.

De Flora, S., Bennicelli, C., Camoirano, A., Serra, D., Romano, M., Rossi, G.A., Morelli, A., and De Flora, A. 1985. *In vivo* effects of *N*-acetylcysteine on glutathione metabolism and on the biotransformation of carcinogenic and/or mutagenic compounds. *Carcinogenesis* **6**: 1735–1745.

De Flora, S., Camoirano, A., Bagnasco, M., Bennicelli, C., van Zandwijk, N., Wigbout, G., Qian, G.S., Zhu, Y.R., and Kensler, T.W. 1996. Smokers and urinary genotoxins: implications for selection of cohorts and modulation of endpoints in chemoprevention trials. *J Cell Biochem Suppl* **25**: 92–98.

De Flora, S., D'Agostini, F., Balansky, R., Camoirano, A., Bennicelli, C., Bagnasco, M., Cartiglia, C., Tampa, E., Longobardi, M.G., Lubet, R.A., and Izzotti, A. 2003. Modulation of cigarette smoke-related end-points in mutagenesis and carcinogenesis. *Mutat Res* **523–524**: 237–252.

De Flora, S., Izzotti, A., D'Agostini, F., and Balansky, R.M. 2001. Mechanisms of *N*-acetylcysteine in the prevention of DNA damage and cancer, with special reference to smoking-related end-points. *Carcinogenesis* **22**: 999–1013.

DiFranza, J.R., Aligne, C.A., and Weitzman, M. 2004. Prenatal and postnatal environmental tobacco smoke exposure and children's health. *Pediatrics* **113**: 1007–1015.

Dockery, D.W., Pope, C.A., 3rd, Xu, X., Spengler, J.D., Ware, J.H., Fay, M.E., Ferris, B.G., Jr., and Speizer, F.E. 1993. An association between air pollution and mortality in six U.S. cities. *N Engl J Med* **329**: 1753–1759.

Durant, J.L., Chen, J., Hemond, H.F., and Thilly, W.G. 1995. Elevated incidence of childhood leukemia in Woburn, Massachusetts: NIEHS Superfund Basic Research Program searches for causes. *Environ Health Perspect* **103**(Suppl 6): 93–98.

Duthie, S.J., Ma, A., Ross, M.A., and Collins, A.R. 1996. Antioxidant supplementation decreases oxidative DNA damage in human lymphocytes. *Cancer Res* **56**: 1291–1295.

Ebelt, S.T., Petkau, A.J., Vedal, S., Fisher, T.V., and Brauer, M. 2000. Exposure of chronic obstructive pulmonary disease patients to particulate matter: relationships between personal and ambient air concentrations. *J Air Waste Manag Assoc* **50**: 1081–1094.

Ehrlich, R.I., Du Toit, D., Jordaan, E., Zwarenstein, M., Potter, P., Volmink, J.A., and Weinberg, E. 1996. Risk factors for childhood asthma and wheezing. Importance of maternal and household smoking. *Am J Respir Crit Care Med* **154**: 681–688.

Engel, R.R., Hopenhayn-Rich, C., Receveur, O., and Smith, A.H. 1994. Vascular effects of chronic arsenic exposure: a review. *Epidemiol Rev* **16**: 184–209.

EPA Integrated Risk Information System. U.S. Environmental Protection Agency. Available at: http://www.epa.gov/iris/subst. Accessed 2000.

EPA. 1988. Special Report on Ingested Inorganic Arsenic. Skin cancer: Nutritional Essentiality. U.S. Environmental Protection Agency. EPA/625/623-687/-613.

EPA. 2002. Health Assessment Document for Diesel Engine Exhaust. U.S. Environmental Protection Agency. EPA/600/608-690/057F.

Everson, R.B., Randerath, E., Santella, R.M., Cefalo, R.C., Avitts, T.A., and Randerath, K. 1986. Detection of smoking-related covalent DNA adducts in human placenta. *Science* **231**: 54–57.

Finette, B.A., O'Neill, J.P., Vacek, P.M., and Albertini, R.J. 1998. Gene mutations with characteristic deletions in cord blood T lymphocytes associated with passive maternal exposure to tobacco smoke. *Nat Med* **4**: 1144–1151.

Fraga, C.G., Motchnik, P.A., Wyrobek, A.J., Rempel, D.M., and Ames, B.N. 1996. Smoking and low antioxidant levels increase oxidative damage to sperm DNA. *Mutat Res* **351**: 199–203.

Gallagher, J., Heinrich, U., George, M., Hendee, L., Phillips, D.H., and Lewtas, J. 1994. Formation of DNA adducts in rat lung following chronic inhalation of diesel emissions, carbon black and titanium dioxide particles. *Carcinogenesis* **15**: 1291–1299.

Garshick, E., Schenker, M.B., Munoz, A., Segal, M., Smith, T.J., Woskie, S.R., Hammond, S.K., and Speizer, F.E. 1988. A retrospective cohort study of lung cancer and diesel exhaust exposure in railroad workers. *Am Rev Respir Dis* **137**: 820–825.

Gilliland, F.D., Li, Y.F., and Peters, J.M. 2001. Effects of maternal smoking during pregnancy and environmental tobacco smoke on asthma and wheezing in children. *Am J Respir Crit Care Med* **163**: 429–436.

Gold, D.R., Burge, H.A., Carey, V., Milton, D.K., Platts-Mills, T., and Weiss, S.T. 1999. Predictors of repeated wheeze in the first year of life: the relative roles of cockroach, birth weight, acute lower respiratory illness, and maternal smoking. *Am J Respir Crit Care Med* **160**: 227–236.

Greenberg, E.R., Baron, J.A., Karagas, M.R., Stukel, T.A., Nierenberg, D.W., Stevens, M.M., Mandel, J.S., and Haile, R.W. 1996. Mortality associated with low plasma concentration of beta carotene and the effect of oral supplementation. *JAMA* **275**: 699–703.

Hansen, C., Asmussen, I., and Autrup, H. 1993. Detection of carcinogen–DNA adducts in human fetal tissues by the 32P-postlabeling procedure. *Environ Health Perspect* **99**: 229–231.

Hei, T.K., Liu, S.X., and Waldren, C. 1998. Mutagenicity of arsenic in mammalian cells: role of reactive oxygen species. *Proc Natl Acad Sci USA* **95**: 8103–8107.

Hou, S.M., Lambert, B., and Hemminki, K. 1995. Relationship between hprt mutant frequency, aromatic DNA adducts and genotypes for GSTM1 and NAT2 in bus maintenance workers. *Carcinogenesis* **16**: 1913–1917.

Howard, D.J., Ota, R.B., Briggs, L.A., Hampton, M., and Pritsos, C.A. 1998. Environmental tobacco smoke in the workplace induces oxidative stress in employees, including increased production of 8-hydroxy-2′-deoxyguanosine. *Cancer Epidemiol Biomarkers Prev* **7**: 141–146.

Hruba, F., Fabianova, E., Koppova and K., and Vandenberg, J.J. 2001. Childhood respiratory symptoms, hospital admissions, and long-term exposure to airborne particulate matter. *J Expo Anal Environ Epidemiol* **11**: 33–40.

Hughes, M.F. 2002. Arsenic toxicity and potential mechanisms of action. *Toxicol Lett* **133**: 1–16.

Hung, J., Kishimoto, Y., Sugio, K., Virmani, A., McIntire, D.D., Minna, J.D., and Gazdar, A.F. 1995. Allele-specific chromosome 3p deletions occur at an early stage in the pathogenesis of lung carcinoma. *JAMA* **273**: 558–563.

International Agency for Research on Cancer. 1987. Overall Evaluation of Carcinogenicity: An updating of IARC Monographs volumes1 to 42. *IARC Monographs on the Evaluation of Carcinogenic Risk to Humans* **7**(Suppl): 100–106.

International Agency for Research on Cancer. 1990. Cromium and Nickel Welding. *IARC Monographs on the Evaluation of Carcinogenic Risks to Humans* **49**.

Iwai, K., Adachi, S., Takahashi, M., Moller, L., Udagawa, T., Mizuno, S., and Sugawara, I. 2000. Early oxidative DNA damages and late development of lung cancer in diesel exhaust-exposed rats. *Environ Res* **84**: 255–264.

Jalili, T., Murthy, G.G., and Schiestl, R.H. 1998. Cigarette smoke induces DNA deletions in the mouse embryo. *Cancer Res* **58**: 2633–2638.

Jha, A.N., Noditi, M., Nilsson, R., and Natarajan, A.T. 1992. Genotoxic effects of sodium arsenite on human cells. *Mutat Res* **284**: 215–221.

Jinot, J., and Bayard, S. 1996. Respiratory health effects of exposure to environmental tobacco smoke. *Rev Environ Health* **11**: 89–100.

Kanojia, R.K., Junaid, M., and Murthy, R.C. 1996. Chromium induced teratogenicity in female rat. *Toxicol Lett* **89**: 207–213.

Kanojia, R.K., Junaid, M., and Murthy, R.C. 1998. Embryo and fetotoxicity of hexavalent chromium: a long-term study. *Toxicol Lett* **95**: 165–172.

Kelly, G.S. 1998. Clinical applications of *N*-acetylcysteine. *Altern Med Rev* **3**: 114–127.

Kishimoto, Y., Sugio, K., Hung, J.Y., Virmani, A.K., McIntire, D.D., Minna, J.D., and Gazdar, A.F. 1995. Allele-specific loss in chromosome 9p loci in preneoplastic lesions accompanying non–small-cell lung cancers. *J Natl Cancer Inst* **87**: 1224–1229.

Kitchin, K.T., and Ahmad, S. 2003. Oxidative stress as a possible mode of action for arsenic carcinogenesis. *Toxicol Lett* **137**: 3–13.

Kurttio, P., Pukkala, E., Kahelin, H., Auvinen, A., and Pekkanen, J. 1999. Arsenic concentrations in well water and risk of bladder and kidney cancer in Finland. *Environ Health Perspect* **107**: 705–710.

Larkin, E.K., Smith, T.J., Stayner, L., Rosner, B., Speizer, F.E., and Garshick, E. 2000. Diesel exhaust exposure and lung cancer: adjustment for the effect of smoking in a retrospective cohort study. *Am J Ind Med* **38**: 399–409.

Lee, B.M., Lee, S.K., and Kim, H.S. 1998. Inhibition of oxidative DNA damage, 8-OHdG, and carbonyl contents in smokers treated with antioxidants (vitamin E, vitamin C, beta-carotene and red ginseng). *Cancer Lett* **132**: 219–227.

Lee, T.C., and Ho, I.C. 1994. Differential cytotoxic effects of arsenic on human and animal cells. *Environ Health Perspect* **102**(Suppl 3): 101–105.

Lippmann, M., Ito, K., Nadas, A., and Burnett, R.T. 2000. Association of particulate matter components with daily mortality and morbidity in urban populations. *Res Rep Health Eff Inst* **95**: 5–72, discussion 73–82.

Liu, S.X., Athar, M., Lippai, I., Waldren, C., and Hei, T.K. 2001. Induction of oxyradicals by arsenic: implication for mechanism of genotoxicity. *Proc Natl Acad Sci USA* **98**: 1643–1648.

Lu, L.J., Disher, R.M., Reddy, M.V., and Randerath, K. 1986. 32P-postlabeling assay in mice of transplacental DNA damage induced by the environmental carcinogens safrole, 4-aminobiphenyl, and benzo(a)pyrene. *Cancer Res* **46**: 3046–3054.

Lu, L.J., and Wang, M.Y. 1990. Modulation of benzo[a]pyrene-induced covalent DNA modifications in adult and fetal mouse tissues by gestation stage. *Carcinogenesis* **11**: 1367–1372.

Lykkesfeldt, J., Christen, S., Wallock, L.M., Chang, H.H., Jacob, R.A., and Ames, B.N. 2000. Ascorbate is depleted by smoking and repleted by moderate supplementation: a study in male smokers and nonsmokers with matched dietary antioxidant intakes. *Am J Clin Nutr* **71**: 530–536.

Mates(II)Study. Available at: http://www.aqmd.gov/matesiidf/matestoc.htm. Accessed 2000.

Mauderly, J.L., Jones, R.K., Griffith, W.C., Henderson, R.F., and McClellan, R.O. 1987. Diesel exhaust is a pulmonary carcinogen in rats exposed chronically by inhalation. *Fundam Appl Toxicol* **9**: 208–221.

McClellan, R.O. 1987. Health effects of exposure to diesel exhaust particles. *Annu Rev Pharmacol Toxicol* **27**: 279–300.

Mitchell, J.R., Thorgeirsson, S.S., Potter, W.Z., Jollow, D.J., and Keiser, H. 1974. Acetaminophen-induced hepatic injury: protective role of glutathione in man and rationale for therapy. *Clin Pharmacol Ther* **16**: 676–684.

Omenn, G.S., Goodman, G.E., Thornquist, M.D., Balmes, J., Cullen, M.R., Glass, A., Keogh, J.P., Meyskens, F.L., Valanis, B., Williams, J.H., Barnhart, S., and Hammar, S. 1996. Effects of a combination of beta carotene and vitamin A on lung cancer and cardiovascular disease. *N Engl J Med* **334**: 1150–1155.

Perera, F.P., Jedrychowski, W., Rauh, V., and Whyatt, R.M. 1999. Molecular epidemiologic research on the effects of environmental pollutants on the fetus. *Environ Health Perspect* **107**(Suppl 3): 451–460.

Pope, C.A., 3rd, Burnett, R.T., Thun, M.J., Calle, E.E., Krewski, D., Ito, K., and Thurston, G.D. 2002. Lung cancer, cardiopulmonary mortality, and long-term exposure to fine particulate air pollution. *JAMA* **287**: 1132–1141.

Pryor, W.A., and Stone, K. 1993. Oxidants in cigarette smoke. Radicals, hydrogen peroxide, peroxynitrate, and peroxynitrite. *Ann NY Acad Sci* **686**: 12–27; discussion 27–18.

Randerath, E., and Randerath, K. 1993. Monitoring tobacco smoke-induced DNA damage by 32P-postlabelling. *IARC Sci Publ* **124**: 305–314.

Rasmussen, R.E., and Menzel, D.B. 1997. Variation in arsenic-induced sister chromatid exchange in human lymphocytes and lymphoblastoid cell lines. *Mutat Res* **386**: 299–306.

Reilly, M., Delanty, N., Lawson, J.A., and FitzGerald, G.A. 1996. Modulation of oxidant stress *in vivo* in chronic cigarette smokers. *Circulation* **94**: 19–25.

Risom, L., Dybdahl, M., Bornholdt, J., Vogel, U., Wallin, H., Moller, P., and Loft, S. 2003. Oxidative DNA damage and defence gene expression in the mouse lung after short-term exposure to diesel exhaust particles by inhalation. *Carcinogenesis* **24**: 1847–1852.

Rossman, T.G., Uddin, A.N., Burns, F.J., and Bosland, M.C. 2001. Arsenite is a cocarcinogen with solar ultraviolet radiation for mouse skin: an animal model for arsenic carcinogenesis. *Toxicol Appl Pharmacol* **176**: 64–71.

RoyChoudhury, A., Das, T., Sharma, A., and Talukder, G. 1996. Dietary garlic extract in modifying clastogenic effects of inorganic arsenic in mice: two-generation studies. *Mutat Res* **359**: 165–170.

Santillan, A.A., Camargo, C.A., Jr., and Colditz, G.A. 2003. A meta-analysis of asthma and risk of lung cancer (United States). *Cancer Causes Control* **14**: 327–334.

Sardas, S., Karahalil, B., Akyol, D., Kukner, S., and Karakaya, A.E. 1995. The effect of smoking on sister chromatid exchange rate of newborn infants born to smoking mothers. *Mutat Res* **341**: 249–253.

Sato, H., Sone, H., Sagai, M., Suzuki, K.T., and Aoki, Y. 2000. Increase in mutation frequency in lung of Big Blue rat by exposure to diesel exhaust. *Carcinogenesis* **21**: 653–661.

Schiestl, R.H., Aubrecht, J., Khogali, F., and Carls, N. 1997. Carcinogens induce reversion of the mouse pink-eyed unstable mutation. *Proc Natl Acad Sci USA* **94**: 4576–4581.

Schins, R.P. 2002. Mechanisms of genotoxicity of particles and fibers. *Inhal Toxicol* **14**: 57–78.

Schwartz, J. 2001. Is there harvesting in the association of airborne particles with daily deaths and hospital admissions? *Epidemiology* **12**: 55–61.

Schwela, D. 2000. Air pollution and health in urban areas. *Rev Environ Health* **15**: 13–42.

Smilkstein, M.J., Knapp, G.L., Kulig, K.W., and Rumack, B.H. 1988. Efficacy of oral N-acetylcysteine in the treatment of acetaminophen overdose. Analysis of the national multicenter study (1976 to 1985). *N Engl J Med* **319**: 1557–1562.

Somers, C.M., McCarry, B.E., Malek, F., and Quinn, J.S. 2004. Reduction of particulate air pollution lowers the risk of heritable mutations in mice. *Science* **304**: 1008–1010.

Stayner, L., Dankovic, D., Smith, R., and Steenland, K. 1998. Predicted lung cancer risk among miners exposed to diesel exhaust particles. *Am J Ind Med* **34**: 207–219.

Stearns, D.M., Belbruno, J.J., and Wetterhahn, K.E. 1995. A prediction of chromium(III) accumulation in humans from chromium dietary supplements. *FASEB J* **9**: 1650–1657.

Steenland, K., Deddens, J., and Stayner, L. 1998. Diesel exhaust and lung cancer in the trucking industry: exposure-response analyses and risk assessment. *Am J Ind Med* **34**: 220–228.

Strachan, D.P., and Cook, D.G. 1998. Health effects of passive smoking. 6. Parental smoking and childhood asthma: longitudinal and case–control studies. *Thorax* **53**: 204–212.

Sun, J.D., Wolff, R.K., and Kanapilly, G.M. 1982. Deposition, retention, and biological fate of inhaled benzo(a)pyrene adsorbed onto ultrafine particles and as a pure aerosol. *Toxicol Appl Pharmacol* **65**: 231–244.

Tang, D., Phillips, D.H., Stampfer, M., Mooney, L.A., Hsu, Y., Cho, S., Tsai, W.Y., Ma, J., Cole, K.J., She, M.N., and Perera, F.P. 2001. Association between carcinogen-DNA adducts in white blood cells and lung cancer risk in the physicians health study. *Cancer Res* **61**: 6708–6712.

Tinwell, H., Stephens, S.C., and Ashby, J. 1991. Arsenite as the probable active species in the human carcinogenicity of arsenic: mouse micronucleus assays on Na and K arsenite, orpiment, and Fowler's solution. *Environ Health Perspect* **95**: 205–210.

Tokiwa, H., Sera, N., Nakanishi, Y., and Sagai, M. 1999. 8-Hydroxyguanosine formed in human lung tissues and the association with diesel exhaust particles. *Free Radic Biol Med* **27**: 1251–1258.

Tondel, M., Rahman, M., Magnuson, A., Chowdhury, I.A., Faruquee, M.H., and Ahmad, S.A. 1999. The relationship of arsenic levels in drinking water and the prevalence rate of skin lesions in Bangladesh. *Environ Health Perspect* **107**: 727–729.

Traber, M.G., van der Vliet, A., Reznick, A.Z., and Cross, C.E. 2000. Tobacco-related diseases. Is there a role for antioxidant micronutrient supplementation? *Clin Chest Med* **21**: 173–187, x.

Tribble, D.L., Giuliano, L.J., and Fortmann, S.P. 1993. Reduced plasma ascorbic acid concentrations in nonsmokers regularly exposed to environmental tobacco smoke. *Am J Clin Nutr* **58**: 886–890.

Tseng, W.P. 1977. Effects and dose–response relationships of skin cancer and blackfoot disease with arsenic. *Environ Health Perspect* **19**: 109–119.

Vahter, M., and Concha, G. 2001. Role of metabolism in arsenic toxicity. *Pharmacol Toxicol* **89**: 1–5.

Valkonen, M.M., and Kuusi, T. 2000. Vitamin C prevents the acute atherogenic effects of passive smoking. *Free Radic Biol Med* **28**: 428–436.

Van Schooten, F.J., Nia, A.B., De Flora, S., D'Agostini, F., Izzotti, A., Camoirano, A., Balm, A.J., Dallinga, J.W., Bast, A., Haenen, G.R., Van't Veer, L., Baas, P., Sakai, H., and Van Zandwijk, N. 2002. Effects of oral administration of *N*-acetyl-L-cysteine: a multi-biomarker study in smokers. *Cancer Epidemiol Biomarkers Prev* **11**: 167–175.

van Zandwijk, N., Dalesio, O., Pastorino, U., de Vries, N., and van Tinteren, H. 2000. EUROSCAN, a randomized trial of vitamin A and *N*-acetylcysteine in patients with head and neck cancer or lung cancer. For the European Organization for Research and Treatment of Cancer Head and Neck and Lung Cancer Cooperative Groups. *J Natl Cancer Inst* **92**: 977–986.

Vincent, J.B. 2004. Recent advances in the nutritional biochemistry of trivalent chromium. *Proc Nutr Soc* **63**: 41–47.

Wang, T.S., and Huang, H. 1994. Active oxygen species are involved in the induction of micronuclei by arsenite in XRS-5 cells. *Mutagenesis* **9**: 253–257.

Wanibuchi, H., Salim, E.I., Kinoshita, A., Shen, J., Wei, M., Morimura, K., Yoshida, K. Kuroda, K., Endo, G., and Fukushima, S. 2004. Understanding arsenic carcinogenicity by the use of animal models. *Toxicol Appl Pharmacol* **198**: 366–376.

Whyatt, R.M., Jedrychowski, W., Hemminki, K., Santella, R.M., Tsai, W.Y., Yang, K., and Perera, F.P. 2001. Biomarkers of polycyclic aromatic hydrocarbon-DNA damage and cigarette smoke exposures in paired maternal and newborn blood samples as a measure of differential susceptibility. *Cancer Epidemiol Biomarkers Prev* **10**: 581–588.

Witschi, H., Joad, J.P., and Pinkerton, K.E. 1997. The toxicology of environmental tobacco smoke. *Annu Rev Pharmacol Toxicol* **37**: 29–52.

Woodson, K., Tangrea, J.A., Barrett, M.J., Virtamo, J., Taylor, P.R., and Albanes, D. 1999. Serum alpha-tocopherol and subsequent risk of lung cancer among male smokers. *J Natl Cancer Inst* **91**: 1738–1743.

Yamanaka, K., Hasegawa, A., Sawamura, R., and Okada, S. 1991. Cellular response to oxidative damage in lung induced by the administration of dimethylarsinic acid, a major metabolite of inorganic arsenics, in mice. *Toxicol Appl Pharmacol* **108**: 205–213.

Yamanaka, K., Hoshino, M., Okamoto, M., Sawamura, R., Hasegawa, A., and Okada, S. 1990. Induction of DNA damage by dimethylarsine, a metabolite of inorganic arsenics, is for the major part likely due to its peroxyl radical. *Biochem Biophys Res Commun* **168**: 58–64.

CHAPTER

13

Endocrine and Paracrine Factors in Carcinogenesis

DAVID HEBER AND PINCHAS COHEN

INTRODUCTION

Endocrine and paracrine factors are modulated by nutritional factors, including deficiency states and obesity, which influence carcinogenesis at molecular, subcellular, cellular, organ, and systemic levels. The insulin-like growth factor 1 (IGF-1) axis, estrogens, androgens, and certain classes of lipids are affected by changes in nutrition and influence tumor cell biology. Hepatic IGF-1 production is subject to complex regulation, and IGF-1 is also produced in peripheral tissues where this peptide can promote carcinogenesis. Reproductive steroids affect the IGF-1 axis, and in turn, steroid hormone production is affected by nutritional status. At a cellular and subcellular level, peptides, steroids, and lipids in the microenvironment of the tumor can affect cell proliferation. Peptide hormones act through membrane receptors, and both steroid hormones and lipids act through cytoplasmic and nuclear receptors. There is emerging evidence for cross-talk between peptide and steroid signals and evidence that some lipids interact with high-capacity/low-affinity receptors, which influence gene expression in the nucleus. Intermittent stimulation by xenobiotics activates metabolic systems through a feed-forward loop and the upregulation of metabolic enzymes that are activated by low-affinity/high-capacity receptors, such as the steroid xenobiotic receptor, and by more specific receptors such as the vitamin D receptor. The study of endocrine and paracrine pathways is vital to an understanding of the processes through which nutrition affects tumor biology and the multistep process of carcinogenesis.

THE IGF AXIS AND ENERGY BALANCE

The IGF axis involves complex regulatory networks that operate at the whole organism, cellular, and subcellular levels. The IGF-1 signaling pathway evolved hundreds of millions of years ago in many different species to regulate cell growth in accord with the availability of nutrients in the environment (Longo and Finch, 2003). This basic function remains in humans because both insulin and IGF-1 have key roles in regulating cell proliferation and apoptosis. The system includes the ligands IGF-1 and IGF-2; the type 1 and type 2 IGF receptors (IGF-1R and IGF-2R); and the IGF-binding proteins (IGF-BPs), in addition to the proteins involved in intracellular signaling triggered by binding of the ligands to IGF-1R, which include members of the insulin-receptor substrate (IRS) family, AKT, target of rapamycin (TOR), and S6 kinase. Most circulating IGFs are produced in the liver.

Hepatic IGF-1 production is subject to complex regulation. Growth hormone (GH), which is produced in the pituitary gland under control of the hypothalamic factors GH-releasing hormone (GHRH) and somatostatin, stimulates IGF-1 production in the liver. Various IGF-BPs are also produced in the liver. In those tissues that respond to IGF, the ligands IGF-1 and IGF-2, as well as IGF-BPs, can be delivered through the circulation from the liver as classical hormones or the IGFs, and IGF-BPs can be locally produced through autocrine or paracrine mechanisms. These mechanisms often involve cell–cell interactions between stromal and epithelial cells.

Nutritional status also influences circulating IGF-1 levels. Starvation reduces both IGF-1 levels (Thissen et al., 1994) and intracellular signaling secondary to IGF-1R activation at the level of TOR (Houghton and Huang, 2004). The nutritional adaptations in the IGF axis may have evolved under conditions where food supplies were scarce and inconsistently available to minimize cellular energy and protein consumption at times of inadequate nutrition through the reduction in cell proliferation rates. The repeated observation that caloric restriction provides protection against carcinogenesis and that this can be reversed by

Copyright © 2006, Elsevier Inc.
All rights of reproduction in any form reserved.

infusing IGF-1 (see later discussion) suggests a significant role for the IGF axis in mediating many of the protective effects of caloric restriction on carcinogenesis.

Other studies indicate that high levels of energy or protein intake are associated with modest increases in IGF-1 levels (Heaney et al., 1999; Holmes et al., 2002; Giovannucci et al., 2003). In several studies, IGF-1 levels were seen to increase with increasing dairy product intake (Holmes et al., 2002; Giovannucci et al., 2003; Gunnell et al., 2003). The underlying mechanism and significance of this relationship deserves further study, particularly as prostate cancer risk has been shown to be associated with both increased IGF-1 levels (Pollak, 2001) and increased dairy food consumption (Chan et al., 2001). Micronutrients such as retinoids also influence circulating IGF-BP3 levels, and this is modified by a genetic polymorphism of IGF-BP3 (Deal et al., 2001).

At a subcellular level, the signaling systems, which translate IGF effects, are highly complex and this brief description should be viewed only as a summary that does not include all the details of complex regulation. The IGF-1R is a tyrosine kinase cell surface receptor that binds either IGF-1 or IGF-2. The local bioavailability of ligands is subject to complex physiological regulation and may be increased in many common forms of cancer. Following ligand binding, intracellular signaling pathways that favor proliferation and cell survival are activated. Initial phosphorylation targets for IGF-1R include IRS proteins, and downstream signaling molecules include phosphatidylinositol 3-kinase, AKT, TOR, S6 kinase, and mitogen-activated protein kinase. IGF-2R preferentially binds IGF-2 but has no intracellular kinase domain and may not act as a signaling molecule.

The IGF-BP family of proteins determines the relative bioavailabilities of IGF-1 and IGF-2 (Firth and Baxter, 2002). At least six IGF-BPs have been found, and their binding affinity for IGF-1 and IGF-2 is similar to that of the IGF-1R. These proteins are present in the circulation and extravascular fluids. IGF-BP3 provides most of the IGF-binding capacity of serum and greatly prolongs the circulating half-life of the IGFs. IGF-BPs in extracellular tissue fluid modulate interactions between IGF ligands and cell surface IGF receptors. IGF-BP3 stimulates apoptosis through direct interaction with nuclear and membrane-bound receptors for IGF-BP3 in prostate cancer cells. The complex actions of IGF-BP proteins are poorly understood. They may increase the half-life of the different IGFs and they may bind directly to nuclear and membrane receptors. IGF-BPs modulate bioavailability of IGFs in both the circulation and the cellular microenvironment. The simplest model postulates that the major biological effect of IGF-BPs is to compete with receptors for ligands. So, under circumstances in which IGF-BP levels are low, free IGF levels are high and there is more proliferative stimulation by IGFs.

Genetic polymorphisms can influence circulating IGF-1 concentration (Harrela et al., 1996). Dozens of proteins are involved in the physiological systems that regulate IGF-1 levels, and polymorphic variation of the genes encoding these has been proposed to influence circulating IGF-1 concentrations. Examples include genes encoding IGF-1 itself; IGF-BPs and their proteases; GH and its receptor; and somatostatin, GHRH, and their receptors. Only a few of these have been studied in the context of their ability to influence IGF-1 levels within the normal range (Deal et al., 2001; LeMarchand et al., 2002; Bonafe et al., 2003; Johnston et al., 2003), but some are mutated in growth disorders associated with abnormal IGF-1 levels (Laron, 1995; Maheshwari et al., 1998). Some (LeMarchand et al., 2002, Wang et al., 2003) but not all (Schernhammer et al., 2003) reports indicate that polymorphic variation within these genes influences cancer risk or prognosis. Common haplotypes might account for much of the variation in circulating levels of IGFs and their binding proteins (Cheng et al., 2004).

Hormones, including endogenous and exogenous steroids, have important influences on IGF-1 regulation. Both tamoxifen and diethylstilbestrol suppress IGF-1 levels (Pollak et al., 1990; Helle et al., 2001). It is believed that estrogens, when administered orally in postmenopausal hormone replacements, reduce circulating levels of IGF-1 by suppressing hepatic production of IGF-1, probably as a consequence of its direct delivery to the liver and suppression of hepatic IGF-1 gene expression (Jernstrom et al., 2001). Estrogen delivery by the transdermal route does not lower circulating IGF-1 levels. In several experimental systems, there is cross-talk between estrogens and IGFs, which may act to stimulate breast cancer growth (Yee and Lee, 2000; Song et al., 2004). Polymorphisms that influence the function of IGF-1R itself (Bonafe et al., 2003; Abuzzahab et al., 2003) or in downstream signaling proteins would also be expected to add complexity to the relation between circulating IGF-1 levels and IGF-1R activation.

The IGF-1 signaling pathway has important roles in regulating cellular proliferation and apoptosis acting in both an endocrine and a paracrine manner. Energy balance affects circulating levels of IGF-1 and IGF-BPs. Obesity is associated with increased IGF-1 and decreased IGF-BP1. Many other intriguing functions have been uncovered in the past 2 decades including effects of IGF-1 on body size, longevity, and various organ functions (Jones and Clemmons, 1995; Nakae et al., 2001; Giudice, 2002; Baserga et al., 2003).

IGF Axis and Cancer

When one considers the aggregate of all knowledge on the relationship between nutrition and cancer, the impact of excess calorie intake on tumorigenesis has been substantiated in more experiments than any other nutritional factor.

The IGF Axis in the Prostate

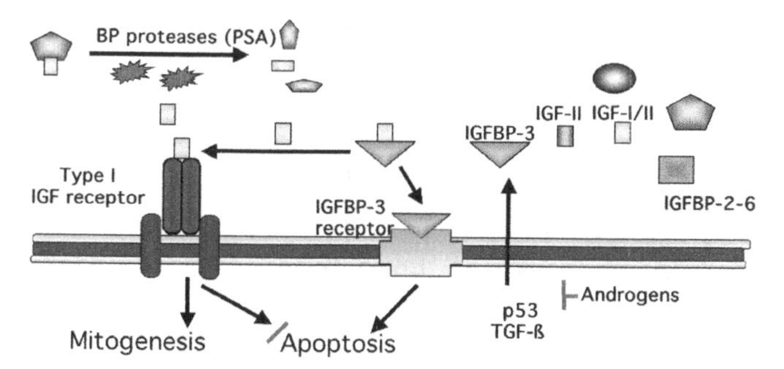

FIGURE 1 The IGF axis in the prostate.

For example, caloric restriction in the TRAMP transgenic mouse model of prostate cancer results in a reduction in IGF-1 and an increase in IGF-BP. The inhibition of tumor growth in this model resulting from caloric restriction can be reversed through provision of IGF-1 intraperitoneally but not by growth hormone. With caloric restriction, increases in IGF-BP result in reduced free IGF levels, and the serum has been shown to stimulate apoptosis through binding of IGF-BP3 to a membrane receptor (Figure 1). In human volunteers (Figure 2) undergoing a 3-week dietary intervention with a very low fat, high-fiber diet, the ability of their serum, when substituted for fetal calf serum, to stimulate prostate cancer cell growth *ex vivo* is reduced. Adding IGF-1 back to the serum samples restores the cell proliferation of cancer cells back to the levels observed with control sera.

Insights from population studies and experimental studies in animals suggest that high levels of circulating IGF-1 are associated with increased risk of several common forms of cancer. The key challenge to researchers in nutritional oncology is to define and clarify the mechanisms through which nutrition affects the IGF axis and to determine the extent to which IGF-1 can influence carcinogenesis. The role of IGF-1 in cell proliferation is of particular relevance to nutritional oncology (Holly, 1998; Burroughs et al., 1999). IGF-1 stimulates cell proliferation and prolongs cell survival *in vitro* (Jones and Clemmons, 1995). In animal models proliferation and metastasis of cancer cells is increased by IGF-1R activation, in relation to either higher levels of circulating IGF-1 in the host or autocrine production of IGF ligands by neoplastic cells (Khandwala et al., 2000).

An association has been observed between elevated circulating levels of IGF-1 and cancer risk in populations. There is significant variation of circulating levels of IGF-1, IGF-2, and IGF-BP concentrations among normal individuals. Although IGF has been measured clinically by endocrinologists to diagnose both GH deficiency and acromegaly and by pediatricians to assess nutritional status, the observations of increased risk are within quartiles spanning the normal range. A number of studies reviewed later in this chapter suggest that the risk of common forms of cancer is increased in individuals who have higher circulating levels of IGF-1, compared with those who have levels at the lower end of the normal range. Significant increases in cancer risk with increasing height have been documented in many studies (Gunnell et al., 2001; Engeland et al., 2003; Lawlor et al., 2003; Mellemkjaer, 2003). Height per se is unlikely to be a risk factor, but the hormonal determinants of height might influence cancer risk. IGF-1 levels are, at most, weakly related to adult height but are related to height early in life (Juul et al., 1994). So, height might be weakly related to the risk in part because it is weakly related to IGF-1 exposure over the first decades of life. Birth weight and size have been associated with risk of breast (Stavola et al., 2000; McCormack et al., 2003), colorectal (Sandhu et al., 2002), prostate (Tibblin et al., 1995), and childhood cancers (Von Behren and Reynolds, 1995) and are positively correlated with cord-blood IGF-1 levels (Vatten et al., 2002a). Conversely, preeclampsia is associated with reduced IGF-1 levels and reduced breast cancer risk (Altinkaynak et al., 2003; Vatten et al., 2002b).

Cancers can be stimulated by IGF-1 or IGF-2 that is synthesized locally in an autocrine or paracrine manner or by responding to changes in circulating levels of these two ligands. One hypothesis worth further investigation is that tumors may initially depend on endocrine or paracrine stimulation, but as the process of carcinogenesis proceeds, the tumor cells acquire the ability to produce IGF, particularly IGF-2, which can stimulate growth via an autocrine loop.

ESTROGENS AND CANCER

Estrogens modulate cellular growth and differentiation (Warner et al., 1999). Its major target organs in females are the mammary gland and uterus, but in both males and females this hormone is essential for maintenance of bone, brain, the cardiovascular system, and the urogenital tract (Ogawa et al., 1998; Simpson, 1998; Wenger, 1999). The biological actions of estrogens are mediated by estrogen binding to one of two specific estrogen receptors ERα and ERβ (Kuiper et al., 1996), which belong to the nuclear receptor superfamily, a family of ligand-regulated transcription factors. ERα and ERβ are products of different genes and exhibit tissue- and cell-type–specific expression.

The characterization of mice lacking ERα, ERβ, or both has revealed that both receptor subtypes have overlapping but also unique roles in estrogen-dependent action *in vivo*. Additionally, ERα and ERβ have different transcriptional activities in certain ligand, cell-type, and promoter contexts. Both receptors, however, are coexpressed in a number of tissues and form functional heterodimers. The biological

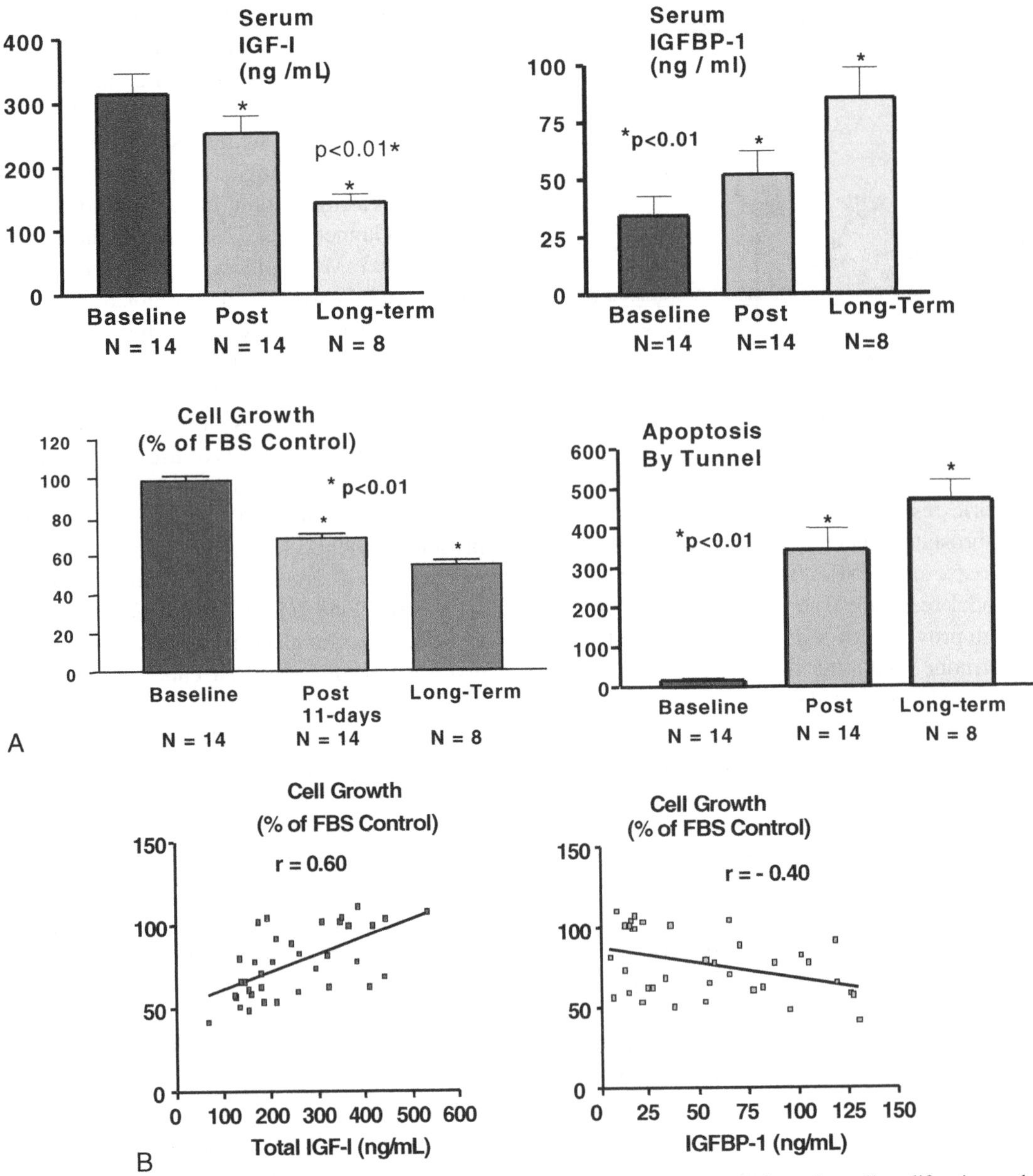

FIGURE 2 (a) Effects of a low-fat diet and exercise on serum IGF-1, IGF-BP1, and *ex vivo* cell proliferation and apoptosis. (b) Correlation of IGF-1 and IGF-BP1 in sera to *ex vivo* effects on LNCaP cell proliferation.

roles of ERα/β heterodimers in the presence of each respective homodimer are unknown. When coexpressed, ERβ exhibits an inhibitory action on ERα-mediated gene expression and in many instances opposes the actions of ERα. A number of ERα and ERβ isoforms have also been described, many of which alter estrogen-mediated gene expression. Uncovering the molecular mechanisms regulating the expression of both ERs and how ERα and ERβ directly or indirectly affect each other's function is critical to understanding the cellular and biological events of estrogen-mediated gene regulation in the process of carcinogenesis and the interaction of nutrients such as soy isoflavones and other plant-based flavonoids, which bind preferentially to ERβ. Estrogen is prominently associated with the induction and growth of breast cancer, which is influenced by obesity and nutritional status. Animal studies have shown that estrogen can induce and stimulate breast cancer, and ovariectomy or administration of antiestrogens opposes this action (Hilakivi-Clarke et al., 1999a,b; Koibuchi et al., 1999; Liao et al., 1998). Because ERα-containing epithelial cells in the normal breast do not express proliferation markers (Clarke et al., 1997a,b; Zeps et al., 1998), the mechanisms through which estrogen induces epithelial growth are not clear. The prevailing concept is that it induces the secretion of growth factors from the stroma and that these agents stimulate epithelial cells to proliferate (Wiesen et al., 1999). There is evidence that ERα is rapidly downregulated in cell lines in response to estradiol treatment (Lonard et al., 2000; Wijayaratne et al., 2001).

In the rodent mammary gland, most of the cells that express the proliferating cell nuclear antigen contain neither ERα nor ERβ (Saji et al., 2000), which suggests that the presence of ERs in epithelial cells restricts their proliferation. Regulation of growth factor receptors in the breast supports this role for ER. In breast cancer cells in culture, loss of ERα is accompanied by an increase in growth factors and growth factor receptors (Clarke et al., 1996; Wosikowski et al., 1997; Nicholson et al., 1999), as well as higher levels of phosphotyrosine residues, indicating increased tyrosine kinase activity (El-Ashry et al., 1997). Expression of ERβ mRNA has been detected by reverse-transcriptase polymerase chain reaction (RT-PCR) in both normal and malignant human breast tissue (Speirs et al., 1999), and full-length ERβ protein (ERβ1) has been identified in human breast tumors by Western blotting (Fuqua et al., 1999). Immunohistochemistry of breast cancer tissue shows that ERβ is often coexpressed with ERα and that the presence of this receptor is associated with negative axillary node status and low tumor grade (Jarvinen et al., 2000). Although it has been suggested that ERβ contributes to the initiation and progression of carcinogenesis (Hu et al., 1998), with expression in breast cancers of higher grades, and acting as a marker for estrogen responsiveness (Dotzlaw et al., 1999), its precise role in breast carcinogenesis remains to be defined.

Clinical studies show that a beneficial response of breast cancer to tamoxifen (Fisher et al., 1998), as well as to other endocrine therapies, including inhibition of aromatase activity (DeSombre and Jensen, 2000), is related to the presence of ERα. Furthermore, breast cancer prevention trials show that there is a reduced incidence of ERα-positive but not ERα-negative cancers in the tamoxifen-treated group (Leygue et al., 1999).

The characterization of ERβ has resulted in a new paradigm for studying the mechanisms underlying estrogen signaling. The fact that estrogen induction of cell proliferation is a crucial step in carcinogenesis of gynecologic target tissues and the mitogenic effects of estrogen in these tissues (e.g., breast, endometrium, ovary) is well documented. There is also an emerging body of evidence that colon and prostate cancer growth may be influenced by estrogens. In all of these tissues, most studies have shown decreased ERβ expression in cancer as compared with benign tumors or normal tissues, whereas ERβ expression persists. The loss of ERβ expression in cancer cells could reflect tumor cell dedifferentiation but may also represent a critical stage in estrogen-dependent tumor progression. Modulation of the expression of ERβ target genes by ERβ or ERβ-specific gene induction could indicate that ERβ has a differential effect on proliferation as compared with ERα. ERβ may exert a protective effect and thus constitute a new target for hormone therapy (e.g., via ligand-specific activation).

ANDROGENS AND CANCER

Androgens are produced by the male gonads and adrenal gland and by the female ovary. They undergo enzymatic conversion in the male and female gonads and in the peripheral tissues where they can be converted to estrogens. In men, 80% of circulating estrogens result from peripheral conversion of androgens to estrogens. Testosterone and dihydrotestosterone are the most potent androgens in terms of binding to the androgen receptor (AR). This receptor (Gregory et al., 1998) is a member of the steroid receptor family that is activated by testicular androgens, and it is the major regulatory transcription factor in normal prostate growth and development and in the growth of androgen-dependent prostate cancer. The AR may also contribute to prostate cancer growth during its recurrence in the androgen-deprived patient. AR has been found in a variety of tissues, including reproductive organs, central nervous system, and skeletal muscle. The role of androgens in breast cancer growth has also been extensively studied but remains less clear and is not further discussed here.

A role for AR-mediated gene activation in recurrent prostate cancer is supported by its expression (Ruizeveld et al., 1991; deVere et al., 1997) together with the expression of androgen-regulated genes. Possible mechanisms for AR reactivation in recurrent prostate cancer include altered growth factor–induced phosphorylation (Culig et al., 1994; Nazareth et al., 1996; Craft et al., 1999; Abreu-Martin et al., 1999; Sadar et al., 1999) and AR mutations (Newmark et al., 1992) that broaden ligand specificity (Tan et al., 1997). AR gene amplification was observed after androgen deprivation in 30% of recurrent prostate cancers (Visakorpi et al., 1995). AR overexpression is associated with increased sensitivity to the growth-stimulating effects of low androgen concentrations in recurrent prostate cancer–derived cell lines (Culig et al., 1999; Gregory et al., 2001).

Steroid hormone action can trigger increased oxidant stress, promoting cell proliferation and DNA damage (Waxman, 1999). Androgens have been demonstrated to increase oxidant stress in prostate cancer cells, and oxidant defense mechanisms have been shown to be impaired early in the cancer process. Fat cells produce paracrine factors and hormones that stimulate the production of steroid hormones in cancer tissue through interactions between stromal and epithelial compartments in tissues. Many of these paracrine factors are cytokines produced by both fat cells and white blood cells. Obesity is associated with increased circulating levels of cytokines and these levels are reduced with weight loss (Storch and Thumser, 2000). The fat cell, the source of many of these so-called *adipocytokines*, may play a significant role in the ability of fat tissue to preserve immune resistance to infections. It has long been recognized that malnutrition is associated with multiple impairments of immune function, including impaired T-helper cell function, so the ability of fat to store calories provides a separate important function to protect immune defenses (Dean et al., 2001). To the extent that cancer and heart disease are replacing infectious diseases as the primary cause of death as obesity becomes more common in developing countries, it is possible that the increased cytokine secretion observed in obesity is simultaneously having a beneficial effect on infectious disease resistance while increasing the risk of cancer.

NUCLEAR RECEPTOR SUPERFAMILIES AND ORPHAN RECEPTORS

At a molecular genetic level, intracellular homeostasis and cellular differentiation are maintained through the complex regulation of nuclear receptors receiving many different signals that are integrated and interact at various levels. The concept of a superfamily of receptors for numerous steroid hormones and some lipids has led to the concept that signaling mechanisms are far more complex than was appreciated at the time when receptors were first isolated and their structure determined. Rather than a single hormone binding to a single receptor to activate gene transcription, nuclear receptors function as ligand-activated transcription factors that regulate the expression of target genes to affect processes that promote cell proliferation, inhibit apoptosis, and stimulate angiogenesis and other aspects of metastatic spread.

Nuclear receptor proteins were first recognized as the mediators of steroid hormone signaling and provided an important link between transcriptional regulation and carcinogenesis (see earlier discussion). In the mid-1980s, the steroid receptors were cloned and found to exhibit extensive sequence similarity. There are 48 members of this receptor superfamily that mediate the action of many steroid hormones, thyroid hormones, and the fat-soluble vitamins A and D. The actions of the steroid hormones are well defined and include estrogen, progesterone, testosterone, cortisol, and all related metabolites. There are also so-called *adopted orphan receptors*. They were formerly orphans without defined hormonal ligands, until they were found to be a group of high-capacity, low-affinity lipid sensors. Exciting progress has been made over the past several years to elucidate the role of these orphan receptors in animal biology.

The most studied of the orphan nuclear receptor subfamilies are the retinoid X receptors (RXR α, β, γ). The identification of the vitamin A derivative, 9-*cis* retinoic acid, as a ligand for the RXRs represented the discovery of the first orphan nuclear receptor ligand and ushered in the age of orphan nuclear receptors. Members of this group include receptors for fatty acids (PPARs), oxysterols (LXRs), bile acids (FXR), and xenobiotics (steroid xenobiotic receptor/pregnane X receptor [SXR/PXR] and constitutive androstane receptor [CAR]). To maintain the cells, the activity of these receptors must be tightly controlled by tissue-specific expression of receptors and ligand availability. Both of these latter processes can be affected by nutrition.

Structure and Action of Nuclear Receptors

The structural organization of nuclear receptors is similar despite wide variation in ligand sensitivity. With few exceptions, these proteins contain an NH2-terminal region that harbors a ligand-independent transcriptional activation function (AF-1); a core DNA-binding domain, containing two highly conserved zinc-finger motifs that target the receptor to specific DNA sequences known as *hormone response elements*; a hinge region that permits protein flexibility for simultaneous receptor dimerization and DNA binding; and a large COOH-terminal region that encompasses the ligand-binding domain, dimerization interface, and a ligand-dependent activation function (AF-2). Upon ligand binding, nuclear receptors undergo a conformational change that coordinately dissociates corepressors and facilitates recruitment of coactivator proteins to enable transcriptional activation (McKenna et al., 1999). Nuclear receptors are important in maintaining the normal physiological state of cells. To maintain a normal physiological state, the spatial and temporal activity of nuclear receptors must be tightly controlled by tissue-specific expression of the receptors, as well as ligand availability. In vertebrates, the steroid receptor system evolved to regulate various crucial metabolic and developmental events, including sexual differentiation, reproduction, carbohydrate metabolism, and electrolyte balance.

The endocrine steroid receptors, their ligands, and the pathways they regulate have been the subject of decades of research, and their mechanism of action is well documented (Wilson and Foster, 1992). The second nuclear receptor paradigm is represented by the adopted orphan nuclear receptors that function as heterodimers with the retinoid X receptor (RXR).

Orphan receptors become adopted when they are shown to bind a physiological ligand. In contrast to the endocrine steroid receptors, the adopted orphan receptors respond to dietary lipids, and therefore, their concentrations cannot be limited by simple negative feedback control. Furthermore, the receptors in this group bind their lipid ligands with lower affinities comparable to physiological concentrations that can be affected by dietary intake (0.1–10 mM). An emerging theme regarding these receptors is that they function as lipid sensors. In keeping with this notion, ligand binding to each of these receptors activates a feed-forward metabolic cascade that maintains nutrient lipid homeostasis by governing the transcription of a common family of genes involved in lipid metabolism, storage, transport, and elimination. Many of the orphan receptors function to elicit gene expression changes to ultimately protect cells from lipid overload.

In addition to the adopted orphan receptors, there are four other RXR heterodimer receptors that do not fit precisely into either the feed-forward or feedback paradigms mentioned. These include the thyroid hormone (TR), retinoic acid (RAR), and the vitamin D (VDR) receptors (Mangelsdorf et al., 1994; Thummel, 1995; Jones et al., 1998; Forrest et al., 2000). The ligands for these three receptors and the pathways they regulate employ elements of both the endocrine and the lipid-sensing receptor pathway. For example, like other RXR heterodimer ligands, retinoic acid is derived from an essential dietary lipid (vitamin A), but it is calorigenic and the transcriptional pathways that this ligand regulates more closely resemble those of the endocrine receptors. Likewise, vitamin D and thyroid hormone require exogenous elements for their synthesis (sunshine for vitamin D, iodine for thyroid hormone), yet the ultimate synthesis of these hormones and the pathways they regulate are under strict endocrine control. Thus, it is possible that these four receptors provide an intermediate case spanning the gap between the endocrine receptors and the adopted orphan receptors that have been shown to be lipid sensors.

Three families of proteins establish a positive feed-forward autoregulatory loop to maintain lipid homeostasis. These families include (i) members of the cytochrome P450 (CYP) enzymes that catalyze various redox reactions to transform lipid ligands into inactive metabolites and facilitate their metabolic clearance (Waxman, 1999); (ii) the intracellular lipid-binding proteins, a family of 14- to 15-kDa proteins that buffer and transport hydrophobic ligands within cells (Storch and Thumser, 2000); and (iii) the ATP-binding cassette (ABC) transporters, which shuttle their lipid ligands and precursors out of the cytosolic compartment into organelles or the extracellular environment (Dean et al., 2001). The coordinated regulation of these three gene families appears to be a particular feature of receptors that function as RXR heterodimers, especially the orphan receptors. Subsequent studies have shown that RXRs also can be activated by a variety of dietary lipids, including docosahexaenoic acid (DHA) (Gigueere, 1999; de Urquiza et al., 2000).

LIPID SENSOR RECEPTORS AND LIPID METABOLISM

The discovery that RXRs function as obligate heterodimer partners for other nuclear receptors was a key finding in this area (Mangelsdorf and Evans, 1995). Thus, RXRs typically do not function alone but serve as master regulators of several crucial regulatory pathways. The evolution of the heterodimeric nuclear receptor has permitted a unique but simple mechanism for expanding the repertoire of lipid signaling pathways. Therefore, it is perhaps not surprising that the lipid-sensing receptors that have been identified thus far are all RXR heterodimers. The recognition that some RXR heterodimers are permissive for activation by RXR ligands has led to the finding that potent synthetic RXR agonists (called *rexinoids*) have dramatic effects on lipid homeostasis (Mukherjee et al., 1998; Repa et al., 2000a).

The peroxisome proliferator-activated receptors (PPAR α, γ, δ) are activated by polyunsaturated fatty acids, eicosanoids, and various synthetic ligands (Willson et al., 2000). Consistent with their distinct expression patterns, gene-knockout experiments have revealed that each PPAR subtype performs a specific function in fatty acid homeostasis (Figure 3).

More than a decade ago, PPARα was found to respond to hypolipidemic drugs, such as fibrates. Subsequently, it was discovered that fatty acids serve as their natural ligands. Together with the analyses of PPARα-null mice, these studies established PPARα as a global regulator of fatty acid catabolism. PPARα target genes function together to coordinate the complex metabolic changes necessary to conserve energy during fasting and feeding. In the fatty acid metabolic cascade, PPARα activation upregulates the transcription of liver fatty acid–binding protein, which buffers intracellular fatty acids and delivers PPARα ligands to the nucleus (Wolfrum et al., 2001). In addition, expression of two members of the adrenoleukodystrophy subfamily of ABC transporters, ABCD2 and ABCD3, is similarly upregulated to promote transport of fatty acids into peroxisomes (Fourcade et al., 2001) where catabolic enzymes promote β-oxidation. The hepatocyte CYP 4A enzymes complete the metabolic cascade by catalyzing γ-oxidation, the final catabolic step in the clearance of PPARα ligands (Lee et al., 1995). PPARγ was identified initially as a key regulator of adipogenesis, but it also plays an important role in cellular differentiation, insulin sensitization, atherosclerosis, and cancer (Rosen and Spiegelman, 2001). Ligands for PPARγ include fatty acids and other arachidonic acid metabolites, antidiabetic drugs (e.g., thiazolidinediones), and triterpenoids. In contrast to PPARα, PPARγ promotes fat storage by increasing adipocyte differentiation and transcription of a number of important lipogenic proteins. Ligand homeostasis is regulated by governing expression of the adipocyte fatty acid–binding protein (A-FABP/aP2) and CYP 4B1 (Way et al., 2001). In macrophages, PPARγ induces the lipid transporter ABCA1 through an indirect mechanism involving the LXR pathway, which in turn promotes cellular efflux of phospholipids and cholesterol into high-density lipoproteins (Chawla et al., 2001; Chinetti et al., 2001). Ligands for

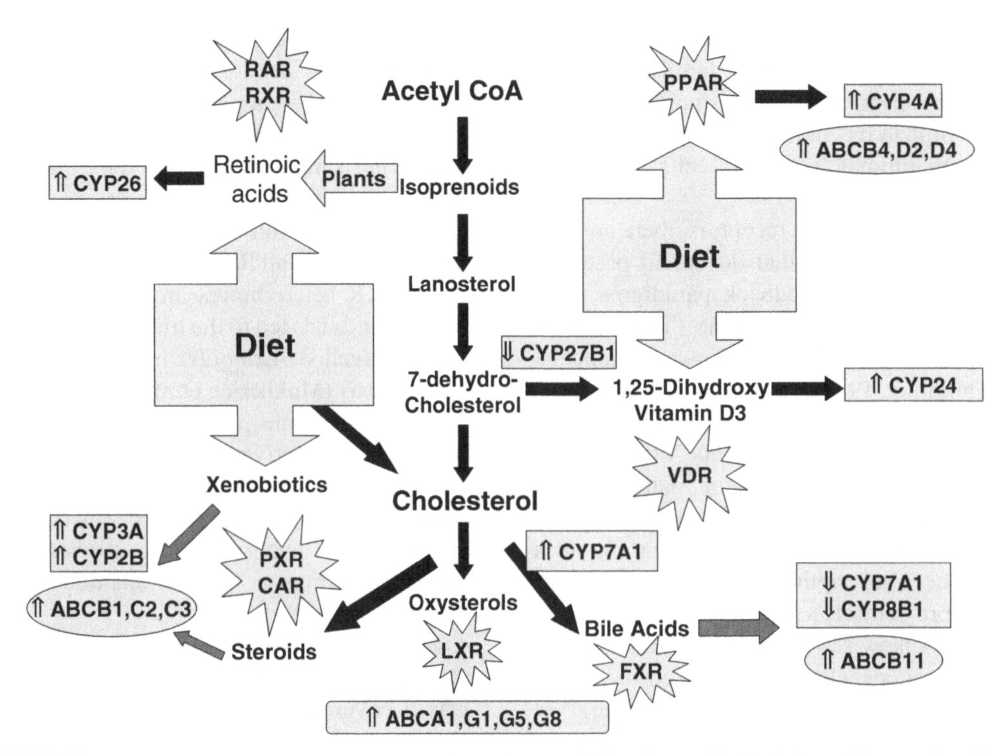

FIGURE 3 Subcellular regulation by lipids and steroids with potential interfaces with diet indicated. See text for abbreviations of receptors, transport proteins, and enzymes. (Adapted from a figure in Chawla et al., 2001.)

PPARδ include long-chain fatty acids and carboprostacyclin. The identification and study of synthetic high-affinity PPARδ ligands also suggest a role for this receptor in lipid metabolism (Oliver et al., 2001; Vosper et al., 2001). Pharmacological activation of PPARδ in macrophages and fibroblasts results in upregulation of the ABCA1 transporter, and because of its widespread expression, PPARδ may affect lipid metabolism in peripheral tissues (Oliver et al., 2001; Vosper et al., 2001). Consistent with this notion, PPARδ-null mice are growth retarded and have reduced adipocyte mass and myelination in their central nervous system (Peters et al., 2000; Barak et al., 2002).

In addition to its expression in the liver, LXRα is also abundantly expressed in other tissues associated with lipid metabolism, including adipose, kidney, intestine, lung, adrenals, and macrophages, whereas LXRβ is ubiquitously expressed (Lu et al., 2001). The LXRs are activated by naturally occurring oxysterols including 24(*S*)-hydroxycholesterol (brain), 22(*R*)-hydroxycholesterol (adrenal), 24(*S*),25-epoxycholesterol (liver), and 27-hydroxycholesterol (human macrophage) (Fu et al., 2001; Lu et al., 2001). Evidence also suggests that LXR activation can be antagonized by other small lipophilic agents, including 22(*S*)-hydroxycholesterol, certain unsaturated fatty acids, and geranylgeranyl pyrophosphate (Gan et al., 2001; Ou et al., 2001; Spencer et al., 2001). LXRs act as cholesterol sensors that respond to elevated sterol concentrations and transactivate a cadre of genes that govern transport, catabolism, and elimination of cholesterol (Lu et al., 2001). LXRs also regulate a number of genes involved in fatty acid metabolism (Repa et al., 2000a; Schultz et al., 2000). In the LXR metabolic cascade, several sterol transporters have been identified as targets, including ABCA1, ABCG1, ABCG4, ABCG5, and ABCG8 (Costet et al., 2000; Repa et al., 2000b; Venkateswaran et al., 2000; Engel et al., 2001). ABCA1 is a monomeric transporter that resides in the plasma membrane of tissues, including liver, intestine, placenta, adipose, and spleen. ABCA1 transports phospholipids and cholesterol and is believed to be the rate-limiting step in reverse cholesterol transport (Tall and Wang, 2000). The dimeric transporters ABCG1, ABCG4, ABCG5, and ABCG8 are likely to be associated with membranes of intracellular organelles and have all been implicated in the intracellular trafficking of sterols in macrophages (for ABCG1 and perhaps ABCG4), as well as in liver and small intestine (for ABCG5 and ABCG8). Mutations in the genes for ABCA1 and ABCG5/G8 result in two disorders in cholesterol metabolism: Tangier disease and sitosterolemia (Berge et al., 2000; Tall and Wang, 2000). These genes, therefore, play pivotal roles in the cellular flux of lipids from macrophages and the biliary secretion and intestinal absorption of sterols. No cytosolic binding proteins have yet been identified as target genes of the LXRs, although one or more of the newly described oxysterol binding proteins may fulfill such a role. However, in rodents, the CYP enzyme cholesterol 7a-hydroxylase (CYP 7A1) has been shown to be an important LXR target gene. CYP 7A1 encodes the rate-limiting enzyme in the neutral bile acid biosynthetic pathway and is one of the principle means for eliminating cholesterol from the body. Mice lacking LXRα fail to increase production of CYP 7A1 and exhibit profound liver accumulation of cholesterol esters (Peet et al., 1998). Mice lacking only LXRβ do not exhibit this alteration in bile acid metabolism, suggesting that the two LXRs may subserve distinct biological roles (Alberti et al., 2001). The human LXRα gene is itself a target of the LXR signaling pathway (Lafitte et al., 2001; Whitney et al., 2001). Particularly in macrophages, the autoregulation of LXRα would be an important way to amplify the cholesterol catabolic cascade.

The FXR is actually misnamed the *farnesoid receptor* because although supraphysiological concentrations of the cholesterol precursor farnesol can weakly activate FXR, the relevant biological ligands for FXR are now known to be certain bile acids, including chenodeoxycholic acid, cholic acid, and their respective conjugated metabolites (Russell, 1999). FXR is highly expressed in the enterohepatic system, where it acts as a bile acid sensor that protects the body from elevated bile acid concentrations. A number of *in vitro* and *in vivo* studies using mouse models have elucidated the FXR gene regulatory cascade (Goodwin et al., 2000; Lu et al., 2000). FXR activation results in the upregulation of ABCB11 (also known as the *bile salt efflux pump* [BSEP]), a bile acid transporter that increases the flow and secretion of these detergent-like molecules into bile, where they are required for the solubilization and absorption of lipids and fat-soluble vitamins in the intestine (Sinal et al., 2000; Ananthanarayanan et al., 2001). In the enterocytes of the ileum, bile acids are efficiently reclaimed for return to the liver. In these ileal enterocytes, bile acids induce the expression of a cytosolic binding protein called ileal bile acid–binding protein (IBABP), another FXR target gene that has been proposed to buffer intracellular bile acids and promote their translocation into the portal circulation (Makishima et al., 1999). In the liver, bile acid activation of FXR represses transcription of the key CYP genes involved in bile acid synthesis. Much of this feedback repression is due to FXR-mediated upregulation of "small heterodimer partner" (SHP), an atypical orphan nuclear receptor that functions as a transcriptional repressor (Goodwin et al., 2000; Lu et al., 2000). SHP interacts with and represses LRH-1, an orphan nuclear receptor that is required for liver-specific expression of CYP 7A1 and sterol 12a-hydroxylase (CYP 8B), the enzyme responsible for the synthesis of trihydroxy-bile acids, such as cholic acid. Thus, FXR uses a rather unique variation on the ligand sensor cascade to maintain bile acid homeostasis.

STEROID AND XENOBIOTIC RECEPTORS

To protect the body against foreign chemicals (xenobiotics) and the buildup of toxic endogenous lipids, two nuclear receptors function to regulate detoxification and elimination. The constitutive androstane receptor (CAR) mediates the response to a narrow range of phenobarbital-like inducers (Tzameli et al., 2001). In contrast, the human steroid xenobiotic receptor (SXR) responds to many prescription drugs, environmental contaminants, steroids, and toxic bile acids (Watkins et al., 2001). Consistent with their role as xenobiotic sensors, both receptors are expressed primarily in liver and small intestine. No cytoplasmic binding proteins have yet been identified that generally bind xenobiotics, although phenobarbital does induce the expression of ABCC3, a member of the multidrug resistance–related protein subfamily (Kiuchi et al., 1998). The CYP 3A enzyme is responsible for metabolizing and clearing >60% of clinically prescribed drugs, and its induction plays a pivotal role in the clearance of hepatotoxic bile salts. CYP 3A gene expression is induced by a large variety of xenobiotic compounds through SXR/PXR activation (Xie et al., 2001).

FEED-FORWARD LOOPS AND UPREGULATION OF METABOLIC ENZYMES

Confirmation that SXR and PXR act as xenobiotic receptors comes from mouse knockouts of the rodent homologue pregnane X receptor (PXR) that abolish both CYP 3A inducibility and the protection of liver from the effects of toxic compounds (Xie et al., 2000; Staudinger et al., 2001). Taken together, the xenobiotic activation of CAR and SXR/PXR induces a positive feed-forward loop that aids in clearance of foreign chemicals and thereby resets the xenosensors for another round of signaling. The vertebrate retinoic acid receptors (RARs) coordinately upregulate two cytosolic binding proteins, cellular retinoic acid–binding protein (CRABPII) and cellular retinol-binding protein (CRBPI), which control the availability and transport of vitamin A–derived ligands (Giguere, 1994). The RARs also upregulate expression of the enzyme CYP-26A1, which deactivates the most potent ligand, all-*trans* retinoic acid (Abu-Abed et al., 1998). Finally, the 1,25-dihydroxyvitamin D receptor (VDR) similarly upregulates expression of a 24-hydroxylase (CYP24), which inactivates the active vitamin D hormone, and downregulates the expression of the 1a-hydroxylase (CYP 27B1), the enzyme that produces the vitamin D hormone (Jones et al., 1998). The remaining RXR heterodimer partner, the thyroid hormone receptor (TR), does not appear to rely on the metabolic cascade and more closely resembles the endocrine steroid receptors in its function.

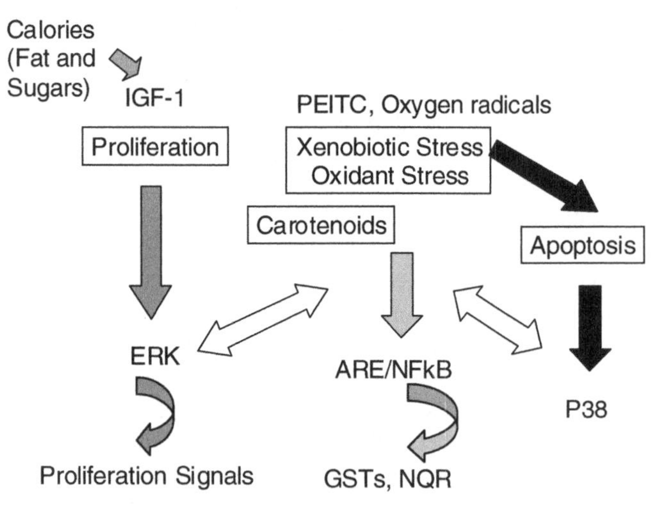

FIGURE 4 Proliferation, xenobiotic stress, oxidant stress, and apoptosis. Three parallel intracellular pathways affect proliferation, the triggering of defense mechanisms through xenobiotic and oxidant stress, and the triggering of apoptosis through prolonged continuous or high dose xenobiotic or oxidant stress.

A THEORETICAL MODEL FOR XENOBIOSIS AND OXIDANT STRESS IN CANCER

The complex pathways evident from this analysis reveal that endocrine and paracrine factors acting at a cellular and subcellular level can affect the process of carcinogenesis. A number of peptides acting through membrane receptors, as well as lipids and steroid hormones acting through nuclear receptors, function as effective regulators of cellular homeostasis by affecting the synthesis of key enzymes that control the intensity, duration, and direction of numerous metabolic steps within the cell. Both the IGF axis and reproductive steroids are critical elements in these systems. Lipids previously thought to function only as nutrients have been found to be potent modulators of cellular function relevant to cellular differentiation, proliferation, and apoptosis.

A theoretical model that expands on the xenobiotic theory of cancer is shown in Figure 4. Excess energy intake both activates the IGF axis and increases steroid production so that proliferation is increased. Xenobiotic and oxidant stress induce metabolic enzymes that counterbalance the oxidant stress resulting from cellular proliferation through the production of protective antioxidant defense systems. However, if these xenobiotic stimuli from carcinogens, oxidants, or radiation are presented continuously or at high doses, apoptotic pathways are activated. This normal function of the cell can be affected by mutagenic events, which alter gene expression so that nutritional homeostasis is no longer maintained. Although not all of the factors promoting carcinogenesis act through these pathways, the study of endocrine and paracrine pathways is vital to an understanding of the processes through which nutrition affects tumor biology and the multistep process of carcinogenesis.

References

Abreu-Martin M.T., Chari A., Palladino A.A., Craft N.A., and Sawyers C.L. 1999. Mitogen-activated protein kinase kinase kinase 1 activates androgen receptor–dependent transcription and apoptosis in prostate cancer. *Mol Cell Biol* **19**: 5143–5154.

Abu-Abed, S.S., Beckett, B.R., Chiba, H., Chithalen, J.V., Jones, G., Metzger, D., Chambon, P., and Petkovich, M. 1998. Mouse P450RAI (CYP26) expression and retinoic acid–inducible retinoic acid metabolism in F9 cells are regulated by retinoic acid receptor gamma and retinoid X receptor alpha. *J Biol Chem* **273**: 2409–2415.

Abuzzahab, M.J., Schneider, A., Goddard, A., Grigorescu, F., Lautier, C., Keller, E., Kiess, W., Klammt, J., Kratzsch, J., Osgood, D., Pfaffle, R., Raile, K., Seidel, B., Smith, R.J., and Chernausek, S.D. 2003. IGF-I receptor mutations resulting in intrauterine and postnatal growth retardation. *N Engl J Med* **349**: 2211–2222.

Alberti, S., Schuster, G., Parini, P., Feltkamp, D., Diczfalusy, U., Rudling, M., Angelin, B., Bjorkhem, I., Pettersson, S., and Gustafsson, J.A. 2001. Hepatic cholesterol metabolism and resistance to dietary cholesterol in LXRbeta-deficient mice. *J Clin Invest* **107**: 565–573.

Altinkaynak, K., Aksoy, H.H., Bakan, E., and Kumtepe, Y. 2003. Serum IGF-I and IGFBP-3 in healthy pregnancies and patients with preeclampsia. *Clin Biochem* **36**: 221–223.

Ananthanarayanan, M., Balasubramanian, N., Makishima, M., Mangelsdorf, D.J., and Suchy, F.J. 2001. Human bile salt export pump promoter is transactivated by the farnesoid X receptor/bile acid receptor. *J Biol Chem* **276**: 28857–28865.

Barak, Y., Liao, D., He, W., Ong, E.S., Nelson, M.C., Olefsky, J.M., Boland, R., and Evans, R.M. 2002. Effects of peroxisome proliferator-activated receptor delta on placentation, adiposity, and colorectal cancer. *Proc Natl Acad Sci USA* **99**: 303–308.

Baserga, R., Peruzzi, F., and Reiss, K. 2003. The IGF-1 receptor in cancer biology. *Int J Cancer* **107**: 873–877.

Berge, K.E., Tian, H., Graf, G.A., Yu, L., Grishin, N.V., Schultz, J., Kwiterovich, P., Shan, B., Barnes, R., and Hobbs, H.H. 2000. Accumulation of dietary cholesterol in sitosterolemia caused by mutations in adjacent ABC transporters. *Science* **290**: 1771–1775.

Bonafe, M., Barbieri, M., Marchegiani, F., Olivieri, F., Ragno, E., Giampieri, C., Mugianesi, E., Centurelli, M., Franceschi, C., and Paolisso, G. 2003. Polymorphic variants of insulin-like growth factor I (IGF-I) receptor and phosphoinositide 3-kinase genes affect IGF-I plasma levels and human longevity: cues for an evolutionarily conserved mechanism of life span control. *J Clin Endocrinol Metab* **88**: 3299–3304.

Burroughs, K.D., Dunn, S.E., Barrett, J.C., and Taylor, J.E. 1999. Insulin-like growth factor-I: a key regulator of human cancer risk? *J Natl Cancer Inst* **91**: 579–581.

Chan, J.M., Stampfer, M.J., Ma, J., Gann, P.H., Gaziano, J.M., and Giovannucci, E.L. 2001. Dairy products, calcium, and prostate cancer risk in the Physicians' Health Study. *Am J Clin Nutr* **74**: 549–554.

Chawla, A., Boisvert, W.A., Lee, C.H., Laffitte, B.A., Barak, Y., Joseph, S.B., Liao, D., Nagy, L., Edwards, P.A., Curtiss, L.K., Evans, R.M., and Tontonoz, P. 2001. A PPAR gamma-LXR-ABCA1 pathway in macrophages is involved in cholesterol efflux and atherogenesis. *Mol Cell* **7**: 161–171.

Chawla, A., Repa, J.J., Evans, R.M., and Mangelsdorf, D.J. 2001. Nuclear receptors and lipid physiology: opening the X-files. *Science* **294**(5548): 1866–1870.

Cheng, I.C. et al. 2004. Haplotype variation in insulin-like growth factor I (IGF-I) and prostate cancer risk: the multiethnic cohort. *Proc Am Assoc Cancer Res* **45**: A4505.

Chinetti, G., Lestavel, S., Bocher, V., Remaley, A.T., Neve, B., Torra, I.P., Teissier, E., Minnich, A., Jaye, M., Duverger, N., Brewer, H.B., Fruchart, J.C., Clavey, V., and Staels, B. 2001. PPAR-alpha and PPAR-gamma activators induce cholesterol removal from human macrophage foam cells through stimulation of the ABCA1 pathway. *Nature Med* **7**: 53–58.

Clarke, R., Skaar, T., Leonessa, F., Branken, H., James, M., Brunner, N., and Lippman, M.E. 1996. Acquisition of an antiestrogen-resistant phenotype in breast cancer: role of cellular and molecular mechanisms. *Cancer Treat Res* **87**: 263–283.

Clarke, R.B., Howell, A., Potten, C.S., and Anderson, E. 1997a. Dissociation between steroid receptor expression and cell proliferation in the human breast. *Cancer Res* **57**: 4987–4991.

Clarke, R.B., Howell, A., and Anderson, E. 1997b. Estrogen sensitivity of normal human breast tissue *in vivo* and implanted into athymic nude mice: analysis of the relationship between estrogen-induced proliferation and progesterone receptor expression. *Breast Cancer Res Treat* **45**: 121–133.

Costet, P., Luo, Y., Wang, N., and Tall, A.R. 2000. Sterol-dependent transactivation of the ABC1 promoter by the liver X receptor/retinoid X receptor. *J Biol Chem* **275**: 28240–28245.

Craft, N., Shostak, Y., Carey, M., and Sawyers, C.L. 1999. A mechanism for hormone-independent prostate cancer through modulation of androgen receptor signaling by the HER-2/*neu* tyrosine kinase. *Nat Med* **5**: 280–285.

Culig, Z., Hobisch, A., Cronauer, M.V., Radmayr, C., Trapman, J., Hittmair, A., Bartsch, G., and Klocker, H. Androgen receptor activation in prostate tumor cell lines by insulin-like growth factor-I, keratinocyte growth factor, and epidermal growth factor. 1994. *Cancer Res* **54**: 5474–5478.

Culig, Z., Hoffmann, J., Erdel, M., Eder, I.E., Hobisch, A., Hittmair, A., Bartsch, G., Utermann, G., Schneider, M.R., Parczyk, K., and Klocker, H. 1999. Switch from antagonist to agonist of the androgen receptor blocker bicalutamide is associated with prostate tumour progression in a new model system. *Br J Cancer* **81**: 242–251.

Deal, C., Ma, J., Wilkin, F., Paquette, J., Rozen, F., Ge, B., Hudson, T., Stampfer, M., and Pollak, M. 2001. Novel promoter polymorphism in insulin-like growth factor-binding protein-3: correlation with serum levels and interaction with known regulators. *J Clin Endocrinol Metab* **86**: 1274–1280.

Dean, M., Hamon, Y., and Chimini, G. 2001. The human ATP-binding cassette (ABC) transporter superfamily. *J Lipid Res* **42**: 1007–1017.

de Urquiza, A.M., Liu, S., Sjoberg, M., Zetterstrom, R.H., Griffiths, W., Sjovall, J., and Perlmann, T. 2000. Docosahexaenoic acid, a ligand for the retinoid X receptor in mouse brain. *Science* **290**: 2140–2144.

DeSombre, E.R., and Jensen, E.V. 2000. *In* "Cancer Medicine" (J.F. Holland, E. Frei, R.C. Bast, D.W. Kufe, R.E. Pollock, and R.R. Weichselbaum, Eds.), pp. 706–714. Decker, Hamilton, ON, Canada.

de Vere White, R., Meyers, F., Chi, S.G., Chamberlain, S., Siders, D., Lee, F., Stewart, S., and Gumerlock, P.H. 1997. Human androgen receptor expression in prostate cancer following androgen ablation. *Eur Urol* **31**: 1–6.

Dotzlaw, H., Leygue, E., Watson, P.H., and Murphy, L.C. 1999. Estrogen receptor-beta messenger RNA expression in human breast tumor biopsies: relationship to steroid receptor status and regulation by progestins. *Cancer Res* **59**: 529–532.

El-Ashry, D., Miller, D.L., Kharbanda, S., Lippman, M.E., and Kern, F.G. 1997. Constitutive Raf-1 kinase activity in breast cancer cells induces both estrogen-independent growth and apoptosis. *Oncogene* **15**: 423–435.

Engel, T., Lorkowski, S., Lueken, A., Rust, S., Schluter, B., Berger, G., Cullen, P., and Assmann, G. 2001. The human ABCG4 gene is regulated by oxysterols and retinoids in monocyte-derived macrophages. *Biochem Biophys Res Commun* **288**: 483–488.

Engeland, A., Tretli, S., and Bjorge, T. 2003. Height, body mass index, and prostate cancer: a follow-up of 950000 Norwegian men. *Br J Cancer* **89**: 1237–1242.

Evans, R.M. 1988. The steroid and thyroid hormone receptor superfamily. *Science* **240**: 889–895.

Firth, S.M., and Baxter, R.C. 2002. Cellular actions of the insulin-like growth factor binding proteins. *Endocr Rev* **23**: 824–854.

Fisher, B., Costantino, J.P., Wickerham, D.L., Redmond, C.K., Kavanah, M., Cronin, W.M., Vogel, V., Robidoux, A., Dimitrov, N., Atkins, J., Daly, M., Wieand, S., Tan-Chiu, E., Ford, L., and Wolmark, N. 1998. Tamoxifen for prevention of breast cancer: report of the National Surgical Adjuvant Breast and Bowel Project P-1 Study. *J Natl Cancer Inst* **90**: 1371–1388.

Forrest, D., and Vennstrom, B. 2000. Functions of thyroid hormone receptors in mice. *Thryoid* **10**: 41–52.

Fourcade, S., Savary, S., Albet, S., Gauthe, D., Gondcaille, C., Pineau, T., Bellenger, J., Bentejac, M., Holzinger, A., Berger, J., and Bugaut, M. 2001. Fibrate induction of the adrenoleukodystrophy-related gene (ABCD2): promoter analysis and role of the peroxisome proliferator-activated receptor PPARalpha. *Eur J Biochm* **268**: 3490–3500.

Fu, X., Menke, J.G., Chen, Y., Zhou, G., MacNaul, K.L., Wright, S.D., Sparrow, C.P., and Lund, E.G. 2001. Orphan nuclear receptors as eLiXiRs and FiXeRs of sterol metabolism. *J Biol Chem* **276**: 38378–38387.

Fuqua, S.A.W., Schiff, R., Parra, I., Friedrichs, W.E., Su, J.L., McKee, D.D., Slentz-Kesler, K., Moore, L.B., Wilson, T.M., and Moore, J.T. 1999. Expression of wild-type estrogen receptor beta and variant isoforms in human breast cancer. *Cancer Res* **59**: 5425–5428.

Gan, X., Kaplan, R., Menke, J.G., MacNaul, K., Chen, Y., Sparrow, C.P., Zhou, G., Wright, S.D., and Cai, T.Q. 2001. Dual mechanisms of ABCA1 regulation by geranylgeranyl pyrophosphate. *J Biol Chem* **276**: 48702–48708.

Giguere, V. 1994. Retinoic acid receptors and cellular retinoid binding proteins: complex interplay in retinoid signaling. *Endocr Rev* **15**: 61–79.

Giovannucci, E., Pollak, M., Liu, Y., Platz, E.A., Majeed, N., Rimm, E.B., and Willett, W.C. 2003. Nutritional predictors of insulin-like growth factor-I and their relationships to cancer in men. *Cancer Epidemiol Biomarkers Prev* **12**: 84–89.

Giudice, L.C. 2002. Maternal-fetal conflict—lessons from a transgene. *J Clin Investig* **110**: 307–309.

Goodwin, B., Jones, S.A., Price, R.R., Watson, M.A., McKee, D.D., Moore, L.B., Galardi, C., Wilson, J.G., Lewis, M.C., Roth, M.E., Maloney, P.R., Willson, T.M., and Kliewer, S.A. 2000. A regulatory cascade of the nuclear receptors FXR, SHP-1, and LRH-1 represses bile acid biosynthesis. *Mol Cell* **6**: 517–526.

Gregory, C.W., Hamil, K.G., Kim, D., Hall, S.H., Pretlow, T.G., Mohler, J.L., and French, F.S. 1998. Androgen receptor expression in androgen-independent prostate cancer is associated with increased expression of androgen regulated genes. *Cancer Res* **58**: 5718–5724.

Gregory, C.W., Johnson, R.T., Mohler, J.L., French, F.S., and Wilson, E.M. 2001. Androgen receptor stabilization in recurrent prostate cancer is associated with hypersensitivity to low androgen. *Cancer Res* **6**: 2892–2898.

Gunnell, D. et al. 2001. Height, leg length, and cancer risk: a systematic review. *Epidemiol Rev* **23**: 313–342.

Gunnell, D. et al. 2001. Are diet–prostate cancer associations mediated by the IGF axis? A cross-sectional analysis of diet, IGF-I and IGFBP-3 in healthy middle-aged men. *Br J Cancer* **88**: 1682–1686.

Harrela, M. et al. 1996. Genetic and environmental components of interindividual variation in circulating levels of IGF-I, IGF-II, IGFBP-1, and IGFBP-3. *J Clin Invest* **98**: 2612–2615.

Heaney, R. et al. 1999. Dietary changes favorably affect bone remodeling in older adults. *J Am Diet Assoc* **99**: 1228–1233.

Helle, S.I. et al. 2001. Alterations in the insulin-like growth factor system during treatment with diethylstilboestrol in patients with metastatic breast cancer. *Br J Cancer* **85**: 147–151.

Hilakivi-Clarke, L., Clarke, R., and Lippman, M. 1999a. The influence of maternal diet on breast cancer risk among female offspring. *Nutrition* **15**: 392–401.

Hilakivi-Clarke, L., Cho, E., Onojafe, I., Raygada, M., and Clarke, R. 1999b. Maternal exposure to genistein during pregnancy increases carcinogen-induced mammary tumorigenesis in female rat offspring. *Oncol Rep* **6**: 1089–1095.

Holly, J.M. 1998. Insulin-like growth factor-I and new opportunities for cancer prevention. *Lancet* **351**: 1373–1375.

Holmes, M.D., Pollak, M.N., Willett, W.C., and Hankinson, S.E. 2002. Dietary correlates of plasma insulin-like growth factor-I and insulin-like growth factor binding protein-3 concentrations. *Cancer Epidemiol Biomarkers Prev* **11**: 852–861.

Houghton, P.J., and Huang, S. 2004. mTOR as a target for cancer therapy. *Curr Top Microbiol Immunol* **279**: 339–359.

Hu, Y.F., Lau, K.M., Ho, S.M., and Russo, J. 1998. Increased expression of estrogen receptor beta in chemically transformed human breast epithelial cells. *Int J Oncol* **12**: 1225–1228.

Jarvinen, T.A.H., Pelti-Huikko, M., Holli, K., and Isola, J. 2000. Estrogen receptor beta is coexpressed with ERalpha and PR and associated with nodal status, grade, and proliferation rate in breast cancer. *Am J Pathol* **156**: 29–35.

Jernstrom, H. et al. 2001. Genetic and non-genetic factors associated with variation of plasma levels of insulin-like growth factor-I and insulin-like growth factor binding protein-3 in healthy premenopausal women. *Cancer Epidemiol Biomarkers* **10**: 377–384.

Johnston, L.B. et al. 2003. Association between insulin-like growth factor 1 (IGF-1) polymorphisms, circulating IGF-1, and pre- and postnatal growth in two European small for gestational age populations. *J Clin Endocrinol Metab* **88**: 4805–4810.

Jones, G., Strugnell, S.A., and DeLuca, H.F. 1998. Current understanding of the molecular actions of vitamin D. *Physiol Rev* **78**: 1193.

Jones, J.I., and Clemmons, D.R. 1995. Insulin-like growth factors and their binding proteins: biological actions. *Endocr Rev* **16**: 3–34.

Juul, A. et al. 1994. The ratio between serum levels of insulin-like growth factor (IGF)-1 and the IGF binding proteins (IGFBP)-1, 2 and 3 decreases with age in healthy adults and is increased in acromegalic patients. *Clin Endocrinol* **41**: 85–93.

Khandwala, H.M., McCutcheon, I.E., Flyvbjerg, A., and Friend, K.E. 2000. The effects of insulin-like growth factors on tumorigenesis and neoplastic growth. *Endocrinol Rev* **21**: 215–244.

Kiuchi, Y., Suzuki, H., Hirohashi, T., Tyson, C.A., Sugiyama, Y. 1998. cDNA cloning and inducible expression of human multidrug resistance associated protein 3 (MRP3). *FEBS Lett* **433**: 149.

Koibuchi, Y., Sugamata, N., Iino, Y., Yokoe, T., Andoh, T., Maemura, M., Takei, H., Horiguchi, J., Matsumoto, H., and Morishita, Y. 1999. The mechanisms of antitumor effects of luteinizing hormone-releasing hormone agonist (buserelin) in 7, 12-dimethylbenz(a)anthracene-induced rat mammary cancer. *Int J Mol Med* **4**: 145–148.

Kuiper, G.G.J.M., Enmark, E., Pelto-Huikko, M., Nilsson, S., and Gustafsson, J.-Å. 1996. Cloning of a novel receptor expressed in rat prostate and ovary. *Proc Natl Acad Sci USA* **93**: 5925–5930.

Laffitte, B.A., Joseph, S.B., Walczak, R., Pei, L., Wilpitz, D.C., Collins, J.L., and Tontonoz, P. 2001. Autoregulation of the human liver X receptor alpha promoter. *Mol Cell Biol* **21**: 7558–7568.

Lee, S.S., Pineau, T., Drago, J., Lee, E.J., Owens, J.W., Kroetz, D.L., Fernandez-Salguero, P.M., Westphal, H., and Gonzalez, F.J. 1995. Targeted disruption of the alpha isoform of the peroxisome proliferator-activated receptor gene in mice results in abolishment of the pleiotropic effects of peroxisome proliferators. *Mol Cell Biol* **15**: 3012.

Lawlor, D.A., Okasha, M., Gunnell, D., Smith, G.D., and Ebrahim, S. 2003. Associations of adult measures of childhood growth with breast cancer: findings from the British Women's Heart and Health Study. *Br J Cancer* **89**: 81–87.

Le Marchand, L. et al. 2002. Association of a common polymorphism in the human *GH1* gene with colorectal neoplasia. *J Natl Cancer Inst* **94**: 454–460.

Leygue, E., Dotzlaw, H., Watson, P.H., and Murphy, L.C. 1999. Expression of estrogen receptor beta1, beta2, and beta5 messenger RNAs in human breast tissue. *Cancer Res* **59**: 1175–1179.

Liao, D.Z., Pantazis, C.G., Hou, X., and Li, S.A. 1998. Promotion of estrogen-induced mammary gland carcinogenesis by androgen in the male Noble rat: probable mediation by steroid receptors. *Carcinogenesis* **19**: 2173–2180.

Lonard, D.M., Nawaz, Z., Smith, C.L., and O'Malley, B.W. 2000. The 26S proteasome is required for estrogen receptor-alpha and coactivator turnover and for efficient estrogen receptor-alpha transactivation. *Mol Cell* **5**: 939–948.

Longo, V.D., and Finch, C.E. 2003. Evolutionary medicine: from dwarf model systems to healthy centenarians? *Science* **299**: 1342–1346.

Lu, T.T., Makishima, M., Repa, J.J., Schoonjans, K., Kerr, T.A., Auwerx, J., Mangelsdorf, D.J. 2000. Molecular basis for feedback regulation of bile acid synthesis by nuclear receptors. *Mol Cell* **6**: 507.

Lu, T.T., Repa, J.J., and Mangelsdorf, D.J. 2001. Orphan nuclear receptors as eLiXiRs and FiXeRs of sterol metabolism. *J Biol Chem* **276**: 37735.

Laron, Z. 1995. Prismatic cases: Laron syndrome (primary growth hormone resistance) from patient to laboratory to patient. *J Clin Endocrinol Metab* **80**: 1526–1531.

Maheshwari, H.G., Silverman, B.L., Dupuis, J., and Baumann, G. 1998. Phenotype and genetic analysis of a syndrome caused by an inactivating mutation in the growth hormone–releasing hormone receptor: Dwarfism of Sindh. *J Clin Endocrinol Metab* **83**: 4065–4074.

Makishima, M., Okamoto, A.Y., Repa, J.J., Tu, H., Learned, R.M., Luk, A., Hull, M.V., Lustig, K.D., Mangelsdorf, D.J., and Shan, B. 1999. Identification of a nuclear receptor for bile acids. *Science* **284**: 1362.

Mangelsdorf, D.J., Umesono, K., and Evans, R.M. 1994. *In* "The Retinoids: Biology, Chemistry, and Medicine" (M.B. Sporn, A.B. Roberts, and D.S. Goodman, Eds.), p. 319. Raven, New York.

Mangelsdorf, D.J., Evans, R.M. 1995. The RXR heterodimers and orphan receptors. *Cell* **83**: 841.

McCormack, V.A. et al. 2003. Fetal growth and subsequent risk of breast cancer: results from long term follow up of Swedish cohort. *Br Med J* **326**: 248.

Sandhu, M.S., Luben, R., Day, N.E., and Khaw, K.T. 2002. Self-reported birth weight and subsequent risk of colorectal cancer. *Cancer Epidemiol Biomarkers Prev* **11**: 935–938.

McKenna, N.J., Lanz, R.B., and O'Malley, B.W. 1999. Nuclear receptor coregulators: cellular and molecular biology. *Endocr Rev* **20**: 321.

Mellemkjaer, L. et al. 2003. Birth weight and risk of early-onset breast cancer (Denmark). *Cancer Causes Control* **14**: 61–64.

Mukherjee, R., Strasser, J., Jow, L., Hoener, P., Paterniti, J.R., Jr., and Heyman, R.A. 1998. RXR agonists activate PPARalpha-inducible genes, lower triglycerides, and raise HDL levels *in vivo*. *Arterioscler Thromb Vasc Biol* **18**: 272.

Nakae, J., Kido, Y., and Accili, D. 2001. Distinct and overlapping functions of insulin and IGF-I receptors. *Endocr Rev* **22**: 818–835.

Nazareth, L.V., and Weigel, N.L. 1996. Activation of the human androgen receptor through a protein kinase A signaling pathway. *J Biol Chem* **271**: 19900–19907.

Newmark, J.R., Hardy, D.O., Tonb, D.C., Carter, B.S., Epstein, J.I., Isaacs, W.B., Brown, T.R., and Barrack, E.R. 1992. Androgen receptor gene mutations in human prostate cancer. *Proc Natl Acad Sci USA* **89**: 6319–6323,

Nicholson, R.I., McClelland, R.A., Robertson, J.F.R., and Gee, J.M.W. 1999. Involvement of steroid hormone and growth factor cross-talk in endocrine response in breast cancer. *Endocrine-Related Cancer* **6**: 373–387.

Ogawa, S., Washburn, T.F., Taylor, J., Lubahn, D.B., Korach, K.S., and Pfaff, D.W. 1998. Modifications of testosterone-dependent behaviors by estrogen receptor-alpha gene disruption in male mice. *Endocrinology* **139**: 5058–5069.

Oliver, W.R., Jr., Shenk, J.L., Snaith, M.R., Russell, C.S., Plunket, K.D., Bodkin, N.L., Lewis, M.C., Winegar, D.A., Sznaidman, M.L., Lambert, M.H., Xu, H.E., Sternbach, D.D., Kliewer, S.A., Hansen, B.C., and Willson, T.M. 2001. A selective peroxisome proliferator-activated receptor delta agonist promotes reverse cholesterol transport. *Proc Natl Acad Sci USA* **98**: 5306.

Ou, J., Tu, H., Shan, B., Luk, A., DeBose-Boyd, R.A., Bashmakov, Y., Goldstein, J.L., and Brown, M.S. 2001. Unsaturated fatty acids inhibit transcription of the sterol regulatory element-binding protein-1c (SREBP-1c) gene by antagonizing ligand-dependent activation of the LXR. *Proc Natl Acad Sci USA* **98**: 6027.

Peet, D.J., Turley, S.D., Ma, W., Janowski, B.A., Lobaccaro, J.M., Hammer, R.E., and Mangelsdorf, D.J. 1998. Cholesterol and bile acid metabolism are impaired in mice lacking the nuclear oxysterol receptor LXR alpha. *Cell* **93**: 693.

Peters, J.M., Lee, S.S., Li, W., Ward, J.M., Gavrilova, O., Everett, C., Reitman, M.L., Hudson, L.D., and Gonzalez, F.J. 2000. Growth, adipose, brain, and skin alterations resulting from targeted disruption of the mouse peroxisome proliferator-activated receptor beta(delta). *Mol Cell Biol* **20**: 5119.

Pollak, M. et al. 1990. Effect of tamoxifen on serum insulin-like growth factor I levels in stage I breast cancer patients. *J Natl Cancer Inst* **82**: 1693–1697.

Pollak, M. 2001. Insulin-like growth factors (IGFs) and prostate cancer. *Epidemiol Rev* **23**: 59–66.

Repa, J.J., Turley, S.D., Lobaccaro, J.A., Medina, J., Li, L., Lustig, K., Shan, B., Heyman, R.A., Dietschy, J.M., and Mangelsdorf, D.J. 2000a. Regulation of absorption and ABC1-mediated efflux of cholesterol by RXR heterodimers. *Science* **289**: 1524.

Repa, J.J., Liang, G., Ou, J., Bashmakov, Y., Lobaccaro, J.M., Shimomura, I., Shan, B., Brown, M.S., Goldstein, J.L., and Mangelsdorf, D.J. 2000b. Regulation of mouse sterol regulatory element-binding protein-1c gene (SREBP-1c) by oxysterol receptors, LXRalpha and LXRbeta. *Genes Dev* **14**: 2819.

Rosen, E.D., and Spiegelman, B.M. 2001. PPARgamma : a nuclear regulator of metabolism, differentiation, and cell growth. *J Biol Chem* **276**: 37731.

Ruizeveld de Winter, J.A., Trapman, J., Vermey, M., Mulder, E., Zegers, N.D., and van der Kwast, T.H. 1991. Androgen receptor expression in human tissues: an immunohistochemical study. *J Histochem Cytochem* **39**: 927–936.

Russell, D.W. 1999. Nuclear orphan receptors control cholesterol catabolism. *Cell* **97**: 539.

Sadar, M.D., Hussain, M., and Bruchovsky, N. 1999. Prostate cancer: molecular biology of early progression to androgen independence. *Endocr Relat Cancer* **6**: 487–502,

Saji, S., Jensen, E.V., Nilsson, S., Rylander, T., Warner, M., and Gustafsson, J.-Å. 2000. Estrogen receptors alpha and beta in the rodent mammary gland. *Proc Natl Acad Sci USA* **97**: 337–342.

Schernhammer, E.S., Hankinson, S.E., Hunter, D.J., Blouin, M.-J., and Pollak, M.N. 2003. Polymorphic variation at the-202 locus in IGFBP3: influence on serum levels of insulin-like growth factors, interaction with plasma retinol and vitamin D and breast cancer risk. *Int J Cancer* **107**: 60–64.

Schultz, J.R., Tu, H., Luk, A., Repa, J.J., Medina, J.C., Li, L., Schwendner, S., Wang, S., Thoolen, M., Mangelsdorf, D.J., Lustig, K.D., and Shan, B. 2000. Role of LXRs in control of lipogenesis. *Genes Dev* **14**: 2831.

Simpson, E.R. 1998. Genetic mutations resulting in estrogen insufficiency in the male. *Mol Cell Endocrinol* **145**: 55–59.

Sinal, C.J., Tohkin, M., Miyata, M., Ward, J.M., Lambert, G., and Gonzalez, F.J. 2000. Targeted disruption of the nuclear receptor FXR/BAR impairs bile acid and lipid homeostasis. *Cell* **102**: 731.

Song, R.X., Barnes, C.J., Zhang, Z., Bao, Y., Kumar, R., and Santen, R.J. 2004. The role of Shc and insulin-like growth factor 1 receptor in mediating the translocation of estrogen receptor alpha to the plasma membrane. *Proc Natl Acad Sci USA* **101**: 2076–2081.

Speirs, V., Parkes, A.T., Kerin, M.J., Walton, D.S., Carleton, P.J., Fox, J.N., and Atkin, S.L. 1999. Coexpression of estrogen receptor alpha and beta: poor prognostic factors in human breast cancer? *Cancer Res.* **59**: 525–528.

Spencer, T.A., Li, D., Russel, J.S., Collins, J.L., Bledsoe, R.K., Consler, T.G., Moore, L.B., Galardi, C.M., McKee, D.D., Moore, J.T., Watson, M.A., Parks, D.J., Lambert, M.H., and Willson, T.M. 2001. Pharmacophore analysis of the nuclear oxysterol receptor LXRalpha. *J Med Chem* **44**: 886.

Staudinger, J.L., Goodwin, B., Jones, S.A., Hawkins-Brown, D., MacKenzie, K.I., LaTour, A., Liu Y., Klaassen, C.D., Brown, K.K., Reinhard, J., Willson, T.M., Koller, B.H., and Kliewer, S.A. 2001. The nuclear receptor PXR is a lithocholic acid sensor that protects against liver toxicity. *Proc Natl Acad Sci USA* **98**: 3369.

Stavola, B.L. et al. 2000. Birthweight, childhood growth and risk of breast cancer in British cohort. *Br J Cancer* **83**: 964–968.

Storch, J.A., and Thumser, A.E.A. 2000. The fatty acid transport function of fatty acid-binding proteins. *Biochim Biophys Acta* **1486**: 28.

Tall, A.R., and Wang, N. 2000. Tangier disease as a test of the reverse cholesterol transport hypothesis. *J Clin Invest* **106**: 1205.

Tan, J.A., Sharief, Y., Hamil, K.G., Gregory, C.W., Zang, D.Y., Sar, M., Gumerlock, P.H., de Vere White, R.W., Pretlow, T.G., Harris, S.E., Wilson, E.M., Mohler, J.L., and French, F.S. 1997. Dehydroepiandrosterone activates mutant androgen receptors expressed in the androgen-dependent human prostate cancer xenograft CWR22 and LNCaP cells. *Mol Endocrinol* **11**: 450–459.

Thissen, J.P., Ketelslegers, J.M., and Underwood, L.E. 1994. Nutritional regulation of the insulin-like growth factors. *Endo Rev* **15**: 80–101.

Thummel, C.S. 1995. From embryogenesis to metamorphosis: the regulation and function of Drosophila nuclear receptor superfamily members. *Cell* **83**: 871.

Tibblin, G., Eriksson, M., Cnattingius, S., and Ekbom, A. 1995. High birthweight as a predictor of prostate cancer risk. *Epidemiology* **6**: 423–424.

Tzameli, I., and Moore, D.D. 2001. Role reversal: new insights from new ligands for the xenobiotic receptor CAR. *Trends Endocrinol Metab* **12**: 7.

Vatten, L.J., Nilsen, S.T., Odegard, R.A., Romundstad, P.R., and Austgulen, R. 2002a. Insulin-like growth factor-I and leptin in umbilical cord plasma and infant birth size at term. *Pediatrics* **109**: 1131–1135.

Vatten, L.J., Romundstad, P.R., Trichopoulos, D., and Skjaerven, R. 2002b. Pre-eclampsia in pregnancy and subsequent risk for breast cancer. *Br J Cancer* **87**: 971–973.

Venkateswaran, A., Repa, J.J., Lobaccaro, J.M., Bronson, A., Mangelsdorf, D.J., and Edwards, P.A. 2000. Human white/murine ABC8 mRNA levels are highly induced in lipid-loaded macrophages. A transcriptional role for specific oxysterols. *J Biol Chem* **275**: 14700.

Visakorpi, T., Hyytinen, E., Koivisto, P., Tanner, M., Keinanen, R., Palmberg, C., Palotie, A., Tammela, T., Isola, J., and Kallioniemi, O.P. 1995. *In vivo* amplification of the androgen receptor gene and progression of human prostate cancer. *Nat Genet* **9**: 401–406.

Von Behren, J., and Reynolds, P. 2003. Birth characteristics and brain cancers in young children. *Int J Epidemiol* **32**: 248–256.

Vosper, H., Patel, L., Graham, T.L., Khoudoli, G.A., Hill, A., Macphee, C.H., Pinto, I., Smith, S.A., Suckling, K.E., Wolf, C.R., and Palmer, C.N. 2001. The peroxisome proliferator-activated receptor delta promotes lipid accumulation in human macrophages. *J Biol Chem* **276**: 44258–44265.

Wang, L. et al. 2003. Insulin-like growth factor-binding protein-3 gene-202 A/C polymorphism is correlated with advanced disease status in prostate cancer. *Cancer Res* **63**: 4407–4411.

Warner, M., Nilsson, S., and Gustafsson, J.-Å. 1999. The estrogen receptor family. *Curr Opin Obstet Gynecol* **11**: 249–254.

Watkins, R.E., Wisely, G.B., Moore, L.B., Collins J.L., Lambert, M.H., Williams, S.P., Willson, T.M., Kliewer, S.A., and Redinbo, M.R. 2001. The human nuclear xenobiotic receptor PXR: structural determinants of directed promiscuity. *Science* **292**: 2329.

Waxman, D.J. 1999. P450 gene induction by structurally diverse xenochemicals: central role of nuclear receptors CAR, PXR, and PPAR. *Arch Biochem Biophys* **369**: 11–23.

Way, J.M., Harrington, W.W., Brown, K.K., Gottschalk, W.K., Sundseth, S.S., Mansfield, T.A,. Ramachandran, R.K., Willson, T.M., and Kliewer S.A. 2001. Comprehensive messenger ribonucleic acid profiling reveals that peroxisome proliferator-activated receptor gamma activation has coordinate effects on gene expression in multiple insulin-sensitive tissues. *Endocrinology* **142**: 1269.

Wenger, N.K. 1999. Postmenopausal hormone use for cardioprotection: what we know and what we must learn. *Curr Opin Cardiol* **14**: 292–297.

Whitney, K.D., Watson, M.A., Goodwin, B., Galardi, C.M., Maglich, J.M., Wilson, J.G., Willson, T.M., Collins, J.L., and Kliewer, S.A. 2001. Liver X receptor (LXR) regulation of the LXRalpha gene in human macrophages. *J Biol Chem* **276**: 43509–43515.

Wilson, J.D., and Foster, D.W., Eds. 1992. "Williams Textbook of Endocrinology," 8th edition. Saunders, Philadelphia, PA.

Willson, T.M., Brown, P.J., Sternbach, D.D., and Henke, B.R. 2000. The PPARs: from orphan receptors to drug discovery. *J Med Chem* **43**: 527.

Wiesen, J.F., Young, P., Werb, Z., and Cunha, G.R. 1999. Signaling through the stromal epidermal growth factor receptor is necessary for mammary ductal development. *Development (Cambridge, UK)* **126**: 335–344.

Wijayaratne, A.L., and McDonnell, D.P. 2001. The human estrogen receptor-alpha is a ubiquitinated protein whose stability is affected differentially by agonists, antagonists, and selective estrogen receptor modulators. *J Biol Chem* **276**: 35684–35692.

Wolfrum, C., Borrmann, C.M., Borchers, T., and Spener, F. 2001. Fatty acids and hypolipidemic drugs regulate peroxisome proliferator-activated receptors alpha- and gamma-mediated gene expression via liver fatty acid binding protein: a signaling path to the nucleus. *Proc Natl Acad Sci USA* **98**: 2323.

Wosikowski, K., Schuurhuis, D., Kops, G.J.P.L., Saceda, M., and Bates, S.E. 1997. Altered gene expression in drug-resistant human breast cancer cells. *Clin Cancer Res* **3**: 2405–2414.

Xie, W., Barwick, J.L., Downes, M., Blumberg, B., Simon, C.M., Nelson, M.C., Neuschwander-Tetri, B.A., Brunt, E.M., Guzelian, P.S., and Evans, R.M. 2000. Humanized xenobiotic response in mice expressing nuclear receptor SXR. *Nature* **406**: 435.

Xie, W., and Evans, R.M. 2001. Orphan nuclear receptors: the exotics of xenobiotics. *J Biol Chem* **276**: 37739.

Yee, D., and Lee, A.V. 2000. Crosstalk between the insulin-like growth factors and estrogens in breast cancer. *J Mammary Gland Biol Neoplasia* **5**: 107–115.

Zeps, N., Bentel, J.M., Papadimitriou, J.M., D'Antuono, M.F., and Dawkins, H.J. 1998. Estrogen receptor-negative epithelial cells in mouse mammary gland development and growth. *Differentiation* **62**: 221–226.

CHAPTER

14

Oxidation and Antioxidation in Cancer

PAUL DAVIS, DAVID HEBER, AND LESTER PACKER

INTRODUCTION

Oxygen comprises ~20% of the air we breathe and the air that bathes the plants that surround us. Both the animal and the plant world use oxygen in many ways but have to defend against its potentially damaging effects, as demonstrated when an apple is cut open and exposed to the air. The browning of an apple in minutes of exposure to air demonstrates that oxidation can proceed within the apple, chemically modifying its sugars once the protective colorful peel is bypassed. Within the cells of our bodies, oxidation reactions occur widely to produce energy within the mitochondria and in enzymatic reactions that detoxify drugs and phytochemicals, or simply in harnessing the energy from the breakdown of key nutrients (e.g., glucose), which often involves unpaired electrons catalyzed by specific enzymes involved in the synthesis and maintenance of complex structures that make life possible. The challenge of managing the potential threat of oxidative damage has led to the development of multiple defense mechanisms against this outcome within all living organisms. Unbalanced oxidation would lead to the destruction of all the critical cellular elements that permit life, including cellular lipids, proteins, and carbohydrates, until they reached their zero ground state incompatible with life.

Oxidation is the loss of electrons, and reduction is the gain of electrons. Oxidation and reduction reactions must occur in pairs (i.e., when one atom or molecule is oxidized, another is reduced to defend against the potentially damaging effects of free radicals). Highly reactive molecules can oxidize molecules (i.e., remove electrons from molecules) that were previously stable and may cause them to become unstable species, such as free radicals. A free radical is a chemical species with an unpaired electron that can be neutral, positively charged, or negatively charged. Although a few stable free radicals are known, most are very reactive. In free radical chain reactions, the radical product of one reaction becomes the starting material for another, propagating free radical damage.

Metabolism is not the only source of free radicals. Environmental pollutants are sources for free radicals including nitrogen dioxide, ozone, cigarette smoke, radiation, halogenated hydrocarbons, heavy metals, and certain pesticides. Alcohol consumption can induce oxidative reactions in the liver. Certain chemotherapeutic agents including doxorubicin, cyclophosphamide, 5-fluorouracil, methotrexate, and vincristine can produce oxygen radicals at doses used in cancer patients. Increased physical activity can generate free radicals as the result of increased oxygen consumption during exercise. Oxygen radicals in the human body react with proteins, lipids, carbohydrates, and nucleotides.

There are three steps to the free radical chain reaction: initiation, propagation, and termination. In the initiation step, free radicals are formed from molecules that readily give up electrons, such as hydrogen peroxide. In the propagation steps, the chain-carrying radicals are alternately consumed and produced. In the termination steps, radicals are destroyed. Thus, without termination by an agent such as an antioxidant, a single free radical can damage numerous molecules.

There are four common reactive oxygen species (ROS) in biological systems that are free radicals: superoxide anion (O_2^-), hydrogen peroxide (H_2O_2), hydroxyl radical (OH^-), and singlet oxygen ($^1O_2$). In addition, peroxynitrite ($ONOO^-$) and nitric oxide (NO) and other reactive nitrogen species (RNS) are called *free radicals*. These free radicals

Copyright © 2006, Elsevier Inc.
All rights of reproduction in any form reserved.

can be generated via a number of mechanisms, including normal physiological processes and processes resulting from external factors. For example, singlet oxygen is generated by photosensitization reactions wherein a molecule absorbs light of a given wavelength, exciting the molecule. This excited molecule transfers the increased energy to molecular oxygen, creating singlet oxygen, which then can attack other cell components. It appears that the primary function of carotenoids, an important class of antioxidants, is to scavenge free radicals, particularly singlet oxygen produced by photosensitization.

A certain amount of oxidative function is necessary for proper health. For example, oxidation processes are used by the body's immune systems to kill microorganisms. Sometimes, however, the level of toxic reactive oxygen intermediates overcomes the antioxidant defenses of the host, resulting in an excess of free radicals and a state called *oxidative stress*. These free radicals can induce local injury by reacting with lipids, proteins, and nucleic acids. The interaction of free radicals with cellular lipids leads to membrane damage and the generation of lipid peroxide byproducts.

The response to this, particularly in the higher animals, is the elaboration of a complex and interdependent network of antioxidants and antioxidant enzymes. The ubiquitous presence, the ever increasing number of compounds, and the increasingly complex interrelationships of oxidants and antioxidants is an area of intense current research interest and multiple reviews have dealt with these (Stanner et al., 2004; Willcox et al., 2004). Cells contain a number of antioxidants that have various roles in protecting against free radical reactions. The major water-soluble antioxidant metabolites are glutathione (GSH) and vitamin C, which reside primarily in the cytoplasm and mitochondria. Many water-soluble enzymes also catalyze these reactions. Glutathione peroxidase catalyzes the reaction between GSH and hydrogen peroxide to form water and oxidized glutathione, which is stable. Vitamin E and the carotenoids are the principal lipid-soluble antioxidants. Vitamin E is the major lipid-soluble antioxidant in cell membranes that can break the chain of lipid peroxidation. Therefore, theoretically, it is the most important antioxidant in preventing oxidation of these fatty acids. Vitamin E is recycled by a reaction with vitamin C. Despite the actions of antioxidant nutrients, oxidative damage occurs inevitably over time in most cells, and accumulation of this damage throughout life is believed to be a major contributing factor to aging and chronic diseases including cancer.

ANTIOXIDANT MECHANISMS

Antioxidants respond to oxidant conditions, and oxidative stress is the most frequently used term to describe the oxidant–antioxidant interaction. As noted earlier in this chapter, ROS and RNS are unavoidably and continuously produced under normal metabolic conditions. ROS/RNS can directly modify DNA, lipids, and proteins, which results in mutations, strand breaks, aldehyde formation, low-density lipoprotein (LDL) oxidation, and alterations in enzyme activities and signal transduction pathways. To minimize these deleterious effects, aerobic organisms have evolved elaborate antioxidant systems, which consist of low-molecular-weight antioxidants and antioxidant enzymes. In some pathological conditions, such as acute or relapsing inflammation or ischemia-reperfusion injury, there is a transient overproduction of ROS/RNS. Under these conditions, the oxidant–antioxidant balance is lost and tissues are exposed to oxidative stress. In such cases, supplementation with antioxidants may be beneficial because they can neutralize the toxic effects of ROS/RNS. The major mechanisms of antioxidant activity in biological systems are shown in Table 1.

TABLE 1 Antioxidant Mechanisms

Activity	Antioxidant effect
Metal chelation	Prevents free radical formation
Free radical scavengers	Removes reactive oxygen/nitrogen species
*Electron and/or proton donors	Chain-breaking, stops free radical propagation *Prevents or delays oxidation of oxidizable substrates
Phase 2 enzyme Induction (e.g., by bioflavonoids, curcumin, sulforaphanes)	Enhances defenses, accelerates oxidant detoxification/excretion
Decrease oxidant burden	Alter genome/proteome expression via pathway selection—"enzyme evolution"

It should be emphasized that ROS/RNS are not merely toxic molecules but are critically involved in normal metabolism, especially in intercellular and intracellular signaling. In these conditions, inadequate antioxidant substances could be deleterious to the overall function of the organism, altering the normal signaling function of ROS/RNS. ROS can act as second messengers. In general, protein kinases are activated by oxidation reactions, whereas protein phosphatases and zinc-finger proteins are inactivated by oxidation reactions, and transcription factor binding is increased by reduction reactions.

Oxidative Stress

Oxidative stress is associated with most pathological disorders and arises from an imbalance between oxidants and antioxidants, which changes the redox status and increases the susceptibility for oxidative damage to cell structure and function.

The interaction of diet and the antioxidant system is complex, and disposal of oxidants and other hazardous natural or xenobiotic compounds is rendered more efficient/less toxic by induction of various phase 2 systems by dietary components (Figure 1). Talalay et al. (2000) have suggested that the definition of phase 2 enzymes be expanded to encompass those proteins with the following characteristics in common: (a) coordinate induction by chemicals reactive with sulfhydryl groups; (b) possess common promoter elements; and (c) reactions are catalyzed with electrophiles and reactive oxygen to produce less toxic products.

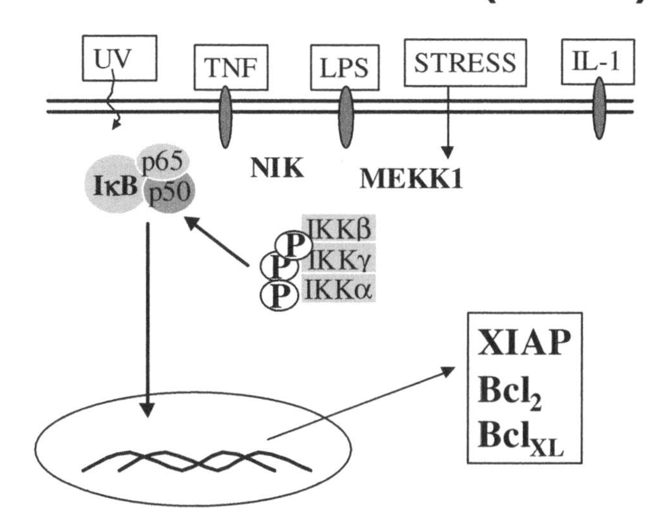

FIGURE 1 Nuclear factor-κB (NFκB) intracellular activation occurs as the result of oxidant stress or activation by ultraviolet light, cytokines, and growth factors. The NFκB p65/p50 dimer is released from its binding protein I κB following its phosphorylation by IKKb, which occurs as part of the signal cascade. The NFκB dimer travels to the nucleus, where it results in the production of numerous mediators of inflammation and when constitutively expressed in antiapoptotic proteins XIAP, Bcl_2, and Bcl_{XL}.

Oxidative Stress, Inflammation, and Cancer in Carcinogenesis

The relationship of oxidants, inflammation, and cancer has been the subject of intense scrutiny (Balkwill and Mantovani, 2001; Aggarwal, 2004). An imbalance among the presence of oxidized and reduced compounds and components (i.e., metabolic oxidative stress) has been linked to a wide variety of degenerative diseases associated with aging, inflammatory diseases, and cancer. In fact, the realization that radicals are a likely link between inflammation and cancer has a long history. More than two millennia ago, Galen first suggested that there was a causal relationship between inflammation and cancer. In the nineteenth century, Virchow revealed the presence of leukocytes in malignant tissues and hypothesized that tumors arose in regions of chronic inflammation. In fact, it is well known that the areas in and around tumors are filled with ROS, proinflammatory cytokines, and chemokines, such as tumor necrosis factor (TNF), interleukin (IL)-1, IL-6, and IL-8, as well as matrix-degrading enzymes and growth factors. These factors often work through nuclear factor-κB (NFκB) so-called by its discoverer, Dr. David Baltimore, because it was a nuclear-binding protein that stimulated kappa-chain transcription in B lymphocytes. It has since been found to be a commonly used pathway for inflammation triggered by oxidant stress, cytokines, and growth factors (Figure 1).

A pro-oxidative state is thought to lead to DNA damage, which can lead to excessive cellular proliferation, cell migration, and angiogenesis with tumor growth. ROS/RNS can also cause DNA damage, which can cause: (1) modification of DNA bases and/or deoxyribose chains, producing mutations, deletions, strand breaks, and gross chromosomal alterations (Cerutti, 1985); (2) inhibition of the DNA repair systems, again producing mutations, deletions, strand breaks, and gross chromosomal alterations; and (3) alterations in cell signaling. The alteration of cell signaling by ROS/RNS can occur through modification of receptors, transcription factors, protein kinases/phosphatases, and calcium homeostasis, which results in genome responses manifested by altered cell growth, differentiation, and apoptosis.

Moreover, there is now convincing evidence that ROS are not merely toxic consequences of cellular metabolism but substances that at low levels are essential to cell signaling and regulation (Figure 2). ROS are implicated in many intracellular signaling pathways leading to changes in gene transcription and protein synthesis and consequently in cell function (Griendling et al., 2000; Reth, 2002; Chiarugi and Cirri, 2003) (Figure 3). Therefore, it is quite plausible that ROS/RNS are involved in the key steps of cancer development.

Nelson et al. (2003) (Figure 4) have made a compelling argument for the involvement of free radicals and inflammation in the development of prostate cancer on the basis of pathological observations in prostate biopsies of the proximity of the premalignant stages of proliferative inflammatory atrophy and prostatic intraepithelial neoplasia to areas of prostatic carcinoma *in situ*.

Although the evidence linking the presence of ROS/RNS to carcinogenesis is considerable, this evidence is based mostly on associations and few studies have directly tested this link. The relationship between radicals/inflammation and cancer has been directly studied by Greten et al. (2004) in a mouse model of colitis-associated cancer. The NFκB signaling system was targeted because its activity is linked to oxidative processes and the NFκB signaling cascade system itself is triggered in response to infectious agents,

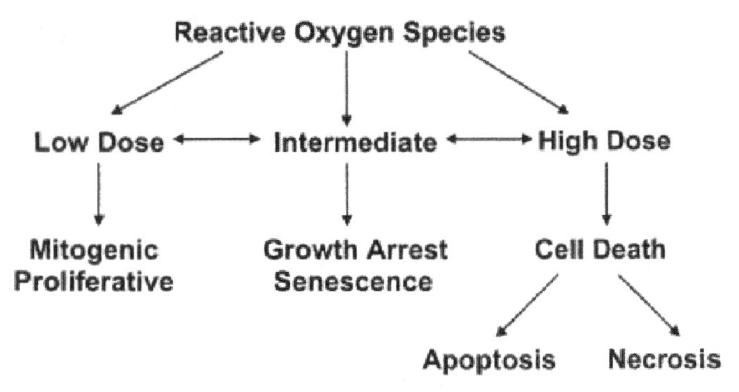

FIGURE 2 At low doses, reactive oxygen species (ROS) stimulate cell proliferation. At intermediate doses, they cause growth arrest of cells or senescence, and at high doses, they cause cell death with associated apoptosis and necrosis.

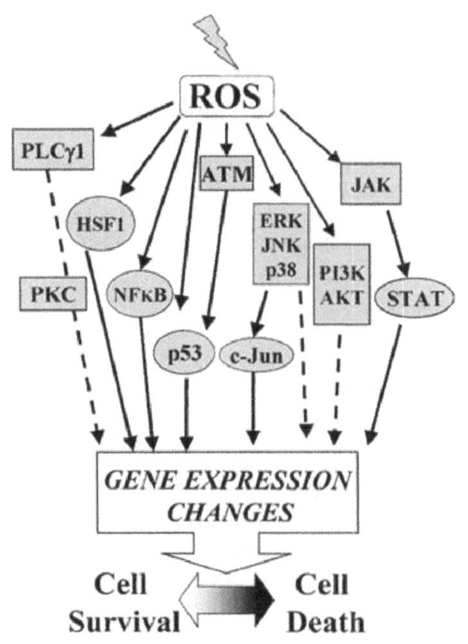

FIGURE 3 In addition to stimulating nuclear factor-κB (NFκB), many other cell signaling pathways can be activated by reactive oxygen species (ROS). As shown, the balance of these can determine cell survival or alternatively stimulate cell death. Failure to proceed normally to cell death is a characteristic of cancer cells, which have mutations in many of these pathways.

proinflammatory cytokines, and colitis-associated cancer (Viatour et al., 2005). In mice with a deletion of IKKbeta—a mediator of the NFκB response to infectious agents and proinflammatory cytokines specifically in intestinal epithelial cells—the absence of the NFκB response due to the loss of IKKbeta leads to a dramatic decrease in tumor incidence without affecting tumor size or tissue inflammation. The decline in tumor incidence was attributed to increased epithelial apoptosis during tumor promotion, reducing the number of cells available for progression to tumors. This effect is consistent with the known role of IKKbeta in the prevention of apoptosis. Thus, IKKbeta deletion in enterocytes tipped the balance between cell survival or apoptosis after damage but did not affect the cells that did survive to become cancerous.

A parallel experiment, using mice that were engineered to specifically delete IKKbeta in the myeloid cells, provided additional evidence. Myeloid cells are responsible for identifying and eliminating tumor cells by producing inflammation. In these mice, deletion of the myeloid IKKbeta produced a significant decrease in tumor size while having no effect on tumor incidence. This was attributed to the diminished expression of proinflammatory cytokines, which function in many cases as trophic factors for tumors.

The observations in these two studies support the notion that oxidation and inflammation play a role in cancer because the IKKbeta deletion led to changes both in enterocytes, which were the target tissues, and on the immune system cells. Therefore, the effects of both oxidation and inflammation are directed at cells and act indirectly via the immune system.

A number of studies conducted in systems examining other disease states support this notion of oxidation and chronic inflammation including hepatitis, gastritis, cystitis, and pancreatitis. All of these conditions are also associated with high incidence of subsequent cancer (Parsonnet, 1997). In these disease conditions, ROS/RNS are continuously produced by phagocytes and likely cause DNA damage. High 8-OHdG levels, markers of DNA oxidative damage, have been found in liver tissue of chronic hepatitis patients (Shimoda et al., 1994), gastric mucosa of *Helicobacter pylori*–infected patients (Baik et al., 1996), and colonic mucosa of patients with inflammatory bowel disease (Wiseman and Halliwell, 1996). The relationship between ROS, inflammation, and cancer is further supported by the association observed between increased body iron stores and increased cancer risk (Toyokuni, 1996). Hemochromatosis patients have high plasma levels of catalytic iron (Grootveld et al., 1989), hepatic DNA damage, and malondialdehyde (MDA)-protein adducts (Carmichael et al., 1995; Houglum et al., 1997) and liver cancer risk >200 times that of the normal population (Niederau et al., 1985). These findings have been replicated in animal studies. For example, a renal cell carcinoma can be induced by multiple injections of an iron complex iron–nitrilotriacetate (Fe-NTA) in A/J mice and Wistar rats (Omenn et al., 1996). Not only do these animals develop cancer but also they demonstrate the elevations in the markers of oxidative damage, such as protein modification by aldehydes (Toyokuni et al., 1994), DNA base modification (Yamaguchi et al., 1996), and strand breakage (Kawabata et al., 1997). Another experimental model of carcinogenesis, the Long-Evans Cinnamon (LEC) rat, has a defect in the expression of a copper-transporting ATPase (Yamaguchi et al., 1994) and therefore accumulates

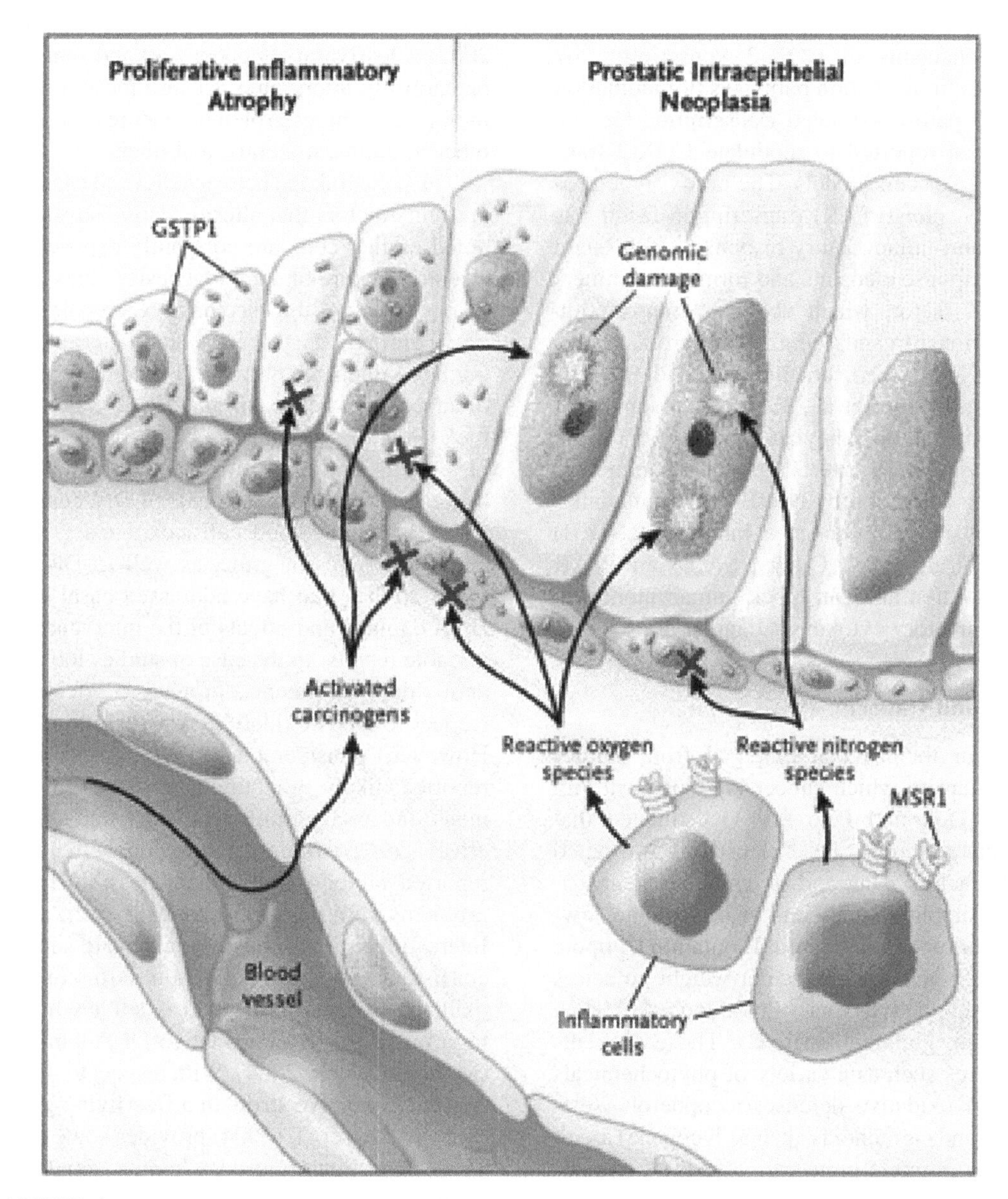

FIGURE 4 Potential role of reactive oxygen species and reactive nitrogen species in prostatic carcinogenesis (from Nelson et al., 2003).

excess copper and iron and spontaneously develops necrotizing hepatitis and hepatocellular carcinoma. Finally, it has been demonstrated that monkey kidney cells can be transformed as the result of stable transfection with hydrogen peroxide–generating rat urate oxidase stimulated by a constitutively active human peroxisomal fatty acylcoenzyme A (acyl-CoA) oxidase gene promoter. The monkey kidney cells transformed in this way demonstrated anchorage-independent growth in cell culture and were able to form adenocarcinomas in nude mice (Chu et al., 1996).

The relationship of inflammation and oxidation to cancer can be demonstrated to be mediated in some systems by cyclooxygenase-2 (COX-2) (O'Leary et al., 2004). COX-2 is induced significantly during inflammation, increased COX-2 levels are found in many colorectal and gastric tumors, and overexpression of COX-2 has been implicated in the pathogenesis of cancer (Eberhart et al., 1994; Ristimaki et al., 1997; Fujita et al., 1998). By their interaction with a number of the oxidant species implicated in inflammation, antioxidants, such as vitamin E and flavonoids, have been studied with respect to their effects on COX-2 or on the formation of arachidonic acid–derived proinflammatory eicosanoids. Vitamin E, with the different stereo-isomers, exhibits different potencies and has been shown to inhibit COX-2 activity in several model systems (Wu et al., 1998, 2000). In addition to directly affecting

COX-2, antioxidants can potentially interfere with COX-2–related mechanisms of COX-2 transcription by interfering with signal transduction pathways or modulation of the inflammatory pathway–related transcription factors. Flavonoids have been reported to modulate COX-2 transcription in a number of cell models. The peroxisome proliferator-activated receptor (PPAR) transcription factor has been implicated in anti-inflammatory responses. PPARs are bound by specific response elements and form heterodimers with the retinoid X factor, which activates transcription in response to various ligands (e.g., nonsteroidal anti-inflammatory drugs (NSAIDs), arachidonic acid metabolites, and some drugs (Keller et al., 1993; Lehmann et al., 1995, 1997). Aspirin, sodium salicylate, and indomethacin, known collectively as *NSAIDs*, exert their anti-inflammatory effects by preventing activation by NFκB of the inflammatory response genes by inhibiting the inhibitor B (IKB) kinase IKK-β (Yin et al., 1998). Other NSAIDs are PPAR ligands such as ibuprofen and can block human monocyte production of inflammatory cytokines (Jiang et al., 1998).

Antioxidant Diets and Cancer

One of the major themes that emerged from studies on cancer is the extent to which cancer is associated with diet and nutrition. Doll and Peto (1981) estimated that ~35% of all cancers could be "plausibly" attributed to dietary/lifestyle factors. Diet and its associated antioxidants include diet-supplied lipid- and water-soluble low-molecular-weight antioxidants (vitamin E, vitamin C, lipoic acid, β-carotene, etc.) and low-molecular-weight cofactors derived from diet-supplied factors (glutathione, NADPH, pyruvate, thioredoxin, glutaredoxin, etc.). Those nutrients and other nonnutrients such as a variety of phytochemicals that are involved in oxidative defense (tocopherols, selenium, polyphenols, and carotenoids such as lycopene) are of current interest. The possible protective effects of antioxidants in food against cancer have been extensively studied, and most studies found statistically significant protective effects from fruit and vegetables, the major source of dietary micronutrients, antioxidants, and inducers of phase 2 proteins against cancer of the lung, esophagus, oral cavity, larynx, stomach, pancreas, colorectal, and bladder (Block et al., 1992). The results of many epidemiological studies consistently show an association of increased cancer risk with low amounts of dietary β-carotene or low plasma β-carotene concentrations (van Poppel, 1995). Ascorbic acid (Block, 1991) and vitamin E (Kline et al., 2004) are also found to be inversely correlated with cancer risk. Both experimental and epidemiological data indicate that vitamin C protects against stomach cancer and esophageal adenocarcinoma (Kono and Hirohata, 1996; Mayne et al., 2001). This conclusion again links cancer and inflammation because oxidative damage from inflammation caused by *H. pylori* infection is a risk factor for stomach cancer (Zhang et al., 2002). Clearly the effects of fruit and vegetables should also be carefully interpreted because these diets are often lower in fat and cholesterol and contain, besides antioxidants, other vitamins, minerals, and fiber.

Thus, the linkage between diet and cancer resides in those nutrients/factors that alter oxidative stress/inflammation. As noted earlier, cells are constantly exposed to oxidants, and a central feature of carcinogenesis is the occurrence of DNA damage, which suggests that DNA repair systems and nutritional antioxidants are important determinants for maintaining DNA damage at low levels and thereby reducing the risk of cancer. Studies examining these systems have monitored the effects of single antioxidants, as well as various vegetables, fruits, and carotenoid- and polyphenolic-rich products using a variety of assessments of DNA damage, such as that found in white blood cells, oxidized DNA-derived bases, and nucleosides in urine, as well as DNA-repair capacity. Other studies that have addressed basal levels of oxidative DNA damage and effects of the interventions have reported variable results. In the case of studies looking at single-dose antioxidant treatments, protective effects were seen with respect to DNA oxidation as assessed in white blood cells. However, considerable variability in results has been reported, likely reflecting differences in populations, regimens, and assays employed. Other studies designed to assess effects of continuous antioxidant treatments have also reported mixed results, again possibly because of various problems with design, statistical power, and period effects. Interestingly, studies using only male subjects have shown consistent antioxidant effects in terms of reduced levels of oxidized pyrimidines, whereas studies in populations with high initial levels of oxidative DNA damage are equivocal (Moller and Loft, 2004). With respect to the linkage between diet and oxidative stress in a free-living population, a study by Smolkova et al. (2004) provides some interesting insight. These investigators used a human population and selected a model that takes advantage of variations over time to provide strong evidence for the connection between diet and oxidative stress. The high incidence in Central/Eastern European countries of diseases connected to inflammation (i.e., cardiovascular disease and certain cancers) was examined and studies assessed whether nutritional imbalances due to a lack of fresh fruit and vegetables in the diet in winter months might produce a seasonally dependent inflammation. The study monitored dietary intake and markers of oxidative stress in urban normolipemics, subjects with heart disease, and a rural control group with minimal swings in dietary intake over a cycle of seasons spanning times of minimum and maximum local availability of fresh fruits and vegetables. Oxidative stress was assessed using plasma MDA (a product of lipid peroxidation) and other antioxidant-related measures (i.e., dietary antioxidants, serum folic acid, homocysteine, total antioxidant status [FRAP], and uric acid). Vegetable consumption in summer/autumn was twice as high as it was in winter/spring, and mean plasma MDA levels for the myocardial infarction (MI) and healthy normolipidemic (NL) groups tracked this pattern, showing high levels in winter/spring and low levels in summer/autumn, whereas the rural control group showed neither the seasonal swings in vegetable consumption nor the fluctuations in MDA levels. Interestingly, the study data showed that high winter MDA levels were seen only in those subjects with relatively low folic acid, suggesting that folic acid might be involved in protection against lipid oxidation.

Other studies have probed the relation between flavonoid intake and subsequent cancer risk among Finnish subjects. An inverse association was observed between the intake of flavonoids and incidence of all sites of cancer combined. The results suggest that flavonoid intake in some circumstances may be involved in the cancer process, resulting in lowered risks (Knekt et al., 1997). This study, and others, provides evidence of the strong link between diet and cancer and suggests that dietary approaches that seek to alter the processes that characterize carcinogenesis are likely to be very important in limiting and reducing cancer. As an example of this potential, Simopoulos (2004) enumerated studies that show that traditional Greek diet is associated with rates of cancer and heart disease lower than any other diet or drug intervention. It was suggested that there are specific features that render the Greek diet so special even relative to other Mediterranean diets; that is, the Greek diet is characterized by an elevated content of bioprotective nutrients, specifically (1) a more balanced intake of EFAs from vegetable, animal, and marine sources; a ratio of n-6 to n-3 fatty acids of 2:1 instead of the 15:1 found in Western and Northern Europe diets and 16.74:1 in the United States; and (2) a diet rich in antioxidants (i.e., high amounts of vitamin C, vitamin E, β-carotene, glutathione, resveratrol, selenium, phytoestrogens, folate, and other phytochemicals from green leafy vegetables); phenolic compounds from wine and olive oil; high intakes of tomatoes, onions, garlic, and herbs, especially oregano, mint, rosemary, parsley, and dill, which contain lycopene and other carotenoids, allyl thiosulfinates, salicylates, indoles, monoterpenes, polyphenols, flavonoids, and other phytochemicals used in cooking vegetables, meat, and fish.

However, although there is overwhelming evidence that fruit and vegetables are protective against most cancers and that effects on oxidation represent a major mechanism, our understanding of all the mechanisms responsible is clearly incomplete. This is put into graphic relief by the almost uniformly disappointing results found in intervention studies that attempted to decrease cancer incidence by supplementation with antioxidants. The daily administration of the combination β-carotene and vitamin A against placebo in 18,314 subjects at high risk of developing lung cancer (i.e., smokers) showed clear evidence of no benefit and substantial evidence of possible harm, in which there were 28% more lung cancers and 17% more deaths in the active intervention group (Omenn et al., 1996). Similar results were obtained in a trial in which the effects of α-tocopherol and β-carotene supplementation on the incidence of lung cancer were studied in heavy smokers. No overall effect was observed for lung cancer following α-tocopherol supplementation, but β-carotene supplementation was associated with increased lung cancer risk (Albanes et al., 1996). Another clinical trial to test the efficacy of β-carotene and vitamins C and E in preventing colorectal adenoma failed to show any evidence that either β-carotene or vitamins C and E reduced the incidence of adenomas (Greenberg et al., 1994). Evidence that antioxidant supplementation improves plasma antioxidant levels or oxidative damage markers is also limited. A study using 2 months of supplementation with vitamin E, ascorbic acid, or coenzyme Q10 did not result in significant changes in the urinary excretion rate of 8-oxodG (Prieme et al., 1997), whereas supplementation for 20 weeks with vitamin C, vitamin E, and β-carotene resulted in a significant decrease in endogenous oxidative base damage in lymphocyte DNA (Duthie et al., 1996). Another study that also demonstrates our lack of understanding is illustrated by the results reported by Dragsted et al. (2004). The study examined the effects of fruit and vegetables on markers of oxidative stress and antioxidative defense in healthy nonsmokers. Their conclusions were that fruit and vegetable consumption increased plasma lipid oxidation lag times and did so more than a supplement containing comparable levels of several known antioxidants. However, other markers of oxidative damage, oxidative capacity, or antioxidant defense were largely unaffected. The authors suggested that the complex interactions observed in their study cannot be explained by a general antioxidant hypothesis of chronic disease prevention. Crucially, the effect of antioxidants when analyzed in terms of a class of compounds does not predict and therefore does not address the fact that different biomarkers used to assess oxidative damage in lipids, proteins, and DNA are in general not well correlated. The authors suggest that redox processes leading to oxidative damage are tightly regulated and localized to specific molecular targets. Another potential reason is that vitamins C and E, β-carotene, and other compounds may also have other direct or indirect biological activities that are not oxidant related but nevertheless are still related to their cancer-preventive properties. They may stimulate immune function, inhibit nitrosamine formation, or enhance cell communication (Traber and Packer 1995; Zhang et al., 2002; Sylvester and Shah 2005). Moreover, oxidants are not merely harmful molecules but have important signaling functions, as discussed earlier. Therefore, it is plausible that inadequate administration of antioxidants may have adverse effects on life.

CONCLUSION

The body's susceptibility to oxidant damage is thought to depend on the balance between the extent of pro-oxidant stress and the antioxidant levels of body tissues. Most antioxidants have large numbers of alternating double bonds that can act as electron traps. In some cases, this quenching reaction can lead to increased oxidation. This occurs when a polyunsaturated fat neutralizes an oxygen radical but becomes a fatty acid radical, which then attacks another lipid leading to a chain reaction. Other antioxidants can also act as pro-oxidants after quenching an oxygen radical. On balance, a number of studies have shown that various antioxidants act as a cooperative system of antioxidant defense. Vitamin C quenches free radicals in aqueous systems and regenerates cellular vitamin E, which helps to control lipid peroxidation. β-Carotene also traps free radicals in concert with vitamin E. The selenium-containing enzyme glutathione peroxidase destroys peroxides before they can damage cell membranes and interacts synergistically with vitamin E. In a number of animal studies, the administration of antioxidants ameliorated damage from experimental oxidant stress. Furthermore, the antioxidant requirement in these studies was directly proportional to the increased tissue concentrations of free radicals. Though not proven, promotion of antioxidation through consumption of antioxidant-rich fruits and vegetables and dietary supplements is a habit many Americans consider health enhancing.

The causative roles of ROS/RNS-mediated oxidation is strongly associated with the pathogenesis of certain forms of cancer, such as radiation-induced, chronic inflammation–associated, and metal overload–associated cancers. In all of these conditions, persistent or recurrent overproduction of ROS/RNS is expected, and elevated levels of oxidatively damaged products have been identified. Nevertheless, a more detailed role of ROS/RNS in carcinogenesis has yet to be established definitively. The importance of ROS/RNS production is less clear in sporadic cancers. Therefore, more research is necessary to determine the mechanisms through which ROS/RNS promote carcinogenesis at a cellular and molecular level. Understanding the exact role of ROS/RNS, as well as associated pathogenic factors, may enable the design of novel nutritional strategies for cancer prevention based on enhancing cellular antioxidant defense mechanisms or reducing oxidant production to prevent common forms of cancer associated with oxidant stress.

On the basis of population studies and animal studies, a number of governmental agencies including the National Research Council, the National Cancer Institute, and the U.S. Department of Agriculture have recommended that Americans eat at least five servings a day of fruits and vegetables in part to increase the intake of beneficial antioxidants. Surveys indicate that only a small fraction of the general population follows this advice, leading some nutrition authorities to recommend dietary supplementation or food fortification with antioxidants to reduce chronic disease incidence. Although there remains some uncertainty about the long-term effects of antioxidant supplementation, there is accumulating evidence that the practice of dietary supplementation may be beneficial.

References

Aggarwal, B.B. 2004. Nuclear factor-kappaB: the enemy within. *Cancer Cell* **6**: 203–208.

Albanes, D., Heinonen, O.P., et al. 1996. Alpha-Tocopherol and beta-carotene supplements and lung cancer incidence in the alpha-tocopherol, beta-carotene cancer prevention study: effects of base-line characteristics and study compliance. *Natl Cancer Inst* **88**: 1560–1570.

Baik, S.C., Youn H.S., et al. 1996. Increased oxidative DNA damage in *Helicobacter pylori*–infected human gastric mucosa. *Cancer Res* **56**: 1279–1282.

Balkwill, F., and Mantovani, A. 2001. Inflammation and cancer: back to Virchow? *Lancet* **357**: 539–545.

Block, G. 1991. Vitamin C and cancer prevention: the epidemiologic evidence. *Am J Clin Nutr* **53**(1 Suppl): 270S–282S.

Block, G., Patterson, B., et al. 1992. Fruit, vegetables, and cancer prevention: a review of the epidemiological evidence. *Nutr Cancer* **18**: 1–29.

Carmichael, P., Hewer, A., et al. 1995. Detection of bulky DNA lesions in the liver of patients with Wilson's disease and primary haemochromatosis. *Mutat Res* **326**: 235–243.

Cerutti, P.A. 1985. Prooxidant states and tumor promotion. *Science* **227**: 375–381.

Chiarugi, P., and Cirri, P. 2003. Redox regulation of protein tyrosine phosphatases during receptor tyrosine kinase signal transduction. *Trends Biochem Sci* **28**: 509–514.

Chu, R., Li., et al. 1996. Transformation of epithelial cells stably transfected with H_2O_2-generating peroxisomal urate oxidase. *Cancer Res* **56**: 4846–4852.

Doll, R., and Peto, R. 1981. The causes of cancer: quantitative estimates of avoidable risks of cancer in the United States today. *J Natl Cancer Inst* **66**: 1191–1308.

Dragsted, L.O., Pedersen, A., et al. 2004. The 6-a-day study: effects of fruit and vegetables on markers of oxidative stress and antioxidative defense in healthy nonsmokers. *Am J Clin Nutr* **79**: 1060–1072.

Duthie, S.J., Ma, A., et al. 1996. Antioxidant supplementation decreases oxidative DNA damage in human lymphocytes. *Cancer Res* **56**: 1291–1295.

Eberhart, C.E., Coffey, R.J., et al. 1994. Up-regulation of cyclooxygenase 2 gene expression in human colorectal adenomas and adenocarcinomas. *Gastroenterology* **107**: 1183–1188.

Fujita, T., Matsui, M., et al. 1998. Size- and invasion-dependent increase in cyclooxygenase 2 levels in human colorectal carcinomas. *Cancer Res* **58**: 4823–4826.

Greenberg, E.R., Baron, J.A., et al. 1994. A clinical trial of antioxidant vitamins to prevent colorectal adenoma. Polyp Prevention Study Group. *N Engl J Med* **331**: 141–147.

Greten, F.R., Eckmann, L., et al. 2004. IKKbeta links inflammation and tumorigenesis in a mouse model of colitis-associated cancer. *Cell* **118**: 285–2896.

Griendling, K.K., Sorescu, D., et al. 2000. Modulation of protein kinase activity and gene expression by reactive oxygen species and their role in vascular physiology and pathophysiology. *Arterioscler Thromb Vasc Biol* **20**: 2175–2183.

Grootveld, M., Bell, J.D., et al. 1989. Non–transferrin-bound iron in plasma or serum from patients with idiopathic hemochromatosis. Characterization by high performance liquid chromatography and nuclear magnetic resonance spectroscopy. *J Biol Chem* **264**: 4417–4422.

Houglum, K., Ramm, G.A., et al. 1997. Excess iron induces hepatic oxidative stress and transforming growth factor beta1 in genetic hemochromatosis. *Hepatology* **26**: 605–610.

Jiang, C., Ting, A.T., et al. 1998. PPAR-gamma agonists inhibit production of monocyte inflammatory cytokines. *Nature* **391**: 82–86.

Kawabata, T., Ma, Y., et al. 1997. Iron-induced apoptosis in mouse renal proximal tubules after an injection of a renal carcinogen, iron-nitrilotriacetate. *Carcinogenesis* **18**: 1389–1394.

Keller, H., Dreyer, C., et al. 1993. Fatty acids and retinoids control lipid metabolism through activation of peroxisome proliferator-activated receptor–retinoid X receptor heterodimers. *Proc Natl Acad Sci USA* **90**: 2160–2164.

Kline, K., Yu, W., et al. 2004. Vitamin E and breast cancer. *J Nutr* **134**(12 Suppl): 3458S–3462S.

Knekt, P., Jarvinen, R., et al. 1997. Dietary flavonoids and the risk of lung cancer and other malignant neoplasms. *Am J Epidemiol* **146**: 223–230.

Kono, S., and Hirohata, T. 1996. Nutrition and stomach cancer. *Cancer Causes Control* **7**: 41–55.

Lehmann, J.M., Lenhard, J.M., et al. 1997. Peroxisome proliferator-activated receptors alpha and gamma are activated by indomethacin and other non-steroidal anti-inflammatory drugs. *J Biol Chem* **272**: 3406–3410.

Lehmann, J.M., Moore, L.B., et al. 1995. An antidiabetic thiazolidinedione is a high affinity ligand for peroxisome proliferator-activated receptor gamma (PPAR gamma). *J Biol Chem* **270**: 12953–12956.

Mayne, S.T., Risch, H.A., et al. 2001. Nutrient intake and risk of subtypes of esophageal and gastric cancer. *Cancer Epidemiol Biomarkers Prev* **10**: 1055–1062.

Moller, P., and Loft, S. 2004. Interventions with antioxidants and nutrients in relation to oxidative DNA damage and repair. *Mutat Res* **551**: 79–89.

Nelson W.G., et al. 2003. Prostate Cancer. *New Engl J Med* **349**: 366–381.

Niederau, C., Fischer, R., et al. 1985. Survival and causes of death in cirrhotic and in noncirrhotic patients with primary hemochromatosis. *N Engl J Med* **313**: 1256–1262.

O'Leary, K.A., de Pascual-Tereasa, S., et al. 2004. Effect of flavonoids and vitamin E on cyclooxygenase-2 (COX-2) transcription. *Mutat Res* **551**: 245–254.

Omenn, G.S., Goodman, G.E., et al. 1996. Effects of a combination of beta carotene and vitamin A on lung cancer and cardiovascular disease. *N Engl J Med* **334**: 1150–1155.

Parsonnet, J. 1997. Molecular mechanisms for inflammation-promoted pathogenesis of cancer—The Sixteenth International Symposium of the Sapporo Cancer Seminar. *Cancer Res* **57**: 3620–3624.

Prieme, H., Loft, S., et al. 1997. No effect of supplementation with vitamin E, ascorbic acid, or coenzyme Q10 on oxidative DNA damage estimated by 8-oxo-7,8-dihydro-2′-deoxyguanosine excretion in smokers. *Am J Clin Nutr* **65**: 503–507.

Reth, M. 2002. Hydrogen peroxide as second messenger in lymphocyte activation. *Nat Immunol* **3**: 1129–1134.

Ristimaki, A., Honkanen, N., et al. 1997. Expression of cyclooxygenase-2 in human gastric carcinoma. *Cancer Res* **57**: 1276–1280.

Shimoda, R., Nagashima, M., et al. 1994. Increased formation of oxidative DNA damage, 8-hydroxydeoxyguanosine, in human livers with chronic hepatitis. *Cancer Res* **54**: 3171–3172.

Simopoulos, A.P. 2004. The traditional diet of Greece and cancer. *Eur J Cancer Prev* **13**: 219–230.

Smolkova, B., Dusinska, M., et al. 2004. Seasonal changes in markers of oxidative damage to lipids and DNA; correlations with seasonal variation in diet. *Mutat Res* **551**: 135–144.

Stanner, S.A., Hughes, J., et al. 2004. A review of the epidemiological evidence for the "antioxidant hypothesis". *Public Health Nutr* **7**: 407–422.

Sylvester, P.W., and Shah, S.J. 2005. Mechanisms mediating the antiproliferative and apoptotic effects of vitamin E in mammary cancer cells. *Front Biosci* **10**: 699–709.

Talalay, P. 2000. Chemoprotection against cancer by induction of phase 2 enzymes. *Biofactors* **12**: 5–11.

Toyokuni, S. 1996. Iron-induced carcinogenesis: the role of redox regulation. *Free Radic Biol Med* **20**: 553–566.

Toyokuni, S., Uchida, K., et al. 1994. Formation of 4-hydroxy-2-nonenal-modified proteins in the renal proximal tubules of rats treated with a renal carcinogen, ferric nitrilotriacetate. *Proc Natl Acad Sci USA* **91**: 2616–2620.

Traber, M.G., and Packer, L. 1995. Vitamin E: beyond antioxidant function. *Am J Clin Nutr* **62**: 1501S–1509S.

van Poppel, G., and Goldbohm, R.A. 1995. Epidemiologic evidence for beta-carotene and cancer prevention. *Am J Clin Nutr* **62**: 1393S–1402S.

Viatour, P., Merville, M.P., et al. 2005. Phosphorylation of NF-kappaB and IkappaB proteins: implications in cancer and inflammation. *Trends Biochem Sci* **30**: 43–52.

Willcox, J.K., Ash, S.L., et al. 2004. Antioxidants and prevention of chronic disease. *Crit Rev Food Sci Nutr* **44**: 275–295.

Wiseman, H., and Halliwell, B. 1996. Damage to DNA by reactive oxygen and nitrogen species: role in inflammatory disease and progression to cancer. *Biochem J* **313**(Pt 1): 17–29.

Wu, D., Meydani, M., et al. 2000. *In vitro* supplementation with different tocopherol homologues can affect the function of immune cells in old mice. *Free Radic Biol Med* **28**: 643–651.

Wu, D., Mura, C., et al. 1998. Age-associated increase in PGE2 synthesis and COX activity in murine macrophages is reversed by vitamin E. *Am J Physiol* **275**(3 Pt 1): C661–C668.

Yamaguchi, R., Hirano, T., et al. 1996. Increased 8-hydroxyguanine levels in DNA and its repair activity in rat kidney after administration of a renal carcinogen, ferric nitrilotriacetate. *Carcinogenesis* **17**: 2419–2422.

Yamaguchi, Y., Heiny, M.E., et al. 1994. Expression of the Wilson disease gene is deficient in the Long-Evans Cinnamon rat. *Biochem J* **301** (Pt 1): 1–4.

Yin, M.J., Yamamoto, Y., et al. 1998. The anti-inflammatory agents aspirin and salicylate inhibit the activity of I(kappa)B kinase-beta. *Nature* **396**: 77–80.

Zhang, Z.W., Abdullahi, M., et al. 2002. Effect of physiological concentrations of vitamin C on gastric cancer cells and *Helicobacter pylori*. *Gut* **50**: 165–169.

CHAPTER

15

Thiols in Cancer

JASON M. HANSEN AND DEAN P. JONES

INTRODUCTION

Thiols have two central roles in cancer biology, one in cancer chemoprevention and the other in cell growth control and cell survival signaling. The former is a well-developed research field from which clear principles have emerged. Most significant among these are the need to maintain an adequate sulfur amino acid intake as a precursor for glutathione (GSH) and good dietary sources of phytochemicals that induce GSH synthesis to aid in elimination of mutagenic chemicals and prevent early steps in chemical carcinogenesis. Additional research is necessary concerning optimal thiol nutrition during cancer therapy because these same nutritional strategies to improve the GSH system can also enhance tumor resistance to radiation and some chemotherapies and promote cell division. Excess sulfur amino acid intake may also pose a risk because of generation of reactive sulfur compounds by colonic flora, but this area has had little investigation.

An understanding of the role of thiols in growth control and cell survival signaling is rapidly developing as a second area of critical importance in nutrition and cancer; clear principles are not yet defined concerning optimized nutritional strategies to maintain normal tissue health without providing a growth advantage to precancerous and cancerous cells. Multiple redox-dependent steps exist in growth control pathways, with both reactive oxygen species (ROS) and thiol compounds promoting growth and cell survival. Because thiol compounds can block ROS signaling and ROS can deplete thiols, no simple conclusions can be made concerning potential benefits or risks from thiol-related components of the diet. Mechanistic studies of dietary effects on redox control and signaling can be expected to clarify the roles of thiols in growth control.

This chapter provides an overview of the roles of thiols in preventing early events of oncogenesis and in growth control in precancerous and cancer tissues. The main dietary and supplemental sources of sulfur amino acids, their conversion to GSH, and other dietary factors affecting GSH homeostasis are provided. Finally, critical questions concerning sulfur amino acid nutrition for support of GSH-dependent detoxification systems and thiol/disulfide redox control are identified with the long-term goal of being able to optimize recommendations for individuals concerning thiol nutrition in cancer prevention and treatment.

SULFUR HAS MULTIPLE BIOLOGICAL ROLES AFFECTING CANCER

Sulfur exists stably in multiple oxidation states, which makes it a versatile component in biological systems. The most highly active and most reduced form of sulfur in biomolecules is the thiol (-SH), present in the amino acid cysteine (Cys). Cys is present in the active site of many proteins and in protein motifs that function in enzyme regulation, protein trafficking, control of gene expression, and receptor signaling. Cys is primarily obtained through dietary protein or through the transsulfuration of the essential dietary amino acid methionine (Met).

Reversible oxidations of sulfur residues are common and fundamentally important in control of cell functions (Gulati et al., 2001; Moran et al., 2001; Dickinson and Forman 2002; Nakashima et al., 2002). Principal regulation occurs via reversible oxidation of thiols in proteins, termed "sulfhydryl switching" mechanisms. There are two types of thiol/disulfide switches: (Type I) where GSSG can interact with a protein thiol, resulting in glutathionylation of the

Copyright © 2006, Elsevier Inc.
All rights of reproduction in any form reserved.

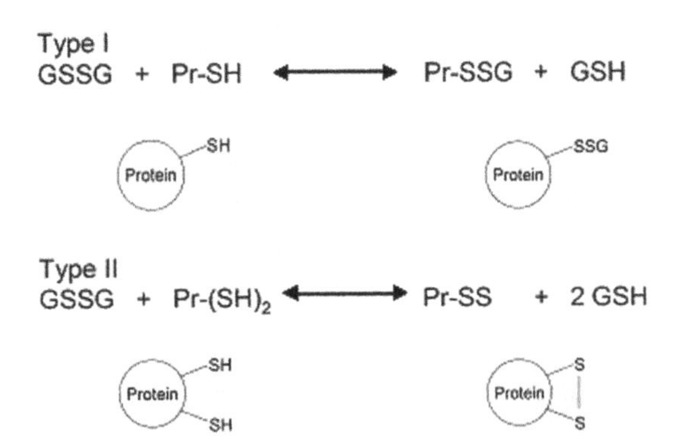

FIGURE 1 Type I and II redox switches. Cysteine modification (type I) or disulfide formation (type II) can lead to an increase or decrease in the activity of the respective protein. Type II switches require larger changes in reducing and oxidizing equivalents than type I switches because of the stoichiometry of the reactions.

protein and (Type II) where GSSG can interact with a protein resulting in the formation of an intramolecular protein disulfide and GSH (Figure 1) (Schafer and Buettner, 2001). Although Cys residues have been largely studied as the focus of redox-mediated mechanisms, the interconversions of Met and methionine sulfoxide can also serve in this capacity. The sulfur in Met is present as a thioether (-CH_2-S-CH_3), which is inherently less reactive, but nonetheless, it is critical for many protein functions and is subject to oxidation that is reversible by methionine sulfide reductases.

Considerable research has focused on regulation and function of proteins through oxidation of cysteines and methionines. In particular, the reversible oxidation of cysteine thiols (-SH) to disulfides (-SS-) or sulfenic acids (-SOH), and the methionine thioethers (S-CH_3) to sulfoxides (-$SOCH_3$), provides mechanistic switches between active and nonactive states in many signaling pathways. Another reversible oxidation occurs at the DNA-binding domains of multiple transcription factors, such as AP-1, nuclear factor-κB (NFκB), p53, and Nrf-2 (Abate et al., 1990; Bloom et al., 2002; Haddad, 2002a,b). These proteins contain critical Cys residues that can be oxidized to a sulfenic acid, thus preventing transcriptional activation, serving as a level of gene regulation (Claiborne et al., 1999). Sulfenic acids are not stable in water but can be stabilized in proteins by the formation of sulfenamides, as found in crystal structure of protein tyrosine phosphatase 1B (van Montfort et al., 2003). A similar oxidation of Met occurs in the protease inhibitor α_1-antitrypsin during oxidative stress. The sulfur in Met is oxidized to a sulfoxide, thereby inactivating the protein and allowing proteolysis to occur. This sulfur oxidation has been implicated in disease states such as emphysema (Johnson and Travis, 1979; Travis et al., 1980). Although both Met and Cys are involved in redox switching, the majority of research in this field has focused on Cys rather than Met, mostly because of Cys reactivity and measurability. With that in mind, the remainder of this chapter concentrates predominantly on Cys-containing proteins and peptides.

THIOLS IN CANCER CHEMOPREVENTION

GSH is the most abundant low-molecular-weight thiol in mammalian tissues, with concentrations ranging from ~1 to 10 mM. The total protein thiol content exceeds the total of low-molecular-weight thiols and is often in the range of 20–40 mM. In the hierarchy of metabolic needs, the availability of Cys for protein synthesis is more fundamental to cell survival than the availability of Cys for GSH synthesis. However, GSH concentrations are easy to measure, change dramatically during chemical exposures and oxidative stress, and correlate with susceptibility to chemical-induced carcinogenesis, as well as overt toxicity and cell death. Considerable literature on GSH was established prior to the development of methods to measure expression of specific proteins. Thus, much of the scientific literature has focused on GSH as a critical defensive factor and ignored the close association of GSH homeostasis with homeostatic regulation of protein synthesis during environmental challenges. With the recognition of the critical roles of regulatory mechanisms requiring rapid protein synthetic responses, a more correct picture may be that GSH status provides a useful biomarker of susceptibility and not the central determinant of susceptibility. Despite this caveat, the wealth of evidence supports the interpretation that the single most important biochemical for cancer prevention is the thiol GSH.

GSH is an effective anticancer agent because it is a nucleophile that readily reacts with electrophilic DNA-damaging agents or with ROS, thereby decreasing potentially mutagenic reactions (Figure 2). GSH is abundant in cells, providing an effective system to scavenge reactive species. Furthermore, a family of enzymes, the GSH *S*-transferases, enhance the reaction of GSH with potentially mutagenic electrophiles.

GSH is a tripeptide composed of glutamate, cysteine, and glycine, with the glutamate linked to the cysteine through the γ-carboxylate, rather than the usual α-carboxylate linkage that is present in proteins (Griffith, 1999). Addition of glutamate to the α-amino group of cysteine decreases the reactivity of the thiol and thereby protects against autooxidation. The unique isopeptide linkage through the γ-carboxyl of glutamate renders GSH (γ-glutamyl-cysteinyl-glycine) resistant to proteases and peptidases that function in protein degradation. GSH synthesis occurs independently of ribosomal protein synthesis and occurs in two distinct steps involving glutamate:cysteine ligase (GCL; formerly known as γ-glutamylcysteine synthetase) and glutathione synthetase, both ATP-dependent enzymes present in the cytosol of all mammalian cells. Degradation of GSH occurs by a unique enzyme, γ-glutamyltransferase (γ-glutamyltranspep-

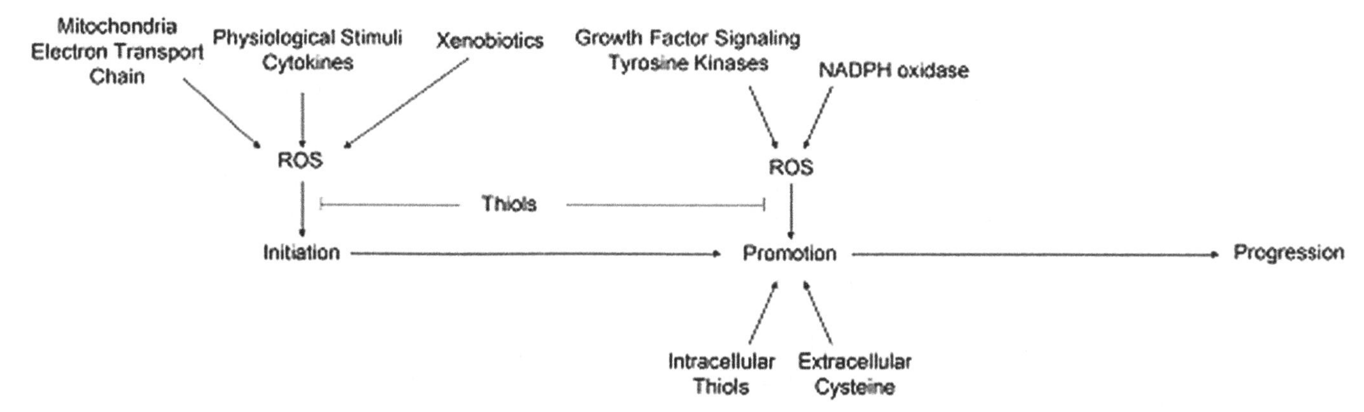

FIGURE 2 Discrete signaling pathways create multiple sets of redox regulation. Reactive oxygen species (ROS) are involved in at least two ways: (1) introduction of mutation in initiation and (2) stimulation of proliferation. Thiols are similarly involved at multiple sites, not only protecting against initiation and mutation by ROS and reactive electrophiles but also decreasing ROS-induced proliferation. *N*-acetylcysteine has been shown to block ROS signaling and proliferation in many model systems. In addition, more reduced extracellular cysteine/cystine redox and increased intracellular redox stimulate cell proliferation.

tidase, γ-GT), found in cell membranes and hydrolyzing extracellular GSH. This enzyme removes glutamate to yield cysteinyl glycine, which is degraded by at least three enzymes with dipeptidase activity, eventually yielding cysteine.

MOST DIETARY AND CHEMICAL CARCINOGENS ARE BIOACTIVATED TO REACTIVE MUTAGENS

As described elsewhere in this volume, environmental and dietary chemicals that are lipophilic are not readily removed by the kidneys and must be converted to more water-soluble derivatives. These processes are controlled by sulfhydryl switching mechanisms and can be functionally important in carcinogenesis because reactive intermediates produced can disrupt other sulfhydryl switches and modify DNA. The liver, kidneys, and barrier epithelia provide primary sites for biotransformation. Lipophilic compounds are converted into more water-soluble derivatives by phase I and phase II drug-metabolizing enzymes. Phase I reactions involve oxidation, reduction, and hydrolysis (esterases, amidases) of the parent molecule; phase II reactions serve as conjugation reactions to add endogenous substrates (glucuronic acid, sulfate, GSH) to phase I metabolites or to reactive groups on the parent molecule. Some chemicals that are not toxic in the parent form are bioactivated to reactive species, often by conversion to electrophiles. These include common dietary components, such as the polycyclic hydrocarbon benzo-a-pyrene (Tierney et al., 1987) found in charbroiled foods, and the fungal toxin aflatoxin B1 (Brodie et al., 1971; Jollow et al., 1974) found in contaminated corn and peanut products. Both of these chemicals are metabolized by CYP oxidases to epoxide intermediates that are reactive with DNA but can be effectively detoxified by GSH-dependent mechanisms. Other electrophilic species include alkyl and aryl halides, carbonium and diazonium ion intermediates, aldehydes, esters, alpha, beta-unsaturated carbon compounds, and compounds containing doubly bound nitrogen (isothiocyanates, isocyanates, quinazolines), and GSH reacts with most of these reactive species as well (Anders et al., 1988; Monks and Lau, 1988).

THE GSH SYSTEM PROTECTS AGAINST CANCER BY DETOXIFICATION OF REACTIVE ELECTROPHILES

The function of GSH in protection against chemically induced cancer has been amply demonstrated in animal studies. Dietary manipulation of sulfur amino acid intake shows that tissue GSH concentrations are decreased by insufficient concentrations of methionine and cysteine, and this deficiency results in increased DNA damage and carcinogenesis from a range of carcinogens (Cesarone et al., 1986; Chung et al., 2005; Komninou, et al., 2005). Similarly, depletion of GSH by treatment with the GSH synthesis inhibitor buthionine sulfoximine (BSO) enhances chemical-induced carcinogenesis (Murata et al., 2001; Chung et al., 2005). Moreover, induction of GSH synthesis and the GSH *S*-transferases decreases chemical-induced carcinogenesis. Thus, in model studies, evidence clearly establishes that GSH is a central component in protection against mutagenic processes that contribute to cancer initiation.

THE LIVER FUNCTIONS TO MAINTAIN SYSTEMIC CYSTEINE SUPPLY THROUGH AN ENTERORGAN GSH/CYSTEINE CYCLE

Although most recognized for detoxification functions, the evolution and conservation of GSH synthetic machinery probably occurred because of a function of GSH in stabilization of Cys supply. A continuous supply of Cys is required for protein synthesis, yet Cys is reactive, continuously lost under aerobic conditions due to irreversible oxidation to cysteine sulfinic and sulfonic acids, and used in higher organisms for biosynthetic functions such as taurine production. In higher organisms, GSH provides a short-term reservoir for Cys, and an interorgan GSH/cysteine cycle allows for constant cysteine supply despite intermittent dietary intake. In this cycle, GSH is released from cells at a rate that is both dependent upon cellular concentrations and modulated by hormones and other homeostatic mechanisms. Under most conditions, the liver is the primary organ responsible for supply of GSH to maintain Cys homeostasis, releasing GSH via transporters such as the multidrug resistance-associated proteins (MRPs) and organic anion transporting polypeptide (Oatp) (Kretzschmar et al., 1992; Ookhtens and Kaplowitz, 1998). With decreased intake of sulfur amino acids, other organ systems become increasingly important to contribute to Cys homeostasis. Nonhepatic tissues can contribute significantly to GSH supply, as evidenced from studies in rats following hepatectomy, where circulating GSH concentrations were found to be ~50% of normal (Kretzschmar et al., 1992).

Studies in rats showed that the GSH release from liver approximated the rate of synthesis, with a turnover time of ~1 hour. Despite this rapid release, the rate of clearance (principally hydrolysis) from the circulation is sufficient so that steady-state concentrations in plasma are in the low micromolar range. Thus, the release and hydrolysis provide a mechanism for cellular GSH to serve as a source of cysteine for the entire body. The human liver content of Cys in GSH approximates the daily sulfur amino acid requirement (~1 g). This pool provides a stable Cys supply despite intermittent Met and Cys consumption. The total amount of cysteine present in GSH in the body is ~3 g, roughly equal to the sulfur amino acid requirement for 3 days (Moriarty and Jones, 2004).

OPTIMAL SULFUR AMINO ACID INTAKE IN HUMANS REMAINS UNCERTAIN

The average American diet contains ~2.4 g of sulfur amino acids per day (i.e., about 2.4 times the recommended daily allowance [RDA]) (Flagg et al., 1994). Intake ranges from <0.5 g to >5 g and is, in general, highly related to animal protein consumption. Sulfur amino acid content in legumes and some nuts is ~20–25% of that in animal protein; other vegetarian food sources often contain only ~10% of that in animal protein. Because protein content is low in foods derived from plants, vegetarians are at risk of being sulfur amino acid deficient. However, sulfur amino acid balance studies are necessary because this effect may be counteracted by a higher content of phytochemicals that induce GSH synthesis and GSH-dependent detoxification systems. Epidemiological studies often show protective effects associated with intake of fruits and vegetables. Thus, if a carcinogenic risk occurs in some individuals due to deficient sulfur amino acid intake, this effect must be restricted to a subgroup rather than to the general population or to specific periods of risk. This can occur, for instance, following illness, surgery, or antitumor therapy that results in prolonged nutritional insufficiency. Increased sulfur amino acid requirements occur during healing, with evidence that individuals with extensive burns have a threefold increase in requirement for sulfur amino acids. To optimize individual health, some individuals may benefit from supplemental sources of sulfur amino acid precursors to protect against mutagenic electrophiles. At present, no clinical tests are available to assess optimal intake of sulfur amino acids.

DIETARY GSH PROVIDES A MEANS TO DECREASE RISK FROM DIRECT-ACTING DIETARY CARCINOGENS

A range of public health regulations and recommendations are designed to minimize carcinogenic chemicals in the food supply, but these are not completely effective (Ames, 1983). Most carcinogens found in food undergo biological activation *in vivo*, but a small number of direct-acting carcinogens are known, which do not require bioactivation for reaction with DNA. Many such chemicals are electrophilic, and the first line of defense against direct-acting carcinogens in the diet occurs in the gastrointestinal (GI) tract, where detoxification by GSH is enhanced by glutathione *S*-transferases. Glutathione *S*-transferase activity is present in the mucus lining the intestinal epithelium, and this activity uses GSH from the bile and diet to detoxify electrophiles before absorption (Samiec et al., 2000). Conjugation also occurs within the epithelial cells lining the GI tract. These cells synthesize GSH, and these cells also have transport mechanisms that allow GSH to be utilized directly from the lumen. Rodent studies with isolated rat enterocytes indicate that up to 80% of the GSH supply in the small intestinal enterocytes can be derived from transport (i.e., from hepatic GSH released into the lumen in bile or from the diet) (Bai and Jones, 1996; Samiec et al., 2000). In addition to detoxification mechanisms within cells, glutathione *S*-transferase activity is present in the mucus lining the intestinal epithelium, and this activity uses GSH from the bile and diet to detoxify electrophiles before absorption. These multiple lines of defense decrease the bioavailability of reactive chemicals and minimize health risks from dietary reactive chemicals. However, one can expect that risk would increase with an imbalance between the detoxification capability and the amounts and reactive character of the electrophiles in foods.

THIOLS IN THE DIET FUNTION TO PROTECT AGAINST DIRECT-ACTING CARCINOGENS IN THE DIET

Glutathione concentrations have been determined in foods listed in the National Cancer Institute's Health Habits and History Questionnaire (Jones et al., 1992). In general, dairy products, cereals, and breads are low in GSH, fruits and vegetables have moderate to high amounts of GSH, and freshly prepared meats are high in GSH. An analysis of association between dietary GSH intake and risk of oral and pharyngeal cancer (Flagg, et al., 1994) in a population-based case-control study showed that the relative risk of cancer was 0.5 among people with the highest quartile of GSH intake (95% confidence interval [CI] 0.3–0.7). However, only GSH from fruit and from vegetables commonly consumed raw (carrots, fresh tomato, cole slaw, lettuce, cucumber, and green pepper) was associated with reduced oral cancer risk (Flagg et al., 1994). These results imply that some additional factors in food, such as chemicals that react with GSH, could interact with GSH and thus could determine the beneficial effect of dietary GSH. Research shows that certain foods contain relatively high contents of GSH-reactive chemicals (He et al., 2004), but the nature of these chemicals has not been identified and defined. The presence of these compounds may decrease the availability of GSH to the intestinal epithelium. Alternatively, if these chemicals include direct-acting carcinogens, then the apparent protective effect of dietary GSH could be a consequence of detoxification of these reactive species by dietary GSH before absorption. These reactive chemicals could also function to disrupt normal sulfhydryl switching mechanisms, as described later. The complexity of the diet and the multiplicity of effects indicate that more comprehensive means are necessary for evaluation of the diet and individual risk of cancer. Comprehensive metabolic profiling by mass spectrometry and nuclear magnetic resonance (NMR) spectroscopy are being developed for such a purpose.

THIOLS IN REDOX SIGNALING AND CONTROL

In addition to supporting GSH synthesis for detoxification of mutagenic electrophiles, dietary sources of sulfur amino acids are critical for the maintenance of intracellular redox balance (the ratio of reducing and oxidizing equivalents). Control of the redox states of the sulfur atoms is critical for normal macromolecule function, affecting lipid integrity, DNA synthesis, and protein folding and stability (Schafer and Buettner, 2001). Moreover, regulation of signal transduction pathways affecting proliferation, differentiation, and apoptosis is also redox mediated. Because the major source of sulfur amino acids is primarily through diet, improper nutrition could alter intracellular redox status, thereby potentiating carcinogenesis. The present section summarizes advances in the understanding of thiol homeostasis and regulation of thiol/disulfide redox state in the initiation and progression of cancer.

Nernst Equation Defines Redox State in Biologic Systems

The energetics of the interactions between thiol/disulfide couples can be described in terms of the tendency to accept or donate electrons, expressed quantitatively by the Nernst equation:

$$E_h = E_o + RT/nF \ln([\text{electron acceptor}]/[\text{electron donor}]),$$

where R is the gas constant, T is the absolute temperature, F is Faraday's constant, and E_o is the standard potential relative to a standard hydrogen electrode. The E_o term provides a measure of the inherent tendency of the molecule to accept or donate electrons at the relevant pH, while the log term expresses the dependence of the energetics on concentrations of the electron donating and accepting forms. This equation takes into account the fact that biological electron transfers do not occur under standard conditions (Schafer and Buettner, 2001) and allows for the comparison of multiple redox couples. Values are given in volts or millivolts (mV), with the more negative redox state defining a more potent reducing force (Jones, 2002).

Cellular Redox Is Primarily Controlled by the Glutathione and Thioredoxin Systems

Although there are a number of components that contribute to intracellular redox status, the two principal systems to maintain cellular thiol/disulfide redox state are GSH and thioredoxin (Trx). These systems are complementary but have overlapping activities that provide a partial redundancy in their functions. While GSH and Trx have many comparable activities, there are some distinct differences between the systems that make them functionally unique. A primary distinction is that the Trx pool size is micromolar, whereas that for GSH is millimolar. At 1000-fold lower concentration, changes mediated by Trx can occur more rapidly in response to substantially lower rates of ROS generation. Preferential use of NADPH for the reduction of oxidized thioredoxin (TrxSS) via TR could allow Trx to be maintained in the reduced state despite extensive oxidation of GSH. Thus, even though the Trx and GSH systems have some overlapping functions, the difference in pool size makes Trx more suitable for redox signaling and GSH more suitable for detoxification. Consequently, an independence of GSH and Trx may allow differential control of specific aspects of redox-sensitive systems and pathways. Quantitative studies of redox responses of the two systems during oxidative stress and redox signaling will greatly aid in delineating these distinct functions.

Another major difference between GSH and Trx is molecular size. GSH has a molecular weight of 307, whereas Trx has a molecular weight of 12 kDa. These differences allow for the redox measurement of subcellular compartments through Trx redox potentials but not GSH. GSH has been shown to affect many nuclear processes, including the regulation of the nuclear matrix organization (Dijkwel and Wenink, 1986); maintenance of cysteine residues on zinc-finger DNA-binding motifs in a reduced and functional state (Klug and Rhodes, 1987); chromosome consolidation (De Capoa, et al., 1982); DNA synthesis (Suthanthiran et al., 1990); DNA protection from oxidative stress (Sandstrom and Marklund 1990); and protection of DNA-binding proteins (Sen and Packer, 1996). However, measurement of nuclear GSH is difficult, as GSH is easily lost during nuclear isolation. Still, some studies of nuclear compartmentalization of GSH provide evidence for differences between nuclear and cytoplasmic compartments (Bellomo et al., 1992; Voehringer et al., 1998; Cotgreave, 2003), but these reports are contradictory, leaving this question largely unanswered.

In contrast, immunohistochemical studies provide strong evidence for distinct nuclear compartmentation of Trx1, with increases in nuclear Trx1 in response to oxidative stress (Tanaka et al., 1997; Hirota et al., 1999). Because of the size of Trx1, the nuclei can be isolated and analyzed not only for relative concentrations but for redox potential as well. These studies have shown that isolated nuclei contain a sizable Trx1 pool as revealed by immunoblot analysis (Watson and Jones, 2003). The presence of Trx reductase in nuclei (Rozell et al, 1988) further indicates that nuclear Trx1 could represent a distinct subcellular pool where redox-sensitive components are controlled independently of the cytoplasmic pool. This likelihood is supported by steady-state redox measurements of cytoplasmic and nuclear Trx1 where cytoplasmic Trx1 is approximately +20 mV more oxidative than Trx1 in the nucleus (Watson and Jones, 2003).

Although the mitochondrial GSH appears to be in equilibrium with the cytosolic fraction, mitochondria appear to maintain a relatively independent GSH as supported toxicological studies showing the preferential depletion of mitochondrial GSH but not cytoplasmic GSH following ethanol exposure (Garcia-Ruiz et al., 1994). Mitochondrial GSH is protective against ROS generation, but other functions have not been well described. Still, the existence of mitochondrial GSH transporters, the 2-oxoglutarate and dicarboxylate carriers, further supports the maintenance of a sequestered, independent mitochondrial GSH pool (Chen and Lash, 1998; Coll et al., 2003).

Although GSH and Trx systems are integral to cellular function and maintenance of many processes, there appears to be little crosstalk between the two systems. Depletion of GSH via glutathione synthesis inhibitors (buthionine sulfoximine [BSO]) had no effect on Trx1 redox status (Hansen et al., 2004). Similarly, during cellular differentiation, where changes in GSH redox potential increased by approximately +50 mV, little effect was observed in the redox status of Trx1 (Nkabyo et al., 2002). Independence of the GSH and Trx systems suggests that they may also autonomously regulate different intracellular processes and pathways.

GSH is an essential endogenous antioxidant system because it functions both directly and indirectly to eliminate toxicants. A direct function to remove harmful reactive oxygen species occurs via a family of GSH peroxidases. GSH also reacts with superoxide and reactive aldehydes generated during lipid peroxidation. Indirect functions include reduction of dehydroascorbate to ascorbate. Free radical termination reactions of ascorbate generate semidehydroascorbate, which in turn, undergoes spontaneous dismutation to form ascorbate and dehydroascorbate. Reduction of dehydroascorbate is key to maintaining the ascorbate pool. Ascorbate, in turn, maintains vitamin E pools by reducing the free radical form of vitamin E generated during radical chain termination by this antioxidant (Buettner, 1993).

The GSH system consists of the redox couple GSH/GSSG; NADPH-dependent glutathione disulfide reductase (GSSG-Rd); and glutaredoxin (Grx), a catalyst for transferring GSH on or off of proteins (Holmgren, 2000). Antioxidant function results in oxidation of GSH to form glutathione disulfide (GSSG). GSSG is subsequently reduced back to GSSG by GSSG-Rd using NADPH as a cofactor. If GSSG accumulates (i.e., during oxidative stress), it can react with protein thiols to form protein disulfides (Pr-SSG), termed *glutathionylation*. Grx is primarily involved in reducing Pr-SSG but has been shown to reduce non-glutathionylated proteins as well (Holmgren, 1989). Pr-SSG formation utilizes available GSH, which depletes the GSH pool and influences protein function (Cappiello et al., 1996; Cotgreave and Gerdes, 1998; Casagrande et al., 2002; Ghezzi et al., 2002).

In 1977, studies began to uncover the etiology of adult T-cell leukemia (ATL), as it was the first cancer found to be caused by a retrovirus, the human T-cell leukemia virus type-I (HTLV-I) (Sasada et al., 1996). ATL cell lines showed the overexpression of IL-2Rα chain, which was attributed to the presence of ATL-derived factor (ADF). Cloning of

ADF showed sequence homology to the bacterial enzyme thioredoxin. In bacteria, thioredoxin had already been characterized as a ribonucleotide reductase, an essential enzyme converting nucleotides to deoxynucleotides, a process critical for DNA synthesis and, subsequently, cell proliferation (Jordan and Reichard, 1998). ADF and Trx were identical, as confirmed by subsequent amino acid sequencing (Tagaya et al., 1989).

The mammalian Trxs are small (~12-kDa) proteins that undergo redox reactions catalyzed by the conserved active site dithiol Cys-Gly-Pro-Cys. In the reduction reactions, Trx(SH) is oxidized to Trx(SS) and then must be recycled by an NADPH-dependent reductase thioredoxin reductase. The thioredoxin reductases are seleno-flavoproteins that maintain the redox state of the Trx(SH)/Trx(SS) couple in a highly reduced state. In mammalian cells, there are two major forms of thioredoxin: Trx1, found in cytoplasm and nucleus, and Trx2, found in mitochondria. A third form has been found to be widely distributed but is not well characterized (Miranda-Vizuete et al., 1998). Trx has numerous functions, including regulation of transcription factors, reduction of protein disulfides and methionine sulfoxides, prevention of apoptosis, antioxidative properties, and DNA synthesis (Watson et al., 2003).

Redox Varies within Cells throughout the Life Cycle

Cellular GSH/GSSG redox state varies in cells in association with proliferation, differentiation, and apoptosis and has been demonstrated in numerous studies. Proliferating cells have GSH/GSSG values ranging from –260 to –230 mV (Kirlin, et al., 1999; Jones, 2002). The mechanistic link between redox and cell cycle has not been completely elucidated, but a redox effect has been identified. For instance, in normal fibroblasts, mRNA levels of *gro*, a gene associated with proliferation, were correlated with the redox environment and the proliferative state of the cells (Hutter and Greene, 2000). The GSH pool becomes oxidized (–220 to –190 mV) during growth arrest because of either differentiation or contact inhibition (Hutter et al., 1997; Kirlin et al., 1999). In normal fibroblasts, an increase in confluency led to an oxidation of the redox state (+34 mV) and the cessation of proliferation, whereas fibrosarcoma cells, which are not affected by contact inhibition, continued to maintain a reduced state and to proliferate despite an increased culture density (Hutter et al., 1997). In human bronchial epithelial cells, growth arrest followed a decrease in intracellular GSH and Cys levels (Atzori et al., 1994). An oxidation of intracellular GSH/GSSG redox and lowered intracellular GSH and GSSG concentrations were observed in contact-inhibited nondividing human retinal pigment epithelial (hRPE) cells (Jiang et al., 2002).

The transition from a proliferating to a differentiating cell also shows a relationship with the oxidation of the intracellular GSH pool. Kirlin et al. (1999) differentiated HT29 cells with sodium butyrate. Concomitant with treatment, GSH redox potentials increased by +50 mV over a 72-hour period and were highly correlative with alkaline phosphatase activity, a measure of cellular differentiation. Using limb bud cultures as a measure for chondrogenesis, total thiol concentrations (primarily GSH) significantly decreased in the differentiative zone (chondrogenic fields) but were elevated in the zone where cells were highly proliferative (Hansen et al., 2001). During apoptosis, GSH export from cells is activated and the redox state is further oxidized to between −170 and −150 mV (Cai et al., 1995; Jiang et al., 2002).

Of considerable interest relative to nutrition, Cys deficiency limits cell growth and is sufficient to result in a marked oxidation of GSH/GSSG redox (Miller et al., 2002). This oxidation indicates that dietary availability of sulfur amino acids may directly determine thiol/disulfide balance in cells. Because Cys is required for protein synthesis, the associated redox change may provide a central mechanism for coupling dietary sulfur amino acid availability to cell growth and tissue homeostasis.

Trx1 redox status, unlike GSH, is relatively unaffected by the transition from a proliferative to differentiative state. In the human colon epithelial cell line (Caco-2), GSH redox shifts typical of the transition between proliferating and differentiating cells were described, increasing by +50 mV (Kirlin et al., 1999; Nkabyo et al., 2002). However, Trx1 protein increased, but the overall Trx1 redox potential did not change during the transition between proliferation and differentiation and was maintained at a constant potential of –280 mV (Nkabyo et al., 2002).

Cysteine and Cystine

Much work has been performed on intracellular redox and has primarily focused on either the GSH or the Trx system. However, there is evidence that cysteine/cystine redox couple may play an equally important role in regulation of redox processes (Jones et al., 2004). Studies show that the extracellular Cys/CySS redox states control the susceptibility to oxidant-induced apoptosis (Jiang et al., 2005) and modulate the sensitivity to epidermal growth factor (EGF)–stimulated activation of p42/44 MAPK (Nkabyo et al., 2005). These studies implicate the extracellular compartment as an important contributor to redox signaling and control.

Plasma cysteine concentrations are ~7–9-fold higher than GSH concentrations, suggesting that it may play a more critical role in extracellular redox processes (Jones et al., 2002). This is supported by findings that plasma cysteine oxidation occurs constantly throughout life, increasing +0.16 mV/yr, but plasma GSH/GSSG redox remains constant until age 45 years and then oxidizes relatively rapidly at a rate of +0.7 mV/yr for the remainder of that individual's life span (Jones et al., 2002). These variations could be important factors in cancer cell growth, with the normal oxidation providing a growth suppression factor that is countered by reductant production in rapidly growing tumors.

SYSTEMS ACT INDEPENDENTLY TO INCREASE THE SPECIFICITY OF REDOX CONTROL

For redox regulation to occur, specificity must be a principal component of redox-sensitive pathways. Glutathione, Trx, and cysteine pools each provide multiple sites for cellular redox control. Global oxidative stress (i.e., addition of exogeneous oxidant), which oxidizes all redox couples to similar extents, may not reflect the intrinsic sensitivities of specific redox-sensitive proteins to regulation by different redox couples. Redox states, in cells, for example, of Trx1, GSH, and cysteine, range from −280, −250, and −145 mV, respectively (Jones et al., 2004), providing a wide range in which redox-sensitive proteins can be regulated through each relevant system. Independence of these three different intracellular redox systems implies that the regulation of redox-sensitive machinery (control of protein activity, protein–protein interaction, protein trafficking, and protein–DNA interaction) can be regulated in a differential manner depending on the redox state of each system (Figure 3). The complexity of redox control by the interactions between these systems is further increased as a result of changes in GSH/GSSG redox states during proliferation, differentiation, and apoptosis.

Different redox systems may be involved in the regulation of a specific protein, interacting with different thiols in the same protein or in specific subcellular compartments. Transcription factors have been studied extensively regarding their redox regulation. Multiple factors have been shown to be regulated by both GSH and Trx1 (Figure 4). For example, nuclear factor (erythroid-derived 2)–like 2 (Nrf2) is a transcription factor that has been described as regulating anticancer and phase II enzyme genes through the antioxidant response element (ARE), including GSH synthesis enzymes and Trx1 (Thimmulappa et al., 2002; Kwak et al., 2003). Inactive Nrf2 is found bound to Keap1 in the cytoplasm. In brief, activation is a result of modifications to cysteine residues on Keap1 that allow for the dissociation of the complex to occur, leaving Nrf2 free to move into the nucleus, bind to the ARE, and upregulate gene expression (Kwak, et al., 2004). GSH, being the most abundant small biothiol in most cells, acts to buffer oxidation of Keap1 residues. This action helps to inhibit Nrf2 activation/nuclear translocation until adequate oxidative signals can overcome the GSH buffer and potentiate signal transduction. Interestingly, Nrf2 has a cysteine (Cys 508) residue in the DNA-binding domain. Upon oxidation of that residue, Nrf2 cannot bind to DNA properly, essentially blocking its ability to upregulate genes even though it has been activated (Bloom et al., 2002). Evidence supports that nuclear Trx1 reduces Cys508 and, therefore, restores gene expression (Hansen et al., 2004). This example shows that two independently regulated redox systems, the GSH and Trx systems, play different roles in the regulation of a single pathway. Other transcription factors, such as NFκB, have shown similar dependence on two (and possibly more) separate redox systems to maintain redox regulation of gene expression as well (Hirota et al., 1999). Similarly, apoptosis signaling kinase 1 (ASK1) has separate GSH- and Trx1-sensitive domains.

OXIDATIVE STRESS AND CARCINOGENESIS

Normal cells effectively balance intracellular redox potential by maintaining pools of reducing (GSH, Trx-$(SH)_2$, cysteine, NADPH, etc.) and oxidizing (GSSG, Trx-SS, cystine, $NADP^+$, etc.) equivalents. *Oxidative stress* is a universal term that typifies an unbalanced ratio between intracellular reducing and oxidizing equivalents, where the pool of oxidizing equivalents is disproportionately large as compared with the reducing pool. Carcinogenesis is a complex process characterized by three stages: initiation, promotion, and progression. Although oxidative stress is implicated in each stage of carcinogenesis (Kovacic and Jacintho, 2001), most studies have centered on oxidative stress' involvement in the initiation of cancer. The initiation of carcinogenesis is, as a general mechanism, the result of mutation in tumor promotion and tumor suppression genes. ROS are mutagenic and can be countered by antioxidants, such as GSH and Trx1. Therefore, alterations in GSH or Trx1 redox states may permit a greater nonlethal concentration of ROS, initiating carcinogenesis.

Promotion, though studied on a smaller scale, has been suggested to be a result of ROS production and/or changes in cellular redox status (Cerutti, 1985). ROS acting as promoters of cell division and growth have been demonstrated in numerous model systems (Giri et al., 1995; Huang et al., 1999; Kamendulis et al., 1999). One chemical promoter that has been well studied is phorbol myristate acetate (PMA). PMA administration is accompanied by ROS production and markers of oxidative stress (Blumberg et al., 1982; Nakamura et al., 1985). Although ROS appear to be a critical component, excessive generation of ROS could prove toxic, suggesting that a proper balance of ROS and antioxidants is necessary for optimal redox growth conditions.

GLUTATHIONE PLAYS OPPOSING ROLES IN CARCINOGENESIS

Glutathione is much more apt at detoxification reactions than Trx1. As a result, the role of GSH in the initiation of

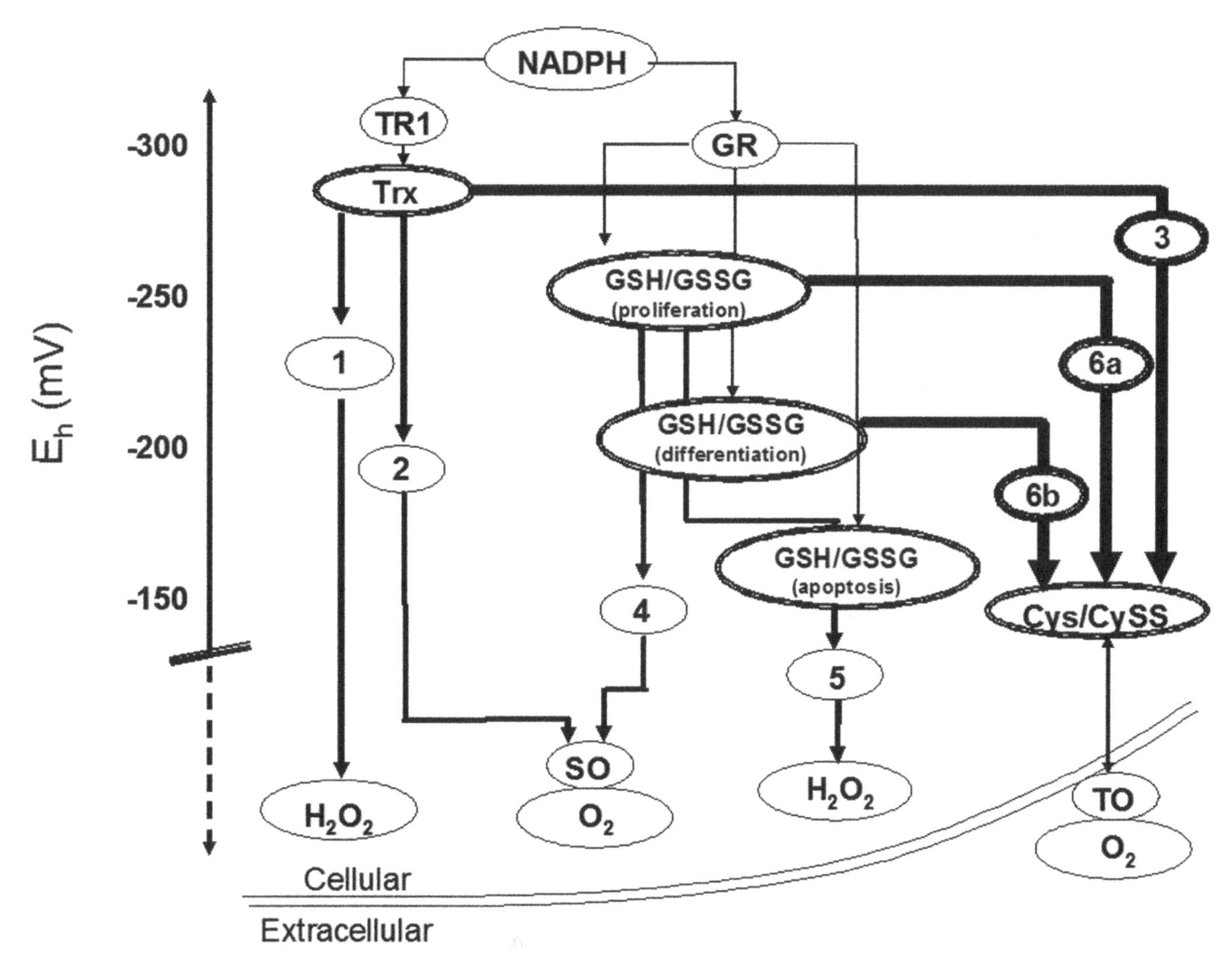

FIGURE 3 Circuitry model for cellular redox signaling and control by reversible oxidation of thiols. Reversible oxidation reduction of possible classes of signaling proteins (labeled 1–6) can occur via combinations of opposing reduction and oxidation reactions. In this scheme, electron flow is from the most reduced component (NADPH) on the top to electron acceptors on the bottom. Reduction is driven by well-characterized NADPH-dependent reductases, thioredoxin reductase 1 (TR1), and glutathione disulfide reductase (GR) through redox control nodes represented by Trx1 and GSH. The Trx1 and GSH are located schematically according to respective measured steady-state redox values, given in the scale on the left. Oxidation of signaling proteins can occur by reactive oxygen species (ROS) or by O_2 catalyzed by sulfhydryl oxidases (SO). The Cys/CySS couple can provide a third thiol/disulfide node for cellular redox signaling in which oxidation can occur without direct coupling to reactive oxygen species (ROS) or O_2. Oxidation of Cys/CySS occurs extracellularly catalyzed by a membranal thiol oxidase (TO). Redox circuits for proteins of classes 1 and 2 include Trx1 as the reducing node and ROS or O_2 as the oxidant, respectively. Redox circuits for proteins of classes 4 and 5 depend on GSH as the reductant and ROS or O_2 as the oxidant. Circuits for proteins of classes 3 and 6 depend on Trx1 and GSH for reduction and are coupled to Cys redox state for oxidation. Because GSH redox state changes as a function of cell growth, proteins with intermediate E_0 values (6a and 6b) could be differentially regulated by the change in GSH/GSSG redox state during cell growth and differentiation.

carcinogenesis is likely due to its ability to actively detoxify ROS and reactive intermediates, protecting the cell from damage that could potentially lead to mutations that could lead to carcinogenesis. Mutations may lead to desensitization of redox-regulation machinery relative to proliferative processes. It has been shown that proliferating cells have a much more reducing intracellular environment than cells that have reached confluence, where redox potentials become more oxidizing (Hutter et al., 1997; Nkabyo et al., 2002). Wild-type fibroblast GSH redox potential was determined to be −247 mV while actively proliferating (Hutter et al., 1997). Upon confluence, proliferation ceases because of contact inhibition, which correlates to a redox potential increase to −213 mV. In fibrosarcoma cells, which are transformed, redox potentials are measured at −238 mV during proliferation. These cells do not exhibit contact inhibition

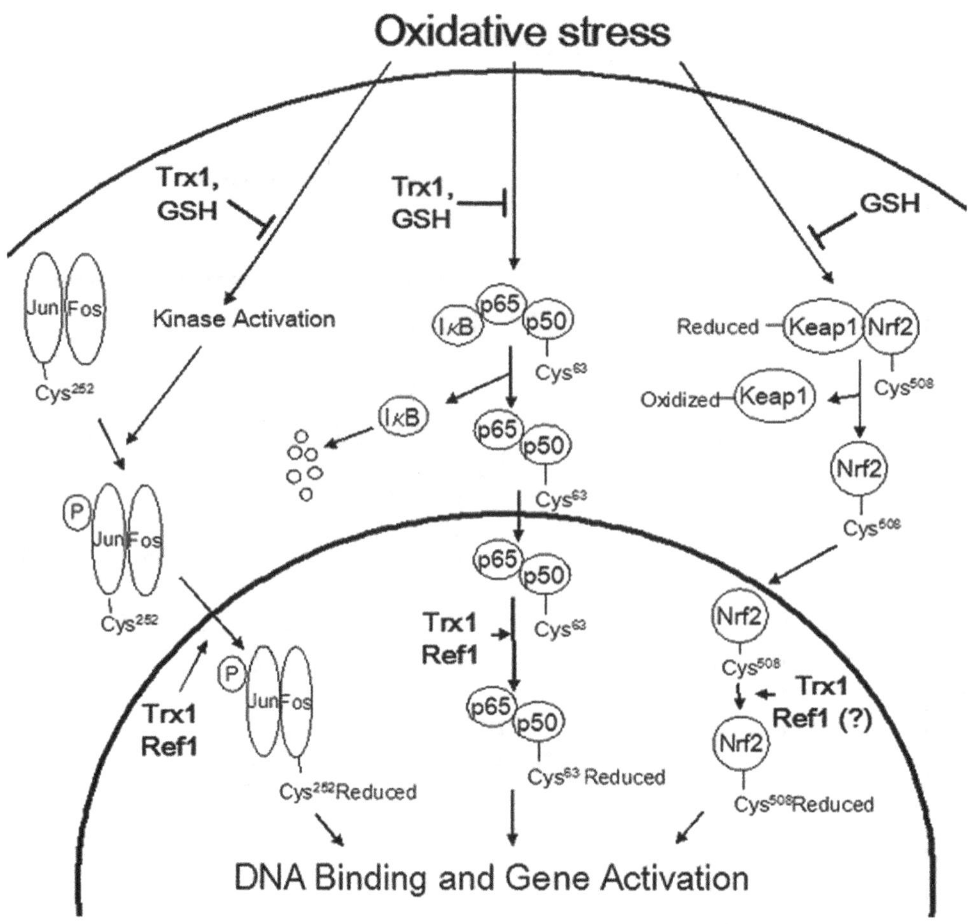

FIGURE 4 Multiple redox couples can act on a single signaling pathway within different compartments. Nuclear and cytoplasmic compartmentation of redox processes in regulation of transcription factors. AP-1, nuclear factor-κB (NFκB), and Nrf2 require an oxidative signal in the cytoplasm to initiate signaling for activation (phosphorylation of Jun or dissociation of NFκB or Nrf2 from inhibitory protein complexes). GSH effectively blocks most oxidative signals that initiate the pathway. After activation and translocation into the nucleus, cysteine residues within the DNA binding domain of each transcription factor are reduced by Trx1 and redox factor-1 (Ref-1). Reduction is a prerequisite for transcription factor binding to DNA and subsequent gene activation. Thus, even though oxidative stress in the cytoplasm signals activation, oxidative stress in the nuclear compartment blocks the process.

and will grow beyond confluence. At confluence, redox potential is unchanged (−238 mV). It is unknown whether low GSH redox potentials can overcome contact inhibition, but it clearly is indicative of changes in proliferation.

THIOREDOXIN IS OVEREXPRESSED IN CANCER

Numerous human tumors have shown an increased level of Trx expression in comparison with normal tissues, including primary cancers of the colon (Berggren et al., 1996), lung (Gasdaska et al., 1994), liver (Kawahara et al., 1996), cervix (Fujii et al., 1991), skin (Barral et al., 2000), and stomach (Grogan et al., 2000). It is hypothesized that Trx may play two roles in cancer: (1) promotion of cell growth and (2) resistance to apoptosis.

Trx1 has been described as having numerous functions, including its secretion and action as a possible growth factor (Teshigawara et al., 1985; Sasada et al., 1996; Powis et al., 2000). Although Trx1 secretion is not entirely understood, it has been linked to the stimulation of many different cell types, including normal fibroblasts, lymphocytes, and various cancer cell lines (Powis et al., 2000). In human subjects with hepatocellular carcinoma, plasma Trx concentrations increased to 147 ng/ml, an increase of 82% compared with subjects without hepatocellular carcinoma (81 ng/ml). Moreover, following tumor removal, Trx concentrations decreased significantly (Miyazaki et al., 1998). Mutation of the redox-active site cysteines decreases Trx's ability to stimulate cell growth in fibroblasts (Oblong et al., 1994). Unfortunately, there is little information about the redox state of plasma Trx, but these findings suggest that stimulation of cell growth via Trx is dependent on the redox state of Trx.

Another primary role that Trx may play in carcinogenesis is its ability to inhibit apoptosis. Injection of Trx-transfected cells into *scid* mice caused an increased tumor growth and a decrease in spontaneous apoptosis compared with mice receiving cells treated with empty vector injections (Powis et al., 2000). Researchers have concluded that unlike overexpression of the oncogene *bcl-2*, which conveys a resistance to apoptosis, Trx overexpression appears to contribute to the resistance to apoptosis while also enhancing growth. Inhibition of apoptosis is, at least partially, due to its antioxidant activities. L-Cysteine and GSH depletion results in oxidative stress (hydrogen peroxide production) and subsequently induces apoptosis after ~24 hours. Transfection with Trx1 inhibited oxidative stress and apoptosis. Interestingly, introduction of oxidized Trx did not show protection against apoptosis (Iwata et al., 1997).

SUMMARY

Albeit contradictory, thiols appear to play multiple roles in cancer: (1) protection against harmful mutagens and (2) the promotion of cell growth. ROS and reactive chemical intermediates are central components in DNA damage and mutation. Protection is primarily conveyed by the ability of small biothiols, such as GSH, to conjugate damaging bioactivated metabolites and electrophiles and is achieved through GST or, in the case of ROS detoxification, GSH peroxidases. ROS detoxification can also be performed by Trx through specifically localized peroxiredoxins as well. In either case, blocking ROS-induced or chemically induced DNA damage is the principal manner in which thiols can inhibit initiation. The contributions of dietary cysteine and methionine clearly inhibit carcinogenesis. Eventual goals will aim to optimize sulfur amino acid dietary intake to increase the overall health of the individual.

Interestingly and counterintuitively, reducing thiol redox states correlate with cell proliferation. Effects of varying redox states are likely due to flipping sulfhydryl switches, where proteins can be activated or deactivated due to cysteine/methionine residue modification. Glutathione redox changes are evident during the natural life cycle of cells (proliferation, differentiation, and apoptosis) and are indicative of environments that promote sulfhydryl switching. Thioredoxin has oxidoreductase activities and, with GSH, appears to be a principal regulator of sulfhydryl switches. There is evidence that cysteine also participates in this regulation as well. It appears that reduced GSH redox potentials promote cell division and proliferation. Comparatively, each redox couple, GSH, Trx, and cysteine have different redox potentials in the cell. Variation between these nodes increases specificity of control of sulfhydryl switches of particular proteins. Examples of proteins that are redox sensitive and have been studied extensively are transcription factors. Differential regulation of transcription factors occurs in different subcellular compartments and by different redox couples. In the case of Trx, overexpression is indicative in many cancers and may promote excessive proliferation. Current cancer chemotherapies are targeting Trx as possible treatments.

Clearly, nutrition and cancer comprise a natural crossroads for study and will be an area of increased interest in cancer biology. Although clear principles are not yet defined, continued effort to define nutritional strategies, including sulfur amino acid supplementation coupled with induction of thiol regulatory machinery by phytochemicals, will be intense. Ideally, these strategies will help us identify optimized thiol values that will inhibit cancer initiation while not affecting the natural cell life cycle and increasing overall health.

References

Abate, C., Patel, L., Rauscher, F.J., 3rd, and Curran, T. 1990. Redox regulation of fos and jun DNA-binding activity *in vitro*. *Science* **249**: 1157–1161.

Ames, B.N. 1983. Dietary carcinogens and anticarcinogens. Oxygen radicals and degenerative diseases. *Science* **221**: 1256–1264.

Anders, M.W., Lash, L., Dekant, W., Elfarra, A.A., and Dohn, D.R. 1988. Biosynthesis and biotransformation of glutathione S-conjugates to toxic metabolites. *Crit Rev Toxicol* **18**: 311–341.

Atzori, L., Dypbukt, J.M., Hybbinette, S.S., Moldeus, P., and Grafstrom, R.C. 1994. Modifications of cellular thiols during growth and squamous differentiation of cultured human bronchial epithelial cells. *Exp Cell Res* **211**: 115–120.

Bai, C., and Jones, D.P. 1996. GSH transport and GSH-dependent detoxication in small intestine of rats exposed *in vivo* to hypoxia. *Am J Physiol* **271**: G701–706.

Barral, A.M., Kallstrom, R., Sander, B., and Rosen, A. 2000. Thioredoxin, thioredoxin reductase and tumour necrosis factor-alpha expression in melanoma cells: correlation to resistance against cytotoxic attack. *Melanoma Res* **10**: 331–343.

Bellomo, G., Vairetti, M., Stivala, L., Mirabelli, F., Richelmi, P., and Orrenius, S. 1992. Demonstration of nuclear compartmentalization of glutathione in hepatocytes. *Proc Natl Acad Sci USA* **89**: 4412–4416.

Berggren, M., Gallegos, A., Gasdaska, J.R., Gasdaska, P.Y., Warneke, J., and Powis, G. 1996. Thioredoxin and thioredoxin reductase gene expression in human tumors and cell lines, and the effects of serum stimulation and hypoxia. *Anticancer Res* **16**: 3459–3466.

Bloom, D., Dhakshinamoorthy, S., and Jaiswal, A.K. 2002. Site-directed mutagenesis of cysteine to serine in the DNA binding region of Nrf2 decreases its capacity to upregulate antioxidant response element-mediated expression and antioxidant induction of NAD(P)H:quinone oxidoreductase1 gene. *Oncogene* **21**: 2191–2200.

Blumberg, P.M., Delclos, K.B., Dunphy, W.G., and Jaken, S. 1982. Specific binding of phorbol ester tumor promoters to mouse tissues and cultured cells. *Carcinog Compr Surv* **7**: 519–535.

Brodie, B.B., Reid, W.D., Cho, A.K., Sipes, G., Krishna, G., and Gillette, J.R. 1971. Possible mechanism of liver necrosis caused by aromatic organic compounds. *Proc Natl Acad Sci USA* **68**: 160–164.

Buettner, G.R. 1993. The pecking order of free radicals and antioxidants: lipid peroxidation, alpha-tocopherol, and ascorbate. *Arch Biochem Biophys* **300**: 535–543.

Cai, J., Sun, W.M., and Lu, S.C. 1995. Hormonal and cell density regulation of hepatic gamma-glutamylcysteine synthetase gene expression. *Mol Pharmacol* **48**: 212–218.

Cappiello, M., Voltarelli, M., Cecconi, I., Vilardo, P.G., Dal Monte, M., Marini, I., Del Corso, A., Wilson, D.K., Quiocho, F.A., Petrash, J.M., and Mura, U. 1996. Specifically targeted modification of human aldose reductase by physiological disulfides. *J Biol Chem* **271**: 33539–33544.

Casagrande, S., Bonetto, V., Fratelli, M., Gianazza, E., Eberini, I., Massignan, T., Salmona, M., Chang, G., Holmgren, A., and Ghezzi, P. 2002. Glutathionylation of human thioredoxin: a possible crosstalk between the glutathione and thioredoxin systems. *Proc Natl Acad Sci USA* **99**: 9745–9749.

Cerutti, P.A. 1985. Prooxidant states and tumor promotion. *Science* **227**: 375–381.

Cesarone, C.F., Scarabelli, L., and Orunesu, M. 1986. Effect of glutathione and N-acetylcysteine on hepatocellular modifications induced by 2-acetylaminofluorene. *Toxicol Pathol* **14**: 445–450.

Chen, Z., and Lash, L.H. 1998. Evidence for mitochondrial uptake of glutathione by dicarboxylate and 2-oxoglutarate carriers. *J Pharmacol Exp Ther* **285**: 608–618.

Chung, F.L., Komninou, D., Zhang, L., Nath, R., Pan, J., Amin, S., and Richie, J. 2005. Glutathione depletion enhances the formation of endogenous cyclic DNA adducts derived from t-4-hydroxy-2-nonenal in rat liver. *Chem Res Toxicol* **18**: 24–27.

Claiborne, A., Yeh, J.I., Mallett, T.C., Luba, J., Crane, E.J., 3rd, Charrier, V., and Parsonage, D. 1999. Protein-sulfenic acids: diverse roles for an unlikely player in enzyme catalysis and redox regulation. *Biochemistry* **38**: 15407–15416.

Coll, O., Colell, A., Garcia-Ruiz, C., Kaplowitz, N., and Fernandez-Checa, J.C. 2003. Sensitivity of the 2-oxoglutarate carrier to alcohol intake contributes to mitochondrial glutathione depletion. *Hepatology* **38**: 692–702.

Cotgreave, I.A. 2003. Analytical developments in the assay of intra- and extracellular GSH homeostasis: specific protein S-glutathionylation, cellular GSH and mixed disulphide compartmentalisation and interstitial GSH redox balance. *Biofactors* **17**: 269–277.

Cotgreave, I.A., and Gerdes, R.G. 1998. Recent trends in glutathione biochemistry—glutathione-protein interactions: a molecular link between oxidative stress and cell proliferation? *Biochem Biophys Res Commun* **242**: 1–9.

De Capoa, A., Ferraro, M., Lavia, P., Pelliccia, F., and Finazzi-Agro, A. 1982. Silver staining of the nucleolus organizer regions (NOR) requires clusters of sulfhydryl groups. *J Histochem Cytochem* **30**: 908–911.

Dickinson, D.A., and Forman, H.J. 2002. Cellular glutathione and thiols metabolism. *Biochem Pharmacol* **64**: 1019–1026.

Dijkwel, P.A., and Wenink, P.W. 1986. Structural integrity of the nuclear matrix: differential effects of thiol agents and metal chelators. *J Cell Sci* **84**: 53–67.

Flagg, E.W., Coates, R.J., Eley, J.W., Jones, D.P., Gunter, E.W., Byers, T.E., Block, G.S., and Greenberg, R.S. 1994. Dietary glutathione intake in humans and the relationship between intake and plasma total glutathione level. *Nutr Cancer* **21**: 33–46.

Flagg, E.W., Coates, R.J., Jones, D.P., Byers, T.E., Greenberg, R.S., Gridley, G., McLaughlin, J.K., Blot, W.J., Haber, M., Preston-Martin, S., et al. 1994. Dietary glutathione intake and the risk of oral and pharyngeal cancer. *Am J Epidemiol* **139**: 453–465.

Fujii, S., Nanbu, Y., Nonogaki, H., Konishi, I., Mori, T., Masutani, H., and Yodoi, J. 1991. Coexpression of adult T-cell leukemia–derived factor, a human thioredoxin homologue, and human papillomavirus DNA in neoplastic cervical squamous epithelium. *Cancer* **68**: 1583–1591.

Garcia-Ruiz, C., Morales, A., Ballesta, A., Rodes, J., Kaplowitz, N., and Fernandez-Checa, J.C. 1994. Effect of chronic ethanol feeding on glutathione and functional integrity of mitochondria in periportal and perivenous rat hepatocytes. *J Clin Invest* **94**: 193–201.

Gasdaska, P.Y., Oblong, J.E., Cotgreave, I.A., and Powis, G. 1994. The predicted amino acid sequence of human thioredoxin is identical to that of the autocrine growth factor human adult T-cell derived factor (ADF): thioredoxin mRNA is elevated in some human tumors. *Biochim Biophys Acta* **1218**: 292–296.

Ghezzi, P., Romines, B., Fratelli, M., Eberini, I., Gianazza, E., Casagrande, S., Laragione, T., Mengozzi, M., Herzenberg, L.A., and Herzenberg, L.A. 2002. Protein glutathionylation: coupling and uncoupling of glutathione to protein thiol groups in lymphocytes under oxidative stress and HIV infection. *Mol Immunol* **38**: 773–780.

Giri, U., Sharma, S.D., Abdulla, M., and Athar, M. 1995. Evidence that in situ generated reactive oxygen species act as a potent stage I tumor promoter in mouse skin. *Biochem Biophys Res Commun* **209**: 698–705.

Griffith, O.W. 1999. Biologic and pharmacologic regulation of mammalian glutathione synthesis. *Free Radic Biol Med* **27**: 922–935.

Grogan, T.M., Fenoglio-Prieser, C., Zeheb, R., Bellamy, W., Frutiger, Y., Vela, E., Stemmerman, G., Macdonald, J., Richter, L., Gallegos, A., and Powis, G. 2000. Thioredoxin, a putative oncogene product, is overexpressed in gastric carcinoma and associated with increased proliferation and increased cell survival. *Hum Pathol* **31**: 475–481.

Gulati, P., Klohn, P.C., Krug, H., Gottlicher, M., Markova, B., Bohmer, F.D., and Herrlich, P. 2001. Redox regulation in mammalian signal transduction. *IUBMB Life* **52**: 25–28.

Haddad, J.J. 2002a. Antioxidant and prooxidant mechanisms in the regulation of redox(y)-sensitive transcription factors. *Cell Signal* **14**: 879–897.

Haddad, J.J. 2002b. Science review: Redox and oxygen-sensitive transcription factors in the regulation of oxidant-mediated lung injury: role for nuclear factor-kappaB. *Crit Care* **6**: 481–490.

Hansen, J.M., Carney, E.W., and Harris, C. 2001. Altered differentiation in rat and rabbit limb bud micromass cultures by glutathione modulating agents. *Free Radic Biol Med* **31**: 1582–1592.

Hansen, J.M., Watson, W.H., and Jones, D.P. 2004. Compartmentation of Nrf-2 redox control: regulation of cytoplasmic activation by glutathione and DNA binding by thioredoxin-1. *Toxicol Sci* **82**: 308–317.

He, M., Openo, K., McCullough, M., and Jones, D.P. 2004. Total equivalent of reactive chemicals in 142 human food items is highly variable within and between major food groups. *J Nutr* **134**: 1114–1119.

Hirota, K., Murata, M., Sachi, Y., Nakamura, H., Takeuchi, J., Mori, K., and Yodoi, J. 1999. Distinct roles of thioredoxin in the cytoplasm and in the nucleus. A two-step mechanism of redox regulation of transcription factor NF-kappaB. *J Biol Chem* **274**: 27891–27897.

Holmgren, A. 1989. Thioredoxin and glutaredoxin systems. *J Biol Chem* **264**: 13963–13966.

Holmgren, A. 2000. Antioxidant function of thioredoxin and glutaredoxin systems. *Antioxid Redox Signal* **2**: 811–820.

Huang, H.S., Chen, C.J., Suzuki, H., Yamamoto, S., and Chang, W.C. 1999. Inhibitory effect of phospholipid hydroperoxide glutathione peroxidase on the activity of lipoxygenases and cyclooxygenases. *Prostaglandins Other Lipid Mediat* **58**: 65–75.

Hutter, D., and Greene, J.J. 2000. Influence of the cellular redox state on NF-kappaB–regulated gene expression. *J Cell Physiol* **183**: 45–52.

Hutter, D.E., Till, B.G., and Greene, J.J. 1997. Redox state changes in density-dependent regulation of proliferation. *Exp Cell Res* **232**: 435–438.

Iwata, S., Hori, T., Sato, N., Hirota, K., Sasada, T., Mitsui, A., Hirakawa, T., and Yodoi, J. 1997. Adult T cell leukemia (ATL)–derived factor/human thioredoxin prevents apoptosis of lymphoid cells induced by L-cystine and glutathione depletion: possible involvement of thiol-mediated redox regulation in apoptosis caused by pro-oxidant state. *J Immunol* **158**: 3108–3117.

Jiang, S., Moriarty-Craige, S.E., Orr, M., Cai, J., Sternberg, P., Jr., and Jones, D.P. 2005. Oxidant-induced apoptosis in human retinal pigment epithelial cells: dependence on extracellular redox state. *Invest Ophthalmol Vis Sci* **46**: 1054–1061.

Jiang, S., Moriarty, S.E., Grossniklaus, H., Nelson, K.C., Jones, D.P., and Sternberg, P., Jr. 2002. Increased oxidant-induced apoptosis in cultured nondividing human retinal pigment epithelial cells. *Invest Ophthalmol Vis Sci* **43**: 2546–2553.

Johnson, D., and Travis, J. 1979. The oxidative inactivation of human alpha-1-proteinase inhibitor. Further evidence for methionine at the reactive center. *J Biol Chem* **254**: 4022–4026.

Jollow, D.J., Mitchell, J.R., Zampaglione, N., and Gillette, J.R. 1974. Bromobenzene-induced liver necrosis. Protective role of glutathione and evidence for 3,4-bromobenzene oxide as the hepatotoxic metabolite. *Pharmacology* **11**: 151–169.

Jones, D.P. 2002. Redox potential of GSH/GSSG couple: assay and biological significance. *Methods Enzymol* **348**: 93–112.

Jones, D.P., Coates, R.J., Flagg, E.W., Eley, J.W., Block, G., Greenberg, R.S., Gunter, E.W., and Jackson, B. 1992. Glutathione in foods listed in the National Cancer Institute's Health Habits and History Food Frequency Questionnaire. *Nutr Cancer* **17**: 57–75.

Jones, D.P., Go, Y.M., Anderson, C.L., Ziegler, T.R., Kinkade, J.M., Jr., and Kirlin, W.G. 2004. Cysteine/cystine couple is a newly recognized node in the circuitry for biologic redox signaling and control. *FASEB J* **18**: 1246–1248.

Jones, D.P., Mody, V.C., Jr., Carlson, J.L., Lynn, M.J., and Sternberg, P., Jr. 2002. Redox analysis of human plasma allows separation of pro-oxidant events of aging from decline in antioxidant defenses. *Free Radic Biol Med* **33**: 1290–1300.

Jordan, A., and Reichard, P. 1998. Ribonucleotide reductases. *Annu Rev Biochem* **67**, 71–98.

Kamendulis, L.M., Jiang, J., Xu, Y., and Klaunig, J.E. 1999. Induction of oxidative stress and oxidative damage in rat glial cells by acrylonitrile. *Carcinogenesis* **20**: 1555–1560.

Kawahara, N., Tanaka, T., Yokomizo, A., Nanri, H., Ono, M., Wada, M., Kohno, K., Takenaka, K., Sugimachi, K., and Kuwano, M. 1996. Enhanced coexpression of thioredoxin and high mobility group protein 1 genes in human hepatocellular carcinoma and the possible association with decreased sensitivity to cisplatin. *Cancer Res* **56**: 5330–5333.

Kirlin, W.G., Cai, J., Thompson, S.A., Diaz, D., Kavanagh, T.J., and Jones, D.P. 1999. Glutathione redox potential in response to differentiation and enzyme inducers. *Free Radic Biol Med* **27**: 1208–1218.

Klug, A., and Rhodes, D. 1987. Zinc fingers: a novel protein fold for nucleic acid recognition. *Cold Spring Harb Symp Quant Biol* **52**: 473–482.

Kovacic, P., and Jacintho, J.D. 2001. Mechanisms of carcinogenesis: focus on oxidative stress and electron transfer. *Curr Med Chem* **8**: 773–796.

Kretzschmar, M., Pfeifer, U., Machnik, G., and Klinger, W. 1992. Glutathione homeostasis and turnover in the totally hepatectomized rat: evidence for a high glutathione export capacity of extrahepatic tissues. *Exp Toxicol Pathol* **44**: 273–281.

Kwak, M.K., Wakabayashi, N., Itoh, K., Motohashi, H., Yamamoto, M., and Kensler, T.W. 2003. Modulation of gene expression by cancer chemopreventive dithiolethiones through the Keap1-Nrf2 pathway. Identification of novel gene clusters for cell survival. *J Biol Chem* **278**: 8135–8145.

Kwak, M.K., Wakabayashi, N., and Kensler, T.W. 2004. Chemoprevention through the Keap1-Nrf2 signaling pathway by phase 2 enzyme inducers. *Mutat Res* **555**: 133–148.

Miller, L.T., Watson, W.H., Kirlin, W.G., Ziegler, T.R., and Jones, D.P. 2002. Oxidation of the glutathione/glutathione disulfide redox state is induced by cysteine deficiency in human colon carcinoma HT29 cells. *J Nutr* **132**: 2303–2306.

Miranda-Vizuete, A., Gustafsson, J.A., and Spyrou, G. 1998. Molecular cloning and expression of a cDNA encoding a human thioredoxin-like protein. *Biochem Biophys Res Commun* **243**: 284–288.

Miyazaki, K., Noda, N., Okada, S., Hagiwara, Y., Miyata, M., Sakurabayashi, I., Yamaguchi, N., Sugimura, T., Terada, M., and Wakasugi, H. 1998. Elevated serum level of thioredoxin in patients with hepatocellular carcinoma. *Biotherapy* **11**: 277–288.

Monks, T.J., and Lau, S.S. 1988. Reactive intermediates and their toxicological significance. *Toxicology* **52**: 1–53.

Moran, L.K., Gutteridge, J.M., and Quinlan, G.J. 2001. Thiols in cellular redox signalling and control. *Curr Med Chem* **8**: 763–772.

Moriarty, S.E., and Jones, D.P. 2004. Extracellular thiols and thiols/disulfide redox in metabolism. *Annu Rev Nutr* **24**: 481–509.

Murata, M., Bansho, Y., Inoue, S., Ito, K., Ohnishi, S., Midorikawa, K., and Kawanishi, S. 2001. Requirement of glutathione and cysteine in guanine-specific oxidation of DNA by carcinogenic potassium bromate. *Chem Res Toxicol* **14**: 678–685.

Nakamura, Y., Colburn, N.H., and Gindhart, T.D. 1985. Role of reactive oxygen in tumor promotion: implication of superoxide anion in promotion of neoplastic transformation in JB-6 cells by TPA. *Carcinogenesis* **6**: 229–235.

Nakashima, I., Kato, M., Akhand, A.A., Suzuki, H., Takeda, K., Hossain, K., and Kawamoto, Y. 2002. Redox-linked signal transduction pathways for protein tyrosine kinase activation. *Antioxid Redox Signal* **4**: 517–531.

Nkabyo, Y.S., Go, Y.M., Ziegler, T.R., and Jones, D.P. 2005. Extracellular cysteine/cystine redox regulates the p44/42 MAPK pathway by metalloproteinase-dependent epidermal growth factor receptor (EGFR) signaling. *Am J Physiol Gastrointest Liver Physiol* **289**: G70–78.

Nkabyo, Y.S., Ziegler, T.R., Gu, L.H., Watson, W.H., and Jones, D.P. 2002. Glutathione and thioredoxin redox during differentiation in human colon epithelial (Caco-2) cells. *Am J Physiol Gastrointest Liver Physiol* **283**: G1352–1359.

Oblong, J.E., Berggren, M., Gasdaska, P.Y., and Powis, G. 1994. Site-directed mutagenesis of active site cysteines in human thioredoxin produces competitive inhibitors of human thioredoxin reductase and elimination of mitogenic properties of thioredoxin. *J Biol Chem* **269**: 11714–11720.

Ookhtens, M., and Kaplowitz, N. 1998. Role of the liver in interorgan homeostasis of glutathione and cyst(e)ine. *Semin Liver Dis* **18**: 313–329.

Powis, G., Mustacich, D., and Coon, A. 2000. The role of the redox protein thioredoxin in cell growth and cancer. *Free Radic Biol Med* **29**: 312–322.

Samiec, P.S., Dahm, L.J., and Jones, D.P. 2000. Glutathione S-transferase in mucus of rat small intestine. *Toxicol Sci* **54**: 52–59.

Sandstrom, B.E., and Marklund, S.L. 1990. Effects of variation in glutathione peroxidase activity on DNA damage and cell survival in human cells exposed to hydrogen peroxide and t-butyl hydroperoxide. *Biochem J* **271**: 17–23.

Sasada, T., Sono, H., and Yodoi, J. 1996. Thioredoxin/adult T-cell leukemia–derived factor (ADF) and redox regulation. *J Toxicol Sci* **21**: 285–287.

Schafer, F.Q., and Buettner, G.R. 2001. Redox environment of the cell as viewed through the redox state of the glutathione disulfide/glutathione couple. *Free Radic Biol Med* **30**: 1191–1212.

Sen, C.K., and Packer, L. 1996. Antioxidant and redox regulation of gene transcription. *FASEB J* **10**: 709–720.

Suthanthiran, M., Anderson, M.E., Sharma, V.K., and Meister, A. 1990. Glutathione regulates activation-dependent DNA synthesis in highly purified normal human T lymphocytes stimulated via the CD2 and CD3 antigens. *Proc Natl Acad Sci USA* **87**: 3343–3347.

Tagaya, Y., Maeda, Y., Mitsui, A., Kondo, N., Matsui, H., Hamuro, J., Brown, N., Arai, K., Yokota, T., Wakasugi, H., et al. 1989. ATL-derived factor (ADF), an IL-2 receptor/Tac inducer homologous to thioredoxin; possible involvement of dithiol-reduction in the IL-2 receptor induction. *EMBO J* **8**: 757–764.

Tanaka, T., Nishiyama, Y., Okada, K., Hirota, K., Matsui, M., Yodoi, J., Hiai, H., and Toyokuni, S. 1997. Induction and nuclear translocation of thioredoxin by oxidative damage in the mouse kidney: independence of tubular necrosis and sulfhydryl depletion. *Lab Invest* **77**: 145–155.

Teshigawara, K., Maeda, M., Nishino, K., Nikaido, T., Uchiyama, T., Tsudo, M., Wano, Y., and Yodoi, J. 1985. Adult T leukemia cells produce a lymphokine that augments interleukin 2 receptor expression. *J Mol Cell Immunol* **2**: 17–26.

Thimmulappa, R.K., Mai, K.H., Srisuma, S., Kensler, T.W., Yamamoto, M., and Biswal, S. 2002. Identification of Nrf2-regulated genes induced by the chemopreventive agent sulforaphane by oligonucleotide microarray. *Cancer Res* **62**: 5196–5203.

Tierney, B., Martin, C.N., and Garner, R.C. 1987. Topical treatment of mice with benzo[a]pyrene or parenteral administration of benzo[a]pyrene diol epoxide-DNA to rats results in fecal excretion of a putative benzo[a]pyrene diol epoxide-deoxyguanosine adduct. *Carcinogenesis* **8**: 1189–1192.

Travis, J., Beatty, K., Wong, P.S., and Matheson, N.R. 1980. Oxidation of alpha 1-proteinase inhibitor as a major, contributing factor in the development of pulmonary emphysema. *Bull Eur Physiopathol Respir* **16**(Suppl): 341–352.

van Montfort, R.L., Congreve, M., Tisi, D., Carr, R., and Jhoti, H. 2003. Oxidation state of the active-site cysteine in protein tyrosine phosphatase 1B. *Nature* **423**: 773–777.

Voehringer, D.W., McConkey, D.J., McDonnell, T.J., Brisbay, S., and Meyn, R.E. 1998. Bcl-2 expression causes redistribution of glutathione to the nucleus. *Proc Natl Acad Sci USA* **95**: 2956–2960.

Watson, W.H., Chen, Y., and Jones, D.P. 2003. Redox state of glutathione and thioredoxin in differentiation and apoptosis. *Biofactors* **17**: 307–314.

Watson, W.H., and Jones, D.P. 2003. Oxidation of nuclear thioredoxin during oxidative stress. *FEBS Lett* **543**: 144–147.

CHAPTER

16

Principles of Tumor Immunology

BENJAMIN BONAVIDA

INTRODUCTION

The immune system has evolved to fight microbial infections and the ability to discriminate between self and nonself. The immune system consists of both the innate and the adaptive responses. Innate immunity is the first defense mechanism and consists of both humoral factors and host immune effector cells. The adaptive immune system consists of both the humoral antibody response and the cell-mediated response, both of which are antigen specific and develop memory. Although immune surveillance is well documented for microbial infections, it has been controversial for its role in cancer. However, it has been recognized that cancer cells can be recognized by the adaptive immune system via the expression of tumor-associated antigens (TAAs) or tumor-specific antigens. The development of cancer has been explained by the failure of the immune system to be generated or for induction of immune tolerance and escape of tumors from immune elimination. Several lines of evidence, both *in vitro* and *in vivo*, strongly suggest that antitumor cytotoxic lymphocytes or antitumor antibodies can participate in tumor destruction and tumor regression. Therefore, patients who do not respond to conventional therapies (e.g., chemotherapy, hormonal therapy, and radiation) have no alternatives for treatment. Immunotherapy is, therefore, considered a good approach for the treatment of such patients. Several antitumor immunotherapeutic manipulations have been developed and tested experimentally and clinically. Antibody-mediated immunotherapy, by passive administration of monoclonal antibodies (mAbs), has resulted in significant successes in the treatment of various tumors. For instance, several antibodies have been approved by the Food and Drug Administration (FDA) for the treatment of non-Hodgkin's lymphoma (NHL) (such as rituximab anti-CD20 mAb), breast cancer (Herceptin anti-Her2/neu mAb), and several other antibodies for the treatment of AML and colon cancer. Cell-mediated immunotherapy has been expanding in an attempt to generate antitumor cytotoxic responses, and such strategies include the adoptive transfer of *in vitro* expanded patients' blood leukocytes or tumor-infiltrating lymphocytes (TILs), vaccines to immunize against TAAs, gene therapy, etc. These various strategies have resulted in the proof of principle (i.e., the ability to generate antitumor cytotoxic T lymphocytes *in vitro* and *in vivo* in cancer patients). However, the clinical response has not been optimized and it may be achieved with better manipulations and/or combination chemotherapy and immunotherapy. Furthermore, it is becoming evident that even in the presence of an adequate antitumor cytotoxic response, the resistant cancer cells may develop mechanisms to resist killing by the cytotoxic lymphocytes. In such cases, sensitizing agents may be required to reverse the resistance of the tumor cells to killing and thus facilitate the cytotoxic activity mediated by immunotherapy. Clearly, significant advances have been made in cancer immunotherapy and new approaches will continue to be developed to achieve a clinical response and tumor elimination. Further advances in deciphering the interplay between the tumor and the host immune system and the microenvironment will undoubtedly lead to the development of new classes of immunotherapeutics.

The thymus-derived (T) dependent cell-mediated immune system recognizes tumor cells by virtue of their receptors by recognizing intracellularly derived protein fragments presented on the cell surface by the Major Histocompatibility Complex (MHC) molecules. The T

Copyright © 2006, Elsevier Inc.
All rights of reproduction in any form reserved.

lymphocytes engage these peptide–MHC complexes through their T-cell receptors. This mechanism allows the immune system to discriminate foreign antigens from self-antigens, as the latter have either induced deletion of self-recognized T cells or developed tolerance. Two types of MHC molecules are involved, namely MHC Class I and MHC Class II. These molecules are displayed on the cell surface and have a peptide-binding domain with a central cleft, where it accommodates a peptide sequence. MHC Class I molecules correspond to human leukocyte antigen (HLA)-A, -B, and -C molecules, and MHC Class II correspond to HLA-D molecules. Circulating T lymphocytes in lymphoid organs, peripheral blood, and nonlymphoid organs search for this specific MHC–peptide complex, and if found, the cytotoxic cell kills the target. There is a polymorphism of the MHC–peptide interaction and a large repertoire of T-lymphocyte specificities. Auto-reactive T cells that recognize dominant self-antigen are deleted in the thymus in a process called *negative selection*. Also, auto-reactive T cells with weak MHC recognition are neglected. These two processes are known as *central tolerance*. Some T cells escape thymic selection and can recognize self under specific conditions. T cells can recognize nonmutated tumor antigens, which are in fact antiself responses (Pardoll, 1999). T-cell activation requires two distinct signals. Signal 1 is delivered by the interaction between the T-cell receptor (TCR) and antigenic peptides presented on MHC molecules. Signal 2 is provided by one of several nonspecific costimulatory molecules such as CD28 on T cells and B7 family molecules on antigen-presenting cells (APCs).

Usually, cancer cells have Signal 1 only, so they can directly induce tolerance or need to be presented by other types of cells to stimulate the immune system. This is achieved by a process called *cross-presentation*, namely, tumor cells or tumor antigens are taken up by APCs, which process the antigens and present them on the APC cell surface restricted for this on MHC Class I and Class II molecules. APCs such as dendritic cells (DCs) can efficiently prime T cells, where they display MHC antigen complexes (Signal 1) together with costimulatory molecules (Signal 2), which activate naïve T cells in a process called *cross-priming*. This process can also cause T-cell unresponsiveness or cross-tolerance (Heath and Carbone, 2001).

Effector Cells

The effector cells of the immune system constitute cells of many types, those with restricted specificities such as CD4 and CD8 and those that are nonrestricted such as natural killer (NK) and NK T cells. The CD4+ T cell's primary role is of a helper type and help APC's activation and maintenance of CD8+ T cells. CD4+ T cells recognize specific peptide sequences presented by MHC Class II. CD8+ T cells are the main effector cells of the adaptive immune response, which mediate antigen-specific MHC-restricted cytotoxic effectors. CD8+ cells recognize peptides presented by MHC Class I molecules through the TCR complex. CD8+ T cells become activated by the TCR–MHC Class I peptide interactions on an APC, together with help from activated CD4+ T cells. This leads to a clonal expansion of antigen-specific cytotoxic T lymphocyte (CTL) that will lyse target cells. Killing by CD8 cells is mediated by the granzyme pathway and the tumor necrosis factor-α (TNF-α) family of ligands and can induce both necrosis and apoptosis.

NK cells are innate effector cells that serve as the first line of defense. They do not express TCRs and are not MHC restricted. However, they express receptors either activating or inhibitory. The NK T cells co-express a TCR and NK 1.1 receptor characteristics of T and NK cells, respectively. They recognize a limited array of peptides and glycolipid antigens presented by the nonpolymorphic MHC-like molecule CD1, which is not widely expressed in most APCs and several tissues (see review by Porcelli and Modlin, 1999).

Auto-Regulation of the Immune System

DCs maintain a balance between immune response and tolerance of tumor antigens. DCs make a decision of what should be presented and recognized as nondangerous self, dangerous self, or nonself (Steinman, 1991; Banchereau and Steinman, 1998). Once T cells are activated, the immune system makes an effort to keep them under control. Lymphocyte expansion after activation and cytokine production are controlled. Cytokine production is balanced by TH1 and TH2 cytokine production. TH1 and TH2 regulate each other. Also, activated T cells undergo apoptosis in the absence of growth factors such as interleukin-2 (IL-2). They also undergo death following antigen recognition by a process called *activation-induced cell death* (Green and Scott, 1994). Another regulatory mechanism is influenced by the costimulatory molecules. CD28 is the ligand for the costimulatory molecules B7.1 (CD80) and B7.2 (CD86), constitutively present on CD4 and CD8 T cells. When these T cells are activated, they upregulate CTLA-4, which is homologous to CD28 but competes and displaces CD28 and attenuates the T-cell response. Cross-linking of B7 with CTLA-4 inhibits T-cell activation. Peripheral T cells with suppressor activity have been the subject of controversy, but a subpopulation of CD4 T cells (5–10%) express CD25 and can suppress auto-reactivity (Shevach, 2001). Tumor cells also develop mechanisms of escape including downregulation of tumor antigen expression or processing, interference with DC presentation, direct inhibition of lymphocyte function, and resistance to apoptosis by immune cells.

The immune system has evolved with various infectious diseases in order to guarantee survival of the host. The immunological effector mechanisms that control microbial infections (bacterial and viral) are primarily dependent on the routes used for entry by the infectious agents. Diseases that are controlled by utilizing antibodies consist of infectious pathogens that spread in the blood such as *Streptococcus pneumoniae*, *Haemophilus influenzae*, Enteroviridae, measles, influenza, and pox viruses (Bachmann and Zinkernagel, 1997; Baumgarth et al., 2000; Ochsenbein, 2002). When the infections target peripheral solid organs with noncytopathic viruses such as hepatitis B and C viruses in humans, these are primarily controlled by the activation of CTLs, which have the ability to extravasate and enter the infected peripheral tissues (Zinkernagel et al., 1996). However, it is well known that both exogenous and endogenous pathogens can illicit both a humoral antibody response and a cell-mediated cytotoxic response. Solid tumors with TAAs may be considered to resemble viral infections of peripheral tissues, so the main effector mechanisms for their control may be through their killing by CTLs (Boon et al., 1997).

IMMUNE SURVEILLANCE OF TUMORS

The immune surveillance theory for tumors was originally proposed by Thomas (1959) and Burnet (1970), and since then, this theory has been challenged by many. The immunological surveillance hypothesis states that tumors arise with similar frequency to infection with pathogens and that the immune system constantly recognizes and rejects these tumors on the basis of the expression of foreign TAAs. The presence of TAAs was based on the finding that tumors induced in animal models were frequently rejected when transplanted into syngeneic hosts, whereas transplants of normal tissues between syngeneic hosts were accepted (Gross, 1943; Foley, 1953; Prehn, 1957). To date, we know that TAAs are the consequences of genetic and epigenetic alterations in cancer cells. A corollary to the original immune surveillance hypothesis is that clinically progressing tumors in all species are not eliminated because they develop active mechanisms of either immune escape or resistance. A fundamental prediction of the immune surveillance hypothesis is that immunodeficient individuals would display a dramatic increase in tumor incidence. This prediction was challenged initially in nude mice whereby there was no increase in spontaneous tumors (Rygaard and Povlsen, 1976; Stutman, 1979). We know that nude mice display an activated NK system that plays an important role in immune surveillance of cancers. Patients with immunodeficiencies revealed a complex pattern of cancer risk (Penn, 1988). There was a significant increase of rare cancers such as Kaposi's sarcoma and lymphoblastic lymphoma, but there was no increase in the common epithelial cancers seen in adulthood (colon cancer, lung cancer, prosthetic cancer, etc.). It became clear that cancers in immunodeficient individuals are primarily virus associated. Thus, immune surveillance indeed protected individuals against certain pathogen (mostly virus)-associated cancers by either preventing infection or clearing chronic infection by viruses that can lead to cancer. The failure to observe an altered incidence in nonvirus (pathogen-associated cancers) was taken as a strong argument against the classic immune-surveillance hypothesis. A caveat of these studies in the immune-deficient individuals is that they tend not to survive past their 30s or 40s and most non–virus-associated cancers arise late in life. Later studies in mice clearly show that various components of the immune system can indeed modify carcinogen-induced and spontaneous carcinogenesis using mice that had been rendered immunodeficient via genetic knockout (Kaplan et al., 1998; Street et al., 2002). For example, in Rag-2-/- mice (necessary for immunoglobulin and TCR gene rearrangement), the tumor incidence was not increased at young age; however, at old age (18 months to 2 years), an increase in tumor incidence was observed. Overall, the findings that the distribution of tumors differs in mice with deletions in different immunoregulatory genes suggests that different components of the immune system may modulate carcinogenesis in different tissues. The emerging evidence for immune surveillance systems of carcinogenic events is counterbalanced by evidence that the normal immune response to tumor antigens is tolerance rather than activation.

DO TUMOR CELLS EXPRESS TUMOR-ASSOCIATED ANTIGENS?

Studies using experimental tumors in animals demonstrate that certain tumors (syngeneic and allogeneic) can be rejected by immunological mechanisms and primarily by a cell-mediated immune response. Therefore, much effort has focused on the identification of TAAs that are recognized by human T lymphocytes (Boon et al., 1997; Rosenberg, 1999). Both CD4+ helper and CD8+ cytotoxic T cells recognize antigens presented as small peptides in the groove of surface HLA molecules. CD8+ cells recognize peptides of 8–10 amino acids in length, derived from intracellular cytoplasmic proteins, digested in proteasomes and presented via the endoplasmic reticulum on cell surface Class I HLA molecules. CD4+ cells use a different intracellular pathway and present engulfed proteins digested to peptides in intracellular endosomes and presented on the cell surface of Class II HLA molecules. These different pathways of antigen processing necessitated the development of separate methodologies to identify tumor antigens. These depend on the ability to generate T lymphocytes that can recognize human cancer cells. Several methods were used to identify tumor antigens recognized by CD8+ lymphocytes. These include transfection of complimentary DNA libraries from tumor cells into target cells expressing the appropriate HLA molecule and then using predetermined antitumor T cells to identify the appropriate transfectants (Boon et al., 1997). Another method consisted of eluting peptides from the surface of human cancer cells, and these were pulsed onto APCs and tested for their activity with specific antitumor lymphocytes (Hunt et al., 1992; Cox et al., 1994). The purification and sequencing of these peptides can then lead to the identification of the parent protein. Another technique referred to as "reverse immunology" has been used successfully to identify whether candidate proteins, selected for their overexpression on human cancer cells, represent cancer antigens (Kawashima et al., 1989). The candidate antigen is used to generate *in vitro* CTLs, and if these CTLs recognize intact human cancer cells, the candidate protein is considered a tumor antigen. These findings demonstrated that it was possible to generate human T cells that recognize melanomas, and most tumor antigens recognized thus far have been derived from melanoma. Other antigens expressed on common epithelial tumors have also been identified. A few examples are listed in Table 1.

Because transfection of cDNA libraries into target cells is not effective because the encoded proteins do not travel to the class II pathway, a new technique involving the screening of cDNA libraries fused to a gene encoding invariant chain sequences and designed to generate the transfected protein into the class II pathway has been adopted (Wang et al., 1999a). Many tumor antigens recognized by CD4+ T cells were also identified (Table 1).

Also, cancer associated with viruses can express antigens recognized by T lymphocytes. These include the E6 and E7 antigens on cervical cancers caused by human papillomaviruses, antigens from Epstein–Barr viruses (EBV) on lymphomas, and human T-cell lymphotropic virus-1 antigens on adult T-cell leukemia (Lowy and Schiller, 2001). Stoler et al. (1999) have estimated thousands (~11,000) of genomic alterations in cancer cells, and these represent candidates for cancer antigens recognized by the immune system. Also, cancers of the hematopoietic system express unique antigens not shared by other cancers such as the unique clonotype on B-cell lymphomas.

TABLE 1 Human Cancer Antigens

Type of antigen	References
Class I—restricted antigens recognized by CD8+ lymphocytes	
A. Melanoma-melanocyte differentiation antigens	
MART-1 (Melan A)	Kawakami et al., 1994a
gp-100 (pmell-17)	Kawakami et al., 1994b
Tyrosinase	Brichard et al., 1993
Tyrosinase related protein-1	Wang et al., 1995
Tyrosinase related protein-2	Wang et al., 1996
Melanocyte stimulatory hormone receptor	Salazar-Onfray et al., 1997
B. Cancer-testis antigens	
MAGE-1	van der Bruggen et al., 1991
MAGE-2	Visseren et al., 1997
MAGE-3	Gaugler et al., 1994
MAGE-12	Panelli et al., 2000
BAGE	Boel et al., 1995
GAGE	Van den Eynde et al., 1995
NY-ESO-1	Jager et al., 1998
C. Mutated antigens	
β-Catenin	Robbins et al., 1996
MUM-1	Chiari et al., 1999
CDK-4	Wolfel et al., 1995
Caspase 8	Mandruzzato et al., 1997
HLA-A2R17d	Brandle et al., 1996
D. Nonmutated shared antigen overexpression in cancers	
α-Fetoprotein	Butterfield et al., 1999
Telomerase catalytic protein	Vonderheide et al., 1999
MUC-1	Jerome et al., 1991
Carcinoembryonic apoptosis	Tsang et al., 1995
p53	Theobald et al., 1995
Her-2/neu	Ioannides et al., 1993
Class II–restricted antigens recognized by CD4+ T lymphocytes	
A. Epitopes for nonmutated protein	
gp-100	Li et al., 1998
MAGE-1	Chaux et al., 1999
MAGE-3	Chaux et al., 1999
Tyrosinase	Topalian et al., 1994
NY-ESO-1	Zeng et al., 2000
B. Epitopes from mutated proteins	
CDC 27	Wang et al., 1999a
LDLR-FUT	Wang et al., 1999b
Triosephosphate isomerase	Pieper et al., 1999

Source: This partial list was derived from Rosenberg (2001).

IMMUNE RESPONSE TO CANCER

Are Tumors Immunogenic in Humans?

Studies in mice have shown that adoptive immunotherapy of lymphocytes from immunized donors were able to transfer antitumor immunity in the recipient (Klein and Sjogren, 1960; Old et al., 1962). In humans, adoptive transfer from tumor-bearing patients of lymphokine-activated killer (LAK) cells with non-HLA restriction were able to recognize and kill cancer cells *in vitro* and some clinical response *in vivo* (Rosenberg et al., 1987). In patients with melanoma, it was possible to obtain TILs and these were grown in large numbers *in vitro* and were capable of specifically recognizing cancer antigens in about one third of patients with melanoma (Muul et al., 1987). TILs adoptively transferred into melanoma patients with IL-2 resulted in an objective response rate in ~35% of patients (Rosenberg et al., 1988). The identification of cancer antigens and their ability to generate an antitumor response was pivotal as it opened the field of cancer immunotherapy and the development of various strategies to generate antitumor cytotoxic responses (see later discussion). The immunogenicity of tumor cells, however, does not explain the failure of the immune system to mount an antitumor response in cancer patients and the seldom demonstration of tumor-specific cytotoxic lymphocytes in cancer patients. If one accepts that cancers are immunogenic, then the failure to generate an immune response must be explained by mechanisms by which the tumor evades the host immune system. Several mechanisms have been reported, and a few are discussed in the following sections.

Tumor Escape from Immunological Responsiveness and Underlying Mechanisms

The lack of clinical responses points to deciphering the mechanisms of tumor escape. Escape mechanisms include loss of antigen expression by the tumor, the local presence of immunosuppressive factors or cells, and the failure of the tumor to activate antitumor responses.

Antigen Expression

Lymphocytes, macrophages, and APCs perform their effector functions as single cells, but to activate CTLs, they need to interact and collaborate in organized lymphoid tissues. These anatomical structures determine the localization of antigen, cytokines, and bystander contacts through costimulatory molecules. The lymph nodes and spleen provide the milieu necessary for lymphoid cell interactions and activation. CTLs respond to antigen that becomes transiently presented within the organized lymphoid tissues for at least 3–5 days. In contrast, T cells do not react against antigens that are continuously present in lymphoid organs (Webb et al., 1990; Moskophidis et al., 1993). Antigen that is continuously present in secondary lymphoid organs would activate and delete all T cells specific for that antigen. The process of activation followed by physical deletion of the T cells is coined *exhaustion*. In summary, (1) a low antigen dose in lymphoid organs is not sufficient to induce a CTL response, and as a consequence, antigens that strictly stay outside lymphoid organs are immunologically ignored, (2) a sufficient antigen dose over a sufficiently long time in lymphoid organs induces a specific CTL response, and (3) a higher amount of antigen continuously present in lymphoid organs tolerizes the specific CTL response (Ochsenbein, 2002). T-cell activation requires two distinct signals. Signal 1 is delivered by the interaction between the TCR and antigenic peptides presented on MHC molecules. The second signal is provided by at least one of several antigen nonspecific costimulatory molecules including the interaction of CD28 on T cells with B7 family molecules on professional APCs (Matzinger, 1994; Chambers and Allison, 1997). Signal 1 alone has been correlated with induction of T-cell energy or deletion. Experimentally, tumors expressing costimulatory molecules are usually rejected more efficiently than control tumors. *In vitro* experiments indicate that DCs process exogenous cell debris and present the peptides on MHC Class I. This cross-priming process may be even more efficient for apoptotic cells than for necrotic cells. Cross-priming has also been shown in *in vivo* experiments (Bevan, 1976). The lack of relevant cross-priming may explain why most peripheral solid tumors do not induce an efficient antitumor response. The T-cell activation state induced by cross-presentation is thought to depend on multiple factors such as T-cell frequency, antigen levels, the maturation stage of DCs presenting the antigen, or the presence of potent CD4+ T-cell help (Spiotto et al., 2003). Increasing data implicate the mechanism of immune deviation as a means by which tumors escape an immune intervention. Mosmann et al. (1986) have shown that fully differentiated T-cell clones exhibited one or two distinct cytokine profiles. TH1 clones produce interferon-γ (IFN-γ) and IL-2, whereas TH2 clones produce IL-4, IL-5, and IL-10. The TH1 response seems to be of primary importance in the cell-mediated immune response that is important for antitumor immunity. Tumors may provoke immune deviation by stimulating a TH2 response.

Downregulation of the antigen-processing machinery and particularly the MHC Class I pathway has been documented in a large variety of human tumors (see review Marincola et al., 2000). Global MHC Class I loss may be due to mutations in combination with deletion of β2-microglobulin genes. Down-modulation of MHC Class I genes can result from down-modulation of the transporter associated with antigen presentation (TAP) genes and components of the immune proteasome (Restifo et al., 1996; Seliger et al., 1996). Other mechanisms of immune resistance mechanisms by tumors include the expression of secreted or cell surface molecules that either kill or inhibit cellular components of the effector immune response, for example, transforming growth factor-β (TGF-β) (Moretti et al., 1997).

IMMUNOTHERAPY

Given the failure of conventional therapeutics to treat resistant metastatic and recurrent cancers and the belief that cancers can respond to the immune system, much attention has been focused on the development of cancer immunotherapy. Several approaches have been considered to improve the immune response to tumors, including peptide vaccines, recombinant viral vaccines, recombinant bacterial vaccines, nucleic acid vaccines, DC vaccines, and the use of heat shock proteins as adjuvant (Pardoll, 1999). Also, adaptive cellular immunotherapy has been considered. Animal models have explored various costimulatory strategies (Hurwitz et al., 2000).

It has been postulated that efficient therapeutic vaccination should aim at triggering naturally occurring specific

T-cell responses to destroy tumor cells. However, there remains a discrepancy between successful findings in animals and the clinical success rate in cancer patients. The identification of tumor antigens and the generation of tumor-reactive lymphocytes are necessary but not sufficient to treatment efficacy. There is evidence for circulating naïve or antigen-specific tumor-reactive T cells in cancer patients (Romero et al., 1998). The mere presence of these cells has fueled hope for the development of therapeutic vaccines. Such experimental vaccination has been shown to induce specific immunity in a considerable number of cancer patients. These responses, however, only sporadically induced tumor regression in patients with metastatic diseases and rarely documented remission and survival (Cranmer et al., 2004). Tumors have also developed mechanisms to escape immune destruction. For instance, tumor cells are embedded in stroma, a network of extracellular matrix that harbors inflammatory cells such as macrophages, granulocytes, and DCs. Such cells produce factors that promote tumorigenesis and angiogenesis and contribute to immune evasion (Ganss et al., 2004). There is a basic assumption that activated tumor-reactive T cells are capable of migrating and destroying the tumor tissue. However, this was not the case in experimental animal models (Ganss et al., 2004). Angiogenesis is a component of the tumor phenotype, is essential for nutrient delivery, and has been neglected in large part by tumor immunologists. Leukocyte extravasation is tightly controlled by blood vessels and contributes to tumors' intrinsic resistance to infiltration. Therefore, effective immune responses require both fully armed effector cells and a tumor microenvironment permissive to infiltration and destruction (Ganss et al., 1999).

A compelling body of evidence argues that vascular components of the tumor stroma, not tumor cells, are indeed the primary targets during immune-mediated tumor rejection. For example, studies by the Blanheister group have reported that the rejection of transplantable tumors by CD4 and CD8 effectors was not mediated by direct tumor cell killing but was correlated with the ability to secrete IFN-γ, which in turn modulates IFN-γ receptor–positive stroma and inhibits angiogenesis (Qin and Blankenstein, 2000; Qin et al., 2003). It appears that angio-immunotherapy is a primary strategy, whereas inflammatory stimuli such as irradiation normalize the vasculature and activate endothelin, thereby promoting effector cell infiltration and antigen-driven tumor cell elimination.

Cell-Mediated Immunotherapy

1. *Cellular adoptive immunotherapy:* Several approaches have been considered for the use and/or activation of antitumor cytotoxic lymphocytes. The ability to successfully immunize patients against defined cancer antigens has facilitated the generation of antitumor T cells that can be expanded and used for adoptive immunotherapy (Rosenberg, 2001). There is also the potential to clone lymphocytes derived from a single cell selected for the high avidity to tumor antigen and to grow them in large numbers for passive adoptive immunotherapy. Also, genetic modification of lymphocytes can be performed to improve their antitumor efficacy and such studies are under active investigation. Peripheral blood mononuclear cells (PBMCs) stimulated *in vitro* with IL-2 generate LAK cells. Adoptive transfer of these cells shows promise in clinical studies but is mostly disappointing. The same findings were also observed with TILs. Expansion and cloning of lymphocytes derived from a single antigen-specific T cell and adoptive transfer after myeloablative conditioning chemotherapy resulted in cell proliferation and persistent clonal repopulation and correlated with tumor regression in patients with melanoma (Dudley et al., 2002).
2. *Cancer vaccines* (Ribas et al., 2003): Whole-cell tumor vaccines with whole-cell tumor lysates have been under clinical investigations for decades. Allogeneic or autologous tumor cells are processed and injected with a powerful adjuvant to attract host APCs. Randomized clinical trials have not been able to reflect an antitumor activity (Mitchell, 1998; Sondak et al., 2002).
3. *Gene-modified tumor vaccines:* These consist of autologous tumor cells stably transfected with an immunostimulating gene like cytokine (Dranoff, 1998). These have been tested in clinical trials (Soiffer et al., 1998).
4. *Peptide-based vaccine:* Tumor-derived peptide epitopes that contain the appropriate HLA-restricted amino acid sequence can be synthetically manufactured and administered with an immune adjuvant. This has led to an enhanced immune response (Rosenberg et al., 1998a).
5. *Naked DNA:* Intramuscular injection of naked DNA sequences results in gene expression and the generation of an immune response. Naked DNA plasmids have low immunological potency for generating antitumor responses to self-antigens in humans (Rosenberg, 2001).
6. *Viral vectors:* A variety of gene therapy vectors have been adapted to cancer immunotherapy. This application has resulted in weak immunological responses in humans (Rosenberg et al., 1998b); however, vectors that carry tumor antigens and costimulatory adhesion with other immune-enhancing molecules are being tested (Abrams and Schlom, 2000).
7. *Prime boost strategy:* The sequential administration of naked DNA and a viral vector has resulted in synergistic immune activation for tumor antigens (Ramshaw and Ramsay, 2000).

8. *Bacterial vectors:* Tumor gene segments have been introduced into bacteria such as *Salmonella* and *Listeria*, resulting in protected immunity in animals (Pan et al., 1995).
9. Ex vivo *APC-based vaccines:*
   a. *DCs:* The ability to generate large quantities of DCs in culture from hematopoietic precursors or peripheral blood allowed extensive testing in clinical trials (Timmerman and Levy, 1999). Immunizations in humans with antigen-loaded DCs resulted in detectable T-cell activation to tumor antigens with occasional clinical responses.
   b. *Immunocytokines:* Local delivery of cytokines to tumors to provide high paracrine levels in order to set a sequence of events leading to recognition of surface molecules on cancer cells (Imboden et al., 2001).
10. *Blockade of tumor-derived suppressor factors:* In the presence of activation of cytotoxic T cells, factors derived from the tumor or the microenvironment can prevent tumor killing. For instance, blocking the immunosuppressive prostaglandin E_2 (Huang et al., 1998) or TGF-β (Fakhrai et al., 1996) resulted in enhancing antitumor response.
11. *Vaccines in clinical trials* (Mocellin et al., 2004): Whole-cell vaccines (autologous or allogeneic): The efficacy of autologous or allogeneic whole-cell vaccines has not been confirmed by Phase III trials done in the therapeutic or adjuvant settings.
   a. *Tumor lysates:* Phase III studies done in the therapeutic or adjuvant setting have not confirmed the efficacy of lysate vaccines (Sondak and Sosman, 2003).
   b. *Heat shock proteins:* There have been encouraging results in humans, as heat shock proteins have been tested in Phase III clinical trials in patients with renal cell carcinoma or with melanoma.
   c. *Antigen-defined vaccines:* There has been little clinical benefit thus far.
   d. *DC vaccines:* There is strong preclinical evidence for the use of DCs in humans for antitumor vaccination, and the results of clinical trials have been conflicting, with a lack of objective tumor response in 12 of 35 trials. A comparative Phase III trial of DC vaccination of patients with advanced cancer is under way.

Antibody-Targeted Immunotherapy (van de Loosdrecht et al., 2004)

There have been successes in the application of engineered antibodies in the treatment of both hematological malignancies and solid tumors. Two basic strategies have been considered, namely, active versus passive immunization. Active immunotherapy refers to the induction of a specific immune response to malignant cells *in vivo*. Passive immunotherapy refers to therapeutic interventions with antibodies that recognize tumor-specific antigens. The development of therapeutic antibodies considers several factors for success, that is, immunogenicity, the nature of the antibody, selection of the appropriate antibody for optimal binding with human effector cells, and selection of target antigens both for induction of apoptosis and/or for regulation of tumor growth (Chinn et al., 2003). Immunogenicity of immune antibodies was initially one of the most striking limitations of using therapeutic antibodies because of the rapid generation of human antimouse antibodies, which prevented the repeated use of the antibody. New recombinant technologies have been developed to reduce the immunogenicity of genetically engineered chimeric antibody in which the antigen-binding region is of murine origin and the remaining sequence of human origin. Humanized antibodies have also been developed. Higher affinity binding to target antigen is a key feature of the antibody, which influences the dose for optimal antigen saturation and efficacy. The ability both to activate host effector functions such as antibody-dependent cellular cytotoxicity (ADCC) and complement-dependent cytotoxicity (CDC) and to induce apoptosis or inhibit survival is also required.

Selection of appropriate antigens for antibody-targeted therapy and the level of antigen expression on neoplastic cells are of significant importance for optimal efficacy. The expression of lineage-specific differentiation antigens in hematological malignancies (e.g., CD20 in B-cell NHL and CD33 in AML) provides unique targets for antibody-targeted therapy. Stable irreversible binding between antibody and antigen should be obtained to maximize host effector cell activity and internalization of antigen by the antibody. Antibody-targeted therapy can be included in an induction phase, during intensification as consolidation therapy with or without autologous or allo-PSCT or as maintenance therapy in a postremission phase of treatment. In addition, antibody-targeted therapy can be included in a treatment program in relapsing diseases or in patients with primary refractory disease.

The expression of the lineage-specific differentiation antigen CD20 has provided a unique target (Chinn et al., 2003). The absence of CD20 on stem cells allows the recovery of normal B cells following treatment, which lends to the destruction of malignant and normal B cells. The absence of CD20 on plasma cells results in only a slight decrease of immunoglobulin. The chimeric anti-CD20 mAb (rituximab; Rituxan) is approved by the FDA for the treatment of B-NHL alone or in combination with chemotherapy (Smith, 2004; Jazirehi and Bonavida, 2005). CD22 is a B-cell–restricted sialo-glycoprotein present in virtually all developing B cells but is detectable on the cell surface only at the mature stages of differentiation. Antibody-targeted therapy with anti-CD22 (Epratuzumab), a humanized immunoglobulin G1 (IgG1) antibody, has been administered in patients with NHL (Cesano and Gayko, 2003). CD33 is a cell surface glycoprotein receptor that is specific for myeloid cells. CD33 is expressed on ~90% of leukemia blasts and leukemic myeloid precursor cells, as well as on normal myeloid precursor cells, but not on CD34+ pluripotent stem cells (van Der Velden et al., 2001). CD33 is internalized after binding with anti-CD33 antibody and is not therapeutically useful. A clinically successful approach used anti-CD33 antibody targeted in combination with an immunotoxin, gemtuzumab ozogamicin (Mylotarg) (Bross et al., 2001). The anti-CD52 mAb CAMPATH-1 is used in patients with CLL given extensive prior therapy (Witzig et al., 1999). In some hematological malignancies, edrecolomab (Panorex) has been approved in Europe for colorectal cancer and trastuzumab (Herceptin) for the treatment of breast cancer in the United States (White et al., 2001). In 2004, the FDA approved bevacizumab anti-vascular endothelial growth factor (VEGF) mAb as first-line therapy for metastatic colorectal cancer (Ferrara et al., 2004). Radioimmunotherapy has been developed in NHL (Chesen, 2002). The most widely used in patients with NHL are directed against CD20 linked to either ^{131}I (tositumomab, Bexxar) or ^{90}Y (ibritumomab, Zevalin).

FUTURE CONSIDERATIONS FOR SUCCESSFUL ANTICANCER IMMUNOTHERAPY

The success of immune-mediated therapies in leukemia and lymphoma and certain solid tumors has stimulated translational research and the development of more effective immunotherapeutic strategies. Promising new approaches will combine classic chemotherapy with tumor-specific targeted immunotherapy. The more we learn about the natural relationship between the endogenous immune system and tumors as they develop, the more effective methods will be developed to manipulate those responses for successful therapeutic antitumor effects. The development of cross-resistance between chemotherapy and immunotherapy requires rethinking about new therapeutic approaches to treat drug-resistant tumor cells. There seems to be the need to develop strategies to overcome tumor cell resistance to apoptotic stimuli by the use, for example, of sensitizing agents and their clinical use in combination with immunotherapy for successful therapeutic results. Thus, treatment of malignant tumors requires at least two complimentary signals for functional complementation using a nontoxic sensitizing agent (Signal 1) that alters the cellular signaling pathways and the expression profile of the apoptotic associated molecules and, hence, facilitates the cytotoxic activity of the therapeutic agent (e.g., chemotherapeutic drugs, radiation, immune cytotoxics) (Signal 2) for the induction of apoptosis (Ng and Bonavida, 2002). Understanding why the endogenous and exogenous immune responses fail to control tumorigenesis is pivotal to improving antitumor immunotherapy. The concept of antigen dose, tumor localization, induction of tolerance, and immunological ignorance must be investigated to decipher the underlying mechanisms that regulate antitumor responses. A vaccine efficiently delivering tumor antigens to secondary lymphoid organs may lead to tumor control, and eradication of the tumor load is neither too great nor too difficult to reach. Only continuous stimulation of endogenous hosts or *in vitro* expanded and adoptively transferred effector T cells will likely be sufficient to lead to rejection of tumors quickly enough before the selection of escaped mutants. Although tumor vaccines have not been clinically efficient *in vivo*, adoptive cell therapy with the expanded *in vitro* tumor-specific effector cells has advantages such as manipulating the host before the autologous cells are transferred, for example, by eliminating host lymphocytes with suppressor activity, thus providing the transfer cells an optimal environment for anticancer therapy.

The realization that immunotherapy may be in large part due to its activity to tumor endothelial cells and the concept of "angio-immunotherapy" are promising, although inflammatory stimuli normalizing the vasculature also activate endothelia, thereby promoting effector cell infiltration and antigen-driven tumor cell elimination. Thus, for future consideration, it is pivotal to understand the complex cascade of events that is necessary to induce angiogenesis and permit effector cells entry into tumors.

It seems likely that the next decade will witness significant advances in the basic science of tumor immunology. The tools available are numerous, including the sequence of the human genome, the development of microarray technologies, the generation of knockout and transgenic animals for studies and *in vivo* imaging techniques, etc. All of these will facilitate the tasks of tumor immunologists. The challenge, though, lies in the clinical application of such knowledge. Clearly, the anticancer potential of adaptive immunity has not been fully exploited. The observation that patients will develop an immunological response to vaccination and they are more likely to benefit from the treatment than those who do not develop such a response raises a challenge to identify the conditions and their underlying basis for the differential response and thus apply them to a larger set of patients. To this aim, multi-parametric comparison of the dynamic immunological variables in patients who respond and those who do not respond by use of high-throughput biotechnology (e.g., DNA microarrays and proteomics) might be useful in the identification of molecular pathways leading to immune rejection in cancer. A better understanding between innate and adaptive immune responses, the discovery of mechanisms underlying immunological tolerance, and acknowledgment of the importance of both cell-mediated and humoral-adaptive immunity for the control of tumor growth are leading to more comprehensive immunotherapeutic approaches that take into consideration the many variables that define an effective antitumor response.

Acknowledgments

This work was supported in part by a grant from the Department of Defense (DOD/U.S. Army DAMD 17-02-1-0023) and a philanthropic contribution from the Jonsson Comprehensive Cancer Center and the Ann C. Rosenfield Fund, under the direction of David A. Leveton.

References

Abrams, S.I., and Schlom, J. 2000. Rational antigen modification as a strategy to upregulate or downregulate antigen recognition. *Curr Opin Immunol* **12**: 85–91.

Bachmann, M.F., and Zinkernagel, R.M. 1997. Neutralizing antiviral B cell responses. *Annu Rev Immunol* **15**: 235–270.

Banchereau, J., and Steinman, R.M. 1998. Dendritic cells and the control of immunity. *Nature* **392**: 245–252.

Baumgarth, N., Herman, O.C., Jager, G.C., Brown, L.E., Herzenberg, L.A., and Chen, J. 2000. B-1 and B-2 cell–derived immunoglobulin M antibodies are nonredundant components of the protective response to influenza virus infection. *J Exp Med* **192**: 271–280.

Bevan, M.J. 1976. Cross-priming for a secondary cytotoxic response to minor H antigens with H-2 congenic cells which do not cross-react in the cytotoxic assay. *J Exp Med* **143**: 1283–1288.

Boel, P., Wildmann, C., Sensi, M.L., Brasseur, R., Renauld, J.C., Coulie, P., Boon, T., and van der Bruggen, P. 1995. BAGE: a new gene encoding an antigen recognized on human melanomas by cytolytic T lymphocytes. *Immunity* **2**: 167–175.

Boon, T., Coulie, P.G., and Van den Eynde, B. 1997. Tumor antigens recognized by T cells. *Immunol Today* **18**: 267–268.

Brandle, D., Brasseur, F., Weynants, P., Boon, T., and Van den Eynde, B. 1996. A mutated HLA-A2 molecule recognized by autologous cytotoxic T lymphocytes on a human renal cell carcinoma. *J Exp Med* **183**: 2501–2508.

Brichard, V., Van Pel, A., Wolfel, T., Wolfel, C., De Plaen, E., Lethe, B., Coulie, P., and Boon, T. 1993. The tyrosinase gene codes for an antigen recognized by autologous cytolytic T lymphocytes on HLA-A2 melanomas. *J Exp Med* **178**: 489–495.

Bross, P.F., Beitz, J., Chen, G., Chen, X.H., Duffy, E., Kieffer, L., Roy, S., Sridhara, R., Rahman, A., Williams, G., and Pazdur, R. 2001. Approval summary: gemtuzumab ozogamicin in relapsed acute myeloid leukemia. *Clin Cancer Res* **7**: 1490–1496.

Burnet, F.M. 1970. The concept of immunological surveillance. *Progress Experimental Tumor Research* **13**: 1–27.

Butterfield, L.H., Koh, A., Meng, W., Vollmer, C.M., Ribas, A., Dissette, V., Lee, E., Glaspy, J.A., McBride, W.H., and Economou, J.S. 1999. Generation of human T-cell responses to an HLA-A2.1–restricted peptide epitope derived from alpha-fetoprotein. *Cancer Res* **59**: 3134–3142.

Cesano, A., and Gayko, U. 2003. CD22 as a target of passive immunotherapy. *Semin Oncol* **30**: 253–257.

Chambers, C.A., and Allison, J.P. 1997. Co-stimulation in T cell responses. *Curr Opin Immunol* **9**: 396–404.

Chaux, P., Vantomme, V., Stroobant, V., Thielemans, K., Corthals, J., Luiten, R., Eggermont, A.M., Boon, T., and van der Bruggen, P. 1999. Identification of MAGE-3 epitopes presented by HLA-DR molecules to CD4(+) T lymphocytes. *J Exp Med* **189**: 767–778.

Cheson, B.D. 2002. Radioimmunotherapy of non-Hodgkin lymphomas. *Blood* **101**: 391–398.

Chiari, R., Foury, F., De Plaen, E., Baurain, J.F., Thonnard, J., and Coulie, P.G. 1999. Two antigens recognized by autologous cytolytic T lymphocytes on a melanoma result from a single point mutation in an essential housekeeping gene. *Cancer Res* **59**: 5785–5792.

Chinn, P., Braslawsky, G., White, C., and Hanna, N. 2003. Antibody therapy of non-Hodgkin's B-cell lymphoma. *Cancer Immunol Immunother* **52**: 257–280.

Cox, A.L., Skipper, J., Chen, Y., Henderson, R.A., Darrow, T.L., Shabanowitz, J., Engelhard, V.H., Hunt, D.F., and Slingluff, C.L., Jr. 1994. Identification of a peptide recognized by five melanoma-specific human cytotoxic T cell lines. *Science* **264**: 716–719.

Cranmer, L.D., Trevor, K.T., and Hersh, E.M. 2004. Clinical applications of dendritic cell vaccination in the treatment of cancer. *Cancer Immunol Immunother* **53**: 275–306.

Dranoff, G. 1998. Cancer gene therapy: connecting basic research with clinical inquiry. *J Clin Oncol* **16**: 2548–2556.

Dudley, M.E., Wunderlich, J.R., Robbins, P.F., Yang, J.C., Hwu, P., Schwartzentruber, D.J., Topalian, S.L., Sherry, R., Restifo, N.P., Hubicki, A.M., Robinson, M.R., Raffeld, M., Duray, P., Seipp, C.A., Rogers-Freezer, L., Morton, K.E., Mavroukakis, S.A., White, D.E., and Rosenberg, S.A. 2002. Cancer regression and autoimmunity in patients after clonal repopulation with antitumor lymphocytes. *Science* **298**: 850–854.

Fakhrai, H., Dorigo, O., Shawler, D.L., Lin, H., Mercola, D., Black, K.L., Royston, I., and Sobol, R.E. 1996. Eradication of established intracranial rat gliomas by transforming growth factor beta antisense gene therapy. *Proc Natl Acad Sci USA* **93**: 2909–2914.

Ferrara, N., Hillan, K.J., Gerber, H.P., and Novotny, W. 2004. Discovery and development of bevacizumab, an anti-VEGF antibody for treating cancer. *Nat Rev Drug Discov* **3**: 391–400.

Foley, E. J. 1953. Antigenic properties of methylcholanthrene-induced tumors in mice of the same strain of origin. *Cancer Res* **13**: 835–837.

Ganss, R., Limmer, A., Sacher, T., Arnold, B., and Hammerling, G.J. 1999. Autoaggression and tumor rejection: it takes more than self-specific T-cell activation. *Immunol Rev* **169**: 263–272.

Ganss, R., Arnold, B., and Hammerling, G.J. 2004. Mini-review: overcoming tumor-intrinsic resistance to immune effector function. *Eur J Immunol* **34**: 2635–2641.

Gaugler, B., Van den Eynde, B., van der Bruggen, P., Romero, P., Gaforio, J.J., De Plaen, E., Lethe, B., Brasseur, F., and Boon, T. 1994. Human gene MAGE-3 codes for an antigen recognized on a melanoma by autologous cytolytic T lymphocytes. *J Exp Med* **179**: 921–930.

Green, D.R., and Scott, D.W. 1994. Activation-induced apoptosis in lymphocytes. *Curr Opin Immunol* **6**: 476–487.

Gross, L. 1943. Intradermal immunization of C3H mice against a sarcoma that originates in an animal of the cell line. *Cancer Res* **3**: 326–333.

Heath, W.R., and Carbone, F.R. 2001. Cross-presentation, dendritic cells, tolerance and immunity. *Annu Rev Immunol* **19**: 47–64.

Huang, M., Stolina, M., Sharma, S., Mao, J.T., Zhu, L., Miller, P.W., Wollman, J., Herschman, H., and Dubinett, S.M. 1998. Non–small cell lung cancer cyclooxygenase-2–dependent regulation of cytokine balance in lymphocytes and macrophages: up-regulation of interleukin 10 and down-regulation of interleukin 12 production. *Cancer Res* **58**: 1208–1216.

Hunt, D.F., Henderson, R.A., Shabanowitz, J., Sakaguchi, K., Michel, H., Sevilir, N., Cox, A.L., Appella, E., and Engelhard, V.H. 1992. Characterization of peptides bound to the class I MHC molecule HLA-A2.1 by mass spectrometry. *Science* **255**: 1261–1263.

Hurwitz, A.A., Kwon, E.D., and van Elsas, A. 2000. Costimulatory wars: the tumor menace. *Curr Opin Immunol* **12**: 589–596.

Imboden, M., Murphy, K.R., Rakhmilevich, A.L., Neal, Z.C., Xiang, R., Reisfeld, R.A., Gillies, S.D., and Sondel, P.M. 2001. The level of MHC class I expression on murine adenocarcinoma can change the antitumor effector mechanism of immunocytokine therapy. *Cancer Res* **61**: 1500–1507.

Ioannides, C.G., Fisk, B., Fan, D., Biddison, W.E., Wharton, J.T., and O'Brian, C.A. 1993. Cytotoxic T cells isolated from ovarian malignant ascites recognize a peptide derived from the HER-2/neu proto-oncogene. *Cell Immunol* **151**: 225–234.

Jager, E., Chen, Y.T., Drijfhout, J.W., Karbach, J., Ringhoffer, M., Jager, D., Arand, M., Wada, H., Noguchi, Y., Stockert, E., Old, L.J., and Knuth, A. 1998. Simultaneous humoral and cellular immune response against cancer-testis antigen NY-ESO-1: definition of human histocompatibility leukocyte antigen (HLA)-A2–binding peptide epitopes. *J Exp Med* **187**: 265–270.

Jazirehi, A., and Bonavida, B. 2005. Cellular and molecular signal transduction pathways modulated by rituximab (Rituxan, anti-CD20 mAb) in non-Hodgkin's lymphoma: implications in chemo-sensitization and therapeutic intervention. *Oncogene* **24**: 2121–2143.

Jerome, K.R., Barnd, D.L., Bendt, K.M., Boyer, C.M., Taylor-Papadimitriou, J., McKenzie, I.F., Bast, R.C., Jr., and Finn, O.J. 1991. Cytotoxic T-lymphocytes derived from patients with breast adenocarcinoma recognize an epitope present on the protein core of a mucin molecule preferentially expressed by malignant cells. *Cancer Res* **51**: 2908–2916.

Kaplan, D.H., Shankaran, V., Dighe, A S., Stockert, E., Aguet, M., Old, L.J., and Schreiber, R.D. 1998. Demonstration of an interferon gamma-dependent tumor surveillance system in immunocompetent mice. *Proc Natl Acad Sci USA* **95**: 7556–7561.

Kawakami, Y., Eliyahu, S., Delgado, C.H., Robbins, P.F., Rivoltini, L., Topalian, S.L., Miki, T., and Rosenberg, S.A. 1994a. Cloning of the gene coding for a shared human melanoma antigen recognized by autologous T cells infiltrating into tumor. *Proc Natl Acad Sci USA* **91**: 3515–3519.

Kawakami, Y., Eliyahu, S., Delgado, C.H., Robbins, P.F., Sakaguchi, K., Appella, E., Yannelli, J.R., Adema, G.J., Miki, T., and Rosenberg, S.A. 1994b. Identification of a human melanoma antigen recognized by tumor-infiltrating lymphocytes associated with *in vivo* tumor rejection. *Proc Natl Acad Sci USA* **91**: 6458–6462.

Kawashima, I., Hudson, S.J., and Sahin, U. 1989. The multi-epitope approach for immunotherapy for cancer: identification of several CTL epitopes from various tumor-associated antigens expressed on solid epithelial tumors. *Hum Immunol* **59**: 1–14.

Klein, E., and Sjogren, H.O. 1960. Humoral and cellular factors in homograft and isograft immunity. *Cancer Res* **20**: 452.

Li, K., Adibzadeh, M., Halder, T., Kalbacher, H., Heinzel S., Muller, C., Zeuthen, J., and Pawelec, G. 1998. Tumour-specific MHC-class-II–restricted responses after *in vitro* sensitization to synthetic peptides corresponding to gp100 and Annexin II eluted from melanoma cells. *Cancer Immunol Immunother* **47**: 32–38.

Lowy, D.R., and Schiller, J.T. 2001. *In* "Cancer Principles & Practice of Oncology" 6th ed. (V.T. DeVita, S. Hellman, and S.A. Rosenberg, Eds.), pp. 3189–3195. Lippincott, Philadelphia.

Mandruzzato, S., Brasseur, F., Andry, G., Boon, T., and van der Bruggen, P. 1997. A CASP-8 mutation recognized by cytolytic T lymphocytes on a human head and neck carcinoma. *J Exp Med* **186**: 785–793.

Marincola, F.M., Jaffee, E.M., Hicklin, D.J., and Ferrone, S. 2000. Escape of human solid tumors from T-cell recognition: molecular mechanisms and functional significance. *Adv Immunol* **74**: 181–273.

Matzinger, P. 1994. Tolerance, danger, and the extended family. *Annu Rev Immunol* **12**: 991–1045.

Mitchell, M.S. 1998. Perspective on allogeneic melanoma lysates in active specific immunotherapy. *Semin Oncol* **25**: 623–635.

Mocellin, S., Mandruzzato, S., Bronte, V., Lise, M., and Nitti, D. 2004. Part I: Vaccines for solid tumours. *Lancet Oncol* **5**: 681–689.

Moretti, S., Pinzi, C., Berti, E., Spallanzani, A., Chiarugi, A., Boddi, V., Reali, U.M., and Giannotti, B. 1997. In situ expression of transforming growth factor beta is associated with melanoma progression and correlates with Ki67, HLA-DR and beta 3 integrin expression. *Melanoma Res* **7**: 313–321.

Moskophidis, D., Lechner, F., Pircher, H., and Zinkernagel, R.M. 1993. Virus persistence in acutely infected immunocompetent mice by exhaustion of antiviral cytotoxic effector T cells. *Nature* **362**: 758–761.

Mosmann, T.R., Cherwinski, H., Bond, M.W., Giedlin, M.A., and Coffman, R.L. 1986. Two types of murine helper T cell clone. I. Definition according to profiles of lymphokine activities and secreted proteins. *J Immunol* **136**: 2348–2357.

Muul, L.M., Spiess, P.J., Director, E.P., and Rosenberg, S.A. 1987. Identification of specific cytolytic immune responses against autologous tumor in humans bearing malignant melanoma. *J Immunol* **138**: 989–995.

Ng, C.P., and Bonavida, B. 2002. A new challenge for successful immunotherapy by tumors that are resistant to apoptosis: two complementary signals to overcome cross-resistance. *Adv Cancer Res* **85**: 145–174.

Ochsenbein, A.F. 2002. Principles of tumor immunosurveillance and implications for immunotherapy. *Cancer Gene Ther* **9**: 1043–1055.

Old, L.J., Boyse, E.A., and Clarke, D.A. 1962. Antigenic properties of chemically induced tumors. *Ann NY Acad Sci* **101**: 80.

Pan, Z.K., Ikonomidis, G., Lazenby, A., Pardoll, D., and Paterson, Y. 1995. A recombinant Listeria monocytogenes vaccine expressing a model tumour antigen protects mice against lethal tumour cell challenge and causes regression of established tumours. *Nat Med* **1**: 471–477.

Panelli, M.C., Bettinotti, M.P., Lally, K., Ohnmacht, G.A., Li, Y., Robbins, P., Riker, A., Rosenberg, S.A., and Marincola, F.M. 2000. A tumor-infiltrating lymphocyte from a melanoma metastasis with decreased expression of melanoma differentiation antigens recognizes MAGE-12. *J Immunol* **164**: 4382–4392.

Pardoll, D.M. 1999. Inducing autoimmune disease to treat cancer. *Proc Natl Acad Sci USA* **96**: 5340–5342.

Penn, I. 1988. Tumors of the immunocompromised patient. *Annu Rev Med* **39**: 63–73.

Pieper, R., Christian, R.E., Gonzales, M.I., Nishimura, M.I., Gupta, G., Settlage, R.E., Shabanowitz, J., Rosenberg, S.A., Hunt, D.F., and Topalian, S.L. 1999. Biochemical identification of a mutated human melanoma antigen recognized by CD4(+) T cells. *J Exp Med* **189**: 757–766.

Porcelli, S.A., and Modlin, R.L. 1999. The CD1 system: antigen-presenting molecules for T cell recognition of lipids and glycolipids. *Annu Rev Immunol* **17**: 297–329.

Prehn, R.T. 1957. Immunity of methylcholanthrene-induced sarcomas. *J Natl Cancer Inst* **18**: 769–778.

Qin, Z., and Blankenstein, T. 2000. CD4+ T cell–mediated tumor rejection involves inhibition of angiogenesis that is dependent on IFN gamma receptor expression by nonhematopoietic cells. *Immunity* **12**: 677–686.

Qin, Z., Schwartzkopff, J., Pradera, F., Kammertoens, T., Seliger, B., Pircher, H., and Blankenstein, T. 2003. A critical requirement of interferon gamma-mediated angiostasis for tumor rejection by CD8+ T cells. *Cancer Res* **63**: 4095–4100.

Ramshaw, I.A., and Ramsay, A.J. 2000. The prime-boost strategy: exciting prospects for improved vaccination. *Immunol Today* **21**: 163–165.

Restifo, N.P., Marincola, F.M., Kawakami, Y., Taubenberger, J., Yannelli, J.R., and Rosenberg, S.A. 1996. Loss of functional beta 2-microglobulin in metastatic melanomas from five patients receiving immunotherapy. *J Natl Cancer Inst* **88**: 100–108.

Ribas, A., Butterfield, L.H., Glaspy, J.A., and Economou, J.S. 2003. Current developments in cancer vaccines and cellular immunotherapy. *J Clin Oncol* **21**: 2415–2432.

Robbins, P.F., El-Gamil, M., Li, Y.F., Kawakami, Y., Loftus, D., Appella, E., and Rosenberg, S.A. 1996. A mutated beta-catenin gene encodes a melanoma-specific antigen recognized by tumor infiltrating lymphocytes. *J Exp Med* **183**: 1185–1192.

Romero, P., Dunbar, P.R., Valmori, D., Pittet, M., Ogg, G.S., Rimoldi, D., Chen, J.L., Lienard, D., Cerottini, J.C., and Cerundolo, V. 1998. Ex vivo staining of metastatic lymph nodes by class I major histocompatibility complex tetramers reveals high numbers of antigen-experienced tumor-specific cytolytic T lymphocytes. *J Exp Med* **188**: 1641–1650.

Rosenberg, S.A. et al. 1987. A progress report on the treatment of 157 patients with advanced cancer using lymphokine activated killer cells and interleukin-2 or high dose interleukin-2 alone. *N Engl J Med* **316**: 889–897.

Rosenberg, S.A. et al. 1988. Use of tumor infiltrating lymphocytes and interleukin-2 in the immunotherapy of patients with metastatic melanoma. Preliminary report. *N Engl J Med* **319**: 1676–1680.

Rosenberg, S.A., Yang, J.C., Schwartzentruber, D.J., Hwu, P., Marincola, F.M., Topalian, S.L., Restifo, N.P., Dudley, M.E., Schwarz, S.L., Spiess, P.J., Wunderlich, J.R., Parkhurst, M.R., Kawakami, Y., Seipp, C.A., Einhorn, J.H., and White, D.E. 1998a. Immunologic and therapeutic evaluation of a synthetic peptide vaccine for the treatment of patients with metastatic melanoma. *Nat Med* **4**: 321–327.

Rosenberg, S.A., Zhai, Y., Yang, J.C., Schwartzentruber, D.J., Hwu, P., Marincola, F.M., Topalian, S.L., Restifo, N.P., Seipp, C.A., Einhorn, J.H., Roberts, B., and White, D.E. 1998b. Immunizing patients with metastatic melanoma using recombinant adenoviruses encoding MART-1 or gp100 melanoma antigens. *J Natl Cancer Inst* **90**: 1894–1900.

Rosenberg, S.A. 1999. A new era for cancer immunotherapy based on the genes that encode cancer antigens. *Immunity* **10**: 281–287.

Rosenberg, S.A. 2001. Progress in human tumour immunology and immunotherapy. *Nature* **411**: 380–384.

Rygaard, J., and Povlsen, C.O. 1976. The nude mouse vs. the hypothesis of immunological surveillance. *Transplant Rev* **28**: 43–61.

Salazar-Onfray, F., Nakazawa, T., Chhajlani, V., Petersson, M., Karre, K., Masucci, G., Celis, E., Sette, A., Southwood, S., Appella, E., and Kiessling, R. 1997. Synthetic peptides derived from the melanocyte-stimulating hormone receptor MC1R can stimulate HLA-A2–restricted cytotoxic T lymphocytes that recognize naturally processed peptides on human melanoma cells. *Cancer Res* **57**: 4348–4355.

Seliger, B., Hohne, A., Knuth, A., Bernhard, H., Ehring, B., Tampe, R., and Huber, C. 1996. Reduced membrane major histocompatibility complex class I density and stability in a subset of human renal cell carcinomas with low TAP and LMP expression. *Clin Cancer Res* **2**: 1427–1433.

Shevach, E.M. 2001. Certified professionals: CD4(+)CD25(+) suppressor T cells. *J Exp Med* **193**: F41–F46.

Smith, M.R. 2003. Rituximab (monoclonal anti-CD20 antibody): mechanisms of action and resistance. *Oncogene* **22**: 7359–7368.

Spiotto, M.T., Fu, Y.X., and Schreiber, H. 2003. Tumor immunity meets autoimmunity: antigen levels and dendritic cell maturation. *Curr Opin Immunol* **15**: 725–730.

Soiffer, R., Lynch, T., Mihm, M., Jung, K., Rhuda, C., Schmollinger, J.C., Hodi, F.S., Liebster, L., Lam, P., Mentzer, S., Singer, S., Tanabe, K.K., Cosimi, A.B., Duda, R., Sober, A., Bhan, A., Daley, J., Neuberg, D., Parry, G., Rokovich, J., Richards, L., Drayer, J., Berns, A., Clift, S., Dranoff, G., et al. 1998. Vaccination with irradiated autologous melanoma cells engineered to secrete human granulocyte-macrophage colony-stimulating factor generates potent antitumor immunity in patients with metastatic melanoma. *Proc Natl Acad Sci USA* **95**: 13141–13146.

Sondak, V.K., Liu, P.Y., Tuthill, R.J., Kempf, R.A., Unger, J.M., Sosman, J.A., Thompson, J.A., Weiss, G.R., Redman, B.G., Jakowatz, J.G., Noyes, R.D., and Flaherty, L.E. 2002. Adjuvant immunotherapy of resected, intermediate-thickness, node-negative melanoma with an allogeneic tumor vaccine: overall results of a randomized trial of the Southwest Oncology Group. *J Clin Oncol* **20**: 2058–2066.

Sondak, V.K., and Sosman, J.A. 2003. Results of clinical trials with an allogenic melanoma tumor cell lysate vaccine: Melacine. *Semin Cancer Biol* **13**: 409–415.

Steinman, R.M. 1991. The dendritic cell system and its role in immunogenicity. *Annu Rev Immunol* **9**: 271–296.

Stoler, D.L., Chen, N., Basik, M., Kahlenberg, M.S., Rodriguez-Bigas, M.A., Petrelli, N.J., and Anderson, G.R. 1999. The onset and extent of genomic instability in sporadic colorectal tumor progression. *Proc Natl Acad Sci USA* **96**: 15121–15126.

Street, S.E., Trapani, J.A., MacGregor, D., and Smyth, M.J. 2002. Suppression of lymphoma and epithelial malignancies effected by interferon gamma. *J Exp Med* **196**: 129–134.

Stutman, O. 1974. Tumor development after 3-methylcholanthrene in immunologically deficient athymic-nude mice. *Science* **183**: 534–536.

Theobald, M.B.J., Dittmer, D., Levine, A.J., and Sherman, L.A. 1995. Targeting p53 as a general tumor antigen. *Proc Natl Acad Sci USA* **92**: 11993–11997.

Thomas, L. 1959. "Discussion of Cellular and Humoral Aspects of the Hypersensitive States." (H.L. Laurence, Ed.). Hoeber-Harper, New York.

Timmerman, J.M., and Levy, R. 1999. Dendritic cell vaccines for cancer immunotherapy. *Annu Rev Med* **50**: 507–529.

Topalian, S.L., Rivoltini, L., Mancini, M., Markus, N.R., Robbins, P.F., Kawakami,Y., and Rosenberg, S.A. 1994. Human CD4+ T cells specifically recognize a shared melanoma-associated antigen encoded by the tyrosinase gene. *Proc Natl Acad Sci USA* **91**: 9461–9465.

Tsang, K.Y., Zaremba, S., Nieroda, C.A., Zhu, M.Z., Hamilton, J.M., and Schlom, J. 1995. Generation of human cytotoxic T cells specific for human carcinoembryonic antigen epitopes from patients immunized with recombinant vaccinia-CEA vaccine. *J Natl Cancer Inst* **87**: 982–990.

van de Loosdrecht, A.A., Huijgens, P.C., and Ossenkoppele, G.J. 2004. Emerging antibody-targeted therapy in leukemia and lymphoma: current concepts and clinical implications. *Anticancer Drugs* **15**: 189–201.

Van den Eynde, B., Peeters, O., De Backer, O., Gaugler, B., Lucas, S., and Boon, T. 1995. A new family of genes coding for an antigen recognized by autologous cytolytic T lymphocytes on a human melanoma. *J Exp Med* **182**: 689–698.

van der Bruggen, P., Traversari, C., Chomez, P., Lurquin, C., De Plaen, E., Van den Eynde, B., Knuth, A., and Boon, T. 1991. A gene encoding an antigen recognized by cytolytic T lymphocytes on a human melanoma. *Science* **254**: 1643–1647.

van Der Velden, V.H., te Marvelde, J.G., Hoogeveen, P.G., Bernstein, I.D., Houtsmuller, A.B., Berger, M.S., and van Dongen, J.J. 2001. Targeting of the CD33-calicheamicin immunoconjugate Mylotarg (CMA-676) in acute myeloid leukemia: *in vivo* and *in vitro* saturation and internalization by leukemic and normal myeloid cells. *Blood* **97**: 3197–3204.

Visseren, M.J., van der Burg, S.H., van der Voort, E.I., Brandt, R.M., Schrier, P.I., van der Bruggen, P., Boon, T., Melief, C.J., and Kast, W.M. 1997. Identification of HLA-A*0201–restricted CTL epitopes encoded by the tumor-specific MAGE-2 gene product. *Int J Cancer* **73**: 125–130.

Vonderheide, R.H., Hahn, W.C., Schultze, J.L., and Nadler, L.M. 1999. The telomerase catalytic subunit is a widely expressed tumor-associated antigen recognized by cytotoxic T lymphocytes. *Immunity* **10**: 673–679.

Wang, R.F., Robbins, P.F., Kawakami, Y., Kang, X.Q., and Rosenberg, S.A. 1995. Identification of a gene encoding a melanoma tumor antigen recognized by HLA-A31–restricted tumor-infiltrating lymphocytes. *J Exp Med* **181**: 799–804.

Wang, R.F., Appella, E., Kawakami, Y., Kang, X., and Rosenberg, S.A. 1996. Identification of TRP-2 as a human tumor antigen recognized by cytotoxic T lymphocytes. *J Exp Med* **184**: 2207–2216.

Wang, R.F., Wang, X., Atwood, A.C., Topalian, S.L., and Rosenberg, S.A. 1999a. Cloning genes encoding MHC class II–restricted antigens: mutated CDC27 as a tumor antigen. *Science* **284**: 1351–1354.

Wang, R.F., Wang, X., and Rosenberg, S.A. 1999b. Identification of a novel major histocompatibility complex class II-restricted tumor antigen resulting from a chromosomal rearrangement recognized by CD4(+) T cells. *J Exp Med* **189**: 1659–1668.

Webb, S., Morris, C., and Sprent, J. 1990. Extrathymic tolerance of mature T cells: clonal elimination as a consequence of immunity. *Cell* **63**: 1249–1256.

White, C.A., Weaver, R.L., and Grillo-Lopez, A.J. 2001. Antibody-targeted immunotherapy for treatment of malignancy. *Annu Rev Med* **52**: 125–145.

Witzig, T.E., White, C.A., Wiseman, G.A., Gordon, L.I., Emmanouilides, C., Raubitschek, A., Janakiraman, N., Gutheil, J., Schilder, R.J., Spies, S., Silverman, D.H., Parker, E., and Grillo-Lopez, A.J. 1999. Phase I/II trial of IDEC-Y2B8 radioimmunotherapy for treatment of relapsed or refractory CD20(+) B-cell non-Hodgkin's lymphoma. *J Clin Oncol* **17**: 3793–3803.

Wolfel, T., Hauer, M., Schneider, J., Serrano, M., Wolfel, C., Klehmann-Hieb, E., De Plaen, E., Hankeln, T., Meyer zum Buschenfelde, K.H., and Beach, D. 1995. A p16INK4a-insensitive CDK4 mutant targeted by cytolytic T lymphocytes in a human melanoma. *Science* **269**: 1281–1284.

Zeng, G., Touloukian, C.E., Wang, X., Restifo, N.P., Rosenberg, S.A., and Wang, R.F. 2000. Identification of CD4+ T cell epitopes from NY-ESO-1 presented by HLA-DR molecules. *J Immunol* **165**: 1153–1159.

Zinkernagel, R.M., Bachmann, M.F., Kundig, T.M., Oehen, S., Pirchet, H., and Hengartner, H. 1996. On immunological memory. *Annu Rev Immunol* **14**: 333–367.

CHAPTER

17

Animal Models in Nutritional Oncology Research

JIN-RONG ZHOU

INTRODUCTION

Epidemiological investigation and experimental studies indicate that nutritional manipulation may play a key role in cancer prevention. The diet contains a diverse array of bioactive components that may have cancer prevention activities. Development of effective dietary and nutritional preventive strategies against cancer requires conclusive evidence of their efficacy in animal models that closely emulate human disease. Carcinogenesis and tumorigenesis is a multistage process, including initiation, promotion, and progression/metastasis. Therefore, tumor models that accurately reflect the different disease stages are necessary to ensure a proper experimental design aimed at increasing our understanding of the biology of the disease and such models are essential tools to accelerate development of nutritional preventive regimens.

Application of clinically relevant animal tumor models to identify nutritional regimens for cancer prevention has been limited, in part due to lack of systematic evaluation of available animal models and inadequate research effort in nutritional prevention studies. This chapter provides an overview of commonly used and well-characterized animal models for specific cancer types and discusses their inherent strengths and weaknesses. Primary emphases are placed on animal models that represent orthotopic tumors and that are designed on the basis of genetic alterations that are frequently found in human cancer. This review should provide a guideline for selecting appropriate animal tumor models and designing research protocols to evaluate the efficacy of nutritional components. In addition, future research directions in further development of tumor models and application of these models to nutritional cancer prevention studies are discussed.

Cancer is a major public health problem in the United States and in the world. Currently, one out of four deaths in the United States is due to cancer (American Cancer Society, 2005). Cancer incidence and mortality demonstrate significant geographic variations. Epidemiological investigations suggest that both lifestyle changes and genetic alterations are responsible for geographic differences of cancer incidence and mortality. In particular, genetic and environmental interactions may play a crucial role in the onset and progression of cancer. Nutritional and dietary alterations have been suggested as major lifestyle factors that influence cancer risk and mortality.

Over the past 2 decades, cancer research has gained major insights into the complexity of tumor development and the cellular and molecular mechanisms that underlie the progressive transformation of normal cells into malignant cells. It is generally agreed that the transformation of a normal cell to a malignant tumor cell is initiated by a small number of genetic alterations, followed by evolution of neoplastic disease, which involves uncontrolled proliferation, impaired programmed cell death, the onset of angiogenesis, invasion of tumor cells into surrounding tissue, and metastatic dissemination of tumor cells to distant organs.

Cancer chemoprevention is the prevention of cancer by administration of one or more chemical compounds, either as individual drugs or as dietary supplements. Prevention of cancer through nutritional and dietary manipulation may offer important means of inhibiting the development and progression of cancer. However, studies to assess the efficacy of potential chemopreventive compounds are difficult to perform in large human populations. Experimental studies, especially animal studies, are imperative to

Copyright © 2006, Elsevier Inc.
All rights of reproduction in any form reserved.

determine the effects of nutritional components and to develop effective nutritional regimens for cancer prevention.

Successful development of nutritional agents for cancer prevention requires conclusive evidence of efficacy in animal models that closely emulate human disease. Because of the complexity of carcinogenesis and tumorigenesis processes, no single animal model can represent all cellular, molecular, and pathological aspects involved in the human cancer. Each animal model may represent a specific phenotype. Therefore, a careful evaluation of animal models can guide appropriate application of different animal models.

The purpose of this chapter is to provide an overview of animal models for specific cancer types, to identify major strengths and limitations of each model, and to discuss how these models could best be applied to determine cancer prevention activity of nutritional and dietary components. An overview of the different types of animal models is first presented, followed by a detailed discussion of animal models for each cancer type. A focus is given to the animal models that are commonly used and well characterized, such as genetically modified animal models and orthotopic xenograft tumor models. Finally, the future directions in animal model development and application for nutritional oncology research are discussed.

AN OVERVIEW OF ANIMAL MODELS

To serve as relevant models, it is essential to focus on animal and cell models that recapitulate the various steps in the natural history of human cancer development and progression. The critical steps in human cancer development and progression involve initiation, promotion, progression, local invasion, and metastasis. A series of animal models have been developed and applied for cancer research. One key emerging use of animal cancer models is as tools to evaluate the efficacy of prevention and intervention agents and define molecular targets.

The tumor models that have been used include ones that are spontaneously developed, are hormone or carcinogen induced, are xenograft transplanted using cells with varying growth and metastatic potential, and are genetically engineered with oncogene overexpression or tumor suppressor gene deletion/mutation. The application of these models requires that they be characterized in ways that demonstrate they possess important similarities to human cancer. The major strengths and limitations of these animal models are summarized in the following sections.

Spontaneous Tumor Models

The spontaneous tumor models are among the first used animal models for cancer research and for evaluation of chemopreventive agents. Different animal species have different susceptibilities to develop spontaneous tumors due to specific genetic backgrounds. The major advantages of spontaneous tumor models are that tumors are developed spontaneously and may represent natural processes of tumor development and progression. However, spontaneous tumors are usually developed over a much longer time than in other tumor models, and tumor incidence is usually low. In addition, spontaneous tumors may be developed at several organs, but not at a specific organ. These limitations in general prevent spontaneous tumor models from being applied for routine evaluation of the efficacy of prevention agents.

Hormone- or Chemical-Induced Tumor Models

Hormone- or chemical carcinogen–induced tumor models have been widely used to deepen our understanding of human tumorigenesis and to provide the *in vivo* systems for the evaluation of innovative preventive and therapeutic modalities. Hormones such as estrogens and androgens have been used, alone or in combination with chemical carcinogens, to emulate carcinogenesis and tumorigenesis processes that may occur in humans. Use of hormones for development of tumor models represents an advantage of these models because estrogens or androgens have been shown to be risk factors for hormone-dependent cancers such as breast and prostate cancers. Another advantage of the hormone- and/or chemical carcinogen–induced tumor model is that tumors are developed through a series of progressive processes involving initiation, promotion, progression, and metastasis, thus providing a suitable model for evaluating the efficacy of dietary and nutritional components in targeting specific stages of carcinogenesis and tumorigenesis. These tumor models have contributed significantly to the development of early chemopreventive and therapeutic agents.

On the other hand, these tumor models have several inherent limitations. Although certain chemical carcinogens are used to develop tumor models, the direct evidence that these chemicals are indeed one of the risk factors has not been adequately established in humans. Both hormones and chemical carcinogens need to be used at high levels and/or with long-term administration. Chemical carcinogens are toxic and may cause harm to those working with them. Tumors present in multiple organs and are not organ specific. These limitations, together with development of other more appropriate tumor models, have resulted in reduced use of these tumor models in cancer prevention research.

Xenograft Tumor Models

Specific cell types derived from human tumors and relevant animal models represent unique molecular and histopathological features related to human cancer development and progression. These cells can be most helpful in delineating the molecular pathways that define cancer development and progression and in developing molecular target-specific preventive and therapeutic regimens. In particular, xenograft tumor models developed from human cancer cells closely represent phenotypes of human disease. Transplantable tumor models derived from murine cells may also share many molecular, histological, and biological features with the particular human cancer they attempt to present.

The xenograft tumor models, in which tumor cells are transplanted subcutaneously or orthotopically (injecting tumor cells into the tissue or organ of their origin) in mice, are usually used for secondary cancer prevention research and particularly for cancer therapeutic research. The advantages of subcutaneously transplantable tumor models are that these models are convenient, faster, and less expensive, and the antitumor activity of testing agents can be established by measuring tumor size. However, subcutaneous tumor models are devoid of natural stromal–epithelial interactions and paracrine growth factor functions that influence tumor growth and metastatic dissemination. Some tumors are difficult to grow subcutaneously, although improved subcutaneous growth of some tumors may be accomplished by injecting cells suspended in Matrigel.

The biological potential of tumor cells is best evaluated at the organ site orthotopic to the tumor cells. Studies have documented site-specific differences in the potential of tumor cell growth. Although many human cancer cells are transplantable, their invasive and metastatic potential depends on both their intrinsic properties and the host environment at the inoculation site. Orthotopic implantation often enhances tumorigenic or metastatic potential (Sato et al., 1997). In comparison with the subcutaneous tumor model, the orthotopic tumor model is more clinically relevant in resembling stromal–epithelial cell interactions, presence of endogenous factors (growth factors, angiogenic factors, etc.), retention of original histological characteristics of the tumor, and presence of extracellular matrix molecules and receptors.

One obvious drawback of xenograft transplantable tumor models is that tumors need to be developed in immune-deficient animals that lack host-versus-graft interactions. Therefore, immune modulation–based regimens related to tumorigenesis and metastasis cannot be evaluated in human cancer cell–based xenograft tumor models. However, the effects of immune modulation agents on tumorigenesis can be evaluated in syngeneic models. Syngeneic models in immunocompetent animals provide the appropriate immunological compatibility between tumor cells and the animal that more closely exemplifies the human and clinical physiology. Another limitation of xenograft tumor models is that because of the *in vitro* culturing process, clones are selected and may not be necessarily similar to the original clones obtained from patients; thus, these models may not necessarily reflect tumor development in humans. Xenograft tumor models, derived in both immune-deficient and syngeneic animals, have been used considerably for testing diverse therapeutic agents and chemopreventive agents.

Genetically Engineered Mouse (GEM) Tumor Models

With advancement of transgenic and knockout technologies, combined with tissue-specific promoters and tissue-specific gene ablation, a new generation of mouse models has emerged. Compared with other tumor models, the GEM tumor models have several distinct advantages. The GEM models develop spontaneous tumors that progress through a well-defined temporal series of stages leading to invasive carcinoma formation, thus allowing evaluation of stage-specific preventive and therapeutic approaches. The GEM models also have intact immune systems, thus permitting evaluation of therapeutic/preventive modalities designed to augment the host immune system surveillance and response to cancer.

The GEM models have been shown to facilitate detailed investigation, such as the identification of a range of discrete molecular and histological stages that occur during tumor initiation and progression. In addition, the GEM models have been utilized increasingly for assessing the inhibitory effects of nutritional and chemopreventive agents on well-defined oncogenic signaling pathways. They are particularly useful for determining cancer stage–specific responses to nutritional and chemopreventive agents.

ORGAN-SPECIFIC ANIMAL TUMOR MODELS

In this section, the animal models for different cancer types, especially for breast and prostate cancers, are discussed for their representative characteristics. Considering that both spontaneous and hormone-/chemical carcinogen–induced tumor models have been extensively reviewed previously by other investigators, the major efforts in this chapter are given to discussion of orthotopic tumor models and genetically engineered animal tumor models, whereas other animal models are briefly summarized.

Animal Models for Breast Cancer (BRCA)

BRCA is a major public health concern in the United States and is the second highest cause of cancer death in women (American Cancer Society, 2005). These statistics highlight the need to further develop methods for the treatment and prevention of BRCA. About two thirds of BRCA are estrogen receptor (ER) positive and depend on estrogens for growth. For estrogen-dependent BRCA, antiestrogens such as tamoxifen (TAM) are effective for prevention and treatment (Fisher et al., 1996, 1998). But these tumors eventually develop TAM-resistant phenotype (Muss, 1992). In addition, not all ER-positive breast tumors respond to TAM treatment. In fact, nearly 40% of ER-positive BRCA does not respond to TAM (Karamura et al., 1989; Jaiyesimi et al., 1995). For ER-negative BRCA, there have been no effective preventive or therapeutic modalities. Thus, chemopreventive agents with the potential to prevent ER-positive, ER-positive but TAM-insensitive, TAM-resistant, and ER-negative BRCA are urgently necessary. Application of clinically relevant animal models that represent these phenotypes is expected to facilitate development of effective regimens for prevention of these BRCA phenotypes.

Hormone- and Chemical Carcinogen–Induced Mammary Tumor Models

Hormone- and chemical carcinogen–induced mammary tumor models have been widely used in preclinical research. 7,12-Dimethylbenz[a]-anthracene–induced mammary tumorigenesis in rats, in particular, has been the most commonly used mammary tumor model. In studies, this model closely recapitulated the disease progression ranging from intraductal proliferation, carcinoma *in situ*, and invasion/metastasis, and the tumors were hormone sensitive (Russo and Russo, 1987). Angiogenic activity was well characterized in this model (Heffelfinger et al., 2000), and progression was known to be dependent on both estrogen stimulation and vascular growth (Heffelfinger et al., 2003, 2004).

The estrogen-induced mammary cancer in female ACI rats appears to be another useful and physiologically relevant animal model for study of BRCA. Ovary-intact ACI rats developed relatively rapid and spontaneous mammary tumors after continuous estradiol treatment (Shull et al., 1997; Shull et al., 2001). Palpable tumors were noted after 14 weeks of estradiol treatment with mean latency of 20 weeks, and all animals developed tumors after 28 weeks (Shull et al., 1997). However, no palpable tumors were found in estradiol-treated ovariectomized ACI rats after 20 weeks, although the mammary tissue of these rats showed hyperplasia treatment (Shull et al., 1997). This observation suggests that ovariectomization may eliminate other critical factors for estrogen-dependent breast tumor development other than estrogens, thus ovariectomization may not be appropriate for manipulating estrogen levels in estrogen-dependent BRCA models.

Orthotopic Breast Tumor Models

Although subcutaneous implantation of tumor cells to develop a tumor model has been widely used, it is generally accepted that implantation of breast tumor cells into mammary fat pads to develop breast tumor is clinically more relevant. Human BRCA cell lines, representing differential phenotypic features, are implanted into the mammary fat pad of immune-deficient animals for development of breast tumor models. Among different human breast cancer cell lines, the MCF-7 cell line is the most widely used to develop an estrogen-dependent breast tumor model. MCF-7 tumors represent the characteristics of estrogen-dependent human breast tumors such as the expression of functional ERs (ER-α and ER-β).

Caution is necessary in using this animal model for estrogen manipulation, especially in mimicking estrogen status of postmenopausal women. Ovariectomization is usually used to manipulate estrogen levels, and circulating estrogen concentrations are similar to those in postmenopausal women. But several lines of evidence suggest that ovariectomization of the mouse bearing the MCF-7 tumor may not be relevant to postmenopausal women with estrogen-dependent BRCA. First, development of the MCF-7 tumor in ovary-intact female mice requires additional estrogens despite that circulating estrogen levels in intact mice are similar to those in premenopausal women (Soule and McGrath, 1980; Zhou et al., 2004a). Much higher circulating estrogen levels in female mice are necessary to support MCF-7 tumor growth (Zhou et al., 2004a), and removal of estrogen pellets in intact female mice stops MCF-7 tumor growth (Soule and McGrath, 1980). Conversely, estrogen-dependent breast tumors develop and progress in postmenopausal women, suggesting that estrogen levels even in postmenopausal women are sufficient to support growth of estrogen-dependent breast tumors. If this effect indicates that tumor-stimulating estrogen bioactivity in mice might be lower than that in women, then clinically relevant animal models of estrogen-dependent breast cancer should contain estrogen levels adequate to support tumor growth. Second, ovariectomization may add another artificial factor to this model. It has been shown that estrogen supplementation induces development of mammary tumors only in the ovary-intact, not in ovariectomized, ACI rats (Shull et al., 1997). Therefore, use of intact animals more closely resembles humans with BRCA. Third, despite reduced circulating estrogen levels in postmenopausal women, adipose tissues such as breast tissue have adequate levels of estrogen because of increased estrogen production via aromatase activity. Indeed, aromatase inhibitors have been shown to be effective, even more effective than TAM, for inhibiting estrogen-dependent breast tumors in postmenopausal women (Winer et al., 2004; Wong et al., 2004), suggesting that localized production of estrogen from adipose tissue may play a more important role in breast tumor growth in postmenopausal women. However, this increased local production of estrogen does not occur in the ovariectomized mouse because of lack of aromatase activity in mouse adipose tissues. These lines of evidence suggest that ovariectomization of MCF-7–bearing mice does not resemble estrogen-dependent BRCA in postmenopausal women, and that clinically relevant animal models for estrogen-dependent BRCA should maintain adequate estrogen levels.

We used a clinically relevant MCF-7 tumor animal model to evaluate the cancer prevention activity of soy and tea components, alone and in combination, on estrogen-dependent breast tumors, and found that the combination of soy and tea bioactive compounds synergistically inhibited the growth of MCF-7 tumors (Zhou et al., 2004a). By using the same animal model, Shao et al. (1998) found that the soy isoflavone genistein significantly inhibited MCF-7 tumor growth, whereas studies using an estrogen-depleted ovariectomized animal model showed that genistein or genistein-containing soy protein stimulated the growth of estrogen-dependent MCF-7 tumors (Hsieh et al., 1998; Ju et al., 2001; Allred et al., 2001a,b).

Transgenic Mouse Models of Multiple-Stage Mammary Carcinogenesis

Transgenic animals, with overexpression or activation of oncogenes and genes implicated to be important in human cancer, have been shown to produce mammary carcinomas that recapitulate human BRCA. One common theme evident from these studies is the complex, multistep nature of all stages of BRCA progression from initiation to metastasis. Several transgenic mouse models for mammary carcinogenesis have been developed and well characterized, and some of them have been applied to evaluate the efficacy of nutritional prevention and intervention regimens. Among those models, three well-characterized transgenic mouse models are discussed here. They are the mouse mammary tumor virus-erbB2 (MMTV-erbB2) transgenic mouse model, the MMTV-Polyma virus middle T (MMTV-PyVT) transgenic mouse model, and the C3(1)-simian virus 40 T antigen (C3(1)/SV40 Tag) transgenic mouse model.

Among transgenic mouse models for BRCA, the epidermal growth factor receptor (EGFR) transgenic mouse model has been the most frequently studied. The EGFR family is composed of four closely related receptors, including EGFR/erbB1, HER2/erbB2, HER3/erbB3, and HER4/erbB4, which use tyrosine kinase activity as the signal transduction trigger. The EGFR pathway contributes to a number of processes involved in tumor survival and growth, including cell proliferation and inhibition of apoptosis, angiogenesis, and metastasis, thus making it an attractive target for cancer prevention and treatment. The MMTV-erbB2 transgenic mouse model develops focal mammary tumors at 4 months of age, with a median incidence of 205 days. Metastasis occurs in most untreated mice by 9 months of age. The MMTV-erbB2 transgenic mouse model has been widely used to evaluate the effects of dietary and nutritional components, such as soy isoflavones (Jin and MacDonald, 2002) and soy meals (Yang et al., 2003), on BRCA prevention. It should be noted that MMTV-erbB2 transgenic mice develop ER-negative mammary tumors (Wu et al., 2002).

The MMTV-PyVT transgenic mouse model, which expresses the PyVT antigen, is one of the most widely used transgenic models of mammary tumorigenesis (Siegel et al., 2000). The model has been used as a surrogate for c-erbB2/HER2 because its middle T gene product functionally mimics erbB2. The PyVT system has exhibited the most rapid neoplastic progression in models using mammary transgenes (Cardiff and Munn, 1995). The PyVT transgenic mice initially developed a normal mammary tree. However, within 5 weeks of birth, the females developed multifocal mammary tumors and ultimately pulmonary metastases. Tumor growth was angiogenesis dependent (LeVoyer et al., 2001), and estrogen regulated angiogenesis in this system (Dabrosin, 2003). However, because tumor induction is so rapid in this transgenic mouse model, this model may not be appropriate for evaluating the efficacy of nutritional prevention regimens.

Another well-characterized transgenic mammary tumor model is the female C3(1)/SV40 Tag transgenic mouse model. This model develops atypia of the mammary ductal epithelium at about 2 months, progressing to mammary intraepithelial neoplasia that resembles human ductal carcinoma *in situ* by 3 months of age (Cardiff et al., 2000). Mammary intraepithelial neoplasia lesions progressed into invasive mammary carcinomas at 4 months of age in 100% of female mice. By 6 months of age, all of the female mice died because of universal development of multifocal mammary adenocarcinomas, with about a 15% incidence of lung metastasis (Maroulakou et al., 1994; Green et al., 2000). Although mammary tumor development appeared hormone responsive at early stages, invasive carcinomas were hormone independent, which corresponded to the loss of ER-α expression during tumor progression. This model can be used to study molecular and biological factors related to mammary tumor progression and to evaluate the efficacy of nutritional intervention and prevention strategies because lesions evolve over a predictable time course.

In summary, a series of animal models have been developed to recapitulate breast carcinogenesis and tumorigenesis processes. The 7,12-dimethylbenz[a]-anthracene–induced mammary tumor model provides a relevant animal model and is among the most commonly used models to evaluate chemopreventive agents. Transplantable breast tumor models, especially orthotopic tumor models, are extensively used in studying secondary preventive effects of chemo or nutritional components on the growth and metastasis of breast tumors. With the development of cancer cell lines that represent differential phenotypic characters, orthotopic implantation tumor models will continue to play a key role in evaluating the effects of nutritional components on the prevention of breast tumors with specific phenotypes. Transgenic mouse models for BRCA play an increasingly important role in evaluating the preventive role of nutritional components in breast tumors at different stages of breast tumorigenesis processes, especially in breast tumors that are initiated and developed by certain genetic alterations. On the other hand, each model has inherited limitations, and care should be taken in selecting appropriate animal models on the basis of specific research purposes.

Animal Models for Prostate Cancer (CaP)

CaP is the most common cancer and the second leading cause of cancer-related death among the U.S. men (American Cancer Society, 2005). In humans, CaP progresses from precursor lesions that are termed *prostatic intraepithelial neoplasia* (PIN) to carcinoma that is confined to the prostate and finally to metastatic disease that often results in lethality. Early, organ-confined disease is typically diagnosed by prostate-specific antigen (PSA) screening and/or digital rectal examination and treated by radical prostatectomy or radiation therapy. Metastatic disease, with primary deposit sites in the skeletal bone but also in lymph nodes and lung, is treated by androgen ablation therapy. Although this hormonal manipulation is palliative in >50% of patients, its effects are usually transient because androgen-independent disease emerges. Androgen-independent, metastatic prostate cancer is refractory to current therapeutic modalities.

The etiology of CaP is largely unknown, rendering disease prevention difficult. The similarity in prevalence of clinically latent carcinomas (Breslow et al., 1977; Guileyardo et al., 1980) and the great differences in the incidence of clinically manifested carcinomas in different areas of the world indicate that nutritional and environmental factors may have important influences on the development and progression of the disease, providing rationale to search for nutritional bioactive components for CaP prevention, especially the prevention of tumor progression. Clinically relevant animal models that represent CaP histopathology are required to facilitate nutritional chemoprevention research. Although PIN occurs in men as young as in their 20s, clinically detectable CaP does not typically arise until the sixth decade; thus, clinical progression is slow and may involve multiple genetic and epigenetic events. Given the heterogeneous and multifocal nature of the disease, as well as difficulties in accessing tissue specimens displaying the earliest stages of prostate carcinogenesis, animal models can provide significant advantages for studying the molecular mechanisms of prostate carcinogenesis and for identifying nutritional chemopreventive agents.

Hormone- or Chemical Carcinogen–Induced Prostate Tumor Models

Among chemical carcinogen- and hormone-induced animal models, the Lobund–Wistar rat model has been commonly used. In this strain of rat, large primary prostate adenocarcinomas are induced at an ~78% incidence rate within an average of 10.7 months after a single dose of *N*-methyl-*N*-nitrosourea, followed by promotion with a pharmacological dose of testosterone (Pollard and Lucker, 1986, 1987). The metastasis rate in these studies was >60%. The Lobund–Wistar rats developed tumors of dorsolateral prostate rather than in the ventral prostate (Pollard and Lucker, 1986, 1987).

Besides *N*-methyl-*N*-nitrosourea, *N*-nitrosobis (2-oxopropyl) amine, 3,2′-dimethyl-4-aminobiphenyl, and 2-amino-1-methyl-6-phenylimidazo [4,5-*b*] pyridine have also been used to induce prostate carcinomas in rodents, and extensive review has been provided by other investigators (Shirai et al., 2000). Although these chemical carcinogen–induced prostate tumor models have provided a diverse array of animal models for CaP and have contributed significantly to CaP research, they usually develop multiorgan tumors and are not prostate specific. In addition, it usually takes a long time for animals to develop tumors and incidence is usually low. These limitations have prevented application of these animal models for future studies.

Orthotopic Prostate Tumor Models

Although subcutaneous implantation is commonly used to develop prostate xenografts, it is well accepted that epithelial–mesenchymal interactions play crucial roles in prostate tumor development and progression. The importance of stromal–epithelial interactions in both normal and abnormal growth of prostate is well recognized, although the precise mechanism has yet to be elucidated. It is widely recognized that a variety of growth factors are implicated in epithelial–stromal interactions. Several orthotopically implanted human prostate tumor models are established that represent diverse phenotypes of CaP. These orthotopic tumor models include ones for androgen-sensitive CaP, for androgen-independent CaP, and for progression of androgen-independent CaP by hormonal manipulation.

Orthotopic Tumor Models for Androgen-Sensitive and Androgen-Independent CaP

Although no animal model provides all of the characteristics of the human disease, androgen-regulated growth and the potential for metastasis are two clinically important characteristics that are captured in orthotopic implant models utilizing the severely combined immune deficient (SCID) mouse and the LNCaP human CaP cell line (Sato et al., 1997; Zhou et al., 2002a). In addition, this model allows the use of serum PSA as a surrogate marker for tumor growth in response to defined dietary and nutritional interventions. Orthotopic implantation of LNCaP cells results in tumor take rate of >85% and lymph nodes and lung metastases of ~50% (Sato et al., 1997; Zhou et al., 2002a). This tumor model has been widely used in our laboratory to evaluate the preventive effects of several dietary components, such as soy components, tea components, and soy and tea combinations, on the growth and metastasis of androgen-sensitive prostate tumors (Zhou et al., 2002a, 2003).

Similar to the development of the androgen-sensitive LNCaP tumor model, androgen-independent human CaP cell lines, such as PC-3 cell line (Waters et al., 1995; Stephenson et al., 1992) and DU 145 cell line (unpublished data in our laboratory), have also been used to develop orthotopic tumor models for androgen-independent CaP. Because PC-3 and DU 145 cells do not produce PSA, other blood markers are necessary to monitor tumor development and growth. One of the markers is interleukin-6 (IL-6). Both cell lines produce IL-6, and our preliminary data indicate that the blood level of IL-6 is correlated with tumor volume and may be used as a marker to monitor the effect of treatment (unpublished data).

An Orthotopic Prostate Tumor Animal Model for Progression of Androgen-Independent CaP by Hormonal Manipulation

In men, most prostate tumors respond to androgen withdrawal but relapse after the initial response. Few, if any, prostate tumors in humans have been cured by hormonal manipulation. Models for the development of experimental therapy are limited. Based on our SCID-LNCaP orthotopic tumor model (Zhou et al., 2002a), we further developed an *in vivo* animal model for human CaP progression from androgen-sensitive to androgen-independent phenotype by surgically castrating SCID mice bearing LNCaP tumors (Zhou et al., 2004b). Tumors responded to androgen ablation initially with growth regression, as measured by serum PSA levels. However, tumors started to grow back after a period of time and developed an androgen-independent phenotype. Progression of androgen-independent prostate tumors was associated with alterations of a series of tumor markers, such as tumor cell proliferation and apoptosis and androgen receptor expression (Zhou et al., 2004b). This orthotopic androgen-independent prostate tumor progression model has been used in our laboratory to evaluate the preventive effects of tea components on delaying this progressive process (Zhou et al., 2002b).

Transgenic Mouse Models of Multistage Prostate Carcinogenesis

Although mice are relatively resistant to the induction of prostatic tumors by chemical carcinogens, several transgenic mouse lines are now available in which prostate carcinomas preferentially occur. Several targeting vectors are successfully used to express heterologous genes to the prostate epithelium of transgenic mice. These include regulatory elements derived from the rat C3 (1) prostate steroid-binding protein gene, rat probasin gene, human PSA gene, and MMTV long terminal repeat. Several transgenic models that are commonly applied and well characterized are discussed. They are the transgenic adenocarcinoma of the mouse prostate (TRAMP) model, the LADY models, and the male C3 (1)/SV40 Tag model.

TRAMP Model

A transgene carrying the rat probasin gene fused to the SV40 early region has been used to generate an independent transgenic autochthonous model for CaP designated the *TRAMP transgenic line of mice* (Greenberg, 1995). The TRAMP model is one such model that mimics progressive forms of human disease. The TRAMP mice develop high-grade PIN within 12 weeks of age and extensive hyperplasia and adenocarcinomas by 18 weeks of age; by 24–30 weeks, all TRAMP male mice develop primary prostate tumors, with about half of them displaying well-differentiated prostatic adenocarcinoma and the other half divided between moderately differentiated and poorly differentiated adenocarcinoma. Metastasis is commonly detected by 30 weeks, primarily to the lungs and lymph nodes and less often to bone, kidneys, and adrenal glands (Greenberg et al., 1995; Gingrich et al., 1996, 1997). Androgen depletion by castration at age 12 weeks resulted in decreased tumor incidence to 80% but subsequently resulted in appearance of androgen-independent disease (Gingrich et al., 1997). Castrated mice developed more poorly differentiated primary tumors and twice the incidence of metastatic disease compared to noncastrated TRAMP controls.

The TRAMP model develops progressive primary prostate tumors much faster than the C3 (1)/SV40 Tag model, so it can offer a quick *in vivo* system for evaluating the preventive effects of chemopreventive agents. On the other hand, since all animals develop PIN and carcinoma of the prostate and metastases in a relatively short period, this model may not be a sensitive system for evaluating preventive activities of agents on CaP progression. This animal model has been used to evaluate the effects of a series of dietary components, such as soy isoflavones (Mentor-Marcel et al., 2001), tea polyphenols (Gupta et al., 2001), and flaxseed (Lin et al., 2002), on CaP prevention.

LADY Models

Several related transgenic lines have been developed in which a large (12-kb) region of prostate-specific rat probasin promoter drives the expression of SV40 large T antigen to the mouse prostate (Kasper et al., 1998; Masumori et al., 2001; Abate-Shen and Shen, 2002). Because this transgene lacks small *t* antigen, disease progression is less aggressive than in TRAMP mice; thus, these mice are collectively named the "LADY" model. The LADY transgenic lines display varying but reproducible rates of tumor formation, ranging from 12 weeks to >20 weeks of age. Each line consistently develops multifocal low-grade PINs that progress to high-grade PINs and early invasive carcinoma, but that generally fail to metastasize (Kasper et al., 1998; Masumori et al., 2001). Furthermore, the remarkable vascularization was accompanied by tumor growth. Similar to the TRAMP model, androgen deprivation of these transgenic mice resulted in temporary regression, followed by the formation of poorly differentiated metastatic carcinomas (Kasper et al., 1998; Masumori et al., 2001).

Compared with the TRAMP model, the "LADY" model has less aggressive disease progression and a longer period of high-grade PIN development. These features make the "LADY" model an appropriate animal model for nutritional prevention studies. In addition, the "LADY" model could serve as an appropriate preclinical model for evaluating the preventive agents that target tumor angiogenesis. However, this model has not been adequately applied in nutritional prevention studies.

Male C3 (1)/SV40 Tag Model

This is a transgenic mouse model for CaP using a recombinant gene expressing the SV40 early-region transforming sequences under the regulatory control of the androgen-responsive rat prostatic steroid binding protein (C3 [1]) gene. Male transgenic mice develop low-grade PIN in the ventral and dorsolateral lobes, which appear identical to those described for the human disease, after ~8 weeks of age (Maroulakou et al., 1994; Shibata et al., 1996). High-grade PIN was found in both lobes by 5 months of age (Shibata et al., 1996). Prostate carcinomas, which appeared to arise from PIN lesions, were found by 7 months of age in the ventral lobe and 11 months of age in the dorsolateral lobe. Metastases were rare (<5%). Apoptosis levels were quite low in normal epithelial cells, moderate in low-grade PIN, and high in high-grade PIN and carcinomas. Levels of expression of proliferating cell nuclear antigen correlated with the degree of severity of the prostate lesions.

One of the advantages of this model is that it provides a well-characterized and reliable prostate tumor progression model from low-grade PIN to high-grade PIN to focal and invasive adenocarcinoma and offers a relatively long time span between the earliest onset of PIN and the development of invasive carcinoma, which may be useful for evaluating the effects of chemopreventive agents on promotion and progression, in addition to initiation. This animal model has been used to determine the effects of several potential chemopreventive agents, including DHEA, 9-cis-retinoic acid, tocopherol acetate, and selenomethionine (Green et al., 2001), on the development and progression of CaP.

In summary, a number of rodent models of prostate carcinoma development have been established to evaluate the preventive potential of nutritional components and to study mechanisms of action. Carcinogens, especially in combination with testosterone, can induce prostate carcinomas in rats, but none are prostate specific, so tumor development in other organs is a complicating factor. Orthotopic tumor models provide clinically relevant models of tumor growth and progression/metastasis. Each of several well-characterized transgenic mouse models has strengths and weaknesses, and it is therefore necessary to select the best model for the purpose of any experimental study. Xenograft/orthotopic tumor models primarily represent late-stage and metastatic disease because cell lines used in these models are typically derived from high-grade CaP or metastatic lesions. In contrast, transgenic mouse models offer the opportunity to study the induction and early stages of prostate tumorigenesis, in addition to late-stage and hormone-refractory CaP. Despite limitations, current animal models should provide suitable *in vivo* systems for preclinical chemoprevention studies to evaluate the efficacy of nutritional components on PIN development, progression, and metastasis.

Animal Models for Bladder Cancers

Bladder cancer comprises a broad spectrum of tumors with various histological types. Transitional cell carcinomas (TCCs) are by far the more prevalent tumors and represent nearly 95% of all bladder cancers in the Western Hemisphere. About 70% of the urinary bladder TCCs are diagnosed at presentation as well-differentiated superficial lesions, and the rest correspond to highly invasive, poorly differentiated tumors with a high risk of progressing to distant metastases, thus posing a major challenge in clinical management. Although patients with superficial disease are initially responsive successfully to transurethral resection via the cystoscope and additional treatment with intravesical chemotherapy or immune therapy, these patients are at high risk (~60%) of developing recurrent superficial bladder cancer. Of those, some (10–40%) progress to invasive or metastatic disease and are, therefore, potentially lethal (Heney et al., 1983).

Bladder cancer mortality varies in different countries. The highest rates are noted in European countries such as Denmark, the United Kingdom, Belgium, and Italy, and the lowest rates come from Asian countries such as Japan, China, and Singapore (Paneau et al., 1992). Populations in Southeast Asia have 4- to 10-fold lower incidence of, and death from, bladder cancer compared with those in the United States (Silverman et al., 1992). Asian people migrating to the United States have an increased risk in one generation to equal that of the Americans (Dunn, 1975). Cigarette smoking is the major risk factor in affluent nations, and exposure to chemical carcinogens in the environment, particularly the workplace, is also a contributing factor (Paneau et al., 1992; Nakata et al., 1995). However, definite etiology for bladder cancer is still unknown.

The role of nutritional manipulation in prevention of bladder cancer has not been well studied, primarily due to lack of appropriate animal models. Although chemical carcinogen–induced bladder tumor models have been primarily applied in bladder cancer research, these models have major weaknesses including low incidence, long periods of carcinogenesis, and tumors not being organ specific. Development of orthotopic bladder tumor models and transgenic mouse models may provide a necessary *in vivo* system to evaluate the chemopreventive role of nutritional components in bladder cancer.

Chemical Carcinogenesis Models

Of the several experimental models of urinary bladder cancer, the *N*-butyl-*N*-(4-hydroxybutyl)nitrosamine (OH-BBN)–induced cancer model has been most widely used for chemoprevention studies. In male C57BL/6 mice, intragastric administration of OH-BBN resulted in the induction of both squamous cell carcinomas (60%) and TCCs (Becci et al., 1978). These carcinomas were highly metastatic; the majority of tumors showed invasion of the bladder muscle wall. Because the majority of human urinary bladder carcinomas are of the transitional cell type, a mouse model in which the induced tumors are TCCs was developed by intragastric administration of OH-BBN to male C57BL/6 × DBA2-F1 mice (Becci et al., 1981). It developed highly invasive urinary bladder carcinomas that are morphologically similar to a human variant of advanced urinary bladder TCC (Becci et al., 1981). However, tumor incidence rate in the C57BL/6 × DBA2-F1 mouse model was only 24% (Grubbs et al., 1993).

Orthotopic Tumor Models

Animal models for orthotopic xenograft bladder tumors have been established previously by using both murine and human bladder cancer cells (Dinney et al., 1995; Jiang and Zhou, 1997; Oshinsky et al., 1995; Wu et al., 2003). Overall, orthotopic implantation of bladder cancer cells results in better tumor take rates and more metastasis, compared with subcutaneous implantation. Human cancer cells that represent different phenotypes of bladder cancer can be used to establish orthotopic tumor models.

Nutritional preventive efficacy on bladder cancer is best evaluated in clinically relevant orthotopic bladder tumor animal models. However, these animal models have not been applied for nutritional prevention studies. We hypothesize that these orthotopic bladder tumor models are particularly relevant for evaluating the efficacy of nutritional components on bladder cancer because dietary bioactive components/metabolites exert their effects via both circulation and direct contact with the mucosa of the bladder. Urinary levels of dietary bioactive components and their metabolites are correlated with dietary levels and could reach much higher than blood levels; thus, bladder cancer may be a unique cancer type that is particularly sensitive to dietary prevention strategies. We used an orthotopic bladder tumor model to evaluate the effects of soy components on prevention of a poorly differentiated human bladder tumor (Zhou et al., 2001; Singh et al., 2006) and found that soy phytochemicals were potent in inhibiting the growth and metastasis of bladder tumors. To our knowledge, this is the first *in vivo* study to use an orthotopic bladder tumor model to evaluate the efficacy of dietary/nutritional components on bladder cancer prevention. This orthotopic human bladder tumor model should provide a clinically relevant experimental tool for assessing the potential preventive activity of other dietary components against bladder tumor growth and metastasis.

Transgenic Mouse Tumor Models

Several genetically modified animal models have been developed that mimic multistep carcinogenesis of bladder cancer. Transgenic mice bearing the SV40 T transgene developed bladder carcinoma *in situ* and invasive and metastatic TCCs, depending on transgene copy numbers (Zhang et al., 1999). In a similar SV40 large T antigen transgenic mouse model, transgenic mice developed highly invasive bladder neoplasms that resemble invasive human bladder TCCs. Stages of disease progression included development of carcinoma *in situ*, stromal invasion, muscle invasion, rapid growth, and intravascular lung metastasis (Grippo and Sandgren, 2000). A transgenic mouse model with urothelial overexpression of EGFR developed hyperplasia but not carcinoma (Cheng et al., 2002). Coexpression of EGFR with the SV40 large T antigen in double transgenic mice accelerated tumor growth and converted the carcinoma *in situ* of the SV40 mice into high-grade bladder carcinomas (Cheng et al., 2002). However, these transgenic mouse models have not been used in evaluating the efficacy of nutritional components on bladder cancer prevention studies.

In summary, chemical-induced bladder carcinogenesis animal models have been the primary *in vivo* systems for studying the role of nutritional components in bladder cancer prevention. Despite availability of a series of human bladder cancer cell lines with different phenotypic features, orthotopic bladder tumor models have not been adequately applied for nutritional prevention studies. Limited studies have been conducted using transgenic mouse models to identify dietary and nutritional components for prevention of bladder cancer. Future application of these models to identify potent nutritional and dietary components is expected to have a significant impact on bladder cancer prevention.

Animal Models for Lung Cancer

Lung cancer is the leading cause of cancer death in both men and women in the United States. Epithelial neoplasms of the lung are pathologically described as either non–small cell lung carcinoma (80%) or small cell carcinoma (20%), and this distinction is important clinically because of their different responses to therapy. The three main types of non–small cell lung carcinoma are adenocarcinoma (30–40%), squamous cell carcinoma (20–25%), and large cell carcinoma (15–20%).

Cigarette smoking is a major etiological factor. Although the lung cancer risk in ex-smokers gradually declines over the years, it remains substantial compared with those who have never been smokers. Thus, approaches to the prevention of lung cancer need to be developed so that they can be implemented to benefit this high-risk population, especially efforts targeted to the progression of preneoplastic and benign neoplastic lesions to more malignant lung tumors. Despite the significant health risk of lung cancer, no effective chemopreventive agent or dietary component has been identified in human trials, in part because of scarcity of information from studies in animals. Successful identification of effective nutritional components for lung cancer prevention, especially for prevention of smoking-related lung carcinogenesis, requires systematic *in vivo* evaluation by using clinically relevant animal models.

Chemical Carcinogen–Induced Lung Cancer Models

The most commonly used animal model for lung cancer is the A/J mouse model. The A/J mouse has a hereditary predisposition for lung cancer, the so-called *pulmonary adenoma susceptibility* gene. This strain is particularly sensitive to develop spontaneous lung tumor (Shimkin, 1955). The A/J mouse is also sensitive to chemical-induced lung cancer. A wide variety of chemicals, such as urethane and constituents of tobacco smoke (polyaromatic hydrocarbons and nitrosamines), stimulated lung tumorigenesis as initiators and/or promoters of lung tumorigenesis by accelerating tumor onset and increasing tumor multiplicity (Shimkin and Stoner, 1975). Because smoke is a major risk factor, the lung tumorigenesis in the A/J mouse induced by tobacco smoke–related chemical carcinogens is considered particularly relevant. The commonly used tobacco smoke constituents include 4-methyl-(nitrosamino)-1-(3-pyridyl)-1-butanone (NNK) and benzo(a)pyrene (BaP). In the A/J mouse induced by NNK and BaP, adenoma appeared during weeks 16–19 after administration of tobacco carcinogens; adenocarcinomas occurred during weeks 28–36 (Hecht et al., 1989; Foley et al., 1991; Belinsky et al., 1993).

The chemical-induced lung tumorigenesis in the A/J mouse model is a well established animal model, and it is the most frequently employed murine model for preclinical chemoprevention studies. This animal model has been used to evaluate the chemopreventive activity of nutritional components, such as black tea extract (Yang et al., 1998), green tea (Lubet et al., 2000), lycopene (Kim et al., 2000), and perillyl alcohol (Lantry et al., 1997) on lung carcinogenesis. On the other hand, since the tumors developed are mainly squamous cell carcinoma, this model may only represent a small proportion of lung cancer. In addition, although tobacco smoke constituents, such as NNK and BaP, are commonly used to induce lung tumors in this model, the gas phase of tobacco smoke, which has markedly reduced levels of NNK and BaP, also induces lung tumorigenesis (Witschi et al., 1997), suggesting that multiple components present in tobacco smoke and their interaction may be responsible for lung tumorigenesis.

The ferret model is another relevant lung carcinogenesis animal model, primarily because of the similarities between ferret and human in absorption and accumulation of some phytochemicals such as carotenoids (Ferreira et al., 2000; Wang et al., 1992), lung architecture, and cigarette smoke–induced lung pathology (Wang et al., 1999). Ferrets exposed to smoke for 9 weeks showed squamous metaplasia lesions (Liu et al., 2003). One of the particularly interesting findings using this animal model is that supplementation of β-carotene to ferrets resulted in increased cell proliferation and squamous metaplasia formation, and these responses were enhanced by exposure to tobacco smoke (Wang et al., 1999). These findings were consistent with the findings in the Beta-Carotene and Retinol Efficacy Trial (CARET) in which β-carotene supplementation to high-risk smokers resulted in a 28% increase in the incidence of lung cancer (Omenn et al., 1996).

Orthotopic Tumor Models

Although subcutaneous implantation is commonly used to establish the lung cancer model for prevention and treatment studies, orthotopic lung tumor models have also been developed. Orthotopic lung tumor animal models were developed by intrapulmonary injection of lung cancer cells representing different phenotypes (Hastings et al., 2000; Yamaura et al., 2000; Chan et al., 2002; Mase et al., 2002; Onn et al., 2003; Kondo et al., 2004) or orthotopic implantation of lung tumors via thoracotomy (Wang et al., 1992). These orthotopic tumor models demonstrate different degrees of metastasis to other organs. In particular, subcutaneous and orthotopic lung tumor models showed differential therapeutic responses to paclitaxel (Onn et al., 2003), suggesting that the orthotopic tumor model is more clinically relevant. However, these orthotopic lung tumor models have not been used to evaluate the chemopreventive effects of nutritional and dietary components.

Transgenic Mouse Models

Human lung carcinogenesis and tumorigenesis is associated with alteration of several genes, such as k-ras, p53, and Ink4A/Arf. Thus, genetically modified lung tumor mouse models are developed on the basis of the function of these genes. In particular, p53 mutations play an important role in tobacco smoke–related carcinogenesis. The p53 mutant transgenic mouse was more susceptible than the wild-type p53 mouse to a number of lung carcinogens, including those from tobacco smoke, NNK, and/or BaP and developed more and larger tumors (Lubet et al., 2000). This NNK-induced lung tumor p53 mutant mouse model was used to determine the chemopreventive effect of green tea (Lubet et al., 2000). The mouse model that was derived from crossing of p53 mutant transgenic mouse and the A/J mouse further increased susceptibility to lung tumor induction (Zhang et al., 2000). This model may be an appropriate lung tumor model for dietary and nutritional prevention studies.

In a similar approach, a double genetically modified mouse model was developed by crossing a p53 transgenic mouse carrying a dominant-negative mutation with the Ink4A/Arf heterozygous–deficient mouse (Wang et al., 2003). Because p53 and Ink4a/Arf mutations are the most prevalent mutations in human lung cancers, the mutant A/J mouse containing alterations with p53 and Ink4a/Arf may serve as a more relevant preclinical system than the standard A/J mouse model to evaluate the efficacy of chemopreventive agents (Lubet et al., 2004).

In summary, despite availability of clinically relevant orthotopic and genetically modified lung tumor animal models, these models have not been adequately applied to identify bioactive dietary and nutritional components for lung cancer prevention. Application of available animal models of lung tumorigenesis should advance identification of potent dietary and nutritional components.

FUTURE RESEARCH DIRECTIONS

It is evident from the models outlined here that it is important to consider many factors when assessing the applicability of a mouse model for cancer research to human cancer. While laboratory animals differ from humans in some respects that may affect responses to hazardous exposure and chemopreventive agents, such models share substantial similarities to humans in genetic, genomic, physiological, biochemical, and metabolic aspects. Animal models with specific phenotypic characteristics have been used and will continue to be used as a major modality to identify chemopreventive agents. On the other hand, it is notable that no current model can recapitulate all features of cancer initiation and progression. The genetically modified animal models are developed on the basis of modification of genes that are involved in the later stages of tumorigenesis. Similarly, orthotopic xenograft models and syngeneic models are more suitable as cancer progression models, rather than cancer initiation or promotion models. With advancement of our understanding of the mechanisms related to cancer initiation and promotion, development of animal models that recapitulate early stages of carcinogenesis and tumorigenesis should be one of the priorities of future research. In addition, future research on nutritional prevention of cancer should emphasize the combined effects of nutritional components. In this section, several future priorities in nutritional oncology research are identified.

Development of New Animal Models for Nutritional Cancer Prevention Research

One of the research priorities should be further development of clinically relevant animal models that recapitulate cancer initiation and promotion processes, based on our understanding of molecular mechanisms that are critical for early development of carcinogenesis. For example, epigenetic alterations are suggested to play a key role in early carcinogenesis, so one of the animal models to be developed should include that in which carcinogenesis is derived by epigenetic alteration. Genetic modification of animals should play a key role in the development of this type of model.

It is commonly investigated that carcinogenesis or tumorigenesis is associated with alterations of multiple genes. Although current genetically modified mouse models are achieved by a single gene modification, it may be more appropriate for models to be developed through modification of multiple genes. Therefore, another type of animal model that needs to be developed should be derived by modification of multiple genes. The crossing of genetically modified animals may provide a useful modality for development of the animal models with multiple genetic modifications.

Evaluation of the Efficacy of Nutritional Cancer Prevention Strategies

One of the future directions is to apply relevant animal models for systematic evaluation of the efficacy of nutritional regimens for cancer prevention. Preclinical efficacy testing of nutritional regimens for cancer prevention should progress through a series of models that include genetically modified animal models and orthotopic tumor models. Genetically modified animal models play a key role in identifying effective regimens for both primary and secondary prevention, while orthotopic tumor models are important for evaluating the efficacy of nutritional regimens on secondary prevention.

Considerable data from animal studies indicate that combinations of agents can be more effective for cancer prevention than any single constituent (Chemoprevention Working Group, 1999). Nutritional modification has long been considered to be an effective regimen for cancer prevention. It is possible that combinations of nutritional components that target different pathways may have a synergistic/additive effect on cancer prevention. However, previous research has mainly focused on the cancer-prevention activity of single nutritional components. Thus, one of the future research priorities should emphasize combined effects of nutritional components in a synergistic manner. Application of the appropriate tumor models derived by targeting multiple genes/pathways should provide a particularly useful modality for evaluating the combined effects of nutritional components that target the modified genes/pathways.

Biomarker Identification and Validation

Along with efficacy evaluation, one of the future research efforts should be identification and validation of the biomarkers that are responsible for the effective cancer prevention activity of the nutritional regimen. Traditional methods of analysis of gene expression patterns have imposed a practical limit on the number of candidate genes. The marriage of mouse tumor models for efficacy evaluation of nutritional regimens with rapidly evolving methods to profile genetic and epigenetic alterations in tumors will provide insight into the key pathways leading to carcinogenesis and tumorigenesis and will hold great promise for identifying relevant biomarkers. Functional analysis of identified genes by application of strategies for short-term or permanent phenotype alteration, such as siRNA and anti-sense, can help to validate the identified biomarkers that may be used as surrogate intermediate markers in the future clinical investigation.

Clinical Prevention Studies

With identification of effective prevention regimens by animal studies, appropriate clinical prevention studies should be considered to assess the effects of these nutritional regimens. The gold standard is still the randomized, double-blinded, and placebo-controlled intervention trial in normal populations. However, the high cost and long duration of this type of trial prohibit common use of this study design. Alternative trials with short and intermediate duration using smaller cohorts of a subgroup of cancer patients or subjects with high risk of developing cancer may provide excellent and cost-effective approaches for efficacy testing. For example, cohorts for CaP prevention may be patients with early-stage cancers scheduled for prostatectomy or patients with PIN. Presurgical BRCA patients and patients with ductal or lobular carcinoma *in situ* may be cohorts for nutritional prevention studies in BRCA. Patients with superficial bladder cancers, such as Ta/T1 with or without carcinoma *in situ*, could be cohorts for studies of nutritional prevention in bladder cancer. These trials are essential in the development of effective nutritional regimens for cancer prevention.

CONCLUSIONS

Chemoprevention through nutritional or dietary manipulation may offer an important means of inhibiting the development and progression of cancer. Development of effective nutritional components for cancer chemoprevention requires conclusive evidence of their efficacy in animal models that closely emulate human disease. We have provided the strengths and limitations of commonly used and well-characterized tumor models. This chapter should provide a guideline for selecting appropriate animal tumor models and for designing research protocols for evaluation of the efficacy of nutritional components that target specific carcinogenesis and tumorigenesis processes.

References

Allred, C.D., Ju, Y.H., Allred, K.F., Chang, J., and Helferich, W.G. 2001a. Dietary genistin stimulates growth of estrogen-dependent breast cancer tumors similar to that observed with genistein. *Carcinogenesis* **22**: 1667–1673.

Allred, C.D., Allred, K.F., Ju, Y.H., Virant, S.M., and Helferich, W.G. 2001b. Soy diets containing varying amounts of genistein stimulate growth of estrogen-dependent (MCF-7) tumors in a dose-dependent manner. *Cancer Res* **61**: 5045–5050.

Abate-Shen, C., and Shen, M.M. 2002. Mouse models of prostate carcinogenesis. *Trends Genet* **18**: S1–S5.

American Cancer Society. 2005. "Cancer Facts and Figures 2005." American Cancer Society, Atlanta, GA.

Becci, P.J., Thompson, H.J., Grubbs, C.J., Squire, R.A., Brown, C.C., Sporn, M.B., *et al.* 1978. Inhibitory effect of 13-cis-retinoic acid on urinary bladder carcinogenesis induced in C57BL/6 mice by N-butyl-N-(4-hydroxybutyl)-nitrosamine. *Cancer Res* **38**: 4463–4466.

Becci, P.J., Thompson, H.J., Strum, J.M., Brown, C.C., Sporn, M.B., and Moon, R.C. 1981. N-butyl-N-(4-hydroxybutyl)nitrosamine-induced urinary bladder cancer in C57BL/6 X DBA/2 F1 mice as a useful model for study of chemoprevention of cancer with retinoids. *Cancer Res* **41**: 927–932.

Belinsky, S.A., Stefanski, S.A., and Anderson, M.W. 1993. The A/J mouse lung as a model for developing new chemointervention strategies. *Cancer Res* **53**: 410–416.

Breslow, N.E., Chan, C.W., Dhom, G., *et al.* 1977. Latent carcinoma of prostate at autopsy in seven areas. *Int J Cancer* **20**: 680–688.

Cardiff, R.D., and Munn, R.J. 1995. Comparative pathology of mammary tumorigenesis in transgenic mice. *Cancer Lett* **90**: 13–19.

Cardiff, R.D., Anver, M.R., Gusterson, B.A., Hennighausen, L., Jensen, R.A., Merino, M.J., *et al.* 2000. The mammary pathology of genetically engineered mice: the consensus report and recommendations from the Annapolis meeting. *Oncogene* **19**: 968–988.

Chan, D.C., Earle, K.A., Zhao, T.L., Helfrich, B., Zeng, C., Baron, A., *et al.* 2002. Exisulind in combination with docetaxel inhibits growth and metastasis of human lung cancer and prolongs survival in athymic nude rats with orthotopic lung tumors. *Clin Cancer Res* **8**: 904–912.

Chemoprevention Working Group. 1999. Prevention of cancer in the next millennium: report of the chemoprevention working group to the American Association for Cancer Research. *Cancer Res* **59**: 4743–4758.

Cheng, J., Huang, H., Zhang, Z.T., Shapiro, E., Pellicer, A., Sun, T.T., *et al.* 2002. Overexpression of epidermal growth factor receptor in urothelium elicits urothelial hyperplasia and promotes bladder tumor growth. *Cancer Res* **62**: 4157–4163.

Dabrosin, C., Palmer, K., Muller, W.J., and Gauldie, J. 2003. Estradiol promotes growth and angiogenesis in polyoma middle T transgenic mouse mammary tumor explants. *Breast Cancer Res Treat* **78**: 1–6.

Dinney, C.P., Fishbeck, R., Singh, R.K., Eve, B., Pathak, S., Brown, N., *et al.* 1995. Isolation and characterization of metastatic variants from human transitional cell carcinoma passaged by orthotopic implantation in athymic nude mice. *J Urol* **154**: 1532–1538.

Dunn, J.E. 1975. Cancer epidemiology in populations of the United States—with emphasis on Hawaii and California—and Japan. *Cancer Res* **35**: 3240–3245.

Ferreira, A.L., Yeum, K.J., Liu, C., Smith, D., Krinsky, N.I., Wang, X.D., *et al.* 2000. Tissue distribution of lycopene in ferrets and rats after lycopene supplementation. *J Nutr* **130**: 1256–1260.

Fisher, B., Dignam, J., Bryant, J., DeCillis, A., Wickerham, D.L., Wolmark, N., *et al.* 1996. Five vs more than five years of tamoxifen therapy for breast cancer patients with negative lymph nodes and estrogen receptor–positive tumors. *J Natl Cancer Inst* **88**: 1529–1542.

Fisher, B., Costantino, J.P., Wickerham, D.L., Redmond, C.K., Kavanah, M., Cronin, W.M., *et al.* (1998). Tamoxifen for prevention of breast cancer: report of the National Surgical Adjuvant Breast and Bowel Project P-1 Study. *J Natl Cancer Inst* **90**: 1371–1388.

Foley, J.F., Anderson, M.W., Stoner, G.D., Gaul, B.W., Hardisty, J.F., and Maronpot, R.R. 1991. Proliferative lesions of the mouse lung: progression studies in strain A mice. *Exp Lung Res* **17**: 157–168.

Gingrich, J.R., Barrios, R.J., Morton, R.A., Boyce, B.F., DeMayo, F.J., Finegold, M.J., *et al.* 1996. Metastatic prostate cancer in a transgenic mouse. *Cancer Res* **56**: 4096–4102.

Gingrich, J.R., Barrios, R.J., Kattan, M.W., Nahm, H.S., Finegold, M.J., and Greenberg, N.M. 1997. Androgen-independent prostate cancer progression in the TRAMP model. *Cancer Res* **57**: 4687–4691.

Green, J.E., Shibata, M.A., Yoshidome, K., Liu, M.L., Jorcyk, C., Anver, M.R., *et al.* 2000. The C3(1)/SV40 T-antigen transgenic mouse model of mammary cancer: ductal epithelial cell targeting with multistage progression to carcinoma. *Oncogene* **19**: 1020–1027.

Green, J.E., Shibata, M.A., Shibata, E., Moon, R.C., Anver, M.R., Kelloff, G., *et al.* 2001. 2-Difluoromethylornithine and dehydroepiandrosterone inhibit mammary tumor progression but not mammary or prostate tumor initiation in C3(1)/SV40 T/t-antigen transgenic mice. *Cancer Res* **61**: 7449–7455.

Greenberg, N.M., DeMayo, F., Finegold, M.J., Medina, D., Tilley, W.D., Aspinall, J.O., *et al.* 1995. Prostate cancer in a transgenic mouse. *Proc Natl Acad Sci USA* **92**: 3439–3443.

Grippo, P.J., and Sandgren, E.P. 2000. Highly invasive transitional cell carcinoma of the bladder in a simian virus 40 T-antigen transgenic mouse model. *Am J Pathol* **157**: 805–813.

Grubbs, C.J., Juliana, M.M., Eto, I., Casebolt, T., Whitaker, L.M., Canfield, G.J., *et al.* 1993. Chemoprevention by indomethacin of N-butyl-N-(4-hydroxybutyl)-nitrosamine–induced urinary bladder tumors. *Anticancer Res* **13**: 33–36.

Guileyardo, J.M., Johnson, W.D., Welsh, R.A., Akazaki, K., and Correa, P. 1980. Prevalence of latent prostate carcinoma in two U.S. populations. *J Natl Cancer Inst* **65**: 311.

Gupta, S., Hastak, K., Ahmad, N., Lewin, J.S., and Mukhtar, H. 2001. Inhibition of prostate carcinogenesis in TRAMP mice by oral infusion of green tea polyphenols. *Proc Natl Acad Sci USA* **98**: 10350–10355.

Hastings, R.H., Burton, D.W., Summers-Torres, D., Quintana, R., Biederman, E., and Deftos, L.J. 2000. Splenic, thymic, bony and lymph node metastases from orthotopic human lung carcinomas in immunocompromised mice. *Anticancer Res* **20**: 3625–3629.

Hecht, S.S., Morse, M.A., Amin, S., Stoner, G.D., Jordan, K.G., Choi, C.I., *et al.* 1989. Rapid single-dose model for lung tumor induction in A/J mice by 4-(methylnitrosamino)-1-(3-pyridyl)-1-butanone and the effect of diet. *Carcinogenesis* **10**: 1901–1904.

Heffelfinger, S.C., Gear, R.B., Taylor, K., Miller, M.A., Schneider, J., LaDow, K., *et al.* 2000. DMBA-induced mammary pathologies are angiogenic *in vivo* and *in vitro*. *Lab Invest* **80**: 485–492.

Heffelfinger, S.C., Gear, R.B., Schneider, J., LaDow, K., Yan, M., Lu, F., *et al.* 2003. TNP-470 inhibits 7,12-dimethylbenz[a]anthracene–induced mammary tumor formation when administered before the formation of carcinoma in situ but is not additive with tamoxifen. *Lab Invest* **83**: 1001–1011.

Heffelfinger, S.C., Yan, M., Gear, R.B., Schneider, J., LaDow, K., and Warshawsky, D. 2004. Inhibition of VEGFR2 prevents DMBA-induced mammary tumor formation. *Lab Invest* **84**: 989–998.

Jaiyesimi, I.A., Buzdar, A.U., Decker, D.A., and Hortobagyi, G.N. 1995. Use of tamoxifen for breast cancer: twenty-eight years later. *J Clin Oncol* **13**: 513–529.

Heney, N.M., Ahmed, S., Flanagan, M.J., Frable, W., Corder, M.P., Hafermann, M.D., *et al.* 1983. Superficial bladder cancer: progression and recurrence. *J Urol* **130**: 1083–1086.

Hsieh, C.-Y., Santell, R.C., Haslam, S.Z., and Helferich, W.G. 1998. Estrogenic effects of genistein on the growth of estrogen receptor–positive human breast cancer (MCF-7) cells *in vitro* and *in vivo*. *Cancer Res* **58**: 3833–3888.

Jiang, F., and Zhou, X.M. 1997. A model of orthotopic murine bladder (MBT-2) tumor implants. *Urol Res* **25**: 179–182.

Jin, Z., and MacDonald, R.S. 2002. Soy isoflavones increase latency of spontaneous mammary tumors in mice. *J Nutr* **132**: 3186–3190.

Ju, Y.H., Allred, C.D., Allred, K.F., Karko, K.L., Doerge, D.R., and Helferich, W.G. 2001. Physiological concentrations of dietary genistein dose-dependently stimulate growth of estrogen-dependent human breast cancer (MCF-7) tumors implanted in athymic nude mice. *J Nutr* **131**: 2957–2962.

Karamura, I., *et al.* 1989. Antiestrogenic and antitumor effects of droloxifene in experimental breast carcinoma. *Arzneimittelforschung* **39**: 889–893.

Kasper, S., Sheppard, P.C., Yan, Y., Pettigrew, N., Borowsky, A.D., Prins, G.S., *et al.* 1998. Development, progression, and androgen-dependence of prostate tumors in probasin-large T antigen transgenic mice: a model for prostate cancer. *Lab Invest* **78**: i–xv.

Kim, D.J., Takasuka, N., Nishino, H., and Tsuda, H. 2000. Chemoprevention of lung cancer by lycopene. *Biofactors* **13**: 95–102.

Kondo, K., Fujino, H., Miyoshi, T., Ishikura, H., Sakiyama, S., and Monden, Y. 2004. Orthotopically implanted SCID mouse model of human lung cancer suitable for investigating metastatic potential and anticancer drug effects. *Oncol Rep* **12**: 991–999.

Lantry, L.E., Zhang, Z., Gao, F., Crist, K.A., Wang, Y., Kelloff, G.J., *et al.* 1997. Chemopreventive effect of perillyl alcohol on 4-(methylnitrosamino)-1-(3-pyridyl)-1-butanone induced tumorigenesis in (C3H/HeJ X A/J)F1 mouse lung. *J Cell Biochem Suppl* **27**: 20–25.

Le Voyer, T., Rouse, J., Lu, Z., Lifsted, T., Williams, M., and Hunter, K.W. 2001. Three loci modify growth of a transgene-induced mammary tumor: suppression of proliferation associated with decreased microvessel density. *Genomics* **74**: 253–261.

Lin, X., Gingrich, J.R., Bao, W., Li, J., Haroon, Z.A., and Demark-Wahnefried, W. 2002. Effect of flaxseed supplementation on prostatic carcinoma in transgenic mice. *Urology* **60**: 919–924.

Liu, C., Lian, F., Smith, D.E., Russell, R.M., and Wang, X.D. 2003. Lycopene supplementation inhibits lung squamous metaplasia and induces apoptosis via up-regulating insulin-like growth factor–binding protein 3 in cigarette smoke-exposed ferrets. *Cancer Res* **63**: 3138–3144.

Lubet, R.A., Zhang, Z., Wiseman, R.W., and You, M. 2000. Use of p53 transgenic mice in the development of cancer models for multiple purposes. *Exp Lung Res* **26**: 581–593.

Lubet, R.A., Zhang, Z., Wang, Y., and You, M. 2004. Chemoprevention of lung cancer in transgenic mice. *Chest* **125**: 144S–147S.

Mase, K., Iijima, T., Nakamura, N., Takeuchi, T., Onizuka, M., Mitsui, T., *et al.* 2002. Intrabronchial orthotopic propagation of human lung adenocarcinoma—characterizations of tumorigenicity, invasion and metastasis. *Lung Cancer* **36**: 271–276.

Masumori, N., Thomas, T.Z., Chaurand, P., Case, T., Paul, M., Kasper, S., *et al.* 2001. A probasin-large T antigen transgenic mouse line develops prostate adenocarcinoma and neuroendocrine carcinoma with metastatic potential. *Cancer Res* **61**: 2239–2249.

Maroulakou, I.G., Anver, M., Garrett, L., and Green, J.E. 1994. Prostate and mammary adenocarcinoma in transgenic mice carrying a rat C3(1) simian virus 40 large tumor antigen fusion gene. *Proc Natl Acad Sci USA* **91**: 11236–11240.

Mentor-Marcel, R., Lamartiniere, C.A., Eltoum, I.E., Greenberg, N.M., and Elgavish, A. 2001. Genistein in the diet reduces the incidence of poorly differentiated prostatic adenocarcinoma in transgenic mice (TRAMP). *Cancer Research* **61**: 6777–6782.

Muss, H.B. 1992. Endocrine therapy for advanced breast cancer: a review. *Breast Cancer Res Treat* **21**: 15–26.

Nakata, S., Sato, J., Ohtake, N., Imai, K., and Yamanaka, H. 1995. Epidemiological study of risk factors for bladder cancer [in Japanese]. *Hinyokika Kiyo Acta Urologica Japonica* **41**: 969–977.

Omenn, G.S., Goodman, G.E., Thornquist, M.D., Balmes, J., Cullen, M.R., Glass, A., *et al.* 1996. Risk factors for lung cancer and for intervention effects in CARET, the Beta-Carotene and Retinol Efficacy Trial. *J Natl Cancer Inst* **88**: 1550–1559.

Onn, A., Isobe, T., Itasaka, S., Wu, W., O'Reilly, M.S., Ki Hong, W., *et al.* 2003. Development of an orthotopic model to study the biology and therapy of primary human lung cancer in nude mice. *Clin Cancer Res* **9**: 5532–5539.

Oshinsky, G.S., Chen, Y., Jarrett, T., Anderson, A.E., and Weiss, G.H. 1995. A model of bladder tumor xenografts in the nude rat. *J Urol* **154**: 1925–1929.

Paneau, C., Schaffer, P., and Bollack, C. 1992. Epidemiology of bladder cancer [in French]. *Annales d Urologie* **26**: 281–293.

Pollard, M., and Luckert, P.H. 1986. Production of autochthonous prostate cancer in Lobund-Wistar rats by treatments with N-nitroso-N-methylurea and testosterone. *Journal of the National Cancer Institute* **77**: 583–587.

Pollard, M., and Luckert, P.H. 1987. Autochthonous prostate adenocarcinomas in Lobund-Wistar rats: a model system. *Prostate* **11**: 219–227.

Russo, J., and Russo, I.H. 1987. Biological and molecular bases of mammary carcinogenesis. *Lab Invest* **57**: 112–137.

Sato, N., Gleave, M.E., Bruchovsky, N., Rennie, P.S., Beraldi, E., and Sullivan, L.D. 1997. A metastatic and androgen-sensitive human prostate cancer model using intraprostatic inoculation of LNCaP cells in SCID mice. *Cancer Res* **57**: 1584–1589.

Shao, Z.-M., Wu, J., Shen, Z.-Z., and Barsky, S.H. 1998. Genistein exerts multiple suppressive effects on human breast carcinoma cells. *Cancer Res* **58**: 4851–4857.

Shibata, M.A., Ward, J.M., Devor, D.E., Liu, M.L., and Green, J.E. 1996. Progression of prostatic intraepithelial neoplasia to invasive carcinoma in C3(1)/SV40 large T antigen transgenic mice: histopathological and molecular biological alterations. *Cancer Res* **56**: 4894–4903.

Shimkin, M.B. 1955. Pulmonary tumors in experimental animals. *Adv Cancer Res* **3**: 223–267.

Shimkin, M.B., and Stoner, G.D. 1975. Lung tumors in mice: application to carcinogenesis bioassay. *Adv Cancer Res* **21**: 1–58.

Shirai, T., Takahashi, S., Cui, L., Futakuchi, M., Kato, K., Tamano, S., *et al.* 2000. Experimental prostate carcinogenesis—rodent models. *Mutat Res* **462**: 219–226.

Shull, J.D., Spady, T.J., Snyder, M.C., Johansson, S.L., and Pennington, K.L. 1997. Ovary-intact, but not ovariectomized female ACI rats treated with 17beta-estradiol rapidly develop mammary carcinoma. *Carcinogenesis* **18**: 1595–1601.

Shull, J.D., Pennington, K.L., Reindl, T.M., Snyder, M.C., Strecker, T.E., Spady, T.J., *et al.* 2001. Susceptibility to estrogen-induced mammary cancer segregates as an incompletely dominant phenotype in reciprocal crosses between the ACI and Copenhagen rat strains. *Endocrinology* **142**: 5124–5130.

Siegel, P.M., Hardy, W.R., Muller, W.J. 2000. Mammary gland neoplasia: insights from transgenic mouse models. *Bioassays* **22**: 554–563.

Silverman, D.T., Hartge, P., Morrison, A.S., and Devesa, S.S. 1992. Epidemiology of bladder cancer. *Hematol Oncol Clin North Am* **6**: 1–30.

Singh, A.V., Franke, A.A., Blackburn, G.L., and Zhou, J.-R. 2006. Soy phytochemicals prevent orthotopic growth and metastasis of bladder cancer in mice by alterations of cancer cell proliferation and apoptosis and tumor angiogenesis. *Cancer Res,* In press.

Soule, H.D., and McGrath, C.M. 1980. Estrogen responsive proliferation of clonal human breast carcinoma cells in athymic mice. *Cancer Lett* **10**: 177–189.

Stephenson, R.A., Dinney, C.P., Gohji, K., Ordonez, N.G., Killion, J.J., and Fidler, I.J. 1992. Metastatic model for human prostate cancer using orthotopic implantation in nude mice. *J Natl Cancer Inst* **84**: 951–957.

Wang, X.D., Krinsky, N.I., Marini, R.P., Tang, G., Yu, J., Hurley, R., *et al.* 1992. Intestinal uptake and lymphatic absorption of beta-carotene in ferrets: a model for human beta-carotene metabolism. *Am J Physiol* **263**: G480–G486.

Wang, X.-D., Liu, C., Bronson, R.T., Smith, D.E., Krinsky, N.I., and and Russell, R.M. 1999. Retinoid signaling and activator protein-1 expression in ferrets given β-carotene supplements and exposed to tobacco smoke. *JNCI* **91**: 60–66.

Wang, X., Fu, X., and Hoffman, R.M. 1992. A patient-like metastasizing model of human lung adenocarcinoma constructed via thoracotomy in nude mice. *Anticancer Res* **12**: 1399–1401.

Wang, Y., Zhang, Z., Kastens, E., Lubet, R.A., and You, M. 2003. Mice with alterations in both p53 and Ink4a/Arf display a striking increase in lung tumor multiplicity and progression: differential chemopreventive effect of budesonide in wild-type and mutant A/J mice. *Cancer Res* **63**: 4389–4395.

Waters, D.J., Janovitz, E.B., and Chan, T.C. 1995. Spontaneous metastasis of PC-3 cells in athymic mice after implantation in orthotopic or ectopic microenvironments. *Prostate* **26**: 227–234.

Winer, E.P., Hudis, C., Burstein, H.J., Wolff, A.C., Pritchard, K.I., Ingle, J.N., *et al.* 2005. American Society of Clinical Oncology technology assessment on the use of aromatase inhibitors as adjuvant therapy for postmenopausal women with hormone receptor–positive breast cancer: status report 2004. *J Clin Oncol* **23**: 619–629.

Witschi, H., Espiritu, I., Maronpot, R.R., Pinkerton, K.E., and Jones, A.D. 1997. The carcinogenic potential of the gas phase of environmental tobacco smoke. *Carcinogenesis* **18**: 2035–2042.

Wong, Z.W., and Ellis, M.J. 2004. First-line endocrine treatment of breast cancer: aromatase inhibitor or antioestrogen? *Br J Cancer* **90**: 20–25.

Wu, K., Zhang, Y., Xu, X.C., Hill, J., Celestino, J., Kim, H.T., *et al.* 2002. The retinoid X receptor-selective retinoid, LGD1069, prevents the development of estrogen receptor–negative mammary tumors in transgenic mice. *Cancer Res* **62**: 6376–6380.

Wu, Q., Mahendran, R., and Esuvaranathan, K. 2003. Nonviral cytokine gene therapy on an orthotopic bladder cancer model. *Clin Cancer Res* **9**: 4522–4528.

Yamaura, T., Murakami, K., Doki, Y., Sugiyama, S., Misaki, T., Yamada, Y., *et al.* 2000. Solitary lung tumors and their spontaneous metastasis in athymic nude mice orthotopically implanted with human non–small cell lung cancer. *Neoplasia* **2**: 315–324.

Yang, C.S., Yang, G.Y., Landau, J.M., Kim, S., and Liao, J. 1998. Tea and tea polyphenols inhibit cell hyperproliferation, lung tumorigenesis, and tumor progression. *Exp Lung Res* **24**: 629–639.

Yang, X., Edgerton, S.M., Kosanke, S.D., Mason, T.L., Alvarez, K.M., Liu, N., *et al.* 2003. Hormonal and dietary modulation of mammary carcinogenesis in mouse mammary tumor virus-c-erbB-2 transgenic mice. *Cancer Res* **63**: 2425–2433.

Zhang, Z.T., Pak, J., Shapiro, E., Sun, T.T., and Wu, X.R. 1999. Urothelium-specific expression of an oncogene in transgenic mice induced the formation of carcinoma in situ and invasive transitional cell carcinoma. *Cancer Res* **59**: 3512–3517.

Zhang, Z., Liu, Q., Lantry, L.E., Wang, Y., Kelloff, G.J., Anderson, M.W., *et al.* 2000. A germ-line p53 mutation accelerates pulmonary tumorigenesis: p53-independent efficacy of chemopreventive agents green tea or dexamethasone/myo-inositol and chemotherapeutic agents taxol or adriamycin. *Cancer Res* **60**: 901–907.

Zhou, J.-R., Yu, L., Zhong, Y., and Blackburn, G.L. 2001. Soybean bioactive components inhibit the orthotopic growth of human bladder carcinoma in mice. *FASEB J* **15**: A61.

Zhou, J.-R., Yu, L., Zhong, Y., Nassr, R.L., Franke, A.A., Gaston, S.M., *et al.* 2002a. Inhibition of orthotopic growth and metastasis of androgen-sensitive human prostate tumors in mice by bioactive soybean components. *Prostate* **53**: 143–153.

Zhou, J.-R., Yu, L., and Blackburn, G.L. 2002b. Only whole black tea significantly inhibits the progression of androgen-independent human prostate tumor in an orthotopic tumor model. *FASEB J Late-Breaking Abstract* **65**: (abst #LB334).

Zhou, J.-R., Yu, L., Zhong, Y., and Blackburn, G.L. 2003. Soy phytochemicals and tea bioactive components synergistically inhibit androgen-sensitive human prostate tumors in mice. *J Nutr* **133**: 516–521.

Zhou, J.-R., Yu, L., Mai, Z., and Blackburn, G.L. 2004a. Combined inhibition of estrogen-dependent human breast carcinoma by soy and tea bioactive components in mice. *Int J Cancer* **108**: 8–14.

Zhou, J.-R., Yu, L., Zerbini, L.F., Libermann, T.A., and Blackburn, G.L. 2004b. Progression to androgen-independent LNCaP human prostate tumors: cellular and molecular alterations. *Int J Cancer* **81**: 800–806.

C H A P T E R

18

The Challenge of Nutrition in Cancer Prevention

PETER GREENWALD AND JOHN MILNER

OVERVIEW OF THE NUTRITION–CANCER RELATIONSHIP

Compelling evidence continues to accumulate to strengthen the link between diet and cancer. Information comes from a wide range of research initiatives, including population-based studies, ecological studies, human metabolic studies, methodology development, investigations of the basic mechanisms of action of dietary constituents, and clinical trials of dietary modification and the chemopreventive potential of individual nutrients or dietary components. In addition, applicable knowledge of genetic, environmental, and molecular influences on carcinogenesis and the interaction of diet or dietary factors with these aspects are providing an interface for cancer prevention researchers to better assess cancer risk and intervene to reduce risk. The relationship between food and cancer and other chronic diseases, such as cardiovascular disease and diabetes, is tremendously complex. Although much progress has been made in understanding this complexity, it seems apparent that the majority of information remains to be discovered and many challenges exist. Possibly the most important lesson for nutrition research in the past decade has been recognizing the need for a new paradigm for discovering the role of nutrition and diet in disease prevention (Greenwald, 2001). This new approach will, by necessity, be more interdisciplinary and will incorporate advances in molecular biology, genetics, metabolic studies, and various other disciplines with clinical trials. By encompassing and integrating lifestyle and medical approaches, cancer prevention researchers will broaden the scope of research activities to develop compelling strategies to improve the public health. Understanding individual variability through enhanced use of emerging technologies and identification of risk profiles to target those who could benefit from lifestyle or medical interventions will fill the need for better research translation.

The new paradigm in nutritional oncology is developing in an environment of change in many fields of science. Advances in our understanding of the changes in the genetic and epigenetic environments after exposure to foods is driving the search for molecular targets and mechanisms that can be altered by dietary modifications, either alone or combined with other lifestyle choices. Along with new approaches to nutritional oncology, new terms have been developed to describe interactions among foods, genes, proteins, and cells (see Box 1). The interrelationships between bioactive food components (BFCs) and cellular processes, as currently understood, are depicted in Figure 1.

Nutritional oncology encompasses prevention of cancer in healthy individuals, prevention of recurring cancer in cancer survivors, and the impact of nutrition among patients undergoing treatment for cancer. Each of these areas is the focus of ongoing research as the role of nutrition in the cancer spectrum of prevention, screening and detection, diagnosis, treatment, and palliative care is determined and strategies developed. There are differences in the approach to nutritional intervention at each step of the spectrum, and health professionals should be aware of differences in recommending dietary or other lifestyle changes, especially before, during, and after cancer treatment (American Cancer Society, 2001; Shattner, 2003; Lada et al., 2004).

Systematic Approaches to Cancer Prevention

The overall research approach for cancer prevention begins with a systematic assessment of what people are

Copyright © 2006, Elsevier Inc.
All rights of reproduction in any form reserved.

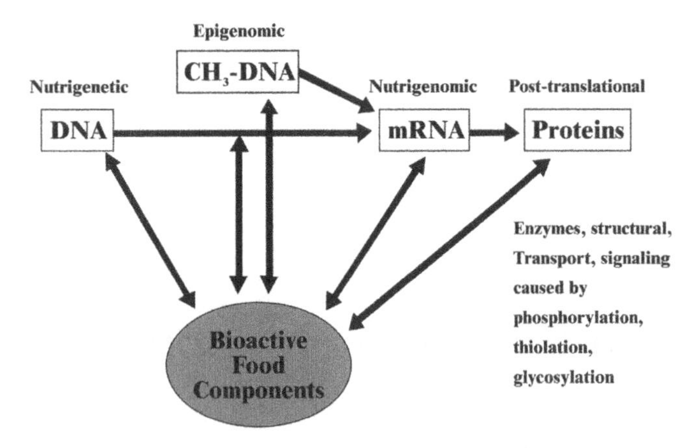

FIGURE 1 The interrelationship of factors that can influence the overall response to food components.

BOX 1 Nutritional Oncology Terminology

Bioactive Food Components
Compounds within foods that have a direct or indirect action on genetic or epigenetic structures and/or processes
Genomics
The study of genes and their functions
Nutrigenomics
The prospective analysis of differences among nutrients regarding the regulation of gene expression
Nutrigenetics
The genetic profile that influences absorption, metabolism, and site of action of the response of genes to bioactive food components
Epigenomics
The study of heritable changes in gene function that cannot be explained by changes in DNA sequence.
Proteomics
The study of protein shape, function, and patterns of expression
Metabolomics
The study of low-molecular-weight fractions of cells, tissues, and body fluids

eating, how nutrients and nonnutrient dietary constituents interact within the body, and other aspects of lifestyle—for example, weight gain, obesity, body mass index (BMI), and physical activity—that are affected by nutrition. One systematic approach, and the approach that is used as the template for this chapter, is the three-D (3-D) approach of *d*iscovery, *d*evelopment, and *d*elivery (von Eschenbach, 2003). The focus of the 3-D approach is on creating a research environment to integrate disparate research communities in an effort to enhance the search for clues to the diet–cancer link and to speed dissemination of research results to the clinician and the public.

- *Discovery* is the process that generates new knowledge about fundamental aspects of cancer-related processes at the genetic, molecular, cellular, organ, person, and population levels.
- *Development* is the process of creating and evaluating tools and interventions to reduce the cancer burden, including the prevention, detection, diagnosis, and treatment of cancer and its sequelae.
- *Delivery* is the process of disseminating, facilitating and promoting evidence-based prevention, detection, diagnosis, and treatment practices and policies to reduce the burden of cancer in all segments of the population. The focus of these efforts is on populations who bear the greatest burden of disease.

The 3-D approach has been developed as a seamless integrated template for initiating and conducting investigations for cancer prevention, not as a sequential approach most common to past research initiatives. Discovery, development, and delivery will be designed to proceed concurrently, with results from each initiative causing adjustments in each of the other initiatives or creation of new research paths. Investigations include both lifestyle and medical approaches, which have provided important clues to the role of nutrition in cancer risk.

Lifestyle Approaches

Nutrition and diet contribute ~35% to cancer risk, approximately the same risk contribution as tobacco smoking (Doll and Peto, 1981). An analysis of worldwide cancer incidence and mortality rates suggests that 3–4 million cancer deaths per year are attributable to dietary factors, with a stronger association among cancers that are not hormonally mediated (stomach and colorectal), compared with those that are (breast and prostate) (Young and LeLeu, 2002) (Table 1). Lifestyle approaches to cancer prevention may begin with changing dietary patterns that may

TABLE 1 Selected Cancers Related to Dietary Factors

Cancer	Estimated percent attributed to dietary factors
Breast	33–50%
Prostate	10–20%
Stomach	66–75%
Colorectal	66–75%
All cancers	30–40%

Source: Young and Le Leu (2002).

be addressed by the complete diet that impacts overall health and cancer, such as obesity. For example, although the U.S. population has decreased the amount of fat in the diet in the past 2 decades, portion sizes (particularly in restaurants), the number of daily calories consumed, the average weight of Americans (especially among adolescents), and the percentage of Americans who are obese have increased. The trend for the increasing prevalence of overweight and obesity is of special concern because of studies that show the negative impact of obesity on cancer risk. In the past decade, the prevalence of overweight (BMI 25.0–29.9) and obesity (BMI ≥30.0) among adults in the United States has increased from 56% to 64% (Flegal et al., 2002). The association between overweight and obesity and a significant risk of cardiovascular mortality has been known for some time; however, the magnitude of the significance for cancer mortality has not been quantified until recently (Calle et al., 1999). A prospective cohort study of more than one million adults in the United States assessed cardiovascular disease mortality and BMI and found a significantly increased risk of death among men (relative risk [RR] = 2.9) and women (RR = 2.37) (Calle et al., 1999). In a subsequent study of cancer mortality in the same cohort, the effect of overweight and obesity was found to contribute to 20% of cancer deaths in women and 14% in men (Calle et al., 2003). For specific cancer sites, there was a linear trend of increasing mortality from lower BMI to higher BMI for cancers of the stomach and prostate in men, and cancers of the breast, uterus, cervix, and ovary in women (Calle et al., 2003). According to this analysis, >90,000 cancer deaths in the United States each year could potentially be prevented if men and women maintained normal weight. Development of effective interventions to reduce the prevalence of overweight and obesity is essential. Research in experimental carcinogenesis models indicates that a regimen of caloric restriction (usually 20–40% relative to *ad libitum* controls), which reduces obesity, may be one of the best broad-based interventions to reduce cancer risk (Hursting et al., 2003), although few consistent data exist in humans. Caloric restriction has a beneficial impact on mechanisms regulated by insulin-like growth factor (IGF)-1, including cell proliferation, apoptosis, and cell cycle regulation. To illustrate, caloric restriction increases the rate of apoptosis by reducing the DNA synthesis, which is necessary to increase the number and volume of preneoplastic lesions (Hursting et al., 2003). Achieving a greater understanding of the relationship between obesity and increased cancer risk will require a concerted effort using an interdisciplinary approach of basic and clinical research.

As the U.S. population becomes heavier and less active, the challenge for modulating the impact of diet on chronic disease risk should become a national priority. Current trends begun in the past decade for "super-sizing" restaurant portions should be viewed as an impediment to a healthy populace. A study of marketplace portion sizes compared actual served portions with recommended federal portion standards and found most marketplace portions are two to eightfold larger than portions used in federal guidelines (Young and Nestle, 2003). A study of trends in portion sizes from national surveys from 1977 to 1996 found that food portion sizes increased both inside and outside the home for all categories except pizza (Nielsen and Popkin, 2003). In addition, energy intake and portion size of salty snacks increased by 93 kcal (60%), soft drinks by 49 kcal (52%), hamburgers by 97 kcal (23%), French fries by 68 kcal (16%), and Mexican food by 133 kcal (27%). A research center study of self-served portions versus larger served portions (double an age-appropriate portion) among children suggests that the larger served portion leads to an increase in entree size by 25% and total energy intakes by 15% (Orlet et al., 2003). A comparison of National Health and Nutrition Examination Survey (NHANES) III (1988–94) data and earlier studies from the 1970s on energy intake among children and adolescents (2–19 years of age) suggests that there has been little increase in energy intake (Troiano et al., 2001). The same study, however, did show that mean percentage of energy from total and saturated fat decreased but remained above recommendations, with overall means of 33.5% of energy from fat and 12.2% of energy from saturated fat. Because overweight and obesity in this age-group has increased over the past decades, some have suggested that decreasing levels of physical activity may account for this finding.

Regular physical activity is one of the most important modifiable risk factors for cancer after dietary choices and smoking. A review of evidence for an association between physical activity and cancer found convincing epidemiological evidence that regular physical exercise, comparing highest to lowest levels, reduces the risk of colon cancer by 40–50% and breast cancer by 30–40% (Friedenreich and Orenstein, 2002). For other cancer sites, this review reported that the association was probable for prostate cancer and possible for cancers of the endometrium and lung. Although the underlying mechanisms for the associations have not been established, possible mechanisms have been proposed. For example, mechanisms that may contribute to a beneficial effect of physical activity on colon cancer include changes in gastrointestinal transit time, altered immune function and prostaglandin levels, and changes in insulin levels, IGFs, bile acid secretion, serum cholesterol, and gastrointestinal and pancreatic hormone profiles (Quadrilatero and Hoffman-Goetz, 2003). Possible mechanisms for a physical activity–breast cancer relationship include decreased levels of exposure to estrogen, increases in the production of sex hormone–binding globulin, and reductions in circulating concentrations of insulin and related growth factors (Friedenreich and Orenstein, 2002). Based on accumulating evidence of the health benefits of physical activity for cancer and cardiovascular disease, the American Cancer Society (2002) and other national organizations have adopted the recommendation that adults should engage in at least moderate activity for ≥30 minutes on 5 or more days of the week. Children and adolescents should engage in ≥60 minutes/day of moderate-to-vigorous physical activity at least 5 days per week.

Medical Approaches

Medical approaches to cancer prevention focus on designing and conducting preclinical and clinical studies to better understand the biological basis of the carcinogenic process and how to influence cancer risk. Chemoprevention (a pharmacological approach to intervention that aims to prevent, arrest, or reverse either the initiation phase of carcinogenesis or the progression of premalignant cells) is an important part of the medical approach developed for cancer prevention and intervention. Laboratory and epidemiological studies have provided the scientific rationale for investigating potential chemopreventive agents (Greenwald et al., 1990). For example, epidemiological studies support an inverse relationship between the intake of vegetables and fruits and cancer risk, and clinical studies have identified possible phytochemical components of these foods (as well as interactions among the components) that might contribute to their ability to reduce cancer risk (Chemoprevention Working Group, 1999; Negri et al., 1991). To illustrate, among the hundreds of phytochemicals and micronutrients with potential chemopreventive effects identified from animal and *in vitro* studies, diallyl sulfide, a phytochemical found in *Allium* vegetables such as garlic and onion, has been associated with a reduced risk of prostate (Hsing et al., 2002) and colorectal and stomach cancers (Fleischauer et al., 2000). A review by Milner (2001a) found garlic protects against carcinogenesis by blocking *N*-nitroso compound formation, suppressing bioactivation of several carcinogens, induces apoptosis, alters the cell cycle, and alters several phase I and II enzymes associated with cancer initiation and progression. Understanding the mechanisms of action of dietary constituents such as garlic with confidence for translating this knowledge into prevention strategies remains a significant challenge.

Dietary Choices and Cancer

Food choices produce dietary patterns that may increase or decrease the risk of cancer (World Cancer Research Fund, 1997). A wealth of information shows that certain specific diets may offer protection against cancer at many sites. The challenge for nutritional science researchers is determining which BFCs, or combinations, are responsible for cancer protection or increased risk and for which cancer sites. The study of the American ("Western") diet and cancer risk has been ongoing for more than 4 decades, with important clues being discovered that suggest research pathways. For example, an analysis of prostate cancer among 3779 men in the NHANES Epidemiological Followup Study Cohort found three distinct dietary patterns in the United States: (1) a "vegetable–fruit" pattern that includes fish and shellfish; (2) a "red meat–starch" pattern that includes salty snacks, cheese, sweets, and desserts; and (3) a "Southern" pattern that includes traditionally Southern foods such as cornbread, grits, sweet potatoes, and okra (Tseng et al., 2004). The only dietary pattern associated with a decreased risk of prostate cancer was the "Southern" pattern (borderline significance), which was seen in both white and black men. Another prospective study of eating patterns and colon cancer found that a diet with high intakes of dietary fiber and folate was protective, especially among older Americans (Slattery et al., 1998). In the same study, a "Western" dietary pattern (high levels of red meat, processed meat, fast food, refined grains, and sugar-containing foods, and low levels of vegetables and fruits) was associated with an increased risk of colon cancer among men and women.

Aside from dietary patterns, a growing base of research exists that indicates specific types of foods or food constituents may reduce the risk of cancer. Table 2 lists selected nutrients that may modify cancer risk. The challenge for nutritional science is to confirm these findings in chemoprevention clinical trials and determine how they should fit into a diet that encourages improved health. Various food choices could satisfy the need for the particular BFCs associated with reduced cancer risk. For example, the carotenoid lycopene has been shown in animal and clinical studies to reduce the risk of prostate cancer by various mechanisms, including acting as an antioxidant, interfering with growth factor receptor signaling and cell cycle progression, and upregulating *connexin 43*, which allows direct intercellular gap junctional communication (Heber and Lu, 2002). A review of tomato products, lycopene, and prostate cancer risk found that eating one serving of lycopene-containing foods per day is associated with lower prostate cancer risk (Miller et al., 2002). In making food choices, lycopene is found in all tomato-based products regardless of processing, grapefruit, watermelon, papaya, and other fruits.

DISCOVERY

Discovery is the initial step in developing hypotheses that can be investigated in clinical investigations and intervention studies. Epidemiological and ecological studies provided clues for avenues of research for elucidating the diet–cancer relationship. In past decades, for example, comprehensive reviews of diet and cancer were published by the U.S. National Academy of Sciences (NAS) and the World Cancer Research Fund (WCRF) (NAS, 1982, 1989; WCRF,

TABLE 2 Selected Examples of Bioactive Food Components That May Modify Cancer Risk

Food source	Class of compound	Bioactive food component (s)
Cruciferous vegetables (arugula, Bok choy, broccoli, Brussels sprouts, cauliflower, collard greens, kale, mustard greens, radishes, rutabaga, turnips)	Isothiocyanate	Benzyl isothiocyanate, 2-phenethyl isothiocyanate, sulforaphane, allyl isothiocyanate, 3-methylsulfinylpropyl isothiocyanate
	Glycosinolate	Indole-3-carbinol, 3,3′-diindoylmethane, indole-3-acetonitrile
Vegetables	Minerals	Calcium, zinc, selenium
	Flavonoids	Quercetin, rutin
	Vitamins	Folic acid, vitamin A, vitamin E, vitamin C
Dark green vegetables (spinach, kale)	Carotenoids	Lutein
	Vitamins	Vitamin A, vitamin C
Vegetables, fruits, black tea	Flavonoid	Anthocyanins
Onions, garlic, scallions, chives	Allium compounds (Organosulfur compounds)	Diallyl sulfide, allylmethyl trisulfide, allyl mercaptan, *S*-allylcysteine
Citrus fruit	Flavonoid	Tangertin, nobiletin, rutin
Citrus fruit (peel), caraway seed oil	Terpenoid Monoterpenes	D-Limonene, perillyl alcohol, geraniol, menthol, carvone
Berries, tomatoes, potatoes, broad beans, broccoli, squash, onions	Flavonoid	Quercetin
Radish, horse radish, kale, endive	Flavonoid	Kaempferol
Tea, chocolate	Polyphenol	Epigallocatechin gallate, epigallocatechin, epicatechin, catechin
Grapes, red wine	Polyphenol	Resveratrol, catechin
Tumeric, curry, mustard fruits, coffee beans, soybeans	Polyphenol	Curcumin, caffeic acid
Strawberries, raspberries, blackberries, walnuts, pecans	Polyphenol	Caffeic acid, ferulic acid, ellagic acid
Cereals, pulses (millet, sorghum, soya beans)	Isoflavone	Genistein
Orange vegetables and fruit	Carotenoid	α- and β-carotene
Tomatoes	Carotenoid	Lycopene
Tea, coffee, cola, cacao (cocoa and chocolate)	Methylxanthines	Caffeine, theophylline, theobromine
Dairy products (milk, cheese, yogurt)	Vitamins	Vitamin D, calcium
Red meat	Vitamins	Iron

Source: Adapted from Manson (2003).

1997), among others. Based on substantive epidemiological and experimental evidence, these reviews indicate strong support for a diet–cancer relationship. In general, these reviews recommended increased intake of fiber and a variety of vegetables and fruits, moderate consumption of alcohol and salt, reduced fat intake, and increased physical activity. To illustrate, the WCRF reported that convincing evidence supported the hypothesis that a diet high in vegetables protects against cancers of the colon and rectum, stomach, lung, esophagus, mouth, and pharynx. Further, vegetables may protect against breast, bladder, pancreas, and larynx cancer, but the evidence was less convincing; and limited evidence suggests that vegetables reduced the risk of prostate, ovary, endometrium, cervix, liver, kidney, and thyroid cancers (WCRF, 1997). In addition, the WCRF proposed that dietary fat, excessive calories, obesity, and alcohol may increase the risk of cancer at various sites, whereas fruits, dietary fiber, and certain micronutrients may protect against cancer. Since the publication of the WCRF review, results from several large population-based epidemiological studies have been reported that provide additional clues to the relationship between nutrition and cancer.

Large-Scale Prospective Studies

Health Professionals Followup Study

The Health Professionals Followup Study (HPFS), begun in 1986 with follow-up in 1990 and 1994, is a prospective cohort study of 47,882 men in the United States that uses a validated 131-item semiquantitative food frequency questionnaire. HPFS analyses of dietary factors and prostate cancer suggests reduced risk with the intake of fish more than three times per week (Augustsson et al., 2003); equivocal findings for the intake of cruciferous vegetables, except for reduced risk among men younger than 65 years and those who reported higher intakes over the 10 years before baseline (Giovannucci et al., 2003a); reduced risk with higher intakes of fructose (>5 vs <1 servings per day) and increased risk with higher intakes of calcium (≥2000 mg/day vs

<500 mg/day) (Giovannucci et al., 1998a); and reduced risk among men younger than 60 years with a BMI ≥30 kg/m^2 compared with men with a BMI ≥23–24.9 kg/m^2 (Giovannucci et al., 2003b). A further analysis by Platz et al. (2003) found a direct association between energy intake and metastatic or fatal prostate cancer (but not prostate cancer incidence) among men who were lean, more physically active, and younger (≤65 years). The HPFS follow-up study will continue until 2007.

Nurses' Health Study

The Nurses' Health Study (NHS), begun in 1976, is a prospective follow-up study of 88,647 women and was originally designed to examine the relationship between contraception and breast cancer. The NHS-II, begun in 1989, was designed to include younger participants than the initial study and to focus on diet and lifestyle in cancer risk. Results of NHS-II and various nested case-control studies within the NHS have contributed important clues about the link between diet and cancer. Participants in the NHS completed a follow-up questionnaire every 2 years, and many of the questions pertained to nutrition and other lifestyle factors. Findings from the NHS indicate that there may be an inverse association between vegetable fat, eggs, and fiber intake and breast cancer (Frazier et al., 2003); fruit and vegetable intake and lung cancer (Feskanich et al., 2000) and colon and rectum cancer (Michels et al., 2000); red meat and all meat and invasive breast cancer (Holmes et al., 2003); folate and colon cancer (at 15 years of follow-up but not at 5 years of follow-up) (Giovannucci et al., 1998b); and folate and hyperplastic polyps of the colon and rectum (Kearney et al., 1995). Direct associations between diet and cancer in the NHS were reported for intake of animal protein and invasive breast cancer (Holmes et al., 2003); alcohol and hyperplastic polyps of the colon and rectum (Kearney et al., 1995); and butter and breast cancer (Frazier et al., 2003). The NHS-II inquired about diet during adolescence of the participants and found inverse associations between vegetable fat, vitamin E, and fiber intake and proliferative benign breast disease (Baer et al., 2003), as well as carbohydrate intake among women with BMI <25 kg/m^2 (Cho et al., 2003). Direct associations in the NHS-II included total animal fat, animal fat, and monosaturated fats, and proliferative benign breast disease (Baer et al., 2003), as well as carbohydrate intake among women with BMI ≥25 kg/m^2 (Cho et al., 2003).

Cancer Prevention Study II Nutrition Cohort

The Cancer Prevention Study II (CPS-II) is a prospective study of cancer incidence and mortality; the Nutrition Cohort is a subgroup of ~86,000 men and 98,000 women from the 1.2 million CPS cohort identified in 1982. Compared with baseline (1992) intakes of whole grains, fruits, and vegetables, results of a 5-year follow-up study indicated that men with the highest vegetable intake had a nonsignificant 30% reduction in risk of colon cancer; men at the lowest quintile of intake of vegetables and fiber had significantly (vegetables RR = 1.79; fiber RR = 1.96) increased risk (McCullough et al., 2003). In addition, women at very low intakes of fruit were at increased risk (RR = 1.86) for colon cancer. Another analysis from CPS-II indicated that postmenopausal women who had gained >70 pounds since age 18 years had double the risk of breast cancer compared with women who had maintained their weight within 5 pounds of their weight at age 18 years (Feigelson et al., 2004).

European Prospective Investigation into Cancer and Nutrition (EPIC)

The EPIC study, the largest study of diet and health ever undertaken, was initiated in 1992 to collect information from >520,000 people in 10 European countries. Recruitment was completed in 1999, and follow-up will continue for 10 years (Riboli and Kaaks, 1997). Preliminary results support the conclusion that increased intakes of fruits and vegetables reduce the incidence of cancers of the colon and rectum and upper aerodigestive tract; preliminary results do not support the protective effect previously found for cancers of the stomach and lung, although this may be due, in part, to the brief follow-up period (Riboli and Lambert, 2002). Other findings include an increase in colon cancer risk with consumption of preserved meats, as well as a significant reduction in colon cancer risk with fish consumption. EPIC also has collected blood samples from most participants for investigations of biomarkers of dietary intake (e.g., levels of vitamins), biomarkers of diet-related factors (e.g., indicators of antioxidant status), and markers of hormones that can be influenced by diet and may be associated with cancer risk (Riboli and Kaaks, 1997).

Black Women's Health Study

The Black Women's Health Study (BWHS), begun in 1995, enrolled 64,500 women in a cohort to assess all aspects of health, including diet, obesity, alcohol consumption, and physical activity, with a focus on breast cancer. This long-term prospective study is collecting data on energy, total fat, saturated fat, protein, carbohydrate, dietary fiber, calcium, iron, vitamin C, folate, β-carotene, and vitamin E using dietary recall, food-frequency questionnaires (FFQs), and daily diaries (Kumanyika et al., 2003). Results will be reported periodically as follow-up data are collected.

Immigrant Studies on Diet and Cancer

Comparison of cancer rates among immigrants in their host country with those in their country of origin has provided important clues to the role of environmental factors in cancer etiology. One of the earliest population-based studies compared gastrointestinal and colon cancer rates, which are related to diet, in the San Francisco area among Japanese, Japanese immigrants, and Japanese Americans (U.S. born) (Dunn, 1977). For gastric cancer, which has a high rate in Japan and low rate in the U.S. population, a stepwise reduction in rates was seen when comparing Japanese rates, rates among Japanese immigrants, and U.S.-born Japanese Americans. For colon cancer, which has a low rate in Japan and a high rate in the U.S. population, a stepwise increase in rates was seen when comparing Japanese rates, rates among Japanese immigrants, and U.S.-born Japanese Americans. A similar pattern of changes was seen for breast, uterine corpus, and ovarian cancer among immigrant women and for prostate cancer rates among immigrant men (Dunn, 1977). A population-based study in Los Angeles of Japanese, non-Spanish–surnamed white, and Spanish-surnamed white immigrants found prostate and breast cancer incident rates were higher than those in homeland populations and approached U.S. rates the longer the immigrant resided in this country (Shimizu et al., 1991). A study in Illinois that investigated the role of acculturation among Mexican and Puerto Rican immigrants indicated that cancer rates for immigrant Puerto Rican males was closer to U.S. rates than for either Puerto Rican females or Mexicans (Mallin and Anderson, 1988). Overall, these results suggested that the quicker an immigrant group becomes acculturated to the host country lifestyle, the quicker the immigrant population transitions to the cancer rates of the host country.

A unique opportunity for nutrition discovery research in an immigrant population is the investigation of cancer rates among the Hmong population, an agrarian people from the mountainous regions of Vietnam, Cambodia, and Laos. The Hmong immigrated to the United States after the Vietnam War, and the U.S. population of Hmong is ~100,000. Population studies in California and Minnesota, where a majority of Hmong immigrants settled, indicate that baseline cancer rates reflective of those from their host country show elevated rates for cancers of the nasopharynx, stomach, liver, pancreas, leukemia, and cervix, as well as non-Hodgkin's lymphoma, and lower rates for cancers of the breast, prostate, and colon/rectum (Mills and Yang, 1997; Ross et al., 2003). This cancer profile is characteristic of rates seen when comparing developing and developed countries. Among the Hmong, cancer rates will be systematically investigated over time not only to determine whether cancer rates become synchronized with U.S. rates, but also to assess which interventions may succeed in interrupting the synchronization. Dietary changes during acculturation will be investigated to assess the role of diet in cancer risk. A study of food habits and food consumption patterns has shown that adult Hmong prefer to maintain strong ties to their native foods and traditional diets, but Hmong adolescents prefer both American and native foods (Story and Harris, 1989). The effect of genetic differences also will be investigated. For example, genotyping studies have found significant differences between the Hmong population and U.S. whites, including significantly lower frequencies of the glutathione *S*-transferase μ1 (GSTM1) and glutathione *S*-transferase theta1 (GSTT1) genes among the Hmong (Kiffmeyer et al., 2004). This information may suggest possible interventions to cancer researchers, including future genetic or proteomic interventions, to reduce cancer risk and increase survival.

Evidence from Animal Models

Animal models offer unique opportunities for discovery related to the process of carcinogenesis, the role of gene–environment interactions, and potential chemoprevention strategies associated with diet and nutrition. Most models for nutrition research assess exposure to specific dietary factors in mice and rats with a predetermined susceptibility to specific types of cancer. These models use tumor development or preneoplastic biomarkers in animals with overexpressed or underexpressed genes as endpoints, often with exposure to exogenous carcinogens such as azomethane (AOM). For example, a review of dietary chemoprevention studies in AOM-induced *Min* mice and other mice with mutations resulting in intestinal tumors found that resveratrol, fish oil, curcumin, folic acid, and caffeic acid phenethyl esters reduced tumor yield by 60–70% (Corpet and Pierre, 2003). This review indicated that similar results occurred in AOM-induced rats. Curcumin also has been shown to reduce the development of adenomas in C57B1/6J *Min*/+ mice, developed as a model for human familial APC (Perkins et al., 2001). In this study, curcumin at 0.1% in the diet had no effect; at 0.2 and 0.5%, however, adenomas were reduced by 39 and 40%, respectively, compared with untreated mice, suggesting that the dose of an agent is important to achieve maximum chemopreventive effect (Perkins et al., 2001). Studies in AOM-induced rats have suggested that almonds and almond fractions reduce aberrant crypt foci in F344 male rats (Davis and Iwahashi, 2001), and dietary whey protein reduces the incidence, though not number or mass, of colon tumors in male offspring of female Sprague–Dawley (S-D) rats (Hakkak et al., 2001). *N*-methyl-*N*-nitrosourea (NMU)–induced mammary tumorigenesis in S-D rats has been reported to be significantly reduced by a diet high in flaxseed, the richest source of plant-based omega-3 fatty acids and dietary lignans, and secoisolariciresinol diglycoside (SDG), a major precursor of mammalian lignan, compared with rats fed a diet lower in these components

(Rickard et al., 1999). Mammary tumorigenesis in S-D rats also is inhibited by exposure to either flaxseed or SDG during suckling (Chen et al., 2003). Male Wistar–Unilever rats treated with NMU and testosterone had a statistically lower risk of dying from prostate cancer on a diet of tomato powder (hazard ratio [HR] = 0.74) or on energy-restricted diets (HR = 0.68) than rats fed diets high in lycopene or *ad libitum* diets (Boileau et al., 2003). Energy (caloric) restriction has been shown to be a viable cancer prevention strategy in several animal models. For example, a review of studies using caloric restriction for spontaneous mammary tumors in various strains of mice found a 55% reduction in mammary tumors in energy-restricted animals compared with controls, regardless of the nutrients used in the studies (Dirx et al., 2003). In addition, a 40% energy-restricted diet in August Copenhagen Irish (ACI) rats treated with 17-estradiol (E2) inhibited mammary carcinogenesis, partly by slowing the progression of atypical hyperplastic foci to carcinoma (Harvell et al., 2001).

The growth of investigations using transgenic animal technology has been significant in the past decade. Transgenic murine models provide insight into mechanisms that contribute to the carcinogenic process. For example, mice develop prostate cancer spontaneously at puberty in the transgenic adenocarcinoma of the mouse prostate (TRAMP) model. Dietary genistein, at levels comparable with those in Asian men on their regular soy diet, significantly reduced the development of prostatic adenocarcinoma in a dose-dependent manner in the TRAMP model (Mentor-Marcel et al., 2001). In addition, the polyphenolic fraction of green tea (GTP) fed to TRAMP mice at a human-equivalent dose of 6 cups of tea/day significantly inhibited prostate cancer development, progression, and metastasis (Gupta et al., 2001).

TRAMP mice fed a diet containing flaxseed for 30 weeks had significantly less aggressive prostate tumors than control mice (Lin et al., 2002). A transgenic murine model also has been developed to investigate the effect of estrogen, antiestrogens, and isoflavones in modifying mammary growth, tumor development, and phenotypic aggression. Female FVB/N-TgN (MMTV-*neu*) transgenic mice were fed a soy-based diet; control mice were fed a casein-based diet (Yang et al., 2003). The FVB mice failed to develop mammary tumors, suggesting that in this *Wt-erbB*-2 transgenic mouse model, tumor development was specifically associated with the transgene. In addition, short-term tamoxifen use at an early stage of development blocked tumor development in 80% of the mice (Yang et al., 2003).

Molecular Targets in Nutrition

To address one of the most compelling questions in nutritional oncology—How does food interact with cellular structures and biological processes to affect genotypic and phenotypic changes?—research has become increasingly more focused on exploring molecular targets of BFCs. Molecular targets may be individual genes, molecules that either result from gene expression or are otherwise affected by gene expression, or any other molecular events that are relevant to the process of carcinogenesis (Milner et al., 2001b). Molecular targets related to cancer risk have been identified and are associated with various nutrients, including vitamin D, calcium, folate, selenium, genistein, and resveratrol (reviewed in Milner et al., 2001b). These nutrients act through various processes to influence hormonal regulation, cell signaling, cell cycle control, apoptosis, differentiation, or carcinogen metabolism. Selenium provides an example of progress being made in understanding the role of molecular targets in nutrition and cancer risk.

Dietary selenium primarily is found in vegetables and fruits, although the amount provided is highly dependent on the soil content. Selenium has been shown to have reduced cancer risk through numerous mechanisms, which include acting as an antioxidant, suppressing cell proliferation, enhancing immune response, altering the metabolism of carcinogens, and inducing apoptosis (reviewed in Fleming et al., 2001). Selenium imposes its biological activity through its numerous compound forms, mainly selenoproteins, which influence various molecular targets and pathways (Ip, 1998). As an antioxidant, selenium takes part in the thioredoxin system, acting as a constituent of the selenoenzyme thioredoxin reductase (TR). TR reduces thioredoxin, which causes reduced activity of nuclear transcription factor-κB (NFκB) activation, an inducible oncogenic factor that causes induction of genes involved in a number of physiological processes, including those associated with cytokines, growth factors, cell adhesion molecules, and immunoreceptors (Milner et al., 2001b). To illustrate, a direct genetic effect of selenium is the inhibition of DNA synthesis and induced DNA strand breakage by increasing cdc2/cdk2 kinase activities and arresting cell growth in $S/G_2/M$ (Sinha et al., 1996). Additionally, selenium is involved in influencing apoptosis by *fas* ligand and *p38* stress kinase induction (Fleming et al., 2001). A study in *Min* mice fed selenium-enriched broccoli investigated gene expression in the mouse liver (Zeng et al., 2003). Results indicated that selenium-enriched broccoli enhanced the binding of transcription factor p53, NFκB, and AP-1 to their *cis*-acting elements, thus reducing tumorigenesis.

Systematic Approach for Biomarkers in Nutrition Research

Discovery in nutrition research through the identification, validation, and application of biomarkers is an emerging strategy for cancer prevention and intervention. Biomarkers are defined as cellular, biochemical, molecular, or genetic alterations that can be recognized or monitored and can be assessed from tissues, cells, or fluids (Verma and Srivastava, 2003). Biomarkers are investigated in nutritional oncology to determine exposure (intake) to BFCs, to assess the response of molecular processes and pathways after exposure to BFCs, to elucidate susceptibility of individuals to specific exposures, and as surrogate endpoints in clinical studies of dietary factors or nutrient-related chemopreventive agents (Srivastava and Gopal-Srivastava, 2002). The National Cancer Institute's (NCI) Early Detection Research Network (EDRN) has initiated a systematic approach for biomarker research that includes the integration of discovery, evaluation, and validation of biomarkers. Detailed information on this approach may be found at the EDRN web site at http://edrn.nci.nih.gov. The use of biomarkers in nutrition represents a considerable challenge because diet-related cancers develop over long periods of time, and changes at the molecular level caused by BFCs appear to be small, with the possible accumulation of these small changes over time being responsible, at least in part, for increases in cancer risk (reviewed in Branca et al., 2001). There are few validated biomarkers for exposure to BFCs or for the effect of BFCs on cancer susceptibility related to diet.

Serum biomarkers have been used for decades to assess dietary intake and to validate information provided on FFQs or other methods for determining dietary habits (Crews et al., 2001). For example, in a study of Michigan breast cancer patients, the Healthy Eating Index (HEI), an analytical measure of compliance with the U.S. Department of Agriculture (USDA) dietary guidelines for daily food consumption, was compared with plasma biomarkers for carotenoids, folate, and vitamin C (Hann et al., 2001). Results indicated that significant correlations existed between HEI scores and biomarkers for carotenoids, except lycopene, and for vitamin C. Serum carotenoids also have been investigated recently in the New York Women's Health Study as a biomarker of fruit and vegetable consumption, with moderate success (van Kappel et al., 2001).

Using biomarkers to identify gene-specific mutations has promise for understanding specific interactions between dietary factors and genetic or epigenetic processes. For example, oxidative DNA damage assessed by 8-hydroxy-2-deoxyguanosine (8OHdG) and the Single Cell Gel Electrophoresis Assay (Comet assay) has been investigated in dietary intervention studies to examine the role of dietary and supplemental antioxidants (Møller and Loft, 2002). They reviewed single-dose, multiple-dose, and natural food product studies and determined that antioxidants generally reduce both 8OHdG concentrations and DNA strand breaks, but variability of study design, length of exposure, and method of assessment differed among studies, making clear associations difficult.

Gene expression profiles have been made possible by the application of emerging technologies in nutritional sciences. The ability to analyze expression patterns of thousands of genes simultaneously is possible by using high-throughput tools such as microarray and chip technology. A study using an oligonucleotide array found that selenium, when added to a culture of synchronized human prostate cells, influences many genes and presents a distinct pattern of expression (Dong et al., 2003). Expression profiles also can be used to determine the effect of BFCs on methylation. Abnormal methylation patterns are almost universally associated with cancer and dietary factors such as folate, choline, and vitamins B6 and B12 limit the availability of methyl groups for DNA methylation (Milner, 2003).

Because nutrition does not generally cause major changes in gene expression, it is important to investigate the many minor changes that occur through nutrient and nonnutrient exposure related to diet. By integrating studies of genomics (the study of genes and their functions), proteomics (the study of protein shape, function, and patterns of expression), and metabolomics (the study of low-molecular-weight fractions of cells, tissues, and body fluids) to identify valid biomarkers associated with the actions of BFCs, the new paradigm for nutritional science may be realized. For example, the use of chromatographic separation technology in a metabolomic study of rats found that >250 diet-dependent compounds could be identified in plasma, which may allow them to be used as biomarkers for the identification of metabolomic genotypes and phenotypes associated with health or disease (Watkins and German, 2002). Proteomic technology has been used to investigate potential prostate cancer biomarkers. Using surface-enhanced laser desorption/ionization time-of-flight (SELDI-TOF) mass spectometry, Zheng et al. (2003) found a protein (PCa-24) present in 16 of 17 prostate carcinoma specimens that may be a potential biomarker for this condition; PCa-24 was not expressed in any of the 12 benign prostatic hyperplasia specimens studied. With the human genome completely sequenced and our improved understanding of the proteins and metabolites involved in gene–nutrient interactions, the challenge for nutrition researchers is to assimilate knowledge from all fields to identify and validate biomarkers that signify changes from good health to clinical cancer.

DEVELOPMENT

Development of nutritional interventions within the 3-D approach to cancer prevention is based on the evaluation of findings from discovery that show promise for reducing the cancer burden (von Eschenbach, 2003). Nutritional components have been under investigation at the NCI for more than 2 decades. Table 3 presents information on selected nutritional components being investigated in NCI chemoprevention trials. Phase I clinical trials are designed to determine the dose-related safety and toxicity of the proposed chemopreventive agent. Phase II clinical trials evaluate agent

TABLE 3 Selected NCI-Sponsored Phase I: II: and III Cancer Prevention Trials of Nutritional Factors

Cancer site	Phase I	Phase II	Phase III
Breast	Soy isoflavones Indole-3-carbinol[b]	EGCG/polyphenon E (green tea extract)	
Colon	Curcumin	Folic acid[a] (2 trials) Vitamin D[a]/calcium	
Lung	*l*-Selenomethionine/vitamin E		Selenized yeast 13-*cis*-retinoic acid[b]
Prostate	Lycopene (3 trials) Soy isoflavones Genistein[b]	Selenized yeast Soy (dietary) Soy isoflavones Vitamin D analogue Selenium[a]	Selenomethionine Selenium/vitamin E [a]Diet low in fat and high in soy, fruits, vegetables, green tea, vitamin E, and fiber
Cervix		9-*cis*-Retinoic acid β-carotene[b]	Folic acid[a]
Bladder			High-dose multivitamins[a]
Anogenital warts + HPV/HIV		Indole-3-carbinol	
Skin	EGCG/polyphenon E (Green tea extract)	Retinol,[a] Retinyl palmitate EGCG[a]/polyphenon E (Green tea extract)	
Head and Neck			β-carotene[a] 13-*cis*-retinoic acid[a] (2 trials)

[a]Accrual completed; study closed to new participants.
[b]Completed.
EGCG, epigallocatechin gallate (polyphenon E).

efficacy in a larger group of participants at high risk for specific cancers and can provide data that characterize dose, safety, and toxicity in the selected population. Phase III clinical trials are randomized, double-blinded, placebo-controlled trials conducted in a large population of participants. Phase III trials have well-defined primary, and often secondary, endpoints that allow investigators to determine the agent's usefulness as a prevention or treatment strategy for a specific cancer type. Development with phase III clinical trials also includes large-scale dietary modification trials that investigate the effect of selected BFCs or groups of BFCs on cancer risk. Modification trials generally have endpoints that address changes in lifestyle, reducing the levels of some dietary factors or increasing others. These trials also offer the opportunity to investigate the overall diet for its effect on biomarkers of exposure and susceptibility.

Large-Scale Phase III Chemoprevention Trials

Selenium and Vitamin E Cancer Prevention Trial (SELECT)

Selenium has been extensively studied in experimental models and has been found to reduce cancer risk through numerous mechanisms, including antioxidant effects, enhancement of immune function, induction of apoptosis, inhibition of cell proliferation, alteration of carcinogen metabolism, cytotoxicity of metabolites, and influence on testosterone production (reviewed in Klein, 2004). SELECT was designed to further clarify findings from previous population-based trials that reported on the possible benefits of selenium and vitamin E. For example, a population-based clinical trial, the Alpha-Tocopherol, Beta-Carotene Cancer Prevention Study (ATBC Study) found in a secondary analysis that men receiving vitamin E had a decrease in prostate cancer mortality (41%) and incidence (36%) (Heinonen et al., 1998). In addition, secondary analysis of the HPFS found that daily use of vitamin E (100 μg/day) decreased the risk of metastatic or fatal prostate cancer 44% compared with nonusers (Chan et al., 1999). Secondary endpoint analyses from a multicenter, double-blind, randomized, placebo-controlled cancer prevention trial indicated that supplemental dietary selenium (200 μg/day) significantly reduced the risk of total cancer mortality by 50% (Clark et al., 1996) and prostate cancer incidence by 63% (Clark et al., 1998). In addition, the Nutrition Intervention Trial in Linxian, China, in a region of low selenium levels in the soil and food, found significant inverse associations between baseline serum selenium and death from esophageal (17% reduction) and gastric cancers (25% reduction) (Wei et al., 2004).

Given these encouraging results, the NCI sponsored SELECT, a randomized, prospective, double-blind study, to determine whether daily supplementation of selenium and vitamin E will decrease the risk of prostate cancer in healthy men (Klein et al., 2001). SELECT is a four-arm intervention trial comparing vitamin E alone (400 mg of racemic α-tocopherol), selenium alone (200 μg of l-selenomethionine), combined vitamin E and selenium, and placebo. The trial is scheduled to provide a 7- to 12-year regimen that includes an optional multivitamin that does not contain selenium or vitamin E. Routine clinical evaluations will include a yearly digital rectal examination and prostate-specific antigen test. SELECT is the largest prostate prevention trial ever conducted, and as of January 2004, ~90% of the targeted goal of 32,400 men had been enrolled. The primary endpoint is diagnosed prostate cancer; secondary endpoints will be the incidence of and survival from lung and colon cancers.

An important role for SELECT in the development of selenium as a chemopreventive agent is the inclusion of a biomarker study within the trial. A nested case-control study within SELECT will assess genetic polymorphisms of four genes, androgen receptor (*AR*), 5α-reductase type II (*SRD5A2*), cytochrome P450c 17α (*CYP17*), and β-hydroxysteroid dehydrogenase (*HSD3*β2), on prostate cancer incidence (Hoque et al., 2001). Substantial discovery efforts involving epidemiological and experimental studies suggest that these biomarkers of risk may affect susceptibility to prostate cancer (Haiman et al., 2001). For example, experimental studies have shown that selenium induces growth inhibition in human prostate cancer cell lines, but only if the cells have a functioning AR (Venkateswaran et al., 2002). Knowing whether the mechanisms of selenium action are dependent on specific AR polymorphisms could assist researchers in developing more specific preventive strategies for populations affected by the relevant AR polymorphisms. In addition, polymorphisms in *CYP17* A1/A1 genotype may confer a significantly higher serum androgen level, which is associated with higher risk of prostate cancer than found in men with either the A1/A2 or A2/A2 genotype (Hoque et al., 2001).

Physicians' Health Study-II

The Physicians' Health Study-II (PHS-II) was designed after the end of PHS-I in 1995, which did not support either benefit or harm from 12 years of β-carotene supplementation on the primary prevention of cancer and cardiovascular disease; the aspirin component of PHS-I was stopped early because of the benefit of aspirin on the risk of a first heart attack (Hennekens et al., 1996). PHS-II is a randomized, double-blind, placebo-controlled trial to investigate the role of vitamin C, vitamin E, β-carotene, and a multivitamin for the primary prevention of total cancer, prostate cancer, and cardiovascular disease (Christen et al., 2000). The trial uses a $2 \times 2 \times 2 \times 2$ factorial design and is the only trial testing the potential benefits of vitamin E in the prevention of prostate cancer and β-carotene on prostate and total cancer; in addition, it is the only primary prevention trial in healthy men testing multivitamins or any single antioxidant vitamin, alone or in combination, on cancer and CVD (Christen et al., 2000). Follow-up is scheduled to begin after 5 years.

Trials of β-Carotene

The Alpha-Tocopherol, Beta-Carotene Cancer Prevention Study (ATBC Study) and the Beta-Carotene and Retinol Efficacy Trial (CARET) have been controversial for the surprising finding that β-carotene was associated with an increased risk of lung cancer among smokers (ATBC Group, 1994; Albanes et al., 1996; Omenn et al., 1996). Both trials were conducted in cigarette smokers, with a 16% increase in lung cancer in the β-carotene group of the ATBC Study and a 28% higher incidence of lung cancer in participants receiving the β-carotene/retinyl palmitate combination in CARET. The ensuing international controversy surrounding these findings has been reviewed by Greenwald (2003); potential issues included dose, timing of the dose, interference by β-carotene in absorption of other carotenoids or antioxidants, and the duration of the studies. Subsequent investigations and reviews have added important information to this controversy. A postintervention follow-up of the ATBC Study found that the beneficial effects of vitamin E (α-tocopherol) and the negative effects of β-carotene disappeared after 4 years postintervention (Virtamo et al., 2003). The authors, representing the ATBC Study Group, continued their recommendation that smokers avoid β-carotene. The *Pooling Project of Prospective Studies of Diet and Cancer* analyzed data from seven cohort studies (~400,000 participants and 3150 cases) of dietary carotenoids and lung cancer (including the ATBC Study) and found that intakes of β-carotene, α-tocopherol, lutein/zeaxanthin, and lycopene were not associated with lung cancer risk (Männistö et al., 2004). Of the carotenoids studied, only β-cryptoxanthin was significantly inversely associated with lung cancer risk.

Large-Scale Dietary Modification Trials

Polyp Prevention Trial

The Polyp Prevention Trial (PPT) is a multicenter, randomized, controlled dietary intervention trial that is examining the effect of a low-fat (20% of calories from fat), high-fiber (18 g/1000 calories), high-vegetable and -fruit (five to eight daily servings, combined) dietary pattern on the recurrence of adenomatous colorectal polyps (APC) (Lanza et al., 1996; Schatzkin et al., 1996). Participants received extensive dietary and behavioral counseling on how to meet dietary goals. Results reported by Shatzkin et al. (2000) indicated that the PPT dietary intervention did not influence the risk of recurrence of APC. A subsequent analysis, however, did show that study participants in the intervention arm of the PPT made sustained significant changes in all PPT goals: reduced fat intake and increases in fiber and fruits and vegetables (Lanza et al., 2001). Intervention participants also reported significantly higher serum carotenoid concentrations and lower body weights than the control group. This finding is of particular importance to cancer prevention researchers as further preventive dietary interventions are designed.

Women's Health Initiative

The Women's Health Initiative (WHI), which began in Fall 1993, is a 15-year, multidisciplinary trial that includes both dietary and chemopreventive interventions. The nutritional components of the WHI include the Low-Fat Dietary Modification Trial (20% of calories from fat) and the Calcium/Vitamin D Supplementation Trial (calcium and vitamin D supplementation) for prevention of cancer, cardiovascular disease, and osteoporosis. A separate WHI initiative on hormone replacement therapy (estrogen plus progestin) was stopped in 2002 because of results indicating an increase in invasive breast cancer (Rossouw et al., 2002). Although disease endpoints are not complete for the nutritional components of the WHI, observational studies suggest that behavioral interventions designed for this trial have resulted in significant dietary changes, especially regarding reduced fat intake (Patterson et al., 2003).

Women's Healthy Eating and Living Study

The Women's Healthy Eating and Living (WHEL) Study, which began in 1996, is a multicenter, randomized dietary intervention trial among breast cancer survivors. The study is investigating the effectiveness of a high-vegetable, low-fat diet in reducing additional breast cancer events and early death in women within 4 years of diagnosis of early-stage invasive breast cancer (Pierce et al., 2002). An important aspect of the study is to investigate the impact of raising circulating carotenoid concentrations through changes in diet. Preliminary results have assessed the methods used in WHEL (FFQ, 24-hour dietary recall, intensive telephone counseling, cooking classes, and print materials) and found that the use of a multimodal, multimethod intervention is beneficial for promoting dietary change (Thomson et al., 2003). The study is scheduled for completion in 2006.

DELIVERY

Delivery is the process of disseminating, facilitating, and promoting evidence-based prevention, detection, diagnosis, and treatment practices and policies to reduce the burden of cancer in all segments of the population (von Eschenbach, 2003). A primary focus of these efforts is to develop strategies for those populations who bear the greatest burden of disease. Delivery works most efficiently when it is part of the processes of "Discovery" and "Development." SELECT is an excellent example of an integrated 3-D approach. Coordinated by the Southwest Oncology Group (SWOG), SELECT includes >400 study sites throughout the United States, Puerto Rico, and Canada. SWOG and many of the other study sites belong to the NCI's Community Clinical Oncology Program (CCOP), which is a creative mechanism designed to improve the accrual of patients to NCI phase III clinical trials while encouraging community-based oncologists to participate in clinical research. In addition, CCOP is one of the most practical means to disseminate new information on state-of-the-art cancer treatment outside the traditional cancer centers and research-oriented medical centers (Kaluzny et al., 1989). Clinicians and the public will receive immediate access to the prevention and treatment strategies that are most relevant to their communities because local researchers and facilities will be developing and participating in research translation efforts at the community level. For example, African American men and those in lower socioeconomic strata (SES) have the highest rates of prostate cancer, with race and SES being independent predictors of stage at diagnosis (Schwartz et al., 2003). Prevention and treatment strategies in SELECT can be immediately integrated and delivered in those CCOP communities that include populations that may benefit the most from intervention.

Understanding the most efficient and successful nutritional strategies to support cancer prevention, screening, and treatment for those individuals or groups that will benefit the most is a significant challenge for cancer researchers. The small and large hospitals, private practices, and groups of organizations or private practices that compose the CCOP network have been invaluable in creating the environment for research translation to health professionals and the public. CCOP includes 51 centers in 34 states, the District of Columbia, and Puerto Rico, as well as 11 Minority-Based CCOP Programs (MB-CCOP) that serve a large population of minorities. The network provides access to cancer clinical trials in 403 community-based hospitals, with >4000 community physicians participating in NCI clinical trials through this network (CCOP web site, 2003). Many of these clinical trials, such as SELECT, are investigating chemoprevention agents that include natural or synthetic nutritional components and contain programs for dissemination.

Challenges in Delivery for Nutritional Oncology

A significant challenge in delivery is determining the benefits within a population of dietary changes and whether lifestyle changes per se offer a greater benefit than treatment, screening, or chemoprevention. The analysis of worldwide cancer incidence and mortality rates mentioned previously confirms that diet influences cancer (Young and LeLeu, 2002), although changes in lifestyle generally take many years to accrue benefits compared with the shorter-term benefits of using treatment or chemoprevention approaches. Risks of treatment or chemoprevention, which are higher than dietary interventions, also must be considered when deciding whether lifestyle approaches should be implemented, especially as nutritional oncology appears to be in a transition period emphasizing the integration of lifestyle and medical approaches to cancer prevention. These issues must be weighted carefully in recommendations for lifestyle or medical approaches.

Medical Education

Delivery of evidence-based practices for the benefit of those most at risk for cancer will depend on improving nutrition education for clinicians and application of proven interventions and programs at the community level. Assessments indicate a lack of time spent on nutrition in our medical training institutions. A survey of medical schools in the United States found that nutrition medical education was required in only ~20% of the programs (Touger-Decker, 2004). A survey of hours of nutrition education in medical schools found that medical schools have an average of only 18 hours of instruction over a 4-year program (Torti et al., 2001). Improving nutrition medical education can encourage delivery of diet-related research results and help integrate delivery into the new nutrition paradigm. There have been calls to provide an integrated nutrition education message within every aspect of medical education so that graduates enter practice with an understanding of the integral role of nutrition in health and disease (Kushner, 2002).

Nutrition Policy

The awareness of the role of nutrition in cancer prevention should be integrated into all policies at the national, state, and local levels. In the past decade, with the maturity of electronic communications systems such as the Internet, cable TV, and home personal computing, information is becoming increasingly more available at every stratum of the population. The same media that bring information to the consumer, however, also bring conflicting information on the role of nutrition and specific diets in maintaining health. The USDA and the U.S. Department of Health and Human Services have the primary role for providing nutrition education and advice at the national level. Development of the Food Pyramid, and subsequent revisions, has provided consumers with science-based information on appropriate food choices. An interactive USDA web site (http://www.mypyramidtracker.gov) allows individuals to assess their diets in context of the amount of physical activity they perform and to set goals for maintaining or losing weight. This type of service adds to the knowledge of those who choose to participate. The movement of policymakers at the national level toward evidence-based national dietary guidelines is promising (Cooper and Zlotkin, 2003).

Application of nutrition-based policy is exemplified by the 5 A Day For Better Health Program (5 A Day), which was begun by the NCI in 1991 but was transferred to the Centers for Disease Control and Prevention. The 5 A Day Program is a cooperative initiative between the federal government and the vegetable and fruit industry to increase the intake of vegetables and fruit to reduce cancer risk. An evaluation of the 5 A Day program indicated that implementing a media campaign, point-of-purchase initiatives, such as use of the "5 A Day" logo on products, and community-level interventions have significantly increased intake from 1991 to 1997 (Stables et al., 2002). The 5 A Day program evaluation report and more about the program can be found by visiting their web site at http://www.5aday.gov/.

References

Albanes, D., Heinonen, O.P., Taylor, P.R., Virtamo, J., Edwards, B.K., Rautalahti, M., Hartman, A.M., Palmgren, J., Freedman, L.S., Haapakoski, J., Barrett, M.J., Pietinen, P., Malila, N., Tala, E., Liippo, K., Salomaa, E.-R., Tangrea, J.A., Teppo, L., Askin, F.B., Taskinen, E., Erozan, Y., Greenwald, P., and Huttunen, J.K. 1996. α-Tocopherol and β-carotene supplements and lung cancer incidence in the Alpha-Tocopherol, Beta-Carotene Cancer Prevention Study: effects of base-line characteristics and study compliance. *J Natl Cancer Inst* **88**: 1560–1570.

Alpha-Tocopherol Beta-Carotene Cancer Prevention Study Group, Heinonen, O.P., Huttunen, J.K., and Albanes, D. 1994. The effect of vitamin E and beta carotene on the incidence of lung cancer and other cancers in male smokers. *N Engl J Med* **330**: 1029–1035.

Augustsson, K., Michaud, D.S., Rimm, E.B., Leitzmann, M.F., Stampfer, M.J., Willett, W.C., and Giovannucci, E. 2003. A prospective study of intake of fish and marine fatty acids and prostate cancer. *Cancer Epidemiol Biomarkers Prev* **12**: 64–67.

Baer, H.J., Schnitt, S.J., Connolly, J.L., Byrne, C., Cho, E., Willett, W.C., and Colditz, G.A. 2003. Adolescent diet and incidence of proliferative benign breast disease. *Cancer Epidemiol Biomarkers Prev* **12**: 1159–1167.

Boileau, T.W., Liao, Z., Kim, S., Lemeshow, S., Erdman, J.W., Jr., and Clinton, S.K. 2003. Prostate carcinogenesis in N-methyl-N-nitrosourea (NMU)-testosterone–treated rats fed tomato powder, lycopene, or energy-restricted diets. *J Natl Cancer Inst* **95**: 1578–1586.

Branca, F., Hanley, A.B., Pool-Zobel, B., and Verhagen, H. 2001. Biomarkers in disease and health. *Br J Nutr* **86**(Suppl 1): S55–S92.

Brown, J., Byers, T., Thompson, K., Eldridge, B., Doyle, C., Williams, A.M.; American Cancer Society Workgroup on Nutrition and Physical Activity for Cancer Survivors. 2001. Nutrition during and after cancer treatment: a guide for informed choices by cancer survivors. *CA Cancer J Clin* **51**: 153–187; quiz 189–192.

Byers, T., Nestle, M., McTiernan, A., Doyle, C., Currie-Williams, A., Gansler, T., Thun, M., and American Cancer Society 2001 Nutrition and Physical Activity Guidelines Advisory Committee. 2002. American Cancer Society guidelines on nutrition and physical activity for cancer prevention. 2002. Reducing the risk of cancer with healthy food choices and physical activity. *CA Cancer J Clin* **52**: 92–119.

Calle, E.E., Thun, M.J., Petrelli, J.M., Rodriguez, C., and Heath, C.W., Jr. 1999. Body-mass index and mortality in a prospective cohort of U.S. adults. *N Engl J Med* **341**: 1097–1105.

Calle, E.E., Rodriguez, C., Walker-Thurmond, K., and Thun, M.J. 2003. Overweight, obesity, and mortality from cancer in a prospectively studied cohort of U.S. adults. *N Engl J Med* **348**: 1625–1638.

CCOP web site. URL: http://www3.cancer.gov/prevention/ccop/. Last visited 02-23-04. 2004. National Cancer Institute.

Chan, J.M., Stampfer, M.J., Ma, J., Rimm, E.B., Willett, W.C., and Giovannucci, E.L. 1999. Supplemental vitamin E intake and prostate cancer risk in a large cohort of men in the United States. *Cancer Epidemiol Biomarkers Prev* **8**: 893–899.

Chemoprevention Working Group, Alberts, D.S., Colvin, O.M., Conney, A.H., Ernster, V.L., Garber, J.E., Greenwald, P., Gudas, L.J., Hong, W.-K., Kelloff, G.J., Kramer, R.A., Lerman, C.E., Mangelsdorf, D.J., Matter, A., Minna, J.D., Nelson, W.G., V, Pezzuto, J.M., Prendergast, F., Rusch, V.W., Sporn, M.B., Wattenberg, L.W., and Weinstein, I.B. 1999. Prevention of cancer in the next millennium: report of the chemoprevention working group to the American Association for Cancer Research. *Cancer Res* **59**: 4743–4758.

Chen, X., Mikhail, S.S., Ding, Y.W., Yang, G., Bondoc, F., and Yang, C.-S. 2000. Effects of vitamin E and selenium supplementation on esophageal adenocarcinogenesis in a surgical model with rats. *Carcinogenesis* **21**: 1531–1536.

Cho, E., Spiegelman, D., Hunter, D.J., Chen, W.-Y., Colditz, G.A., and Willett, W.C. 2003. Premenopausal dietary carbohydrate, glycemic index, glycemic load, and fiber in relation to risk of breast cancer. *Cancer Epidemiol Biomarkers Prev* **12**: 1153–1158.

Christen, W.G., Gaziano, J.M., and Hennekens, C.H. 2000. Design of Physicians' Health Study IICa randomized trial of beta-carotene, vitamins E and C, and multivitamins, in prevention of cancer, cardiovascular disease, and eye disease, and review of results of completed trials. *Ann Epidemiol* **10**: 125–134.

Clark, L.C., Combs, G.F., Jr., Turnbull, B.W., Slate, E.H., Chalker, D.K., Chow, J., Davis, L.S., Glover, R.A., Graham, G.F., Gross, E.G., Krongrad, A., Lesher, J.L., Jr., Park, H.K., Sanders, B.B., Jr., Smith, C.L., and Taylor, J.R. 1996. Effects of selenium supplementation for cancer prevention in patients with carcinoma of the skin. A randomized controlled trial. Nutritional Prevention of Cancer Study Group. *JAMA* **276**: 1957–1963.

Clark, L.C., Dalkin, B., Krongrad, A., Combs, G.F., Jr., Turnbull, B.W., Slate, E.H., Witherington, R., Herlong, J.H., Janosko, E., Carpenter, D., Borosso, C., Falk, S., and Rounder, J. 1998. Decreased incidence of prostate cancer with selenium supplementation: results of a double-blind cancer prevention trial. *Br J Urol* **81**: 730–734.

Cooper, M.J., and Zlotkin, S.H. 2003. An evidence-based approach to the development of national dietary guidelines. *J Am Diet Assoc* **103**: S28–S33.

Corpet, D.E., and Pierre, F. 2003. Point: From animal models to prevention of colon cancer. Systematic review of chemoprevention in min mice and choice of the model system. *Cancer Epidemiol Biomarkers Prev* **12**: 391–400.

Crews, H., Alink, G., Andersen, R., Braesco, V., Holst, B., Maiani, G., Ovesen, L., Scotter, M., Solfrizzo, M., van den, B.R., Verhagen, H., and Williamson, G. 2001. A critical assessment of some biomarker approaches linked with dietary intake. *Br J Nutr* **86**: S5–35.

Davis, P.A., and Iwahashi, C.K. 2001. Whole almonds and almond fractions reduce aberrant crypt foci in a rat model of colon carcinogenesis. *Cancer Lett* **165**: 27–33.

Dirx, M.J., Zeegers, M.P., Dagnelie, P.C., van den, B.T., and van den Brandt, P.A. 2003. Energy restriction and the risk of spontaneous mammary tumors in mice: a meta-analysis. *Int J Cancer* **106**: 766–770.

Doll, R., and Peto, R. 1981. The causes of cancer: quantitative estimates of avoidable risks of cancer in the United States today. *J Natl Cancer Inst* **66**: 1191–1308.

Dong, Y., Zhang, H., Hawthorn, L., Ganther, H.E., and Ip, C. 2003. Delineation of the molecular basis for selenium-induced growth arrest in human prostate cancer cells by oligonucleotide array. *Cancer Res* **63**: 52–59.

Dunn, J.E., Jr. 1977. Breast cancer among American Japanese in the San Francisco Bay area. *Natl Cancer Inst Monogr* **47**: 157–160.

Feigelson, H.S., Jonas, C.R., Teras, L.R., Thun, M.J., and Calle, E.E. 2004. Weight gain, body mass index, hormone replacement therapy, and postmenopausal breast cancer in a large prospective study. *Cancer Epidemiol Biomarkers Prev* **13**: 220–224.

Feskanich, D., Ziegler, R.G., Michaud, D.S., Giovannucci, E.L., Speizer, F.E., Willett, W.C., and Colditz, G.A. 2000. Prospective study of fruit and vegetable consumption and risk of lung cancer among men and women. *J Natl Cancer Inst* **92**: 1812–1823.

Flegal, K.M., Carroll, M.D., Ogden, C.L., and Johnson, C.L. 2002. Prevalence and trends in obesity among US adults, 1999–2000. *JAMA* **288**: 1723–1727.

Fleischauer, A.T., and Arab, L. 2001. Garlic and cancer: a critical review of the epidemiologic literature. *J Nutr* 131: 1032S–1040S.

Fleming, J., Ghose, A., and Harrison, P.R. 2001. Molecular mechanisms of cancer prevention by selenium compounds. *Nutr Cancer* **40**: 42–49.

Frazier, A.L., Ryan, C.T., Rockett, H., Willett, W.C., and Colditz, G.A. 2003. Adolescent diet and risk of breast cancer. *Breast Cancer Res* **5**: R59–R64.

Friedenreich, C.M., and Orenstein, M.R. 2002. Physical activity and cancer prevention: etiologic evidence and biological mechanisms. *J Nutr* **132**: 3456S–3464S.

Giovannucci, E., Rimm, E.B., Wolk, A., Ascherio, A., Stampfer, M.J., Colditz, G.A., and Willett, W.C. 1998a. Calcium and fructose intake in relation to risk of prostate cancer. *Cancer Res* **58**: 442–447.

Giovannucci, E., Stampfer, M.J., Colditz, G.A., Hunter, D.J., Fuchs, C., Rosner, B.A., Speizer, F.E., and Willett, W.C. 1998b. Multivitamin use, folate, and colon cancer in women in the Nurses' Health Study. *Ann Intern Med* **129**: 517–524.

Giovannucci, E., Rimm, E.B., Liu, Y., Stampfer, M.J., and Willett, W.C. 2003a. A prospective study of cruciferous vegetables and prostate cancer. *Cancer Epidemiol Biomarkers Prev* **12**: 1403–1409.

Giovannucci, E., Rimm, E.B., Liu, Y., Leitzmann, M., Wu, K., Stampfer, M.J., and Willett, W.C. 2003b. Body mass index and risk of prostate cancer in U.S. health professionals. *J Natl Cancer Inst* **95**: 1240–1244.

Greenwald, P., Nixon, D.W., Malone, W.F., Kelloff, G.J., Stern, H.R., and Witkin, K.M. 1990. Concepts in cancer chemoprevention research. *Cancer* **65**: 1483–1489.

Greenwald, P., Milner, J.A., and Clifford, C.K. 2000. Creating a new paradigm in nutrition research within the National Cancer Institute. *J Nutr* **130**: 3103–3105.

Greenwald, P. 2003. Beta-carotene and lung cancer: a lesson for future chemoprevention investigations? *J Natl Cancer Inst* **95**: E1.

Gupta, S., Hastak, K., Ahmad, N., Lewin, J.S., and Mukhtar, H. 2001. Inhibition of prostate carcinogenesis in TRAMP mice by oral infusion of green tea polyphenols. *Proc Natl Acad Sci USA* **98**: 10350–10355.

Haiman, C.A., Hankinson, S.E., Colditz, G.A., Hunter, D.J., and De Vivo, I. 2001. A polymorphism in *CYP17* and endometrial cancer risk. *Cancer Res* **61**: 3955–3960.

Hakkak, R., Korourian, S., Ronis, M.J., Johnston, J.M., and Badger, T.M. 2001. Dietary whey protein protects against azoxymethane-induced colon tumors in male rats. *Cancer Epidemiol Biomarkers Prev* **10**: 555–558.

Hann, C.S., Rock, C.L., King, I., and Drewnowski, A. 2001. Validation of the Healthy Eating Index with use of plasma biomarkers in a clinical sample of women. *Am J Clin Nutr* **74**: 479–486.

Harvell, D.M., Strecker, T.E., Xie, B., Buckles, L.K., Tochacek, M., McComb, R.D., and Shull, J.D. 2001. Diet-gene interactions in estrogen-induced mammary carcinogenesis in the ACI rat. *J Nutr* **131**: 3087S–3091S.

Heber, D., and Lu, Q.Y. 2002. Overview of mechanisms of action of lycopene. *Exp Biol Med (Maywood)* **227**: 920–923.

Heinonen, O.P., Albanes, D., Virtamo, J., Taylor, P.R., Huttunen, J.K., Hartman, A.M., Haapakoski, J., Malila, N., Rautalahti, M., Ripatti, S., Maenpaa, H., Teerenhovi, L., Koss, L., Virolainen, M., and Edwards, B.K. 1998. Prostate cancer and supplementation with α-tocopherol and β-carotene: Incidence and mortality in a controlled trial. *J Natl Cancer Inst* **90**: 440–446.

Hennekens, C.H., Buring, J.E., Manson, J.E., Stampfer, M., Rosner, B., Cook, N.R., Belanger, C., LaMotte, F., Gaziano, J.M., Ridker, P.M., Willett, W., and Peto, R. 1996. Lack of effect of long-term supplementation with beta carotene on the incidence of malignant neoplasms and cardiovascular disease. *N Engl J Med* **334**: 1145–1149.

Holmes, M.D., Colditz, G.A., Hunter, D.J., Hankinson, S.E., Rosner, B., Speizer, F.E., and Willett, W.C. 2003. Meat, fish and egg intake and risk of breast cancer. *Int J Cancer* **104**: 221–227.

Hoque, A., Albanes, D., Lippman, S.M., Spitz, M.R., Taylor, P.R., Klein, E.A., Thompson, I.M., Goodman, P., Stanford, J.L., Crowley, J.J., Coltman, C.A., and Santella, R.M. 2001. Molecular epidemiologic studies within the Selenium and Vitamin E Cancer Prevention Trial (SELECT). *Cancer Causes Control* **12**: 627–633.

Hsing, A.W., Chokkalingam, A.P., Gao, Y.-T., Madigan, M.P., Deng, J., Gridley, G., and Fraumeni, J.F., Jr. 2002. Allium vegetables and risk of prostate cancer: a population-based study. *J Natl Cancer Inst* **94**: 1648–1651.

Hursting, S.D., Lavigne, J.A., Berrigan, D., Perkins, S.N., and Barrett, J.C. 2003. Calorie restriction, aging, and cancer prevention: mechanisms of action and applicability to humans. *Annu Rev Med* **54**: 131–152.

Ip, C. 1998. Lessons from basic research in selenium and cancer prevention. *J Nutr* **128**: 1845–1854.

Kaluzny, A.D., Ricketts, T., III, Warnecke, R., Ford, L., Morrissey, J., Gillings, D., Sondik, E.J., Ozer, H., and Goldman, J. 1989. Evaluating organizational design to assure technology transfer: the case of the Community Clinical Oncology Program. *J Natl Cancer Inst* **81**: 1717–1725.

Kearney, J., Giovannucci, E., Rimm, E.B., Stampfer, M.J., Colditz, G.A., Ascherio, A., Bleday, R., and Willett, W.C. 1995. Diet, alcohol, and smoking and the occurrence of hyperplastic polyps of the colon and rectum (United States). *Cancer Causes Control* **6**: 45–56.

Kiffmeyer, W.R., Langer, E., Davies, S.M., Envall, J., Robison, L.L., and Ross, J.A. 2004. Genetic polymorphisms in the Hmong population: implications for cancer etiology and survival. *Cancer* **100**: 411–417.

Klein, E.A., Thompson, I.M., Lippman, S.M., Goodman, P.J., Albanes, D., Taylor, P.R., and Coltman, C. 2001. SELECT: the next prostate cancer prevention trial. Selenium and Vitamin E Cancer Prevention Trial. *J Urol* **166**: 1311–1315.

Klein, E.A. 2004. Selenium: epidemiology and basic science. *J Urol* **171**: S50–S53.

Kumanyika, S.K., Mauger, D., Mitchell, D.C., Phillips, B., Smiciklas-Wright, H., and Palmer, J.R. 2003. Relative validity of food frequency questionnaire nutrient estimates in the Black Women's Health Study. *Ann Epidemiol* **13**: 111–118.

Kushner, R.F. 2003. Denon Institute Award for Excellence in Medical/Dental Nutrition Education Lecture, 2002. Will there be a tipping point in medical nutrition education? *Am J Clin Nutr* **77**: 288–291.

Ladas, E.J., Jacobson, J.S., Kennedy, D.D., Teel, K., Fleischauer, A., and Kelly, K.M. 2004. Antioxidants and cancer therapy: a systematic review. *J Clin Oncol* **22**: 517–528.

Lanza, E., Schatzkin, A., Ballard-Barbash, R., Clifford, D.C., Paskett, E., Hayes, D., Bote, E., Caan, B., Shike, M., Weissfeld, J., Slattery, M., Mateski, D., and Daston, C. 1996. The Polyp Prevention Trial II: dietary intervention program and participant baseline dietary characteristics. *Cancer Epidemiol Biomarkers Prev* **5**: 385–392.

Lanza, E., Schatzkin, A., Daston, C., Corle, D., Freedman, L., Ballard-Barbash, R., Caan, B., Lance, P., Marshall, J., Iber, F., Shike, M., Weissfeld, J., Slattery, M., Paskett, E., Mateski, D., and Albert, P. 2001. Implementation of a 4-y, high-fiber, high-fruit-and-vegetable, low-fat dietary intervention: results of dietary changes in the Polyp Prevention Trial. *Am J Clin Nutr* **74**: 387–401.

Lin, X., Gingrich, J.R., Bao, W., Li, J., Haroon, Z.A., and Demark-Wahnefried, W. 2002. Effect of flaxseed supplementation on prostatic carcinoma in transgenic mice. *Urology* **60**: 919–924.

Mallin, K., Anderson, K. 1988. Cancer mortality in Illinois Mexican and Puerto Rican immigrants, 1979–1984. *Int J Cancer* **41**: 670–676.

Männistö, S., Smith-Warner, S.A., Spiegelman, D., Albanes, D., Anderson, K., van den Brandt, P.A., Cerhan, J.R., Colditz, G., Feskanich, D., Freudenheim, J.L., Giovannucci, E., Goldbohm, R.A., Graham, S., Miller, A.B., Rohan, T.E., Virtamo, J., Willett, W.C., and Hunter, D.J. 2004. Dietary carotenoids and risk of lung cancer in a pooled analysis of seven cohort studies. *Cancer Epidemiol Biomarkers Prev* **13**: 40–48.

Manson, M.M. 2003. Cancer prevention—the potential for diet to modulate molecular signaling. *Trends Mol Med* **9**: 11–18.

McCullough, M.L., Robertson, A.S., Chao, A., Jacobs, E.J., Stampfer, M.J., Jacobs, D.R., Diver, W.R., Calle, E.E., and Thun, M.J. 2003. A prospective study of whole grains, fruits, vegetables and colon cancer risk. *Cancer Causes Control* **14**: 959–970.

Mentor-Marcel, R., Lamartiniere, C.A., Eltoum, I.E., Greenberg, N.M., and Elgavish, A. 2001. Genistein in the diet reduces the incidence of poorly differentiated prostatic adenocarcinoma in transgenic mice (TRAMP). *Cancer Res* **61**: 6777–6782.

Michels, K.B., Edward, G., Joshipura, K.J., Rosner, B.A., Stampfer, M.J., Fuchs, C.S., Colditz, G.A., Speizer, F.E., and Willett, W.C. 2000. Prospective study of fruit and vegetable consumption and incidence of colon and rectal cancers. *J Natl Cancer Inst* **92**: 1740–1752.

Miller, E.C., Giovannucci, E., Erdman, J.W., Jr., Bahnson, R., Schwartz, S.J., and Clinton, S.K. 2002. Tomato products, lycopene, and prostate cancer risk. *Urol Clin North Am* **29**: 83–93.

Mills, P.K., and Yang, R. 1997. Cancer incidence in the Hmong of Central California, United States, 1987–94. *Cancer Causes Control* **8**: 705–712.

Milner, J.A. 2001a. A historical perspective on garlic and cancer. *J Nutr* **131**: 1027S–1031S.

Milner, J.A., McDonald, S.S., Anderson, D.E., and Greenwald, P. 2001b. Molecular targets for nutrients involved with cancer prevention. *Nutr Cancer* **41**: 1–16.

Milner, J.A. 2003. Incorporating basic nutrition science into health interventions for cancer prevention. *J Nutr* **133**: 3820S–3826S.

Møller, P., and Loft, S. 2002. Oxidative DNA damage in human white blood cells in dietary antioxidant intervention studies. *Am J Clin Nutr* **76**: 303–310.

National Academy of Sciences, National Research Council. 1982. "Diet, Nutrition and Cancer." National Academy Press, Washington, DC.

National Academy of Sciences, National Research Council, Commission on Life Sciences, Food and Nutrition Board. 1989. "Diet and Health. Implications for Reducing Chronic Disease Risk." National Academy Press, Washington, D.C.

Negri, E., La Vecchia, C.L., Franceschi, S., D'Avanzo, B., and Parazzini, F. 1991. Vegetable and fruit consumption and cancer risk. *Int J Cancer* **48**: 350–354.

Nielsen, S.J., and Popkin, B.M. 2003. Patterns and trends in food portion sizes, 1977–1998. *JAMA* **289**: 450–453.

Omenn, G.S., Goodman, G., Thornquist, M., Grizzle, J., Rosenstock, L., Barnhart, S., Balmes, J., Cherniack, M.G., Cullen, M.R., Glass, A., Keogh, J., Meyskens, F.L., Jr., Valanis, B., and Williams, J., Jr. 1994. The beta-carotene and retinol efficacy trial (CARET) for chemoprevention of lung cancer in high risk populations: smokers and asbestos-exposed workers. *Cancer Res* **54**: 2038–2043.

Orlet, F.J., Rolls, B.J., and Birch, L.L. 2003. Children's bite size and intake of an entree are greater with large portions than with age-appropriate or self-selected portions. *Am J Clin Nutr* **77**: 1164–1170.

Patterson, R.E., Kristal, A., Rodabough, R., Caan, B., Lillington, L., Mossavar-Rahmani, Y., Simon, M.S., Snetselaar, L., and Van Horn, L. 2003. Changes in food sources of dietary fat in response to an intensive low-fat dietary intervention: early results from the Women's Health Initiative. *J Am Diet Assoc* **103**: 454–460.

Perkins, S., Verschoyle, R.D., Hill, K., Parveen, I., Threadgill, M.D., Sharma, R.A., Williams, M.L., Steward, W.P., and Gescher, A.J. 2002. Chemopreventive efficacy and pharmacokinetics of curcumin in the min/+ mouse, a model of familial adenomatous polyposis. *Cancer Epidemiol Biomarkers Prev* **11**: 535–540.

Pierce, J.P., Faerber, S., Wright, F.A., Rock, C.L., Newman, V., Flatt, S.W., Kealey, S., Jones, V.E., Caan, B.J., Gold, E.B., Haan, M., Hollenbach, K.A., Jones, L., Marshall, J.R., Ritenbaugh, C., Stefanick, M.L., Thomson, C., Wasserman, L., Natarajan, L., Thomas, R.G., and Gilpin, E.A. 2002. A randomized trial of the effect of a plant-based dietary pattern on additional breast cancer events and survival: the Women's Healthy Eating and Living (WHEL) Study. *Control Clin Trials* **23**: 728–756.

Platz, E.A., Leitzmann, M.F., Michaud, D.S., Willett, W.C., and Giovannucci, E. 2003. Interrelation of energy intake, body size, and physical activity with prostate cancer in a large prospective cohort study. *Cancer Res* **63**: 8542–8548.

Poirier, L.A. 2002. The effects of diet, genetics and chemicals on toxicity and aberrant DNA methylation: an introduction. *J Nutr* **132**: 2336S–2339S.

Quadrilatero, J., and Hoffman-Goetz, L. 2003. Physical activity and colon cancer. A systematic review of potential mechanisms. *J Sports Med Phys Fitness* **43**: 121–138.

Riboli, E., and Kaaks, R. 1997. The EPIC Project: rationale and study design. European Prospective Investigation into Cancer and Nutrition. *Int J Epidemiol* **26**(Suppl 1): S6–14.

Riboli, E., and Lambert, R., Eds. 2002. "Nutrition and Lifestyle: Opportunities for Cancer Prevention." International Agency for Research on Cancer, Lyon, France.

Rickard, S.E., Yuan, Y.V., Chen, J., and Thompson, L.U. 1999. Dose effects of flaxseed and its lignan on N-methyl-N-nitrosourea–induced mammary tumorigenesis in rats. *Nutr Cancer* **35**: 50–57.

Ross, J.A., Xie, Y., Kiffmeyer, W.R., Bushhouse, S., and Robison, L.L. 2003. Cancer in the Minnesota Hmong population. *Cancer* **97**: 3076–3079.

Rossouw, J.E., Anderson, G.L., Prentice, R.L., LaCroix, A.Z., Kooperberg, C., Stefanick, M.L., Jackson, R.D., Beresford, S.A., Howard, B.V., Johnson, K.C., Kotchen, J.M., and Ockene, J. 2002. Risks and benefits of estrogen plus progestin in healthy postmenopausal women: principal results From the Women's Health Initiative randomized controlled trial. *JAMA* **288**: 321–333.

Schattner, M. 2003. Enteral nutritional support of the patient with cancer: route and role. *J Clin Gastroenterol* **36**: 297–302.

Schatzkin, A., Lanza, E., Freedman, L.S., Tangrea, J., Cooper, M.R., Marshall, J.R., Murphy, P.A., Selby, J.V., Shike, M., Schade, R.R., Burt, R.W., Kikendall, J.W., and Cahill, J. 1996. The Polyp Prevention Trial I: rationale, design, recruitment, and baseline participant characteristics. *Cancer Epidemiol Biomarkers Prev* **5**: 375–383.

Schatzkin, A., Lanza, E., Corle, D., Lance, P., Iber, F., Caan, B., Shike, M., Weissfeld, J., Burt, R., Cooper, M.R., Kikendall, J.W., and Cahill, J. 2000. Lack of effect of a low-fat, high-fiber diet on the recurrence of colorectal adenomas. Polyp Prevention Trial Study Group. *N Engl J Med* **342**: 1149–1155.

Schwartz, K.L., Crossley-May, H., Vigneau, F.D., Brown, K., and Banerjee, M. 2003. Race, socioeconomic status and stage at diagnosis for five common malignancies. *Cancer Causes Control* **14**: 761–766.

Shimizu, H., Ross, R.K., Bernstein, L., Yatani, R., Henderson, B.E., and Mack, T.M. 1991. Cancers of the prostate and breast among Japanese and white immigrants in Los Angeles County. *Br J Cancer* **63**: 963–966.

Sinha, R., Said, T.K., and Medina, D. 1996. Organic and inorganic selenium compounds inhibit mouse mammary cell growth in vitro by different cellular pathways. *Cancer Lett* **107**: 277–284.

Slattery, M.L., Boucher, K.M., Caan, B.J., Potter, J.D., and Ma, K.-N. 1998. Eating patterns and risk of colon cancer. *Am J Epidemiol* **148**: 4–16.

Srivastava, S., and Gopal-Srivastava, R. 2002. Biomarkers in cancer screening: a public health perspective. *J Nutr* **132**: 2471S–2475S.

Stables, G.J., Subar, A.F., Patterson, B.H., Dodd, K., Heimendinger, J., Van Duyn, M.A., and Nebeling, L. 2002. Changes in vegetable and fruit consumption and awareness among US adults: results of the 1991 and 1997 5 A Day for Better Health Program surveys. *J Am Diet Assoc* **102**: 809–817.

Story, M., and Harris, L.J. 1989. Food habits and dietary change of Southeast Asian refugee families living in the United States. *J Am Diet Assoc* **89**: 800–803.

Thomson, C.A., Giuliano, A., Rock, C.L., Ritenbaugh, C.K., Flatt, S.W., Faerber, S., Newman, V., Caan, B., Graver, E., Hartz, V., Whitacre, R., Parker, F., Pierce, J.P., and Marshall, J.R. 2003. Measuring dietary change in a diet intervention trial: comparing food frequency questionnaire and dietary recalls. *Am J Epidemiol* **157**: 754–762.

Torti, F.M., Jr., Adams, K.M., Edwards, L.J., Lindell, K.C., and Zeisel, S.H. 2001. Survey of nutrition education in U.S. medical schools—an instructor-based analysis. Source http://www.med-ed-online.org/pdf/res00023.pdf. *Med Educ Online* [serial online] **6**: 8, 1–6.

Touger-Decker, R. 2004. Nutrition education of medical and dental students: innovation through curriculum integration. *Am J Clin Nutr* **79**: 198–203.

Troiano, R.P., Briefel, R.R., Carroll, M.D., and Bialostosky, K. 2000. Energy and fat intakes of children and adolescents in the united states: data from the national health and nutrition examination surveys. *Am J Clin Nutr* **72**: 1343S–1353S.

Tseng, M., Breslow, R.A., DeVellis, R.F., and Ziegler, R.G. 2004. Dietary patterns and prostate cancer risk in the National Health and Nutrition Examination Survey Epidemiological Follow-up Study cohort. *Cancer Epidemiol Biomarkers Prev* **13**: 71–77.

van Kappel, A.L., Steghens, J.P., Zeleniuch-Jacquotte, A., Chajes, V., Toniolo, P., and Riboli, E. 2001. Serum carotenoids as biomarkers of fruit and vegetable consumption in the New York Women's Health Study. *Public Health Nutr* **4**: 829–835.

Venkateswaran, V., Klotz, L.H., and Fleshner, N.E. 2002. Selenium modulation of cell proliferation and cell cycle biomarkers in human prostate carcinoma cell lines. *Cancer Res* **62**: 2540–2545.

Verma, M., and Srivastava, S. 2003. New cancer biomarkers deriving from NCI early detection research. *Recent Results Cancer Res* **163**: 72–84.

Virtamo, J., Pietinen, P., Huttunen, J.K., Korhonen, P., Malila, N., Virtanen, M.J., Albanes, D., Taylor, P.R., and Albert, P. 2003. Incidence of cancer and mortality following alpha-tocopherol and beta-carotene supplementation: a postintervention follow-up. *JAMA* **290**: 476–485.

von Eschenbach, A.C. 2003. NCI sets goal of eliminating suffering and death due to cancer by 2015. *J Natl Med Assoc* **95**: 637–639.

Watkins, S.M., and German, J.B. 2002. Toward the implementation of metabolomic assessments of human health and nutrition. *Curr Opin Biotechnol* **13**: 512–516.

Wei, W.-Q., Abnet, C.C., Qiao, Y.-L., Dawsey, S.M., Dong, Z.-W., Sun, X.-D., Fan, J.-H., Gunter, E.W., Taylor, P.R., and Mark, S.D. 2004. Prospective study of serum selenium concentrations and esophageal and gastric cardia cancer, heart disease, stroke, and total death. *Am J Clin Nutr* **79**: 80–85.

World Cancer Research Fund. 1997. "Food, Nutrition and the Prevention of Cancer: A Global Perspective." American Institute for Cancer Research, Washington, DC.

Yang, X., Edgerton, S.M., Kosanke, S.D., Mason, T.L., Alvarez, K.M., Liu, N., Chatterton, R.T., Liu, B., Wang, Q., Kim, A., Murthy, S., and Thor,

A.D. 2003. Hormonal and dietary modulation of mammary carcinogenesis in mouse mammary tumor virus-c-erbB-2 transgenic mice. *Cancer Res* **63**: 2425–2433.

Young, G.P., and Le Leu, R.K. 2002. Preventing cancer: dietary lifestyle or clinical intervention? *Asia Pacific J Clin Nutr* **11**(Suppl): S618–S631.

Young, L.R., and Nestle, M. 2003. Expanding portion sizes in the US marketplace: implications for nutrition counseling. *J Am Diet Assoc* **103**: 231–234.

Zeng, H., Davis, C.D., and Finley, J.W. 2003. Effect of selenium-enriched broccoli diet on differential gene expression in min mouse liver(1,2). *J Nutr Biochem* **14**: 227–231.

Zheng, Y., Xu, Y., Ye, B., Lei, J., Weinstein, M.H., O'Leary, M.P., Richie, J.P., Mok, S.C., and Liu, B.-C. 2003. Prostate carcinoma tissue proteomics for biomarker discovery. *Cancer* **98**: 2576–2582.

C H A P T E R

19

Dietary Assessment

CATHERINE L. CARPENTER

INTRODUCTION

Over the past 25 years, dietary assessment methodology has made significant progress in identifying associations between patterns of dietary consumption and cancer risk. Although it is not yet possible to quantify specific cancer risks related to specific foods or dietary patterns, there is considerable evidence that certain foods are associated with increased cancer risk. For example, epidemiological studies have identified a clear association of increased red meat intake with an increased risk for colorectal cancer (Chao et al., 2005; Willett, 2005).

The choice of optimal dietary assessment methods depends on the research question being asked, the cancer site under study, the research study design, and the metabolic/biochemical measurements available for characterizing dietary intake. Moreover, factors intrinsic to the dietary assessment instruments have been shown to affect the results obtained. These include the quality of nutrient and food composition databases, the sensitivity of specific assessment instruments to differences in nutrient intake, and the flexibility of the assessment instrument for diverse dietary intakes. A number of these methodological constraints that can lead to inconsistent results on the association of diet and cancer risk have appeared in published studies from different groups of investigators.

STUDY DESIGN AND ASSESSMENT

Dietary Pattern Assessment

Measurements of dietary patterns are generally conducted using recall methods (Tarasuk and Brooker, 1997). Recall of subjects' dietary histories are meant to approximate dietary exposures before cancer induction. Because cancer tends to develop very slowly over a 20–30 year period, memories of subjects' diets long ago are often inaccurate.

Recall bias can occur for many reasons. One example of recall bias is reporting of dietary intake by obese subjects, which is different from reporting of dietary habits by lean subjects. Many obese subjects omit mentioning those foods they know they should not be eating. Patients suffering from cancer malnutrition may be weakened, or even cachectic, so their ability to recall foods may be impaired in comparison to healthy controls. Controls reporting higher consumption with a particular food relative to cases that are cachectic may distort associations toward a preventive or risk-enhancing direction, leading to false conclusions.

Prospective Longitudinal Study Designs

The major advantage of conducting a prospective cohort study is measurement of dietary intake before disease onset, which can provide important insight into causal relationships between dietary patterns and cancer. However, determination of the relevant etiological time period for dietary assessment can be challenging (Tarasuk and Brooker, 1997).

Major disadvantages for conducting a prospective cohort study include lengthy time of study, large sample sizes required to detect associations with rare cancer outcomes, the higher costs associated with subject recruitment and measurement over time, and specialized composition of cohorts that limit generalizability.

Nutrigenetics and Nutrigenomics

Genetic and molecular epidemiological study designs such as case–case and gene-association studies are

Copyright © 2006, Elsevier Inc.
All rights of reproduction in any form reserved.

beginning to evaluate interactions between dietary intake and genetic polymorphisms, as well as interactions between dietary intake and gene expression. Genetic polymorphisms are a function of inheritance and can be considered fixed exposures over the lifetime, whereas gene expression and epigenetic changes vary over the lifetime.

Both acquired genetic changes and inherited susceptibility, coupled with environmental exposures, are responsible for development of cancer. The technology for measuring gene expression and epigenetic changes such as DNA methylation in relationship to nutritional intake and cancer has only been developed recently. A study of DNA methylation of gastric tumors was conducted among 58 male patients who completed food frequency questionnaires (FFQs) and lifestyle questionnaires. Tumors were categorized according to methylation status, and dietary factors were compared in relationship to methylation. The study found an association between CDX2 gastric tumor methylation and decreased intake of green tea and cruciferous vegetables (Yuasa et al., 2005).

Gene-association studies examine relationships between polymorphisms of inherited genes, environmental exposures, and risk of disease. Dietary intake and gene association studies in relationship to cancer risk can be conducted prospectively or retrospectively, using cross-sectional, case-control, or prospective cohort designs. One example is a report of serum biomarkers of carotenoids that were studied in relationship to DNA repair gene (XRCC1) haplotypes and breast cancer risk in the Nurses' Health Study (Han et al., 2003). The study found a marginally significant reduction in breast cancer risk among women who carried at least one 194Trp allele compared wtih noncarriers. One of the haplotypes of the XRCC1 gene, Arg194Trp, modified the inverse associations of plasma α-carotene level and plasma β-carotene level with breast cancer risk (Han et al., 2003).

METHODS OF DIETARY ASSESSMENT

Dietary assessment is used to identify and monitor types and amounts of foods and beverages consumed by individuals and groups of individuals. Results of dietary assessments, in turn, shape public health policy and programs. Identifying dietary patterns or food constituents that clearly contribute to or prevent development of cancer is a primary goal and challenge of diet and cancer research.

Accurate estimation of nutritional intake is fundamental to studies of diet and cancer. Various methods exist for assessment of dietary intake in free-living individuals. The three main approaches are 24-hour recalls, diet records, and FFQs. Both 24-hour recalls and diet records allow for free-form open-ended recording of food intake. FFQs have pre-assigned lists of foods and set categories for amount of food consumed.

An ideal dietary assessment instrument should provide an accurate, objective, unbiased, and quantitative measure of long-term exposure to dietary constituents. The accuracy of dietary assessment depends, in part, on the accuracy of available food composition data; the need for expanded composition data for commonly eaten foods is widely recognized. Epidemiological surveys, controlled feeding, metabolic studies, and clinical trials of dietary modification all use dietary assessment methods.

The general-purpose instruments used to estimate nutrient intake in populations are not well suited to assessing the modest dietary changes that might result from a dietary intervention. Even within an intervention, different instruments might be used for assessment at baseline versus after intervention because of significant changes in consumption and food preparation techniques.

Controlled feeding and metabolic studies, in which all foods are provided, permit close monitoring of food and nutrient intake, as well as biological and metabolic responses that result from dietary change. Such studies are important for development of validated standardized nutritional biomarkers, which may be useful adjuncts to traditional dietary assessment instruments. Selection of the dietary survey methodology, among other things, is dependent on the study design and timing of dietary exposure measurement (Barrett-Connor, 1991; Sempos et al., 1999).

Twenty-four Hour Recall

Twenty-four hour recalls ask individuals to describe, in either an in-person or telephone interview with a nutritionist or trained interviewer, what they have eaten during the previous 24 hours (Willett et al., 1985; World Cancer Research Fund [WCRF], 1997).

This method has the advantages of requiring minimal effort on the part of the study participant (Willett, 1987). Although single 24-hour recalls are highly accurate and reliable measures of recent intake, they do not account for day-to-day variability in an individual's diet and generally are not recommended for use in longitudinal large-scale cohort studies (Willett et al., 1985; Willett, 1987; WCRF, 1997). On the other hand, 24-hour recall methods have better reliability for assessing current and immediate dietary patterns for validation of biomarkers that characterize the intake of particular nutrients, as well as assessing dietary compliance in dietary intervention studies.

Using data from a carefully designed validation study conducted by Willett et al. (1985), Byar and Freedman (1989) argue that one reason the precision of subjective dietary assessment methods such as FFQs and dietary records is limited or compromised is that individuals are not aware of what they eat. Willett's validation study included 173 female nurses who were asked to record everything they ate for 7 days on four separate occasions ~3 months apart. The same subjects also completed a semiquantitative FFQ on two separate occasions. In this case, the dietary food records served as the "gold standard" against which the questionnaire data were validated.

Quintiles of intake from the FFQ were then cross-classified with quintiles from the 7-day food records. If the two methods were measuring the same intakes with no measurement error, a one-to-one direct correlation (a correlation of 1) between the same quintiles of intake would result. Interestingly, however, only 53% of individuals in the first quintile for the questionnaire data also were in the first quintile for the food record data. Correlations were even lower for the other quintile comparisons. Such data provide insight into how well, or poorly, one assessment method compares with another. Whether participants actually provide different dietary profiles in the different instruments, or whether questionnaires and recall methods do not adequately match items described in personal food diaries, warrants further investigation.

The new multiple-pass method for collecting 24-hour dietary recalls maintains related systems and databases and is designed to engage the respondent more completely to provide more accurate recalls than earlier methods (Dwyer et al., 2001). These types of 24-hour recalls have been consistently used to characterize food intakes of large population groups such as those surveyed in the National Health and Nutrition Examination Survey (NHANES) (U.S. Department of Health and Human Services, 2005). The Continuing Survey of Food Intakes by Individuals (CSFII) and the NHANES have become integrated (Dwyer et al., 2001). The integrated survey has been administered as part of the NHANES that began in 2002.

Another well-respected automated 24-hour recall is the Nutrition Data System for Research (NDS-R), developed by the Nutrition Coordinating Center from the University of Minnesota (Nutrition Coordinating Center, 2005). The computer-based application allows entry of dietary data in a standardized fashion and uses a multiple-pass approach for dietary data collection that prompts for complete food descriptions, food preparation methods, and diverse amount descriptions. The Nutrition Data System links to an extensive database that contains values for 136 nutrients, nutrient ratios, and other food components and includes >18,000 foods, with many ethnic foods and >8000 brand-name products (Nutrition Coordinating Center, 2005).

Food Records

Food records or diaries are detailed descriptions of types and amounts of foods and beverages consumed over a prescribed period, usually 3–7 days. The record or diary may be a special form or booklet that contains prompts or suggested categories of foods for each day. In some applications, subjects measure food with scales using specific procedures (Willett, 1990).

Maintaining a food diary requires meticulous record keeping; sustaining these activities over even a relatively short period requires highly motivated literate individuals. Recording daily intakes often increases subjects' awareness of what they are eating, which in turn can lead to immediate alterations in the diet. Because of this reactive effect of the participant changing his or her dietary intake by omitting foods to simplify record-keeping, dietary records often do not represent actual intake (Willett, 1987; Bingham and Paul, 1998). In dietary intervention studies, a heightened awareness can be instilled in subjects to enhance the accuracy of diet records, and diet records become a teaching device within the intervention (Willett, 1990).

In general, dietary record keeping is expensive and inappropriate for studies focused on past intake. Unlike most other methods, however, food diaries do not depend heavily on memory and thus are relatively free from recall bias, compared with other methods. Food records also reduce day-to-day variation in diet by averaging intake over a number of days and can control for differential intakes between weekdays and weekends. Furthermore, record-keeping methods that require foods and beverages to be weighed or measured dramatically reduce errors associated with estimating portion size (Willett, 1987). Food records can be invaluable tools to monitor group compliance in dietary intervention trials; however, the possibility that compliance may be good during the period of recall and poor otherwise may promote biases in reporting. Diet records are one of the several methods for validating FFQs (Willett, 1990).

Food records are being used in large-scale prospective studies to measure diet at various intervals over time. The Data Into Nutrients for Epidemiological Research (DINER) system program is a computerized software system for entry of 7-day diaries in the EPIC-Norfolk cohort (Welch et al., 2001). A food list of 9000 food items and values for 24,000 portion sizes have been incorporated into the database. Daily food intake is recorded in a food diary booklet that is entered into the DINER system using a series of pull-down menus that record time of day and meal, food item, amount of food, method of preparation, and so forth. Food items are then merged to an extensive database that converts the food items to nutrients and food groups (Welch et al., 2001).

There are possible drawbacks to recording and inferring usual intake from 7-day food records (Gersovitz et al., 1978; Willett, 1990; Flegal, 1999). Seven-day food records require a high degree of respondent cooperation that may be difficult to achieve in a large study (Flegal, 1999). Moreover, food records tend to become less accurate after the first 4 days of record keeping (Gersovitz et al., 1978). Other limitations to food records include inability to fully represent usual dietary intake and the requirement that the respondent population be motivated, literate, and cooperative (Willett,

1990). Food records collected over specified time intervals in a prospective design can, however, be a relatively accurate and unbiased method for assessing dietary intake and risk of disease (Barrett-Connor, 1991).

Food Frequency Questionnaires

FFQs are designed to assess frequencies with which food items are consumed during a specified time (Tarasuk and Brooker, 1997). FFQs generally provide a listing of foods and include categories to mark, indicating how often a food item is consumed on a monthly, weekly, or daily basis. The underlying principle of the food frequency approach is that average long-term diet, for example, consumption over months or years, is the conceptually important exposure rather than intake on a few specific days, such as what is measured in 24 hours (Willett, 1990). Although recall of diet >20 years ago is impractical, the food frequency approach may approximate crude underlying dietary patterns that have been present over the long term. Two well-known FFQs, among others, have been used extensively in epidemiological studies of diet and cancer (Willett et al., 1985; Block et al., 1986). In a comparability study of nutrient estimation among subjects who completed both the Willett Food Frequency Questionnaire (Willett et al., 1985) and the Block Food Frequency Questionnaire (Block et al., 1986), both questionnaires were found to be, on the average, interchangeable with respect to estimates of nutrients in the overall diet (McCann et al., 1999).

FFQ data may be affected by the educational level of research subjects. Completion of FFQs requires cognitive ability to distinguish how often foods are consumed, remembering which foods are consumed, and recording in such a way that responses reflect usual intake (Flegal, 1999). Portion size estimation also requires that respondents modify and adjust their frequency responses according to, in some cases, prespecified portion sizes (Willett, 1987). Being able to specify portion size is another demanding cognitive task. The challenges of completing FFQs may lead to inaccurate reporting of usual intake.

The dietary assessment method selected may impact the associations of diet and cancer risk observed. In one example, diet was assessed with both an FFQ and a detailed 7-day food diary. This study was conducted in the EPIC-Norfolk cohort among 13,070 women (Bingham et al., 2003). Total fat measured by the 7-day food diaries was positively associated with increased breast cancer risk (p for trend = 0.05), whereas total fat measured by the FFQ was not associated with breast cancer risk (p for trend = 0.14). An even stronger difference in measurement methodology was seen for saturated fat intake, where saturated fat measured by 7-day diaries was strongly associated with breast cancer risk (p for trend = 0.005) and saturated fat measured by the FFQ was not (p for trend = 0.23). Models were adjusted for weight, height, menopausal status, parity, hormone replacement therapy, and nonfat energy (Bingham et al., 2003).

NUTRITIONAL BIOMARKERS

Nutritional biomarkers are biological consequences of dietary intake or dietary patterns resulting in the presence of components or metabolic byproducts (Consensus Group for Biomarkers in Cancer Chemoprevention, 2001; Potischman and Freudenheim, 2003). Exposure biomarkers may include endogenous or exogenous agents and their metabolites or adducts in tissues or body products, whether in physiological or pathological amounts. Structural changes in the cell or organism that reflect exposure are also included (Consensus Group for Biomarkers in Cancer Chemoprevention, 2001). Biomarkers have the capacity to improve risk estimation and define mechanisms of exposure–disease linkages. Furthermore, utility of biomarkers in population and prevention studies is continuous; that is, some markers are more informative than others, depending on how they are being used, with a gradation from extremely useful to artifactual (Groopman, 2005).

Biomarkers can be sorted into functional use categories (Consensus Group for Biomarkers in Cancer Chemoprevention, 2001), which include the following:

1. Validation of dietary instruments
2. Surrogate indicator of dietary intake
3. Integrated measure of nutritional status for a particular nutrient
4. Measurement of nutrient metabolism or interaction metabolic byproduct with other factors

Biomarkers and Dietary Assessment

Biomarkers as Validation Tools for Dietary Assessments

Biomarker measurement can provide complementary information to help assess performance of different dietary assessment methods. The objectivity of biomarkers makes reliance on subjects' memory or cooperativeness less important (Consensus Group for Biomarkers in Cancer Chemoprevention, 2001). The use of randomized controlled feeding trials is one method for validating dietary assessments. Controlled feeding studies in healthy humans have been used to establish quantitative requirements and confirm functional levels of nutrients. These studies rely on small sample sizes with intensive control, including restriction of calories or feeding of specific nutrients with determination of biological availability in specific tissues (Lampe, 2004). Small-scale intensive feeding studies can be enormously useful in describing hypothesized mechanisms observed in large population-based studies.

An example of validation by feeding trial results is a study that measured the effect of vegetable intake on plasma carotenoid concentrations (Martini et al., 1995). High vegetable diets consisted of a control diet plus either carrots and spinach (carotenoid diet), broccoli and cauliflower (cruciferous diet), or tofu and a textured vegetable protein product (soy diet). The control diet consisted of commonly consumed foods and was essentially carotenoid free. Participants consumed each of the experimental diets for 9 days, with at least a 10-day washout period between diets, and were instructed to consume no other foods or beverages. Carotenoid intakes of all diets were calculated using the updated carotenoid food composition database developed by Mangels et al. (1993). When compared with the control diet, mean plasma concentration for α-carotene, β-carotene, and lutein were 5.2, 3.3, and 2.2 times higher on the carotenoid diet, respectively; plasma lutein concentrations were 2.1 times higher on the cruciferous diet. Plasma concentrations of β-cryptoxanthin and lycopene did not differ among diets. Carotenoids are widespread in vegetables and fruits. These data indicate that plasma carotenoid concentrations may be useful exposure markers for total vegetable and fruit intake in a free-living population and might be useful compliance markers in dietary interventions that emphasize vegetable and fruit intake (Martini et al., 1995).

Another example of the application of controlled feeding studies involves a comprehensive investigation that compared results of 12 dietary intervention studies using 7-day food records with data from controlled feeding studies for the same individuals (Mertz et al., 1991). Free-living participants were trained by dietitians to keep 7-day food records. Subsequently, participants received diets of conventional foods for 45 days; these diets were adjusted so that each individual maintained his or her body weight. Participants reported intakes using 7-day food records; the estimated energy intake from the food records was compared with the actual intake determined to maintain weight. These comparisons found that 81% of the total subject population reported usual energy intakes that were ~700 kcal below the intake subsequently determined to maintain body weight; 8% reported a higher intake (by ~400 kcal); and 11% reported and calculated intakes that were within 100 kcal of each other. The mean difference between recorded and determined intakes was equally underreported (by ~18%) for both men and women; age had no effect on reporting (Mertz et al., 1991).

Use of the doubly labeled water technique, a validated reference method that permits a precise measure of energy expenditure in free-living populations, confirmed the aforementioned finding that subjects recording diet records may underestimate their usual intake substantially (Black et al., 1993; Hebert et al., 1995; Martin et al., 1996; Sawaya et al., 1996). A review of studies in randomly recruited men and women that compared dietary energy intake, as assessed from weighed diet records, with total energy expenditure, as measured by doubly labeled water, reported that energy intake was only 82% (men) and 81% (women) of energy expenditure (Black et al., 1993). A comparison of food records with data from the doubly labeled water method found a similar underreporting of ~20% in a subset of women participating in the Canadian Diet and Breast Cancer Prevention Trial (Black et al., 1993).

Such analyses suggest that a large proportion of individuals consistently underestimate caloric intake, even those who have received training in keeping accurate food records. The exact reasons for this inaccuracy have not been determined, although the tendency of an individual to convey an image in keeping with social norms (e.g., low-fat vs high-fat diets) and to avoid criticism in a testing situation could bias self-reported dietary intake (Hebert et al., 1995). In any event, caution should be used when interpreting epidemiological survey data and the results of other epidemiological studies that use self-reported dietary assessment instruments to collect food data and estimate nutrient intake, even those that use multiple-day food records.

Other validation studies using doubly labeled water found that both men and women underreported energy and protein intakes on 24-hour recalls and FFQs (Subar et al., 2003). In a partnered publication, attenuation of relative risk estimates by FFQs was lessened by adjusting for energy intake using nutrient density or nutrient residuals (Kipnis et al., 2003), suggesting that caution is warranted in interpreting results from epidemiological studies that rely on FFQs to estimate the effects of dietary intake. However, energy adjustment can correct to some degree the imprecision in estimating the true underlying association between intake and cancer risk. In a commentary on both studies, it was noted that the doubly labeled water technique itself is error prone, suggesting that validation biomarkers carry their own level of imprecision (Willett, 2003). Most importantly doubly labeled water sampling needs to be done over several time points to account for within-subject variation. FFQs are designed to assess usual intake, whereas 24-hour recalls and daily food records are designed to assess proximate and immediate intake. It is assumed that individuals' food intake varies over time, and that it is important to reliably estimate the effect of foods during the 20–30 year cancer induction period.

Biomarkers Used in Combination with Dietary Assessment

Despite ongoing improvements in dietary assessment methods, errors inherent in these tools persist. The search for more objective measures of intake is leading researchers to utilize biomarkers that reflect dietary intake in combination with those that predict disease outcome or status. Such biomarkers ideally should (see Pearce et al., 1995; Consensus Group for Biomarkers in Cancer Chemoprevention, 2001)

1. be inexpensive to collect and analyze,
2. be present in small amounts of a biological specimen that can be obtained using a minimally invasive collection method,
3. persist for an extended period and reflect all routes of exposure,
4. be specific and highly predictive of the exposure of interest,
5. be measurable using a sensitive, specific, and reliable assay, and
6. be present in low concentrations in unexposed populations at baseline.

Although it is difficult to meet all of these criteria, there are several promising biomarkers of intake. For example, tissue and serum long-chain n-3 and n-6 polyunsaturated fatty acids have been reported to be reflective of dietary intake of fish, n-3, and n-6 fatty acids (Lands, 1995; Marckmann et al., 1995; Andersen et al., 1996; Connor, 1996; Bagga et al., 1997; Kohlmeier, 1997) and may be indicative of risk for breast (Kohlmeier, 1997) and prostate (Godley et al., 1996) cancers. Serum levels of β-carotene have been positively associated with intake of carotenoid-rich fruits and vegetables (Mangels et al., 1993; Campbell et al., 1994; Drewnowski et al., 1997). Several studies also corroborate the use of vitamin E (α-tocopherol) concentrations in serum and adipose tissue as measures of external intake (both dietary and supplemental) of that nutrient (Riemersma et al., 1991; Rimm et al., 1993).

A convincing body of evidence similarly suggests a direct relationship between consumption of a variety of soy-based products, lignans, isoflavones, isoflavonoid phytoestrogens, and plasma and urinary concentrations (Adlercreutz et al., 1993; Morton et al., 1994; Hutchins et al., 1995a,b; Kelly et al., 1995; Gross et al., 1996). Wu et al. (2004) showed a direct correlation between self-reported soy isoflavone intake from a FFQ and plasma isoflavone levels drawn from a subset of both cases and controls in a population-based study of breast cancer among Asian American women living in Los Angeles County. These findings suggested that, in this instance, breast cancer cases and controls were reliably able to recall their usual soy intake without selective recall biases (Wu et al., 2004).

Although biomarkers appear to be a promising method that could replace food frequency methods, it is important to understand that not all foods have biomarkers of intake. Moreover, several studies have shown a weak association between dietary intake and biological markers of intake (Polsinelli et al., 1998; Crews et al., 2001; El-Sohemy et al., 2002; IARC Working Group on the Evaluation of Cancer-Preventive Strategies, 2003). Well-designed studies of dietary intake and cancer risk ought to include both dietary recall methods and specific biomarkers of intake.

Biomarkers as Measures of Dietary Exposure

In instances in which specific biomarkers of intake exist such as serum lycopene level as a marker of tomato product intake, accuracy of dietary exposure measurement can be improved by use of biomarkers. Results of epidemiological studies of fruit, vegetables, and breast cancer risk have been inconsistent and serve as a good example for how biomarkers can potentially increase the accuracy of dietary exposure measurement.

Fruits and vegetables contain numerous compounds that have demonstrated anticarcinogenic effects, including carotenoids (Sato et al., 2002), flavonoids (Le, 2002), and isothiocyanates (ITCs) (Fowke et al., 2003). Self-reported dietary intake results from population-based case-control studies of breast cancer all demonstrate a protective association at the highest category of fruit and vegetable consumption (Hirose et al., 2003; Malin et al., 2003; Shannon et al., 2003), whereas eight prospective cohort studies, when summarized together, report a null association (Smith-Warner et al., 2001). Most epidemiological studies rely on FFQs to measure dietary intake. The increased variability introduced by self-reported intake has been suggested by several reviews (WCRF, 1997; Smith-Warner et al., 2001; Riboli and Norat, 2003) as one of the reasons for inconsistent results of fruits and vegetables and breast cancer risk observed across studies.

Inverse associations observed for biomarkers of fruit and vegetable intake have strengthened biological evidence for fruit and vegetable consumption and reduction of breast cancer risk. Two nested case-control studies found protective associations between serum biomarkers of carotenoids and breast cancer risk (Toniolo et al., 2001; Sato et al., 2002). A protective association was observed for urinary ITCs and breast cancer risk in a case-control study of Shanghai Chinese (Fowke et al., 2003). Dietary intake of soy (flavonoid family) that was later validated by plasma isoflavone was found to be protective for breast cancer risk in a case-control study of Asian Americans conducted in Los Angeles County (Wu et al., 2002, 2004).

Protective associations between biomarkers of fruit and vegetable intake and other diseases such as lung cancer have also been found. Observational studies have consistently shown that elevated intake of vegetables reduces the risk of lung cancer (Ziegler et al., 1984, 1986, 1992; Fontham et al., 1988; Le et al., 1989; Dorgan et al., 1993; Alpha-Tocopherol, 1994; Mayne et al., 1994; Omenn et al., 1996; Speizer et al., 1999). A report of fruit and vegetable consumption in two prospective cohorts found the strongest protective association from cruciferous vegetables, citrus fruits, and foods high in total carotenoids (Feskanich et al., 2000). Other large-scale population-based studies have also shown overall inverse associations between cruciferous vegetable intake and lung cancer risk (Le et al., 1989; Verhoeven et al., 1996; Speizer et al., 1999). ITC, a marker for cruciferous vegetable consumption and metabolism found in urine specimens, was inversely related to lung cancer risk in a population (Shanghai) that consumes high levels of cruciferous vegetables. The protective effect was greatest in subjects genetically deficient in glutathione-*S*-transferase M1 (GSTM1) (London et al., 2000). This observation has been confirmed in a U.S. Texas population (Spitz et al., 2000) and in Singapore Chinese (Zhao et al., 2001) using dietary questionnaire data.

A pooled analysis of eight cohort studies did not find an association with consumption of broccoli or cabbage and lung cancer risk (Smith-Warner et al., 2003). On the other hand, a metaanalysis of cohort studies conducted by the IARC Working Group on the Evaluation of Cancer Preventive Strategies reported an odds ratio of 0.86 (95% confidence interval [CI] = 0.75–0.98) for the association between ITCs either measured directly in urine or calculated from dietary intake reports (IARC Working Group on the Evaluation of Cancer-Preventive Strategies, 2004).

SUMMARY

As research of diet and cancer moves forward, it is clear that no one method of dietary assessment is ideal. The type of nutrients under investigation, the study design, the study hypothesis, and cancer site under investigation will help determine the optimal assessment instrument and whether biomarkers of intake should be included. If study design permits, use of biomarkers and dietary assessment together appears to be the most accurate and comprehensive method for measurement of diet in relationship to cancer risk.

Acknowledgment

This research was supported by the National Cancer Institute (1 P01 CA 42710), California Breast Cancer Research Program (9PB-0117), and the UCLA Center for Human Nutrition.

References

Adlercreutz, H., Fotsis, T., Lampe, J., Wahala, K., Makela, T., Brunow, G., and Hase, T. 1993. Quantitative determination of lignans and isoflavonoids in plasma of omnivorous and vegetarian women by isotope dilution gas chromatography-mass spectrometry. *Scand J Clin Lab Invest* Suppl **215**: 5–18.

Alpha-Tocopherol B-CCPSG. 1994. The effect of vitamin E and beta-carotene on the incidence of lung cancer and other cancers in male smokers. *N Engl J Med* **330**: 1029–1035.

Andersen, L.F., Solvoll, K., and Drevon, C.A. 1996. Very-long-chain n-3 fatty acids as biomarkers for intake of fish and n-3 fatty acid concentrates. *Am J Clin Nutr* **64**: 305–311.

Bagga, D., Capone, S., Wang, H.J., Heber, D., Lill, M., Chap, L., Glaspy, J.A. 1997. Dietary modulation of omega-3/omega-6 polyunsaturated fatty acid ratios in patients with breast cancer. *J Natl Cancer Inst* **89**: 1123–1131.

Barrett-Connor, E. 1991. Nutrition epidemiology: how do we know what they ate? *Am J Clin Nutr* **54**: 182S–187S.

Bingham, S.A., Nelson, M. and Paul, A.A. Methods for data collection at an individual level. 1998. In, "Manual on Methodology for Food Consumption Studies" (Cameron ME and Van Stayern WA, eds). Oxford University Press, New York, New York.

Bingham, S.A., Luben, R., Welch, A., Wareham, N., Khaw, K.T., and Day, N. 2003. Are imprecise methods obscuring a relation between fat and breast cancer? *Lancet* **362**: 212–214.

Black, A.E., Prentice, A.M., Goldberg, G.R., Jebb, S.A., Bingham, S.A., Livingstone M.B., and Coward W.A. 1993. Measurements of total energy expenditure provide insights into the validity of dietary measurements of energy intake. *J Am Diet Assoc* **93**: 572–579.

Block, G., Hartman, A.M., Dresser, C.M., Carroll, M.D., Gannon, J., and Gardner, L. 1986. A data-based approach to diet questionnaire design and testing. *Am J Epidemiol* **124**: 453–469.

Byar, D.P., and Freedman, L.S. 1989. Clinical trials in diet and cancer. *Prev Med* **18**: 203–219

Campbell, D.R., Gross, M.D., Martini, M.C., Grandits, G.A., Slavin, J.L., and Potter, J.D. 1994. Plasma carotenoids as biomarkers of vegetable and fruit intake. *Cancer Epidemiol Biomarkers Prev* **3**: 493–500.

Chao, A., Thun, M.J., Connell, C.J., McCullough, M.L., Jacobs, E.J., Flanders, W.D., Rodriguez, C., Sinha, R., and Calle, E.E. 2005. Meat consumption and risk of colorectal cancer. *JAMA* **293**: 172–182.

Connor, S.L. 1996. Biomarkers and dietary intake data are mutually beneficial. *Am J Clin Nutr* **64**: 379–380.

Consensus Group for Biomarkers in Cancer Chemoprevention. 2001. Biomarkers in cancer chemoprevention, a working report. International Agency for Research on Cancer. Biomarkers in Cancer Chemoprevention, IARC Scientific Publications, Lyon, France.

Crews, H., Alink, G., Andersen, R., Braesco, V., Holst, B., Maiani, G., Ovesen, L., Scotter, M., Solfrizzo, M., van den Berg, R., Verhagen, H., and Williamson, G. 2001. A critical assessment of some biomarker approaches linked with dietary intake. *Br J Nutr* **86**(Suppl 1): S5–35.

Dorgan, J.F., Ziegler, R.G., Schoenberg, J.B., Hartge, P., McAdams, M.J., Falk, R.T., Wilcox, H.B., and Shaw, G.L. 1993. Race and sex differences in associations of vegetables, fruits, and carotenoids with lung cancer risk in New Jersey (United States). *Cancer Causes Control* **4**: 273–281.

Drewnowski, A., Rock, C.L., Henderson, S.A., Shore, A.B., Fischler, C., Galan, P., Preziosi, P., and Hersberg, S. 1997. Serum beta-carotene and vitamin C as biomarkers of vegetable and fruit intakes in a community-based sample of French adults. *Am J Clin Nutr* **65**: 1796–1802.

Dwyer, J., Ellwood, K., Leader, N.P., Moshfegh, A.J., and Johnson, C.L. 2001. Integration of the Continuing Survey of Food Intakes by Individuals and the National Health And Nutrition Examination Survey. *J Am Diet Assoc* **101**: 1142–1143.

El-Sohemy, A., Baylin, A., Kabagambe, E., Ascherio, A., Spiegelman, D., and Campos, H. 2002. Individual carotenoid concentrations in adipose tissue and plasma as biomarkers of dietary intake. *Am J Clin Nutr* **76**: 172–179.

Feskanich, D., Ziegler, R.G., Michaud, D.S., Giovannucci, E.L., Speizer, F.E., Willett, W.C., and Colditz, G.A. 2000. Prospective study of fruit and vegetable consumption and risk of lung cancer among men and women. *J Natl Cancer Inst* **92**: 1812–1823.

Flegal, K.M. 1999. Evaluating epidemiologic evidence of the effects of food and nutrient exposures. *Am J Clin Nutr* **69**: 1339S–1344S.

Fontham, E.T., Pickle, L.W., Haenszel, W., Correa, P., Lin, Y.P., Falk, R.T. 1988. Dietary vitamins A and C and lung cancer risk in Louisiana. *Cancer* **62**: 2267–2273.

Fowke, J.H., Chung, F.L., Jin, F., Qi, D., Cai, Q., Conaway, C., Cheng, J.R., Shu, X.O., Gao, Y.T., and Zheng, W. 2003. Urinary isothiocyanate levels, brassica, and human breast cancer. *Cancer Res* **63**: 3980–3986.

Gersovitz, M., Madden, J.P., and Smiklas-Wright, H. 1978. Validity of the 24-hr. dietary recall and seven-day record for group comparisons. *J Am Diet Assoc* **73**: 48–55.

Godley, P.A., Campbell, M.K., Miller, C., Gallagher, P., Martinson, F.E., Mohler, J.L., and Sandler, R.S. 1996. Correlation between biomarkers of omega-3 fatty acid consumption and questionnaire data in African American and Caucasian United States males with and without prostatic carcinoma. *Cancer Epidemiol Biomarkers Prev* **5**: 115–119.

Grandesso, F., Sanderson, F., Kruijt, J., Koene, T., and Brown, V. 2005. Mortality and malnutrition among populations living in South Darfur, Sudan: results of 3 surveys, September 2004. *JAMA* **293**: 1490–1494.

Groopman, J.D. 2005. "Validation Strategies for Biomarkers: Old and New. 2005." American Association of Cancer Research. AACR Education Book, Philadelphia, PA.

Gross, M., Pfeiffer, M., Martini, M., Campbell, D., Slavin, J., Potter, J. 1996. The quantitation of metabolites of quercetin flavonols in human urine. *Cancer Epidemiol Biomarkers Prev* **5**: 711–720.

Han, J., Hankinson, S.E., De, V.I., Spiegelman, D., Tamimi, R.M., Mohrenweiser, H.W., Colditz, G.A., and Hunter, D.J. 2003. A prospective study of XRCC1 haplotypes and their interaction with plasma carotenoids on breast cancer risk. *Cancer Res* **63**: 8536–8541.

Hebert, J.R., Clemow, L., Pbert, L., Ockene, I.S., Ockene, J.K. 1995. Social desirability bias in dietary self-report may compromise the validity of dietary intake measures. *Int J Epidemiol* **24**: 389–398.

Hirose, K., Takezaki, T., Hamajima, N., Miura, S., Tajima, K. 2003. Dietary factors protective against breast cancer in Japanese premenopausal and postmenopausal women. *Int J Cancer* **107**: 276–282.

Hutchins, A.M., Lampe, J.W., Martini, M.C., Campbell, D.R., Slavin, J.L. 1995a. Vegetables, fruits, and legumes: effect on urinary isoflavonoid phytoestrogen and lignan excretion. *J Am Diet Assoc* **95**: 769–774.

Hutchins, A.M., Slavin, J.L., and Lampe, J.W. 1995b. Urinary isoflavonoid phytoestrogen and lignan excretion after consumption of fermented and unfermented soy products. *J Am Diet Assoc* **95**: 545–551.

IARC Working Group on the Evaluation of Cancer-Preventive Strategies. 2003. Fruits and Vegetables. "IARC Handbook of Cancer Prevention," Vol. 8. International Agency for Research on Cancer, Lyon, France.

IARC Working Group on the Evaluation of Cancer-Preventive Strategies. 2004. Cruciferous Vegetables, Isothiocyanates and Indoles. "IARC Handbook of Cancer Prevention," Vol. 9. International Agency for Research on Cancer. Lyon, France.

Kelly, G.E., Joannou, G.E., Reeder, A.Y., Nelson, C., and Waring, M.A. 1995. The variable metabolic response to dietary isoflavones in humans. *Proc Soc Exp Biol Med* **208**: 40–43.

Kipnis, V., Subar, A.F., Midthune, D., Freedman, L.S., Ballard-Barbash, R., Troiano, R.P., Bingham, S., Schoeller, D.A., Schatzkin, A., and Carroll, R.J. 2003. Structure of dietary measurement error: results of the OPEN biomarker study. *Am J Epidemiol* **158**: 14–21.

Kohlmeier, L. 1997. Biomarkers of fatty acid exposure and breast cancer risk. *Am J Clin Nutr* **66**: 1548S–1556S.

Lampe, J.W. 2004. Nutrition and cancer prevention: small-scale human studies for the 21st century. *Cancer Epidemiol Biomarkers Prev* **13**: 1987–1988.

Lands, W.E. 1995. Long-term fat intake and biomarkers. *Am J Clin Nutr* **61**: 721S–725S.

Le, M.L. 2002. Cancer preventive effects of flavonoids—a review. *Biomed Pharmacother* **56**: 296–301.

Le, M.L., Yoshizawa, C.N., Kolonel, L.N., Hankin, J.H., and Goodman, M.T. 1989. Vegetable consumption and lung cancer risk: a population-based case-control study in Hawaii. *J Natl Cancer Inst* **81**: 1158–1164.

London, S.J., Yuan, J.M., Chung, F.L., Gao, Y.T., Coetzee, G.A., Ross, R.K., and Yu, M.C. 2000. Isothiocyanates, glutathione S-transferase M1 and T1 polymorphisms, and lung-cancer risk: a prospective study of men in Shanghai, China. *Lancet* **356**: 724–729.

Malin, A.S., Qi, D., Shu, X.O., Gao, Y.T., Friedmann, J.M., Jin, F., and Zheng, W. 2003. Intake of fruits, vegetables and selected micronutrients in relation to the risk of breast cancer. *Int J Cancer* **105**: 413–418.

Mangels, A.R., Holden, J.M., Beecher, G.R., Forman, M.R., Lanza, E. 1993. Carotenoid content of fruits and vegetables: an evaluation of analytic data. *J Am Diet Assoc* **93**: 284–296.

Marckmann, P., Lassen, A., Haraldsdottir, J., and Sandstrom, B. 1995. Biomarkers of habitual fish intake in adipose tissue. *Am J Clin Nutr* **62**: 956–959.

Martin, L.J., Su, W., Jones, P.J., Lockwood, G.A., Tritchler, D.L., and Boyd, N.F. 1996. Comparison of energy intakes determined by food records and doubly labeled water in women participating in a dietary-intervention trial. *Am J Clin Nutr* **63**: 483–490.

Martini, M.C., Campbell, D.R., Gross, M.D., Grandits, G.A., Potter, J.D., and Slavin, J.L. 1995. Plasma carotenoids as biomarkers of vegetable intake: the University of Minnesota Cancer Prevention Research Unit Feeding Studies. *Cancer Epidemiol Biomarkers Prev* **4**: 491–496.

Mayne, S.T., Janerich, D.T., Greenwald, P., Chorost, S., Tucci, C., Zaman, M.B., Melamed, M.R., Kiely, M., McKneally, M.F. 1994. Dietary beta carotene and lung cancer risk in U.S. nonsmokers. *J Natl Cancer Inst* **86**: 33–38.

McCann, S.E., Trevisan, M., Priore, R.L., Muti, P., Markovic, N., Russell, M., Chan, A.W., and Freudenheim, J.L. 1999. Comparability of nutrient estimation by three food frequency questionnaires for use in epidemiological studies. *Nutr Cancer* **35**: 4–9.

Mertz, W., Tsui, J.C., Judd, J.T., Reiser, S., Hallfrisch, J., Morris, E.R., Steele, P.D., and Lashley, E. 1991. What are people really eating? The relation between energy intake derived from estimated diet records and intake determined to maintain body weight. *Am J Clin Nutr* **54**: 291–295.

Morton, M.S., Wilcox, G., Wahlqvist, M.L., Griffiths, K. 1994. Determination of lignans and isoflavonoids in human female plasma following dietary supplementation. *J Endocrinol* **142**: 251–259.

Moyad, M.A. 2002. Dietary fat reduction to reduce prostate cancer risk: controlled enthusiasm, learning a lesson from breast or other cancers, and the big picture. *Urology* **59**: 51–62.

Nutrition Coordinating Center. 2005. University of Minnesota. Nutrition Data System for Research (NDS-R): Food and Nutrient Database and Interview System, version 8.04. Available at: http://www.ncc.umn.edu/ [accessed April 2005].

Omenn, G.S., Goodman, G.E., Thornquist, M.D., Balmes, J., Cullen, M.R., Glass, A., Keogh, J.P., Meyskens, F.L., Jr., Valanis, B., Williams, J.H., Jr., Barnhart, S., Cherniack, M.G., Brodkin, C.A., and Hammar, S. 1996. Risk factors for lung cancer and for intervention effects in CARET, the Beta-Carotene and Retinol Efficacy Trial. *J Natl Cancer Inst* **88**: 1550–1559.

Pearce, N., de Sanjose, S., Boffetta, P., Kogevinas, M., Saracci, R., and Savitz, D. 1995. Limitations of biomarkers of exposure in cancer epidemiology. *Epidemiology* **6**: 190–194.

Polsinelli, M.L., Rock, C.L., Henderson, S.A., Drewnowski, A. 1998. Plasma carotenoids as biomarkers of fruit and vegetable servings in women. *J Am Diet Assoc* **98**: 194–196.

Potischman, N., Freudenheim, J.L. 2003. Biomarkers of nutritional exposure and nutritional status: an overview. *J Nutr* **133** Suppl 3: 873S–874S.

Riboli, E., and Norat, T. 2003. Epidemiologic evidence of the protective effect of fruit and vegetables on cancer risk. *Am J Clin Nutr* **78**: 559S–569S.

Riemersma, R.A., Wood, D.A., Macintyre, C.C., Elton, R.A., Gey, K.F., and Oliver, M.F. 1991. Risk of angina pectoris and plasma concentrations of vitamins A, C, and E and carotene. *Lancet* **337**: 1–5.

Rimm, E.B., Stampfer, M.J., Ascherio, A., Giovannucci, E., Colditz, G.A., and Willett, W.C. 1993. Vitamin E consumption and the risk of coronary heart disease in men. *N Engl J Med* **328**: 1450–1456.

Sato, R., Helzlsouer, K.J., Alberg, A.J., Hoffman, S.C., Norkus, E.P., and Comstock, G.W. 2002. Prospective study of carotenoids, tocopherols, and retinoid concentrations and the risk of breast cancer. *Cancer Epidemiol Biomarkers Prev* **11**: 451–457.

Sawaya, A.L., Tucker, K., Tsay, R., Willett, W., Saltzman, E., Dallal, G.E., and Roberts, S.B. 1996. Evaluation of four methods for determining energy intake in young and older women: comparison with doubly labeled water measurements of total energy expenditure. *Am J Clin Nutr* **63**: 491–499.

Sempos, C.T., Liu, K., and Ernst, N.D. 1999. Food and nutrient exposures: what to consider when evaluating epidemiologic evidence. *Am J Clin Nutr* **69**: 1330S–1338S.

Shannon, J., Cook, L.S., Stanford, J.L. 2003. Dietary intake and risk of postmenopausal breast cancer (United States). *Cancer Causes Control* **14**: 19–27.

Smith-Warner, S.A., Spiegelman, D., Yaun, S.S., Adami, H.O., Beeson, W.L., van den Brandt, P.A., Folsom, A.R., Fraser, G.E., Freudenheim, J.L., Goldbohm, R.A., Graham, S., Miller, A.B., Potter, J.D., Rohan, T.E., Speizer, F.E., Toniolo, P., Willett, W.C., Wolk, A., Zeleniuch-Jacquotte, A., and Hunter, D.J. 2001. Intake of fruits and vegetables and risk of breast cancer: a pooled analysis of cohort studies. *JAMA* **285**: 769–776.

Smith-Warner, S.A., Spiegelman, D., Yaun, S.S., Albanes, D., Beeson, W.L., van den Brandt, P.A., Feskanich, D., Folsom, A.R., Fraser, G.E., Freudenheim, J.L., Giovannucci, E., Goldbohm, R.A., Graham, S., Kushi, L.H., Miller, A.B., Pietinen, P., Rohan, T.E., Speizer, F.E., Willett, W.C., and Hunter, D.J. 2003. Fruits, vegetables and lung cancer: a pooled analysis of cohort studies. *Int J Cancer* **107**: 1001–1011.

Speizer, F.E., Colditz, G.A., Hunter, D.J., Rosner, B., and Hennekens, C. 1999. Prospective study of smoking, antioxidant intake, and lung cancer in middle-aged women (USA). *Cancer Causes Control* **10**: 475–482.

Spitz, M.R., Duphorne, C.M., Detry, M.A., Pillow, P.C., Amos, C.I., Lei, L., de Andrade, M., Gu, X., Hong, W.K., and Wu, X. 2000. Dietary intake of isothiocyanates: evidence of a joint effect with glutathione S-transferase polymorphisms in lung cancer risk. *Cancer Epidemiol Biomarkers Prev* **9**: 1017–1020.

Subar, A.F., Kipnis, V., Troiano, R.P., Midthune, D., Schoeller, D.A., Bingham, S., Sharbaugh, C.O., Trabulsi, J., Runswick, S., Ballard-Barbash, R., Sunshine, J., and Schatzkin, A. 2003. Using intake biomarkers to evaluate the extent of dietary misreporting in a large sample of adults: the OPEN study. *Am J Epidemiol* **158**: 1–13.

Tarasuk, V.S., and Brooker, A.S. 1997. Interpreting epidemiologic studies of diet–disease relationships. *J Nutr* **127**: 1847–1852

Toniolo, P., van Kappel, A.L., Akhmedkhanov, A., Ferrari, P., Kato, I., Shore, R.E., and Riboli, E. 2001. Serum carotenoids and breast cancer. *Am J Epidemiol* **153**: 1142–1147.

U.S. Department of Health and Human Services. 2005. NHANES III, II, I, and NHES 1. [http://www.cdc.gov/nchs/nhanes.htm]. National Center for Health Statistics. Accessed, June 14, 2005.

Verhoeven, D.T., Goldbohm, R.A., van Poppel, G., Verhagen, H., and van den Brandt, P.A. 1996. Epidemiological studies on brassica vegetables and cancer risk. *Cancer Epidemiol Biomarkers Prev* **5**: 733–748.

Welch, A.A., McTaggart, A., Mulligan, A.A., Luben, R., Walker, N., Khaw, K.T., Day, N.E., and Bingham, S.A. 2001. DINER (Data Into Nutrients for Epidemiological Research)—a new data-entry program for nutritional analysis in the EPIC-Norfolk cohort and the 7-day diary method. *Public Health Nutr* **4**: 1253–1265.

Willett, W.C., Sampson, L., Stampfer, M.J., Rosner, B., Bain, C., Witschi, J., Hennekens, C.H., and Speizer, F.E. 1985. Reproducibility and validity of a semiquantitative food frequency questionnaire. *Am J Epidemiol* **122**: 51–65.

Willett, W. 1987. Nutritional epidemiology: issues and challenges. *Int J Epidemiol* **16**: 312–317.

Willett, W.C. 1990. "Nutritional Epidemiology," 1st edition. Oxford University Pressk, New York.

Willett, W. 2003. Invited Commentary: OPEN Questions. *Am J Epidemiol* **158**: 22–24.

World Cancer Research Fund (WCRF). 1997. Food, Nutrition and the Prevention of Cancer: A Global Perspective. American Institute for Cancer Research, Washington, D.C.

Wu, A.H., Wan, P., Hankin, J., Tseng, C.C., Yu, M.C., and Pike, M.C. 2002. Adolescent and adult soy intake and risk of breast cancer in Asian-Americans. *Carcinogenesis* **23**: 1491–1496.

Wu, A.H., Yu, M.C., Tseng, C.C., Twaddle, N.C., and Doerge, D.R. 2004. Plasma isoflavone levels versus self-reported soy isoflavone levels in Asian-American women in Los Angeles County. *Carcinogenesis* **25**: 77–81.

Yuasa, Y., Nagasaki, H., Akiyama, Y., Sakai, H., Nakajima, T., Ohkura, Y., Takizawa, T., Koike, M., Tani, M., Iwai, T., Sugihara, K., Imai, K., and Nakachi, K. 2005. Relationship between CDX2 gene methylation and dietary factors in gastric cancer patients. *Carcinogenesis* **26**: 193–200.

Zhao, B., Seow, A., Lee, E.J., Poh, W.T., The, M., Eng, P., Wang, Y.T., Tan, W.C., Yu, M.C., and Lee, H.P. 2001. Dietary isothiocyanates, glutathione S-transferase -M1, -T1 polymorphisms and lung cancer risk among Chinese women in Singapore. *Cancer Epidemiol Biomarkers Prev* **10**: 1063–1067.

Ziegler, R.G., Mason, T.J., Stemhagen, A., Hoover, R., Schoenberg, J.B., Gridley, G., Virgo, P.W., Altman, R., and Fraumeni, J.F., Jr. 1984. Dietary carotene and vitamin A and risk of lung cancer among white men in New Jersey. *J Natl Cancer Inst* **73**: 1429–1435.

Ziegler, R.G., Mason, T.J., Stemhagen, A., Hoover, R., Schoenberg, J.B., Gridley, G., Virgo, P.W., and Fraumeni, J.F., Jr. 1986. Carotenoid intake, vegetables, and the risk of lung cancer among white men in New Jersey. *Am J Epidemiol* **123**: 1080–1093.

Ziegler, R.G., Subar, A.F., Craft, N.E., Ursin, G., Patterson, B.H., and Graubard, B.I. 1992. Does beta-carotene explain why reduced cancer risk is associated with vegetable and fruit intake? *Cancer Res* **52**: 2060s–2066s.

CHAPTER

20

Prostate Cancer

HOWARD PARNES, ASHRAFUL HOQUE, DEMETRIUS ALBANES, PHILIP TAYLOR, AND SCOTT LIPPMAN

INTRODUCTION

Prostate cancer is the most common noncutaneous malignancy in U.S. men and remains the second leading cause of cancer death despite advances in screening, early detection, and treatment (Jemal et al., 2005). Prostate cancer represents 33% of all newly diagnosed cancers, with 230,000 new cases and 30,000 deaths expected in 2004 (Jemal et al., 2004). Although most newly diagnosed patients present with nonmetastatic disease, the primary treatments available such as radical prostatectomy and radiation therapy continue to have a significant 30–50% failure rate (Trapasso et al., 1994; Khuntia et al., 2004). Further, treatment of localized disease may adversely affect quality of life and there are no known cures for advanced epithelial cancers, regardless of primary site.

The probability of developing prostate cancer increases with age, such that only 1 in nearly 13,000 men younger than 40 years will be diagnosed with prostate cancer, versus 1 in 44 in men 40–59 years of age, 1 in 7 in men 60–79 years of age, and finally 1 in 6 in men older than 70 years. Accordingly, >70% of prostate cancers are diagnosed in men older than 65 years; it is the third leading cause of cancer death in men aged 60–79 years and the second leading cause of cancer death in men 80 years or older (Jemal et al., 2004).

Race or ethnicity as a predictor for prostate cancer is most clearly demonstrated in African American men. The incidence of prostate cancer in African American men is ~1.5 times higher than among white men and is 2.7 times higher than among Asian/Pacific Islander men (U.S. Cancer Statistics Working Group, 2003). In addition, a higher prevalence of more aggressive disease and higher prostate-specific antigen (PSA) levels at diagnosis have been noted in African American men versus white men (Moul et al., 1995; Presti et al., 1997). Accordingly, some screening guidelines recommend that African American men begin annual PSA and digital rectal examination (DRE) screening at age 45 years rather than at age 50 years.

The risk for Hispanic men is not as clear. Surveillance, epidemiology, and end results (SEER) data from 11 geographic areas in 1992–1996 show a lower incidence of prostate cancers among Hispanic men compared with white men (Canto and Chu, 2000). Results from the Prostate Cancer Outcomes Study, a population-based longitudinal study initiated in 1994 by the National Cancer Institute (NCI) using SEER data from six cancer registries, demonstrated that Hispanic men were more likely than white men to present with clinically advanced stage disease (Hoffman et al., 2001), suggesting that Hispanic men might be at greater risk for more advanced disease. However, the difference between the groups was no longer significant after adjustment for socioeconomic factors. Studies of other ethnic groups have also shown that environmental factors can affect risk profiles: One study found that duration of residence in North America independently increased prostate cancer incidence in Asian-born men living in the United States and Canada (Whittemore et al., 1995), while a second found that mortality from prostate cancer in Japanese-born men living in the United States tends to match the higher rates seen in the overall U.S. population rather than the lower rates seen in the overall Japanese population (Locke and King, 1980). Although the precise mechanisms remain unclear, these data clearly indicate that the effects of diet, lifestyle, and other factors on the development of prostate cancer cannot be overlooked.

The third primary risk factor, family history, has also been shown to affect the risk of prostate cancer development.

Copyright © 2006, Elsevier Inc.
All rights of reproduction in any form reserved.

Hereditary prostate cancer that is attributable to high-penetrance gene mutations and is reflected in obvious family clustering accounts for ~5%–10% of cases in the entire population and for up to 40% in men younger than 55 years (Hsieh and Albertsen, 2003). Data from a population-based case–control study of 563 men younger than 70 years with prostate cancer and 703 age-matched controls with no history of disease indicate that the risk of prostate cancer varies depending on the number of first-degree relatives affected and on the relationship of the affected family members to the case (Lesko et al., 1996). Men with a single relative with a history of prostate cancer had a 2.2-fold risk of cancer, whereas those with two or more relatives with a history of prostate cancer had a 3.9-fold risk of cancer; the risk was higher if the brother had prostate cancer than if the father had prostate cancer (Lesko et al., 1996).

Of note, early age at onset of prostate cancer in the affected family members increased the risk, with the highest risk seen in those with family members diagnosed at younger than 60 years (Lesko et al., 1996). Because of this increased risk, the American Cancer Society guidelines recommend that men with a strong family history of prostate cancer initiate regular screening 5 years earlier than the general population, at age 45 years (Smith et al., 2004).

As with other epithelial cell cancers, somatic genetic alterations underlie prostate cancer development. A wide variety of alterations have been identified in patients with prostate cancer, but the heterogeneity of these mutations has made study of the genetic underpinnings of prostate cancer challenging. In addition, genetic alterations have been shown to accumulate over time, suggesting that environmental factors not only affect risk profiles and disease incidence rates but can also induce further somatic genetic abnormalities (DeMarzo et al., 2004). The link between prostate cancer and gene–nutrient interaction remains unconfirmed (see discussion later in this chapter), but data clearly suggest that both genetic and nutritional factors play a role in prostate cancer development and progression.

Although epidemiological studies strongly suggest that environmental factors contribute to prostate cancer risk, the major risk factors for this disease (age, race, and family history) are not modifiable. Thus, efforts directed at prostate cancer prevention would appear to hold the greatest promise for reducing death and suffering from this disease in the future. The study of finasteride, a drug that inhibits 5α-reductase, while demonstrating an overall beneficial effect, resulted in significant side effects both positive and negative.

There are observations suggesting that obesity, a Western dietary pattern, and certain types of fat in the diet may influence prostate cancer incidence and mortality. Nutrition researchers have focused on a number of individual vitamins and a number of antioxidant nutrients in an attempt to identify specific dietary elements that can be used to delay disease development and/or progression. The most work in this area has been conducted with tomato-based products and lycopene, vitamin E, selenium, and vitamin D. The NCI-funded Selenium and Vitamin E Cancer Prevention Trial (SELECT) is the largest trial ever launched in prostate cancer chemoprevention and will provide answers related to the impact of selenium and vitamin E in primary prevention. Future research on gene–nutrient interaction using specific transgenic animal models and translational research promise to advance the field of prostate cancer prevention through nutrition.

INTERNATIONAL EPIDEMIOLOGICAL OBSERVATIONS

Although latent or clinically insignificant prostate cancer occurs at equal rates in autopsy studies among men in Asia and the United States (~30% of men older than 50 years), the incidence of clinically significant prostate cancer is 15-fold higher in the United States than in Asian countries (Muir et al., 1991).

Chinese and Japanese men who immigrate to the United States have a higher incidence of and mortality from prostate cancer than Chinese and Japanese men in their native country (Shimizu et al., 1991; Whittemore et al., 1995). The incidence of prostate cancer in Japan has also been increasing at a time when Western diets and lifestyles are being adopted into that country (Wynder et al., 1991). These data suggest that a significant proportion of prostate cancers may be caused by and, conversely, prevented by changes in the environment. Substantial data suggest that obesity, secondary to dietary patterns and the sedentary lifestyle in Western developed countries, may play an important role in the development, progression, and mortality from prostate cancer.

PROSTATE ANATOMY, PHYSIOLOGY, AND PATHOGENESIS OF PROSTATE CANCER

The prostate is a walnut-sized gland located in front of the rectum and underneath the urinary bladder. It contains gland cells that produce some of the seminal fluid, which protects and nourishes sperm cells in semen. Just behind the prostate gland are the seminal vesicles that produce most of the fluid for semen. The prostate surrounds the first part of the urethra, the tube that carries urine from the bladder and semen out of the body through the penis. Male hormones stimulate the prostate gland to develop in the fetus. The prostate continues to grow as a man reaches adulthood and is maintained after it reaches normal size as long as male hormones are produced. If male hormone levels are low, the prostate gland will not fully develop. In older men, the part of the prostate around the urethra often continues to grow, a condition called *benign prostatic hypertrophy* or *benign prostatic hyperplasia*. This can cause problems with urinating. Prostate cancer, however, develops in the dorsal prostate epithelium.

Pathological and molecular biology studies (Nelson et al., 2004) have led to the hypothesis that chronic or recurrent prostate inflammation may initiate and promote prostate cancer development. The case for prostate inflammation as a cause of prostate cancer is compelling. Epidemiological data have correlated prostatitis and sexually transmitted infections with increased prostate cancer risk and intake of anti-inflammatory drugs and antioxidants with decreased prostate cancer risk.

GENE–NUTRIENT INTERACTION IN PROSTATE CANCER

Genetic studies have identified susceptibility genes for familial prostate cancer, which encode an interferon-inducible ribonuclease and subunits of the macrophage scavenger receptor. Somatic silencing of a glutathione *S*-transferase (GSTP1), capable of defending against oxidant cell and genome damage, has been found in almost all prostate cancer cases. Proliferative inflammatory atrophy (PIA) lesions are found adjacent to prostatic intraepithelial neoplasia and carcinoma in situ. These PIA lesions contain activated inflammatory cells, and proliferating epithelial cells appear likely to be precursors to prostatic intraepithelial neoplasia lesions and prostatic carcinomas. Emerging hints that prostate inflammation may contribute to prostatic carcinogenesis provide additional research directions for examining the effects of diet and exercise, altering dietary patterns, or adding antioxidant nutrients to the diet.

Nutritional Factors

Prostate cancer appears to be associated with certain nutritional risk factors on the basis of evidence from epidemiological data (variation of prostate cancer incidence according to various regions of the world, modification of these incidences in relation to migratory flows of certain populations) and eating habit studies. These findings are the basis for a number of studies designed to determine the ideal diet to prevent and, if possible, contribute to, the treatment of prostate cancer. Obesity, fat intake, type of fat, vitamins, trace elements, and antioxidants (lycopene, vitamin E) may all constitute nutritional factors involved in prostatic carcinogenesis. However, although some populations appear to be more effectively protected than others by their cultural consumption of particular substances, the link with efficacy, in terms of prevention, of a diet based on this substance administered to another population has yet to be demonstrated. Although the ideal diet is unknown, some of these ingredients appear to be good candidates.

Obesity and Prostate Cancer

The association of obesity with prostate cancer is somewhat controversial, most likely due to misassignment of body mass index (BMI) and prostate cancer. In one study among men in China, it was found that men in the highest quartile of waist-to-hip ratio (WHR) had an almost threefold increased risk for developing prostate cancer, suggesting a relationship to metabolic syndrome and insulin resistance, as discussed later in this chapter (Hsing et al., 2000).

Although the relationship between obesity and prostate cancer risk is unclear, the relationship between obesity and progression and mortality from prostate cancer is well established (Snowdon et al., 1984; Andersson et al., 1996; Rodriguez et al., 2001, 2003). One the basis of this evidence, obese men are more likely to have higher grade disease, and obesity is likely to be an independent predictor of prostate cancer recurrence following radical prostatectomy.

In 1959 and 1982, the American Cancer Society enrolled a cohort of patients for longitudinal studies on cancer, known as the Cancer Prevention Study (CPS) I and II, respectively. Men were then followed for 13 years in CPS-I and 14 years in CPS-II. Together these studies followed 816,268 men, during which time there were 5212 prostate cancer deaths. Both CPS-I and CPS-II reported that obese men (BMI > 30 kg/m^2) were significantly more likely to die from prostate cancer with a 27% increased risk of prostate cancer death from CPS-I and a 21% increased risk of death from CPS-II (Rodriguez et al., 2005). More details regarding CPS-II were published, which showed that severely obese men (BMI > 35 kg/m^2) were at even greater risk of dying from prostate cancer, with a 34% higher risk of prostate cancer death relative to normal weight men (Abu-Abid et al., 2002). The data linking obesity with prostate cancer progression and mortality support the urgent need for more research in this area.

HORMONES, OBESITY, AND PROSTATE CANCER

Studies regarding obesity and prostate cancer are complicated by the fact that obesity is associated not only with excess body fat, but also with altered serum levels of numerous hormones including testosterone, estrogen, insulin, insulin-like growth factor-1 (IGF-1), and leptin, all of which have, to some degree, been linked to prostate cancer.

Androgens act in the prostate by binding and activating the androgen receptor, resulting in enhanced transcription of genes involved in cellular proliferation such as the mitogenic growth factors epidermal growth factor (EGF) and IGF-1 (Ho et al., 2004). Studies in animal models of prostate cancer further support the role for androgens in the development of prostate cancer (McCormick et al., 1998). Of interest, obese men are known to have decreased free testosterone levels (Vermeulen, 1996; Niskanen et al., 2004). As discussed later, this fact may explain why obese men have higher-grade prostate cancers.

An important advance in the prevention of prostate cancer was the observation from the Prostate Cancer Prevention Trial (PCPT) that finasteride, an inhibitor of 5α-reductase (the enzyme that converts testosterone to the major intraprostatic androgen dihydrotestosterone), reduced the 7-year period prevalence of prostate cancer by 24.8% compared with a placebo control group (18.4% vs 24.4%, $p < .001$). However, this highly beneficial effect was accompanied by a small but significant increase in the period prevalence of high-grade disease among the men randomized to receive finasteride (6.4% vs 5.1%, $p = .005$). Although it is not clear whether this represents a true increase in high-grade disease or is a consequence of detection bias (finasteride reduces prostate gland size by 25%, thus potentially enhancing detection of high-grade disease), there is clearly a need for additional approaches to prevention of this common and often fatal disease. The men exposed to finasteride had more poorly differentiated tumors than the control group, possibly because of lower prostate dihydrotestosterone levels (Thompson et al., 2003).

Data from retrospective studies suggest that testosterone may exert a differentiating effect on prostate cancer and decreased serum testosterone levels have been associated with more advanced and poorly differentiated tumors at presentation (Massengill et al., 2003; Schatzl et al., 2003). Thus, the lower free testosterone levels found in obese men may predispose them to developing more poorly differentiated advanced prostate cancers and explain the higher mortality of prostate cancer among obese men (Freedland and Aronson, 2005).

Obese men are known to have increased serum estradiol levels because of peripheral conversion in adipocytes of testosterone to estradiol by aromatase. In fact, 80% of circulating estradiol in men is derived from the peripheral conversion of androgens to estrogens in fat tissue, whereas only 20% is due to intratesticular conversion of testosterone to estradiol. The exact role of estrogen in prostate cancer development and progression is unclear, but animal and experimental studies suggest that elevated estradiol levels may play an important role in testosterone-induced carcinogenesis. Studies in mice with genetically altered aromatase or estrogen receptor expression found that estradiol combined with testosterone plays an important role in regulating proliferation and apoptosis of prostate cells (McPherson et al., 2001). Leav et al. (1989) demonstrated that testosterone needed to be combined with estrogen to develop proliferative lesions in mouse prostate tissue. In addition, other investigators demonstrated that chronic combined administration of testosterone with estrogens to the Noble rat model resulted in a high incidence of prostate tumors after 52 weeks of treatment, with precancerous lesions seen as early as 16 weeks (Drago, 1984; Bosland et al., 1995).

On the basis of these experimental data, it is possible that elevated levels of estradiol in obese men may enhance the growth-promoting effect of testosterone on prostate cancer. Of importance, a short-term low-fat diet and exercise weight-loss program has previously been shown to reduce serum estradiol in men by 48% (Rosenthal et al., 1985).

Metabolic Syndrome and the IGF Axis

Obesity is associated with insulin resistance and non–insulin-dependent diabetes mellitus. Increasing evidence suggests that adipose tissue not only stores excess fat but also can function as an endocrine organ. Adipocytes produce multiple polypeptide hormones, of which leptin is the best characterized. Metabolic syndrome is associated with increased intraabdominal fat and a genetic predisposition to diabetes, hypertension, and hyperlipidemia. This syndrome was initially described as an aggregation of risk factors for the development of coronary artery disease with insulin resistance and compensatory hyperinsulinemia and elevated levels of fatty acids and adipocyte-derived peptides as pathogenic factors. IGF-1 levels are increased in the metabolic syndrome associated with abdominal obesity in men. IGF-1 is also a potent mitogen for the growth of androgen-responsive and androgen-independent human prostate cancer cell lines (Iwamura et al., 1993; Yu and Rohan, 2000).

Epidemiological investigations have found a positive correlation between elevated serum IGF-1 levels and the risk of developing prostate cancer (Mantzoros et al., 1997; Chan et al., 1998; Wolk et al., 1998; Stattin et al., 2000). Tissue levels of IGF-1 appear to be a critically important factor during initiation and progression of prostate cancer (Kaplan et al., 1999).

Animal studies have demonstrated that caloric restriction decreases growth of prostate tumors and decreases serum IGF-1 levels (Dunn et al., 1997; Mukherjee et al., 1999).

The activity of IGF-1 is modulated by high-affinity IGF-binding proteins (IGF-BPs) (IGF-BPs 1–6) (Ferry et al., 1999). Circulating levels of IGF-BP1 and IGF-BP2 vary in response to nutritional status and in response to changes in energy metabolism (Yu and Rohan, 2000). In the energy-restricted state, circulating levels of IGFBP1 and IGF-BP2 are increased (Thissen et al., 1994; Donaghy and Baxter, 1996). Overeating and obesity, on the other hand, lead to hyperinsulinemia and decreased levels of IGFBP1, although the effect of insulin on serum IGF-BP2 levels in humans is less clear. Research is necessary to clarify the role of energy balance through decreased caloric intake and increased physical activity on the IGF axis, prostate cancer risk, and progression.

Red Meat and Type of Dietary Fat

Epidemiological research has demonstrated that residence in North America increases the risk of prostate cancer incidence in Asian-born men within a single generation (Whittemore et al., 1995). One hypothesis to explain this observation is that a "Western-style" diet (i.e., high in dietary fats and red meat) may be a contributing factor. Cooked meats contain aromatic hydrocarbons, which can promote prostate carcinogenesis, but red meats are also rich sources of dietary fats and may contribute to obesity and hormonal imbalance (see previous discussion) (Freedland et al., 2004).

Prospective data from the National Health and Nutrition Examination Survey Epidemiological Follow-up Study (NHANES) cohort of 3779 men followed for 10 years showed that α-linolenic acid, which is present in some vegetable oils and nuts, leafy vegetables, and animal fats, is an independent risk factor for advanced prostate cancer (Giovannucci et al., 1993). Specifically, after adjusting for potentially confounding variables, the relative risk of advanced prostate cancer conferred by α-linolenic acid from meat, dairy, and nonanimal sources was 1.92; the relative risk went up to 2.12 when evaluating the effect of α-linolenic acid on death from prostate cancer (Leitzmann et al., 2004). On the other hand, increased consumption of fish oils, specifically eicosapentaenoic acid and docosahexaenoic acid, was inversely correlated with the risk of prostate cancer and advanced prostate cancer, such that each additional daily intake of 0.5 g of fish oils from food was associated with a 24% decreased risk of metastatic prostate cancer. Data from the same cohort after 4 years of follow-up demonstrated that total fat intake, and particularly animal fat intake, directly correlated with increased risk of advanced prostate cancer. When analyzed by food group, red meat intake had the strongest association, whereas fat from dairy foods showed no association. At 10 years of follow-up, both red meat and dairy foods showed an association with advanced disease, but after controlling for known risk factors such as calcium and α-linolenic acid, much of the risk was attenuated (Michaud et al., 2001).

Two other large epidemiological studies found little to no association between the different types of fat and prostate cancer. A review of data from The Netherlands Cohort Study of 58,279 men after 6.3 years of follow-up showed no associations between prostate cancer and intake of total fat, total saturated fatty acids, or total trans-unsaturated fatty acids (Schuurman et al., 1999). Nonsignificant associations were seen with oleic acid and linolenic acid, whereas no associations were seen with eicosapentaenoic acid or docosahexaenoic acid. Similarly, in a study of 25,708 Norwegian men followed for 15 years, no associations were found between prostate cancer and energy-adjusted intake of total fat, saturated fat, monounsaturated fat, or polyunsaturated fat (Veierod et al., 1997). At this point, it seems probable that dietary fat intake, particularly that from animal sources, does play some role in prostate cancer development. Whether the effect is strictly due to the already identified components or to other components remains to be explored.

Tomato-Based Foods and Lycopene

Data from the Health Professionals Follow-Up Study, a prospective cohort study of 51,529 male health professionals aged 40–75 years in 1986, demonstrated that increased consumption of lycopene-rich tomato-based foods conferred a 35% reduction in the risk of prostate cancer and a 54% reduction in the risk of advanced disease on the basis of data culled from a questionnaire at baseline (Giovannucci et al., 1995). Updated results after 6 years showed that the reduction in prostate cancer risk was durable, but decreased to 17%, with increased consumption of lycopene-rich tomato-based products; after 12 years, although the reduction remained significant, it decreased to 16% (Giovannucci et al., 2002).

Specifically, following previous research suggesting that the benefits of tomato-based foods result from the increased bioavailability of lycopene and other compounds when the foods are heated (Giovannucci et al., 1995), the researchers noted that increased consumption of tomato sauce was associated with a 44% reduction in the risk of prostate cancer at baseline and remained significant after 12 years of follow-up, with a 23% reduction noted in men who consumed at least two servings per week (Giovannucci et al., 2002). Of note, after 12 years of follow-up, men who consumed at least two servings of tomato sauce per week demonstrated a 36% lower risk of metastatic disease and a 35% lower risk in locally advanced disease.

A prospective analysis of plasma lycopene in patients enrolled in the Physicians' Health Study, a randomized placebo-controlled trial of aspirin and β-carotene in 22,071 men, demonstrated an ~40% reduction in the risk of prostate cancer in men with the highest levels of plasma lycopene among those assigned to placebo rather than to β-carotene. In contrast, a possible benefit of β-carotene with regard to prostate cancer risk was only evident among men with the lowest lycopene levels. These results suggest that there is a ceiling to the benefit that can be achieved from the carotenoids, and that this maximum benefit can be achieved by either food intake or supplementation (Gann et al., 1999).

Tomatoes contain not only lycopene, which was measured in the blood in the aforementioned study, but a mixture of related compounds including phytoene, phytofluene, vitamin C, and vitamin E. Newer studies suggest that these other components of the tomato may also have a preventive benefit. Carcinogen and hormone-treated rats fed whole tomato powder showed a significant decrease in the risk of developing prostate cancer, but those fed a crystalline-pure lycopene supplement did not (Boileau et al., 2003). These results reinforce the notion that a family of related compounds is more effective than a single isolated compound. There may well be complex interactions among the multiple elements and compounds found in foods, and because processing of foods can alter their absorption, it might not be possible to achieve the risk reduction seen with foods by supplementation of purified single compounds alone. Supplements based on extraction of whole tomatoes, juice supplements, and other food-based strategies might be necessary for an effective preventive approach to prostate cancer (Gann and Khachik, 2003). Further research into the benefits of supplementation relative to food-based intake will help better define the optimal nutritional preventive strategy.

Vitamin D

On the basis of laboratory and epidemiological data, it has been proposed that 1,25-dihydroxyvitamin D_3 (1,25$[OH]_2$ D_3), the active metabolite of vitamin D, inhibits prostate carcinogenesis, and that by lowering levels of this metabolite, calcium, in turn, minimizes its protective effects (Giovannucci, 1998).

Substantial experimental evidence indicates that the hormonal form of vitamin D promotes the differentiation and inhibits the proliferation, invasiveness, and metastasis of human prostatic cancer cells. Vitamin D receptor (VDR), a member of the steroid/thyroid hormone nuclear receptor family, is bound by the steroid hormone 1,25-dihydroxyvitamin D_3, which is thought to play a role in the etiology and progression of prostate cancer. Polymorphisms in the VDR gene have been associated with prostate cancer risk.

Results from epidemiological studies of vitamin D status and/or VDR polymorphisms and prostate cancer risk have been mixed. John et al. (2005) conducted a population-based case–control study of advanced prostate cancer among men aged 40–79 years from the San Francisco Bay area. Interview data on lifetime sun exposure and other risk factors were collected for 905 non-Hispanic White men (450 cases and 455 controls). Using a reflectometer, constitutive skin pigmentation was measured on the upper underarm (a sun-protected site) and facultative pigmentation on the forehead (a sun-exposed site) and a sun exposure index was calculated from these measurements. Biospecimens were collected for 426 cases and 440 controls. Genotyping was done for VDR polymorphisms in the 5′ regulatory region (Cdx-2), exon 2 (FokI), and the 3′ region (TaqI and BglI). Reduced risk of advanced prostate cancer was associated with high sun exposure determined by reflectometry (odds ratio [OR], 0.51; 95% confidence interval [CI], 0.33–0.80) and high occupational outdoor activity (OR, 0.73; 95% CI, 0.48–1.11). Significant risk reductions with the high-activity alleles FokI FF or Ff, TaqI tt, and BglI BB genotypes and a nonsignificant reduction with Cdx-2 AG or AA genotype were observed in the presence of high sun exposure, with ORs ranging from 0.46 to 0.67. These findings support the hypothesis that sun exposure and VDR polymorphisms together play important roles in the etiology of prostate cancer most likely via production and subsequent actions of vitamin D.

Vitamin E

The tocopherols and tocotrienols encompass vitamin E and are a class of naturally occurring and synthetic lipid-soluble compounds essential for normal mammalian reproduction (Evans, 1922). There are eight forms of vitamin E (four tocopherols and four tocotrienols) with varying levels of biological activity (Brigelius-Flohe et al., 1999). The richest sources of vitamin E in the U.S. diet are vegetable oils and foods made from vegetable oils, such as salad dressings and mayonnaise, with smaller amounts in grains, nuts, and meats (Eitenmiller, 1995). Estimated average daily dietary intake among U.S. women and men is between 8 and 10 mg, respectively (NHANES, 1999–2000), which is substantially lower than the current Dietary Reference Intake of 15 mg recommended for both men and women (Food and Nutrition Board, 2000).

The strongest evidence in support of a preventive effect of vitamin E supplementation comes from a large intervention trial conducted in Finland, the Alpha-Tocopherol, Beta-Carotene Cancer Prevention (ATBC) Study. This randomized, double-blind, placebo-controlled trial of synthetic all rac-α-tocopheryl acetate (50 mg daily) and β-carotene (20 mg daily) among 29,133 male smokers 50–69 years old suggested that chronic supplementation with vitamin E can reduce prostate cancer incidence and mortality (Heinonen et al., 1998). During the 5–8 years of intervention and follow-up, there were 246 new cases of and 64 deaths from prostate cancer. Among those assigned to the α-tocopherol (AT) supplementation arm of the trial ($n = 14,564$), 99 incident prostate cancers were diagnosed, compared with 147 cases among those assigned to the non-AT arm ($n = 14,569$), representing a statistically significant 32% reduction in prostate cancer incidence (95% CI, 12–47%; $p = .002$) (Heinonen et al., 1998). The observed preventive effect appeared stronger in clinically evident prostate cancer cases (i.e., stages B–D) for which the incidence was decreased 40% in subjects receiving vitamin E (95% CI, 20–55%). Prostate cancer mortality was 41% lower in the vitamin E group (95% CI, 1–64%); however, vitamin E supplementation did not affect survival time after diagnosis. Although prostate cancer was prespecified only as a secondary endpoint in this trial, these findings suggested a potentially substantial impact of AT in reducing prostate cancer incidence and mortality, thus offering an important lead that warranted further evaluation.

AT may influence the development of cancer through several plausible mechanisms. AT is a potent antioxidant of highly reactive and genotoxic electrophiles (e.g., hydroxyl, superoxide, lipid peroxyl and hydroperoxyl, and nitrogen radicals) that prevents the propagation of free radical damage in biological membranes and decreases mutagenesis and carcinogenesis (Burton and Ingold, 1981). Vitamin E also blocks nitrosamine formation. AT inhibits protein kinase C activity (Boscoboinik et al., 1991a; Tasinato et al., 1995) and the proliferation of smooth muscle cells (Boscoboinik et al., 1991b; Tasinato et al., 1995) and melanoma cells (Ottino and Duncan, 1997), thus possibly affecting tumor growth or aggressiveness. Vitamin E also induces the detoxification enzyme NADPH:quinone reductase in cancer cell lines (Wang and Higuchi, 1995) and inhibits arachidonic acid and prostaglandin metabolism (Rimbach et al., 2002). Vitamin E effects on hormones that can increase cellular oxidative stress and proliferative activity and on cell-mediated immunity have also been reported (Rimbach et al., 2002). Reductions of serum testosterone and androstenedione were observed in the ATBC Study in response to daily supplementation with AT, 50 mg daily, supporting a highly relevant mechanism of action on prostate carcinogenesis in this study (Hartman et al., 2001).

The most biologically active form of vitamin E is AT, which also is the predominant form in human tissues, including the prostate (Brigelius-Flohe and Traber, 1999; Freeman et al., 2000). AT in capsules must be esterified for stability, but esters are hydrolyzed in the intestinal lumen and absorption does not vary among different esters (Traber and Wuller, 1993). AT is also available in the pure RRR configuration, but absorption does not differ between pure RRR and all racemic forms of vitamin E, and once dose is adjusted to account for the 50% of all racemic AT that is biologically active, the formulations are biologically equivalent (Food and Nutrition Board, 2000).

In vitro and *in vivo* experimental data suggest that vitamin E may inhibit carcinogenesis by a variety of mechanisms. Vitamin E can inhibit the growth of human cancer cell lines, including prostate, lung, melanoma, oral carcinoma, and breast (Dieber-Rotheneder et al., 1991; Traber, 1997; Traber and Arai, 1999), and animal experiments show prevention of various chemically induced tumors, including hormonally mediated tumors. In addition, vitamin E has been shown to slow the growth of prostate tumors in rats receiving various doses of chemotherapeutic agents.

Other trial data supporting the evaluation of vitamin E and AT in cancer prevention include lower colorectal cancer incidence in the AT arm of the ATBC Study (relative risk 0.78, 95% CI, 0.55–1.09) (Albanes et al., 2000), a finding consistent with some prior epidemiological research of vitamin E supplement use (described later in this chapter). Additionally, although only a negligible 1% decrease in lung cancer incidence occurred overall during this study within the vitamin E group (compared with the non–vitamin E group), a supplementation duration analysis showed an increased reduction of lung cancer with longer trial participation (e.g., >3 years), culminating in a 10–15% reduction in risk between the fifth and eighth years in the AT group (Albanes et al., 1996). Further support of the potential effectiveness of vitamin E supplementation in nonprostatic cancers was reported from the first Nutrition Intervention Trial conducted in China. This trial tested a combination of vitamin E, β-carotene, and selenium and found a 21% lower mortality from stomach cancer and a 13% reduction in total cancer mortality in a population of >29,000 individuals, ages 40–69 years, who were at high risk of developing esophageal/gastric cardia cancer (Blot et al., 1993). The study did not specifically examine prostate cancer, and the specific efficacy of vitamin E or any other compound (or combination) could not be determined because the agents were not tested separately.

Observational data also suggest that vitamin E may also protect against lung (Comstock et al., 1992; Shibata et al., 1992; Knekt et al., 1991; Yong et al., 1997) and colorectal cancer (Longnecker et al., 1992). In contrast to lung cancer, no association with colorectal cancer risk has been seen for dietary intake levels of vitamin E, although a lower risk of colorectal cancer has been observed among those taking vitamin E supplements at >200 mg daily (Bostick et al., 1993; Ferraroni et al., 1994). Nevertheless, such observational data should be considered hypothesis generating, rather than definitive, given the possibility of measurement error (particularly for dietary vitamin E intake), selection and recall biases, and unrecognized confounding factors.

Lung cancer studies have reported lower prediagnostic serum vitamin E (AT) levels among cancer cases compared with noncases (Knekt et al., 1991; Comstock et al., 1992; Shibata, 1992; Yong et al., 1997) or a weak protective association for supplemental vitamin E (Shibata et al., 1992). Five prospective studies showed an inverse association between serum AT and colorectal cancer, with a pooled estimate of a 40% lower relative risk for the highest compared with the lowest categories (Longnecker et al., 1992). Although no association with colorectal cancer risk has been seen for dietary intake levels of vitamin E, a lower risk was observed for vitamin E supplement use (i.e., ≥200 IU daily) (Bostick et al., 1993; Ferraroni et al., 1994). Inherent to such observational studies are problems with measurement error (particularly for dietary vitamin E intake), selection and recall biases, and confounding factors.

The epidemiological data supporting a beneficial association between vitamin E and prostate and other cancers are based on assessments of the relationship between cancer development and estimated dietary and supplemental vitamin E intake and AT blood levels. Some prospective studies reported lower serum or plasma vitamin E concentrations among prostate cancer cases years before diagnosis, compared with these concentrations among noncases, although dose–response relationships were not observed (Willett et al., 1984; Knekt et al., 1988; Hsing et al., 1990; Eichholzer et al., 1999; Helzlsouer et al., 2000). One study of 3000 subjects over a 17-year follow-up found that low-serum AT concentrations were associated with a higher prostate cancer risk (Eichholzer, 1999), and a trial-based cohort analysis suggested a protective effect from prostate cancer for total vitamin E intake among men who received AT supplementation (Hartman et al., 1998). A study of 117 prostate cancer cases and 223 matched control subjects conducted in Washington county, Maryland, showed a stronger inverse association for γ-tocopherol then for α-tocopherol (Helzlsouer et al., 2000). However, an analysis of 100 cases and 200 matched controls from the ATBC Study cohort revealed a slightly stronger inverse association for α-tocopherol than for γ-tocopherol (Weinstein et al., 2005).

A long history of research supports the safety AT supplementation in humans (NIH/ODS, 2005). The tolerable upper limit of vitamin E intake has been set at 1000 mg/day, and the dose required to kill 50% of test animals (LD_{50}) for AT acetate is in excess of 2000 mg/kg for rats, mice, and rabbits (Food and Nutrition Board, 2000). No significant adverse effects were reported, with the exception of elevated risk of hemorrhagic stroke among male smokers in the ATBC Study (Alpha Tocopherol Beta Carotene CPSG, 1994), a finding that was subsequently isolated to the subgroup of men with uncontrolled hypertension (Leppala et al., 2000). Thus, poorly controlled hypertension is an exclusion criterion for the SELECT trial (see later discussion), as is the use of anticoagulant medication, with the exception of cardioprotective doses of aspirin.

Selenium

Selenium is an essential trace element whose principal dietary sources include seafood, meats, and grain products (El-Bayoumy, 1991). Most dietary selenium is in organic form, primarily selenomethionine and selenocysteine (Combs, 1984). Typical dietary intake of selenium in the United States is in the range of 80–165 μg/day (Schrauzer, 2000), and the Recommended Dietary Allowance is 55 μg/day for adult North Americans (Food and Nutrition Board, 2000). The safe upper limit of intake is considered 400 μg/day (Food and Nutrition Board, 2000).

There are extensive *in vitro* animal experimental and human epidemiological data supporting an association of selenium with reduced prostate cancer risk. *In vitro*, selenium has antiproliferative and proapoptotic effects (Redman et al., 1997, 1998; Menter, 2000), can alter carcinogen metabolism (Shimada et al., 1997), and can influence several aspects of immune function (Taylor, 1995; Field et al., 2002). More than 60 published animal studies in 10 organ systems have demonstrated that selenium inhibits tumor formation in chemical, viral, and transplantable tumor models (Medina and Morrison, 1988; Combs, 1991; El-Bayoumy, 1991; Shibata et al., 1992; NCI, 1996). Observational studies in humans, conducted throughout the United States and in many other countries, have also generally found inverse associations between selenium status and cancer risk (Combs, 1997, 2001).

Some of this research, however, is weak. Any study based on dietary selenium intake rather than serum or toenail selenium concentration is suspect because selenium intake cannot be measured using standard dietary assessment instruments. Further, case-control studies of serum selenium are difficult to interpret because sequestration of selenium by tumor cells and poor nutritional status may contribute to reduced selenium levels among patients with advanced cancer (Willett, 1986). Thus, the best epidemiological evidence on selenium and prostate cancer is currently from nine prospective cohort studies (Willett et al., 1983; Coates et al., 1988; Knekt et al., 1990; Yoshizawa et al., 1998; Helzlsouer et al., 2000; Nomura et al., 2000; Brooks et al., 2001; Goodman et al., 2001; Steiner et al., 2002). Early studies, published from 1983 to 1991, hinted at a benefit for higher selenium levels but had such small sample sizes (cases from all four studies totaled only 81) that they were largely uninformative. Subsequently, five larger studies with 53–249 cases each (and a total of 834 cases) have provided substantially more information. Although one study reported no association between plasma selenium concentration and prostate cancer risk (Brooks et al., 2002), four studies reported selenium levels that were 3–15% lower in cases than controls, as well as relative risk reductions of 50–76% contrasting the high versus low quantile of serum or toenail selenium.

The most compelling evidence for selenium as a potential chemopreventive agent comes from the secondary findings of the Nutritional Prevention of Cancer Study (Clark et al., 1996). In this double-blind clinical trial completed between 1983 and 1991, 1312 patients with prior basal or squamous cell skin cancer were randomized to receive 200 μg/day of selenium as high-selenium yeast versus placebo, with a mean time on study of 4.5 years. The primary endpoint of the trial was the incidence of nonmelanoma skin cancer, and secondary endpoints, added in 1990, included all-cause mortality, total cancer mortality, total cancer incidence, and the incidences of lung, prostate, and colon cancer. Although the incidence of skin cancer was modestly increased among participants randomized to the selenium arm (hazard ratio [HR] = 1.17; 95% CI, 1.02–1.34), primarily because of an elevated risk of squamous cell cancer (HR = 1.25; 95% CI, 1.03–1.51) (Duffield-Lillico et al., 2003), those who received selenium through 1993 had a significant reduction in total (HR = 0.75; 95% CI, 0.58–0.97) and prostate cancer incidence (HR = 0.48; 95% CI, 0.28–0.80) (Duffield-Lillico et al., 2002). The magnitude of reduced prostate cancer risk depended on baseline selenium levels and was largest among men with low baseline selenium and absent among those with high baseline selenium. Two other large randomized trials have reported findings supporting a protective role of selenium supplementation, but in both, selenium was given in combination with other nutrients, thus precluding evaluation of selenium as an independent agent, and the number of prostate cancers was too small to be separately evaluated (Blot et al., 1993; Li et al., 1993; Mark et al., 2000).

There are a variety of potential mechanisms whereby selenium could reduce cancer risk. The best defined biological role for selenium is as an essential constituent of selenoenzymes such as the glutathione peroxidases, where it is incorporated into the active site of the enzyme as the substituted amino acid selenocysteine. This may not account for the antitumor effects of selenium because glutathione peroxidase activity is maximal at physiological selenium levels and the function of this enzyme does not correlate well with tissue selenium levels at cancer-inhibitory doses (NCI, 1996). However, because the glutathione peroxidases are highly polymorphic, selenium supplements may affect enzyme activity in subgroups of men with genetic variants in selenoproteins. Selenium likely has other activity independent of its incorporation into proteins. Both selenite and selenomethionine are metabolized via different pathways to selenide, which is then converted to the highly antitumorigenic monomethylated form, methylselenol. Ip et al. (2000) showed that the antitumor activity of selenocompounds is directly related to their ability to generate methylselenol.

In December 1998, a panel of nationally recognized selenium experts was consulted to provide advice on the dose and form of selenium to be used in SELECT. The panel members were unanimous in recommending 200 μg/day as the optimal dose based on the available efficacy and safety data. However, identifying the optimal formulation was more controversial. Although there was considerable interest in several of the newer selenium compounds due to their rapid conversion to the putative active moiety methylselenol, the absence of phase I data in humans with these forms of selenium effectively excluded them from further consideration. Consideration was also given to the inorganic forms, selenite and selenate; however, this option was rejected because of concerns regarding stability, bioavailability, and potential for genotoxicity. Thus, the choice was essentially limited to the two available organic forms of selenium, selenomethionine and high-selenium yeast. Most panel members favored selenomethionine; however, the Data and Safety Monitoring Committee asked that this recommendation be reconsidered given the fact that the strongest data in favor of a prostate cancer preventive effect came from a study (the NPC trial) using the yeast formulation. Therefore, the preliminary decision to use selenomethionine was reexamined by an expanded panel of selenium experts, and reaffirmed in July and October 2000.

The SELECT Trial

SELECT is a randomized, placebo-controlled, phase III trial of selenium (200 μg/day of selenomethionine) and/or vitamin E (400 IU/day of DL-α-tocopheryl acetate) for prostate cancer prevention (Lippman et al., 2005). Eligibility requirements included the following: age older than 55 years (50 years or older for African Americans due to the earlier age at onset in this group), nonsuspicious DRE results, and a PSA level of ≤4 ng/ml within 1 year of entry. Participants were randomized to one of four study arms: selenium + vitamin E placebo, vitamin E + selenium placebo, selenium + vitamin E, or two placebos and are expected to remain on their assigned treatment for 7–12 years. The primary study endpoint is the clinical incidence of prostate cancer detected by routine clinical practice. Between July 25, 2001, and June 24, 2004, 35,534 men from >400 sites in the United States, Puerto Rico, and Canada were accrued to this trial, making SELECT the largest cancer chemoprevention study ever conducted.

A panel of experts considered selenomethionine a well-characterized chemically discrete compound that would facilitate future *in vitro* mechanistic and pharmacokinetic analyses. In addition, selenomethionine had demonstrated activity in cell lines (Redman et al., 1997, 1998) and some experimental animal models (Yan et al., 1999). The relative inefficiency with which selenomethionine is metabolized to methylselenol was considered unlikely to be consequential in well-nourished individuals who received prolonged supplementation.

In contrast, the primary advantage of selenium yeast is that it would provide the most direct comparison with the Clark trial, which was the major impetus for studying selenium in a large-scale, phase III clinical trial. In addition, selenium yeast contains unidentified selenium metabolites that could potentially generate methylselenol directly, leading to an earlier reduction in cancer risk than would be anticipated for selenomethionine. However, the uniformity of the selenium yeast used throughout the Clark trial and the degree of similarity between that yeast product and currently available selenium yeast formulations was unknown. To address these issues, speciation analyses were undertaken to evaluate four representative yeast tablet lots from the Clark trial in conjunction with a currently available commercial selenium yeast product.

Analysis of the currently available selenium yeast product showed good batch-to-batch uniformity and indicated that 69% of its selenium content was selenomethionine. However, archived sample tablets of the selenium yeast used in the Clark trial analyzed by the same procedure had substantial sample-to-sample differences in both the presence and the relative levels of specific organoselenium compounds, some of which seemed to involve oxidation products of selenomethionine. These differences were not readily attributable to the time of manufacture or duration of storage. In some cases, released selenomethionine content was as low as 7% and substantial percentages of other organoselenium compounds were found, as yet incompletely characterized (Block et al., 2004; Pter Uden, personal communication).

The panel also considered data produced by Menter et al. (2000) on the effects of both inorganic (sodium selenite) and organic (selenomethionine) selenium on monolayer and anchorage-independent growth of normal prostate and prostate cancer cell lines. Differential dose-dependent growth inhibition, apoptosis, and cell cycle arrest were observed in prostate cancer cells versus normal cells. These changes were most pronounced in androgen-sensitive cells and were observed with *in vitro* concentrations of selenium within the range achieved with pharmacological selenium use. The *in vitro* selenium results have subsequently been confirmed by other investigators (Venkateswaran et al., 2002; Wan et al., 2003).

Given these considerations, the panel recommended selenomethionine over selenium yeast for use in the SELECT by a vote of 6 to 1. This decision was supported by data in men randomized to selenomethionine or placebo during the 4–6 week preprostatectomy period, indicating significant accumulation of selenium in the prostate gland and preferential accumulation in the prostate gland versus seminal vesicles (Sabichi et al., 2002).

The formulation of vitamin E being used in SELECT, *all rac*-α-tocopheryl acetate, encompasses the eight possible stereoisomers (*RRR, RRS, RSR* . . . *SSS*) of the AT molecule resulting from methyl group positioning at the 2′, 4′, and 8′ asymmetrical carbon atoms of the chromanol ring. Naturally occurring AT is exclusively in the *RRR* configuration, and only the four *2-R* sterisomers in synthetic AT are incorporated into lipoproteins and thus considered biologically active. This form was used in the ATBC study and is also the most common formulation used in dietary supplements. There are alternative formulations of AT supplements, but for various reasons, these were not relevant when designing SELECT.

A report from the Heart Outcomes Prevention Evaluation (HOPE) trial, a randomized, double-blind, placebo-controlled trial of AT, 400 mg a day, in patients at high cardiac risk, revealed no significant increase in the primary endpoint of major cardiovascular events (Lonn et al., 2005). However, an increase in heart failure (RR = 1.13; 95% CI, 1.01–1.26; $p = .03$) and hospitalizations for heart failure (RR = 1.21; 95% CI, 1.00–1.47; $p = .045$) among participants randomized to the AT arm was noted on secondary analyses (Lonn et al., 2005). A meta-analysis of 19 randomized controlled studies of vitamin E, reported shortly after SELECT had reached its accrual goal, suggested that high-dose vitamin E, up to 2000 mg/day, may be associated with an increase in all-cause mortality (Miller et al., 2005). These new data on vitamin E were submitted to the SELECT Data and Safety Monitoring Committee (as had been the increased risk of nonmelanoma skin cancer observed on the selenium arm of the NPC trial, discussed earlier [Duffield-Lillico et al., 2003]), and the appropriate measures have been taken to inform participants of the potential risks and to ensure their safety through careful monitoring of adverse events.

Although there was general support among the SELECT investigators for using the *all rac*-α-tocopheryl formulation of vitamin E, the optimal choice of vitamin E dosage was less clear. Some investigators supported using 50 mg to specifically confirm the results of the ATBC, which also used 50 mg. This low dose was rejected, however, in deference to AT's favorable safety profile and the possibility that higher doses might be required to obtain other health benefits, most notably protection against cardiac disease (Rimm et al., 1993), Alzheimer's disease (Sano et al., 1997), and macular degeneration (Age-Related Eye Disease Research Group, 2001). In addition, data from the ATBC showed greater benefit for AT supplementation with regard to the reduction in prostate and lung cancer incidence among subjects with higher baseline and thus, overall, AT levels.

Secondary Endpoints

Prespecified secondary endpoints were a major design consideration of SELECT. A trial of this size allows the inclusion of numerous, hypothesis-generating secondary endpoints. The effects of selenium and/or vitamin E on lung cancer incidence and survival and colon cancer incidence and survival are especially prominent secondary endpoints of the trial. Other prespecified endpoints chosen for prospective secondary evaluation are prostate cancer–specific survival, overall survival, all-cancer incidence and survival, and cardiovascular deaths. In addition, several substudies with clearly specified entry criteria and requiring separate informed consent have been nested within the parent trial. These substudies will explore the potential role of selenium and vitamin E, either alone or in combination, for the prevention of Alzheimer's disease, macular degeneration, chronic obstructive lung disease, and colonic polyps.

Translational Ancillary Endpoints

SELECT is a unique opportunity not only to evaluate prespecified secondary endpoints but also to incorporate prespecified translational ancillary studies previously unknown to very large-scale phase III trials. The SELECT biorepository of prospectively collected prostate biopsy tissue, white blood cells, red blood cells, and plasma for correlative mechanistic study also is unique to trials of the SELECT's scale. The trial will permit studies of diet/nutrient levels, molecular epidemiology, other molecular/cellular biomarkers, and quality of life, using these valuable specimens and/or prospectively collected clinical and questionnaire data.

Prospective collection of blood for research is the key to examining genetic/nutrient background, factors that may affect prostate cancer incidence in various intervention groups. Blood studies will include measurement of micronutrients and hormones in plasma, as well as hemoglobin adducts in red blood cells. Particular emphasis will be placed on the examination of genetic polymorphisms in DNA extracted from lymphocytes. This will allow the conduct of nested case-control studies to determine the relative contribution of genetic polymorphisms to the risk of prostate cancer with the ultimate goal of developing molecular risk profiles for prostate cancer in general and for aggressive prostate cancer in particular. SELECT biospecimens will be available for the best future science to identify highest risk men for prevention and screening and to identify novel molecular targets.

Nutrition-Related Ancillary Studies

A comprehensive set of nutrition-related measures were added to SELECT to support ancillary studies of the associations between prostate cancer risk and diet and dietary supplement use. There are three primary motives for these ancillary studies. First, we are motivated by the basic nutrient character of both agents, which occur naturally in foods, as added fortification in some foods, and in multivitamins and single supplements. The SELECT will allow a comprehensive understanding of the results of selenium and AT supplementation based on analyses that examine total and long-term exposure to these agents. Second, other nutritional exposures, from supplements or foods, could modify the effects of supplemental selenium and AT. Third, this is a large study of a common and important cancer, and there are many questions about associations of dietary patterns with prostate cancer risk that can be addressed within this trial.

Two specific aims will examine whether supplement use or dietary patterns modify the effects of the experimental agents. Specifically, we will evaluate the effects of the duration and dose of prior supplemental AT and selenium, as well as the usual intake of nutrients and foods potentially associated with prostate cancer risk (e.g., fat, lycopene, soy, red meat, and vegetables). Three additional specific aims will examine questions about the relationship of nutrient-related exposures with prostate cancer risk. These will test whether prostate cancer risk is associated with use of dietary supplements other than selenium and AT, nutrient intake (in particular dietary fat, specific fatty acids and lycopene), and specific dietary patterns (consumption of red meat, soy products, and fruits and vegetables).

Nutrient-related measures will include (1) at baseline, a 10-year history of dietary supplement use using a self-administered questionnaire; usual nutrient intake over the past year using a food frequency questionnaire; and nutrient concentrations from blood and toenail samples; and (2) at each annual visit, use of dietary supplements over the previous year. Planned biochemical analyses include tissue, serum and toenail selenium and zinc, phospholipid fatty acids, and serum folate, carotenoids, and tocopherols. Results from these studies can be used to better understand the study's primary outcomes and will be important in formulating public health recommendations for prostate cancer prevention.

Molecular Epidemiology

One of the most exciting tertiary objectives of SELECT is to conduct timely molecular epidemiological investigations on the basis of blood specimens collected at baseline from all participants and from a subsample annually. The SELECT molecular epidemiology design was reviewed in detail previously (Hoque et al., 2001) and is outlined more briefly here. These studies will generate unprecedented data with the potential to have a substantial impact on generations to come. These studies will permit the examination of the main effects of the interventions on individuals with particular genetic backgrounds and may help to identify those men who may benefit the most (or the least) from the study interventions. In addition to assessing the effects of these supplements on prostate cancer incidence among men with a specific genotype, for example, short androgen receptor (CAG)n repeat length, variations in risk according to the presence or absence of other risk factors, such as high-fat diet, can also be examined. Thus, the molecular epidemiological studies will be critical to fully assessing the potential benefit of SELECT interventions. Identification of any subgroups of men for whom these interventions significantly reduce prostate cancer incidence may enhance our understanding of the underlying molecular defects and environmental exposures that may affect prostate cancer risk. This knowledge may be important for the development of new cancer prevention strategies.

The assembly of this large cohort also provides an excellent opportunity to evaluate molecular/genetic markers that contribute to the development of prostate cancer. Nested case-control studies will be performed, with incident cancer patients being matched to participants who are free of disease at the time of the cases' diagnoses. Because all SELECT enrollees will have blood drawn at baseline and be on the study for up to 12 years, the nested case-control design is highly efficient and affords the advantage of providing sample-based risk estimates that are as stable as those generated from analysis of the entire cohort.

Approximately 1500–2000 prostate cancers are expected to occur in this population during the 12-year study. The certainty that new hypotheses regarding prostate carcinogenesis will evolve over time; the identification of new candidate genes and other exposures that may influence susceptibility; and biotechnological improvements in the efficiency of analysis, sensitivity, and reproducibility of assays argue in favor of a flexible analytical plan for these investigations. Planned analysis include evaluation of polymorphisms in androgen metabolism genes (e.g., *AR*, *CYP17*, *HSD3B2*, *SRD5A1* and *2*); genes coding for growth factors (e.g., *IGF-1* and *IGFBP3*); and carcinogen metabolism genes (e.g., *CYP1A1*, *GSTM1*, and *GSTP1*); DNA repair (e.g., *hMLH1* and *2*, *OGG1*, *XRCC1*, and *XRCC3*); and oxidative stress genes (e.g., *MPO*, *ecNOS*, *MnSOD*, *GPX1*). The role of environmental exposures (e.g., chemicals, dietary intake) can be explored by measuring carcinogen–DNA or carcinogen–protein adducts, as well as plasma nutrients. Tissue-based studies of tumor markers will also be conducted in SELECT.

With its activation on July 25, 2001, the SELECT joined an historical march of large-scale phase III cancer chemoprevention trials, beginning in the 1980s. Although most completed phase III trials were negative, chemoprevention finally reached its stride in 1998, when the Breast Cancer Prevention Trial produced a dramatic positive result leading to the U.S. Food and Drug Administration approval of tamoxifen for breast cancer risk reduction in high-risk healthy women.

A hallmark of phase III trials is to generate provocative secondary and tertiary translational data that in turn generate new hypotheses for future trials and biological studies. Whatever its primary outcome, the SELECT undoubtedly will spawn new trials, just as the ATBC and NPC studies spawned SELECT. The SELECT was designed prospectively to maximize provocative translational study opportunities of large-scale interventions, in contrast with most (if not all) other large trials, which implemented post hoc methods for biological study. An invaluable biorepository of SELECT blood samples and toenails and prostate biopsy tissue samples will be collected. All these samples will be used in future correlative and other molecular/cellular biological studies of prostate cancer and other disease processes. The SELECT promises to contribute to our understanding of cancer risk and development for generations to come.

CONCLUSION AND FUTURE DIRECTIONS OF RESEARCH

Increased research on prostate cancer over the past decade has led to many new insights into the role of nutrition in the pathogenesis and prevention of prostate cancer. At this time, our understanding of how the various phytochemicals and micronutrients interact is incomplete.

At a basic science level, there remains much work to be done on gene–nutrient interaction and the specification of where bioactive compounds have their impact. The ability to modify the expression of specific genes in the mouse through genetic engineering technologies allows the generation of previously unavailable models for prostate cancer prevention research. Although animal models have existed for some time for the study of prostate cancer prevention (primarily in the rat), it is uncertain whether the mechanisms that drive prostate carcinogenesis in these models are relevant to those in human prostate cancer.

Cell culture studies are of limited usefulness because the conditions are inherently artificial. Factors such as relevant physiological concentrations and metabolism of putative chemoprevention compounds are difficult to model in an *in vitro* system. These studies also preclude the types of interactions known to occur between multiple cell types *in vivo*. In addition, all prostate cancer cell lines are already highly progressed and are not representative of the type of cells to which most preventive strategies would be targeted.

Due to the advent of transgenic mouse (TgM) models, there are now models of prostate cancer that are dependent on molecular mechanisms already implicated in human prostate carcinogenesis. With these models, it is possible to perform a variety of experiments that could previously only be done in cell culture or in prostate cancer cell line xenografts. These experiments can specify pathways that examine nutrient–nutrient interactions and take into account the metabolism of bioactive compounds into active metabolites. This work will require a combination of expertise from multiple disciplines coordinated around specific issues to advance the field. Then it will be possible using the insights gained from the SELECT to power future studies appropriately through the cooperative group mechanism to ultimately determine optimal nutritional strategies for the prevention of prostate cancer and the prevention of prostate cancer recurrence.

Acknowledgments

The SELECT trial is supported by a grant from the NCI (U 10 CA 37429) to the Southwest Oncology Group. Heber and Aronson's work is supported by the UCLA Clinical Nutrition Research Unit (NCI Grant No 1 P30 CA42710) and the UCLA Prostate Cancer SPORE Nutrition Project (NCI Grant No. 1P50 CA92131).

References

Abu-Abid, S., Szold, A., and Klausner, J. 2002. Obesity and cancer. *J Med* **33**: 73–86.

Age-Related Eye Disease Research Group. 2001. A randomized, placebo-controlled, clinical trial of high-dose supplementation with vitamins C and E, beta carotene, and zinc for age-related macular degeneration and vision loss: AREDS report No. 8. *Arch Ophthalmol* **119**: 1417–1436.

Albanes, D., et al. 1996. Alpha-Tocopherol and beta-carotene supplements and lung cancer incidence in the alpha-tocopherol, beta-carotene cancer prevention study: effects of base-line characteristics and study compliance. *J Natl Cancer Inst* **88**: 1560–1570.

Albanes, D., et al. 2000. Effects of supplemental alpha-tocopherol and beta-carotene on colorectal cancer: results from a controlled trial (Finland). *Cancer Causes Control* **11**: 197–205.

The Alpha-Tocopherol, Beta Carotene Cancer Prevention Study Group. 1994. The effect of vitamin E and beta carotene on the incidence of lung cancer and other cancers in male smokers. *N Engl J Med* **330**: 1029–1035.

Andersson, S.O., Wolk, A., Bergstrom, R., Giovannucci, E., Lindgren, C., Baron, J., and Adami, H.O. 1996. Energy, nutrient intake and prostate cancer risk: a population-based case-control study in Sweden. *Int J Cancer* **11**: 716–722.

Block, E., Glass, R.S., Jacobsen, N.E., Johnson, S., Kahakachchi, C., Kamiski, R., Skowroska, A., Boakye, H.T., Tyson, J.F., Uden, P.C. 2004. Identification and synthesis of a novel selenium-sulfur amino acid found in selenized yeast: rapid indirect detection NMR methods for characterizing low-level organoselenium compounds in complex matrices. *J Agric Food Chem* **52**: 3761–3771.

Blot, W.J., et al. 1993. Nutrition intervention trials in Linxian, China: supplementation with specific vitamin/mineral combinations, cancer incidence, and disease-specific mortality in the general population. *J Natl Cancer Inst* **85**: 1483–1492.

Boileau, T.W., Liao, Z., Kim, S., Lemeshow, S., Erdman, J.W., Jr., and Clinton, S.K. 2003. Prostate carcinogenesis in N-methyl-N-nitrosourea (NMU)-testosterone-treated rats fed tomato powder, lycopene, or energy-restricted diets. *J Natl Cancer Inst* **95**, 1578–1586.

Boscoboinik, D., Szewczyk, A., and Azzi, A. 1991a. Alpha-tocopherol (vitamin E) regulates vascular smooth muscle cell proliferation and protein kinase C activity. *Arch Biochem Biophys* **286**: 264–269.

Boscoboinik, D., et al. 1991b. Inhibition of cell proliferation by alpha-tocopherol. Role of protein kinase C. *J Biol Chem* **266**: 6188–6194.

Bosland, M.C., Ford, H., and Horton, L. 1995. Induction at high incidence of ductal prostate adenocarcinomas in NBL/Cr and Sprague-Dawley Hsd:SD rats treated with a combination of testosterone and estradiol-17 beta or diethylstilbestrol. *Carcinogenesis.* **16**: 1311–1317

Bostick, R.M., et al. 1993. Reduced risk of colon cancer with high intake of vitamin E: the Iowa Women's Health Study. *Cancer Res* **53**: 4230–4237.

Brigelius-Flohe, R., and Traber, M.G. 1999. Vitamin E: function and metabolism. *FASEB J* **13**: 1145–1155.

Brooks, J.D., et al. 2001. Plasma selenium level before diagnosis and the risk of prostate cancer development. *J Urol* **166**: 2034–2038.

Burton, G., and Ingold, K.U. 1981. Autoxidation of biological molecules. 1. The antioxidant activity of vitamin E and related chain-breaking phenolic antioxidants *in vitro*. *J Am Chem Soc* **103**: 6472.

Canto, M.T., and Chu, K.C. 2000. Annual cancer incidence rates for Hispanics in the United States: surveillance, epidemiology, and end results, 1992–1996. *Cancer* **88**: 2642.

Chan, J.M., Stampfer, M.J., Giovannucci, E., Gann, P.H., Ma, J., Wilkinson, P., Hennekens, C.H., and Pollak, M. 1998. Plasma insulin-like growth factor-I and prostate cancer risk: a prospective study. *Science* **279**: 563–566.

Clark, L.C., et al. 1996. Effects of selenium supplementation for cancer prevention in patients with carcinoma of the skin. A randomized controlled trial. Nutritional Prevention of Cancer Study Group. *JAMA* **276**: 1957–1963.

Coates, R.J., et al. 1988. Serum levels of selenium and retinol and the subsequent risk of cancer. *Am J Epidemiol* **128**: 515–523.

Combs, G.F., Jr., and Combs, S.B. 1984. The nutritional biochemistry of selenium. *Ann Review Nutrition* **4**: 257–280.

Combs, G.F. 1991. Selenium in Nutrition. *In* "Encyclopedia of Human Biology", pp 789–800. Academic Press, San Diego.

Combs, G.F. 1997. Selenium and Cancer Prevention. *In* "Antioxidants and Disease Prevention" (H.S. Garewal, Ed.), CRC Press, Boca Raton.

Combs, G.F. 2001. Selenium in global food systems. *Br J Nutr* **85**: 517–547.

Comstock, G.W., Bush, T.L., and Helzlsouer, K. 1992. Serum retinol, beta-carotene, vitamin E, and selenium as related to subsequent cancer of specific sites. *Am J Epidemiol* **135**: 115–121.

DeMarzo, A.M., DeWeese, T.L., Platz, E.A., et al. 2004. Pathological and molecular mechanisms of prostate carcinogenesis: implications for diagnosis, detection, prevention, and treatment. *J Cell Biochem* **91**: 459–477.

Dieber-Rotheneder, M., et al. 1991. Effect of oral supplementation with D-alpha-tocopherol on the vitamin E content of human low density lipoproteins and resistance to oxidation. *J Lipid Res* **32**: 1325–1332.

Donaghy, A.J., and Baxter, R.C. 1996. Insulin-like growth factor bioactivity and its modification in growth hormone resistant states. *Baillieres Clin Endocrinol Metab* **10**: 421–446.

Drago, J.R. 1984. The induction of NB rat prostatic carcinomas. *Anticancer Res* **4**: 255–256.

Duffield-Lillico, A.J., et al. 2002. Baseline characteristics and the effect of selenium supplementation on cancer incidence in a randomized clinical trial: a summary report of the Nutritional Prevention of Cancer Trial. *Cancer Epidemiol Biomarkers Prev* **11**: 630–639.

Duffield-Lillico, A.J., et al. 2003. Selenium supplementation and secondary prevention of nonmelanoma skin cancer in a randomized trial. *J Natl Cancer Inst* **95**: 1477–1481.

Dunn, S.E., Kari, F.W., French, J., Leininger, J.R., Travlos, G., Wilson, R., and Barrett, J.C. 1997. Dietary restriction reduces insulin-like growth factor I levels, which modulates apoptosis, cell proliferation, and tumor progression in p53-deficient mice. *Cancer Res* **57**: 4667–4672.

Eichholzer, M., et al. 1999. Smoking, plasma vitamins C, E, retinol, and carotene, and fatal prostate cancer: seventeen-year follow-up of the prospective basel study. *Prostate* **38**: 189–198.

Eitenmiller, S. 1995. "Tocopherols and tocotrienols in key foods in the U.S. diet" (L. Packer, Ed.), pp. 327–342. AOCS Press, Champaign.

El-Bayoumy, K. 1991. The role of selenium in cancer prevention. *In* "Cancer Prevention" (H.S. DeVita, and S.A. Rosenberg, Eds.), pp. 1–15. Lippincott, Philadelphia.

Evans, H.M., and Bishop, K.S. 1922. On the existence of a hitherto unrecognized dietary factor essential for reproduction. *Science* **56**: 650–651.

Ferraroni, M., et al. 1994. Selected micronutrient intake and the risk of colorectal cancer. *Br J Cancer* **70**: 1150–1155.

Ferry, R.J., Jr., Katz, L.E.L., Grimberg, A., Cohen, P., and Weinzimer, S.A. 1999. Cellular actions of insulin-like growth factor binding proteins. *Horm Metab Res* **31**: 192–202.

Field, C.J., Johnson, J.R., and Schley, P.D. 2002. Nutrients and their role in host resistance to infection. *J Leukoc Biol* **71**: 16–32.

Food and Nutrition Board, Institute of Medicine. 2000. "Dietary Reference Intakes for Vitamin C, Vitamin E, Selenium and Carotenoids: A Report of the Panel on Dietary Antioxidants and Related Compounds," pp. 186–283. National Academy Press, Washington, DC.

Freedland, S.J., Aronson, W.J., Kane, C.J., et al. 2004. Impact of obesity on biochemical control following radical prostatectomy for clinically localized prostate cancer. *J Clin Oncol* **22**: 446–453.

Freedland, S.J., and Aronson, W.J. 2005. Obesity and Prostate Cancer. *Urology* **65**: 433–439.

Freeman, V.L., et al. 2000. Prostatic levels of tocopherols, carotenoids, and retinol in relation to plasma levels and self-reported usual dietary intake. *Am J Epidemiol* **151**: 109–118.

Gann, P.H., and Khachik, F. 2003. Tomatoes or lycopene versus prostate cancer: is evolution anti-reductionist? *J Natl Cancer Inst* **95**: 1563–1565.

Gann, P.H., Ma, J., Giovannucci, E., et al. 1999. Lower prostate cancer risk in men with elevated plasma lycopene levels: results of a prospective analysis. *Cancer Res* **59**: 1225–1230.

Giovannucci, E., Rimm, E.B., Colditz, G.A., et al. 1993. A prospective study of dietary fat and risk of prostate cancer. *J Natl Cancer Inst* **85**: 1571–1579.

Giovannucci, E. 1998. Dietary influences of 1,25(OH)2 vitamin D in relation to prostate cancer: a hypothesis. *Cancer Causes Control* **9**: 567–582.

Giovannucci, E., Rimm, E.B., Liu, Y., Stampfer, M.J., and Willett, W.C. 2002. A prospective study of tomato products, lycopene, and prostate cancer risk. *J Natl Cancer Inst* **94**: 391–398.

Goodman, G.E., et al. 2001. Predictors of serum selenium in cigarette smokers and the lack of association with lung and prostate cancer risk. Cancer *Epidemiol Biomarkers Prev* **10**: 1069–1076.

Hartman, T.J., et al. 1998. The association between baseline vitamin E, selenium, and prostate cancer in the alpha-tocopherol, beta-carotene cancer prevention study. *Cancer Epidemiol Biomarkers Prev* **7**: 335–340.

Hartman, T.J., Dorgan, J.F., Woodson, K., Virtamo, J., Tangrea, J.A., Heinonen, O.P., Taylor, P.R., Barrett, M.J., Albanes, D. 2001. Effects of long-term γ-tocopherol supplementation on serum sex hormones in older men. *Prostate* **45**: 1–6.

Heinonen, O.P., et al. 1998. Prostate cancer and supplementation with alpha-tocopherol and beta-carotene: incidence and mortality in a controlled trial. *J Natl Cancer Inst* **90**: 440–446.

Helzlsouer, K.J., et al. 2000. Association between alpha-tocopherol, gamma-tocopherol, selenium, and subsequent prostate cancer. *J Natl Cancer Inst* **92**: 2018–2023.

Ho, E., Boileau, T.W., and Bray, T.M. 2004. Dietary influences on endocrine-inflammatory interactions in prostate cancer development. *Arch Biochem Biophys* **428**: 109–117.

Hoffman, R.M., Gilliland, F.D., Eley, J.W., et al. 2001. Racial and ethnic differences in advanced-stage prostate cancer: the Prostate Cancer Outcomes Study. *J Natl Cancer Inst* **93**: 388–395.

Hoque, A., et al. 2001. Molecular epidemiologic studies within the Selenium and Vitamin E Cancer Prevention Trial (SELECT). *Cancer Causes Control* **12**: 627–633.

Hsieh, K., and Albertsen, P.C. 2003. Populations at high risk for prostate cancer. *Urol Clin North Am* **30**: 669–676.

Hsing, A.W., et al. 1990. Serologic precursors of cancer. Retinol, carotenoids, and tocopherol and risk of prostate cancer. *J Natl Cancer Inst* **82**: 941–946.

Hsing, A.W., Deng, J., Sesterhenn, I.A., Mostofi, F.K., Stanczyk, F.Z., Benichou, J., Xie, T., and Gao, Y.T. 2000. Body size and prostate cancer: a population-based case-control study in China. *Cancer Epidemiol Biomarkers Prev* **9**: 1335–1341.

Ip, C., et al. 2000. In vitro and *in vivo* studies of methylseleninic acid: evidence that a monomethylated selenium metabolite is critical for cancer chemoprevention. *Cancer Res* **60**: 2882–2886.

Iwamura, M., Sluss, P.M., Casamento, J.B., and Cockett, A.T. 1993. Insulin-like growth factor I: action and receptor characterization in human prostate cancer cell lines. *Prostate* **22**: 243–252.

Jemal, et al. 2005. Cancer statistics, 2005. *CA Cancer J Clin* **55**: 10–30.

Jemal, A., Clegg, L.X., Ward, E., Ries, L.A., Wu, X., Jamison, P.M., Wingo, P.A., Howe, H.L., Anderson, R.N., and Edwards, B.K. 2004. Annual report to the nation on the status of cancer, 1975–2001, with a special feature regarding survival. *Cancer* **101**: 3–27.

John, E.M., Schwartz, G.G., Koo, J., Van Den Berg, D., and Ingles, S.A. 2005. Sun exposure, vitamin D receptor gene polymorphisms, and risk of advanced prostate cancer. *Cancer Res* **65**: 5470–5479.

Kaplan, P.J., Mohan, S., Cohen, P., Foster, B., and Greenberg, N. 1999. The insulin-like growth factor axis and prostate cancer: lessons from the transgenic adenocarcinoma of mouse prostate (TRAMP) model. *Cancer Res* **59**: 2203–2209.

Khuntia, D., Reddy, C.A., Mahadevan, A., Klein, E.A., and Kupelian, P.A. 2004. Recurrence-free survival rates after external-beam radiotherapy for patients with clinical T1-T3 prostate carcinoma in the prostate-specific antigen era: what should we expect? *Cancer* **100**: 1283–1292.

Knekt, P., et al. 1988. Serum vitamin E and risk of cancer among Finnish men during a 10-year follow-up. *Am J Epidemiol* **127**: 28–41.

Knekt, P., et al. 1990. Serum selenium and subsequent risk of cancer among Finnish men and women. *J Natl Cancer Inst* **82**: 864–868.

Knekt, P., et al. 1991. Vitamin E and cancer prevention. *Am J Clin Nutr* **53**(1 Suppl): 283S–286S.

Leav, I., Merk, F.B., Kwan, P.W., and Ho, S.M. 1989. Androgen-supported estrogen-enhanced epithelial proliferation in the prostates of intact Noble rats. *Prostate* **15**: 23–40.

Leitzmann, M.F., Stampfer, M.J., Michaud, D.S., et al. 2004. Dietary intake of n-3 and n-6 fatty acids and the risk of prostate cancer. *Am J Clin Nutr* **80**: 204–216.

Leppala, J.M., et al. 2000. Controlled trial of alpha-tocopherol and beta-carotene supplements on stroke incidence and mortality in male smokers. *Arterioscler Thromb Vasc Biol* **20**: 230–235.

Lesko, S.M., Rosenberg, L., and Shapiro, S. 1996. Family history and prostate cancer risk. *Am J Epidemiol* **144**: 1041–1047.

Li, J.Y., et al. 1993. Nutrition intervention trials in Linxian, China: multiple vitamin/mineral supplementation, cancer incidence, and disease-specific mortality among adults with esophageal dysplasia. *J Natl Cancer Inst* **85**: 1492–1498.

Lippman, S.M., et al. 2005. Designing the Selenium and Vitamin E Cancer Prevention Trial (SELECT). *J Natl Cancer Inst* **97**: 94–102.

Locke, F.B., and King, H. 1980. Cancer mortality risk among Japanese in the United States. *J Natl Cancer Inst* **65**: 1149–1156.

Longnecker, M.P., et al. 1992. Serum alpha-tocopherol concentration in relation to subsequent colorectal cancer: pooled data from five cohorts. *J Natl Cancer Inst* **84**: 430–435.

Lonn, E., et al. 2005. Effects of long-term vitamin E supplementation on cardiovascular events and cancer: a randomized controlled trial. *JAMA* **293**: 1338–1347.

Mantzoros, C.S., Tzonou, A., Signorello, L.B., Stampfer, M., Trichopoulos, D., and Adami, H.O. 1997. Insulin-like growth factor 1 in relation to prostate cancer and benign prostatic hyperplasia. *Br J Cancer* **7**: 1115–1118.

Mark, S.D., et al. 2000. Prospective study of serum selenium levels and incident esophageal and gastric cancers. *J Natl Cancer Inst* **92**: 1753–1763.

Massengill, J.C., Sun, L., Moul, J.W., Wu, H., McLeod, D.G., Amling, C., Lance, R., Foley, J., Sexton, W., Kusuda, L., Chung, A., Soderdahl, D., and Donahue, T. 2003. Pretreatment total testosterone level predicts pathological stage in patients with localized prostate cancer treated with radical prostatectomy. *J Urol* **169**: 1670–1675.

McCormick, D.L., Rao, K.V., Dooley, L., Steele, V.E., Lubet, R.A., Kelloff, G.J., and Bosland, M.C. 1998. Influence of N-methyl-N-nitrosourea, testosterone, and N-(4-hydroxyphenyl)-all-trans-retinamide on prostate cancer induction in Wistar-Unilever rats. *Cancer Res* **58**: 3282–3288.

McPherson, S.J., Wang, H., Jones, M.E., Pedersen, J., Iismaa, T.P., Wreford, N., Simpson, E.R., and Risbridger, G.P. 2001. Elevated androgens and prolactin in aromatase-deficient mice cause enlargement, but not malignancy, of the prostate gland. *Endocrinology* **142**: 2458–2467.

Medina, D., and Morrison, D.G. 1988. Current ideas on selenium as a chemopreventive agent. *Pathol Immunopathol Res* **7**: 187–199.

Menter, D.G., Sabichi, A.L., and Lippman, S.M. 2000. Selenium effects on prostate cell growth. *Cancer Epidemiol Biomarkers Prev* **9**: 1171–1182.

Michaud, D.S., Augustsson, K., Rimm, E.B., Stampfer, M.J., Willet, W.C., and Giovannucci, E. 2001. A prospective study on intake of animal products and risk of prostate cancer. *Cancer Causes Control*. **12**: 557–567.

Miller, E.R., et al. 2005. Meta-analysis: high-dosage vitamin E supplementation may increase all-cause mortality. *Ann Intern Med* **142**: 37–46.

Moul, J.W., Sesterhenn, I.A., Connelly, R.R., et al. 1995. Prostate-specific antigen values at the time of prostate cancer diagnosis in African-American men. *JAMA* **274**: 1277.

Muir, C.S., Nectoux, J., and Staszewski, J. 1991. The epidemiology of prostatic cancer. Geographical distribution and time-trends. *Acta Oncol* **30**: 133–140.

Mukherjee, P., Sotnikov, A.V., Mangian, H.J., Zhou, J.R., Visek, W.J., and Clinton, S.K. 1999. Energy intake and prostate tumor growth, angiogenesis, and vascular endothelial growth factor expression. *JNCI* **91**: 512–523.

National Cancer Institute, Chemoprevention Branch. 1996. Clinical development plan: selenomethionine. *J Cell Biochem* **26S**: 202–218.

National Institutes of Health/Office of Dietary Supplements. 2005. Vitamin E. Available at: http://ods.od.nih.gov/factsheets/vitamine.asp; accessed July 18, 2005.

Nelson, W.G., De Marzo, A.M., DeWeese, T.L., and Isaacs, W.B. 2004. The role of inflammation in the pathogenesis of prostate cancer. *J Urol* **172**: S6–S11.

Niskanen, L., Laaksonen, D.E., Punnonen, K., Mustajoki, P., Kaukua, J., and Rissanen, A. 2004. Changes in sex hormone-binding globulin and testosterone during weight loss and weight maintenance in abdominally obese men with the metabolic syndrome. *Diabetes Obes Metab* **6**: 208–215.

Nomura, A.M., et al. 2000. Serum selenium and subsequent risk of prostate cancer. *Cancer Epidemiol Biomarkers Prev* **9**: 883–887.

Ottino, P., and Duncan, J.R. 1997. Effect of alpha-tocopherol succinate on free radical and lipid peroxidation levels in BL6 melanoma cells. *Free Radic Biol Med* **22**: 1145–1151.

Presti, J.C., Jr., Hovey, R., Bhargava, V., Carroll, P.R., and Shinohara, K. 1997. Prospective evaluation of prostate specific antigen and prostate specific antigen density in the detection of carcinoma of the prostate: ethnic variations. *J Urol* **157**: 907.

Redman, C., et al. 1997. Involvement of polyamines in selenomethionine induced apoptosis and mitotic alterations in human tumor cells. *Carcinogenesis* **18**: 1195–202.

Redman, C., et al. 1998. Inhibitory effect of selenomethionine on the growth of three selected human tumor cell lines. *Cancer Lett* **125**: 103–110.

Rimbach, G., et al. 2002. Regulation of cell signalling by vitamin E. *Proc Nutr Soc* **61**: 415–425.

Rimm, E.B., et al. 1993. Vitamin E consumption and the risk of coronary heart disease in men. *N Engl J Med* **328**: 1450–1456.

Rodriguez, C., Patel, A.V., Calle, E.E., Jacobs, E.J., Chao, A., and Thun, M.J. 2001. Body mass index, height, and prostate cancer mortality in two large cohorts of adult men in the United States. *Cancer Epidemiol Biomarkers Prev* **10**: 345–353.

Rodriguez, C., McCullough, M.L., Mondul, A.M., Jacobs, E.J., Fakhrabadi-Shokoohi, D., Giovannucci, E.L., Thun, M.J., and Calle, E.E. 2003. Calcium, dairy products, and risk of prostate cancer in a prospective cohort of United States men. *Cancer Epidemiol Biomarkers Prev* **12**: 597–603.

Rodriguez, C., Patel, A.V., Mondul, A.M., Jacobs, E.J., Thun, M.J., and Calle, E.E. 2005. Diabetes and risk of prostate cancer in a prospective cohort of U.S. men. *Am J Epidemiol* **15**: 147–152.

Rosenthal, M.B., Barnard, R.J., Rose, D.P., Inkeles, S., Hall, J., and Pritikin, N. 1985. Effects of a high-complex-carbohydrate, low-fat, low-cholesterol diet on levels of serum lipids and estradiol. *Am J Med* **78**: 23–27.

Sabichi, A., Lee, J.J., Taylor, R.J., Thompson, I.M., Jr., Miles, B.J., Basler, J.W., et al. 2002. Selenium accumulates in prostate tissue of prostate cancer patients after short-term administration of l-selenomethionine. *Proc Am Assoc Cancer Res* **43**: 1007.

Sano, M., et al. 1997. A controlled trial of selegiline, alpha-tocopherol, or both as treatment for Alzheimer's disease. The Alzheimer's Disease Cooperative Study. *N Engl J Med* **336**: 1216–1222.

Schatzl, G., Madersbacher, S., Haitel, A., Gsur, A., Preyer, M., Haidinger, G., Gassner, C., Ochsner, M., and Marberger, M. 2003. Associations of serum testosterone with microvessel density, androgen receptor density and androgen receptor gene polymorphism in prostate cancer. *J Urol* **169**: 1312–1315.

Schuurman, A.G., van den Brandt, P.A., Dorant, E., Brants, H.A., and Goldbohm, R.A. 1999. Association of energy and fat intake with prostate carcinoma risk: results from The Netherlands Cohort Study. *Cancer* **86**: 1019–1027.

Shibata, A., et al. 1992. Intake of vegetables, fruits, beta-carotene, vitamin C and vitamin supplements and cancer incidence among the elderly: a prospective study. *Br J Cancer* **66**: 673–679.

Shimada, T., et al. 1997. Inhibition of human cytochrome P450-catalyzed oxidations of xenobiotics and procarcinogens by synthetic organoselenium compounds. *Cancer Res* **57**: 4757–4764.

Shimizu, H., Ross, R.K., Bernstein, L., Yatani, R., Henderson, B.E., and Mack, T.M. 1991. Cancers of the prostate and breast among Japanese and white immigrants in Los Angeles County *Br J Cancer* **63**: 963–966.

Smith, R.A., Cokkinides, V., Eyre, H.J., and the American Cancer Society. 2004. American Cancer Society guidelines for the early detection of cancer *CA Cancer J Clin* **54**: 41–52.

Snowdon, D.A., Phillips, R.L., and Choi, W. 1984. Diet, obesity, and risk of fatal prostate cancer. *Am J Epidemiol* **120**: 244–250.

Stattin, P., Bylund, A., Rinaldi, et al. 2000. Plasma insulin-like growth factor-I, insulin-like growth factor-binding proteins, and prostate cancer risk: a prospective study. *JNCI* **92**: 1910–1917.

Steiner, M.S., Pound, C.R., and Gingrich, J.R. 2002. Acapodene (Gtx-006) reduces high grade prostatic intrepithelial neoplasia (HGPIN) in a phase II clinical trial. *Proc AACR* 105A.

Tasinato, A., et al. 1995. d-alpha-tocopherol inhibition of vascular smooth muscle cell proliferation occurs at physiological concentrations, correlates with protein kinase C inhibition, and is independent of its antioxidant properties. *Proc Natl Acad Sci USA* **92**: 12190–12194.

Taylor, E.W. 1995. Selenium and cellular immunity. Evidence that selenoproteins may be encoded in the +1 reading frame overlapping the human CD4, CD8, and HLA-DR genes. *Biol Trace Elem Res* **49**: 85–95.

Thissen, J.P., Ketelslegers, J.M., and Underwood, L.E. 1994. Nutritional regulation of the insulin-like growth factors. *Endocr Rev* **15**: 80–101.

Thompson, I.M., Goodman, P.J., Tangen, C.M., Lucia, M.S., Miller, G.J., Ford, L.G., Lieber, M.M., Cespedes, R.D., Atkins, J.N., Lippman, S.M., Carlin, S.M., Ryan, A., Szczepanek, C.M., Crowley, J.J., and Coltman, C.A., Jr. 2003. The influence of finasteride on the development of prostate cancer. *N Engl J Med* **349**: 215–224.

Traber, M.G., and Wuller, D.P. 1993. "Vitamin E in Health and Disease" (F.J. Packer, Ed.), pp. 35–51. Marcel Dekker, New York.

Traber, M.G. 1997. Regulation of human plasma vitamin E. *Adv Pharmacol* **38**: 49–63.

Traber, M.G., and Arai, H. 1999. Molecular mechanisms of vitamin E transport. *Annu Rev Nutr* **19**: 343–355.

Trapasso, J.G., deKernion, J.B., Smith, R.B., and Dorey, F. 1994. The incidence and significance of detectable levels of serum prostate specific antigen after radical prostatectomy. *J Urol* **152**: 1816

U.S. Cancer Statistics Working Group. 2003. United States Cancer Statistics: 2000 Incidence. Department of Health and Human Services, Centers for Disease Control and Prevention and National Cancer Institute, Atlanta.

Veierod, M.B., Laake, P., and Thelle, D.S. 1997. Dietary fat intake and risk of prostate cancer: a prospective study of 25,708 Norwegian men. *Int J Cancer* **73**: 634–638.

Venkateswaran, V., Klotz, L.H., and Fleshner, N.E. 2002. Selenium modulation of cell proliferation and cell cycle biomarkers in human prostate carcinoma cell lines. *Cancer Res* **62**: 2540–2545.

Vermeulen, A. 1996. Decreased androgen levels and obesity in men. *Ann Med.* **28**: 13–15.

Wan, X.S., et al. 2003. *In vitro* evaluation of chemopreventive agents using cultured human prostate epithelial cells. *Oncol Rep* **10**: 2009–2014.

Wang, W., and Higuchi, C.M. 1995. Induction of NAD(P)H:quinone reductase by vitamins A, E and C in Colo205 colon cancer cells. *Cancer Lett* **98**: 63–69.

Weinstein, S.J., Wright, M.E., Pietinen, P., King, I., Tan, C., Taylor, P.R., Virtamo, J., Albanes, D. 2005. Serum α-tocopherol and γ-tocopherol concentrations in relation to prostate cancer risk in a prospective study. *J Natl Cancer Inst* **97**: 396–398.

Whittemore, A.S., Kolonel, L.N., Wu, A.H., John, E.M., Gallagher, R.P., Howe, G.R., Burch, J.D., Hankin, J., Dreon, D.M., West, D.W., et al. 1995. Prostate cancer in relation to diet, physical activity, and body size in blacks, whites, and Asians in the United States and Canada. *J Natl Cancer Inst* **87**: 652–661.

Willett, W.C., et al. 1983. Prediagnostic serum selenium and risk of cancer. *Lancet* **2**: 130–134.

Willett, W.C., et al. 1984. Relation of serum vitamins A and E and carotenoids to the risk of cancer. *N Engl J Med* **310**: 430–434.

Willett, W.C., et al. 1986. Selenium and human cancer: Epidemiological aspects and implications for clinical trials. *J Am Coll Toxicol* **5**: 29–36.

Wolk, A., Mantzoros, C.S., Andersson, S.O., Bergstrom, R., Signorello, L.B., Lagiou, P., Adami, H.O., and Tricdhopoulos, D. 1998. Insulin-like growth factor 1 and prostate cancer risk: a population-based, case–control study. *J Natl Cancer Inst* **90**: 911–915.

Wynder, E.L., Fujita, Y., Harris, R.E., Hirayama, T., and Hiyama, T. 1991. Comparative epidemiology of cancer between the United States and Japan. A second look. *Cancer* **1**: 746–763.

Yan, L., et al. 1999. Dietary supplementation of selenomethionine reduces metastasis of melanoma cells in mice. *Anticancer Res* **19**: 1337–1342.

Yong, L.C., et al. 1997. Intake of vitamins E, C, and A and risk of lung cancer. The NHANES I epidemiologic followup study. First National Health and Nutrition Examination Survey. *Am J Epidemiol* **146**: 231–243.

Yoshizawa, K., et al. 1998. Study of prediagnostic selenium level in toenails and the risk of advanced prostate cancer. *J Natl Cancer Inst* **90**: 1219–1224.

Yu, H., and Rohan, T. 2000. Role of the insulin-like growth factor family in cancer development and progression. *J Natl Cancer Inst* **92**: 1472–1488.

CHAPTER

21

Breast Cancer

DAVID HEBER AND GEORGE BLACKBURN

INTRODUCTION

Breast cancer is the most common form of cancer in women and is the second most common cause of cancer-related deaths among women. In fact, breast cancer accounts for 22% of all female cancers and 15% of cancer deaths among women (Edwards et al., 2002; Stewart et al., 2004). In the United States, which currently accounts for ~20% of the one million cases occurring worldwide, there has been an increase in breast cancer incidence over the past 20 years with an overall slight decrease in mortality. Therefore, although treatment and early diagnosis has made some modest inroads, much more needs to be done in primary breast cancer prevention and prevention of breast cancer recurrence in the breast cancer survivor. Gene–nutrient interaction plays a key role in breast cancer, and the factors that influence susceptibility to breast cancer from an environmental and genetic standpoint remain poorly understood. There is an urgency to this research because there is a global trend in developing countries of an increase in breast cancer incidence as Western diets and lifestyles are spreading around the world.

The etiology of breast cancer has been studied extensively using several different but complementary approaches. Our understanding of the possible etiological factors has been obtained by considering information derived from epidemiological studies, including genetic epidemiology studies and information derived over 7 decades on the basic physiology, anatomy, and cellular signaling within the cellular matrix of breast tissue. Intraductal epithelial cells account for the vast majority of breast cancer (Russo et al., 2001). Physiological studies in animals and humans have provided a valuable framework in which to consider the etiology of breast cancer by describing the growth, differentiation, and involution of breast tissue at menopause and the critical role of the breast ductal cell microenvironment.

BREAST ANATOMY AND PHYSIOLOGY

The breast is a mass of glandular, fatty, and fibrous tissues positioned over the pectoral muscles of the chest wall and attached to the chest wall by fibrous strands called *Cooper's ligaments*. A layer of fatty tissue surrounds the breast glands and extends throughout the breast. The fatty tissue gives the breast a soft consistency. The breast functions to produce milk and is composed of 15–20 sections called *lobes*, with each lobe ending in many smaller lobules also known as the *terminal ductal lobular units* (TDLUs). The lobules terminate in many tiny bulbs that produce milk during lactation. The lobes, lobules, and bulbs are all linked by the ducts. The breast tissues consist of connective or stromal tissues surrounding the complex ductal system opening into about nine orifices on each breast nipple. These openings in the areolae are usually blocked with dried secretions except during lactation (Figure 1).

The breast tissue forms in women at about age 8–10 years in a process called *thelarche*. This process is influenced by hormones related to the onset of puberty and occurs earlier in societies with a Western diet and a higher incidence of obesity (Sales et al., 2003). The stage of thelarche in humans corresponds to the short period of ~7 days around the time of terminal end-bud formation in rodents when the administration of a carcinogen such as DMBA will result in tumor formation in 100% of animals. In order for tumor formation

Copyright © 2006, Elsevier Inc.
All rights of reproduction in any form reserved.

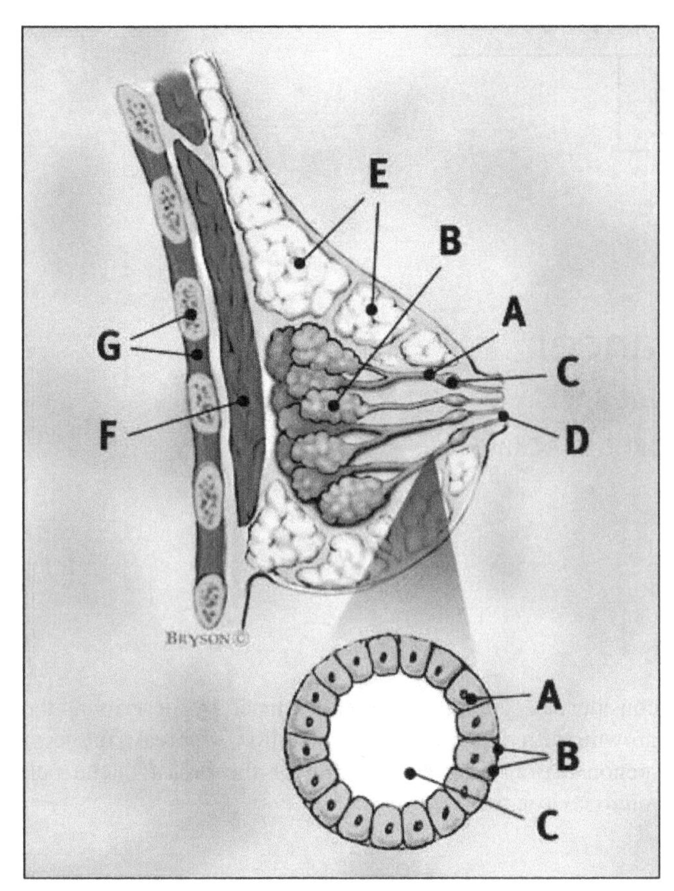

FIGURE 1 Breast anatomy. (A) Ducts; (B) lobules; (C) dilated section of duct to hold milk; (D) nipple; (E) fat; (F) pectoralis major muscle; (G) chest wall/ribcage. Enlargement: (A) normal duct cells; (B) basement membrane; (C) lumen (center of duct). www.breastcancer.org.

to occur, the DMBA must be administered at 55 days of age. If administered before 48 days of age or after 62 days of age, carcinogenesis is not initiated. Histological studies have shown high rates of DNA synthesis in the terminal end buds at about 55 days of age, suggesting that the cells are dividing and vulnerable to carcinogens in the environment including diet at this stage of breast development (Klurfeld et al., 1989a).

Following initiation in these animal models, the effects of diet on breast tumor growth and angiogenesis are well documented. A high-fat diet promotes the growth of the initiated breast cancers so that they appear at an earlier time and with greater frequency by comparison to animals fed a low-fat diet (Klurfeld et al., 1989b). A number of other dietary factors have been examined, but energy balance and obesity can be demonstrated to affect the incidence of breast cancer in these animal models (Klurfeld et al., 1991). Animals trained to exercise have a reduced rate of growth of tumors compared with sedentary animals, and genetically obese animals have an inherently increased incidence of breast cancer compared with wild-type animals. In humans, exercise in adolescence reduces breast cancer, whereas adult weight gain and obesity are associated with an increased incidence of breast cancer, as discussed in more detail in Chapter 9.

Breast cancer forms in the epithelial ductal cells, which are shed into ductal fluid, which is an apocrine secretion containing a number of peptide and steroid hormones, as well as lipids and proteins. Three major proteins present in breast gross cystic disease fluid (Selim et al., 2001) and expressed by the cyst lining apocrine epithelium are gross cystic disease fluid protein-15 (GCDFP-15), apolipoprotein-D (APO-D; GCDFP-24) and zinc α_2-glycoprotein (ZnGP; GCDFP-44). These proteins can be identified in breast ductal fluid expressed from the nonlactating breast nipple by simple negative pressure aspiration using a suction pump. APO-D can bind with low affinity to a number of steroids and lipids including a number of reproductive hormones, but its function in the ductal fluid microenvironment is not understood.

Ductal fluid production has been proposed as an additional risk factor for breast cancer and is related genetically to the ability to produce liquid ear secretions (Tice et al., 2005). Asians have reduced breast ductal fluid production and dry earwax secretions. Breast ductal fluid production is also reduced after menopause but can be obtained for study by aspiration after cleaning the breast nipple surface. Furthermore, these ducts can be cannulated and infused with contrast material and exfoliated breast ductal cells can be obtained by ductal lavage. Atypia of these cells correlates with breast pathology. Pregnancy results in a differentiation of breast ducts to enable the secretion of milk proteins, and this is driven by reproductive hormones including progesterone and estrogens (Pike et al., 1993). As discussed later, pregnancy is protective by comparison to nulliparity.

EPIDEMIOLOGICAL STUDIES

There are five- to ten-fold differences in the incidence and mortality of breast cancer between low-risk and high-risk countries internationally (Ziegler et al., 1993). The developing economies of the world in Asia, Africa, and South America, when compared with developed economies of North America and Northern Europe, demonstrated a difference that was linearly related to dietary fat as a percentage of total dietary intake based on crude food disappearance data (Carroll, 1992). These classical observations first made >30 years ago are striking but likely do not indicate a direct cause-and-effect relationship. In fact, the associations observed may have been due to more than simply dietary fat but to differences in dietary patterns, physical activity, and lifestyle. The large variation of breast cancer incidence among or within different regions of the world may also be attributed to genetic differences among populations that interact with differences in lifestyle, including diet and environmental exposures (McPherson et al., 2000; Robert et al., 2004).

Studies of individuals who migrate from a country with low breast cancer incidence (e.g., Japan) to one with higher breast cancer incidence (the United States) have demonstrated an increased risk of breast cancer within a single generation (Ziegler et al., 1993). Environmental and lifestyle factors may largely explain the observed differences in breast cancer risk in different countries, but this observation may not mean that the effects are entirely independent of the genetic influences on breast cancer risk (McPherson et al., 2000). Environmental influences can be passed on via *in utero* effects on genetic programming to subsequent generations, which assume the breast cancer risk of the new country for several generations, sometimes to an increased extent compared wtih the first generation of immigrants.

Interestingly, women with a higher socioeconomic status (SES) or from urban communities are at slightly increased risk for breast cancer than women who have a low SES or come from rural communities, respectively (relative risks [RR] are 1.20 and 1.17 in that order) (Robert et al., 2004). These differences may relate to differences in physical activity and diet, considered elsewhere.

ENDOCRINOLOGY OF BREAST CANCER

Mammary epithelial cell proliferation is correlated with serum ovarian hormonal levels. Proliferation rates are low in the follicular phase of the menstrual cycle, when estradiol and progesterone levels are low as well, whereas during the luteal phase, proliferation rates are twofold higher and correlate with the significantly increased ovarian hormone levels (Feigelson and Henderson, 1996). Increased rates of breast epithelial cellular proliferation have been proposed to expose the DNA in the breast epithelial cell to increased risk of mutagenesis via the action of endogenous oxidants, carcinogens, and exogenous carcinogens (Berkey et al., 1999).

Metabolism of endogenous androgens and estrogens, interaction with sex hormone–binding globulin (SHBG), insulin, and insulin-like growth factors (IGFs) all influence the net stimuli to the breast epithelial cell signaling such events as cellular proliferation, differentiation, and apoptosis. Prolonged exposure of breast epithelium to estrogens and progesterone due to earlier regular ovulatory menstrual cycles (Kelsey et al., 1993) has been proposed to increase the lifetime risk of breast cancer.

The age at which menarche occurs, the age at first full-term pregnancy, number of pregnancies, and age at menopause all determine lifetime exposure to estrogens (Brinton et al., 1988; Titus-Ernstoff et al., 1998; Bernstein, 2002; Michels and Willett, 2004). Increase in lifetime exposure to estrogens increases breast cancer risk, as evidenced by the risk increase noted with onset of menarche at younger than 12 years in comparison with onset after 14 years of age. The earlier age at onset of menarche has been associated with an increase in breast cancer risk of ~10–20% (Titus-Ernstoff et al., 1998).

Circulating levels of estradiol are higher in women with early menarche during their adolescence. These women have higher follicular, but not luteal, phase estradiol levels and lower SHBG levels as well. Lower SHBG levels are associated with a greater fraction of total estradiol being available to breast cells (Titus-Ernstoff et al., 1998).

Later onset of menopause results in a greater lifetime number of ovulatory cycles and has been proposed to lead to an increased breast cancer risk. It has been estimated that breast cancer risk is increased by 3% for every 1-year delay beyond average in the onset of menopause (Titus-Ernstoff et al., 1998). Surgically induced menopause (ovariectomy or hysterectomy) before the age of 35 years results in a 40% decreased risk by comparison with women experiencing natural menopause (Kreiger et al., 1999). Lower ovarian hormone levels are associated with a reduced risk of breast cancer, as demonstrated by the fact that unilateral ovariectomy before the age of 45 years is associated with a reduced risk of breast cancer (Kreiger et al., 1999).

After menopause, ovarian hormone is reduced and the androgen-to-estrogen ratio changes with a concomitant substantial decrease in mammary epithelial cell proliferation (Russo et al., 2000). Numerous prospective epidemiological studies provide strong evidence for the role of circulating estrogens, which can be derived from fat cell aromatization of circulating androgens as a key mechanism for increasing breast cancer risk in this age group. Postmenopausal women who develop breast cancer have, on average, 15% higher levels of circulating estradiol than postmenopausal women who do not develop breast cancer (Pathak et al., 2000).

Because of the effects of pregnancy on breast ductal cell differentiation, early pregnancy has a protective effect against breast cancer (Lambe et al., 1994; Kreiger et al., 1999; Lipworth et al., 2000; Russo et al., 2000; Pathak et al., 2000; Beral, 2002; Bernstein et al., 2002; Helewa et al., 2002). Women who have their first full-term pregnancy before age 20 years have a lower risk of breast cancer compared with women with their first full-term pregnancy after 30 years of age, as do women with an early second pregnancy (Titus-Ernstoff et al., 1998). Women with multiple pregnancies have half the risk of breast cancer of nulliparous women. Women with their first birth after age 35 years are at higher risk than nulliparous women (Titus-Ernstoff et al., 1998) for reasons that are not clear. Exposure to high levels of estrogens during pregnancy, as evidenced by serious nausea and vomiting during pregnancy (Titus-Ernstoff et al., 1998), are at higher risk for developing breast cancer.

Prolonged lactation has been demonstrated to be protective as well (Lambe et al., 1994). There is a 4.3% decrease in the RR of breast cancer for every 12 months of breast feeding, in addition to a decrease of 7.0% for each birth (Helewa et al., 2002). Some of the mechanisms explaining the protective effect of pregnancy have been explored in animal models of breast cancer. One mechanism may involve a markedly reduced susceptibility of the fully differentiated mammary gland to carcinogens due to, at least in part, a decrease in proliferative activity of parous epithelium. Another possibility is that the decrease of the risk is due to the altered hormonal environment during pregnancy (specific molecular changes induced by estrogen and progesterone, decrease in circulating growth hormone, etc.) (Lipworth et al., 2000).

The decrease of breast cancer risk due to prolonged lactation may be explained in part by the reduction of total number of ovulatory menstrual cycles and consequently cumulative ovarian hormone exposure. The radiographic density of the breast ducts and associated connective tissues is increased in women taking hormone replacement therapy (HRT) during menopause compared with women who do not. It has been shown that HRT users are more than twice as likely to have high-risk increased breast density patterns on mammography in comparison with nonusers (Sala et al., 2000). In addition, any hormones that stimulate breast cell proliferation can stimulate mammographic density. Mammographic density is a well-established risk factor for breast cancer in both premenopausal and postmenopausal women. The Breast Cancer Detection Demonstration Project (Brinton et al., 1995) and the Canadian National Breast Screening Study (Boyd et al., 1995) have shown that women with >75% increased breast density on the mammography have an approximately fivefold increase in the risk of developing breast cancer by comparison to women with <5% increased breast density. Both premenopausal and postmenopausal nulliparous women, as well as thinner women, frequently have increased breast density (Biglia et al., 2004). Nulliparity and high breast density seem to act synergistically since the breast cancer risk goes up to sevenfold when they are both present in the same woman (van Gils et al., 2000). History of benign breast disease is also known to increase the risk of developing breast cancer. Women with severe atypical epithelial hyperplasia have a fourfold to fivefold increased breast cancer risk when compared with women without proliferative changes in their breasts.

Bone density is a risk factor for developing breast cancer because it is a biomarker related to systemic long-term estrogen stimulation. Studies in postmenopausal women have found a positive correlation between increased bone density and high breast cancer risk, with RR varying from 2.0 to 3.5 (van Gils et al., 2000). This correlation may be explained by an increased total amount of estrogen (endogenous and exogenous) available for target tissues, including the breasts (Cauley et al., 1994).

Adult height is a biomarker of prepubertal growth rates and is an independent factor that has been consistently shown to have a modest contribution to the risk for breast cancer in postmenopausal women (RR is between 1.07 and 1.10 per height increment of 5 cm) (van den Brandt et al., 2000; Lahmann et al., 2004). A metaanalysis of epidemiological studies on IGF-1 and one of its binding proteins, IGF-BP3, demonstrated a significant correlation between high circulating concentrations of IGF-1 and IGF-BP3 and increased breast cancer risk in premenopausal women (Renehan et al., 2004). Furthermore, a synergistic effect of IGF-1 or IGF-BP3 with estrone or testosterone on breast cancer risk has been observed among both premenopausal and postmenopausal women (Yu et al., 2003).

Prolactin has been proposed to contribute to breast cancer risk, but the association is weak. A correlation was first noted in case-control studies (Clevenger et al., 2003). A twofold increase of breast cancer risk in premenopausal women with high plasma levels of prolactin (Hankinson et al., 1999) was found in the large Nurses' Health Study cohort. Interestingly, there are also effects of peptide hormones, cytokines, and other steroid hormones on breast cancer biology, and these are discussed elsewhere because most of these associations have not been evaluated in population-based studies.

EXOGENOUS HORMONES AND BREAST CANCER RISK

HRT before and after menopause increases breast cancer risk depending on the duration of exposure and whether the estrogen is used alone or in combination with progestins (Ross et al., 2000). On the other hand, administration of antiestrogens (e.g., tamoxifen) reduces breast cancer incidence in women at increased risk of breast cancer (Fisher et al., 1998).

Long-term HRT has been associated with excess breast tumors over those expected in women who have not used HRT. For women between the ages of 50 and 70 years, there is an increase of 2, 6, and 12 more cases for every 1000 women taking HRT for 5, 10, and 15 years, respectively, compared with women who have not taken HRT (Collaborate Group on Hormonal Factors in Breast Cancer, 1997). Use of popular conjugated equine estrogens alone increased breast cancer risk by ~2.2% per year of use (Kelsey et al., 1993). Data from the Women's Health Initiative (WHI) (Rossouw et al., 2003), as well as three other previous large studies (Magnusson et al., 1999; Ross et al., 2000; Schairer et al., 2000), have indicated that addition of a progestin to estrogen regimens increases breast cancer risk after 5 years of use from 10% (estrogen alone) to 30% (combined HRT).

This difference would account for an excess of eight breast cancers per 10,000 women per year of use (Rossouw et al., 2002).

The association of oral contraceptive (OC) use with breast cancer risk has been studied extensively, but the data are more robust for the older higher-dose OC used prior to 1975. More studies are necessary on the more recently employed OCs containing lower doses of estrogens and progestogens. The Collaborative Group on Hormonal Factors conducted a metaanalysis of 54 epidemiological studies showing a statistically significant increase of breast cancer risk in women taking combined OC with estrogens and progestogens, independent of dose, age at first use, length of use, age at diagnosis, or family history of breast cancer (Magnusson et al., 1999). The greatest increase in risk was observed in current users of oral contraceptives. These women had a 24% increase in breast cancer risk. If OC use is stopped, the risk decreases, and 10 years after stopping OC use there is no detectable increase in risk. Using OC before age 20 years is associated with a greater increase in breast cancer risk than using OCs at later ages (Collaborative Group on Hormonal Factors in Breast Cancer, 1996). Use of combination OC prior to 1975, when higher estrogen doses were used routinely, increased risk threefold in women with a family history of breast cancer in a first-degree relative, and a similar trend was found in women with the BRCA1 mutation (Grabrick et al., 2000; Heimdal et al., 2002).

MACRONUTRIENT INTAKES, DIET, ENERGY BALANCE, AND BREAST CANCER RISK

A Western dietary pattern is simultaneously associated with increased dietary fat intake; increased intake of refined carbohydrates, sugar, and starch; and decreased intake of fruits, vegetables, whole grains, and dietary fiber. This dietary pattern has repeatedly been associated with an increased risk of breast cancer, starting with the classic international epidemiological studies of Carroll (1968) in the 1960s, which were based entirely on food disappearance data. Although dietary fat intakes were the focus of these reports, the large international variation in fat intakes also belied many other differences in lifestyle and diet. For example, at that time in Japan, fat intakes were estimated to be ~10–15% of total energy. U.S. intakes at the same time were about 40%. The risk of breast cancer in Japan was one-fourth that in the United States at a time in line with the linear correlation Carroll proposed. This remarkable and striking correlation led to decades of work in humans examining the role of dietary fat in breast cancer risk.

In animals, it was possible to separate the effects of dietary fat and total caloric intake, but in humans fat is the least satiating macronutrient and is easily hidden in foods where excess calorie intake occurs without compensation in terms of energy expenditure leading to weight gain. Among the most widely used cohorts for the analysis of dietary factors affecting incidence is the Nurses' Health Study (Colditz and Hankinson, 2005) carried out at the Harvard School of Public Health.

The dietary analysis tool used for this cohort is normalized per 1000kcal intake per day in order to be able to discern effects of vitamins and minerals. However, fat cannot be considered separately from total caloric intake in humans and the balance of physical activity is not measured by questionnaires. In analyses in which fat intake is normalized to total energy intake, the effects of dietary fat on breast cancer risk are not seen. However, when total fat intake is considered independent of energy intake, there is a statistically significant association (Kushi et al., 1992). This analysis raises one possible explanation for the absence of significant associations in the Nurses' Health Study between fat intake normalized to total energy intake and breast cancer risk.

In the 1980s, the low-fat hypothesis led to the development of diets that were low in fat but enriched in refined carbohydrates and sugars, so with these dietary interventions, there was little weight loss except in those individuals in whom high-fat foods were responsible for the majority of excess calorie intake (Henderson et al., 1990). In the 1990s, the counterreaction, especially to restriction of red meat intake, was a high-fat and high-protein diet that restricted carbohydrates, including fruits and vegetables. Extensive epidemiological data, including a metaanalysis published by the American Institute of Cancer Research and the World Cancer Research Fund (1997), documented the impact of increased fruit and vegetable intake on cancer risk and the National Cancer Institute began a campaign to encourage the intake of five or more servings of fruits and vegetables per day for cancer prevention (http://5aday.gov/homepage/index_content.html). The recommendations have been changed to encourage seven servings per day in women and in teenagers.

Dietary factors cannot be considered absent an analysis of the effects of energy balance and obesity. Obesity and physical activity in breast cancer are the subjects of a separate chapter and are not considered in detail here. In summary, it is clear that obesity has a complex relationship with breast cancer risk modulated by menopausal status and fat distribution, as well as physical activity. Large studies conducted both in the United States and Europe have demonstrated that obesity and weight gain increase breast cancer risk among postmenopausal women. Risk is particularly evident among obese women who do not use HRT, with RRs up to 2 (Harris et al., 1992; Huang et al., 1997; Trentham-Dietz et al., 2000; Friedenreich, 2001). For each

5 kg of weight gain above minimum adult weight, breast cancer risk is estimated to be increased by 8% (Trentham-Dietz et al., 2000). A primary mechanism through which postmenopausal obesity increases the risk for developing breast cancer is through higher levels of endogenous estrogen in obese women, as adipose tissue is an important converter of androgens from the adrenal to estrogens (McTiernan et al., 2003). In contrast, obesity in premenopausal women has been associated with a decrease of breast cancer risk before menopause, but the mechanism is still unclear (Huang et al., 1997; Trentham-Dietz et al., 2000; Friedenreich, 2001; McTiernan et al., 2003).

Physical activity in the form of exercise or sports participation, especially in adolescence, has a profound effect on breast cancer risk. A metaanalysis of 19 case–control and four cohort studies investigating the relationship between physical activity and breast cancer risk has shown a consistent 20% reduction associated with physical activity performed in adolescence and young adulthood (12–24 years old) (Lagerros et al., 2004). For each 1-hour increase in recreational physical activity per week during adolescence, the breast cancer risk drops by 3% (Lagerros et al., 2004). Physical activity may reduce risk by delaying onset of menarche and by modifying bioavailable estrogen levels (Hankinson et al., 2004).

The human diet contains a large number of bioactive substances (Sugimura, 2000) that can affect breast cancer risk via blocking of carcinogen activation, inducing enzymes that inactivate carcinogens, and affecting metabolism and bioavailability of carcinogenic substances and hormones. In addition, some substances have been implicated in directly increasing cancer risk. For example, consumption of meat cooked at high temperatures has been associated with increased breast cancer risk (Zheng et al., 1998), probably due to production of heterocyclic aromatic amines (HAAs) during the cooking of the meat. The fat from meat drips onto either charcoals or other highly heated surfaces, and volatile aromatic hydrocarbons are produced in the meat itself. Precooking the meat at lower temperatures so that the inside is cooked and then browning for only a short time can significantly reduce the production of aromatic hydrocarbons.

Increased intake of unsaturated fatty acids has been reported to be weakly associated with an increased breast cancer risk (Velie et al., 2000). In particular, omega-3 polyunsaturated fatty acids (PUFAs) found in ocean-caught fish and in certain grains have been found to be protective (Bartsch et al., 1999; Saadatian-Elahi et al., 2004). These effects are thought to be mediated via effects on the generation of prostaglandins such that the balance is in either a proinflammatory or an anti-inflammatory direction. Use of aspirin or other nonsteroidal anti-inflammatory drugs that inhibit the cyclooxygenase enzymes that generate prostaglandins and thromboxanes from free arachidonic acid have been found to be inversely correlated with the incidence of breast cancer (Arun and Goss, 2004).

INSULIN RESISTANCE AND BREAST CANCER: PROPOSED MECHANISMS

An estimated 10–40% of breast cancer cases are attributed to obesity, as discussed in Chapter 9. Excess adipose tissue, a central feature of obesity, increases the release of free fatty acids and certain cytokines, which leads to hyperinsulinemia and insulin resistance. Chronic hyperinsulinemia is associated with an increased risk of breast (Kaaks, 1996; Stoll, 1999) cancer, but more studies are necessary to validate a causal relationship (Goodwin et al., 2002).

Hyperinsulinemia, through its negative effect on proper cell functioning, appears to play a role in the etiology of breast cancer. Most breast cancer cells overexpress the IR (Papa et al., 1990; Papa and Belfiore, 1996) and the IGF-1R (Papa et al., 1993), which contribute to the pathophysiology of breast cancer (Cullen et al., 1990; Milazzo et al., 1992; Papa and Belfiore, 1996). Insulin and IGF-1 regulate cell proliferation via a tyrosine kinase growth factor cascade in breast cancer (Zhang and Yee, 2002), which may explain evidence of insulin's tumorigenic effects (Cullen et al., 1990; Papa and Belfiore, 1996; Zhang and Yee, 2002).

ABDOMINAL OBESITY AND BREAST CANCER RECURRENCE AND SURVIVAL

Obesity, particularly abdominal obesity, plays a role in the biology of breast cancer by increasing circulating concentrations of androgens, as well as insulin, IGF-1, and other growth factors. Obesity is also associated with steroid hormonal profiles thought to favor breast cancer growth (McTiernan et al., 2003), including higher concentrations of female hormones in postmenopausal women who are estrogen receptor positive and increased risk of breast cancer in women older than 50 years.

Weight also influences breast cancer survival. Women who are overweight, obese, or who gain weight after diagnosis have poorer survival from breast cancer compared with women who maintain an appropriate body mass index (BMI) (Goodwin and Boyd, 1990; McTiernan et al., 2003). Race is another important factor. Obesity and obesity-related disorders, including breast cancer, are more prevalent in African American women (Heck et al., 1997; Kumanyika, 1997) than in their white counterparts, a disparity even more pronounced among middle-aged women (55% vs 28%, respectively) (National Center for Health Statistics, 1985). African American women develop breast cancer an average of 10 years earlier than white women. They also present at a higher stage, with an increased number of positive nodes

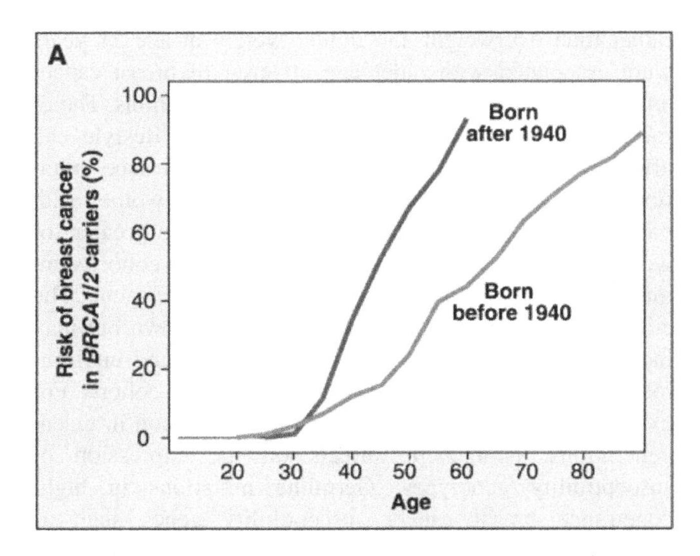

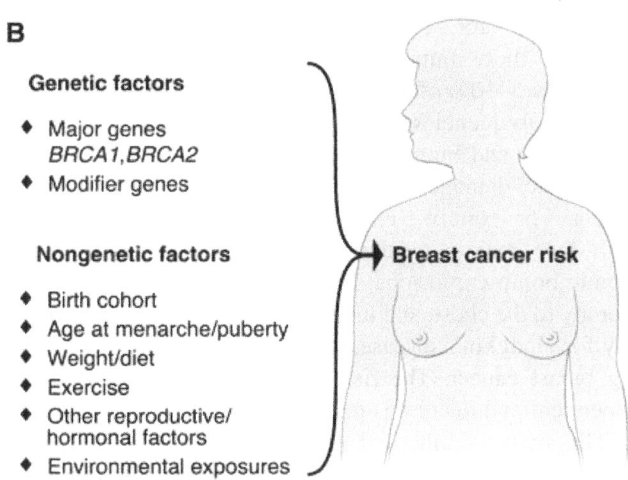

FIGURE 2 (A) Risk of breast cancer in *BRCA1/2* carriers born before and after 1940. (B) Genetic and nongenetic factors and breast cancer risk (from Levy-Lahad and Plon, 2003).

and more estrogen receptor–/progesterone receptor–negative tumors (Aziz et al., 1999). African American women appear to be at greatest risk for weight gain in their second and third decades of life.

Metabolic syndrome, in which excess weight is a central feature, is common among minority women. The prevalence among African American women is ~57% higher than in African American men. Hispanic women have a prevalence ~26% higher than their male counterparts (Ford et al., 2002) (Figure 2). Finally, African American women have poorer outcomes from breast cancer than their white counterparts. These racial disparities in survival may stem from hormonal and genetic differences in African American women that affect their response to breast cancer therapy (Aziz et al., 1999).

Data from the Women's Intervention Nutrition Study (WINS) suggest that a low-fat diet may affect breast cancer outcome. The evidence linking breast cancer and dietary fat, particularly saturated and unsaturated fatty acids, was strong enough to warrant intervention through WINS and other studies such as the Women's Health Initiative (WHI) and the Women's Healthy Eating Lifestyle study (WHEL). Launched in 1987, WINS is a National Cancer Institute–funded trial investigating the effect of a low-fat diet on the recurrence of breast cancer in postmenopausal women with stage I and II disease. Participants were randomized either to a diet in which 15% of caloric intake is from fat or to a nonintervention group (control diet) in which ~30% of caloric intake is from fat (Chlebowski et al., 1993). All had previously received currently recommended treatment with tamoxifen or chemotherapy. The study accrued 2500 participants at 30 participating cancer centers. Dietary intake was assessed by the mean of three recalls (one weekend and two weekdays) using the multiple-pass 24-hour recall system previously shown to be useful in this population (Buzzard et al., 1996). Women in the low-fat diet arm experienced a 24% reduction in recurrence risk over 5 years compared with their control counterparts (Chlebowski, et al., 2005).

ALCOHOL AND FOLATE INTAKE IN BREAST CANCER

Numerous epidemiological studies have found a positive association between alcohol intake and the risk of developing breast cancer in both premenopausal and postmenopausal women with an overall risk of 1.6 (Singletary and Gapstur, 2001). The risk increases linearly in a dose-dependent manner up to an intake of 60 g (~two to five drinks)/day. For every 10-g increment (~0.75–1.0 drink) increase in daily consumption of alcohol the risk increases by 9% (Smith-Warner et al., 1998).

Although the exact mechanisms by which alcohol can cause breast cancer have not been elucidated completely, breakthrough has been made. Alcohol can act indirectly through its first metabolite acetaldehyde, a well-characterized carcinogen and mutagen, or can be a tumor promoter, leading to enhanced procarcinogen activation (Ginsburg et al., 1995; Onland-Moret et al., 2004; Poschl and Seitz, 2004). Another mechanism of particular interest for breast cancer is the significant increase of estrogen levels in both premenopausal (especially in the periovulatory phase of menstrual cycle) (Reichman et al., 1993; Coutelle et al., 2004) and postmenopausal (Ginsburg et al., 1995; Onland-Moret et al., 2004) women associated with alcohol consumption. Also, alcohol causes an increased exposure to endogenous androgens (Singletary and Gapstur, 2001). Furthermore, alcohol causes alterations of the immune system and nutritional deficiencies including, but not limited to, folate, pyridoxal phosphate (vitamin B6—linked to methyl group synthesis and transfer), vitamin B12, vitamin D, vitamin A and retinoids, vitamin E, zinc, and selenium, all of which impair the ability of the human body to fight carcinogenesis (Smith-Warner et al., 1998).

At the molecular level, alterations of the cell cycle leading to hyperproliferation, modulation of cellular regeneration, or induction of cytochrome P450 2E1 (CYP 2E1), leading to generation of reactive oxygen species (ROS), are just a few mechanisms that may explain the correlation between alcohol intake and increased breast cancer risk (Smith-Warner et al., 1998). It has been demonstrated that postmenopausal women who have a higher alcohol and low folate intake have an increased risk of developing estrogen receptor–negative tumors (Sellers et al., 2002). Folate deficiency may increase the risk of malignancy by causing DNA hypomethylation or inducing uracil misincorporation during DNA synthesis, therefore leading to deficiencies in the DNA repair process (DNA strand breaks) (Duthie, 1999). In contrast, increased folate intake may play a role in the prevention of breast cancer in women who consume alcohol (Zhang, 2004).

GENETICS, NONGENETIC FACTORS, AND GENE–NUTRIENT INTERACTION IN BREAST CANCER

Most breast cancers are sporadic, but some are the result of inherited predisposition. Women born with mutations in BRCA1 and BRCA2 are at significantly higher risk than the general population for both breast and ovarian cancer (King et al., 2005). In families with multiple affected members used to clone these genes, the lifetime risk with either mutation is >80% for breast cancer, and for ovarian cancer it is 40% for BRCA1 and 65% for BRCA2 carriers. The New York Breast Cancer Study Group selected 1008 cases of breast cancer regardless of whether other family members were affected. They found that with this method the overall lifetime risk of breast cancer in the entire cohort was 82% regardless of whether other family members were affected. Risk of breast cancer in relatives of individuals with BRCA1 or BRCA2 mutations was 20% by age 40, 55% by age 60, and 80% by age 80 (Levy-Lahad and Plon, 2003).

Nongenetic factors were also able to greatly affect risk even in the presence of this high penetrance gene for breast cancer. Two modifiable risk factors were significantly associated with delayed onset of breast cancer among women with BRCA1 or BRCA2 mutations. First, there was lower risk if women were physically active as adolescents, as evidenced by a history of regular exercise in sports, dance, or casual exercise as compared with those who were not physically active. Second, a normal body weight at menarche rather than overweight and lighter weight at age 21 years were associated with older age at onset of breast cancer among women with BRCA1 and BRCA 2 mutations. Therefore, nongenetic factors including diet and lifestyle can affect the penetrance of even these high penetrance mutations. Although breast cancer risk was high for women with these mutations born before 1940, it was even greater for women born after 1940. These effects of birth cohort were much larger than those of any reported modifier gene. The etiology of these nongenetic effects is not known but may include the dietary, hormonal, reproductive, and environmental differences over time between these two cohorts. For example, early age at menarche is more common in recent generations. Nongenetic effects on the expression of susceptibility genotypes. Germline mutations in high-penetrance breast cancer susceptibility genes such as BRCA1, BRCA2, p53, ATM, or PTEN confer a high individual risk for developing hereditary breast cancer. However, these mutations have been shown to account for up to only 5–10% of all breast cancers, probably because of their low frequencies in the population (Easton et al., 1993; Oesterreich and Fuqua, 1999).

Genetic damage can also increase the risk of breast cancer. For example, exposure of the mammary gland to high-dose ionizing radiation, as occurs in survivors of atomic bomb explosions, individuals treated with radiation therapy to the chest, and individuals treated with chemotherapy for Hodgkin's disease, have increased risks of developing breast cancer. The risk of radiation exposure is dose dependent and decreases gradually over time.

The study of inherited genes in populations that affect breast cancer risk has uncovered both high-penetrance and low-penetrance breast cancer susceptibility genes. These genes interact with the environment and a number of the aforementioned factors in a complex way. Relatively common low-penetrance cancer susceptibility genes, acting together with endogenous and lifestyle risk factors, are likely to account for most of the sporadic breast cancers, which comprise the majority of all breast cancers (Johnson-Thompson and Guthrie, 2000). Inherited breast cancers usually arise earlier in life and are frequently bilateral, whereas sporadic breast cancers generally occur first in one breast and have a later age at onset (Rebbeck, 1999).

As with other common forms of cancer, gene–nutrient interactions have to be studied in order to develop and evaluate new biomarkers of the overall risk of breast tumorigenesis. Necessarily, this will involve nutritional genetics, nutritional genomics, and phenotyping of individual women in order to optimize the nutritional approach to prevention and treatment.

Although mutations in BRCA1 and BRCA2 are responsible for ~80–90% of all hereditary breast cancers, these mutations are not at all common in sporadic breast cancers (deJong et al., 2002). Interestingly, the normal expression of the wild-type BRCA1 gene is reduced in most sporadic breast cancers, further implicating this gene in breast carcinogenesis (Deng and Brodie, 2000).

The p53 gene was the first tumor suppressor gene linked to hereditary breast cancer and is localized on chromosome 17p13. p53 is one of the most commonly mutated genes, being mutated in ~50% of all human cancers (Malkin, 1994). Germline p53 mutations have been identified in patients with Li-Fraumeni cancer susceptibility syndrome, an autosomal dominant disorder characterized by a markedly increased risk of breast cancer with early onset, among other types of cancers (sarcomas, leukemias, brain tumors, adrenocortical carcinomas, etc.) (Malkin, 1994). Affected women have an 18-fold higher risk for developing breast cancer before age 45 years as compared with the general population, and the risk declines with age (maximum is before age 20 years) (Garber et al., 1991). PTEN germline mutations are present in 80% of patients with Cowden syndrome, a rare hereditary breast and thyroid cancer predisposition syndrome associated with a 25–50% lifetime breast cancer risk (de Jong et al., 2002) (general population has an 8–10% lifetime risk).

Ataxia telangiectasia (AT) is an autosomal recessive genetic disease caused by mutations in the ATM gene. AT carriers, who are heterozygous for ATM mutations, appear to be at an increased risk of developing breast cancer (deJong et al., 2002), estimated at 11% by the age of 50 years and 30% by the age of 70 years (Easton, 1994). Germline missense mutations (resulting in a stable but functionally abnormal protein that acts in a dominant negative fashion and inhibits the normal ATM protein), rather than truncating mutations (resulting in an unstable, abnormal ATM protein), confer the high breast cancer risk found in AT carriers (deJong et al., 2002).

Polymorphisms in breast cancer susceptibility genes with low penetrance (but present in a high percentage of individuals) have a greater contribution to breast tumorigenesis in combination with exogenous (e.g., diet, pollution) and endogenous (e.g., hormones) exposures (Rothman et al., 2001). Low-penetrance susceptibility genes can be identified by studying the biochemical or physiological pathways that are postulated to be involved in breast carcinogenesis.

Candidate polymorphic genes include those encoding for enzymes implicated in the metabolism of estrogen or various carcinogens, detoxification of reactive oxygen species emerging from these reactions, alcohol, and one-carbon metabolism pathways, or proteins that play a role in DNA repair or cell signaling processes.

Enzymes from different metabolic pathways can be divided into phase I enzymes that metabolically activate carcinogens (e.g., the CYP family proteins) and phase II enzymes that metabolically inactivate carcinogens (e.g., NAT and GST family proteins). Polymorphisms in both phase I and II enzyme genes involved in xenobiotic and endobiotic metabolism, therefore, may modulate the RR of breast cancer for an individual (Okobia and Bunker, 2003).

CYP 1A1 encodes aryl hydrocarbon hydroxylase (AHH), an enzyme that activates cigarette smoke constituents and polycyclic aromatic hydrocarbons (PAHs) leading to electrophilic carcinogenic molecules (Bartsch et al., 2000). In addition, it also catalyzes the 2-hydroxylation of estradiol in several extrahepatic tissues, including the breast (Hellmold et al., 1998). Members of the glutathione-*S*-transferase (GST) superfamily catalyze the conjugation of glutathione (GSH) to a variety of electrophiles, increasing their water solubility and excretability (Strange and Fryer, 1999). Polymorphisms leading to the absence of different GST isoenzymes affect the tolerance of the organism to chemical challenges and may influence cancer susceptibility. A pooled analysis of studies on GSTM1 null genotype (homozygous deletion) has found a small and only marginally significant association with increased breast cancer risk. GSTP1 is expressed consistently in both normal and tumor breast tissues (Albin et al., 1993). A metaanalysis study found that an isoleucine to valine substitution at codon 105, which may reduce the conjugating activity of the enzyme (Gudmundsdottir et al., 2001), has been associated with a moderately increased breast cancer risk in homozygous carriers.

Polymorphisms in the rate-limiting enzyme involved in alcohol oxidation, alcohol dehydrogenase (ADH), may modulate breast cancer risk, as alcohol is a well-documented risk factor. Premenopausal women with homozygous for ADH1C*1 allele have been found to be at a 1.8 times higher risk for breast cancer than women with the other two possible genotypes (Freudenheim et al., 1999).

Folate metabolism is directly related to methylation of genes, which can lead to silencing of genes or gene activation. Two polymorphisms in MTHFR gene, C677T and A1298C, which have decreased enzyme activity in carriers of these genetic variations, are associated with an increased risk of developing breast cancer (Campbell et al., 2002; Ergul et al., 2003).

DNA repair genes constitute another low-penetrance cancer susceptibility gene group. Polymorphisms in these genes leading to attenuated DNA repair capacities, especially after the exposure to endogenous and exogenous genotoxic agents, may contribute to breast cancer risk (Duell et al., 2001; Smith et al., 2003; Goode et al., 2002).

Breast cancer is a complex disease, and a variety of risk factors are involved in the etiology and development of breast cancer. Mutations in high-penetrance cancer susceptibility genes, such as BRCA1 and BRCA2, p53, PTEN, and ATM, are responsible for a high proportion of the hereditary breast cancers. Various polymorphisms in low-penetrance genes like CYP 1A1, CYP 2D6, CYP 19, GSTM1 and GSTP1, and MTHFR have been associated with either an increased or a decreased breast cancer risk.

Chemopreventive agents such as tamoxifen, aromatase inhibitors, or COX-2 inhibitors can be used in women at high risk of developing breast cancer to reduce their risk and have effects in combination with a healthy diet and energy balance that could favorably influence breast cancer risk. There is a clear need for further research on how nutrition affects the identification of phenotypic and genetic traits that account for the increase in breast cancer seen in the past century. An understanding of gene–nutrient interaction in breast cancer can help to enhance these efforts.

References

Albin, N., Massaad, L., Toussaint, C., Mathieu, M.C., Morizet, J., et al. 1993. Main drug-metabolizing enzyme systems in human breast tumors and peritumoral tissues. *Cancer Res* **53**: 3541–3546.

Arun, B., and Goss, P. 2004. The role of COX-2 inhibition in breast cancer treatment and prevention. *Semin Oncol* **31**: 22–29.

Aziz, H., Hussain, F., Sohn, C., Mediavillo, R., Saitta, A., Hussain, A., Brandys, M., Homel, P., and Rotman, M. 1999. Early onset of breast carcinoma in African American women with poor prognostic factors. *Am J Clin Oncol* **22**: 436–440.

Bartsch, H., Nair, J., and Owen, R.W. 1999. Dietary polyunsaturated fatty acids and cancers of the breast and colorectum: emerging evidence for their role as risk modifiers. *Carcinogenesis* **20**: 2209–2218.

Bartsch, H., Nair, U., Risch, A., Rojas, M., Wikman, H., and Alexandrov, K. 2000. Genetic polymorphism of CYP genes, alone or in combination, as a risk modifier of tobacco-related cancers, *Cancer Epidemiol Biomarkers Prev* **9**: 3–28.

Beral, V. 2002. Breast cancer and breastfeeding: collaborative reanalysis of individual data from 47 epidemiological studies in 30 countries, including 50302 women with breast cancer and 96973 women without the disease. *Lancet* **360**: 187–195.

Berkey, C.S., Frazier, A.L., Gardner, J.D., and Colditz, G.A. 1999. Adolescence and breast carcinoma risk. *Cancer* **85**: 2400–2409.

Bernstein, L. 2002. Epidemiology of endocrine-related risk factors for breast cancer. *J Mammary Gland Biol Neoplasia* **7**: 3–15.

Biglia, N., Defabiani, E., Ponzone, R., Mariani, L., Marenco, D., and Sismondi, P. 2004. Management of risk of breast carcinoma in postmenopausal women. *Endocr Relat Cancer* **11**: 69–83.

Boyd, N.F., Byng, J.W., Jong, R.A., Fishell, E.K., Little, L.E., Miller, A.B., Lockwood, G.A., Tritchler, D.L., and Yaffe, M.J. 1995. Quantitative classification of mammographic densities and breast cancer risk: results from the Canadian National Breast Screening Study. *J Natl Cancer Inst* **87**: 670–675.

Brinton, L.A., Schairer, C., Hoover, R.N., and Fraumeni, J.F., Jr. 1988. Menstrual factors and risk of breast cancer. *Cancer Invest* **6**: 245–254.

Brinton, L.A., Hoover, R., and Haile, R, 1995. Mammographic features and breast cancer risk: effects with time, age, and menopause status. *J Natl Cancer Inst* **87**: 1622–1629.

Buzzard, I.M., Faucett, C.L., Jeffery, R.W., McBane, L., McGovern, P., Baxter, J.S., Shapiro, A.C., Blackburn, G.L., Chlebowski, R.T., Elashoff, R.M., and Wynder, E.L. 1996. Monitoring dietary change in low-fat diet intervention study: advantages of using 24-hour recalls versus food records. *J Am Diet Assoc* **96**: 574–579.

Campbell, I.G., Baxter, S.W., Eccles, D.M., and Choong, D.Y. 2002. Methylenetetrahydrofolate reductase polymorphism and susceptibility to breast cancer. *Breast Cancer Res* **4**: R14.

Carroll, K.K., Gammal, E.B., and Plunkett, E.R. 1968. Dietary fat and mammary cancer. *Can Med Assoc J* **98**: 590–594.

Carroll, K.K. 1992. Dietary fat and breast cancer. *Lipids* **27**: 793–797.

Cauley, J.A., Gutai, J.P., Kuller, L.H., Scott, J., and Nevitt, M.C. 1994. Black–white differences in serum sex hormones and bone mineral density. *Am J Epidemiol* **139**: 1035–1046.

Chlebowski, R.T., Blackburn, G.L., Buzzard, I.M., Rose, D.P., Martino, S., Khandekar, J.D., York, R.M., Jeffery, R.W., Elashoff, R.M., and Wynder, E.L. 1993. Adherence to a dietary fat intake reduction program in postmenopausal women receiving therapy for early stage breast cancer. *J Clin Oncol* **11**: 2072–2080.

Chlebowski, R.T., Blackburn, G.L., Elashoff, R.M., et al. 2005. Dietary fat reduction in postmenopausal women with primary breast cancer: Phase III Women's Intervention Nutrition Study (WINS). *Proc Am Soc Clin Oncol* **24**: 10.

Clevenger, C.V., Furth, P.A., Hankinson, S.E., and Schuler, L.A. 2003. The role of prolactin in mammary carcinoma. *Endocr Rev* **24**: 1–27.

Colditz, G.A., and Hankinson, S.E. 2005. The Nurses' Health Study: lifestyle and health among women. *Nat Rev Cancer* **5**: 388–396.

Collaborative Group on Hormonal Factors in Breast Cancer. 1996. Breast cancer and hormonal contraceptives: further results. *Contraception* **54**: 1S–106S.

Collaborative Group on Hormonal Factors in Breast Cancer. 1997. Breast cancer and hormone replacement therapy: collaborative reanalysis of data from 51 epidemiological studies of 52,705 women with breast cancer and 108,411 women without breast cancer. *Lancet* **350**: 1047–1059.

Coutelle C., Hohn B., Benesova M., Oneta C.M., Quattrochi P., et al. 2004. Risk factors in alcohol associated breast cancer: alcohol dehydrogenase polymorphism and estrogens. *Int J Oncol* **25**: 1127–1132.

Cullen, K.J., Yee, D., Sly, W.S., Perdue, J., Hampton, B., Lippman, M.E., and Rosen, N. 1990. Insulin-like growth factor receptor expression and function in human breast cancer. *Cancer Res* **50**: 48–53.

de Jong, M.M., Nolte, I.M., te Meerman, G.J., van der Graaf, W.T., Oosterwijk, J.C., et al. 2002. Genes other than BRCA1 and BRCA2 involved in breast cancer susceptibility. *J Med Genet* **39**: 225–242.

Deng, C.X., and Brodie, S.G. 2000. Roles of BRCA1 and its interacting proteins. *Bioessays* **22**: 728–737.

Duell, E.J., Millikan, R.C., Pittman, G.S., Winkel, S., Lunn, R.M., et al. 2001. Polymorphisms in the DNA Repair Gene XRCC1 and Breast Cancer, *Cancer Epidemiol Biomarkers Prev* **10**: 217–222.

Duthie, S.J. 1999. Folic acid deficiency and cancer: mechanisms of DNA instability. *Br Med Bull* **55**: 578–592.

Easton, D., Ford, D., and Peto, J. 1993. Inherited susceptibility to breast cancer. *Cancer Surv* **18**: 95–113.

Easton, D.F. 1994. The inherited component of cancer. *Br Med Bull* **50**: 527–535.

Eat 5 to 9 A Day for Better Health. Available at: http://5aday.gov/homepage/index_content.html; accessed May 25, 2005.

Edwards, B.K., Howe, H.L., Ries, L.A., Thun, M.J., Rosenberg, H.M., Yancik, R., Wingo, P.A., Jemal, A., Ergul, E., Sazci, A., Utkan, Z., and Canturk, N.Z. 2003. Polymorphisms in the MTHFR gene are associated with breast cancer. *Tumour Biol* **24**: 286–290.

Feigal, E.G. 2002. Annual report to the nation on the status of cancer, 1973–1999, featuring implications of age and aging on U.S. cancer burden. *Cancer* **94**: 2766–2792.

Feigelson, H.S., and Henderson, B.E. 1996. Estrogens and breast cancer. *Carcinogenesis* **17**: 2279–2284.

Fisher, B., Costantino, J.P., Wickerham, D.L., Redmond, C.K., Kavanah, M., et al. 1998. Tamoxifen for prevention of breast cancer: report of the National Surgical Adjuvant Breast and Bowel Project P-1 Study. *J Natl Cancer Inst* **90**: 1371–1388.

Ford, E.S., Giles, W.H., and Dietz, W.H. 2002. Prevalence of the metabolic syndrome among US adults: findings from the Third National Health and Nutrition Examination Survey. *JAMA* **287**: 356–359.

Freudenheim, J., Ambrosone, C.B., Moysich, K.B., Vena, J.E., Graham, S., et al. 1999. Alcohol dehydrogenase 3 genotype modification of the association of alcohol consumption with breast cancer risk. *Cancer Causes Control* **10**: 369–377.

Friedenreich, C.M. 2001. Review of anthropometric factors and breast cancer risk. *Eur J Cancer Prev* **10**: 15–32.

Garber, J.E., Goldstein, A.M., Kantor, A.F., Dreyfus, M.G., Fraumeni, J.F., Jr., and Li, F.P. 1991. Follow-up study of twentyfour families with Li-Fraumeni syndrome. *Cancer Res* **51**: 6094–6097.

Ginsburg, E.S., Walsh, B.W., Gao, X., Gleason, R.E., Feltmate, C., and Barbieri, R.L. 1995. The effect of acute ethanol ingestion on estrogen levels in postmenopausal women using transdermal estradiol. *J Soc Gynecol Investig* **2**: 26–29.

Goode, E.L., Ulrich, C.M., and Potter, J.D. 2002. Polymorphisms in DNA Repair Genes and Associations with Cancer Risk. *Cancer Epidemiol Biomarkers Prev* **11**: 1513–1530.

Goodwin, P.J., and Boyd, N.F. 1990. Body size and breast cancer prognosis: a critical review of the evidence. *Breast Cancer Res Treat* **16**: 205–214.

Goodwin, P.J., Ennis, M., Pritchard, K.I., Trudeau, M.E., Koo, J., Madarnas, Y., Hartwick, W., Hoffman, B., and Hood, N. 2002. Fasting insulin and outcome in early-stage breast cancer: results of a prospective cohort study. *J Clin Oncol* **20**: 42–51.

Grabrick, D.M., Hartmann, L.C., Cerhan, J.R., Vierkant, R.A., Therneau, T.M., et al. 2000. Risk of breast cancer with oral contraceptive use in women with a family history of breast cancer. *JAMA* **284**: 1791–1798.

Gudmundsdottir, K., Tryggvadottir, L., and Eyfjord, J.E. 2001. GSTM1, GSTT1, and GSTP1 genotypes in relation to breast cancer risk and frequency of mutations in the p53 gene. *Cancer Epidemiol Biomarkers Prev* **10**: 1169–1173.

Hankinson, S.E., Willett, W.C., Michaud, D., Manson, J.E., Colditz, G.A., et al. 1999. Plasma prolactin levels and subsequent risk of breast cancer in postmenopausal women. *J Natl Cancer Inst* **91**: 629–634.

Hankinson, S.E., Colditz, G.A., and Willett, W.C. 2004. Towards an integrated model for breast cancer etiology: the lifelong interplay of genes, lifestyle, and hormones. *Breast Cancer Res* **6**: 213–218.

Harris, R., Namboodiri, K.K., and Wynder, E.L. 1992. Breast cancer risk: effects of estrogen replacement therapy and body mass. *J Natl Cancer Inst* **84**: 1575–1582.

Heck, K.E., Wagener, D.K., Schatzkin, A., Devesa, S.S., and Breen, N. 1997. Socioeconomic status and breast cancer mortality, 1989 through 1993: an analysis of education data from death certificates. *Am J Public Health* **87**: 1218–1222.

Heimdal, K., Skovlund, E., and Moller, P. 2002. Oral contraceptives and risk of familial breast cancer, *Cancer Detect Prev* **26**: 23–27.

Helewa, M., Levesque, P., Provencher, D., Lea, R.H., Rosolowich, V., and Shapiro, H.M. 2002. Breast cancer, pregnancy, and breastfeeding. *J Obstet Gynaecol Can* **24**: 164–180.

Hellmold, H., Rylander, T., Magnusson, M., Reihner, E., Warner, M., and Gustafsson, J.A. 1998. Characterization of cytochrome P450 enzymes in human breast tissue from reduction mammaplasties. *J Clin Endocrinol Metab* **83**: 886–895.

Henderson, M.M., Kushi, L.H., Thompson, D.J., Gorbach, S.L., Clifford, C.K., Insull, W., Jr., Moskowitz, M., and Thompson, R.S. 1990. Feasibility of a randomized trial of a low-fat diet for the prevention of breast cancer: dietary compliance in the Women's Health Trial Vanguard Study. *Prev Med* **19**: 115–133.

Huang, Z., Hankinson, S.E., Colditz, G.A., Stampfer, M.J., Hunter, D.J., et al. 1997. Dual effects of weight and weight gain on breast cancer risk. *JAMA* **278**: 1407–1411.

Johnson-Thompson, M.C., and Guthrie, J. 2000. Ongoing research to identify environmental risk factors in breast carcinoma *Cancer* **88**: 1224–1229.

Kaaks, R. 1996. Nutrition, hormones, and breast cancer: is insulin the missing link? *Cancer Causes Control* **7**: 605–625.

Kelsey, J.L., Gammon, M.D., and John, E.M. 1993. Reproductive factors and breast cancer. *Epidemiol Rev* **15**: 36–47.

King, M.-C., Marks, J.H., and Mandell, J.B., for the New York Breast Cancer Study Group. 2005. Breast and ovarian cancer risks due to inherited mutations in BRCA1 and BRCA2. *Science* **302**: 643–646.

Klurfeld, D.M., Welch, C.B., Davis, M.J., and Kritchevsky, D. 1989a. Determination of degree of energy restriction necessary to reduce DMBA-induced mammary tumorigenesis in rats during the promotion phase. *J Nutr* **119**: 286–291.

Klurfeld, D.M., Welch, C.B., Lloyd, L.M., and Kritchevsky, D. 1989b. Inhibition of DMBA-induced mammary tumorigenesis by caloric restriction in rats fed high-fat diets. *Int J Cancer* **15**: 922–925.

Klurfeld, D.M., Lloyd, L.M., Welch, C.B., Davis, M.J., Tulp, O.L., and Kritchevsky, D. 1991. Reduction of enhanced mammary carcinogenesis in LA/N-cp (corpulent) rats by energy restriction. *Proc Soc Exp Biol Med* **196**: 381–384.

Kolonel, L.N., Horn-Ross, P.L., and Rosenthal, J.F. 1993. Migration patterns and breast cancer risk in Asian-American women. *J Natl Cancer Inst* **85**: 1819–1827.

Kreiger, N., Sloan, M., Cotterchio, M., and Kirsh, V. 1999. The risk of breast cancer following reproductive surgery. *Eur J Cancer* **35**: 97–101.

Kumanyika, S.K. 1997. The impact of obesity on hypertension management in African Americans. *J Health Care Poor Underserved* **8**: 352–364.

Kushi, L.H., Sellers, T.A., Potter, J.D., Nelson, C.L., Munger, R.G., Kaye, S.A., and Folsom, A.R. 1992. Dietary fat and postmenopausal breast cancer. *J Natl Cancer Inst* **84**: 1092–1009.

Lagerros, Y.T., Hsieh, S.F., and Hsieh, C.C. 2004. Physical activity in adolescence and young adulthood and breast cancer risk: a quantitative review. *Eur J Cancer Prev* **13**: 5–12.

Lahmann, P.H., Hoffmann, K., Allen, N., van Gils, C.H., Khaw, K.T., Tehard, B., et al. 2004. Body size and breast cancer risk: findings from the European Prospective Investigation into Cancer And Nutrition (EPIC). *Int J Cancer* **111**: 762–771.

Lambe, M., Hsieh, C., Trichopoulos, D., Ekbom, A., Pavia, M., and Adami, H.O. 1994. Transient increase in the risk of breast cancer after giving birth. *N Engl J Med* **331**: 5–9.

Levy-Lahad, E., and Plon, S.E. 2003. A risky business—assessing breast cancer risk. *Science* **302**: 574–575.

Lipworth, L., Bailey, L.R., and Trichopoulos, D. 2000. History of breast-feeding in relation to breast cancer risk: a review of the epidemiologic literature. *J Natl Cancer Inst* **92**: 302–312.

Magnusson, C., Baron, J., Correia, N., Bergstrom, R., Adami, H.O., and Persson, I. 1999. Breast-cancer risk following long-term oestrogen- and oestrogen-progestin-replacement therapy. *Int J Cancer* **81**: 339–344.

Malkin, D. 1994. Germline p53 mutations and heritable cancer. *Ann Rev Genet* **28**: 443–465.

McPherson, K., Steel, C.M., and Dixon, J.M. 2000. ABC of breast diseases. Breast cancer—epidemiology, risk factors, and genetics. *BMJ* **321**: 624–628.

McTiernan, A., Rajan, K.B., Tworoger, S., Irwin, M., Bernstein, L., et al. 2003. Adiposity and Sex Hormones in Postmenopausal Breast Cancer Survivors. *J Clin Oncol* **21**: 1961–1966.

Michels, K.B., and Willett, W.C. 2004. Breast cancer—early life matters. *N Engl J Med* **14**: 1619–1626.

Milazzo, G., Giorgino, F., Damante, G., Sung, C., Stampfer, M.R., Vigneri, R., Goldfine, I.D., and Belfiore, A. 1992. Insulin receptor expression and function in human breast cancer cell lines. *Cancer Res* **52**: 3924–3930.

National Center for Health Statistics, Public Health Service. 1985. Health Promotion and Disease Prevention: United States, 1985. Vital and Health Statistics. US Government Printing Office, Hyattsville, MD.

Oesterreich, S., and Fuqua, S.A. 1999. Tumor suppressor genes in breast cancer. *Endocr Relat Cancer* **6**: 405–419.

Okobia, M.N., and Bunker, C.H. 2003. Molecular epidemiology of breast cancer: a review. *Afr J Reprod Health* **7**: 17–28.

Onland-Moret, N.C., Peeters, P.H., van der Schouw, Y.T., Grobbee, D.E., and van Gils, C.H. 2004. Alcohol and endogenous sex steroid levels in postmenopausal women: a cross-sectional study. *J Clin Endocrinol Metab* **90**: 1414–1419.

Papa, V., Pezzino, V., Constantino, A., Belfiore, A., Giuffrida, D., Frittitta, L., Vannelli, G.B., Brand, R., Goldfine, I.D., and Vigneri, R. 1990. Elevated insulin receptor content in human breast cancer. *J Clin Invest* **86**: 1503–1510.

Papa, V., Gliozzo, B., Clark, G.M., McGuire, W.L., Moore, D., Fujita-Yamaguchi, Y., Vigneri, R., Goldfine, I.D., and Pezzino, V. 1993. Insulin-like growth factor-I receptors are overexpressed and predict a low risk in human breast cancer. *Cancer Res* **53**: 3736–3740.

Papa, V., and Belfiore, A. 1996. Insulin receptors in breast cancer: biological and clinical role. *J Endocrinol Invest* **19**: 324–333.

Pathak, D.R., Osuch, J.R., and He, J. 2000. Breast carcinoma etiology: current knowledge and new insights into the effects of reproductive and hormonal risk factors in black and white populations. *Cancer* **88**: 1230–1238.

Pike, M.C., Spicer, D.V., Dahmoush, L., and Press, M.F. 1993. Estrogens, progestogens, normal breast cell proliferation, and breast cancer risk. *Epidemiol Rev* **15**: 17–35.

Poschl, G., and Seitz, H.K. 2004. Alcohol and cancer. *Alcohol* **39**: 155–165.

Rebbeck, T.R. 1999. Inherited genetic predisposition in breast cancer. A population-based perspective. *Cancer* **86**: 2493–2501.

Reichman, M.E., Judd, J.T., Longcope, C., Schatzkin, A., Clevidence, B.A., et al. 1993. Effects of alcohol consumption on plasma and urinary hormone concentrations in premenopausal women. *J Natl Cancer Inst* **85**: 722–727.

Remington, P.L. 2004. Socioeconomic risk factors for breast cancer: distinguishing individual- and community-level effects. *Epidemiology* **15**: 442–450.

Renehan, A.G., Zwahlen, M., Minder, C., O'Dwyer, S.T., Shalet, S.M., and Egger, M. 2004. Insulin-like growth factor (IGF)-I,IGF binding protein-3, and cancer risk: systematic review and meta-regression analysis. *Lancet* **363**: 1346–1353.

Robert, S.A., Strombom, I., Trentham-Dietz, A., Hampton, J.M., McElroy, J.A., Newcomb, P.A., and Remington, P.L. 2004. Socioeconomic risk factors for breast cancer: distinguishing individual- and community-level effects. *Epidemiology* **15**: 442–450.

Ross, R.K., Paganini-Hill, A., Wan, P.C., and Pike, M.C. 2000. Effect of hormone replacement therapy on breast cancer risk: estrogen versus estrogen plus progestin. *J Natl Cancer Inst* **92**: 328–332.

Rossouw, J.E., Anderson, G.L., Prentice, R.L., LaCroix, A.Z., et al. 2002. Risks and benefits of estrogen plus progestin in healthy postmenopausal women: principal results from the Women's Health Initiative randomized controlled trial. *JAMA* **288**: 321–333.

Rothman, N., Wacholder, S., Caporaso, N.E., Garcia-Closas, M., Buetow, K., and Fraumeni, J.F. 2001. The use of common genetic polymorphisms to enhance the epidemiologic study of environmental carcinogens. *Biochimica et Biophysica Acta (BBA) Reviews on Cancer* **1471**: C1–C10.

Russo, J., Hu, Y.F., Yang, X., and Russo, I.H. 2000. Developmental, cellular, and molecular basis of human breast cancer. *J Natl Cancer Inst Monogr* **27**: 17–37.

Russo, J., and Russo, I.H. 2001. The pathway of neoplastic transformation of human breast epithelial cells. *Radiat Res* **155**: 151–154.

Saadatian-Elahi, M., Norat, T., Goudable, J., and Riboli, E. 2004. Biomarkers of dietary fatty acid intake and the risk of breast cancer: a meta-analysis. *Int J Cancer* **111**: 584–591.

Sala, E., Warren, R., McCann, J., Duffy, S., Luben, R., and Day, N. 2000. High-risk mammographic parenchymal patterns, hormone replacement therapy and other risk factors: a case–control study. *Int J Epidemiol* **29**: 629–636.

Sales, D.S., Moreira, A.C., Camacho-Hubner, C., Ricco, R.G., Daneluzzi, J.C., Campos, A.D., and Martinelli, C.E., Jr. 2003. Serum insulin-like growth factor (IGF)-I and IGF-binding protein-3 in girls with premature thelarche. *J Pediatr Endocrinol Metab* **16**: 827–833.

Schairer, C., Lubin, J., Troisi, R., Sturgeon, S., Brinton, L., and Hoover, R. 2000. Menopausal estrogen and estrogen-progestin replacement therapy and breast cancer risk. *JAMA* **283**: 485–491.

Selim, A.A., El-Ayat, G., and Wells, C.A. 2001. Immunohistochemical localization of gross cystic disease fluid protein-15, -24 and -44 in ductal carcinoma in situ of the breast: relationship to the degree of differentiation. *Histopathology* **39**: 198–202.

Sellers, T.A., Vierkant, R.A., Cerhan, J.R., Gapstur, S.M., Vachon, C.M., et al. 2002. Interaction of dietary folate intake, alcohol, and risk of hormone receptor-defined breast cancer in a prospective study of postmenopausal women. *Cancer Epidemiol Biomarkers Prev* **11**: 1104–1107.

Singletary, K.W., and Gapstur, S.M. 2001. Alcohol and breast cancer: review of epidemiologic and experimental evidence and potential mechanisms *JAMA* **286**: 2143–2151.

Smith, T.R., Levine, E.A., Perrier, N.D., Miller, M.S., Freimanis, R.I., et al. 2003. *Cancer Epidemiol Biomarkers Prev* **12**: 1200–1204.

Smith-Warner, S.A., Spiegelman, D., Yaun, S.S., van den Brandt, P.A., Folsom, A.R., et al. 1998. Alcohol and breast cancer in women: a pooled analysis of cohort studies. *JAMA* **279**: 535–540.

Stewart, S.L., King, J.B., Thompson, T.D., Friedman, C., and Wingo, P.A. 2004. Cancer mortality surveillance—United States, 1990–2000, MMWR. *Surveill Summ* **53**: 1–108.

Stoll, B.A. 1999. Western nutrition and the insulin resistance syndrome: a link to breast cancer. *Eur J Clin Nutr* **53**: 83–87.

Strange, R.C., and Fryer, A.A. 1999. The glutathione S-transferases: influence of polymorphism on cancer susceptibility. *IARC Sci Publ* **148**: 231–249.

Sugimura, T. 2000. Nutrition and dietary carcinogens. *Carcinogenesis* **21**: 387–395.

Tice, J.A., Miike, R., Adduci, K., Petrakis, N.L., King, E., and Wrensch, M.R. 2005. Nipple aspirate fluid cytology and the Gail model for breast cancer risk assessment in a screening population. *Cancer Epidemiol Biomarkers Prev* **14**: 324–328.

Titus-Ernstoff, L., Longnecker, M.P., Newcomb, P.A., Dain, B., Greenberg, E.R., Mittendorf, R., Stampfer, M., and Willett, W. 1998. Menstrual factors in relation to breast cancer risk. *Cancer Epidemiol Biomarkers Prev* **7**: 783–789.

Trentham-Dietz, A., Newcomb, P.A., Egan, K.M., Titus-Ernstoff, L., Baron, J.A., et al. 2000. Weight change and risk of postmenopausal breast cancer (United States). *Cancer Causes Control* **11**: 533–542.

van den Brandt, P.A., Spiegelman, D., Yaun, S.S., Adami, H.O., Beeson, L., et al. 2000. Pooled Analysis of Prospective Cohort Studies on Height, Weight, and Breast Cancer Risk. *Am J Epidemiol* **152**: 514–527.

van Gils, C.H., Hendriks, J.H., Otten, J.D., Holland, R., and Verbeek, A.L. 2000. Parity and mammographic breast density in relation to breast cancer risk: indication of interaction. *Eur Cancer Prev* **9**: 105–111.

Velie, E., Kulldorff, M., Schairer, C., Block, G., Albanes, D., and Schatzkin, A. 2000. Dietary fat, fat subtypes, and breast cancer in postmenopausal women: a prospective cohort study. *J Natl Cancer Inst* **92**: 833–839.

World Cancer Research Fund & American Institute for Cancer Research. 1997. "Food, Nutrition, and the Prevention of Cancer: A Global Perspective." American Institute for Cancer Research, Washington, DC.

Yu, H., Shu, X.O., Li, B.D.L., Dai, Q., Gao, Y.T., Jin, F., and Zheng, W. 2003. Joint effect of insulin-like growth factors and sex steroids on breast cancer risk. *Cancer Epidemiol Biomarkers Prev* **12**: 1067–1073.

Zhang, S.M. 2004. Role of vitamins in the risk, prevention, and treatment of breast cancer. *Curr Opin Obstet Gynecol* **16**: 19–25.

Zhang, X., and Yee, D. 2002. Tyrosine kinase signalling in breast cancer: insulin-like growth factors and their receptors in breast cancer. *Breast Cancer Res Treat* **2**: 170–175.

Zheng, W., Gustafson, D.R., Sinha, R., Cerhan, J.R., Moore, D., et al. 1998. Well-done meat intake and the risk of breast cancer *J Natl Cancer Inst* **90**: 1724–1729.

Ziegler, R.G., Hoover, R.N., Pike, M.C., Hildesheim, A., Nomura, A.M., West, D.W., et al. 1993. Migration patterns and breast cancer risk in Asian-American Women. *J Natl Cancer Inst* **85**: 1819–1827.

CHAPTER

22

Skin Cancer

HOMER S. BLACK

INTRODUCTION

The skin represents one of the largest organ systems of the human body, constituting about one-twelfth of total body weight. Situated at the interface between the body and its environment, and acting as a barrier to the harmful effects of an expansive array of extrinsic agents, the skin consequently provides the foremost target for environmental insult (Thody and Friedmann, 1986). Consequently, skin cancer is the most frequently occurring malignant neoplasm in the United States, accounting for an estimated 900,000–1,200,000 new cases annually (Miller and Weinstock, 1994). Using age-adjusted incidence data based on the 2000 population standard of the United States, the American Cancer Society projected that more than a million new cases of skin cancer will have been diagnosed in 2004.

Major milestones in the study of cancer development have been achieved through investigations of the carcinogenic potential of various agents on skin (Berenblum, 1954, 1979; Boutwell, 1964) because this target tissue provides a model with obvious advantage for cancer studies.

Although Sir Percival Pott (1775) was the first to associate excessive exposure to an external agent (soot) and the unusually high skin cancer incidence of chimney sweeps, it was not until 1915 that Yamagiwa and Ichikawa (1918) first successfully produced cancer (skin) in experimental animals with coal tar—a study that helped launch the investigative era of carcinogenesis. Insight into the carcinogenic process was advanced with development of the two-stage theory, operationally defined as initiation and promotion (Berenblum, 1941; Rous and Kidd, 1941). Tumor initiation is generally regarded as a permanent alteration of the cell genotype that is brought about by a single or sequential exposure to a subthreshold dose of a carcinogenic agent, whereas promotion has been described as "the process whereby an initiated tissue or organ develops focal proliferations, one or more which may act as precursors for subsequent steps in the carcinogenic process" (Farber, 1982). This factitious segmentation of the carcinogenic continuum has been invaluable in allowing dissection and definition of the biochemical steps in the cancer process, and confirmation of the two-stage theory with the so-called "reverse" experiment of Berenblum and Haran (1955) demonstrated that initiation and promotion stages were actually descriptive of the process occurring in mouse skin. It was from these early studies that the concept of a multistage carcinogenic process developed.

Even though the perception prevails that interest in environmental agents as causal factors in human cancer represents a more recent shift in emphasis (Higginson and Muir, 1976; Weisburger et al., 1977), it should be clear from the foregoing that the study of cancer and the carcinogenic process has been driven by early recognition that environmental and occupational factors played a paramount role in the occurrence of cancer (Haagensen, 1931). Foremost among those factors are chemicals, viruses, radiation, and diet. Although there are >200 types of skin cancer, and much of our knowledge gleaned of the carcinogenic process has been obtained from studies with carcinogenic chemicals, exposure to ultraviolet (UV) radiation accounts for ~90% of nonmelanoma skin cancer incidence (Elmets and Mukhtar, 1996).

This chapter deals primarily with two of the major extrinsic factors that can influence the development of skin cancer, namely, UV radiation, the primary causal agent, and diet, a potential modifier. Also provided are: (1) a brief historical

Copyright © 2006, Elsevier Inc.
All rights of reproduction in any form reserved.

preface and an overview of the status of our current understanding of the relationship of how diet may influence skin cancer from both an experimental and clinical prospect; (2) suggestions for future research directions; and (3) general dietary guidelines, based on our current knowledge, proposed for the prevention and/or management of skin cancer. The chapter is not intended to be a complete bibliographic reference source of skin cancer.

Many major contributions have been made to our understanding of the carcinogenic process in skin, as already noted, through studies with an array of chemicals and even combined with some dietary factors. Only from an historical perspective are some of the early contributions recognized. But we focus on the carcinogenic agent, UV, with the knowledge that many of the chemical studies are irrelevant to most human skin cancers. For example, UV involves no activation or detoxification of the presumed carcinogenic species; no competitive chemical inhibition, no binding to target molecules, and no transport to respective target sites. Changing the chemical milieu through dietary modification could have an impact on any of these activities. Thus, it is fortuitous, in this respect, that the primary causal agent of skin cancer (UV) is a complete physical carcinogen, allowing examination of the underlying mechanisms of dietary modification of the skin cancer process.

THE NATURE OF ULTRAVIOLET RADIATION

Solar radiant energy includes a broad region of the electromagnetic spectrum containing UV, visible (light), and infrared radiation (International Agency for Research on Cancer [IARC], 1992). UV radiation is generally considered to include wavelengths between 10 and 400 nm, with the extreme UV extending from 10 to 100 nm; far UV from 100 to 180 nm; middle UV from 180 to 300 nm; and near UV from 300 to 400 nm. Those wavelengths reaching the earth's surface are usually limited to 290 nm and greater, as shorter wavelengths are absorbed by stratospheric ozone. The photobiological designations (UV radiation of biological importance) of the Commission Internationale de l'Eclairage (CIE, International Commission on Illumination, Vienna, Austria) are reflected in Figure 1, with the exceptions that 320 nm, rather than 315 nm, has been used to define the upper limit of UVB, and UVA has been further segmented into UVA1 and UVA2 based on the recommendations of a task force impanelled at the first conference on the biological effects of UVA (Harber, 1986). Thus, UVC is defined as 100–280 nm; UVB as 280–320 nm; and UVA as 320–400 nm.

Although electromagnetic radiation is propagated in the form of waves, radiation may alternatively be considered composed of a very large number of small packets of energy called *quanta* or *photons* (Tarrant, 1989). The energy content

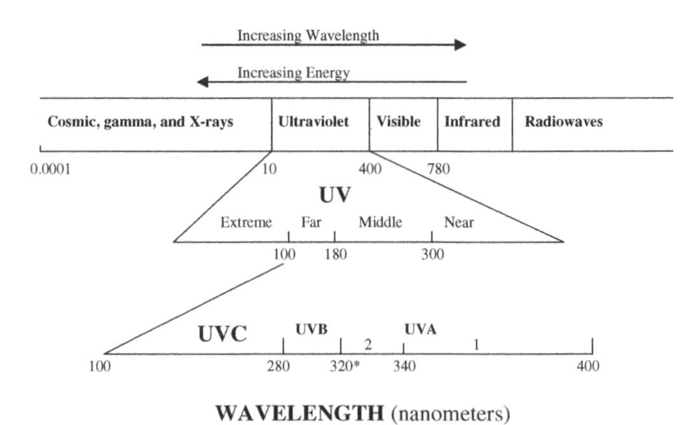

FIGURE 1 The electromagnetic spectrum with expanded scale of biologically relevant ultraviolet wavelengths.

of a photon is inversely proportional to the wavelength. Photons of the UVB band, at 280–320 nm, exhibit energies from 3.9 to 4.4 eV, whereas those of the longer UVA band range from 3.1 to 3.9 eV (Grossweiner, 1989). In general, photon energy, or wavelength, determines the nature of the photochemical/photobiological process initiated, whereas the "exposure dose" (the energy falling upon a unit surface area of an object and expressed as joules per square meter) limits the rate at which the process takes place. Implicit in this is the requirement that photons are absorbed by a suitable target molecule (chromophore) before the process or response can occur—known as the First Law of Photochemistry. Thus, a photobiological response, per unit exposure of UV radiation, varies with the wavelength of radiation and is dependent on the efficacy of interaction between target molecules and the incident photons. A quantitative plot of this spectral variation is known as an "action spectrum."

When radiation strikes the skin, part of it may be reflected, part may be absorbed in outer layers of the skin, and part may be transmitted inward to deeper layers where the energy of the photon is absorbed (Morison, 1991). Depth of penetration is wavelength dependent. Many chromophores, such as nucleic acids and proteins, absorb the shorter wavelengths, and scattering of shorter wavelengths is normally more pronounced. In a fair-skinned individual, only ~15% of the UVB radiation reaches the dermis, whereas ~50 % of the longer UVA wavelengths penetrate to the dermis.

The more energetic UVB band is also the most biologically active portion of the solar spectrum, ~1000 times more so than UVA with regard to erythema (sunburn). With regard to carcinogenesis, Forbes (1984) concluded that wavelengths >330 nm had an average relative efficiency for carcinogenesis in mice of <0.002, relative to 1.0 at 297 nm. Using a similar animal model, van Weelden et al. (1986)

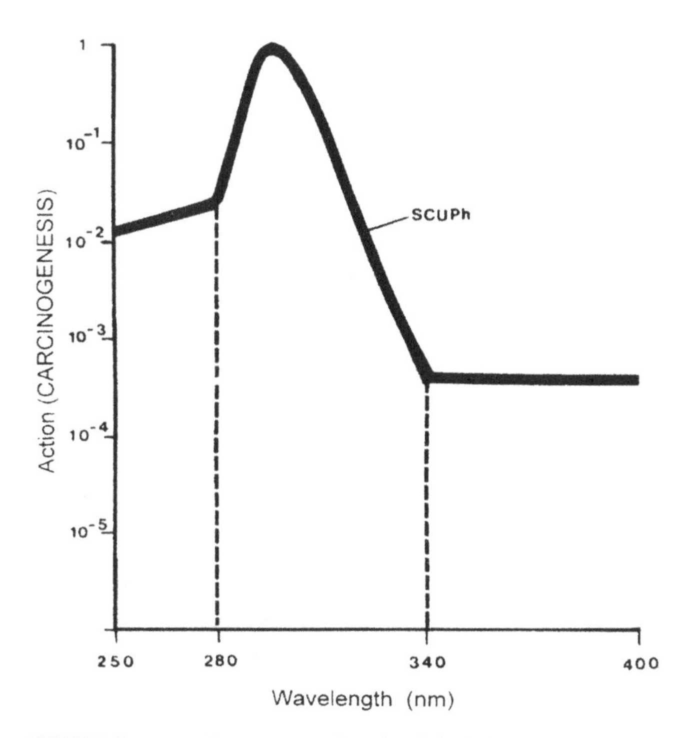

FIGURE 2 An action spectrum for ultraviolet-induced skin cancer in humans. This action spectrum, based on available data and with qualifying caveats in the CIE Technical Committee (TC-32) report "Action Spectrum for Photocarcinogenesis (Non-Melanoma Skin Cancers)," has been recommended as a CIE standard.

found that to produce tumors in 1% of the animals, 1000 times more UVA exposure was required compared with UVB. The greater efficacy of UVB in carcinogenesis is readily apparent in Figure 2, which represents an action spectrum for human nonmelanoma skin cancer. This action spectrum was derived from experiments with hairless mice and adjusted for humans by correcting for optical differences between murine and human epidermis (deGruijl et al., 1993; deGruijl and van der Leun, 1994). Nevertheless, there is ~20–30 times more UVA radiant energy in sunlight than UVB, and it is clear from the action spectrum that wavelengths >340 nm may contribute, in no small part, to the carcinogenic action of UV radiation. Thus, the risks from additional UVA exposure, such as from tanning parlors or excessively prolonged sun exposure of individuals protected with effective UVB sunscreens, cannot be ignored, although the latter concern may be unfounded (Urbach, 1992–1993).

THE ETIOLOGICAL ROLE OF UV RADIATION IN SKIN CANCER

More than 100 years after Potter (1962) had associated excessive exposure to soot with skin cancer occurrence, Unna (1894) associated the severe degenerative changes of the sun-exposed areas of the skin of sailors with the development of skin cancer, "Carcinome der Seemannshaut" (Urbach, 1997). Shortly thereafter, Dubreuilh (1896) confirmed the association of "la lumiere solaire" (sunlight) exposure with keratoses and skin cancer exhibited by vineyard workers in southern France. The predisposition to skin cancer of light-skinned individuals, especially of Celtic origin, and living in geographical areas of high insolation, was also observed by Shield (1899).

Experimental proof of the causal role of UV irradiation in skin cancer was provided by Findlay (1928) when he demonstrated that UV radiation delivered daily from a quartz mercury-vapor lamp produced skin cancers in mice. Roffo (1939) demonstrated that skin cancer in rats could be induced by radiation from both a mercury arc lamp and natural sunlight. In addition, he showed that the principal offending UV wavelengths were excluded by clear window glass, thus setting an approximate limit of effectiveness in producing skin cancer to those wavelengths of ≤320 nm.

Between 1941 and 1975, Blum and his collaborators (1941, 1975; Blum, 1959) conducted important and extensive quantitative studies on the carcinogenic effects of UV radiation. They concluded that (1) repeated, but not single, doses of UV are required to produce tumors within the lifetime of an animal, and (2) tumor growth is accelerated by successive doses of UV radiation. Development time, a measure of tumor induction, was defined as the time from the application of the first dose of UV to the appearance of a tumor of defined volume. They also found that (3) differences in dose, intensity, or interval between doses did not alter the shape or the slope of the dose–time response but only moved the relative position of the response curve along the dose axis, and (4) reciprocity of the carcinogenic response held until doses of UV became too small to result in tumors during the lifetime of the animal. Other aspects of Blum's experimental model of UV carcinogenesis have been summarized (Blum, 1948; Urbach et al., 1976; Black and Chan, 1977).

Roffo (1939) was the first to conduct an epidemiological study of skin cancer in humans, a study in which skin cancer occurrence was analyzed with respect to anatomical site, gender, nationality, and occupation. Whereas the question of an etiological role of sunlight in human skin cancer does not lend itself to direct experimentation, it is nevertheless firmly based on extensive observation and supported with animal experimentation. The evidence has been summarized as follows (Urbach, 1969; Emmett, 1973; Urbach et al., 1974):

- Skin cancers occur most frequently on the head, neck, arms, and hand—those parts of the body habitually exposed to sunlight.
- Members of pigmented races who sunburn less readily than light-skinned individuals have much less skin cancer.

When skin cancer does occur in pigmented races, it affects those areas exposed most frequently to sunlight (Mulay, 1963; Quisenberry, 1963; Segi, 1963).

- There appears to be much greater incidence of skin cancer among those Caucasians who spend more time outdoors than those who work predominantly indoors (Gellin et al., 1966).
- Skin cancer is more common in light-skinned people living in areas of greatest insolation (Silverstone and Searle, 1970; Mason et al., 1975).
- An exceptionally high risk of skin cancer exists among those individuals with genetic diseases characterized by intolerance to sunlight (Cleaver, 1968).
- Skin cancer is readily produced in mice and rats upon repeated exposure to UV radiation (Roffo, 1939, Blum et al., 1941; Winkelmann et al., 1963).

EXPERIMENTAL DATA ON NUTRITIONAL EFFECTS

Background to Nutritional Aspects of Experimental Cancer

The fact that diet, and particularly food quantity, could influence cancer was recognized by early physicians who advocated "fames cura," or a starvation diet, as treatment for cancer. It was surmised that this disease, as others to which humans were subjected, proceeded from the food they ate (Garrison, 1929). Thus, many of the earlier experimental studies examined the growth-inhibiting effect of undernourishment observed on both development of neoplasms and the effects on growth of existing tumors (Stern and Willheim, 1943). This growth-inhibiting effect was widely observed for numerous animal tumor transplants. For example, Bischoff et al. (1935) found that marked caloric restriction (50 %), a caloric intake adequate for maintenance of the animals' general health, resulted in a 10-fold retardation in tumor growth of transplanted mouse sarcoma 180, whereas a 20% reduction resulted in no significant effect. In a carefully controlled experiment employing semipurified diets, Visscher et al. (1942) found the incidence of spontaneous mammary carcinoma dropped from 67% in control animals fed *ad libitum* to zero in animals fed a diet adequate in protein, vitamins, and minerals but in which carbohydrates and fats were each reduced to approximately one third of the total calories ingested. Two important observations were noted around this period. First, animals on a restricted caloric diet exhibited greater longevity (Tannenbaum, 1940b), and second, short-term starvation was much less effective in restricting tumor growth than chronic undernourishment—a result that paralleled the clinical experience and undoubtedly tended to relegate dietary treatment of cancer as ineffective. Thus, the practical significance of caloric restriction appeared to lie in prevention or at least a delay in time of appearance of neoplasms.

Tannenbaum (1942a) demonstrated that underfeeding, again a 33–50% caloric restriction, resulted in both a marked delay in appearance of 3,4-benzpyrene–induced skin cancers and a decrease in total number of cancers. He also observed that caloric restriction exerted its main effect on the developmental (postinitiation) stage of carcinogenesis (Tannenbaum, 1944a). This influence of caloric restriction on induced primary tumor formation set the stage for a more analytical approach to the evaluation of the role of dietary factors in carcinogenesis. There seems little doubt that caloric restriction could play an important role in prevention of a wide range of human cancers (Albanes, 1987; Hocman, 1988; Weindruch et al., 1991).

Early studies to determine the influence of dietary fat on cancer also began with observations on the development of transplanted tumors (Sugiura and Benedict, 1930). Mixed results were obtained, as exemplified by the finding that with Flexnor-Jobling rat carcinoma, the percentage of positive tumor inoculations (takes) and tumor growth rates were diminished, whereas the number of tumor regressions increased when the host animals were fed high-fat (butter fat) diets. However, the indictment of lipid as a dietary constituent that potentiated carcinogenesis resulted from the studies of Watson and Mellanby (1930) in which dietary fat (12.5–25.0% butterfat) was shown to enhance coal tar–induced skin tumors in mice. This observation was followed with intense investigation of the effect of dietary fat on carcinogenesis in the 1940s and 1950s (Tannenbaum, 1953, 1959). Lavik and Baumann (1941) made several intriguing observations that provided early insight into the nature of the fat effect. First, the presence of lipid peroxides did not alter tumor-promoting power of fat. Both oxygenated and UV-irradiated samples, although exhibiting a high peroxide number, were relatively inactive in their influence on carcinogenesis. In their studies, heated (300°C for 1 hour) fat samples exhibiting lower peroxide numbers were most effective in promoting carcinogenesis. In this regard, it is interesting to note that Haven (1936) found the growth rate of rat carcinoma 256 was lower in animals receiving a diet containing cod liver oil (Iodine number 145–180) than in those fed coconut oil (Iodine number 8–9.5). This was determined to be related to the presence of longer chain fatty acids in cod liver oil, no doubt the long-chain n-3 fatty acids that are now known to exhibit anticarcinogenic effects. The second noteworthy observation in their studies was that mice seldom survived diets with ≥25% fat. A fat level of 15% (lard, butter, or vegetable oils) was adequate to demonstrate an effect on tumor formation, and 10% gave a measurable response. Finally, they observed that the most effective period for enhancing skin carcinogenesis by feeding high fat was 1.5–3.0 months after the beginning of application of methyl chloranthane (MCA). These observations suggest that the degree of saturation of the dietary lipid was less important than the level and/or fatty acid composition of the dietary lipid source; that the percentage change in level of fat required to elicit a response was considerably less than the percentage of caloric restriction required to produce a similar response; and that the fat effect occurred in the postinitiation or promotion stage of carcinogenesis. Indeed, Tannenbaum (1944b) clearly demonstrated that the dietary fat effect occurred during the postinitiation stage of chemical-induced carcinogenesis. Contemporary studies of that time (Tannenbaum, 1942b; Lavik and Baumann, 1943; Rusch et al., 1945) suggested that although most of the accelerating action of fat on tumor formation could be explained on the basis of an increased calorie intake, fat, per se, increased the rate of tumor formation, particularly when the total intake of calories was restricted. Despite the many methodological problems suffered by the early experimental studies, they clearly pointed to caloric restriction and dietary fat reduction as two important dietary avenues to prevent or moderate the course of cancer for several organ sites and established fertile lines for future investigation. It is interesting to note that nearly 65 years after Tannenbaum (1940a) observed that "persons of average weight or less are not so likely to develop the disease [cancer] as those who are overweight," Calle et al. (2003), in a large prospective study, found that "increased body weight was associated with increased death rates for all cancers combined and for cancers at multiple sites." Tannenbaum had suggested "that a caloric restricted and low-fat diet may aid in the prevention of human cancer, or at least delay its onset."

UV-INDUCED SKIN CANCER AND DIETARY MODIFICATION

Roffo (1929), who had provided early evidence for the role of UV irradiation in the etiology of skin cancer, had also recognized the importance of lipids in cancer development. He had hypothesized that cholesterol was an "heliotropic" substance that migrated and accumulated at anatomical sites routinely exposed to UV rays of the sun. Subsequent degradation of cholesterol resulted in substances with carcinogenic activity (Roffo, 1933). This presented an attractive theory because cholesterol is naturally occurring and widely distributed in biological tissues and, thus, could provide a basis for the biogenic origin of cancer. Indeed, a flurry of investigative activity continued through the 1950s in search of carcinogenic cholesterol derivatives and/or evidence of cholesterol involvement in cancer development (Fieser, 1954). It was just such an investigation that resulted in the observation that dietary fat had an influence on UV carcinogenesis (Baumann and Rusch, 1939). These investigators, in an effort to examine the purported role of cholesterol in the carcinogenic process, used a fat-enhanced (5% hydrogenated cottonseed oil) ration to ensure sterol absorption. In addition, a second group of animals were fed a high-fat ration containing 30% cottonseed oil. Tumor latency of animals receiving cholesterol-supplemented diets was found to be no different from that of animals receiving a stock ration, whereas latency was shortened by about 4 weeks for animals receiving the high-fat diet. Thus, although failing to find supporting evidence for the role of cholesterol in UV-induced skin cancer, and despite that their experimental design failed to control the usual nutritional variables, as did many of the early investigations, they were the first to demonstrate the potential influence of dietary lipid on UV-induced skin cancer.

Pursuant to the potential involvement of cholesterol in UV-induced carcinogenesis, a putative carcinogen, 5α,6α-cholesterol epoxide, was identified in UV-irradiated skin from among several photooxidation products of the parent sterol (Black and Lo, 1971). Using the hairless mouse model (Black, 1983), cholesterol epoxide formation was shown to be UV dose dependent, and levels of this compound increased eightfold in chronically irradiated animals (Black and Douglas, 1972, 1973). This increase preceded the appearance of squamous cell carcinomas. Although suggestive, no definitive evidence for the causal involvement of this compound in UV carcinogenesis was forthcoming. In addition, cholesterol feeding studies did not indicate a role for this sterol in UV carcinogenesis, although a slight but statistically significant protective effect was observed (Black et al., 1979).

As the formation of cholesterol epoxide was the result of photooxidative reactions, it seemed reasonable that these reactions might be inhibited by antioxidants. This concept was explored by feeding mice a closed formula ration containing a 2% (w/w) antioxidant mixture composed of 1.2% ascorbic acid, 0.5% butylated hydroxytoluene (BHT), 0.2% DL-α-tocopherol (acetate), and 0.1% reduced glutathione. At various intervals, cutaneous antioxidant levels were determined. When skin at the various feeding intervals was irradiated with UV and cholesterol epoxide levels measured, an inverse relationship with antioxidant content was observed (Lo and Black, 1973). Thus, antioxidants, known to impede lipid peroxidation, were shown to inhibit the photochemical conversion of skin cholesterol to its epoxide and provided evidence for peroxidative involvement in carcinogenesis. These findings suggested possible prophylactic effects of systemic antioxidants not only on the formation of this putative carcinogen but also on the subsequent pathological conditions that might result from, or concurrently with, its formation (Black, 1987). Indeed, when fed the same antioxidant mixture and chronically irradiated, animals demonstrated significantly fewer actinic lesions and tumors than control animals (Black, 1974; Black and Chan, 1975). Pauling et al. (1982) corroborated the observations concerning the inhibitory effect of the antioxidant mixture on

UV carcinogenesis. Subsequent studies demonstrated that BHT, at concentrations in the antioxidant mixture, was the most active principal (Black et al., 1978), although a second study from Pauling's group (Dunham et al., 1982) found that higher levels of ascorbic acid, alone, could significantly inhibit UV carcinogenesis.

Other antioxidants and singlet oxygen quenchers have been shown to provide significant protection against UV carcinogenesis. β-Carotene, a carotenoid that is widely distributed in nature, was shown to provide significant protection (Epstein, 1977; Mathews-Roth, 1982; Mathews-Roth and Krinsky, 1985). The protective effect was thought to be related to quenching of specific reactive oxygen species. β-Carotene also acts as an antioxidant (Krinsky, 1987). However, under certain conditions β-carotene may exhibit autocatalytic, prooxidant effects (Burton and Ingold, 1984). Indeed, β-carotene supplementation has been shown to *exacerbate* UV carcinogenic expression, causing an increase in tumor multiplicity and a shortened tumor latent period (Black, 1998). The exacerbative response was found to be dependent on the type of dietary ration administered (i.e., closed-formula vs semidefined rations) (Black et al., 2000). On the basis of the redox potential of interacting antioxidants, a mechanism was proposed by which β-carotene participated with vitamins E and C to repair oxyradicals (Edge et al., 1998; Edge and Truscott, 2000). The β-carotene radical cation, itself a strong oxidizing agent, was an intermediate in the redox schema and, if left unrepaired, could be responsible for the exacerbative effect of β-carotene. According to the schema, repair of the carotenoid radical cation was dependent on vitamin C. However, in subsequent studies in which experimental animals were fed β-carotene–supplemented semidefined diets with varying levels of vitamin C, no effect on UV carcinogenic expression was observed (Black and Gerguis, 2003). It is suspected that the noninjurious or protective effect of β-carotene found in the previous studies employing closed-formula rations might be dependent on interaction with other dietary factors that are absent in the semidefined diet. At present, β-carotene use as a dietary supplement for photoprotection should be approached cautiously (Black, 2004). Nevertheless, strong indirect evidence for reactive oxygen species and radical involvement comes from studies in which UV carcinogenesis has been inhibited by a wide range of natural and synthetic agents exhibiting antioxidant properties (Black, 1974; Epstein, 1977; Dunham et al., 1982; Bissett et al., 1991; Wang et al., 1991; Burke et al., 1992; Gerrish and Gensler, 1993).

As a corollary to antioxidant-inhibited UV carcinogenesis, any condition that limits the level of radical susceptible targets should, likewise, modulate the UV carcinogenic process. Unsaturated fatty acids are a prime center for free radical attack and, therefore, prime candidates for manipulation of radical susceptible targets. Thus, it was nearly 45 years after Baumann and Rusch (1939) first reported that dietary lipid could influence UV carcinogenesis that this seminal observation was to again receive attention, albeit from a somewhat different perspective (Black et al., 1983).

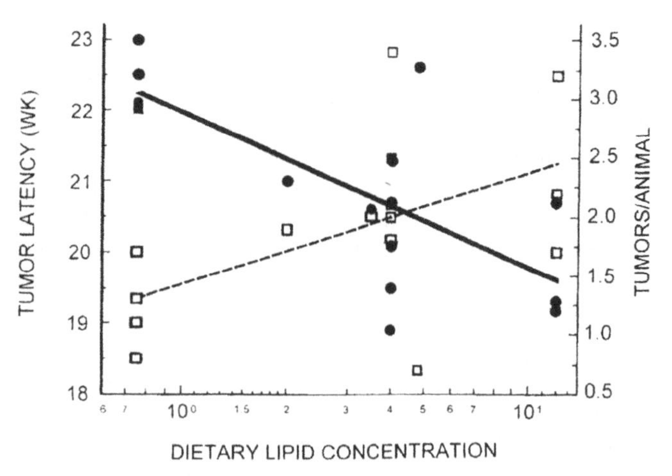

FIGURE 3 Relationship of ultraviolet (UV)–carcinogenic parameters, tumor latency, and tumor multiplicity to lipid level intake (corn oil). Regression lines are derived from 15 observations from six experiments evaluated in an incomplete block design. Solid line and circles indicate the tumor latency period; dashed line and open squares indicate tumor multiplicity. Tumor latency period decreases and tumor multiplicity increases as the level of corn oil intake increases. (Reprinted with permission from Black, 1993.)

Indeed, an approximate linear relationship between polyunsaturated lipid (corn or soybean oil) intake and UV carcinogenic expression was observed (Black et al., 1985), with the lowest lipid level resulting in a significantly longer tumor latent period. In addition, with increased lipid intake, the number of tumors per animal (tumor multiplicity) increased. The relationship between level of dietary lipid intake and carcinogenic parameters is reflected in Figure 3 (Black, 1993). Interestingly, dietary antioxidants produced an inhibitory effect almost equal to the degree of exacerbation of UV carcinogenesis evoked by increasing dietary lipid levels.

Reeve et al. (1988) found that feeding a diet supplying totally saturated sunflower oil (catalytically hydrogenated) completely abolished the UV carcinogenic response, whereas those animals fed polyunsaturated sunflower oil exhibited 100% tumor incidence. When the diet of the animals receiving hydrogenated fat was reconstituted to a normal mixed fat diet, large numbers of skin tumors rapidly appeared, suggesting that tumor initiation had not been prevented by lack of polyunsaturated fat but that an essential fatty acid deficiency held the tumors in abeyance, that is, at the promotion stage. It was subsequently shown that the principal effect of high dietary fat (corn oil) occurs at the promotion stage of UV carcinogenesis and that by replacing a high-fat diet with one of low fat immediately after UV initiation, the exacerbating effect of high fat could be negated (Black et al., 1992). Further support for a polyunsaturated fat requirement for UV carcinogenic expression was obtained when animals were fed constant levels of fat with graded proportions of polyunsaturated sunflower oil mixed with hydrogenated cottonseed oil (Reeve et al., 1996). The UV carcinogenic response was of increasing severity as the polyunsaturated content of the mixed dietary fat was increased.

That degree of dietary fatty acid saturation was an important determinant of carcinogenesis was suggested at an earlier period in nutritional carcinogenesis studies when Miller et al. (1944) found that diets composed almost entirely of saturated fatty acids would retard chemically induced hepatomas in rats. Similarly, Carroll and Kohr (1971) and Carroll and Hopkins (1979) found that rats fed unsaturated lipids developed more mammary tumors than those fed the same levels of saturated lipid. The polyunsaturated fatty acid, linoleic acid, appears to be a requirement for mammary carcinogenesis (Ip et al., 1985). In an earlier study of UV carcinogenesis, partially hydrogenated (60%) corn oil was found to inhibit UV carcinogenesis compared with animals fed 4% or 12% corn oil diets (Black et al., 1983). On careful inspection, those data suggest that a more complex relationship exists between degree of lipid saturation and UV carcinogenesis. The 60% hydrogenated corn oil would have had approximately the same level of linoleic acid (18:2), the principal polyunsaturated fatty acid in corn oil, as that of the 4% corn oil diet, yet, by comparison, significantly inhibited UV carcinogenesis. Potential products of catalytic hydrogenation, such as *trans* fatty acids or conjugated linoleic acid, have not been examined for effect in UV carcinogenesis. Moreover, when animals were fed a diet employing menhaden oil as lipid source, a polyunsaturated lipid rich in eicosapentaenoic and other n-3 fatty acids, UV carcinogenic expression was not enhanced but markedly inhibited (Orengo et al., 1989). These observations would suggest that degree of dietary fatty acid saturation alone is not a determinant in modulation of UV carcinogenic expression.

POSSIBLE MODE OF ACTION OF DIETARY FATTY ACIDS IN MODULATION OF UV CARCINOGENESIS

From the foregoing, it should be apparent that both essential n-6 (particularly linoleic acid) and n-3 fatty acids are important modulators of the carcinogenic process. Both types of fatty acids are important determinants of prostanoid metabolism as well. Prostaglandins (PG), particularly of the 2-series, are recognized as important participants in the inflammatory response to UV, and indeed, it has been demonstrated that omega-3 fatty acid supplementation in humans not only results in a small but significant rise in the sunburn threshold (the inflammatory response to UV irradiation) (Orengo et al., 1992; Rhodes et al., 1994, 2000) but also reduces the basal and UVB-induced PGE_2 levels in skin (Rhodes et al., 1995). Prostaglandins also act as physiological immunoregulators (Plescia and Racis, 1988). With respect to the latter, some studies suggest that the promotion stage of carcinogenesis, the point at which certain dietary lipids exert maximal influence, may be modulated immunologically (Vitale and Broitman, 1981). Indeed, it has been shown that suppressor T-cell function is PGE_2 dependent (Chung et al., 1986). These investigators have demonstrated that UV-induced immunosuppression is abrogated by treatment with an inhibitor (indomethacin) of PG synthesis. Indomethacin treatment has also been reported to convey a protective effect to UV carcinogenesis (Reeve et al., 1995). In addition, celecoxib, a rather specific inhibitor of cyclooxygenase-2, one of the isozymes involved in PG synthesis, has been shown to be an effective inhibitor of UV carcinogenesis (Fischer et al, 1999; Pentland et al., 1999; Orengo et al., 2002).

UV not only is immunosuppressive but also is known to activate epidermal enzymes responsible for facilitating PG synthesis from arachidonic acid (AA) through the cyclooxygenase pathway. Omega-3 fatty acids compete for reactive sites on the cyclooxygenase enzyme and may shunt PG precursors through the lipoxygenase path, in effect reducing proinflammatory PG levels. PG synthesis may also be suppressed by reducing the level of hydroperoxide activator, possibly achieved by free radical scavengers or antioxidants that impede lipid peroxidation (Lands et al., 1982). Thus, n-3 fatty acids not only act competitively with cyclooxygenase substrates to reduce PG levels, but n-3 fatty acids exhibit a high requirement for hydroperoxide activator, an *in vivo* level that may normally be insufficient to promote rapid PG synthesis. Indeed, Henderson et al. (1989) have shown that diets containing menhaden oil dramatically suppress plasma and cutaneous PGE_2 levels. Furthermore, plasma PGE_2 levels exhibit a near linear relationship to the log of corn oil intake, with lower levels of plasma PGE_2 present in animals receiving low-fat diets (Fischer and Black, 1991). Epidermal capacity to metabolize AA via the cyclooxygenase pathway is also potentiated by n-6 dietary fatty acid intake and is drastically inhibited in animals receiving dietary n-3 fatty acids.

It has been shown that dietary fat can suppress the T-cell–mediated immune status in UV-irradiated mice, both with respect to contact hypersensitivity (CH) and delayed-type hypersensitivity (DTH) (Black et al., 1995a; Reeve et al., 1996). Two questions arise with respect to the relevance of these findings to carcinogenesis. First, is the timing of these influences on specific immune responses compatible with the time (i.e., postinitiation) at which high levels of dietary fat (n-6 fatty acids) are known to exacerbate UV carcinogenesis? Second, does dietary fat affect these specific immune responses via T-cell–mediated immunological pathways common with those related to carcinogenesis? Some evidence suggests that they do not, at least for DTH. High dietary fat intake results in DTH suppression, even before UV exposure (Black et al., 1995a). UV irradiation hastens the complete suppression of this response in animals receiving high-fat diets. However, the DTH response rebounds by the time tumors appear in chronically irradiated animals. Thus, the temporal profile of DTH response does not conform to the time at which dietary fat exerts its principal influence on UV carcinogenesis. In contrast, when tumor transplantation studies were undertaken, with animals receiving various periods of UV radiation, tumor rejection was significantly greater in animals fed low-fat diets—but only at a time when the complete tumor-initiating UV dose had been delivered. This, of course, is the time (post-initiation) when dietary fat does exert its influence on carcinogenesis.

In conclusion, it is clear that high levels of dietary fat exert profound influence (suppression) over specific immune responses, some of which occur when high dietary fat exacerbates UV carcinogenic expression. High dietary fat has been shown to elevate PGE_2 levels, the latter known to act as an immunoregulator of T-cell function and to modulate UV carcinogenesis. These observations make a strong circumstantial case that high dietary fat, especially those rich in essential fatty acids, potentiates UV carcinogenesis via regulation of prostanoid metabolism in a manner that consequently suppresses immune responses that control the outgrowth of UV-induced tumors.

CLINICAL STUDIES OF NUTRITIONAL EFFECTS

Nonmelanoma Skin Cancer

The magnitude of the skin cancer problem is readily apparent when comparing its occurrence with that of other forms of cancer. As noted earlier, Miller and Weinstock (1994) estimated that the most common nonmelanoma skin cancers—basal and squamous cell carcinomas—account for 900,000–1,200,000 new cases annually in the United States. An estimate of new cases in the United States of all forms of cancer (exclusive of nonmelanoma skin cancer, which is usually not recorded in population-based registries) for 1997 is 1,400,000 (Parker et al., 1997). Thus, the incidence of nonmelanoma skin cancer is approximately equal to the combined incidence of all other cancers. Alarmingly, population-based studies indicate that there has been a steady increase in incidence of nonmelanoma skin cancer over the past 2 decades (Glass and Hoover, 1989; Weinstock, 1989; Gallagher et al., 1990). This increase occurs in regions of both high and low insolation for both basal and squamous cell carcinomas and appears to affect all age-groups.

Epidemiological studies indicate that at least 90% of basal and squamous cell carcinomas can be attributed to UV exposure (Mason et al., 1975; Committee on Chemistry and Physics of Ozone Depletion, 1982; Scotto et al., 1983). Koh et al. (1995) have updated and summarized the evidence linking solar exposure to nonmelanoma skin cancer. It is estimated that >50% of the total lifetime dose of solar UV is received in childhood and adolescence (Marks et al., 1990). In accord with this, it has also been estimated that the regular use of an SPF-15 sunscreen during the first 18 years of life would reduce the lifetime incidence of basal and squamous cell carcinomas by 78% (Stem et al., 1986). About 95% of basal cell carcinomas in men occur after the age of 40 years, whereas squamous cell carcinoma primarily (75–80%) affects men older than 60 years (Scotto et al., 1983). These studies point to the relatively long latent period between time of exposure to solar UV adequate to induce nonmelanoma skin cancer and its actual appearance. Further, when prevention measures are ineffective or fail, it points to a need to develop intervention strategies, a potential role to be filled by dietary modification.

Role of Diet in Nonmelanoma Skin Cancer: Epidemiological and Clinical Studies

Analytical epidemiological studies have provided the principal evidence associating dietary factors with cancer (Armstrong and Doll, 1975). These associations, even when supported by experimental animal studies or clinical observations, have not always proved to be clinically pertinent (Rackett et al., 1993), as noted from the examples in the following subsections.

β-Carotene

On the basis of existing epidemiological data, it was suggested that individuals with an above average intake of β-carotene might experience a lower incidence of cancer (Peto et al., 1981). A case-control study found that the incidence of skin cancer was inversely related to the level of serum β-carotene (Kune et al., 1992). In addition, as previously noted, β-carotene had been shown to inhibit UV-induced skin cancer incidence in experimental animals (Mathews-Roth, 1982). Thus, β-carotene was examined as a skin cancer preventative agent in a controlled clinical trial. A total of 1805 patients who were diagnosed with a recent nonmelanoma skin cancer were given either 50 mg of oral β-carotene daily or placebo (Greenberg et al., 1990). Adherence to the prescribed treatment was good, determined by annual plasma β-carotene levels. In fact, β-carotene supplementation resulted in about a 10-fold increase of the plasma carotenoid level. However, after 5 years, there was no significant difference between treatment and control groups in any of the predefined primary endpoints (i.e., the mean number of new nonmelanoma skin cancers per patient or with time delay before new tumor occurrence). Under the conditions of the clinical trial, the investigators concluded that β-carotene supplementation was inefficacious with respect to reducing the occurrence of nonmelanoma skin cancer. Subsequent evaluations from nested case-control studies indicated that β-carotene supplementation had no effect in any of the controlled patient subgroups, that is, numbers of previous skin cancers, age, gender, smoking, skin type, or baseline β-carotene levels (Greenberg et al., 1996; Karagas et al., 1997). A clinical study has confirmed that β-carotene supplementation has no effect on risk of monmelanoma skin cancer among men with low baseline plasma β-carotene (Schaumberg et al., 2004). Interestingly, it was found, in the Greenberg and Karagas studies, that those persons in the study who were in the highest quartile of the initial plasma β-carotene level had a lower risk of death from all causes, although β-carotene supplementation did not affect mortality.

A second randomized trial, the Nambour Skin Cancer Prevention Trial, examined the influence of daily (30 mg/day) β-carotene supplementation, over a 4-year period, on the incidence of basal and squamous cell carcinomas (Green et al., 1999). A small (1508 vs 1146 per 100,000) but statistically insignificant increase in the incidence of squamous cell carcinoma was indicated with β-carotene supplementation when compared with placebo. The investigators concluded that there was no beneficial or harmful effect on skin cancer rates as a result of β-carotene supplementation.

More disturbing than finding no beneficial effect of β-carotene supplementation on cancer occurrence, and despite overwhelming epidemiological evidence for a cancer-preventive effect of the carotenoid, were results from the 8-year intervention trial of the α-tocopherol, β-Carotene Cancer Prevention Study Group (1996) in which an 18% increase in lung cancer incidence occurred among β-carotene–supplemented (20 mg/day) smokers. The IARC working group (1998), after extensive review of the epidemiological and intervention trials, concluded: "Until further insight is gained, β-carotene should not be recommended for use in cancer prevention in the general population and it should not be assumed that β-carotene is responsible for the cancer protecting effects of diets rich in carotenoid-containing fruits and vegetables."

Isotretinoin

Despite reports of positive responses to treatment of basal and squamous cell carcinomas with oral retinoids, these agents have not proved to be efficacious in prevention of nonmelanoma skin cancer. A total of 981 patients with two or more previously confirmed basal cell carcinomas were randomly assigned to receive either 10 mg of isotretinoin or a placebo daily. After 3 years of treatment, no statistically significant difference in either cumulative percent of patients with an occurrence of basal cell carcinoma or annual rate of basal cell carcinoma formation was observed between treatment and placebo groups (Tangrea et al., 1992). There was, however, significant toxicity associated with the low-dose regimen of retinoid. Another randomized, double-blind, controlled trial of oral retinol (25,000 units) or isotretinoin (5–10 mg) also found no differences in the incidence of nonmelanoma skin cancer in high-risk patients between either treatment or placebo groups (Levine et al., 1997). Noncompliance in a large percentage of patients enrolled in retinol chemoprevention studies was due to symptoms consistent with vitamin A ingestion (Cartmel et al., 2000).

Therapeutically, oral treatment of acquired immunodeficiency syndrome (AIDS)–related Kaposi sarcoma (KS) with 9-cis-retinoic acid has shown moderate activity with durable responses, but, again, substantial toxicity limits its use as an anti-KS therapy (Aboulafia et al., 2003).

Selenium

Selenium is another dietary factor that has been studied as a nonmelanoma skin cancer preventative. Clark et al. (1984), in a case-control study, examined the association between plasma selenium level and nonmelanoma skin cancer. Plasma selenium levels were significantly lower in the skin cancer patients. In a subsequent phase III randomized study of 1300 skin cancer patients, supplemental yeast-based selenium was administered for up to 10 years. Although there was a significant reduction in new cases of colon cancer in the patients randomized to the selenium-supplemented group, there were no significant effects on the occurrence of nonmelanoma skin cancer (Clark et al., 1996). A report that summarizes the entire blinded treatment period that ended in 1996, in which associations between treatment and time to first nonmelanoma skin cancer diagnosis and time to multiple skin tumors overall were analyzed, continued to show no statistically significant association of selenium supplementation with the risk of basal cell carcinoma. However, selenium supplementation was significantly associated with an elevated risk of squamous cell carcinoma. Overall, the results from the National Prevention of Cancer Trial demonstrate that selenium supplementation is ineffective at preventing basal cell carcinoma and that it *increases* the risk of squamous cell carcinoma and total nonmelanoma skin cancer (Duffield-Lillico et al., 2003).

Tea

A number of experimental studies have shown that tea, both green and black teas, contains several constituents that are effective inhibitors of UV carcinogenesis (Wang et al., 1991; Bickers and Athar, 2000). These constituents, monomeric and polymeric polyphenols, exhibit strong antioxidant properties and are capable of inhibiting UV-induced erythema in human skin (Katiyar et al., 1999). Tea polyphenols are absorbed and enter the circulation quickly after ingestion, significantly increasing the plasma antioxidant capacity (Benzie et al., 1999). Epidemiological studies have generally failed to provide convincing evidence that the consumption of tea polyphenols contribute to a reduction in human neoplastic disease, although these agents may exert a site-specific effect with respect to skin cancer (Linden et al., 1988; LaVecchia et al., 1992; Goldbohm, et al., 1996; Black and Rhodes, 2001). Indeed, in a population-based case-control study, Hakim et al. (2000c) found no association between general tea consumption and skin squamous cell carcinoma. However, after adjusting for brewing time, the association between skin squamous cell carcinoma and hot black tea consumption indicated a significantly lower risk in consumers of hot tea compared with nonconsumers.

Fat

Results from epidemiological and experimental studies regarding the influence of dietary fat on skin cancer have often been in conflict. Whereas experimental studies previously discussed clearly demonstrate a strong influence of dietary fat upon UV-induced skin cancer expression, both case-control and prospective cohort studies have failed to find a relationship of skin cancer incidence with dietary fat intake or specific vitamin supplementation (Graham, 1983; Hunter et al., 1992; van Dam et al., 2000; Davies et al., 2002). The larger prospective study involved a cohort of 73,366 women during a 4-year follow-up. Thind (1986), in an international study, found a positive association of dietary fat with skin cancer incidence but was unaware of a biological basis for these findings and cautioned against the pitfalls of international databases and broad correlation studies. Indeed, these types of studies are fraught with methodological difficulties because of (1) the complexity of the human diet in a free-living population; (2) the difficulties in measuring food intake and analyzing dietary information; in particular, dietary history questionnaires and surveys, although availing epidemiologists with large sample sizes, lack validation procedures that would demonstrate that the method measures what it is intended to measure; (3) the nutritionist seeks methods that accurately reflect current food intake, as opposed to the epidemiologist who requires assessment of dietary patterns that are stable over long periods, usually years if cancer induction is under study (Lyon et al., 1992). Some of the limitations of observational studies of diet and cancer can be circumvented by randomized intervention designs whereby direct answers to the question of dietary impact upon cancer incidence can be obtained (Henderson, 1992).

The rationale for undertaking a dietary intervention to modify nonmelanoma skin cancer occurrence rests upon several factors: (1) First, experimental animal studies had shown that high dietary fat intake exacerbated UV carcinogenesis, principally during the postinitiation period. (2) Further, changing from a high-fat to a low-fat diet, after a cancer-causing dose of UV had been administered, negated the exacerbating effect of high-fat intake (Black et al., 1992). This suggested that dietary modification, even after one had been exposed to skin cancer–inducing doses of UV, could represent a potentially important intervention strategy. Furthermore, (3) the high prevalence of skin cancer and the identification of the relative risks of skin cancer patients developing subsequent skin cancers within 2 years (28% cumulative rate; Karagas, 1994) made it practical to make significant comparisons within a relatively short-term study; and, in addition, (4) an intervention design creates a dietary difference, which, followed with frequent dietary assessment, averts many of the problems associated with epidemiological studies and allows direct comparisons of dietary fat exposure and disease status.

Such an intervention trial has been undertaken by Black et al. (1994). Of 133 skin cancer patients (basal or squamous cell carcinomas) recruited for the 2-year clinical intervention trial, 115 successfully completed the study. Fifty-eight patients were randomly assigned to the control arm in which no dietary changes were introduced. The 57 patients assigned to the intervention arm learned how to adopt low-fat eating habits to their food preferences and lifestyles, each patient given a "fat gram goal" that defined the grams of fat that would provide 20% of calories from fat. Baseline and follow-up dietary data were compiled from 7-day food records, from which 4 days were selected for analysis. Food records were verified for types of foods, amounts, and methods of preparation. Nutrient analyses were performed using the Minnesota Nutrition Data System. As the study was specifically designed to examine the influence of dietary fat on nonmelanoma skin cancer, stability of body weight and calorie intake was required to prevent any possible confounding effect due to these variables. Thus, patients in the intervention arm consumed higher levels of complex carbohydrate to compensate for the reduction in fat. The success of the dietary intervention protocol, with respect to meeting the goal of 20% of calories from fat, is reflected in Figure 4. Patients in the intervention group had reduced their percentage of calories from fat from 39% to 21%, a level maintained during the remainder of the 2-year study.

The potential for a low-fat intervention became apparent early in the study after only 76 patients had completed it. A clear and significant difference in number of actinic keratoses (premalignant lesions) between groups occurred after 8–12 months, with patients in the control group diagnosed with new keratoses four times as often as those in the low-fat group. Based on diet alone, patients in the control group consuming high levels of fat were found to be at 4.7 times greater risk of having one or more actinic keratoses during the 2-year period than similar patients in the low-fat inter-

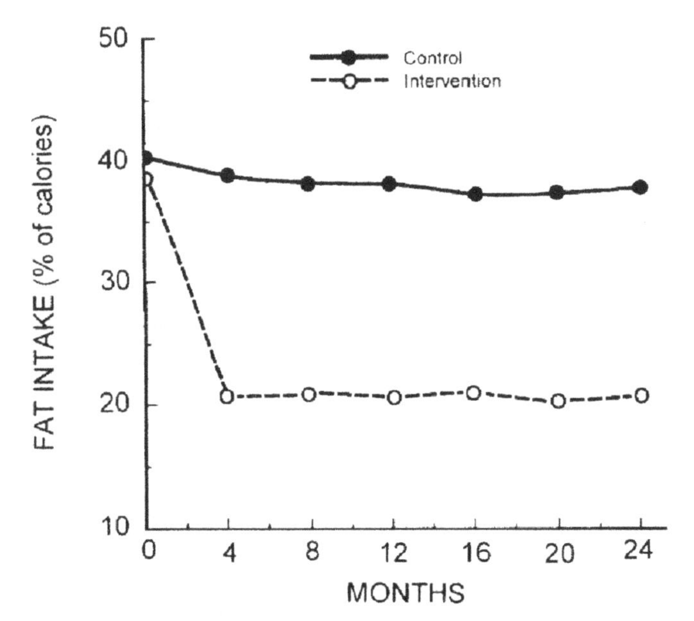

FIGURE 4 Dietary fat intake (fat as percentage of calories) of skin cancer patients in control group (solid circles) and in a low-fat intervention group (open circles). (Reprinted with permission from Jaax et al., 1997.)

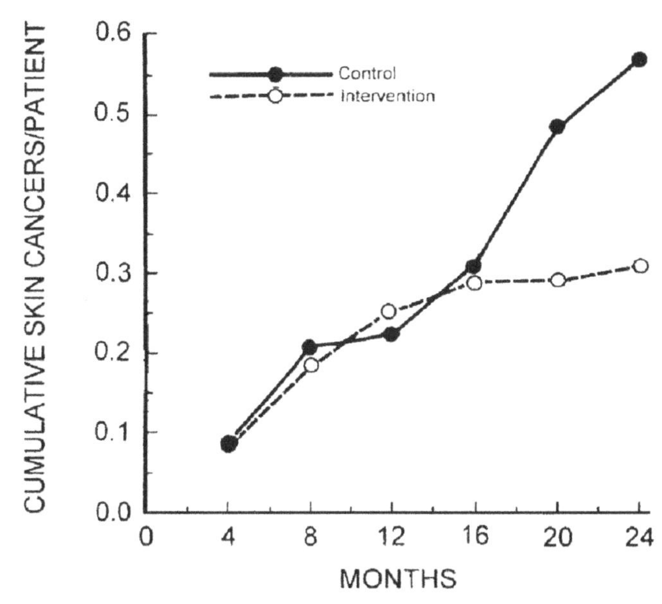

FIGURE 5 Influence of dietary fat intake on nonmelanoma skin cancer occurrence in control (solid circles) and low-fat dietary intervention (open circles) groups. Data points reflect cumulative numbers of nonmelanoma skin cancers per patient at each 4-month follow-up period. (Reprinted with permission from Jaax et al., 1997.)

vention group. The predisposing factors for actinic keratosis are similar to those for basal and squamous cell carcinomas (Marks et al., 1988).

Indeed, the influence of reduction in the percentage of calories as fat on nonmelanoma skin cancer occurrence (basal and squamous cell carcinomas) was observed after 101 patients had completed the study (Black et al., 1995b) and became even stronger after all 115 patients had completed it (Table 1). When skin cancer occurrence was examined in 8-month intervals across the 2-year study, occurrence in the control group did not change significantly from the baseline period. However, cancer occurrence in the intervention group was significantly lower ($p < .02$) in the last 8-month evaluation period. The cumulative rate of occurrence of nonmelanoma skin cancer (cumulative skin cancers/patient/time period) was 0.21 and 0.19 during the first 8-month period of the study and 0.26 and 0.02 during the last 8-month period for control and intervention groups, respectively (Figure 5).

With regard to diet, there were no significant differences in total caloric intake between the two groups, but there was a 47% reduction in the percentage of calories consumed as fat in the intervention group. To compensate the total caloric intake of the intervention group, there was a 36% increase in carbohydrates compared with the control group. A small but significant increase in percentage of calories from protein was observed. No difference in percentage of calories from alcohol was observed between groups (Jaax et al., 1997). Dietary parameters are shown in Table 2.

TABLE 1 Effect of Low-Fat Diet on Incidence and Occurrence of Nonmelanoma Skin Cancer (NMSK)[a]

Treatment	N	NMSK/Patient	Patients with NMSK	Improvement
Control	58	0.26	9	$9 \rightarrow 9$ *NS*
		$p < 0.01$	$p < 0.02$	
Intervention	57	0.02	1	$9 \rightarrow 1$ $p < 0.05$

[a]Numbers of new confirmed skin cancers (basal and squamous cell carcinomas) per patient were totaled in 8-month intervals of a 2-year study period. Each of the last two 8-month periods, within each dietary group, was compared with their respective initial 8-month period. In addition, the corresponding 8-month periods of the two dietary groups were compared. Cancer occurrence (nonmelanoma skin cancer [NMSK]/patient) in the dietary intervention group declined by the last 8-month period compared with the control group (0.02 vs 0.26 cancers/patient). The incidence (numbers of patients with NMSK) in the intervention group was less in the last 8-month period than in the control group. This is reflected as a significant improvement in those patients in the intervention group (i.e., the control and intervention groups each had nine patients with NMSK in the first 8-month period). The control group also had nine patients with NMSK in the last 8-month period, with only one patient with NMSK in the intervention group for this period.

Overall, the methods for controlling fat intake permitted considerable flexibility in food choices because foods with little or no fat were emphasized, although higher-fat foods could be included as long as the fat gram goal was not exceeded. Thus, a singular strategy of reducing fat intake,

TABLE 2 Major Dietary Variables of Control and Low-Fat Dietary Intervention Groups[a]

Dietary variable	Baseline	Within study	p
Total calories (kcal)			
Control	2265 ± 659	2196 ± 615	
Intervention	2400 ± 629	1995 ± 564	NS
% of calories from:			
FAT			
Control	39.9 ± 4.4	37.8 ± 4.1	
Intervention	38.9 ± 3.4	20.7 ± 5.5	0.0001
CARBOHYDRATE			
Control	42.7 ± 8.1	44.6 ± 6.9	
Intervention	44.2 ± 5.4	60.3 ± 6.3	0.0001
PROTEIN			
Control	15.5 ± 2.9	15.7 ± 2.4	
Intervention	15.6 ± 2.3	17.7 ± 2.2	0.0001
ALCOHOL			
Control	3.2 ± 4.5	3.2 ± 3.9	
Intervention	2.8 ± 3.8	3.2 ± 3.4	NS

[a]Baseline values represent values ±SD of diets at the time of randomization into the study. Within the study, values are the mean values from 4 months through 24 months. There were no statistically significant differences in any of the parameters at the time of randomization. *p* values are shown for the within-study differences between groups.

Source: Data taken from Jaax et al., 1997, with permission.

with the goal of 20% of calories from fat, could be an effective aid in the management and prophylaxis of nonmelanoma skin cancer. Moreover, the influence of caloric restriction on cancer development should not be ignored. A diet in which the level of fat intake has been reduced, as in the study described, but in which no effort is made to maintain initial caloric intake or body weight, might be expected to convey even greater protection to nonmelanoma skin cancer and certainly to provide collateral health benefits as well.

Not only level, but also composition, of dietary fat must be considered as a potentiator of skin cancer. A considerable body of evidence has previously been discussed on the influence of polyunsaturated fatty acids on UV carcinogenesis. However, it is now clear that a distinction must be made between omega-6 and omega-3 fatty acids with regard to their influence on carcinogenesis. Studies discussed previously have clearly demonstrated that omega-3 fatty acids can elevate the erythema threshold in humans, and it is reasoned that this is the result of the anti-inflammatory properties of these fatty acids (Jackson et al., 2002). An assessment of early genotoxic markers in humans indicates that omega-3 fatty acid protects against UV-induced genotoxicity and suggests that longer-term supplementation might reduce skin cancer occurrence (Rhodes et al., 2003). Hakim et al. (2000a), in a population-based case-control study, have found a consistent tendency for a lower risk of squamous cell carcinoma with higher intakes of omega-3 fatty acids. Their data also suggested a tendency toward a decreased risk of squamous cell carcinoma with increased intake of diets with high omega-3/omega-6 fatty acid ratios.

The preceding discussion suggests that human dietary manipulation, with respect to dietary lipid, offers a safe intervention approach for protection against UV-induced effects that lead to skin cancer. Specific strategies such as a reduction in total fat and omega-3 fatty acid supplementation both show promise in protecting against nonmelanoma skin cancer.

Melanoma

It would be remiss not to consider melanoma in a discussion of skin cancer, although the etiology of this type of skin cancer is not clearly understood. In addition, not until recently have there been animal models to study the role of UV in the etiology of melanoma (Ley et al., 1989; Setlow et al., 1993; Noonan et al., 2001), only one of which lends itself easily to dietary manipulation.

Cutaneous melanoma is a cancer of the pigment producing cells (melanocytes) that reside primarily in the basal layer of the epidermis (Koh, 1991). The incidence rate of malignant melanoma has nearly tripled in the past 40 years (Rigel et al., 1987; Glass and Hoover, 1989; Grin-Jorgensen et al., 1992) and currently ranks as the eighth most common cancer among whites in the United States (Koh et al., 1995), where it is the most common cancer among whites between the ages of 25–29 years, although the median age at occurrence is 53 years. In 1993, ~32,000 new cases of melanoma were diagnosed in the United States (Boring et al., 1993). That number was projected to rise to 40,300 new cases in 1997 (Parker et al., 1997), consistent with the 5% increase per annum observed earlier (Glass and Hoover, 1989). It was estimated that by year 2000, malignant melanoma will have afflicted 1 in 90 white Americans (Rigel et al., 1987). The American Cancer Society estimated that >55,000 new cases will have been diagnosed in 2004.

Unlike nonmelanocytic skin cancer, the precise causal agent(s) of melanoma is unknown. Nevertheless, examination of worldwide latitude gradients, in association with melanoma rates, provided the first evidence that sunlight might be a causal agent of melanoma (Grin-Jorgensen et al., 1992). Although cumulative UV exposure does not seem to explain the occurrence of melanoma as it does for nonmelanoma skin cancer, there is some evidence that frequent intermittent UV exposure is involved. In addition, anatomical site of occurrence does not conform to those areas of the body habitually exposed to UV, although patients with malignant melanoma tend to have lighter complexions and spend more time outdoors (Gellin et al., 1969). Koh et al. (1990) have summarized the evidence for UV involvement, as well as that which disputes such a role. Other potential etiological factors, including an immunological role, have been discussed (Lee and Merrill, 1970; Longstreth et al., 1992). To date, little evidence supports a role for diet in development of melanoma (Koh et al., 1995; Lew et al., 1995), although a number of factors have been examined.

Retinol, Vitamins E and C, Carotenoids, and Alcohol

In a clinic-based case-control study of nutritional factors and risk of malignant melanoma involving 204 patients and 248 controls, little or no evidence was found for a protective effect of increased plasma levels of retinol, α-tocopherol (vitamin E), or carotenoids (Stryker et al., 1990). Alcohol consumption (>10 g/day) exhibited a moderate trend of increasing risk. Even though vitamin E supplementation provided no association with decreased risk, there was a consistent increased risk in persons with low vitamin E intake. Millen et al. (2004) also found that high alcohol consumption was associated with increased risk for melanoma but that high carotenoid levels were associated with reduced risk. In a large cohort of U.S. women, vitamins A, C, and E were found to have no association with lower risk of melanoma (Feskanich et al., 2003). Interestingly, higher risks of melanoma were associated with greater intakes of vitamin C from food, as well as a significant positive response with frequency of orange juice consumption. Contrary to this finding with melanoma, Hakim et al. (2000b), in a case-control study, found no association between overall consumption of citrus juices and squamous cell carcinoma. They did, however, observe a dose–response relationship between higher citrus peel intake and degree of risk lowering for squamous cell carcinoma. Citrus peel is a major source of limonene.

Vitamin D

Speculation regarding the potential preventative effects of vitamin D on melanoma grew from laboratory studies that demonstrated that this vitamin inhibited the growth of cultured melanoma cells. Weinstock et al. (1992) examined the relationship between vitamin D and melanoma risk in a case-control study. Vitamin D intake was assessed by food-frequency questionnaires in 165 melanoma patients and 209 controls. They found no association of melanoma risk with total vitamin D intake, calorie-adjusted vitamin D intake, vitamin D intake from foods, or consumption of milk or vitamin D supplements. Thus, no evidence was found to support the contention that vitamin D protects against melanoma. Millen et al. (2004), on the other hand, concluded that diets consisting of foods rich in vitamin D may be associated with a reduction in risk for melanoma. Obviously, the relationship of vitamin D and melanoma remains uncertain.

Dietary Fat

In 1974, Mackie observed an unusual increase in incidence of melanoma (five patients over a 12-week period) in his clinical practice in Sydney. After an interview with a dietitian, it was determined that all five patients had altered their diets 10 months or more before onset of their melanoma and had enthusiastically replaced saturated fat sources, such as butter, with polyunsaturated fat substitutes. Mackie suggested that the increased intake of polyunsaturated fat may have predisposed patients to the development of melanoma. In a subsequent study involving 142 melanoma patients and 82 controls, dietary questionnaires were administered to assess dietary habits, and fatty acid analysis of subcutaneous adipose tissue was employed as a marker for the percentage of linoleic acid ingestion in the preceding 3 years. No significant differences in linoleic acid intake, use of cooking oils, frequency of cooking habit, meals out, or intake of antioxidants were found (Mackie et al., 1980). This study failed to control for racial differences in which dietary habits might have been influential, and a second study was undertaken with 100 melanoma patients and 100 matched controls. The polyunsaturated fat content of adipose tissue was significantly higher in melanoma patients than in controls and there were significantly more controls than patients who had a low percentage of linoleic acid in the triglyceride fraction of subcutaneous adipose tissue (Mackie et al., 1987). Although the critical studies have not yet been undertaken, these preliminary findings suggest a potential role for diet in the prevention of melanoma (Mackie and Mackie, 1990).

A retrospective study compared 5-year melanoma survival rates of patients receiving Gerson's diet therapy with survival rates in the medical literature (Hildenbrand et al., 1995). The alternative Gerson's therapy includes a lactovegetarian diet that is low in fat. The 5-year survival rates for patients on this therapy were considerably higher than those reported elsewhere. It would be enlightening to know whether a low-fat diet, such as that used in the nonmelanoma study, would be a beneficial adjunct (in terms of survival rates) to conventional therapies employed in the treatment of melanoma.

CONCLUSIONS

- Experimental animal data clearly demonstrate that dietary lipid and certain antioxidants can have significant influence on UV-induced carcinogenic expression.
- Degree of saturation, per se, appears not to have as important an influence on carcinogenic response in skin as level of the dietary fat and its fatty acid composition.
- A clinical dietary intervention trial indicates that a decrease in percentage of calories consumed as fat reduces

the occurrence of premalignant actinic keratosis and nonmelanoma skin cancer.

- Reduction in skin cancer occurrence was observed after 1 year of the low-fat dietary intervention.
- Reduction in dietary fat reduces the occurrence of basal cell carcinomas in humans and of squamous cell carcinomas in animals.
- Results from the clinical trial validate the relevancy of the hairless mouse/UV dietary model.
- *In toto*, these data suggest that implementation of a low-fat diet and omega-3 fatty acid supplementation show the greatest promise as dietary strategies for the management and prevention of the highly prevalent nonmelanoma skin cancer. Single antioxidant supplementation, in contrast, should be approached with caution.

Acknowledgments

The author's research has been sponsored by grants from the National Cancer Institute; the National Institutes of Health; the American Institute for Cancer Research; and medical research funds from the Department of Veterans Affairs.

References

Aboulafia, D.M., Norris, D., Henry, D., Grossman, R.J., Thommes, J., Bundow, D., Yocum, R.C., and Stevens, V. 2003. 9-cis-retinoic acid capsules in the treatment of AIDS-related Kaposi sarcoma: results of a phase 2 multicenter clinical trial. *Arch Dermatol* **139**: 178–186.

Albanes, D. 1987. Caloric intake, body weight, and cancer: a review. *Nutr Cancer* **9**: 199–217.

Armstrong, B., and Doll, R. 1975. Environmental factors and cancer incidence and mortality in different countries, with special reference to dietary practices. *Int J Cancer* **15**: 617–631.

Baumann, C.A., and Rusch, H.P. 1939. Effect of diet on tumors induced by ultraviolet light. *Am J Cancer* **35**: 213–221.

Benzie, I.F.F., Szeto, Y.T., Strain, J.J., and Tomlinson, B. 1999. Consumption of green tea causes rapid increase in plasma antioxidant power in humans. *Nutr Cancer* **34**: 83–87.

Berenblum, I. 1941. The mechanism of carcinogenesis: a study of the significance of cocarcinogenic action and related phenomena. *Cancer Res* **1**: 807–814.

Berenblum, I. 1954. Carcinogenesis and tumor pathogenesis. *Adv Cancer Res* **11**: 129–175.

Berenblum, I. 1979. Theoretical and practical aspects of the two-stage mechanism of carcinogenesis. *In* "Carcinogens: Identification and Mechanisms of Action" (A.C. Griffin and C.R. Shaw, Eds.), pp. 25–36. Raven Press, New York.

Berenblum, I., and Haran, N. 1955. The significance of the sequence of initiating and promoting actions in the process of skin carcinogenesis in the mouse. *Br J Cancer* **9**: 268–271.

Bischoff, R., Long, M.L., and Maxwell, L.C. 1935. Influence of caloric intake upon the growth of sarcoma 180. *Am J Cancer* **24**: 549–553.

Bissett, D.L., Chatterjee, R., and Hannon, D.P. 1991. Chronic ultraviolet radiation-induced increase in skin iron and the photoprotective effect of topically applied iron chelators. *Photochem Photobiol* **54**: 215–223.

Black, H.S. 1974. Effects of dietary antioxidants on actinic tumor induction. *Res Commun Chem Pathol Pharmacol* **7**: 783–786.

Black, H.S. 1983. Utility of the skin/UV-carcinogenesis model for evaluating the role of nutritional lipids in cancer. *In* "Diet, Nutrition, and Cancer: From Basic Research to Policy Implications" (D.A. Roe, Ed.), pp. 49–60. Liss, New York.

Black, H.S. 1987. Photocarcinogenesis and diet. *Fed Proc Fed Am Soc Exp Biol* **46**: 1901–1905.

Black, H.S. 1993. Role of dietary factors in UV-carcinogenesis. *Cancer Bull* **45**: 232–237.

Black, H.S. 1998. Radical interception by carotenoids and effects on UV carcinogenesis. *Nutr Cancer* **31**: 212–217.

Black, H.S. 2004. Pro-carcinogenic activity of β-carotene, a putative systemic photoprotectant. *Photochem Photobiol* Sci. **3**: 753–758.

Black, H.S., and Chan, J.T. 1975. Suppression of ultraviolet light induced tumor formation by dietary antioxidants. *J Invest Dermatol* **65**: 412–414.

Black, H.S., and Chan, J.T. 1977. Experimental ultraviolet light-carcinogenesis. *Photochem Photobiol* **26**: 183–199.

Black, H.S., Chan, J.T., and Brown, G.E. 1978. Effects of dietary constituents on ultraviolet light-mediated carcinogenesis. *Cancer Res* **38**: 1384–1387.

Black, H.S., and Douglas, D.R. 1972. A model system for the evaluation of the role of cholesterol a-oxide in ultraviolet carcinogenesis. *Cancer Res* **32**: 2630–2632.

Black, H.S., and Douglas, D.R. 1973. Formation of a carcinogen of natural origin in the etiology of ultraviolet light-induced carcinogenesis. *Cancer Res* **33**: 2094–2096.

Black, H.S., and Lo, W.B. 1971. Formation of a carcinogen in human skin irradiated with ultraviolet light. *Nature (London)* **234**: 306–308.

Black, H.S., and Gerguis, J. 2003. Modulation of dietary vitamins E and C fails to ameliorate β-carotene exacerbation of UV-carcinogenesis in mice. *Nutr Cancer* **45**: 36–45.

Black, H.S., Henderson, S.V., Kleinhans, C.M., Phelps, A.W., and Thornby, J.I. 1979. The effect of dietary cholesterol on ultraviolet light-carcinogenesis. *Cancer Res* **39**: 5022–5027.

Black, H.S., Herd, J.A., Goldberg, L.H., Wolf, J.E., Thomby, J.I., Rosen, T., Bruce, S., Tschen, J.A., Foreyt, J.P., Scott, L.W., and Jaax, S. 1994. Effect of a low-fat diet on the incidence of actinic keratosis. *N Engl J Med* **330**: 1272–1275.

Black, H.S., Lenger, W., Phelps, A.W., and Thomby, J.I. 1983. Influence of dietary lipid upon ultraviolet light-carcinogenesis. *Nutr Cancer* **5**: 59–68.

Black, H.S., Lenger, W., Gerguis, J., and Thomby, J.I. 1985. Relation of antioxidants and level of dietary lipid to epidermal lipid peroxidation and ultraviolet carcinogenesis. *Cancer Res* **45**: 6254–6259.

Black, H.S., Okotie-Eboh, G., Gerguis, J., Urban, J.I., and Thomby, J.I. 1995a. Dietary fat modulates immunoresponsiveness in UV-irradiated mice. *Photochem Photobiol* **62**: 964–969.

Black, H.S., Okotie-Eboh, G., Gerguis, J. 2000. Diet potentiates the UV-carcinogenic response to β-carotene. *Nutr Cancer* **37**: 55–60.

Black, H.S., and Rhodes, L.E. 2001. Systemic photoprotection: dietary intervention and therapy. *In* "Sun Protection in Man" (P.U. Giacomoni, Ed.), pp. 573–591. Elsevier, Amsterdam.

Black, H.S., Thomby, J.I., Gerguis, J., and Lenger, W. 1992. Influence of dietary omega-6, -3 fatty acid sources on the initiation and promotion stages of photocarcinogenesis. *Photochem Photobiol* **56**: 195–199.

Black, H.S., Thornby, J.I., Wolf, J.E., Goldberg, L.H., Herd, J.A., Rosen, T., Bruce, S., Tschen, J.A., Scott, L.W., Jaax, S., Foreyt, J.P., and Reusser, B. 1995b. Evidence that a low-fat diet reduces the occurrence of non-melanoma skin cancer. *Int J Cancer* **62**: 165–169.

Blum, H.F. 1948. Sunlight as a causal factor in cancer of the skin of man. *J Natl Cancer Inst (US)* **9**: 247–258.

Blum, H.F. 1959. "Carcinogenesis by Ultraviolet Light." Princeton University Press, Princeton, NJ.

Blum, H.F., Kirby-Smith, J.S., and Grady, H.G. 1941. Quantitative induction of tumors in mice with ultraviolet radiation. *J Natl Cancer Inst (US)* **2**: 259–268.

Blum, H.F., McVaugh, J., Ward, M., and Bush, H.L., Jr. 1975. Epidermal hyperplasia is induced by ultraviolet radiation: error and uncertainty of measurement. *Photochem Photobiol* **21**: 255–260.

Boring, C.C., Squires, T.S., and Tong, T. 1993. Cancer Statistics, 1993. *CA Cancer J Clin* **43**: 7–26.

Boutwell, R.K. 1964. Some biological aspects of skin carcinogenesis. *Prog Exp Tumor Res* **4**: 207–250.

Burke, K.E., Combs, G.F., Goss, E.G., Bhuyan, K.C., and Abu-Libdeh, H. 1992. The effects of topical and oral L-selenomethionine on pigmentation and skin cancer induced by ultraviolet irradiation. *Nutr Cancer* **17**: 123–137.

Burton, G.W., and Ingold, K.U. 1984. Beta-carotene: an unusual type of lipid antioxidant. *Science* **224**: 569–573.

Calle, E.E., Rodriguez, C., Walker-Thurmond, K., Thun, M.J. 2003. Overweight, obesity, and mortality from cancer in a prospectively studied cohort of U.S. adults. *N Engl J Med* **348**: 1625–1638.

Carroll, K.K., and Hopkins, G.T. 1979. Dietary polyunsaturated fat versus saturated fat in relation to mammary carcinogenesis. *Lipids* **14**: 155–158.

Carroll, K.K., and Khor, H.T. 1971. Effects of level and type of dietary fat on the incidence of mammary tumors induced in female Sprague-Dawley rats by 7,12-dimethylbenz[a]anthracene. *Lipids* **6**: 415–420.

Cartmel, B., Moon, T.E., Levine, N., Rodney, S., and Alberts, D. 2000. Predictors of inactivation and reasons for participant inactivation during a skin cancer chemoprevention study. *Cancer Epidemiol Biomarkers Prev* **9**: 999–1002.

Chung, H.T., Bumham, D.K., Robertson, B., Roberts, L.K., and Daynes, R.A. 1986. Involvement of prostaglandins in the immune alterations caused by the exposure of mice to ultraviolet radiation. *J Immunol* **137**: 2478–2484.

Clark, L.C., Graham, G.E., Crounse, R.G., Grimson, R., Hulka, B., and Shy, C.M. 1984. Plasma selenium and skin neoplasms: a case-control study. *Nutr Cancer* **6**: 13–21.

Clark, L.C., Combs, G.R., Tumbull, B.W., Slate, E.H., Chalker, D.K., Chow, J., Davis, L.S., Glover, R.A., Graham, G.R., Gross, E.G., Krongrad, A., Lesher, J.L., Park, H.K., Sanders, B.B., Smith, C.L., and Taylor, J.R. 1996. Effects of selenium supplementation for cancer prevention in patients with carcinoma of the skin. *JAMA* **276**: 1957–1963.

Cleaver, J.E. 1968. Defective repair replication of DNA in Xeroderma pigmentosum. *Nature (London)* **218**: 652–656.

Committee on Chemistry and Physics of Ozone Depletion and the Committee on Biological Effects of Increased Solar Ultraviolet Radiation. 1982. "Causes and Effects of Stratospheric Ozone Reduction: An Update." National Academy Press, Washington, DC.

Davies, T.W., Treasure, F.P., Welch, A.A., and Day, N.E. 2002. Diet and basal cell skin cancer: results from the EPIC-Norfolk cohort. *Br J Dermatol* **146**: 1017–1022.

deGruijl, F.R., and van der Leun, J.C. 1994. Estimate of wavelength dependence of ultraviolet carcinogenesis in humans and its relevance to the risk assessment of a stratospheric ozone depletion. *Health Phys* **67**: 314–325.

deGruijl, F.R., Sterenborg, H.J.C.M., Forbes, P.D., Davies, R.E., Cole, C., Kelfkens, G., van Weelden, H., Slaper, H., and van der Leun, J.C. 1993. Wavelength dependence of skin cancer induction by ultraviolet irradiation of albino hairless mice. *Cancer Res* **53**: 53–60.

Dubreuilh, W. 1896. Des hyperkeratoses circonscrites. *Ann Dermatol Syphiligra* **7**: 1158–1204.

Duffield-Lillico, A.J., Slate, E.H., Reid, M.E., Turnbull, B.W., Wilkins, P.A., Combs, G.F. Jr., Park, H.K., Gross, E.G., Graham, G.F., Stratton, M.S., Marshall, J.R., and Clark, L.C.; Nutritional Prevention of Cancer Study Group. 2003. Selenium supplementation and secondary prevention of nonmelanoma skin cancer in a randomized trial. *J Natl Cancer Inst* **95**: 1477–1481.

Dunham, W.B., Zuckerkandl, E., Reynolds, R., Willoughby, R., Marcuson, R., Barth, R., and Pauling, L. 1982. Effects of intake of L-ascorbic acid on the incidence of dermal neoplasms induced in mice by ultraviolet light. *Proc Natl Acad Sci USA* **79**: 7532–7536.

Edge, R., Land, E.J., McGarvey, D., Mulroy, L., and Truscott, T.G. 1998. Relative one-electron reduction potentials of carotenoid radical cations and the interactions of carotenoids with the vitamin E radical cation. *J Am Chem Soc* **120**: 4087–4090.

Edge, R., and Truscott, T.G. 2000. Carotenoids—free radical interactions. *Spectrum* **13**: 12–20.

Elmets, C.A., and Mukhtar, H. 1996. Ultraviolet radiation and skin cancer: progress in pathophysiologic mechanisms. *Prog Dermatol* **30**: 1–16.

Emmett, E.A. 1973. Ultraviolet radiation as a cause of skin tumors. *CRC Crit Rev Toxicol* **2**: 211–255.

Epstein, J.H. 1977. Effects of beta-carotene on ultraviolet light induced cancer formation in the hairless mouse skin. *Photochem Photobiol* **25**: 211–213.

Farber, E. 1982. Chemical carcinogenesis: a biologic perspective. *Am J Pathol* **106**: 269–296.

Feskanich, D., Willett, W.C., Hunter, D.J. and Colditz, G.A. 2003. Dietary intakes of vitamins A, C, and E and risk of melanoma in cohorts of women. *Br J Cancer* **88**: 1381–1387.

Fieser, L.F. 1954. Some aspects of the chemistry and biochemistry of cholesterol. *Science* **119**: 710–716.

Findlay, G.M. 1928. Ultra-violet light and skin cancer. *Lancet* **2**: 1070–1073.

Fischer, M.A., and Black, H.S. 1991. Modification of membrane composition, eicosanoid metabolism, and immunoresponsiveness by dietary omega-3 and omega-6 fatty acid sources, modulators of ultraviolet-carcinogenesis. *Photochem Photobiol* **54**: 381–387.

Fischer, S.M., Lo, H., Gordon, G.B., Seibert, K., Kelloff, G., Lubert, A., and Conti, C.J. 1999. Chemopreventive activity of celecoxib a specific cylooxygenase-2 inhibitor, against UV-induced skin carcinogenesis. *Mol Carcinogen* **25**: 231–240.

Forbes, P.D. 1984. Relative effectiveness of UVA and UVB for photocarcinogenesis. *In* "The Biological Effects of UVA Radiation" (F. Urbach and R.W. Gange, Eds.), pp. 111–121. Praeger, New York.

Gallagher, R.P., Ma, B., McLean, D.I., Yang, C.P., Ho, V., Carruthers, J.A., and Warshawski, L.M. 1990. Trends in basal cell carcinoma, squamous cell carcinoma, and melanoma of the skin from 1973 through 1987. *J Am Acad Dermatol* **23**: 413–421.

Garrison, F.H. 1929. "An Introduction to the History of Medicine," p. 31. Saunders, Philadelphia.

Gellin, G.A., Kopf, A.W., and Garfinkel, L. 1966. Basal cell epithelioma: a controlled study of associated factors. *Adv Biol Skin* **7**: 329–344.

Gellin, G.A., Kopf, A.W., and Garfinkel, L. 1969. Malignant melanoma: a controlled study of possible associated factors. *Arch Dermatol* **99**: 43–48.

Gerrish, K.E., and Gensler, H.L. 1993. Prevention of photocarcinogenesis by dietary vitamin E. *Nutr Cancer* **19**: 125–133.

Glass, A.G., and Hoover, R.N. 1989. The emerging epidemic of melanoma and squamous cell skin cancer. *JAMA* **262**: 2097–2100.

Goldbohm, R.A., Hertog, M.G.L., Brants, H.A.M., van Poppel, G., and van der Brandt, P.A. 1996. Consumption of black tea and cancer risk: a prospective cohort study. *J Natl Cancer Inst* **88**: 93–100.

Graham, S. 1983. Results of case-controlled studies of diet and cancer in Buffalo, New York. *Cancer Res* **43**(Suppl): 2409–2413.

Green, A., Williams, G., Neale, R., Hart, V., Leslie, D., Parsons, P., Marks, G.C., Gaffney, P., Battistutta, D., Frost, C., Lang, C., and Russell, A. 1999. Daily sunscreen application and betacarotene supplementation in prevention of basal-cell and squamous-cell carcinomas of the skin: a randomized controlled trial. *Lancet* **354**: 723–729.

Greenberg, E.F., Baron, J.A., Stukel, T.A., Stevens, M.M., Mandel, J.S., Spencer, S.K., Elias, P.M., Lowe, N., Nierenberg, D.W., Bayrd, G., Vance, J.C., Freeman, D.H., Clendenning, W.E., and Kwan, T. 1990. A clinical trial of beta carotene to prevent basal-cell and squamous cell cancers of the skin. *N Engl J Med* **323**: 789–795.

Greenberg, E.F., Baron, J.A., Karagas, M.R., Stukel, T.A., Nierenberg, D.W., Stevens, M.M., Mandel, J.S., and Haile, R.W. 1996. Mortality associated with low plasma concentration of beta carotene and the effect of oral supplementation. JAMA **275**: 699–703.

Grin-Jorgensen, C.M., Rigel, D.S., and Friedman, R.J. 1992. The worldwide incidence of malignant melanoma. *In* "Cutaneous Melanoma" (C.M. Balch, A.N. Houghton, G.W. Milton, A.J. Sober, and S.J. Soong, Eds.), 2nd edition, pp. 27–39. Lippincott, Philadelphia.

Grossweiner, L.I. 1989. Photophysics. *In* "The Science of Photobiology" (K.C. Smith, Ed.), pp. 1–45. Plenum, New York.

Haagensen, C.D. 1931. Occupational neoplastic disease. *Am J Cancer* **15**: 641–703.

Hakim, I.A., Harris, R.B., and Ritenbaugh, C. 2000a. Fat intake and risk of squamous cell carcinoma of the skin. *Nutr Cancer* **36**: 155–162.

Hakim, I.A. Harris, R.B., and Ritenbaugh, C. 2000b. Citrus peel use is associated with reduced risk of squamous cell carcinoma of the skin. *Nutr Cancer* **37**: 161–168.

Hakim, I.A., Harris, R.B., and Weisgerber, U.M. 2000c. Tea intake and squamous cell carcinoma of the skin: influence of type of tea beverages. *Cancer Epidemiol Biomarkers Prev* **9**: 727–731.

Harber, L. 1986. Recommendations for future research and possible actions. *In* "The Biologic Effects of UVA Radiation" (F. Urbach and R.W. Gange, Eds.), p. 314. Praeger, New York.

Haven, F.L. 1936. The effect of cod-liver oil on tumor growth. *Am J Cancer* **27**: 95–9S.

Henderson, C.D., Black, H.S., and Wolf, J.E., Jr. 1989. Influence of omega-3 and omega-6 fatty acid sources on prostaglandin levels in mice. *Lipids* **24**: 502–505.

Henderson, M.M. 1992. Role of intervention trials in research on nutrition and cancer. *Cancer Res* **52**(Suppl): 2030–2034.

Higginson, J., and Muir, C.S. 1976. The role of epidemiology in elucidating the importance of environmental factors in human cancer. *Cancer Detect Prev* **1**: 79–105.

Hildenbrand, G.L., Hildenbrand, L.C., Bradford, K., and Calvin, S.W. 1995. Five-year survival rates of melanoma patients treated by diet therapy after the manner of Gerson: a retrospective review. *Altern Ther Health Med* **1**: 29–37.

Hocman, G. 1988. Prevention of cancer: restriction of nutritional energy intake (Joules). *Comp Biochem Physiol A* **91A**: 209–220.

Hunter, D.J., Colditz, G.A., Stampfer, M.J., Rosner, B., Willett, W.C., and Speizer, F.E. 1992. Diet and risk of basal cell carcinoma of the skin in a prospective cohort of women. *Ann Epidermal* **2**: 231–239.

International Agency for Research on Cancer. 1992. Solar and ultra violet radiation. IARC Monogr. *Eval Carcinog Risks Hum* **55**: 43–72.

International Agency for Research on Cancer. 1998. "IARC Working Group on the Evaluation of Cancer-Preventive Agents, Carotenoids. IARC Handbooks of Cancer Prevention," Vol. 2. IARC, Lyon.

Ip, C., Carter, C.A., and Ip, M.M. 1985. Requirement of essential fatty acid for mammary tumorigenesis in the rat. *Cancer Res* **45**: 1997–2001.

Jaax, S., Scott, L.W., Wolf, J.E., Thornby, J.I., and Black, H.S. 1997. General guidelines for a low-fat diet effective in the management and prevention of nonmelanoma skin cancer. *Nutr Cancer* **27**: 150–156.

Jackson, M.J., Jackson, M.J., McArdle, F., Storey, A, Jones, S.A., McArdle, A., and Rhodes, L.E. 2002. Effects of micronutrient supplements on UV-induced skin damage. *Proc Nutr Soc* **61**: 187–189.

Karagas, M.R. 1994. Occurrence of cutaneous basal cell and squamous cell malignancies among those with a prior history of skin cancer. *J Invest Dermatol* **102**(Suppl): 10–13.

Karagas, M.R., Greenberg, E.R., Nierenberg, D., Stukel, T.A., Morris, J.S., Stevens, M.M., and Baron, J.A. 1997. Risk of squamous cell carcinoma of the skin in relation to plasma selenium, α-tocopherol, β-carotene, and retinol: a nested case-control study. *Cancer Epidemiol Biomarkers Prev* **6**: 25–29.

Katiyar, S.K., Matsui, M.S., Elmets, C.A., and Mukhtar, H. 1999. Polyphenolic antioxidant (–)-epigalloocatechin-3-gallate from green tea reduces UVB-induced inflammatory responses and infiltration of leukocytes in human skin. *Photochem Photobiol* **69**: 148–153.

Kinden, L.J., Willows, A.N., Goldblatt, P, and Yudkin, J. 1988. Tea consumption and cancer. *Br J Cancer* **58**: 397–401.

Koh, H.K. 1991. Cutaneous melanoma. *N Engl J Med* **325**: 171–182.

Koh, H.K., Kligler, B.E., and Lew, R.A. 1990. Sunlight and cutaneous malignant melanoma: evidence for and against causation. *Photochem Photobiol* **51**: 765 –779.

Koh, H.K., Lew, R.A., Geller, A.C., Miller, D.R., and Davis, B.E. 1995. Skin cancer: prevention and control. *In* "Cancer Prevention and Control" (P. Greenwald, B.S. Kramer, and D.L. Weed, Eds.), pp. 611–640. Dekker, New York.

Krinsky, N.I. 1987. Mechanisms of inactivation of oxygen species by carotenoids. *In* "Anticarcinogenesis and Radiation Protection" (P.A. Cerutti, O.F. Nygaard, and M.G. Simic, Eds.), pp. 41–46. Plenum, New York.

Kune, G.A., Bannerman, S., Field, B., Watson, L.F., Cleland, H., Merenstein, D., and Vitetta, L. 1992. Diet, alcohol, smoking, serum β-carotene, and vitamin A in male nonmelanocytic skin cancer patients and controls. *Nutr Cancer* **18**: 237–244.

Lands, W.E.M., Kulmacz, R.J., Marshall, P.J. 1982. Lipid peroxide actions in the regulation of prostaglandin biosynthesis. *In* "Free Radicals in Biology" (W.A. Pryor, Ed.), Vol. 6, pp. 39–61. Academic Press, New York.

LaVecchia, C., Negri, E., Franceschi, S., D'Avanzo, B., and Boyle, P. 1992. Tea consumption and cancer risk. *Nutr Cancer* **17**: 27–31.

Lavik, P.S., and Baumann, C.A. 1941. Dietary fat and tumor formation. *Cancer Res* **1**: 181–187.

Lavik, P.S., and Baumann, C.A. 1943. Further studies on the tumor-promoting action of fat. *Cancer Res* **3**: 749–756.

Lee, J.A.H., and Merrill, J.M. 1970. Sunlight and the aetiology of malignant melanoma: a synthesis. *Med J Aust* **2**: 846–851.

Levine, N., Moon, T.E., Cartmel, B., Bangert, J.L., Rodney, S., Dong, Q., Peng, Y., and Alberts, D.S. 1997. Trial of retinol and isotretinoin in skin cancer prevention: a randomized, double-blind, controlled trial. Southwest Skin Cancer Prevention Study Group. *Cancer Epidemiol Biomarkers Prev* **6**: 957–961.

Lew, R.A., Koh, H.K., and Sober, A.J. 1985. Epidemiology of cutaneous melanoma. *Dermatol Clin* **3**: 257–269.

Ley, R.D., Applegate, L.A., Padilla, R.S., and Stuart, T.D. 1989. Ultraviolet radiation–induced malignant melanoma in Monodelphia domestica. *Photochem Photobiol* **50**: 1–5.

Lo, W.B., and Black, H.S. 1973. Inhibition of carcinogen formation in skin irradiated with ultraviolet light. *Nature (London)* **246**: 489–491.

Longstreth, J.D., Lea, C.S., and Kripke, M.L. 1992. Ultraviolet radiation and other putative causes of melanoma. *In* "Cutaneous Melanoma" (C.M. Balch, A.N. Houghton, G.W. Milton, A.J. Sober, and S.J. Soong, Eds.), 2nd edition, pp. 46–58. Lippincott, Philadelphia.

Lyon, J.L., Gardner, J.W., West, D.W., and Mahoney, A.M. 1992. Methodological issues in epidemiological studies of diet and caner. *Cancer Res* **52**(Suppl): 2040–2048.

Mackie, B.S. 1974. Malignant melanoma and diet. *Med J Aust* **1**: 810.

Mackie, B.S., and Mackie, L.E. 1990. Prevention of melanoma. *Nutr Cancer* **14**: 81–83.

Mackie, B.S., Johnson, A.R., Mackie, L.E., Fogerty, A.C., Ferris, M., and Baxter, R.I. 1980. Dietary polyunsaturated fats and malignant melanoma. *Med J Aust* **1**: 159–163.

Mackie, B.S., Mackie, L.E., Curtin, L.D., and Bourne, D.J. 1987. Melanoma and dietary lipids. *Nutr Cancer* **9**: 219–226.

Marks, R., Rennie, G., and Selwood, T. 1988. The relationship of basal cell carcinomas and squamous cell carcinomas to solar keratoses. *Arch Dermatol* **124**: 1039–1042.

Marks, R., Jolley, D., Lectsas, S., and Foley, P. 1990. The role of childhood exposure to sunlight in the development of solar keratoses and non-melanocytic skin cancer. *Med J Aust* **152**: 62–66.

Mason, T.J., McKay, F.W., Hoover, R., Blot, W.J., and Fraumeni, J.F., Jr. 1975. "Atlas of Cancer Mortality for U.S. Counties: 1950–1969," DHEW Publication No. (NIH) 75-780. Washington, DC.

Mathews-Roth, M.M. 1982. Antitumor activity of β-carotene, canthaxanthin, and phytoene. *Oncology* **39**: 33–37.

Mathews-Roth, M.M., and Krinsky, N.I. 1985. Carotenoid dose level and protection against UV-B–induced skin tumors. *Photochem Photobiol* **42**: 35–38.

Miller, D.L., and Weinstock, M.A. 1994. Nonmelanoma skin cancer in the United States: Incidence. *J Am Acad Dermatol* **30**: 774–778.

Millen, A.E., Tucker, M.A., Hartge, P., Halpern, A., Elder, D.E., Guerry, D., 4th, Holly, E.A., Sagebiel, R.W., and Potischman, N. 2004. Diet and melanoma in a case-control study. *Cancer Epidemiol Biomarkers Prev* **1**: 1042–1051.

Miller, J.A., Kline, B.E., Rusch, H.P., and Baumann, C.A. 1944. The effect of certain lipids on the carcinogenicity of *p*-dimethylaminoazobenzene. *Cancer Res* **4**: 756–761.

Morison, W.L. 1991. "Phototherapy and Photochemotherapy of Skin Disease," pp. 10–36. Raven Press, New York.

Mulay, D.M. 1963. Skin cancer in India. *Natl Cancer Inst Monogr* **10**: 215–223.

Noonan, F.P., Recio, J.A., Takayama, H., Duray, P., Anver, M.R., Rush, W.L., DeFabo, E.C., and Merlino, G. 2001. Neonatal sunburn and melanoma in mice. *Nature,* **413**: 271–272.

Orengo, I. F, Black, H.S., Kettler, A.H., and Wolf, J.E., Jr. 1989. Influence of dietary menhaden oil upon carcinogenesis and various cutaneous responses to ultraviolet radiation. *Photochem Photobiol* **49**: 71–77.

Orengo, I.F., Black, H.S., and Wolf, J.E. 1992. Influence of fish oil supplementation on the minimal erythema dose in humans. *Arch Dermatol Res.* **284**: 219–221.

Orengo, I.F., Gerguis, J., Phillips, R., Guevara, A., Lewis, A.T., and Black, H.S. 2002. Celecoxib, a cyclooxygenase 2 inhibitor as a potential chemopreventive to UV-induced skin cancer. *Arch Dermatol* **138**: 751–755.

Parker, S.L., Tong, T., Bolden, S., and Wingo, P.A. 1997. Cancer statistics, 1997. *CA Cancer J Clin* **47**: 5–27.

Pauling, L., Willoughby, R., Reynolds, R., Blaisdell, B.E., and Lawson, S. 1982. Incidence of squamous cell carcinoma in hairless mice irradiated with ultraviolet light in relation to intake of ascorbic acid (vitamin C) and D,L-α-tocopheryl acetate (vitamin E). *Int J Vitam Nutr Res* **23**: 53–82.

Pentland, A.P., Schoggins, J.W., Scott, G.A., Khan, K.N.M., and Han, R. 1999. Reduction of UV-induced skin tumors in hairless mice by selective COX-2 inhibition. *Carcinogenesis* **20**: 1939–1944.

Peto, R., Doll, R., Buckley, J.D., and Spom, M.D. 1981. Can dietary β-carotene materially reduce human cancer rates? *Nature (London)* **290**: 201–208.

Plescia, O.J., and Racis, S. 1988. Prostaglandins as physiological immunoregulators. *Prog Allergy* **44**: 153–171.

Pott, P. 1775. "Chirurgical Observations," pp. 63–68. Hawes, Clarke, and Collins, London [as reproduced in *Natl Cancer Inst Monogr* **10**: 1–13 (1963)].

Potter, M. 1962. Percivall Pott's contribution to cancer research. *Natl Cancer Inst Monogr* **10**: 1–13.

Quisenberry, W.B. 1963. Ethnic differences in skin cancer in Hawaii. *Natl Cancer Inst Monogr* **10**: 181–189.

Rackett, S.C., Rothe, M.J., and Grant-Kels, J.M. 1993. Diet and dermatology. *J Am Acad Dermatol* **29**: 447–461.

Reeve, V.E., Matheson, M.J., Greenoak, G.E., Canfield, P.J., Boehm-Wilcox, C., and Gallagher, C.H. 1988. Effect of dietary lipid on UV light carcinogenesis in the hairless mouse. *Photochem Photobiol* **48**: 689–696.

Reeve, V.E., Matheson, M.J., Bosnic, M., and Boehm-Wilcox, C. 1995. The protective effect of indomethacin on photocarcinogenesis in hairless mice. *Cancer Lett* **95**: 213–219.

Reeve, V.E., Bosnic, M., and Boehm-Wilcox, C. 1996. Dependence of photocarcinogenesis and photoimmunosuppression in the hairless mouse on dietary polyunsaturated fat. *Cancer Lett* **108**: 271–279.

Rhodes, L.E., Azurdia, R.M., Dean, M.P., Moison, R., Steenwinkel, N.J., Beijersbergen van Henegouwen, G.M.J., and Vink, A.A. 2000. Systemic eicosapentaenoic acid reduces UVB-induced erythema and p53 induction in skin, while increasing oxidative stress, in a double-blind randomised study. *Br J Dermatol* **142**: 601–602.

Rhodes, L.E., Durham, B.H., Fraser, W.D., and Friedmann, P.S. 1995. Dietary fish oil reduces basal and ultraviolet B-generated PGE_2 levels in skin and increases the threshold to provocation of polymorphic light eruption. *J Invest Dermatol* **105**: 532–535.

Rhodes, L.E., O'Farrell, S., Jackson, M.J., and Friedmann, P.S. 1994. Dietary fish-oil supplementation in humans reduces UVB-erythemal sensitivity but increases epidermal lipid peroxidation. *J Invest Dermatol* **103**: 151–154.

Rhodes, L.E., Shahbakhti, H., Azurdia, R.M., Moison, R.M., Steenwinkel, M.J., Homburg, M.I., Dean, M.P., McArdle, F., Beijersbergen van Henegouwen, G.M.J., Epe, B., and Vink, A.A. 2003. Effect of eicosapentaenoic acid, an omega-3 polyunsaturated fatty acid, on UVR-related cancer risk in humans. An assessment of early genotoxic markers. *Carcinogenesis* **24**: 919–925.

Rigel, D.S., Kopf, A.W., and Friedman, R.J. 1987. The rate of malignant melanoma in the United States: Are we making an impact? *J Am Acad Dermatol* **17**: 1050–1053.

Roffo, A.H. 1929. La nutricion y el desarrollo de los tumores. Importanciade las lipoides. *Bol Inst Med Exp Estud Trat Cancer Buenos Aires* **5**: 170.

Roffo, A.H. 1933. Heliotropism of cholesterol in relation to skin cancer. *Am J Cancer* **17**: 42–57.

Roffo, A.H. 1939. Uber die physikalische-chemische atiologie der krebskrankheit. *Stralentherapie* **66**: 328–350.

Rous, P., and Kidd, J.G. 1941. Conditional neoplasms and subthreshold neoplastic states. *J Exp Med* **73**: 365–390.

Rusch, H.P., Kline, B.E., and Baumann, C.A. 1945. The influence of caloric restriction and of dietary fat on tumor formation with ultraviolet radiation. *Cancer Res* **5**: 431–435.

Schaumberg, D.A., Frieling, U.M., Rifai, N., and Cook, N. 2004. No effect of beta-carotene supplementation on risk of nonmelanoma skin cancer among men with low baseline plasma beta-carotene. *Cancer Epidemiol Biomarkers Prev* **13**: 1079–1080.

Scotto, J., Fears, T.R., and Fraumeni, J.F., Jr. 1983. "Incidence of Nonmelanoma Skin Cancer in the United States," NIH Publication No. 83-2433.U.S. Department of Health and Human Services, National Cancer Institute, Bethesda, MD.

Segi, M. 1963. World incidence and distribution of skin cancer. *Natl Cancer Inst Monogr* **10**: 245–255.

Setlow, R.B., Grist, E., Thompson, K., and Woodhead, A. 1993. Wavelengths effective in induction of malignant melanoma. *Proc Natl Acad Sci USA* **90**: 6666–6670.

Shield, A.M. 1899. A remarkable case of multiple growths of the skin caused by exposure to the sun. *Lancet* **1**: 22–23.

Silverstone, H., and Searle, J.H.A. 1970. The epidemiology of skin cancer in Queensland: The influence of phenotype and environment. *Br J Cancer* **24**: 235–252.

Stern, K.G., and Willheim, R. 1943. "The Biochemistry of Malignant Tumors," pp. 389–460. Reference Press, Brooklyn, NY.

Stern, R.S., Weinstein, M.C., and Baker, S.G. 1986. Risk reduction for nonmelanoma skin cancer with childhood sunscreen use. *Arch Dermatol* **122**: 537–545.

Stryker, W.S., Stampfer, M.J., Stein, E.A., Kaplan, L., Louis, T.A., Sober, A., and Willett, W.C. 1990. Diet, plasma levels of beta-carotene and alpha-tocopherol, and risk of malignant melanoma. *Am J Epidemiol* **131**: 597–611.

Sugiura, K., and Benedict, S.R. 1930. The influence of high fat diets on growth of carcinoma and sarcoma in rats. *J Cancer Res* **14**: 311–318.

Tangrea, J.A., Edwards, B.K., Taylor, P.R., Hartman, A.M., Peck, G.L., Salasche, S.J., Menon, P.A., Benson, P.M., Mellette, J.R., Guill, M.A., Robinson, J.K., Guin, J.D., Stoll, H.L., Granski, W.J., and Winton, G.B. 1992. Long-term therapy with low-dose isotretinoin for prevention of basal cell carcinoma: a multicenter clinical trial. *J Natl Cancer Inst* **84**: 328–332.

Tannenbaum, A. 1940a. Relationship of body weight to cancer incidence. *Arch Pathol* **30**: 509–517.

Tannenbaum, A. 1940b. The initiation and growth of tumors. I. Effects of underfeeding. *Am J Cancer* **38**: 335–350.

Tannenbaum, A. 1942a. The genesis and growth of tumors. II. Effects of caloric restriction per se. *Cancer Res* **2**: 460–467.

Tannenbaum, A. 1942b. The genesis and growth of tumors. III. Effects of a high-fat diet. *Cancer Res* **2**: 468–475.

Tannenbaum, A. 1944a. The dependence of the genesis of induced skin tumors on the caloric intake during different stages of carcinogenesis. *Cancer Res* **4**: 673–677.

Tannenbaum, A. 1944b. The dependence of the genesis of induced skin tumors on the fat content of the diet during different stages of carcinogenesis. *Cancer Res* **4**: 683–687.

Tannenbaum, A. 1953. Nutrition and cancer. *In* "The Physiopathology of Cancer" (F. Homburger and W.H. Fishman, Eds.), pp. 392–437. Harper (Hoeber), New York.

Tannenbaum, A. 1959. Nutrition and cancer. *In* "The Physiopathology of Cancer" (F. Homburger, ed.), 2nd edition, pp. 517–562. Harper (Hoeber), New York.

Tarrant, A.W.S. 1989. Basic principles of light measurement. *In* "Radiation Measurement in Photobiology" (B.L. Diffey, Ed.), pp. 1–21. Academic Press, London.

The α-Tocopherol, β-Carotene Cancer Prevention Study Group. 1996. The effect of vitamin E and β-Carotene on the incidence of lung cancer and other cancers in male smokers. *N Engl J Med* **330**: 1029–1035.

Thind, I.S. 1986. Diet and cancer—an international study. *Int J Epidemiol* **15**: 160–163.

Thody, A.J., and Friedmann, P.S. 1986. Functions of the skin. *In* "Scientific Basis of Dermatology" (A.J. Thody and P.S. Friedmann, Eds.), pp. 1–5. Churchill-Livingstone, Edinburgh.

Unna, P. 1894. "Histopathologie der Hautkrankheiten," pp. 719–724. Hirschwald, Berlin.

Urbach, F. 1969. Geographic pathology of skin cancer. *In* "The Biologic Effects of Ultraviolet Radiation" (F. Urbach, Ed.), pp. 635–650. Pergamon, Oxford.

Urbach, F. 1992–1993. Ultraviolet A transmission by modem sunscreens: Is there a real risk? *Photodermatol Photoimmunol Photomed* **9**: 237–241.

Urbach, F. 1997. Photocarcinogenesis: from the widow's coif to the p53 gene. *Photochem Photobiol* **65S**: 129S–133S.

Urbach, F., Epstein, J.H., and Forbes P.D. 1974. Ultraviolet carcinogenesis: experimental, global, and genetic aspects. *In* "Sunlight and Man" (T.B. Fitzpatrick, M.A. Pathak, L.C. Harber, M. Sieji, and A. Kukita, Eds.), pp. 259–283. University of Tokyo Press, Tokyo.

Urbach, F., Forbes, P.D., Davies, R.E., and Berger, D. 1976. Cutaneous photobiology: past, present and future. *J Invest Dermatol* **67**: 209–224.

van Dam, R.M., Huang, Z., Giovannucci, E., Rimm, E.B., Hunter, D.J., Colditz, G.A., Stampfer, M.J., and Willett, W.C. 2000. Diet and basal cell carcinoma of the skin in a prospective cohort of men. *Am J Clin Nutr* **71**: 135–141.

van Weelden, H., de Gruiji, F.R., and van der Leun, J.C. 1986. Carcinogenesis by UVA, with an attempt to access the carcinogenic risk of tanning with UVA and UVB. *In* " The Biological Effects of UVA Radiation" (F. Urbach and R.W. Gange, Eds.), pp. 137–146. Praeger, New York.

Visscher, M.B., Ball, Z.B., Bames, R.H., and Sivertsen, I. 1942. The influence of caloric restriction upon the incidence of spontaneous mammary carcinoma in mice. *Surgery (St. Louis)* **11**: 48–55.

Vitale, J.J., and Broitman, S.A. 1981. Lipids and immune function. *Cancer Res* **41**: 3706–3710.

Wang, Z.Y., and Agarwal, R., Bickers, D.R., and Muktar, H. 1991. Protection against ultraviolet B radiation–induced photocarcinogenesis in hairless mice by green tea polyphenols. *Carcinogenesis (London)* **12**: 1527–1530.

Watson, A.F., and Mellanby, E. 1930. Tar cancer in mice. II. The condition of the skin when modified by external treatment or diet, as a factor in influencing this cancerous reaction. *Br J Exp Pathol* **11**: 311–322.

Weindruch, R., Albanes, D., and Kritchevsky, D. 1991. *Hematol/Oncol Clin North Am* **5**: 79–89.

Weinstock, M.A. 1989. The epidemic of squamous cell carcinoma. *JAMA* **262**: 2138–2140.

Weinstock, M.A., Stampfer, M.J., Lew, R.A., Willett, W.C., and Sober, A.J. 1992. Case-control study of melanoma and dietary vitamin D: implications for advocacy of sun protection and sunscreen use. *J Invest Dermatol* **98**: 809–811.

Weisburger, J.H., Cohen, L.A., and Wynder, E.L. 1977. On the etiology and metabolic epidemiology of the main human cancers. *In* "Origins of Human Cancer" (H.H. Hiatt et al., Eds.), pp. 567–602. Cold Spring Harbor.

Winkelmann, R.K., Zollman, P.E., and Baldes, E.J. 1963. Squamous cell carcinoma produced by ultraviolet light in hairless mice. *J Invest Dermatol* **40**: 217–224.

Yamagiwa, K., and Ichikawa, K. 1918. Experimental study of the pathogenesis of carcinoma. *J. Cancer Res* **3**: 1–29.

CHAPTER

23

Colon Cancer

LEO TREYZON, GORDON OHNING, AND DAVID HEBER

INTRODUCTION

Colorectal cancer (CRC) is the third most common cancer in both men and women. It is the second leading cause of cancer death in the United States and is usually lethal when diagnosed at later stages of progression. In essentially all economically developed countries, the incidence of CRC is high. Both the number of new cases and the death rates are approximately equal for men and women. In the United States in 2005, 56,290 CRC deaths were projected to occur (American Cancer Society [ACS], 2005). It accounts for 10% of all new cases of cancer and 10% of all cases of cancer death. There were projected to be 145,300 new cases of CRC diagnosed in 2005. Of these cancers, 72% (104,950) occur in the colon and 28% (40,340) in the rectum.

Survival from CRC remains poor because precancerous polyps and early cancers are often asymptomatic, resulting in many cases being diagnosed at an advanced stage. This cancer is a highly preventable disease if precancerous lesions are diagnosed early because CRCs develop from adenomas, which are readily identified by colonoscopy. Surveillance research shows that the age-adjusted death rates have been declining for cancers of the colon and rectum since the late 1940s (ACS, 2005). The existing strategies for CRC prevention include dietary prevention, chemoprevention, and endoscopic prevention. Beginning at age 50 years, men and women who are at average risk for developing CRC are advised to begin screening. Fecal occult blood testing has demonstrated the ability to detect CRC, whereas virtual colonoscopy and fecal DNA analysis have yet to achieve adequate sensitivity to become primary screening tools. Flexible sigmoidoscopy and colonoscopy are recommended preventive measures that can detect and diagnose colonic polyps, which can then be removed, thus preventing the development of a cancer. Although distal colon polyps are poor predictors of subsequent polyps and cancer in the upper colon, the finding of a polyp should motivate changes in lifestyle and diet.

In 1981, two investigators (Doll and Peto, 1981), using international comparisons of exposure prevalences and disease rates, estimated that up to 90% of colon cancers may be related to diet and lifestyle. A number of hypotheses attempting to explain these patterns continue to be evaluated in observational and intervention studies. As with other common forms of cancer, the primary risk factor for CRC is age. More than 90% of diagnosed cases are in individuals older than 50 years (ACS, 2005). Risk is increased by a personal or family history of colon cancer and/or polyps or a personal history of long-standing inflammatory bowel disease. The main nutritional factors believed to influence the risk of this disease include obesity, red meat intake, calcium, vitamin D, folic acid, alcohol, fiber, phytonutrients, and the dietary fatty acids. Interactions of dietary factors that can neutralize mutagenic secondary bile acids have revealed interesting nutrient–nutrient interactions. Epidemiological studies have also uncovered interesting interactions among nutrients, such as alcohol and folic acid, which affect colon cancer risk.

The development of the Vogelstein model for multistep carcinogenesis is based on the progression of adenomatous colon polyps to cancer, providing insights into the epigenetic changes that occur in this process and providing molecular targets for cancer prevention strategies. The adenoma–carcinoma sequence of colorectal carcinogenesis consists of a progressive loss of differentiation and normal morphology

Copyright © 2006, Elsevier Inc.
All rights of reproduction in any form reserved.

in a growing lesion in association with the acquisition of somatic mutations and of aberrant methylation of CpG islands, leading to gene silencing. These molecular events are accompanied by functional changes, including increased mitosis and loss of apoptosis. Studies of families at increased risk of colon cancer have led to the discovery of inherited abnormalities of DNA mismatch repair enzymes and even to common genetic polymorphisms of metabolic enzymes such as GSTM1, which may affect individual responses to preventive phytochemicals. These nutrigenetics models in combination with the emerging evidence on nutrigenomics of phytochemicals in the colonic epithelium promise to provide important new insights helpful in designing strategies for colon cancer prevention through changes in diet and lifestyle.

Diet and lifestyle are most likely related to colon cancer etiology through overconsumption of energy, coupled with inadequate intakes of protective substances, including micronutrients, dietary fiber, and a variety of phytochemicals. The latter are biologically active secondary plant metabolites, many of which modify cell proliferation and induce apoptosis *in vitro*. There is growing evidence that such effects also occur *in vivo* and that they can suppress the progress of neoplasia. The risk of carcinomas of the colon appears to be reduced by diets rich in fruits and vegetables, but no definitive evidence has been provided by intervention trials. In fact, the largest such trial (see later discussion) did not demonstrate a reduction in polyp number with a global intervention based on reducing fat, increasing fiber, and increasing fruits and vegetables. Nonetheless, plant foods contain a variety of components including micronutrients, polyunsaturated fatty acids, and secondary metabolites such as glucosinolates and flavonoids, many of which can inhibit cell proliferation and induce apoptosis, and which may well act synergistically when combined in the human diet. The future challenge is to fully characterize and evaluate these effects at the cellular and molecular level, to exploit their full potential as protective mechanisms for the population as a whole. The power of early diagnosis via colonoscopy and the preventive potential of healthy diets and lifestyles should lead to further decreases in the incidence of colon cancer.

THE MULTISTEP PROCESS OF COLORECTAL CARCINOGENESIS

Colorectal carcinogenesis is a stepwise process. Through a series of nonlinear genetic alterations, carcinogenesis is characterized by changes from normal mucosa through early and advanced adenomas to invasive carcinoma (Vogelstein et al., 1988). Fearon and Vogelstein (1991) have proposed a phenomenological model of colorectal carcinogenesis correlating specific genetic events with evolving tissue morphology. This conceptual approach describes a system that proceeds linearly from normal mucosa to a small polyp to a large polyp to an invasive cancer, with each step driven by well-defined alterations in the genome. Some investigators regard this progression as "the adenoma–carcinoma sequence" (Renehan et al., 2002). Formation of a malignant tumor requires mutation of a cascade of genes (Figure 1). The first event is inactivation of the adenomatous polyposis coli (APC) gene in both chromosomes. APC, a tumor-suppressor gene, is inactivated by mutation and the mutagenesis cascade is initiated. Then, mutation in the oncogene k-*ras* and further mutation of other tumor-suppressing genes SMAD4 and TP53 occurs (Fodde et al., 2001). Other genetic events become important as well, for example, modulation of DNA methylation in CpG sequences of the promoter regions of tumor-suppressor and DNA-repair genes, leading to inactivation, or DNA amplification as a mechanism of oncogene activation (Kinsler and Vogelstein, 1996). These genetic insults are associated with the development of pre-neoplastic lesions such as aberrant crypt foci, polyps, and adenomas (Takayama et al., 1998). Up to 10% of all sporadic cancer types feature an additional pattern that is characterized by development of deficient DNA repair; this leads to genetic instability and, therefore, to an increased rate of mutation (Hawkins and Ward, 2001). This type of tumor often has k-*ras* mutations.

Increased cell proliferation occurs within the colonic crypt as one of the earliest events in the neoplastic process, as first suggested by Dukes (1932). An increased colonic epithelial proliferation rate and an expansion of the cryptal proliferative zone have been the object of extensive research as potential markers of increased susceptibility to colon cancer. An immunohistochemical method using 5-bromodeoxyuridine (BrdU) can measure the proliferation rate of colonic mucosa. Fresh endoscopic colonic biopsy specimens are incubated with BrdU and then processed for immunohistochemistry (IHC) using a monoclonal antibody. The proliferation rate is then expressed as the labeling index (LI). The mean LI in healthy controls has been found to be significantly lower than in patients with colonic polyps and in those with colon cancer. Often, controls are those referred for colonoscopy in whom no lesions are found. Although this method was promising for screening persons at risk for colon cancer and was thought to be of great potential in performing dietary intervention studies in high-risk subjects, results with dietary interventions have been disappointing. Since then, many investigators have found increased cellular proliferation in colonic crypts representing the earliest step in this sequence (Jass et al., 1997). However, many newer studies, using newer techniques, have failed to substantiate the initial literature (Jass et al., 1997).

It is now appreciated that the process of apoptosis is vital for normal crypt homeostasis. Its impairment may be an early event in the neoplastic process and this event is marked

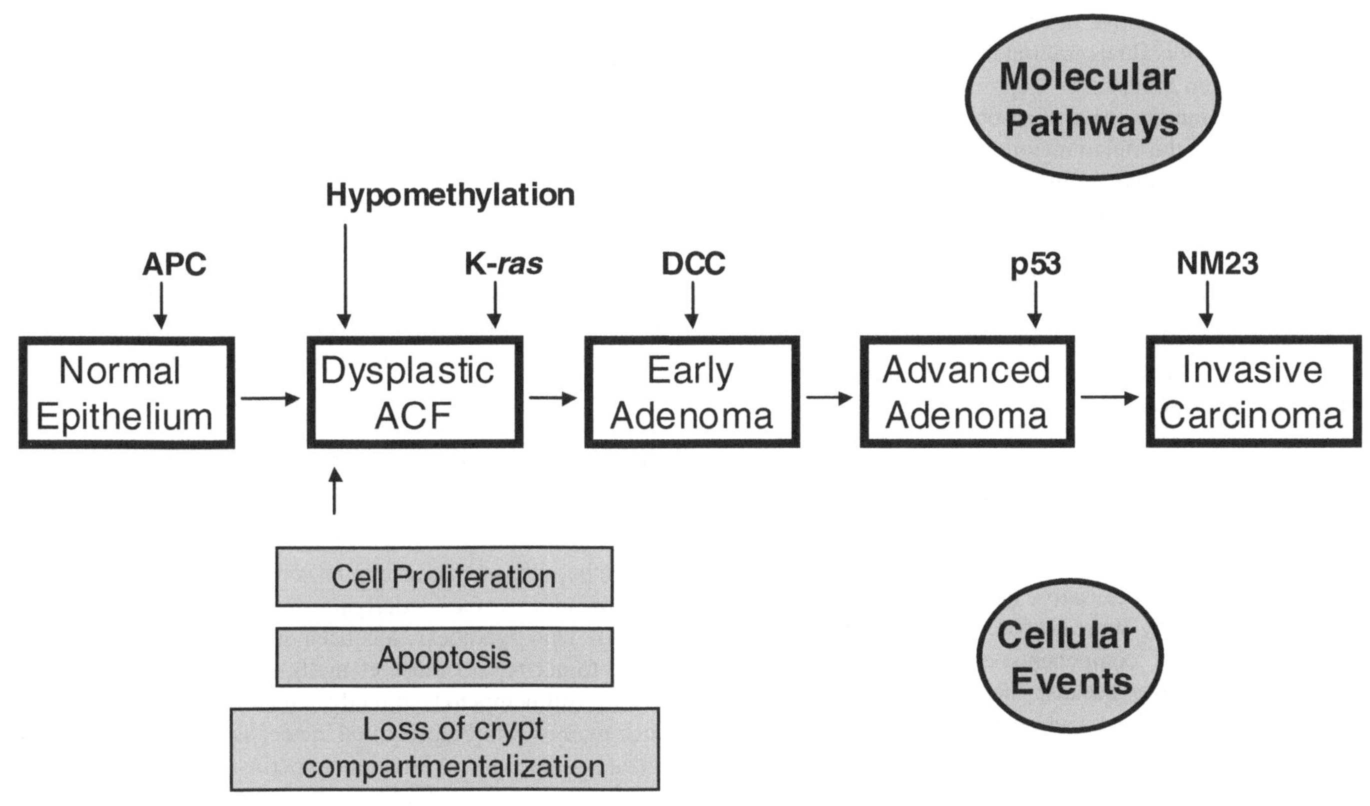

FIGURE 1 Aberrant crypt focus: adenoma–carcinoma sequence.

by the occurrence of aberrant crypt foci (ACFs) (Renehan et al., 2002). Two ACF types are identifiable: hypercellular and dysplastic. Hypercellular ACFs are more common and are never dysplastic. Increased proliferative activity may be seen in both. The dysplastic entity is most relevant to carcinogenesis. Both animal and human studies support the notion that ACFs grow by crypt fission, leading to formation of microadenoma (Renehan et al., 2002). Adenomas are monoclonal expansions of a disrupted cell, but very early lesions may be polyclonal. Distinction between hyperplastic and dysplastic aberrant crypts has important consequences for the use of biomarkers.

INHERITED AND SPONTANEOUS COLON CANCER

Inheritance of genetic alterations accounts for up to 20% of colorectal tumors (Berlau et al., 2004). The best-described genetic contributions include the syndrome familial adenomatous polyposis (FAP) and hereditary nonpolyposis colorectal cancer (HNPCC, or Lynch syndrome). HNPCC is a dominantly inherited syndrome characterized by the development of CRC, endometrial cancer, and other cancers, as well as the presence of microsatellite instability (MSI) in tumors. The Bethesda guidelines have been proposed for the identification of families suspected of having HNPCC that require further molecular analysis. The loss of mismatch repair (MMR) protein detected by IHC of CRC and endometrial cancer correlates with the presence of MSI and/or an MMR gene mutation. The Bethesda criteria, with a few modifications, are appropriate to identify families eligible for genetic testing. In addition, MSI and IHC analysis of CRC using antibodies against MLH1, MSH2, MSH6, and PMS2 proteins is equally effective for identifying carriers of the known MMR gene defects. Because other putative MMR genes in hereditary CRC have not been elucidated, IHC analysis cannot completely replace MSI. MSI analysis is still the first step in families suspected of HNPCC. In contrast, in families in which the probability of detecting a mutation is relatively high, IHC is the first diagnostic step because the result might predict the specific underlying MMR gene mutation (Vasen et al., 2004).

The identification of HNPCC is important because it makes it possible to target effective preventative measures. MSI and IHC analysis of CRC and endometrial cancer are reliable, cost-effective tools that can be used to identify patients with HNPCC. Such identification may make it more feasible to conduct dietary intervention trials in smaller numbers of subjects and to increase the likelihood of uncovering preventive interventions than when low-risk and high-risk individuals are randomly assigned to control and intervention groups.

Colorectal tumors are also associated with predisposing factors, namely the inflammatory bowel diseases (Crohn's disease and ulcerative colitis). The great percentage of colorectal tumors develop sporadically or are caused by exposure to environmental factors. Diet and lifestyle factors (discussed later in this chapter) may modulate genetic and biochemical processes that culminate in initiation, promotion, and progression of carcinogenesis. The evidence from epidemiological and limited intervention trials is reviewed in the following section.

NUTRITIONAL FACTORS IN COLON CANCER

Our knowledge of causative factors in colon carcinogenesis is supported by several epidemiological observations. Direct-acting food components could contribute to the occurrence of cancer because there is a direct interaction between food constituents and the mucosa.

Physiological traits, such as obesity, decreased physical activity level, and increased body mass index (BMI), have been reported to be involved in the promotion of colorectal tumorigenesis (Reddy, 1981). Physical inactivity might be associated with diminished mechanical stimulation of the colon, leading to less rapid defection. This increases the time that the mucosa is exposed to potential toxic metabolites. In addition to direct mechanisms, metabolites might also act indirectly to enhance lipid peroxidation (Berlau et al., 2004).

Energy Balance and Obesity

As previously mentioned, colon cancer rates are highly correlated with economic development or "Westernization." Although several factors related to the Western lifestyle may contribute to colon cancer, a large and growing body of evidence implicates energy balance. Many studies, including prospective studies, have found that obesity, usually assessed by BMI, is associated with an increased risk of colon cancer (Wu et al., 1987; Giovannucci et al., 1995; Martinez et al., 1997). The association appears to be stronger for men than for women, possibly because the relationship becomes weaker in women postmenopause (Terry et al., 2001). Evidence also suggests that a tendency for the central distribution of adipose (visceral adiposity) increases risk independently of BMI. For example, in a study of men (Giovannucci et al., 1995), when comparing upper to lower quintiles, the relative risk for colon cancer was about 3.5 in men with a high waist-to-hip ratio compared with those with a low ratio.

Physical Activity

Whereas obesity increases risk, physical activity is associated with a decrease in risk. Although physical activity is difficult to measure in epidemiological studies, >50 studies in diverse populations show that more physically active individuals are at lower risk for colon cancer, though not for rectal cancer (Giovannucci, 2002). Although physical activity is often associated with other lifestyle factors that may be related to colon cancer risk (Giovannucci et al., 1995), the inverse association between colon cancer risk and physical activity appears to be independent of confounders.

Hyperinsulinemia and IGF-1

The consistent findings for obesity, central obesity, and physical inactivity as risk factors for colon cancer have led to the hypothesis that insulin resistance and resulting hyperinsulinemia is the underlying risk factor (Giovannucci, 1995). This hypothesis has been supported by studies that have found type 2 diabetes mellitus (Hu et al., 1999) and hyperinsulinemia to be directly associated with colon cancer risk many years before colon cancer is diagnosed (Schoen et al., 1999). In addition to hyperinsulinemia, high concentrations of insulin-like growth factors (IGFs) also appear to increase risk of colorectal neoplasia. For example, acromegaly, a condition characterized by chronically elevated growth hormone levels resulting from a pituitary adenoma and IGF-1 hypersecretion, is associated with increased colonic epithelial cell proliferation (Cats et al., 1996) and elevated risk of benign and malignant colon tumors (Jenkins et al., 1997). Prospective studies have found high but normal circulating levels of IGF-1 related to elevated risk of colorectal neoplasia (Ma et al., 1999; Giovannucci et al., 2000).

Fruits, Vegetables, and Fiber

Most of the case-control studies (>15 studies) show an inverse association between intake of vegetables, and possibly fruits, and colon cancer risk (Giovannucci, 2002). Trock et al. (1990) conducted a metaanalysis of six case-control studies and found that a high intake of vegetables was associated with approximately half the risk for colon cancer, and high fiber was associated with an approximately 40% reduction in risk (Trock et al., 1990). Some studies fail to show a relationship for total fruits and vegetables (Michels et al., 2000). A randomized intervention study in which total servings of fruits and vegetables were increased without regard to the type of fruit or vegetable being eaten and using recurrent adenomas as the endpoint did not find a preventive effect of increasing fruit and vegetable intake (Schatzkin et al., 2000).

Dietary fiber has been the focus of numerous studies since it was first introduced as a potentially protective dietary component by Burkitt (1971). He observed that diseases of the bowel, including colon cancer, were rare in Africa where a high-fiber diet was consumed. Many correlational and case-control epidemiological studies support this hypothesis (Freudenheim et al., 1990; Martinez et al., 1997; Negri et al., 1998); however, several prospective studies have yielded equivocal results (Platz et al., 1997; Fuchs et al., 1999).

For the most part, relationships observed in well-designed observational studies have not been supported by interventional trials. The results of two randomized clinical trials failed to show a protective effect of increased fiber and/or decreased fat in the diet on the risk of adenomatous polyp recurrence (Alberts et al., 2000; Jacobs et al., 2002). In the Polyp Prevention Trial, there was no reduction in risk of colorectal adenoma recurrence with consumption of a low-fat, high-fiber diet (Jacobs et al., 2002). In one trial there was no difference in the rate of recurrent adenomatous polyps between those randomized to consume a high-fiber supplement as compared with those in the low-fiber group (Alberts et al., 2000). The additional studies that do not point to a cancer-preventive role of fiber include the Finnish ATBC study with >27,000 male volunteers older than 8 years (Pietinen et al., 1999), a cohort study with >45,000 female volunteers (Mai et al., 2003), and intervention trials with patients with existing colonic adenomas and prevention of recurrence by means of increased fiber intake (McKeown-Eyssen et al., 1994; Bonithon-Kopp et al., 2000; Schatzkin et al., 2000; Jacobs et al., 2002).

A Cochrane metaanalysis by Asano and McLeod (2002) found no evidence that increased dietary fiber reduces either incidence or recurrence of adenomatous polyps within a 2–4 year period. However, the largest single study performed (European EPIC study—performed with >500,000 volunteers in 22 European centers) revealed an inverse relationship between fiber intake and risk of developing colon cancer (Bingham et al., 2003). High fiber intake (>30 g/day) was associated with a 25% reduction in colon cancer risk (Bingham et al., 2003). Another study showed that for subjects with colonic adenoma fiber intake was lower, particularly from grains, cereals, and fruit (Peters et al., 2003).

It is clear that these data are conflicting. Explanations of these contradictory results might lie in the definition of low and high fiber intake. Compared with the last two studies, the fiber intake in the other studies was not exceptionally high. Moreover, it might not be the fiber itself that has the protective effect, but the whole pattern of a diet that provides less saturated and animal fat and more antioxidants, trace minerals, and phytoestrogens, which might be the real protective elements (Ferguson and Harris, 2003).

Red Meat

Early prospective cohort studies have been inconsistent with regard to implicating red meat intake with an increased risk of colon cancer risk (Bjelke, 1980; Phillips and Snowdon, 1984; Stemmermann et al., 1984). A number of prospective studies have shown statistically significant or suggestive positive associations for intake of processed meats and the risk of colon cancer (Bostick et al., 1994; Giovannucci et al., 1994; Goldbohm et al., 1994). Data from the prospective Health Professionals Follow-up Study (Giovannucci et al., 1994) and the Nurses' Health Study (Willett et al., 1990) showed a direct association between red meat consumption and risk of colon cancer, but no association was observed with other sources of fat or meats such as chicken or fish.

The cytotoxic effect of dietary heme has been proposed as a potential mechanism by which red meat increases CRC risk because of higher heme content in red meat compared with poultry and fish (Sesink et al., 1999; Cross et al., 2003). Heme damages the colonic mucosa and stimulates epithelial proliferation in animal studies (Sesink et al., 1999). Both ingestion of red meat and heme iron supplementation have been shown to increase fecal concentrations of N-nitroso compounds (Cross et al., 2003) and DNA adducts in human colonocytes (Hughes et al., 2001, 2002). Non–red meat sources of animal protein—including low-fat dairy products, fish, and poultry—have typically been associated with a lower risk of colon cancer or adenoma (Bostick et al., 1994; Giovannucci et al., 1994). The mechanism for this potential benefit is unknown, however. Diets high in these sources of protein, in contrast to red meat, may also be associated with other healthful behaviors. Regardless of the mechanism, the studies in general tend to support substitution of other protein sources for red meat. Few studies have examined risk in relation to long-term meat intake or the association of red meat with rectal cancer. In 2005, Chao et al. examined 185,000 patients in the CPS-II cohort and found that a high intake of red and processed meats was associated with a higher risk of colon cancer after adjusting for age and energy intake but not after further adjustment for BMI, cigarette smoking, and other covariates.

Results of some studies suggest that risk of colon cancer may be increased among meat eaters who consume meat with a heavily browned surface, but not among those who consume meat with a medium or lightly browned surface (Chen et al., 1998; Singh and Fraser, 1998). When meat undergoes prolonged frying, grilling, or broiling at high temperatures, mutagenic heterocyclic aromatic amines are formed from creatinine reacting with amino acids (Hsing et al., 1998). A metaanalysis of the epidemiological literature implicated processed meats as opposed to fresh meats (Thun et al., 1992). Ongoing and future investigations should substantiate whether levels of heterocyclic amines caused by cooking or nitrate compounds in processed meats present carcinogenic risks in humans.

Dietary Fats and Fatty Acids

Both the type and the amount of dietary fats consumed have been implicated in colon cancer etiology. Studies have demonstrated that n-3 polyunsaturated fatty acids (PUFAs), commonly found in fish oil, could prevent colon cancer development. Evidence shows that n-3 PUFAs act at different stages of cancer development and through several mechanisms including the modulation of arachidonic acid–derived prostaglandin synthesis, and Ras protein and protein kinase C expression and activity. As a result, n-3 PUFAs limit tumor cell proliferation, increase apoptotic potential along the crypt axis, promote cell differentiation, and possibly limit angiogenesis. The modulatory actions of n-3 PUFAs on the immune system and their anti-inflammatory effects might also play a role in reducing colon carcinogenesis. There remains, nevertheless, some ambiguity over the safety of n-3 PUFAs with respect to secondary tumor formation.

Epidemiological studies revealed a significantly lower incidence of CRC in Greenland Eskimo populations eating their traditional diet compared with reference populations in the West (Byers, 1996). This population consumed substantial amounts (>10.0 g/day) of long-chain n-3 PUFAs (EPA, DHA, and docosapentaenoic acid). In contrast, the Western diet contains approximately only 1–2 g/day of n-3 PUFAs, mostly as ALNA with long-chain n-3 PUFAs contributing <0.25 g/day (British Nutrition Foundation, 1992; British Nutrition Foundation, 1999). Japanese migrants to the United States who adopt an American diet have an increased colon cancer incidence compared with their counterparts in Japan, where long-chain n-3 PUFA consumption is high (Bingham, 1998). Analyses of data from 24 European countries indicate that a low ratio of n-3 to n-6 PUFAs in the diet is a risk factor for colon cancer (Caygill and Hill, 1995). Numerous studies conducted in rodents indicate that the incidence of chemically induced colon tumors is significantly lower in those animals fed fish oil–enriched diets than in those fed saturated fat– or vegetable oil–enriched diets. A fish oil–enriched diet has also decreased the growth of implanted murine colon tumors in mice (Cannizzo and Broitman, 1989) and human colon tumors in athymic mice (Calder et al., 1998) and has reduced tumor burden in a multiple intestinal neoplasia mouse model ($Apc^{Min/+}$) (Petrik et al., 2000). In a study of fish oil supplementation providing 4.1 g EPA and 3.6 g DHA per day in patients with sporadic adenomatous colorectal polyps, the percentage of cells in the S phase was reduced in the upper crypt of the rectal mucosa (Anti et al., 1992).

Vegetarian Diet

Vegetarians have an overall lower cancer rate compared with the general population, but it is not clear to what extent this is due to diet. When nondietary cancer risk factors are considered in the analysis, overall cancer rates between vegetarians and nonvegetarians are greatly reduced, although marked differences remain in rates of certain cancers. An analysis from the Adventist Health Study that controlled for age, sex, and smoking found no differences between vegetarians and nonvegetarians for lung, breast, uterine, or stomach cancer but did find that nonvegetarians had a 54% increased risk for prostate cancer and an 88% increased risk for CRC (Fraser, 1999). Other research has shown lower rates of colon cell proliferation in vegetarians compared with nonvegetarians (Lipkin et al., 1985) and lower levels of serum IGF-1, thought to be involved in the etiology of several cancers, in vegans compared with both nonvegetarians and lacto-ovo-vegetarians (Allen et al., 2000).

Multivitamins and Colon Cancer

Acute deficiencies of vitamins and minerals are rare in developed countries, but suboptimal nutrient intake—less than the recommended daily allowance (RDA)—is a widespread problem. Considerable metabolic damage can still occur when nutrient intake levels fall below the RDA—even though they might not cause acute disease.

Evidence indicates that deficiencies of iron and zinc and the vitamins folate, B12, B6, and C can cause DNA damage and lead to cancer. Reduced folate intake has been associated with cancer. Folate, B6, and B12 deficiencies cause the incorporation of deoxyuracil into DNA, leading to DNA breakage, and could promote tumorigenesis.

The relationship of vitamin and mineral deficiencies and cancer is extremely complex. An integrated analysis of the findings from epidemiological, animal model, metabolic, and intervention studies, as well as from genetic polymorphism research, is required. Approaches to eliminating micronutrient deficiencies include improving diet, fortifying foods, and providing multivitamin and mineral supplements. Prevention strategies such as these could have a significant impact on cancer and public health, with minimal risk being involved (Ames and Wakimoto, 2002).

Calcium

Calcium might reduce colon cancer risk by binding secondary bile acids and ionized fatty acids to form insoluble soaps in the lumen of the colon, thereby reducing the proliferative stimulus of these compounds on colon mucosa (Newmark et al., 1984; Van der Meer and de Vries, 1985). Calcium may also directly influence the proliferative activity of the colonic mucosa (Lipkin and Newmark., 1985).

Data from the large prospective studies are consistent in showing weak, nonsignificant inverse associations, although there is little evidence of a dose–response relationship (Martinez et al., 1998). The results of an intervention trial of calcium supplementation (1200 mg of elemental calcium vs placebo) among 913 participants found a statistically significant reduction in risk of adenoma recurrence, although this association was moderate (Baron et al., 1999). The adenoma recurrence rate in the calcium treatment group was 31%, and that of the placebo group was 38%. Similar results, though not statistically significant, were observed in the smaller European Calcium Fiber Polyp Prevention trial (Faivre et al., 1999). An analysis of cases from the Nurses' Health Study and the Health Professionals Follow-Up Study found that calcium reduced the risk of distal colon cancer but not of proximal colon cancer (Wu et al., 2002). The study also suggested a threshold effect whereby most of the benefit is achieved by reaching intakes of 700–800 mg/day. An interesting result from the Physicians' Health Study indicated that calcium exerts its protective influence primarily in men who have relatively high circulating concentrations of IGF-1; this result needs confirmation, however (Ma et al., 2001). To date, the results strongly suggest that avoiding a low intake of calcium is important for minimizing the risk of colon cancer; however, whether high intakes of calcium lower the risk is not clear.

Vitamin D

Vitamin D may have a role in the control of cell proliferation beyond that associated with the maintenance of blood-calcium concentrations. Cell culture studies consistently have shown decreases in cell proliferation in the presence of elevated vitamin D and calcium concentrations (Colston et al., 1981; Buset et al., 1986). There are several possible mechanisms of action. $1,25(OH)_2D$ induces cell differentiation and inhibits cell proliferation. It induces changes in gene expression involved in the control of cell proliferation. These include cyclin D1, Kip1, and WAF1, as well as c-Fos, c-Myc, cyclin C, c-Jun, and members of the TGF-beta family (Lamprecht and Lipkin, 2003). Cell differentiation and apoptosis are promoted by $1,25(OH)_2D$ through changes in gene expression (Diaz et al., 2000). Together, these mechanisms are potent regulators of cell proliferation and may have a strong antitumor activity.

Several animal studies have shown a reduction in colonic cell proliferation with the administration of vitamin D (Beaty et al., 1993; Mokady et al., 2000). Colonic cell proliferation was enhanced with the intake of a stress diet (low calcium and high phosphorus-to-calcium ratio). This effect was abrogated by the administration of supplemental dietary vitamin D. Moreover, the vitamin D supplement reduced formation of 1,2-dimethylhydrazine–induced tumors (Mokady et al., 2000). One study suggested an interaction between dietary calcium and vitamin D was necessary for a reduction in cell proliferation and colonic tumors (Beaty et al., 1993).

Epidemiological Studies

The results of epidemiological studies are mixed, with several finding a significant inverse relation between vitamin D/calcium and several colon cancer–related endpoints (Grau et al., 2003) and others not finding any association (Bostick et al., 1993). A nested case-control study found a higher risk of colorectal adenomas among subjects with the lowest plasma concentrations of $1,25(OH)_2D$ and 25(OH)D (Platz et al., 2000). The concentration–risk relations were not entirely consistent but generally showed lower risk with higher vitamin D concentrations. A Swedish study (569 cases) found significant inverse associations between dietary vitamin D and the risk of CRC (Protchard et al., 1996). A large U.S. cohort did not find an association between dietary calcium or vitamin D and the risk of colorectal adenomas (Kampman et al., 1994). A large case-control study (1953 cases) found an inverse association between dietary intakes of calcium and vitamin D with the risk of CRC (La Vecchia et al., 1997). A calcium supplementation study found significant interactions between calcium and vitamin D in the prevention of colorectal adenoma recurrence (Grau et al., 2003). The supplemented group was given 1200 mg of calcium per day for 4 years. A significant reduction in adenoma occurrence was found in the supplemented group. Serum 25(OH)D concentrations were inversely associated with a protective effect but only in the treatment group. No association was found between serum 25(OH)D concentrations and colorectal adenoma recurrence in the placebo group. The findings suggest that the vitamin D effect occurred only in the presence of high dietary calcium intakes and that vitamin D did not have an independent effect. Taken together, these results suggest the possible presence of unmeasured confounders and the possible dependence of a response on background diet, genetics, and other population characteristics (Gross, 2005).

New Approaches for Vitamin D, Calcium, and Colon Cancer

Studies in this area may benefit from better measures of exposure, a better understanding of interactions between mechanisms of vitamin D and calcium action, and characterization of *in vivo* cellular responses and intermediary markers. The measures of exposure would be improved by incorporation of 25(OH)D measurements. This measure was incorporated into several studies and may be expanded for the inclusion of replicate measurements to reduce misclassification of exposure and to provide an indication of the timeframe for changes in exposure. Additional mechanistic studies may define the circumstances required for interactions between vitamin D and calcium in the regulation of cell proliferation. These experiments could be performed with cell culture and animal models.

Further characterization of *in vivo* cellular responses may provide insights regarding the relation between calcium, vitamin D, and the risk of colon cancer. The mainstay of this area has been polyp formation and recurrence. The main limitation of this indicator is the slow rate of recurrence and formation. Vitamin D and calcium also may alter cell proliferation, apoptosis, and cell differentiation. The *in vivo* effects of vitamin D and calcium remain largely unknown for these colon cancer–related parameters (Gross 2005). Measurement of intermediary markers may provide a basis for understanding the inconsistent relations between vitamin D, calcium, and colon cancer in human populations.

Cruciferous Vegetables and Gene–Nutrient Interaction

The ability to upregulate detoxification systems is a defense mechanism to counteract damage of the colorectal mucosa by reactive compounds (Hoensch and Hartmann, 1981; Roediger and Babidge, 1997).

Essential is the glutathione (GSH)/glutathione *S*-transferase (GST) detoxification system, which comprises antioxidant reduced GSH and GSTs (EC 2.5.1.18); a family of phase II enzymes, which, in humans, consists of four main subgroups: alpha (α) mu (μ), pi, and theta (υ). Because this system plays an important role in detoxification of a broad range of carcinogens (Hayes and Pulford, 1995), high GST enzyme activity has been suggested as being beneficial to cancer prevention (Peters et al., 1991). Considering the low GST enzyme activity in the colon and rectum compared with tissues in which cancer occurs less frequently, it has been hypothesized previously that GST enzyme activity might be critically low and related to high rates of carcinogenesis (Peters et al., 1993).

Colonic GST enzyme activity and GST protein levels vary considerably among individuals (Coles et al., 2002; Ebert et al., 2003), which may be related to differential susceptibility to CRC. Individuals with homozygous deletions of *GSTM1* or *GSTT1* (null genotype) do not have detectable GSTM1 or GSTT1 enzyme activity, respectively, and were postulated to be at higher risk of CRC. However, no consistent associations of *GSTM1* and *GSTT1* null polymorphisms with risk of CRC have been observed (Cotton et al., 2000). Apart from inherited polymorphisms in GSTs, individuals may differ in GST enzyme activity because of differential exposure to bioactive compounds.

In vivo and *in vitro* studies have shown that a variety of dietary compounds or their metabolites can induce the GSH/GST detoxification system. These include glucosinolate metabolites and dithiolthiones present in Brassica vegetables, diallyl sulfides present in allium vegetables, limonoids and flavonoids present in citrus fruits (Hayes and Pulford, 1995), and butyrate produced by colonic fermentation of fiber (Ebert et al., 2003).

Evidence for induction of the human rectal GSH/GST detoxification system was found in a crossover study among 10 volunteers consuming 300 g/day of cooked Brussels sprouts during 7 days. This yielded 30 and 15% increases of GST-α and GSTP1-1 protein levels, respectively. However, no effect upon GST enzyme activity was found (Nijhoff et al., 1995), and taking 3 g/day of broccoli supplements for 14 days also did not influence GST enzyme activity in lymphocytes or colon mucosa (Clapper et al., 1997).

Nonetheless, indications of the upregulation of GST enzyme activity by Brassica and allium vegetables were found in blood plasma, urine, and saliva (Wark et al., 2004). Moreover, duodenal GST-α and GST-π protein levels were higher among subjects consuming vegetables at least four times a week, and antral GSTT1 protein levels were higher among subjects consuming fruits at least four times a week compared with those who consumed these products less frequently. However, no associations between frequency of consumption of fruits and vegetables and GST enzyme activity were found in these tissues (Hoensch et al., 2002).

Induction of the GSH/GST detoxification system by fruits and vegetables may partially account for the observed inverse associations between their consumption and risk of CRC (Steinmetz and Potter, 1996; Lampe et al., 2000).

NUTRIENT–NUTRIENT INTERACTIONS

Red meat, fat, and alcohol are suspected of increasing the formation of free radicals in the bowel, especially reactive oxygen species (Slattery et al., 1997). Free oxygen radicals and lipid degradation products (e.g., 4-hydroxyalkenals, aldehydes) are genotoxic (Bardou, 2002). In 1997, Erhardt demonstrated enhanced formation of hydroxyl radicals in feces from subjects consuming a diet rich in fat and meat but poor in fiber, in comparison with feces from those consuming a vegetarian diet (Erhardt et al., 1997). These radicals can react directly with DNA resulting in oxidized bases and, ultimately, mutations after replication (Nagata et al., 1982). Furthermore, free radicals could enhance the formation of secondary toxic metabolites, such as the very reactive degradation products of fatty acids (Owen et al., 2000).

Alcohol could enhance the tumor risk by being metabolized to the toxic metabolite acetaldehyde (Owen et al., 2000). Low folate uptake, combined with high alcohol intake, might pose yet another risk (Erhardt et al., 1997). For instance, lack of folate leads indirectly to physiologically disturbed DNA methylation, which might inhibit transcription of tumor suppressor genes (gene silencing) or increase transcription of protooncogenes (gene activation) (Nagata et al., 1982). Possible risk substances also include nitroso compounds, which can be formed in the gut after meat uptake (Esterbauer et al., 1990). High-temperature cooking, frying, and barbecuing of meat products can lead to the formation of contaminating products, which are mutagenic or carcinogenic (e.g., heterocyclic amines) (Homann et al., 1997). Unfortunately, our knowledge of which specific substances are actually responsible for molecular alterations in cell transformation is still fragmentary, and adequate toxicological assessment of relevant endogenous risk factors is usually still missing.

ANTIOXIDANTS AND PHYTOCHEMICALS

Vegetables and fruits are the major sources of most dietary antioxidants, so the weak results in studies raise doubt about the importance of dietary antioxidants for decreasing the risk of colon cancer. Some of the important dietary antioxidants, including vitamins C and E, carotenoids, and selenium, have also been evaluated in chemoprevention trials of adenoma recurrence. In general, antioxidant nutrients have yielded mixed results for the development of CRC (Alpha-Tocopherol Beta-Carotene Cancer Prevention Study Group, 1994; Clark et al., 1996) or adenoma recurrence (Paganelli et al., 1992; Greenberg et al., 1994; MacLennan et al., 1995); however, a >50% reduction in CRC incidence was shown for a selenium (in the form of brewer's yeast) intervention in the Nutritional Prevention of Skin Cancer (Clark et al., 1996). Because these results were based on secondary endpoint data among a population of selenium-deficient areas in the United States, it is believed that a large trial is necessary to confirm this provocative finding. In 2005, there was insufficient evidence to support recommendations that individuals obtain supplementary sources of antioxidants to reduce their risk of colon cancer.

One possible way to achieve a well-balanced diet is to increase the proportion of plant foods, fruits, and vegetables (Heber and Bowerman, 2001). Phytonutrients are substances that plants make for their own benefit but, when consumed by humans, lead to apparent reductions in incidence of chronic diseases, including CRC. Protective factors from plants, fruits, and vegetables have physical effects such as higher stool volume, decreased transit time, and absorption of mutagens to the fiber itself. They can also affect the release of certain beneficial fermentation products by the gut flora and plant substances with antioxidative potential and other chemoprotective properties (Priebe et al., 2002).

One of the defenses of the colonic epithelium is its mucinous layer. This has been reported to have capacity to detoxify reactive substances (Takayama et al., 1989). Despite the protective mucinous layer, colonocytes are still susceptible to damage from toxins. Compared with hepatocytes, colonocytes express relatively smaller amounts of phase II enzymes such as GST, which inactivate many genotoxic carcinogens (Takahashi et al., 1991). Plant substances or fermentation products (butyrate) from the gut can, however, induce these protective enzyme systems (Ochiai, 1991). Thus, it might be possible to maintain this mechanism of chemoprevention on a continuous optimal level by means of health-promoting nutrition. Results from animal experiments show that phytoprotectants and chemoprotectants such as ethoxyquin, butylated hydroxyanisole, butylated hydroxytoluene, oltipraz and indole-3-carbinol (Langouet et al., 2002), and high-amylose starch, which alters the fermentation profile and the composition of the gut microflora (Takahashi et al., 1991), induce GST-α and GST-π in non-transformed rat colon cells. These studies support the hypothesis that nutrition, by affecting the gut flora, can induce this potentially protective and important class of phase II enzymes in important tumor-target cells. This induction is supposed to provide increased protection from genotoxic carcinogens, as has been demonstrated experimentally for the liver (Pool-Zobel and Leucht, 1997).

CONCLUSION

Colon cancer is a diet-related cancer. Most incident colon cancer is preventable through modulation of nutritional choices over a lifetime. As far as this disease is the second leading cause of cancer death in the United States, with >56,000 projected deaths in 2005, it represents a high-priority area for further investigation. Survival remains poor because most cases are diagnosed at an advanced stage. The existing strategies for CRC prevention include dietary prevention, chemoprevention, and endoscopic prevention. Although distal colon polyps are poor predictors of subsequent polyp and cancer in the upper colon, the finding of a polyp should motivate changes in lifestyle and diet.

The main nutritional factors believed to influence the risk of this disease include obesity, increased red meat intake, calcium, vitamin D, folic acid, alcohol, fiber, phytonutrients, and dietary fatty acids. Epidemiological studies have also uncovered interesting interactions among nutrients such as alcohol and folic acid, which affect colon cancer risk.

Although the relative contributions of these individual dietary factors on colon carcinogenesis are still in question, it remains clear that healthy nutritional choices constitute the main prescription for colon cancer prevention at the societal level. Insofar as the prescription for avoidance of these harmful constituents and consumption of the beneficial ones is associated with prevention of other chronic diseases such as atherosclerotic heart disease, it can be assumed that there are health benefits that this prescription carries beyond colon cancer prevention.

The Vogelstein model for multistep colon carcinogenesis has provided insights into the epigenetic changes that occur in the process and has provided molecular targets for cancer prevention strategies. Nutritional factors have been shown to be effective at ameliorating transition at each of these steps.

Studies of families at increased risk of colon cancer have led to the discovery of inherited abnormalities of DNA mismatch repair enzymes and even to common genetic polymorphisms of metabolic enzymes such as GSTM1, which may affect individual responses to preventive phytochemicals. These nutrigenetic models in combination with the emerging evidence on nutrigenomics of phytochemicals in the colonic epithelium promise to provide important new insights helpful in designing strategies for colon cancer prevention through changes in diet and lifestyle.

Carcinomas of the colon appear to be partially preventable by diets rich in fruits and vegetables. Plant foods contain a variety of components including micronutrients, PUFAs, and secondary metabolites such as glucosinolates and flavonoids, many of which can inhibit cell proliferation and induce apoptosis and may act synergistically when combined in the human diet.

The challenge is to fully characterize and evaluate these effects at the cellular and molecular level to exploit their full potential as protective mechanisms for the population as a whole. The power of early diagnosis via colonoscopy, fecal DNA analysis, and the preventive potential of healthy diets and lifestyles should lead to further decreases in incident colon cancer.

References

ATBC Study Group. 1994. The effect of vitamin E and beta carotene on the incidence of lung cancer and other cancers in male smokers. The Alpha-Tocopherol, Beta Carotene Cancer Prevention Study Group. *N Engl J Med* **330**: 1029–1035.

Alberts, D.S., Martinez, M.E., et al. 2000. Lack of effect of a high-fiber cereal supplement on the recurrence of colorectal adenomas. Phoenix Colon Cancer Prevention Physicians' Network. *N Engl J Med* **342**: 1156–1162.

Allen, N.E., Appleby, P.N., et al. 2000. Hormones and diet: low insulin-like growth factor-I but normal bioavailable androgens in vegan men. *Br J Cancer* **83**: 95–97.

American Cancer Society [online] Cancer Facts and Figures. 2005. http://www.cancer.org [accessed 3.7.05]

Ames, B.N., and Wakimoto, P. 2002. Are vitamin and mineral deficiencies a major cancer risk? *Nat Rev Cancer* **2**: 694–704.

Anti, M., Marra, G., et al. 1992. Effect of omega-3 fatty acids on rectal mucosal cell proliferation in subjects at risk for colon cancer. *Gastroenterology* **103**: 883–891.

Asano, T., and McLeod, R.S. 2002. Dietary fibre for the prevention of colorectal adenomas and carcinomas. *Cochrane Database Syst Rev*(2), CD003430.

Bardou, M., Montembault, S., et al. 2002. Excessive alcohol consumption favours high risk polyp or colorectal cancer occurrence among patients with adenomas: a case control study. *Gut* **50**: 38–42.

Baron, J.A., Beach, M., et al. 1999. Calcium supplements for the prevention of colorectal adenomas. Calcium Polyp Prevention Study Group. *N Engl J Med* **340**: 101–107.

Beaty, M.M., Lee, E.Y., et al. 1993. Influence of dietary calcium and vitamin D on colon epithelial cell proliferation and 1,2-dimethylhydrazine-induced colon carcinogenesis in rats fed high fat diets. *J Nutr* **123**: 144–152.

Berlau, J., Glei, M., et al. 2004. Colon cancer risk factors from nutrition. *Anal Bioanal Chem* **378**: 737–743.

Bingham, S.A. 1998. Epidemiology of colorectal cancer. *In* "Encyclopedia of human nutrition" (J. Strain, M. Sadler, and B. Caballero, Eds.), Vol. 1, pp. 230–235. Academic Press, New York.

Bingham, S.A., Day, N.E., et al. 2003. Dietary fibre in food and protection against colorectal cancer in the European Prospective Investigation into Cancer and Nutrition (EPIC): an observational study. *Lancet* **361**: 1496–1501.

Bjelke, E. 1980. Epidemiology of colorectal cancer, with emphasis on diet. *In* "Human cancer. Its Characterization and Treatment" (W. Davis, K.R. Harrup, and G. Stathopoulos, Eds.), pp. 158–174. Amsterdam Exerpta Medica, Int, Amsterdam.

Bonithon-Kopp, C., Kronborg, O., et al. 2000. Calcium and fibre supplementation in prevention of colorectal adenoma recurrence: a randomised intervention trial. European Cancer Prevention Organisation Study Group. *Lancet* **356**: 1300–1306.

Bostick, R.M., Potter, J.D., et al. 1993. Calcium and colorectal epithelial cell proliferation: a preliminary randomized, double-blinded, placebo-controlled clinical trial. *J Natl Cancer Inst* **85**: 132–141.

Bostick, R.M., Potter, J.D., et al. 1994. Sugar, meat, and fat intake, and non-dietary risk factors for colon cancer incidence in Iowa women (United States). *Cancer Causes Control* **5**: 38–52.

British Nutrition Foundation. 1992. "Unsaturated Fatty Acids—Nutritional and Physiological Significance." British Nutrition Foundation, London.

British Nutrition Foundation. 1999. "Briefing Report: n-3 Fatty Acids and Human Health." British Nutrition Foundation, London.

Burkitt, D.P. 1971. Epidemiology of cancer of the colon and rectum. *Cancer* **28**: 3–13.

Buset, M., Lipkin, M., et al. 1986. Inhibition of human colonic epithelial cell proliferation in vivo and in vitro by calcium. *Cancer Res* **46**: 5426–5430.

Byers, T. 1996. Nutrition and cancer among American Indians and Alaska Natives. *Cancer* **78**: 1612–1616.

Calder, P.C., Davis, J., et al. 1998. Dietary fish oil suppresses human colon tumour growth in athymic mice. *Clin Sci (Lond)* **94**: 303–311.

Cannizzo, F., and Broitman, S.A. 1989. Postpromotional effects of dietary marine or safflower oils on large bowel or pulmonary implants of CT-26 in mice. *Cancer Res* **49**: 4289–4294.

Cats, A., Dullaart, R.P., et al. 1996. Increased epithelial cell proliferation in the colon of patients with acromegaly. *Cancer Res* **56**: 523–526.

Caygill, C.P., and Hill, M.J. 1995. Fish, n-3 fatty acids and human colorectal and breast cancer mortality. *Eur J Cancer Prev* **4**: 329–332.

Chao, A., Thun, M.J., et al. 2005. Meat consumption and risk of colorectal cancer. *JAMA* **293**: 172–182.

Chen, J., Stampfer, M.J., et al. 1998. A prospective study of N-acetyltransferase genotype, red meat intake, and risk of colorectal cancer. *Cancer Res* **58**: 3307–3311.

Clapper, M.L., Szarka, C.E., et al. 1997. Preclinical and clinical evaluation of broccoli supplements as inducers of glutathione S-transferase activity. *Clin Cancer Res* **3**: 25–30.

Clark, L.C., Combs, Jr.G.F., et al. 1996. Effects of selenium supplementation for cancer prevention in patients with carcinoma of the skin. A randomized controlled trial. Nutritional Prevention of Cancer Study Group. *JAMA* **276**: 1957–1963.

Coles, B.F., Chen, G., et al. 2002. Interindividual variation and organ-specific patterns of glutathione S-transferase alpha, mu, and pi expression in gastrointestinal tract mucosa of normal individuals. *Arch Biochem Biophys* **403**: 270–276.

Colston, K., Colston, M.J., et al. 1981. 1,25-dihydroxyvitamin D3 and malignant melanoma: the presence of receptors and inhibition of cell growth in culture. *Endocrinology* **108**: 1083–1086.

Comer, P.F., Clark, T.D., et al. 1993. Effect of dietary vitamin D3 (cholecalciferol) on colon carcinogenesis induced by 1,2-dimethylhydrazine in male Fischer 344 rats. *Nutr Cancer* **19**: 113–124.

Cotton, S.C., Sharp, L., et al. 2000. Glutathione S-transferase polymorphisms and colorectal cancer: a HuGE review. *Am J Epidemiol* **151**: 7–32.

Cross, A.J., Pollock, J.R., et al. 2003. Haem, not protein or inorganic iron, is responsible for endogenous intestinal N-nitrosation arising from red meat. *Cancer Res* **63**: 2358–2360.

Diaz, G.D., Paraskeva, C., et al. 2000. Apoptosis is induced by the active metabolite of vitamin D3 and its analogue EB1089 in colorectal adenoma and carcinoma cells: possible implications for prevention and therapy. *Cancer Res* **60**: 2304–2312.

Doll, R., and Peto, R. 1981. The causes of cancer: quantitative estimates of avoidable risks of cancer in the United States today. *J Natl Cancer Inst* **66**: 1191–1308.

Dukes, C. 1932. The classification of cancer of the rectum. *J Pathol Bacteriol* **35**: 323–333.

Ebert, M.N., Klinder, A., et al. 2003. Expression of glutathione S-transferases (GSTs) in human colon cells and inducibility of GSTM2 by butyrate. *Carcinogenesis* **24**: 1637–1644.

Erhardt, J.G., Lim, S.S., et al. 1997. A diet rich in fat and poor in dietary fiber increases the in vitro formation of reactive oxygen species in human feces. *J Nutr* **127**: 706–709.

Esterbauer, H., Eckl, P., et al. 1990. Possible mutagens derived from lipids and lipid precursors. *Mutat Res* **238**: 223–233.

Faivre, J., Bonithon-Kopp, C., Medicinne CINE FD. A randomized trial of calcium and fiber supplementation in the prevention of recurrence of colorectal adenomas. Presented at the American Gastroenterological Association Annual Meeting. Orlando, 1999.

Ferguson, L.R., and Harris, P.J. 2003. The dietary fibre debate: more food for thought. *Lancet* **361**: 1487–1488.

Fodde, R., Smits, R., et al. 2001. APC, signal transduction and genetic instability in colorectal cancer. *Nat Rev Cancer* **1**: 55–67.

Fraser, G.E. 1999. Associations between diet and cancer, ischemic heart disease, and all-cause mortality in non-Hispanic white California Seventh-Day Adventists. *Am J Clin Nutr* **70**: 532S–538S.

Freudenheim, J.L., Graham, S., et al. 1990. Risks associated with source of fiber and fiber components in cancer of the colon and rectum. *Cancer Res* **50**: 3295–3300.

Fuchs, C.S., Giovannucci, E.L., et al. 1999. Dietary fiber and the risk of colorectal cancer and adenoma in women. *N Engl J Med* **340**: 169–176.

Giovannucci, E. 1995. Insulin and colon cancer. *Cancer Causes Control* **6**: 164–179.

Giovannucci, E. 2002. Modifiable risk factors for colon cancer. *Gastroenterol Clin North Am* **31**: 925–943.

Giovannucci, E., Ascherio, A., et al. 1995. Physical activity, obesity, and risk for colon cancer and adenoma in men. *Ann Intern Med* **122**: 327–334.

Giovannucci, E., Pollak, M.N., et al. 2000. A prospective study of plasma insulin-like growth factor-1 and binding protein-3 and risk of colorectal neoplasia in women. *Cancer Epidemiol Biomarkers Prev* **9**: 345–349.

Giovannucci, E., Rimm, E.B., et al. 1994. Intake of fat, meat, and fiber in relation to risk of colon cancer in men. *Cancer Res* **54**: 2390–2397.

Goldbohm, R.A., van den Brandt, P.A., et al. 1994. A prospective cohort study on the relation between meat consumption and the risk of colon cancer. *Cancer Res* **54**: 718–723.

Grau, M.V., Baron, J.A., et al. 2003. Vitamin D, calcium supplementation, and colorectal adenomas: results of a randomized trial. *J Natl Cancer Inst* **95**: 1765–1771.

Greenberg, E.R., Baron, J.A., et al. 1994. A clinical trial of antioxidant vitamins to prevent colorectal adenoma. Polyp Prevention Study Group. *N Engl J Med* **331**: 141–147.

Gross, M.D. 2005. Vitamin D and calcium in the prevention of prostate and colon cancer: new approaches for the identification of needs. *J Nutr* **135**: 326–331.

Hawkins, N.J., and Ward, R.L. 2001. Sporadic colorectal cancers with microsatellite instability and their possible origin in hyperplastic polyps and serrated adenomas. *J Natl Cancer Inst* **93**: 1307–1313.

Hayes, J.D., and Pulford, D.J. 1995. The glutathione S-transferase supergene family: regulation of GST and the contribution of the isoenzymes to cancer chemoprotection and drug resistance. *Crit Rev Biochem Mol Biol* **30**: 445–600.

Heber, D., and Bowerman, S. 2001. "What Color Is Your Diet?" Harper Collins, New York.

Hoensch, H., Morgenstern, I., et al. 2002. Influence of clinical factors, diet, and drugs on the human upper gastrointestinal glutathione system. *Gut* **50**: 235–240.

Hoensch, H.P., and Hartmann, F. 1981. The intestinal enzymatic biotransformation system: potential role in protection from colon cancer. *Hepatogastroenterology* **28**: 221–228.

Homann, N., Jousimies-Somer, H., et al. 1997. High acetaldehyde levels in saliva after ethanol consumption: methodological aspects and pathogenetic implications. *Carcinogenesis* **18**: 1739–1743.

Hsing, A.W., McLaughlin, J.K., et al. 1998. Risk factors for colorectal cancer in a prospective study among U.S. white men. *Int J Cancer* **77**: 549–553.

Hu, F.B., Manson, J.E., et al. 1999. Prospective study of adult onset diabetes mellitus (type 2) and risk of colorectal cancer in women. *J Natl Cancer Inst* **91**: 542–547.

Hughes, R., Cross, A.J., et al. 2001. Dose-dependent effect of dietary meat on endogenous colonic N-nitrosation. *Carcinogenesis* **22**: 199–202.

Hughes, R., Pollock, J.R., et al. 2002. Effect of vegetables, tea, and soy on endogenous N-nitrosation, fecal ammonia, and fecal water genotoxicity during a high red meat diet in humans. *Nutr Cancer* **42**: 70–77.

Jacobs, E.T., Giuliano, A.R., et al. 2002. Intake of supplemental and total fiber and risk of colorectal adenoma recurrence in the wheat bran fiber trial. *Cancer Epidemiol Biomarkers Prev* **11**: 906–914.

Jass, J.R., Ajioka, Y., et al. 1997. Failure to detect colonic mucosal hyperproliferation in mutation positive members of a family with hereditary non-polyposis colorectal cancer. *Histopathology* **30**: 201–207.

Jenkins, P.J., Fairclough, P.D., et al. 1997. Acromegaly, colonic polyps and carcinoma. *Clin Endocrinol (Oxf)* **47**: 17–22.

Kampman, E., Giovannucci, E., et al. 1994. Calcium, vitamin D, dairy foods, and the occurrence of colorectal adenomas among men and women in two prospective studies. *Am J Epidemiol* **139**: 16–29.

Kato, I., Akhmedkhanov, A., et al. 1997. Prospective study of diet and female colorectal cancer: the New York University Women's Health Study. *Nutr Cancer* **28**: 276–281.

Kinzler, K.W., and Vogelstein, B. 1996. Lessons from hereditary colorectal cancer. *Cell* **87**: 159–170.

La Vecchia, C., Braga, C., et al. 1997. Intake of selected micronutrients and risk of colorectal cancer. *Int J Cancer* **73**: 525–530.

Lampe, J.W., Chen, C., et al. 2000. Modulation of human glutathione S-transferases by botanically defined vegetable diets. *Cancer Epidemiol Biomarkers Prev* **9**: 787–793.

Lamprecht, S.A., and Lipkin, M. 2003. Chemoprevention of colon cancer by calcium, vitamin D and folate: molecular mechanisms. *Nat Rev Cancer* **3**: 601–614.

Langouet, S., Paehler, A., et al. 2002. Differential metabolism of 2-amino-1-methyl-6-phenylimidazo[4,5-b]pyridine in rat and human hepatocytes. *Carcinogenesis* **23**: 115–122.

Lipkin, M., and Newmark, H. 1985. Effect of added dietary calcium on colonic epithelial-cell proliferation in subjects at high risk for familial colonic cancer. *N Engl J Med* **313**: 1381–1384.

Lipkin, M., Uehara, K., et al. 1985. Seventh-Day Adventist vegetarians have a quiescent proliferative activity in colonic mucosa. *Cancer Lett* **26**: 139–144.

Ma, J., Pollak, M.N., et al. 1999. Prospective study of colorectal cancer risk in men and plasma levels of insulin-like growth factor (IGF)-I and IGF-binding protein-3. *J Natl Cancer Inst* **91**: 620–625.

MacLennan, R., Macrae, F., et al. 1995. Randomized trial of intake of fat, fiber, and beta carotene to prevent colorectal adenomas. *J Natl Cancer Inst* **87**: 1760–1766.

Mai, V., Flood, A., et al. 2003. Dietary fibre and risk of colorectal cancer in the Breast Cancer Detection Demonstration Project (BCDDP) follow-up cohort. *Int J Epidemiol* **32**: 234–239.

Martinez, M.E., Giovannucci, E., et al. 1997. Leisure-time physical activity, body size, and colon cancer in women. Nurses' Health Study Research Group. *J Natl Cancer Inst* **89**: 948–955.

Martinez, M.E., McPherson, R.S., et al. 1997. A case-control study of dietary intake and other lifestyle risk factors for hyperplastic polyps. *Gastroenterology* **113**: 423–429.

Martinez, M.E., and Willett, W.C. 1998. Calcium, vitamin D, and colorectal cancer: a review of the epidemiologic evidence. *Cancer Epidemiol Biomarkers Prev* **7**: 163–168.

McKeown-Eyssen, G.E., Bright-See, E., et al. 1994. A randomized trial of a low fat high fibre diet in the recurrence of colorectal polyps. Toronto Polyp Prevention Group. *J Clin Epidemiol* **47**: 525–536.

Michels, K.B., Edward, G., et al. 2000. Prospective study of fruit and vegetable consumption and incidence of colon and rectal cancers. *J Natl Cancer Inst* **92**: 1740–1752.

Mokady, E., Schwartz, B., et al. 2000. A protective role of dietary vitamin D3 in rat colon carcinogenesis. *Nutr Cancer* **38**: 65–73.

Negri, E., Franceschi, S., et al. 1998. Fiber intake and risk of colorectal cancer. *Cancer Epidemiol Biomarkers Prev* **7**: 667–671.

Newmark, H.L., Wargovich, M.J., et al. 1984. Colon cancer and dietary fat, phosphate, and calcium: a hypothesis. *J Natl Cancer Inst* **72**: 1323–1325.

Nijhoff, W.A., Grubben, M.J., et al. 1995. Effects of consumption of Brussels sprouts on intestinal and lymphocytic glutathione S-transferases in humans. *Carcinogenesis* **16**: 2125–2128.

Ochiai, M., Ogawa, K., et al. 1991. Induction of intestinal adenocarcinomas by 2-amino-1-methyl-6-phenylimidazo[4,5-b]pyridine in Nagase analbuminemic rats. *Jpn J Cancer Res* **82**: 363–366.

Owen, R.W., Spiegelhalder, B., et al. 2000. Generation of reactive oxygen species by the faecal matrix. *Gut* **46**: 225–232.

Paganelli, G.M., Biasco, G., et al. 1992. Effect of vitamin A, C, and E supplementation on rectal cell proliferation in patients with colorectal adenomas. *J Natl Cancer* **84**: 47–51.

Peters, U., Sinha, R., et al. 2003. Dietary fibre and colorectal adenoma in a colorectal cancer early detection programme. *Lancet* **361**: 1491–1495.

Peters, W.H., Kock, L., et al. 1991. Biotransformation enzymes in human intestine: critical low levels in the colon? *Gut* **32**: 408–412.

Peters, W.H., Roelofs, H.M., et al. 1993. Glutathione and glutathione S-transferases in Barrett's epithelium. *Br J Cancer* **67**: 1413–1417.

Petrik, M.B., McEntee, M.F., et al. 2000. Antagonism of arachidonic acid is linked to the antitumorigenic effect of dietary eicosapentaenoic acid in Apc(Min/+) mice. *J Nutr* **130**: 1153–1158.

Phillips, R.L., and Snowdon, D.A. 1983. Association of meat and coffee use with cancers of the large bowel, breast, and prostate among Seventh-Day Adventists: preliminary results. *Cancer Res* **43**: 2403s–2408s.

Phillips, R.L., and Snowdon D.A. 1985. Dietary relationships with fatal colorectal cancer among Seventh-Day Adventists. *J Natl Cancer Inst* **74**: 307–317.

Pietinen, P., Malila, N., et al. 1999. Diet and risk of colorectal cancer in a cohort of Finnish men. *Cancer Causes Control* **10**: 387–396.

Platz, E.A., Giovannucci, E., et al. 1997. Dietary fiber and distal colorectal adenoma in men. *Cancer Epidemiol Biomarkers Prev* **6**: 661–670.

Platz, E.A., Hankinson, S.E., et al. 2000. Plasma 1,25-dihydroxy- and 25-hydroxyvitamin D and adenomatous polyps of the distal colorectum. *Cancer Epidemiol Biomarkers Prev* **9**: 1059–1065.

Pool-Zobel, B.L., and Leucht, U. 1997. Induction of DNA damage by risk factors of colon cancer in human colon cells derived from biopsies. *Mutat Res* **375**: 105–115.

Priebe, M.G., Vonk, R.J., et al. 2002. The physiology of colonic metabolism. Possibilities for interventions with pre- and probiotics. *Eur J Nutr* **41**: 2–10.

Pritchard, R.S., Baron, J.A., et al. 1996. Dietary calcium, vitamin D, and the risk of colorectal cancer in Stockholm, Sweden. *Cancer Epidemiol Biomarkers Prev* **5**: 897–900.

Reddy, B.S. 1981. Diet and excretion of bile acids. *Cancer Res* **41**: 3766–3768.

Reddy, B.S., and Sugie, S. 1988. Effect of different levels of omega-3 and omega-6 fatty acids on azoxymethane-induced colon carcinogenesis in F344 rats. *Cancer Res* **48**: 6642–6647.

Renehan, A.G., O'Dwyer, S.T., et al. 2002. Early cellular events in colorectal carcinogenesis. *Colorectal Dis* **4**: 76–89.

Roediger, W.E., and Babidge, W. 1997. Human colonocyte detoxification. *Gut* **41**: 731–734.

Schatzkin, A., Lanza, E., et al. 2000. Lack of effect of a low-fat, high-fiber diet on the recurrence of colorectal adenomas. Polyp Prevention Trial Study Group. *N Engl J Med* **342**: 1149–1155.

Schoen, R.E., Tangen, C.M., et al. 1999. Increased blood glucose and insulin, body size, and incident colorectal cancer. *J Natl Cancer Inst* **91**: 1147–1154.

Sesink, A.L., Termont, D.S., et al. 1999. Red meat and colon cancer: the cytotoxic and hyperproliferative effects of dietary heme. *Cancer Res* **59**: 5704–5709.

Singh, P.N., and Fraser, G.E. 1998. Dietary risk factors for colon cancer in a low-risk population. *Am J Epidemiol* **148**: 761–774.

Sitrin, M.D., Halline, A.G., et al. 1991. Dietary calcium and vitamin D modulate 1,2-dimethylhydrazine-induced colonic carcinogenesis in the rat. *Cancer Res* **51**: 5608–5613.

Slattery, M.L., Benson, J., et al. 1997. Dietary sugar and colon cancer. *Cancer Epidemiol Biomarkers Prev* **6**: 677–685.

Steinmetz, K.A., and Potter, J.D. 1996. Vegetables, fruit, and cancer prevention: a review. *J Am Diet Assoc* **96**: 1027–1039.

Stemmermann, G.N., Nomura, A.M., et al. 1984. Dietary fat and the risk of colorectal cancer. *Cancer Res* **44**: 4633–4637.

Takahashi, S., Ogawa, K., et al. 1991. Induction of aberrant crypt foci in the large intestine of F344 rats by oral administration of 2-amino-1-methyl-6-phenylimidazo[4,5-b]pyridine. *Jpn J Cancer Res* **82**: 135–137.

Takayama, K., Yamashita, K., et al. 1989. DNA modification by 2-amino-1-methyl-6-phenylimidazo[4,5-b]pyridine in rats. *Jpn J Cancer Res* **80**: 1145–1148.

Takayama, T., Katsuki, S., et al. 1998. Aberrant crypt foci of the colon as precursors of adenoma and cancer. *N Engl J Med* **339**: 1277–1284.

Talalay, P., Fahey, J.W., et al. 1995. Chemoprotection against cancer by phase 2 enzyme induction. *Toxicol Lett* **82**: 173–179.

Terry, P., Giovannucci, E., et al. 2001. Body weight and colorectal cancer risk in a cohort of Swedish women: relation varies by age and cancer site. *Br J Cancer* **85**: 346–349.

Thun, M.J., Calle, E.E., et al. 1992. Risk factors for fatal colon cancer in a large prospective study. *J Natl Cancer Inst* **84**: 1491–1500.

Tisdale, M.J., and Dhesi, J.K. 1990. Inhibition of weight loss by omega-3 fatty acids in an experimental cachexia model. *Cancer Res* **50**: 5022–5026.

Trock, B., Lanza, E., et al. 1990. Dietary fiber, vegetables, and colon cancer: critical review and meta-analyses of the epidemiologic evidence. *J Natl Cancer Inst* **82**: 650–661.

Van der Meer, R., and De Vries, H.T. 1985. Differential binding of glycine- and taurine-conjugated bile acids to insoluble calcium phosphate. *Biochem J* **229**: 265–268.

Vasen, H.F., Hendriks, Y., et al. 2004. Identification of HNPCC by molecular analysis of colorectal and endometrial tumors. *Dis Markers* **20**: 207–213.

Vogelstein, B., Fearon, E.R., et al. 1988. Genetic alterations during colorectal-tumor development. *N Engl J Med* **319**: 525–532.

Willett, W.C., Stampfer, M.J., et al. 1990. Relation of meat, fat, and fiber intake to the risk of colon cancer in a prospective study among women. *N Engl J Med* **323**: 1664–1672.

Wu, A.H., Paganini-Hill, A., et al. 1987. Alcohol, physical activity and other risk factors for colorectal cancer: a prospective study. *Br J Cancer* **55**: 687–694.

Wu, K., Willett, W.C., et al. 2002. Calcium intake and risk of colon cancer in women and men. *J Natl Cancer Inst* **94**: 437–446.

CHAPTER

24

Gastric Cancer

NAI-CHIEH YUKO YOU AND ZUO-FENG ZHANG

INTRODUCTION

Gastric cancer is the fourth leading cancer incidence in the world. It ranks second in cancer incidence for men, only behind lung cancer, and kills more than half a million people a year according to Globocan 2000. The incidence and mortality rates of gastric cancer have steadily declined worldwide in the past few decades. The reasons for the decline in incidence and mortality rates are not fully understood; however, dietary and lifestyle factors may be associated with the phenomena, including better refrigeration, reduced consumption of preserved foods, increased intake of fruits and vegetables, improved living standards, and a decline in the prevalence of *Helicobacter pylori* infection. A multifactorial model of human gastric carcinogenesis is currently suggested in which different dietary and nondietary factors, including genetic susceptibility of the host and *H. pylori* infection, are involved at different stages in the cancer process. Twin studies and immigrant studies have also suggested that dietary factors play an important role in the development of gastric cancer. Dietary modifications may potentially reduce the risk of gastric cancer. In this chapter, we review the epidemiological and animal experimental evidence regarding specific dietary factors in the etiology and prevention of gastric cancer. We discuss the major findings of chemoprevention trials for gastric cancer and the future directions for gastric cancer prevention and control research.

BACKGROUND

Gastric cancer ranks fourth in cancer incidence in the world for both sexes according to Globocan 2000 (Parkin et al., 2001a); however, it ranks second in cancer incidence for men, only behind lung cancer (Parkin et al., 2001a). The estimated number of new cases in 2000 was 876,300 worldwide, including 558,500 men and 317,900 women (Parkin et al., 2001a). It is the second leading cause of death from cancer. The estimated number of deaths in the year 2000 was 646,600 (Parkin et al., 2001a), accounting for >10% of all cancer deaths in the world. There is a great geographic variation observed in gastric cancer case distribution. Almost two-thirds of the cases occur in developing countries (Parkin et al., 2001b). High-risk areas include Japan, Central and South America, and Eastern Asia; however, significant differences are observed even within these areas. Incidence rates are low in Southern Asia, North and East Africa, and North America (Parkin et al., 2001b).

In the United States, gastric cancer is the fourteenth most common cancer in terms of incidence and the thirteenth most common cause of death from cancer (Jemal et al., 2003). The estimated numbers of new cases in 2003 were 13,400 men and 9000 women. The estimated number of deaths from gastric cancer was 12,100 (Jemal et al., 2003).

The survival rate for gastric cancer is moderately good only in Japan (52%) and ranges from 10 to 25% elsewhere (Parkin, 2001). The reason that Japan has the highest gastric cancer survival rate is that mass screening by photofluoroscopy has been practiced in the population since the 1960s (Parkin, 2001).

The incidence and mortality rates of gastric cancer have steadily declined in most countries (Parkin et al., 2001b). The estimated incidence rates in 2000 were ~11% lower than those for 1990 (Parkin, 2001), and there has been a 4–5% decrease in age-adjusted risk (Parkin et al., 1999). The decrease may be due to the improvements in preservation

Copyright © 2006, Elsevier Inc.
All rights of reproduction in any form reserved.

and storage of foods and the changes in the prevalence of *H. pylori* by birth cohort (Parkin, 2001). In contrast to the overall decreasing trend, there has been an increasing trend in cancers localized to the cardia of the stomach observed in several populations (Parkin, 2001; Parkin et al., 2001b). The reason is still not clear; however, these changes parallel the increased prevalence of Barrett's esophagus and adenocarcinoma of the lower third of the esophagus (Parkin, 2001; Parkin et al., 2001b).

The incidence rate of gastric cancer rises progressively with age (Lam, 1999; Kelley and Duggan, 2003). The age at which gastric cancer starts to appear is lower in Eastern Asians (~30 years of age) compared with the Western population (~50 years of age) (Lam, 1999). The risk of gastric cancer is higher in men than women (Parkin et al., 2001a; Kelley and Duggan, 2003). Gastric cancer prevalence varies with ethnic distribution, even for those living in the same region (Kelley and Duggan, 2003). Migrants from high-risk to low-risk regions tend to maintain the high-risk patterns of the population of origin (Kono and Hirohata, 1996; Parkin et al., 2001b). Low socioeconomic status is associated with a general increase in gastric cancer risk (Kono and Hirohata, 1996; Kelley and Duggan, 2003). First-degree relatives of patients with gastric cancer histories are at increased risk of about two to threefold (Kelley and Duggan, 2003). This may indicate that familial genetic abnormalities may alter individual susceptibility to gastric cancer carcinogens (Lam, 1999). Body mass index (BMI) above the lowest quartile is responsible for the 19.2% (95% confidence interval [CI], 4.9–52.0%) of gastric cardia adenocarcinoma (Engel et al., 2003).

Infection with *H. pylori* is considered an important risk factor for noncardia gastric cancers (Mayne and Navarro, 2002). The International Agency for Research on Cancer (IARC) accepted *H. pylori* infection as being carcinogenic for humans in 1994 (Parkin, 1998; Parkin et al., 2001b; Gonzalez, 2002). Meta-analyses have found that the infection increases the risk of noncardia gastric cancer by two to sixfold compared with noninfected control populations (Huang et al., 1998; Eslick et al., 1999; Xue et al., 2001). *H. pylori* may be responsible for causing ~40% of all gastric cancer cases worldwide (Parkin et al., 2001b).

In a twin study (Lichtenstein, 2000; O'Brien, 2000), model fitting found that inherited genes contributed 28% (95% CI, 0–51%), shared environmental factors 10% (95% CI, 0–34%), and environmental factors 62% (95% CI, 0–76%) to the etiology of gastric cancer. The results provide evidence that environmental and lifestyle patterns play major roles in gastric cancer. The constant decline in stomach cancer has been attributed to improved food preservation practices and better nutrition (Reed, 1993; Parkin et al., 2001b). The wide availability of refrigeration has changed the way of preserving food (Reed, 1993; Kono and Hirohata, 1996; Gonzalez, 2002; Kelley and Duggan, 2003); specifically, refrigeration may reduce the use of salt as a food preservative and decrease the likelihood of mold growth in food (Reed, 1993; Parkin et al., 2001b; Kelley and Duggan, 2003). Smoking weakly increased the risk of gastric cancer (Kono and Hirohata, 1996; Ogimoto et al., 2000; Parkin et al., 2001b; Mayne and Navarro, 2002; Kelley and Duggan, 2003). Other factors that may be associated with gastric cancer risk include blood type A, gastric surgery, gastric polyps, peptic ulcer disease, Epstein–Barr virus (EBV) infection, pernicious anemia (Kelley and Duggan, 2003), obesity (Mayne and Navarro, 2002), chronic reflux (Mayne and Navarro, 2002), use of table salt (Boeing et al., 1991b), the frequency of eating hot meals (Boeing et al., 1991b), irregular eating patterns (Boeing et al., 1991b), ionizing radiation, and asbestos exposure (Kelley and Duggan, 2003).

Studies provide evidence that some dietary factors and micronutrients may protect against gastric cancer. In this chapter, we review the epidemiological evidence regarding specific dietary factors in the etiology of gastric cancer. Furthermore, we also discuss the findings of previous and ongoing chemoprevention trials for gastric cancer.

DIETARY FACTORS AND GASTRIC CANCER

Fruit and Vegetable Consumption

The dominant dietary hypothesis is that fresh fruits and vegetables, or contained micronutrients and antioxidants, are protective against gastric cancer (Kelley and Duggan, 2003). Epidemiological studies have consistently found a decreased risk of gastric cancer associated with frequent consumption of fresh fruits and vegetables independent of other dietary factors. Most of the cohort studies showed a relative risk (RR) of 0.5–0.9, and case–control studies showed an odds ratio (OR) of 0.1–0.8 (Lam, 1999). The results are still remarkable even after adjustment for total caloric intake (Kono and Hirohata, 1996). The World Cancer Research Fund/American Institute of Cancer Research (WCRF/AICR) 1997 report and the COMA 1998 report concluded that there was moderate consistent evidence of the protective effect of vegetable and fruit consumption on gastric cancer (Ogimoto et al., 2000; Gonzalez, 2002). They also considered that some of those findings might be confounded by *H. pylori* infection. However, the strength of association, dose–response relationship, and consistency of results from those studies went against their doubts (Gonzalez, 2002). Furthermore, WCRF/AICR suggests that ~66–75% of gastric cancer risk could be reduced with high intake of fruits and vegetables in the past decade (Ogimoto et al., 2000; Gonzalez, 2002). The meta-analysis suggests that 40–50% of gastric cancer incidence could be prevented with high intake of fruits and vegetables (Steinmetz and Potter, 1991; Norat and Riboli, 2002).

Several studies consistently found that high vegetable intake, especially when consumed raw, may decrease gastric cancer risk (Jedrychowski et al., 1986; Kono et al., 1988; Gonzalez et al., 1991; Kono and Hirohata, 1996; Gao et al., 1999; Gonzalez, 2002). A Hawaiian study (Haenszel et al., 1972) observed a 40–50% decrease in gastric cancer risk among those who consumed high levels of each of the following Western-style vegetables: tomatoes, celery, corn, lettuce, and onions. A Polish study (Boeing et al., 1991b) found that increased consumption of vegetables and fruits, especially onions and radishes, decreased risk. For leeks, a Belgian study showed a protective effect against gastric cancer (Tuyns et al., 1992). Finally, a Chinese study suggested that tomato consumption may decrease risk (Gao et al., 1999).

Animal studies and *in vitro* studies that have suggested that garlic and onion extracts, compounds or their synthetically prepared analogues, may inhibit the development of several tumors (Dorant et al., 1993) provide evidence of the anticarcinogenic potential of several bioactive compounds in allium vegetables (Fleischauer and Arab, 2001). Interest has grown in the protective roles and mechanisms that allium vegetables may have in the etiology of stomach cancer. The allium genus of vegetables includes garlic, onions, leeks, scallions, chives, and shallots. These vegetables are characterized by a composition that is high in flavonols and organosulfur compounds (Fleischauer and Arab, 2001). A study in China (You et al., 1989) found that persons in the highest quartile of intake of total consumption of all allium vegetables (garlic, garlic stalks, leeks, Chinese chives and onions) experienced only 40% risk of those in the lowest quartile. Another Chinese study found that in a high-incidence area for gastric cancer, frequent intake of allium vegetables (including garlic, onion, Welsh onion, and Chinese chives) was inversely associated with the risk of gastric cancer (Gao et al., 1999). Garlic is the most studied allium vegetable. In a meta-analysis of the protective effect of garlic on the risk of gastric cancer, the RR estimate was 0.53 (95% CI, 0.31–0.92) (Fleischauer et al., 2000). However, when it comes to garlic products, low study power and lack of product variety limit the reliability of conclusions (Fleischauer et al., 2000). Onions are also a popular allium vegetable; however, the findings are inconsistent (Kono and Hirohata, 1996). A possible explanation for this inconsistency is that the preparation and serving methods of onions vary in different countries, and the effective contents of the vegetable may decrease depending on the cooking method.

Starchy Food

High gastric cancer risk regions (Japan, China, and Korea) also have been characterized as "high starchy food intake areas" (Mettlin, 1986); therefore, researchers have raised the possibility that starchy foods may be a risk factor for gastric cancer. Cereals, rice, wheat, noodles, pastas, breads, potatoes, and millets are classified as high-starch foods. One hypothesis is that high-starch, low-protein diets may favor acid-catalyzed nitrosation in the stomach as a result of the poor buffering capacity of such diets (Kono and Hirohata, 1996). Low-protein diets may decrease gastric mucous production and enhance carcinogen absorption (Kono and Hirohata, 1996). They may also cause mechanical damage in the gastric mucosa (Kono and Hirohata, 1996). Another hypothesis is that monotonous diets high in starchy food pose an increased risk, probably because they are deficient in protective dietary constituents (Parkin et al., 2001b). For example, there is an inverse colinearity association observed between dairy product consumption and starchy food consumption (Kono and Hirohata, 1996).

It is not easy to compare the studies among different countries or regions because of the huge variation in type and amount of starchy food consumed. Starchy food consumption is higher and less varied in most Asian countries compared with Western countries (Kono and Hirohata, 1996). Therefore, the findings of studies of high-starch food intake on gastric cancer risk are not as consistent as those of fresh fruits and vegetables or salty food intake (Kono and Hirohata, 1996). Most studies found that high consumption of carbohydrates, starch, or cereals increases the risk of gastric cancer (Bjelke, 1974; Modan et al., 1974; Risch et al., 1985; Trichopoulos et al., 1985; Graham et al., 1990; Buiatti et al., 1990; Tuyns et al., 1992; Ramon et al., 1993; Ji et al., 1996; Mathew et al., 2000), whereas other studies found opposite results (Correa et al., 1985; Gonzalez et al., 1991; Memik et al., 1992; Hansson et al., 1994). In the WCRF/AICR 1997 report, for instance, Ogimoto et al. (2000) suggested that whole-grain intake may be a protective factor for gastric cancer. For individual foods, pasta was found to increase the risk of cancer in Greece (Trichopoulos et al., 1985) and Italy (La Vecchia et al., 1987; Munoz et al., 1997). Rice consumption may increase gastric cancer risk of cancer in India (Mathew et al., 2000), Hawaii (among those of Japanese descent) (Haenszel et al., 1972), and Portugal (Azevedo et al., 1999), but not in Japan (Masaki et al., 2003) and China (You et al., 1988). For bread, several studies found that white bread consumption may increase risk (Wu-Williams et al., 1990; Tuyns et al., 1992; Memik et al., 1992; Ji et al., 1996; Munoz et al., 1997), while whole meal bread or nonwhite bread was found to reduce risk (Jedrychowski et al., 1986; Boeing et al., 1991a,b; Hansson et al., 1994).

Salt and Salty Food

The hypothesis that excess salt intake could be involved in the etiology of stomach cancer was first presented in 1965. It was postulated that the continuous use of high doses of salt would result in early atrophic gastritis, thereby increasing the later risk of stomach cancer (Joossens et al., 1996; Kelley and Duggan, 2003). Although salt is not a carcinogen by itself, it was hypothesized that salt may serve as a co-initiator and promoter in gastric carcinogenesis (Kono and Hirohata, 1996). The mechanism by which salt may be a co-initiator is by irritating gastric mucosa and initial lesions and, thereby, introducing superficial gastritis and atrophic gastritis. The mechanism of the promoting effect is by damaging stomach mucosa and thereby increasing DNA synthesis and cell proliferation, and thus increasing the possibility of endogenous mutation. These mechanisms were demonstrated by animal models (Kono and Hirohata, 1996).

Most of the studies estimated salt intake by measuring intake of salted fish, cured meat, and salted vegetables; only a few studies quantitatively estimated total salt intake (Kono and Hirohata, 1996; Ogimoto et al., 2000). Of the studies exploring the association between total salt intake and gastric cancer risk, six of them found positive associations (La Vecchia et al., 1987; Graham et al., 1990; Ramon et al., 1993; Nazario et al., 1993; Sriamporn et al., 2002; van den Brandt et al., 2003), and only one did not (Risch et al., 1985). The results suggest that heavy use of salt is compatible with a 50% increase in gastric cancer risk (Reed, 1993). For studies of salted fish, cured meat, and salted vegetable intake, almost all of them found an increased risk of gastric cancer (Kono and Hirohata, 1996). However, because of the huge variety of these preserved foods, the results may be confounded by other components of the foods.

Nitrite, Nitrate, and *N*-nitroso Compounds

N-nitroso compounds are known animal carcinogens, including *N*-nitrosodimethylamine and *N*-nitrosodiethylamine, which are classified as group 2A carcinogens. There is extensive evidence that they are carcinogenic to the stomach and other organs in animals (Mirvish, 1983; Lam, 1999). Such compounds may be formed in the human stomach from dietary nitrites or nitrates (Kelley and Duggan, 2003). Nitrate reacts with amines, amides, and other proteins and may be reduced bacterially to nitrites with the subsequent formation of *N*-nitroso compounds (Forman, 1989; Kono and Hirohata, 1996; Lam, 1999). The reduction of nitrates to highly reactive nitrites occurs through the action of nitrate-reducing bacteria in the saliva and hypoacidic stomach (Reed, 1993). However, endogenous *N*-nitroso compounds may also occur under normal gastric conditions (Reed, 1993). The major sources of nitrites and nitrates exposure for humans are vegetables, cured meat, and drinking water (Kono and Hirohata, 1996).

However, the evidence from epidemiological studies on dietary nitrates and gastric cancer is relatively weak. Of 15 ecological studies of nitrate exposure and gastric cancer risk in 10 countries, one-third showed increased risks, one-third showed decreased risks, and another third showed no association (Forman, 1989). Similar results were found in case-control studies. Seven found that nitrate may increase gastric cancer risk, but the associations were relatively weak (Risch et al., 1985; Correa et al., 1985; Buiatti et al., 1990; Boeing et al., 1991a; Palli et al., 1992; Gonzalez et al., 1994; Mayne et al., 2001; Kim et al., 2002), whereas others observed an inverse association (Hansson et al., 1994; Palli et al., 2001).

There are some factors that may confound the association between nitrates and gastric cancer. Concomitant intake of vitamin C and α-tocopherol in vegetables may counteract the increased risk of nitrates in vegetables (Lam, 1999). Many studies have evaluated nitrate exposure by evaluating cured meat or nitrate-cured food consumption. However, the results also may be due to other preservation compounds contained in those foods. Another issue is that nitrate intake may be an index of vegetable intake (Kono and Hirohata, 1996). Since vegetable intake is considered a protective factor for gastric cancer, the effect of nitrates may be obscured. In conclusion, more research and better dose evaluation methods are necessary to address this relation.

Soybean Products

Interest in soybean products and their role in gastric cancer prevention has increased among researchers in East Asian countries. Soybeans are an abundant source of isoflavones, which are antioxidants and possess other antitumor activities, including inhibition of angiogenesis, topoisomerase, and tyrosine kinase (Wu et al., 2000). There are two main categories of traditional soy foods: nonfermented and fermented. The main nonfermented soy foods include soy milk, tofu (bean curd), soybeans, and soy nuts. The main fermented soy foods include soy paste (miso in Japan) and fermented soybeans (natto in Japan) (Wu et al., 2000). The gastric cancer estimates for nonfermented soy foods were 0.61 (95% CI, 0.38–0.98) for the cohort studies and 0.73 (95% CI, 0.63–0.83) for the case-control studies (Wu et al., 2000). The meta-analysis estimates for fermented soy foods and gastric cancer risk were 1.13 (95% CI, 0.85–1.49) for cohort studies and 1.30 (95% CI, 1.13–1.50) for case-control studies (Wu et al., 2000). These results suggest that nonfermented soy food consumption may decrease risk of gastric cancer, whereas fermented soy foods or other compounds may increase risk.

Green Tea

The relation between tea consumption and gastric cancer has been addressed in many studies. The active components in green tea are polyphenols and mainly epigallocatechin gallate. The tea leaf polyphenol oxidase mediates oxidation to oolong and black tea, yielding other polyphenols, theaflavin and thearubigins (Weisburger and Chung, 2002). Experimental studies reveal that many polyphenolic compounds have demonstrated anticarcinogenic activities in animal models (Yang et al., 1997). Black tea was also effective, although the activity was weaker than green tea in some experiments. Decaffeinated tea preparations were also active in many model systems (Yang et al., 1997). The possible protective mechanisms of green tea on gastric cancer are (1) its action as an antioxidant, (2) the specific induction of detoxifying enzymes (including cytochrome P450 1A1, 1A2 and 2B1, and glucuronosyl transferase), (3) its molecular regulatory functions on cellular growth, development, and apoptosis (Hayakawa et al., 2001), and (4) a selective improvement in the function of the intestinal bacterial flora (Weisburger and Chung, 2002).

There is no conclusive result on gastric cancer when combining the observations on black tea and green tea (Lam, 1999). Looking at green tea only, six case-control studies (Kono et al., 1988; Yu et al., 1995; Ji et al., 1996; Inoue et al., 1998; Setiawan et al., 2001; Mu et al., 2003) observed a reduced risk of gastric cancer with a high level of green tea consumption, whereas prospective studies did not (Galanis et al., 1998; Tsubono et al., 2001; Hoshiyama et al., 2002). For black tea, most of the studies found no association with the risk of gastric cancer. The difference between green tea and black tea is the length of the fermentation process (Weisburger and Chung, 2002). Black tea is fermented for a longer time than green tea; therefore, in black tea some active components may be reduced or changed by the additional process.

Alcohol

Although drinking alcohol is an established cancer risk factor, ethanol per se is not a carcinogen. Although several possible mechanisms have been proposed (Blot, 1992), the mechanism by which alcohol induces cancer is not clear. The main components of all alcoholic beverages are ethanol and water; beer also contains substantial amounts of carbohydrates (IARC, 1988). The hypothesized mechanism is that ethanol could act as a syncarcinogen or a cocarcinogen. High concentrations of ethanol may cause local irritation in the upper gastrointestinal tract in humans after consumption of alcoholic beverages. Furthermore, ethanol will be oxidized to acetaldehyde, resulting in increased levels of acetaldehyde in the liver and blood. Acetaldehyde is a recognized animal carcinogen (IARC, 1985) and is suspected to be the key substance in alcohol-related cancer (IARC, 1988).

A 1994 review by Franceschi and La Vecchia of the experimental, descriptive, and analytical evidence relating to alcohol and gastric cancer found little to support an association. However, a meta-analysis found that alcohol consumption may elevate gastric cancer risk: ORs were 1.07 (95% CI, 1.04–1.10), 1.15 (95% CI, 1.09–1.22), and 1.32 (95% CI, 1.18–1.49) with alcohol intake of >25 g/day, 50 g/day, and 100 g/day, respectively (Bagnardi et al., 2001a,b). The results suggest that alcohol may be an important risk factor for gastric cancer.

Dietary Fat and Animal Protein

There is limited evidence that dietary fat and animal protein is associated with gastric cancer risk. Most of these studies found that fat and animal protein consumption may increase risk of gastric cancer (Zhang et al., 1997b; Lopez-Carrillo et al., 1999; De Stefani et al., 2001; Mayne et al., 2001; Palli et al., 2001; Chen et al., 2002; Thomson et al., 2003), whereas other studies failed to observe similar results (Reed, 1993; Ogimoto et al., 2000). Animal protein and fat consumption may induce reflux symptoms (Terry et al., 2000) and well-done meat may contain carcinogens (de Meester and Gerber, 1995). Japanese studies report a significantly positive association between grilled fish consumption and gastric cancer risk and suggest that grilled fish intake may be a risk factor for Japanese gastric cancer (Ogimoto et al., 2000).

Other Dietary Factors

Several studies have found that dietary fiber consumption was inversely associated with risk of gastric cancer (Tzonou et al., 1996; Zhang et al., 1997b; Terry et al., 2001; Chen et al., 2002). A Korean study (Kim et al., 2002) found that kimchi (prepared with salted Chinese cabbage and red pepper, etc.) consumption may protect against gastric cancer. Two case-control studies conducted in Mexico (Lopez-Carrillo et al., 1994, 2003) reported that chili pepper consumption may increase the risk of gastric cancer. Some studies suggest that milk consumption may be related to increased gastric cancer risk (Kneller et al., 1991; Memik et al., 1992; Hansson et al., 1993). Conversely, Boeing et al. (1991b) found that consumption of cheese products was associated with decreased gastric cancer risk. Self-reported use of supplemental calcium/Tums was found to be associated with a significant increase in the risk of gastric cancer because it may be associated with gastroesophageal reflux disease (GERD) (Mayne et al., 2001). A Swedish population-based case-control study (Akre et al., 2001) observed that aspirin users had a moderately reduced risk of stomach cancer (RR = 0.7), however, there was a significant inverse trend in risk with frequency of use.

MICRONUTRIENTS

With consistent observations that fresh fruit and vegetable intake may protect against gastric cancer, researchers hypothesize that the effect may be due to the micronutrients they contain. Vegetables and fruits are rich in vitamin C and carotenoids, and vegetables are also major sources of vitamin E and selenium (Kono and Hirohata, 1996). All of these micronutrients have antioxidative properties with different mechanisms. To further understand the protective mechanisms of fruits and vegetables, many studies have evaluated the effect of individual micronutrients in several populations.

Vitamin C

The current U.S. recommended daily allowance (RDA) for vitamin C for adults (>19 years) is 90 mg/day for men and 75 mg/day for women (Frei and Trabe, 2001). Vitamin C is widely distributed in fresh fruits and vegetables. It is present in fruits like oranges, lemons, grapefruits, watermelons, papayas, strawberries, cantaloupe, mangoes, pineapples, raspberries, and cherries. It is also found in green leafy vegetables, tomatoes, broccoli, green and red peppers, cauliflower, and cabbage (Naidu, 2003).

Most prospective and case-control studies have found a significant protective effect of dietary vitamin C intake on gastric cancer (Risch et al., 1985; Correa et al., 1985; La Vecchia et al., 1987; You et al., 1988; Buiatti et al., 1990; Boeing et al., 1991a; Ramon et al., 1993; Hansson et al., 1994; Gonzalez et al., 1994; De Stefani et al., 2001; Mayne et al., 2001; Palli et al., 2001). Vitamin C is an important dietary antioxidant; it significantly decreases the adverse effect of free radical species, which can cause oxidative damage to macromolecules such as lipids, DNA, and proteins (Naidu, 2003). Oxidative damage is implicated in chronic diseases including cardiovascular disease, stroke, cancer, neurodegenerative diseases, and cataractogenesis (Naidu, 2003). Another potential mechanism of vitamin C protection against gastric cancer is its function as a free radical scavenger and inhibitor of the formation of potentially carcinogenic *N*-nitroso compounds in the stomach (Naidu, 2003).

Vitamin E

The term *vitamin E* covers eight forms that are produced by plants alone: α-, β-, γ-, and δ-tocopherol and α-, β-, γ-, and δ-tocotrienol (Brigelius-Flohe et al., 2002). Tocotrienols have an unsaturated side chain, whereas tocopherols contain a phytyl tail with three chiral centers that naturally occur in the RRR configuration (Brigelius-Flohe et al., 2002). The mechanism of vitamin E on gastric cancer is the same as that for vitamin C. It acts as an antioxidant and may also inhibit the formation of *N*-nitroso compounds in the stomach. Vitamin C reduces *N*-nitroso compounds in the aqua phase, whereas vitamin E reduces *N*-nitroso compounds in the lipid phase.

The association between vitamin E and gastric cancer requires further research, as only three case-control studies (Buiatti et al., 1990; Hansson et al., 1994; Nomura et al., 2003) show significant inverse associations between vitamin E and gastric cancer.

Selenium

The antioxidative effect of selenium is linked with the activity of glutathione peroxidase, which acts against oxidative tissue damage (Kono and Hirohata, 1996). In animal studies, selenium can inhibit the development of several types of tumors (Kono and Hirohata, 1996). Dietary assessment of selenium intake is difficult because selenium content within food depends on the selenium content in soil (Kono and Hirohata, 1996). Vegetables and fruits contain selenium as well; therefore, it may influence the result of intervention trials. The selenium-rich fruits and vegetables include bananas, kiwi, strawberry, lima beans, peas, mushrooms, kale, and nuts. Epidemiological studies using serum selenium levels to estimate previous exposure show that low serum selenium levels are associated with increased gastric cancer risk (Knekt et al., 1990; Pawlowicz et al., 1991; Kabuto et al., 1994; Mark et al., 2000).

β-Carotene, Vitamin A, and Retinol

β-Carotene, like vitamins C and E, is a well-known free radical–trapping agent (Ferguson, 1999). β-Carotene, a violet to yellow plant pigment, can be converted to vitamin A by enzymes in the intestinal wall and liver. Retinol is an alcohol chemical form of vitamin A (Ferguson, 1999). Retinol is converted to retinal by metabolic oxidation and is biologically essential for light perception in the retina. Retinol is further transformed into retinoic acid by strictly controlled metabolic oxidation (Kakizoe, 2003).

Vitamin A and its analogues play important roles in cellular processes related to carcinogenesis (Ferguson, 1999). The important biological function of vitamin A is mainly through retinoic acid, which has a close relationship with important cellular functions such as morphogenesis, cellular proliferation, and cellular differentiation (Kakizoe, 2003) and may prevent the malignant transformation of cells (Kono and Hirohata, 1996).

Most case-control studies support the protective role of β-carotene on the risk of gastric cancer (Risch et al., 1985; La Vecchia et al., 1987; You et al., 1988; Buiatti et al., 1990; Ramon et al., 1993; Hansson et al., 1994; Kaaks et al., 1998; Azevedo et al., 1999; Ekstrom et al., 2000; Mayne et al., 2001; Jedrychowski et al., 2001; Nomura et al., 2003). There are also studies that found that retinol (Risch et al., 1985; Hansson et al., 1994; Jedrychowski et al., 2001), vitamin A (Azevedo et al., 1999; De Stefani et al., 2000), and β-carotene (De Stefani et al., 2000) intake have inverse associations with gastric cancer risk.

Other Micronutrients

Several studies have examined the association between other micronutrients and the risk of gastric cancer. The micronutrients that may have a protective effect are folate (Mayne et al., 2001; Nomura et al., 2003), vitamin B6 (Kaaks et al., 1998; Mayne et al., 2001), vitamins B1 and B3 (Kaaks et al., 1998), and lycopene (De Stefani et al., 2000). Those that may increase gastric cancer risk are vitamins B12 (Mayne et al., 2001) and B2 (Kaaks et al., 1998).

PREVENTION TRIALS FOR GASTRIC CANCER

Several chemoprevention trials have been done or are currently ongoing for gastric cancer prevention in the general population. Chemoprevention is defined as the use of specific agents to suppress or reverse carcinogenesis and thereby to prevent the development of cancers (Greenwald and Kelloff, 1996). Those trials are all focused on evaluating the effect of micronutrients that may reduce gastric cancer risk in several high-risk populations. The results from those trials may provide more insight into how these micronutrients prevent gastric cancer.

Nutrition Intervention Trials in Linxian, China

Linxian, China, has one of the highest gastric cancer rates in the world. In 1985, 29,584 healthy adults aged 40–69 years were recruited from four Linxian communes for a trial in which they received daily vitamin and mineral supplements. Mortality and cancer incidence were ascertained from March 1986 to May 1991 (Blot et al., 1993). This design enabled testing for the effects of four combinations of nutrients: (1) retinol and zinc, (2) riboflavin and niacin, (3) vitamin C and molybdenum, and (4) β-carotene, vitamin E, and selenium. Doses ranged from one to two times the U.S. RDAs. Total mortality was 13% lower among those receiving supplementation with β-carotene, vitamin E, and selenium (Blot et al., 1993). Gastric cancer incidence was 16% lower, and mortality was 21% lower. The prevalence of gastric cancer among participants receiving retinol and zinc was 62% lower than among those not receiving those supplements (Taylor et al., 1994). The pretrial serum micronutrient level analysis showed that the highest quartile of selenium was strongly associated with a reduced risk of gastric cancer (RR = 0.47; 95% CI, 0.33–0.65). The α-tocopherol level was also associated with reduced gastric cancer, but was not significant. The serum β-carotene and γ-tocopherol levels were not associated with the incidence of gastric cancer (Taylor et al., 2003).

The Alpha-Tocopherol, Beta-Carotene Study in Finland

In the Alpha-Tocopherol, Beta-Carotene (ATBC) study, 29,133 male smokers aged 50–69 years received either α-tocopherol (50 mg), β-carotene (20 mg), both agents, or a placebo daily for 5–8 years (The ATBC Cancer Prevention Study Group, 1994). Ascertainment of cancer cases during the intervention phase was via the Finnish Cancer Registry, which provides almost 100% case coverage. Neither α-tocopherol nor β-carotene supplementation had any association with end-of-trial prevalence of gastric cancer (Varis et al., 1998). However, the incidence of gastric cancer was slightly higher among men receiving β-carotene than among those not receiving it. Subgroup analyses by histological type suggested an increased risk of intestinal-type cancers with β-carotene. There were no differences across anatomical locations (cardia/noncardia) in the effects of α-tocopherol or β-carotene supplementation (Malila et al., 2002).

Randomized β-Carotene Trial of Male Physicians in the United States

A randomized, double-blind, placebo-controlled trial of β-carotene (50 mg on alternate days) recruited 22,071 male physicians, 40–84 years of age, in the United States (Hennekens et al., 1996). The trial began in 1982 to December 31, 1995. Less than 1% had been lost to follow-up, and compliance was 78% in the group that received β-carotene. Among 11,036 physicians randomly assigned to receive β-carotene and 11,035 assigned to receive placebo, virtually no difference was observed in the incidence of gastric cancer.

Other Trials

Several prevention trials are still ongoing. Hong initiated the first clinical trials of green tea extract with humans in the United States, in a population that did not previously consume green tea regularly. In 1997, the U.S. Food and Drug Administration (FDA) approved a phase I clinical trial with green tea capsules (Kakizoe, 2003). Another randomized trial is in progress to assess the effects of diet supplementation with β-carotene and vitamin C on the development of gastric cancer for high-risk persons with chronic atrophic gastritis in Akita, Japan, the region with the highest mortality from gastric cancer in Japan (Kakizoe, 2003).

The development of gastric cancer progresses from chronic gastritis to gastric atrophy, intestinal metaplasia, dysplasia, and finally invasive cancer (Correa, 1992). Several chemoprevention trials focus on a gastric premalignant lesion instead of gastric cancer. A chemoprevention trial in Columbia (Correa et al., 2000) with 1219 volunteers was assigned to receive anti–*H. pylori* triple therapy and/or dietary supplementation with ascorbic acid, β-carotene, or their corresponding placebos. The results found that all three interventions resulted in a significantly protective effect by increasing the rate of regression of cancer precursor lesions in the gastric mucosa. The results from those trials may provide more clues regarding gastric cancer prevention.

CONCLUSION AND FUTURE PERSPECTIVES

In conclusion, many present epidemiological studies provide evidence for the role of nutrition and diet on the risk of gastric cancer. However, the limitations of different study designs need to be considered. Although animal studies provide important evidence regarding the mechanisms involved, evidence regarding humans is still based primarily on case-control studies, which are susceptible to recall and selection bias. Prospective studies may provide better evidence, but such studies require long-term follow-up. Some prospective and case-control studies use serum levels to estimate current micronutrient consumption. The metabolism and half-life of these metabolites must be considered. Furthermore, any retrospective studies of gastric cancer must consider the health consequences of gastric cancer. Nutrient absorption may decrease as a result of gastric cancer. Gupta and Ihmaidat (2003) found an average of 15% weight loss, reduced indices of body fat, body protein, serum albumin, and total iron-binding capacity in gastric cancer patients.

Another issue pertaining to nutrition factors and gastric cancer research is the role of *H. pylori* infection. Not only is it an important risk factor, but it may interact with several micronutrients. *H. pylori* may be associated with various micronutrient deficiencies, including vitamins A, E, C, and B12 (Lacy and Rosemore, 2001; Yakoob et al., 2003) in both children and adults. Moreover, *in vitro* studies show that vitamin C may inhibit the growth of *H. pylori in vitro* and *in vivo* (Zhang et al., 1997a; Wang et al., 2000).

Interest in how dietary and micronutrient factors play preventive roles in gastric cancer is still growing. More well-designed epidemiological studies and clinical trials are necessary to clarify the mechanisms involved. Future perspectives of gastric cancer studies may focus on the study of molecular markers and gene–nutrient interaction epidemiology studies. The results may help to improve our understanding of genetic aspects of nutrition and gastric cancer and to aid in the future planning and designing of an appropriate intervention study to help establish prevention strategies for both high-risk and general populations.

References

Akre, K., Ekstrom, A.M., Signorello, L.B., Hansson, L.E., and Nyren, O. 2001. Aspirin and risk for gastric cancer: a population-based case–control study in Sweden. *Br J Cancer* **84**: 965–968.

Azevedo, L.F., Salgueiro, L.F., Claro, R., Teixeira-Pinto, A., and Costa-Pereira, A. 1999. Diet and gastric cancer in Portugal—a multivariate model. *Eur J Cancer Prev* **8**: 41–48.

Bagnardi, V., Blangiardo, M., La Vecchia, C., and Corrao, G. 2001a. A meta-analysis of alcohol drinking and cancer risk. *Br J Cancer* **85**: 1700–1705.

Bagnardi, V., Blangiardo, M., La Vecchia, C., and Corrao, G. 2001b. Alcohol consumption and the risk of cancer: a meta-analysis. *Alcohol Res Health* **25**: 263–270.

Bjelke, E. 1974. Epidemiologic studies of cancer of the stomach, colon, and rectum; with special emphasis on the role of diet. *Scand J Gastroenterol Suppl* **31**: 1–235.

Blot, W.J. 1992. Alcohol and cancer. *Cancer Res* **52**: 2119s–2123s.

Blot, W.J., Li, J.Y., Taylor, P.R., Guo, W., Dawsey, S., Wang, G.Q., Yang, C.S., Zheng, S.F., Gail, M., and Li, G.Y. 1993. Nutrition intervention trials in Linxian, China: supplementation with specific vitamin/mineral combinations, cancer incidence, and disease-specific mortality in the general population [see comments]. *J Natl Cancer Inst* **85**: 1483–1492.

Boeing, H., Frentzel-Beyme, R., Berger, M., Berndt, V., Gores, W., Korner, M., Lohmeier, R., Menarcher, A., Mannl, H.F., Meinhardt, M., et al. 1991a. Case–control study on stomach cancer in Germany. *Int J Cancer* **47**: 858–864.

Boeing, H., Jedrychowski, W., Wahrendorf, J., Popiela, T., Tobiasz-Adamczyk, B., and Kulig, A. 1991b. Dietary risk factors in intestinal and diffuse types of stomach cancer: a multicenter case–control study in Poland. *Cancer Causes Control* **2**: 227–233.

Brigelius-Flohe, R., Kelly, F.J., Salonen, J.T., Neuzil, J., Zingg, J.M., and Azzi, A. 2002. The European perspective on vitamin E: current knowledge and future research. *Am J Clin Nutr* **76**: 703–716.

Buiatti, E., Palli, D., Decarli, A., Amadori, D., Avellini, C., Bianchi, S., Bonaguri, C., Cipriani, F., Cocco, P., Giacosa, A., et al. 1990. A case–control study of gastric cancer and diet in Italy: II. Association with nutrients. *Int J Cancer* **45**: 896–901.

Chen, H., Tucker, K.L., Graubard, B.I., Heineman, E.F., Markin, R.S., Potischman, N.A., Russell, R.M., Weisenburger, D.D., and Ward, M.H. 2002. Nutrient intakes and adenocarcinoma of the esophagus and distal stomach. *Nutr Cancer* **42**: 33–40.

Correa, P. 1992. Human gastric carcinogenesis: a multistep and multifactorial process—First American Cancer Society Award Lecture on Cancer Epidemiology and Prevention. *Cancer Res* **52**: 6735–6740.

Correa, P., Fontham, E., Pickle, L.W., Chen, V., Lin, Y.P., and Haenszel, W. 1985. Dietary determinants of gastric cancer in south Louisiana inhabitants. *J Natl Cancer Inst* **75**: 645–654.

Correa, P., Fontham, E.T., Bravo, J.C., Bravo, L.E., Ruiz, B., Zarama, G., Realpe, J.L., Malcom, G.T., Li, D., Johnson, W.D., and Mera, R. 2000. Chemoprevention of gastric dysplasia: randomized trial of antioxidant supplements and anti–*Helicobacter pylori* therapy. *J Natl Cancer Inst* **92**: 1881–1888.

de Meester, C., and Gerber, G.B. 1995. The role of cooked food mutagens as possible etiological agents in human cancer. A critical appraisal of recent epidemiological investigations. *Rev Epidemiol Sante Publique* **43**: 147–161.

De Stefani, E., Boffetta, P., Brennan, P., Deneo-Pellegrini, H., Carzoglio, J.C., Ronco, A., and Mendilaharsu, M. 2000. Dietary carotenoids and risk of gastric cancer: a case–control study in Uruguay. *Eur J Cancer Prev* **9**: 329–334.

De Stefani, E., Ronco, A., Brennan, P., and Boffetta, P. 2001. Meat consumption and risk of stomach cancer in Uruguay: a case–control study. *Nutr Cancer* **40**: 103–107.

Dorant, E., van den Brandt, P.A., Goldbohm, R.A., Hermus, R.J., and Sturmans, F. 1993. Garlic and its significance for the prevention of cancer in humans: a critical view. *Br J Cancer* **67**: 424–429.

Ekstrom, A.M., Serafini, M., Nyren, O., Hansson, L.E., Ye, W., and Wolk, A. 2000. Dietary antioxidant intake and the risk of cardia cancer and noncardia cancer of the intestinal and diffuse types: a population-based case–control study in Sweden. *Int J Cancer* **87**: 133–140.

Engel, L.S., Chow, W.H., Vaughan, T.L., Gammon, M.D., Risch, H.A., Stanford, J.L., Schoenberg, J.B., Mayne, S.T., Dubrow, R., Rotterdam, H., West, A.B., Blaser, M., Blot, W.J., Gail, M.H., and Fraumeni, J.F., Jr. 2003. Population attributable risks of esophageal and gastric cancers. *J Natl Cancer Inst* **95**: 1404–1413.

Eslick, G.D., Lim, L.L., Byles, J.E., Xia, H.H., and Talley, N.J. 1999. Association of *Helicobacter pylori* infection with gastric carcinoma: a meta-analysis. *Am J Gastroenterol* **94**: 2373–2379.

Ferguson, L.R. 1999. Prospects for cancer prevention. *Mutat Res* **428**: 329–338.

Fleischauer, A.T., and Arab, L. 2001. Garlic and cancer: a critical review of the epidemiologic literature. *J Nutr* **131**: 1032S–1040S.

Fleischauer, A.T., Poole, C., and Arab, L. 2000. Garlic consumption and cancer prevention: meta-analyses of colorectal and stomach cancers. *Am J Clin Nutr* **72**: 1047–1052.

Forman, D. 1989. Are nitrates a significant risk factor in human cancer? *Cancer Surv* **8**: 443–458.

Franceschi, S., and La Vecchia, C. 1994. Alcohol and the risk of cancers of the stomach and colon-rectum. *Dig Dis* **12**: 276–289.

Frei, B., and Trabe, M.G. 2001. The new US Dietary Reference Intakes for vitamins C and E. *Redox Rep* **6**: 5–9.

Galanis, D.J., Kolonel, L.N., Lee, J., and Nomura, A. 1998. Intakes of selected foods and beverages and the incidence of gastric cancer among the Japanese residents of Hawaii: a prospective study. *Int J Epidemiol* **27**: 173–180.

Gao, C.M., Takezaki, T., Ding, J.H., Li, M.S., and Tajima, K. 1999. Protective effect of allium vegetables against both esophageal and stomach cancer: a simultaneous case-referent study of a high-epidemic area in Jiangsu Province, China. *Jpn J Cancer Res* **90**: 614–621.

Gonzalez, C.A. 2002. Vegetable, fruit and cereal consumption and gastric cancer risk. *IARC Sci Publ* **156**: 79–83.

Gonzalez, C.A., Riboli, E., Badosa, J., Batiste, E., Cardona, T., Pita, S., Sanz, J.M., Torrent, M., and Agudo, A. 1994. Nutritional factors and gastric cancer in Spain. *Am J Epidemiol* **139**: 466–473.

Gonzalez, C.A., Sanz, J.M., Marcos, G., Pita, S., Brullet, E., Saigi, E., Badia, A., and Riboli, E. 1991. Dietary factors and stomach cancer in Spain: a multi-centre case–control study. *Int J Cancer* **49**: 513–519.

Graham, S., Haughey, B., Marshall, J., Brasure, J., Zielezny, M., Freudenheim, J., West, D., Nolan, J., and Wilkinson, G. 1990. Diet in the epidemiology of gastric cancer. *Nutr Cancer* **13**: 19–34.

Greenwald, P., and Kelloff, G.J. 1996. The role of chemoprevention in cancer control. *IARC Sci Publ* 13–22.

Gupta, R., and Ihmaidat, H. 2003. Nutritional effects of oesophageal, gastric and pancreatic carcinoma. *Eur J Surg Oncol* **29**: 634–643.

Haenszel, W., Kurihara, M., Segi, M., and Lee, R.K. 1972. Stomach cancer among Japanese in Hawaii. *J Natl Cancer Inst* **49**: 969–988.

Hansson, L.E., Nyren, O., Bergstrom, R., Wolk, A., Lindgren, A., Baron, J., and Adami, H.O. 1993. Diet and risk of gastric cancer. A population-based case–control study in Sweden. *Int J Cancer* **55**: 181–189.

Hansson, L.E., Nyren, O., Bergstrom, R., Wolk, A., Lindgren, A., Baron, J., and Adami, H.O. 1994. Nutrients and gastric cancer risk. A population-based case–control study in Sweden. *Int J Cancer* **57**: 638–644.

Hayakawa, S., Kimura, T., Saeki, K., Koyama, Y., Aoyagi, Y., Noro, T., Nakamura, Y., and Isemura, M. 2001. Apoptosis-inducing activity of high molecular weight fractions of tea extracts. *Biosci Biotechnol Biochem* **65**: 459–462.

Hennekens, C.H., Buring, J.E., Manson, J.E., Stampfer, M., Rosner, B., Cook, N.R., Belanger, C., LaMotte, F., Gaziano, J.M., Ridker, P.M., Willett, W., and Peto, R. 1996. Lack of effect of long-term supplementation with beta carotene on the incidence of malignant neoplasms and cardiovascular disease. *N Engl J Med* **334**: 1145–1149.

Hoshiyama, Y., Kawaguchi, T., Miura, Y., Mizoue, T., Tokui, N., Yatsuya, H., Sakata, K., Kondo, T., Kikuchi, S., Toyoshima, H., Hayakawa, N., Tamakoshi, A., Ohno, Y., and Yoshimura, T. 2002. A prospective study of stomach cancer death in relation to green tea consumption in Japan. *Br J Cancer* **87**: 309–313.

Huang, J.Q., Sridhar, S., Chen, Y., and Hunt, R.H. 1998. Meta-analysis of the relationship between *Helicobacter pylori* seropositivity and gastric cancer. *Gastroenterology* **114**: 1169–1179.

Inoue, M., Tajima, K., Hirose, K., Hamajima, N., Takezaki, T., Kuroishi, T., and Tominaga, S. 1998. Tea and coffee consumption and the risk of digestive tract cancers: data from a comparative case-referent study in Japan. *Cancer Causes Control* **9**: 209–216.

International Agency for Research on Cancer. 1985. Allyl compounds, aldehyde, epoxides and peroxides, IARC monographs on the evaluation of the carcinogenic risk of chemicals to humans. IARC monographs on the evaluation of the carcinogenic risks to humans 36. IARC, Lyon, France.

International Agency for Research on Cancer. 1988. Alcohol drinking. IARC monographs on the evaluation of the carcinogenic risks to humans 44. IARC, Lyon, France.

Jedrychowski, W., Popiela, T., Steindorf, K., Tobiasz-Adamczyk, B., Kulig, J., Penar, A., and Wahrendorf, J. 2001. Nutrient intake patterns in gastric and colorectal cancers. *Int J Occup Med Environ Health* **14**: 391–395.

Jedrychowski, W., Wahrendorf, J., Popiela, T., and Rachtan, J. 1986. A case–control study of dietary factors and stomach cancer risk in Poland. *Int J Cancer* **37**: 837–842.

Jemal, A., Murray, T., Samuels, A., Ghafoor, A., Ward, E., and Thun, M.J. 2003. Cancer statistics, 2003. *CA Cancer J Clin* **53**: 5–26.

Ji, B.T., Chow, W.H., Yang, G., McLaughlin, J.K., Gao, R.N., Zheng, W., Shu, X.O., Jin, F., Fraumeni, J.F., Jr., and Gao, Y.T. 1996. The influence of cigarette smoking, alcohol, and green tea consumption on the risk of carcinoma of the cardia and distal stomach in Shanghai, China. *Cancer* **77**: 2449–2457.

Joossens, J.V., Hill, M.J., Elliott, P., Stamler, R., Lesaffre, E., Dyer, A., Nichols, R., and Kesteloot, H. 1996. Dietary salt, nitrate and stomach cancer mortality in 24 countries. European Cancer Prevention (ECP) and the INTERSALT Cooperative Research Group. *Int J Epidemiol* **25**: 494–504.

Kaaks, R., Tuyns, A.J., Haelterman, M., and Riboli, E. 1998. Nutrient intake patterns and gastric cancer risk: a case–control study in Belgium. *Int J Cancer* **78**: 415–420.

Kabuto, M., Imai, H., Yonezawa, C., Neriishi, K., Akiba, S., Kato, H., Suzuki, T., Land, C.E., and Blot, W.J. 1994. Prediagnostic serum selenium and zinc levels and subsequent risk of lung and stomach cancer in Japan. *Cancer Epidemiol Biomarkers Prev* **3**: 465–469.

Kakizoe, T. 2003. Chemoprevention of cancer—focusing on clinical trials. *Jpn J Clin Oncol* **33**: 421–442.

Kelley, J.R., and Duggan, J.M. 2003. Gastric cancer epidemiology and risk factors. *J Clin Epidemiol* **56**: 1–9.

Kim, H.J., Chang, W.K., Kim, M.K., Lee, S.S., and Choi, B.Y. 2002. Dietary factors and gastric cancer in Korea: a case–control study. *Int J Cancer* **97**: 531–535.

Knekt, P., Aromaa, A., Maatela, J., Alfthan, G., Aaran, R.K., Hakama, M., Hakulinen, T., Peto, R., and Teppo, L. 1990. Serum selenium and subsequent risk of cancer among Finnish men and women. *J Natl Cancer Inst* **82**: 864–868.

Kneller, R.W., McLaughlin, J.K., Bjelke, E., Schuman, L.M., Blot, W.J., Wacholder, S., Gridley, G., CoChien, H.T., and Fraumeni, J.F., Jr. 1991. A cohort study of stomach cancer in a high-risk American population. *Cancer* **68**: 672–678.

Kono, S., and Hirohata, T. 1996. Nutrition and stomach cancer. *Cancer Causes Control* **7**: 41–55.

Kono, S., Ikeda, M., Tokudome, S., and Kuratsune, M. 1988. A case–control study of gastric cancer and diet in northern Kyushu, Japan. *Jpn J Cancer Res* **79**: 1067–1074.

La Vecchia, C., Negri, E., Decarli, A., D'Avanzo, B., and Franceschi, S. 1987. A case–control study of diet and gastric cancer in northern Italy. *Int J Cancer* **40**: 484–489.

Lacy, B.E., and Rosemore, J. 2001. *Helicobacter pylori*: ulcers and more: the beginning of an era. *J Nutr* **131**: 2789S–2793S.

Lam, S.K. 1999. 9th Seah Cheng Siang Memorial Lecture: gastric cancer—where are we now? *Ann Acad Med Singapore* **28**: 881–889.

Lopez-Carrillo, L., Hernandez, A.M., and Dubrow, R. 1994. Chili pepper consumption and gastric cancer in Mexico: a case–control study. *Am J Epidemiol* **139**: 263–271.

Lopez-Carrillo, L., Lopez-Cervantes, M., Robles-Diaz, G., Ramirez-Espitia, A., Mohar-Betancourt, A., Meneses-Garcia, A., Lopez-Vidal, Y., and Blair, A. 2003. Capsaicin consumption, *Helicobacter pylori* positivity and gastric cancer in Mexico. *Int J Cancer* **106**: 277–282.

Lopez-Carrillo, L., Lopez-Cervantes, M., Ward, M.H., Bravo-Alvarado, J., and Ramirez-Espitia, A. 1999. Nutrient intake and gastric cancer in Mexico. *Int J Cancer* **83**: 601–605.

Malila, N., Taylor, P.R., Virtanen, M.J., Korhonen, P., Huttunen, J.K., Albanes, D., and Virtamo, J. 2002. Effects of alpha-tocopherol and beta-carotene supplementation on gastric cancer incidence in male smokers (ATBC Study, Finland). *Cancer Causes Control* **13**: 617–623.

Mark, S.D., Qiao, Y.L., Dawsey, S.M., Wu, Y.P., Katki, H., Gunter, E.W., Fraumeni, J.F., Jr., Blot, W.J., Dong, Z.W., and Taylor, P.R. 2000. Prospective study of serum selenium levels and incident esophageal and gastric cancers. *J Natl Cancer Inst* **92**: 1753–1763.

Masaki, M., Sugimori, H., Nakamura, K., and Tadera, M. 2003. Dietary patterns and stomach cancer among middle-aged male workers in Tokyo. *Asian Pac J Cancer Prev* **4**: 61–66.

Mathew, A., Gangadharan, P., Varghese, C., and Nair, M.K. 2000. Diet and stomach cancer: a case–control study in South India. *Eur J Cancer Prev* **9**: 89–97.

Mayne, S.T., and Navarro, S.A. 2002. Diet, obesity and reflux in the etiology of adenocarcinomas of the esophagus and gastric cardia in humans. *J Nutr* **132**: 3467S–3470S.

Mayne, S.T., Risch, H.A., Dubrow, R., Chow, W.H., Gammon, M.D., Vaughan, T.L., Farrow, D.C., Schoenberg, J.B., Stanford, J.L., Ahsan, H., West, A.B., Rotterdam, H., Blot, W.J., and Fraumeni, J.F., Jr. 2001. Nutrient intake and risk of subtypes of esophageal and gastric cancer. *Cancer Epidemiol Biomarkers Prev* **10**: 1055–1062.

Memik, F., Nak, S.G., Gulten, M., and Ozturk, M. 1992. Gastric carcinoma in northwestern Turkey: epidemiologic characteristics. *J Environ Pathol Toxicol Oncol* **11**: 335–338.

Mettlin, C. 1986. Dietary factors for cancer of specific sites. *Surg Clin North Am* **66**: 917–929.

Mirvish, S.S. 1983. The etiology of gastric cancer. Intragastric nitrosamide formation and other theories. *J Natl Cancer Inst* **71**: 629–647.

Modan, B., Lubin, F., Barell, V., Greenberg, R.A., Modan, M., and Graham, S. 1974. The role of starches in etiology of gastric cancer. *Cancer* **34**: 2087–2092.

Mu, L.N., Zhou, X.F., Ding, B.G., Wang, R.H., Zhang, Z.F., Jiang, Q.W., and Yu, S.Z. 2003. [Study on the protective effect of green tea on gastric, liver and esophageal cancers]. *Zhonghua Yu Fang Yi Xue Za Zhi* **37**: 171–173.

Munoz, S.E., Ferraroni, M., La Vecchia, C., and Decarli, A. 1997. Gastric cancer risk factors in subjects with family history. *Cancer Epidemiol Biomarkers Prev* **6**: 137–140.

Naidu, K.A. 2003. Vitamin C in human health and disease is still a mystery? An overview. *Nutr J* **2**: 7.

Nazario, C.M., Szklo, M., Diamond, E., Roman-Franco, A., Climent, C., Suarez, E., and Conde, J.G. 1993. Salt and gastric cancer: a case–control study in Puerto Rico. *Int J Epidemiol* **22**: 790–797.

Nomura, A.M., Hankin, J.H., Kolonel, L.N., Wilkens, L.R., Goodman, M.T., and Stemmermann, G.N. 2003. Case–control study of diet and other risk factors for gastric cancer in Hawaii (United States). *Cancer Causes Control* **14**: 547–558.

Norat, T., and Riboli, E. 2002. Fruit and vegetable consumption and risk of cancer of the digestive tract: meta-analysis of published case–control and cohort studies. *IARC Sci Publ* **156**: 123–125.

O'Brien, J.M. 2000. Environmental and heritable factors in the causation of cancer: analyses of cohorts of twins from Sweden, Denmark, and Finland, by P. Lichtenstein, N.V. Holm, P.K. Verkasalo, A. Iliadou, J. Kaprio, M. Koskenvuo, E. Pukkala, A. Skytthe, and K. Hemminki. *N Engl J Med* **343**: 78–84, 2000. *Surv Ophthalmol* **45**: 167–168.

Ogimoto, I., Shibata, A., and Fukuda, K. 2000. World Cancer Research Fund/American Institute of Cancer Research 1997 recommendations: applicability to digestive tract cancer in Japan. *Cancer Causes Control* **11**: 9–23.

Palli, D., Bianchi, S., Decarli, A., Cipriani, F., Avellini, C., Cocco, P., Falcini, F., Puntoni, R., Russo, A., Vindigni, C., et al. 1992. A case–control study of cancers of the gastric cardia in Italy. *Br J Cancer* **65**: 263–266.

Palli, D., Russo, A., and Decarli, A. 2001. Dietary patterns, nutrient intake and gastric cancer in a high-risk area of Italy. *Cancer Causes Control* **12**: 163–172.

Parkin, D.M. 1998. The global burden of cancer. *Semin Cancer Biol* **8**: 219–235.

Parkin, D.M. 2001. Global cancer statistics in the year 2000. *Lancet Oncol* **2**: 533–543.

Parkin, D.M., Bray, F., Ferlay, J., and Pisani, P. 2001a. Estimating the world cancer burden: Globocan 2000. *Int J Cancer* **94**: 153–156.

Parkin, D.M., Bray, F.I., and Devesa, S.S. 2001b. Cancer burden in the year 2000. The global picture. *Eur J Cancer* **37**(Suppl 8): S4–66.

Parkin, D.M., Pisani, P., and Ferlay, J. 1999. Global cancer statistics. *CA Cancer J Clin* **49**: 33–64.

Pawlowicz, Z., Zachara, B.A., Trafikowska, U., Maciag, A., Marchaluk, E., and Nowicki, A. 1991. Blood selenium concentrations and glutathione peroxidase activities in patients with breast cancer and with advanced gastrointestinal cancer. *J Trace Elem Electrolytes Health Dis* **5**: 275–277.

Ramon, J.M., Serra, L., Cerdo, C., and Oromi, J. 1993. Dietary factors and gastric cancer risk. A case–control study in Spain. *Cancer* **71**: 1731–1735.

Reed, P.I. 1993. Diet and gastric cancer. *Adv Exp Med Biol* **348**: 123–132.

Risch, H.A., Jain, M., Choi, N.W., Fodor, J.G., Pfeiffer, C.J., Howe, G.R., Harrison, L.W., Craib, K.J., and Miller, A.B. 1985. Dietary factors and the incidence of cancer of the stomach. *Am J Epidemiol* **122**: 947–959.

Setiawan, V.W., Zhang, Z.F., Yu, G.P., Lu, Q.Y., Li, Y.L., Lu, M.L., Wang, M.R., Guo, C.H., Yu, S.Z., Kurtz, R.C., and Hsieh, C.C. 2001. Protective effect of green tea on the risks of chronic gastritis and stomach cancer. *Int J Cancer* **92**: 600–604.

Sriamporn, S., Setiawan, V., Pisani, P., Suwanrungruang, K., Sirijaichingkul, S., Mairiang, P., and Parkin, D.M. 2002. Gastric Cancer: the Roles of Diet, Alcohol Drinking, Smoking and *Helicobacter pylori* in Northeastern Thailand. *Asian Pac J Cancer Prev* **3**: 345–352.

Steinmetz, K.A., and Potter, J.D. 1991. Vegetables, fruit, and cancer. I. Epidemiology. *Cancer Causes Control* **2**: 325–357.

Taylor, P.R., Li, B., Dawsey, S.M., Li, J.Y., Yang, C.S., Guo, W., and Blot, W.J. 1994. Prevention of esophageal cancer: the nutrition intervention trials in Linxian, China. Linxian Nutrition Intervention Trials Study Group. *Cancer Res* **54**: 2029s–2031s.

Taylor, P.R., Qiao, Y.L., Abnet, C.C., Dawsey, S.M., Yang, C.S., Gunter, E.W., Wang, W., Blot, W.J., Dong, Z.W., and Mark, S.D. 2003. Prospective study of serum vitamin E levels and esophageal and gastric cancers. *J Natl Cancer Inst* **95**: 1414–1416.

Terry, P., Lagergren, J., Wolk, A., and Nyren, O. 2000. Reflux-inducing dietary factors and risk of adenocarcinoma of the esophagus and gastric cardia. *Nutr Cancer* **38**: 186–191.

Terry, P., Lagergren, J., Ye, W., Wolk, A., and Nyren, O. 2001. Inverse association between intake of cereal fiber and risk of gastric cardia cancer. *Gastroenterology* **120**: 387–391.

The ATBC Cancer Prevention Study Group. 1994. The alpha-tocopherol, beta-carotene lung cancer prevention study: design, methods, participant characteristics, and compliance. *Ann Epidemiol* **4**: 1–10.

Thomson, C.A., LeWinn, K., Newton, T.R., Alberts, D.S., and Martinez, M.E. 2003. Nutrition and diet in the development of gastrointestinal cancer. *Curr Oncol Rep* **5**: 192–202.

Trichopoulos, D., Ouranos, G., Day, N.E., Tzonou, A., Manousos, O., Papadimitriou, C., and Trichopoulos, A. 1985. Diet and cancer of the stomach: a case–control study in Greece. *Int J Cancer* **36**: 291–297.

Tsubono, Y., Nishino, Y., Komatsu, S., Hsieh, C.C., Kanemura, S., Tsuji, I., Nakatsuka, H., Fukao, A., Satoh, H., and Hisamichi, S. 2001. Green tea and the risk of gastric cancer in Japan. *N Engl J Med* **344**: 632–636.

Tuyns, A.J., Kaaks, R., Haelterman, M., and Riboli, E. 1992. Diet and gastric cancer. A case–control study in Belgium. *Int J Cancer* **51**: 1–6.

Tzonou, A., Lipworth, L., Garidou, A., Signorello, L.B., Lagiou, P., Hsieh, C., and Trichopoulos, D. 1996. Diet and risk of esophageal cancer by histologic type in a low-risk population. *Int J Cancer* **68**: 300–304.

van den Brandt, P.A., Botterweck, A.A., and Goldbohm, R.A. 2003. Salt intake, cured meat consumption, refrigerator use and stomach cancer incidence: a prospective cohort study (Netherlands). *Cancer Causes Control* **14**: 427–438.

Varis, K., Taylor, P.R., Sipponen, P., Samloff, I.M., Heinonen, O.P., Albanes, D., Harkonen, M., Huttunen, J.K., Laxen, F., and Virtamo, J. 1998. Gastric cancer and premalignant lesions in atrophic gastritis: a controlled trial on the effect of supplementation with alpha-tocopherol and beta-carotene. The Helsinki Gastritis Study Group. *Scand J Gastroenterol* **33**: 294–300.

Wang, X., Willen, R., and Wadstrom, T. 2000. Astaxanthin-rich algal meal and vitamin C inhibit *Helicobacter pylori* infection in BALB/cA mice. *Antimicrob Agents Chemother* **44**: 2452–2457.

Weisburger, J.H., and Chung, F.L. 2002. Mechanisms of chronic disease causation by nutritional factors and tobacco products and their prevention by tea polyphenols. *Food Chem Toxicol* **40**: 1145–1154.

Wu, A.H., Yang, D., and Pike, M.C. 2000. A meta-analysis of soyfoods and risk of stomach cancer: the problem of potential confounders. *Cancer Epidemiol Biomarkers Prev* **9**: 1051–1058.

Wu-Williams, A.H., Yu, M.C., and Mack, T.M. 1990. Life-style, workplace, and stomach cancer by subsite in young men of Los Angeles County. *Cancer Res* **50**: 2569–2576.

Xue, F.B., Xu, Y.Y., Wan, Y., Pan, B.R., Ren, J., and Fan, D.M. 2001. Association of *H. Pylori* infection with gastric carcinoma: a Meta analysis. *World J Gastroenterol* **7**: 801–804.

Yakoob, J., Jafri, W., and Abid, S. 2003. *Helicobacter pylori* infection and micronutrient deficiencies. *World J Gastroenterol* **9**: 2137–2139.

Yang, C.S., Lee, M.J., Chen, L., and Yang, G.Y. 1997. Polyphenols as inhibitors of carcinogenesis. *Environ Health Perspect* **105**(Suppl 4): 971–976.

You, W.C., Blot, W.J., Chang, Y.S., Ershow, A., Yang, Z.T., An, Q., Henderson, B.E., Fraumeni, J.F., Jr., and Wang, T.G. 1989. Allium vegetables and reduced risk of stomach cancer. *J Natl Cancer Inst* **81**: 162–164.

You, W.C., Blot, W.J., Chang, Y.S., Ershow, A.G., Yang, Z.T., An, Q., Henderson, B., Xu, G.W., Fraumeni, J.F., Jr., and Wang, T.G. 1988. Diet and high risk of stomach cancer in Shandong, China. *Cancer Res* **48**: 3518–3523.

Yu, G.P., Hsieh, C.C., Wang, L.Y., Yu, S.Z., Li, X.L., and Jin, T.H. 1995. Green-tea consumption and risk of stomach cancer: a population-based case–control study in Shanghai, China. *Cancer Causes Control* **6**: 532–538.

Zhang, H.M., Wakisaka, N., Maeda, O., and Yamamoto, T. 1997a. Vitamin C inhibits the growth of a bacterial risk factor for gastric carcinoma: *Helicobacter pylori*. *Cancer* **80**: 1897–1903.

Zhang, Z.F., Kurtz, R.C., Yu, G.P., Sun, M., Gargon, N., Karpeh, M., Jr., Fein, J.S., and Harlap, S. 1997b. Adenocarcinomas of the esophagus and gastric cardia: the role of diet. *Nutr Cancer* **27**: 298–309.

CHAPTER

25

Pancreatic Cancer

DIANE M. HARRIS, MANISH C. CHAMPANERIA, AND VAY LIANG W. GO

INTRODUCTION

Pancreatic cancer is one of the most devastating of all malignancies. It is the fourth leading cause of cancer death in both males and females in the United States, with the lowest survivability rates of any cancer (American Cancer Society [ACS], 2004). The poor prognosis is in large part due to the fact that most pancreatic cancer patients are diagnosed with advanced disease. However, in spite of its lethality, pancreatic cancer has been insufficiently studied at the basic and clinical levels. In 2001, the National Cancer Institute (NCI) convened an expert Progress Review Group that set an agenda for research priorities in pan-creatic cancer (see the report at http://prg.nci.nih.gov/pancreatic/pancreatic.pdf) (Kern et al., 2001). Among their conclusions was that a critical component in battling pancreatic cancer is understanding environmental risk factors and gene–environmental interactions to identify and treat premalignant lesions and high-risk candidates for prevention. A subsequent workshop held at the National Institutes of Health (NIH) in 2002 was entitled "Nutritional Links to Plausible Mechanisms Underlying Pancreatic Cancer" (Hine et al., 2003). Among the dietary factors discussed were vegetable and fruit intake, as well as related health and lifestyle factors such as alcohol intake, long-standing diabetes, and body mass index (BMI).

This chapter outlines the current understanding of the pathogenesis of pancreatic cancer, particularly the identification of the preneoplastic lesion PanIN and some of the most common genetic alterations that have been described in this process. The known and postulated dietary and related lifestyle risk factors are reviewed, and where possible, their relevance to particular molecular targets in the carcinogenesis process is described.

BACKGROUND

In the United States, ~30,000 cases of pancreatic cancer are diagnosed yearly, with an equal number of deaths (ACS, 2004). In 2004, the expected incidence rates of pancreatic cancer ranked it ninth and tenth among the cancer sites in women and men, respectively. However, the expected rate of deaths from pancreatic cancer place it fourth among men and fifth in women because of the very low survival rates of untreated patients. For all stages combined, the 1-year survival rate is 19% and the 5-year survival rate is 4% (Yeo et al., 2002). This grave prognosis is a consequence of the late development of clinical symptoms in the progression of the disease, so 80% of cases are metastatic at the time of diagnosis. Around 15–20% of patients have potentially resectable pancreatic cancer (including no evidence of extra-pancreatic involvement of the tumor, demonstration of fully patent superior mesenteric/portal veins, and no evidence of tumor encroachment on the arterial celiac axis or the superior mesenteric artery); however, even in optimally staged patients, the 5-year survival rate is only 20% (Li et al., 2004a). Therefore, most patients die of pancreatic cancer a short time after diagnosis, making this truly a devastating disease.

The majority (80–90%) of pancreatic cancers are ductal adenocarcinomas, although other rarer pancreatic neoplasms are found, including acinar cell carcinoma, pseudopapillary neoplasm, pancreatoblastoma, serous cystadenoma, mucinous cystadenocarcinoma, intraductal papillary-mucinous neoplasm, and undifferentiated carcinoma with osteoclast-like giant cells (Hansel et al., 2003). There is extensive interaction between the endocrine and exocrine portions of the pancreas during pancreatic carcinogenesis; however, malignancies rarely derive from the acinar cells that form the bulk

Copyright © 2006, Elsevier Inc.
All rights of reproduction in any form reserved.

of the pancreas, and islet cell carcinomas account for <2% of all pancreatic cancers (Hine et al., 2003). Emerging evidence shows that ductal adenocarcinomas arise from normal ductal epithelial cells of the exocrine portion of the pancreas in a multistage process very analogous to that first described for colorectal cancer. Pathological analysis shows ductal adenocarcinomas are characterized by abnormal gland formation with desmoplastic stroma, and cells of the lesions fall within a spectrum from well-differentiated to poorly differentiated. Pancreatic ductal adenocarcinoma is a highly aggressive neoplasm, frequently associated with vascular, lymphatic, and perineural invasion (Hansel et al., 2003).

The pathogenesis of pancreatic ductal adenocarcinoma is postulated to be similar to other epithelial cancers in that a diffuse genomic instability after exposure to damaging agents (inflammation, toxins, etc.) and increased epithelial hyperplasia is the initiating act. A single basal cell may develop one or more mutations of a number of critical oncogenic or tumor suppressor genes, allowing escape from regulatory controls on position, differentiation, and growth (Boone and Kelloff, 2004). Neoplastic clonal expansion of transformed cells starts at one or more sites in an epithelium and progresses independently at different sites. This leads to the development of preinvasive intraepithelial neoplasia, or a multicellular mass that tends to distort surrounding normal cells. The onset of intraepithelial neoplasia is initiated by a monoclonal expansion that progresses via clonal evolution; that is, the different mutated cell types with the fastest growth rate overtake all others as they expand. This neoplastic promotion leads to increases in both total mass and extent of dissemination (known clinically as increase in stage and grade of the neoplasm with time) (Boone and Kelloff, 2004). The host tissue environment, particularly through the action of hormones and cytokines emanating from the stroma around the developing epithelial tumor, influences the tumor's development. Eventually the mass progresses to an invasive neoplasia defined by the presence of stromal invasion, and possibly subsequent metastasis to distant sites (Go et al., 2001).

Figure 1 shows the multistage carcinogenesis pathway that has been described for pancreatic cancer. A standardized classification scheme for the preinvasive lesions has been designated the pancreatic intraepithelial neoplasia (PanIN) system. PanINs are lesions composed of mucin-producing epithelia with varying degrees of cytological and architectural atypia that involve the small ducts of the pancreas. PanINs can be flat (PanIN-1A), papillary without atypia (PanIN-1B), papillary with atypia (PanIN-2), or meet the histopathological criteria for carcinoma *in situ* (PanIN-3) (see the PanIN web site at http://pathology.jhu.edu/pancreas_panin/ for a comprehensive description of the morphology of each stage). Specific alterations in genes and gene expression patterns have been described in each of the PanIN stages (Maitra et al., 2003). Because pancreatic cancers are usually diagnosed late in the progression of the disease, PanINs are infrequently seen. However, it is hoped that by understanding the genetic and cellular alterations characteristic in this multistage process, new tests to diagnose early pancreatic cancers or their precursors can be devised and used not only for diagnosis, but also to monitor responsiveness to both pharmacological and dietary interventions. Enhancing early detection and prevention of carcinogenesis are critical strategies to reduce pancreatic cancer mortality (Hine et al., 2003).

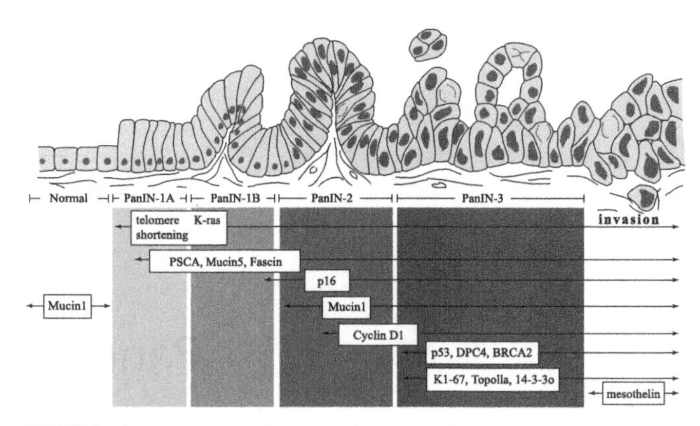

FIGURE 1 Schematic diagram of PanINs illustrating current understanding of the molecular changes in the multistep progression model of pancreas adenomas (reprinted with permission from Takaori et al., 2004.)

As with most epithelial tumors, the latency period from undetected lesions, multifocal and multiclonal, until clinical diagnosable cancer can span years (Figure 2). Pathological changes associated with PanINs may occur for as long as 15–20 years before the diagnosis of carcinoma. Although certain familial patterns of pancreatic cancer exist, these are thought to account for only 10–15% of pancreatic cancer cases (Hine et al., 2003) and have a comparable age at onset as sporadic cases in the general population, unlike familial cancer syndromes for breast, colon, and melanoma (Bardeesy and DePinho, 2002). The fact that most pancreatic cancer cases occur sporadically implies a large environmental influence, and coupled with the postulated lengthy latency period during which multiple carcinogenic hits are probable, we can surmise that chemoprevention and environmental modification are practical measures that can be taken to modify the etiology of pancreatic cancer.

GENES ALTERED IN SPORADIC DUCTAL ADENOCARCINOMAS

As mentioned earlier and in Figure 1, a defined set of alterations in genes and gene expression patterns have been described for pancreatic cancer in each of the PanIN stages. This illustrates that pancreatic tumorigenesis is a multistep

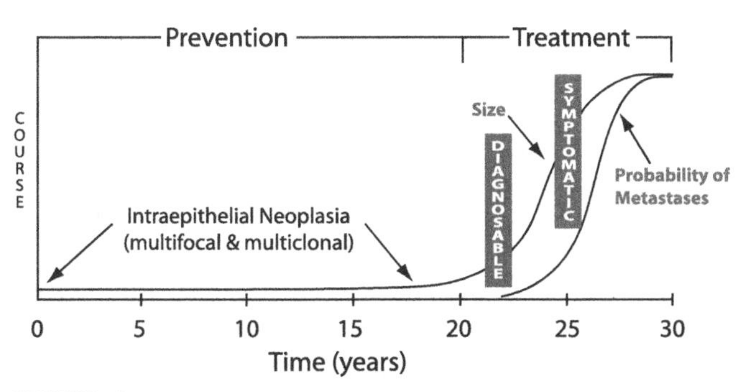

FIGURE 2 Clinical course of epithelial tumors over time, from the intraepithelial neoplasia stage to metastases (reprinted with permission from Go et al., 2003.)

process, and these steps reflect a succession of genetic changes, each of which confers a growth advantage that drives the progressive transformation of normal human cells into highly malignant cells. Hanahan and Weinberg (2000) have postulated that the vast array of cancer cell genotypes can be defined as a manifestation of six essential alterations in cell physiology that cumulatively lead to malignant growth. These six changes are (1) self-sufficiency in growth signals; (2) insensitivity to growth-inhibitory signals; (3) evasion of programed cell death (apoptosis); (4) acquisition of limitless replicative potential; (5) sustained angiogenesis; and (6) ability to invade tissue and metastasize. The authors propose that these six capabilities are shared by most and perhaps all types of human tumors and represent successful breaching of protective mechanisms normally in place to prevent uncontrolled growth. However, their analysis does not consider additional factors that predispose to these cellular alterations, including inflammation, carcinogen detoxification by xenobiotic metabolizing enzymes, and epigenetic events.

In pancreatic cancer, important genetic and metabolic changes include activation of the K-*ras* oncogene, silencing of tumor suppressor genes (including *p16*, *MADH4*, and *p53*), shortening of telomeres, alterations in DNA methylation, amplification of certain oncogenes, overexpression of growth factors, inactivation of DNA mismatch repair genes, and stimulation of matrix metalloproteinases (MMPs) that facilitate early pancreatic tumor invasion and metastasis (Jaffee et al., 2002; Hine et al., 2003). New techniques, such as serial analysis of gene expression (SAGE) and gene microarray technologies, can comprehensively profile gene expression patterns of pancreatic cancer leading to identification of unique genes and sets of genes that are overexpressed in pancreatic cancers (Iacobuzio-Donahue and Hruban, 2003). For example, mesothelin is highly expressed in nearly all, and prostate stem cell antigen in most, ductal adenocarcinomas of the pancreas (Jaffee et al., 2002). Proteomics takes into account information that cannot be predicted simply from nucleic acid sequences, such as gene amplification, alternative RNA splicing, cotranslational modification, post-translation modifications, and differential stability and secretion of proteins. Singular serum markers, such as sialylated Lewis blood group antigen CA19-9, have had limited usefulness as a diagnostic marker because of lack of specificity and sensitivity; therefore, proteomic studies have focused on identifying unique cell protein network signatures associated with stages of disease and response to therapy (Goggins, 2005; Posadas et al., 2005). Perhaps the ultimate functional analysis is at the level of metabolomics, which incorporates the total relationship of enzymes, cofactors, substrates, metabolites, and enzyme kinetics influencing metabolic networks and fluxes (Go et al., 2005a). Application of each of these high-dimensional approaches has the potential to develop new diagnostic tests, and identify novel therapeutic targets and biomarkers of disease incidence and progression (see the section "Future Directions," later in this chapter).

Although ongoing research continues to document these pancreatic cancer–specific fingerprints, the role of nutrients and diet in affecting these genotypic–phenotypic relationships, often called *nutrigenomics*, has not been well studied (Go et al., 2005a). For instance, the multitude of growth factors that promote pancreatic cancer cell growth and their signaling pathways have been extensively investigated, but the effects of specific nutrients or dietary patterns on these pathways have not. Similarly, several pharmacological agents that inhibit pancreatic tumor angiogenesis have been identified (MacKenzie, 2004), but few of the plant-derived bioactive compounds, called *phytochemicals*, which are known to be antiangiogenic in other cancers types (such as genistein from soy and epigallocatechin gallate [EGCG] from green tea), have been investigated in pancreatic tumor development (Bisacchi et al., 2003). What is known about molecular targets in pancreatic carcinogenesis is briefly outlined here; for further information, a number of excellent reviews are available (Hruban et al., 1999; Bardeesy and DePinho, 2002; Hansel et al., 2003; Li et al., 2004a; Schneider et al., 2005).

Genetic Alterations

Oncogenes

K-*ras*: The most prevalent gene mutations in pancreatic cancer are mutations in the K-*ras* oncogene, which are considered a marker of pancreatic neoplasia. Activating K-*ras* mutations seem to be the first genetic changes detected in the earliest lesions; these mutations are seen in all PanIN stages and increase in frequency with disease progression (Bardeesy and DePinho, 2002). Pancreatic cancer has the highest frequency (>85%) of K-*ras* mutations among all human cancers (Li et al., 2004a). Most of the mutations change codon 12 from glycine (wild type) to aspartic acid or valine. Other mutations, such as in codons 13 and 61, occur less frequently (Bardeesy and DePinho, 2002). Mutant K-*ras* genes shed from PanINs have been identified in bile, stool, pancreatic brushings, duodenal aspirate, and pancreatic juice samples (Caldas, 1999; O'Mahony and Sreedharan, 2001). *Ras* mutations have been associated with cigarette smoking, as well as alcohol and coffee consumption (Li and Jiao, 2003; Li et al., 2004a). However, because K-*ras* mutations are also found in a significant minority of patients with chronic pancreatitis—the main differential diagnosis for pancreatic cancer—the utility of this approach can be questioned (O'Mahony and Sreedharan, 2001).

Ras proteins are involved in cell growth and differentiation and serve as connectors between signals generated at the plasma membrane and nuclear effectors, which eventually affect the production and regulation of other key proteins. Specifically, K-*ras* mutations impair guanosine triphosphatase (GTPase) activity, thus inhibiting the hydrolysis of guanosine triphosphate (GTP), which in turn keeps the protein constitutively active. The constant *ras* signaling function activates downstream targets, thus mimicking steady mitogenic stimulus. Waf1/p21 also seems to be coordinately induced with the onset of K-*ras* mutations, perhaps because of activation of the mitogen-activated protein kinase (MAPK) pathway (Bardeesy and DePinho, 2002).

Activation of *ras* family oncogenes leads to induction of proliferation, survival, and invasion processes through stimulation of a number of downstream pathways. One mechanism includes stimulation of autocrine epidermal growth factor (EGF) signaling. Overexpression of EGF family ligands and receptors is seen in low-grade PanINs, indicating that upregulation of EGF signaling may be an early event in the carcinogenesis pathway (Bardeesy and DePinho, 2002). Oncogenic *ras* also induces gastrin gene expression via activation of the Raf-MEK-ERK signal transduction pathway (Hine et al., 2003).

Tumor Suppressors

Loss of tumor suppressor genes occurs at later stages in the PanIN classification system and facilitates rapid growth of the transformed clone. The commonly silenced tumor suppressor genes include *p16*, *p21*, *p53*, *MADH4*, and *BRCA2*.

1. *p16*: The most commonly mutated tumor suppressor gene in pancreatic cancer is *p16*. It is located on chromosome 9p and is inactivated in 95% of pancreatic ductal cell carcinomas. The *p16* gene is a member of the cyclin-dependent kinase (CDK) inhibitor family and functions to prevent the phosphorylation of retinoblastoma protein (Rb-1) by CDKs 4 and 6, leading to failure of cell cycle control and unchecked proliferation (Hansel et al., 2003). Loss of *p16* in pancreatic ductal adenocarcinomas occurs through a variable set of alterations, including homozygous deletion, single allelic loss coupled with an intragenic mutation in the second allele, and promoter hypermethylation (Hansel et al., 2003).
2. *p53*: The p53 tumor suppressor gene is mutated, primarily by missense alterations in the DNA-binding domain, in >50% of pancreatic adenocarcinomas (Bardeesy and DePinho, 2002). Mutations in the p53 gene arise in later stage PanINs that have acquired significant dysplastic characteristics, indicating that loss of p53 promotes malignant progression. The p53 gene, located on chromosome 17p, encodes a transcription factor protein that participates in the upregulation of cell cycle arrest in G_1 and G_2 following DNA damage or apoptosis pathways. Under genotoxic stress, p53 forms a tetramer, binds to DNA, and upregulates genes involved with cell cycle arrest or apoptosis pathways (Hansel et al., 2003). Loss of p53 allows cell cycle progression in the presence of DNA damage and undoubtedly promotes the rampant genetic instability that characterizes pancreatic adenocarcinoma; pancreatic tumors exhibit aneuploidy and complex cytogenetic rearrangements, as well as cytological heterogeneity within tumors, consistent with ongoing genomic rearrangements (Bardeesy and DePinho, 2002). This mechanism may involve dysfunction of telomeres, as pancreatic tumors have shortened telomere length and activation of telomerase is a late event (Bardeesy and DePinho, 2002).
3. *TGF-β/DPC4*: The Deleted in Pancreatic Cancer 4 (DPC4; also called SMAD4 or MADH4) gene is a tumor suppressor gene that maps to chromosome 18q21 and is mutated or homozygously deleted in ~55% of pancreatic ductal cancers (Hansel et al., 2003). DPC4 seems to be a progression allele for pancreatic adenocarcinoma, as its loss occurs only in later stage PanINs (Bardeesy and DePinho, 2002). Although patients that inherit a germline DPC4 mutation do not have a strong predisposition to pancreatic adenocarcinoma, loss of DPC4 is a predictor of decreased survival in spontaneous adenocarcinoma (Bardeesy and DePinho, 2002).

   Mothers Against Decapentaplegic homolog (SMAD) proteins are responsible for the signaling pathways of the transforming growth factor-β (TGF-β) superfamily. In a normal epithelial cell, exposure to TGF-β signaling stops cell proliferation by blocking the G_1/S cell cycle transition and promotes apoptosis (Bardeesy and DePinho, 2002). Loss of SMAD4 interferes with intracellular signaling cascades downstream from TGF-β and activin, resulting in decreased growth inhibition via loss of proapoptotic signaling or inappropriate G_1/S transition (Hansel et al., 2003).
4. *BRCA2*: Family-associated pancreatic cancer accounts for some 10–15% of pancreatic cancers. A number of different genes have been implicated in familial

syndromes of pancreatic cancer. For example, pancreatic cancer is seen in some breast cancer families carrying mutations in breast cancer genes BRCA1 and BRCA2 (Ghadirian et al., 2003). The cumulative risk of pancreatic cancer to age 75 years among BRCA2 gene carriers in the Ashkenazi Jewish population is reported to be ~7%, compared with 85% risk of breast cancer among carriers of BRCA1 and BRCA2 mutations (Ozcelik et al., 1997).

Inflammation and Eicosanoid Pathways

Inflammation is a significant factor in the development of a number of solid tumor malignancies. The risk of pancreatic cancer development is enhanced in patients with hereditary and sporadic forms of pancreatitis (Farrow and Evers, 2002). Modulators of the inflammatory response include prostaglandins and other hormone-like members of the eicosanoid pathway, which are thought to induce carcinogenesis through action on nuclear transcription sites and downstream gene products important in the control of cell proliferation. Eicosanoids are locally acting hormone-like compounds derived predominantly from arachidonic acid in tissue cells and tumor-infiltrating leukocytes (Wargovich et al., 2001). The best known eicosanoids, the prostaglandins, are produced by the action of the cyclooxygenases (COX), but the lipoxygenase group of enzymes produce the leukotrienes and hydroperoxyeicosatetraenoic acids, which also have important proinflammatory effects (Wallace, 2002). Substantial evidence from animal studies and human epidemiological and clinical trials shows that nonsteroidal anti-inflammatory drugs (NSAIDs), which are inhibitors of COX, are associated with reduced risk of a number of cancers, including those of the colon-rectum, esophagus, stomach, breast, lung, prostate, bladder, brain, and cervix (Wallace, 2002). At least six epidemiological studies have investigated aspirin and other NSAID use in relation to pancreatic cancer risk, and although the epidemiological data are not consistent, experimental data suggest that NSAIDs inhibit pancreatic cancer cell proliferation (Michaud, 2004).

COX-2 has been shown to contribute to the malignant phenotype via various activities, including suppressing the host immune system, conferring resistance to apoptosis, stimulating cancer cell growth and invasion, and recruiting new blood vessels in angiogenesis (Eibl et al., 2004). COX-2 expression is regulated in part by the transcription factor nuclear factor-κB (NF-κB), a ubiquitously expressed transcription factor that regulates the expression of a number of inflammatory, apoptotic, and oncogenic genes (Farrow and Evers, 2002). COX-2 in normal pancreas is only detectable in pancreatic islets but is found in preinvasive PanINs and is overexpressed in most invasive pancreatic cancers in the cancer cells themselves and not in the tumor stroma (Eibl et al., 2004). Selective COX-2 inhibitors (termed *coxibs*) used *in vivo* suppress pancreatic cancer growth in an orthotopic (Tseng et al., 2002) and a chemically induced cancer model (Schuller et al., 2002; Furukawa et al., 2003).

However, chronic NSAID use in patients leads to toxicities, including gastric ulceration, perforation, or obstruction, which limit their therapeutic use (Wallace, 2002). Newer selective coxibs have been postulated to be safer, but the voluntary worldwide recall of several of these drugs, including Merck's product rofecoxib (Vioxx), illustrates that the long-term safety of these drugs has yet to be established (U.S. Food and Drug Administration [FDA], 2005). Therefore, research has focused on identifying and understanding the bioactivity of a number of natural nontoxic agents to control inflammatory eicosanoids. Those agents that have been studied in various cancers include the omega-3 polyunsaturated fatty acids (PUFA), eicosapentaenoic acid (EPA), and docosahexaenoic acid (DHA) such as from fish oils, vitamin A, vitamin E, and a number of botanically derived anti-inflammatory agents, including boswellic acids, bromelain, curcumin, resveratrol, quercetin, and EGCG (Wallace, 2002). One mechanism of action of these compounds is via inhibition of NFκB, which is activated by proinflammatory signals and upregulates COX-2 expression (Bremner and Heinrich, 2002).

Eibl et al. (2004) proposed that the COX and the peroxisome proliferator-activated receptor (PPAR) pathways can interact in pancreatic cancer, and they provide evidence that coxibs have effects on COX-independent pathways, particularly the PPAR system, which either augment or even reverse the expected action of the COX inhibitors (Eibl et al., 2004). Although the exact role of PPARγ, the best characterized member of the PPAR family, in tumorigenesis is ambiguous, it has been shown that PPARγ is overexpressed in pancreatic tumors (Motomura et al., 2000; Itami et al., 2001). In addition, PPARγ ligands induce cell cycle arrest with terminal differentiation (Hashimoto et al., 2002; Kawa et al., 2002; Ohta et al., 2002; Toyota et al., 2002; Tsujie et al., 2003a) and apoptosis (Eibl et al., 2001; Hashimoto et al., 2002) and decrease cellular invasion (Hashimoto et al., 2002; Farrow et al., 2003; Motomura et al., 2004). Coxibs may either increase or decrease PPARγ transcription through different mechanisms, and the model of Eibl et al. (2004) postulates that the overall effect of coxibs on PPARγ activity is a balance between positive and negative influences (Eibl et al., 2004). This also implies that the effect of coxibs on PPARγ activation is likely to depend on COX-2 status of the pancreatic cancer cell. Stimulation of PPAR activity by coxibs (with hypothetically protumorigenic results) in COX-2–positive pancreatic cancers may be offset by inhibition of the production of protumorigenic prostaglandins. However, 10–40% of human pancreatic ductal adenocarcinomas are COX-2 negative, and in these cancers, the PPARγ-activating effects of coxibs may dominate. This conflicting mechanism implies that further study of pharmaceutical and natural COX-2 inhibitors in cancer prevention needs to include the possibility of PPARγ activation and enhanced tumor growth in COX-2–negative cancers, making genotyping of tumors prior to initiation of treatment necessary.

The other arm of the eicosanoid pathway consists of the lipoxygenases (LOX), termed 5-, 12-, and 15-LOX in humans. Expression of 5-LOX is shown to also be upregulated in human pancreatic cancer tissue, as confirmed by immunohistochemistry (Hennig et al., 2002). The staining of the 5-LOX protein was especially evident in the ductal components of more differentiated tumors, but not present in ductal cells from normal pancreatic tissues. Also, hepatic metastases had higher levels of 5-LOX expression than primary tumors. Use of pharmacological inhibitors of the 5-LOX pathway inhibits growth of pancreatic tumor xenografts in athymic nude mice via induction of apoptosis (Tong et al., 2002). In cell culture, the general LOX inhibitor nordihydroguaiaretic acid (NDGA), the specific 5-LOX inhibitor Rev5901, and the 12-LOX inhibitor baicalein all induced apoptosis in pancreatic cancer lines, as well as increased intracellular carbonic anhydrase activity, a marker of cell differentiation (Ding et al., 1999). Also, the 5-LOX pathway inhibitor MK886 diminished pancreatic carcinogenesis induced by transplacental exposure to ethanol and the tobacco carcinogen NNK in hamsters (Schuller et al., 2002). Further studies to validate the role in pancreatic cancer of other LOX enzymes, including 15-LOX, are required. A number of natural compounds found in foods and spices have anti-LOX activities, and some have dual anti-COX and anti-LOX activities, including quercetin, curcumin, and resveratrol, making them potentially attractive anti-inflammatory and anticancer agents (Wallace, 2002; Schneider and Bucar, 2005).

Oxidative Stress

Cells are normally in a balance between oxidant stress, as evidenced through the generation of reactive oxygen species (ROS, also called *oxygen radicals*) and other electrophilic species, and antioxidant mechanisms, which deactivate the reactive species. Generation of ROS occurs during acute and chronic pancreatitis, and increased cellular ROS have been associated with carcinogenesis (Sanfey et al., 1984). ROS, including superoxide and hydroxyl radicals and hydrogen peroxide, are products of cellular metabolism and respiration that at high concentrations cause oxidative damage to cellular DNA, protein, and lipids (such as in membranes). Antioxidant systems include the enzymes superoxide dismutase, catalase, and peroxidase, of which glutathione peroxidase is the most prominent (Benzie, 2000). In addition, a number of nutrients, such as the vitamins C and E and selenium, as well as the dietary constituents β-carotene, quercetin, resveratrol, and genistein and a host of other phytochemicals, have antioxidant properties (Valko et al., 2004).

Expression of the antioxidant enzymes has been shown to progressively decrease in pancreatic cells from normal pancreas to chronic pancreatitis to pancreatic cancer in human histology samples, showing that capacity to disable ROS decreases as cells undergo oncogenic transformation (Cullen et al., 2003a). Overexpression of one antioxidant enzyme, MnSOD, attenuated the growth of human pancreatic cancer cells (Cullen et al., 2003b). Furthermore, growth factor stimulation (by serum, insulin-like growth factor-1 [IGF-1], or fibroblast growth factor-2) of pancreatic cancer cells generated ROS via nonmitochondrial NAD(P)H oxidase (Vaquero et al., 2004). This ROS protects cells from apoptosis, demonstrating that ROS are prosurvival antiapoptotic factors in pancreatic cancer cells and suggesting a mechanism for the general resistance to induction of apoptosis by chemotherapy and radiotherapy of pancreatic malignancy.

However, increased intake of antioxidant nutrients can diminish the ROS pool and presumably carcinogenesis. High intake of selenium has been shown to reduce the numbers of histologically diagnosed cancerous pancreatic lesions in a hamster model (Kise et al., 1990). Adenomas and carcinomas of the pancreas were significantly reduced in azaserine-treated rats with diets supplemented with β-carotene, vitamin C, or selenium, but not vitamin E (Woutersen et al., 1999). This effect was most prominent during the promotion phase of the carcinogenic process (Appel and Woutersen, 1996b). Similar studies in BOP-induced pancreatic tumors in hamsters were contradictory. In one, vitamin A and C diminished incidence of pancreatic cancer and decreased levels of superoxide dismutase (Wenger et al., 2001), whereas in another study of longer duration, vitamin C did diminish the number of advanced ductular lesions, but vitamin E, β-carotene, or selenium had no effect on tumor development (Appel et al., 1996). In pancreatic cell lines, treatment with vitamins A and D, but not E and K, decreased cell number (Ohlsson et al., 2004). In humans, however, a supplementation trial determining the effects of β-carotene or α-tocopherol on cancer incidence in male smokers showed no effect on the rate of incidence of pancreatic carcinoma or the rate of mortality caused by the disease; this negative result is perhaps explainable by the lack of statistical power because of the small number of pancreatic cancer cases in this cohort (Rautalahti et al., 1999).

DNA Methylation

A key role of nutrient action is epigenetic, referring to changes in the phenotype that are not due to changes in the genotype, or in other words, changes in gene expression that are transmissible through mitosis but do not involve mutations of the primary DNA sequence itself (Jaenisch and Bird,

2003). A critical mechanism for epigenetic gene regulation involves alterations in patterns of DNA methylation. DNA methylation, or the covalent addition of a methyl group to the 5-position of cytosine within CpG dinucleotides, is particularly important in epigenetic control by nutrients. Tumors commonly exhibit widespread global DNA hypomethylation, region-specific hypermethylation, and increased activity of *Dnmt* enzymes, which catalyze the transfer of methyl groups from *S*-adenosylmethionine (SAM) to cytosine residues in DNA. Global genomic hypomethylation is linked to induction of chromosomal instability, whereas hypermethylation is associated with inactivation of most pathways of carcinogenesis, including DNA repair, cell cycle regulation, and apoptosis (Ross, 2003). In pancreatic cancer, a number of genes have been shown to be hypermethylated in promoter regions, including *p16*, RAS association domain family 1A gene (RASSF1A), heparin sulfate *D*-glucosaminyl 3-*O*-sulfotransferase-2 (3-OST-2), cyclin D2, suppressor of cytokine signaling-1 (SOCS-1), retinoic acid receptor-β (RARβ), and adenomatous polyposis coli (APC) genes. Promoter hypermethylation in serum DNA may be used as a marker for the early detection of pancreatic cancer cells, and demethylating agents have potential as therapeutic agents (Kuroki et al., 2004).

Dietary factors may influence DNA methylation patterns in several ways. First, nutrient inadequacies will influence the supply of methyl groups for the formation of SAM. Dietary factors that are involved in one-carbon metabolism that influence the availability of SAM include folate, vitamin B12 (cobalamin), vitamin B6 (pyroxidine), vitamin B2 (riboflavin), methionine, and choline; excess alcohol intake is known to deplete these nutrients (Lieber, 2000). Other nutrients including zinc, selenium, and retinoic acid will affect global DNA hypomethylation (Ross, 2003). A second way diet alters methylation is by regulating the use of methyl groups, including modifying DNA methyltransferase activity via *Dnmt* enzymes. Higher *Dnmt* activity has been observed in tumor cells compared with normal cells, and activity of these enzymes is upregulated with chronic methyl deficiency in an apparent attempt to compensate for diminished SAM supply. In addition, the DNA demethylation process, previously assumed to be passive, may be a regulated activity (Ross, 2003). The subsequent changes in methylation patterns can influence activity of specific genes; this likely occurs through modifying transcription factor–gene interactions through methyl DNA–binding proteins (Ross, 2003). DNA hypomethylation was associated with overexpression of a number of genes known to be upregulated in pancreatic adenocarcinoma, including claudin 4, lipocalin 2, 14-3-3 sigma, trefoil factor 2, S100A4, mesothelin, and prostate stem cell antigen, as measured in pancreatic cancer cell lines and primary carcinomas (Sato et al., 2003).

The effects of manipulating dietary levels of several methyl donors have been tested in animal models. Methionine enhanced atrophic change of pancreatic acinar cells in hamsters given BOP, indicating that the inhibitory effects on the post-initiation stage of BOP-induced pancreatic carcinogenesis in hamsters could be generally linked to suppression of growth (Furukawa et al., 2000). The effects of choline-deficient diets on carcinogenesis in azaserine-treated rats are inconsistent. In one study an increased incidence of neoplasms in the choline-deficient diet was attributed to the high fat content (20%) of the experimental diet compared with the control diet (5%) (Roebuck et al., 1981). In a separate study, the incidence of azaserine-induced focal hyperplasia was lower in a choline-deficient diet than in a control choline-sufficient group in a study at the same level of fat (14%) (Shinozuka et al., 1978). In another study, results showed an increased incidence of azaserine-induced focal hyperplasia in rats fed a choline-deficient diet compared with a group fed a choline-deficient diet against a high-fat (30%) background in a short-term study (Andry et al., 1990); however, in contrasting results from another study in rats fed choline-deficient or choline-sufficient high-fat diets, the incidence of spontaneously occurring acinar cell neoplasms was similar in the two groups (Longnecker et al., 1991).

These experimental studies suggest that perturbations in DNA methylation can alter cellular differentiation in the pancreas and contribute to toxic injury that predisposes to pancreatic carcinogenesis. As discussed earlier, folate metabolism is integral to epigenetic regulation of genes important in the carcinogenesis pathway. Therefore, the contribution of folate and other methyl donor nutrients is of interest in interpreting the role of diet in pancreatic cancer risk, but few epidemiological studies have explored this relationship. In the Alpha-Tocopherol, Beta-Carotene Cancer Prevention Study cohort, the adjusted hazards ratio for pancreatic cancer comparing the highest with the lowest quintile of dietary folate intake was 0.52, demonstrating the importance of folate intake on pancreatic cancer risk. Dietary methionine, alcohol intake, and smoking history did not modify this relation, and no significant associations were observed between dietary methionine, vitamins B6 and B12, or alcohol intake and pancreatic cancer risk (Stolzenberg-Solomon et al., 1999). However, results from two large prospective cohorts did not support a strong association between energy-adjusted folate intake and risk of pancreatic cancer (Skinner et al., 2004). Because of the presence of well-defined polymorphisms in the enzymes involved in folate metabolism, study populations probably need to be stratified by genotype. For example, there is an interaction of genotype of 5,10-methylenetetrahydrofolate reductase (MTHFR) that catalyzes the conversion of 5,10-methylenetetrahydrofolate into 5-methyltetrahydrofolate (the major circulating form of folate), with pancreatic cancer risk; those with the least frequent TT genotype displayed increased risk of pancreatic cancer, and a positive interaction between the TT genotype and heavy smoking or heavy alcohol consumption was detected (Li et al., 2005).

Genetic Susceptibility to Xenobiotic Exposure

Metabolic activation is required for the effect of many carcinogens, including those of dietary sources, and substantial interindividual variation exists in the metabolic capacity of carcinogen activation and inactivation. Polymorphisms are present in a number of metabolic genes, including cytochrome P450 (CYP isoforms 1A1, 1B1, and 2E1), *N*-acetyltransferase (NAT1 and NAT2), and glutathione *S*-transferase (GST M1 and GST T1); no significant main effect of these genes on pancreatic cancer risk is observed. However, a possible gene–environment interaction among individuals with specific environmental exposures (e.g. dietary heterocyclic amine intake and smoking) was observed (Li and Jiao, 2003).

In addition to carcinogen-metabolizing enzymes, DNA repair capability after genotoxic insult has a critical interaction with cancer susceptibility. X-ray repair cross-complementing group 1 (XRCC1) is a base excision repair protein that plays a central role in repair of DNA strand breaks and base damage from various exogenous and endogenous agents including oxidants and DNA alkylating agents (Li and Jiao, 2003). The Arg399Gln polymorphism of XRCC1 is significantly associated with the risk of pancreatic cancer among smokers (Duell et al., 2002). Other DNA repair genes, O^6-alkylguanine DNA transferase (AGT) and 8-oxoguanine DNA glycosylase/DNA-AP lyase (hOGG1), are being studied in the context of pancreatic cancer (Li and Jiao, 2003).

Polymorphisms in the genes involved with metabolic activation, detoxification, and repair have all been shown to confer variable susceptibility to a number of cancers. For example, hOGG1 polymorphisms are associated with increased risk for cancers of lung, prostate, and esophagus (Weiss et al., 2005). We are just beginning to understand the interaction of these polymorphisms with dietary factors. In colon cancer, broccoli consumption in combination with the GST M1 null genotype is associated with a lower prevalence of colorectal adenomas because of higher isothiocyanate levels (Lin et al., 1998). Furthermore, potential interactions of the DNA repair system with flavonoids are being explored (Ferguson, 2001). These types of studies linking dietary factors with interindividual variation in the function of gene products, termed *gene–nutrient interactions*, are critical to understanding individual susceptibility to cancer and potential individualized recommendations for pancreatic disease prevention and management.

THE IMPORTANCE OF DIET

The strongest risk factor for pancreatic cancer is age at diagnosis; >80% of cases are diagnosed in individuals between 60 and 80 years of age (Ghadirian et al., 2003). There are racial/ethnic/gender disparities within the U.S. population in incidence and mortality rates of pancreatic cancer, with generally higher rates among males relative to females, African Americans relative to white Americans, and people of Jewish heritage (Hine et al., 2003). The other established probable risk factors for pancreatic cancer include (1) cigarette smoking; (2) long-standing diabetes; (3) chronic and hereditary pancreatitis; and (4) family history of pancreatic cancer. Possible risk factors include (1) noncigarette tobacco use; (2) other medical conditions (gallbladder disease/cholecystectomy, gastrectomy/peptic ulcer); (3) occupational exposures (e.g., organochlorine compounds [DDT, PCBs] and chlorinated hydrocarbon solvents); (4) low socioeconomic status; (5) "heavy" alcohol consumption; (6) dietary factors (e.g., infrequent intake of vegetables, high intake of grilled or charred meats, positive energy balance, and high BMI); and (7) high caloric intake and frequent meals per day (Hine et al., 2003; Li et al., 2004a). Undoubtedly, many of the listed risk factors are interrelated. Disorders of the exocrine pancreas, such as chronic and acute pancreatitis and pancreatic adenocarcinoma, can induce endocrine pancreatic disorders such as diabetes mellitus and islet cancer. In turn, diabetes and glucose intolerance are often associated with exocrine pancreatic dysfunction and may participate in pancreatic carcinogenesis. Epidemiological studies confirm that glucose intolerance is a risk factor for pancreatic cancer, therefore the association is unlikely due to an adverse impact of early pancreatic cancer on β-cell function and insulin may act as a promoter for pancreatic carcinogenesis (Go and Wang, 2005). In fact, insulin resistance may be the unifying factor linking hyperglycemia, diabetes, obesity, and nutrition in pancreatic cancer development (Michaud et al., 2002; Hine et al., 2003).

Relative to other cancer sites, fewer studies have been undertaken to explore associations between particular dietary factors and risk for pancreatic cancer. Given the intimate role of the pancreas in digestion and nutrient absorption, however, one can predict that diet may have a large role in pancreatic cancer development and prevention. Unlike other organs of the gastrointestinal tract, the pancreas is not directly exposed to ingested or absorbed nutrients. Therefore, the effects of diet on carcinogenesis are via changes in the metabolic environment of the pancreas and/or exposure to bloodborne agents (World Cancer Research Fund and American Institute for Cancer Research, 1997). In the 1997 review of diet and cancer prepared by the American Institute for Cancer Research/World Cancer Research Fund, the contribution of dietary factors to development of pancreatic cancer is estimated to be 35%. For most dietary constituents, the findings at the time of the committee's review were equivocal, with insufficient data to determine association (World Cancer Research Fund and American Institute for Cancer Research, 1997). However, newer data are being examined and publication of new judgments by the committee is anticipated in 2007.

Several limitations in conducting research in pancreatic cancer have slowed progress in understanding risk factors in development of this disease. First, there are few relevant preclinical models of pancreatic cancer. The ideal model should provide morphological, clinical, and genetic alterations comparable with those found in human cases (Ulrich et al., 2002). However, some models exhibit tumor formation in cell types other than ductal epithelial cells or lack mutations in genes associated with human cancers. As mentioned previously, one of the most widely studied animal models for pancreatic duct carcinoma is the use of the carcinogen *N*-nitrosobis(2-oxopropyl)amine (BOP) in Syrian golden hamsters (*Mesocricetus auratus*), although other carcinogens, such as azaserine, have also been used to induce pancreatic cancer in hamsters and rats. In the BOP/hamster model, invasive pancreatic adenocarcinomas develop in 80–100% of treated animals, with a tumor latency as short as 8 weeks after a single subcutaneous injection. The most common tumors in this model are ductal adenocarcinomas, which display perineural lymphatic invasion and a pronounced desmoplastic reaction similar to the human disease (Hotz et al., 2000). In addition, hamsters with pancreatic cancer exhibit weight loss, diarrhea, jaundice, ascites, vascular thrombosis, and abnormal glucose metabolism, signs that are similar to those displayed clinically in human pancreatic cancer patients. However, certain human cancer biomarkers, such as carcinoembryonic antigen, pancreatic oncofetal antigen, α-fetoprotein, and DU-PAN-2, are infrequently or not expressed by hamster pancreatic cancer cells (Standop et al., 2001).

An alternative approach to generation of animal models involves use of implanted human tumor cell xenografts in immunodeficient mice, including nude mice and severe combined immunodeficient (SCID) mice. These methods of tumor induction include direct injection of human pancreatic cancer cells into the pancreas (orthotopic implant), transplantation of tumor fragments from tumors grown in donor animals (ectopic implant), and transplantation of tumor fragments obtained from resected human tumors (Hotz et al., 2000). All of these techniques have shortcomings; for example, direct injection of tumor cells into the pancreas may result in cell loss into the peritoneal cavity, where abdominal organs may be seeded with tumor cells (Hotz et al., 2000). Cell lines have variable characteristics and can exhibit genetic instability in grafts, and the tumors produced generally are necrotic toward the center of the graft. A refined procedure involves implantation of small tumor fragments into surgically prepared tissue pockets in the pancreatic parenchyma (Hotz et al., 2003). The limitation of all immunodeficient mouse models is that the impact of the host immune system is negated; however, they do provide a reliable and reasonably reproducible model for evaluating treatment strategies.

Few transgenic mice models of spontaneous pancreatic ductal adenocarcinoma are available, but more are in development (Leach, 2004). Transgenic mice with the elastase promoter SV40 early antigen construct (Ela-1-SV40 T) and variations on this construct develop focal acinar cell lesions that develop into carcinomas with a high incidence after 3–6 months (Standop et al., 2001). The mechanism of T-antigen transformation involves inactivation of the tumor suppressor genes p53 and Rb. However, the tumors formed do not carry K-*ras* mutations. A mouse model of PanIN has been developed through targeted mutation of $KRAS^{G12D}$ in progenitor cells of mouse pancreas (Hingorani et al., 2003). In this model ductal lesions are induced to recapitulate the full spectrum of human PanIN and progress to fully metastatic disease. These models hold much promise for study of gene–nutrient interactions in pancreatic carcinogenesis.

In vitro and animal studies are very useful in exploring mechanistic aspects, but the ability to generalize findings from preclinical studies to human populations needs to be evaluated specifically in epidemiological and dietary intervention studies (Gold, 1995). In human studies, attempts to link pancreatic cancer to diet are hampered by the fact that the clinical course of the disease is rapid. Most studies of risk factors for pancreatic cancer are case-control studies, with fewer prospective cohort diet studies, which record diet and food intake in healthy patients before disease development (Hine et al., 2003). At the time of determination of an affected individual, many patients are either at a late stage of the disease, too late for interventions, or even too late to provide accurate detailed answers on dietary questionnaires; proxy respondents, such as close relatives, are often used but are notoriously inaccurate (Howe and Burch, 1996). In addition, there is a lack of biomarkers for preclinical and clinical pancreatic cancer, making early detection and evaluation of the effectiveness of intervention regimens difficult.

The following sections review the data for the relationship between selected dietary and lifestyle factors and pancreatic cancer risk in epidemiological studies and nutrient modulation of pancreatic carcinogenesis in preclinical models. Although smoking is a clearly identified and very important risk factor for pancreatic cancer, the contribution of this lifestyle factor has been reviewed previously (Schuller, 2002) and is not discussed here.

Obesity, Physical Activity, and Diabetes

Several prospective cohort studies have reported elevated risks of pancreatic cancer among overweight and obese individuals. In the ACS study of a very large cohort of >900,000 U.S. adults monitored over 16 years, death rates from pancreatic cancer, as well as for a number of other cancers, were increased as BMI increased; relative risks for individuals with BMIs >30 kg/m^2 were 1.49 for men and 2.76 for women (Calle et al., 2003). Further analysis showed that after adjusting for BMI, risk of pancreatic cancer was independently increased among men and women who reported a tendency for central weight gain compared with men and women reporting a tendency for peripheral weight gain; accumulation of intraabdominal fat is particularly associated with development of insulin resistance (Patel et al., 2005). In another prospective analysis of two large cohort studies of 163,689 men and women showed that tall height and greater BMI were independently and positively associated with pancreatic cancer (Michaud et al., 2001). In a Swedish cohort study, a 46% increase in risk was observed among individuals who had gained ≥12 kg as adults, compared with those who gained 2–5 kg (Isaksson et al., 2002). However, several case-control studies have also shown no correlations between BMI or weight and pancreatic cancer; a meta-analysis of these studies illustrates the heterogeneity among results of different studies, which may be linked to such factors as use of proxy respondents, self-reporting of anthropometric measures, and lack of adjustment for potential confounding factors of diabetes or smoking (Berrington de Gonzalez et al., 2003).

Physiological mechanisms accounting for the relationship between excess adiposity and enhancement of pancreatic cancer growth are unclear. The mature adipocyte is an active endocrine and metabolic organ known to secrete a number of peptide hormones, such as leptin, tumor necrosis factor-α (TNF-α), resistin, and adiponectin—collectively termed adipocytokines—as well as nonesterified fatty acids (NEFAs), which in numerous cancer cell types stimulate proliferation. *In vitro* studies, however, demonstrate that leptin *inhibits*, rather than promotes, proliferation of MIA-PaCa and PANC-1 ductal cancer cells; the mechanism and significance of this effect is unknown (Somasundar et al., 2003). Increased release of NEFA, resistin, and TNF-α, as well as reduced release of adiponectin, gives rise to insulin resistance and compensatory hyperinsulinemia (Calle and Kaaks, 2004). Chronic hyperinsulinemia is associated with increased risk of pancreatic cancer (Weiderpass et al., 1998; Silverman, 2001). Elevated insulin stimulates IGF-1 production and activity (McCarty, 2001). High serum levels of IGF-1 and one of its binding proteins IGF binding protein-3 (IGF-BP3) have been associated with increased risk of pancreatic cancer in some studies (Lin et al., 2004), and *in vitro* exposure to insulin and IGF-1 stimulates pancreatic cancer cell proliferation and inhibits apoptosis (Ohmura et al., 1990; Takeda and Escribano, 1991; Bergmann et al., 1995; Flossmann-Kast et al., 1998; Nair et al., 2001; Yao et al., 2002).

The association between diabetes mellitus and pancreatic cancer is not entirely clear, as clinical diabetes can be one of the early manifestations of pancreatic cancer. A meta-analysis published in 1995 suggested that diabetics have about a twofold increased risk of pancreatic cancer (Everhart and Wright, 1995). A subsequent population-based case-control study of pancreatic cancer in three U.S. cancer registries showed that a diagnosis of diabetes at least 10 years before diagnosis conferred 50% increased risk for pancreatic cancer (Silverman et al., 1999). This association held within each level of BMI. In a prospective cohort study, a group of >35,000 men and women in the Chicago area were monitored for 25 years (Gapstur et al., 2000). Insulin sensitivity was measured at baseline and at incidence of pancreatic cancer during the 25 years of follow-up. They found that risk for pancreatic cancer increased in proportion to the 2-hour serum glucose values measured during the glucose tolerance test. Furthermore, a meta-analysis of 17 case-control and 19 cohort or nested case-control studies showed that the age and sex-adjusted odds ratio for pancreatic cancer was increased by 50% in individuals who had type II diabetes diagnosed within 4 years of pancreatic cancer diagnosis (Huxley et al., 2005). These findings suggest that development of pancreatic cancer is associated with abnormality of islet cell function and glucose intolerance precedes the onset of pancreatic cancer.

As discussed earlier in this chapter, plasma insulin and postload plasma glucose may be associated with risk of pancreatic cancer. One measure of the ability of individual foods to raise postprandial glycemia and hence blood insulin levels is the glycemic index (GI). This measure classifies the carbohydrate content of individual foods according to their postfeeding glycemic effects relative to a standard glucose load. Consumption of high GI diets is associated with hyperinsulinemia (Augustin et al., 2002). A perhaps more accurate portrayal is glycemic load, which multiplies the GI by the carbohydrate content of an individual food to take into account carbohydrate density of foods. The relationship between GI, glycemic load, and intake of fructose with pancreatic cancer risk was most apparent among those women participating in the U.S. Nurses' Health Study with elevated BMI or with low physical activity, suggesting a diet high in glycemic load may increase pancreatic cancer risk in women who already have an underlying degree of insulin resistance (Michaud et al., 2002). However, GI and glycemic load, as well as total sugar and total carbohydrate intake, were not associated with pancreatic cancer risk in a Canadian population (Silvera et al., 2005). Overall, the association of diabetes in pancreatic cancer remains unclear, and the fact that 20–30% of pancreatic cancer patients do not develop a glucose metabolic abnormality suggests multiple mechanisms of diabetes in the development of human pancreatic cancer (Saruc and Pour, 2003).

In animal models, decreasing insulin levels seem to inhibit pancreatic carcinogenesis. For example, pretreatment of hamsters with streptozotocin (a pancreatic β-cell toxin) reduces the incidence of carcinogen-induced pancreatic cancer (Bell et al., 1988, 1989; Fisher et al., 1996). Also, caloric restriction, which decreases daily insulin secretion, inhibits pancreatic cancer induction in hamsters (Roebuck et al., 1993). Conversely, high-fat–fed hamsters have increased insulin levels but normal glucose levels and subsequently increased islet cell proliferation and pancreatic carcinogenesis. Administration of metformin, an oral antihyperglycemic drug, normalized insulin levels and the rate of islet cell turnover (Schneider et al., 2001).

Physical activity is associated with a decreased risk of pancreatic cancer, especially among overweight people. The inverse relationship was observed for moderate physical activity, specifically for walking or hiking outdoors for ≥4 hours/wk, but not for vigorous activity (Michaud et al., 2001). In another study, mild obesity (BMI 25–30), adult weight gain, sedentary work, and low physical activity during leisure time were all associated with increased risk of pancreatic cancer (Isaksson et al., 2002). Among Canadian men, men in the highest quartile of the composite moderate and strenuous physical activity index were at a reduced risk of pancreatic cancer, with a trend toward the same relationship in women (Hanley et al., 2001). However, in a study of 32,687 subjects with data on physical activity and BMI collected serially over time, neither physical activity or BMI significantly predicted pancreatic cancer mortality (Lee et al., 2003), nor was there any difference in pancreatic cancer incidence rates between men and women who were most active at baseline compared with those who reported no recreational activity in the ACS Cancer Prevention Cohort (Patel et al., 2005). The mechanisms for any observed effect are unclear, except that exercise helps to maintain normal body weight, again illustrating the interaction between insulin resistance, overweight, and lack of physical activity in cancer risk.

Fruit and Vegetable Intake

A growing body of evidence suggests that diets high in fruits and vegetables may be protective against pancreatic cancer. Fruits and vegetables contain a multitude of anticancer agents such as fiber, carotenoids, vitamins C and E, selenium, flavonoids, and plant sterols (Hart, 1999; International Agency for Research on Cancer [IARC] Working Group on the Evaluation of Cancer-Preventive Strategies, 2003). Several reviews have summarized the epidemiological evidence on fruit and vegetables intake and pancreatic cancer prevention (Block et al., 1992; Howe and Burch, 1996; World Cancer Research Fund and American Institute for Cancer Research, 1997). Overall, the pattern is very consistent, showing decreasing risk with increasing consumption of fruits and vegetables. However, there is quite a bit of variation in the specific food items showing protective relationships, suggesting perhaps that there are multiple active food components that contribute to this apparent protective effect. Another more recent case-control study differentiated among three dietary patterns in subjects using food frequency questionnaires: Western (characterized by high intake of processed meats, sweets and desserts, refined grains, and potatoes), drinker (high consumption of liquor, wine, and beer), and the potentially beneficial high fruit and vegetable intake pattern (characterized by high intake of fresh fruits and cruciferous vegetables). After adjustment for various anthropometric and demographic factors (age, BMI, smoking, physical activity, socioeconomic factors, etc.), the high fruit and vegetable intake pattern was associated with a 49% reduction in pancreatic cancer risk among men when comparing the highest and lowest quartile of dietary pattern scores (Nkondjock et al., 2005b).

Specific phytochemicals have been implicated in the anticancer action of vegetable intake. Studies have shown that genistein, a phytoestrogen and the predominant isoflavonoid of the soy plant, inhibits cell growth in pancreatic cancer cells *in vitro* and *in vivo* (Boros et al., 2001; Mouria et al., 2002; Buchler et al., 2003). In an orthotopic nude mouse model, genistein significantly improved survival, almost completely inhibited metastasis, and increased apoptosis (Buchler et al., 2003). When genistein was combined with the tumor necrosis factor–related apoptosis-inducing ligand/Apo2 ligand (TRAIL/Apo2L), the combination of the two agents decreased cell proliferation *in vitro* and tumor volume *in vivo* and increased the number of apoptotic cells to a greater extent than with either agent alone (Nozawa et al., 2004). The constitutively activated signal transducer and activator of transcription-3 protein (STAT3), a mediator of several hormone and growth factors, was modulated by genistein, as well as indole-3-carbinol (I3C; a breakdown product of glucosinolates, which are found primarily in cruciferous vegetables, as described later in this chapter), in pancreatic tumor cell lines (Panc-1 and MIA PaCa-2) (Lian et al., 2004). STAT3 constitutive activation is inhibited at 10 μM of genistein or I3C. Induction of apoptosis by I3C was also shown. Boros et al. (2001) reported that genistein regulates cell tumor proliferation by regulating glucose oxidation and inhibiting synthesis of nucleic acid ribose from glucose through nonoxidative steps of the pentose cycle, which is necessary for nucleic acid synthesis and salvage pathways of purine and pyrimidine bases.

Biochanin A, the 4′-methyl ether of genistein found in various legumes, has been reported to inhibit metastasis in breast cancer and colon cancer (Peterson and Barnes, 1996; Wang et al., 1998). A study of two pancreatic adenocarcinoma cell lines, one derived from a male and the other a female patient, found that biochanin A inhibited growth in both male and female tumor cells (Lyn-Cook et al., 1999b). However, two other phytoestrogens, equol and coumestrol, which are found in alfalfa sprouts, clover sprouts, and beans, were found to inhibit cancer cell proliferation only in the female cell lines, primarily through downregulation of K-*ras* expression (Lyn-Cook et al., 1999b).

The effects of several food-derived polyphenols were compared in *in vivo* and *in vitro* models of pancreatic cancer (Mouria et al., 2002). Quercetin (a flavonoid with widespread distribution in vegetables and fruits, including onions, apples, and teas) decreased primary tumor growth, increased apoptosis, and prevented metastasis in nude mice implanted with human pancreatic cells. In human MIA PACa-2 and rat BSp73AS pancreatic cancer cell lines, quercetin and trans-resveratrol (enriched in red wine and grapes) markedly enhanced apoptosis, causing mitochondrial depolarization and cytochrome *c* release followed by caspase-3 activation; however, the flavonol glycoside of quercetin, rutin, did not. In addition, the effect of a combination of quercetin and trans-resveratrol on mitochondrial cytochrome *c* release and caspase-3 activity was greater than the expected additive response. The inhibition of mitochondrial permeability transition prevented cytochrome *c* release, caspase-3 activation, and apoptosis caused by polyphenols. The activity of NFκB was inhibited by quercetin and trans-resveratrol, but not genistein, indicating that this transcription factor is not the only mediator of the polyphenols' effects on apoptosis. These results suggest that food-derived polyphenols inhibit pancreatic cancer growth and prevent metastasis by inducing mitochondrial dysfunction, resulting in cytochrome *c* release, caspase activation, and apoptosis. An additional study confirmed the antiproliferative and proapoptotic effect of resveratrol on human pancreatic cancer cell lines PANC-1 and AsPC-1 (Ding and Adrian, 2002).

Vegetables of the *Brassica oleracea* species (e.g., cabbage, broccoli, cauliflower, Brussels sprouts, kohlrabi, and kale; also called *cruciferous vegetables*) and many other genera that include a variety of food plants (e.g., arugula, radish, daikon, watercress, horseradish, and wasabi) are known to be rich in glucosinolates (β-thioglycoside-*N*-hydroxysulfates). These compounds are hydrolyzed by myrosinase, a plant enzyme released when plants are cut, ground, or chewed, releasing the biologically active isothiocyanates (ITCs). Some naturally occurring forms of this phytochemical include 2-phenethyl isothiocyanate (PEITC), benzyl isothiocyanate, and sulforaphanes (Kris-Etherton et al., 2002). ITCs are known to induce expression of phase I and phase II enzymes and, to a lesser extent, directly inhibit the P450s; the effect is dependent on the individual ITC. PEITC has been shown to inhibit pancreatic carcinogenesis in terms of incidence of atypical hyperplasias and multiplicity of pancreatic proliferative lesions including adenocarcinomas in BOP-treated hamsters given PEITC during the initiation phase (i.e., administered concomitantly with the carcinogen) (Nishikawa et al., 1996) but not in the post-initiation phase (i.e., PEITC administered after BOP) (Nishikawa et al., 1999). The mechanisms of PEITC on cell kinetics were further investigated in BOP-treated hamsters (Nishikawa et al., 1997). PEITC seems to exert its chemopreventive activity against BOP initiation of carcinogenesis by decreasing cell turnover and DNA methylation in the target organs, and by influencing hepatic xenobiotic-metabolizing phase I enzymes (Nishikawa et al., 1997, 2004). Similar studies with other synthetic ITCs with longer alkyl chains showed that 3-phenylpropyl ITC (PPITC) is not effective in BOP-induced pancreatic cancers, in contrast to lung cancers (Nishikawa et al., 1996), whereas 4-phenylbutyl ITC (PBITC) did inhibit the development of pancreatic atypical hyperplasias and adenocarcinomas of ductal origin (Son et al., 2000). In cell culture benzyl ITC (BITC), also derived from cruciferous vegetables, inhibits growth of BxPC-3 pancreatic cancer cells in a concentration-dependent manner with an IC_{50} of ~8 μM, a concentration achievable in plasma with regular dietary intake of cruciferous vegetables (Srivastava and Singh, 2004). The mechanism of this action involves G_2/M cell cycle arrest and induction of apoptosis, which is associated with inhibition of NFκB activation. Sulforaphane, another ITC, also induced G_2/M arrest and apoptosis, and cellular toxicity was correlated with a decrease in cellular glutathione levels *in vitro*; treatment of a xenograft mouse model of pancreatic cancer with sulforaphane resulted in a decrease in mean tumor volume by 40% relative to controls (Pham et al., 2004).

Curcumin, a yellow pigment chemical present in the spice turmeric (*Curcuma longa*), has been shown to inhibit pancreatic cancer growth *in vitro* (Hidaka et al., 2002; Li et al., 2004b). Furthermore, curcumin ameliorates ethanol- and non-ethanol–induced experimental pancreatitis, which may be a precursor condition for pancreatic cancer development (Gukovsky et al., 2003). The mechanism of curcumin's inhibition of inflammation and cell growth, as well as stimulation of apoptosis, involves downregulation of NFκB, which is constitutively activated in pancreatic cells, and growth control molecules (e.g., prostaglandin E_2 [PGE_2]) induced by NFκB in human pancreatic cells (Gukovsky et al., 2003; Li et al., 2004b). Furthermore, production of cytokines (and their receptors) such as interleukin-6 (IL-6) and TNF-α, as well as the chemokines IL-8 and KC (a rodent analog of IL-8/GROa) and inducible nitric oxide synthase (iNOS) in pancreas, are diminished by curcumin (Gukovsky et al., 2003; Hidaka et al., 2002). The effectiveness of curcumin in inhibiting pancreatic carcinogenesis in animal models has apparently not been tested.

Carotenoids have various cancer preventive activities, including antioxidant activity, enhancement of immune function, stimulation of gap junctional intercellular communication, induction of detoxifying enzymes, and inhibition of cellular proliferation (Heber and Lu, 2002). Rich sources of carotenoids (such as α- and β-carotenes, lutein, and lycopene) include tomatoes, carrots, cantaloupes, sweet potatoes, and spinach, as well as many leafy greens and yellow-red fruits and vegetables. A case-control study in a Canadian population explored the relationship between dietary carotenoid intake and pancreatic cancer risk (Nkondjock et al., 2005a). It was found that (after adjusting for age, Canadian province of residence, BMI, smoking educational attainment, dietary folate, and total energy intake), lycopene provided primarily by tomatoes was associated with a 31% reduction in pancreatic cancer risk among men.

Meats and Fats

Numerous case-control and international mortality and food pattern studies have shown a positive correlation between the average amount of oil and fat consumption and cancer of the pancreas (Baghurst et al., 1991; Ghadirian et al., 1991a,b; Howe et al., 1992; Stolzenberg-Solomon et al., 2002). Similarly, a number of studies have associated consumption of meat, eggs, and milk with an increased risk of pancreatic cancer (reviewed in World Cancer Research Fund and American Institute for Cancer Research, 1997; Howe and Burch, 1996; Michaud, 2004). This trend is illustrated in a Japanese case-control study that showed that intake of meats and animal viscera increased pancreatic cancer risk, whereas vegetables and the traditional Japanese foods (e.g., tofu and raw fish) reduced the risk (Ohba et al., 1996). The responsible component in dietary patterns with high meat intake is unknown but may include total fat or saturated fat, cholesterol, protein, and *N*-nitroso or heterocyclic aromatic compounds produced in meats by high-temperature cooking (Howe and Burch, 1996; World Cancer Research Fund and American Institute for Cancer Research, 1997).

A number of studies in rats and hamsters have demonstrated potentiation of carcinogen-induced carcinogenesis by high-fat diets, particularly those high in lard (a saturated fat) or corn oil (high in PUFAs, especially linoleic acid—an omega-6 fatty acid) (reviewed in Roebuck, 1992; Zhang and Go, 1996). Furthermore, an experimental "Western diet"—high in fat and protein and low in calcium—increases pancreatic epithelial cell hyperproliferation in mice (Xue et al., 1996, 1999). Conversely, dietary restriction does not inhibit pancreatic carcinogenesis induced by BOP in the hamster, at least in one study (Birt et al., 1997), and voluntary physical exercise does not ameliorate the effects of a high-fat diet in promoting pancreatic carcinogenesis in the BOP-treated hamster (Kazakoff et al., 1996).

A potential mechanism of the carcinogenesis-promoting effect of PUFA involves the production of various reactive intermediates. ROS are generated during lipid peroxidation and can arise directly from linoleic acid hydroperoxide decomposition (Zhang and Go, 1996). Consequently these oxygen free radicals can damage DNA and produce mutations that are associated with the initiation and progression of human cancer. Z'graggen et al. (2001) showed that a high-fat, high-protein diet promoted tumor development in 7,12-dimethylbenzanthracene (DMBA)–induced ductal pancreatic cancer, possibly through faulty gene repair mechanisms or delayed natural regression of early lesions. The authors postulated that a high-fat diet may cause K-*ras* gene mutations by increasing COX-2 and *ras*-p21 expression, as well as membrane localization of *ras*-p21, which is essential for proper *ras* protein function, phenomena that have been demonstrated in colon cancer (Z'graggen et al., 2001).

Another mechanism linking meat intake to pancreatic cancer risk may involve carcinogens produced in grilled meat products. Heterocyclic amines (HCAs) and polycyclic aromatic hydrocarbons are carcinogens formed during cooking of meat in a time- and temperature-dependent manner. A case-control study found that grilled red meat intake specifically was a risk factor for pancreatic cancer, and that method of meat preparation in addition to total intake is important in assessing the effects of meat consumption (Anderson et al., 2002). One study in an animal model of pancreatic cancer has confirmed the carcinogenicity of certain HCAs. Several HCAs were tested in a "rapid-production" model of pancreatic carcinogenesis in hamsters, whereby carcinogenesis was initiated with BOP, then augmentation pressure was exerted through treatment with DL-ethionine and methionine and feeding of a choline-deficient diet (Yoshimoto et al., 1999). Out of eight HCAs tested, two compounds, 3-amino-1,4-dimethyl-5*H*-pyrido[4,3-*b*]indole (Trp-P-1) and 2-amino-3,4,8-trimethylimidazo [4,5-*f*]quinoxaline (4,8-DiMeIQx), enhanced pancreatic carcinogenesis in this model.

As described earlier in this chapter, diets rich in PUFAs stimulate pancreatic cancer development. In contrast, supplements of long-chain omega-3 PUFA, such as DHA and EPA, which are enriched in fish oils, exert suppressive effects in several cancer models, particularly breast cancer (Terry et al., 2003). A fish oil–enriched nutritional supplement reverses weight loss in patients with pancreatic cancer cachexia (Barber et al., 1999) by diminishing production of IL-6, increasing serum insulin, and decreasing the cortisol-to-insulin ratio and the proportion of patients excreting proteolysis-inducing factor (associated with cancer-associated cachexia) (Barber et al., 2001).

The first experiments investigating the effect of omega-3 fatty acids in animal models showed that a 20% menhaden fish oil diet fed for 4 months produced a significant decrease in the development of both the size and the number of preneoplastic lesions when compared with a 20% corn oil diet rich in omega-6 fatty acids in male azaserine-treated rats (O'Connor et al., 1985). Follow-up studies showed that as the ratio of dietary omega-3 to omega-6 fatty acids increased in a diet totaling 20% by weight of fat, the development of preneoplastic atypical acinar cell nodules (AACN) decreased significantly (O'Connor et al., 1989). In addition, serum levels of PGE_2, thromboxane B_2 (TXB_2), and 6-keto-prostaglandin $F_{1\alpha}$ (6-keto-$PGF_{1\alpha}$) decreased significantly. Intervention of the omega-6 fatty acid–rich diet with the omega-3 fatty acid–rich diet significantly decreased focal development when given after carcinogen exposure. However, in a 6-month study using the MaxEPA product, which contains 9.4% fish oil, in a high-linoleic acid background diet did not protect against the increased number and size of pancreatic atypical acinar cell foci stimulated by the high-fat diet in azaserine-treated rats, although cell proliferation in atypical acinar cell foci and prostaglandin levels was decreased (Appel and Woutersen, 1994). In a follow-up 12-month study of MaxEPA feeding, a dose-dependent increase of preneoplastic AACNs was seen with an induction of eicosanoids PGE_2, $PGF_{2\alpha}$, and TXB_2 (Appel and Woutersen, 1996a). In BOP-treated hamsters, increasing doses of MaxEPA in a high-fat diet had little effect, although pancreatic levels of PGE_2, 6-keto-$PGF_{1\alpha}$, and $PGF_{2\alpha}$ decreased significantly with increasing dietary MaxEPA (Appel and Woutersen, 1995). The reason for these anomalous results is unclear but may involve the linoleic acid content of the high-fat diets, which could overwhelm any protective effect of the omega-3 PUFA. However, linoleic acid in the BOP-induced pancreatic cancer did not enhance pancreatic tumor growth, even though levels of lipid peroxidation were increased and activity of glutathione peroxidase decreased in pancreatic intratumoral tissue (Kilian et al., 2002; Kilian et al., 2003).

Tea and Coffee

An early study from 1981 found that coffee drinkers consuming three or more cups of coffee per day had a relative risk of pancreatic cancer of 2.7 compared with noncoffee drinkers (MacMahon et al., 1981), stimulating interest in a potential link between coffee consumption and pancreatic cancer. A cohort study of >110,000 Japanese subjects reported that heavy coffee consumption (>4 cups/day) may increase risk of pancreatic cancer (Lin et al., 2002). However, a number of other studies have concluded no association (Heuch et al., 1983; Mack et al., 1986; Howe et al., 1992; Gold, 1995; Isaksson et al., 2002). One confounder in these studies could be cigarette smoking, as not all studies control for this factor or self-reporting in subjects is inaccurate (Porta et al., 2000).

Interestingly, though, in the Spanish PANKRAS II case-control study, an association between coffee consumption and K-*ras* mutations was identified. Among 121 cases, K-*ras* mutations were significantly more common in tumors of regular coffee drinkers than in nonregular coffee drinkers. The odds of a mutated tumor increased in approximately linear manner with increasing level of coffee consumption (Porta et al., 1999). It is not clear whether caffeine, other coffee compounds, or other factors with which coffee drinking is associated may modulate K-*ras* activation. Potentially, coffee components can induce or inhibit relevant metabolic pathways that are involved with activation or inactivation of carcinogenic molecules. Alternatively, these compounds can inhibit DNA repair mechanisms. However, another study conducted in California did not show a significant association between K-*ras* mutational pattern or p53 staining and coffee drinking (caffeinated coffee, decaffeinated coffee, and total coffee drinking) (Slebos et al., 2000). One limitation of this study may be that the questionnaire used evaluated average total coffee consumption habits during the year before diagnosis, which may not capture the etiologically relevant exposure period. Although the results of these studies are inconsistent and the mechanisms underlying the associations between K-*ras* mutation and diet are not understood, these studies illustrate the potential for identifying important gene–nutrient interactions in pancreatic cancer.

Inhibition of tumorigenesis in animal models by green or black tea preparations has been demonstrated for a number of organ sites, such as skin, lung, oral cavity, esophagus, forestomach, stomach, small intestine, colon, mammary gland, and pancreas. Epidemiological studies, however, are not as clear concerning the protective effects of tea consumption against cancer formation in humans (Yang et al., 2002). Very limited epidemiological evidence from several studies suggests an inverse association between tea consumption and pancreatic cancer in humans (Bushman, 1998). A population-based case-control study in Shanghai indicated a reduction in risk of colorectal and pancreatic cancer in both men and women with consistent green tea consumption (Ji et al., 1997). However, in the Iowa Women's Study, a prospective cohort study of some 34,000 postmenopausal women, no relationship between tea intake and pancreatic cancer incidence was demonstrated (Harnack et al., 1997).

In vitro data support a cancer-inhibiting effect of EGCG, the major polyphenol component of green tea. EGCG inhibits growth of three pancreatic carcinoma cell lines (PANC-1, MIA PaCa-2, and BxPC-3) in a dose-dependent manner (Takada et al., 2002). Further study included black and green tea extracts and components of these extracts to determine their effect on tumor cell growth *in vitro*. Fractions studied included a mixture of polyphenols from green tea (GTP), mixtures of polyphenols (BTP) and of theaflavins (MF) from black tea, and the purified components epicatechin-3-gallate (ECG) and EGCG. Results showed inhibition (~90%) of cell growth in HPAC pancreatic adenocarcinoma cells by black and green tea extracts (0.02%). GTP (10 μg/ml) and MF (100 μg/ml) significantly inhibited growth (~90%); ECG and EGCG inhibited growth as well (~95%).

Black and green tea extracts, GTP, and EGCG decreased the expression of the K-*ras* gene. Green and black tea extracts decreased the multidrug-resistant gene (*mdr-1*), although GTP and EGCG increased expression (Lyn-Cook et al., 1999a). Other studies explored the molecular mechanism of EGCG action in pancreatic cancer cells *in vitro*. Takada et al. (2002) showed that EGCG treatment resulted in significant suppression of the invasive ability of these lines but did not affect the cell cycle protein cyclin D1. Qanungo et al. (2005) showed that the antiproliferative action of EGCG is mediated through induction of apoptosis, invoked by oligomerization of Bcl-2–associated X (Bax) protein, depolarization of mitochondrial membranes to facilitate cytochrome *c* release into the cytosol and downregulation of X Chromosome-Linked Inhibitor of Apoptosis Protein (XIAP). In addition, EGCG elicited production of intracellular ROS, as well as activation of *c*-Jun *N*-terminal kinase (JNK). Blocking these pathways with an inhibitor of JNK signaling and the antioxidant *N*-acetyl-*L*-cysteine (NAC) blocked EGCG-induced apoptosis, implicating the involvement of ROS-mediated JNK activation in the apoptotic response.

Pancreatic carcinogenesis and tumor promotion were inhibited in two hamster models with feeding of green tea extract, demonstrating an *in vivo* effect (Hiura et al., 1997). In addition, when green tea polyphenols were combined with palm carotene, which consists of 60% β-carotene, 30% α-carotene, 3% γ-carotene, and 4% lycopene, the same effect was seen in diminishing pancreatic preneoplastic lesions and duct epithelial hyperplasia and atypical hyperplasia (Majima et al., 1998). Therefore, compelling preclinical evidence with tea extracts and isolated tea components suggests that tea intake may inhibit pancreatic carcinogenesis, although much further research is warranted.

Alcohol

The results of numerous prospective cohort and case-control studies for alcohol consumption and pancreatic cancer risk have been inconsistent, with many confounding variables present in various studies. However, heavy alcohol consumption has been known to be a major cause of acute and chronic pancreatitis; in the United States and other developed countries, 60–90% of cases of chronic pancreatitis are linked to alcohol consumption (Durbec and Sarles, 1978; Dufour and Adamson, 2003; Swaroop et al., 2004). The chronic inflammation of pancreatitis accelerates the pancreatic oncogenic processes, and chronic pancreatitis has been linked to pancreatic cancer (Gordis and Gold, 1984; Lowenfels et al., 1993). It is thought that chronic heavy alcohol consumption potentiates other risk factors such as smoking in pancreatic and other cancers. In fact, according to the Eleventh Annual Report on Carcinogens by the U.S. National Toxicology Program (http://ntp.niehs.nih.gov/ntp/roc/toc11.html), alcoholic beverage consumption has been classified as a human carcinogen since 2000 (U.S. Department of Health and Human Services, 2005).

An important mediator of the deleterious effects of ethanol consumption is acetaldehyde, which is produced in the pancreas through oxidative metabolism of ethanol via alcohol dehydrogenase, as well as CYP 2E1. Acetaldehyde is mutagenic and carcinogenic *in vitro* and *in vivo* (Poschl and Seitz, 2004). The molecular mechanisms by which alcohol and its metabolites such as acetaldehyde and fatty acid ethyl esters induce inflammation and carcinogenesis have been studied and are reviewed by Go et al. (2005b). In summary, these mechanisms include (1) premature activation of zymogens; (2) induction of the inflammatory response through activation of nuclear transcription factors (including NFκB) and activation protein 1 (AP-1); (3) increased production of ROS resulting in oxidative DNA damage and altered effect of dietary antioxidants; (4) activation of pancreatic stellate cells that lead to fibrosis; (5) gene mutation in enzymes related to CYP, glutathione *S*-transferase, aldehyde dehydrogenase, cationic trypsinogen, and pancreatic secretory trypsin inhibitor (PST1); (6) effects on metabolism of tobacco carcinogen NNK; and (7) dysregulation of proliferation and apoptosis. In addition to direct effects of ethanol, a number of factors including genetics, intestinal infection, and dietary factors may make the pancreas more susceptible to damage induced by alcohol consumption.

Dietary fat appears to potentiate the development of alcoholic pancreatitis by modulating oxidative stress. For example, unsaturated fat (corn oil) potentiated development of alcoholic pancreatitis in female Wistar rats fed high levels of ethanol. This effect was mediated through oxidative stress as measured by radical adducts in pancreatic secretions and levels of lipid peroxidation in the pancreas (Kono et al., 2001). However, saturated fat (medium-chain triglycerides) attenuated the injury and blunted oxidative stress.

Isoprenoids

Various other phytochemicals found in plants also have antitumor or anticarcinogenic effects. Isoprenoids are non-nutritive dietary phytochemicals found in the essential oils of citrus fruits, cherry, spearmint, dill, caraway, and other plants. Bioactive isoprenoids include limonene, perillyl alcohol, geraniol, and farnesol. The important mechanistic activities of this class of compounds are as regulators of the mevalonate pathway, which produces essential sterols, ubiquinones, retinoids, and isoprenoids, which are essential to cell survival. Several of these compounds are required intermediates for the post-translational modification of small G proteins, including *ras*, nuclear lamins, and growth factor receptors. Suppressors of activities providing and transferring mevalonate-derived substrates for the modifications of these growth-associated proteins diminish cellular growth (Mo and Elson, 2004).

A number of pharmacological inhibitors of the mevalonate pathway show promising activities in inhibiting pancreatic carcinogenesis in preclinical studies. For example, lovastatin, a competitive inhibitor of 3-hydroxy-3-methylglutaryl coenzyme A (HMG-CoA) reductase activity, inhibited the proliferation of human and hamster pancreatic tumor cells in culture (Sumi et al., 1994; Muller et al., 1998) and of pancreatic tumor xenografts implanted in nude mice (Sumi et al., 1992). However, these types of nondiscriminate inhibitors of the mevalonate pathway may have dose-limiting toxicities. Mevalonate-derived isoprenoids from natural sources post-transcriptionally downregulate HMG-CoA reductase activity with specificity for tumors and may have greater potential in pancreatic tumor chemoprevention (Mo and Elson, 2004). Significant inhibition of human pancreatic tumor cells *in vitro* (60–90%) is attained by administration of farnesol, geranyl geraniol, perillyl amine, geraniol, and perillyl alcohol (Burke et al., 1997). In the same report, hamsters fed geraniol or farnesol at 20 g/kg diet exhibited complete inhibition of BOP-induced pancreatic tumor growth. Both farnesol and geraniol were more potent than perillyl alcohol, which inhibited tumor growth by 50% at 40 g/kg diet with no effects on plasma cholesterol levels (Burke et al., 1997). *In vitro*, farnesol, geraniol, and perillyl alcohol increased apoptosis and proapoptotic Bak levels (Stayrook et al., 1997; Burke et al., 2002). Similarly, *in vivo* treatment during the promotion/progression phase of BOP-induced pancreatic carcinogenesis with perillyl alcohol or farnesol resulted in hyperplastic pancreatic ductal neoplasms with higher apoptotic rates, increased Bak protein expression, diminished expression of the antiapoptotic protein Bcl-XL, and lowered rates of DNA synthesis (Burke et al., 2002). Interestingly, farnesylation of H-*ras*, but not K-*ras*, was inhibited by perillyl alcohol in pancreatic tumor cells transformed with either *ras* isoform; similarly, the downstream effector MAP kinase phosphorylation was inhibited in H-*ras* tumor cells only (Stayrook et al., 1998). Farnesol mimetics *S*-trans, trans-farnesylthiosalicylic acid (FTS) inhibited the proliferation of Panc-1 cells and the growth of Panc-1 xenograft in nude mice (Weisz et al., 1999). Geranyl geraniol and menaquinone-4 (vitamin K2; a mixed isoprenoid with a geranyl geraniol side chain) inhibited the proliferation of MIA PaCa-2 cells and induced apoptosis (Shibayama-Imazu et al., 2003).

Retinoids and Vitamin D: Differentiation Agents

The vitamin A metabolite, retinoic acid, has been shown to have chemopreventive and therapeutic activity against several cancers. These effects are the results of induction of differentiation and growth arrest, which are mediated through retinoid nuclear receptors termed *retinoic acid receptors* (RARs) and retinoic X receptors (RXRs) (Niles, 2004). In cell culture, treatment with several retinoids, including all-*trans*-retinoic acid, 9-*cis*-retinoic acid, and 13-*cis*-retinoic acid, results in a time- and dose-dependent growth inhibition in ductal but not acinar pancreatic tumor cells, although results for individual ligands are not consistent among studies (Rosewicz et al., 1995; Bold et al., 1996; Vickers et al., 1997; Albrechtsson et al., 2002). One report (El-Metwally et al., 2005a) showed that natural all-*trans*-retinoic acid inhibited proliferation in 10 human pancreatic adenocarcinoma cell lines with varying degrees of differentiation, some of which were characterized previously as retinoid resistant. Retinoid treatment *in vitro* induces a differentiated phenotype, as evidenced by cellular morphology and expression of differentiation-specific genes such as carbonic anhydrase II (Rosewicz et al., 1995; El-Metwally et al., 2005b). In addition, 9-*cis* retinoic acid enhanced the G_1 cell cycle arrest induced by troglitazone, a PPARγ ligand, implicating the action of the RXRα/PPARγ pathway in growth inhibition (Tsujie et al., 2003b). Retinoids also induce apoptosis and decrease the Bcl-2/Bax ratio in pancreatic adenocarcinoma cells, activity that requires RARα (Pettersson et al., 2002; El-Metwally et al., 2005a). Additional targets for retinoic acid action identified in pancreatic cancer cells include protein kinase C (Rosewicz et al., 1996), stromelysin 3 (an MMP) (von Marschall Z. et al., 1998), kinesin-related protein HsEg5 (important for spindle assembly and function during mitosis) (Kaiser et al., 1999), α_6,β_1-integrin receptor (modulates cell adhesion to laminin) (Rosewicz et al., 1997), MUC4 (mucin; high molecular weight glycoprotein overexpressed in pancreatic tumors) (Choudhury et al., 2000), c-Met (hepatocyte growth factor receptor) (Leelawat et al., 2005), and TGF-β protein and EGF receptor (autocrine growth factor pathways) (El-Metwally et al., 2005b).

On the basis of promising *in vitro* data, a number of studies evaluated retinoic acid action in animal models. In azaserine-initiated pancreatic carcinogenesis in rats, long-term treatment with various synthetically derived retinoids inhibited progression of pancreatic carcinomas (Longnecker et al., 1982, 1983); similar results were born out in short-term studies looking at number and size of acidophilic foci, believed to be precancerous lesions (preceding the definition of PanIN) (Roebuck et al., 1984). The inhibitory effect of low-dose retinoids could be enhanced to a small degree by addition of selenium to the diet (Curphey et al., 1988). Results of retinoid action in BOP-induced carcinogenesis are not as clear. In this model there was either little to no effect (Longnecker et al., 1983, 1986) or a small enhancing effect of retinoids on BOP-induced carcinogenesis (Birt et al., 1981, 1983).

Based on these findings, clinical trials have been initiated, but with disappointing results. Phase II studies have been conducted on retinoic acid co-administered with interferon-α (IFN-α) in patients with advanced unresectable pancreatic carcinoma, without impressive results (Moore et al., 1995; Brembeck et al., 1998). In another study, retinoids were added to chemotherapy plus IFN-β treatment in patients with metastatic pancreatic cancer. However, there was not a large effect on survival, and moreover the incidence of toxicities was high (Recchia et al., 1998). Therefore, the prospect of retinoic acid as a therapeutic agent is not great; however, there still may be applications in prevention.

Another differentiation agent, vitamin D and analogs thereof, shows growth inhibitory effects in pancreatic cancer cells (Kawa et al., 1996; Zugmaier et al., 1996; Colston et al., 1997; Pettersson et al., 2000; Albrechtsson et al., 2003), and these effects interact with those of retinoids (Zugmaier et al., 1996; Pettersson et al., 2000). Most pancreatic cancer cells express the vitamin D receptor (Kawa et al., 1996; Colston et al., 1997; Albrechtsson et al., 2003), as well as the enzyme 25-hydroxyvitamin D-1α-hydroxylase that converts the vitamin prohormone to the most active form (Schwartz et al., 2004). Vitamin D analogs block the G_1/S transition by upregulating p21 and p27 proteins (Kawa et al., 1997; Schwartz et al., 2004). A Western-style diet (high fat, calcium, and vitamin D) fed to mice induces hyperproliferation of epithelial cells of the exocrine pancreas, but the effect is ameliorated by replacement of dietary calcium and vitamin D (Xue et al., 1996, 1999). A phase II trial of a non-hypercalcemic vitamin D analog Seocalcitol (EB1089) has been conducted in patients with inoperable pancreatic cancer; the drug was well tolerated, but no cytostatic activity was seen in this trial (Evans et al., 2002). Further research is warranted to determine the therapeutic potential of vitamin D analogs in less advanced pancreatic cancer and in prevention of pancreatic carcinogenesis.

METABOLIC HYPOTHESIS FOR PANCREATIC CANCER

Pancreatic tumor cells are characterized by poor differentiation and a high glucose-utilizing phenotype. Boros et al. (2002) have hypothesized that a specific metabolic phenotype is associated with tumor cells relative to normal cells. Tumor cells assume their unique characteristics according to their diverse genetic aberrations. Their invasive and proliferative characteristics, however, are limited by the availability of substrates, nutrients, and metabolic pathway enzyme activities. On the basis of these factors, tumor cells exhibit distinct metabolic phenotypes determining the rate of proliferation, apoptosis, cell cycle arrest, and differentiation. Hormones, signaling pathways, environmental factors, and nutritional habits have a strong influence on these metabolic phenotypes. Cell transformation and tumor growth are associated with the activation of metabolic enzymes that increase glucose carbon utilization for nucleic acid synthesis, whereas enzymes of the lipid and amino acid synthesis pathways are activated in tumor growth inhibition. Furthermore, phosphorylation and allosteric and transcriptional regulation of intermediary metabolic enzymes and their substrate availability together mediate and sustain cell transformation from one condition to another. Metabolic profiling of cancer cells using labeled tracers have shown opposite changes in metabolic phenotypes induced by TGF-β, which is a cell-transforming agent (Boros et al., 2000), and tumor growth–inhibiting phytochemicals such as genistein, as outlined earlier in this chapter (Boros et al., 2001).

The authors illustrate that understanding adaptive metabolic changes in glycolysis and anabolic reactions in response to tumor growth–modulating agents is fundamental to the understanding of tumor pathophysiology in the pancreas. The proposed metabolic hypothesis of tumor cell growth and death permits a wide range of basic and clinical studies in developing new strategies to revert tumor-specific metabolic changes. Complex metabolic networks of key regulatory metabolic enzymes offer a large number of targets for direct intervention. This new class of metabolic regulators offers a potentially effective alternative to current gene therapeutics, chemotherapeutics, and signal pathway regulators to achieve the same endpoint effect of reducing cell proliferation through limiting glucose carbon use for nucleic acid synthesis (Boros et al., 2002).

FUTURE DIRECTIONS

Progress in the understanding of the genome has been paralleled by development in the understanding of the process of carcinogenesis. As outlined in this chapter, cancer is now considered a genetic disease; tumor cells result from multiple genetic defects caused by exposure to environmental and infectious agents, as well as dietary and various lifestyle factors (Go et al., 2003). Knowledge of the genetic signatures and molecular markers of tumorigenesis provides us with the opportunity to use approaches such as dietary intervention to prevent cancer development. High-dimensional technologies to assay genetic and metabolic changes within the cell on a global basis are new weapons in the scientific arsenal that allow nutrition scientists to move forward beyond the reductionist method of investigating single nutrient effects on an isolated biological pathway toward a more holistic approach of exploring the molecular details of food and nutrient effects on an entire biological organism.

As these concepts are evolving, so has the very definition of a *nutrient*. The classic definition of a *nutrient* is a constituent of food necessary for normal physiological function and *essential nutrients* are those required for optimal health (Go et al., 2003). With our expanding working knowledge of the role of nutrients in gene expression and cellular response to changes in nutrient availability, the pursuit of a definitive definition of the term *nutrient* is a work in progress. Young (2002) defined the term *nutrient* in the postgenomic era as a "fully characterized (physical, chemical, physiological) constituent of a diet, natural or designed, that serves as a significant energy yielding substrate or a precursor for the synthesis of macromolecules or of other components needed for normal cell differentiation, growth, renewal, repair, defense and/or maintenance or a required signaling molecule, cofactor or determinant of normal molecular structure/function and/or promoter of cell and organ integrity." In addition, nutrients can catalyze reactions and promote the assembly of mechanistic structures. Nutrient–genome interactions may differ according to the life cycle of the organism and have a profound influence on health maintenance and disease (cancer) prevention. Within this mechanistic definition of nutrients, one must consider that the requirement range of a particular nutrient is contingent upon the functionality of the cell and organism, that the required amount may vary depending on whether the nutrient is necessary for normal cell growth or cancer prevention, and that certain nutrients may also be harmful in supernormal doses.

The new definition of *nutrients* can provide the appropriate mode of gene–nutrient analysis needed at the genome, transcriptome, proteome, metabolome, physiome/phenome, and populome level to generate appropriate biomarkers (Figure 3). With the development of novel technologies and the advent of nutritional genomics, proteomics, metabolomics, and other so-called "-omics" sciences, there is renewed interest in dietary components that affect global gene expression and the integrative physiological and metabolic functions of an organism. Nutrition science has thus evolved into a multidisciplinary field that applies molecular biochemistry and integration of individual health to epidemiological investigation and population health (German et al., 2004). Therefore, there exists ample justification for creating an innovative research model to further explore the role of diet in health promotion and disease prevention, including pancreatic cancer.

The implications of our broadening knowledge of the impact of nutrient intake on cancer biology are that we can hope to utilize nutritional interventions to slow the progression of tumor development in the intraepithelial hyperplasia phase before tumor size becomes large enough for diagnosis and probability of metastasis increases (Figure 2). Opportunity exists to stretch this prevention phase so that symptom-free life of the future cancer patient is prolonged. Because the median age at cancer diagnosis in the United Sates is 70 years, and the average life expectancies are 74 years for men and 79 years for women, cancer delay may result in total prevention for many people (Lippman and Hong, 2002).

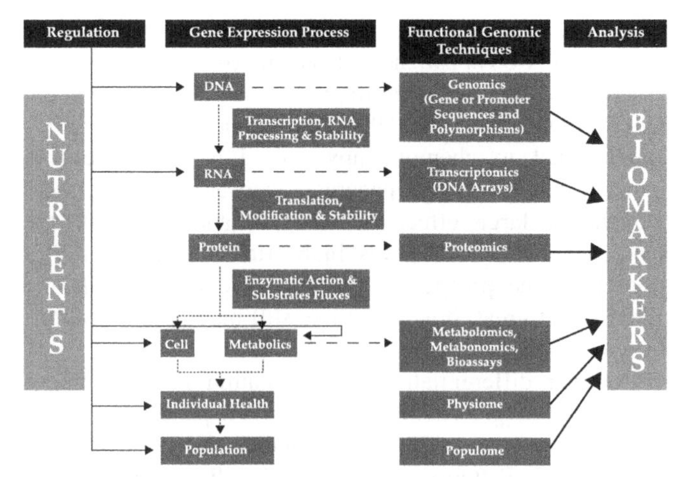

FIGURE 3 Nutritional genomics and biomarker discovery. The steps involved in gene expression (center); the stages at which diet, represented by nutrients, can modulate these processes from cell to population (left); and the functional genomics techniques used to analyze each stage, with appropriate biomarkers (reprinted with permission from Go et al., 2003.)

The results of new approaches will be to facilitate molecular analysis of nutrient action and identification of appropriate biomarkers that target individuals who are at risk and predisposed to pancreatic cancer. Ever-increasing evidence, including that presented in this volume, substantiates the beneficial effects of certain nutrients and interactions between nutrients in the carcinogenesis pathway, paving the way for modification of nutritional requirements as a cancer prevention strategy. In the future, diet, nutrition, and cancer prevention will be included in public health programs that target cancer risk management in the population at large, as well as on individual programs that focus on particular cancer risk profiles. Concomitantly, agricultural sciences will continue to develop improved plants through both traditional breeding techniques and genetic modification, and food industries will provide functional foods enriched with beneficial nutrients (Milner et al., 2001). Targeting pancreatic cancer prevention with specific foods and/or bioactive components is a relatively nontoxic and cost-effective strategy for reducing cancer burden. However, the complexity of the human diet coupled with individual variation in the carcinogenesis process will make continued research in the area of diet and pancreatic cancer prevention mandatory (Milner, 2002).

Toward this end, we would like to highlight the following research priorities for identifying gene–nutrient interactions in pancreatic cancer (Kern et al., 2001; Hine et al., 2003):

- Strengthening the evidence base linking dietary and lifestyle factors with cancer risk via epidemiological studies, especially where associations between specific genetic and metabolic alterations and dietary factors can be examined

- Identification of physiologically relevant polymorphisms in genes related to metabolism and detoxification of food-derived agents, both anticarcinogens and procarcinogens, and relate these individual variations to pancreatic cancer risk
- Refinement of relevant biomarkers and/or imaging systems for pancreatic cancer, especially present in the early PanIN stages, to identify affected individuals and to track impact of nutritional intervention on carcinogenesis
- Further development of animal models of pancreatic ductal adenocarcinoma, especially of transgenic models that recapitulate the human disease
- Validate use of high-dimensional analysis systems, including genomics, proteomics, and metabolomics, as biomarkers of pancreatic disease and to discriminate among subtypes to develop most effective intervention regimens.

Acknowledgment

Funding provided by the National Cancer Institute (NCI)/UCLA Clinical Nutrition Research Unit (CA42710) and NCI/National Center for Complementary and Alternative Medicine (AT1535). The authors recognize Yu Wang, Raymond Gonzales, Debra Wong, and Anita Stein for their expert editorial and technical assistance and Drs. Guido Eibl and Huanbiao Mo for critical review of the manuscript.

References

Albrechtsson, E., Jonsson, T., Moller, S., Hoglund, M., Ohlsson, B., and Axelson, J. 2003. Vitamin D receptor is expressed in pancreatic cancer cells and a vitamin D_3 analogue decreases cell number. *Pancreatology* **3**: 41–46.

Albrechtsson, E., Ohlsson, B., and Axelson, J. 2002. The expression of retinoic acid receptors and the effects in vitro by retinoids in human pancreatic cancer cell lines. *Pancreas* **25**: 49–56.

American Cancer Society. 2004. "Cancer Facts and Figures 2004." American Cancer Society, Atlanta, GA.

Anderson, K.E., Sinha, R., Kulldorff, M., Gross, M., Lang, N.P., Barber, C., Harnack, L., DiMagno, E., Bliss, R., and Kadlubar, F.F. 2002. Meat intake and cooking techniques: associations with pancreatic cancer. *Mutat Res* **506–507**: 225–231.

Andry, C.D., Kupchik, H.Z., and Rogers, A.E. 1990. L-azaserine induced preneoplasia in the rat pancreas. A morphometric study of dietary manipulation (lipotrope deficiency) and ultrastructural differentiation. *Toxicol Pathol* **18**: 10–17.

Appel, M.J., Garderen-Hoetmer, A., and Woutersen, R.A. 1996. Lack of inhibitory effects of β-carotene, vitamin C, vitamin E and selenium on development of ductular adenocarcinomas in exocrine pancreas of hamsters. *Cancer Lett* **103**: 157–162.

Appel, M.J., and Woutersen, R.A. 1994. Modulation of growth and cell turnover of preneoplastic lesions and of prostaglandin levels in rat pancreas by dietary fish oil. *Carcinogenesis* **15**: 2107–2112.

Appel, M.J., and Woutersen, R.A. 1995. Effects of dietary fish oil (MaxEPA) on *N*-nitrosobis(2-oxopropyl)amine (BOP)–induced pancreatic carcinogenesis in hamsters. *Cancer Lett* **94**: 179–189.

Appel, M.J., and Woutersen, R.A. 1996a. Dietary fish oil (MaxEPA) enhances pancreatic carcinogenesis in azaserine-treated rats. *Br J Cancer* **73**: 36–43.

Appel, M.J., and Woutersen, R.A. 1996b. Effects of dietary β-carotene and selenium on initiation and promotion of pancreatic carcinogenesis in azaserine-treated rats. *Carcinogenesis* **17**: 1411–1416.

Augustin, L.S., Franceschi, S., Jenkins, D.J., Kendall, C.W., and La, V.C. 2002. Glycemic index in chronic disease: a review. *Eur J Clin Nutr* **56**: 1049–1071.

Baghurst, P.A., McMichael, A.J., Slavotinek, A.H., Baghurst, K.I., Boyle, P., and Walker, A.M. 1991. A case-control study of diet and cancer of the pancreas. *Am J Epidemiol* **134**: 167–179.

Barber, M.D., Fearon, K.C., Tisdale, M.J., McMillan, D.C., and Ross, J.A. 2001. Effect of a fish oil-enriched nutritional supplement on metabolic mediators in patients with pancreatic cancer cachexia. *Nutr Cancer* **40**: 118–124.

Barber, M.D., Ross, J.A., Voss, A.C., Tisdale, M.J., and Fearon, K.C. 1999. The effect of an oral nutritional supplement enriched with fish oil on weight-loss in patients with pancreatic cancer. *Br J Cancer* **81**: 80–86.

Bardeesy, N., and DePinho, R.A. 2002. Pancreatic cancer biology and genetics. *Nat Rev Cancer* **2**: 897–909.

Bell, R.H., Jr., McCullough, P.J., and Pour, P.M. 1988. Influence of diabetes on susceptibility to experimental pancreatic cancer. *Am J Surg* **155**: 159–164.

Bell, R.H., Jr., Sayers, H.J., Pour, P.M., Ray, M.B., and McCullough, P.J. 1989. Importance of diabetes in inhibition of pancreatic cancer by streptozotocin. *J Surg Res* **46**: 515–519.

Benzie, I.F. 2000. Evolution of antioxidant defence mechanisms. *Eur J Nutr* **39**: 53–61.

Bergmann, U., Funatomi, H., Yokoyama, M., Beger, H.G., and Korc, M. 1995. Insulin-like growth factor I overexpression in human pancreatic cancer: evidence for autocrine and paracrine roles. *Cancer Res* **55**: 2007–2011.

Berrington de Gonzalez, A., Sweetland, S., and Spencer, E. 2003. A meta-analysis of obesity and the risk of pancreatic cancer. *Br J Cancer* **89**: 519–523.

Birt, D.F., Davies, M.H., Pour, P.M., and Salmasi, S. 1983. Lack of inhibition by retinoids of bis(2-oxopropyl)nitrosamine-induced carcinogenesis in Syrian hamsters. *Carcinogenesis* **4**: 1215–1220.

Birt, D.F., Pour, P.M., Nagel, D.L., Barnett, T., Blackwood, D., and Duysen, E. 1997. Dietary energy restriction does not inhibit pancreatic carcinogenesis by N-nitrosobis-2-(oxopropyl)amine in the Syrian hamster. *Carcinogenesis* **18**: 2107–2111.

Birt, D.F., Sayed, S., Davies, M.H., and Pour, P. 1981. Sex differences in the effects of retinoids on carcinogenesis by N-nitrosobis(2-oxopropyl)amine in Syrian hamsters. *Cancer Lett* **14**: 13–21.

Bisacchi, D., Benelli, R., Vanzetto, C., Ferrari, N., Tosetti, F., and Albini, A. 2003. Anti-angiogenesis and angioprevention: mechanisms, problems and perspectives. *Cancer Detect Prev* **27**: 229–238.

Block, G., Patterson, B., and Subar, A. 1992. Fruit, vegetables, and cancer prevention: a review of the epidemiological evidence. *Nutr Cancer* **18**: 1–29.

Bold, R.J., Ishizuka, J., Townsend, C.M., Jr., and Thompson, J.C. 1996. All-*trans*-retinoic acid inhibits growth of human pancreatic cancer cell lines. *Pancreas* **12**: 189–195.

Boone, C.W., and Kelloff, G.J. 2004. Cancer chemoprevention: subject cohorts with early neoplasia, agents, and intermediate marker endpoints in clinical trials evaluated by computer-assisted image analysis. *In* "Nutritional Oncology" (D. Heber, G.L. Blackburn, and V.L. Go, Eds), Vol. 22, pp. 343–378. Academic Press, San Diego.

Boros, L.G., Bassilian, S., Lim, S., and Lee, W.N. 2001. Genistein inhibits nonoxidative ribose synthesis in MIA pancreatic adenocarcinoma cells: a new mechanism of controlling tumor growth. *Pancreas* **22**: 1–7.

Boros, L.G., Lee, W.N., and Go, V.L. 2002. A metabolic hypothesis of cell growth and death in pancreatic cancer. *Pancreas* **24**: 26–33.

Boros, L.G., Torday, J.S., Lim, S., Bassilian, S., Cascante, M., and Lee, W.N. 2000. Transforming growth factor β_2 promotes glucose carbon incorporation into nucleic acid ribose through the nonoxidative pentose cycle in lung epithelial carcinoma cells. *Cancer Res* **60**: 1183–1185.

Brembeck, F.H., Schoppmeyer, K., Leupold, U., Gornistu, C., Keim, V., Mossner, J., Riecken, E.O., and Rosewicz, S. 1998. A phase II pilot trial of 13-*cis* retinoic acid and interferon-α in patients with advanced pancreatic carcinoma. *Cancer* **83**: 2317–2323.

Bremner, P., and Heinrich, M. 2002. Natural products as targeted modulators of the nuclear factor-κB pathway. *J Pharm Pharmacol* **54**: 453–472.

Buchler, P., Gukovskaya, A.S., Mouria, M., Buchler, M.C., Buchler, M.W., Friess, H., Pandol, S.J., Reber, H.A., and Hines, O.J. 2003. Prevention of metastatic pancreatic cancer growth *in vivo* by induction of apoptosis with genistein, a naturally occurring isoflavonoid. *Pancreas* **26**: 264–273.

Burke, Y.D., Ayoubi, A.S., Werner, S.R., McFarland, B.C., Heilman, D.K., Ruggeri, B.A., and Crowell, P.L. 2002. Effects of the isoprenoids perillyl alcohol and farnesol on apoptosis biomarkers in pancreatic cancer chemoprevention. *Anticancer Res* **22**: 3127–3134.

Burke, Y.D., Stark, M.J., Roach, S.L., Sen, S.E., and Crowell, P.L. 1997. Inhibition of pancreatic cancer growth by the dietary isoprenoids farnesol and geraniol. *Lipids* **32**: 151–156.

Bushman, J.L. 1998. Green tea and cancer in humans: a review of the literature. *Nutr Cancer* **31**: 151–159.

Caldas, C. 1999. Biliopancreatic malignancy: screening the at risk patient with molecular markers. *Ann Oncol* **10**(Suppl 4): 153–156.

Calle, E.E., and Kaaks, R. 2004. Overweight, obesity and cancer: epidemiological evidence and proposed mechanisms. *Nat Rev Cancer* **4**: 579–591.

Calle, E.E., Rodriguez, C., Walker-Thurmond, K., and Thun, M.J. 2003. Overweight, obesity, and mortality from cancer in a prospectively studied cohort of U.S. adults. *N Engl J Med* **348**: 1625–1638.

Choudhury, A., Singh, R.K., Moniaux, N., El-Metwally, T.H., Aubert, J.P., and Batra, S.K. 2000. Retinoic acid-dependent transforming growth factor-β_2-mediated induction of MUC4 mucin expression in human pancreatic tumor cells follows retinoic acid receptor-α signaling pathway. *J Biol Chem* **275**: 33929–33936.

Colston, K.W., James, S.Y., Ofori-Kuragu, E.A., Binderup, L., and Grant, A.G. 1997. Vitamin D receptors and anti-proliferative effects of vitamin D derivatives in human pancreatic carcinoma cells *in vivo* and *in vitro*. *Br J Cancer* **76**: 1017–1020.

Cullen, J.J., Mitros, F.A., and Oberley, L.W. 2003a. Expression of antioxidant enzymes in diseases of the human pancreas: another link between chronic pancreatitis and pancreatic cancer. *Pancreas* **26**: 23–27.

Cullen, J.J., Weydert, C., Hinkhouse, M.M., Ritchie, J., Domann, F.E., Spitz, D., and Oberley, L.W. 2003b. The role of manganese superoxide dismutase in the growth of pancreatic adenocarcinoma. *Cancer Res* **63**: 1297–1303.

Curphey, T.J., Kuhlmann, E.T., Roebuck, B.D., and Longnecker, D.S. 1988. Inhibition of pancreatic and liver carcinogenesis in rats by retinoid- and selenium-supplemented diets. *Pancreas* **3**: 36–40.

Ding, X.Z., and Adrian, T.E. 2002. Resveratrol inhibits proliferation and induces apoptosis in human pancreatic cancer cells. *Pancreas* **25**: e71–e76.

Ding, X.Z., Kuszynski, C.A., El-Metwally, T.H., and Adrian, T.E. 1999. Lipoxygenase inhibition induced apoptosis, morphological changes, and carbonic anhydrase expression in human pancreatic cancer cells. *Biochem Biophys Res Commun* **266**: 392–399.

Duell, E.J., Holly, E.A., Bracci, P.M., Wiencke, J.K., and Kelsey, K.T. 2002. A population-based study of the Arg399Gln polymorphism in X-ray repair cross-complementing group 1 (XRCC1) and risk of pancreatic adenocarcinoma. *Cancer Res* **62**: 4630–4636.

Dufour, M.C., and Adamson, M.D. 2003. The epidemiology of alcohol-induced pancreatitis. *Pancreas* **27**: 286–290.

Durbec, J.P., and Sarles, H. 1978. Multicenter survey of the etiology of pancreatic diseases. Relationship between the relative risk of developing chronic pancreaitis and alcohol, protein and lipid consumption. *Digestion* **18**: 337–350.

Eibl, G., Reber, H.A., Hines, O.J., and Go, V.L. 2004. COX and PPAR: possible interactions in pancreatic cancer. *Pancreas* **29**: 247–253.

Eibl, G., Wente, M.N., Reber, H.A., and Hines, O.J. 2001. Peroxisome proliferator-activated receptor-γ induces pancreatic cancer cell apoptosis. *Biochem Biophys Res Commun* **287**: 522–529.

El-Metwally, T.H., Hussein, M.R., Pour, P.M., Kuszynski, C.A., and Adrian, T.E. 2005a. Natural retinoids inhibit proliferation and induce apoptosis in pancreatic cancer cells previously reported to be retinoid resistant. *Cancer Biol Ther* **4**: 474–483.

El-Metwally, T.H., Hussein, M.R., Pour, P.M., Kuszynski, C.A., and Adrian, T.E. 2005b. High concentrations of retinoids induce differentiation and late apoptosis in pancreatic cancer cells *in vitro*. *Cancer Biol Ther* **4**: 602–611.

Evans, T.R., Colston, K.W., Lofts, F.J., Cunningham, D., Anthoney, D.A., Gogas, H., de Bono, J.S., Hamberg, K.J., Skov, T., and Mansi, J.L. 2002. A phase II trial of the vitamin D analogue Seocalcitol (EB1089) in patients with inoperable pancreatic cancer. *Br J Cancer* **86**: 680–685.

Everhart, J., and Wright, D. 1995. Diabetes mellitus as a risk factor for pancreatic cancer. A meta-analysis. *JAMA* **273**: 1605–1609.

Farrow, B., and Evers, B.M. 2002. Inflammation and the development of pancreatic cancer. *Surg. Oncol.* **10**: 153–169.

Farrow, B., O'Connor, K.L., Hashimoto, K., Iwamura, T., and Evers, B.M. 2003. Selective activation of PPARg inhibits pancreatic cancer invasion and decreases expression of tissue plasminogen activator. *Surgery* **134**: 206–312.

Ferguson, L.R. 2001. Role of plant polyphenols in genomic stability. *Mutat Res* **475**: 89–111.

Fisher, W.E., Boros, L.G., and Schirmer, W.J. 1996. Insulin promotes pancreatic cancer: evidence for endocrine influence on exocrine pancreatic tumors. *J Surg Res* **63**: 310–313.

Flossmann-Kast, B.B., Jehle, P.M., Hoeflich, A., Adler, G., and Lutz, M.P. 1998. Src stimulates insulin-like growth factor I (IGF-I)–dependent cell proliferation by increasing IGF-I receptor number in human pancreatic carcinoma cells. *Cancer Res* **58**: 3551–3554.

Furukawa, F., Nishikawa, A., Lee, I.S., Kanki, K., Umemura, T., Okazaki, K., Kawamori, T., Wakabayashi, K., and Hirose, M. 2003. A cyclooxygenase-2 inhibitor, nimesulide, inhibits postinitiation phase of *N*-nitrosobis(2-oxopropyl)amine–induced pancreatic carcinogenesis in hamsters. *Int J Cancer* **104**: 269–273.

Furukawa, F., Nishikawa, A., Lee, I.S., Son, H.Y., Nakamura, H., Miyauchi, M., Takahashi, M., and Hirose, M. 2000. Inhibition by methionine of pancreatic carcinogenesis in hamsters after initiation with *N*-nitrosobis(2-oxopropyl) amine. *Cancer Lett* **152**: 163–167.

Gapstur, S.M., Gann, P.H., Lowe, W., Liu, K., Colangelo, L., and Dyer, A. 2000. Abnormal glucose metabolism and pancreatic cancer mortality. *JAMA* **283**: 2552–2558.

German, J.B., Bauman, D.E., Burrin, D.G., Failla, M.L., Freake, H.C., King, J.C., Klein, S., Milner, J.A., Pelto, G.H., Rasmussen, K.M., and Zeisel, S.H. 2004. Metabolomics in the opening decade of the 21st century: building the roads to individualized health. *J Nutr* **134**: 2729–2732.

Ghadirian, P., Lynch, H.T., and Krewski, D. 2003. Epidemiology of pancreatic cancer: an overview. *Cancer Detect Prev* **27**: 87–93.

Ghadirian, P., Simard, A., Baillargeon, J., Maisonneuve, P., and Boyle, P. 1991a. Nutritional factors and pancreatic cancer in the Francophone community in Montreal, Canada. *Int J Cancer* **47**: 1–6.

Ghadirian, P., Thouez, J.P., and PetitClerc, C. 1991b. International comparisons of nutrition and mortality from pancreatic cancer. *Cancer Detect Prev* **15**: 357–362.

Go, V.L., Butrum, R.R., and Wong, D.A. 2003. Diet, nutrition, and cancer prevention: the postgenomic era. *J Nutr* **133**: 3830S–3836S.

Go, V.L., Nguyen, C.T., Harris, D.M., and Lee, W.N. 2005a. Nutrient–gene interaction: Metabolic genotype-phenotype relationship. *J Nutr* **135**: 3016S–3020S.

Go, V.L., Wong, D.A., and Butrum, R. 2001. Diet, nutrition and cancer prevention: where are we going from here? *J Nutr* **131**: 3121S–3126S.

Go, V., Gukovskaya, A., and Pandol, S. 2005b. Alcohol and pancreatic cancer. *Alcohol* **35**: 205–211.

Go, V., and Wang, Y. 2005. Pancreatic exocrine–endocrine interactions. *In* "Toxicology of the Pancreas" (P.M. Pour, ed.). Taylor and Francis Books Ltd, London, U.K.

Goggins, M. 2005. Molecular markers of early pancreatic cancer. *J Clin Oncol* **23**: 4524–4531.

Gold, E.B. 1995. Epidemiology of and risk factors for pancreatic cancer. *Surg Clin North Am* **75**: 819–843.

Gordis, L., and Gold, E.B. 1984. Epidemiology of pancreatic cancer. *World J Surg* **8**: 808–821.

Gukovsky, I., Reyes, C.N., Vaquero, E.C., Gukovskaya, A.S., and Pandol, S.J. 2003. Curcumin ameliorates ethanol and nonethanol experimental pancreatitis. *Am J Physiol Gastrointest Liver Physiol* **284**: G85–G95.

Hanahan, D., and Weinberg, R.A. 2000. The hallmarks of cancer. *Cell* **100**: 57–70.

Hanley, A.J., Johnson, K.C., Villeneuve, P.J., and Mao, Y. 2001. Physical activity, anthropometric factors and risk of pancreatic cancer: results from the Canadian enhanced cancer surveillance system. *Int J Cancer* **94**: 140–147.

Hansel, D.E., Kern, S.E., and Hruban, R.H. 2003. Molecular pathogenesis of pancreatic cancer. *Annu Rev Genomics Hum Genet* **4**: 237–256.

Harnack, L.J., Anderson, K.E., Zheng, W., Folsom, A.R., Sellers, T.A., and Kushi, L.H. 1997. Smoking, alcohol, coffee, and tea intake and incidence of cancer of the exocrine pancreas: the Iowa Women's Health Study. *Cancer Epidemiol Biomarkers Prev* **6**: 1081–1086.

Hart, A.R. 1999. Pancreatic cancer: any prospects for prevention? *Postgrad Med J* **75**: 521–526.

Hashimoto, K., Ethridge, R.T., and Evers, B.M. 2002. Peroxisome proliferator-activated receptor-g ligand inhibits cell growth and invasion of human pancreatic cancer cells. *Int J Gastrointest Cancer* **32**: 7–22.

Heber, D., and Lu, Q.Y. 2002. Overview of mechanisms of action of lycopene. *Exp Biol Med Maywood* **227**: 920–923.

Hennig, R., Ding, X.Z., Tong, W.G., Schneider, M.B., Standop, J., Friess, H., Buchler, M.W., Pour, P.M., and Adrian, T.E. 2002. 5-Lipoxygenase and leukotriene B_4 receptor are expressed in human pancreatic cancers but not in pancreatic ducts in normal tissue. *Am J Pathol* **161**: 421–428.

Heuch, I., Kvale, G., Jacobsen, B.K., and Bjelke, E. 1983. Use of alcohol, tobacco and coffee, and risk of pancreatic cancer. *Br J Cancer* **48**: 637–643.

Hidaka, H., Ishiko, T., Furuhashi, T., Kamohara, H., Suzuki, S., Miyazaki, M., Ikeda, O., Mita, S., Setoguchi, T., and Ogawa, M. 2002. Curcumin inhibits interleukin-8 production and enhances interleukin 8 receptor expression on the cell surface: Impact on human pancreatic carcinoma cell growth by autocrine regulation. *Cancer* **95**: 1206–1214.

Hine, R.J., Srivastava, S., Milner, J.A., and Ross, S.A. 2003. Nutritional links to plausible mechanisms underlying pancreatic cancer: a conference report. *Pancreas* **27**: 356–366.

Hingorani, S.R., Petricoin, E.F., Maitra, A., Rajapakse, V., King, C., Jacobetz, M.A., Ross, S., Conrads, T.P., Veenstra, T.D., Hitt, B.A., Kawaguchi, Y., Johann, D., Liotta, L.A., Crawford, H.C., Putt, M.E., Jacks, T., Wright, C.V., Hruban, R.H., Lowy, A.M., and Tuveson, D.A. 2003. Preinvasive and invasive ductal pancreatic cancer and its early detection in the mouse. *Cancer Cell* **4**: 437–450.

Hiura, A., Tsutsumi, M., and Satake, K. 1997. Inhibitory effect of green tea extract on the process of pancreatic carcinogenesis induced by *N*-nitrosobis-(2-oxypropyl)amine (BOP) and on tumor promotion after transplantation of *N*-nitrosobis-(2-hydroxypropyl)amine (BHP)–induced pancreatic cancer in Syrian hamsters. *Pancreas* **15**: 272–277.

Hotz, H.G., Hines, O.J., Foitzik, T., and Reber, H.A. 2000. Animal models of exocrine pancreatic cancer. *Int J Colorectal Dis* **15**: 136–143.

Hotz, H.G., Reber, H.A., Hotz, B., Yu, T., Foitzik, T., Buhr, H.J., Cortina, G., and Hines, O.J. 2003. An orthotopic nude mouse model for evaluating pathophysiology and therapy of pancreatic cancer. *Pancreas* **26**: e89–e98.

Howe, G.R., and Burch, J.D. 1996. Nutrition and pancreatic cancer. *Cancer Causes Control* **7**: 69–82.

Howe, G.R., Ghadirian, P., Bueno de Mesquita, H.B., Zatonski, W.A., Baghurst, P.A., Miller, A.B., Simard, A., Baillargeon, J., de Waard, F., Przewozniak, K., McMichael, A.J., Jain, M., Hsteh, C.C., Maisonneure, P., Boyle, P., and Walker, A.M. 1992. A collaborative case–control study of nutrient intake and pancreatic cancer within the SEARCH programme. *Int J Cancer* **51**: 365–372.

Hruban, R.H., Petersen, G.M., Goggins, M., Tersmette, A.C., Offerhaus, G.J., Falatko, F., Yeo, C.J., and Kern, S.E. 1999. Familial pancreatic cancer. *Ann Oncol* **10**(Suppl 4): 69–73.

Huxley, R., Ansary-Moghaddam, A., Berrington de, G.A., Barzi, F., and Woodward, M. 2005. Type-II diabetes and pancreatic cancer: a meta-analysis of 36 studies. *Br J Cancer* **92**: 2076–2083.

Iacobuzio-Donahue, C.A., and Hruban, R.H. 2003. Gene expression in neoplasms of the pancreas: applications to diagnostic pathology. *Adv Anat Pathol* **10**: 125–134.

IARC Working Group on the Evaluation of Cancer-Preventive Strategies. 2003. "Fruits and Vegetables." IARC Handbooks of Cancer Prevention. Vol. 8. (H. Vainio and F. Bianchini, eds). IARC Press, Lyon, France,

Isaksson, B., Jonsson, F., Pedersen, N.L., Larsson, J., Feychting, M., and Permert, J. 2002. Lifestyle factors and pancreatic cancer risk: a cohort study from the Swedish Twin Registry. *Int J Cancer* **98**: 480–482.

Itami, A., Watanabe, G., Shimada, Y., Hashimoto, Y., Kawamura, J., Kato, M., Hosotani, R., and Imamura, M. 2001. Ligands for peroxisome proliferator-activated receptor γ inhibit growth of pancreatic cancers both *in vitro* and *in vivo*. *Int J Cancer* **94**: 370–376.

Jaenisch, R., and Bird, A. 2003. Epigenetic regulation of gene expression: how the genome integrates intrinsic and environmental signals. *Nat Genet* **33**(Suppl): 245–254.

Jaffee, E.M., Hruban, R.H., Canto, M., and Kern, S.E. 2002. Focus on pancreas cancer. *Cancer Cell* **2**: 25–28.

Ji, B.T., Chow, W.H., Hsing, A.W., Mclaughlin, J.K., Dai, Q., Gao, Y.T., Blot, W.J., and Fraumeni, J.F., Jr. 1997. Green tea consumption and the risk of pancreatic and colorectal cancers. *Int J Cancer* **70**: 255–258.

Kaiser, A., Brembeck, F.H., Nicke, B., Wiedenmann, B., Riecken, E.O., and Rosewicz, S. 1999. All-*trans*-retinoic acid-mediated growth inhibition involves inhibition of human kinesin-related protein HsEg5. *J Biol Chem* **274**: 18925–18931.

Kawa, S., Nikaido, T., Aoki, Y., Zhai, Y., Kumagai, T., Furihata, K., Fujii, S., and Kiyosawa, K. 1997. Vitamin D analogues up-regulate p21 and p27 during growth inhibition of pancreatic cancer cell lines. *Br J Cancer* **76**: 884–889.

Kawa, S., Nikaido, T., Unno, H., Usuda, N., Nakayama, K., and Kiyosawa, K. 2002. Growth inhibition and differentiation of pancreatic cancer cell lines by PPAR-γ ligand troglitazone. *Pancreas* **24**: 1–7.

Kawa, S., Yoshizawa, K., Tokoo, M., Imai, H., Oguchi, H., Kiyosawa, K., Homma, T., Nikaido, T., and Furihata, K. 1996. Inhibitory effect of 22-oxa-1,25-dihydroxyvitamin D_3 on the proliferation of pancreatic cancer cell lines. *Gastroenterology* **110**: 1605–1613.

Kazakoff, K., Cardesa, T., Liu, J., Adrian, T.E., Bagchi, D., Bagchi, M., Birt, D.F., and Pour, P.M. 1996. Effects of voluntary physical exercise on high-fat diet–promoted pancreatic carcinogenesis in the hamster model. *Nutr Cancer* **26**: 265–279.

Kern, S., Hruban, R., Hollingsworth, M.A., Brand, R., Adrian, T.E., Jaffee, E., and Tempero, M.A. 2001. A white paper: the product of a pancreas cancer think tank. *Cancer Res* **61**: 4923–4932.

Kilian, M., Mautsch, I., Gregor, J.I., Heinichen, D., Jacobi, C.A., Schimke, I., Guski, H., Muller, J.M., and Wenger, F.A. 2003. Influence of conjugated and conventional linoleic acid on tumor growth and lipid peroxidation in pancreatic adenocarcinoma in hamster. *Prostaglandins Leukot Essent Fatty Acids* **69**: 67–72.

Kilian, M., Mautsch, I., Gregor, J.I., Stahlknecht, P., Jacobi, C.A., Schimke, I., Guski, H., and Wenger, F.A. 2002. Influence of conjugated vs. conventional linoleic acid on liver metastasis and hepatic lipidperoxidation in BOP-induced pancreatic cancer in Syrian hamster. *Prostaglandins Leukot Essent Fatty Acids* **67**: 223–228.

Kise, Y., Yamamura, M., Kogata, M., Uetsuji, S., Takada, H., Hioki, K., and Yamamoto, M. 1990. Inhibitory effect of selenium on hamster pancreatic cancer induction by *N*′-nitrosobis(2-oxopropyl)amine. *Int J Cancer* **46**: 95–100.

Kono, H., Nakagami, M., Rusyn, I., Connor, H.D., Stefanovic, B., Brenner, D.A., Mason, R.P., Arteel, G.E., and Thurman, R.G. 2001. Development of an animal model of chronic alcohol-induced pancreatitis in the rat. *Am J Physiol Gastrointest Liver Physiol* **280**: G1178–G1186.

Kris-Etherton, P.M., Hecker, K.D., Bonanome, A., Coval, S.M., Binkoski, A.E., Hilpert, K.F., Griel, A.E., and Etherton, T.D. 2002. Bioactive compounds in foods: their role in the prevention of cardiovascular disease and cancer. *Am J Med* **113**(Suppl 9B): 71S–88S.

Kuroki, T., Tajima, Y., and Kanematsu, T. 2004. Role of hypermethylation on carcinogenesis in the pancreas. *Surg Today* **34**: 981–986.

Leach, S.D. 2004. Mouse models of pancreatic cancer: the fur is finally flying! *Cancer Cell* **5**: 7–11.

Lee, I.M., Sesso, H.D., Oguma, Y., and Paffenbarger, R.S., Jr. 2003. Physical activity, body weight, and pancreatic cancer mortality. *Br J Cancer* **88**: 679–683.

Leelawat, K., Ohuchida, K., Mizumoto, K., Mahidol, C., and Tanaka, M. 2005. All-*trans* retinoic acid inhibits the cell proliferation but enhances the cell invasion through up-regulation of *c*-met in pancreatic cancer cells. *Cancer Lett* **224**: 303–310.

Li, D., Ahmed, M., Li, Y., Jiao, L., Chou, T.H., Wolff, R.A., Lenzi, R., Evans, D.B., Bondy, M.L., Pisters, P.W., Abbruzzese, J.L., and Hassan, M.M. 2005. 5,10-Methylenetetrahydrofolate reductase polymorphisms and the risk of pancreatic cancer. *Cancer Epidemiol Biomarkers Prev* **14**: 1470–1476.

Li, D., and Jiao, L. 2003. Molecular epidemiology of pancreatic cancer. *Int J Gastrointest Cancer* **33**: 3–14.

Li, D., Xie, K., Wolff, R., and Abbruzzese, J.L. 2004a. Pancreatic cancer. *Lancet* **363**: 1049–1057.

Li, L., Aggarwal, B.B., Shishodia, S., Abbruzzese, J., and Kurzrock, R. 2004b. Nuclear factor-κB and IκB kinase are constitutively active in human pancreatic cells, and their down-regulation by curcumin (diferuloylmethane) is associated with the suppression of proliferation and the induction of apoptosis. *Cancer* **101**: 2351–2362.

Lian, J.P., Word, B., Taylor, S., Hammons, G.J., and Lyn-Cook, B.D. 2004. Modulation of the constitutive activated STAT3 transcription factor in pancreatic cancer prevention: effects of indole-3-carbinol (I3C) and genistein. *Anticancer Res* **24**: 133–137.

Lieber, C.S. 2000. Alcohol: its metabolism and interaction with nutrients. *Annu Rev Nutr* **20**: 395–430.

Lin, H.J., Probst-Hensch, N.M., Louie, A.D., Kau, I.H., Witte, J.S., Ingles, S.A., Frankl, H.D., Lee, E.R., and Haile, R.W. 1998. Glutathione transferase null genotype, broccoli, and lower prevalence of colorectal adenomas. *Cancer Epidemiol Biomarkers Prev* **7**: 647–652.

Lin, Y., Tamakoshi, A., Kawamura, T., Inaba, Y., Kikuchi, S., Motohashi, Y., Kurosawa, M., and Ohno, Y. 2002. Risk of pancreatic cancer in relation to alcohol drinking, coffee consumption and medical history: findings from the Japan collaborative cohort study for evaluation of cancer risk. *Int J Cancer* **99**: 742–746.

Lin, Y., Tamakoshi, A., Kikuchi, S., Yagyu, K., Obata, Y., Ishibashi, T., Kawamura, T., Inaba, Y., Kurosawa, M., Motohashi, Y., and Ohno, Y. 2004. Serum insulin-like growth factor-I, insulin-like growth factor binding protein-3, and the risk of pancreatic cancer death. *Int J Cancer* **110**: 584–588.

Lippman, S.M., Hong, W.K. 2002. Cancer prevention by delay. Commentary re: J.A. O'Shaughnessy et al., Treatment and prevention of intraepithelial neoplasia: An important target for accelerated new agent development. *Clin Cancer Res* **8**: 314–346, 2002. *Clin Cancer Res* **8**: 305–313.

Longnecker, D.S., Chandar, N., Sheahan, D.G., Janosky, J.E., and Lombardi, B. 1991. Preneoplastic and neoplastic lesions in the pancreas of rats fed choline-devoid or choline-supplemented diets. *Toxicol Pathol* **19**: 59–65.

Longnecker, D.S., Curphey, T.J., Kuhlmann, E.T., and Roebuck, B.D. 1982. Inhibition of pancreatic carcinogenesis by retinoids in azaserine-treated rats. *Cancer Res* **42**: 19–24.

Longnecker, D.S., Curphey, T.J., Kuhlmann, E.T., Roebuck, B.D., and Neff, R.K. 1986. Effects of retinoids in *N*-nitrosobis(2-oxopropyl)amine–treated hamsters. *Pancreas* **1**: 224–231.

Longnecker, D.S., Kuhlmann, E.T., and Curphey, T.J. 1983. Effects of four retinoids in *N*-nitrosobis(2-oxopropyl)amine–treated hamsters. *Cancer Res* **43**: 3226–3230.

Lowenfels, A.B., Maisonneuve, P., Cavallini, G., Ammann, R.W., Lankisch, P.G., Andersen, J.R., DiMagno, E.P., ndren-Sandberg, A., and Domellof, L. 1993. Pancreatitis and the risk of pancreatic cancer. International Pancreatitis Study Group. *N Engl J Med* **328**: 1433–1437.

Lyn-Cook, B.D., Rogers, T., Yan, Y., Blann, E.B., Kadlubar, F.F., and Hammons, G.J. 1999a. Chemopreventive effects of tea extracts and various components on human pancreatic and prostate tumor cells *in vitro*. *Nutr Cancer* **35**: 80–86.

Lyn-Cook, B.D., Stottman, H.L., Yan, Y., Blann, E., Kadlubar, F.F., and Hammons, G.J. 1999b. The effects of phytoestrogens on human pancreatic tumor cells *in vitro*. *Cancer Lett* **142**: 111–119.

Mack, T.M., Yu, M.C., Hanisch, R., and Henderson, B.E. 1986. Pancreas cancer and smoking, beverage consumption, and past medical history. *J Natl Cancer Inst* **76**: 49–60.

MacKenzie, M.J. 2004. Molecular therapy in pancreatic adenocarcinoma. *Lancet Oncol* **5**: 541–549.

MacMahon, B., Yen, S., Trichopoulos, D., Warren, K., and Nardi, G. 1981. Coffee and cancer of the pancreas. *N Engl J Med* **304**: 630–633.

Maitra, A., Adsay, N.V., Argani, P., Iacobuzio-Donahue, C., De Marzo, A., Cameron, J.L., Yeo, C.J., and Hruban, R.H. 2003. Multicomponent analysis of the pancreatic adenocarcinoma progression model using a pancreatic intraepithelial neoplasia tissue microarray. *Mod Pathol* **16**: 902–912.

Majima, T., Tsutsumi, M., Nishino, H., Tsunoda, T., and Konishi, Y. 1998. Inhibitory effects of β-carotene, palm carotene, and green tea polyphenols on pancreatic carcinogenesis initiated by *N*-nitrosobis(2-oxopropyl)amine in Syrian golden hamsters. *Pancreas* **16**: 13–18.

McCarty, M.F. 2001. Insulin secretion as a determinant of pancreatic cancer risk. *Med Hypotheses* **57**: 146–150.

Michaud, D.S. 2004. Epidemiology of pancreatic cancer. *Minerva Chir* **59**: 99–111.

Michaud, D.S., Giovannucci, E., Willett, W.C., Colditz, G.A., Stampfer, M.J., and Fuchs, C.S. 2001. Physical activity, obesity, height, and the risk of pancreatic cancer. *JAMA* **286**: 921–929.

Michaud, D.S., Liu, S., Giovannucci, E., Willett, W.C., Colditz, G.A., and Fuchs, C.S. 2002. Dietary sugar, glycemic load, and pancreatic cancer risk in a prospective study. *J Natl Cancer Inst* **94**: 1293–1300.

Milner, J.A. 2002. Strategies for cancer prevention: the role of diet. *Br J Nutr* **87**(Suppl 2): S265–S272.

Milner, J.A., McDonald, S.S., Anderson, D.E., and Greenwald, P. 2001. Molecular targets for nutrients involved with cancer prevention. *Nutr Cancer* **41**: 1–16.

Mo, H., and Elson, C.E. 2004. Studies of the isoprenoid-mediated inhibition of mevalonate synthesis applied to cancer chemotherapy and chemoprevention. *Exp Biol Med (Maywood)* **229**: 567–585.

Moore, D.F., Jr., Pazdur, R., Sugarman, S., Jones, D., III, Lippman, S.M., Bready, B., and Abbruzzese, J.L. 1995. Pilot phase II trial of 13-*cis*-retinoic acid and interferon-α combination therapy for advanced pancreatic adenocarcinoma. *Am J Clin Oncol* **18**: 525–527.

Motomura, W., Nagamine, M., Tanno, S., Sawamukai, M., Takahashi, N., Kohgo, Y., and Okumura, T. 2004. Inhibition of cell invasion and morphological change by troglitazone in human pancreatic cancer cells. *J Gastroenterol* **39**: 461–468.

Motomura, W., Okumura, T., Takahashi, N., Obara, T., and Kohgo, Y. 2000. Activation of peroxisome proliferator-activated receptor-γ by troglitazone inhibits cell growth through the increase of $p27^{KiP1}$ in human pancreatic carcinoma cells. *Cancer Res* **60**: 5558–5564.

Mouria, M., Gukovskaya, A.S., Jung, Y., Buechler, P., Hines, O.J., Reber, H.A., and Pandol, S.J. 2002. Food-derived polyphenols inhibit pancreatic cancer growth through mitochondrial cytochrome *C* release and apoptosis. *Int J Cancer* **98**: 761–769.

Muller, C., Bockhorn, A.G., Klusmeier, S., Kiehl, M., Roeder, C., Kalthoff, H., and Koch, O.M. 1998. Lovastatin inhibits proliferation of pancreatic cancer cell lines with mutant as well as with wild-type *K*-ras oncogene but has different effects on protein phosphorylation and induction of apoptosis. *Int J Oncol* **12**: 717–723.

Nair, P.N., De Armond, D.T., Adamo, M.L., Strodel, W.E., and Freeman, J.W. 2001. Aberrant expression and activation of insulin-like growth factor-1 receptor (IGF-1R) are mediated by an induction of IGF-1R promoter activity and stabilization of IGF-1R mRNA and contributes to growth factor independence and increased survival of the pancreatic cancer cell line MIA PaCa-2. *Oncogene* **20**: 8203–8214.

Niles, R.M. 2004. Signaling pathways in retinoid chemoprevention and treatment of cancer. *Mutat Res* **555**: 81–96.

Nishikawa, A., Furukawa, F., Kasahara, K., Tanakamaru, Z., Miyauchi, M., Nakamura, H., Ikeda, T., Imazawa, T., and Hirose, M. 1999. Failure of phenethyl isothiocyanate to inhibit hamster tumorigenesis induced by *N*-nitrosobis(2-oxopropyl)amine when given during the post-initiation phase. *Cancer Lett* **141**: 109–115.

Nishikawa, A., Furukawa, F., Lee, I.S., Tanaka, T., and Hirose, M. 2004. Potent chemopreventive agents against pancreatic cancer. *Curr Cancer Drug Targets* **4**: 373–384.

Nishikawa, A., Furukawa, F., Uneyama, C., Ikezaki, S., Tanakamaru, Z., Chung, F.L., Takahashi, M., and Hayashi, Y. 1996. Chemopreventive effects of phenethyl isothiocyanate on lung and pancreatic tumorigenesis in *N*-nitrosobis(2-oxopropyl)amine–treated hamsters. *Carcinogenesis* **17**: 1381–1384.

Nishikawa, A., Lee, I.S., Uneyama, C., Furukawa, F., Kim, H.C., Kasahara, K., Huh, N., and Takahashi, M. 1997. Mechanistic insights into chemopreventive effects of phenethyl isothiocyanate in *N*-nitrosobis(2-oxopropyl)amine–treated hamsters. *Jpn J Cancer Res* **88**: 1137–1142.

Nkondjock, A., Ghadirian, P., Johnson, K.C., and Krewski, D. 2005a. Dietary intake of lycopene is associated with reduced pancreatic cancer risk. *J Nutr* **135**: 592–597.

Nkondjock, A., Krewski, D., Johnson, K.C., and Ghadirian, P. 2005b. Dietary patterns and risk of pancreatic cancer. *Int J Cancer* **114**: 817–823.

Nozawa, F., Itami, A., Saruc, M., Kim, M., Standop, J., Picha, K.S., Cowan, K.H., and Pour, P.M. 2004. The combination of tumor necrosis factor-related apoptosis-inducing ligand (TRAIL/Apo2L) and genistein is effective in inhibiting pancreatic cancer growth. *Pancreas* **29**: 45–52.

O'Connor, T.P., Roebuck, B.D., Peterson, F., and Campbell, T.C. 1985. Effect of dietary intake of fish oil and fish protein on the development of *L*-azaserine–induced preneoplastic lesions in the rat pancreas. *J Natl Cancer Inst* **75**: 959–962.

O'Connor, T.P., Roebuck, B.D., Peterson, F.J., Lokesh, B., Kinsella, J.E., and Campbell, T.C. 1989. Effect of dietary omega-3 and omega-6 fatty acids on development of azaserine-induced preneoplastic lesions in rat pancreas. *J Natl Cancer Inst* **81**: 858–863.

O'Mahony, S., and Sreedharan, A. 2001. Does detection of *K*-ras mutations in pancreatic juice influence clinical decision making? *Eur J Gastroenterol Hepatol* **13**: 1141–1142.

Ohba, S., Nishi, M., and Miyake, H. 1996. Eating habits and pancreas cancer. *Int J Pancreatol* **20**: 37–42.

Ohlsson, B., Albrechtsson, E., and Axelson, J. 2004. Vitamins A and D but not E and K decreased the cell number in human pancreatic cancer cell lines. *Scand J Gastroenterol* **39**: 882–885.

Ohmura, E., Okada, M., Onoda, N., Kamiya, Y., Murakami, H., Tsushima, T., and Shizume, K. 1990. Insulin-like growth factor I and transforming growth factor-α as autocrine growth factors in human pancreatic cancer cell growth. *Cancer Res* **50**: 103–107.

Ohta, T., Elnemr, A., Yamamoto, M., Ninomiya, I., Fushida, S., Nishimura, G., Fujimura, T., Kitagawa, H., Kayahara, M., Shimizu, K., Yi, S., and Miwa, K. 2002. Thiazolidinedione, a peroxisome proliferator-activated receptor-γ ligand, modulates the E-cadherin/β-catenin system in a human pancreatic cancer cell line, BxPC-3. *Int J Oncol* **21**: 37–42.

Ozcelik, H., Schmocker, B., Di, N.N., Shi, X.H., Langer, B., Moore, M., Taylor, B.R., Narod, S.A., Darlington, G., Andrulis, I.L., Gallinger, S., and Redston, M. 1997. Germline BRCA2 6174delT mutations in Ashkenazi Jewish pancreatic cancer patients. *Nat Genet* **16**: 17–18.

Patel, A.V., Rodriguez, C., Bernstein, L., Chao, A., Thun, M.J., and Calle, E.E. 2005. Obesity, recreational physical activity, and risk of pancreatic cancer in a large U.S. Cohort. *Cancer Epidemiol Biomarkers Prev* **14**: 459–466.

Peterson, G., and Barnes, S. 1996. Genistein inhibits both estrogen and growth factor-stimulated proliferation of human breast cancer cells. *Cell Growth Differ* **7**: 1345–1351.

Pettersson, F., Colston, K.W., and Dalgleish, A.G. 2000. Differential and antagonistic effects of 9-*cis*-retinoic acid and vitamin D analogues on pancreatic cancer cells *in vitro*. *Br J Cancer* **83**: 239–245.

Pettersson, F., Dalgleish, A.G., Bissonnette, R.P., and Colston, K.W. 2002. Retinoids cause apoptosis in pancreatic cancer cells via activation of RAR-γ and altered expression of Bcl-2/Bax. *Br J Cancer* **87**: 555–561.

Pham, N.A., Jacobberger, J.W., Schimmer, A.D., Cao, P., Gronda, M., and Hedley, D.W. 2004. The dietary isothiocyanate sulforaphane targets pathways of apoptosis, cell cycle arrest, and oxidative stress in human pancreatic cancer cells and inhibits tumor growth in severe combined immunodeficient mice. *Mol Cancer Ther* **3**: 1239–1248.

Porta, M., Malats, N., Alguacil, J., Ruiz, L., Jariod, M., Carrato, A., Rifa, J., and Guarner, L. 2000. Coffee, pancreatic cancer, and *K*-ras mutations: updating the research agenda. *J Epidemiol Community Health* **54**: 656–659.

Porta, M., Malats, N., Guarner, L., Carrato, A., Rifa, J., Salas, A., Corominas, J.M., Andreu, M., and Real, F.X. 1999. Association between coffee drinking and K-ras mutations in exocrine pancreatic cancer. PANKRAS II Study Group. *J Epidemiol Community Health* **53**: 702–709.

Posadas, E.M., Simpkins, F., Liotta, L.A., MacDonald, C., and Kohn, E.C. 2005. Proteomic analysis for the early detection and rational treatment of cancer—realistic hope? *Ann Oncol* **16**: 16–22.

Poschl, G., and Seitz, H.K. 2004. Alcohol and cancer. *Alcohol Alcohol* **39**: 155–165.

Qanungo, S., Das, M., Haldar, S., and Basu, A. 2005. Epigallocatechin-3-gallate induces mitochondrial membrane depolarization and caspase-dependent apoptosis in pancreatic cancer cells. *Carcinogenesis* **26**: 958–967.

Rautalahti, M.T., Virtamo, J.R., Taylor, P.R., Heinonen, O.P., Albanes, D., Haukka, J.K., Edwards, B.K., Karkkainen, P.A., Stolzenberg-Solomon, R.Z., and Huttunen, J. 1999. The effects of supplementation with α-tocopherol and β-carotene on the incidence and mortality of carcinoma of the pancreas in a randomized, controlled trial. *Cancer* **86**: 37–42.

Recchia, F., Sica, G., Casucci, D., Rea, S., Gulino, A., and Frati, L. 1998. Advanced carcinoma of the pancreas: phase II study of combined chemotherapy, β-interferon, and retinoids. *Am J Clin Oncol* **21**: 275–278.

Roebuck, B.D. 1992. Dietary fat and the development of pancreatic cancer. *Lipids* **27**: 804–806.

Roebuck, B.D., Baumgartner, K.J., and MacMillan, D.L. 1993. Caloric restriction and intervention in pancreatic carcinogenesis in the rat. *Cancer Res* **53**: 46–52.

Roebuck, B.D., Baumgartner, K.J., Thron, C.D., and Longnecker, D.S. 1984. Inhibition by retinoids of the growth of azaserine-induced foci in the rat pancreas. *J Natl Cancer Inst* **73**: 233–236.

Roebuck, B.D., Yager, J.D., Jr., and Longnecker, D.S. 1981. Dietary modulation of azaserine-induced pancreatic carcinogenesis in the rat. *Cancer Res* **41**: 888–893.

Rosewicz, S., Brembeck, F., Kaiser, A., Marschall, Z.V., and Riecken, E.O. 1996. Differential growth regulation by all-*trans* retinoic acid is determined by protein kinase Cα in human pancreatic carcinoma cells. *Endocrinology* **137**: 3340–3347.

Rosewicz, S., Stier, U., Brembeck, F., Kaiser, A., Papadimitriou, C.A., Berdel, W.E., Wiedenmann, B., and Riecken, E.O. 1995. Retinoids: effects on growth, differentiation, and nuclear receptor expression in human pancreatic carcinoma cell lines. *Gastroenterology* **109**: 1646–1660.

Rosewicz, S., Wollbergs, K., Von Lampe, B., Matthes, H., Kaiser, A., and Riecken, E.O. 1997. Retinoids inhibit adhesion to laminin in human pancreatic carcinoma cells via the α6β1-integrin receptor. *Gastroenterology* **112**: 532–542.

Ross, S.A. 2003d. Diet and DNA methylation interactions in cancer prevention. *Ann NY Acad Sci* **983**: 197–207.

Sanfey, H., Bulkley, G.B., and Cameron, J.L. 1984. The role of oxygen-derived free radicals in the pathogenesis of acute pancreatitis. *Ann Surg* **200**: 405–413.

Saruc, M., and Pour, P.M. 2003. Diabetes and its relationship to pancreatic carcinoma. *Pancreas* **26**: 381–387.

Sato, N., Maitra, A., Fukushima, N., van Heek, N.T., Matsubayashi, H., Iacobuzio-Donahue, C.A., Rosty, C., and Goggins, M. 2003. Frequent hypomethylation of multiple genes overexpressed in pancreatic ductal adenocarcinoma. *Cancer Res* **63**: 4158–4166.

Schneider, G., Siveke, J.T., Eckel, F., and Schmid, R.M. 2005. Pancreatic cancer: basic and clinical aspects. *Gastroenterology* **128**: 1606–1625.

Schneider, I., and Bucar, F. 2005. Lipoxygenase inhibitors from natural plant sources. Part 1: Medicinal plants with inhibitory activity on arachidonate 5-lipoxygenase and 5-lipoxygenase/cyclooxygenase. *Phytother Res* **19**: 81–102.

Schneider, M.B., Matsuzaki, H., Haorah, J., Ulrich, A., Standop, J., Ding, X.Z., Adrian, T.E., and Pour, P.M. 2001. Prevention of pancreatic cancer induction in hamsters by metformin. *Gastroenterology* **120**: 1263–1270.

Schuller, H.M. 2002. Mechanisms of smoking-related lung and pancreatic adenocarcinoma development. *Nat Rev Cancer* **2**: 455–463.

Schuller, H.M., Zhang, L., Weddle, D.L., Castonguay, A., Walker, K., and Miller, M.S. 2002. The cyclooxygenase inhibitor ibuprofen and the FLAP inhibitor MK886 inhibit pancreatic carcinogenesis induced in hamsters by transplacental exposure to ethanol and the tobacco carcinogen NNK. *J Cancer Res Clin Oncol* **128**: 525–532.

Schwartz, G.G., Eads, D., Rao, A., Cramer, S.D., Willingham, M.C., Chen, T.C., Jamieson, D.P., Wang, L., Burnstein, K.L., Holick, M.F., and Koumenis, C. 2004. Pancreatic cancer cells express 25-hydroxyvitamin D_{1a}-hydroxylase and their proliferation is inhibited by the prohormone 25-hydroxyvitamin D_3. *Carcinogenesis* **25**: 1015–1026.

Shibayama-Imazu, T., Sakairi, S., Watanabe, A., Aiuchi, T., Nakajo, S., and Nakaya, K. 2003. Vitamin K_2 selectively induced apoptosis in ovarian TYK-nu and pancreatic MIA PaCa-2 cells out of eight solid tumor cell lines through a mechanism different from geranylgeraniol. *J Cancer Res Clin Oncol* **129**: 1–11.

Shinozuka, H., Katyal, S.L., and Lombardi, B. 1978. Azaserine carcinogenesis: organ susceptibility change in rats fed a diet devoid of choline. *Int J Cancer* **22**: 36–39.

Silvera, S.A., Rohan, T.E., Jain, M., Terry, P.D., Howe, G.R., and Miller, A.B. 2005. Glycemic index, glycemic load, and pancreatic cancer risk (Canada). *Cancer Causes Control* **16**: 431–436.

Silverman, D.T. 2001. Risk factors for pancreatic cancer: a case–control study based on direct interviews. *Teratog Carcinog Mutagen* **21**: 7–25.

Silverman, D.T., Schiffman, M., Everhart, J., Goldstein, A., Lillemoe, K.D., Swanson, G.M., Schwartz, A.G., Brown, L.M., Greenberg, R.S., Schoenberg, J.B., Pottern, L.M., Hoover, R.N., and Fraumeni, J.F., Jr. 1999. Diabetes mellitus, other medical conditions and familial history of cancer as risk factors for pancreatic cancer. *Br J Cancer* **80**: 1830–1837.

Skinner, H.G., Michaud, D.S., Giovannucci, E.L., Rimm, E.B., Stampfer, M.J., Willett, W.C., Colditz, G.A., and Fuchs, C.S. 2004. A prospective study of folate intake and the risk of pancreatic cancer in men and women. *Am J Epidemiol* **160**: 248–258.

Slebos, R.J., Hoppin, J.A., Tolbert, P.E., Holly, E.A., Brock, J.W., Zhang, R.H., Bracci, P.M., Foley, J., Stockton, P., McGregor, L.M., Flake, G.P., and Taylor, J.A. 2000. *K*-ras and p53 in pancreatic cancer: association with medical history, histopathology, and environmental exposures in a population-based study. *Cancer Epidemiol Biomarkers Prev* **9**: 1223–1232.

Somasundar, P., Yu, A.K., Vona-Davis, L., and McFadden, D.W. 2003. Differential effects of leptin on cancer *in vitro*. *J Surg Res* **113**: 50–55.

Son, H.Y., Nishikawa, A., Furukawa, F., Lee, I.S., Ikeda, T., Miyauchi, M., Nakamura, H., and Hirose, M. 2000. Modifying effects of 4-phenylbutyl isothiocyanate on *N*-nitrosobis(2-oxopropyl)amine-induced tumorigenesis in hamsters. *Cancer Lett* **160**: 141–147.

Srivastava, S.K., and Singh, S.V. 2004. Cell cycle arrest, apoptosis induction and inhibition of nuclear factor-Kappa B activation in anti-proliferative activity of benzyl isothiocyanate against human pancreatic cancer cells. *Carcinogenesis* **25**: 1701–1709.

Standop, J., Schneider, M.B., Ulrich, A., and Pour, P.M. 2001. Experimental animal models in pancreatic carcinogenesis: lessons for human pancreatic cancer. *Dig Dis* **19**: 24–31.

Stayrook, K.R., McKinzie, J.H., Barbhaiya, L.H., and Crowell, P.L. 1998. Effects of the antitumor agent perillyl alcohol on *H*-Ras vs. *K*-Ras farnesylation and signal transduction in pancreatic cells. *Anticancer Res* **18**: 823–828.

Stayrook, K.R., McKinzie, J.H., Burke, Y.D., Burke, Y.A., and Crowell, P.L. 1997. Induction of the apoptosis-promoting protein Bak by perillyl alcohol in pancreatic ductal adenocarcinoma relative to untransformed ductal epithelial cells. *Carcinogenesis* **18**: 1655–1658.

Stolzenberg-Solomon, R.Z., Albanes, D., Nieto, F.J., Hartman, T.J., Tangrea, J.A., Rautalahti, M., Sehlub, J., Virtamo, J., and Taylor, P.R. 1999. Pancreatic cancer risk and nutrition-related methyl-group availability indicators in male smokers. *J Natl Cancer Inst* **91**: 535–541.

Stolzenberg-Solomon, R.Z., Pietinen, P., Taylor, P.R., Virtamo, J., and Albanes, D. 2002. Prospective study of diet and pancreatic cancer in male smokers. *Am J Epidemiol* **155**: 783–792.

Sumi, S., Beauchamp, R.D., Townsend, C.M., Jr., Pour, P.M., Ishizuka, J., and Thompson, J.C. 1994. Lovastatin inhibits pancreatic cancer growth regardless of RAS mutation. *Pancreas* **9**: 657–661.

Sumi, S., Beauchamp, R.D., Townsend, C.M., Jr., Uchida, T., Murakami, M., Rajaraman, S., Ishizuka, J., and Thompson, J.C. 1992. Inhibition of pancreatic adenocarcinoma cell growth by lovastatin. *Gastroenterology* **103**: 982–989.

Swaroop, V.S., Chari, S.T., and Clain, J.E. 2004. Severe acute pancreatitis. *JAMA* **291**: 2865–2868.

Takada, M., Nakamura, Y., Koizumi, T., Toyama, H., Kamigaki, T., Suzuki, Y., Takeyama, Y., and Kuroda, Y. 2002. Suppression of human pancreatic carcinoma cell growth and invasion by epigallocatechin-3-gallate. *Pancreas* **25**: 45–48.

Takaori, K., Hruban, R.H., Maitra, A., and Tanigawa, N. 2004. Pancreatic intraepithelial neoplasia. *Pancreas* **28**: 257–262.

Takeda, Y., and Escribano, M.J. 1991. Effects of insulin and somatostatin on the growth and the colony formation of two human pancreatic cancer cell lines. *J Cancer Res Clin Oncol* **117**: 416–420.

Terry, P.D., Rohan, T.E., and Wolk, A. 2003. Intakes of fish and marine fatty acids and the risks of cancers of the breast and prostate and of other hormone-related cancers: a review of the epidemiologic evidence. *Am J Clin Nutr* **77**: 532–543.

Tong, W.G., Ding, X.Z., Witt, R.C., and Adrian, T.E. 2002. Lipoxygenase inhibitors attenuate growth of human pancreatic cancer xenografts and induce apoptosis through the mitochondrial pathway. *Mol Cancer Ther* **1**: 929–935.

Toyota, M., Miyazaki, Y., Kitamura, S., Nagasawa, Y., Kiyohara, T., Shinomura, Y., and Matsuzawa, Y. 2002. Peroxisome proliferator-activated receptor-γ reduces the growth rate of pancreatic cancer cells through the reduction of cyclin D1. *Life Sci* **70**: 1565–1575.

Tseng, W.W., Deganutti, A., Chen, M.N., Saxton, R.E., and Liu, C.D. 2002. Selective cyclooxygenase-2 inhibitor rofecoxib (Vioxx) induces expression of cell cycle arrest genes and slows tumor growth in human pancreatic cancer. *J Gastrointest Surg* **6**: 838–843.

Tsujie, M., Nakamori, S., Okami, J., Hayashi, N., Hiraoka, N., Nagano, H., Dono, K., Umeshita, K., Sakon, M., and Monden, M. 2003a. Thiazolidinediones inhibit growth of gastrointestinal, biliary, and pancreatic adenocarcinoma cells through activation of the peroxisome proliferator-activated receptor γ/retinoid X receptor α pathway. *Exp Cell Res* **289**: 143–151.

Tsujie, M., Nakamori, S., Okami, J., Takahashi, Y., Hayashi, N., Nagano, H., Dono, K., Umeshita, K., Sakon, M., and Monden, M. 2003b. Growth inhibition of pancreatic cancer cells through activation of peroxisome proliferator-activated receptor γ/retinoid X receptor α pathway. *Int J Oncol* **23**: 325–331.

U.S. Department of Health and Human Services, Public Health Service, National Toxicology Program. 2005. Report on Carcinogens. Eleventh Edition. Available at: http://ntp.niehs.nih.gov/ntp/roc/toc11.html.

U.S. Food and Drug Administration. 2005. Vioxx (rofecoxib) Drug Information Page. Available at: http://www.fda.gov/cder/drug/infopage/vioxx/default.htm

Ulrich, A.B., Schmied, B.M., Standop, J., Schneider, M.B., and Pour, P.M. 2002. Pancreatic cell lines: a review. *Pancreas* **24**: 111–120.

Valko, M., Izakovic, M., Mazur, M., Rhodes, C.J., and Telser, J. 2004. Role of oxygen radicals in DNA damage and cancer incidence. *Mol Cell Biochem* **266**: 37–56.

Vaquero, E.C., Edderkaoui, M., Pandol, S.J., Gukovsky, I., and Gukovskaya, A.S. 2004. Reactive oxygen species produced by NAD(P)H oxidase inhibit apoptosis in pancreatic cancer cells. *J Biol Chem* **279**: 34643–34654.

Vickers, S.M., Sampson, L.K., Ying, W., and Phillips, J.O. 1997. Receptor-dependent growth inhibition of human pancreatic cancer by 9-*cis* retinoic acid. *J Gastrointest Surg* **1**: 174–181.

von Marschall Z., Riecken, E.O., and Rosewicz, S. 1998. Stromelysin 3 is overexpressed in human pancreatic carcinoma and regulated by retinoic acid in pancreatic carcinoma cell lines. *Gut* **43**: 692–698.

Wallace, J.M. 2002. Nutritional and botanical modulation of the inflammatory cascade—eicosanoids, cyclooxygenases, and lipoxygenases—as an adjunct in cancer therapy. *Integr Cancer Ther* **1**: 7–37.

Wang, M., Abbruzzese, J.L., Friess, H., Hittelman, W.N., Evans, D.B., Abbruzzese, M.C., Chiao, P., and Li, D. 1998. DNA adducts in human pancreatic tissues and their potential role in carcinogenesis. *Cancer Res* **58**: 38–41.

Wargovich, M.J., Woods, C., Hollis, D.M., and Zander, M.E. 2001. Herbals, cancer prevention and health. *J Nutr* **131**: 3034S–3036S.

Weiderpass, E., Partanen, T., Kaaks, R., Vainio, H., Porta, M., Kauppinen, T., Ojajarvi, A., Boffetta, P., and Malats, N. 1998. Occurrence, trends and environment etiology of pancreatic cancer. *Scand J Work Environ Health* **24**: 165–174.

Weiss, J.M., Goode, E.L., Ladiges, W.C., and Ulrich, C.M. 2005. Polymorphic variation in hOGG1 and risk of cancer: al review of the functional and epidemiologic literature. *Mol Carcinog* **42**: 127–141.

Weisz, B., Giehl, K., Gana-Weisz, M., Egozi, Y., Ben-Baruch, G., Marciano, D., Gierschik, P., and Kloog, Y. 1999. A new functional Ras antagonist inhibits human pancreatic tumor growth in nude mice. *Oncogene* **18**: 2579–2588.

Wenger, F.A., Kilian, M., Ridders, J., Stahlknecht, P., Schimke, I., Guski, H., Jacobi, C.A., and Muller, J.M. 2001. Influence of antioxidative vitamins A, C and E on lipid peroxidation in BOP-induced pancreatic cancer in Syrian hamsters. *Prostaglandins Leukot Essent Fatty Acids* **65**: 165–171.

World Cancer Research Fund and American Institute for Cancer Research. 1997. "Food, Nutrition and the Prevention of Cancer: A Global Perspective." American Institute for Cancer Research, Washington, D.C.

Woutersen, R.A., Appel, M.J., van Garderen-Hoetmer, A., and Wijnands, M.V. 1999. Dietary fat and carcinogenesis. *Mutat Res* **443**: 111–127.

Xue, L., Lipkin, M., Newmark, H., and Wang, J. 1999. Influence of dietary calcium and vitamin D on diet-induced epithelial cell hyperproliferation in mice. *J Natl Cancer Inst* **91**: 176–181.

Xue, L., Yang, K., Newmark, H., Leung, D., and Lipkin, M. 1996. Epithelial cell hyperproliferation induced in the exocrine pancreas of mice by a Western-style diet. *J Natl Cancer Inst* **88**: 1586–1590.

Yang, C.S., Maliakal, P., and Meng, X. 2002. Inhibition of carcinogenesis by tea. *Annu Rev Pharmacol Toxicol* **42**: 25–54.

Yao, Z., Okabayashi, Y., Yutsudo, Y., Kitamura, T., Ogawa, W., and Kasuga, M. 2002. Role of Akt in growth and survival of PANC-1 pancreatic cancer cells. *Pancreas* **24**: 42–46.

Yeo, T.P., Hruban, R.H., Leach, S.D., Wilentz, R.E., Sohn, T.A., Kern, S.E., Iacobuzio-Donahue, C.A., Maitra, A., Goggins, M., Canto, M.I., Abrams, R.A., Laheru, D., Jaffee, E.M., Hidalgo, M., and Yeo, C.J. 2002. Pancreatic cancer. *Curr Probl Cancer* **26**: 176–275.

Yoshimoto, M., Tsutsumi, M., Iki, K., Sasaki, Y., Tsujiuchi, T., Sugimura, T., Wakabayashi, K., and Konishi, Y. 1999. Carcinogenicity of heterocyclic amines for the pancreatic duct epithelium in hamsters. *Cancer Lett* **143**: 235–239.

Young, V.R. 2002. 2001 W.O. Atwater Memorial Lecture and the 2001 ASNS President's Lecture: Human nutrient requirements: the challenge of the post-genome era. *J Nutr* **132**: 621–629.

Z'graggen, K., Warshaw, A.L., Werner, J., Graeme-Cook, F., Jimenez, R.E., and Fernandez-del Castillo, C. 2001. Promoting effect of a high-fat/high-protein diet in DMBA-induced ductal pancreatic cancer in rats. *Ann Surg* **233**: 688–695.

Zhang, J., and Go, V. 1996. High fat diet, lipid peroxidation, and pancreatic carcinogenesis. *In* "Dietary Fats, Lipids, Hormones, and Tumorigenesis" (D. Heber, and D. Kritchevsky, eds), Vol. 13, pp. 165–172. Plenum Press, New York.

Zugmaier, G., Jager, R., Grage, B., Gottardis, M.M., Havemann, K., and Knabbe, C. 1996. Growth-inhibitory effects of vitamin D analogues and retinoids on human pancreatic cancer cells. *Br J Cancer* **73**: 1341–1346.

CHAPTER

26

Bladder Cancer

ALLAN J. PANTUCK, RON LIEBERMAN, KELLY KAWAOKA, OLEG SHVARTS, AND DONALD LAMM

BACKGROUND

Bladder cancer, which currently ranks the fourth most common cancer site in men and the eighth most leading site in women (Jemal et al., 2003), represents an important health problem in the United States. An estimated 57,400 new cases of bladder cancer will be diagnosed in the United States, with ~12,500 estimated cancer deaths (Jemal et al., 2003). The highest incidence of new cases in the United States is estimated to be in California (5300 cases, or nearly 10%). The expected male-to-female ratio is 2.6:1.0, the disease is more common in whites than blacks, and the average age at diagnosis is 65 years. There has been a slow rise in the total number of new cases in the past 20 years. Approximately 90% of bladder tumors arise from the urothelial lining, and transitional cell carcinoma (TCC) is the most common histological type in cases arising in the United States. Exogenous risk factors appear to play a pivotal role in the development of bladder cancer. Cigarette smoking represents the single most significant preventable cause of bladder cancer in the United States.

The process of bladder tumor carcinogenesis results from the interaction of environmental exposures and genetic susceptibility. The molecular pathology of bladder cancer begins not with the appearance of visually aberrant lesions, but with altered biochemical and genetic processes. Clinically and pathologically, one can separate bladder tumors into two entities: low-grade papillary lesions and high-grade *in situ* or invasive malignancies. Most bladder tumors (70–80%) are classified as superficial. Papillary tumors that are confined to the mucosa can be cured by surgical resection; however, there may be changes elsewhere in the bladder that are not clinically detectable that can lead to disease recurrence. Additionally, genetic changes may occur and induce the development of higher-grade papillary lesions that result in the transformation of low-grade lesions to higher-grade, more aggressive lesions. Between 50 and 70% of patients with superficial tumors will develop new superficial TCC, often within 12 months of diagnosis, and 10–20% progress to infiltrate muscle (Heney et al., 1982). There is increasing evidence to support the concept of histopathological and molecular biochemical field disease occurring years in advance of overt malignancy in bladder cancer (Rao et al., 1999), offering an ample latency period and opportunity for cancer preventive strategies. The development of biomarkers of susceptibility, exposure, and effect establishes a powerful paradigm for individual risk assessment. Although primary prevention is ideal, the premalignant field serves as a useful target for chemoprevention by targeting functional pathways relevant to apoptosis, proliferation, differentiation, and cytotoxicity. Drugs, biologics, or nutrients that halt, slow, or reverse the carcinogenic process are likely to be effective when administered before the emergence of genetic instability.

SMOKING AND BLADDER CANCER

TCCs of the bladder are clearly related to occupational, chemical, and environmental exposures, such as aniline dyes, arsenic, nitrates, and certain analgesics. In the past, occupational exposures have been estimated to account for 20% of the cases of bladder cancer in the United States with long latency periods of 30–50 years (Cole et al., 1972). Occupations that have been associated with exposures to bladder carcinogens include autoworkers, painters, truck

Copyright © 2006, Elsevier Inc.
All rights of reproduction in any form reserved.

drivers, drill-press operators, leather workers, metalworkers, machinists, dry cleaners, paper manufacturers, rope and twine makers, dental technicians, barbers and beauticians, plumbers, apparel manufacturers, and physicians (Morrison, 1984; Silverman et al., 1989). Today, tobacco smoke represents the most important exogenous risk factor for bladder cancer. Smokers are at least two to three times more at risk for developing TCC of the bladder than nonsmokers (Hoover and Cole, 1971), with heavy smokers being at five times the risk (Wynder and Goldsmith, 1977). Furthermore, it has been estimated that up to 50% of all bladder tumors are directly attributable to cigarette smoking (Wynder and Goldsmith, 1977). A dose–effect relationship appears to be present because increasing the number of packs smoked per day increases the risk ratio of the individual (Morrison et al., 1984). It has been estimated that smoking two or more packs of cigarettes can increase the risk to about seven times that for nonsmokers (Morrison et al., 1984). More than 3000 chemicals are present in tobacco smoke, including at least 60 known carcinogens such as nitrosamines and polycyclic aromatic hydrocarbons (PAHs). Tobacco contains many urothelial carcinogens, including 4-amino-biphenyl, acrolein, and oxygen free radicals (Bartsch et al., 1993a).

The exact mechanism of bladder carcinogenicity remains unknown, but data support the arylamines, including the amino-biphenyls, as the major carcinogen in smoking-induced bladder carcinogenesis (Zang and Wynder, 1996). Mutations in the p53 tumor suppressor gene have also been associated with smoking (Curigliano et al., 1996). Furthermore, Thompson et al. (1987) demonstrated a positive correlation between smoking history and histological grade, stage, number, and size of bladder tumors. All three variables were increased in smokers. Other studies suggest that bladder cancers that develop in association with cigarette smoking lead to higher mortality with survival data, suggesting that 40% of smokers versus 27% of nonsmokers died of their disease (Raitanen et al., 1995). Estimates suggest that ~50% of adults are former smokers, including 44 million in the United States (U.S. Department of Health and Human Services, 1993). From the current smoking trends, former smokers will account for a growing percentage of all bladder cancer cases. Conflicting data exist on the prognostic value of smoking cessation (Thompsin et al., 1987; Carpenter, 1989; Castelao et al., 2001). The risk of developing bladder cancer is not precipitously reduced by smoking cessation, and former smokers still have a higher bladder cancer risk than nonsmokers. A decrease in smoking-related incidence of bladder cancer to a rate equal to that of nonsmokers may not occur until after 15 years of abstinence (Wynder and Goldsmith, 1977). A dose response between smoking and DNA adduct formation has been confirmed, and the slow and fast acetylation NAT2 genes relate to adduct formation in cigarette exposure, but do not necessarily result in a biological effect (Vineis et al., 1990). An understanding of the procarcinogens related to bladder cancer development permits a better understanding of the genetic polymorphisms in phase I and phase II enzymes, which may play an important role in activating mutagens, as well as repair of DNA damage and detoxification and excretion of mutagens. Furthermore, this knowledge opens avenues of exploration for the identification of nutritional factors that may modulate the balance between detoxification and cancer formation.

INTRINSIC GENETIC SUSCEPTIBILITY FACTORS IN BLADDER CANCER

No inherited syndromes have pointed to specific genes involved in bladder carcinogenesis in the way that familial adenopolyposis has identified a sequence for colon cancer (Kinzler and Vogelstein, 1996). However, Lynch syndrome involving multiple inherited cancer, which manifests as hereditary nonpolyposis colon cancer (HNPCC), involves bladder cancer frequently and identifies the importance of DNA repair genes in the process of carcinogenesis (Schulte, 1988). There are multiple genes that could potentially contribute to the network of signaling pathways related directly or indirectly to DNA repair in addition to the specific enzyme pathways, which have been defined and concisely summarized by Larminat et al. (1995). Enzymes related to the activation and inactivation of xenobiotics also may function as biomarkers of genetic susceptibility. These may be assayed by defining the genetic polymorphisms or from phenotypic functional assays. In most circumstances, the two approaches provide similar data, but the genetic analysis does not reflect the influence of subtle endogenous and exogenous factors influencing the metabolism of the xenobiotic.

GSTM1

Glutathione *S*-transferase (GST) M1 belongs to a family of phase II detoxification enzymes (Awasthi et al., 1994). GSTM1 detoxifies reactive chemical species, by catalyzing their conjugation to glutathione (Bell et al., 1993a). Deficiency in enzyme activity is caused by homozygous deletion of the GSTM1 gene. The frequency of homozygous deletion of the GSTM1 (i.e., GSTM1 null or 0/0 genotype) gene is about 50% in white populations and 30–70% in other racial/ethnic groups. Bell et al. (1993) studied 229 patients with TCCs of the bladder and 211 control subjects and reported that GSTM1 0/0 genotype conferred a 70% increased risk of bladder cancer (95% confidence interval [CI], 1.2–2.5), compared with individuals with at least one copy of the gene. Subsequent studies have confirmed this finding. A study in Spain by Lafuente et al. (1993) reported a twofold increased risk of bladder cancer in smokers for this polymorphic alteration. Daly et al. (1993) reported that odds ratios for bladder cancer associated with homozygous deletion of GSTM1 were 1.4 and 3.8, compared with hospitalized and healthy controls, respectively. Brockmoller et al. (1994) reported an odds ratio of 1.4 (95% CI, 1.0–1.9) for GSTM1 0/0 genotype and reported an etiological fraction of 17% for bladder cancer in Germany. In a pilot study, 175 patients with TCC and 162 cancer-free controls were assessed for GSTM1 genotype. The odds ratio was 1.7 for homozygous deletion of the GSTM1 gene.

GSTP1

GSTP1 belongs to the Pi class of the GST family. GSTP1-1 is the only member of the Pi class of GSTs expressed in humans. GSTP1 catalyzes the detoxification of polycyclic aromatic hydrocarbons (Strange et al., 1999). GSTP1 demonstrated an A-G polymorphism at codon 104, which has been indicated in bladder, testicular, and prostate cancer. Harries et al. (1997) reported that two variant GST cDNAs have been described at the GSTP1 locus, which differ by a single base pair (A-G) substitution at nucleotide 313 of the GSTP1 cDNA (GSTP1a and GSTP1b). This results in an amino acid substitution, which alters the function of the enzyme. The Pi-class GST has been associated with preneoplastic and neoplastic changes (Esteller et al., 1998).

N-Acetyltransferase

N-Acetyltransferase (NAT) activity in humans is coded by two distinct genes named *NAT1* and *NAT2*. NAT2 displayed polymorphism in humans, which results in the detection of individuals with slow and rapid *N*-acetylating phenotypes (Bartsch et al., 1993b). Slow acetylators have been found to be associated with higher incidence of bladder cancer, but fast acetylators are associated with higher incidence of colon cancer, which suggests that acetyltransferase polymorphism is related to both metabolic activation and deactivation of carcinogenic arylamines (Hein et al., 1993). The *N*-hydroxy metabolite of arylamine interacts with DNA and initiates tumorigenesis. The detoxification and elimination of carcinogens at this stage is through *N*-acetylation by *N*-acetyltransferase (Vineis et al., 1990). It has been estimated that slow acetylators are 55% of Caucasian populations and 41% in African American population (Bell et al., 1993b).

CHEMOPREVENTION OF BLADDER CANCER

Bladder cancer is an ideal organ system for testing chemoprevention strategies. The urinary bladder is easily accessible and can be monitored by various noninvasive or minimally invasive surveillance techniques. The entire mucosal surface at risk can be visually examined by cystoscopy, and if necessary, biopsy specimens can be taken. The accessibility of the voided urine for noninvasive longitudinal sampling is suitable for mass screening studies, and the accessibility of the bladder for cystoscopic observation and pathological sampling provides tissue and cells for longitudinal follow-up and allows the process of bladder carcinogenesis to be followed. Thus, the bladder can be evaluated easily for evidence of early or premalignant lesions. Furthermore, the mean time from the initial carcinogen exposure to the development of overt TCC is close to 20 years, a lengthy period that provides ample opportunity to apply chemopreventive measures. The past 10 years have revealed the potential of chemoprevention in the reduction of mortality associated with common epithelial cancers (Hong and Sporn, 1997). Despite this fact, few large-scale trials have been performed for bladder cancer prevention. Currently, there are very few bladder cancer chemoprevention trials actively enrolling patients for study. From a clinical standpoint, chemopreventive agents should be easy to administer, have minimal side effects to encourage compliance, should be specific to tumor tissue, and have no deleterious effects on normal tissue. Thus, chemoprevention measures should target people who are generally healthy, at high risk for bladder cancer, have precancerous lesions, or other cancer histories but have not yet developed the disease.

Dietary Aspects for the Chemoprevention of Bladder Cancer

There is an urgent need for research on dietary phytochemicals, which may prevent cancer through antioxidation and via gene–nutrient interactions, or which may be useful adjuncts in the prevention of cancer recurrence among successfully treated cancer survivors where prevention of cancer recurrence is vital. The role of nutrition in the development and course of bladder cancer and other malignancies is expanding rapidly but was recognized by early ancestors. Most research in bladder cancer has evaluated specific substances such as the various vitamins or specific foods such as green tea or garlic, but there is a vast starry-sky array of micronutrients in fruits and vegetables that are only beginning to be characterized. A meta-analysis of 38 articles on six dietary variables shows that the risk of bladder cancer is increased by diets low in fruits and vegetables or high in fat with an estimated relative risk (RR) of 0.7 for high vegetable and 0.8 for high fruit in the diet (Steinmaus et al., 2000). Future reviews will undoubtedly extol the enhanced benefits of micronutrients that are not appreciated today.

Caloric Intake

Numerous studies have investigated the impact of diet upon the incidence of various malignancies. One aspect of

TABLE 1 Bladder cancer prevention clinical trials

Agent	Group/location	Study	Result
DFMO	ILEX Oncology, University of Wisconsin	450 patients randomized, double-blind DFMO or placebo	In progress; accrual completed
Pyridoxine	Byar and Blackard, 1977	121 patients in a multicenter trial comparing pyridoxine or thiotepa with placebo	No significant difference
Vitamin C	Shibata et al., 1992	Cohort study of 11,590 patients over 9 years with diets high in vitamin C	0.59 relative risk for bladder cancer patients
High-dose combination multivitamins	Lamm et al., 1994	65 patients given BCG and multivitamins	Decreased recurrence compared with MDR
Celecoxib	M.D. Anderson; University of Texas	Patients receive BCG and are randomized to either celecoxib or placebo	In progress
Tarceva and green tea polyphenol extract	UCLA and Mayo Clinics	330 high-risk former smokers randomized to three arms	In progress

these dietary studies has been the role of caloric intake. Animal studies with mice have demonstrated that a reduction in total calories consumed decreased the development of numerous cancers including prostate and breast carcinoma (Cohen et al., 1988; Weindruch, 1992). The growth of bladder tumors was also demonstrated to decrease through caloric restriction in a mouse model (Dunn et al., 1992). A human study also demonstrated that higher caloric intake was associated with a higher incidence of bladder cancer in American men younger than 65 years (Vena et al., 1993). The effect of caloric intake on tumorigenesis appears to be related to insulin-like growth factor (IGF). Animal studies have demonstrated that the decrease in the growth of bladder tumors seen in calorically restricted mice was reversed when these mice were given IGF-1 (Dunn et al., 1992). Similarly, a human study also demonstrated that people with the highest quartile of plasma IGF-1 were three times more likely to develop bladder cancer (Zhao et al., 2003).

Fluid Intake

Increased fluid intake has also been isolated as a potential dietary method of decreasing the risk of bladder cancer. Studies focused on fluid intake as a result of the theory that the development of bladder cancer was related to the duration of time during which the bladder urothelium is exposed to carcinogens, as well as the concentration of the carcinogens within the urine (Oyasu and Hupp, 1974). Most bladder carcinogens are thought to exert their effect by direct contact with the urothelium through excretion in the urine. Increased fluid intake, in theory, should shorten this exposure time and decrease the risk of subsequent development of bladder cancer by diluting metabolites and increasing the frequency of voiding. The largest cohort study to date assessing this question was the Health Professionals' Follow-up Study, which followed 48,000 men for 10 years (Michaud et al., 1999a). The study demonstrated that fluid consumption was inversely correlated with the risk of bladder cancer. Those men meeting the criteria for the highest quintile of fluid consumption (2531 ml/day) demonstrated approximately half the risk of developing bladder cancer as those men whose fluid consumption placed them in the lowest quintile (1290 ml/day) (Michaud et al., 1999a). Water consumption, in particular, resulted in a significantly lower RR of 0.49 for those men drinking more than six cups a day as compared with those drinking only a single cup per day (Michaud et al., 1999a). The consumption of all other fluids also demonstrated an inverse, though not statistically significant, relationship with the development of bladder cancer in this population.

Other case-control studies have, in contrast, demonstrated a positive correlation between the consumption of some beverages and the incidence of bladder cancer. A pooled analysis of case-control studies, for example, reported a significant increase in bladder cancer in those people drinking large amounts of coffee (≥10 cups/day) (Sala et al., 2000). Other studies have demonstrated that increased intake of any fluids, including tap water, led to an increased incidence of bladder cancer, whereas still others have argued that fluid intake has no impact on bladder cancer, either positive or negative (Kunze et al., 1986; Geoffroy-Perez et al., 2001). Overall, the evidence on fluid intake and bladder cancer risk remains controversial, with results ranging from increased risk, to inverse risk, to no association. The inconsistencies in these studies may result from the difficulty in measuring total fluid intake. Furthermore, the source and purity of the water may also be important, with metals such as arsenic or disinfectants such as chlorine adversely affecting the overall protective effect of increased fluid intake. More data are necessary before definite recommendations regarding this potential preventative strategy can be made.

Fat Consumption

Restriction of dietary fat has also been proposed as a method of bladder cancer prevention. Numerous studies have correlated dietary fat intake with carcinogenesis through such mechanisms as oxidative stress and the formation of free radicals (Fleshner and Klotz, 1998–1999). Studies have demonstrated an increased incidence of bladder cancer in people with high-fat diets. A multicenter case-control study from Spain demonstrated that men with the highest intake of saturated fat had a significantly increased risk of bladder cancer, with an RR of 2.25 (Riboli et al., 1991). In addition, Steineck et al. (1990) demonstrated a dose–response relationship between fat consumption and bladder cancer incidence. Other case-control studies have verified these results, correlating an increased risk of bladder cancer with greater ingestion of saturated fats and fried foods (Bruemmer et al., 1996). Still other studies have demonstrated that the ingestion of meat, in particular, is associated with an increased risk of bladder cancer (Mills et al., 1991). Whether the increased risk demonstrated by these studies is attributable to increased intake of fat rather than to merely increased calories is yet to be determined. Nonetheless, reduction of dietary fat should be advised as a potential method of reducing the risk of bladder cancer and other malignancies.

Consumption of Fruits and Vegetables

In 1997, an international review panel concluded that there was convincing evidence that high intake of vegetables decreased the risk of cancers of the mouth, pharynx, esophagus lung, stomach, colon, and rectum, and that it probably decreases the risk of cancers of the larynx, pancreas, breast, and bladder (World Cancer Research Fund, 1997). Numerous studies have evaluated the effect of fruit and vegetable consumption on the risk of developing bladder cancer, and most of these studies have reported a lower risk of bladder cancer in subjects with high consumption (Negri and La Vecchia, 2001). A meta-analysis of 38 articles on six dietary variables shows that the risk of bladder cancer is increased by diets low in fruits and vegetables or high in fat, with an estimated RR of 0.7 for high vegetable and 0.8 for high fruit in the diet (Steinmaus et al., 2000). A large prospective study from Japan of 39,000 atomic bomb survivors in Japan (Nagano et al., 2000) demonstrated that regular fruit and vegetable consumption led to up to a 50% decreased risk of the future development of bladder cancer. Similarly, the Health Professionals' Follow-up Study, based on 252 cases of bladder cancer, reported an inverse, though not significant, relationship between fruit and vegetable consumption and bladder cancer (Michaud et al., 1999). Further analysis from these studies demonstrated that vegetables appeared to have a greater protective effect against bladder cancer than fruits. The Health Professionals' Follow-up Study reported that only the consumption of cruciferous vegetables had a significant impact on the risk of developing bladder cancer when comparing study participants with the greatest versus the least consumption of these vegetables (Michaud et al., 1999b). Also, whereas all cruciferous vegetables in the diet were associated with a decreased risk of bladder cancer, only broccoli and cabbage were found to have a statistically significant impact when comparing people with intakes less than once a week to those with intake of at least once per week. The study by Nagano et al. (2000) also reported the greatest effect from green and yellow vegetables. Interestingly, while tomatoes and tomato products have been demonstrated to have a preventative role in prostate cancer secondary to their lycopene contents, no such association has been found in relation to bladder cancer (Michaud et al., 1999b). Also, studies have reported that the risk reduction provided by vegetables seems have the greatest impact on nonsmokers (Michaud et al., 1999b). Nonetheless, dietary fruit consumption, particularly that of green vegetables, has definitely been demonstrated to serve some benefit in preventing bladder cancer and deserves mention during counseling of at-risk patients.

Garlic

Garlic, in use before recorded history, was known to have medicinal properties by ancient health professionals, including Hippocrates (Rivlin, 2001). Epidemiological studies have found reduced risk of stomach cancer (You et al., 1989) and prostate cancer (Hsing et al., 2002). Scientific study dates from the 1950s when Weisberger and Pensky (1958) demonstrated *in vitro* and *in vivo* that thiosulfinate extracts of garlic inhibited the growth of malignant cells and prevented growth of sarcoma 180 ascites tumor. Since that time, garlic has been shown in animal models to have antitumor activity in sarcoma, mammary carcinoma, hepatoma, colon cancer, and squamous cell carcinoma of the skin and esophagus (Lau et al., 1990). The activity of garlic in reducing the growth of bladder cancer in animals is quite striking. In 1986, Lau et al. compared intralesional and intraperitoneal garlic extract therapy with effective immunotherapies for bladder cancer: BCG, *Corynebacterium parvum* (CP, now termed *Propionibacter acnes*), and keyhole limpet hemocyanin (KLH) in the transplantable murine bladder tumor model MBT2. Intralesional garlic significantly inhibited the growth of transplanted bladder carcinoma. This efficacy was subsequently confirmed when Marsh (1987) reported intralesional garlic to be more effective and less toxic than BCG. Lamm, who has championed BCG therapy, was skeptical of these results and found that in his hands BCG could provide superior protection, but both intralesional and oral garlic significantly inhibited the growth of murine bladder cancer and prolonged survival. Clinical trials of garlic have not been reported (Lamm and Riggs, 2001).

Green Tea Polyphenols

Flavonoids found in green tea and available as botanical dietary supplements may play a role in bladder cancer protection and have been shown to have potent antioxidant and antitumor effects. Direct effects on cells and effects on enzyme systems, which inactivate carcinogens or act as part of the antioxidant response of cells, may mediate the effects of green tea. Tea is the most widely consumed beverage in the world and is a complex mixture of many substances including caffeine (2–4%), amino acids (4%), lignin (6.5%), organic acids (1.5%), protein (15%), chlorophyll (0.5%), and polyphenols (8–12%). Green tea contains 35–52% catechins and flavonols combined. Catechins belong to the general natural product class of flavonoids. The four major catechins in green tea are (−)-epicatechin, (−)-epicatechin-3-gallate, (−)-epigallocatechin, and (−)-epigallocatechin-3-gallate (EGCG). These catechins, which are believed to be the key active constituents in green tea polyphenol preparations, are potent antioxidants, which have been shown to reduce tumor growth, metastatic capacity, and angiogenesis in several studies. EGCG is the primary component, accounting for 40% of the total polyphenolic mixture, but it is not clear that this is the only component important in the action of green tea. One cup of green tea usually contains ~300–400 mg of polyphenols, and commercial preparations are now available that have reduced caffeine content and are enriched to contain 60–80% or more dry weight polyphenols. Numerous *in vitro*, human, and animal studies have identified these antioxidant polyphenols, in particular EGCG, as cancer-chemoprevention agents (Komori et al., 1993; Mukhtar et al., 1994). Preliminary work suggests that these polyphenols protect DNA to a much greater extent than either vitamin E or β-carotene in the retro-Ames assay. EGCG has been predicted to guard against carcinogenesis by blocking cell membrane receptors, repressing the catalytic activities of several cytochrome P450 (CYP) enzymes including CYP 1A and CYP 2B1, and enhancing cancer-detoxification enzymes. In *in vitro* studies, green tea polyphenols blocked nitrosamines and suppressed carcinogenic activity in lung, breast, colon, melanoma (Khan et al., 1992; Chung et al., 1993), and bladder cancers (Sato, 1999).

Human studies suggest that green tea polyphenols may have anticarcinogenic effects on nitrosation (Xu et al., 1993) and chromosome damage (Shim et al., 1995). In humans (Xu et al., 1993), the urinary excretion of *N*-nitrosoproline is decreased with consumption of green tea extract, showing evidence of decreased nitrosation *in vivo*. Blood samples, cultures, and chromosome spreads have been examined and have shown an inverse incidence with tea intake (Shim et al., 1995). Moreover, urinary excretion of polyphenols can be measured and may be useful in quantifying tea ingestion and polyphenol exposure in humans (Lee et al., 1995). There is increasing evidence of an inverse association with various cancers, in particular pancreatic (Ji et al., 1997), colon, stomach, and urinary bladder cancers.

Of note, the incidence of bladder cancer in Japan and elsewhere in Asia is very low compared with the incidence in the United States and western Europe. The occurrence of bladder cancer in Japanese families emigrating from Japan to the United States beyond the second generation is twice that seen in natives remaining in Japan (Heuper, 1969). A number of epidemiological and human studies have shown an inverse association between green tea consumption and the risk of bladder cancer (Bushman, 1998; Bianchi, 2000). In preclinical studies, green tea has been shown to dose-dependently inhibit bladder tumor growth in animal models, including the induction of bladder tumors by *N*-butyl-*N*-(4-hydroxybutyl)-nitrosamine in rats (Sato, 1999). In addition to its antioxidant and antiangiogenic effects, *in vivo* studies have shown that green tea polyphenols are capable of inhibiting the enzymatic activity of ornithine decarboxylase (ODC), the rate-limiting enzyme in the pathway of mammalian polyamine synthesis (Steele et al., 2000) and an enzyme that appears to play an important role in the process of tumor promotion. Polyamines affect DNA, RNA, and protein synthesis. For these reasons, ODC activity is said to be closely associated with tumor promotion. Green tea polyphenols have been demonstrated to inhibit ODC induction caused by tumor promoters in a number of tissues (Gupta et al., 1999). The inhibition of ODC results in a decrease in polyamine synthesis and cell growth. The biological properties of bladder cancer may render it susceptible to the effects of ODC blockade. Although normal and malignant human bladder epithelial cells have similar baseline ODC activities, activity of this enzyme is preferentially inducible by epidermal growth factor (EGF) in TCC (Messing et al., 1987). Also, ODC activity is significantly higher in TCC than in normal urothelium (Messing et al., 1995). Furthermore, human bladder cancer cell lines have been shown to be quite sensitive to the specific inhibitor of ornithine decarboxylase, α-difluoromethylornithine (DFMO) (Messing et al., 1988). DFMO has already been identified by the National Cancer Institute (NCI) as a promising bladder cancer chemopreventive agent for these capabilities (Malone et al., 1987). A phase II study of a green tea polyphenol extract is under way at the David Geffen School of Medicine at UCLA.

Soy Products

Soy products have been found to be beneficial in protection from numerous disease processes. Studies have demonstrated an association between higher intake of soy products and a lower risk of malignancies of the breast, colon, and prostate (Messina and Barnes, 1991). Experimental evidence has also demonstrated that soy products may affect the growth of bladder cancer cells *in vitro* and *in vivo*. The mechanism behind this effect appears to be cell cycle arrest, induction of apoptosis, and reduction of angiogenesis by means of interaction of various isoflavones such as genistein (Zhou et al., 1998; Su et al., 2000). Given that isoflavones are excreted in the urine with ingestion of soy products, the direct contact of these compounds with the bladder urothelium may prevent the development of bladder tumors (Seow et al., 1998). Very few epidemiological and clinical studies have investigated the role of soy in bladder cancer prevention. A small study of 40 patients by Lu et al. (1999) reported a small, insignificant decrease in bladder cancer risk in people who regularly consumed soy juice. This benefit was further reduced when adjustments were made for confounding variables. Similarly, Garcia et al. (1999) also failed to demonstrate a relationship between flavonoid intake and reduction of bladder cancer risk.

Vitamins

Vitamins that have been implicated by chemical, epidemiological, physiological, immunological, or clinical trial evidence to be potentially beneficial in bladder cancer include vitamins A, B6, C, D, and E. Each of these are briefly discussed as they related to bladder cancer, but it important to emphasize that the key to nutritional therapy in bladder cancer is balance rather than bullet: Combinations of beneficial nutrients working together will likely produce superior results to an approach based on single factors.

Vitamin A

As early as 1972 clinical evidence suggested that vitamin A was effective in bladder cancer. Evard and Bolag (1972) gave an oral dose of 100 mg of vitamin A to 15 patients and reported 26.7% complete and 46.7% partial response in the treatment of existing TCCs in the bladder. Vitamin A and its analogs, especially the retinoids, are among the best-studied chemopreventive agents in bladder cancer. Vitamin A is important for cell differentiation and has been found to enhance the differentiation of normal and neoplastic cells in tissue culture (Lotan, 1980). The reported biological actions of vitamin A analogs include antioxidant activity and immunoenhancement. In addition to their effects on singlet oxygen, carotenoids are also thought to suppress oxygen free radicals. All-trans-retinoic acid causes acute promyelocytic leukemia blasts to differentiate into polymorphonuclear leukocytes *in vitro* and has been observed to significantly improve response in controlled trials when used in combination with chemotherapy in acute promyelocytic leukemia (Chomienne et al., 1991).

Epidemiological data regarding vitamin A remain conflicting. Studies that favor a protective role include that of Mettlin and Graham (1979), who compared retrospective data from 569 bladder cancer patients and 1025 age-matched an increase in sex-adjusted RR for bladder cancer with lower levels of vitamin A intake. In another study of 2974 men followed for 17 years, low mean plasma levels of carotene were associated with increased overall mortality from cancer (Eichholzer et al., 1996). Both serum carotene and serum retinol levels are significantly reduced in patients with bladder cancer when compared with controls (Hicks, 1983). However, a meta-analytical review of epidemiological studies linking six dietary factors to bladder cancer demonstrated no increased risks for diets low in retinol (RR = 1.01, 95% CI, 0.83, 1.23) or β-carotene (RR = 1.10, 95% CI, 0.93, 1.30) intake (Steinmaus et al., 2000). The effect of low vitamin A serum levels is often lost when corrected for smoking.

Retinoids are potent suppressors of neoplastic transformation induced by various carcinogens, including viral, chemical, and radioactive agents, and antitumor activity against carcinogen-induced cancer of the skin, mammary gland, urinary bladder, esophagus, cervix, and liver has been demonstrated in animal models (Sporn and Newton, 1979). Like most chemopreventive agents, retinoids are most effective when given before or shortly after the inciting carcinogen, but efficacy in preventing bladder cancer is reported even when treatment is delayed (Becci et al., 1979).

Hypervitaminosis A inhibits keratinization and squamous metaplasia in bladder lesions induced by the carcinogen *N*-butyl-*N*-4-hydroxybutyl nitrosamine (BBN) and reduces incidence of transitional cell carcinoma and papilloma of the urinary bladder ($p < .02$) (Miyata et al., 1978). Becci et al. (1978) further showed that 13-*cis*-retinoic acid can reduce the incidence, average number, and grade of TCCs, as well as hyperplasia and cellular atypia in BBN-exposed mice urinary bladders even when the treatment was delayed by 9 weeks (Becci et al., 1978). Similar results have been reported with β-carotene. Mice supplemented with β-carotene for 5 weeks before receiving the carcinogen and maintained on β-carotene for an additional 26 weeks developed significantly fewer tumors than did control mice (Mathews-Roth et al., 1991). Using DNA flow cytometry as an intermediate endpoint, Decensi et al. (1992) demonstrated a reversion to normal cytology with the administration of 4-HPR to patients with previously suspicious or positive DNA flow cytometry. Although 4-HPR and other retinoids have been touted as "superior chemopreventive agents," clinical trials such as the CARROT and Finnish study suggest that a combination of retinoids, as well as other vitamins, may be preferable.

Studies combining retinoids with BCG have shown improved efficacy and suggest that the activity of retinoids may be potentiated by nonspecific immune stimulation. Treatment of mice with a combination of the retinoid Ro 10-

9359 and BCG results in an 83.3% incidence of complete tumor regression within 80 days (Pang and Morales, 1983). Similar findings have also been noted when combining retinoids with interferons (IFNs). Furthermore, it has been shown that human tumor-induced inhibition of IFN *in vitro* can be reversed by the β-carotene (Rhodes et al., 1983). Further support for immune-mediated response is demonstrated by the reduction of insulin-like growth factor 2 (IGF-II) (an important factor in IGFs in the pathogenesis of different solid tumors) by 16% with fenretinide treatment (Torrisi et al., 2000).

Clinical trials of retinoids in bladder cancer have been generally remarkably successful but largely ignored. In one of the earliest human trials Evard and Bolag in 1972 gave 15 patients 100 mg of vitamin A orally and found complete response in 26.7% and partial response in 46.7% (Evard and Bolag, 1972). A controlled clinical trial by the National Bladder Cancer Collaborative Group A of 13-cis-retinoic acid in patients with rapidly recurring bladder cancer refractory to other treatments closed early and failed to show any benefit (Prout and Barton, 1992). However, this study in patients who had failed multiple prior treatments would not be expected to show benefit of chemoprevention.

Another form of vitamin A, etretinate, was reported in two independent studies to be an effective chemopreventive for superficial bladder tumors. Thirty patients were enrolled in a double-blind, placebo-controlled study using etretinate in grade 1–2 Ta or T1 lesions. With duration of treatment ranging from 10 to 26 months, the recurrences were reduced from 87% to 60% ($p < .01$) in patients given etretinate (Alfthan et al., 1983). This report stimulated further larger studies with conforming results. Studer et al. (1995) studied 79 eligible patients with superficial (Ta, T1) papillary bladder tumor in a prospective double-blind multicenter trial. These patients were randomized to receive either 25 mg/day of etretinate orally or a placebo. Although the time to first recurrence was similar in both groups (13.5 and 13.6 months in the placebo and etretinate groups, respectively), the mean interval to subsequent tumor recurrence was 20.3 months in the etretinate group as compared with 12.7 months in the placebo arm ($p = .006$). A longer time to recurrence resulted in a decrease in the number of transurethral resections per patient-year from 2.1 in the control arm to 0.95 in the etretinate arm ($p < .001$). The side effects of etretinate were acceptable to most patients.

Vitamin B

Vitamin B6 (pyridoxine, pyridoxal, and pyridoxamine) and its metabolites are coenzymes for multiple pathways including tryptophan metabolism. Metabolites of tryptophan have been observed to have carcinogenic properties, and studies of human families suggest a clustering of abnormal tryptophan metabolism in patients with bladder cancer. Kynurenine, 3-hydroxy-anthranilic acid, and other tryptophan breakdown products can be elevated in the urine of patients with bladder cancer, and in animal models, these substances induce bladder cancer (Brown et al., 1960). Pyridoxine shifts the metabolism of tryptophan away from the carcinogenic derivatives and, therefore, prevents recurrences of superficial bladder cancers. The benefit observed with vitamin B6 may also be related to its effect on augmentation of immunity because elevated levels of vitamin B6 stimulate lymphocyte response in the geriatric population, suppress tumor growth, and boost anti-tumor immunity in mice (Gridley et al., 1987; Talbott et al., 1997).

Two large human trials have been instituted with conflicting results. In 1977, Byar et al. (1977) studied 118 patients with stage I bladder cancer randomized to placebo, pyridoxine 25 mg orally, or intravesical thiotepa. Tumor recurrence rate was 60% of the controls, 46% in the pyridoxine group, and 47% in the thiotepa group. If events during the first 10 months were excluded from analysis (allowing for time to action of pyridoxine), pyridoxine was as effective as thiotepa and significantly better than placebo ($p = .03$) (Byar et al., 1977). Another trial by the EORTC GU group failed to show an advantage for pyridoxine therapy. In this double-blind randomized trial comparing 20 mg/day of pyridoxine with placebo in 291 patients, no difference in time to first recurrence or the recurrence rate was observed. Adjusting for prognostic factors such as the recurrence rate or number of tumors before entry, the tumor grade or the levels of tryptophan metabolites did not change the results (Newling et al., 1995).

Vitamin C

Vitamin C is a major circulating water-soluble antioxidant and free radical scavenger. *In vitro* studies show it to decrease chromosome damage in lymphocytes induced by exposure to bleomycin (Pohl and Reidy, 1989). Diets high in vitamin C are associated with lower risk for oral, gastrointestinal, and lung cancers. For gastric and esophageal cancer, there is evidence that this association is due to an inhibition of *in vivo* *N*-nitroso compound formation (Mirvish, 1986). Vitamin C reduces the *in vivo* formation of *N*-nitroso compounds, including 3-hydroxanthranilic acid and nitrosamines, which are implicated as potential causative agents in bladder cancers (Schlegel, 1975; Kakizoe et al., 1988).

Bladder cancer decreases with increasing levels of vitamin C intake ($p = .03$). Nomura et al. (1991) reported that the odds ratio for the highest quartile of vitamin C intake compared with the lowest quartile was 0.4. In a similar study, Shibata et al. (1992) followed 11,580 residents of a retirement community who were initially free from cancer. With 8 years of follow-up, 1335 cancer cases were diagnosed. After adjusting for age and smoking, there was an inverse association between vitamin C supplementation and bladder cancer risk (Shibata et al., 1992).

Some studies have hinted that sodium L-ascorbate and L-ascorbic acid might promote urinary bladder carcinogenesis in a dose-related manner (Birt, 1986), but studies are again inconsistent (Fukushima et al., 1987). The cytotoxic effects of ascorbic acid on the sensitive cell lines are time and dosage dependent (Kao and Meyer, 1993). It has been suggested that there is a threshold dose beyond which vitamin C has carcinogen-promoting effect (Fukushima et al., 1983) and that cancer cells may exist in two forms, one sensitive to inhibition by ascorbic acid and the other resistant to its anticarcinogenic effect. It may be best to limit the dose of vitamin C to moderate doses of 2000 mg daily until further data are available.

Vitamin D

In a study of ultraviolet B (UVB) radiation and U.S. cancer mortality rates, decreased sunlight was associated with increased risk of cancer of the bladder and other tumors including breast, colon, ovary, prostate, kidney, and lung (Grant, 2002). Vitamin D inhibits the proliferation of various tumor cells in tissue culture, including human bladder cancer cell lines, and *in vivo* inhibits the growth of *N*-methyl nitrosourea–induced bladder cancer in rats (Konety et al., 2001).

Vitamin E

Vitamin E is a major lipid-soluble antioxidant and free radical scavenger and acts as an antioxidant, protecting unsaturated lipids in cell membranes and metabolic enzymes from free radical oxidation damage. Diets high in vitamin E are associated with a lower risk of cancer (Byers and Guerrero, 1995). Nitrosamines, occurring in tobacco products, certain industrial chemicals, and nitrite-cured meat and other foods, have been implicated in cancers of the stomach, esophagus, nasopharynx, urinary bladder, and colon (Mirvish, 1995). In a cohort study of 991,522 U.S. adults in which 1289 bladder cancer deaths occurred, long-term vitamin E consumption, but not vitamin C consumption, significantly reduced mortality from bladder cancer (Jacobs et al., 2002). Vitamin E inhibits *N*-nitroso compound formation and produces 30–60% inhibition of induced carcinogenesis in most animal experiments (Mirvish et al., 1986). It is also possible that vitamin E provides protection from cancer by stimulating antitumor immunity. Supplementation of vitamin E enhances resistance to infection, reticuloendothelial system activity, and delayed cutaneous hypersensitivity response and antibody production (Beisel et al., 1981). Studies of thymidine incorporation have shown that vitamin E supplementation reduces DNA synthesis and causes fragmentation leading to apoptosis and, thus, inhibits cancer cell growth in a dose-dependent fashion. Cells vary in sensitivity to this effect, with breast and prostate cancer cells being most sensitive (Sigounas et al., 1997).

Selenium

Conflicting data exist as to the potential role of selenium in preventing bladder cancer. This essential trace mineral has been extensively investigated by numerous studies through the measurement and comparison of serum and toenail selenium levels of bladder cancer patients and controls. Helzlsouer et al. (1989) reported on a population of 25,802 people followed for 12 years and found to have 35 cases of bladder cancer. In this population, serum selenium was found to be significantly lower in patients with bladder cancer than in controls. In contrast, in the Nurses' Health Study, selenium levels were measured from toenail clippings of more than 62,500 women, and women with bladder cancer were actually found to have higher selenium levels than controls (Garland et al., 1995). Also, an overall higher cancer risk was also found in those women taking selenium supplements. In another large trial of selenium supplementation, a nonsignificant association was reported between selenium supplementation and bladder cancer risk (Clark et al., 1996). More study is necessary before dietary or supplemental selenium can be recommended for the prevention of bladder cancer.

Combination Vitamins

Lamm et al. (1994) studied the effect of a megadose vitamin combination in a double-blind randomized trial. Sixty-five patients with biopsy-confirmed TCC of the bladder were randomized to receive either the RDA of multiple vitamins or the RDA plus 40,000 IU vitamin A, 100 mg vitamin B6, 2000 mg vitamin C, and 400 IU vitamin E and 90 mg zinc. As might be expected from a chemoprevention trial, curves for time to recurrence for the two groups were identical for the first 10 months but diverged significantly thereafter. Five-year estimates of tumor recurrence were 91% in the RDA arm and 41% in the high-dose vitamin arm ($p = .0014$). Overall recurrence was 80% (25/30) in the RDA arm and 40% (14/35) in the high-dose vitamin arm ($p = .0011$). Stratifying the patients according to tumor stage showed a statistically significant ($p = .003$) benefit of a 42% reduction in tumor recurrence in those with stage Ta or T1 TCC. Stratifying the patients according to tumor grade also showed a statistically significant ($p = .007$) benefit of 53% in those with low grade (G1, G2) TCC. The high-dose vitamins were generally well tolerated, with mild nausea being the most common side effect.

THE FUTURE OF BLADDER CANCER CHEMOPREVENTION: A RATIONAL STRATEGY FOR THE IDENTIFICATION AND TESTING OF NEW AGENTS

Development of newer or more effective preventive strategies for bladder cancer is of critical importance. Chemoprevention lies at an interesting intersection between disease management and health promotion, and competing values play a role in determining the nature and magnitude of the risks and benefits of chemoprevention of cancer.

Ethical questions related to these trials concern the enrollment of healthy or "at-risk" individuals rather than cancer patients, and one has to balance competing benefits and toxicities of treatment. Many authorities question the validity of current recommendations for nutritional chemoprevention against bladder cancer. The reason for this skepticism revolves around the wide variations reported in epidemiological studies that are in the nature of observational studies. Observation dietary studies have been limited in their conclusions because the protection afforded by the consumption of a particular nutrient may be multifactorial, with different components of the food exerting potential chemopreventive effects. Furthermore, measuring levels of nutrients in the food intake of populations is confounded by factors that might affect these levels and the incidence of cancer. In addition, chemoprevention studies using dietary strategies may be expected to have mild effects, and large studies may be required to confirm statistical significance. Therefore, prospective randomized trials with a large sample size, longer follow-up, an extended duration of treatment, and validated biomarkers of risk, effect, and prognosis are necessary to clarify the association between micronutrients and cancer protection. The final section of this chapter explores key issues related to the prospective testing of new agents for bladder cancer prevention.

A Strategy for Developing Interventions for Superficial TCC: The ABCD Matrix

The design and conduct of investigational studies for the prevention and management of superficial bladder cancer involves the rational integration of several key factors including (1) *agents* (pharmaceuticals, biologics, and natural products); (2) *biomarkers* (intermediate endpoints that reflect biological activity and cancer risk reduction); (3) *cohorts* (well-defined individuals with high risk for recurrence and progression); (4) *designs* (efficient randomized controlled trials linked to the phase of Food and Drug Administration–guided drug development); and (5) *endpoints* (meaningful clinical outcomes such as reduction of cancer recurrence and progression). Because patients with superficial TCC typically present with early-stage disease (Ta, T1, CIS) that frequently recurs and is readily accessible and monitored through serial cystoscopies and urine cytology, superficial bladder cancer can serve as a prototypical clinical model for conducting prevention and adjuvant treatment trials.

Clinical Models and Trial Designs for Evaluating Nutritional, Biological, and Chemopreventive Agents

Prevention of Recurrence of Superficial TCC

The design most frequently employed to demonstrate clinical and biological activity is to administer the experimental agent(s) after the initial or recurrent lesion is surgically removed (TURBT) as adjuvant therapy. Because recurrences can represent a new second primary tumor or can reflect recurrence of the original clonal outgrowth, interventions in this setting are also considered to be secondary prevention. The cohort is typically a patient with low to intermediate grade Ta or T1 lesions. However, with the FDA approval of intravesical BCG immunotherapy initially for the treatment of carcinoma in situ (CIS) and more recently for an expanded indication to include adjunct treatment of resected stage Ta or T1 tumors, an increasing number of patients with high grade (grade 2 or 3) Ta and T1 lesions that are multifocal and larger than 3 cm are also managed after TURBT with BCG induction and/or maintenance therapy. Based on current recommendations of the FDA, definitive clinical response would be assessed by the 2-year recurrence rate and longer term follow-up of disease progression (Hirsch, personal communication, 2004).

Neoadjuvant Treatment Prior to Definitive TURBT

A practical design that has gained popularity for several cancers (e.g., prostate and breast) is to administer the experimental agent(s) in the window of opportunity between the diagnostic or surveillance positive cystoscopy and definitive treatment (TURBT for superficial or cystectomy for muscle invasive disease). An advantage of this approach is the clinical histological response of the index lesion(s) and the effect on the field changes (dysplasia), and intermediate endpoint biomarkers in the bladder and urine can be concurrently assessed over a relatively shorter interval (3 weeks to 3 months). This approach should allow for more rapid screening of promising agents.

Intravesical Administration

Another strategy that is feasible is the intralesional or intravesical administration of experimental agents including immunological vaccines, chemopreventive, chemotherapeutic, and gene therapy. This approach would appear to be well suited for the evaluation of the prevention of low-grade recurrent disease implantation, as well as adjuvant treatment of CIS in combination with BCG or as salvage treatment of BCG failures (e.g., valrubicin).

Intermediate Endpoint Biomarkers: The Search for Surrogate Endpoints

Validation of Surrogate Endpoints and Accelerated Drug Development

A major goal of chemoprevention is the validation of surrogate endpoints (SEs) for bladder cancer incidence reduction. The rationale for identifying SEs to evaluate efficacy relates to the improved efficiency and predictability by reduced sample size, decreased duration to conduct clinical trials, and more cost-effective drug development for pharmaceutical and biotechnology sponsors of phase 3 clinical trials organized to gain FDA approval for marketing.

Validation can be achieved during phase 3 randomized controlled trials by incorporating candidate SEs and correlating changes in the SE with the primary clinical endpoint of cancer incidence reduction. In this context, information should be elucidated regarding the relationship between the SE and the causal pathway of bladder carcinogenesis. Once validated, an SE of bladder cancer carcinogenesis can accelerate new agent development because it may now be used as the primary endpoint versus the clinical endpoint of bladder cancer recurrence in phase 2b/3 trials under current FDA clinical guidelines. However, no SE has been prospectively validated as a substitute for cancer incidence/recurrence in bladder cancer.

Categories of Intermediate Endpoint Biomarkers

Currently, several types of intermediate endpoint biomarkers (IEBs) are under active evaluation or have been proposed as candidate SEs. These include (1) histological markers such as IEN and nuclear histomorphometric indices in the urothelium at risk; these histological-based markers can be quantitated by nuclear morphometric analysis; (2) tissue and cellular markers such as apoptosis, proliferation, angiogenesis, inflammation, and differentiation; (3) genetic markers such as specific mutations, aneuploidy, loss of heterozygosity, microsatellite analysis, and cDNA gene expression microarrays; (4) markers associated with signal transduction pathways such as overexpression or loss of function of oncogenes and tumor suppressor genes; (5) markers associated with regulatory and cell cycle control; (6) markers of inflammation and oxidative stress; (7) markers associated with proteomics patterns and protein products in the serum, urine, and bladder washings; (8) markers based on epigenetics (methylated DNA) in the serum and urine; and (9) markers associated with functional imaging.

Although the FDA has approved five bladder cancer markers including NMP-22, BLCA-4, and BTA, the clinical gold standard for confirming bladder cancer incidence and recurrence remains cystoscopic surveillance with examination of bladder washings and urine cytology. Several promising urine markers include MSA, survivin, telomerase, and methylated genes.

Evidence-Based Leads for Identifying New Agents

Molecular Epidemiology, Pharmacogenomics, and Nutritional Science

Epidemiology and nutritional science continue to provide promising leads for identifying populations at risk and novel interventions. This would include subjects with polymorphisms in known antioxidant/anticarcinogen defense mechanisms related to cytochrome P450 metabolism (i.e., GSTM1 null variants), acetylator phenotypes (i.e., NAT2 slow acetylator), DNA repair enzymes (i.e., hMSH2), and gene–environment interactions with carcinogens in tobacco, common drugs such as nonsteroidal anti-inflammatory drugs (NSAIDs), and dietary exposures to micronutrient antioxidants (i.e., carotenoids, selenium, vitamin E, and phytochemicals such as soy isoflavones, green tea polyphenols, and garlic).

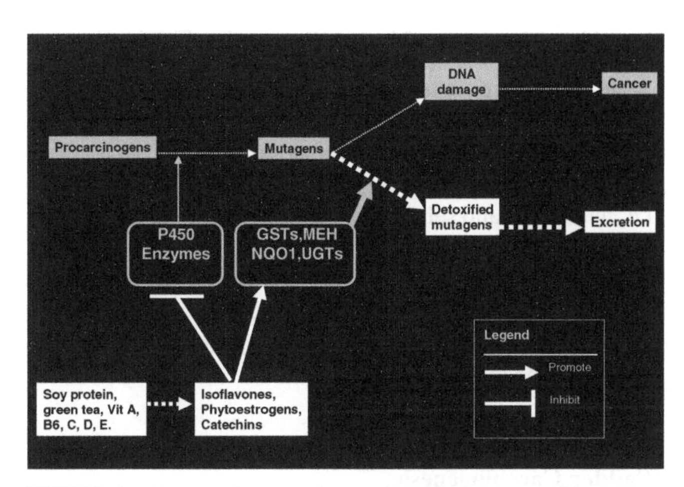

FIGURE 1 Gene–environment interactions: Diet may modify enzyme metabolism and subsequent risk of cancer development.

Adjuvant Trials

Successful adjuvant and secondary prevention trials using intravesical administration as noted earlier have been the gold standard to identify agents such as BCG and KLH that could be applied earlier in superficial bladder cancer. Furthermore, the realization of significant limitations in the ability to prevent recurrences and especially progression to muscle invasive disease in CIS and high-grade Ta and T1 lesions with these intravesical agents alone underscores the need for other modes of administration including chronic systemic approaches. In this regard, the successful experience with systemic adjuvant treatment regimens for other epithelial cancers such as breast and colon cancer is relevant. This strategy to use chronically administered oral agents is being pursued through several collaborations among the NCI, pharmaceutical/nutriceutical industry, and academia. One innovative design is a three-arm randomized controlled trial using two promising oral agents (i.e., extracts derived from green tea [polyphenon E] and the selective EGF receptor [EGFR] inhibitor [erlotinib]). This trial is actually two parallel randomized trials that use a common control group (Belldegrun, personal communication).

Secondary Analyses of Large Prevention Trials

Historically, post hoc analyses of large prevention trials have proven informative in hypothesis generation, which can be tested in prospective randomized controlled trials. Two antioxidant nutrients for prostate cancer prevention (i.e., vitamin E and selenium) were identified in this way and are now undergoing clinical evaluation in a large primary chemoprevention trial for prostate cancer known as SELECT. Thus, even negative phase 3 trials for bladder cancer chemoprevention (e.g., DFMO) could provide new leads thru secondary analyses.

***In Vitro* and *In Vivo* Experimental Models of Bladder Carcinogenesis**

Chemopreventive activity has been identified for several classes of agents including NSAIDs and their derivatives, synthetic and natural retinoids, phase 2 enzyme inducers, antioxidant nutrients, phytochemical natural products, immune modulators, and molecularly targeted agents such as EGFR inhibitors. Experimental model systems include *in vitro* human bladder cell lines, human xenografted rodent models, carcinogen (OH-BBN) rodent models of bladder carcinogenesis, and new transgenic murine models of bladder cancer using p53 heterozygotes. These models have yielded positive results and have led to randomized controlled trials (e.g., DFMO, 4-HPR, celecoxib, green tea extracts, and EGFR inhibitors).

CONCLUSIONS

Preclinical and limited clinical data demonstrate that bladder cancer is responsive to primary and secondary preventive efforts. Furthermore, epidemiological studies imply that natural products, such as vitamins and herbal compounds, may provide preventive benefit, but these agents have not been prospectively studied. Bladder cancer is an attractive target for prevention efforts because renal excretion of agents enables prolonged exposure to high concentrations of drugs in the urine. Additionally, the urothelium is easily evaluated and monitored with strategies that are highly successful and relatively noninvasive. The frequent recurrence of superficial bladder cancer with low occurrence of muscle-invasive disease permits the safe and efficient assessment of strategies to prevent secondary bladder cancers with a modest number of patients and short follow-up. Although improved understanding of the pathways of bladder carcinogenesis presents new targets for prevention, the lack of identifiable high-risk populations and SEBs (for both malignancies) limits our ability to implement prevention studies. The development of validated surrogate endpoints will facilitate the future evaluation of novel chemopreventive agents and strategies.

References

Alfthan, O., Tarkkanen, J., Grohn, P., Heinonen, E., Pyrhonen, S., and Saila, K. 1983. Tigason (etretinate) in prevention of recurrence of superficial bladder tumors. A double-blind clinical trial. *Eur Urol* **9**(1): 6.

Awasthi, Y.C., Sharma, R., and Singhal, S.S. 1994. Human glutathione S-transferases. *Int J Biochem* **26**: 295–308.

Bartsch, H., Castegnaro, M., Camus, A.M., Schouft, A., Geneste, O., Rojas, M., et al. 1993a. Analysis of DNA adducts in smokers' lung and urothelium by 32P-postlabelling: metabolic phenotype dependence and comparisons with other exposure markers. IARC Scientific Publications pp. 331–340.

Bartsch, H., Malaveille, C., Friesen, M., Kadlubar, F.F., and Vineis, P. 1993b. Black (air-cured) and blond (flue-cured) tobacco cancer risk. IV: Molecular dosimetry studies implicate aromatic amines as bladder carcinogens. *Eur J Cancer* **29A**: 1199–1207.

Becci, P.J., Thompson, H.J., Grubbs, C.J., Brown, C.C., and Moon, R.C. 1979. Effect of delay in administration of 13-cis-retinoic acid on the inhibition of urinary bladder carcinogenesis in the rat. *Cancer Res* **39**(8): 3141.

Becci, P.J., Thompson, H.J., Grubbs, C.J., Squire, R.A., Brown, C.C., Sporn, M.B., and Moon, R.C. 1978. Inhibitory effect of 13-cis-retinoic acid on urinary bladder carcinogenesis induced in C57BL/6 mice by *N*-butyl-*N*-(4-hydroxybutyl)-nitrosamine. *Cancer Res* **38**(12): 4463.

Beisel, W.R., Edelman, R., Nauss, K., and Suskind, R.M. 1981. Single nutrient effects on immunologic functions. Report of a workshop sponsored by the Department of Food and Nutrition and its nutrition advisory group of the American Medical Association. *JAMA* **245**: 53.

Bell, D.A., Taylor, J.A., Paulson, D.F., Robertson, C.N., Mohler, J.L., and Lucier, G.W. 1993a. Genetic risk and carcinogen exposure: a common inherited defect of the carcinogen-metabolism gene glutathione *S*-transferase M1 (GSTM1) that increases susceptibility to bladder cancer. *J Nat Cancer Inst* **85**: 1159–1164.

Bell, D.A., Taylor, J.A., Butler, M.A., Stephens, E.A., Wiest, J., Brubaker, L.H., et al. 1993b. Genotype/phenotype discordance for human arylamine *N*-acetyltransferase (NAT2) reveals a new slow-acetylator allele common in African-Americans. *Carcinogenesis* **14**: 1689–1692.

Bianchi, G.D., Cerhan, J.R., Parker, A.S., Putnam, S.D., See, W.A., Lynch, C.F., et al. 2000. Tea consumption and risk of bladder and kidney cancers in a population-based case–control study. *Am J Epidemiol* **151**: 377–383.

Birt, D.F. 1986. Update on the effects of vitamins A, C, and E and selenium on carcinogenesis. *Proc Soc Exp Biol Med* **183**: 311.

Byers, T., and Guerrero, N. 1995. Epidemiologic evidence for vitamin C and vitamin E in cancer prevention. *Am J Clin Nutr* **62**(6 Suppl): 1385S.

Brockmoller, J., Kerb, R., Drakoulis, N., Staffeldt, B., and Roots, I. 1994. Glutathione *S*-transferase M1 and its variants A and B as host factors of bladder cancer susceptibility: a case-control study. *Cancer Res* **54**: 4103–4111.

Brown, R.R., Price, J.M., Satter, E.J., and Wear, J.B. 1960. The metabolism of tryptophan in patients with bladder cancer. *Acta Un Int Cancer* **16**: 299.

Bruemmer, B., White, E., Vaughn, T., and Cheney, C. 1996. Nutrient intake in relation to bladder cancer among middle aged men and women. *Am J Epidemiol* **144**: 485.

Bushman, J.L. 1998. Green tea and cancer in humans: a review of the literature. *Nutr Cancer* **31**: 151–159.

Byar, D., and Blackard, C. 1977. Comparisons of placebo, pyridoxine, and topical thiotepa in preventing recurrence of stage I bladder cancer. *Urology* **10**(6): 556.

Carpenter, A.A. 1989. Clinical experience with transitional cell carcinoma of the bladder with special reference to smoking. *J Urol* **141**: 527–528.

Castelao, J.E., Yuan, J.M., Skipper, P.L., Tannenbaum, S.R., Gago-Dominguez, M., Crowder, J.S., et al. 2001. Gender- and smoking-related bladder cancer risk. *J Natl Cancer Inst* **93**: 538–545.

Chomienne, C., Balitrand, N., Ballerini, P., Castaigne, S., de The, H., and Degos, L. 1991. All-trans retinoic acid modulates the retinoic acid receptor-alpha in promyelocytic cells. *Clin Invest* **88**(6): 2150–2154.

Chung, F.L., Morse, M.A., Eklind, K.I., and Xu, Y. 1993. Inhibition of tobacco-specific nitrosamine-induced lung tumorigenesis by compounds derived from cruciferous vegetables and green tea. *Ann NY Acad Sci* **686**: 186–201; discussion 201–202.

Clark, L., Combs, G., Turnbull, B., et al. 1996. Effects of selenium supplementation for cancer prevention in patients with carcinoma of the skin: a randomized controlled trial. *JAMA* **276**: 1957.

Cohen, L., Choi, K., and Wang, C. 1988. Influence of dietary fat, caloric restriction, and voluntary exercise in *N*-nitrosomethylurea–induced mammary tumorigenesis in rats. *Cancer Res* **48**: 4276.

Cole, P., Hoover, R., and Friedell, G. 1972. Occupation and cancer of the lower urinary tract. *Cancer* **29**: 1250.

Curigliano, G., Zhang, Y.J., Wang, L.Y., Flamini, G., Alcini, A., Ratto, C., et al. 1996. Immunohistochemical quantitation of 4-aminobiphenyl-DNA adducts and p53 nuclear overexpression in T1 bladder cancer of smokers and nonsmokers. *Carcinogenesis* **17**: 911–916.

Daly, A.K., Thomas, D.J., Cooper, J., Pearson, W.R., Neal, D.E., and Idle, J.R. 1993. Homozygous deletion of gene for glutathione *S*-transferase M1 in bladder cancer. *BMJ* **307**: 481–482.

Decensi, A., Bruno, S., Giaretti, W., et al. 1992. Activity of 4-HPR in superficial bladder cancer using DNA flow cytometry as an intermediate endpoint. *J Cell Biochem* **16I**: 139.

Dunn, S., Kari, F., French, J., et al. 1992. Dietary restriction reduces insulin0like growth factor I levels, which modulates apoptosis, call proliferation and tumor progression in p53 deficient mice. *Cancer Res* **57**: 4667.

Eichholzer, M., Bernasconi, F., Ludin, E., Gey, K.F., and Stahelin, H.B. 1996. Prediction of male cancer mortality by plasma levels of interacting vitamins: 17-year follow-up of the prospective Basel study. *Int J Cancer* **66**(2): 145.

Esteller, M., Corn, P.G., Urena, J.M., Gabrielson, E., Baylin, S.B., and Herman, J.G. 1998. Inactivation of glutathione S-transferase P1 gene by promoter hypermethylation in human neoplasia. *Cancer Res* **58**: 4515–4518.

Evard, J.P., and Bolag, W. 1972. Konservative behandlung der rezidivierenden harnblasenpapillomatose mit vitamin-A-saure. Vorlafige Mitteilung. *Schweiz Med Wochenschr* **102**: 1880.

Fleshner, N, and Klotz, L. 1998–1999. Diet, androgens, oxidative stress, and prostate cancer susceptibility. *Cancer Metastasis Rev* **17**: 325.

Fukushima, S., Imaida, K., Sakata, T., OkamUra, T., Shibata, M., and Ito, N. 1983. Promoting effects of sodium L-ascorbate on two-stage urinary bladder carcinogenesis in rats. *Cancer Res* **43**: 4454.

Fukushima, S., Ogiso, T., Kurata, Y., Shibata, M.A., and Kakizoe, T. 1987. Absence of promotion potential for calcium L-ascorbate, L-ascorbic dipalmitate, L-ascorbic stearate and erythorbic acid on rat urinary bladder carcinogenesis. *Cancer Lett* **35**: 17.

Garcia, R., Gonzalez, C., Agudo, A., et al. 1999. High intake of specific carotenoids and flavonoids does not reduce the risk of bladder cancer. *Nutr Cancer* **35**: 212.

Garland, M., Morris, J., Stampfer, M., et al. 1995. Prospective study of toenail selenium levels and cancer among women. *J Natl Cancer Inst* **87**: 497.

Geoffroy-Perez, B., and Cordier, S. 2001. Fluid consumption and the risk of bladder cancer: results of a multicenter case–control study. *Int J Cancer* **93**: 880.

Grant, W.B. 2002. An estimate of premature cancer mortality in the U.S. due to inadequate doses of solar ultraviolet-B radiation. *Cancer* **94**(6): 1867–1875.

Gridley, D.S., Stickney, D.R., Nutter, R.L., Slater, J.M., and Shultz, T.D. 1987. Suppression of tumor growth and enhancement of immune status with high levels of dietary vitamin B6 in BALB/c mice. *J Natl Caner Inst* **78**: 951.

Gupta, S., Ahmad, N., Mohan, R.R., Husain, M.M., and Mukhtar, H. 1999. Prostate cancer chemoprevention by green tea: *in vitro* and *in vivo* inhibition of testosterone-mediated induction of ornithine decarboxylase. *Cancer Res* **59**: 2115–2120.

Harries, L.W., Stubbins, M.J., Forman, D., Howard, G.C., and Wolf, C.R. 1997. Identification of genetic polymorphisms at the glutathione *S*-transferase Pi locus and association with susceptibility to bladder, testicular and prostate cancer. *Carcinogenesis* **18**: 641–644.

Hein, D.W., Doll, M.A., Gray, K., Rustan, T.D., and Ferguson, R.J. 1993. Metabolic activation of *N*-hydroxy-2-aminofluorene and *N*-hydroxy-2-acetylaminofluorene by monomorphic *N*-acetyltransferase (NAT1) and polymorphic *N*-acetyltransferase (NAT2) in colon cytosols of Syrian hamsters congenic at the NAT2 locus. *Cancer Res* **53**: 509–514.

Helzlsouer, K., Comstock, G., and Morris, J. 1989. Selenium, lycopene, alpha-tocopherol, beta-carotene, retinol and subsequent bladder cancer. *Cancer Res* **49**: 6144.

Heney, N.M., Nocks, B.N., Daly, J.J., Prout, G.R., Newall, J.B., Griffin, P.P., et al. 1982. Ta and T1 bladder cancer: location, recurrence and progression. *Br J Urol* **54**: 152–157.

Heuper, W.G. 1969. Cancers of urinary system. *In* "Occupational and Environmental Cancers of the Urinary System" (W.G. Heuper, ed.), pp. 1–67. Yale University Press, New Haven, CT.

Hicks, R.M. 1983. The scientific basis for regarding vitamin A and its analogues as anti-carcinogenic agents. *Proc Nutr Soc* **42**(1): 83.

Hong, W.K., and Sporn, M.B. 1997. Recent advances in chemoprevention of cancer. *Science* **278**: 1073–1077.

Hoover, R., and Cole, P. 1971. Population trends in cigarette smoking and bladder cancer. *Am J Epidemiol* **94**: 409–418.

Hsing, A.W., Chokkalingam, A.P., Gao, Y.T., Madigan, M.P., Deng, J., Gridley, G., and Fraumeni, J.F., Jr. 2002. Allium vegetables and risk of prostate cancer: a population-based study. *J Natl Cancer Inst* **94**(21): 1648–1651.

Jacobs, E.J., Henion, A.K., Briggs, P.J., Connell, C.J., McCullough, M.L., Jonas, C.R., Rodriguez, C., Calle, E.E., and Thun, M.J. 2002. Vitamin C and vitamin E supplement use and bladder cancer mortality in a large cohort of US men and women. *Am J Epidemiol* **156**(11): 1002–1010.

Jemal, A., Murray, T., Samuels, A., Ghafoor, A., Ward, E., and Thun, M. 2003. Cancer statistics 2003. *CA Cancer J Clin* **53**: 5.

Ji, B.T., Chow, W.H., Hsing, A.W., McLaughlin, J.K., Dai, Q., Gao, Y.T., et al. 1997. Green tea consumption and the risk of pancreatic and colorectal cancers. *Int J Cancer* **70**: 255–258.

Kakizoe, T., Takai, K., Tobisu, K., Ohtani, M., and Sato, S. 1988. Validity of short-term examination for antipromoters of bladder carcinogenesis *Jpn J Cancer Res* **79**: 231.

Kao, T.L., Meyer, W.J., 3rd, and Post, J.F. 1993. Inhibitory effects of ascorbic acid on growth of leukemic and lymphoma cell lines. *Cancer Lett* **70**: 101.

Khan, S.G., Katiyar, S.K., Agarwal, R., and Mukhtar, H. 1992. Enhancement of antioxidant and phase II enzymes by oral feeding of green tea polyphenols in drinking water to SKH-1 hairless mice: possible role in cancer chemoprevention. *Cancer Res* **52**: 4050–4052.

Kinzler, K.W., and Vogelstein, B. 1996. Lessons from hereditary colorectal cancer. *Cell* **87**: 159–170.

Komori, A., Yatsunami, J., Okabe, S., Abe, S., Hara, K., Suganuma, M., et al. 1993. Anticarcinogenic activity of green tea polyphenols. *Jpn J Clin Oncol* **23**: 186–190.

Konety, B.R., Lavelle, J.P., Pirtskalaishvili, G., Dhir, R., Meyers, S.A., Nguyen, T.S., Hershberger, P., Shurin, M.R., Johnson, C.S., Trump, D.L., Zeidel, M.L., and Getzenberg, R.H. 2001. Effects of vitamin D (calcitriol) on transitional cell carcinoma of the bladder *in vitro* and *in vivo*. *J Urol* **165**(1): 253–258.

Kunze, E., Chang-Clause, J., and Frentzel-Beyme, R. 1986. Life style and occupational risk factors in cancer of the lower urinary tract. *Am J Epidemiol* **124**: 578.

Lafuente, A., Pujol, F., Carretero, P., Villa, J.P., and Cuchi, A. 1993. Human glutathione *S*-transferase mu (GST mu) deficiency as a marker for the susceptibility to bladder and larynx cancer among smokers. *Cancer Lett* **68**: 49–54.

Lamm, D.L., and Riggs, D.R. 2001. Enhanced immunocompetence by garlic: role in bladder cancer and other malignancies. *J Nutr* **131**(3s): 1067S–1070S.

Lamm, D.L., Riggs, D.R., Shriver, J.S., Vanguilder, P.F., Rach, J.F., and DeHaven, J.I. 1994. Megadose vitamins in bladder cancer: a double-blind clinical trial. *J Urol* **151**: 21.

Larminat, F., Beecham, E.J., Link, C.J., May, A., and Bohr, V.A. 1995. DNA repair in the endogenous and episomal amplified c-*myc* oncogene loci in human tumor cells. *Oncogene* **10**: 1639–1645.

Lau, B.H.S., Tadi, P.P., and Tosk, J.M. 1990. Allium sativum (garlic) and cancer prevention. *Nutr Res* **10**: 937–948.

Lau, B.H., Woolley, J.L., Marsh, C.L., Barker, G.R., Koobs, D.H., and Torrey, R.R. 1986. Superiority of intralesional immunotherapy with corynebacterium parvum and allium sativum in control of murine transitional cell carcinoma. *J Urol* **136**: 701–705.

Lee, M.J., Wang, Z.Y., Li, H., Chen, L., Sun, Y., Gobbo, S., et al. 1995. Analysis of plasma and urinary tea polyphenols in human subjects. *Cancer Epidemiol Biomarkers Prev* **4**: 393–399.

Lotan, R. 1980. Effects of vitamin A and its analogs (retinoids) on normal and neoplastic cells. *Biochim Biophys Acta* **605**: 33.

Lu, C., Lan, S., Lee, Y., et al. 1999. Tea consumption, fluid intake, and bladder cancer risk in Southern Taiwan. *Urology* **54**: 823.

Malone, W.F., Kelloff, G.J., Pierson, H., and Greenwald, P. 1987. Chemoprevention of bladder cancer. *Cancer* **60**(3 Suppl): 650–657.

Marsh, C.L., Torrey, R.R., Woolley, J.L., Barker, G.R., and Lau, B.H. 1987. Superiority of intravesical immunotherapy with corynebacterium parvum and allium sativum in control of murine bladder cancer. *J Urol* **137**: 359–362.

Mathews-Roth, M.M., Lausen, N., Drouin, G., Richter, A., and Krinsky, N.I. 1991. Effects of carotenoid administration on bladder cancer prevention. *Oncology* **48**(3): 177.

Messina, M., and Barnes, S. 1991. The role of soy products in reducing risk of cancer. *J Natl Cancer Inst* **83**: 541.

Messing, E.M., Hanson, P., and Reznikoff, C.A. 1988. Normal and malignant human urothelium: *in vitro* response to blockade of polyamine synthesis and interconversion. *Cancer Res* **48**: 357–361.

Messing, E.M., Hanson, P., Ulrich, P., and Erturk, E. 1987. Epidermal growth factor—interactions with normal and malignant urothelium: *in vivo* and *in situ* studies. *J Urol* **138**: 1329–1335.

Messing, E.M., Verma, A., Bram, L., and Storer, B.R.S. 1995. Ornithine decarboxylase activity in normal and malignant urothelium. *J Urol* **153**: 523A.

Mettlin, C., and Graham, S. 1979. Dietary risk factors in human bladder cancer. *Am J Epidemiol* **110**(3): 255.

Michaud, D., Spiegelman, D., Clinton, S., Rimm, E., Willett, W., and Giovannucci, E. 1999a. Fluid intake and rhe risk of bladder cancer in men. *N Engl J Med* **340**: 1390.

Michaud, D., Spiegelman, D., Clinton, S., et al. 1999b. Fruit and vegetable intake and incidence of bladder cancer in a male prospective cohort. *J Natl Cancer Inst* **91**: 605.

Mills, P., Beeson, W., Phillips, R., and Fraser, G. 1991. Bladder cancer in a low risk population: results from the Adventist Health Study. *Am J Epidemiol* **133**: 230.

Mirvish, S.S. 1986. Effects of vitamins C and E on *N*-nitroso compound formation, carcinogenesis, and cancer. *Cancer* **58**: 1842.

Mirvish, S.S. 1995. Role of *N*-nitroso compounds (NOC) and *N*-nitrosation in etiology of gastric, esophageal, nasopharyngeal and bladder cancer and contribution to cancer of known exposures to NOC. *Cancer Lett* **93**(1): 17.

Miyata, Y., Tsuda, H., Matayoshi-Miyasato, K., Fukushima, S., Murasaki, G., Ogiso, T., and Ito, N. 1978. Effect of vitamin A acetate on urinary bladder carcinogenesis induced by N-butyl-N-(4-hydroxybutyl)-nitrosamine in rats. *Gann* **69**(6): 845.

Morrison, A. 1984. Advances in the etiology of urothelial cancer. *Urol Clin North Am* **11**: 557.

Morrison, A.S., Buring, J.E., Verhoek, W.G., Aoki, K., Leck, I., Ohno, Y., et al. 1984. An international study of smoking and bladder cancer. *J Urol* **131**: 650–654.

Mukhtar, H., Katiyar, S.K., and Agarwal, R. 1994. Green tea and skin—anticarcinogenic effects. *J Investig Dermatol* **102**: 3–7.

Nagano, J., Kono, S., Preston, D., et al. 2000. Bladder cancer incidence in relation to vegetable and fruit consumption: a prospective study of atomic bomb survivors. *Int J Cancer* **86**: 132.

Negri, E., and La Vecchia, C. 2001. Epidemiology and prevention of bladder cancer. *Eur J Cancer Prev* **10**: 7–14.

Newling, D.W., Robinson, M.R., Smith, P.H., Byar, D., Lockwood, R., Stevens, I., De Pauw, M., and Sylvester, R. 1995. Tryptophan metabolites, pyridoxine (vitamin B6) and their influence on the recurrence rate of superficial bladder cancer. Results of a prospective, randomized phase III study performed by the EORTC GU Group. *Eur Urol* **27**(2): 110.

Nomura, A.M., Kolonel, L.N., Hankin, J.H., and Yoshizawa, C.N. 1991. Dietary factors in cancer of the lower urinary tract. *Int J Cancer* **48**: 199.

Oyasu, R., and Hupp, M. 1974. The etiology of cancer of the bladder. *Surg Gynecol Obstet* **138**: 97.

Pang, A.S., and Morales, A. 1983. Chemoimmunoprophylaxis of an experimental bladder cancer with retinoids and *Bacillus* Calmette-Guérin. *J Urol* **130**(1): 166.

Pohl, H., and Reidy, J.A. 1989. Vitamin C intake influences the bleomycin-induced chromosome damage assay: implications for detection of cancer susceptibility and chromosome breakage syndromes. *Mutat Res* **224**(2): 247.

Prout, G.R., Jr., and Barton, B.A. 1992.13-*cis*-retinoic acid in chemoprevention of superficial bladder cancer. The National Bladder Cancer Group. *J Cell Biochem Suppl* **16I**: 148.

Raitanen, M.P., Nieminen, P., and Tammela, T.L. 1995. Impact of tumour grade, stage, number and size, and smoking and sex, on survival in patients with transitional cell carcinoma of the bladder. *Br J Urol* **76**: 470–474.

Rao, J.Y., Jin, Y.S., Zheng, Q., Cheng, J., Tai, J., and Hemstreet, G.P. 1999. Alterations of the actin polymerization status as an apoptotic morphological effector in HL-60 cells. *J Cell Biochem* **75**: 686–697.

Rhodes, J., Stokes, P., and Abrams, P. 1984. Human tumour-induced inhibition of interferon action *in vitro*: reversal of by beta-carotene (provitamin A). *Cancer Immunol Immunother* **16**(3): 189–192.

Riboli, E., Gonzalez, C., Lopez-Abente, G., et al. 1991. Diet and bladder cancer in a low risk population: a multi-center case-control study. *Int J Cancer* **49**: 214.

Rivlin, R.S. 2001. Historical perspective on the use of garlic. *J Nutr* **131**(3s): 951S–954S.

Sala, M., Cordier, S., Chang-Claude, J., Donato, F., Escolar-Pujolar, A., Fernandez, F., et al. 2000. Coffee consumption and bladder cancer in nonsmokers: a pooled analysis of case-control studies in European countries. *Cancer Causes Control* **11**: 925.

Sato, D. 1999. Inhibition of urinary bladder tumors induced by *N*-butyl-*N*-(4-hydroxybutyl)-nitrosamine in rats by green tea. *Int J Urol* **6**: 93–99.

Schlegel, J.U. 1975. Proposed uses of ascorbic acid in the prevention of bladder carcinoma. *Ann NY Acad Sci* **258**: 432.

Schulte, P.A. 1988. The role of genetic factors in bladder cancer. *Cancer Detect Prev* **11**: 379–388.

Seow, A., Shi, C., Franke, A., et al. 1998. Isoflavonoid levels in spot urine are associated with frequency of dietary soy intake in a population-based sample of middle-aged and older Chinese in Singapore. *Cancer Epidemiol Biomark Prev* **7**: 135.

Shibata, A., Paganini-Hill, A., Ross, R.K., and Henderson, B.E. 1992. Intake of vegetables, fruits, beta-carotene, vitamin C and vitamin supplements and cancer incidence among the elderly: a prospective study. *Br J Cancer* **66**: 673.

Shim, J.S., Kang, M.H., Kim, Y.H., Roh, J.K., Roberts, C., and Lee, I.P. 1995. Chemopreventive effect of green tea (Camellia sinensis) among cigarette smokers. *Cancer Epidemiol Biomarkers Prev* **4**: 387–391.

Sigounas, G., Steiner, M., and Anagnostou, A. 1997. DL-alpha-tocopherol induces apoptosis in erythroleukemia, prostate, and breast cancer cells. *Nutr Cancer* **28**(1): 30.

Silverman, D., Levin, L., and Hoover, R. 1989. Occupational risks of bladder cancer in the United States II. Nonwhite men. *J Natl Cancer Inst* **81**: 1480.

Sporn, M.B., and Newton, D.L. 1979. Chemoprevention of cancer with retinoids. *Fed Proc* **38**(11): 2528–2534.

Steele, V.E., Kelloff, G.J., Balentine, D., Boone, C.W., Mehta, R., Bagheri, D., et al. 2000. Comparative chemopreventive mechanisms of green tea, black tea and selected polyphenol extracts measured by *in vitro* bioassays. *Carcinogenesis* **21**: 63–67.

Steineck, G., Haugman, U., Gerhardsson, M., et al. 1990. Vitamin A supplements, fried foods, fat, and urothelial cancer: a case-referent study in Stockholm in 1985–87. *Int J Cancer* **45**: 1006.

Steinmaus, C.M., Nunez, S., and Smith, A.H. 2000. Diet and bladder cancer: a meta-analysis of six dietary variables. *Am J Epidemiol* **151**(7): 693–702.

Strange, R.C., and Fryer, A.A. 1999. The glutathione S-transferases: influence of polymorphism on cancer susceptibility. *IARC Sci Pub* **148**: 231–249.

Studer, U.E., Jenzer, S., Biedermann, C., Chollet, D., Kraft, R., von Toggenburg, H., and Vonbank, F. 1995. Adjuvant treatment with a vitamin A analogue (etretinate) after transurethral resection of superficial bladder tumors. Final analysis of a prospective, randomized multicenter trial in Switzerland. *Eur Urol* **28**(4): 284.

Su, S., Yeh, T., Lei, H., and Chow, N. 2000. The potential of soybean foods as a chemoprevention approach for human urinary tract cancer. *Clin Cancer Res* **6**: 230.

Talbott, M.C., Miller, L.T., and Kerkvliet, N. 1997. Pyridoxine supplementation: effect on lymphocyte responses in elderly persons. *Am J Clin Nutr* **46**: 659.

Thompson, I.M., Peek, M., and Rodriguez, F.R. 1987. The impact of cigarette smoking on stage, grade and number of recurrences of transitional cell carcinoma of the bladder. *J Urol* **137**: 401–403.

Torrisi, R., Mezzetti, M., Johansson, H., Barreca, A., Pigatto, F., Robertson, C., and Decensi, A. 2000. Time course of fenretinide-induced modulation of circulating insulin-like growth factor (IGF)-I, IGF-II and IGFBP-3 in a bladder cancer chemoprevention trial. *Int J Cancer* **87**(4): 601–605.

Vena, J., Graham, S., Freudenheim, J., Marshall, J., Zielezny, M., Swanson, M., et al. 1993. Diet in the epidemiology of bladder cancer in western New York. *Nutr Cancer* **48**: 191.

Vineis, P., Caporaso, N., Tannenbaum, S.R., Skipper, P.L., Glogowski, J., Bartsch, H., et al. 1990. Acetylation phenotype, carcinogen-hemoglobin adducts, and cigarette smoking. *Cancer Res* **50**: 3002–3004.

Weindruch, R. 1992. Effect of caloric restriction on age associated cancers. *Exp Gerontol* **27**: 575.

Weisberger, A.S., and Pensky, J. 1958. Tumor inhibition by a sulfhydryl-blocking agent related to an active principle of garlic (*Allium sativum*). *Cancer Res* **18**: 1301–1308.

World Cancer Research Fund. 1997. "Food, Nutrition and the Prevention of Cancer: A Global Perspective." American Institute for Cancer Research, Washington, D.C.

Wynder, E.L., and Goldsmith, R. 1977. The epidemiology of bladder cancer: a second look. *Cancer* **40**: 1246–1268.

Xu, G.P., Song, P.J., and Reed, P.I. 1993. Effects of fruit juices, processed vegetable juice, orange peel and green tea on endogenous formation of N-nitrosoproline in subjects from a high-risk area for gastric cancer in Moping County, China. *Eur J Cancer Prev* **2**: 327–335.

You, W.C., Blot, W.J., Chang, Y.S., Ershow, A., Yang, Z.T., An, Q., Henderson, B.E., Fraumeni, J.F., Jr., and Wang, T.G. 1989. Allium vegetables and reduced risk of stomach cancer. *J Natl Cancer Inst* **81**: 162–164.

Zang, E.A., and Wynder, E.L. 1996. Differences in lung cancer risk between men and women: examination of the evidence. *J Natl Cancer Inst* **88**: 183–192.

Zhao, H., Grossman, H., Spitz, M., Lerner, S., Zhang, K, and Wu, X. 2003. Plasma levels of insulin-like-growth-factor 1 and binding protein 3 and their association with bladder cancer risk. *J Urol* **169**: 714.

Zhou, J., Mukherjee, P., and Gugger, E., et al. 1998. Inhibition of murine bladder tumorigenesis by soy isoflavones via alterations in the cell cycle, apoptosis, and angiogenesis. *Cancer Res* **58**: 5231.

CHAPTER

27

Differentiation Induction in Leukemia and Lymphoma

SVEN DE VOS AND H. PHILLIP KOEFFLER

INTRODUCTION

Leukemia can be divided into four major subtypes: lymphoid and myeloid, each of which can be either chronic or acute. The median age at diagnosis of patients with chronic lymphocytic leukemia (CLL) is 60–65 years, with a steadily increasing incidence with age. Individuals with this disease often survive in excess of 7–10 years. CLL is characterized by a clonal expansion of mature, long-lived, and functionally defective lymphocytes. Acute lymphocytic leukemia (ALL) is the most common leukemia in children. With aggressive chemotherapy, long-term disease-free survival (DFS) rates of 70–75% are possible. In contrast, ALL is less common and less curable in adults. Only 20% of all adult acute leukemias are ALL, and the 5-year survival rates reach only 25–35%. Chronic myelocytic leukemia (CML) is a clonal stem cell disorder characterized by a balanced translocation between the long arms of chromosome 9 and 22 (t[9;22], known as Philadelphia chromosome). CML is very rare in children; the median age at presentation is 50–60 years. The medium survival is 5–7 years. Initially the myeloid cells are expanded in number but mature correctly. However, toward the end of the disease, additional chromosomal changes besides the Philadelphia chromosome occur and the leukemia evolves into blast crisis, which is nearly impossible to cure. Acute myelogenous leukemias (AMLs) occur at all ages. The World Health Organization (WHO) classification (WHO) distinguishes (a) AMLs with recurrent cytogenetic translocations, (b) AMLs with multilineage dysplasia, (c) therapy-related AML, (d) AMLs not otherwise characterized, and (e) biphenotypic leukemias that display features of ALL and AML. Chromosomal abnormalities are the most important prognostic factors in patients with newly diagnosed AML. The best outcomes occur in patients with acute promyelocytic leukemia (APL) harboring the t(15;17) translocation. Overall, long-term survival or cure rates vary between 20 and 40%.

Myelodysplastic syndrome (MDS) is characterized by peripheral blood cytopenias, and a bone marrow (BM) that shows ineffective hematopoiesis. Karyotypic and genetic marker data indicate that MDS results from a preneoplastic transformation at a pluripotent stem cell level (Koeffler, 1996). The MDS clone has a selective growth advantage over the normal stem cells compartment, perhaps in part mediated by a maturational block. The mechanism of this maturational block is unknown. Treatment of MDS has long been frustrating for the physician. Although it represents a preleukemic state in some patients, therapy with standard antileukemic chemotherapy is excessively toxic. Cytokines, transfusions, and antibiotics for infections have been the mainstays of patient management. Theoretically the use of differentiation therapy to induce normal maturation of the aberrant clone of cells is an interesting approach (Koeffler 1983). The goal of this therapy is not to eliminate the dysplastic clone of cells but to induce the defective hematopoietic progenitors to acquire more normal maturational and functional characteristics. Differentiation therapy attempts to improve the ability of the abnormal progenitors to produce functional blood cells.

The WHO classifies lymphomas as either B-cell neoplasms, T/NK-cell neoplasms, or Hodgkin's lymphoma. The classification and further subdivisions are based on the integration of morphological, immunophenotypic, genetic, and clinical features. Low-grade lymphomas are frequently responsive to a variety of treatments but remain fairly resistant to cure. Still, patients usually achieve long survival

Copyright © 2006, Elsevier Inc.
All rights of reproduction in any form reserved.

times. Patients with high-grade lymphomas are potentially curable with aggressive chemotherapy regimens including high-dose chemotherapy with peripheral stem cell transplantation. Today, most patients with Hodgkin's lymphoma can expect to be cured with combination chemotherapy regimen. The current emphasis in clinical research is to maintain this treatment success with less long-term toxicities.

No clear association exists between nutrition and the development of leukemias and lymphomas. Occasionally, some nutritional deficiencies can be confused with either preleukemia or leukemia. For example, individuals with severe vitamin B12 or folate deficiency display BM abnormalities that resemble a preleukemia or erythroleukemia. These individuals respond dramatically to replacement therapy with vitamin B12 or folate and do not have an increased incidence of leukemias or lymphomas. However, evidence points to a possible role of folate deficiency in the development of childhood or adult ALL. Considerable epidemiological evidence suggests that a low folate intake confers a higher risk of several types of cancers (Ames and Wakimoto, 2002). A polymorphism (C677T) in the gene encoding methylene-THF reductase (MTHFR) reduces its enzymatic function resulting in decreased uracil incorporation and increased occurrence of chromosome breaks (Ames and Wakimoto, 2002). Both adult (Skibola et al., 1999) and childhood ALL (Wiemels et al., 2001) have an inverse relationship with the C677T homozygous MTHFR-TT genotype, suggesting that folate deficiency might promote ALL. Pan et al. (2004), in line with earlier publications, has observed an increased risk of cancer associated with obesity, including non-Hodgkin's lymphoma (Wolk et al., 2001), leukemia (Moller et al., 1994), and multiple myeloma (Friedman et al., 1994). The mechanistic link between obesity and these hematological malignancies remains elusive, although speculations point to impaired immune responses (Stallone, 1994; Chandra, 1997) and lower intake of antioxidants and nutrients (Hotzel, 1986).

RETINOIDS

Mechanism of Action

Retinoids are a family of molecules important for many biological processes such as embryonal morphogenesis, epidermal cell growth, and hematopoiesis *in vivo* and *in vitro*. The natural retinoids, 9-cis-retinoic acid (RA), 13-cis-RA (cRA), and their genomic isomer, all-trans-RA (ATRA), constitute a group of structurally similar compounds with diverse profiles of pharmacokinetics, therapeutic, and adverse effects.

Retinoids affect the transcription of various genes critical to cellular proliferation and differentiation. Upon entering the cell, retinoids must be transported to the nucleus to exert their effect. The cellular responses to RA are mediated by two families of transcription factors, which include the RA receptors (RARs) and the retinoid X receptors (RXRs). ATRA crosses the cell membrane by passive diffusion. It can be bound by cellular RA-binding protein (CRABP) and degraded by cytochrome P450 (CYP) enzymes in the endoplasmic reticulum. Only unbound ATRA or its isomers enter the cell nucleus and bind to RARs or to RXRs. After dimerization (homodimer or heterodimer), these RA-activated receptors bind with high affinity to specific DNA segments (RA response elements) and effect the transcription of messenger RNA of target genes. Binding of retinoids to these receptors increases the DNA-binding affinity of other nuclear receptors including vitamin D receptor (VDR), thyroid hormone receptor (THR), and peroxisome proliferation-activating receptor (PPAR). Each of these nuclear receptors has its own specific ligand (Mangelsdorf et al., 1990). Each retinoid receptor superfamily consists of several receptor isoforms: RARα (Petkovich et al., 1987), RARβ (Brand et al., 1988), RARγ (Krust et al., 1989), and RXRα,β,γ (Mangelsdorf et al., 1992). RARs and RXRs act as transacting enhancer factors and modulate transcription of target genes by binding as either heterodimers (RAR/RXR) or homodimers (RAR/RAR and RXR/RXR) to RA-responsive elements (RAREs). The consensus DNA sequences recognized by RAR are represented by a tandem repeat of the sequence AGGTCA separated by five nucleotides (Umesono et al., 1991). In contrast, the consensus sequences recognized by RXR consist of the same tandem repeats separated by only one nucleotide (Mangelsdorf et al., 1991).

Retinoids and Hematopoiesis

Selective vitamin A deprivation induces anemia in humans and rats that is reversible by readministering retinol (Hodges et al., 1978; Mejia et al., 1979). Progenitor cells capable of giving rise to erythroid colonies in the presence of erythropoietin are termed *erythroid burst-forming units* (BFUs-E). The addition of 10^{-8} to 10^{-7}M of either ATRA, 13-cRA, or 9-cRA to BM cells or peripheral blood cells in methylcellulose cultures containing erythropoietin increases BFU-E formation (Douer and Koeffler, 1982a,b; Sakashita et al., 1993). Retinoids have a similar effect on myeloid colony formation. Bone marrow mononuclear cells contain a population of committed progenitors termed *granulocyte-monocyte colony-forming units* (GM-CFUs), which are capable of producing myeloid colonies *in vitro* in the presence of colony-stimulating factors (CSFs). Colony formation by GM-CFU in methylcellulose or soft agar containing CFUs is enhanced by either ATRA, 13-cRA, or 9-cRA (10^{-8} to 10^{-7}M) (Douer and Koeffler, 1982a,b; Sakashita et al., 1993).

Retinoids and Leukemia Cells

Cultured in the presence of retinoids, the late myeloid-promyelocytic cell lines HL-60 and NB4 are induced to differentiate down the granulocytic pathway (Breitman et al., 1980; Lanotte et al., 1991). A dose-dependent increase in HL-60 differentiation is observed with exposure to ATRA concentrations between 10^{-9} and 10^{-6}M. The monoblastic cell lines THP-1 and U937 are induced to undergo monocytic differentiation by retinoids (Olsson et al., 1984; Hemmi and Breitman, 1985). This process is accompanied by the progressive loss of proliferative capacity. On the other hand, the myeloblastic cell lines KG1 and KG1a and many fresh leukemia samples are growth inhibited but not induced to differentiate when exposed to RA (Douer and Koeffler, 1982a,b). The erythroid cell line HEL undergoes differentiation with RA and is growth inhibited (Suedhoff et al., 1990), whereas the K562 cell line is not affected by retinoids but differentiates down the erythroid pathway when cultured with hemin and butyrate (Miller et al., 1984).

Fresh cells from 21 patients with either acute myelocytic leukemia (AML) or chronic myelogenous leukemia (CML) in blast crisis were incubated in the presence of ATRA (10^{-6}M) for 5–7 days (Breitman et al., 1981). Differentiation was seen only in cells obtained from two patients with APL. A subsequent study confirmed the differentiating activity of RA on cells from APL patients (Honma et al., 1983) (Figure 1).

Therefore, retinoid concentrations capable of enhancing the proliferation of normal myeloid progenitors inhibit the clonal growth of myeloid leukemia cell lines. Retinoid-induced leukemia cell differentiation is invariably accompanied by loss of proliferative capacity, whereas growth inhibition need not be attended by morphological or functional changes.

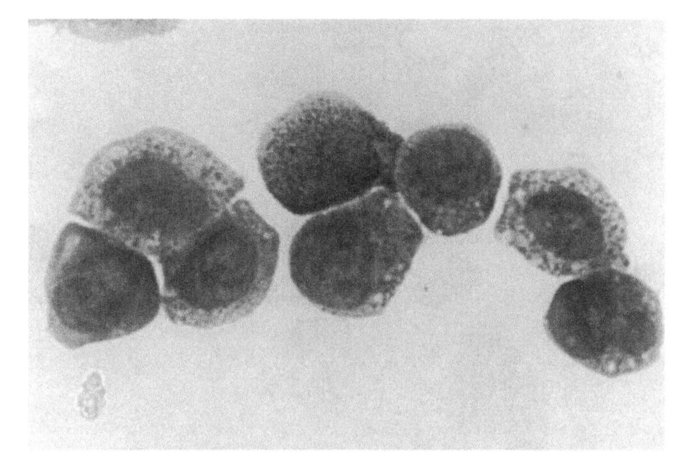

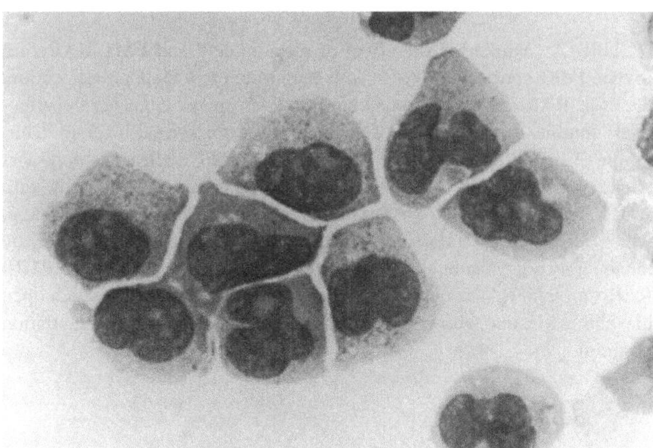

FIGURE 1 **Morphological changes of acute promyelocytic leukemia cells treated with all-trans-RA.** Cells were cultured for 7 days in (A) culture medium and (B) culture medium containing 10^{-7}M all-trans-RA. Control cells (A) demonstrate prominent azurophilic granules, and a fine nuclear chromatin pattern. All-trans-RA–treated cells (B) show loss of primary granules and appearance of secondary granulation, nuclear condensation and segmentation.

Retinoid Therapy of Acute Promyelocytic Leukemia

Mechanism of Action in APL

The leukemia cells from almost all APL patients possess the reciprocal translocation t(15;17). The gene on chromosome 17 that is disrupted by this rearrangement encodes RARα (Borrow et al., 1990). The translocation eliminates the promoter region and exon 1 of RARα and fuses the remainder of the gene to the PML gene present on chromosome 15 (de The et al., 1991). The fusion gene encodes a chimeric protein that retains the RARα domain capable of binding the retinoid ligand and the DNA. The resulting PML-RARα fusion protein is present in all APL patients with the reciprocal translocation t(15;17) and likely contributes to the pathogenesis of the disease. This concept is supported by studies showing that artificial expression of the PML-RARα fusion protein in myelocytic or erythrocytic leukemic cell lines blocks differentiation induced by vitamin D3 (VD3), VD3 and transforming growth factor-1 (TGF-1) in combination, or hemin (Grignani et al., 1993, 1995). Furthermore, the ability of the PML-RARα product to transform chicken hematopoietic progenitor cells *in vitro* and to induce acute leukemias further demonstrates its oncogenic potential (Altabef et al., 1996). The PML-RARα protein suppresses transcription of RARE-containing genes to a greater degree than RARα protein in the absence of ligand (Kakizuka et al., 1991). The transcriptional repression by PML-RARα can be attributed to the recruitment of nuclear co-repressors that inhibits transactivation from RARα target genes through recruitment of molecules sin3, Dnmt1, and Dnmt3a (Di Croce et al., 2002), and histone deacetylases (HDs) (Grignani et al., 1998; He et al., 1998; Lin et al., 1998). HDs deacetylate histones and keep the DNA in a state inaccessible for the transcription machinery, effectively shutting down the expression of genes needed for further

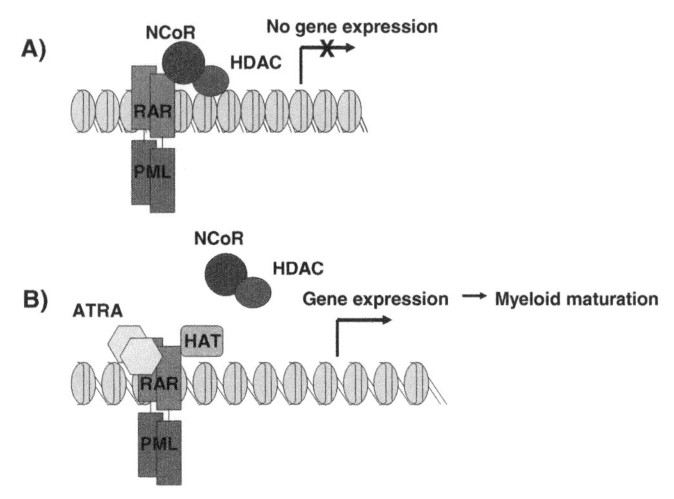

FIGURE 2 **Model for the effect of retinoic acid and PML-RARα on myeloid differentiation.** (A) In cells harboring the t(15;17) translocation, the PML-RARα chimeric protein binds to RA response elements and effectively inhibits the expression of genes required for normal myeloid maturation. This is facilitated by the recruitment of nuclear corepressors (NCoRs) and histone deacetylases (HDs). (B) When treating cells with ATRA, ATRA binds to the RARα part of the PML-RARα chimeric protein, which results in the release of the transcriptional repressor complex by inducing a conformational change of RARα and degradation of the PML-RARα protein. RARα now attracts histone acetylases (HATs), which open the chromatin and allow the expression of the myeloid differentiation program.

maturation of promyelocytes. ATRA binds to RARα of the PML-RARα chimeric protein and induces a conformational change that releases the nuclear co-repressor and HDs. Consequently, the differentiation program is expressed again leading to the rapid and simultaneous maturation of the promyelocytes (Figure 2).

PML-RARα also plays a role in the induction of differentiation and maturation of leukemic cells by RA. Immunohistochemical studies of PML and PML-RARα show that they co-localize in an APL-specific microparticulate structure, whereas in normal cells, PML displays a punctuate pattern (POD) (Dyck et al., 1994). Treatment with RA reconstitutes the normal POD pattern in APL cells, suggesting that deranged PML function may also play a role in the pathophysiology of APL. These data show that retinoids induce APL cells to mature by reversing the oncogenic properties of PML-RARα. An additional mechanism by which retinoids induce differentiation of APL cells involves retinoid-induced degradation of PML-RARα, and thus releasing the suppressive activity of PML-RARα (Raelson et al., 1996).

Clinical Trials

APL (M3 in the French-American-British (FAB) classification) (Bennett et al., 1985) is characterized as a proliferation of cells blocked at the promyelocytic differentiation stage and is complicated in its clinical course by disseminated intravascular coagulation (DIC). PML-RARα is the central leukemia-inducing lesion in APL and is directly targeted by ATRA and by arsenic, both compounds able to induce complete remissions by overcoming the differentiation block. In rare cases, the translocation fuses other partners rather than the PML gene with the RARα gene, namely promyelocytic leukemia zinc-finger gene (PLZF), nucleophosmin (NMP), nuclear mitotic apparatus (NUMA), and STAT5b (Melnick and Licht, 1999). Usually, these alternative chimeric–protein expressing leukemias are insensitive to differentiation therapy with ATRA. Unique to APL compared with other AML subtypes is the occurrence of life-threatening DIC (Barbui and Falanga, 2001) and the achievement of complete remissions (CRs) in ~90% of patients treated with ATRA (Degos and Wang, 2001) or 75–90% of patients treated with low-dose arsenic trioxide (Lengfelder et al., 2003). Although APL is very sensitive to chemotherapy, in early clinical experience, 10–20% of the patients died of fatal hemorrhage resulting from DIC (Bauer and Rosenberg, 1984).

Treatment with oral 13-cRA (100 mg/m^2/day) for various durations resulted in either clinical improvement (Flynn et al., 1983) or CR in APL patients (Fontana et al., 1986). The first trial of ATRA for APL patients was reported from China (Huang et al., 1988). Twenty-four APL patients were treated with ATRA (45–100 mg/m^2/day). Of these, eight cases had been resistant to prior chemotherapy; the other 16 cases were previously untreated. All but one patient achieved a CR with 20–119 days of continuous treatment. During the course of therapy, DIC either disappeared rapidly or was not observed after the onset of treatment. All but six complete responders received various types of consolidation chemotherapy. In spite of this, eight patients relapsed after 2–5 months of remission.

Two subsequent studies have confirmed the promising result of the initial Chinese trial. A French center treated 22 APL patients with ATRA (45 mg/m^2/day) for 90 days (Castaigne et al., 1990). Fourteen patients (including patients in relapse) had a complete response in 30–90 days after starting therapy, four patients had a transient response, one patient had no response, and three patients died <2 weeks after RA treatment. Whether maintenance treatment consisted of low-dose chemotherapy or ATRA, early relapses were observed. An American trial reported that 9 of the 11 APL patients treated with ATRA (45 mg/m^2/day) entered a CR (Warrell et al., 1991).

One small study (Chomienne et al., 1989) compared the efficacy of 13-cRA and ATRA in four APL patients. Two patients received 13-cRA, and two were given ATRA at the same dose (45 mg/m^2/day) for 30 days. Only the patients receiving the ATRA responded and achieved CR. Although both ATRA and 13-cRA at 10^{-6} M induce differentiation of

TABLE 1 Comparison between All-trans-RA Followed by Intensive Chemotherapy versus Chemotherapy Alone in Newly Diagnosed APL

All-trans-RA followed by chemotherapy			Chemotherapy alone	
Investigators	**No. of patients**	**Results**	**Type of comparison**	**Results**
Fenaux et al., 1994	26	CR rate: 96% EFS: 62% at 4 yr Survival: 77% at 4 yr	Historical (29 cases)	CR rate: 76% EFS: 28% at 4 yr Survival: 40% at 4 yr
Soignet et al., 1997	65	CR rate: 83% Median CR > 40 mo Median survival > 43 mo	Historical (80 cases)	Median CR 14 mo Median survival 17 mo

APL, acute promyelocytic leukemia; CR, complete remission; EFS, event-free survival.

APL cells, only ATRA is effective at 10^{-7}M. A review published in 1993 showed that ATRA was able to induce CR in 84% of 565 APL patients (Warrell et al., 1993). These studies demonstrate a dramatic achievement for differentiation therapy. This therapy has now become the first choice in the treatment of APL. Nevertheless, most patients treated solely with the retinoid relapsed shortly after a complete response is attained and remained unresponsive to reinduction with ATRA. The treatment programs using ATRA for induction followed by several cycles of cytotoxic chemotherapy as consolidation yielded superior overall survival compared with chemotherapy alone (Tables 1).

Clinical results show that the combination of ATRA and cytosine arabinoside (CA) chemotherapy can increase the CR rate to >90%, and patients presenting with high leukocyte counts seem to benefit particularly from this combination therapy (Fenaux and Degos, 1996). ATRA followed by chemotherapy also reduced the incidence of relapse (particularly early relapse) as compared with chemotherapy alone. In a randomized trial of 93 European centers, APL patients with an initial white blood cell (WBC) count <5000/mm^3 were randomized to either ATRA followed by CA or ATRA with CA started on day 3 (Table 2). More relapses occurred in the "ATRA followed by CA" group than in those receiving concurrent ATRA and CA, but no significant differences in the CR rate, event-free survival, and survival between these two groups were observed (Fenaux et al., 1999). However, CA may not be required for induction or consolidation therapy in APL. Two retrospective studies could not demonstrate improved CR rates when CA was added to daunorubicin (Marty et al., 1984; Petti et al., 1987). The PETHEMA trial demonstrated high CR rates in APL patients receiving just ATRA plus idarubicin (Sanz et al., 1999). The standard approach is concomitant ATRA and anthracycline chemotherapy. To prevent early DIC, provided that the initial WBC count is not too high, the ATRA can be given for 2–4 days to induce promyelocyte differentiation before adding chemotherapy. Because some patients still relapse after ATR plus chemotherapy, prognostic factors predisposing to relapse need to be precisely determined. They certainly include persistence or reappearance of the PML-RARs fusion gene. This molecular marker can be conveniently followed using reverse-transcriptase polymerase chain reaction (RT-PCR) (Diverio et al., 1998).

TABLE 2 Prospective Randomized Trials of ATRA in APL

Trial	N	Induction	CR (%)	ED (%)	DFS/EFS 2–3 yr (%)
APL91 (Fenaux	54	ATRA (+Chemo)	97	9	79
et al., 1993)	47	Chemo	81	8	50
APL93 (Fenaux	109	ATRA → Chemo	95	8	75
et al., 1999)	99	ATRA + Chemo	94	7	86
No. Am. Intergroup	172	ATRA	72	11	69
(Tallman et al., 1997)	174	Chemo	69	14	29
MRC (Burnett et al., 1999)	119	ATRA 95d) → Chemo	70	23	59
	120	ATRA + Chemo	87	12	78

APL, acute promyelocytic leukemia; DFS, disease-free survival; MRC, Medical Research Council; CR, complete remission; ED, early death; EFS, event-free survival.

Usually, patients receive at least two courses of anthracycline-based consolidation chemotherapy. Further, two randomized prospective trials showed the benefit of maintenance therapy with ATRA. A North American Intergroup study reported a 5-year DFS rate of 74% in patients who received ATRA during both the induction and the maintenance phase (Tallman et al., 1997). The European APL93 trial reported lowest relapse rates in patients who received a combination of ATRA and 6-mercaptopurine/methotrexate for maintenance (Fenaux et al., 1999).

Retinoic Acid Side Effects in APL

In this form of treatment, leukemic cells undergo terminal differentiation and lose the capacity to proliferate. The clinical response to ATRA includes an increase in the number of abnormal neutrophils, which is caused by the maturation of leukemic cells during the induction of remission. This beneficial effect can usually be achieved with low morbidity and only mild side effects, such as dryness of the skin and mucosa, bone pain, or elevated liver enzymes, but some patients have had adverse events from the rapid development of hyperleukocytosis, called *RA syndrome* (Chen et al., 1991). RA syndrome presents with fever, respiratory distress, pleural or pericardial effusions, peripheral edema, hypotension, and sometimes renal failure. It is a major cause of early death in ATRA treatment for APL patients and has been reported to cause a 15–30% mortality rate in those patients who develop the syndrome (Frankel et al., 1992). These serious complications of the RA syndrome have been almost entirely eliminated with the institution of a short course of high-dose corticosteroids with the first suggestive signs or symptoms (Vahdat et al., 1994). Another approach is either to add chemotherapy at the onset of ATRA treatment when the patients present with high WBC counts or to give the chemotherapy if the WBC count increases at the initiation of ATRA (Fenaux et al., 1993; Ohno 1994).

Resistance to Retinoids

Despite an excellent initial response, APL cells develop resistance to RA and relapses occur in APL patients treated with RA alone. Several mechanisms for this acquired ATRA resistance have been postulated, including accelerated *in vivo* clearance of ATRA (Muindi et al., 1992) and increased levels of cellular RA-binding protein (CRABP) (Delva et al., 1993). However, cells from a number of RA-resistant patients have been shown to be completely refractory *in vitro* to high concentrations of retinoids, including 9-cRA that does not bind CRABP well (Miller et al., 1995).

Another mechanism for acquired ATRA resistance includes additional genetic mechanisms, such as mutations of the nuclear retinoid receptors, as previously found in embryonal carcinoma (Pratt et al., 1990). RA-resistant HL-60 subclones have been reported with mutations in the ligand-binding domain of RARα (Robertson et al., 1992). The mutant RARα gene may be either homozygous or coexpressed with the wild-type RARα, thus displaying a dominant negative activity. Also, a point mutation could result in a protein that is unable to form RXR-RARα heterodimers, does not bind to retinoid response elements, and thus might not inhibit transcription as a dominant negative factor (Dore and Momparler, 1996). In the RA-resistant NB4 promyelocytic subclone, RA resistance is caused by a point mutation found in the PML-RARα fusion gene, not in the RARα gene (Shao et al., 1997). This mutation mediates a retinoid-independent dominant negative inhibition of the coexpressed wild-type RARα.

In rare cases, the translocation fuses other partners than the PML gene with the RARα gene, namely PLZF (Chen et al., 1993a,b), nucleophosmin (NMP), nuclear mitotic apparatus (NUMA), and STAT5b (Melnick and Licht, 1999). Usually, these alternative chimeric protein expressing leukemias are insensitive to differentiation therapy with ATRA. APL cells harboring a t(11;17) causing a PLZF-RARα fusion protein are morphologically indistinguishable from APL caused by PML-RARα, but in contrast they are usually unresponsive to retinoids. PLZF-RARα has a retinoid-independent corepressor-binding domain in the amino terminus (poxvirus and zinc-finger [POZ] domain) of PLZF, which may be the cause for retinoid resistance of these APL cells both *in vivo* and *in vitro* (Chen et al., 1993a,b).

Treatment of Relapsed or ATRA Refractory-APL

Continuing the success of Chinese ancient medicine in APL, arsenic trioxide is the treatment of choice for patients with relapsed or ATRA-refractory disease (Zhu et al., 2002). Studies from China and two confirmatory studies demonstrated high CR rates in this difficult patient population (Zhang et al., 1996; Soignet et al., 1998, 2001; Niu et al., 1999).

New Retinoids and Combination Therapy

Although ATRA therapy induces a high CR rate in patients with APL, these CRs are only short lived and most patients subsequently relapse and develop RA-resistant leukemia. Therefore, the establishment of new therapies for patients with ATRA-resistant APL is an important clinical goal. A natural ligand of RXRs, 9-cRA, has since been identified (Heyman et al., 1992). RXRs are known to act as cofactors for RARs and vitamin D, thyroid hormone, and PPARs (Mangelsdorf et al., 1990). Unlike ATRA, which binds RARs but not RXRs, 9-cRA can bind and activate both receptor families. In fact, the DNA-binding affinity of RAR/RXR heterodimers is markedly increased relative to homodimers of either receptor (Zhang et al., 1992). In early studies with HL-60 leukemia cells, 9-cRA proved more potent than ATRA in inducing myeloid differentiation (Kizaki et al., 1993; Sakashita et al., 1993). Seven patients with APL who had previously relapsed from a remission induced by ATRA were treated with 9-cRA at daily oral doses ranging from 30 to 220 mg/m^2 (Miller et al., 1995). Only one of the seven patients achieved CR, corroborating *in vitro* studies of blasts from three of the nonresponders that showed a relatively equivalent degree of resistance to both

ATRA and 9-cRA. Thus, 9-cRA probably does not offer much therapeutic advantage over ATRA.

The efficacy of a new synthetic retinoid, Am80 (4[(5,6,7,8-tetrahydro-5,5,8,8-tetramethyl-2-naphthalenyl) carbamoyl]benzoic acid), was tested in a prospective multicenter study in APL patients who had relapsed from CR induced by ATRA (Tobita et al., 1997). Am80 is ~10 times more potent than ATRA as an *in vitro* inducer of differentiation in NB4 and HL-60 cells. It is chemically more stable to light, heat, and oxidation than ATRA, has low affinity for CRABP, and does not bind to RARγ (Hashimoto et al., 1995). Therefore, Am80 might have therapeutic effectiveness in patients with ATRA-resistant APL with increased CRABP and may have fewer adverse drug reactions related to RARγ, which is the major RAR in the dermal epithelium (Zelent et al., 1989). Tobita et al. (1997) treated patients with Am80 (6 mg/m^2/day) orally alone until CR was achieved. Of 24 evaluable patients, 14 (58%) achieved CR between 20 and 58 days after the start of therapy. The clinical response was fairly well correlated with the *in vitro* response to 10^{-8} M Am80. Adverse events included RA syndrome, hyperleukocytosis, xerosis, cheilitis, hypertriglyceridemia, and hypercholesterolemia, but these side effects were generally milder than those of individuals receiving ATRA, which all patients had received previously (Tobita et al., 1997). In an update on this study, durable CRs exceeding 4 years in selected patients have been reported (Shinjo et al., 2000). No clinical trial data have been reported to date combining Am80 with chemotherapy in patients with APL.

RETINOID THERAPY OF MYELODYSPLASTIC SYNDROME

MDSs are a heterogeneous group of clonal hematopoietic disorders characterized by alterations in cell maturation in the BM that lead to abnormalities in the peripheral blood, such as anemia, thrombocytopenia, and granulocytopenia. MDS has also been called "preleukemia" as a subset of MDS evolves into acute myeloid leukemia. The main treatment of MDS has been to provide supportive care with blood transfusions and antibiotics for infections. Chemotherapy, BM transplantation, hormone therapy, and differentiating agents have been tried (Cheson, 1990). For this latter approach, retinoids have been administered in an attempt to overcome the phenotypic block in differentiation of the dysplastic clone.

In many trials, 13-cRA has been used for treatment of MDS, but complete or partial response to the drug has been described only in a small percentage of patients with no prolongation of overall survival. In the first trial, 17 MDS patients were treated with 13-cRA (20–125 mg/m^2/day) for a minimum of 7 weeks, and 5 of the 15 evaluable patients showed an improvement of at least one hematological parameter after 3 weeks of treatment (Gold et al., 1983). In a multicenter study, a double-blind randomized trial of 68 patients who were assigned to either 13-cRA 100 mg/m^2/day or placebo for 6 months, the drug dose was relatively high and not well tolerated, which led to the discontinuation of the treatment in a number of cases (Koeffler et al., 1988). Nevertheless, no significant differences in leukemic transformation, hematological response, or disease progression were noted between the two groups. Another large trial treated 66 transfusion-dependent MDS patients with 13-cRA alone (21 patients) or 13-cRA combined with α-tocopherol (45 patients); the latter drug was added to reduce skin toxicity (Besa et al., 1990). Of the first 21 patients, four responded to 13-cRA, but because of considerable toxicity, discontinuation of the treatment occurred frequently. In the second group, the addition of α-tocopherol improved the tolerability of the drug at higher doses (median 98 vs 60 mg/m^2/day), allowing a prolonged duration of treatment. However, no significant difference in treatment outcome was observed between the two groups. Taken together, these studies suggest that although 13-cRA might have a moderate effect for 20–30% of MDS patients, it requires long-term treatment and only selected patients with nonaggressive disease might benefit.

In vitro studies have shown that the combination of agents that operate through disparate cellular pathways may enhance differentiation in an additive or synergistic fashion. In a phase II study, 14 MDS patients were treated with a combination of 13-cRA (60 mg/m^2/day) and low-dose CA (5 mg/m^2/12 h subcutaneously) for 14 days. Only one partial response was obtained, indicating that this combined therapy did not produce better results than either agent used alone (Ho et al., 1987). In contrast, a multicenter study reported that 9 of 18 MDS patients treated with interferon-α (IFN-α) (3 3 10^6 U/day) combined with RA and vitamin D had a partial clinical response, suggesting that IFN-α might potentiate the effect of other differentiating agents (Hellstrom et al., 1988).

Despite the success obtained with ATRA as a differentiating agent in APL, the results obtained in MDS have been unsatisfactory. In a multicenter prospective study, 12 patients were treated with ATRA at 45 mg/m^2/day for a minimum of 4 weeks (Ohno, 1994). Three patients (two RAEB and one RAEB-T) had a partial response with an increase of their granulocyte counts; however, their response was not durable, lasting <5 weeks despite the continuation of ATRA treatment. In another study, two patients with preleukemia (refractory anemia with excess blasts) were treated with ATRA for 8–10 weeks, and an improvement of hematological parameters was observed in both patients after 2 weeks of therapy, indicating that a prolonged administration period is not necessary for a response (Visani et al., 1992). Thirty-nine MDS patients were treated with ATRA at doses of 10, 25, 50, 100, 150, and 200 mg/m^2/day for 8 weeks, including at least three patients in each group (Kurzrock et al., 1993). The maximum tolerated dose was 150 mg/m^2/day. Of 29 evaluable patients, only 1 patient who received 150 mg/m^2/day showed an improvement of platelet and neutrophil counts but remained red blood cell transfusion dependent; however, the response lasted only 5 months.

In vitro studies on leukemia cell lines have shown an induction of differentiation with the combination of retinoids and growth factors. Therefore, 15 MDS patients were treated with ATRA (45 mg/m^2/day) for 12 weeks combined with granulocyte-CSF (G-CSF) (5 mg/kg/day) for 8 weeks of therapy (Ganser et al., 1989, 1994). A bilineage response was observed with an increase in platelet and neutrophil counts in three patients. Platelet counts were elevated only during the first half of the G-CSF treatment (Ganser et al., 1994). In 1995, the same group published the results of two studies on 18 MDS patients: The first used ATRA plus G-CSF (Study 1), and the second administered ATRA plus G-CSF/erythropoietin/tocopherol (Study 2). In both studies, the investigators observed an increase in the absolute neutrophil count in 95% of patients, although an improvement of the other hematological parameters and decreased requirement of RBC transfusion were observed in 40% of patients (Maurer et al., 1995). In addition, this group reported that ATRA, IFN-α, and G-CSF as combination therapy in 17 patients with low-risk MDS was effective in about six patients (35%) and induced CR in a single case (Hofmann et al., 1999).

ADULT T-CELL LEUKEMIA AND RETINOIDS

Adult T-cell leukemia (ATL) is a malignancy of mature T cells that is associated with human T lymphotropic virus type 2 (HTLV-2) (Hinuma et al., 1981). The interleukin-2 receptor (IL-2R, p55, CD25, also known as *Tac*) is overexpressed on these leukemic cells (Depper et al., 1984; Uchiyama et al., 1985). Incubation of HTLV-2–positive T-cell lines for 48 hours with either 13-cRA or ATRA resulted in marked inhibition of cell growth and in downregulation of CD25 expression (Miyatake and Maeda, 1997). RA produced neither growth inhibition nor downregulation of CD25 in the HTLV-2–negative T-cell lines or in normal lymphocytes. According to a single case report, ATRA treatment of a chemotherapy-resistant acute ATL patient resulted in a clinical remission (Toshima et al., 2000). In a 2004 report, N-(4-hydroxyphenyl)-retinamide (HPR), a synthetic retinoid, induced growth arrest and apoptosis in HTLV-1–transformed cells, whereas no effect was observed on resting or activated normal lymphocytes. These results suggest that retinoids may have a potential role in developing novel therapies for patients with ATL (Darwiche et al., 2004).

CUTANEOUS T-CELL LYMPHOMA AND RETINOIDS

Bexarotene (Targretin), or LGD1069 (4-{1-(3,5,5,8,8-pentamethyl-5,6,7,8-tetrahydro-2-naphthyl)ethenyl}benzoic acid), is a synthetic compound that bears little resemblance to the natural retinoids, except in its isoprene backbone. It was identified as a highly selective RXR (RXRα, RXRβ, RXRγ) agonist with low affinity for RARs. RXRs can form heterodimers with various receptor partners such as RARs, VDR, thyroid receptor, and PPARs. Once activated, these receptors function as transcription factors that regulate the expression of genes that control cellular differentiation and proliferation. The exact mechanism of action of bexarotene in the treatment of cutaneous T-cell lymphoma (CTCL) is unknown. Interestingly, the compound directly induced apoptosis in a variety of *in vivo* and *in vitro* models, especially human tumor xenografts of head and neck carcinomas; however, it had no differentiation effects on human leukemic promyelocytes (Mehta et al., 1996). Fifty-two patients including nine with T-cell lymphoma received LGD1069 administered orally once daily at doses ranging from 5 to 500 mg/m^2 for 1 to 41 weeks (Miller et al., 1997). Two of nine patients with cutaneous T-cell lymphoma had a major improvement by day 29. The durations of these responses were 3.5 and 4.5 months, respectively.

Bexarotene was evaluated in 152 patients with advanced and early-stage cutaneous T-cell lymphoma (CTCL) in two multicenter, open-label, historically controlled clinical studies conducted in the United States, Canada, Europe, and Australia. At the initial dose of 300 mg/m^2/day, 1 (1.6%) of 62 patients had a complete clinical tumor response and 19 patients (30%) had a partial tumor response. The rate of relapse in the 20 patients who had a tumor response was 6 (30%) over a median duration of observation of 21 weeks, and the median duration of tumor response had not been reached. Responses were seen as early as 4 weeks, and new responses continued to be seen at later visits (Duvic et al., 2001). In summary, Bexarotene is indicated for the treatment of cutaneous manifestations of cutaneous T-cell lymphoma in patients who are refractory to at least one prior systemic therapy.

Because bexarotene has little BM toxicity, it is an excellent candidate for combination therapy with other modalities useful in the treatment of cutaneous T-cell lymphoma.

1,25-DIHYDROXYVITAMIN D_3

Mechanism of Action

The active metabolite of VD3, choleciferol (25-hydroxycholecalciferol 1,25-dihydroxycholecalciferol), is capable of regulating many genes that are critical for development and cell differentiation. The VDR belongs to the superfamily of steroid-thyroid receptors; it mediates the action of its ligand 1,25$(OH)_2D_3$ and regulates gene transcription by binding to specific vitamin D–responsive elements (VDREs) as a heterodimer with RXR (Pike 1985; Carlberg et al., 1993).

1,25$(OH)_2D_3$ and Hematopoiesis

Normal human BM committed stem cells cultured in soft agar with 1,25$(OH)_2D_3$ (10^{-7}M) or liquid culture with 1,25$(OH)_2D_3$ (5×10^{-9}M for 5 days) and monocytes cultured in serum-free medium with 1,25$(OH)_2D_3$ (10^{-8}M for 7 days) differentiate into macrophages (Koeffler et al., 1984). Furthermore, the terminal differentiation of monocytes into mature macrophages can be obtained *in vitro* by culturing these cells in the presence of serum or in a serum-free medium with addition of VD3 compounds (Choudhuri et al., 1990).

1,25$(OH)_2D_3$ appears to be able to regulate many lymphokines. 1,25$(OH)_2D_3$ is able to inhibit IL-2 synthesis and the proliferation of peripheral blood lymphocytes (Lemire et al., 1985). The expression of GM-CSF is regulated by 1,25$(OH)_2D_3$ through cellular VDR by a process independent of IL-2 production (Tobler et al., 1987).

1,25$(OH)_2D_3$ and Leukemia Cells

The role of 1,25$(OH)_2D_3$ in cell differentiation was first described in the murine leukemia cell line M1, which was induced to differentiate into more mature cells by 1,25$(OH)_2D_3$ (Abe et al., 1981). 1,25$(OH)_2D_3$ and related VD3 compounds have a similar potent effect on inducing differentiation and inhibiting proliferation of several acute myeloid leukemia cell lines such as HL-60, U937, THP-1, HEL, and NB4. In contrast, more immature myeloid leukemia cell lines such as HL-60 blasts, KG1, KG1a, and K562 do not respond to the metabolites. HL-60 cells treated with 1,25$(OH)_2D_3$ acquire the morphology and functional characteristics of macrophages, which contrasts with the granulocytic differentiation induced by retinoids. They become adherent to charged surfaces, develop pseudopodia, stain positively for nonspecific esterase (NSE) with a reduction of nitroblue tetrazolium test (NBT), and acquire the ability to phagocytose yeast during incubation with 1,25$(OH)_2D_3$ (10^{-10} to 10^{-7}M for 7 days) (Mangelsdorf et al., 1984). The proliferation of HL-60 cells is also inhibited by 1,25$(OH)_2D_3$; in fact, colony formation in soft agar is reduced by 50% (ED_{50}) in the presence of $\sim 10^{-9}$M 1,25$(OH)_2D_3$ (Munker et al., 1986). Cells of other leukemia cell lines are also inhibited in their clonal growth, such as U937, HEL, THP-1, and M1 after exposure to 1,25$(OH)_2D_3$ with ED_{50} in the range of 4×10^{-9}M to 3×10^{-8}M (Munker et al., 1986).

Because of the potential toxicity of 1,25$(OH)_2D_3$ at the concentrations required *in vivo*, various attempts have been made to combine 1,25$(OH)_2D_3$ with another compound that might act synergistically for an antileukemic effect capable of promoting cell differentiation with an acceptable toxicity. VD3 compounds may cooperate with other differentiating agents such as retinoids, TPA, and IFNs. For example, 1,25$(OH)_2D_3$ can potentiate IFN to induce the expression of CD11b and CD14. Also, the combination of 1,25$(OH)_2D_3$ and either ATRA or 9-cRA can enhance the terminal differentiation process of HL-60 cells down the monocyte/macrophage pathway (Elstner et al., 1996). These findings have also been demonstrated by other investigators (Brown et al., 1994). Cells cultured in the presence of the combination of 1,25$(OH)_2D_3$ and ATRA developed atypically, having a neutrophilic morphology, but in other properties were typical of monocytes including expression of CD14 and sodium fluoride–inhibited NSE (Elstner et al., 1996).

Leukemic cells from AML patients respond to VD3 compounds when cultured *in vitro*; however, they are often less sensitive than the cell lines. They are still able to undergo monocytic differentiation assessed by NBT reduction, morphology, and phagocytic ability, and their clonal growth is often inhibited, but all of these are blunted compared with 1,25$(OH)_2D_3$–sensitive cell lines (Koeffler et al., 1984).

1,25$(OH)_2D_3$ and Therapy of MDS

A number approaches to differentiation therapy have been attempted or contemplated including the use of a secosteroid such as a retinoid or 1.25$(OH)_2$-vitamin D_3 (1,25$[OH]_2D_3$). Although ATRA and 9-cRA therapy has worked exceedingly well for APL, which has the PML/RAR_ fusion gene, they have not been helpful in MDS (Koeffler et al., 1988; Ganser et al., 1994, 1996; Hofmann et al., 1999). Although 1,25$(OH)_2D_3$ appears to work well in AML cell lines (Abe et al., 1981; Tanaka et al., 1982; Mangelsdorf et al., 1984), clinical investigations in MDS show only limited activity (Mehta et al., 1984; Koeffler et al., 1985; Richard et al., 1986; Motomura et al., 1991).

Previously, we treated 18 MDS patients with increasing doses of 1,25$(OH)_2D_3$, up to a maximum of 2 μg/day for 12 weeks. Nine patients developed hypercalcemia, which was the dose-limiting toxicity. The clinical responses were transitory in nature. These lackluster results of orally administered 1,25$(OH)_2$-vitamin D3 to MDS patients may have occurred because plasma concentrations of the secosteroid that were required for the observed activity *in vitro* could not be achieved *in vivo* without concomitant hypercalcemia (Koeffler et al., 1985). Therefore, research activities have been redirected at finding new 1,25$(OH)_2D_3$ analogs with a more favorable therapeutic index, that is to say, a compound with potent increased ability to induce differentiation without causing hypercalcemia (Zhou et al., 1990; Jung et al., 1994; Asou et al., 1998; Kubota et al., 1998; Hisatake et al., 1999; Shiohara et al., 2001).

In another clinical study, 30 MDS patients were divided into two different groups. One group received 1α-OH-vitamin D_3 at 4–6 mg/day and another group received placebo; the patients were treated for a median of 17 weeks (Motomura et al., 1991). An improvement of hematological parameters was detected in only one patient, but the authors felt that the treated group had a greater proportion of patients who did not progress to leukemia as compared with the control group. Hypercalcemia and increased serum creatinine were observed in two patients, but these toxicities disappeared with dose reductions. A case has been reported of an individual with chronic myelomonocytic leukemia (subtype of MDS) who achieved a CR with 25-OH-vitamin D3 therapy for 15 months, and this remission was sustained for 15 months after the end of the treatment (Mellibovsky et al., 1993). These results were surprising because 25-OH-vitamin D3 has less activity than 1α-OH-vitamin D3 and has only little antileukemic activity *in vitro*.

Combination differentiating therapy for MDS was studied in an Italian phase II trial. Fifty-three MDS patients were treated with a low-dose combination of cRA (20–40 mg/day) and cholecalciferol or calcifediol (25-hydroxycholecalciferol 1,25-dihydroxycholecalciferol) (1–1.5 micrograms/day) ± intermittent 6-thioguanine (30 mg/m^2/day). The latter was reserved for patients with BM blast excess (≥5%). The treatment was well tolerated, without major toxicity. Among 25 patients with BM blasts <5%, the population not receiving additional 6-thioguanine, one complete, eight partial, and four minor responses were observed, with a total response rate of 52% and a median response duration of 8 months. A reduction in the transfusion need was observed in 53% of those patients without blast excess (Ferrero et al., 1996).

Another trial of vitamin D in low- to intermediate-risk MDS evaluated 19 patients. Seven had refractory anemia with ringed sideroblasts, five had refractory anemia, one had refractory anemia with excess of blasts, and six had chronic myelomonocytic leukemia. Responders were defined as a granulocyte or platelet count increased by 50% or hemoglobin increase of 1.5 g/dl or a decrease of transfusion requirements by 50%. The first five patients received 266 μg of calcifediol three times a week, and the other 14 received calcitriol (1,25-dihydroxycholecalciferol) (0.25–0.75 μg/day). Responses were observed in 11 patients. In the calcifediol-treated group, one case responded, three were nonresponders, and one showed progression. In the calcitriol group, 10 were responders (two with major response) and four were nonresponders. No hypercalcemia was observed (Mellibovsky et al., 1998).

The vitamin D analog 19-nor-1,25(OH)$_2$-vitamin D_2 (paricalcitol, Zemplar) was approved by the Food and Drug Administration (FDA) for the treatment of secondary hyperparathyroidism. This compound has very little calcemic potential, as shown by several controlled randomized clinical trials (Llach et al., 1998; Martin et al., 1998). Antiproliferative *in vitro* effects of 19-nor-1,25(OH)$_2$D$_2$ were reported against human AML and prostate cancer cells (Chen et al., 2000; Kumagai et al., 2003). We found that this compound was probably 10–1,000 fold more potent in inducing differentiation and inhibiting proliferation of leukemic cells *in vitro* and had at least 10-fold less ability to cause hypercalcemia *in vivo* than 1,25(OH)$_2$-D$_3$ (Kumagai et al., 2003). Since paricalcitol had this activity on myeloid leukemic cells, it possibly could be of use in MDS, a disease characterized by a block in cell maturation. Therefore, we initiated a small clinical trial of oral paricalcitol to 12 MDS patients whose disease varied between an IPSS of low to high. Therapy began at 8 μg/day (q.d.) and increased at 2-week intervals until serum calcium was slightly above normal level, at which point dose was decreased by 4–8 μg q.d. The dose of paricalcitol varied between 8 μg every other day (q.o.d.) and 54 μg q.d (average 16 μg q.d.). The drug was well tolerated in all patients. Two of the twelve individuals had a clinical response. One patient's platelet counts rose from 50,000 to 120,000/μl blood over 5 weeks; however, the patient succumbed to a fatal fungal infection. The second patient responded by a decrease in RBC transfusions associated with a rise in his hemoglobin, which lasted for ~5 months. Eventually, his hemoglobin began to fall, and erythropoietin therapy was substituted for paricalcitol. In summary, high doses of paricalcitol were well tolerated in all patients. Two individuals had a partial clinical response. In general, paricalcitol given as a single agent to MDS patients is not therapeutically very efficacious; further trials of the vitamin D analog should be considered in combination with other approaches.

New Vitamin D Analogs

Calcipotriol (MC903) has a cyclopropyl group at the end of the side chain formed by the fusion of the 26th and 27th carbons, a hydroxyl group at carbon 24, and a double bond at carbon 22. Exposure of the transformed diffuse large B-cell lymphoma cell lines SU-DUL4 and SU-DUL5, carrying the t(14;18), to MC903, resulted in an inhibition of proliferation only at high concentrations of the compound (10^{-7} M) (Hickish et al., 1993). At the same time, it was 100-fold less active than 1,25(OH)$_2$D$_3$ at inducing hypercalcemia and mobilizing bone calcium in rats (Rebel et al., 1992).

1,25(OH)$_2$-16ene-23yne-D3 is four times more potent than 1,25(OH)$_2$D$_3$ in blocking HL-60 clonal growth (Pakkala et al., 1995). An ATRA-resistant HL-60 clone was >20-fold more sensitive to inhibition of proliferation by 1,25(OH)$_2$-16ene-23yne-D$_3$ than by 1,25(OH)$_2$D$_3$. In addition, the induction of differentiation of these cells by

$1,25(OH)_2$-16ene-23yne-D_3 was much more pronounced in these cells compared with wild-type HL-60 cells (Pakkala et al., 1995). This compound administered to vitamin D–deficient chicken is ~30 times less active than $1,25(OH)_2D_3$ in stimulating intestinal calcium absorption and ~50 times less effective in inducing bone calcium mobilization (Brown et al., 1994). A synergistic antineoplastic effect of this compound combined with ATRA has been shown in HL-60 cells (Dore et al., 1993). Furthermore, in a murine leukemia model, the administration of $1,25(OH)_2$-16ene-23yne-D_3 eliminated the leukemia in ~30–40% of animals (Zhou et al., 1990).

Another analog is $1,25(OH)_2$-16ene-D_3, which is >1000-fold more active than $1,25(OH)_2D_3$ in inhibiting clonal growth of HL-60 cells and 5-fold more potent in inducing their differentiation (Jung et al., 1994). This compound has a high binding affinity for VDR and has ~50-fold lower affinity for the D-binding proteins present in serum, therefore increasing the availability of this compound to target tissues. However, the ability of this compound to induce hypercalcemia in mice was comparable with that of $1,25(OH)_2D_3$ (Jung et al., 1994).

A study suggested that $1,25(OH)_2$-20-epi-D_3 is an exceedingly potent VD3 compound at inhibiting the clonal growth of HL-60 cells and inducing cell differentiation. In fact, it is ~2600-fold more potent than $1,25(OH)_2D_3$ in suppressing the clonal growth of HL-60 cells and ~5000-fold more active than $1,25(OH)_2D_3$ in preventing clonal growth of fresh human leukemic myeloid cells (Elstner et al., 1994). The $1,25(OH)_2$-20-epi-D_3 exerts its effects by binding directly to VDR. Furthermore, this compound was a powerful inhibitor of an HTLV-transformed T-cell line that expresses VDR.

KH1060 is a potent VD3 20-epi analog with an oxygen at carbon 22 of the side chain, and three additional carbons are present on the side chain. It is ~14,000-fold more potent than $1,25(OH)_2D_3$ in inhibiting the clonal growth of U937 (Pakkala et al., 1995). However, the analog has the same hypercalcemic activity and the same receptor-binding affinity as $1,25(OH)_2D_3$. Additional *in vivo* studies should help define its clinical potential.

VITAMIN K

Physiologically, the natural K vitamins (phylloquinone [vitamin K_1], menaquinone [vitamin K_2]) are known to act as cofactors for γ-carboxylation of selected glutamates at the N-terminus of prothrombin and other vitamin K–dependent coagulation factors (Suttie 1985; Buitenhuis et al., 1990). Surprisingly, vitamin K2 and its derivatives showed a strong leukemic cell-killing effect, and when combined with ATRA, they resulted in enhancement of the apoptosis-inducing effect of APL cells (Yaguchi et al., 1997). These observations deserve further studies.

ASCORBIC ACID

Ascorbic acid (vitamin C) has been suggested to be a protective agent against development of cancer and a therapeutic agent against cancer. An initial *in vitro* study using primary acute nonlymphocytic leukemia (ANLL) cells from patients suggested that growth of leukemic cells may be inhibited by ascorbic acid (Park et al., 1980a,b). This prompted a larger *in vitro* study of 163 ANLL samples. In 53 samples (33%), the leukemic colony formation was increased and in 28 cases (17%) suppressed by L-ascorbic acid (0.3 mM) (Park, 1985). No colony growth stimulation of 34 normal bone marrow samples in response to L-ascorbic acid was observed. It decreased the growth of two T-cell lymphocyte cell lines (M4 and C7) in a time- and dosage-dependent manner, but a myeloma cell line (CLL 155) was unaffected by the presence of 0.1% ascorbic acid (Kao et al., 1993). Taken together, the *in vitro* studies suggest that ascorbic acid does not have a clearly defined effect on leukemia cell growth and determining which cases will be stimulated and which will be inhibited requires further study.

FUTURE PERSPECTIVE

What is the future of differentiation therapy? Clearly, the therapeutic breakthrough of retinoids in APL has raised the hope to replicate the successful story of differentiation therapy in other hematological malignancies. Unfortunately, over the past 20 years, we have learned that the abnormal cells from most MDS and AML patients rarely undergo terminal differentiation either *in vitro* or *in vivo* with "differentiation-inducing agents." Gleevec is an active drug in CML because it targets the defining genetic lesion of CML, the BCR/ABL tyrosine kinase. RA works as a differentiation agent in APL because it is the ligand for the defining genetic abnormality, the fusion gene PML/RARα. We have to elucidate the aberrant pathways causing MDS, AML, and lymphoma in order to devise target-specific therapies. Having these "roadmaps," we can find ways to reverse the abnormality or manipulate genes that are downstream of the genetic alteration. These novel pathways then may or may not include differentiation-inducing strategies. A cancer cell often has several aberrant complementary pathways, including those that provide self-sufficiency in growth signals, insensitivity to antigrowth signals, limitless replicative potential, and ability to evade apoptosis, as well as the capacity for tissue invasion and sustained angiogenesis (Hanahan and Weinberg, 2000). Corrections of any one of these abnormal pathways may either partially or completely reverse the growth advantage of the transformed cells as compared with their normal counterparts. However, the simultaneous attack of several aberrant pathways should have enhanced potency, for example, a compound that inhibits an inappropriately expressed kinase and another agent that stimulates either the apoptotic or the differentiation pathway may be more effective than either alone. Likely, the most efficacious therapies will simultaneously attack several abnormal pathways in the malignant cells.

Acknowledgments

Dr. Koeffler acknowledges support by the National Institutes of Health, U.S. Army Grants, Parker Hughes Trust, the Tom Collier Fund, and the Sheryl & David Weissberg Trust. He holds the Mark Goodson Endowed Chair of Oncology Research. Both Drs. De Vos and Koeffler thank the generous support of the Lymphoma Research Foundation (LRF).

References

Abe, E., Miyaura, C., Sakagami, H., Takeda, M., Konno, K., Yamazaki, T., Yoshiki, S., and Suda, T. 1981. Differentiation of mouse myeloid leukemia cells induced by 1 alpha,25-dihydroxyvitamin D3. *Proc Natl Acad Sci USA* **78**(8): 4990–4994.

Altabef, M., Garcia, M., Lavau, C., Bae, S.C., Dejean, A., and Samarut, J. 1996. A retrovirus carrying the promyelocyte-retinoic acid receptor PML-RARalpha fusion gene transforms haematopoietic progenitors *in vitro* and induces acute leukaemias. *EMBO J* **15**(11): 2707–2716.

Ames, B.N., and Wakimoto, P. 2002. Are vitamin and mineral deficiencies a major cancer risk? *Nat Rev Cancer* **2**(9): 694–704.

Asou, H., Koike, M., Elstner, E., Cambell, M., Le, J., Uskokovic, M.R., Kamada, N., and Koeffler, H.P. 1998. 19-nor vitamin-D analogs: a new class of potent inhibitors of proliferation and inducers of differentiation of human myeloid leukemia cell lines. *Blood* **92**(7): 2441–2449.

Barbui, T., and Falanga, A. 2001. Disseminated intravascular coagulation in acute leukemia. *Semin Thromb Hemost* **27**(6): 593–604.

Bauer, K.A., and Rosenberg, R.D. 1984. Thrombin generation in acute promyelocytic leukemia. *Blood* **64**(4): 791–776.

Bennett, J.M., Catovsky, D., Daniel, M.T., Flandrin, G., Galton, D.A., Gralnick, H.R., and Sultan, C. 1985. Criteria for the diagnosis of acute leukemia of megakaryocyte lineage (M7). A report of the French-American-British Cooperative Group. *Ann Intern Med* **103**(3): 460–462.

Besa, E.C., Abrahm, J.L., Bartholomew, M.J., Hyzinski, M., and Nowell, P.C. 1990. Treatment with 13-cis-retinoic acid in transfusion-dependent patients with myelodysplastic syndrome and decreased toxicity with addition of alpha-tocopherol. *Am J Med* **89**(6): 739–747.

Borrow, J., Goddard, A.D., Sheer, D., and Solomon, E. 1990. Molecular analysis of acute promyelocytic leukemia breakpoint cluster region on chromosome 17. *Science* **249**(4976): 1577–1580.

Brand, N., Petkovich, M., Krust, A., Chambon, P., de The, H., Marchio, A., Tiollais, P., and Dejean, A. 1988. Identification of a second human retinoic acid receptor. *Nature* **332**(6167): 850–853.

Breitman, T.R., Collins, S.J., and Keene, B.R. 1981. Terminal differentiation of human promyelocytic leukemic cells in primary culture in response to retinoic acid. *Blood* **57**(6): 1000–1004.

Breitman, T.R., Selonick, S.E., and Collins, S.J. 1980. Induction of differentiation of the human promyelocytic leukemia cell line (HL-60) by retinoic acid. *Proc Natl Acad Sci USA* **77**(5): 2936–2940.

Brown, A.J., Dusso, A., and Slatopolsky, E. 1994. Selective vitamin D analogs and their therapeutic applications. *Semin Nephrol* **14**(2): z156–174.

Brown, G., Bunce, C.M., Rowlands, D.C., and Williams, G.R. 1994. All-trans retinoic acid and 1 alpha,25-dihydroxyvitamin D3 co-operate to promote differentiation of the human promyeloid leukemia cell line HL60 to monocytes. *Leukemia* **8**(5): 806–815.

Buitenhuis, H.C., Soute, B.A., and Vermeer, C. 1990. Comparison of the vitamins K1, K2 and K3 as cofactors for the hepatic vitamin K–dependent carboxylase. *Biochim Biophys Acta* **1034**(2): 170–175.

Burnett, A.K., Grimwade, D., Solomon, E., Wheatley, K., and Goldstone, A.H. 1999. Presenting white blood cell count and kinetics of molecular remission predict prognosis in acute promyelocytic leukemia treated with all-trans retinoic acid: result of the Randomized MRC Trial. *Blood* **93**(12): 4131–4143.

Carlberg, C., Bendik, I., Wyss, A., Meier, E., Sturzenbecker, L.J., Grippo, J.F., and Hunziker, W. 1993. Two nuclear signalling pathways for vitamin D. *Nature* **361**(6413): 657–660.

Castaigne, S., Chomienne, C., Daniel, M.T., Ballerini, P., Berger, R., Fenaux, P., and Degos, L. 1990. All-trans retinoic acid as a differentiation therapy for acute promyelocytic leukemia.I. Clinical results. *Blood* **76**(9): 1704–1709.

Chandra, R.K. 1997. Nutrition and the immune system: an introduction. *Am J Clin Nutr* **66**(2): 460S–463S.

Chen, Z., Brand, N.J., Chen, A., Chen, S.J., Tong, J.H., Wang, Z.Y., Waxman, S., and Zelent, A. 1993a. Fusion between a novel Kruppel-like zinc finger gene and the retinoic acid receptor-alpha locus due to a variant t(11;17) translocation associated with acute promyelocytic leukaemia. *EMBO J* **12**(3): 1161–1167.

Chen, S.J., Zelent, A., Tong, J.H., Yu, H.Q., Wang, Z.Y., Derre, J., Berger, R., Waxman, S., and Chen, Z. 1993b. Rearrangements of the retinoic acid receptor alpha and promyelocytic leukemia zinc finger genes resulting from t(11;17)(q23;q21) in a patient with acute promyelocytic leukemia. *J Clin Invest* **91**(5): 2260–2267.

Chen, T.C., Schwartz, G.G., Burnstein, K.L., Lokeshwar, B.L., and Holick, M.F. 2000. The *in vitro* evaluation of 25-hydroxyvitamin D3 and 19-nor-1alpha,25-dihydroxyvitamin D2 as therapeutic agents for prostate cancer. *Clin Cancer Res* **6**(3): 901–908.

Chen, Z.X., Xue, Y.Q., Zhang, R., Tao, R.F., Xia, X.M., Li, C., Wang, W., Zu, W.Y., Yao, X.Z., and Ling, B.J. 1991. A clinical and experimental study on all-trans retinoic acid-treated acute promyelocytic leukemia patients. *Blood* **78**(6): 1413–1419.

Cheson, B.D. 1990. The myelodysplastic syndromes: current approaches to therapy. *Ann Intern Med* **112**(12): 932–941.

Chomienne, C., Ballerini, P., Balitrand, N., Amar, M., Bernard, J.F., Boivin, P., Daniel, M.T., Berger, R., Castaigne, S., and Degos, L. 1989. Retinoic acid therapy for promyelocytic leukaemia. *Lancet* **2**(8665): 746–747.

Choudhuri, U., Adams, J.A., Byrom, N., McCarthy, D.M., and Barrett, J. 1990. 1,25-Dihydroxyvitamin D3 induces normal mononuclear blood cells to differentiate in the direction of monocyte-macrophages. *Haematologia (Budap)* **23**(1): 9–19.

Darwiche, N., Hatoum, A., Dbaibo, G., Kadara, H., Nasr, R., Abou-Lteif, G., Bazzi, R., Hermine, O., de The, H., and Bazarbachi, A. 2004. N-(4-hydroxyphenyl)retinamide induces growth arrest and apoptosis in HTLV-I–transformed cells. *Leukemia* **18**(3): 607–615.

de The, H., Lavau, C., Marchio, A., Chomienne, C., Degos, L., and Dejean, A. 1991. The PML-RAR alpha fusion mRNA generated by the t(15;17) translocation in acute promyelocytic leukemia encodes a functionally altered RAR. *Cell* **66**(4): 675–684.

Degos, L., and Wang, Z.Y. 2001. All trans retinoic acid in acute promyelocytic leukemia. *Oncogene* **20**(49): 7140–7145.

Delva, L., Cornic, M., Balitrand, N., Guidez, F., Miclea, J.M., Delmer, A., Teillet, F., Fenaux, P., Castaigne, S., Degos, L., et al. 1993. Resistance to all-trans retinoic acid (ATRA) therapy in relapsing acute promyelocytic leukemia: study of *in vitro* ATRA sensitivity and cellular retinoic acid binding protein levels in leukemic cells. *Blood* **82**(7): 2175–2181.

Depper, J.M., Leonard, W.J., Kronke, M., Waldmann, T.A., and Greene, W.C. 1984. Augmented T cell growth factor receptor expression in HTLV-1–infected human leukemic T cells. *J Immunol* **133**(4): 1691–1695.

Di Croce, L., Raker, V.A., Corsaro, M., Fazi, F., Fanelli, M., Faretta, M., Fuks, F., Lo Coco, F., Kouzarides, T., Nervi, C., Minucci, S., and

Pelicci, P.G. 2002. Methyltransferase recruitment and DNA hypermethylation of target promoters by an oncogenic transcription factor. *Science* **295**(5557): 1079–1082.

Diverio, D., Rossi, V., Avvisati, G., De Santis, S., Pistilli, A., Pane, F., Saglio, G., Martinelli, G., Petti, M.C., Santoro, A., Pelicci, P.G., Mandelli, F., Biondi, A., and Lo Coco, F. 1998. Early detection of relapse by prospective reverse transcriptase-polymerase chain reaction analysis of the PML/RARalpha fusion gene in patients with acute promyelocytic leukemia enrolled in the GIMEMA-AIEOP multicenter AIDA trial. GIMEMA-AIEOP Multicenter AIDA Trial. *Blood* **92**(3): 784–789.

Dore, B.T., and Momparler, R.L. 1996. Mutation in the ligand-binding domain of the retinoic acid receptor alpha in HL-60 leukemic cells resistant to retinoic acid and with increased sensitivity to vitamin D3 analogs. *Leuk Res* **20**(9): 761–769.

Dore, B.T., Uskokovic, M.R., and Momparler, R.L. 1993. Interaction of retinoic acid and vitamin D3 analogs on HL-60 myeloid leukemic cells. *Leuk Res* **17**(9): 749–757.

Douer, D., and Koeffler, H.P. 1982a. Retinoic acid. Inhibition of the clonal growth of human myeloid leukemia cells. *J Clin Invest* **69**(2): 277–283.

Douer, D., and Koeffler, H.P. 1982b. Retinoic acid enhances growth of human early erythroid progenitor cells *in vitro*. *J Clin Invest* **69**(4): 1039–1041.

Duvic, M., Martin, A.G., Kim, Y., Olsen, E., Wood, G.S., Crowley, C.A., and Yocum, R.C. 2001. Phase 2 and 3 clinical trial of oral bexarotene (Targretin capsules) for the treatment of refractory or persistent early-stage cutaneous T-cell lymphoma. *Arch Dermatol* **137**(5): 581–593.

Dyck, J.A., Maul, G.G., Miller, W.H., Jr., Chen, J.D., Kakizuka, A., and Evans, R.M. 1994. A novel macromolecular structure is a target of the promyelocyte-retinoic acid receptor oncoprotein. *Cell* **76**(2): 333–343.

Elstner, E., Lee, Y.Y., Hashiya, M., Pakkala, S., Binderup, L., Norman, A.W., Okamura, W.H., and Koeffler, H.P. 1994. 1 alpha,25-Dihydroxy-20-epi-vitamin D3: an extraordinarily potent inhibitor of leukemic cell growth *in vitro*. *Blood* **84**(6): 1960–1967.

Elstner, E., Linker-Israeli, M., Umiel, T., Le, J., Grillier, I., Said, J., Shintaku, I.P., Krajewski, S., Reed, J.C., Binderup, L., and Koeffler, H.P. 1996. Combination of a potent 20-epi-vitamin D3 analogue (KH 1060) with 9-cis-retinoic acid irreversibly inhibits clonal growth, decreases bcl-2 expression, and induces apoptosis in HL-60 leukemic cells. *Cancer Res* **56**(15): 3570–3576.

Fenaux, P., Chastang, C., Chevret, S., Sanz, M., Dombret, H., Archimbaud, E., Fey, M., Rayon, C., Huguet, F., Sotto, J.J., Gardin, C., Makhoul, P.C., Travade, P., Solary, E., Fegueux, N., Bordessoule, D., Miguel, J.S., Link, H., Desablens, B., Stamatoullas, A., Deconinck, E., Maloisel, F., Castaigne, S., Preudhomme, C., and Degos, L. 1999. A randomized comparison of all transretinoic acid (ATRA) followed by chemotherapy and ATRA plus chemotherapy and the role of maintenance therapy in newly diagnosed acute promyelocytic leukemia. The European APL Group. *Blood* **94**(4): 1192–1200.

Fenaux, P., and Degos, L. 1996. Treatment of acute promyelocytic leukaemia. *Baillieres Clin Haematol* **9**(1): 107–128.

Fenaux, P., Le Deley, M.C., Castaigne, S., Archimbaud, E., Chomienne, C., Link, H., Guerci, A., Duarte, M., Daniel, M.T., Bowen, D., et al. 1993. Effect of all transretinoic acid in newly diagnosed acute promyelocytic leukemia. Results of a multicenter randomized trial. European APL 91 Group. *Blood* **82**(11): 3241–3249.

Fenaux, P., Wattel, E., Archimbaud, E., Sanz, M., Hecquet, B., Fegueux, N., Guerci, A., Link, H., Fey, M., Castaigne, S., et al. 1994. Prolonged follow-up confirms that all-trans retinoic acid followed by chemotherapy reduces the risk of relapse in newly diagnosed acute promyelocytic leukemia. The French APL Group. *Blood* **84**(2): 666–667.

Ferrero, D., Bruno, B., Pregno, P., Stefani, S., Larizza, E., Ciravegna, G., Luraschi, A., Vietti-Ramus, G., Schinco, P., Bazzan, M., Gallo, E., and Pileri, A. 1996. Combined differentiating therapy for myelodysplastic syndromes: a phase II study. *Leuk Res* **20**(10): 867–876.

Flynn, P.J., Miller, W.J., Weisdorf, D.J., Arthur, D.C., Brunning, R., and Branda, R.F. 1983. Retinoic acid treatment of acute promyelocytic leukemia: *in vitro* and *in vivo* observations. *Blood* **62**(6): 1211–1217.

Fontana, J.A., Rogers, J.S., 2nd, and Durham, J.P. 1986. The role of 13 cis-retinoic acid in the remission induction of a patient with acute promyelocytic leukemia. *Cancer* **57**(2): 209–217.

Frankel, S.R., Eardley, A., Lauwers, G., Weiss, M., and Warrell, R.P., Jr. 1992. The retinoic acid syndrome in acute promyelocytic leukemia. *Ann Intern Med* **117**(4): 292–296.

Friedman, G.D., and Herrinton, L.J. 1994. Obesity and multiple myeloma. *Cancer Causes Control* **5**(5): 479–483.

Ganser, A., Maurer, A., Contzen, C., Seipelt, G., Ottmann, O.G., Schadeck-Gressel, C., Kolbe, K., Haas, R., Zander, C., Reutzel R., and Hoelzer, D. 1996. Improved multilineage response of hematopoiesis in patients with myelodysplastic syndromes to a combination therapy with all-trans-retinoic acid, granulocyte colony-stimulating factor, erythropoietin and alpha-tocopherol. *Ann Hematol* **72**(4): 237–244.

Ganser, A., Seipelt, G., Verbeek, W., Ottmann, O.G., Maurer, A., Kolbe, K., Hess, U., Elsner, S., Reutzel, R., Wormann, B., et al. 1994. Effect of combination therapy with all-trans-retinoic acid and recombinant human granulocyte colony-stimulating factor in patients with myelodysplastic syndromes. *Leukemia* **8**(3): 369–375.

Ganser, A., Volkers, B., Greher, J., Ottmann, O.G., Walther, F., Becher, R., Bergmann, L., Schulz, G., and Hoelzer, D. 1989. Recombinant human granulocyte-macrophage colony-stimulating factor in patients with myelodysplastic syndromes—a phase I/II trial. *Blood* **73**(1): 31–37.

Gold, E.J., Mertelsmann, R.H., Itri, L.M., Gee, T., Arlin, Z., Kempin, S., Clarkson, B., and Moore, M.A. 1983. Phase I clinical trial of 13-cis-retinoic acid in myelodysplastic syndromes. *Cancer Treat Rep* **67**(11): 981–986.

Grignani, F., De Matteis, S., Nervi, C., Tomassoni, L., Gelmetti, V., Cioce, M., Fanelli, M., Ruthardt, M., Ferrara, F.F., Zamir, I., Seiser, C., Lazar, M.A., Minucci, S., and Pelicci, P.G. 1998. Fusion proteins of the retinoic acid receptor-alpha recruit histone deacetylase in promyelocytic leukaemia. *Nature* **391**(6669): 815–818.

Grignani, F., Ferrucci, P.F., Testa, U., Talamo, G., Fagioli, M., Alcalay, M., Mencarelli, A., Peschle, C., Nicoletti, I., et al. 1993. The acute promyelocytic leukemia–specific PML-RAR alpha fusion protein inhibits differentiation and promotes survival of myeloid precursor cells. *Cell* **74**(3): 423–431.

Grignani, F., Testa, U., Fagioli, M., Barberi, T., Masciulli, R., Mariani, G., Peschle, C., and Pelicci, P.G. 1995. Promyelocytic leukemia–specific PML-retinoic acid alpha receptor fusion protein interferes with erythroid differentiation of human erythroleukemia K562 cells. *Cancer Res* **55**(2): 440–443.

Hanahan, D., and Weinberg, R.A. 2000. The hallmarks of cancer. *Cell* **100**(1): 57–70.

Hashimoto, Y., Kagechika, H., Kawachi, E., Fukasawa, H., Saito, G., and Shudo, K. 1995. Correlation of differentiation-inducing activity of retinoids on human leukemia cell lines HL-60 and NB4. *J Cancer Res Clin Oncol* **121**(11): 696–698.

He, L.Z., Guidez, F., Tribioli, C., Peruzzi, D., Ruthardt, M., Zelent, A., and Pandolfi, P.P. 1998. Distinct interactions of PML-RARalpha and PLZF-RARalpha with co-repressors determine differential responses to RA in APL. *Nat Genet* **18**(2): 126–135.

Hellstrom, E., Robert, K.H., Gahrton, G., Mellstedt, H., Lindemalm, C., Einhorn, S., Bjorkholm, M., Grimfors, G., Uden, A.M., Samuelsson, J., et al. 1988. Therapeutic effects of low-dose cytosine arabinoside, alpha-interferon, 1 alpha-hydroxyvitamin D3 and retinoic acid in acute leukemia and myelodysplastic syndromes. *Eur J Haematol* **40**(5): 449–459.

Hemmi, H., and Breitman, T.R. 1985. Induction of functional differentiation of a human monocytic leukemia cell line (THP-1) by retinoic acid and cholera toxin. *Jpn J Cancer Res* **76**(5): 345–351.

Heyman, R.A., Mangelsdorf, D.J., Dyck, J.A., Stein, R.B., Eichele, G., Evans, R.M., and Thaller, C. 1992. 9-cis retinoic acid is a high affinity ligand for the retinoid X receptor. *Cell* **68**(2): 397–406.

Hickish, T., Cunningham, D., Colston, K., Millar, B.C., Sandle, J., Mackay, A.G., Soukop, M., and Sloane, J. 1993. The effect of 1,25-dihydroxyvitamin D3 on lymphoma cell lines and expression of vitamin D receptor in lymphoma. *Br J Cancer* **68**(4): 668–672.

Hinuma, Y., Nagata, K., Hanaoka, M., Nakai, M., Matsumoto, T., Kinoshita, K.I., Shirakawa, S., and Miyoshi, I. 1981. Adult T-cell leukemia: antigen in an ATL cell line and detection of antibodies to the antigen in human sera. *Proc Natl Acad Sci USA* **78**(10): 6476–6480.

Hisatake, J., Kubota, T., Hisatake, Y., Uskokovic, M., Tomoyasu, S., and Koeffler, H.P. 1999. 5,6-trans-16-ene-vitamin D3: a new class of potent inhibitors of proliferation of prostate, breast, and myeloid leukemic cells. *Cancer Res* **59**(16): 4023–4029.

Ho, A.D., Martin, H., Knauf, W., Reichardt, P., Trumper, L., and Hunstein, W. 1987. Combination of low-dose cytarabine and 13-cis retinoic acid in the treatment of myelodysplastic syndromes. *Leuk Res* **11**(11): 1041–1044.

Hodges, R.E., Sauberlich, H.E., Canham, J.E., Wallace, D.L., Rucker, R.B., Mejia, L.A., and Mohanram, M. 1978. Hematopoietic studies in vitamin A deficiency. *Am J Clin Nutr* **31**(5): 876–885.

Hofmann, W.K., Ganser, A., Seipelt, G., Ottmann, O.G., Zander, C., Geissler, G., Hoffmann, K., Hoffken, K., Fischer, J.T., Isele, G., and Hoelzer, D. 1999. Treatment of patients with low-risk myelodysplastic syndromes using a combination of all-trans retinoic acid, interferon alpha, and granulocyte colony-stimulating factor. *Ann Hematol* **78**(3): 125–130.

Honma, Y., Fujita, Y., Kasukabe, T., Hozumi, M., Sampi, K., Sakurai, M., Tsushima, S., and Nomura, H. 1983. Induction of differentiation of human acute non-lymphocytic leukemia cells in primary culture by inducers of differentiation of human myeloid leukemia cell line HL-60. *Eur J Cancer Clin Oncol* **19**(2): 251–261.

Hotzel, D. 1986. Suboptimal nutritional status in obesity (selected nutrients). *Bibl Nutr Dieta* (37): 36–41.

Huang, M.E., Ye, Y.C., Chen, S.R., Chai, J.R., Lu, J.X., Zhoa, L., Gu, L.J., and Wang, Z.Y. 1988. Use of all-trans retinoic acid in the treatment of acute promyelocytic leukemia. *Blood* **72**(2): 567–572.

Jung, S.J., Lee, Y.Y., Pakkala, S., de Vos, S., Elstner, E., Norman, A.W., Green, J., Uskokovic, M., and Koeffler, H.P. 1994. 1,25(OH)2-16ene-vitamin D3 is a potent antileukemic agent with low potential to cause hypercalcemia. *Leuk Res* **18**(6): 453–463.

Kakizuka, A., Miller, W.H., Jr., Umesono, K., Warrell, R.P., Jr., Frankel, S.R., Murty, V.V., Dmitrovsky, E., and Evans, R.M. 1991. Chromosomal translocation t(15;17) in human acute promyelocytic leukemia fuses RAR alpha with a novel putative transcription factor, PML. *Cell* **66**(4): 663–674.

Kao, T.L., Meyer, W.J., 3rd, and Post, J.F. 1993. Inhibitory effects of ascorbic acid on growth of leukemic and lymphoma cell lines. *Cancer Lett* **70**(1–2): 101–106.

Kizaki, M., Ikeda, Y., Tanosaki, R., Nakajima, H., Morikawa, M., Sakashita, A., and Koeffler, H.P. 1993. Effects of novel retinoic acid compound, 9-cis-retinoic acid, on proliferation, differentiation, and expression of retinoic acid receptor-alpha and retinoid X receptor-alpha RNA by HL-60 cells. *Blood* **82**(12): 3592–3599.

Koeffler, H.P. 1983. Induction of differentiation of human acute myelogenous leukemia cells: therapeutic implications. *Blood* **62**(4): 709–721.

Koeffler, H.P. 1996. Myelodysplastic syndromes. *Semin Hematol* **33**(2): 87–94.

Koeffler, H.P., Amatruda, T., Ikekawa, N., Kobayashi, Y., and DeLuca, H.F. 1984. Induction of macrophage differentiation of human normal and leukemic myeloid stem cells by 1,25-dihydroxyvitamin D3 and its fluorinated analogues. *Cancer Res* **44**(12 Pt 1): 5624–5628.

Koeffler, H.P., Heitjan, D., Mertelsmann, R., Kolitz, J.E., Schulman, P., Itri, L., Gunter, P., and Besa, E. 1988. Randomized study of 13-cis retinoic acid v placebo in the myelodysplastic disorders. *Blood* **71**(3): 703–708.

Koeffler, H.P., Hirji, K., and Itri, L. 1985. 1,25-Dihydroxyvitamin D3: *in vivo* and *in vitro* effects on human preleukemic and leukemic cells. *Cancer Treat Rep* **69**(12): 1399–1407.

Krust, A., Kastner, P., Petkovich, M., Zelent, A., and Chambon, P. 1989. A third human retinoic acid receptor, hRAR-gamma. *Proc Natl Acad Sci USA* **86**(14): 5310–5314.

Kubota, T., Koshizuka, K., Koike, M., Uskokovic, M., Miyoshi, I., and Koeffler, H.P. 1998. 19-nor-26,27-bishomo-vitamin D3 analogs: a unique class of potent inhibitors of proliferation of prostate, breast, and hematopoietic cancer cells. *Cancer Res* **58**(15): 3370–3375.

Kumagai, T., O'Kelly, J., Said, J.W., and Koeffler, H.P. 2003. Vitamin D2 analog 19-nor-1,25-dihydroxyvitamin D2: antitumor activity against leukemia, myeloma, and colon cancer cells. *J Natl Cancer Inst* **95**(12): 896–905.

Kurzrock, R., Estey, E., and Talpaz, M. 1993. All-trans retinoic acid: tolerance and biologic effects in myelodysplastic syndrome. *J Clin Oncol* **11**(8): 1489–1495.

Lanotte, M., Martin-Thouvenin, V., Najman, S., Balerini, P., Valensi, F., and Berger, R. 1991. NB4, a maturation inducible cell line with t(15;17) marker isolated from a human acute promyelocytic leukemia (M3). *Blood* **77**(5): 1080–1086.

Lemire, J.M., Adams, J.S., Kermani-Arab, V., Bakke, A.C., Sakai, R., and Jordan, S.C. 1985. 1,25-Dihydroxyvitamin D3 suppresses human T helper/inducer lymphocyte activity *in vitro*. *J Immunol* **134**(5): 3032–3035.

Lengfelder, E., Gnad, U., Buchner, T., and Hehlmann, R. 2003. Treatment of relapsed acute promyelocytic leukemia. *Onkologie* **26**(4): 373–379.

Lin, R.J., Nagy, L., Inoue, S., Shao, W., Miller, W.H., Jr., and Evans, R.M. 1998. Role of the histone deacetylase complex in acute promyelocytic leukaemia. *Nature* **391**(6669): 811–814.

Llach, F., Keshav, G., Goldblat, M.V., Lindberg, J.S., Sadler, R., Delmez, J., Arruda, J., Lau, A., and Slatopolsky, E. 1998. Suppression of parathyroid hormone secretion in hemodialysis patients by a novel vitamin D analogue: 19-nor-1,25-dihydroxyvitamin D2. *Am J Kidney Dis* **32**(2 Suppl 2): S48–S54.

Mangelsdorf, D.J., Borgmeyer, U., Heyman, R.A., Zhou, J.Y., Ong, E.S., Oro, A.E., Kakizuka, A., and Evans, R.M. 1992. Characterization of three RXR genes that mediate the action of 9-cis retinoic acid. *Genes Dev* **6**(3): 329–344.

Mangelsdorf, D.J., Koeffler, H.P., Donaldson, C.A., Pike, J.W., and Haussler, M.R. 1984. 1,25-Dihydroxyvitamin D3-induced differentiation in a human promyelocytic leukemia cell line (HL-60): receptor-mediated maturation to macrophage-like cells. *J Cell Biol* **98**(2): 391–398.

Mangelsdorf, D.J., Ong, E.S., Dyck, J.A., and Evans, R.M. 1990. Nuclear receptor that identifies a novel retinoic acid response pathway. *Nature* **345**(6272): 224–229.

Mangelsdorf, D.J., Umesono, K., Kliewer, S.A., Borgmeyer, U., Ong, E.S., and Evans, R.M. 1991. A direct repeat in the cellular retinol-binding protein type II gene confers differential regulation by RXR and RAR. *Cell* **66**(3): 555–561.

Martin, K.J., Gonzalez, E.A., Gellens, M., Hamm, L.L., Abboud, H., and Lindberg, J. 1998. 19-Nor-1-alpha-25-dihydroxyvitamin D2 (Paricalcitol) safely and effectively reduces the levels of intact parathyroid hormone in patients on hemodialysis. *J Am Soc Nephrol* **9**(8): 1427–1432.

Marty, M., Ganem, G., Fischer, J., Flandrin, G., Berger, R., Schaison, G., Degos, L., and Boiron, M. 1984. [Acute promyelocytic leukemia: retrospective study of 119 patients treated with daunorubicin]. *Nouv Rev Fr Hematol* **26**(6): 371–378.

Maurer, A.B., Ganser, A., Seipelt, G., Ottmann, O.G., Mentzel, U., Geissler, G.R., and Hoelzer, D. 1995. Changes in erythroid progenitor cell and accessory cell compartments in patients with myelodysplastic syndromes during treatment with all-trans retinoic acid and haemopoietic growth factors. *Br J Haematol* **89**(3): 449–456.

Mehta, A.B., Kumaran, T.O., Marsh, G.W., and McCarthy, D.M. 1984. Treatment of advanced myelodysplastic syndrome with alfacalcidol. *Lancet* **2**(8405): 761.

Mehta, K., McQueen, T., Neamati, N., Collins, S., and Andreeff, M. 1996. Activation of retinoid receptors RAR alpha and RXR alpha induces differentiation and apoptosis, respectively, in HL-60 cells. *Cell Growth Differ* **7**(2): 179–186.

Mejia, L.A., Hodges, R.E., and Rucker, R.B. 1979. Clinical signs of anemia in vitamin A–deficient rats. *Am J Clin Nutr* **32**(7): 1439–1444.

Mellibovsky, L., Diez, A., Aubia, J., Nogues, X., Perez-Vila, E., Serrano, S., and Recker, R.R. 1993. Long-standing remission after 25-OH D3 treatment in a case of chronic myelomonocytic leukaemia. *Br J Haematol* **85**(4): 811–812.

Mellibovsky, L., Diez, A., Perez-Vila, E., Serrano, S., Nacher, M., Aubia, J., Supervia, A., and Recker, R.R. 1998. Vitamin D treatment in myelodysplastic syndromes. *Br J Haematol* **100**(3): 516–520.

Melnick, A., and Licht, J.D. 1999. Deconstructing a disease: RARalpha, its fusion partners, and their roles in the pathogenesis of acute promyelocytic leukemia. *Blood* **93**(10): 3167–3215.

Miller, C.W., Young, K., Dumenil, D., Alter, B.P., Schofield, J.M., and Bank, A. 1984. Specific globin mRNAs in human erythroleukemia (K562) cells. *Blood* **63**(1): 195–200.

Miller, V.A., Benedetti, F.M., Rigas, J.R., Verret, A.L., Pfister, D.G., Straus, D., Kris, M.G., Crisp, M., Heyman, R., Loewen, G.R., Truglia, J.A., and Warrell, R.P., Jr. 1997. Initial clinical trial of a selective retinoid X receptor ligand, LGD1069. *J Clin Oncol* **15**(2): 790–795.

Miller, W.H., Jr., Jakubowski, A., Tong, W.P., Miller, V.A., Rigas, J.R., Benedetti, F., Gill, G.M., Truglia, J.A., Ulm, E., Shirley, M., et al. 1995. 9-cis retinoic acid induces complete remission but does not reverse clinically acquired retinoid resistance in acute promyelocytic leukemia. *Blood* **85**(11): 3021–3027.

Miyatake, J.I., and Maeda, Y. 1997. Inhibition of proliferation and CD25 down-regulation by retinoic acid in human adult T cell leukemia cells. *Leukemia* **11**(3): 401–407.

Moller, H., Mellemgaard, A., Lindvig, K., and Olsen, J.H. 1994. Obesity and cancer risk: a Danish record-linkage study. *Eur J Cancer* **30A**(3): 344–350.

Motomura, S., Kanamori, H., Maruta, A., Kodama, F., and Ohkubo, T. 1991. The effect of 1-hydroxyvitamin D3 for prolongation of leukemic transformation-free survival in myelodysplastic syndromes. *Am J Hematol* **38**(1): 67–68.

Muindi, J., Frankel, S.R., Miller, W.H., Jr., Jakubowski, A., Scheinberg, D.A., Young, C.W., Dmitrovsky, E., and Warrell, R.P., Jr. 1992. Continuous treatment with all-trans retinoic acid causes a progressive reduction in plasma drug concentrations: implications for relapse and retinoid resistance in patients with acute promyelocytic leukemia. *Blood* **79**(2): 299–303.

Munker, R., Norman, A., and Koeffler, H.P. 1986. Vitamin D compounds. Effect on clonal proliferation and differentiation of human myeloid cells. *J Clin Invest* **78**(2): 424–430.

Niu, C., Yan, H., Yu, T., Sun, H.P., Liu, J.X., Li, X.S., Wu, W., Zhang, F.Q., Chen, Y., Zhou, L., Li, J.M., Zeng, X.Y., Yang, R.R., Yuan, M.M., Ren, M.Y., Gu, F.Y., Cao, Q., Gu, B.W., Su, X.Y., Chen, G.Q., Xiong, S.M., Zhang, T., Waxman, S., Wang, Z.Y., Chen, S.J., et al. 1999. Studies on treatment of acute promyelocytic leukemia with arsenic trioxide: remission induction, follow-up, and molecular monitoring in 11 newly diagnosed and 47 relapsed acute promyelocytic leukemia patients. *Blood* **94**(10): 3315–3324.

Ohno, R. 1994. Differentiation therapy of myelodysplastic syndromes with retinoic acid. *Leuk Lymphoma* **14**(5–6): 401–409.

Olsson, I.L., Sarngadharan, M.G., Breitman, T.R., and Gallo, R.C. 1984. Isolation and characterization of a T lymphocyte-derived differentiation inducing factor for the myeloid leukemic cell line HL-60. *Blood* **63**(3): 510–517.

Pakkala, S., de Vos, S., Elstner, E., Rude, R.K., Uskokovic, M., Binderup, L., and Koeffler, H.P. 1995. Vitamin D3 analogs: effect on leukemic clonal growth and differentiation, and on serum calcium levels. *Leuk Res* **19**(1): 65–72.

Pan, S.Y., Johnson, K.C., Ugnat, A.M., Wen, S.W., and Mao, Y. 2004. Association of obesity and cancer risk in Canada. *Am J Epidemiol* **159**(3): 259–268.

Park, C.H. 1985. Biological nature of the effect of ascorbic acids on the growth of human leukemic cells. *Cancer Res* **45**(8): 3969–3973.

Park, C.H., Amare, M., Savin, M.A., Goodwin, J.W., Newcomb, M.M., and Hoogstraten, B. 1980a. Prediction of chemotherapy response in human leukemia using an *in vitro* chemotherapy sensitivity test on the leukemic colony-forming cells. *Blood* **55**(4): 595–601.

Park, C.H., Amare, M., Savin, M.A., and Hoogstraten, B. 1980b. Growth suppression of human leukemic cells *in vitro* by L-ascorbic acid. *Cancer Res* **40**(4): 1062–1065.

Petkovich, M., Brand, N.J., Krust, A., and Chambon, P. 1987. A human retinoic acid receptor which belongs to the family of nuclear receptors. *Nature* **330**(6147): 444–450.

Petti, M.C., Avvisati, G., Amadori, S., Baccarani, M., Guarini, A.R., Papa, G., Rosti, G.A., Tura, S., and Mandelli, F. 1987. Acute promyelocytic leukemia: clinical aspects and results of treatment in 62 patients. *Haematologica* **72**(2): 151–155.

Pike, J.W. 1985. Intracellular receptors mediate the biologic action of 1,25-dihydroxyvitamin D3. *Nutr Rev* **43**(6): 161–168.

Pratt, M.A., Kralova, J., and McBurney, M.W. 1990. A dominant negative mutation of the alpha retinoic acid receptor gene in a retinoic acid-nonresponsive embryonal carcinoma cell. *Mol Cell Biol* **10**(12): 6445–6453.

Raelson, J.V., Nervi, C., Rosenauer, A., Benedetti, L., Monczak, Y., Pearson, M., Pelicci, P.G., and Miller, W.H., Jr. 1996. The PML/RAR alpha oncoprotein is a direct molecular target of retinoic acid in acute promyelocytic leukemia cells. *Blood* **88**(8): 2826–2832.

Rebel, V.I., Ossenkoppele, G.J., van de Loosdrecht, A.A., Wijermans, P.W., Beelen, R.H., and Langenhuijsen, M.M. 1992. Monocytic differentiation induction of HL-60 cells by MC 903, a novel vitamin D analogue. *Leuk Res* **16**(5): 443–451.

Richard, C., Mazo, E., Cuadrado, M.A., Iriondo, A., Bello, C., Gandarillas, M.A., and Zubizarreta, A. 1986. Treatment of myelodysplastic syndrome with 1.25-dihydroxy-vitamin D3. *Am J Hematol* **23**(2): 175–178.

Robertson, K.A., Emami, B., and Collins, S.J. 1992. Retinoic acid–resistant HL-60R cells harbor a point mutation in the retinoic acid receptor ligand-binding domain that confers dominant negative activity. *Blood* **80**(8): 1885–1889.

Sakashita, A., Kizaki, M., Pakkala, S., Schiller, G., Tsuruoka, N., Tomosaki, R., Cameron, J.F., Dawson, M.I., and Koeffler, H.P. 1993. 9-cis-retinoic acid: effects on normal and leukemic hematopoiesis *in vitro*. *Blood* **81**(4): 1009–1016.

Sanz, M.A., Martin, G., Rayon, C., Esteve, J., Gonzalez, M., Diaz-Mediavilla, J., Bolufer, P., Barragan, E., Terol, M.J., Gonzalez, J.D., Colomer, D., Chillon, C., Rivas, C., Gomez, T., Ribera, J.M., Bornstein, R., Roman, J., Calasanz, M.J., Arias, J., Alvarez, C., Ramos, F., and Deben, G. 1999. A modified AIDA protocol with anthracycline-based consolidation results in high antileukemic efficacy and reduced toxicity in newly diagnosed PML/RARalpha-positive acute promyelocytic leukemia. PETHEMA group. *Blood* **94**(9): 3015–3021.

Shao, W., Benedetti, L., Lamph, W.W., Nervi, C., and Miller, W.H., Jr. 1997. A retinoid-resistant acute promyelocytic leukemia subclone expresses a dominant negative PML-RAR alpha mutation. *Blood* **89**(12): 4282–4289.

Shinjo, K., Takeshita, A., Ohnishi, K., Sakura, T., Miyawaki, S., Hiraoka, A., Takeuchi, M., Tomoyasu, S., Wakita, H., Ata, K., Fukutani, H., Ueda, R., and Ohno, R. 2000. Good prognosis of patients with acute promyelocytic leukemia who achieved second complete remission (CR) with a new retinoid, Am80, after relapse from CR induced by all-trans-retinoic acid. *Int J Hematol* **72**(4): 470–473.

Shiohara, M., Uskokovic, M., Hisatake, J., Hisatake, Y., Koike, K., Komiyama, A., and Koeffler, H.P. 2001. 24-Oxo metabolites of vitamin D3 analogues: disassociation of their prominent antileukemic effects from their lack of calcium modulation. *Cancer Res* **61**(8): 3361–3368.

Skibola, C.F., Smith, M.T., Kane, E., Roman, E., Rollinson, S., Cartwright, R.A., and Morgan, G. 1999. Polymorphisms in the methylenetetrahydrofolate reductase gene are associated with susceptibility to acute leukemia in adults. *Proc Natl Acad Sci USA* **96**(22): 12810–12815.

Soignet, S., Fleischauer, A., Polyak, T., Heller, G., and Warrell, R.P., Jr. 1997. All-trans retinoic acid significantly increases 5-year survival in patients with acute promyelocytic leukemia: long-term follow-up of the New York study. *Cancer Chemother Pharmacol* **40**(Suppl): S25–S29.

Soignet, S.L., Frankel, S.R., Douer, D., Tallman, M.S., Kantarjian, H., Calleja, E., Stone, R.M., Kalaycio, M., Scheinberg, D.A., Steinherz, P., Sievers, E.L., Coutre, S., Dahlberg, S., Ellison, R., and Warrell, R.P., Jr. 2001. United States multicenter study of arsenic trioxide in relapsed acute promyelocytic leukemia. *J Clin Oncol* **19**(18): 3852–3860.

Soignet, S.L., Maslak, P., Wang, Z.G., Jhanwar, S., Calleja, E., Dardashti, L.J., Corso, D., DeBlasio, A., Gabrilove, J., Scheinberg, D.A., Pandolfi, P.P., and Warrell, R.P., Jr. 1998. Complete remission after treatment of acute promyelocytic leukemia with arsenic trioxide. *N Engl J Med* **339**(19): 1341–1348.

Stallone, D.D. 1994. The influence of obesity and its treatment on the immune system. *Nutr Rev* **52**(2 Pt 1): 37–50.

Suedhoff, T., Birckbichler, P.J., Lee, K.N., Conway, E., and Patterson, M.K., Jr. 1990. Differential expression of transglutaminase in human erythroleukemia cells in response to retinoic acid. *Cancer Res* **50**(24): 7830–7834.

Suttie, J.W. 1985. Vitamin K–dependent carboxylase. *Annu Rev Biochem* **54**: 459–477.

Tallman, M.S., Andersen, J.W., Schiffer, C.A., Appelbaum, F.R., Feusner, J.H., Ogden, A., Shepherd, L., Willman, C., Bloomfield, C.D., Rowe, J.M., and Wiernik, P.H. 1997. All-trans-retinoic acid in acute promyelocytic leukemia. *N Engl J Med* **337**(15): 1021–1028.

Tanaka, H., Abe, E., Miyaura, C., Kuribayashi, T., Konno, K., Nishii, Y., and Suda, T. 1982. 1 alpha,25-Dihydroxycholecalciferol and a human myeloid leukaemia cell line (HL-60). *Biochem J* **204**(3): 713–719.

Tobita, T., Takeshita, A., Kitamura, K., Ohnishi, K., Yanagi, M., Hiraoka, A., Karasuno, T., Takeuchi, M., Miyawaki, S., Ueda, R., Naoe, T., and Ohno, R. 1997. Treatment with a new synthetic retinoid, Am80, of acute promyelocytic leukemia relapsed from complete remission induced by all-trans retinoic acid. *Blood* **90**(3): 967–973.

Tobler, A., Gasson, J., Reichel, H., Norman, A.W., and Koeffler, H.P. 1987. Granulocyte-macrophage colony-stimulating factor. Sensitive and receptor-mediated regulation by 1,25-dihydroxyvitamin D3 in normal human peripheral blood lymphocytes. *J Clin Invest* **79**(6): 1700–1705.

Toshima, M., Nagai, T., Izumi, T., Tarumoto, T., Takatoku, M., Imagawa, S., Komatsu, N., and Ozawa, K. 2000. All-trans-retinoic acid treatment for chemotherapy-resistant acute adult T-cell leukemia. *Int J Hematol* **72**(3): 343–345.

Uchiyama, T., Hori, T., Tsudo, M., Wano, Y., Umadome, H., Tamori, S., Yodoi, J., Maeda, M., Sawami, H., and Uchino, H. 1985. Interleukin-2 receptor (Tac antigen) expressed on adult T cell leukemia cells. *J Clin Invest* **76**(2): 446–453.

Umesono, K., Murakami, K.K., Thompson, C.C., and Evans, R.M. 1991. Direct repeats as selective response elements for the thyroid hormone, retinoic acid, and vitamin D3 receptors. *Cell* **65**(7): 1255–1266.

Vahdat, L., Maslak, P., Miller, W.H., Jr., Eardley, A., Heller, G., Scheinberg, D.A., and Warrell, R.P., Jr. 1994. Early mortality and the retinoic acid syndrome in acute promyelocytic leukemia: impact of leukocytosis, low-dose chemotherapy, PMN/RAR-alpha isoform, and CD13 expression in patients treated with all-trans retinoic acid. *Blood* **84**(11): 3843–3849.

Visani, G., Cenacchi, A., Tosi, P., Finelli, C., Fogli, M., Gamberi, B., Martinelli, G., and Tura, S. 1992. All-trans retinoic acid improves erythropoiesis in myelodysplastic syndromes: a case report. *Br J Haematol* **81**(3): 444–446.

Warrell, R.P., Jr., de The, H., Wang, Z.Y., and Degos, L. 1993. Acute promyelocytic leukemia. *N Engl J Med* **329**(3): 177–189.

Warrell, R.P., Jr., Frankel, S.R., Miller, W.H., Jr., Scheinberg, D.A., Itri, L.M., Hittelman, W.N., Vyas, R., Andreeff, M., Tafuri, A., Jakubowski, A., et al. 1991. Differentiation therapy of acute promyelocytic leukemia with tretinoin (all-trans-retinoic acid). *N Engl J Med* **324**(20): 1385–1393.

Wiemels, J.L., Smith, R.N., Taylor, G.M., Eden, O.B., Alexander, F.E., and Greaves, M.F. 2001. Methylenetetrahydrofolate reductase (MTHFR) polymorphisms and risk of molecularly defined subtypes of childhood acute leukemia. *Proc Natl Acad Sci USA* **98**(7): 4004–4009.

Wolk, A., Gridley, G., Svensson, M., Nyren, O., McLaughlin, J.K., Fraumeni, J.F., and Adam, H.O. 2001. A prospective study of obesity and cancer risk (Sweden). *Cancer Causes Control* **12**(1): 13–21.

Yaguchi, M., Miyazawa, K., Katagiri, T., Nishimaki, J., Kizaki, M., Tohyama, K., and Toyama, K. 1997. Vitamin K2 and its derivatives induce apoptosis in leukemia cells and enhance the effect of all-trans retinoic acid. *Leukemia* **11**(6): 779–787.

Zelent, A., Krust, A., Petkovich, M., Kastner, P., and Chambon, P. 1989. Cloning of murine alpha and beta retinoic acid receptors and a novel receptor gamma predominantly expressed in skin. *Nature* **339**(6227): 714–717.

Zhang, P., Wang, S., and Hu, X. 1996. Treatment of 72 caese of acute promyelocytic leukemia with intravenous arsenic trioxide. *Chinese Journal of Hematology* **17**: 58–62.

Zhang, X.K., Lehmann, J., Hoffmann, B., Dawson, M.I., Cameron, J., Graupner, G., Hermann, T., Tran, P., and Pfahl, M. 1992. Homodimer formation of retinoid X receptor induced by 9-cis retinoic acid. *Nature* **358**(6387): 587–591.

Zhou, J.Y., Norman, A.W., Chen, D.L., Sun, G.W., Uskokovic, M., and Koeffler, H.P. 1990. 1,25-Dihydroxy-16-ene-23-yne-vitamin D3 prolongs survival time of leukemic mice. *Proc Natl Acad Sci USA* **87**(10): 3929–3932.

Zhu, J., Chen, Z., Lallemand-Breitenbach, V., and de The, H. 2002. How acute promyelocytic leukaemia revived arsenic. *Nat Rev Cancer* **2**(9): 705–713.

CHAPTER

28

Dietary Supplements in Cancer Prevention and Therapy

MARY FRANCES PICCIANO, BARBARA E. COHEN, AND PAUL R. THOMAS

INTRODUCTION

Dietary supplements are regulated in the United States by the Food and Drug Administration (FDA) under authority of the Federal Food, Drug, and Cosmetic Act (FFDCA). An amendment to the FFDCA, the Dietary Supplement Health and Education Act of 1994 (DSHEA), defines a dietary supplement as a product that is intended to supplement the diet and contains at least one or more of certain dietary ingredients, such as a vitamin, mineral, herb or other botanical, or an amino acid. These products may not be represented as conventional foods and are marketed in forms that include capsules, tablets, gelcaps, softgels, and powders. Although manufacturers are required to have evidence to support their claims of a dietary supplement's safety and efficacy, FDA approval is not required before a product is marketed.

The passage of DSHEA played a role in increasing the use of supplements in the United States by ensuring consumer access to a wide range of such products (U.S. Congress, 1994). The legislation also created the Office of Dietary Supplements within the National Institutes of Health (NIH) with the mission "to strengthen knowledge and understanding of dietary supplements by evaluating scientific information, stimulating and supporting research, disseminating research results, and educating the public to foster an enhanced quality of life and health for the U.S. population" (Office of Dietary Supplements, 2004).

Dietary supplements are commonly purchased and consumed in the United States even though they may not have proven benefits for the general population and, for some, may have harmful effects. However, the possibility that supplements help to prevent cancer development, progression, or reoccurrence attracts many people. A rigorous approach must be taken to determine the circumstances under which dietary supplements may have beneficial health effects on cancer or on any other disease or medical disorder. Special attention must be given to the circumstances that could influence the effects of dietary supplements, including the timing of supplement use, dose and dose–response, the role of specific supplement components, and the impact of interactive factors. This chapter addresses these issues with selected examples. Although it is beyond the scope of this chapter to address these issues for all supplements, the points made here are relevant to almost all categories of dietary supplements.

PREVALENCE OF DIETARY SUPPLEMENT USAGE AMONG PEOPLE WITH CANCER AND THE GENERAL POPULATION

As many people are motivated to change their food-intake behaviors with the hope of improving their health, they also are using a variety of alternative strategies including the consumption of vitamin, mineral, herbal, and botanical supplements (Halsted, 2003). The following two subsections present the most recent data on the prevalence of and reasons for dietary supplement use, first in the general population and then among people diagnosed with cancer.

Dietary Supplement Use in the General Population

Data from the latest National Health and Nutrition Examination Survey (NHANES) indicate that 52% of the U.S.

Copyright © 2006, Elsevier Inc.
All rights of reproduction in any form reserved.

adult population took some sort of dietary supplement in 1999–2000, most commonly a multivitamin and multimineral supplement (35%) (Radimer et al., 2004). The 1987 National Health Interview Survey (NHIS), conducted by the Centers for Disease Control and Prevention, found that 51.1% of U.S. adults used a vitamin or mineral supplement, but only 23.1% on a daily basis (Subar and Block, 1990). The daily use of vitamin or mineral supplements increased to 33.9% in the 2000 NHIS, and 6% of the respondents reported using nonvitamin or nonmineral supplements (Millen et al., 2004). The 2002 NHIS indicated that 38.2 million American adults (~19%) use nonvitamin nonmineral supplements, primarily botanical products (Barnes et al., 2004). Market data show that in 2004 the sale of vitamins, herbs and botanicals, sports nutrition supplements, minerals, meal supplements, and other specialty supplements totaled $20.33 billion, representing a $4.27 billion (26.6%) increase since 1999 (*Nutrition Business Journal*, 2005). The 2004 sales of vitamins and minerals, in either a multivitamin-multimineral or single-nutrient form, were 42% of all sales ($8.63 billion).

Data from NHANES and other research efforts have also been useful in identifying characteristics of supplement users and the reasons for supplement use. These findings indicate that the highest usage of vitamin and mineral supplements is associated with being female, having an education beyond high school, having a higher income, being non-Hispanic white, and being older (Steward et al., 1985; Koplan et al., 1986; Medeiros et al., 1989; Moss et al., 1989; Subar and Block, 1990; Bender et al., 1992; Slesinski et al., 1995; Lyle et al., 1998; Newman et al., 1998). This profile is similar to that for people using herbal supplements, with a few exceptions. Herbal use does not increase with age, and although those with health insurance are more likely to use vitamins or minerals, those without health insurance are more likely to use herbs (Fennell, 2004). Nationally representative data from NHANES indicate that although an increase in the use of supplements has occurred since the passage of DSHEA, usage patterns among various demographic groups are similar to those reported by researchers using nonrepresentative population samples.

Reasons cited for usage of dietary supplements by various subgroups suggest that a large segment of people living in the United States is adopting a health-promotion strategy that includes seeking alternative forms of medicine (Slesinski et al., 1995; Eliason et al., 1997; Eisenberg et al., 1998; Patterson et al., 1998; Gilbert, 1999; Hensrud et al., 1999; Radimer et al., 2000; Greger, 2001). Supplements are used to improve nutrition, make up for nutrients missing in the diet, decrease susceptibility to or severity of disease, increase energy (vitality), or improve performance. Herbal and botanical preparations are frequently used to supplement conventional medical treatments. Those most commonly used by the general population before 1995 were garlic and lecithin (Radimer et al., 2000). In 2003, the top-selling herbals were weight-loss blends with and without ephedra and glucosamine/chondroitin sulfate (*Nutrition Business Journal*, 2004). It is interesting that many dietary supplement users report that they do not discuss their supplement use with their physicians because they believe that physicians are biased against, and not knowledgeable enough about, supplements (Hensrud et al., 1999).

Dietary Supplement Use among People with Cancer

Given the prevalence and usage trends of dietary supplements in the general population, it is not surprising to see similar trends among people who have been diagnosed with cancer. However, the majority of prevalence studies do not collect data on supplement use before cancer diagnosis but only provide information on supplement use after diagnosis. This disallows inferences to be made on the role of a cancer diagnosis as a motivator for dietary supplement use. In general, motivators for supplement use among cancer patients include maintenance of health, increased well-being, prevention of recurrence, and alleviation of symptoms. Tables 1, 2, and 3 summarize studies published since 2000 that provide prevalence data on dietary supplement use among people with cancer. Table 1 summarizes studies with data from pools of cancer patients, generally adults. The range of any supplement use in this set of studies is between 29 and 80%. Multivitamins were the most frequently used supplement; vitamins A, B, C, and E were the most frequently used single vitamins; calcium and selenium were the most frequently used single minerals; garlic, ginseng, and soy were the most frequently used botanicals; and shark cartilage, hydrazine sulfate, and coenzyme Q10 (CoQ10) the most frequently used nonbotanical dietary supplements. However, the list of other supplements used by any proportion of the study samples is extensive. Table 2 focuses on studies with data from people with specific cancer diagnoses (in which the range of supplement use is between 35 and 64%), and Table 3 presents two studies published on pediatric cancer patients.

Among studies on the general adult cancer patient population, two compared dietary supplement usage by people with cancer to people not diagnosed with cancer. The first of these analyzed data from the NHIS in 1987 and 1992 (McDavid et al., 2001). Among both populations in this nationally representative survey, multivitamins were more commonly used than other supplements (taken by 75%), although ~50% of both groups reported taking vitamin C. It is important to note that this is not necessarily daily use, but any use during the period for which data were collected. Unfortunately, the small sample size of the cancer cohort (689 people) provided little power to test differences between this group and those not reporting a diagnosis of

TABLE 1 Prevalence of Dietary Supplement Use among People Diagnosed with Cancer

Reference	Type of study	Location	Population	N	Results
McDavid et al., 2001	Cross-sectional, nationally representative probability household survey	Entire United States	Male and female cancer survivors (median age 63 years) and individuals with no reported history of cancer (median age 40 years)	33,456 (689 cancer survivors and 32,767 without cancer)	Vitamin and mineral supplement use similar in both groups; >75% took multivitamins and almost half took vitamin C; among cancer survivors, calcium use was significantly higher among women (34.9%) than men (13.8%), and vitamin A use was higher among men (9.0%) than women (7.6%)
Metz et al., 2001	Prospective evaluation of consecutive patients at a university cancer center	Philadelphia, Pennsylvania	Patients with a malignancy at first visit; median age 61 years	196 (133 men and 63 women)	79 individuals reported use of "unconventional medical therapies"; among them, 46% took megavitamins (especially high-dose vitamin C [at >10 g/day] and vitamin E), 34% took herbal supplements (23 identified), and 16% took other supplements (such as shark cartilage and hydrazine sulfate); admitting use of unconventional therapies increased from 7% to 40% when patients directly queried
Kumar et al., 2002	Retrospective chart review of consecutive patients at a university cancer center	Tampa, Florida	Patients ranging in age from younger than 30 years (4% of total) to older than 60 years (56% of total)	237 (120 men and 117 women)	139 individuals took multivitamins/mineral supplements, 205 used individual vitamins (vitamins E and C most frequently), 104 used botanical supplements (typically garlic, ginseng, soy, ginkgo, and echinacea), and 67 used individual minerals (calcium, followed by iron and selenium)
Greenlee et al., 2004	Cross-sectional cohort study of participants in the Vitamins and Lifestyle (VITAL) study	Western Washington State	Men and women 50–76 years of age	75,083 (10,857 cancer survivors and 64,226 cancer-free controls)	Both groups took similar numbers of supplements. Among cancer survivors, 47.3% and 54.5% of men and women, respectively, took a multivitamin, 41.0% and 57.5% had high use (two or more per day) of vitamin and mineral supplements, and 16.0% and 20.7% had high use of herbal and specialty supplements; strongest positive associations were found for cranberry pills with bladder cancer, zinc with ovarian cancer, soy with prostate cancer, melatonin with cervical cancer, and vitamin D with thyroid cancer
Hedderson et al., 2004	Telephone survey of randomly selected cancer patients in state surveillance system	Washington State	Individuals 20–70 years of age diagnosed with breast, colon, or prostate cancer	356 (178 men and 178 women)	54.5% of men and 72.5% of women took any vitamin or mineral supplement beyond a basic multi; 32.6% of men and 42.7% of women took any herbal or other type of supplement; conclusion: men and women "differ considerably" in their use of complementary and alternative medicine, including use of dietary supplements
Jazieh et al., 2004	Cross-sectional study of cancer patients at a veterans' hospital oncology clinic	Cincinnati, Ohio	Military veterans with a malignancy; median age 68 years	200 (196 men and 4 women)	Most commonly used supplements were multivitamins (80.3%) and minerals (40.6%); 10 took herbal supplements. 74% of users reported benefits, including improved health and energy; 38% did not disclose supplement use to their physicians

TABLE 2 Prevalence of Dietary Supplement Use by Diagnosis of Breast, Prostate, and Colorectal Cancer

Reference	Type of study	Location	Population	N	Results
Lengacher et al., 2002	Descriptive cross-sectional survey	Tampa, Florida	Convenience sample of women with diagnosis of breast cancer; mean age 59 years	105	On regular basis, 64% used vitamin and mineral supplements, 33% took antioxidants, and 13% used herbs; more than half did not take supplements before diagnosis, and majority discussed supplement use with doctor
Hall et al., 2003	Descriptive survey of responses to mailed questionnaire	Charlottesville, Virginia	Men treated for prostate cancer at a medical center	238	84 took vitamins (53 used vitamin E), 52 took a multivitamin, and 29 used an herbal supplement (most commonly lycopene and saw palmetto); many believed supplements helped cure their cancer and helped them to feel better
Patterson et al., 2003	Telephone survey of randomly selected patients in state surveillance system	Washington State	Adults with breast, prostate, or colorectal cancer	356 (126 with breast cancer, 116 with colorectal cancer, and 114 with prostate cancer	48% took new supplements after diagnosis (primarily multivitamins, vitamins E and C, calcium, garlic, and echinacea); women were 2.2 times more likely to do this than men; >90% reported that supplement use improved health and well-being
Rock et al., 2004	Multisite, randomized controlled trial	Sites in California, Arizona, and Oregon	Women with history of early-stage breast cancer	3,008	At enrollment, 58% took multivitamins, 46% vitamin E (17% of them at intakes ≥500 mg/day), 42% vitamin C (24% at intakes ≥1000 mg/day), 11% vitamin A and carotenoids, and ~10% antioxidant mixtures; trend toward use of multi-ingredient products containing herbs; supplements commonly used for general health and "to feel better"
Salminen et al., 2004	Responses to questionnaires administered to patients on site	Melbourne, Australia and Turku, Finland	Women with newly diagnosed breast cancer	354 (215 from Australia and 139 from Finland)	50% of the Australians and 47% of the Finns took supplements, primarily vitamins and minerals

cancer. The second such study offering comparative statistics was the Vitamins and Lifestyle (VITAL) study, composed of a self-selected sample of adults in western Washington State, most of whom took at least one vitamin supplement at the start (Greenlee et al., 2004). This study, which focused on supplement use at least five times weekly, showed little difference among cancer patients and those without cancer with respect to both multivitamin, single vitamin or mineral supplement, and herbal supplement use. Differences among prevalence rates reported in these and the remaining four studies in Table 1 reflect variation in study design and outcome indicators (Metz et al., 2001; Kumar et al., 2002; Hedderson et al., 2004; Jazieh et al., 2004).

The differences in results reported in Table 2 also reflect the variation in study design, sample selection, and outcome variables. Patterson et al. (2003) only report on new supplements taken after a diagnosis of breast, prostate, and colorectal cancer and do not include usual supplements taken before and after diagnosis. Hall et al. (2003) limited their study to men with prostate cancer, and Lengacher et al. (2002) and Salminen et al. (2004) limited their studies to

TABLE 3 Prevalence of Dietary Supplement Use among Pediatric Cancer Patients

Reference	Type of study	Location	Population	N	Results
Neuhouser et al., 2001b	Telephone survey of parents of randomly selected patients in state surveillance system	Western Washington State	Pediatric cancer patients 18 years or younger	75	After cancer diagnosis, subjects took miscellaneous supplements (n = 28; including antioxidant mixtures and shark cartilage), herbal supplements (14), single-nutrient supplements (13), vitamin C (7), and echinacea (6); majority used supplements to maintain health or to treat noncancer symptoms like cold and flu
Ball et al., 2005	Convenience sample of parents of chronically ill patients who completed questionnaire at clinic	Salt Lake City, Utah	Children and adolescents with solid-tumor cancer or leukemia (mean age ~9 years)	100 (50 with each type of cancer)	50% took supplements (typically without doctor's knowledge), primarily vitamins, botanicals, and minerals; most common reasons: improve health, supplement diet, and prevent disease; supplements were discontinued within past year by one third of parents

women with breast cancer. Rock et al. (2004) presented comparative data from a study conducted with breast cancer patients and one with the general population. Reported multivitamin use in women with a history of early-stage breast cancer in the Women's Healthy Eating and Living (WHEL) Study (n = 3,088) was 58%, with 42% using vitamin C.

The two studies of children with cancer (Table 3) also use different outcome measures. Ball et al. (2005) reported on the prevalence of dietary supplement use separately for children with leukemia and solid tumors (42% and 50%, respectively, used vitamins; 10% and 16% used minerals; and 18% and 24% used botanicals). Neuhouser et al. (2001b) did not differentiate by type of cancer and reported 29% use of single vitamin supplements, 15% use of vitamin and mineral mixtures, and 35% use of herbal supplements. Most parents of the children in this study reported perceived improvement from single vitamin use (76.9%) and herbal supplement use (85.7%). Motivators for dietary supplement use included treating side effects or symptoms of cancer or cancer treatment (47.2%), preventing recurrence or spread of cancer (33.3%), preventing or treating noncancer symptoms such as a cold or flu (51.4%), and maintaining general good health (72.2%).

Despite the variations in populations, study design, sample size, and outcome variables, it is clear that significant proportions of people who have been diagnosed with cancer are using dietary supplements. This underscores the need for additional information on the efficacy and safety of these supplements for people with different types of cancers, undergoing different types of treatments, and at varying stages of life.

Importance of Evidence-Based Research

Any recommendations for supplementation must be based on scientific evidence that the supplements are both effective and safe. Ideally, a rigorous systematic research approach (Table 4) is carried out and the results are evaluated to assess the health benefits of a dietary supplement and whether its use is recommended. The review begins with preclinical (*in vitro* and *in vivo* studies) and epidemiological evidence. Although these lines of evidence may provide insight into anticipated outcomes, it is important that research be taken to the next level of clinical trials. Before the conduct of human clinical trials, however, all available evidence must be reviewed thoroughly and objectively to determine whether data on efficacy and safety justify proceeding to clinical trials. Such evidence-based reviews differ from traditional opinion-based narrative reviews in that they systematically attempt to reduce bias by the comprehensiveness and reproducibility of the search for and selection of articles for review. Systematic reviews also assess the methodological quality of the included studies and evaluate the overall strength of the body of evidence (Agency for Healthcare Research and Quality [AHRQ], 2002). When the body of evidence on safety and efficacy justifies proceeding to clinical trials, the trials are usually conducted in three

TABLE 4 Evaluating Dietary Supplements: A Research Approach

BASIC BIOMEDICAL LABORATORY RESEARCH
(*In vitro* experiments and *in vivo* animal experiments)

↓

HUMAN OBSERVATIONAL EPIDEMIOLOGICAL STUDIES
(Identify possible links between dietary supplements and cancer prevention)

↓

HYPOTHESIS DEVELOPMENT
(Evaluation of existing laboratory and epidemiological evidence on dietary supplement safety and effectiveness: as related to cancer prevention and therapy)

↓

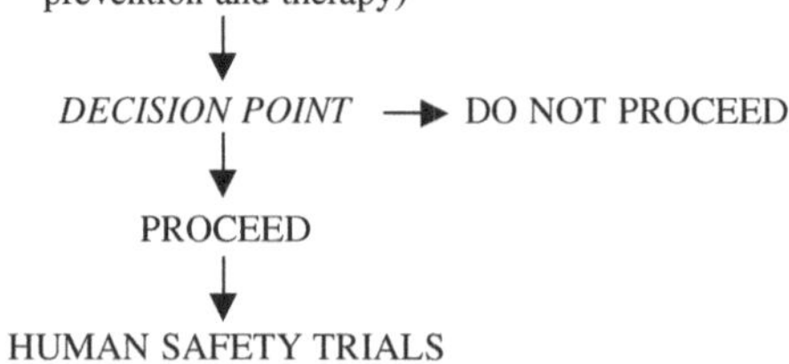

DECISION POINT → DO NOT PROCEED

↓

PROCEED

↓

HUMAN SAFETY TRIALS
(Identify adverse side effects: safe dosage: and potential interactions)

↓

SMALL TRIALS IN DEFINED POPULATIONS
(Measure supplement effectiveness at various safe doses)

↓

LARGE-SCALE: DOUBLE-BLIND: PLACEBO-CONTROLLED: RANDOMIZED CLINICAL INTERVENTION TRIALS
(Test whether supplementation has the hypothesized human health benefit)

↓

DEVELOP SUPPLEMENTATION RECOMMENDATION

phases: human safety trials, small efficacy trials (usually in defined target groups), and large-scale trials that are essential in moving from basic and observational science to evidence-based public health recommendations that have human benefits.

The large-scale, double-blind, randomized, placebo-controlled clinical trial, which is designed to eliminate all possible bias, is considered the gold standard of scientific intervention research. In such trials, some people receive the substance being tested and some receive an inactive placebo. These trials may not be possible in all circumstances, however, because of ethical issues that make it inappropriate to withhold the substance being tested from any trial participants. For example, after it was observed that low folate intake by pregnant women was linked to neural tube defects, a placebo-controlled intervention trial to test the validity of this association would not have been ethical. In such cases, all available evidence from *in vitro* laboratory research and *in vivo* animal studies, as well as epidemiological studies and surveys, must be reviewed systematically and objectively to draw conclusions about the possible effectiveness and safety of the supplement of interest and to make recommendations for supplementation.

Two evidence-based reviews have been conducted on the effect of specific supplements on cancer prevention. The first was a review by the U.S. Preventive Services Task Force (PSTF) on routine vitamin supplementation to prevent cancer and cardiovascular disease. For cancer, the PSTF recommended against the use of β-carotene supplements, either alone or in combination, and concluded that insufficient evidence exists either for or against the use of supplements of vitamins A, C, or E, multivitamins with folic acid, or antioxidant combinations for the prevention of cancer (PSTF, 2003). The second systematic review by the AHRQ on the use of the antioxidant vitamins C and E and CoQ10 supported the PSTF recommendations for vitamins C and E and determined that the literature does not support the use of CoQ10 supplements to help prevent or treat cancer (AHRQ, 2003). The AHRQ recognized that a few individual trials did report benefits in patients with bladder cancer and that other trials reported beneficial intermediate outcomes, such as colonic crypt cell proliferation with vitamin C and E supplementation.

Although clinical trials provide a wealth of information, various interactions must be accounted for when interpreting the results and developing public health recommendations. These factors include a person's stage of life, general health status, genetic makeup, and health and lifestyle behaviors. Each may influence the absorption, usefulness, and need for any particular dietary supplement. For example, the results of a large randomized clinical trial, the Alpha-Tocopherol, Beta-Carotene Cancer Prevention (ATBC) study conducted in Finland suggested a substantial benefit of vitamin E in reducing prostate cancer (Heinonen et al., 1998). However, almost all the participants were current or past smokers.

Another major concern associated with clinical trials designed to evaluate the health effects of dietary supplements is that participants might take additional supplements, which could influence trial outcomes. In the Prostate Cancer Prevention Trial (PCPT) of the drug finasteride, for example, almost half of the participants reported using a multivitamin supplement, about a third used single supplements of either vitamin C or E, and one in five used calcium supplements. Limitations to the study included the lack of control for dosage amount, frequency of intake, type of supplement, and the limited data on micronutrient intake from fortified foods (Neuhouser et al., 2001a). Very little evidence is available about how individual micronutrients might interact with one another to influence health outcomes. The Selenium and Vitamin E Prevention Trial (SELECT) is expected to help clarify the association of dietary supplement use with prostate and other cancers. SELECT is a randomized, prospective, double-blind study designed to determine whether selenium and vitamin E reduce the risk of prostate cancer in healthy men (Klein et al., 2003). The vitamin E supplement will be a higher dose than that used in the ATBC study (400 vs 50 mg), and final results are expected in 2013.

The following section explores the relationship of these interactive factors with respect to the role of dietary supplements and cancer.

ROLE OF DIETARY SUPPLEMENTS IN CANCER PREVENTION AND DURING THERAPY

To understand the potential role of dietary supplements in the prevention of cancer, scientists have developed models of molecular mechanisms through which nutrient and nonnutrient supplements might affect metabolic processes that lead to cancer. Potential mechanisms include inhibiting carcinogen uptake, inhibiting the formation or activation of carcinogens, and preventing dietary carcinogen binding to DNA (American Institute for Cancer Research, 2000). Different supplements use different pathways to influence carcinogenesis. For example, antioxidants neutralize free radicals, preventing them from damaging other molecules, which over time may lead to cancer. In addition to the well-known antioxidants (vitamin C, vitamin E, and β-carotene), other substances such as mistletoe extract exhibit antioxidant properties. Calcium inhibits carcinogen uptake most often in conjunction with vitamin D. Folic acid helps to synthesize and repair DNA, potentially preventing cancer development. Phytoestrogens, the most common of which (genistein and daidzein) come from soy products, may inhibit the growth of estrogen receptor (ER)-positive and ER-negative breast cancer cells (Jennings, 1995; Peterson and Barnes, 1996). These are only a few supplement-related mechanisms that have been or are being studied.

Researchers have also investigated additional factors that might influence the involvement of dietary supplements in the prevention of cancer. They include the timing of supplement use, the effect of dose and dose–response, the role of specific supplement components, and the impact of interactive factors. Each factor is discussed in the following subsections with examples.

Timing

The issue of timing in dietary supplement use with respect to cancer prevention and treatment reflects on the age of the person and the time within the course of the disease that supplements are taken. A better understanding of these issues may help explain some of the conflicting results from epidemiological and clinical studies on dietary supplement use. Calcium and the soy isoflavone genistein provide examples of the importance of timing in supplement use.

Timing with the Framework of a Day: The Example of Calcium

Calcium has been investigated for its role in cancer prevention because it participates in multiple molecular signaling pathways and alterations of gene expression associated with cancer and for its role in many other key biological processes, such as bone formation and proper functioning of the nervous system (NIH Consensus Conference, 1994; Patton et al., 2003). However, the time of supplementation may influence its impact. Ingesting calcium supplements between meals supports calcium bioavailability because some foods contain compounds such as oxalates that reduce calcium absorption (NIH Consensus Conference, 1994). Also, high intakes of calcium from foods or supplements taken with meals may inhibit nonheme iron absorption and negatively affect the redox and antioxidant availability of iron (NIH Consensus Conference, 1994; Whiting, 1995).

Timing with the Lifespan: The Example of Phytoestrogens

Another example of timing is exposure during different periods of life. Throughout the lifespan, estrogens increase mammary cell proliferation, but other factors, such as hormonal levels, may influence estrogens' ability to induce differentiation or affect mammary growth by other means. Thus, estrogens can have a different impact on the breast if the exposure occurs *in utero*; during childhood, puberty, or pregnancy; premenopausally; or during postmenopause (Hilakivi-Clarke and Clarke, 1998). There is evidence that genistein also has different effects on the breast depending on the timing of exposure. For example, studies in rats have shown that prepubertal exposure to genistein protects against chemically induced mammary tumors, possibly because genistein increases cellular differentiation at early stages of mammary development (Lamartiniere et al., 2002). During the reproductive years, genistein increases mammary gland proliferation, as has been shown in both animal and human studies (Petrakis et al., 1996; Hsieh et al., 1998; McMichael-Phillips et al., 1998). Differences have been noted in the effect of genistein premenopausally and postmenopausally. Although there is no evidence that genistein promotes breast cancer in premenopausal women, animal studies suggest that it may play a role in the growth of cancer cells in postmenopausal women (Hsieh et al., 1998; Trock et al., 2000). It is possible that the different impact of genistein on premenopausal and postmenopausal women reflects the increased likelihood that postmenopausal women already have malignant cells in their breasts and that genistein, acting as an estrogenic agent, proliferates mammary cell growth, be it healthy or malignant cells (Bouker and Hilakivi-Clarke, 2000).

Dose and Dose–Response

Because dietary supplements are ingested to add to or replace dietary factors generally found in food products, issues of dose and bioavailability are important in discussions of their efficacy and safety. Often, the dose of a dietary supplement is greater than the amount normally found in food and may equal or exceed recommended levels of intake. For example, the recommendation for vitamin C is 75 mg/day for adults older than 18 years, but an average dose of a vitamin C supplement is 500 mg. Although dietary recommendations suggest the value of eating large amounts of fruits and vegetables, which contain vitamin C and other antioxidants, research is necessary to determine the levels of specific nutrient or nonnutrient components of these foods, which when used as supplements will have an impact on carcinogenesis.

Vitamin A and β-Carotene

For example, both the α-Tocopherol, β-Carotene Cancer Prevention (ATBC) Study and the β-Carotene and Retinol Efficacy Trial (CARET) reported that the use of β-carotene supplements in smokers may promote lung cancer (ATBC Study Group, 1994; Omenn et al., 1996). Among the explanations for these results is that the dose of β-carotene in the trial was 5–10 times greater than that supplied by a healthy diet; this higher dose may have inhibited the absorption of other antioxidants with cancer-preventive properties (Greenwald, 2003). In addition, tissues of trial participants supplemented with β-carotene showed a 50-fold higher concentration than those of individuals who consumed large amounts of fruits and vegetables (Borrás et al., 2003).

Dose–response to vitamin A also is dependent on the vitamin A status of cells. Vitamin A circulates in the body after binding to a retinol-binding protein (RBP), which is accumulated in the liver, and homeostasis results in extra retinol being stored for future use. When cells are deficient in vitamin A, the liver accumulates large amounts of RBP in anticipation of future availability of the vitamin (Russell, 2000). Ingesting vitamin A through the diet or by supplement in a vitamin A–deficient state causes a rapid large rise in serum retinol that is short-lived. Vitamin A ingestion when cells are not deficient results in a slower and smaller rise in serum retinol, with extra amounts being stored for later use (Russell, 2000).

Vitamin E and Its Constituents

The two subgroups of vitamin E are tocopherols and tocotrienols. Tocotrienols have been shown to have potent anticancer activity at doses that do not appear to affect normal cell growth or function. Their antitumor activity is independent of antioxidant activity. Dose–response studies show that growth-inhibitory doses of tocotrienols are five to six times lower than their corresponding lethal doses, suggesting that different mechanisms control their antiproliferative and cytotoxic effects (Sylvester and Shah, 2005).

Folic Acid

Epidemiological studies suggest that dose and dose–response are important factors in folate supplementation to reduce cancer risk, especially for colon cancer and colorectal adenoma. A 35–40% risk reduction was observed in those with the highest folate intake compared with those with the lowest intake (Kim, 1999). A randomized study of patients with recurrent polyps reported that supplementation with 2 mg of folate significantly decreased colonic mucosal-cell proliferation in the treatment group compared with controls (no supplementation) (Khosraviani et al., 2002).

Calcium and Vitamin D

Calcium, which has the potential to reduce the risk of colon cancer, also has been shown to exhibit a dose–response relationship (Wu et al., 2002). Data from the Nurses' Health Study (Martínez et al., 1996) and Health Professionals Follow-up Study (Kearney et al., 1996) indicate that higher calcium intake is associated with a reduced risk of distal colon cancer. The incremental benefit of additional calcium intake >700 mg/day was minimal. Interestingly, it has been shown that the relationship between calcium and vitamin D is important in their associations with cancer risk (Milner et al., 2001). Results of the Calcium Polyp Prevention Study show that vitamin D status strongly influenced the impact of calcium supplementation on adenoma recurrence (Grau et al., 2003). Calcium supplements only lowered the risk of adenoma in subjects with 25-hydroxyvitamin D levels above the median. Similarly, 25-hydroxyvitamin D was associated with reduced risk only among those supplemented with calcium. It was concluded that vitamin D and calcium supplements appear to act together, not separately, on colorectal carcinogenesis.

Interactive Impacts: Environment, Gender, Genetic Differences

Environmental, genetic, and other differences may determine whether benefit or harm is derived from the use of dietary supplements in healthy individuals, populations at risk for certain diseases, and patients undergoing disease therapy. Selenium, folate, genistein, and zinc are examples of dietary supplements that have been investigated for their association with environmental, genetic, and hormonal factors and cancer risk.

Environmental Factors

Epidemiological studies suggest an increase in colon cancer in areas where selenium levels are low in the soil (Clark et al., 1991). Because the amount of selenium provided by the diet is dependent on the amount found in the soil used to grow food products, the level of intake among populations is varied, especially when most food consumed comes from a single geographic source. Clinical trial results from Linxian, China, an area characterized by epidemic rates of squamous esophageal and adenomatous gastric-cardia cancers, indicated a significant inverse association of serum selenium levels with these cancers when the highest-to-lowest quartiles of serum selenium were compared (Mark et al., 2000). Selenium supplementation has been associated with a reduction in prostate, lung, and colorectal cancers (Greenwald et al., 2002).

Genetic Factors

Genetic variability and selenium intake may both play important roles in reducing cancer risk. A large randomized phase III trial, The Selenium and Vitamin E Cancer Prevention Trial (SELECT), is investigating the effect of supplementation with selenium and vitamin E, alone or in combination, on prostate cancer incidence. A nested case-control study within SELECT will assess genetic polymorphisms of four genes (androgen receptor [*AR*], 5α-reductase type II [*SRD5A2*], cytochrome P450c 17α [*CYP17*], and β-hydroxysteroid dehydrogenase [*HSD3β2*]) on prostate cancer incidence (Hoque et al., 2001). *CYP17* is of particular interest because previous studies have suggested that the A1/A1 genotype confers a significantly higher serum androgen level than is found in men with either the A1/A2 or the A2/A2 genotype.

Folate provides another example of genetic differences that can influence the potential benefits of supplementation. Methylenetetrahydrofolate reductase (MTHFR) is a critical enzyme that regulates the metabolism of folate by converting 5,10-methylenetetrahydrofolate (methyleneTHF) to 5-methyltetrahydrofolate (methylTHF), the major form of circulating folate in plasma. A common polymorphism of the *MTHFR* gene (677C→T) results in an alanine→valine substitution in the enzyme and, subsequently, in significantly decreased activity (Greenwald et al., 2002). This results in increased methyleneTHF, which results in reduced incorporation of uracil in DNA, which leads to fewer chromosome breaks and possibly reduced cancer risk (Greenwald et al., 2001).

Studies of data from the Health Professionals Follow-Up Study and the Physician's Health Study on the 677→6T *MTHFR* polymorphism and dietary intake of folate in colorectal tumorigenesis found that when the dietary methyl supply was high, individuals with the *MTHFR* polymorphism were at reduced risk of colorectal cancer. Interestingly, alcohol consumption reversed this association—possibly by depletion of the dietary methyl supply and folate breakdown by acetaldehyde—and suggests that individuals with this genotype may be more susceptible to the carcinogenic effects of alcohol (Greenwald et al., 2001).

Epidemiological studies report that zinc deficiency is associated with an increased risk of esophageal squamous cell carcinoma in high incidence areas of China and Iran (Fong et al., 2003). Abnormalities in the *p53* tumor suppressor gene, which causes a loss of function leading to increased tumor proliferation and decreased apoptosis, has been studied in zinc-deficient mice exposed to the carcinogen N-nitromethylbenzylamine (NMBA). An investigation of esophageal NMBA-induced tumor proliferation in *p53–/–* zinc-deficient mice suggests that zinc modulates genetic susceptibility to cancer caused by *p53* inactivation (Fong et al., 2003).

Hormonal Factors

The relationship between genistein and hormones in the lifespan of women was described in the section "Timing with the Lifespan: The Example of Phytoestrogens." In men, epidemiological and experimental evidence suggests that genistein may inhibit prostate tumor growth through various mechanisms, including cell proliferation and increased apoptosis (Greenwald et al., 2002). In a study in LNCaP prostate cancer cells, genistein completely inhibited expression of prostate-regulated transcript 1 (*PART-1*), an androgen-induced gene that may represent a novel tumor marker for prostate cancer (Yu et al., 2003). In a small study of patients with prostate cancer, a dietary supplement of red-clover isoflavones, including genistein, was administered before surgery. After prostatectomy, apoptosis in cells from treated patients was significantly higher than in cells from controls, specifically in regions of low- to moderate-grade cancer (Jarred et al., 2002).

Therapeutic Interactions

Just as there are many mechanisms through which dietary supplements influence the prevention of cancer, so are there a variety of ways in which they influence cancer treatment. The following highlights some of the mechanisms that have an impact on the efficacy of treatment and its side effects. This is not meant to be a complete list of all influential factors, but a highlight of examples of potential interactions.

Antioxidants

Chemotherapeutic agents include alkylating agents (cyclophosphamides), anthracycline antibiotics (doxorubicin), platinum compounds (cisplatin), mitotic inhibitors (vincristine), antimetabolites (5-fluorouracil), camptothecin derivatives (topotecan), biological response modifiers (interferon), and hormonal therapies (tamoxifen). Anticancer therapies that may potentially be influenced by antioxidants include: alkylating agents (cyclophosphamide and iphosphamide), platinum compounds (cisplatin), antibiotics (doxorubicin and bleomycin), topoisomerase II inhibitors (etoposide), and radiation (Conklin, 2000). However, the evidence with respect to the impact of antioxidants on chemotherapy or radiation is controversial. Studies show both that antioxidants are safe and effective enhancers of chemotherapy and that they interfere with the oxidative breakdown of cellular DNA and cell membranes needed for the chemotherapy to be effective (Norman et al., 2003). Although most clinical trials have not shown significant impacts of antioxidant supplementation on chemotherapy or radiation, some have reported either the potentiation or the inhibition of these therapies by antioxidants (Weiger et al., 2002). Three clinical trials indicate that melatonin (an antioxidant) enhances the efficacy of radiation therapy and chemotherapy (Lissoni et al., 1996, 1997, 1999). Animal studies indicate that the impact of antioxidants may depend on dosage and timing of administration with respect to radiation (Sakamoto and Sakka, 1973).

Phytoestrogens

As was discussed in the section "Timing with the Lifespan: The Example of Phytoestrogens," soy isoflavonoids, particularly genistein and daidzein, have both positive and negative estrogenic effects on breast tissue. In a review of 26 animal studies, soy was found to have a positive effect in most cases (Messina et al., 1994). However, other animal studies suggest the need for concern that soy supplementation in women with breast cancer, particularly with ER-positive tumors, may cause a proliferation of the cancerous cells (Weiger et al., 2002). A review addressed this dichotomous role and concluded that the data are not strong enough on either side to support the use or nonuse of soy supplements (Messina and Loprinzi, 2001). Additional effects of soy on cancer treatments have also been examined. Animal study data indicate that genistein can negate the inhibitory effect of tamoxifen on breast cancer growth (Ju et al., 2002). Given its antioxidant activity, there is also concern with respect to the use of soy supplementation during radiation or chemotherapy (Wiseman, 1996).

Other Supplements

Supplements that are neither antioxidants nor phytoestrogens also may affect treatment. Blood levels of medications may be influenced by the use of St. John's wort. This herb is an inducer of the cytochrome P450 enzyme system and drug-transporting P glycoprotein. Studies have found that St. John's wort reduces levels of drugs such as cyclosporine and indinavir, as well as levels of the active metabolite of irinotecan, a chemotherapeutic agent (Mathijssen et al., 2002; Weiger et al., 2002).

CONCLUSIONS

Despite varied results with respect to specific foods and specific cancers, results of observational, ecological, and clinical studies provide strong evidence that diets high in vegetables, fruits, and plant-based foods and low in animal fats lower the risk for cancer. The specific agents responsible for cancer protection are unknown (World Cancer Research Fund, 1997). At best, the evidence is mixed that dietary supplements taken for health promotion and disease prevention actually provide the benefits expected by consumers and patients. However, given the high rate of dietary supplement use among the general population and those diagnosed with cancer, a better understanding of possible differences between a dietary factor in food and the same factor as a supplement is necessary. As new molecular and technological approaches are developed to study the nutritional sciences, investigations can be designed to elucidate the mechanisms of action of dietary factors in both forms. Experimental and animal models must be developed to help assess the safety and efficacy of the multitude of vitamins, minerals, and botanicals in the marketplace. Also, identification and use of intermediate outcomes as endpoints in future clinical research could provide a more cost-effective method for gauging the efficacy of dietary supplements. Furthermore, attention should be directed toward possible confounding effects of supplement use by participants in clinical trials for cancer prevention and control. From a broader research perspective, there is a need to investigate dietary supplement use in the context of health disparities and cultural, ethnic, and demographic determinants. A better understanding of supplement timing, dose and dose–response, and vulnerability of specific populations is essential for providing scientifically sound information on the use of dietary supplements.

Important issues to be addressed in research aimed at determining the effects of dietary supplements on cancer include developing better methods to measure the contribution of dietary supplements for various population groups and to monitor these usage trends over time. Although data are available on the prevalence of dietary supplement use among people with cancer, the data collection is not systematic and the data are not collected both before and after cancer diagnosis. The majority of information is collected on people who have been diagnosed with cancer. This makes inferences to the role of supplements in cancer prevention difficult, if not impossible. Although some of the nationally representative survey data provide comparisons between cancer patients and individuals not diagnosed with cancer, the number of cancer patients is too small, limiting the strength of the comparative results. Additionally, although some studies collect data on new supplement use (post diagnosis), most do not ask about length of time for which supplements have been used.

The systematic collection of prevalence data could include the development of a set of core prevalence indicators that include definitions of *cancer patient* or *survivor*, frequency of supplement use (daily, regularly, ever), length of time a supplement has been used, supplement dose (low to high for each supplement), motivators for use, perceived benefits, and other user characteristics. Such systematic prevalence data could assist researchers, healthcare professionals, and policymakers in identifying the supplements most frequently used and the characteristics of those most likely to use them, helping to set an agenda for future research. Along with ensuring that prevalence data on supplements includes botanicals and other nonbotanical nonmicronutrient products, additional work is necessary to understand how best to ask people questions about these supplements, given the different languages and names used in their sale, the multitude of herbal combinations used, and the variety of forms in which people take them (e.g., prepared teas, concentrated drinks, powders, and tablets).

Taking dietary supplements is likely to remain a significant strategy used by consumers and patients to improve health and combat diseases such as cancer. The scientific community must respond by providing guidance about the responsible use of these products to the public, medical professionals, and policymakers that is based on sound scientific evidence. Research—experimental, epidemiological, and clinical—on nutrition and cancer is the best way to identify dietary factors that show promise as cancer prevention or control agents. This approach will allow scientists to either confirm or refute the growing amount of consumer information on the benefits and risks of dietary supplement use. Physicians and healthcare providers need to openly discuss the use of dietary supplements with their patients, especially because many supplement users get most of their information about these products from friends, family, the media, and other word-of-mouth sources. Patients need to understand the potential positive and negative impacts of the supplements they may choose to use and need to be informed that supplements should not be used as a substitute for medical therapies. Healthcare providers should encourage patients to enumerate the various supplements they take and provide expert advice about using these products responsibly. The NIH Office of Dietary Supplements, for example, provides helpful materials for this purpose, including a consumer-friendly brochure titled "What Dietary Supplements Are You Taking? Does Your Health Care Provider Know? It Matters and Here's Why" (Office of Dietary Supplements, 2005).

References

Agency for Healthcare Research and Quality. 2002. Systems to rate the strength of scientific evidence. Agency for Healthcare Research and Quality, Rockville, MD. Evidence Report/Technology Assessment No. 47. AHRQ Publication No. 02-E016.

Agency for Healthcare Research and Quality. 2003. Effect of the supplemental use of antioxidants vitamin C, vitamin E, and coenzyme Q10 for the prevention and treatment of cancer. Agency for Healthcare Research and Quality, Rockville, MD. Evidence Report/Technology Assessment No. 75. AHRQ Publication No. 03-E047.

Alpha-Tocopherol, Beta-Carotene Cancer Prevention Study Group. 1994. The effect of vitamin E and beta carotene on the incidence of lung cancer and other cancers in male smokers. *N Engl J Med* **330**: 1029–1035.

American Institute for Cancer Research. 2000. "Nutrition of the Cancer Patient." American Institute for Cancer Research, Washington, D.C.

Ball, S.D., Kertesz, D., and Moyer-Mileur, L.J. 2005. Dietary supplement use is prevalent among children with a chronic illness. *J Am Diet Assoc* **105**: 78–84.

Barnes, P.M., Powell-Griner, E., McFann, K., and Nahin, R. 2004. Complementary and alternative medicine use among adults: United States, Advance Data, No. 343. National Center for Health Statistics. (PHS) 2004–1250.

Bender, M.M., Levy, A.S., Schucker, R.E., and Yetley, E.A. 1992. Trends in prevalence and magnitude of vitamin and mineral supplement usage and correlation with health status. *J Am Diet Assoc* **92**: 1096–1101.

Borrás, E., Zaragozá, R., Morante, M., Garcia, C., Gimeno, A., López-Rodas, G., Barber, T., Miralles, V.J., Viña, J.R., and Torres, L. 2003. *In vivo* studies of altered expression patterns of p53 and proliferative control genes in chronic vitamin A deficiency and hypervitaminosis. *Eur J Biochem* **270**: 1493–1501.

Bouker, K.B., and Hilakivi-Clarke, L. 2000. Genistein: does it prevent or promote breast cancer? *Environ Health Perspect* **108**: 701–708.

Clark, L.C., Cantor, K.P., and Allaway, W.H. 1991. Selenium in forage crops and cancer mortality in U.S. counties. *Arch Environ Health* **46**: 37–42.

Conklin, K.A. 2000. Dietary antioxidants during cancer therapy: impact on chemotherapeutic effectiveness and development of side effects. *Nutr Cancer* **37**: 1–18.

Eisenberg, D.M., Davis, R.B., Ettner, S.L., and Appel, S. 1998. Trends in alternative medicine use in the United States, 1990–1997: results of a follow-up national survey. *JAMA* **280**:1569–1574.

Eliason, B.C., Kruger, J., Mark, D., and Rasmann, D.N. 1997. Dietary supplement users: demographics, product use, and medical system interaction. *J Am Board Fam Pract* **10**: 265–271.

Fennell, D. 2004. Determinants of supplement usage. *Prev Med* **39**: 932–939.

Fong, L.Y., Ishii, H., Nguyen, V.T., Vecchione, A., Farber, J.L., Croce, C.M., and Huebner, K. 2003. *P53* deficiency accelerates induction and progression of esophageal and forestomach tumors in zinc-deficient mice. *Cancer Res* **63**: 186–195.

Gilbert, L. 1999. "HealthFocus Trend Report." HealthFocus, Des Moines, IA.

Grau, M.V., Baron, J.A., Sandler, R.S., Haile, R.W., Beach, M.L., Church, T.R., and Heber, D. 2003. Vitamin D, calcium supplementation, and colorectal adenomas: results of a randomized trial. *J Natl Cancer Inst* **95**: 1765–1771.

Greger, J.L. 2001. Dietary supplement use: consumer characteristics and interests. *J Nutr* **131**: 1339S–1343S.

Greenlee, H., White, E., Patterson, R.E., and Kristal, A.R. 2004. Supplement use among cancer survivors in the Vitamins and Lifestyle (VITAL) study cohort. *J Altern Complement Med* **10**: 660–666.

Greenwald, P. 2003. Beta-carotene and lung cancer: a lesson for future chemoprevention investigations? *J Natl Cancer Inst* **95**: E1.

Greenwald, P., Clifford, C.K., and Milner, J.A. 2001. Diet and cancer prevention. *Eur J Cancer* **37**: 948–965.

Greenwald, P., Milner, J.A., Anderson, D.E., and McDonald, S.S. 2002. Micronutrients in cancer chemoprevention. *Cancer Metastas Rev* **21**: 217–230.

Hall, J.D., Bissonette, E.A., Boyd, J.C., and Theodorescu, D. 2003. Motivations and influences on the use of complementary medicine in patients with localized prostate cancer treated with curative intent: results of a pilot study. *BJU Int* **91**: 603–607.

Halsted, C.H. 2003. Dietary supplements and functional foods: 2 sides of a coin? *Am J Clin Nutr* **77**: 1001S–1007S.

Hedderson, M.M., Patterson, R.E., Neuhouser, M.L., Schwartz, S.M., Bowen, D.J., Standish, L.J., and Marshall, L.M. 2004. Sex differences in motives for use of complementary and alternative medicine among cancer patients. *Altern Ther Health Med* **10**(5): 58–64.

Heinonen, O.P., Albanes, D., Virtamo, J., Taylor, P.R., Huttunen, J.K., Hartman, A.M., Haapakoski, J., Malila, N., Rautalahti, M., Riatti, S., Maenpaa, H., Teerenhovi, L., Koss, L., Virolainen, M., and Edwards, B.K. 1998. Prostate cancer and supplementation with alpha-tocopherol and beta-carotene: incidence and mortality in a controlled trial. *J Natl Cancer Inst* **90**: 440–446.

Hensrud, D.D., Engle, D.D., and Scheitel, S.M. 1999. Underreporting the use of dietary supplements and nonprescription medications among patients undergoing periodic health examination. *Mayo Clin Proc* **74**: 443–447.

Hilakivi-Clarke, L., and Clarke, R. 1998. Timing of dietary fat exposure and mammary tumorigenesis: role of estrogen receptor and protein kinase C activity. *Mol Cell Biochem* **188**: 5–12.

Hoque, A., Albanes, D., Lippman, S.M., Spitz, M.R., Taylor, P.R., Klein, E.A., Thompson, I.M., Goodman, P., Stanford, J.L., Crowley, J.J., Coltman, C.A., and Santella, R.M. 2001. Molecular epidemiologic studies within the Selenium and Vitamin E Cancer Prevention Trial (SELECT). *Cancer Causes Control* **12**: 627–633.

Hsieh, C.Y., Santell, R.C., Haslam, S.Z., and Helferich, W.G. 1998. Estrogenic effects of genistein on the growth of estrogen receptor-positive human breast cancer (MCF-7) cells *in vitro* and *in vivo*. *Cancer Res* **58**: 3833–3838.

Jarred, R.A., Keikha, M., Dowling, C., McPherson, S.J., Clare, A.M., Husband, A.J., Pedersen, J.S., Frydenberg, M., and Risbridger, G.P. 2002. Induction of apoptosis in low to moderate-grade human prostate carcinoma by red clover-derived dietary isoflavones. *Cancer Epidemiol Biomarkers Prev* **11**: 1689–1696.

Jazieh, A.R., Kopp, M., Foraida, M., Ghouse, M., Khalil, M., Savidge, M., Sethuraman, G. 2004. The use of dietary supplements by veterans with cancer. *J Altern Complement Med* **10**: 560–564.

Jennings, E. 1995. Folic acid as a cancer preventing agent. *Med Hypotheses* **45**: 297–303.

Ju, Y.H., Doerge, D.R., Allred, K.F., Allred, C.D., and Helferich, W.G. 2002. Dietary genistein negates the inhibitory effect of tamoxifen on growth of estrogen-dependent human breast cancer (MCF-7) cells implanted in athymic mice. *Cancer Res* **62**: 2474–2477.

Kearney, J., Giovannucci, E., Rimm, E.B., Ascherio, A., Stampfer, M.J., Colditz, G.A., Wing, A., Kampman, E., and Willett, W.C. 1996. Calcium, vitamin D, and dairy foods and the occurrence of colon cancer in men. *Am J Epidemiol* **143**: 907–917.

Khosraviani, K., Weir, H.P., Hamilton, P., Moorehead, J., and Williamson, K. 2002. Effect of folate supplementation on mucosal cell proliferation in high risk patients for colon cancer. *Gut* **51**: 195–199.

Kim, Y.I. 1999. Folate and cancer prevention: a new medical application of folate beyond hyperhomocysteinemia and neural tube defects. *Nutr Rev* **57**: 314–321.

Klein, E.A., Thompson, I.M., Lippman, S.M., Goodman, P.J., Albanes, D., Taylor, P.R., and Coltman, C. 2003. The selenium and vitamin E cancer prevention trial. *Semin Urol Oncol* **21**: 59–65.

Koplan, J.P., Annest, J.L., Layde, P.M., and Rubin, G.L. 1986. Nutrient intake and supplementation in the United States (NHANES II). *Am J Public Health* **76**: 287–289.

Kumar, N.B., Hopkins, K., Allen, K., Riccardi, D., Besterman-Dahan, K., and Moyers, S. 2002. Use of complementary/integrative nutritional therapies during cancer treatment: implications in clinical practice. *Cancer Control* **9**: 236–243.

Lamartiniere, C.A., Cotroneo, M.S., Fritz, W.A., Wang, J., Mentor-Marcel, R., and Elgavish, A. 2002. Genistein chemoprevention: timing and mechanisms of action in murine mammary and prostate. *J Nutr* **132**: 552S–558S.

Lengacher, C.A., Bennett, M.P., Kip, K.E., Keller, R., LaVance, M.S., Smith, L.S., and Cox, C.E. 2002. Frequency of use of complementary and alternative medicine in women with breast cancer. *Oncol Nurs Forum* **29**: 1445–1452.

Lissoni, P., Barni, S., Mandala, M., Ardizzoia, A., Paolorossi, F., Vaghi, M., Longarini, R., Malugani, F., and Tancini, G. 1999. Decreased toxicity and increased efficacy of cancer chemotherapy using the pineal hormone melatonin in metastatic solid tumour patients with poor clinical status. *Eur J Cancer* **35**: 1688–1692.

Lissoni, P., Meregalli, S., Nosetto, L., Barni, S., Tancini, G., Fossati, V., and Maestroni, G. 1996. Increased survival time in brain glioblastomas by a radioneuroendocrine strategy with radiotherapy plus melatonin compared to radiotherapy alone. *Oncology* **53**: 43–46.

Lissoni, P., Paolorossi, F., Ardizzoia, A., Barni, S., Chilelli, M., Mancuso, M., Tancini, G., Conti, A., and Maestroni, G.J. 1997. A randomized study of chemotherapy with cisplatin plus etoposide versus chemoendocrine therapy with cisplatin, etoposide and the pineal hormone melatonin as a first-line treatment of advanced non–small cell lung cancer patients in a poor clinical state. *J Pineal Res* **23**: 15–19.

Lyle, B., Mares-Perlman, J., Klein, B., Klein, R., and Greger, J.L. 1998. Supplement users differ from nonusers in demographic, lifestyle, dietary and health characteristics. *J Nutr* **128**: 2855–2862.

Mark, S.D., Qiao, Y.L., Dawsey, S.M., Wu, Y.P., Katki, H., Gunter, E.W., Fraumeni, J.F. Jr, Blot, W.J., Dong, Z.W., and Taylor, P.R. 2000. Prospective study of serum selenium levels and incident esophageal and gastric cancers. *J Natl Cancer Inst* **92**: 1753–1763.

Martínez, M.E., Giovannucci, E.L., Colditz, G.A., Stampfer, M.J., Hunter, D.J., Speizer, F.E., Wing, A., and Willett, W.C. 1996. Calcium, vitamin D, and the occurrence of colorectal cancer among women. *J Natl Cancer Inst* **88**: 1375–1382.

Mathijssen, R.H., Verweij, J., de Bruijn, P., Loos, W.J., and Sparreboom, A. 2002. Effects of St. John's wort on irinotecan metabolism. *J Natl Cancer Inst* **94**: 1247–1249.

McDavid, K., Breslow, R.A., and Radimer, K. 2001. Vitamin/mineral supplementation among cancer survivors: 1987 and 1992 National Health Interview Surveys. *Nutr Cancer* **41**: 29–32.

McMichael-Phillips, D.F., Harding, C., Morton, M., Robert, S.A., Howell, A., Potten, C.S., and Bundred, N.J. 1998. Effects of soy-protein supplementation on epithelial proliferation in the histologically normal human breast. *Am J Clin Nutr* **68**: 1431S–1436S.

Medeiros, D.M., Bock, M.A., Ortiz, M., Raab, C., Read, M., Schutz, H.G., Sheehan, E.T., and Williams, D.K. 1989. Vitamin and mineral supplementation practices of adults in seven western states. *J Am Diet Assoc* **89**: 383–386.

Metz, J.M., Jones, H., Devine, P., Hahn, S., and Glatstein, E. 2001. Cancer patients use unconventional medical therapies far more frequently than standard history and physical examination suggest. *Cancer J* **7**: 149–154.

Messina, M. J., and Loprinzi, C. L. 2001. Soy for breast cancer survivors: a critical review of the literature. *J Nutr* **131**: 3095S–3108S.

Messina, M. J., Persky, V., Setchell, K. D., and Barnes, S. 1994. Soy intake and cancer risk: a review of the *in vitro* and *in vivo* data. *Nutr Cancer* **21**: 113–131.

Millen, A.E., Dodd, K.W., and Subar, A.F. 2004. Use of vitamin, nonvitamin, and nonmineral supplements in the United States: The 1987, 1992, and 2000 National Health Interview Survey results. *J Am Diet Assoc* **104**: 942–950.

Milner, J.A., McDonald, S.S., Anderson, D.E., and Greenwald, P. 2001. Molecular targets for nutrients involved with cancer prevention. *Nutr Cancer* **41**: 1–16.

Moss, A.J., Levy, A.S., Kim, I., and Park, Y.K. 1989. Use of vitamin and mineral supplements in the United States: current users, types of products, and nutrients. National Center for Health Statistics. Advance Data, No. 174.

Neuhouser, M.L., Kristal, A.R., Patterson, R.E., and Thompson, I. 2001a. Dietary supplement use in the Prostate Cancer Prevention Trial: implications for prevention trials. *Nutr Cancer* **39**: 12–18.

Neuhouser, M.L., Patterson, R.E., Schwartz, S.M., Hedderson, M.M., Bowen, D.J., and Standish, L.J. 2001b. Use of alternative medicine by children with cancer in Washington State. *Prev Med* **33**: 347–354.

Newman, V., Rock, C.L., Faerber, S., Flatt, S.W., Wright, F.A., and Pierce, J.P. 1998. Dietary supplement use by women at risk for breast cancer recurrence: the Women's Healthy Eating and Living Study Group. *J Am Diet Assoc* **98**: 285–292.

NIH Consensus Conference. 1994. Optimal calcium intake. National Institutes of Health Consensus Development Panel on Optimal Calcium Intake. *JAMA* **272**: 1942–1948.

Norman, H.A., Butrum, R.R., Feldman, E., Heber, D., Nixon, D., Picciano, M.F., Rivlin, R., Simopoulos, A., Wargovich, M.J., Weisburger, E.K., and Zeisel, S.H. 2003. The role of dietary supplements during cancer therapy. *J Nutr* **133**:3794S–3799S.

Nutrition Business Journal. 2004. Top 100 selling supplements sales and growth 1997–2003. Available at: http://www.nutritionbusiness.com. Accessed September 29, 2004.

Nutrition Business Journal. 2005. Annual industry overview. *Nutrition Business J* **10**(5–6): 1–11.

Office of Dietary Supplements. 2004. Promoting quality science in dietary supplement research, education, and communication: a strategic plan for the Office of Dietary Supplements 2004–2009. National Institutes of Health. Publication No. 04-5533. Available at: http://ods.od.nih.gov/strategicplan2004. Accessed August 3, 2005.

Office of Dietary Supplements. 2005. What dietary supplements are you taking? Does your health care provider know? It matters and here's why. Available at: http://ods.od.nih.gov/pubs/partnersbrochure.asp. Accessed August 3, 2005.

Omenn, G.S., Goodman, G.E., Thornquist, M.D., Balmes, J., Cullen, M.R., Glass, A., Keogh, J.P., Meyskens, F.L., Jr., Valanis, B., Williams, J.H., Jr., Barnhart, S., and Hammar, S. 1996. Effects of a combination of beta carotene and vitamin A on lung cancer and cardiovascular disease. *N Engl J Med* **334**: 1150–1155.

Patterson, R.E., Neuhouser, M.L., Hedderson, M.M., Schwartz, S.M., Standish, L.J., and Bowen, D.J. 2003. Changes in diet, physical activity, and supplement use among adults diagnosed with cancer. *J Am Diet Assoc* **103**: 323–328.

Patterson, R.E., Neuhouser, M.L., White, E., Hunt, J.R., and Kristal, A.R. 1998. Cancer-related behavior of vitamin supplement users. *Cancer Epidemiol Biomarkers Prev* **7**: 79–81.

Patton, A.M., Kassis, J., Doong, H., and Kohn, E.C. 2003. Calcium as a molecular target in angiogenesis. *Curr Pharm Des* **9**: 543–551.

Peterson, G., and Barnes, S. 1996. Genistein inhibits both estrogen and growth factor–stimulated proliferation of human breast cancer cells. *Cell Growth Differ* **7**: 1345–1351.

Petrakis, N.L., Barnes, S., King, E.B., Lowenstein, J., Wiencke, J., Lee, M.M., Miike, R., Kirk, M., and Coward, L. 1996. Stimulatory influence of soy protein isolate on breast secretion in pre- and postmenopausal women. *Cancer Epidemiol Biomarkers Prev* **5**: 785–794.

Radimer, K., Bindewald, B., Hughes, J., Ervin, R., Swanson, C., and Picciano, M.F. 2004. Dietary supplement use by US adults: data from the National Health and Nutrition Examination Survey, 1999–2000. *Am J Epidemiol* **160**: 339–349.

Radimer, K.L., Subar, A.F., and Thompson, F.E. 2000. Nonvitamin, nonmineral dietary supplements: issues and findings from NHANES III. *J Am Diet Assoc* **100**: 447–454.

Rock, C.L., Newman, V.A., Neuhouser, M.L., Major, J., and Barnett, M.J. 2004. Antioxidant supplement use in cancer survivors and the general population. *J Nutr* **134**: 3194S–3195S.

Russell, R.M. 2000. The vitamin A spectrum: from deficiency to toxicity. *Am J Clin Nutr* **71**: 878–884.

Sakamoto, K., and Sakka, M. 1973. Reduced effect of irradiation on normal and malignant cells irradiated *in vivo* in mice pretreated with vitamin E. *Br J Radiol* **46**: 538–540.

Salminen, E., Bishop, M., Poussa, T., Drummond, R., and Salminen, S. 2004. Dietary attitudes and changes as well as use of supplements and complementary therapies by Australian and Finnish women following the diagnosis of breast cancer. *Eur J Clin Nutr* **58**: 137–144.

Slesinski, M.J., Subar, A.F., and Kahle, L.L. 1995. Trends in use of vitamin and mineral supplements in the United States: the 1987 and 1992 National Health Interview Surveys. *J Am Diet Assoc* **95**: 921–923.

Steward, M.L., McDonald, J.T., Schucker, R.E., and Henderson, D.P. 1985. Vitamin/mineral supplement use: a telephone survey of adults in the United States. *J Am Diet Assoc* **85**: 1585–1590.

Subar, A.F., and Block, G. 1990. Use of vitamin and mineral supplements: demographics and amounts of nutrients consumed in the 1987 Health Interview Survey. *Am J Epidemiol* **132**: 1091–1101.

Sylvester, P.W., and Shah, S.J. 2005. Mechanisms mediating the antiproliferative and apoptotic effects of vitamin E in mammary cancer cells. *Front Biosci* **10**: 699–709.

Trock, B., White, B.L., Clarke, R., and Hilakivi-Clarke, L. 2000. Meta-analysis of soy intake and breast cancer risk. *J Nutr* **130**: 653S–680S.

U.S. Congress. 1994. Dietary Supplement Health and Education Act (DSHEA). Public Law 103-417. U.S. Government Printing Office, Washington, D.C.

U.S. Preventive Services Task Force. 2003. Routine vitamin supplementation to prevent cancer and cardiovascular disease: recommendations and rationale. *Ann Intern Med* **139**: 51–55.

Weiger, W.A., Smith, M., Boon, H., Richardson, M.A., Kaptchuk, T.J., and Eisenberg, D.M. 2002. Advising patients who seek complementary and alternative medical therapies for cancer. *Ann Intern Med* **137**: 889–903.

Whiting, S.J. 1995. The inhibitory effect of dietary calcium on iron bioavailability: a cause for concern? *Nutr Rev* **53**: 77–80.

Wiseman, H. 1996. Role of dietary phyto-oestrogens in the protection against cancer and heart disease. *Biochem Soc Trans* **24**: 795–800.

World Cancer Research Fund. 1997. "Food, Nutrition, and the Prevention of Cancer: A Global Perspective." American Institute for Cancer Research, Washington, DC.

Wu, K., Willett, W.C., Fuchs, C.S., Colditz, G.A., and Giovannucci, E.L. 2002. Calcium intake and risk of colon cancer in women and men. *J Natl Cancer Inst* **94**: 437–446.

Yu, L., Blackburn, G.L., and Zhou, J.R. 2003. Genistein and daidzein downregulate prostate androgen-regulated transcript-1 (PART-1) gene expression induced by dihydrotestosterone in human prostate LNCaP cancer cells. *J Nutr* **133**: 389–392.

CHAPTER

29

Dietary Fiber and Carbohydrates

MARÍA ELENA MARTÍNEZ AND ELIZABETH T. JACOBS

INTRODUCTION

Various dietary factors have long been suspected to play a prominent role in the etiology of cancer. A substantial amount of research has been carried out in attempts to identify the specific risk factors. Dietary hypotheses comprise several macronutrients and micronutrients, as well as other dietary constituents. Although little focus has been placed on the direct effect of carbohydrates in general, a great deal of effort has been spent on identifying the specific role of dietary fiber and its food sources as potential protective factors for various cancers. However, the overall contribution of fiber to cancer risk is unclear. This uncertainty is due to a variety of reasons, including the chemical complexity of dietary fiber, the lack of direct evidence regarding the exact mechanism of action specific to each type of fiber, and our limited understanding of the carcinogenic process. This chapter focuses on malignancies for which the effect of carbohydrates and dietary fiber has been investigated. Although the data suggest some consistent patterns for some malignancies, some uncertainties are also evident. An attempt is made to outline plausible new and existing mechanisms of action for these effects. Overall, the complexities inherent in the study of diet and cancer, which involve complex biological mechanisms and human behavior, create an enormous and exciting challenge for future investigations.

CARBOHYDRATE CLASSIFICATION AND METABOLISM

Carbohydrates are classified as monosaccharides, disaccharides, and polysaccharides (Table 1). Whereas monosaccharides cannot be hydrolyzed to a simpler form, disaccharides may be hydrolyzed to give two molecules of the same or different monosaccharides, and polysaccharides yield >10 units. Carbohydrates are absorbed through the intestinal mucosa as monosaccharides, primarily glucose, with minor quantities of other sugars. All carbohydrates are then carried in the portal blood to the liver, after which they are utilized in one of several ways. The principal function of carbohydrates is to serve as a major source of energy for the body. The body tissues require a constant daily supply of carbohydrates in the form of glucose in all metabolic reactions. Much of the glucose is used for immediate energy needs via oxidation to CO_2 and water. Part is stored as glycogen in the liver and muscle tissue, and some is converted to fatty acids and possibly stored as triglycerides in fat tissue. A small amount is converted to other necessary carbohydrates and some becomes the carbon skeletons for the production by the body of the nonessential amino acids.

Carbohydrates that escape digestion and absorption in the small intestine and yield short-chain fatty acids in the large intestine are mainly the nonstarch polysaccharides (NSPs) and the resistant starches. Cellulose and other insoluble indigestible carbohydrates aid in normal elimination by stimulating the peristaltic movements of the gastrointestinal (GI) tract and absorbing water to give bulk to the intestinal contents.

DIETARY FIBER

Definition and Physiological Effects

Dietary fiber is defined as the endogenous components of plant materials in the diet that are resistant to digestion by

Copyright © 2006, Elsevier Inc.
All rights of reproduction in any form reserved.

TABLE 1 Classification of Carbohydrates

		Polysaccharides	
Monosaccharides	**Disaccharides**	**Digestible**	**Nonresistant starch**
Glucose	Sucrose	Starch	Cellulose
Galactose	Lactose	Resistant starch	Hemicellulose
Fructose	Maltose	Dextrins	Pectin
		Glycogen	Gums
		Inulin	Mucilages
		Mannosans	
		Raffinose	
		Stachyose	
		Pentosans	

the enzymes produced by intestinal flora (Trowell et al., 1985; Cummings and Bingham, 1987; Pilch, 1987; Kritchevsky, 1988). Fibers in foods are complex carbohydrates; however, due to their chemical complexity, they are poorly defined. Fiber consists of a heterogeneous mixture of complex polysaccharides and nonpolysaccharide polymers mostly made up of plant cell wall carbohydrate and NSP. By its definition, dietary fiber reaches the colon intact and is a major source of energy for colonic bacteria. Analytical methods have determined that dietary fiber is composed of at least six general components, which include cellulose, hemicellulose, pectins, gums, mucilages, and lignin (Table 1). According to the definition given by Trowell et al. (1985), dietary fiber is the sum of lignin and the plant polysaccharides that are not digested by the endogenous secretions of the human digestive tract. Thus, lignin, a noncarbohydrate, can be included in this definition. Lignin, a highly polymeric substance occurring in woody plant tissues, is virtually indigestible. Values for lignins (enterolactone and enterodiol) can be obtained from published sources (Thompson et al., 1991).

The physiological effects of dietary fiber depend largely on the type of fiber. Thus, these effects differ whether reference is made to foods rich in fiber such as grain products, legumes, fruit, and vegetables or isolated fibers such as cellulose, pectin, or lignin. Although several types of fiber have been identified, for purposes of their mechanistic protective action in carcinogenesis, they can be classified into two general types according to water solubility. Soluble fibers are present in fruit, vegetables, and certain grains, such as oats. These include the gel-forming fibers such as pectins, gums, and mucilages. This type of fiber undergoes metabolism in the small intestine and especially in the large intestine, as bacterial enzymes convert it to products that increase stool size. The function of the pectins is mainly to absorb water, form gel, and increase bulk. Another important function of soluble fiber is its potential to slow down glucose absorption and lower serum cholesterol. These polysaccharides can prevent the absorption of nutrients such as carbohydrates and lipids from the gut (Jenkins et al., 1978; Blackburn and Johnson, 1981; Sandberg et al., 1983). In most cases, this results from slowing of absorption rather than an inhibition in amount absorbed; this action also involves delayed gastric emptying and slowed small bowel absorption (Jenkins et al., 1978). Enzymes in the intestinal flora do not substantially metabolize insoluble fibers, present in considerable amounts in bran cereals (i.e., wheat, rice). These fibers, which include cellulose, lignin, and some hemicelluloses, are insoluble and nonfermentable. Among these, cellulose is not hydrolyzed, whereas hemicellulose forms bulk and roughage. Such fibers increase stool size substantially through several mechanisms, including water retention. Therefore, these affect intestinal function by retaining water in the stool, thereby increasing fecal bulk and decreasing GI transit time. The larger bulk generated by the action of these fibers dilutes carcinogens, especially tumor promoters such as secondary bile acids, which may result in lower risk of some cancers, such as colon cancer. The fermentable soluble fibers are also capable of decreasing intestinal transit time by stimulating microbial growth in the intestine resulting in higher fecal bacterial mass.

The total amount of dietary fiber varies markedly in different foods. Furthermore, each type of fiber is composed of different proportions and combinations of the six basic components and no two are the same in their action in the GI tract. Although the exact action of dietary fiber depends on the type and amount of fiber ingested, most of this is limited to the large intestine. Adding to its complexity, the physiological effects of dietary fiber depend not only on the type of fiber ingested but also on the composition of the rest of the meal or diet and the unique physiology of the individual.

Analysis of Fiber in Foods

No method of dietary intake assessment is without flaws. Earlier animal research related to fiber focused on crude fiber and other methods that did not allow complete analysis of fiber in foods for human studies (Goering and van Soest, 1970; van Soest and van Soest, 1973). However, crude fiber consists mainly of lignin and cellulose, whereas dietary fiber contains these plus other components (hemicellulose, gums, pectin, etc.). Subsequently, analysis methods described by Southgate (1969, 1976) and Englyst (1980) evolved and became more applicable to studies in humans. The problems of isolating dietary polysaccharides (which are equivalent to dietary fiber) have been the objective of more recent methods for measuring fiber in food (Asp et al., 1992; Li, 1995). However, controversy regarding the most appropriate method of chemical analysis continues.

Dietary fiber, chemically speaking, is a polysaccharide and, in terms of food composition, is best seen as such. Currently, there is no one accepted definition or method of analysis for dietary fiber. Englyst and Cummings (1988) define it as a component of NSP. In this method of analysis, starch is removed enzymatically, after solubilization, and NSP is measured as the sum of constituent sugars released by acid hydrolysis. The Southgate method provides data on total dietary fiber and individual fiber components (cellulose, lignin, etc.); thus, the Englyst method is considered a modified Southgate method. The Association of Analytical Chemists (AOAC) describes *fiber* as endogenous plant food material from the diet that is resistant to human digestive secretions but that is substantially fermented in the colon (Prosky et al., 1985). This method relies on an enzymatic gravimetric system of analysis and has been suggested to be the most practical and simplest approach to measuring the major components of dietary fiber as a single unit (Dreher, 1987). The AOAC method is the most accepted in the United States, whereas that of Englyst is preferred in European countries. When data on dietary fiber and disease are reported using different analytical techniques, comparison across studies may be difficult. Thus, standardized analytical chemical techniques of fiber content in foods are imperative.

CARBOHYDRATES AND CANCER

Relatively few studies have focused solely on the effects of carbohydrate and its role in cancer risk. For colon cancer, results of correlational studies show a strong inverse association between intake of starch and risk of this malignancy (Cassidy et al., 1994). In analytical epidemiological studies, for the most part, investigators have focused on various food sources of carbohydrate, although analyses of total carbohydrate and colorectal adenoma and cancer were conducted in a large cohort of >34,000 women. The results showed no association between total carbohydrate intake and risk of colorectal adenoma (Oh et al., 2004) but did find an increased risk for colorectal cancer with higher carbohydrate intake (Higginbotham et al., 2004). A higher risk of colon cancer has been shown for higher intake of starch in countries such as Japan, where rice is the main source (Wynder et al., 1969); southern Europe, where pasta, rice, bread, polenta, potatoes, and cereals are the major sources (Macquart-Moulin et al., 1986; La Vecchia et al., 1988; Benito et al., 1990; Bidoli, et al., 1992; Centonze et al., 1994); Australia (Steinmetz and Potter, 1993); and Russia (Zaridze et al., 1985).

Because of its low incidence rate, investigations of diet and pancreatic cancer are few. Furthermore, most of the evidence relies on data from retrospective studies, many of which use proxy information on the case individuals. The largest data set comes from five case-control studies conducted simultaneously by the International Agency for Research on Cancer (IARC) SEARCH program (Howe et al., 1992). A main objective for the implementation of these studies was for the combination of the data in a pooled analysis. The data comprise >800 case and 2000 control individuals. For carbohydrate intake, four (Bueno de Mesquita et al., 1990; Howe et al., 1990b; Baghurst et al., 1991; Zatonoski et al., 1991) of the five case-control studies show positive associations with pancreatic cancer, although only one (Baghurst et al., 1991) was statistically significant. A combined analysis of these studies shows a significant positive association (odds ratio [OR] = 1.74; 95% confidence interval [CI], 1.26–2.40). However, data from two case-control studies not included in the SEARCH pooled analysis (Kalapothaki et al., 1993) do not support these findings. Thus, the evidence for the effect of carbohydrate- or starch-rich foods on risk of pancreatic cancer is inconsistent across studies. Furthermore, no biological mechanism has been identified.

As in the case of pancreatic cancer, epidemiological data on diet and gastric cancer have mainly derived from case-control studies. Although intake of fruit and vegetables is inversely correlated with risk of stomach cancer (Kono and Hirohata, 1996), the results for diets high in carbohydrate are less clear. Various case-control studies (Bjelke, 1974; Modan et al., 1974; Correa et al., 1985; Trichopoulos et al., 1985; Buiatti et al., 1990; Graham et al., 1990; Tuyns et al., 1992; Ramon et al., 1993) and one cohort study (Kneller et al., 1991) support a positive association between carbohydrate intake and risk of stomach cancer, although a small number did not (Correa et al., 1985; Gonzalez et al., 1991; Hansson et al., 1993). Among individual food sources of carbohydrate, pasta (Trichopoulos et al., 1985; La Vecchia et al., 1987) and rice (Haenszel et al., 1972; Nomura et al., 1990) consumption have been shown to increase risk; however, in countries where sufficient interindividual variation may be lacking, such an association is nonexistent (Hirayama, 1971; Haenszel et al., 1976; Hirohata, 1983; You et al., 1988; Kono et al., 1988). Thus, current data are inconclusive as to whether high-carbohydrate diets confer an increased risk for gastric cancer.

SIMPLE SUGARS AND CANCER

Investigations on the relationship between sucrose and the simple sugars and cancer have mainly been focused on colorectal malignancies. Biologically plausible mechanisms for an enhanced risk for colorectal cancer with higher intake of sucrose have been published (Bostick et al., 1994). Sucrose increases colonic epithelial cell proliferation and increases microadenoma formation (Corpet et al., 1990; Stamp et al., 1993) in rodents. In humans, a high sucrose diet increases mouth-to-anus transit time despite decreasing the mouth-to-cecum time and increases fecal concentration of both total and secondary bile acids (Kruis et al., 1991). At least 11 case-control studies (Phillips, 1975; Manousos et al., 1983; Miller et al., 1983; Pickle et al., 1984; Bristol et al., 1985; Macquart-Moulin et al., 1986; La Vecchia et al., 1988; Tuyns et al., 1988; Benito et al., 1990; Bidoli et al., 1992; Peters et al., 1992) and one cohort study (Bostick et al., 1994) have reported results on the relation of sucrose intake and colon cancer; of these, 10 (Phillips, 1975; Miller et al., 1983; Pickle et al., 1984; Bristol et al., 1985; Macquart-Moulin et al., 1986; La Vecchia et al., 1988; Tuyns et al., 1988; Benito et al., 1990; Bidoli et al., 1992; Bostick et al., 1994) indicate an association in the direction of increased risk with results being significant in three (Bristol et al., 1985; Tuyns et al., 1988; Bostick et al., 1994). In particular, in the Iowa Women's Health Study (Bostick, et al., 1994), the relative risk (RR) for the upper versus the lower quintile of sucrose-containing foods was 1.74 (95% CI, 1.06–2.87).

Few studies have investigated the association of sugar and other malignancies. Results of four case-control studies of pancreatic cancer (Raymond et al., 1987; Bueno de Mesquita et al., 1990; Baghurst et al., 1991; Kalapothaki et al., 1993) showed one null finding, one of a nonsignificant slightly elevated risk, and two of significant positive associations. In a cohort investigation conducted among women in the Nurses' Health Study, sucrose was not associated with increased risk of pancreatic cancer, although fructose appeared to be associated with increased risk, particularly among overweight and sedentary women (Michaud et al., 2002). However, data on this malignancy continue to be sparse and inconclusive.

GLYCEMIC INDEX AND CANCER

Glycemic index and glycemic load in the diet are among the new methodologies to assess the role of carbohydrates in disease etiology. Glycemic index uses a system whereby carbohydrates are ranked according to their acute effects on blood glucose levels. For example, the highest glycemic indexes are assigned to carbohydrates that are quickly broken down, whereas those that are more slowly metabolized are assigned a lower index score. Glycemic load takes into account the amount of carbohydrates by multiplying the grams of carbohydrates in the serving of food by its glycemic index.

High intake of highly refined carbohydrates has been recognized as a risk factor for a variety of chronic diseases, including type 2 diabetes, cardiovascular disease, obesity, and some cancers (Liu et al., 2000; Jenkins et al., 2002; Willett et al., 2002). Glycemic index represents a dietary indicator used to classify carbohydrate content of foods. Diets high in glycemic index or glycemic load have been associated with increased risk of colon cancer in some (Slattery et al., 1997; Franceschi, Dal Maso et al., 2001) but not all (Terry et al., 2003; Michaud et al., 2005) studies. In the Women's Health Study (Higginbotham et al., 2004), dietary glycemic load was statistically significantly associated with an increased risk of colorectal cancer (adjusted RR = 2.85; 95% CI, 1.40–5.80), comparing high versus low quintiles of dietary glycemic load.

High glycemic diets have also been investigated in relation to breast cancer risk. Results of a prospective study (Silvera et al., 2004) showed a positive association between glycemic index and postmenopausal breast cancer (RR = 1.87; 95% CI, 1.18–2.97). However, results of both the Cancer Prevention Study II (Jonas et al., 2003) and the Nurses' Health Study (Holmes et al., 2004) do not support this association. Other malignancies where glycemic index or load have been shown to be positively associated with risk include prostate cancer (Augustin et al., 2004) and pancreatic cancer (Michaud et al., 2002). Clearly, this active area of research is still in its infancy. As is the case with any observational study, reproducibility of findings from large studies, especially those prospective in nature, will be necessary before firm conclusions can be drawn regarding high glycemic diets and cancer risk.

FIBER AND CANCER

The malignancy most closely linked to fiber consumption is that of the colorectum. The observations by Burkitt in 1971 of lower incidence rates of colon cancer in African populations than in Western countries led to the hypothesis of an association of this malignancy with fiber intake. Correlational studies (Schrauzer, 1976; IARC, Intestinal Microecology Group, 1977; Liu et al., 1979) later supported this hypothesis. However, these studies also alluded to the complexity of exposure assessment, as the associations were often attenuated when other nutrients such as fat and cholesterol were taken into account (Greenwald et al., 1987). Correlational data comparing areas with high colon cancer rates and low fiber intake (e.g., New York) and those with low rates and high fiber intake (e.g., Finland) suggest that dietary fiber may account for the differences in the rates, given the similarities in dietary fat consumption (MacLennan et al., 1978).

Results of analytical epidemiological studies of a retrospective nature strongly support the fiber–colon cancer hypothesis. The results of a meta-analysis of 13 case-control studies of colon cancer showed a combined OR of 0.58 ($p < 0.001$) between the upper and lower quintile of fiber intake (Howe et al., 1992). Giovannucci and Willett (1994a) noted that most case-control studies have found an inverse association between total fiber and risk of colon cancer, although a stronger case can be made for the protective effect of fruit and/or vegetable consumption. Results of prospective studies (Heilbrun et al., 1989; Willett et al., 1990; Thun et al., 1992; Giovannucci et al., 1994; Steinmetz et al., 1994), on the other hand, are less convincing. Although an inverse association is shown when comparing highest with lowest categories of intake, the dose–response relationship is nonexistent, except for the American Cancer Society (ACS) study of colon cancer mortality (Thun et al., 1992). In this study, the exposure factor (the combination of vegetables, citrus, and high-fiber grain consumption) was inversely related to risk of fatal colon cancer (RR < 0.76; 95% CI, 0.57–1.02; p for trend < 0.031). Heilbrun et al. (1989) also showed a protective effect for dietary fiber and colon cancer risk; however, assessment of diet was made using a single 24-hour recall. The reasons for the inconsistency in the findings of the retrospective and prospective studies are not clear. It is possible that bias related to the difference in study design may account for the discrepancies. Also, early epidemiological studies focused on foods and food groups high in fiber only or used a measure of crude fiber rather than dietary fiber. Of interest, among the case-control studies reviewed by Giovannucci and Willett (1994a) published prior to 1990, only two of the nine reviewed show a significant reduction by dietary fiber on colon cancer risk, whereas the majority published in or after 1990 show a significant inverse association. Because issues related to the measurement and definition of fiber have only been recently addressed, future studies utilizing standard definitions and approaches should help clarify this field of research.

Although many studies appear to support a benefit of fiber, a puzzling observation has been that cereal fiber, generally the major determinant of fecal mass and determinant of transit time (Cummings et al., 1978), has not been related consistently to colon cancer risk in analytical epidemiological studies. Results of case-control studies that have examined the role of grain fiber or cereal fiber generally show intake to be unrelated or positively related to risk of colon cancer (Giovannucci and Willett, 1994a). Furthermore, only one prospective study (Thun et al., 1992) has shown a significant reduction in colon cancer risk associated with intake of high-fiber grains. In fact, vegetables and fruits, important contributors of water-soluble fibers, have historically been more consistently associated with reduced risk. Nonetheless, two large cohort studies of >135,000 men and women from the Nurses' Health Study and the Health Professionals' Follow-Up Study failed to find a protective effect of fruit and vegetable consumption on colorectal cancers (Michels et al., 2000). The RR for colon cancer associated with one extra serving of fruit per day was 1.02 (95% CI, 0.98–1.05), whereas for an additional vegetable serving, it was 1.03 (95% CI, 0.97–1.09). Results from the Nurses' Health Study also failed to show any impact of dietary fiber overall on colorectal cancers or adenomas (Fuchs et al., 1999), as discussed later in this chapter.

TABLE 2 Baseline Characteristics in the Wheat Bran Fiber and Polyp Prevention Trials

Characteristic	Wheat Bran Fiber Trial	Polyp Prevention Trial
Age (mean ± sd)	65.9 ± 8.8	61.1 ± 9.9
Gender (male)	874 (67%)	1228 (64%)
Family history of colorectal cancer (yes)	220 (17%)	479 (25%)
Previous adenomas (yes)	452 (35%)	334 (18%)
Aspirin use (yes)	368 (28.2)	438 (23%)
Folate (μg/day)	326.5 ± 136.6	304.4 ± 122.0
Calcium (mg/day)	892.3 ± 379.2	843.9 ± 433.9
Fiber (g/day)	21.9 ± 9.9	17.8 ± 7.8
Alcohol (g/day)	7.2 ± 14.9	7.1 ± 12.4
Energy (kcal/day)	1927.2 ± 699.0	1923.1 ± 582.7
Fat (g/day)	69.2 ± 30.5	76.9 ± 31.2

TABLE 3 Results from the Wheat Bran Fiber and Polyp Prevention Trials

	Recurrence (%)		
	Low fiber	High fiber	Relative risk (95% confidence interval)
Wheat Bran Fiber Trial	51.2	47.0	0.88 (0.70–1.11)
Polyp Prevention Trial	39.5	39.7	1.00 (0.90–1.12)

Further adding to the equivocal results in the literature, two large clinical trials of fiber and colorectal adenoma recurrence showed that fiber appeared to have no protective effect. Table 2 presents selected baseline characteristics of the participants in these trials.

The Wheat Bran Fiber Trial (Alberts et al., 2000) tested the effect of a high-fiber cereal supplement (13.5 g/day) and a low-fiber supplement (2.0 g/day) on adenoma recurrence over 3 years of supplementation among patients who had recently had an adenoma removed at colonoscopy (Alberts et al., 2000). No difference was observed between the treatment groups for adenoma recurrence (Table 3). Upon further analysis of this trial, there was a suggestion that, in those who were already consuming relatively high amounts of fiber at baseline, the fiber intervention did result in protection from adenoma recurrence (Jacobs et al., 2002), but these results must be further explored. The Polyp Prevention Trial (PPT) was a multicenter study conducted by the National Cancer Institute to evaluate whether a dietary intervention aimed at decreasing fat intake and increasing consumption of fiber, fruits, and vegetables reduced the rate of adenoma recurrence when compared with a usual diet after 4 years of follow-up (Schatzkin et al., 2000). As shown in Table 3, no reduction in risk was observed for adenoma recurrence (Schatzkin et al., 2000).

Following the publication of these two clinical trials, two large prospective investigations reported that higher intake of fiber was indeed associated with a significantly decreased risk of colorectal adenoma (Peters et al., 2003) and cancer (Bingham et al., 2003).

In the study conducted within the Prostate, Lung, Colorectal, and Ovarian (PLCO) Cancer Screening Trial, participants in the highest quintile of total dietary fiber intake had a 27% decreased risk of adenoma compared with those in the lowest quintile (p trend = 0.002). The European Prospective Investigation into Cancer and Nutrition (EPIC) study results showed that the highest quintile of dietary fiber intake was associated with a relative risk of 0.75 (95% CI, 0.59–0.95) for colorectal cancer compared with the lowest quintile of intake. Again, the reasons for the discrepant results are unclear. One possibility is related to differences in fiber intake in the populations under study. For example, participants in the highest quartile of the PLCO and EPIC studies, in which a protective effect of fiber was observed, had a median fiber intake of ~31 g/day (Figure 1). In contrast, those in the highest quartile of the Nurses' Health Study, in which no protection from fiber was reported, were consuming a comparatively lower 25 g/day (Figure 1). These results suggest that the amount of fiber necessary for protection from colorectal neoplasia may be higher than has been attained in clinical trials thus far. Equivocal results between the cohort studies and the clinical intervention trials might relate to limitations inherent in intervention studies of adenoma recurrence (Martinez, 2001); these include short intervention phase as well as the fact that these studies are assessing recurrence of the premalignant lesion rather than cancer. Lifetime intake of a variety of foods high in fiber may be necessary for protection from colorectal neoplasia. Therefore, a negative finding from clinical trials of adenoma recurrence does not necessarily translate into a lack of efficacy of the intervention.

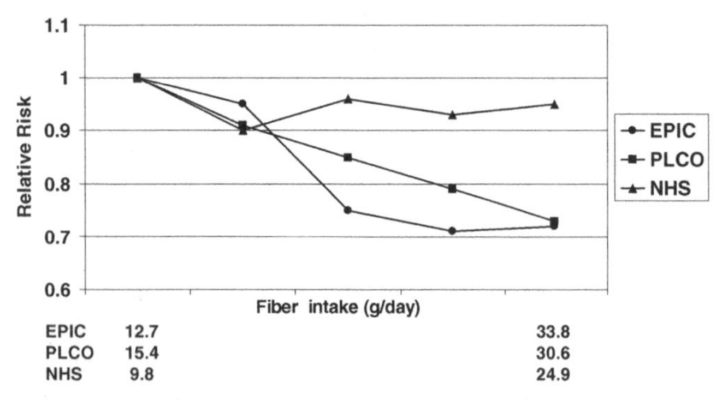

FIGURE 1 Association between dietary fiber and colon cancer (European Prospective Investigation into Cancer and Nutrition [EPIC] and Nurses' Health Study) or colorectal adenoma (Prostate, Lung, Colorectal, and Ovarian [PLCO).

Potential Mechanisms of Action

There are several, not mutually exclusive, mechanisms by which dietary fiber may modify colon cancer risk. One important mechanism involves the physiochemical capacity of fiber to bind cytotoxic bile acids, which may act as tumor promoters, thereby making them unavailable for metabolic activity (Jacobs, 1988). Fibers, particularly insoluble fibers, modify the enzyme activities of the intestinal bacterial flora, usually yielding a lower level of such enzymes (Weisburger et al., 1993). Some of the fibers also generate a lower intestinal pH such that the hydrolytic enzymes are not in a medium. An important aspect of intestinal biochemistry stemming from fiber, particularly insoluble fiber, is the lower rate of conversion of primary bile acids produced in the liver and secreted in the bile. Primary bile acids are converted to secondary bile acids through the action of enzymes from the bacterial flora, the activity of which is a function of intestinal fiber content. Most studies that have investigated the effect of wheat bran fiber dietary supplementation on the concentration and excretion of fecal bile acids have shown an increase in total and/or secondary fecal bile acid excretion, as well as a significant decrease in fecal bile acid concentrations (Reddy et al., 1977; Hill, 1991). Results of a published double-blinded phase II trial of wheat bran fiber (2.0 or 13.5 g/day) and calcium carbonate (250 or 1500 mg/day) showed that high-dose wheat bran fiber supplement was associated with a significant reduction in total and secondary fecal bile acid concentrations after 9 months of intervention (Alberts et al., 1996). These results suggest that one important mechanism by which wheat bran fiber may reduce colon cancer risk is through the reduction in concentration of secondary bile acids.

Given the international variations in breast cancer rates, it has been suggested that diet and differences in endogenous estrogen metabolism and excretion may play a role in the development of this malignancy (Miller and Bulbrook, 1986; Parkin et al., 1993). Although a modest number of studies have assessed the role of fiber or its components in breast cancer risk, a protective effect is largely supported by results of case-control studies (Lubin et al., 1986; Rohan et al., 1988; Howe et al., 1990a; Van'T Veer et al., 1990; Graham et al., 1991; Lee et al., 1991; Baghurst and Rohan, 1994; Yuan et al., 1995; Freudenheim et al., 1996; De Stefani et al., 1997; Bonilla-Fernandez et al., 2003; Mattisson et al., 2004). Howe et al. (1990a) conducted a combined analysis of 12 case-control studies carried out in Argentina, Australia, Canada, China, Greece, Hawaii, Israel, and Italy. These results also support a modest protective effect for dietary fiber and risk of breast cancer, with an increase of 20 g of fiber per day associated with RRs of 0.89 ($p < 0.15$) for premenopausal and 0.83 ($p < .02$) for postmenopausal women. Of some concern, however, are data from the few published cohort studies (Kushi et al., 1992; Willett et al., 1992) less prone to recall and selection bias, which do not support an inverse association between dietary fiber and breast cancer.

Among the proposed mechanisms for the protective effect of fiber on breast carcinogenesis, the most widely accepted is that of the alteration of estrogen levels by dietary fiber (Adlercreutz, 1990). The exact mechanism responsible for this action is unclear. It is suggested that fiber may affect the enterohepatic circulation of estrogens and the actions of fiber-associated phytoestrogens (Rose, 1990; Rose et al., 1991). Based on this hypothesis, intervention studies have been conducted to assess the indirect effect of various fiber components on mammary tumors. Although the results of these studies have demonstrated the potential for change in estrogen levels by means of interventions consisting of high-fiber or low-fat diets, they do not provide clear evidence for these effects (Adlercreutz et al., 1989; Woods et al., 1989, 1996; Rose et al., 1991; Goldin et al., 1994).

Overall, data concerning the relationship between dietary fiber and breast cancer indicate that the degree of protection due to fiber intake is unclear, and that the exact mechanism by which fiber may act is unknown. The potential for a protective effect of fiber on breast cancer risk is of great public health importance, given that most recognized risk factors for this disease are not modifiable.

Data on the relation between fiber and pancreatic cancer are consistent with a protective effect of this nutrient in all (Bueno de Mesquita et al., 1990, 1991; Howe et al., 1990b; Baghurst et al., 1991; Ji et al., 1995), with one of the studies (Zatonoski et al., 1991) reporting data on fiber. The association was significant in most studies (Bueno de Mesquita et al., 1990; Howe et al., 1990b, 1991). Consequently, the pooled analysis of the five SEARCH studies showed a significant association (OR = 0.42; 95% CI, 0.12–0.63; *p* for trend < 0.01). Simultaneous adjustment for saturated, monounsaturated, and polyunsaturated fat, protein, carbohydrate, cholesterol, fiber, and vitamin C showed an even stronger effect for fiber where an increase of 26 g/day was associated with an OR of 0.37 (95% CI, 0.25–0.55). From the SEARCH data, it is suggested that dietary fiber, as well as fruit and vegetable consumption, may play an important role in decreasing risk of pancreatic cancer.

Additional Plausible Mechanisms

Dietary carbohydrate is heterogeneous in nature, and therefore a simple carbohydrate– or even a fiber–cancer hypothesis may be unjustified. The various existing proposed biological mechanisms for the specific carbohydrates and their constituents have been addressed earlier in this chapter. A strong case can also be made for two additional hypotheses: One is based on existing data based on the correlation of fiber and carbohydrates with other nutrients known to be related to cancer risk, and the second is from a proposal by Giovannucci (1995) dealing with insulin resistance.

Giovannucci (1995) proposed that exposure to elevated blood-insulin levels may promote the growth of colon tumors. Thus, hyperinsulinemia or its determinants may increase the occurrence of colon cancer. If this hypothesis is correct, the determinants of both fasting and postprandial serum insulin levels should have an effect on colon cancer risk. As discussed earlier, epidemiological data suggest that a diet high in refined carbohydrates and low in water-soluble fiber increases risk of colon cancer. These same factors lead to the rapid absorption of glucose into the blood and cause postprandial hyperinsulinemia. Among dietary factors, simple sugars, easily digestible starch, low water-soluble fiber, and extensive food processing, which contribute to a high glycemic load, result in hyperinsulinemia and a subsequent increase in risk of colon cancer.

Among all fibers, water-soluble fibers appear to be most effective in leveling off blood glucose response and moderating insulin levels (Riccardi and Riverllese, 1991; Wolever et al., 1991) in response to carbohydrate intake. Therefore, it is plausible that the carcinogenic or protective action of carbohydrates and/or its constituents in colon carcinogenesis might involve the effect of these nutrients or their sources on insulin levels. This mechanism may involve the stimulation of growth of colon tumors by insulin's action as a growth factor of colonic epithelial cells (Koenuma et al., 1989). Based on present knowledge, it can be further hypothesized that the carcinogenic mechanism of action differs depending on the type of fiber. If focus is placed on insoluble fiber, particularly that derived from wheat bran, its action is known to be mediated through the direct effect on bile acid metabolism and excretion. However, if emphasis is placed on fruit and vegetables, rich sources of soluble fiber, their anticarcinogenic effect may be mediated through their action on insulin levels. It must be emphasized, however, that sufficient direct evidence is lacking to support the various proposed steps. Clearly, much research needs to take place before we can put all the pieces of this complex puzzle together.

There are many future directions for elucidating the relationship between fiber and colorectal neoplasia. The effect of fiber may vary by age, gender, and fiber intake throughout life, and each of these factors may in turn have effects on different areas of the colorectum. Further, the actions of fiber related to the development of more advanced neoplasia are unknown. Single trials that have been conducted may not have sufficient statistical power to investigate these issues in depth. Therefore, large studies are under way to combine data from multiple large trials to investigate the role of fiber in colorectal neoplasia in more detail.

SUMMARY AND CONCLUSIONS

The role of carbohydrate, per se, in the carcinogenic process is difficult to assess because of its chemical diversity and the physiological effects specific to each type of carbohydrate. Furthermore, few studies have assessed carbohydrate intake without focusing on individual food sources or specific types of polysaccharides, especially the NSP. Therefore, it is not possible to ascertain any direct contribution of carbohydrate consumption on cancer risk. As a result, public health recommendations (National Academy of Sciences, 1989; World Health Organization, 1990) emphasize a higher consumption of complex carbohydrates, whole-grain foods and cereal products, and dietary fiber and limitation of sugar consumption.

Although many studies of dietary fiber and cancer have been conducted, the evidence for its protective effect is not clear. The epidemiological evidence suggests some consistent patterns along with some apparent disparities. Some of the inconsistent findings have been attributed to insufficient variation in fiber intake plus inadequate dietary instruments in analytical studies. In addition, the chemical complexity of fiber, inconsistency in its definition, and our limited understanding of its chemical characteristics make it difficult to define its overall contribution to cancer risk. These contradictions may also reflect our incomplete understanding of the carcinogenic process. A conservative interpretation of the data suggests that some component of plant products, especially those present in fruit and vegetables, may reduce the risk of cancer of the colon. Although a plausible biological mechanism for the action of fiber on breast cancer risk has been identified, the overall evidence is inconsistent. For pancreatic cancer, although there is some consistency in the findings supporting a protective effect of fiber, it is unclear whether this effect is due to the effect of fiber or to the nutrients or dietary components associated with fiber. For all other cancers, there is little or no evidence to support the role of fiber. Further investigations focusing on the proposed relationships with special attention on types and sources of fiber, as well as a full consideration of other factors in fruit and vegetables, are warranted. As large prospective studies continue to mature, their results will be extremely valuable in providing more concise evidence, particularly for rare cancers.

References

Adlercreutz, H. 1990. Western diet and Western diseases: some hormonal and biochemical mechanisms and associations. *Scand J Clin Lab Invest* **50**(Suppl 201): 3–23.

Adlercreutz, H., Hamalainen, E., et al. 1989. Diet and plasma androgens in postmenopausal vegetarian and omnivorous women and postmenopausal women with breast cancer. *Am J Clin Nutr* **49**: 433–442.

Alberts, D.S., Martinez, M.E., et al. 2000. Lack of effect of a high-fiber cereal supplement on the recurrence of colorectal adenomas. *N Engl J Med* **342**: 1156–1162.

Alberts, D.S., Ritenbaugh, C., et al. 1996. Randomized, double-blinded, placebo-controlled study of effect of wheat bran fiber and calcium on fecal bile acids in patients with resected adenomatous colon polyps. *J Natl Cancer Inst* **88**: 81–92.

Asp, N.-G., Schweizer, T.F., et al. 1992. "Dietary Fibre—A Component of Food-Nutritional Function in Health and Disease." ILSI Europe Workshop, Springer Verlag, New York.

Augustin, L.S., Gallus, S., et al. 2004. Glycemic index, glycemic load and risk of gastric cancer. *Ann Oncol* **15**(4): 581–584.

Baghurst, P.A., McMichael, A.J., et al. 1991. A case–control study of diet and cancer of the pancreas. *Am J Epidemiol* **134**: 167–179.

Baghurst, P.A., and Rohan, T.E. 1994. High-fiber diets and reduced risk of breast cancer. *Int J Cancer* **56**: 173–176.

Benito, E., Obrador, A., et al. 1990. A population-based case–control study of colorectal cancer in Majorca. I. Dietary factors. *Int J Cancer* **45**: 69–76.

Bidoli, E., Franceschi, S., et al. 1992. Food consumption and cancer of the colon and rectum in north-eastern Italy. *Int J Cancer* **50**: 223–229.

Bingham, S.A., Day, N.E., et al. 2003. Dietary fibre in food and protection against colorectal cancer in the European Prospective Investigation into Cancer and Nutrition (EPIC): an observational study. *Lancet* **361**: 1496–1501.

Bjelke, E. 1974. Epidemiologic studies of cancer of the stomach, colon and rectum; with special emphasis on the role of diet. *Scand J Gastroenterol (Suppl)* **31**: 1–235.

Blackburn, N.A., and Johnson, I.T. 1981. The effect of guar gum on the viscosity of the gastrointestinal contents and on glucose uptake from the perfused jejunum of the rat. *Br J Nutr* **46**: 239–246.

Bonilla-Fernandez, P., Lopez-Cervantes, M., et al. 2003. Nutritional factors and breast cancer in Mexico. *Nutr Cancer* **45**(2): 148–155.

Bostick, R.M., Potter, J.D., et al. 1994. Sugar, meat, and fat intake, and non-dietary risk factors for colon cancer incidence in Iowa women (United States). *Cancer Causes Control* **5**: 38–52.

Bristol, J.B., Emmett, P.M., et al. 1985. Sugar, fat, and the risk of colorectal cancer. *Br Med J Clin Res Ed* **291**: 1467–1470.

Bueno de Mesquita, H.B., Maisonneuve, P., et al. 1991. Intake of foods and nutrients and cancer of the exocrine pancreas: a population-based case–control study in the Netherlands. *Int J Cancer* **48**: 540–549.

Bueno de Mesquita, H.B., Moerman, C.J., et al. 1990. Are energy and energy-providing nutrients related to exocrine carcinoma of the pancreas? *Int J Cancer* **45**: 435–444.

Buiatti, E., Palli, D., et al. 1990. A case–control study of gastric cancer and diet in Italy. II. Association with nutrients. *Int J Cancer* **45**: 896–901.

Burkitt, D.P. 1971. Epidemiology of cancer of the colon and rectum. *Cancer* **28**: 3–13.

Centonze, S., Boeing, H., et al. 1994. Dietary habits and colorectal cancer in a low-risk area. Results from a population-based case–control study in Southern Italy. *Nutr Cancer* **21**: 233–246.

Corpet, D., Stamp, D., et al. 1990. Promotion of colonic microadenoma growth in mice and rats fed cooked sugar or cooked casein and fat. *Cancer Res* **50**: 6955–6958.

Correa, P., Fonthorn, E., et al. 1985. Dietary determinants of gastric cancer in South Louisiana inhabitants. *J Natl Cancer Inst* **75**: 645–653.

Cummings, J.H., and Bingham, S.A. 1987. Dietary fiber, fermentation and large bowel cancer. *Cancer Res* **6**: 601–621.

Cummings, J.H., Branch, W., et al. 1978. Colonic response to dietary fiber from carrot, cabbage, apple, bran and guar gum. *Lancet* **1**: 5–9.

De Stefani, E., Correa, P., et al. 1997. Dietary fiber and risk of breast cancer: a case–control study in Uruguay. *Nutr Cancer* **28**: 14–19.

Dreher, M. 1987. "Handbook of Dietary Fiber: An Applied Approach." Marcel Drekker, New York.

Englyst, H. 1980. The determination of carbohydrate and its composition in plant materials. *In* "Methods for the Measurement of Dietary Fiber" (O. Theander and W.P.T. James, eds). Marcel Dekker, London.

Englyst, H.N., and Cummings, J.H. 1988. Improved method for measurement of dietary fiber as non starch polysaccharides in plant foods. *J Assoc Off Anal Chem* **71**: 808–814.

Franceschi, S., Dal Maso, L., et al. 2001. Dietary glycemic load and colorectal cancer risk. *Ann Oncol* **12**(2): 173–178.

Freudenheim, J.L., Marshall, J.R., et al. 1996. Premenopausal breast cancer risk and intake of vegetables, fruits, and related nutrients. *J Natl Cancer Inst* **88**: 340–348.

Fuchs, C.S., Giovannucci, E.L., et al. 1999. Dietary fiber and the risk of colorectal cancer and adenoma in women. *N Engl J Med* **340**: 169–176.

Giovannucci, E. 1995. Insulin and colon cancer. *Cancer Causes and Control* **6**: 164–179.

Giovannucci, E., Rimm, E.B., et al. 1994. Intake of fat, meat, and fiber in relation to risk of colon cancer in men. *Cancer Res* **54**: 2390–2397.

Giovannucci, E., and Willett, W.C. 1994a. Dietary factors and risk of colon cancer. *Ann Med* **26**: 443–452.

Giovannucci, E., and Willett, W.C. 1994b. Dietary lipids and colon cancer. *Princip Practice Oncol* **9**: 1–12.

Goering, H.K., and van Soest, P.J. 1970. "Forage Fiber Analysis (Apparatus, Reagents, Procedures and some Applications)." Agricultural Research Service, USDA, Washington, D.C.

Goldin, B.R., Woods, M.N., et al. 1994. The effect of dietary fat and fiber on serum estrogen concentrations in premenopausal women under controlled dietary conditions. *Cancer* **74**: 1125–1131.

Gonzalez, C.A., Sanz, J.M., et al. 1991. Dietary factors and stomach cancer in Spain: a multi-centre case–control study. *Int J Cancer* **49**: 513–519.

Graham, S., Haughey, B., et al. 1990. Diet in the epidemiology of gastric cancer. *Nutr Cancer* **13**: 19–34.

Graham, S., Hellmann, R., et al. 1991. Nutritional epidemiology of postmenopausal breast cancer in western New York. *Am J Epidemiol* **134**: 552–556.

Greenwald, P., Lanza, E., et al. 1987. Dietary fiber in the reduction of colon cancer risk. *J Am Diet Assoc* **87**: 1178–1188.

Haenszel, W., Kurihara, M., et al. 1976. Stomach cancer in Japan. *J Natl Cancer Inst* **56**: 265–278.

Haenszel, W., Kurihara, M., et al. 1972. Stomach cancer among Japanese in Hawaii. *J Natl Cancer Inst* **49**: 969–988.

Hansson, L.E., Nyren, O., et al. 1993. Diet and risk of gastric cancer. A population-based case–control study in Sweden. *Int J Cancer* **55**(2): 181–189.

Heilbrun, L., Nomura, A., et al. 1989. Diet and colorectal cancer with special reference to fiber intake. *Int J Cancer* **44**: 1–6.

Higginbotham, S., Zhang, Z.F., et al. 2004. Dietary glycemic load and risk of colorectal cancer in the Women's Health Study. *J Natl Cancer Inst* **96**(3): 229–233.

Hill, M.J. 1991. Bile acids and colorectal cancer: hypothesis. *Eur J Cancer Prev* **1**(Suppl 2): 69–74.

Hirayama, T. 1971. Epidemiology of stomach cancer. *Gann Monogr Cancer Res* **11**: 3–19.

Hirohata, T. 1983. A case–control study of stomach cancer. Proceedings of the 21st General Congress of Japan Medical Association.

Holmes, M.D., Liu, S., et al. 2004. Dietary carbohydrates, fiber, and breast cancer risk. *Am J Epidemiol* **159**(8): 732–739.

Howe, G.R., Benito, E., et al. 1992. Dietary intake of fiber and decreased risk of cancers of the colon and rectum: evidence from the combined analysis of 13 case–control studies. *J Natl Cancer Inst* **84**: 1887–1896.

Howe, G.R., Ghadirian, P., et al. 1992. A collaborative case–control study of nutrient intake and pancreatic cancer within the SEARCH programme. *Int J Cancer* **51**: 365–372.

Howe, G.R., Hirohata, T., et al. 1990a. Dietary factors and risk of breast cancer: combined analysis of 12 case–control studies. *J Natl Cancer Inst* **82**: 561–569.

Howe, G.R., Jain, M., et al. 1990b. Dietary factors and risk of pancreatic cancer: results of a Canadian population-based case–control study. *Int J Cancer* **45**: 604–608.

International Agency for Research on Cancer Intestinal Microecology Group. 1977. Dietary fibre, transit time, faecal bacteria, steroids and colon cancer in two Scandinavian populations. *Lancet* **2**: 207–211.

Jacobs, E.T., Giuliano, A.R., et al. 2002. Baseline dietary fiber intake and colorectal adenoma recurrence in the wheat bran fiber randomized trial. *J Natl Cancer Inst* **94**(21): 1620–1625.

Jacobs, L. 1988. Fiber and colon cancer. *Gastroenterol Clin North Am* **17**: 747–760.

Jenkins, D.J., Kendall, C.W., et al. 2002. Glycemic index: overview of implications in health and disease. *Am J Clin Nutr* **76**(1): 266S–273S.

Jenkins, D.J.A., Wolever, T.M.S., et al. 1978. Dietary fibers, fiber analogues and glucose tolerance importance of viscosity. *Br Med J* **1**: 1392–1394.

Ji, B.T., Chow, W.H., et al. 1995. Dietary factors and the risk of pancreatic cancer: a case–control study in Shanghai China. *Cancer Epidemiol Biomarkers Prev* **4**: 885–893.

Jonas, C.R., McCullough, M.L., et al. 2003. Dietary glycemic index, glycemic load, and risk of incident breast cancer in postmenopausal women. *Cancer Epidemiol Biomarkers Prev* **12**(6): 573–577.

Kalapothaki, V., Tzonou, A., et al. 1993. Nutrient intake and cancer of the pancreas: a case–control study in Athens, Greece. *Cancer Causes Control* **4**: 383–389.

Kneller, R.W., McLaughlin, J.K., et al. 1991. A cohort study of stomach cancer in a high-risk American population. *Cancer* **68**: 672–678.

Koenuma, M., Yamori, T., et al. 1989. Insulin and insulin-like growth factor 1 stimulate proliferation of metastatic variants of colon carcinoma 26. *Jpn J Cancer Res* **80**: 51–58.

Kono, S., and Hirohata, T. 1996. Nutrition and stomach cancer. *Cancer Causes Control* **7**: 41–55.

Kono, S., Ikeda, M., et al. 1988. A case–control study of gastric cancer and diet in northern Kyushu, Japan. *Jpn J Cancer Res* **79**: 1067–1074.

Kritchevsky, D. 1988. Dietary fiber. *Ann Rev Nutr* **8**: 301–328.

Kruis, W., Forstmaier, G., et al. 1991. Effect of diets low and high in refined sugars on gut transit, bile acid metabolism, and bacterial fermentation. *Gut* **32**: 367–371.

Kushi, L.H., Sellers, T.A., et al. 1992. Dietary fat and postmenopausal breast cancer. *J Natl Cancer Inst* **84**: 1092–1099.

La Vecchia, C., Negri, E., et al. 1987. A case–control study of diet and gastric cancer in northern Italy. *Int J Cancer* **40**: 484–489.

La Vecchia, C., Negri, E., et al. 1988. A case–control study of diet and colorectal cancer in northern Italy. *Int J Cancer* **41**: 492–498.

Lee, H.P., Gourley, L., et al. 1991. Dietary effects on breast cancer risk in Singapore. *Lancet* **337**: 1197–1200.

Li, B.W. 1995. Determination of total dietary fiber in foods and food products by using a single-enzyme, enzymatic-gravimetric method: interlaboratory study. *J Assoc Off Anal Chem Int* **78**: 1440–1444.

Liu, K., Stamler, J., et al. 1979. Dietary cholesterol, fat and fibre, and colon cancer mortality. *Lancet* **2**: 782–785.

Liu, S., Willett, W.C., et al. 2000. A prospective study of dietary glycemic load, carbohydrate intake, and risk of coronary heart disease in US women. *Am J Clin Nutr* **71**(6): 1455–1461.

Lubin, F., Wax, Y., et al. 1986. Role of fat, animal protein, and dietary fiber in breast cancer etiology: A case–control study. *J Natl Cancer Inst* **77**: 605–612.

MacLennan, R., Jensen, O.M., et al. 1978. Diet, transit time, stool weight, and colon cancer in two Scandinavian populations. *Am J Clin Nutr* **31**: S239–S242.

Macquart-Moulin, G., Riboli, E., Cornee, J., Charnay, B., and Berthezene, P. 1986. Case–control study on colorectal cancer and diet in Marseilles. *Int J Cancer* **38**: 183–191.

Manousos, O., Day, N.E., et al. 1983. Diet and colorectal cancer: a case–control study in Greece. *Int J Cancer* **32**: 1–5.

Martinez, M.E. 2001. Hormone replacement therapy and adenoma recurrence: implications for its role in colorectal cancer risk. *J Natl Cancer Inst* **93**: 1764–1765.

Mattisson, I., Wirfalt, E., et al. 2004. Intakes of plant foods, fibre and fat and risk of breast cancer—a prospective study in the Malmo Diet and Cancer cohort. *Br J Cancer* **90**(1): 122–127.

Michaud, D.S., Fuchs, C.S., et al. 2005. Dietary glycemic load, carbohydrate, sugar, and colorectal cancer risk in men and women. *Cancer Epidemiol Biomarkers Prev* **14**(1): 138–147.

Michaud, D.S., Liu, S., et al. 2002. Dietary sugar, glycemic load, and pancreatic cancer risk in a prospective study. *J Natl Cancer Inst* **94**(17): 1293–1300.

Michels, K., Giovannucci, E., et al. 2000. Prospective study of fruit and vegetable consumption and incidence of colon and rectal cancers. *J Natl Cancer Inst* **92**: 1740–1752.

Miller, A.B., Howe, G.R., et al. 1983. Food items and food groups as risk factors in a case–control study of diet and colo-rectal cancer. *Int J Cancer* **32**: 155–161.

Miller, B.A., and Bulbrook, R.D. 1986. UICC multidisciplinary project on breast cancer: The epidemiology, etiology and prevention of breast cancer. *Int J Cancer* **37**: 173–177.

Modan, B., Lubin, F., et al. 1974. The role of starches in the etiology of gastric cancer. *Cancer* **34**: 2087–2092.

National Academy of Sciences. 1989. "Diet, Nutrition and Cancer." National Academy Press, Washington, D.C.

Nomura, A., Grove, J.S., et al. 1990. A prospective study of stomach cancer and its relation to diet, cigarettes, and alcohol consumption. *Cancer Res* **50**: 627–631.

Oh, K., Willett, W.C., et al. 2004. Glycemic index, glycemic load, and carbohydrate intake in relation to risk of distal colorectal adenoma in women. *Cancer Epidemiol Biomarkers Prev* **13**(7): 1192–1198.

Parkin, D.M., Pisani, P., et al. 1993. Estimates of the worldwide incidence of eighteen major cancers in 1985. *Int J Cancer* **54**: 594–606.

Peters, R.K., Pike, M.C., et al. 1992. Diet and colon cancer in Los Angeles County, California. *Cancer Causes Control* **3**: 457–473.

Peters, U., Sinha, R., et al. 2003. Dietary fibre and colorectal adenoma in a colorectal cancer early detection programme. *Lancet* **361**: 1491–1495.

Phillips, R.L. 1975. Role of life-style and dietary habits in risk of cancer among Seventh-Day Adventists. *Cancer Res* **35**: 3513–3522.

Pickle, L.W., Green, M.H., et al. 1984. Colorectal cancer in rural Nebraska. *Cancer Res* **44**: 363–369.

Pilch, S. 1987. "Physiological Effects and Health Consequences of Dietary Fiber." Life Sciences Research, Bethesda, MD.

Prosky, L., Asp, N., et al. 1985. Determination of total dietary fiber and food products: Collaborative study. *J Assoc Off Anal Chem* **68**:677–679.

Ramon, J.M., Serra, L., et al. 1993. Dietary factors and gastric cancer risk: a case–control study in Spain. *Cancer* **71**: 1731–1735.

Raymond, L., Infante, F., et al. 1987. Alimentation et cancer du pancreas. *Gastroenterol Clin Biol* **11**: 488–492.

Reddy, B.S., Watanabe, K., et al. 1977. Promoting effect of bile acids in colon carcinogenesis in germ-free and conventional F344 rats. *Cancer Res* **37**: 3238–3242.

Riccardi, G., and Riverllese, A.A. 1991. Effects of dietary fiber and carbohydrate on glucose and lipoprotein metabolism in diabetic patients. *Diabetes Care* **14**: 1115–11125.

Rohan, T.E., McMichael, A.J., et al. 1988. A population-based case–control study of diet and breast cancer in Australia. *Am J Epidemiol* **128**: 478–489.

Rose, D.P. 1990. Dietary fiber and breast cancer. *Nutr Cancer* **13**: 1–8.

Rose, D.P., Goldman, M., et al. 1991. High-fiber diet reduces estrogen concentrations in premenopausal women. *Am J Clin Nutr* **54**: 520–525.

Sandberg, A.S., Ahdeerinne, R., et al. 1983. The effect of citrus pectin on the absorption of nutrients in the small intestine. *Hum Nutr Clin Nutr* **37**: 171–183.

Schatzkin, A., Lanza, E., et al. 2000. Lack of effect of a low-fat, high-fiber diet on the recurrence of colorectal adenomas. Polyp Prevention Trial Study Group. *N Engl J Med* **342**: 1149–1155.

Schrauzer, G.N. 1976. Cancer mortality correlation studies II. Regional associations of mortalities with the consumptions of foods and other commodities. *Med Hypoth* **2**: 39–43.

Silvera, S.A., Jain, M., et al. 2004. Dietary carbohydrates and breast cancer risk: A prospective study of the roles of overall glycemic index and glycemic load. *Int J Cancer* **114**(4): 653–658.

Slattery, M.L., Benson, J., et al. 1997. Dietary sugar and colon cancer. *Cancer Epidemiol Biomarkers Prev* **6**(9): 677–685.

Southgate, D.A., Bailey, B., et al. 1976. A guide to calculating intakes of dietary fiber. *J Hum Nutr* **30**: 303–313.

Southgate, D.A.T. 1969. Determination of carbohydrates in foods. II Unavailable carbohydrates. *J Sci Fd Agric* **20**: 331–335.

Stamp, D., Zhang, X.M., et al. 1993. Sucrose enhancement of the early steps of colon carcinogenesis in mice. *Carcinogenesis* **14**: 777–779.

Steinmetz, K.A., Kushi, L.H., et al. 1994. Vegetables, fruit, and colon cancer in the Iowa Women's Health Study. *Am J Epidemiol* **139**: 1–15.

Steinmetz, K.A., and Potter, J.D. 1993. Food-group consumption and colon cancr in the Adelaide Case–Control Study. *Int J Cancer* **53**: 711–719.

Terry, P.D., Jain, M., et al. 2003. Glycemic load, carbohydrate intake, and risk of colorectal cancer in women: a prospective cohort study. *J Natl Cancer Inst* **95**(12): 914–916.

Thompson, L.U., Robb, P., et al. 1991. Mammalian lignan production from various foods. *Nutr Cancer* **16**: 43–52.

Thun, M.J., Calle, E.E., et al. 1992. Risk factors for fatal colon cancer in a large prospective study. *J Natl Cancer Inst* **84**: 1491–1500.

Trichopoulos, D., Ouranos, G., et al. 1985. Diet and cancer of the stomach: a case–control study in Greece. *Int J Cancer* **37**: 837–842.

Trowell, H., Burkitt, D., et al. 1985. "Dietary Fibre, Fibredepleted Foods and Disease." San Diego, Academic Press.

Tuyns, A.J., Kaaks, R., et al. 1988. Colorectal cancer and the consumption of foods: a case–control study of Belgium. *Nutr Cancer* **11**: 189–204.

Tuyns, A.J., Kaaks, R., et al. 1992. Diet and gastric cancer: a case–control study in Belgium. *Int J Cancer* **51**: 1–6.

van Soest, H.K., and van Soest, P.J. 1973. The chemistry and estimation of fibre. *Proc Nutr Soc* **32**: 123.

Van'T Veer, P., Kolb, C.M., et al. 1990. Dietary fiber, beta-carotene and breast cancer: results from a case–control study. *Int J Cancer* **45**: 825–828.

Weisburger, J.H., Reddy, F.S., et al. 1993. Protective mechanisms of dietary fiber in nutritional carcinogenesis. *Basic Life Sci* **61**: 45–63.

Willett, W., Manson, J., et al. 2002. Glycemic index, glycemic load, and risk of type 2 diabetes. *Am J Clin Nutr* **76**(1): 274S–280S.

Willett, W.C., Hunter, D.J., et al. 1992. Dietary fat and fiber in relation to risk of breast cancer: An eight year follow-up. *J Am Med Assoc* **268**: 2037–2044.

Willett, W.C., Stampfer, M.J., et al. 1990. Relation of meat, fat, and fiber intake to the risk of colon cancer in a prospective study among women. *N Engl J Med* **323**: 1664–1672.

Wolever, T.M.S., Jenkins, D.J., et al. 1991. The glycemic index: methodology and clinical implications. *Am J Clin Nutr* **54**: 846–854.

Woods, M.N., Barnett, J., et al. 1996. Hormone levels during dietary changes in premenopausal African-American women. *J Natl Cancer Inst* **88**: 1369–1374.

Woods, M.N., Gorbach, S.L., et al. 1989. Low-fat, high-fiber diet and serum estrone sulfate in premenopausal women. *Am J Clin Nutr* **49**: 1179–1193.

World Health Organization. 1990. "Diet, Nutrition, and the Prevention of chronic Diseases." World Health Organization, Geneva.

Wynder, E.L., Kajitani, T., et al. 1969. Environmental factors of cancer of the colon and rectum. II. Japanese epidemiological data. *Cancer* **23**: 1210–1220.

You, W.C., Blot, W.J., et al. 1988. Diet and high risk of stomach cancer in Shandong, China. *Cancer Res* **48**: 3518–3523.

Yuan, J.M., Wang, Q.S., et al. 1995. Diet and breast cancer in Shanghai and Tianjin, China. *Br J Cancer* **71**: 1353–1358.

Zaridze, D.G., Muir, C.S., et al. 1985. Diet and cancer: value of different types of epidemiological studies. *Nutr Cancer* **7**: 155–166.

Zatonoski, W., Przewozniak, K., et al. 1991. Nutritional factors and pancreatic cancer: a case–control study from south-west Poland. *Int J Cancer* **48**: 390–394.

CHAPTER

30

Dietary Lipids

HUSEYIN AKTAS, MICHAEL CHOREV, AND J.A. HALPERIN

INTRODUCTION

A combination of epidemiological, case-control, and cohort studies in the second half of the past century underscored the possibility that high dietary intake of n-3 polyunsaturated fatty acids (n-3 PUFAs) could have a protective effect against cancer. Although the results of those studies were controversial and not uniformly embraced in the field of nutritional epidemiology (Willett, 1997), the notion that n-3 PUFAs may exert anticancer properties was strongly supported by extensive experimental studies documenting an anticancer effect both in cancer cells *in vitro* and in animal models of experimental cancer. These studies opened the door to more detailed experimental work aimed at elucidating the cellular and molecular mechanism of the putative anticancer properties of n-3 PUFAs. In this chapter, we summarize the sometimes-inconsistent nomenclature of fatty acids, the basic biochemistry needed to understand the principal biological differences between n-3 and n-6 PUFAs, and the mechanisms proposed to explain the putative anticancer properties of n-3 PUFAs. Finally, we summarize our work that led to include n-3 PUFAs among an emerging class of anticancer agents generally known as *inhibitors of translation initiation* (Clemens and Bommer, 1999; Palakurthi et al., 2000). The chapter focuses only on putative anticancer effects of n-3 PUFAs; other postulated health benefits are acknowledged but are not discussed.

FATTY ACID BIOSYNTHESIS

Metabolism of both dietary and *de novo* synthesized fatty acids generates the fatty acids required for normal physiology. Many physiologically relevant fatty acids have linear, even-numbered chains of 18 carbons or longer and are polyunsaturated, presenting several sequential double bonds separated by single methylene units. These double bonds are exclusively in the *cis* configuration in which the two substituting hydrogens are on one side while the two substituting methylenes are on the opposite side of the double bond (Table 1).

Because they lack the enzymes required to introduce double bonds within the last seven carbons proximate to the methyl end of the molecule, mammals can neither synthesize linoleic (18:2 n-6) or linolenic acid (18:3 n-3) nor interconvert one to the other. These two fatty acids must be obtained from the diet and are, therefore, termed *essential*; they are extremely important constituents of the membrane lipids and indispensable precursors in the biosynthesis of eicosanoids such as prostaglandins, thromboxanes, leukotrienes, and 5-hydroxyeicosatetraenoic acid (Hansen et al., 1958; Collins et al., 1971; Paulsrud et al., 1972; Holman et al., 1982).

Nomenclature

The systematic nomenclature of fatty acids is based on the length of the carbon chain, the number of double bonds, their location relative to the carboxyl end, and the geometric configuration. For example, the systematic name for arachidonic acid, the precursor of many eicosanoid signaling molecules, is *cis,cis,cis,cis*-5,8,11,14-eicosatetraenoic acid. In addition to the trivial and systematic names, there are two numerical systems that describe attributes of PUFAs. In one of these numerical systems, arachidonic acid is denoted "20:4 n-6," meaning that it contains 20 carbons, 4

Copyright © 2006, Elsevier Inc.
All rights of reproduction in any form reserved.

TABLE 1 Fatty Acids Structure and Nomenclature

Fatty acid	Structure	n-Designation[a]	Δ-Designation[b]
Saturated fatty acids			
Caprylic acid	CO_2H	8:0	8:0
Caproic acid	CO_2H	10:0	10:0
Lauric acid	CO_2H	12:0	12:0
Myristic acid	CO_2H	14:0	14:0
Palmitic acid	CO_2H	16:0	16:0
Stearic acid	CO_2H	18:0	18:0
***cis* Monounsaturated fatty acids**			
Myristoleic acid	CO_2H	14:1 n-5	14:1 Δ9
Palmitoleic acid	CO_2H	16:1 n-7	16:1 Δ9
Vaccenic acid	CO_2H	18:1 n-7	18:1 Δ11
Oleic acid	CO_2H	18:1 n-9	18:1 Δ9
Eicosanoic acid	CO_2H	20:1 n-9	20:1 Δ9
Erucic acid	CO_2H	22:1 n-9	22:1 Δ9
Primary n-6 polyunsaturated fatty acids[c]			
Linoleic acid	CO_2H	18:2 n-6	18:2 Δ9,12
γ-Linolenic acid	CO_2H	18:3 n-6	18:3 Δ6,9,12
Dihomo-γ-linolenic acid	CO_2H	20:3 n-6	20:3 Δ8,11,14
Arachidonic acid	CO_2H	20:4 n-6	20:4 Δ5,8,11,14
Adrenic acid	CO_2H	22:4 n-6	22:4 Δ7,10,13,16
Docosapentaenoic acid	CO_2H	22:5 n-6	22:5 Δ4,7,10,13,16
n-3 polyunsaturated fatty acids[d]			
α-Linolenic acid	CO_2H	18:3 n-3	18:3 Δ9,12,15
Eicosapentaenoic acid	CO_2H	20:5 n-3	20:5 Δ5,8,11,14,17
Docosapentaenoic acid	CO_2H	22:5 n-3	22:5 Δ7,10,13,16,17
Docosahexaenoic acid	CO_2H	22:6 n-3	22:6 Δ4,7,10,13,16,19

[a]Carbon numbering starts from the methyl terminal useful to link diet with tissue fatty acid metabolism.
[b]Carbon numbering starts from the carboxyl terminal useful to describe biochemistry of fatty acid metabolism.
[c]Also called ω6-polyunsaturated fatty acids.
[d]Also called ω3-polyunsaturated fatty acids.

double bonds, and the first double bond is located between carbons 6 (n-6) and 7 counting from the methyl end of the molecule (Table 1). In the other system, arachidonic acid is denoted "20:4 Δ5,8,11,14," meaning that it contains 20 carbons with 4 double bonds, and that the first double bond is between carbons 5 (Δ) and 6 starting from the carboxyl end, and the other 3 double bonds start at carbons 8, 11, and 14, from the same end. The first numerical system indicates the relatedness to the essential fatty acid from which a given PUFA is derived: n-6 PUFAs are derived from linoleic (18:2 n-6) and n-3 PUFAs from linolenic acid (18:3 n-3). The second numeric system reflects the biochemistry of a given fatty acid metabolism. Table 1 lists the trivial names, structures, and designations for some of the more abundant series of saturated fatty acids, monosaturated fatty acids, and PUFAs in mammalian biology.

Metabolism of Essential Fatty Acids

The 20-carbon or longer polyunsaturated n-6 or n-3 fatty acids are, respectively, derived from linoleic (18:2 n-6) or linolenic (18:3 n-3) acid (Figure 1). Linoleic acid is

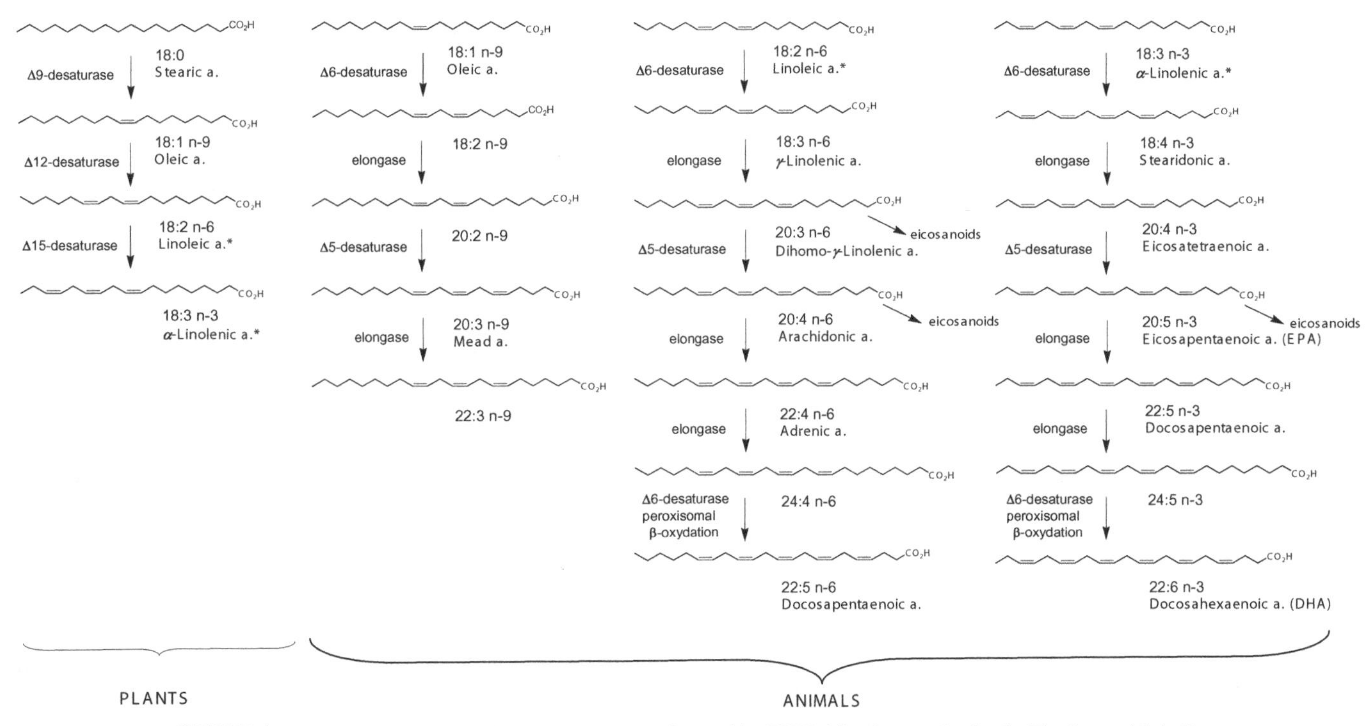

FIGURE 1 Biosynthetic pathways for polyunsaturated fatty acids (PUFAs) in plants and animals. The fatty acids indicated by an asterisk (*) are the essential PUFAs in the animal diet.

metabolized by a Δ6-desaturase that adds a double bond between carbons 6 and 7 from the carboxyl group generating γ-linolenic acid (18:3 n-6). This is followed by elongase generating the dihomo-γ-linolenic acid (20:3 n-6), which is longer by two carbons added in proximity to the carboxyl group. A subsequent modification by Δ5-desaturase adds another double bond between carbons 5 and 6 from the carboxyl group yielding arachidonic acid (20:4 n-6). Arachidonic acid is a substrate for prostaglandin synthases, which produce the two double-bond–containing prostanoids: prostaglandins, prostacyclin, and thromboxanes, and for lipoxygenases, which produce hydroxyeicosatetraenoic acids and the four double bonds containing leukotrienes.

α-Linolenic acid (18:3 n-3) is similarly metabolized to eicosapentaenoic acid (20:5 n-3; EPA), the precursor of the three double bonds containing prostanoids (Needleman et al., 1979; Fischer and Weber, 1984) and the 5 double bonds containing leukotrienes such as LTA_5, LTB_5, and LTC_5 (Lee et al., 1984; Prescott, 1984; Strasser et al., 1985).

Although the metabolism of both n-6 and n-3 PUFA series utilizes the same elongase and desaturase enzymes, some observations suggest that the desaturase has a higher affinity for n-3 than for n-6 PUFAs (Brenner, 1974). As a result, dietary n-3 PUFAs reduce the synthesis of arachidonic acid and the eicosanoids derived from it (Chen and Nilsson, 1993; Emken, 1994; Sauerwald et al., 1996; Emken et al., 1998, 1999).

Animals cannot interconvert n-3 and n-6 PUFAs and lack the Δ12- and Δ15-desaturases necessary to convert oleic acid (18:1 n-9) to linoleic (18:2 n-6) and α-linolenic (18:3 n-3) acids, the two essential fatty acids. In contrast, algae have the full repertoire of enzymes to synthesize stearic (18:0 n-9) and oleic (18:1 n-9) acids and to convert oleic acid to linoleic acid (18:2 n-6) by Δ12-desaturase and subsequently to α-linolenic acid (18:3 n-3) by Δ15-desaturase (Sayanova and Napier, 2004) (Figure 1). Fish obtain both n-6 and n-3 fatty acids from the food available to them, and the n-6/n-3 fatty acid distribution of fish oils is determined in great part by the availability of n-3 fatty acids producing microalgae in the marine food chain in the geographic location of their habitat. Humans obtain their n-3 fatty acids by dietary intake of fish or fish oils. n-3 PUFAs are more abundant in cold-water fatty fish than in warm-water lean fish. It is also important to highlight that because the n-3 PUFA content of the fish fat is dependent on the fishes' food source, aquaculture fish fed with processed food tend to have a lower content of n-3 PUFAs as a percentage of the total fat.

EPIDEMIOLOGICAL, PROSPECTIVE, AND EXPERIMENTAL STUDIES

The incidence of some cancers in different populations around the world shows dramatic variation. For example, the incidence of prostate and breast cancer is much higher in the United States and northern Europe than in Asia. This difference cannot be explained by ethnic or racial differences because one-to-two generations after Asian men or women migrate to the United States, the age-adjusted risk of prostate and breast cancer rises to reach the risk of the white American population (Ziegler et al., 1993; Deapen et al., 2002). Because dietary habits are prominent among the major differences in the lifestyles of Western and Asian societies, the regional distribution of breast and prostate cancers, together with other comparable observations, fueled the speculation that dietary factors, especially the amount of fat consumed and its dietary origin, critically influence the genesis and/or progression of some cancers. A classical example frequently quoted in support of the fat–cancer risk connection is that populations such as Alaskan Eskimos and Greenland populations, whose diets are based almost exclusively on cold-water fish rich in n-3 PUFAs, reportedly have a low incidence of prostate and breast cancer (Bjarnason et al., 1974; Karmali et al., 1987; Bruce et al., 2000a,b). Another example is that in countries historically considered to have low incidence of cancer, cancer rates are increasing coincidentally with the adoption of more Westernized diets, including a higher fat intake (Nielson and Hansen, 1980; Lanier, 1996; Lanier et al., 1996a; Tsuji et al., 1996; You et al., 2002). In Japan, for example, parallel to a progressive increase in the incidence of breast cancer, the average fat consumption increased from 9% of total energy in 1955 to 25% in 1987 (Hirayama, 1978; Karmali et al., 1987; Wynder et al., 1991).

Increasing attention has been paid to a connection between cancer risk and the intake of specific fatty acids rather than total fat intake, and notable among these have been marine fatty acids. This is because most of those populations mentioned earlier, with apparent low rates of cancer, derive a very significant part of their diet from fish and marine animals, whose fat contains large amounts of n-3 PUFA, and the progressive increase in cancer risk parallels a decline in the intake of n-3 PUFAs concomitant with an increased intake of n-6 PUFAs (Bjarnason et al., 1974; Armstrong and Doll, 1975; Jansson et al., 1975; Nielson and Hansen, 1980; Kaizer et al., 1989; Sasaki et al., 1993; Lanier et al., 1996b).

Although ecological studies of special populations seem to support a negative association between dietary n-3 PUFA intake and cancer risk, it is worth noting that the epidemiological evidence is purely inferential and correlative, and its interpretation is difficult because of other confounding factors.

For example, factors such as early age at menarche and at first pregnancy, and prolonged lactation, known to reduce the risk of breast cancer, are also prevalent among most of the populations shown to have low incidence of breast cancer and high consumption of n-3 PUFAs. These behavioral/cultural patterns may also be changing in response to Western influence. In summary, although nutritional epidemiology studies have intrinsic problems related to both methodology and multifactorial confounding factors that are difficult to control, they were useful in bringing to the forefront the notion that dietary fat in general and the relative intake of n-3 marine fatty acids in particular could exert a protective effect against some cancers.

Case–control and cohort studies provide another approach to analyze possible correlations between diet and the risk of cancer. In case-control studies, the diet and lifestyle of the cancer patients are compared with those of control subjects, whereas in cohort studies a group of healthy individuals is followed for an extended period and the incidence of cancer and dietary habits among the participants is compared at the end of the study period.

In contrast with the frequently quoted ecological studies mentioned earlier, most case-control studies do not support a potential cancer-protective effect of consuming a predominantly fish-based diet (reviewed by Willett, 1997). In an extensive review of epidemiological, case-control, and cohort studies examining the association between consumption of fish and risk of breast cancer, prostate cancer, and other hormone-dependent cancers published by Terry et al. (2003), the authors concluded that ". . . the development and progression of breast and prostate cancer appear to be affected by a process in which eicosapentaenoic acid (EPA) and docosahexaenoic acid (DHA) play important roles; yet whether the consumption of fish containing marine fatty acids can alter the risk of these or of other cancers is unclear." Importantly, these authors point out some critical factors that could have clouded the results of those studies. For example, the concentration of EPA and DHA contained in fish varies among species. Relatively high concentrations are found in wild cold-water fatty fish such as salmon, mackerel, sardines, and herring, whereas warm-water lean fish usually have lower concentrations of n-3 PUFAs and sometimes higher content of arachidonic acid (n-6 FA). Thus, case-control or cohort studies that analyzed only total fish consumption in relation to cancer risk regardless of the type of fish may generate conflicting results. Terry et al. (2003) also point out that an analysis of published studies indicates that the duration of the follow-up period may also affect the results of a study because stronger inverse associations between cancer risk and fish/n-3 PUFA consumption were found in studies with the longest follow-up periods. It seems, therefore, that a clearer picture of the potential association between fatty acid intake and cancer risk would emerge from studies and a long follow-up period, with repeated assessment of diet during that period, would provide information on cancers at various stages of growth and progression.

This was the case in a report within the Health Professionals' Follow-up Study that examined prospectively consumption of fish and marine oil intake in relation to risk of prostate cancer in a cohort of 50,000 men followed for 12 years. The participants responded to a semiquantitative food frequency questionnaire mailed four times during the 12-year period. The food questionnaire was validated measuring actual food intake for a week among a sample of 127 cohort members, and dietary intake of n-3 PUFAs verified by analysis of the relative composition of fatty acids in a subcutaneous fat aspirate taken from a sample of men from this cohort. The results, adjusted for other dietary and nondietary risk factors, showed that men consuming more than three servings of fish per week had almost half the risk of metastatic prostate cancer as compared with rare or nonconsumers of fish (Augustsson et al., 2003). Even more remarkable in that study is the finding that each additional daily intake of 0.5 g of marine oil further reduced the risk of metastatic prostate cancer by 24%. Interestingly, no association was found between fish intake and the overall risk (incidence) of prostate cancer among the cohort, suggesting that the intake of fish or marine oils affects tumor progression and metastatic potential rather than the malignant transformation.

Experimental studies have provided more consistent data showing that both EPA and DHA, the main n-3 fatty acids in fish oils, exert anticancer properties in cancer cell lines *in vitro* and in animal xenograft models of human cancer (Falconer et al., 1994; Grammatikos et al., 1994; Rose et al., 1996; Calviello et al., 1998; Whelan et al., 2002). In our laboratory, daily oral administration of EPA doubled the life expectancy of $p53^{-/-}$ mice, which develop multiple cancers with 100% penetrance and die at ~40 weeks of age (unpublished observation).

Taken together, studies in humans, animals, and cells indicate that n-3 PUFAs may exert a protective anticancer effect that deserves further investigation. Critical for such future studies is defining the cellular and molecular mechanism(s) underlying the anticancer effects of n-3 PUFAs, and deriving from this research much-needed mechanism-specific biomarkers to be used in human studies.

Proposed Mechanisms of Anti-cancer Activity of n-3 PUFAs

Effect on Membrane Structure and Function

Because n-3 PUFAs incorporate into and are an integral part of membrane phospholipids, they can exert profound effects on membrane physical properties, including permeability, lateral diffusion, lipid packing, and domain formation, and thereby affect the function of membrane proteins intimately involved in intracellular signaling. Consistently, n-3 PUFAs have been shown to influence G protein–coupled receptor and receptor tyrosine kinase signaling pathways (Zhang et al., 1999; Mitchell et al., 2003), as well as ion channels (Xiao et al., 2001), a diversity of cellular effects believed to contribute to their anticancer properties.

Inhibition of Eicosanoid Production from Arachidonic Acid

Eicosanoids, including prostaglandins, leukotrienes, and thromboxanes, which are derived from 20-carbon PUFAs, affect a wide variety of cellular processes, including cell proliferation, differentiation, and apoptosis. Arachidonic acid, a 20-carbon fatty acid abundant in cell membrane phospholipids, is the major precursor of two double-bond–containing prostanoids. Cyclooxygenase (COX) catalyzes the first step in the conversion of arachidonic acid to prostaglandins and thromboxanes, and lipoxygenase catalyzes its conversion to four double-bond–containing leukotrienes.

Increased expression of COX and overproduction of some eicosanoids have been implicated in both the development of cancers and the promotion of angiogenesis. Prostaglandins derived from arachidonic acid by the COX-2 enzyme, notably prostaglandin E_2 (PGE_2), have been linked to carcinogenesis in studies of the proliferation of breast and prostate cancer cell lines *in vitro*, in experimental animal models leading to the development of mammary tumors, and in human studies on the effect of fish oil intake on epithelial cell proliferation rates (Rose and Connolly, 1999).

Increasing the dietary intake of n-3 PUFAs reduces the production of arachidonic acid (Christiansen et al., 1991) and thereby the generation of arachidonic acid–derived eicosanoids. In addition, both EPA and DHA can displace arachidonic acid in cell membrane phospholipids (Rose et al., 1994) and in diacylglycerols (Madani et al., 2004) and have been shown to inhibit COX-2 (Rose and Connolly, 1999) and lipoxygenase. Thus, replacement and reduced formation of arachidonic acid, as well as inhibition of key enzymes in the eicosanoid synthesis pathways, are proposed mechanisms underlying the anticancer effects of n-3 PUFAs, a view supported in part by the apparent inhibitory effect on cancer cells' growth of some nonsteroidal anti-inflammatory drugs that inhibit COX activity.

Effect on Estrogen and Testosterone Metabolism

17β-Estradiol, the main natural estrogen, stimulates normal mammary development and promotes the neoplastic transformation of breast cells. Estradiol is metabolized along two major pathways, one generating 16-hydroxyestrone and the other 2-hydroxyestrone. 16-Hydroxyestrone is considered more bioactive than the 2-estrone metabolites. 16-Hydroxyestrone produces aberrant hyperproliferation in mammary explants and is considered a mediator of estrogen-induced transformation of breast epithelial cells

(Chajes et al., 1995); also, clinical studies suggest that an elevated C16-hydroxylation of estradiol may provide a biomarker for breast cancer risk (Telang et al., 1997). Osborne et al. (1988) reported that feeding an n-3 fatty acid–rich fish-oil supplement to women reduced the extent of C16-hydroxylation, suggesting that a reduced production of 16-hydroxyestrone and perhaps increased generation of 2-hydroxyestrone may contribute to an anticancer effect of n-3 PUFAs in breast cancer.

Testosterone promotes proliferation and neoplastic transformation of prostate cells. It has also been shown that both n-3 and n-6 PUFAs interfere with testosterone metabolism by inhibiting the enzyme 5α-reductase and thereby the conversion of testosterone to dihydrotestosterone (Liang and Liao, 1992). However, the anticancer properties of PUFAs in prostate cancer seem to be limited to the n-3 series. Also, finasteride, a specific inhibitor of the 5α-reductase that lowers 5-dihydrotestosterone to the castrate levels and is clinically used for treatment of benign prostate hyperplasia, was shown to significantly increase the risk of high-grade prostate cancers in a large prospective study. This study argues against the 5α-reductase as the primary target of the n-3 PUFAs, which appear to decrease the incidence of aggressive prostate cancer (Augustsson et al., 2003).

Effect of Lipid Peroxidation

The long-chain PUFAs are highly susceptible to lipid peroxidation, and peroxidation products of the marine fatty acids have been proposed as mediators of their anticancer effects (Gonzalez, 1995; Welsch, 1997). For example, in breast cancer cell lines, DHA increased lipid peroxides and enhanced the toxicity of anthracyclines (agents that generate oxidative stress); both effects were inhibited by the antioxidant vitamin E (Gonzalez et al., 1993). Similar results have been reported in animal models of experimental breast cancer (Gonzalez et al., 1991). However, the mechanisms by which these oxidation products of n-3 PUFAs inhibit cancer cell growth are still uncertain (Welsch, 1995). Thus, although effects on the cell membrane, eicosanoid formation, estrogen and testosterone metabolism, and lipid peroxidation have been proposed as potential mediators of the anticancer effects of marine fish oils, these mechanisms are not embraced because of the lack of stringent and direct evidence for their causative role.

THE TRANSLATION INITIATION CONNECTION

Work has identified translation initiation as a molecular target of the anticancer effects of n-3 PUFAs. Translation, the cellular process by which mRNAs are translated into proteins, is operationally divided in three phases: initiation, elongation, and termination. Translation initiation, a highly regulated process, requires the concerted participation of >20 proteins/cellular factors known as *eukaryotic translation initiation factors* (eIFs), plays a critical role in the control of growth and division in eukaryotic cells. This is because structural features in the mRNAs' coding for most proto-oncogenic and cell cycle–regulatory proteins make their translation rather inefficient and critically dependent on the activity of translation initiation factors such as eIF2, eIF4E, eIF4A, and eIF4G. Indeed, experimental evidence indicates that the rate of translation controls the expression of most cell growth–regulatory proteins. For example, early mitogenic signals that turn on the transcription of cell growth–regulatory genes simultaneously activate translation initiation factors such as eIF2 and eIF4E that are rate limiting for translation initiation. In this manner, extracellular signals that stimulate cell proliferation couple transcription with translation, resulting in a dramatic increase in the expression of growth regulatory proteins at the G_0–G_1 transition and during the G_1 phase of the cell cycle. Consistently, we and others have shown experimentally that reducing the rate of translation initiation preferentially inhibits the synthesis and expression of oncogenic proteins and cell growth regulatory proteins such as the G_1-cyclins (cyclin D1, cyclin E, and cyclin A), whereas other "housekeeping" proteins are minimally affected (Aktas et al., 1998). The tight translational control of proteins that promote cell proliferation represents a key physiological restraint to cell growth, and uncontrolled translation results in malignant transformation (Lazaris-Karatzas et al., 1990; Koromilas et al., 1992a; Donze et al., 1995).

Translation Initiation and Cancer

Cancer cells proliferate disregarding the checkpoints that restrain growth in normal cells. This ability is acquired through mutations that lead to inactivation of growth inhibitory genes such as Rb (retinoblastoma) or of tumor suppressor genes such as p53, and/or to activation of proto-oncogenes such as cyclin D1, c-myc, or Ras. Products of these genes regulate specific events in cell growth and division. Interestingly, overexpression of proteins that regulate translation initiation causes neoplastic transformation because the consequent increase in the rate of protein synthesis leads to a disproportionately higher translation of oncogenic proteins such as cyclin D1 and c-myc, which are overexpressed in a large number of human cancers (Lazaris-Karatzas et al., 1990; Duan et al., 1995; Shilatifard et al., 1996).

In human cancers, overexpression of the translation initiation factor eIF2α correlates with neoplastic transformation of mammary epithelial cells and with the aggressiveness of non-Hodgkin's lymphomas (Raught et al., 1996; Wang et al., 1999). Overexpression of eIF4E reportedly is a prognostic tumor marker for breast cancers (Li et al., 2002), a predictor of recurrence in head and neck tumors (Nathan et al., 1997; Rosenwald et al., 2001), and is abundant in breast (Li et al., 1998), head and neck (Nathan et al., 2002), primary bladder (Crew et al., 2000) and colon carcinomas (Berkel et al., 2001), as well as non-Hodgkin's lymphomas (Wang et al., 1999). Also, in many human cancers, the translational efficiency of oncogenic proteins and growth factors such as c-myc, vascular endothelial growth factor (VEGF), or transforming growth factor-β (TGF-β) is significantly enhanced through variations that simplify the structure of their mRNA, thus enabling them to escape tight control of translation initiation (Scott et al., 1998). For example, the mRNA for TGF-β has two alternative splicing forms: one with an 1100-nucleotide-long and highly structured 5′UTR and the other with a 230-nucleotide-long and simpler 5′UTR that has sevenfold higher translational efficiency. The shorter, translationally stronger, and upregulated TGF-β mRNA is almost exclusively seen in cancers and is believed to contribute to the metastatic potential of some breast cancers (Arrick et al., 1994).

In contrast, inhibition of translation initiation interferes with both cell growth and malignant transformation (Sonenberg, 1994; Graff et al., 1995; Rousseau et al., 1996). For instance, attenuation of translation initiation by overexpression of the inhibitory eIF4E-binding protein or interferons suppresses cancer cell and tumor growth (Rastinejad et al., 1993; Davis and Watson, 1996; Rousseau et al., 1996).

The previous paragraphs highlight the critical role played by translation initiation in the physiological control of cell growth, as well as in both malignant transformation and in maintenance of transformed phenotypes. The cellular translation initiation machinery, therefore, represents an attractive target for cancer treatment (Clemens and Bommer, 1999), and translation initiation inhibitors are now recognized as an emerging class of anticancer agents (Dua et al., 2001).

Inhibition of Translation Initiation Mediates the Anticancer Effect of EPA

In the following sections, we briefly describe the translation initiation process and summarize the experimental evidence generated in our laboratories demonstrating that the anticancer effects of EPA are mediated by inhibition of translation initiation.

In the initiation phase of mRNA translation, the translation initiation factor eIF2 forms a ternary complex with GTP and the initiating methionyl-tRNA (Met-tRNAi). The eIF2·GTP·Met-tRNAi ternary complex recruits the 40S ribosomal subunit forming the 43S preinitiation complex, which then binds to the mRNA cap with the help of other translation initiation factors. The preinitiation complex scans the 5′ untranslated region (5′UTR) of mRNA for the initiator AUG codon, a process that requires the participation of several translation initiation factors including eIF4E, eIF4G, and the RNA helicase eIF4A. At the AUG codon, the 60S ribosomal subunit is recruited to form the 80S ribosome. Concomitantly, GTP associated with eIF2 is hydrolyzed to GDP, which must be exchanged for GTP to initiate a new cycle of translation. This GDP–GTP exchange is catalyzed by the multisubunit guanine nucleotide exchange factor eIF2B and is inhibited when the alpha subunit of eIF2 (eIF2α) is phosphorylated. The higher affinity of phosphorylated eIF2α for eIF2B sequesters it from the cytosol so it cannot catalyze the GDP-GTP exchange (Pain, 1996). In other words, phosphorylated eIF2α is a competitive inhibitor of eIF2B. Because the stoichiometric ratio of eIF2B to eIF2 in the cytosol is quite low (i.e., molecules of eIF2 are far more abundant than molecules of eIF2B), even partial phosphorylation of eIF2α is sufficient to eliminate the free eIF2B necessary to recycle the eIF2·GDP into the functional eIF2·GTP and reduce the overall rate of translation initiation (Brostrom et al., 1989; Srivastava et al., 1995). Figure 2 summarizes the translation initiation process.

The enzymes that phosphorylate eIF2α on its serine 51 residue are known as *eIF2α kinases*. At least two eIF2α kinases, interferon-inducible double-stranded RNA-dependent protein kinase R (PKR) and PKR-like ER-resident kinase (PERK), are activated by signals from a "stressed" endoplasmic reticulum (ER) triggering a cascade of events generally termed the *ER-stress response*. Most proteins synthesized in the cytoplasm are translocated to the ER for folding and post-translational modifications. Increased or accelerated protein synthesis that overwhelms the ER capacity for folding or other perturbations that prevent protein

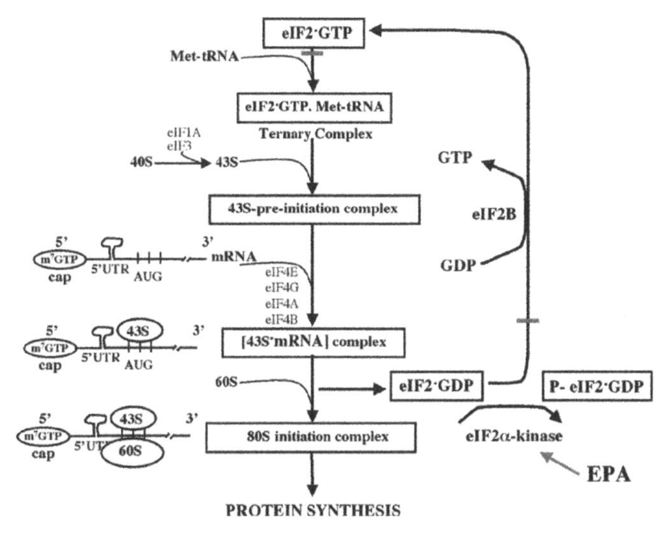

FIGURE 2 Schematic representation of translation initiation highlighting the sites of action of the n-3 polyunsaturated fatty acids.

folding or transport induce ER stress (Kaufman, 1999; Harding et al., 2000b). Another ER stressor is the partial depletion of intracellular calcium stores (Kaufman, 1999; Harding et al., 2000b). Indeed, it is well established that partial depletion of ER Ca^{2+} stores rapidly activates eIF2α kinases that phosphorylate eIF2α, thus limiting the rate of translation initiation and protein synthesis (Brostrom et al., 1989; Aktas et al., 1998). The exact mechanism by which reduction of intracellular Ca^{2+} activates eIF2α kinases is not clearly understood (Figure 2 identifies the putative sites for EPA action on the translation initiation process).

EPA Depletes Intracellular Ca^{2+} Stores

Binding of many physiological agonists of cell processes such as hormones, growth factors, or cytokines to their cognate cell membrane receptors induces a transient rise in cytosolic Ca^{2+} following its release from intracellular stores. When Ca^{2+} is released from intracellular stores, Ca^{2+} channels in the plasma membrane, known as *store-operated calcium* (SOC) *channels,* open to refill the intracellular stores by capacitative Ca^{2+} entry from the extracellular medium, thus reestablishing cellular Ca^{2+} homeostasis (Berridge, 1995; Putney, 1997).

EPA has a dual effect on intracellular Ca^{2+} homeostasis. On the one hand, it induces Ca^{2+} release from the intracellular Ca^{2+} stores, and on the other, it inhibits Ca^{2+} influx through SOC in the plasma membrane; these cellular effects require peroxidation of EPA because they are blocked by vitamin E (Palakurthi et al., 2000). By releasing Ca^{2+} from the ER stores while simultaneously closing SOC, EPA partially depletes intracellular Ca^{2+} stores (Figure 3A). Depletion of the intracellular Ca^{2+} stores by EPA was confirmed by transfecting cells with ER-targeted "cameleon" proteins that monitor the ER calcium content in real time. Figure 3B shows the ER calcium–depleting effect of EPA.

As mentioned earlier, depletion of intracellular Ca^{2+} stores activates eIF2α kinases and inhibits translation initiation. Inhibition of translation initiation by EPA was demonstrated by sucrose density gradient centrifugation of cell lysates followed by determination of the cell polysome profile. Treatment of cells with EPA shifts the polysome profile from heavy polyribosomal fractions towards light polysomes and free ribosomal subunits (Palakurthi et al., 2000) (Figure 4). This shift of the cell polysome profile toward lighter fractions is recognized as the hallmark of inhibition of translation initiation.

Phosphorylation of eIF2α Mediates Inhibition of Translation Initiation by EPA

Inhibition of translation initiation by EPA is mediated by activation of eIF2α kinase–dependent phosphorylation of eIF2α. This conclusion is based on the experimental findings in cancer cell lines treated with EPA: (a) EPA causes phosphorylation of eIF2α (inset to Figure 4); (b) it inhibits translation initiation in wild-type cells but not in cells expressing a dominant-negative mutant of PKR; and (c) cells transfected with a constitutively active but phosphorylation-resistant mutant of eIF2α (eIF2α-S51A) are resistant to the effects of EPA on translation initiation, protein synthesis, and cell growth (Palakurthi et al., 2000).

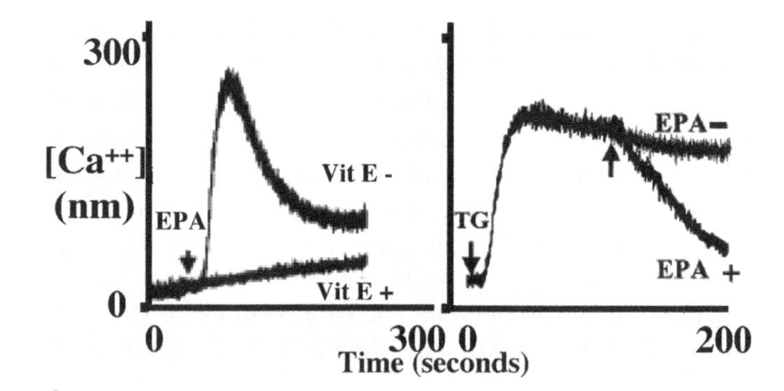

A

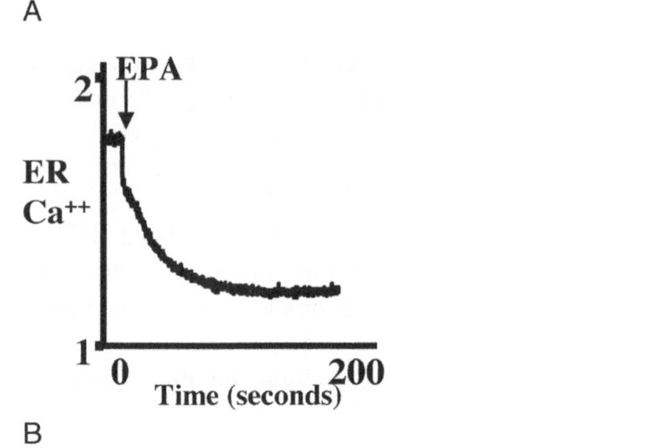

B

FIGURE 3 Eicosapentaenoic acid (EPA) releases Ca^{2+} from ER stores and closes store-operated calcium (SOC) channels. Fura-2–loaded cells were treated with EPA in the presence or absence of vitamin E (A) in Ca^{2+}-free media or with thapsigargin (TG) in Ca^{2+}-containing media to open SOC channels and then treated with or without EPA (Palakurthi, 2000). (B) ER-targeted Ca^{2+}-sensitive cameleon-expressing cells were treated with EPA excited at 440 nm and fluorescence resonance energy transfer (FRET) was measured by determining the emission ratio at 530 nm (Yellow Fluorescent Protein) versus 480 nm (Cyan Fluorescent Protein) (C).

EPA Downregulates G_1 Cyclins and Blocks Cell Cycle Progression in the G_1 Phase

Phosphorylation of eIF2α results in preferential downregulation of oncogenes and G_1 cyclins. It is well established that several structural features influence the translational efficiency of individual mRNAs. For example, long and complex 5′UTRs are associated with inefficient translation probably because in the presence of stable secondary structures, ribosomes cannot scan efficiently the entire 5′UTR to reach the AUG initiation codon (Koromilas et al., 1992b; Rousseau et al., 1996b). In contrast, mRNAs with simple, less structured 5′UTRs are translated more efficiently.

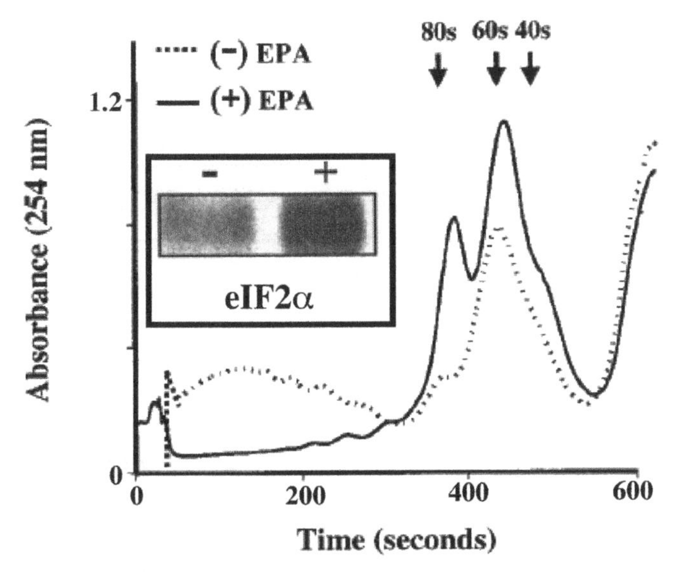

FIGURE 4 Eicosapentaenoic acid (EPA) shifts the cell polysome profile from heavy to lighter polysomes. Lysates of exponentially growing cells were processed by sucrose density gradient centrifugation and then read from the bottom at 214 nm. The inset shows phosphorylation of eIF2α by EPA.

Interestingly, the leader sequences of ~90% of vertebrate mRNAs are between 10 and 200 bases long, mostly without a complex secondary structure, and are efficiently translated ("strong" mRNAs). On the other hand, most mRNAs encoding for cell growth regulatory proteins or proto-oncogenes contain atypical 5′UTRs, which are >200 bases long and complex, which restricts their translational efficiency and renders their translation highly dependent on the activity of translation initiation factors ("weak" mRNAs) (Kozak, 1991). This translational inefficiency of proteins that regulate cell proliferation probably plays a crucial role in the maintenance of proper restraints on cell growth; unrestricted translation due to overexpression or dysregulation of translation initiation factors mostly increases the expression of oncogenic proteins and results in malignant transformation. For the reasons summarized earlier, interventions that restrict the rate of translation initiation by targeting translation initiation factors (such as eIF2) preferentially decrease the expression of growth-promoting and oncogenic proteins and can thereby inhibit the growth and metastatic potential of cancers (Graff et al., 1995; Rosenwald, 1996; Willis, 1999).

Consistently, EPA-mediated phosphorylation of eIF2α limits the rate of translation initiation and results in a preferential translational downregulation of G_1 cyclins. Figure 5A shows that EPA inhibits the synthesis and expression of cyclin D1, cyclin E, and Ras while minimally affecting the synthesis and expression of housekeeping proteins such as β-actin or ubiquitin. Figure 5B shows that cyclin D1 expression is downregulated at the level of translation. In this experiment, cells were made quiescent by serum withdrawal for 18 hours and then stimulated with basic fibroblast growth factor (bFGF). The figure shows that in quiescent cells there is no cyclin D1 mRNA. Eight hours after mitogenic stimulation with bFGF, the expression of cyclin D1 mRNA is fully induced, and the cyclin D1 protein is synthesized at a high level. In contrast, cells stimulated with bFGF in the presence of EPA show full expression of cyclin D1 mRNA but reduced synthesis of cyclin D1 protein. This experiment confirms that EPA inhibits cyclin D1 synthesis and expression at the level of translation. Importantly, this experiment also shows that EPA does not inhibit the bFGF-induced mitogenic signal upstream from the transcriptional activation of cyclin D1. Furthermore, EPA also downregulated cyclin D1 expression in the tumors *in vivo*. Taken together, these data indicate that EPA inhibits preferentially the translation initiation of cell cycle–regulatory but not of housekeeping proteins that may account for the potent anticancer effects of EPA with low toxicity. Downregulation of G_1 cyclins by EPA causes cell cycle arrest in the G_1 phase, as would have been expected from an agent that inhibits expression of G_1 cyclins (Palakurthi et al., 2000).

EPA Induces the Translation of ER-stress Genes Including Expression of Proapoptotic Proteins

EPA induces the translation of the activating transcription factor-4 (ATF-4)–regulated gene cluster. As previously discussed, treatment of cells with EPA limits the availability of the eIF2·GTP·Met-tRNAi ternary complex and decreases the overall rate of translation initiation. Scarcity of the ternary complex has different consequences for the translation of the various mRNAs. Under conditions of limited ternary complex availability, the translation of mRNAs' coding for housekeeping proteins such as β-actin and ubiquitin is minimally affected, while the translation of mRNAs' coding for oncogenic proteins such as cyclin D1 is dramatically reduced. Paradoxically, the translational efficiency of another subset of mRNAs is significantly enhanced when the ternary complex is scarce. Among these is the mRNA encoding for activating ATF-4, which regulates the transcription of the ER-stress response gene cluster (Harding et al., 2000a; Scheuner et al., 2001). The ATF-4 mRNA is more efficiently translated under conditions of limited ternary complex availability because its 5′UTR contains several upstream open reading frames (uORFs) that render its translation highly inefficient when the ternary complex is abundant but significantly more efficient when the ternary complex is scarce. When the 43S preinitiation complex binds to the 5′ end of the ATF-4 mRNA, it scans the 5′UTR and initiates translation at the AUG codon of the first uORF (exemplified in the schematic mRNA represented in Figure 5D). By recognizing the initiation codon of the first uORF, the ribosomal machinery is primed to also recognize its stop codon and dissociate. However, a small fraction of

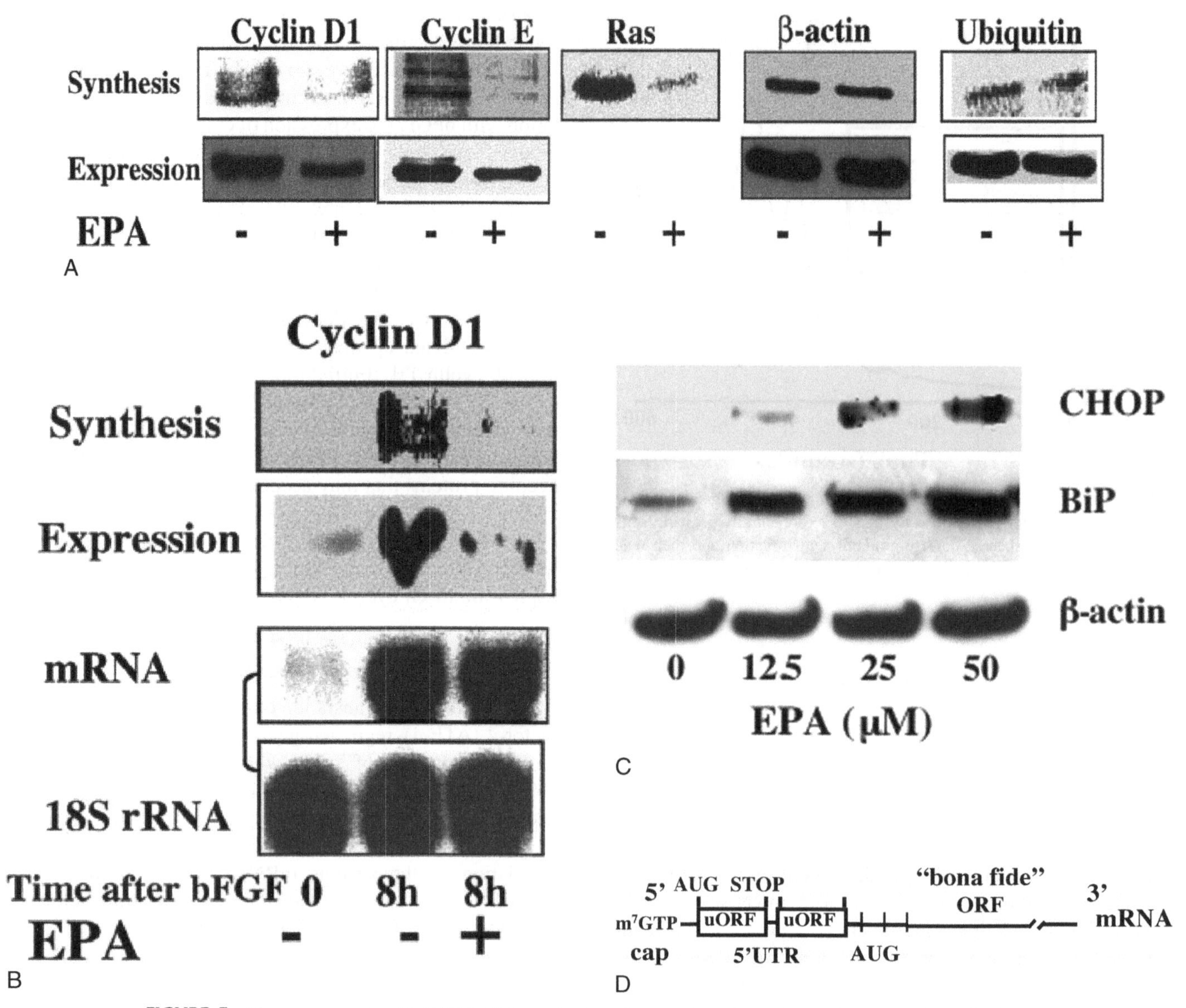

FIGURE 5 Eicosapentaenoic acid (EPA) inhibits synthesis and expression of growth-regulatory proteins at the level of translation initiation. (A) Exponentially growing cells were pulsed with [^{35}S]Met-Cys with or without 30 mM EPA for 1 hour, and equal protein-containing cell lysates immunoprecipitated with anti-cyclin D1, cyclin E, Ras, β-actin, or ubiquitin antibodies. Immunocomplexes were separated by sodium dodecyl sulfate–polyacrylamide gel electrophoresis (SDS-PAGE) and visualized by PhosphorImager (synthesis) or by Western blot (expression). (B) Quiescent NIH 3T3 cells were stimulated with bFGF (5 ng/ml)/0.1% calf serum for 8 hours with or without 30 mM EPA, and total RNA was extracted and Northern blotted with a cyclin D1–specific probe using 18S mRNA as loading control. Parallel cultures were pulse-labeled with [35 S]Met-Cys, and cell lysates were immunoprecipitated with anti-cyclin D1 antibodies. (C) MCF-7 breast cancer cells treated with EPA increase the expression of BiP and CHOP. (D) Schematic representation of an mRNA with several uORFs that restrict its translational efficacy when the ternary complex is abundant but increase its translation when the ternary complex is scarce.

the 40S ribosomal subunit that remains associated with the mRNA continues scanning toward the 3′ end, restarting initiation and falling off at the subsequent initiation and stop codons, respectively. In summary, the probability of reaching the initiation codon of the ATF-4 bona fide uORF is very low when the ternary complex is abundant. In contrast, when the ternary complex is scarce, the probability that the ribosomal machinery would translate the uORFs is reduced, and the probability that the 43S subunit would reach and translate the bona fide uORF of ATF4 is enhanced several-fold (Harding et al., 2000a). As a consequence, stimuli like EPA treatment that induce phosphorylation of eIF2α limit the

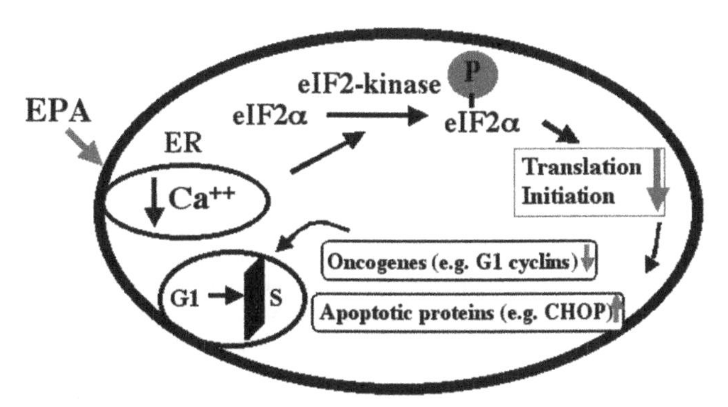

FIGURE 6 Schematic representation of the effect of eicosapentaenoic acid (EPA) on translation initiation. EPA induces Ca^{2+} release from ER calcium stores and closes SOC thus reducing the Ca content of the ER stores. Partial depletion of calcium in the ER activates eIF2α kinases, which phosphorylate eIF2α and thereby inhibit translation initiation. Inhibition of translation initiation by eIF2α phosphorylation has a differential effect on the translation of mRNAs that depends in part on the structure of their 5′UTR. Most are minimally affected; oncogenic and cell growth–regulatory proteins such the G1 cyclins are translationally downregulated; proteins such as BiP and the proapoptotic CHOP, which are under the transcriptional control of ATF-4, are upregulated. This results in interruption of the cell cycle in the G1 phase and in activation of proapoptotic pathways.

availability of the ternary complex, translationally upregulate the expression of ATF-4, and increase the transcription and expression of ATF-4 target genes such as chaperon binding protein (BiP) and C/EBP-homologous protein (CHOP). Indeed, treatment of cancer cells with EPA induces the expression of both BiP and proapoptotic CHOP (Figure 5C), providing a molecular explanation for the increased apoptotic rate reportedly seen in cancer cells upon prolonged treatment with EPA. Together with downregulation of oncogenic proteins and the blockade of cell cycle progression in the G_1 phase, increased apoptosis would also contribute to the anticancer properties of EPA.

In summary, we have identified the molecular mechanism of the anticancer activity of n-3 PUFAs such as EPA *in vitro* and most likely *in vivo*. By partially depleting ER Ca^{2+} stores, these natural dietary products inhibit translation initiation and preferentially downregulate the synthesis and expression of oncogenic proteins, thereby blocking the progression of the cell cycle in G_1, in association with increased apoptosis, mediated, at least in part, by upregulation of ER-stress response genes. Figure 6 summarizes the proposed mechanism of the anticancer effect of n-3 PUFAs such as EPA.

CONCLUSION

n-3 PUFAs were readily available nutrients in the primitive food chain. The effect of n-3 PUFAs on the translational regulation of genes that control cell proliferation and survival can be conceived as an environmental clue to maintain a correct restraint on physiological cell growth. Evolutionary and cultural changes have shifted the human diet over time toward a lower n-3 to n-6 PUFA ratio to the point that the modern Western diet is overwhelmingly rich in n-6 PUFAs. The observed increase in cancer rates in populations that until recently relied on n-3 PUFA-rich diets may be a reflection of the potential impact of the dietary transition from n-3 to n-6 PUFA–rich diets.

Efforts to reintroduce an adequate balance of n-3 to n-6 PUFAs in the modern diet might be hampered by the precipitous decline of marine fish stocks. Indeed, it seems that current marine sources would not be capable of sustaining a progressively increasing demand for dietary n-3 PUFAs by the world population. Fish produced in aquaculture farms do not represent a viable alternative to increase the n-3 PUFA content of the modern human diet because the fish diet contains vegetable oil that is rich in n-6 PUFAs. These fish will be low in n-3 PUFAs, relative to the population in the wild. There may be hope, however, because genes that can convert n-6 to n-3 fatty acids such as *fat-1* can be transgenically introduced into both plants and animals, as reported in mice (Kang et al., 2004).

Thus, given the magnitude of the potential public health benefits that could derive from increasing n-3 PUFAs in the human diet, and the multifactorial economic, cultural, and practical difficulties implicated in achieving that goal, extensive intervention studies are needed to determine conclusively whether n-3 PUFA–rich diets reduce cancer risk in a manner that justifies the effort. The conduction and success of such human trials critically depends on the availability of biomarkers that will provide clear-cut and efficient endpoints, thus limiting their duration and facilitating the interpretation of their results. The generation of such biomarkers is an important contribution of the research summarized in this chapter. Indeed, preliminary results in human cancer patients indicate that administration of EPA-rich fish oils induces phosphorylation of eIF2α *in vivo*. Thus, the theoretical and practical tools needed are now available for the design of prospective trials to validate first the translation initiation machinery as the molecular target of the putative effects of n-3 PUFAs in human cancers and, if confirmed, conduct adequate trials to assess the preventive and perhaps therapeutic effects of these nutrients, an approach recently advocated in *The Lancet* by Professor David Horrobin, a pioneer investigator on the potential therapeutic effects of n-3 PUFAs (Horrobin, 2003a, b).

References

Aktas, H., Fluckiger, R., Acosta, J.A., Savage, J.M., Palakurthi, S.S., and Halperin, J.A. 1998. Depletion of intracellular Ca^{2+} stores, phosphorylation of eIF2alpha, and sustained inhibition of translation initiation mediate the anticancer effects of clotrimazole. *Proc Natl Acad Sci USA* **95**: 8280–8285.

Armstrong, B., and Doll, R. 1975. Environmental factors and cancer incidence and mortality in different countries, with special reference to dietary practices. *Int J Cancer J Int Du Cancer* **15**: 617–631.

Arrick, B.A., Grendell, R.L., and Griffin, L.A. 1994. Enhanced translational efficiency of a novel transforming growth factor beta 3 mRNA in human breast cancer cells. *Mol Cell Biol* **14**: 619–628.

Augustsson, K., Michaud, D.S., Rimm, E.B., Leitzmann, M.F., Stampfer, M.J., Willett, W.C., and Giovannucci, E. 2003. A prospective study of intake of fish and marine fatty acids and prostate cancer. *Cancer Epidemiol Biomarkers Prev* **12**: 64–67.

Berkel, H.J., Turbat-Herrera, E.A., Shi, R., and de Benedetti, A. 2001. Expression of the translation initiation factor eIF4E in the polyp-cancer sequence in the colon. *Cancer Epidemiol Biomarkers Prev* **10**: 663–666.

Berridge, M.J. 1995. Capacitative calcium entry. *Biochem J* **312**: 1–11.

Bjarnason, O., Day, N., Snaedal, G., and Tulinius, H. 1974. The effect of year of birth on the breast cancer age-incidence curve in Iceland. *Int J Cancer* **13**: 689–696.

Brenner, R.R. 1974. The oxidative desaturation of unsaturated fatty acids in animals. *Mol Cell Biochem* **3**: 41–52.

Brostrom, C.O., Chin, K.V., Wong, W.L., Cade, C., and Brostrom, M.A. 1989. Inhibition of translational initiation in eukaryotic cells by calcium ionophore. *J Biol Chem* **264**: 1644–1649.

Bruce, W.R., Giacca, A., and Medline, A. 2000a. Possible mechanisms relating diet and risk of colon cancer. *Cancer Epidemiol Biomarkers Prev* **9**: 1271–1279.

Bruce, W.R., Wolever, T.M., and Giacca, A. 2000b. Mechanisms linking diet and colorectal cancer: the possible role of insulin resistance. *Nutr Cancer* **37**: 19–26.

Calviello, G., Palozza, P., Piccioni, E., Maggiano, N., Frattucci, A., Franceschelli, P., and Bartoli, G.M. 1998. Dietary supplementation with eicosapentaenoic and docosahexaenoic acid inhibits growth of Morris hepatocarcinoma 3924A in rats: effects on proliferation and apoptosis. *Int J Cancer* **75**: 699–705.

Chajes, V., Sattler, W., Stranzl, A., and Kostner, G.M. 1995. Influence of n-3 fatty acids on the growth of human breast cancer cells in vitro: relationship to peroxides and vitamin-E. *Breast Cancer Res Treat* **34**: 199–212.

Chen, Q., and Nilsson, A. 1993. Desaturation and chain elongation of n-3 and n-6 polyunsaturated fatty acids in the human CaCo-2 cell line. *Biochim Biophys Acta* **1166**: 193–201.

Christiansen, E.N., Lund, J.S., Rortveit, T., and Rustan, A.C. 1991. Effect of dietary n-3 and n-6 fatty acids on fatty acid desaturation in rat liver. *Biochim Biophys Acta* **1082**: 57–62.

Clemens, M.J., and Bommer, U.A. 1999. Translational control: the cancer connection. *Int J Biochem Cell Biol* **31**: 1–23.

Collins, F.D., Sinclair, A.J., Royle, J.P., Coats, D.A., Maynard, A.T., and Leonard, R.F. 1971. Plasma lipids in human linoleic acid deficiency. *Nutr Metab* **13**: 150–167.

Crew, J.P., Fuggle, S., Bicknell, R., Cranston, D.W., de Benedetti, A., and Harris, A.L. 2000. Eukaryotic initiation factor-4E in superficial and muscle invasive bladder cancer and its correlation with vascular endothelial growth factor expression and tumour progression. *Br J Cancer* **82**: 161–166.

Davis, S., and Watson, J.C. 1996. In vitro activation of the interferon-induced, double-stranded RNA- dependent protein kinase PKR by RNA from the 3′ untranslated regions of human alpha-tropomyosin. *Proc Natl Acad Sci USA* **93**: 508–513.

Deapen, D., Liu, L., Perkins, C., Bernstein, L., and Ross, R.K. 2002. Rapidly rising breast cancer incidence rates among Asian-American women. *Int J Cancer* **99**: 747–750.

Donze, O., Jagus, R., Koromilas, A.E., Hershey, J.W., and Sonenberg, N. 1995. Abrogation of translation initiation factor eIF-2 phosphorylation causes malignant transformation of NIH 3T3 cells. *EMBO J* **14**: 3828–3834.

Dua, K., Williams, T.M., and Beretta, L. 2001. Translational control of the proteome: relevance to cancer. *Proteomics* **1**: 1191–1199.

Duan, D.R., Pause, A., Burgess, W.H., Aso, T., Chen, D.Y., Garrett, K.P., Conaway, R.C., Conaway, J.W., Linehan, W.M., and Klausner, R.D. 1995. Inhibition of transcription elongation by the VHL tumor suppressor protein. *Science* **269**: 1402–1406.

Emken, E.A. 1994. Metabolism of dietary stearic acid relative to other fatty acids in human subjects. *Am J Clin Nutr* **60**: 1023S–1028S.

Emken, E.A., Adlof, R.O., Duval, S.M., and Nelson, G.J. 1998. Effect of dietary arachidonic acid on metabolism of deuterated linoleic acid by adult male subjects. *Lipids* **33**: 471–480.

Emken, E.A., Adlof, R.O., Duval, S.M., and Nelson, G.J. 1999. Effect of dietary docosahexaenoic acid on desaturation and uptake in vivo of isotope-labeled oleic, linoleic, and linolenic acids by male subjects. *Lipids* **34**: 785–791.

Falconer, J.S., Ross, J.A., Fearon, K.C., Hawkins, R.A., O'Riordain, M.G., and Carter, D.C. 1994. Effect of eicosapentaenoic acid and other fatty acids on the growth in vitro of human pancreatic cancer cell lines. *Br J Cancer* **69**: 826–832.

Fischer, S., and Weber, P.C. 1984. Prostaglandin I3 is formed *in vivo* in man after dietary eicosapentaenoic acid. *Nature* **307**: 165–168.

Gonzalez, M.J. 1995. Fish oil, lipid peroxidation and mammary tumor growth. *J Am Coll Nutr* **14**: 325–335.

Gonzalez, M.J., Schemmel, R.A., Dugan, L., Jr., Gray, J.I., and Welsch, C.W. 1993. Dietary fish oil inhibits human breast carcinoma growth: a function of increased lipid peroxidation. *Lipids* **28**: 827–832.

Gonzalez, M.J., Schemmel, R.A., Gray, J.I., Dugan, L., Jr, Sheffield, L.G., and Welsch, C.W. 1991. Effect of dietary fat on growth of MCF-7 and MDA-MB231 human breast carcinomas in athymic nude mice: relationship between carcinoma growth and lipid peroxidation product levels. *Carcinogenesis* **12**: 1231–1235.

Graff, J.R., Boghaert, E.R., De Benedetti, A., Tudor, D.L., Zimmer, C.C., Chan, S.K., and Zimmer, S.G. 1995. Reduction of translation initiation factor 4E decreases the malignancy of ras-transformed cloned rat embryo fibroblasts. *Int J Cancer* **60**: 255–263.

Grammatikos, S.I., Subbaiah, P.V., Victor, T.A., and Miller, W.M. 1994. n-3 and n-6 fatty acid processing and growth effects in neoplastic and non-cancerous human mammary epithelial cell lines. *Br J Cancer* **70**: 219–227.

Hansen, A.E., Haggard, M.E., Boelsche, A.N., Adam, D.J., and Wiese, H.F. 1958. Essential fatty acids in infant nutrition. III. Clinical manifestations of linoleic acid deficiency. *J Nutr* **66**: 565–576.

Harding, H.P., Novoa, I., Zhang, Y., Zeng, H., Wek, R., Schapira, M., and Ron, D. 2000a. Regulated translation initiation controls stress-induced gene expression in mammalian cells. *Mol Cell* **6**: 1099–1108.

Harding, H.P., Zhang, Y., Bertolotti, A., Zeng, H., and Ron, D. 2000b. Perk is essential for translational regulation and cell survival during the unfolded protein response. *Mol Cell* **5**: 897–904.

Hirayama, T. 1978. Epidemiology of breast cancer with special reference to the role of diet. *Prev Med* **7**: 173–195.

Holman, R.T., Johnson, S.B., and Hatch, T.F. 1982. A case of human linolenic acid deficiency involving neurological abnormalities. *Am J Clin Nutr* **35**: 617–623.

Horrobin, D.F. 2003a. Are large clinical trials in rapidly lethal diseases usually unethical? *Lancet* **361**: 695–697.

Horrobin, D.F. 2003b. A low toxicity maintenance regime, using eicosapentaenoic acid and readily available drugs, for mantle cell lymphoma and other malignancies with excess cyclin D1 levels. *Med Hypotheses* **60**: 615–623.

Jansson, B., Seibert, B., and Speer, J.F. 1975. Gastrointestinal cancer. Its geographic distribution and correlation to breast cancer. *Cancer* **36**: 2373–2384.

Kaizer, L., Boyd, N.F., Kriukov, V., and Tritchler, D. 1989. Fish consumption and breast cancer risk: an ecological study. *Nutr Cancer* **12**: 61–68.

Kang, J.X., Wang, J., Wu, L., and Kang, Z.B. 2004. Transgenic mice: fat-1 mice convert n-6 to n-3 fatty acids. *Nature* **427**: 504.

Karmali, R.A., Reichel, P., Cohen, L.A., Terano, T., Hirai, A., Tamura, Y., and Yoshida, S. 1987. The effects of dietary υ-3 fatty acids on the DU-145 transplantable human prostatic tumor. *Anticancer Res* **7**: 1173–1180.

Kaufman, R.J. 1999. Stress signaling from the lumen of the endoplasmic reticulum: coordination of gene transcriptional and translational controls. *Genes Dev* **13**: 1211–1233.

Koromilas, A.E., Lazaris-Karatzas, A., and Sonenberg, N. 1992b. mRNAs containing extensive secondary structure in their 5′ non-coding region translate efficiently in cells overexpressing initiation factor eIF-4E. *EMBO J* **11**: 4153–4158.

Koromilas, A.E., Roy, S., Barber, G.N., Katze, M.G., and Sonenberg, N. 1992a. Malignant transformation by a mutant of the IFN-inducible dsRNA-dependent protein kinase. *Science* **257**: 1685–1689.

Kozak, M. 1991. An analysis of vertebrate mRNA sequences: intimations of translational control. *J Cell Biol* **115**: 887–903.

Lanier, A., Kelly, J., Smith, B., Harpster, A., Tanttila, H., Amadon, C., Beckworth, D., Key, C., and Davidson, A. 1996a. Alaska Native cancer update: incidence rates 1989–1993. *Cancer Epidemiol Biomarkers Prev* **5**: 749–751.

Lanier, A.P. 1996. Cancer in Circumpolar Inuit. Background information for Alaska. *Acta Oncol* **35**: 523–525.

Lanier, A.P., Kelly, J.J., Smith, B., Harpster, A.P., Tanttila, H., Amadon, C., Beckworth, D., Key, C., and Davidson, A.M. 1996b. Alaska Native cancer update: incidence rates 1989–1993. *Cancer Epidemiol Biomarkers Prev Publ Am Assoc Cancer Res Cosponsored Am Soc Prev Oncol* **5**: 749–751.

Lazaris-Karatzas, A., Montine, K.S., and Sonenberg, N. 1990. Malignant transformation by a eukaryotic initiation factor subunit that binds to mRNA 5′ cap. *Nature* **345**: 544–547.

Lee, T.H., Menica-Huerta, J.M., Shih, C., Corey, E.J., Lewis, R.A., and Austen, K.F. 1984. Characterization and biologic properties of 5,12-dihydroxy derivatives of eicosapentaenoic acid, including leukotriene B5 and the double lipoxygenase product. *J Biol Chem* **259**: 2383–2389.

Li, B.D., Gruner, J.S., Abreo, F., Johnson, L.W., Yu, H., Nawas, S., McDonald, J.C., and DeBenedetti, A. 2002. Prospective study of eukaryotic initiation factor 4E protein elevation and breast cancer outcome. *Ann Surg* **235**: 732–739.

Li, B.D., McDonald, J.C., Nasssar, R., and DeBenedetti, A. 1998. Clinical outcome in stage I to III breast carcinoma and eIF4E overexpression. *Ann Surg* **227**: 756–763.

Liang, T., and Liao, S. 1992. Inhibition of steroid 5 alpha-reductase by specific aliphatic unsaturated fatty acids. *Biochem J* **285**: 557–562.

Madani, S., Hichami, A., Charkaoui-Malki, M., and Khan, N.A. 2004. Diacylglycerols containing omega 3 and omega 6 fatty acids bind to RasGRP and modulate MAP kinase activation. *J Biol Chem* **279**: 1176–1183.

Mitchell, D., Niu, S., and Litman, B. 2003. DHA-rich phospholipids optimize G-protein–coupled signaling. *J Pediatr* **143**: S80–S86.

Nathan, C.A., Amirghahri, N., Rice, C., Abreo, F.W., Shi, R., and Stucker, F.J. 2002. Molecular analysis of surgical margins in head and neck squamous cell carcinoma patients. *Laryngoscope* **112**: 2129–2140.

Nathan, C.A., Carter, P., Liu, L., Li, B.D., Abreo, F., Tudor, A., Zimmer, S.G., and De Benedetti, A. 1997. Elevated expression of eIF4E and FGF-2 isoforms during vascularization of breast carcinomas. *Oncogene* **15**: 1087–1094.

Needleman, P., Raz, A., Minkes, M.S., Ferrendelli, J.A., and Sprecher, H. 1979. Triene prostaglandins: prostacyclin and thromboxane biosynthesis and unique biological properties. *Proc Natl Acad Sci USA* **76**: 944–948.

Nielson, N.H., and Hansen, J.P. 1980. Breast cancer in Greenland—selected epidemiological, clinical, and histological features. *Clin Oncol* **1980**: 287–299.

Osborne, C.K. 1988. Effects of estrogens and antiestrogens on cell proliferation: implications for the treatment of breast cancer. *Cancer Treat Res* **39**: 111–129.

Pain, V.M. 1996. Initiation of protein synthesis in eukaryotic cells. *Eur J Biochem* **236**: 747–771.

Palakurthi, S.S., Fluckiger, R., Aktas, H., Changolkar, A.K., Shahsafaei, A., Harneit, S., Kilic, E., and Halperin, J.A. 2000. Inhibition of translation initiation mediates the anticancer effect of the n-3 polyunsaturated fatty acid eicosapentaenoic acid. *Cancer Res* **60**: 2919–2925.

Paulsrud, J.R., Pensler, L., Whitten, C.F., Stewart, S., and Holman, R.T. 1972. Essential fatty acid deficiency in infants induced by fat-free intravenous feeding. *Am J Clin Nutr* **25**: 897–904.

Prescott, S.M. 1984. The effect of eicosapentaenoic acid on leukotriene B production by human neutrophils. *J Biol Chem* **259**: 7615–7621.

Putney, J.W., Jr. 1997. Type 3 inositol 1,4,5-trisphosphate receptor and capacitative calcium entry. *Cell Calcium* **21**: 257–261.

Rastinejad, F., Conboy, M.J., Rando, T.A., and Blau., H.M. 1993. Tumor suppression by RNA from the 3′ untranslated region of α-tropomyosin. *Cell* **75**: 1107–1117.

Raught, B., Gingras, A.-C., James, A., Medina, D., Sonenberg, N., and Rosen, J.M. 1996. Expression of a translationally regulated, dominant-negative CCAAT/enhancer-binding protein β isoform and up-regulation of the eukaryotic translation initiation factor 2α are correlated with neoplastic transformation of Mammary epithelial cells. *Cancer Res* **56**: 4382–4386.

Rose, D.P., and Connolly, J.M. 1999. Omega-3 fatty acids as cancer chemopreventive agents. *Pharmacol Ther* **83**: 217–244.

Rose, D.P., Connolly, J.M., and Coleman, M. 1996. Effect of omega-3 fatty acids on the progression of metastases after the surgical excision of human breast cancer cell solid tumors growing in nude mice. *Clin Cancer Res Off J Am Assoc Cancer Res* **2**: 1751–1756.

Rose, D.P., Rayburn, J., Hatala, M.A., and Connolly, J.M. 1994. Effects of dietary fish oil on fatty acids and eicosanoids in metastasizing human breast cancer cells. *Nutr Cancer* **22**: 131–141.

Rosenwald, I.B. 1996. Deregulation of protein synthesis as a mechanism of neoplastic transformation. *Bioessays* **18**: 243–250.

Rosenwald, I.B., Hutzler, M.J., Wang, S., Savas, L., and Fraire, A.E. 2001. Expression of eukaryotic translation initiation factors 4E and 2alpha is increased frequently in bronchioloalveolar but not in squamous cell carcinomas of the lung. *Cancer* **92**: 2164–2171.

Rousseau, D., Gingras, A.C., Pause, A., and Sonenberg, N. 1996. The eIF4E-binding proteins 1 and 2 are negative regulators of cell growth. *Oncogene* **13**: 2415–2420.

Rousseau, D., Kaspar, R., Rosenwald, I., Gehrke, L., and Sonenberg, N. 1996b. Translation initiation of ornithine decarboxylase and nucleocytoplasmic transport of cyclin D1 mRNA are increased in cells overexpressing eukaryotic initiation factor 4E. *Proc Natl Acad Sci USA* **93**: 1065–1070.

Sasaki, S., Horacsek, M., and Kesteloot, H. 1993. An ecological study of the relationship between dietary fat intake and breast cancer mortality. *Prev Med* **22**: 187–202.

Sauerwald, T.U., Hachey, D.L., Jensen, C.L., Chen, H., Anderson, R.E., and Heird, W.C. 1996. Effect of dietary alpha-linolenic acid intake on incorporation of docosahexaenoic and arachidonic acids into plasma phospholipids of term infants. *Lipids* **31**(Suppl): S131–S135.

Sayanova, O.V., and Napier, J.A. 2004. Eicosapentaenoic acid: biosynthetic routes and the potential for synthesis in transgenic plants. *Phytochemistry* **65**: 147–158.

Scheuner, D., Song, B., McEwen, E., Liu, C., Laybutt, R., Gillespie, P., Saunders, T., Bonner-Weir, S., and Kaufman, R.J. 2001. Translational control is required for the unfolded protein response and in vivo glucose homeostasis. *Mol Cell* **7**: 1165–1176.

Scott, P.A., Smith, K., Poulsom, R., De Benedetti, A., Bicknell, R., and Harris, A.L. 1998. Differential expression of vascular endothelial growth factor mRNA vs protein isoform expression in human breast cancer and relationship to eIF-4E. *Br J Cancer* **77**: 2120–2128.

Shilatifard, A., Lane, W.S., Jackson, K.W., Conaway, R.C., and Conaway, J.W. 1996. An RNA polymerase II elongation factor encoded by the human ELL gene. *Science* **271**: 1873–1876.

Sonenberg, N. 1994. mRNA translation: influence of the 5′ and 3′ untranslated regions. *Curr Opin Genet Dev* **4**: 310–315.

Srivastava, S.P., Davies, M.V., and Kaufman, R.J. 1995. Calcium depletion from the endoplasmic reticulum activates the double-stranded RNA-dependent protein kinase (PKR) to inhibit protein synthesis. *J Biol Chem* **270**: 16619–16624.

Strasser, T., Fischer, S., and Weber, P.C. 1985. Leukotriene B5 is formed in human neutrophils after dietary supplementation with icosapentaenoic acid. *Proc Natl Acad Sci USA* **82**: 1540–1543.

Telang, N.T., Katdare, M., Bradlow, H.L., and Osborne, M.P. 1997. Estradiol metabolism: an endocrine biomarker for modulation of human mammary carcinogenesis. *Environ Health Perspect* **105**: 559–564.

Terry, P.D., Rohan, T.E., and Wolk, A. 2003. Intakes of fish and marine fatty acids and the risks of cancers of the breast and prostate and of other hormone-related cancers: a review of the epidemiologic evidence. *Am J Clin Nutr* **77**: 532–543.

Tsuji, K., Harashima, E., Nakagawa, Y., Urata, G., and Shirataka, M. 1996. Time-lag effect of dietary fiber and fat intake ratio on Japanese colon cancer mortality. *Biomed Environ Sci* **9**: 223–228.

Wang, S., Rosenwald, I.B., Hutzler, M.J., Pihan, G.A., Savas, L., Chen, J.J., and Woda, B.A. 1999. Expression of the eukaryotic translation initiation factors 4E and 2alpha in non-Hodgkin's lymphomas. *Am J Pathol* **155**: 247–255.

Welsch, C. 1997. The role of lipid peroxidation in growth suppression of human breast carcinoma by dietary fish oil. *Adv Exp Med Biol* **400B**: 849–860.

Welsch, C.W. 1995. Review of the effects of dietary fat on experimental mammary gland tumorigenesis: role of lipid peroxidation. *Free Radic Biol Med* **18**: 757–773.

Whelan, J., Petrik, M.B., McEntee, M.F., and Obukowicz, M.G. 2002. Dietary EPA reduces tumor load in ApcMin/+ mice by altering arachidonic acid metabolism, but conjugated linoleic acid, gamma- and alpha-linolenic acids have no effect. *Adv Exp Med Biol* **507**: 579–584.

Willett, W.C. 1997. Specific fatty acids and risks of breast and prostate cancer: dietary intake. *Am J Clin Nutr* **66**: 1557S–1563S.

Willis, A.E. 1999. Translational control of growth factor and proto-oncogene expression. *Int J Biochem Cell Biol* **31**: 73–86.

Wynder, E.L., Fujita, Y., Harris, R.E., Hirayama, T., and Hiyama, T. 1991. Comparative epidemiology of cancer between the United States and Japan. A second look. *Cancer* **67**: 746–763.

Xiao, Y.-F., Ke, Q., Wang, S.-Y., Auktor, K., Yang, Y., Wang, G.K., Morgan, J.P., and Leaf, A. 2001. Single point mutations affect fatty acid block of human myocardial sodium channel alpha subunit Na+ channels. *PNAS* **98**: 3606–3611.

You, W.C., Jin, F., Devesa, S., Gridley, G., Schatzkin, A., Yang, G., Rosenberg, P., Xiang, Y.B., Hu, Y.R., and Li, Q. 2002. Rapid increase in colorectal cancer rates in urban Shanghai, 1972–97, in relation to dietary changes. *J Cancer Epidemiol Prev* **7**: 143–146.

Zhang, Y.W., Morita, I., Yao, X.S., and Murota, S. 1999. Pretreatment with eicosapentaenoic acid prevented hypoxia/reoxygenation-induced abnormality in endothelial gap junctional intercellular communication through inhibiting the tyrosine kinase activity. *Prostaglandins Leukot Essent Fatty Acids* **61**: 33–40.

Ziegler, R.G., Hoover, R.N., Pike, M.C., Hildesheim, A., Nomura, A.M., West, D.W., Wu-Williams, A.H., Kolonel, L.N., Horn-Ross, P.L., Rosenthal, J.F., and et al. 1993. Migration patterns and breast cancer risk in Asian-American women. *J Natl Cancer Inst* **85**: 1819–1827.

C H A P T E R

31

Calcium and Vitamin D

JOELLEN WELSH

OVERVIEW: CALCIUM, VITAMIN D, AND CANCER

Epidemiological, molecular, and cellular studies have implicated vitamin D, a fat-soluble vitamin, in the development or progression of cancer. The activation of vitamin D in the body is intricately linked to dietary calcium, another nutrient that has been associated with cancer risk in epidemiological studies. Although the physiology of calcium and vitamin D are intricately connected, particularly in maintenance of skeletal health, it is now recognized that these nutrients also exert independent effects on cell behavior, including proliferation, differentiation, and apoptosis. This chapter focuses on the cellular and molecular mechanisms whereby calcium and vitamin D might have an impact on cancer risk and briefly discusses supportive data from epidemiological and clinical studies.

VITAMIN D AND CALCIUM METABOLISM: INTERPLAY OF ENDOCRINOLOGY AND NUTRITION

Forms, Functions, and Metabolism of Vitamin D

The term *vitamin D* refers to *calciferols*, steroid compounds originally identified as lipid-soluble compounds that could ameliorate the childhood bone disease rickets. Indeed, the best-characterized role of vitamin D is maintenance of extracellular calcium homeostasis, and rickets results from impaired bone mineralization secondary to insufficient calcium availability to the growing skeleton. Normally, low calcium availability induces transient hypocalcemia that stimulates secretion of parathyroid hormone (PTH) and enhances metabolic activation of vitamin D. Vitamin D in turn promotes absorption of dietary calcium in enterocytes, release of calcium from bone, and reabsorption of calcium in the kidney, processes mediated by the vitamin D receptor (VDR) (Holick, 2003). Once calcium influx restores normocalcemia, PTH secretion is diminished in a classic endocrine negative feedback loop. Under normal circumstances, therefore, this endocrine system maintains extracellular calcium homeostasis and allows for normal bone mineralization as long as sufficient calcium and vitamin D are available.

The two naturally occurring forms of vitamin D are cholecalciferol (vitamin D_3, from animal sources) and ergocalciferol (vitamin D_2, from plant sources); both forms require metabolism for biological activity. For simplicity, this review focuses on vitamin D_3 (Figure 1), but the metabolism and functions of vitamin D_2 are similar. Vitamin D_3 can be synthesized from a cholesterol derivative (7-dehydrocholesterol) in the epidermis, a conversion that requires ultraviolet B (UVB) radiation. Vitamin D_3 can also be obtained from natural and fortified foods and supplements (discussed in the section "Diet, Sunlight, and Vitamin D," later in this chapter) and is absorbed along with other dietary lipids. Regardless of source (endogenous synthesis or diet), the initial step in metabolism of vitamin D_3 is hepatic hydroxylation at the 25 position, generating 25-hydroxyvitamin D_3 (25[OH]D_3). 25(OH)D_3 is the major circulating form, which is also stored in adipose tissue and is the most accurate biomarker of overall vitamin D_3 status. Further metabolism of 25(OH)D_3 generates two metabolites: 24,25-dihydroxyvitamin D_3 (24,25[OH]$_2D_3$) or 1α,25-

Copyright © 2006, Elsevier Inc.
All rights of reproduction in any form reserved.

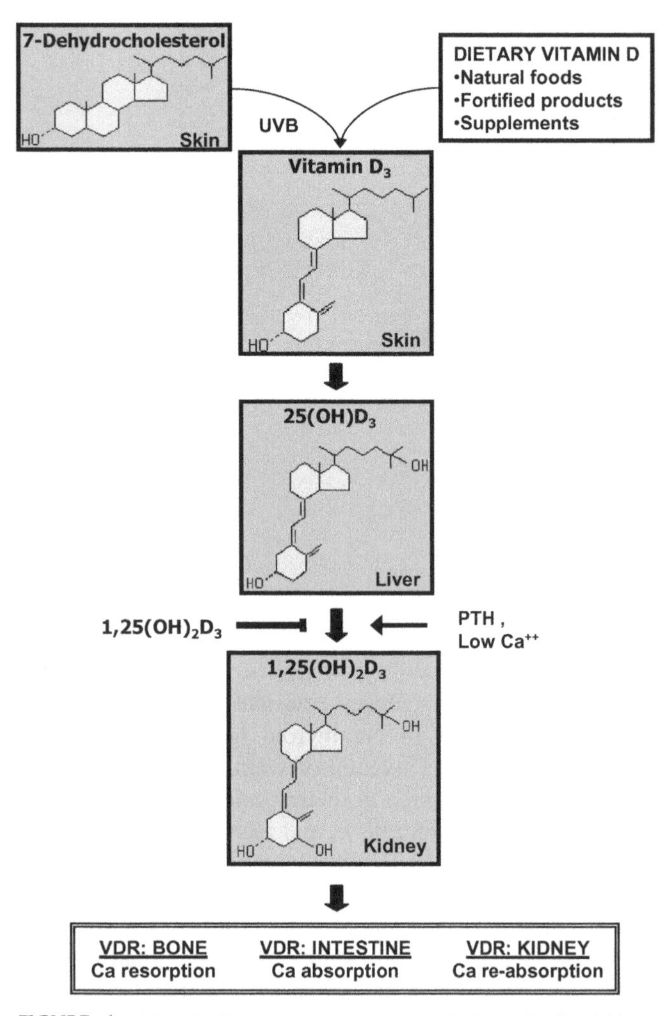

FIGURE 1 **Vitamin D3: structures and metabolism.** Cholecalciferol (vitamin D_3) can be endogenously synthesized in the epidermis upon exposure to ultraviolet B (UVB) radiation from sunlight, indoor tanning, or other sources. UVB energy cleaves the B ring in 7-dehydrocholesterol, creating the flexible A ring characteristic of cholecalciferol (D_3). Cholecalciferol can also be obtained from the diet, either from foods or from supplements; therefore, this compound was initially labeled a vitamin, and 7-dehydrocholesterol a previtamin. In the liver, cholecalciferol is metabolically converted to 25-hydroxycholecalciferol or $25(OH)D_3$ (the prohormone form) by the microsomal 25-hydroxylase enzyme. Production of the hormonal form, 1,25-dihydroxycholecalciferol or $1,25(OH)_2D_3$, in the proximal renal tubules is catalyzed by the mitochondrial 1α-hydroxylase, whose activity is tightly controlled by parathyroid hormone (PTH), calcium, and $1,25(OH)_2D_3$ itself. The metabolism of vitamin D_2 (ergocalciferol) is similar. In the classic endocrine control of calcium homeostasis, both $1,25(OH)_2D_3$ and $1,25(OH)_2D_2$ act as ligand for the vitamin D receptor (VDR) to mediate calcium influx into the circulation from bone, intestine, and kidney.

dihydroxyvitamin D_3 ($1,25[OH]_2D_3$). Production of $24,25(OH)_2D_3$ is catalyzed by the $25(OH)D_3$ 24-hydroxylase (also termed *CYP24* or *P450C24*), an enzyme present in the majority of vitamin D target tissues. The $24,25(OH)_2D_3$ metabolite does not readily bind VDR, and its production is considered the first step in degradation of $25(OH)D_3$. Production of $1,25(OH)_2D_3$, the biologically active vitamin D_3 metabolite, is mediated by the $25(OH)D_3$ 1α-hydroxylase (also termed *CYP27B1* or *P450C1*), an enzyme that is highly expressed in renal proximal tubules (Miller and Portale, 2003). $1,25(OH)_2D_3$, or *calcitriol*, is the ligand for the VDR and is a potent calcium-elevating hormone.

Because the kidney 1α-hydroxylase produces $1,25(OH)_2D_3$ for the systemic circulation, its activity reflects calcium availability. If calcium demand is increased, renal 1α-hydroxylase activity is induced and more $1,25(OH)_2D_3$ is generated (it is this activation step that is enhanced by PTH). Elevated circulating $1,25(OH)_2D_3$ subsequently interacts with VDR in target tissues such as kidney, intestine, and bone to mobilize calcium. Conversely, when calcium demands are low, the renal 1α-hydroxylase is suppressed and the 24-hydroxylase is enhanced, leading to formation of $24,25(OH)_2D_3$ and initiation of catabolism. These regulatory concepts of $25(OH)D_3$ hydroxylation are based on the renal enzymes and control of extracellular calcium homeostasis and are not likely to be applicable to regulation of these enzymes in other tissues. This issue is discussed further in the section "Uptake and Metabolism of Vitamin D Metabolites in Novel Target Tissues," later in this chapter, in the context of control of epithelial cell turnover by $1,25(OH)_2D_3$.

Diet, Sunlight, and Vitamin D Deficiency

Natural foods, with the exception of certain fish, are relatively low in calciferols, and epidermal synthesis is highly variable. For this reason, milk and other products are fortified with vitamin D_3 in the United States, Canada, and many other countries (Tangpricha et al., 2003). It should be noted, however, that fortification is voluntary, and the actual vitamin D_3 content of fortified milk is often less than the stated 400IU/quart (Holick et al., 1992). Despite the fortification of vitamin D_3 in foods and endogenous synthesis, the prevalence of vitamin D insufficiency, as defined by low circulating 25(OH)D, is surprisingly common, especially in populations living in northern climates and in the elderly (Lips, 2001; Zittermann, 2003). More than 50% of patients admitted to Massachusetts General Hospital in a 1998 sample were diagnosed as vitamin D deficient (Thomas et al., 1998), and >40% of healthy young men in Boston had serum 25(OH)D levels in the insufficient range at the end of winter (Tangpricha et al., 2002). Similar rates of vitamin D insufficiency were reported for middle-aged men in Finland (Ahonen et al., 2000). A study conducted in Boston reported that 24% of healthy adolescents were vitamin D deficient as defined by low serum 25(OH)D levels (Gordon et al., 2004). Factors associated with low vitamin D status include limited epidermal synthesis of cholecalciferol (because of infrequent exposure to sunlight, living in geographic areas with low solar radiation, dark pigmentation, and liberal use of sunscreen), liver or kidney disease, certain medications, poor diet, and aging. Indeed the current recommended daily allowance for vitamin D increases with age (200 IU for those younger than 50 years, 400 IU for those 51–70 years, and 600 IU for those 71 years or older).

The increasing number of reports of vitamin D insufficiency has prompted reevaluation of the recommended dietary allowances, which were designed to prevent rickets. There is fairly compelling evidence that prolonged subclinical vitamin D deficiency, which may not be associated with hypocalcemia but could limit availability of vitamin D metabolites to tissues, contributes to chronic disease in human populations (Zwittermann, 2003). However, relevant biomarkers of vitamin D status that reflect newly identified actions in target tissues such as colon, prostate, and breast (as discussed below) remain to be identified.

In most cases, overt vitamin D deficiency can be prevented or cured by dietary adjustments or use of a daily multivitamin supplement (Tangpricha et al., 2002; Zittermann, 2003). There are a number of hereditary defects in humans that impair bioactivation or utilization of vitamin D, and these are not cured by vitamin D itself. These vitamin D–resistant syndromes are rare and have been well characterized at the biochemical and molecular levels (Malloy and Feldman, 2003). Mouse models of hereditary vitamin D–resistance syndromes have become powerful research tools for identification of new functions of vitamin D (Li et al., 1997; Dardenne et al., 2001).

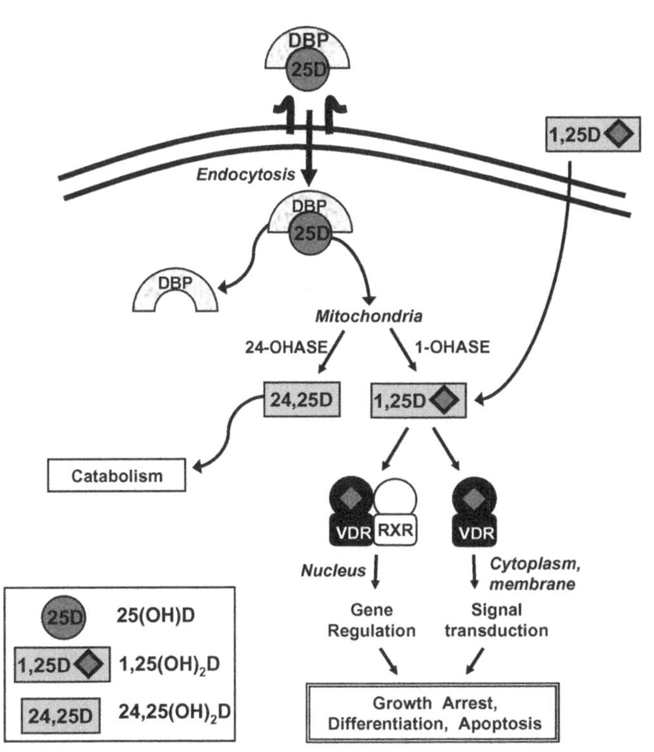

FIGURE 2 **Cellular pathways of vitamin D signaling.** Vitamin D metabolites circulate as free steroids and in complex with vitamin D binding protein (DBP). Free steroids, including $1,25(OH)_2D_3$, diffuse through the plasma membrane, whereas DBP containing bound vitamin D metabolites such as $25(OH)D_3$ is imported via receptor-mediated endocytosis. Inside cells, $25(OH)D_3$ is released from DBP and transported into mitochondria, likely via intracellular binding proteins that act as chaperones (not shown). Metabolism of $25(OH)D_3$ to $24,25(OH)_2D_3$ or $1,25(OH)_2D_3$ depends on the relative activities of the 24-hydroxylase (24-OHASE) and 1α-hydroxylase (1-OHASE) mitochondrial enzymes. Generation of $24,25(OH)_2D_3$ is considered the first step in a catabolism pathway, whereas $1,25(OH)_2D_3$, whether generated in mitochondria or taken up from the circulation, acts as ligand for the vitamin D receptor (VDR). VDR can mediate transcriptional regulation (as a heterodimer with RXR or other nuclear receptors) or nongenomic effects on membrane-initiated or cytoplasmic signal transduction pathways, leading to growth arrest, differentiation, and apoptosis.

CELLULAR MECHANISMS OF VITAMIN D ACTION

Uptake and Metabolism of Vitamin D Metabolites in Novel Target Tissues

The identification of the VDR in tissues that do not participate in control of extracellular calcium homeostasis prompted studies of vitamin D metabolism and action in additional cell types (Figure 2). Vitamin D metabolites, including $25(OH)D_3$ and $1,25(OH)_2D_3$, circulate in the free form, as well as bind to the vitamin D binding protein (DBP), a member of the albumin gene family. Free steroids, in particular $1,25(OH)_2D_3$, which has relatively low affinity for DBP, are presumed to enter cells via diffusion through the plasma membrane. In contrast, $25(OH)D_3$ bound to DBP enters renal cells via receptor-mediated endocytosis, facilitated by the megalin–cubulin complex (Willnow and Nykjaer, 2002). Though not yet demonstrated experimentally, it is likely that $25(OH)D_3$ bound to DBP can also be imported into nonrenal cells that express megalin. If so, the metabolic fate of $25(OH)D_3$ would depend on the relative expression/activity of $25(OH)D_3$–metabolizing enzymes. In cells with high levels of the $25(OH)D_3$ 24-hydroxylase, catabolism would predominate, whereas in cells with functional $25(OH)D_3$ 1α-hydroxylase, activation to $1,25(OH)_2D_3$ would occur. Examples of nonrenal cell types that express 25(OH)D 1α-hydroxylase include keratinocytes, macrophages, and epithelial cells derived from the prostate, breast, pancreas, and colon (Rizk-Rabin et al., 1994; Chen et al., 2003; Cross et al., 2003; Hewison et al., 2003; Welsh et al., 2003; Schwartz et al., 2004). The presence of 1α-hydroxylase in extrarenal tissues suggests that concentrations of $1,25(OH)_2D_3$ sufficient to elicit effects on cell proliferation could be generated from $25(OH)D_3$. In support of this possibility, some epithelial cells that express 1α-hydroxylase are growth inhibited by physiological concentrations of $25(OH)D_3$ *in vitro*, presumably due to its bioactivation to $1,25(OH)_2D_3$ (Hsu et al., 2001; Welsh et al.,

2003). This new concept of tissue-specific vitamin D metabolism and action indicates that the optimal serum levels of $25(OH)D_3$ will need to be redefined in terms of maintenance of local $1,25(OH)_2D_3$ generation.

These observations have thus identified two distinct pathways of vitamin D biosynthesis and action: an *endocrine* pathway geared toward maintenance of calcemia via circulating $1,25(OH)_2D_3$ (Figure 1) and an *autocrine* pathway (Figure 2), which mediates tissue-specific cell-regulatory effects via local generation of $1,25(OH)_2D_3$. The implication of the autocrine pathway is that cellular production of $1,25(OH)_2D_3$ would likely be regulated in a tissue-specific fashion independently of systemic calcium homeostasis. Similarly, the actions of locally produced $1,25(OH)_2D_3$ would be confined to the immediate cellular environment and would not necessarily affect body calcium homeostasis. Existence of the autocrine pathway implies that circulating $25(OH)D_3$ becomes the critical determinant of cellular vitamin D activity.

The Vitamin D Receptor

Whether generated in cells from $25(OH)D_3$ or taken up from the circulation, $1,25(OH)_2D_3$ binds to the VDR, a member of the steroid receptor family of ligand-dependent transcription factors that modulate gene expression in a tissue-specific manner (Carlberg, 2003; Christakos et al., 2003). Gene regulation by the liganded VDR requires dimerization, most often with the retinoid X receptor (RXR) family, and binding to specific DNA sequences in target gene promoters (Figure 2). Although a variety of structurally distinct vitamin D–responsive elements have been identified, the best characterized is a hexanucleotide direct repeat separated by three variable base pairs (DR3) to which VDR:RXR heterodimers bind. However, the recognition that VDR also functions as a homodimer or as a heterodimer with partners other than RXR and can bind diverse DNA sequences suggests enormous flexibility to the genomic pathways regulated by vitamin D. VDR can also influence gene expression via interactions with other transcription factors such as Sp1. In addition, the VDR is subject to post-translational modifications, including phosphorylation, which affect its transcriptional activity.

In addition to genomic signaling, $1,25(OH)_2D_3$ can exert rapid effects on signal transduction pathways, leading to biological responses at the plasma membrane or in the cytoplasm (Figure 2). Identification of an alternative binding pocket in the VDR for ligands that mediate rapid effects (Mizwicki et al., 2004) suggests that the VDR mediates some of these nongenomic effects, a suggestion supported by studies with cells from VDR-null mice (Erben et al., 2002; Zanello and Norman, 2004). Localization of the nuclear VDR protein to caveolae, specialized signaling complexes present in plasma membrane, further supports this concept (Huhtakangas et al., 2004). Examples of nontranscriptional effects of the $1,25(OH)_2D_3$–VDR complex with potential relevance to cancer cell regulation include calcium uptake, protein kinase C activation, interaction with β-catenin, and activation of protein phosphatases PP1c and PP2Ac (Palmer et al., 2001; Bettoun et al., 2002; Norman et al., 2002). The possibility that alternative receptors for vitamin D metabolites, which have been linked to rapid responses (Farach-Carson and Nemere, 2003), may contribute to cancer cell regulation by $1,25(OH)_2D_3$ has yet to be thoroughly investigated. Thus, the relative contributions of genomic and nongenomic signaling in mediating the diverse biological effects of $1,25(OH)_2D_3$, particularly in relation to its anticancer properties, remain to be fully clarified.

Newly Identified Vitamin D Target Cells

Although originally identified based on its role in bone homeostasis, vitamin D signaling has an impact on many cell types, including leukemic cells, osteoblasts, keratinocytes, and mammary, colon, and prostate epithelial cells. In an early study, 23 of 33 established human cancer cell lines surveyed expressed VDR (Frampton et al., 1982). In most VDR-positive cells, $1,25(OH)_2D_3$ mediates antiproliferative effects, and it may subsequently trigger differentiation or apoptosis. Importantly, studies with cells from VDR-null mice have demonstrated that the VDR is required for the growth-regulatory effects of $1,25(OH)_2D_3$ in transformed epithelial cells (Zinser et al., 2003). Expression profiling of breast, prostate, colon, and squamous carcinoma cells has identified $1,25(OH)_2D_3$–responsive gene clusters involved in regulation of cell cycle, differentiation, cell adhesion, and immune responses, indicating a diverse and broad range of VDR targets potentially involved in cell regulation (Palmer et al., 2001; Lin et al., 2002; Swami et al., 2003; Krishnan et al., 2004). The mechanisms by which $1,25(OH)_2D_3$ mediates growth-regulatory effects are briefly described; more details can be found in several reviews (Mork-Hansen et al., 2001; Lowe et al., 2003; Welsh et al., 2003).

Cell Regulatory Effects of $1,25(OH)_2D_3$

Cell Cycle Regulation

The antiproliferative effects of $1,25(OH)_2D_3$ result from alterations in key cell cycle regulators, which culminate in dephosphorylation of the retinoblastoma protein (Liu et al., 1996; Simboli-Campbell et al., 1997; Flanagan et al., 2003) and arrest of cells in G_0/G_1 (Munker et al., 1986; Zhuang and Burnstein, 1998; Park et al., 2000b). The cyclin-dependent kinase inhibitors p21 and p27 are genomic targets of the $1,25(OH)_2D_3$–VDR complex in many cell types (Liu et al., 1996; Park et al., 2000b; Scaglione-Sewell et al., 2000; Hager et al., 2001; Liu et al., 2002). In colon cancer cells, liganded VDR activates protein phosphatases PP1c and PP2Ac, leading to dephosphorylation of S6 kinase, which prevents progression from G_1 to S phase (Bettoun et al., 2002). In leukemic cells, $1,25(OH)_2D_3$–mediated growth arrest is paralleled by activation of Erk, JNK, and p38 mitogen-activated protein kinase pathways (Pepper et al., 2003). Thus, although the mechanisms vary with cell type, a common feature of vitamin D signaling is to prevent transition of cells from G_1 into S phase.

In addition to direct regulation of cell cycle modulators, $1,25(OH)_2D_3$ blocks mitogenic signaling, including that of estrogen, epidermal growth factor (EGF), insulin-like growth factor-1 (IGF-1), and KGF (Tong et al., 1999; Xie et al., 1999; Crescioli et al., 2000), and upregulates negative growth factors such as transforming growth factor-β (TGF-β) (Mehta et al., 1997; Jung et al., 1999; Yang et al., 2001). Although the tumor suppressor p53 mediates cell cycle arrest in response to many stimuli, $1,25(OH)_2D_3$ inhibits growth of cells that express mutant p53 (Eisman et al., 1989), indicating that functional p53 is not required for the antiproliferative effects of vitamin D. This notion is consistent with data indicating that $1,25(OH)_2D_3$–mediated activation of the p21 gene promoter is p53 independent (Liu et al, 1996).

Induction of Differentiation

In many cells, $1,25(OH)_2D_3$ has been shown to induce differentiation markers, suggesting that a major function of $1,25(OH)_2D_3$ in normal cells may be maintenance of the differentiated phenotype. The best studied example of vitamin D–induced differentiation is the keratinocyte (Bikle et al., 1993). In keratinocytes, $1,25(OH)_2D_3$–mediated differentiation is dependent on increases in intracellular calcium and induction of the calcium sensing receptor and phospholipase C (Bikle et al., 2003). The ability of vitamin D compounds to mediate keratinocyte differentiation has become important therapeutically, as vitamin D–based drugs are effective against psoriasis, a hyperproliferative skin disorder. Furthermore, skin from VDR-null mice exhibits abnormal differentiation (Xie et al., 2002) and is highly sensitive to tumor formation in response to chemical carcinogens (Zinser et al., 2002b).

Cancer cells that retain the ability to differentiate may be programmed to do so in response to $1,25(OH)_2D_3$. Examples include induction of β-casein in breast cancer cells (Lazzaro et al., 2000; Wang et al., 2001) and modulation of β-catenin signaling in colon cancer cells (Palmer et al., 2001). In leukemic cell lines such as HL-60, NB4, and U937 cells, $1,25(OH)_2D_3$ induces differentiation along the macrophage/monocyte pathway (Elstner et al., 1997). Genes identified as targets of $1,25(OH)_2D_3$ in leukemic cells include p21 and the homeobox gene HOXA10 (Liu et al., 1996; Rots et al., 1998). Numerous signaling pathways have been implicated in $1,25(OH)_2D_3$–induced monocytic differentiation, including nuclear factor-κB (NFkB), protein kinase C, ERKs, JNK, and p38 MAP kinases (Pepper et al., 2003). There is evidence that the induction of differentiation by $1,25(OH)_2D_3$ in NB4 leukemic cells is mediated, at least partially, through nongenomic pathways involving protein kinase C, changes in intracellular calcium, calpain activation, and NFkB signaling (Norman et al., 2002).

Activation of Apoptotic Cell Death

In some transformed cells, $1,25(OH)_2D_3$ induces apoptotic cell death via generation of reactive oxygen species, dissipation of the mitochondrial membrane potential, and cytochrome *c* release (Welsh et al., 1995; Narvaez and Welsh, 2001; Guzey et al., 2002; Flanagan et al., 2003), features of the intrinsic (mitochondrial) pathway of apoptosis. Cell lines reported to undergo apoptosis in response to $1,25(OH)_2D_3$ or various synthetic analogs include those derived from breast cancer, prostate cancer, colon carcinoma, squamous carcinoma, myeloma, retinoblastoma, neuroblastoma, and glioma (Simboli-Campbell et al., 1996; Diaz et al., 2000; Park et al., 2000a; McGuire et al., 2001; Audo et al., 2003; Elias et al., 2003; Wagner et al., 2003). Furthermore, $1,25(OH)_2D_3$ exerts additive or synergistic effects in combination with other triggers of apoptosis, such as radiation and chemotherapeutic agents (Chaudhry et al., 2001; Posner et al., 2001; Sundaram et al., 2003).

Sensitivity to $1,25(OH)_2D_3$–mediated apoptosis reflects the relative expression and/or subcellular localization of the Bcl-2 family of proapoptotic and antiapoptotic proteins, although the specific proteins involved and their modulation vary with cell type. In breast cancer cells, $1,25(OH)_2D_3$ downregulates the antiapoptotic protein Bcl-2 and induces redistribution of the proapoptotic protein Bax from cytosol to mitochondria (Narvaez and Welsh, 2001; Flanagan et al., 2003; Narvaez et al., 2003; Wagner et al., 2003). Furthermore, overexpression of Bcl-2 renders prostate and breast cancer cells resistant to $1,25(OH)_2D_3$–mediated apoptosis (Mathiasen et al., 1999; Blutt et al., 2000; Guzey et al., 2002).

The role of caspases and other proteases in $1,25(OH)_2D_3$–mediated cell death appears to vary with cell type. Activation of caspases 3 and 9 occurs during $1,25(OH)_2D_3$–induced apoptosis in some cells, and caspase inhibition can prevent some features of $1,25(OH)_2D_3$–mediated apoptosis (Park et al., 2000a; McGuire et al., 2001; Narvaez and Welsh, 2001; Guzey et al., 2002; Pepper et al., 2003). However, caspase inhibitors do not prevent

$1,25(OH)_2D_3$–mediated death (Mathiasen et al., 1999; Narvaez and Welsh, 2001; Pirianov and Colston, 2001; Guzey et al., 2002). Another protease pathway implicated in $1,25(OH)_2D_3$–mediated apoptosis involves calcium release from the endoplasmic reticulum and activation of μ-calpain (Mathiasen et al., 2002). In this study, $1,25(OH)_2D_3$–mediated apoptosis could be prevented by either calpain inhibitors or calcium-buffering agents such as calbindin D28K, indicating a requirement for both enzyme activation and calcium signaling (Mathiasen et al., 2002). Collectively, these studies indicate that a wide variety of signaling pathways, apoptotic-regulatory proteins, and proteases may contribute to $1,25(OH)_2D_3$–mediated apoptosis depending on the specific cell type or context.

MODULATION OF CELL TURNOVER AND CARCINOGENESIS BY VITAMIN D *IN VIVO*: ANIMAL STUDIES

Additional evidence that vitamin D can have an impact on both prevention and treatment of several common cancers has come from animal feeding studies. Rodents fed Western-style diets (low in vitamin D and calcium, high in saturated fat) developed hyperproliferation and/or enhanced rates of tumor formation in colon, prostate, and mammary gland compared with rats fed adequate calcium and vitamin D (Pence and Buddingh, 1988; Jacobson et al., 1989; Newmark et al., 1990; Xue et al., 1997, 1999). In mammary gland organ culture, $1,25(OH)_2D_3$ inhibits hormone-driven proliferation (Zinser et al., 2002a) and reduces the number of carcinogen-initiated preneoplastic lesions during both the initiation and the promotion stages (Mehta et al., 1997), indicating that vitamin D signaling can exert direct antineoplastic effects at multiple steps in the carcinogenesis process. VDR agonists have also been shown to inhibit angiogenesis, invasion, and metastasis (Hansen et al., 1994; Schwartz et al., 1997; Bernardi et al., 2002; Flanagan et al., 2003), indicating a potential benefit of vitamin D on later stages of cancer progression.

In addition to dietary manipulation, the effects of $1,25(OH)_2D_3$ and synthetic forms of vitamin D have been studied in animal models of cancer. In 1987, Eisman et al. presented the first evidence that $1,25(OH)_2D_3$ could inhibit growth of human colon carcinoma xenografts in immune-suppressed mice (Eisman et al., 1987). In most subsequent *in vivo* studies, synthetic vitamin D compounds have been utilized in attempts to avoid the hypercalcemic effects associated with chronic $1,25(OH)_2D_3$ administration. Pharmaceutical firms have since developed thousands of vitamin D analogs, some of which display enhanced cell-regulatory effects with reduced calcemic activity (Carlberg, 2003; Guyton et al., 2003; Pinette et al., 2003). Although their specific mechanisms of action are not completely understood, most vitamin D analogs that display antiproliferative effects bind to and activate VDR. Many synthetic analogs of vitamin D delay tumor formation in chemical carcinogenesis models and inhibit growth of established tumors in xenograft models (James et al., 1998; VanWeelden et al., 1998; Polek et al., 2001; Kumagai et al., 2003). Both $1,25(OH)_2D_3$ and a synthetic analog reduced polyp formation and tumor burden in the Apc/min mouse, a spontaneous model of hereditary colon cancer (Huerta et al., 2002). Analysis of regressing tumors indicated that vitamin D analogs induce growth arrest and apoptosis *in vivo* (James et al., 1998; VanWeelden et al., 1998; Audo et al., 2003), similar to that observed with VDR agonists *in vitro*. Vitamin D analogs have also been shown to reduce the number of secondary tumors and experimental metastasis in nude mouse models of breast and prostate cancer (Lokeshwar et al., 1999; El Abdaimi et al., 2000; Flanagan et al., 2003).

Newer studies with VDR-null mice have demonstrated that VDR status can modulate proliferation and carcinogenesis in normal tissues including mammary gland, colon, and skin (Kallay et al., 2001; Zinser et al., 2002a,b). VDR ablation significantly delays apoptotic remodeling of normal breast tissue during postlactational involution (Zinser and Welsh, 2004), providing the first evidence that vitamin D signaling has an impact on physiological apoptosis *in vivo*. VDR status alters tumor incidence in a transgenic model of breast cancer (MMTV-neu mice) and in chemically induced skin carcinogenesis (Zinser et al., 2002b; Zinser and Welsh, 2004). Collectively, these and other animal studies (summarized in Tables 1 and 2) have confirmed that the effects of vitamin D signaling observed *in vitro* translate to effects on cell proliferation, differentiation, and apoptosis *in vivo* that are of sufficient magnitude to have an impact on the carcinogenic process.

TABLE 1 Vitamin D and Prevention of Cancer

- Inverse associations reported between biomarkers of sunlight exposure, dairy products, and/or dietary vitamin D and risk of colon, prostate, and breast cancer
- Low circulating $25(OH)D_3$ and/or $1,25(OH)_2D_3$ associated with enhanced cancer risk and/or disease activity
- Amplification of $25(OH)D_3$ 24-hydroxylase in breast and esophageal cancers
- Vitamin D receptor (VDR) polymorphisms linked to cancer risk and/or metastatic progression
- VDR and $25(OH)D_3$ hydroxylases are expressed in normal epithelial tissues
- $1,25(OH)_2D_3$ inhibits carcinogen induced preneoplastic lesions in organ culture
- VDR-null mice exhibit abnormal cell turnover in colon, mammary gland, and epidermis
- VDR status correlates with carcinogenesis susceptibility in animal studies

TABLE 2 Vitamin D in Cancer Therapy

- Vitamin D receptor (VDR) is expressed in transformed cell lines and in human tumor biopsies.
- Natural and synthetic VDR agonists induce G_1 arrest, apoptosis, and/or differentiation *in vivo* and *in vitro*.
- $1,25(OH)_2D_3$ inhibits angiogenesis and invasion via effects on tumor cells, endothelial cells, and extracellular matrix proteases.
- Synthetic vitamin D analogs inhibit growth of carcinogen-induced tumors and human xenografts in absence of weight loss or hypercalcemia.
- Clinical trials indicate vitamin D–based drugs are well tolerated with some antitumor efficacy.

CALCIUM AND CANCER RISK

Calcium Intakes and Calcium Status

The majority of dietary calcium is derived from dairy products, although the mineral is also present in reasonable concentrations in certain vegetables, nuts, grains, and beans. Because of increased awareness that calcium intakes are frequently low, calcium-fortified foods (such as orange juice) and calcium supplements are encouraged. Although most attention has been paid to the role of calcium in protection against osteoporosis, the mineral has also been linked to protection against cancer of the colon and possibly other tissues (see the next subsection). Because of the tight homeostatic controls exerted by the PTH–vitamin D axis, which allow the body to adapt to a wide range of calcium intakes, *calcium deficiency* is not easy to define. Adaptation to chronic low dietary calcium is associated with compensatory increases in circulating PTH, which maintains serum calcium at the expense of calcium release from bone. Thus, unless severe or accompanied by vitamin D deficiency, low dietary calcium is not usually associated with changes in serum calcium.

Potential Mechanisms of Cancer Prevention by Calcium

In general, animal studies have supported the concept that high dietary calcium can inhibit colon, and possibly breast, cancer (Lipkin and Newmark, 1999; Lamprecht and Lipkin, 2003). Feeding a Western-style diet (low in calcium and vitamin D but high in saturated fat) induces hyperplasia and aberrant cell proliferation in colon and other tissues that is prevented by supplemental calcium (Richter et al., 1995). In the colonic lumen, calcium may bind lipids and/or bile acids and minimize damage to mucosal epithelial cells. In support of this concept, high dietary calcium reduces both incidence and multiplicity of cholic acid–promoted colon tumors in rats, an effect that correlates with inhibition of ornithine decarboxylase (Pence et al., 1995).

In some studies, interdependent effects of calcium and vitamin D on growth control have been identified. The ability of $1,25(OH)_2D_3$ to inhibit proliferation, induce differentiation, and activate apoptosis in colon cancer cells has been linked to changes in intracellular calcium (Zhao and Feldman, 1993; Vandewalle et al., 1995). In rodents, dietary vitamin D modulated the intracellular calcium gradient normally present along the colonic crypt–villus axis (Brenner et al., 1998).

Other evidence supports direct effects of calcium on epithelial cells (Lamprecht and Lipkin, 2003). Low extracellular calcium increases caco-2 cell proliferation via induction of c-myc (Hulla et al., 1995), and high calcium media inhibits proliferation and induces differentiation in many cell types (Lipkin and Newmark, 1999). The calcium-sensing receptor, originally identified in cells of the parathyroid gland, has been linked to calcium-mediated growth control. The calcium-sensing receptor is expressed in many cell types, including breast, ovarian, and intestinal epithelial cells and keratinocytes (Rodland, 2004). The calcium-sensing receptor is a G protein–coupled receptor in the plasma membrane that responds to physiological changes in extracellular calcium concentration by activating downstream signal transduction pathways involving phospholipase Cβ, inositol triphosphate, and diacylglycerol. Ultimately, these signals provoke calcium release from the endoplasmic reticulum, leading to elevated intracellular calcium and activation of protein kinase C. In colon cancer cells, calcium-sensing receptor signaling induces E-cadherin and suppresses B-catenin signaling (Chakrabarty et al., 2003), and resistance to calcium-mediated growth suppression correlates with loss of the calcium-sensing receptor (Rodland, 2004). The calcium-sensing receptor is also present in normal human breast cells, where it co-localizes with the vitamin D–dependent calcium-binding protein calbindin D28K, suggesting potential crosstalk between $1,25(OH)_2D_3$ and calcium signaling in this signal transduction pathway (Cheng et al., 1998; Parkash et al., 2004). Collectively, these data indicate that the calcium-sensing receptor represents a molecular link among extracellular calcium, intracellular calcium signaling, and growth control.

EPIDEMIOLOGICAL AND CLINICAL STUDIES ON VITAMIN D, CALCIUM, AND CANCER

Overview

Motivated by the cellular, molecular, and whole animal studies demonstrating antitumor effects of calcium and vitamin D, multiple studies have addressed the impact of these nutrients on cancer risk, particularly for breast, colon, and prostate carcinoma, in human populations. Because most cells that give rise to cancer express functional VDR and are sensitive to calcium-mediated signaling, it is envisioned that optimization of these pathways may actually prevent cancer development (Table 1). This concept has not yet been adequately tested in large-scale intervention trials in humans, although the ongoing Women's Health Initiative is addressing the effect of supplemental calcium and vitamin D on colon cancer development (Jackson et al., 2003).

The available evidence linking vitamin D and calcium to breast, prostate, and colon cancers is briefly reviewed in the following subsections, and readers are encouraged to consult the references cited in each section for more specific information. There are many similarities among these three common carcinomas: All are derived from epithelial tissues that normally express VDR and are independently growth inhibited by calcium and $1,25(OH)_2D_3$. All three tissues express 25(OH)D 1α-hydroxylase, highlighting the probability of local $1,25(OH)_2D_3$ production acting in an autocrine fashion to regulate cellular proliferation, differentiation, or apoptosis. Potentially relevant to cancer etiology, transformation may be associated with reduced function of the 25(OH)D 1α-hydroxylase (Ma et al., 2004) and amplification of the 25(OH)D 24-hydroxylase, which can inactivate both 25(OH)D and $1,25(OH)_2D_3$ (Albertson et al., 2000; Mimori et al., 2004). Furthermore, biopsies indicate that the majority of human colonic, breast, and prostate tumors retain expression of the VDR, highlighting the possibility that VDR agonists may have therapeutic value (Table 2).

Breast Cancer

Several studies have reported inverse associations between indices of vitamin D status (such as intake, sunlight exposure, solar radiation, and/or latitude) and breast cancer incidence or mortality (Garland et al., 1990; Knekt et al., 1996; John et al., 1999; Grant, 2002). A review of the epidemiological literature concluded that although there is no consistent correlation between dairy product intake and breast cancer risk (Moorman and Terry, 2004), there are inverse correlations between certain forms of dietary calcium and breast cancer (Shin et al., 2002; Boyapati et al., 2003). In a 2004 study, Berube et al. demonstrated that high dietary intakes of calcium and vitamin D are associated with reduced mammographic breast density, a strong risk factor for development of breast cancer.

Although no differences in serum $1,25(OH)_2D_3$ were found between breast cancer cases and controls 15 years prior to diagnosis (Hiatt et al., 1998), low levels of $1,25(OH)_2D_3$ were associated with increased breast cancer risk or disease progression in two case-control studies (Mawer et al., 1997; Janowsky et al., 1999). A high percentage of breast cancers express VDR, but there is no significant correlation between VDR expression and estrogen receptor expression, lymph node status, or tumor grade (Freake et al., 1984; Eisman et al., 1986; Berger et al., 1987, 1991). Tumor VDR status is not related to overall survival or to survival after relapse, but women with VDR-negative tumors relapsed earlier than women with VDR-positive tumors (Colston et al., 1989; Berger et al., 1991).

A few small clinical trials with vitamin D analog therapy have included patients with advanced breast cancer. Topical treatment with a rapidly metabolized analog (calcipotriol) was assessed in women with locally advanced or cutaneous metastatic disease (Bower et al., 1991), and ~20% of the participants showed partial responses. Similarly, disease stabilization was observed in some patients with breast cancer who received the low calcemic vitamin D analog EB1089 orally (Gulliford et al., 1998). Although no clear antitumor effects have been observed, these and other trials have demonstrated proof of principle that chronic administration of vitamin D analogs can be tolerated in breast cancer patients.

Prostate Cancer

Like breast cancer, prostate cancer risk is inversely correlated with solar radiation (Hanchette and Schwartz, 1992, Grant, 2002). Two studies have found a higher risk for early onset and/or more aggressive prostate cancer in young men with low serum $25(OH)D_3$ (Ahonen et al., 2000). Interestingly, high consumption of dairy foods or calcium (>2000 mg/day) may enhance prostate cancer incidence and mortality (Chan et al., 2001), an effect postulated to be secondary to inhibition of $1,25(OH)_2D_3$ production. However, no differences in serum $1,25(OH)_2D_3$ or $25(OH)D_3$ were found between prostate cancer cases and controls in another prospective study (Platz et al., 2004).

A number of phase I and II clinical trials with $1,25(OH)_2D_3$ have been conducted in patients with androgen-responsive and androgen-unresponsive prostate cancer (Johnson et al., 2002; Beer et al., 2003; Krishnan et al., 2003). These trials have evaluated toxicity, administration schedules, and changes in prostate-specific antigen (PSA), a serum biomarker of tumor responsiveness. In general, these studies have demonstrated reduction or stabilization of serum PSA level in a subset of patients, with limited toxicity particularly with intermittent $1,25(OH)_2D_3$ administration. Furthermore, combination therapy of $1,25(OH)_2D_3$ with other drugs such as paclitaxel and dexamethasone was associated with less toxicity, suggesting that simultaneously targeting vitamin D signaling and conventional cytotoxic pathways may be a more effective approach clinically.

Colon Cancer

Studies that combine multiple sources of vitamin D (intakes, supplements, and solar UV radiation) or measure serum 25(OH)D levels have generally reported inverse associations between vitamin D status and colon cancer risk

(Peters et al., 2001; Feskanich et al., 2004; Grant and Garland, 2004). In one human trial, calcium in milk products was shown to precipitate bile acids and increase their excretion (Govers et al., 1996). More significantly, supplemental dietary calcium inhibited colonic epithelial cell proliferation in subjects at high risk for colon cancer (Lipkin and Newmark, 1985). Several cohort and case-control studies support the association between dietary calcium and reduction of colon cancer risk (Schatzkin and Peters, 2004). Furthermore, two randomized, placebo-controlled clinical trials have shown that calcium supplements modestly decrease risk of colorectal adenoma recurrence (Baron et al., 1999; Grau et al., 2003). In the Calcium Polyp Prevention Study, 1200 mg elemental calcium reduced recurrence rate 19% within 1 year of intervention and had an even more pronounced effect on advanced colorectal lesions (Baron et al., 1999; Wallace et al., 2004). In studies that have addressed the role of both calcium and vitamin D, data strongly suggest that these nutrients interact to reduce the risk of colon carcinoma (Grau et al., 2003; Peters et al., 2004; Slattery et al., 2004).

VDR Gene Variants May Modify Cancer Risk

A number of common variants, or polymorphisms, in the human VDR gene have been studied in relation to cancer risk (Uitterlinden et al., 2004). VDR polymorphisms are distributed throughout the gene, including within the extensive promoter region (*Cdx-2* site), the coding sequence (*Fok*I, *Bsm*I, *Apa*I, and *Taq*I sites), and the 3'UTR (polyA repeat variants). Although the majority of VDR polymorphisms do not alter the amount, structure, or function of the VDR protein, the *Fok*I variation may have functional significance because individuals carrying the *Fok*I site produce a shorter VDR, which may be less active than the full-length VDR (Jurutka et al., 2000). More than a dozen studies have reported associations between one or more VDR polymorphisms and incidence or progression of breast, prostate, and colon cancer. Not unexpectedly, many studies report that associations between VDR polymorphisms and disease are highly dependent on other factors, including dietary calcium, ethnicity, UV radiation, and tumor histopathology (Habuchi et al., 2000; Kim et al., 2001; Hamasaki et al., 2002; Guy et al., 2003). Although more research is necessary to determine whether VDR genotypes have an impact on cancer risk, these studies highlight the importance of identifying the role of individual genetic variability in the response to dietary factors such as calcium and vitamin D.

SUMMARY

In this review, the possible relationship between vitamin D status, calcium intake, and cancer risk has been discussed on the basis of available evidence. Although the data are predominantly supportive that these nutrients can reduce cancer risk, many questions remain to be answered. For example, to what degree does individual genetic variation in components of the calcium or vitamin D signaling pathways alter the effectiveness of dietary interventions? Are specific subtypes of tumors (i.e., those harboring particular mutations) or patients (those with hereditary cancer syndromes) more or less responsive to dietary factors? Can biomarkers for vitamin D and calcium signaling at the cellular level be identified that can be used to define optimal status and the intakes necessary to achieve such status? Once these questions have been satisfactorily answered, public health measures to increase calcium and vitamin D intake via diet, food fortification, or supplementation might be warranted.

Acknowledgments

The author is indebted to her excellent research team at the University of Notre Dame, consisting of Lindsay Barnett, Belinda Byrne, Carly Kemmis, Carmen J. Narvaez, Matthew Rowling, Meggan Valrance, and Glendon Zinser, who contributed significantly to the studies and concepts discussed in this review. Work in the author's laboratory is supported by the National Cancer Institute, the Susan G. Komen Foundation, and the Department of Defense Breast Cancer Research Program.

References

Ahonen, M.H., Tenkanen, L., Teppo, L., Hakama, M., and Tuohimaa, P. 2000. Prostate cancer risk and prediagnostic serum 25-hydroxyvitamin D levels (Finland). *Cancer Causes Control* **11**: 847–852.

Albertson, D.G., Ylstra, B., Segraves, R., Collins, C., Dairkee, S.H., Kowbel, D., Kuo, W.L., Gray, J.W., and Pinkel, D. 2000. Quantitative mapping of amplicon structure by array CGH identifies CYP24 as a candidate oncogene. *Nat Genet* **25**: 144–146.

Audo, I., Darjatmoko, S.R., Schlamp, C.L., Lokken, J.M., Lindstrom, M.J., Albert, D.M., and Nickells, R.W. 2003. Vitamin D analogues increase p53, p21, and apoptosis in a xenograft model of human retinoblastoma. *Investig Ophthalmol Visual Sci* **44**: 4192–4199.

Baron, J.A., Beach, M., Mandle, J.S., van Stolk, R.U., Haile, R.W., Sandler, R.S., Rothstein, R., Summers, R.W., Snover, D.C., Beck, G.J., Bond, J.H., and Greenberg, E.R. 1999. Calcium supplements for the prevention of colorectal adenomas. *N Engl J Med* **340**: 101–107.

Beer, T.M., Lemmon, D., Lowe, B.A., and Henner, W.D. 2003. High-dose weekly oral calcitriol in patients with a rising PSA after prostatectomy or radiation for prostate carcinoma. *Cancer* **97**: 1217–1224.

Berger, U., McClelland, R.A., Wilson, P., Greene, G.L., Haussler, M.R., Pike, J.W., Colston, K., Easton, D., and Coombes, R.C. 1991. Immunocytochemical determination of estrogen receptor, progesterone receptor, and 1,25-dihydroxyvitamin D3 receptor in breast cancer and relationship to prognosis. *Cancer Res* **51**: 239–244.

Berger, U., Wilson, P., McClelland, R.A., Colston, K., Haussler, M.R., Pike, J.W., and Coombes, R.C. 1987. Immunocytochemical detection of 1,25-dihydroxyvitamin D3 receptor in breast cancer. *Cancer Res* **47**: 6793–6799.

Bernardi, R.J., Johnson, C.S., Modzelewski, R.A., and Trump, D.L. 2002. Antiproliferative effects of 1alpha,25-dihydroxyvitamin D(3) and vitamin D analogs on tumor-derived endothelial cells. *Endocrinology* **143**: 2508–2514.

Berube, S., Diorio, C., Verhoek-Oftedahl, W., and Brisson, J. 2004. Vitamin D, calcium and mammographic breast densities. *Cancer Epidemiol Biomarkers Prev* **13**: 1466–1472.

Bettoun, D.J., Buck, D.W., Lu, J., Khalifa, B., Chin, W.W., and Nagpal, S. 2002. A vitamin D receptor-Ser/Thr phosphatase-p70 S6 kinase complex and modulation of its enzymatic activities by the ligand. *J Biol Chem* **277**: 24847–24850.

Bikle, D.D., Gee, E., and Pillai, S. 1993. Regulation of keratinocyte growth, differentiation, and vitamin D metabolism by analogs of 1,25-dihydroxyvitamin D. *J Investig Dermatol* **101**: 713–718.

Bikle, D.D., Tu, C.L., Xie, Z., and Oda, Y. 2003. Vitamin D regulated keratinocyte differentiation: role of coactivators. *J Cell Biochem* **88**: 290–295.

Blutt, S.E., McDonnell, T.J., Polek, T.C., and Weigel, N.L. 2000. Calcitriol-induced apoptosis in LNCaP cells is blocked by overexpression of Bcl-2. *Endocrinology* **141**: 10–17.

Bower, M., Colston, K.W., Stein, R.C., Hedley, A., Gazet, J.-C., Ford, H.T., and Coombes, R.C. 1991. Topical calcipotriol treatment in advanced breast cancer. *Lancet* **337**: 701–702.

Boyapati, S.M., Shu, X.O., Jin, F., Dai, Q., Ruan, Z., Gao, Y.T., and Zheng, W. 2003. Dietary calcium intake and breast cancer risk among Chinese women in Shanghai. *Nutr Cancer* **46**: 38–43.

Brenner, B.M., Russell, N., Albrecht, S., and Davies, R.J. 1998. The effect of dietary vitamin D3 on the intracellular calcium gradient in mammalian colonic crypts. *Cancer Lett* **127**: 43–53.

Carlberg, C. 2003. Current understanding of the function of the nuclear vitamin D receptor in response to its natural and synthetic ligands. *Recent Results Cancer Res* **164**: 29–42.

Chakrabarty, S., Radjendirane, V., Appelman, H., and Varani, J. 2003. Extracellular calcium and the calcium sensing receptor function in human colon carcinomas: promotion of E-cadherin expression and suppression of β-catenin/TCF activation. *Cancer Res* **63**: 67–71.

Chan, J.M., Stampfer, M.J., Ma, J., Gann, P.H., Gaziano, J.M., and Giovannucci, E.L. 2001. Dairy products, calcium, and prostate cancer risk in the Physicians' Health Study. *Am J Clin Nutr* **74**: 549–554.

Chaudhry, M., Sundaram, S., Gennings, C., Carter, H., and Gewirtz, D.A. 2001. The vitamin D3 analog, ILX-23-7553, enhances the response to adriamycin and irradiation in MCF-7 breast tumor cells. *Cancer Chemother Pharmacol* **47**: 429–436.

Chen, T.C., Wang, L., Whitlatch, L.W., Flanagan, J.N., and Holick, M.F. 2003. Prostatic 25-hydroxyvitamin D-1alpha-hydroxylase and its implication in prostate cancer. *J Cell Biochem* **88**: 315–322.

Cheng, I., Klingensmith, M.E., Chattopadhyay, N., Kifor, O., Butters, R.R., Soybel, D.I., and Brown, E.M. 1998. Identification and localization of the extracellular calcium sensing receptor in human breast. *J Clin Endocrinol Metab* **83**: 703–707.

Christakos, S., Dhawan, P., Liu, Y., Peng, X., and Porta, A. 2003. New insights into the mechanisms of vitamin D action. *J Cell Biochem* **88**: 695–705.

Colston, K.W., Berger, U., and Coombes, R.C. 1989. Possible role for vitamin D in controlling breast cancer cell proliferation. *Lancet* **1**: 188–191.

Crescioli, C., Maggie, M., Vannelli, G.B., Luconi, M., Salerno, R., Barni, T., Gulisano, M., Forti, G., and Serio, M. 2000. Effect of a vitamin D3 analogue on keratinocyte growth factor-induced cell proliferation in benign prostate hyperplasia. *J Clin Endocrinol Metab* **85**: 2576–2583.

Cross, H.S., Kallay, E., Farhan, H., Weiland, T., and Manhardt, T. 2003. Regulation of extrarenal vitamin D metabolism as a tool for colon and prostate cancer prevention. *Recent Results Cancer Res* **164**: 413–425.

Dardenne, O., Prud-homme, J., Arabian, A., Glorieux, F.H., and St. Arnaud, R. 2001. Targeted inactivation of the 25-hydroxyvitamin D(3)-1(alpha)-hydroxylase gene (CYP27B1) creates an animal model of pseudovitamin D–deficiency rickets. *Endocrinology* **142**: 3135–3141.

Diaz, G.D., Paraskeva, C., Thomas, M.G., Binderup, L., and Hague, A. 2000. Apoptosis is induced by the active metabolite of vitamin D3 and its analogue EB1089 in colorectal adenoma and carcinoma cells: possible implications for prevention and therapy. *Cancer Res* **60**: 2304–2312.

Eisman, J.A., Barkla, D.H., and Tutton, P.J. 1987. Suppression of *in vivo* growth of human cancer solid tumor xenografts by 1,25-dihydroxyvitamin D3. *Cancer Res* **47**: 21–25.

Eisman, J.A., Sutherland, R.L., McMenemy, M.L., Fragonas, J.C., Musgrove, E.A., and Pang, G.Y. 1989. Effects of 1,25-dihydroxyvitamin D3 on cell-cycle kinetics of T 47D human breast cancer cells. *J Cell Physiol* **138**: 611–616.

Eisman, J.A., Suva, L.J., and Martin, T.J. 1986. Significance of 1,25-dihydroxyvitamin D3 receptor in primary breast cancers. *Cancer Res* **46**: 5406–5408.

El Abdaimi, K., Dion, N., Papavasiliou, V., Cardinal, P.E., Binderup, L., Goltzman, D., Ste-Marie, L.G., and Kremer, R. 2000. The vitamin D analogue EB1089 prevents skeletal metastasis and prolongs survival time in nude mice transplanted with human breast cancer cells. *Cancer Res* **60**: 4412–4418.

Elias, J., Marian, B., Edling, C., Lachmann, B., Noe, C.R., Rolf, S.H., and Schuster, I. 2003. Induction of apoptosis by vitamin D metabolites and analogs in a glioma cell line. *Recent Results Cancer Res* **164**: 319–332.

Elstner, E., Linker-Israeli, M., Le, J., Umiel, T., Michl, P., Said, J.W., Binderup, L., Reed, J.C., and Koeffler, H.P. 1997. Synergistic decrease of clonal proliferation, induction of differentiation, and apoptosis of acute promyelocytic leukemia cells after combined treatment with novel 20-epi vitamin D3 analogs and 9-cis retinoic acid. *J Clin Invest* **99**: 349–360.

Erben, R.G., Soegiarto, D.W., Weber, K., Zeitz, U., Lieberherr, M., Gniadecki, R., Moller, G., Adamski, J., and Balling, R. 2002. Deletion of deoxyribonucleic acid binding domain of the vitamin D receptor abrogates genomic and nongenomic functions of vitamin D. *Mol Endocrinol* **16**: 1524–1537.

Farach-Carson, M.C., and Nemere, I. 2003. Membrane receptors for vitamin D steroid hormones: potential new drug targets. *Curr Drug Targets* **4**: 67–76.

Feskanich, D., Ma, J., Fuchs, C.S., Kirkner, G.J., Hankinson, S.E., Hollis, B.W., and Giovannucci, E. 2004. Plasma vitamin D metabolites and risk of colorectal cancer in women. *Cancer Epidemiol Biomarkers Prev* **13**: 1502–1508.

Flanagan, L., Packman, K., Juba, B., O-Neill, S., Tenniswood, M., and Welsh, J. 2003. Efficacy of Vitamin D compounds to modulate estrogen receptor negative breast cancer growth and invasion. *J Steroid Biochem Mol Biol* **84**: 181–192.

Frampton, R.J., Suva, L.J., Eisman, J.A., Findlay, D.M., Moore, G.E., Moseley, J.M., and Martin, T.J. 1982. Presence of 1,25-dihydroxyvitamin D3 receptors in established human cancer cell lines in culture. *Cancer Res* **42**: 1116–1119.

Freake, H.C., Abeyasekera, G., Iwasaki, J., Marcocci, C., MacIntyre, I., McClelland, R.A., Skilton, R.A., Easton, D.F., and Coombes, R.C. 1984. Measurement of 1,25-dihydroxyvitamin D3 receptors in breast cancer and their relationship to biochemical and clinical indices. *Cancer Res* **44**: 1677–1681.

Garland, F.C., Garland, C.F., Gorham, E.D., and Young, J.F. 1990. Geographic variation in breast cancer mortality in the United States: a hypothesis involving solar radiation. *Prev Med* **19**: 614–622.

Gordon, C.M., DePeter, K.C., Feldman, H.A., Grace, E., and Emans, S.J. 2004. Prevalence of vitamin D deficiency among healthy adolescents. *Arch Pediatr Adolesc Med* **158**: 531–537.

Govers, M.J., Termont, D.S., Lapre, J.A., Kleibeuker, J.H., Vonk, R.J., and Van der Meer, R. 1996. Calcium in milk products precipitates intestinal fatty acids and secondary bile acids and thus inhibits colonic cytotoxicity in humans. *Cancer Res* **56**: 3270–3275.

Grant, W.B. 2002. An ecologic study of dietary and solar ultraviolet-B links to breast carcinoma mortality rates. *Cancer* **94**: 272–281.

Grant, W.B., and Garland, C.F. 2004. A critical review of studies on vitamin D in relation to colorectal cancer. *Nutr Cancer* **48**: 115–123.

Grau, M.V., Baron, J.A., Sandler, R.S., Haile, R.W., Beach, M., Church, T.R., and Heber, D. 2003. Vitamin D, calcium supplementation, and colorectal adenomas: results of a randomized trial. *J Natl Cancer Inst* **95**: 1765–1771.

Gulliford, T., English, J., Colston, K.W., Menday, P., Moller, S., and Coombes, R.C. 1998. A phase I study of the vitamin D analogue EB1089 in patients with advanced breast and colorectal cancer. *Br J Cancer* **78**: 6–13.

Guy, M., Lowe, L.C., Bretherton-Watt, D., Mansi, J.L., and Colston, K.W. 2003. Approaches to evaluating the association of vitamin D receptor gene polymorphisms with breast cancer risk. *Recent Results Cancer Res* **164**: 43–54.

Guyton, K.Z., Kensler, T.W., and Posner, G.H. 2003. Vitamin D and vitamin D analogs as cancer chemopreventive agents. *Nutr Rev* **61**: 227–238.

Guzey, M., Kitada, S., and Reed, J.C. 2002. Apoptosis induction by 1alpha,25-dihydroxyvitamin D3 in prostate cancer. *Mol Cancer Ther* **1**: 667–677.

Habuchi, T., Suzuki, T., Sasaki, R., Wang, L., Sato, K., Satoh, S., Akao, T., Tsuchiya, N., Shimoda, N., Wada, Y., Koizumi, A., Chihara, J., Ogawa, O., and Kato, T. 2000. Association of vitamin D receptor gene polymorphism with prostate cancer and benign prostatic hyperplasia in a Japanese population. *Cancer Res* **60**: 305–308.

Hager, G., Formanek, M., Gedlicka, C., Thurnher, D., Knerer, B., and Kornfehl, J. 2001. 1,25(OH)2 vitamin D3 induces elevated expression of the cell cycle–regulating genes P21 and P27 in squamous carcinoma cell lines of the head and neck. *Acta Oto-Laryngol* **121**: 103–109.

Hamasaki, T., Inatomi, H., Katoh, T., Ikuyama, T., and Matsumoto, T. 2002. Significance of vitamin D receptor gene polymorphism for risk and disease severity of prostate cancer and benign prostatic hyperplasia in Japanese. *Urol Int* **68**: 226–231.

Hansen, C.M., Frandsen, T.L., Brunner, N., and Binderup, L. 1994. 1 alpha,25-Dihydroxyvitamin D3 inhibits the invasive potential of human breast cancer cells *in vitro*. *Clin Exp Metastasis* **12**: 195–202.

Hewison, M., Kantorovich, V., Liker, H.R., Van-Herle, A.J., Cohan, P., Zehnder, D., and Adams, J.S. 2003. Vitamin D–mediated hypercalcemia in lymphoma: evidence for hormone production by tumor-adjacent macrophages. *J Bone Min Res* **18**: 579–582.

Hiatt, R.A., Krieger, N., Lobaugh, B., Drezner, M.K., Vogelman, J.H., and Orentreich, N. 1998. Prediagnostic serum vitamin D and breast cancer. *J Natl Cancer Inst* **90**: 461–463.

Holick, M.F. 2003. Vitamin D: A millennium perspective. *J Cell Biochem* **88**: 296–307.

Holick, M.F., Shao, Q., Liu, W.W., and Chen, T.C. 1992. The vitamin D content of fortified milk and infant formula. *N Engl J Med* **326**: 1178–1181.

Hsu, J.Y., Feldman, D., McNeal, J.E., and Peehl, D.M. 2001. Reduced 1alpha-hydroxylase activity in human prostate cancer cells correlates with decreased susceptibility to 25-hydroxyvitamin D3–induced growth inhibition. *Cancer Res* **61**: 2852–2856.

Huerta, S., Irwin, R.W., Heber, D., Go, V.L., Koeffler, H.P., Uskokovic, M.R., and Harris, D.M. 2002. 1alpha,25-(OH)(2)-D(3) and its synthetic analogue decrease tumor load in the Apc(min) Mouse. *Cancer Res* **62**: 741–746.

Huhtakangas, J.A., Olivera, C.J., Bishop, J.E., Zanello, L.P., and Norman, A.W. 2004. The vitamin D receptor is present in caveolae-enriched plasma membranes and binds 1α,25(OH)2-vitamin D3 *in vivo* and *in vitro*. *Mol Endocrinol* **18**: 2660–2671.

Hulla, W., Kallay, E., Krugluger, W., Peterlik, M., and Cross, H.S. 1995. Growth control of human colon-adenocarcinoma–derived Caco-2 cells by vitamin-D compounds and extracellular calcium *in vitro*: relation to c-myc-oncogene and vitamin-D-receptor expression. *Int J Cancer* **62**: 711–716.

Jackson, R.D., LaCroix, A.Z., Cauley, J.A., and McGowan, J. 2003. The Women's Health Initiative calcium-vitamin D trial: overview and baseline characteristics of participants. *Ann Epidemiol* **13**.

Jacobson, E.A., James, K.A., Newmark, H.L., and Carroll, K.K. 1989. Effects of dietary fat, calcium and vitamin D on growth and mammary tumorigenesis induced by 7,12-dimethylbenz(a)anthracene in female Sprague-Dawley rats. *Cancer Res* **49**: 6300–6303.

James, S.Y., Mercer, E., Brady, M., Binderup, L., and Colston, K.W. 1998. EB1089, a synthetic analogue of vitamin D, induces apoptosis in breast cancer cells *in vivo* and *in vitro*. *Br J Pharmacol* **125**: 953–962.

Janowsky, E.C., Lester, G.E., Weinberg, C.R., Millikan, R.C., Schildkraut, J.M., Garrett, P.A., and Hulka, B.S. 1999. Association between low levels of 1,25-dihydroxyvitamin D and breast cancer risk. *Public Health Nutr* **2**: 283–291.

John, E.M., Schwartz, G.G., Dreon, D.M., and Koo, J. 1999. Vitamin D and breast cancer: the NHANES I epidemiologic follow-up study, 1971–1975 to 1992. *Cancer Epidemiol Biomarkers Prev* **8**: 399–406.

Johnson, C.S., Hershberger, P.A., and Trump, D.L. 2002. Vitamin D–related therapies in prostate cancer. *Cancer Metastasis Rev* **21**: 147–158.

Jung, C.W., Kim, E.S., Seol, J.G., Park, W.H., Lee, S.J., Kim, B.K., and Lee, Y.Y. 1999. Antiproliferative effect of a vitamin D3 analog, EB1089, on HL-60 cells by the induction of TGF-beta receptor. *Leuk Res* **23**: 1105–1112.

Jurutka, P.W., Remus, L.S., Whitfield, G.K., Thompson, P.D., Hsieh, J.C., Zitzer, H., Tavakkoli, P., Galligan, M.A., Dang, H.T., Haussler, C.A., and Haussler, M.R. 2000. The polymorphic N terminus in human vitamin D receptor isoforms influences transcriptional activity by modulating interaction with transcription factor IIB. *Mol Endocrinol* **14**: 401–420.

Kallay, E., Pietschmann, P., Toyokuni, S., Bajna, E., Hahn, P., Mazzucco, K., Bieglmayer, C., Kato, S., and Cross, H.S. 2001. Characterization of a vitamin D receptor knockout mouse as a model of colorectal hyperproliferation and DNA damage. *Carcinogenesis* **22**: 1429–1435.

Kim, H.S., Newcomb, P.A., Ulrich, C.M., Keener, C.L., Bigler, J., Farin, F.M., Bostick, R.M., and Potter, J.D. 2001. Vitamin D receptor polymorphism and the risk of colorectal adenomas: evidence of interaction with dietary vitamin D and calcium. *Cancer Epidemiol Biomarkers Prev* **10**: 869–874.

Knekt, P., Jarvinen, R., Seppanen, R., Pukkala, E., and Aromaa, A. 1996. Intake of dairy products and risk of breast cancer. *Br J Cancer* **73**: 687–691.

Krishnan, A.V., Peehl, D.M., and Feldman, D. 2003. The role of vitamin D in prostate cancer. *Recent Results Cancer Res* **164**: 205–221.

Krishnan, A.V., Shinghal, R., Raghavachari, N., Brooks, J.D., Peehl, D.M., and Feldman, D. 2004. Analysis of vitamin D–regulated gene expression in LNCaP human prostate cancer cells using cDNA microarrays. *Prostate* **59**: 243–251.

Kumagai, T., O-Kelly, J., Said, J.W., and Koeffler, H.P. 2003. Vitamin D2 analog 19-nor-1,25-dihydroxyvitamin D2: antitumor activity against leukemia, myeloma, and colon cancer cells. *J Natl Cancer Inst* **95**: 896–905.

Lamprecht, S.A., and Lipkin, M. 2003. Chemoprevention of colon cancer by calcium, vitamin D and folate: molecular mechanisms. *Nat Rev Cancer* **3**: 601–614.

Lazzaro, G., Agadir, A., Qing, W., Poria, M., Mehta, R.R., Moriarty, R.M., Das-Gupta, T.K., Zhang, X.K., and Mehta, R.G. 2000. Induction of differentiation by 1alpha-hydroxyvitamin D(5) in T47D human breast cancer cells and its interaction with vitamin D receptors. *Eur J Cancer* **36**: 780–786.

Li, Y.C., Pirro, A.E., Amling, M., Delling, G., Baron, R., Bronson, R., and Demay, M.B. 1997. Targeted ablation of the vitamin D receptor: an animal model of vitamin D–dependent rickets type II with alopecia. *Proc Natl Acad Sci USA* **94**: 9831–9835.

Lin, R., Nagai, Y., Sladek, R., Bastien, Y., Ho, J., Petrecca, K., Sotiropoulou, G., Diamandis, E.P., Hudson, T.J., and White, J.H. 2002. Expression profiling in squamous carcinoma cells reveals pleiotropic effects of vitamin D3 analog EB1089 signaling on cell proliferation, differentiation, and immune system regulation. *Mol Endocrinol* **16**: 1243–1256.

Lipkin, M., and Newmark, H.L. 1985. Effect of added dietary calcium on colonic epithelial cell proliferation in subjects at high risk for familial colon cancer. *N Engl J Med* **313**: 1381–1384.

Lipkin, M., and Newmark, H.L. 1999. Vitamin D, calcium and prevention of breast cancer: a review. *J Am Coll Nutr* **18**: 392S–397S.

Lips, P. 2001. Vitamin D deficiency and secondary hyperparathyroidism in the elderly: consequences for bone loss and fractures and therapeutic implications. *Endocr Rev* **22**: 477–501.

Liu, M., Lee, M.H., Cohen, M., Bommakanti, M., and Freedman, L.P. 1996. Transcriptional activation of the Cdk inhibitor p21 by vitamin D3 leads to the induced differentiation of the myelomonocytic cell line U937. *Genes Dev* **10**: 142–153.

Liu, W., Asa, S.L., Fantus, I.G., Walfish, P.G., and Ezzat, S. 2002. Vitamin D arrests thyroid carcinoma cell growth and induces p27 dephosphorylation and accumulation through PTEN/akt-dependent and -independent pathways. *Am J Pathol* **160**: 511–519.

Lokeshwar, B.L., Schwartz, G.G., Selzer, M.G., Burnstein, K.L., Zhuang, S.H., Block, N.L., and Binderup, L. 1999. Inhibition of prostate cancer metastasis *in vivo*: a comparison of 1,23-dihydroxyvitamin D (calcitriol) and EB1089. *Cancer Epidemiol Biomarkers Prev* **8**: 241–248.

Lowe, L., Hansen, C.M., Senaratne, S., and Colston, K.W. 2003. Mechanisms implicated in the growth regulatory effects of vitamin D compounds in breast cancer cells. *Recent Results Cancer Res* **164**: 99–110.

Ma, J.F., Nonn, L., Campbell, M.J., Hewison, M., Feldman, D., and Peehl, D.M. 2004. Mechanisms of decreased vitamin D 1α-hydroxylase activity in prostate cancer cells. *Mol Cell Endocrinol* **221**: 67–74.

Malloy, P.J., and Feldman, D. 2003. Hereditary 1,25-Dihydroxyvitamin D–resistant rickets. *Endocr Dev* **6**: 175–199.

Mathiasen, I.S., Lademann, U., and Jaattela, M. 1999. Apoptosis induced by vitamin D compounds in breast cancer cells is inhibited by Bcl-2 but does not involve known caspases or p53. *Cancer Res* **59**: 4848–4856.

Mathiasen, I.S., Sergeev, I.N., Bastholm, L., Elling, F., Norman, A.W., and Jaattela, M. 2002. Calcium and calpain as key mediators of apoptosis-like death induced by vitamin D compounds in breast cancer cells. *J Biol Chem* **277**: 30738–30745.

Mawer, E.B., Walls, J., Howell, A., Davies, M., Ratcliffe, W.A., and Bundred, N.J. 1997. Serum 1,25-dihydroxyvitamin D may be related inversely to disease activity in breast cancer patients with bone metastases. *J Clin Endocrinol Metab* **82**: 118–122.

McGuire, T.F., Trump, D.L., and Johnson, C.S. 2001. Vitamin D(3)–induced apoptosis of murine squamous cell carcinoma cells. Selective induction of caspase-dependent MEK cleavage and up-regulation of MEKK-1. *J Biol Chem* **276**: 26365–26373.

Mehta, R.G., Moriarty, R.M., Mehta, R.R., Penmasta, R., Lazzaro, G., Constantinou, A., and Guo, L. 1997. Prevention of preneoplastic mammary lesion development by a novel vitamin D analogue, 1alpha-hydroxyvitamin D5. *J Natl Cancer Inst* **89**: 212–218.

Miller, W.L., and Portale, A.A. 2003. Vitamin D biosynthesis and vitamin D 1 alpha-hydroxylase deficiency. *Endocr Dev* **6**: 156–174.

Mimori, K., Tanaka, Y., Yoshinaga, K., Masuda, T., Yamashita, K., Okamoto, M., Inoue, H., and Mori, M. 2004. Clinical significance of the overexpression of the candidate oncogene CYP24 in esophageal cancer. *Ann Oncol* **15**: 236–241.

Mizwicki, M.T., Keidel, D., Bula, C.M., Bishop, J.E., Zanello, L.P., Wurtz, J., Moras, D., and Norman, A.W. 2004. Identification of an alternative ligand-binding pocket in the nuclear vitamin D receptor and its functional importance in 1α,25(OH)$_2$-vitamin D$_3$ signaling. *Proc Natl Acad Sci USA* **101**: 12876–12881.

Moorman, P.G., and Terry, P.D. 2004. Consumption of dairy products and the risk of breast cancer: a review of the literature. *Am J Clin Nutr* **80**: 5–14.

Mork-Hansen, C., Binderup, L., Hamberg, K.J., and Carlberg, C. 2001. Vitamin D and cancer: effects of 1,25(OH)2D3 and its analogs on growth control and tumorigenesis. *Front Biosci* **6**: D820–D848.

Munker, R., Norman, A., and Koeffler, H.P. 1986. Vitamin D compounds. Effect on clonal proliferation and differentiation of human myeloid cells. *J Clin Invest* **78**: 424–430.

Narvaez, C.J., Byrne, B.M., Romu, S., Valrance, M., and Welsh, J. 2003. Induction of apoptosis by 1,25-dihydroxyvitamin D(3) in MCF-7 vitamin D(3)–resistant variant can be sensitized by TPA. *J Steroid Biochem Mol Biol* **84**: 199–209.

Narvaez, C.J., and Welsh, J. 2001. Role of mitochondria and caspases in vitamin D–mediated apoptosis of MCF-7 breast cancer cells. *J Biol Chem* **276**: 9101–9107.

Newmark, H.L., Lipkin, M., and Maheswari, N. 1990. Colonic hyperplasia and hyperproliferation induced by a nutritional stress diet with four components of Western-style diet. *J Natl Cancer Inst* **82**: 491–496.

Norman, A.W., Bishop, J.E., Bula, C.M., Olivera, C.J., Mizwicki, M.T., Zanello, L.P., Ishida, H., and Okamura, W.H. 2002. Molecular tools for study of genomic and rapid signal transduction responses initiated by 1 alpha,25(OH)(2)-vitamin D(3). *Steroids* **67**: 457–466.

Palmer, H.G., Gonzalez-Sancho, J.M., Espada, J., Berciano, M.T., Puig, I., Baulida, J., Quintanilla, M., Cano, A., de-Herreros, A.G., Lafarga, M., and Munoz, A. 2001. Vitamin D(3) promotes the differentiation of colon carcinoma cells by the induction of E-cadherin and the inhibition of beta-catenin signaling. *J Cell Biol* **154**: 369–387.

Park, W.H., Seol, J.G., Kim, E.S., Hyun, J.M., Jung, C.W., Lee, C.C., Binderup, L., Koeffler, H.P., Kim, B.K., and Lee, Y.Y. 2000a. Induction of apoptosis by vitamin D3 analogue EB1089 in NCI-H929 myeloma cells via activation of caspase 3 and p38 MAP kinase. *Br J Haematol* **109**: 576–583.

Park, W.H., Seol, J.G., Kim, E.S., Jung, C.W., Lee, C.C., Binderup, L., Koeffler, H.P., Kim, B.K., and Lee, Y.Y. 2000b. Cell cycle arrest induced by the vitamin D(3) analog EB1089 in NCI-H929 myeloma cells is associated with induction of the cyclin-dependent kinase inhibitor p27. *Exp Cell Res* **254**: 279–286.

Parkash, J., Chaudhry, M.A., and Rhoten, W.B. 2004. Calbindin D28K and calcium sensing receptor cooperate in MCF-7 human breast cancer cells. *Int J Oncol* **24**: 1111–1119.

Pence, B.C., and Buddingh, F. 1988. Inhibition of dietary fat promoted colon carcinogenesis in rats by supplemental calcium or vitamin D. *Carcinogenesis* **9**: 187–190.

Pence, B.C., Dunn, D.M., Zhao, C., Landers, M., and Wargovich, M.J. 1995. Chemopreventive effects of calcium but not aspirin supplementation in cholic acid–promoted colon carcinogenesis: correlation with intermediate endpoints. *Carcinogenesis* **16**: 757–765.

Pepper, C., Thomas, A., Hoy, T., Milligan, D., Bentley, P., and Fegan, C. 2003. The vitamin D3 analog EB1089 induces apoptosis via a p53-independent mechanism involving p38 MAP kinase activation and suppression of ERK activity in B-cell chronic lymphocytic leukemia cells *in vitro*. *Blood* **101**: 2454–2460.

Peters, U., Hayes, R.B., Chatterjee, N., Shao, W., Schoen, R.E., Pinsky, P., Hollis, B.W., and McGlynn, K.A. 2004. Circulating vitamin D metabolites, polymorphism in vitamin D receptor, and colorectal adenoma risk. *Cancer Epidemiol Biomarkers Prev* **13**: 546–552.

Peters, U., McGlynn, K.A., Chatterjee, N., Gunter, E., Garcia-Closas, M., Rothman, N., and Sinha, R. 2001. Vitamin D, calcium, and vitamin D receptor polymorphism in colorectal adenomas. *Cancer Epidemiol Biomarkers Prev* **10**: 1267–1274.

Pinette, K.V., Yee, Y.K., Amegadzie, B.Y., and Nagpal, S. 2003. Vitamin D receptor as a drug discovery target. *Mini Rev Med Chem* **3**: 193–204.

Pirianov, G., and Colston, K.W. 2001. Interactions of vitamin D analogue CB1093, TNFalpha and ceramide on breast cancer cell apoptosis. *Mol Cell Endocrinol* **172**: 69–78.

Platz, E.A., Leitzmann, M.F., Hollis, B.W., Willet, W.C., and Giovannucci, E. 2004. Plasma 1,25-dihydroxy- and 25-hydroxyvitamin D and subsequent risk of prostate cancer. *Cancer Causes Control* **15**: 255–265.

Polek, T.C., Murthy, S., Blutt, S.E., Boehm, M.F., Zou, A., Weigel, N.L., and Allegretto, E.A. 2001. Novel nonsecosteroidal vitamin D receptor modulator inhibits the growth of LNCaP xenograft tumors in athymic mice without increased serum calcium. *Prostate* **49**: 224–233.

Posner, G.H., Crawford, K.R., Peleg, S., Welsh, J.E., Romu, S., Gewirtz, D.A., Gupta, M.S., Dolan, P., and Kensler, T.W. 2001. A non-calcemic sulfone version of the vitamin D(3) analogue seocalcitol (EB 1089): chemical synthesis, biological evaluation and potency enhancement of the anticancer drug adriamycin. *Bioorganic Medicinal Chem* **9**: 2365–2371.

Richter, F., Newmark, H.L., Richter, A., Leung, D., and Lipkin, M. 1995. Inhibition of Western-diet induced hyperproliferation and hyperplasia in mouse colon by two sources of calcium. *Carcinogenesis* **16**: 2685–2689.

Rizk-Rabin, M., Zineb, R., Zhor, B., Michele, G., and Jana, P. 1994. Synthesis of and response to 1,25 dihydroxycholecalciferol by subpopulations of murine epidermal keratinocytes: existence of a paracrine system for 1,25 dihydroxycholecalciferol. *J Cell Physiol* **159**: 131–141.

Rodland, K. 2004. The role of the calcium-sensing receptor in cancer. *Cell Calcium* **35**: 291–295.

Rots, N.Y., Liu, M., Anderson, E.C., and Freedman, L.P. 1998. A differential screen for ligand-regulated genes: identification of HoxA10 as a target of vitamin D3 induction in myeloid leukemic cells. *Mol Cell Biol* **18**: 1911–1918.

Scaglione-Sewell, B.A., Bissonnette, M., Skarosi, S., Abraham, C., and Brasitus, T.A. 2000. A vitamin D3 analog induces a G1-phase arrest in CaCo-2 cells by inhibiting cdk2 and cdk6: roles of cyclin E, p21Waf1, and p27Kip1. *Endocrinology* **141**: 3931–3939.

Schatzkin, A., and Peters, U. 2004. Advancing the calcium-colorectal cancer hypothesis. *J Natl Cancer Inst* **96**: 893–894.

Schwartz, G.G., Eads, D., Rao, A., Cramer, S.D., Willingham, M.C., Chen, T.C., Jamieson, D.P., Wang, L., Burnstein, K.L., Holick, M.F., and Koumenis, C. 2004. Pancreatic cancer cells express 25-hydroxyvitamin D-1 alpha-hydroxylase and their proliferation is inhibited by the prohormone 25-hydroxyvitamin D3. *Carcinogenesis* **25**: 1015–1026.

Schwartz, G.G., Wang, M.H., Zang, M., Singh, R.K., and Siegal, G.P. 1997. 1 alpha,25-Dihydroxyvitamin D (calcitriol) inhibits the invasiveness of human prostate cancer cells. *Cancer Epidemiol Biomarkers Prev* **6**: 727–732.

Shin, M.J., Holmes, M.D., Hankinson, S.E., Wu, K., Colditz, G.A., and Willet, W.C. 2002. Intake of dairy products, calcium and vitamin D and risk of breast cancer. *J Natl Cancer Inst* **94**: 1301–1310.

Simboli-Campbell, M., Narvaez, C.J., Tenniswood, M., and Welsh, J. 1996. 1,25-Dihydroxyvitamin D3 induces morphological and biochemical markers of apoptosis in MCF-7 breast cancer cells. *J Steroid Biochem Mol Biol* **58**: 367–376.

Simboli-Campbell, M., Narvaez, C.J., vanWeelden, K., Tenniswood, M., and Welsh, J. 1997. Comparative effects of 1,25(OH)2D3 and EB1089 on cell cycle kinetics and apoptosis in MCF-7 breast cancer cells. *Breast Cancer Res Treatment* **42**: 31–41.

Slattery, M.L., Neuhausen, S., Hoffman, M., Caan, B., Curtin, K., Ma, K.N., and Samowitz, W. 2004. Dietary calcium, vitamin D, VDR genotypes and colorectal cancer. *Int J Cancer* **111**: 750–756.

Sundaram, S., Sea, A., Feldman, S., Strawbridge, R., Hoopes, P.J., Demidenko, E., Binderup, L., and Gewirtz, D.A. 2003. The combination of a potent vitamin D(3) analog, EB 1089, with ionizing radiation reduces tumor growth and induces apoptosis of MCF-7 breast tumor xenografts in nude mice. *Clinical Cancer Res* **9**: 2350–2356.

Swami, S., Raghavachari, N., Muller, U.R., Bao, Y.P., and Feldman, D. 2003. Vitamin D growth inhibition of breast cancer cells: gene expression patterns assessed by cDNA microarray. *Breast Cancer Res Treat* **80**: 49–62.

Tangpricha, V., Koutkia, P., Rieke, S.M., Chen, T.C., Perez, A.A., and Holick, M.F. 2003. Fortification of orange juice with vitamin D: a novel approach for enhancing vitamin D nutritional health. *Am J Clin Nutr* **77**: 1478–1483.

Tangpricha, V., Pearce, E.N., Chen, T.C., and Holick, M.F. 2002. Vitamin D insufficiency among free-living healthy young adults. *Am J Med* **112**: 659–662.

Thomas, M.K., Lloyd-Jones, D.M., Thadhani, R.I., Shaw, A.C., Deraska, D.J., Kitch, B.T., Vamvakas, E.C., Dick, I.M., Prince, R.L., and Finkelstein, J.S. 1998. Hypovitaminosis D in medical inpatients. *N Engl J Med* **338**: 777–783.

Tong, W.M., Hofer, H., Ellinger, A., Peterlik, M., and Cross, H.S. 1999. Mechanism of antimitogenic action of vitamin D in human colon carcinoma cells: relevance for suppression of epidermal growth factor-stimulated cell growth. *Oncol Res* **11**: 77–84.

Uitterlinden, A.G., Fang, Y., VanMeurs, J.B., Pols, H.A., and VanLeeuwen, J.P. 2004. Genetics and biology of vitamin D receptor polymorphisms. *Gene* **338**: 143–156.

Vandewalle, B., Wattez, N., and Lefebvre, J. 1995. Effects of vitamin D3 derivatives on growth, differentiation and apoptosis in tumoral colonic HT 29 cells: possible implication of intracellular calcium. *Cancer Lett* **97**: 99–106.

VanWeelden, K., Flanagan, L., Binderup, L., Tenniswood, M., and Welsh, J. 1998. Apoptotic regression of MCF-7 xenografts in nude mice treated with the vitamin D3 analog, EB1089. *Endocrinology* **139**: 2102–2110.

Wagner, N., Wagner, K.D., Schley, G., Badiali, L., Theres, H., and Scholz, H. 2003. 1,25-dihydroxyvitamin D3–induced apoptosis of retinoblastoma cells is associated with reciprocal changes of Bcl-2 and bax. *Exp Eye Res* **77**: 1–9.

Wallace, K., Baron, J.A., Cole, B.F., Sandler, R.S., Karagas, M.R., Beach, M.A., Haile, R.W., Burke, C.A., Pearson, L.H., Mandel, J.S., Rothstein, R., and Snover, D.C. 2004. Effect of calcium supplementation on the risk of large bowel polyps. *J Natl Cancer Inst* **96**: 921–925.

Wang, Q., Lee, D., Sysounthone, V., Chandraratna-RAS, Christakos, S., Korah, R., and Wieder, R. 2001. 1,25-dihydroxyvitamin D3 and retinoic acid analogues induce differentiation in breast cancer cells with function- and cell-specific additive effects. *Breast Cancer Res Treat* **67**: 157–168.

Welsh, J., Simboli-Campbell, M., Narvaez, C.J., and Tenniswood, M. 1995. Role of apoptosis in the growth inhibitory effects of vitamin D in MCF-7 cells. *Adv Exp Med Biol* **375**: 45–52.

Welsh, J., Wietzke, J.A., Zinser, G.M., Byrne, B., Smith, K., and Narvaez, C.J. 2003. Vitamin D-3 receptor as a target for breast cancer prevention. *J Nutr* **133**: 2425S–2433S.

Willnow, T.E., and Nykjaer, A. 2002. Pathways for kidney-specific uptake of the steroid hormone 25-hydroxyvitamin D3. *Current Opinion Lipidol* **13**: 255–260.

Xie, S.P., Pirianov, G., and Colston, K.W. 1999. Vitamin D analogues suppress IGF-I signalling and promote apoptosis in breast cancer cells. *Eur J Cancer* **35**: 1717–1723.

Xie, Z., Komuves, L., Yu, Q.C., Elalieh, H., Ng, D.C., Leary, C., Chang, S., Crumrine, D., Yoshizawa, T., Kato, S., and Bikle, D.D. 2002. Lack of the vitamin D receptor is associated with reduced epidermal differentiation and hair follicle growth. *J Invest Dermatol* **118**: 11–16.

Xue, L.X., Lipkin, M., and Newmark, H.L. 1997. Induced hyperproliferation in epithelial cells of mouse prostate by a Western-style diet. *Carcinogenesis* **18**.

Xue, L.X., Lipkin, M., Newmark, H.L., and Wang, J. 1999. Influence of dietary calcium and vitamin D on diet-induced epithelial cell hyperproliferation in mice. *J Natl Cancer Inst* **91**.

Yang, L., Yang, J., Venkateswarlu, S., Ko, T., and Brattain, M.G. 2001. Autocrine TGFbeta signaling mediates vitamin D3 analog–induced growth inhibition in breast cells. *J Cell Physiol* **188**: 383–393.

Zanello, L.P., and Norman, A.W. 2004. Rapid modulation of osteoblast ion channel responses by 1(alpha),25(OH)2-vitamin D3 requires the presence of a functional vitamin D nuclear receptor. *Proc Natl Acad Sci USA* **101**: 1589–1594.

Zhao, X., and Feldman, D. 1993. Regulation of vitamin D receptor abundance and responsiveness during differentiation of HT-29 human colon cancer cells. *Endocrinology* **132**: 1808–1814.

Zhuang, S.H., and Burnstein, K.L. 1998. Antiproliferative effect of 1alpha,25-dihydroxyvitamin D3 in human prostate cancer cell line LNCaP involves reduction of cyclin-dependent kinase 2 activity and persistent G1 accumulation. *Endocrinology* **139**: 1197–1207.

Zinser, G., Packman, K., and Welsh, J. 2002a. Vitamin D(3) receptor ablation alters mammary gland morphogenesis. *Development* **129**: 3067–3076.

Zinser, G.M., McEleney, K., and Welsh, J. 2003. Characterization of mammary tumor cell lines from wild type and vitamin D(3) receptor knockout mice. *Mol Cell Endocrinol* **200**: 67–80.

Zinser, G.M., Sundberg, J.P., and Welsh, J. 2002b. Vitamin D(3) receptor ablation sensitizes skin to chemically induced tumorigenesis. *Carcinogenesis* **23**: 2103–2109.

Zinser, G.M., and Welsh, J.E. 2004. Accelerated mammary gland development during pregnancy and delayed post-lactational involution in vitamin D3 receptor null mice. *Mol Endocrinol* **18**: 2208–2223.

Zinser, G.M., and Welsh, J.E. (in press). Vitamin D receptor status alters mammary gland morphology and tumorigenesis in MMTV-neu mice. *Carcinogenesis* **25**: 2361–2372.

Zittermann, A. 2003. Vitamin D in preventive medicine: are we ignoring the evidence? *Br J Nutr* **89**: 552–572.

C H A P T E R

32

Soy Isoflavones

STEPHEN BARNES, JEEVAN PRASAIN, TRACY D'ALESSANDRO, CHAO-CHENG WANG, HUANG-GE ZHANG, AND HELEN KIM

INTRODUCTION

The value of soy as an important part of the diet has been known for several millennia. Systematic research over the past 30–40 years has established a beneficial role of soy foods and their constituents in several chronic diseases, including cancer. Soy's presence in foods has risen over the past 10–20 years in the United States and Western Europe, mostly in the form of increasingly purified protein preparations. This is in contrast to the use of soy in Southeast Asia, where it more commonly appears in forms prepared from whole soybeans using fermentation techniques. Several constituents of soy (isoflavones, protease inhibitors, phytosterols, and inositol phosphates) have been shown to have biological activity in models of cancer. The isoflavones have an estrogen-like activity (hence, the term *phytoestrogen*), but this is not their only mode of action. Unlike many other bioflavonoids, isoflavones are well absorbed, although they undergo substantial metabolism. It is possible that a bacterial metabolite, equol, has unique biochemical properties, giving advantage to those who can form it. A new class of bioactive compounds from soy may include unique peptides that can pass intact into the blood circulation.

The link between diet and lowered risk of several chronic diseases is well recognized. It has stimulated groups of investigators to pursue cancer-prevention hypotheses on the basis of the roles of specific foods and compounds derived from them. In this chapter, we examine the connection between soy food consumption and lowered risk of several cancers, as well as one class of the phytochemicals in soybeans, the isoflavones. We explore the historical aspects of soy foods, their modern forms, and apparent influence on cancer risk, and the biochemistry, chemistry, metabolism, and mode of action of the soy isoflavones.

HISTORY OF SOY

The soybean is a plant (*Glycine max*) that originated in Southeast Asia. The seeds of the soybean were mentioned as a medicine in the writings of the Chinese Emperor Cheng-Nung in 2838 BC. They were used by monks in Japan in the second through sixth centuries AD to prepare an alternative to salted meat garnishes. This fermented product is *soy sauce*, now commonly used as a condiment in meals in many countries of the world. Soybeans were brought to Europe and America in the eighteenth century by traders who traveled to and from Southeast Asia. In the years leading up to the American Revolution of 1776, soybeans were cultivated as a crop in South Carolina (Hymowitz, 1990). However, the agricultural use of soybeans did not occur for more than 100 years. In the period from 1890 to 1900, the U.S. Department of Agriculture (USDA) systematically investigated the selection of soybean strains for the different growing conditions in each agricultural state. Since then, soybeans have become an important crop in the United States. Ironically, the United States has become a major provider of soybeans to Japan and other Asian countries, although over the past 25 years it has faced increasing competition from new soybean suppliers in countries such as Brazil.

FOOD MATERIALS DERIVED FROM SOYBEANS

The soybean is processed to provide a number of different foods and food products (Figure 1). *Soy milk* is prepared by grinding soybeans and extracting them with water. Soy milk is an advantage to Asians because many of them lack

Copyright © 2006, Elsevier Inc.
All rights of reproduction in any form reserved.

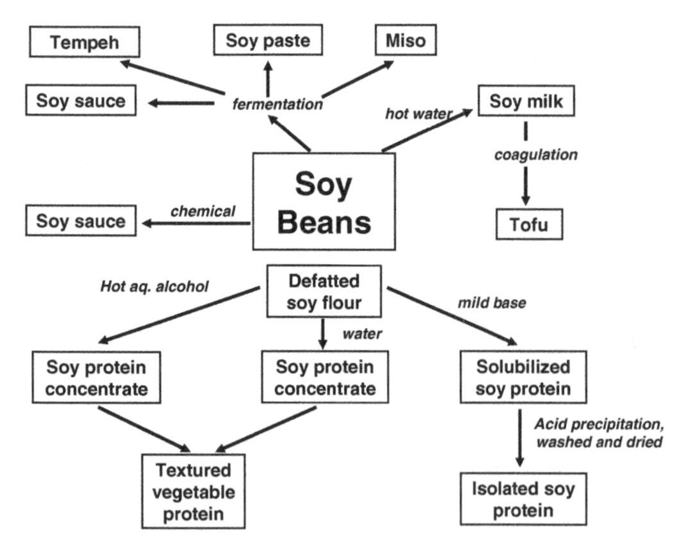

FIGURE 1 **Processing of soybeans to produce soy foods.** In the upper part of this diagram, soy foods that are common in the Asian diet are shown. Extraction of proteins from soybeans with water creates a liquid form of soy that takes the place of cow's milk. This soy milk is converted to a semisolid form, tofu, by coagulation. Miso, soy paste, tempeh, and soy sauce are each fermented products of soybeans. The remaining items represent soy products prepared in the United States, mostly those enriched in soy proteins. There is a transition soy food, soy sauce, prepared by acid hydrolysis.

intestinal lactase and, thereby, cannot digest lactose in cow's milk (Simoons, 1978). It is also an alternative for those infants who are intolerant to cow's milk, and it is used in infant milk formula. The sales of soy milk have risen sharply in the past 15–20 years, and it is sold in the United States in full-fat and low-fat varieties. *Tofu* (or bean curd) is a protein fraction prepared from soy milk by calcium-induced coagulation, although it can also be formed by weak acids in a closed sterile container, thereby giving an extended shelf life. It comes in several forms by reducing the water content by pressing the curd in a filter. *Silken* tofu can be blended with other ingredients in puddings, whereas *firm* tofu is often a separate protein dish in a meal. Fermented soy products such as soybean paste are common in Asia. In Korea, soybean paste is combined with peppers to produce a hot sauce. In Japan, the fermentation is carried out slowly with barley and wheat to produce *miso*. Miso is widely used as a condiment and in soups. In Indonesia, intact soybeans are incubated with microorganisms to produce *Tempeh*, a fermented food with a meatlike appearance.

In the United States, soybeans were initially largely grown as a source of cooking oil, with the residual protein fraction being used as an animal feed. However, there was an early interest in creating novel products from soybeans. Henry Ford explored the use of soybeans to make plastics. In the second half of the twentieth century, food chemists created protein fractions (soy flour, textured soy protein, and isolated soy protein) that have appeared in a wide variety of food products. Defatted soy flour is the protein fraction (50% of solids) left after the extraction of the oil fraction with hexane. It is prepared in various forms dependent on the extent of heating used to denature the enzymes left after extraction. The roasted form is the one fed to livestock. Treatment of soy flour with hot water or hot aqueous ethanol removes the soluble carbohydrates (some of these, raffinose and stachyose, are poorly hydrolyzed in the gut). The alcoholic wash also removes other low molecular weight compounds such as the isoflavones (see Table 1 for data on the isoflavone content of soy foods). The protein content of the washed *soy protein concentrate* is ~70%. Extruded soy protein concentrate is textured soy protein. If the defatted soy flour is treated with a mild alkaline solution, the protein fraction is largely solubilized, leaving behind the insoluble complex carbohydrate fraction. The protein-rich extract is treated with acid to pH 4–5 to precipitate the protein fraction. It is washed and dried to form *soy protein isolate,* a fraction containing 90–92% protein and <0.5% lipid. This material is used as the basis for many new low-fat soy products that have appeared in grocery stores.

CHEMISTRY AND BIOSYNTHESIS OF ISOFLAVONES

Isoflavones are members of a large family of polyphenols formed in many plants. The latter include many bioflavonoids, stilbenes, coumestanes, and lignans (Figure 2). The bioflavonoids are formed by the conversion of phenylalanine into trans-4-hydroxycinnamoyl coenzyme A (CoA) and its subsequent condensation catalyzed by chalcone synthase with three molecules of malonyl CoA to form naringenin, a chalcone (Figure 3). Naringenin is a substrate for many flavonoids and has a phenyl group (B ring) in the 2-position of the benzopyran moiety (A and C rings). The isoflavonoids are formed by the action of the enzyme chalcone isomerase that moves the phenyl group to the 3-position of the benzopyran. This enzyme has a restricted range, being largely limited to tropical members of the *Leguminoseae* family. The best known member of this family is the soybean. However, there are other significant sources of isoflavonoids. These include the subterranean red clover *Trifolium pratense* (Schultz, 1965), found in Western Australia, the tubers of the American groundnut *Apios americana* (Barnes et al., 2002), a longstanding part of the diet of the Eastern American Indians, and the Japanese ivy *Pueraria lobata*, more commonly known as the kudzu, that literally covers most of the trees and vegetation in Southeast United States. Extracts of kudzu root have long been used as a traditional medicine in Southeast Asia (Foster, 1994). Kudzu isoflavones are available as a dietary supplement in the United States and are a component in preparations of isoflavones being used as a phytoestrogen alternative to the equine estrogen product Premarin.

TABLE 1 Mean Isoflavone Concentrations (mg/g)[a] Found in Common American and Asian Foods

	Daidzein		Genistein	
Food name	**Conjugated**	**Unconjugated**	**Conjugated**	**Unconjugated**
American foods				
Soy nuts	0.521[b]	0.054[b]	0.868[b]	0.066[b]
Soybean chips	0.202[b]	0.065[b]	0.223[b]	0.052[b]
Soy flour (defatted)	0.355[c]	n.d.	0.463[c]	0.015[c]
Soy protein concentrate (water washed)	0.720[c]	0.039[c]	0.878[c]	0.033[c]
Soy protein concentrate (alcohol washed) (water washed)	0.039[c]	0.004[c]	0.054[c]	0.004[c]
Textured vegetable protein				
Isolated soy protein	0.170[c]	0.102[c]	0.368[c]	0.189[c]
Asian foods				
Soy sauce	n.d.	0.054[b]	n.d.	0.036[b]
Soy paste	0.055[b]	0.404[b]	0.100[b]	0.514[b]
Miso	0.033[b]	0.516[b]	0.041[b]	0.745[b]
Soy milk	0.816[b]	0.141[b]	1.050[b]	0.098[b]
Tofu	0.924[b]	0.113[b]	1.304[b]	0.116[b]
Tempeh	0.063[b]	0.298[b]	0.185[b]	0.434[b]

Note: [a]The concentrations are given as isoflavone aglycon equivalents and are expressed as mg isoflavone/g of dry weight[b] or protein[c]. They are adapted from Coward et al. (1993).

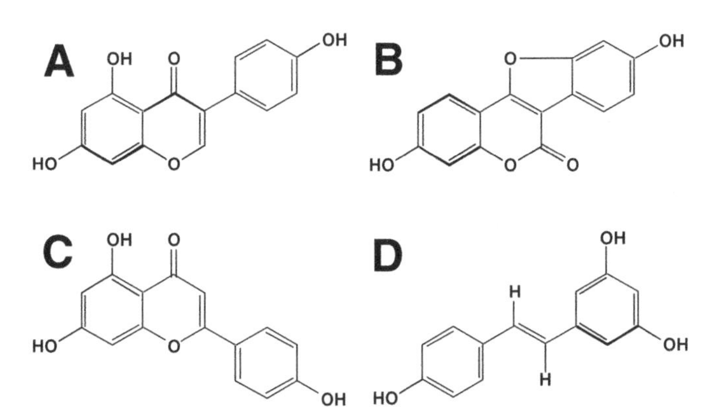

FIGURE 2 **Examples of dietary polyphenols with biological activity.** Genistein (A) is an isoflavonoid from soy with estrogenic activity among many other properties; coumestrol (B) is a coumestane with strong estrogenic effects *in vivo*; apigenin (C) is the flavonoid isomer of genistein with weak estrogenic activity; and resveratrol (D) is a stilbene found in red grapes (and hence red wine).

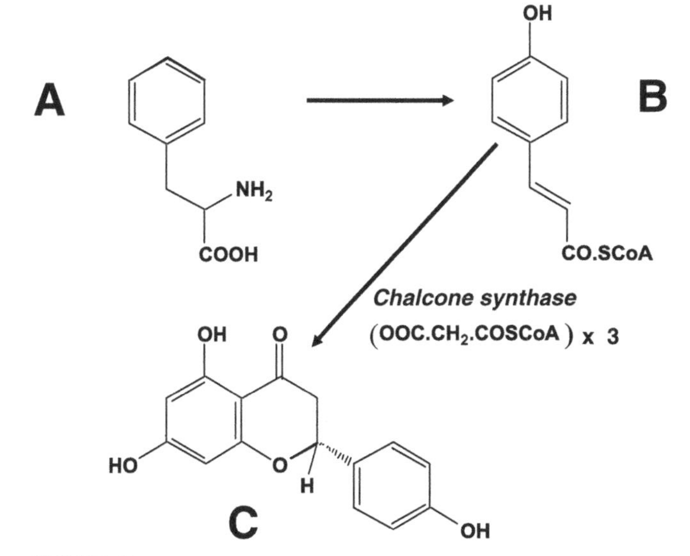

FIGURE 3 **Chalcone synthase: the key step in the biosynthesis of flavonoids.** Phenylalanine (A) is converted via several enzymatic steps to cleave the amine group, 4-hydroxylate cinnamic acid and form cinnamoyl coenzyme A (CoA) (B). This intermediate reacts with three molecules of malonyl CoA to form a polyketide that then undergoes rearrangement to yield (−)naringenin (C). The formation of isoflavones comes as the result of migration of the phenyl ring from the 2-position to the 3-position catalyzed by the enzyme chalcone isomerase.

Isoflavone Concentrations in Soy Foods

Table 1 contains data on the concentrations of daidzein and genistein and their β-glycoside conjugates from a study published in 1993 (Coward et al., 1993). It demonstrates that the concentrations in the soybean before processing are in the range from 0.2 to 0.8 mg/g, of which 90% or greater are the β-glycosides. The higher figures for soy nuts are probably a reflection of removal of moisture. Removing the fat with hexane does not lead to a loss of isoflavones—indeed, the concentration per gram goes up. A further increase per gram is also observed for soy protein concentrate, but aqueous alcohol extraction rather than water extraction drastically lowers (>95%) the isoflavone content. The preparation of isolated soy protein leads to a loss of isoflavones, particularly the β-glycosides. Interestingly, the unconjugated isoflavones are increased, suggesting that the process causes hydrolysis of the conjugated isoflavones. Changes in the process of preparing isolated soy protein occurred in the mid-1990s and materials used in many clinical studies contained isoflavone concentrations in excess of 1.0 mg/g dry weight.

Miso, soy paste, and tempeh each have total isoflavone concentrations that are comparable to unprocessed soybeans or soy flakes. However, the fermentation processes used in their preparation convert the β-glycosides to the unconjugated isoflavones. Soy foods in which other materials are added (barley, rice, or wheat) have a lower isoflavone content per gram. Soy milk and tofu have a high isoflavone content per gram, mostly as β-glycosides.

Thus, it is critical in a preclinical or clinical study to carefully determine the isoflavones composition and concentrations. Because of differences in absorption of each of the isoflavone forms, the isoflavones that enter the systemic circulation, and thus, the tissues, will be a function of the composition of the soy preparation used. A large database of the isoflavone content of a wide variety of foods is available at http://www.nal.usda.gov/fnic/foodcomp/Data/isoflav/isoflav.html. Because soy protein is added to many foods and dietary or energy-producing supplements, investigators should not rely on dietary questionnaires to assess isoflavone intake but instead collect urine samples and perform isoflavone analysis (Horn-Ross et al., 1997). An example of an unusual source of isoflavones is in certain brands of canned tuna in which a protein (soy) broth is added to the fish (Horn-Ross et al., 2000).

Importance of Glycoside Conjugates in Isoflavone Chemistry and Biological Action

In the soybean and red clover, isoflavones are converted to their *O*-glycosides by *O*-glycosyltransferases and then to 6-*O*-malonate esters of the glycosides (Kudou et al., 1991). The *O*-glycoside conjugates are formed by a carbon–oxygen bond between the C-1 carbon of the sugar moiety and (generally) the O-7 oxygen of the isoflavones. The majority of the isoflavones in Kudzu root are unusual *C*-glycosides (Prasain et al., 2003). These conjugates are formed by a carbon–carbon bond between the C-1 carbon of the sugar moiety and the C-8 carbon of the isoflavones. In the groundnut, *A. americana*, a 7-*O*-glycosylglycoside conjugate of genistein is the principal isoflavone in the edible tuber of this plant (N. Barnes and S. Barnes, unpublished observations).

When soybeans are extracted with hot water or pressurized steam to produce soy milk and tofu, there is substantial hydrolysis of the malonyl esters to form the simple β-glycosides of the isoflavones (Barnes et al., 1994b) (Figure 4). This also occurred when analytical chemists used hot aqueous-organic solvent mixtures to extract isoflavones from plant and food materials (Barnes et al., 1994b). To avoid this analytical complication, extraction should be carried out at 4°C (Coward et al., 1998). Once extracted, the solution should be kept cold. We found that the isoflavone β-glycoside malonyl esters in such extracts when placed on a high-performance liquid chromatography (HPLC) autosampler slowly degrade (M. Smith-Johnson and S. Barnes, unpublished observations). A cooled sample tray prevents this problem.

Processing of the soybeans with hexane to recover soy oil does not damage the isoflavone conjugates. However, post-extraction heating leads to the well-known decarboxylation of the malonyl group to an acetyl group (Figure 4). Thus, defatted toasted soy flakes/flour have substantial amounts of 6′-*O*-acetyl-β-glycoside conjugates of isoflavones (Barnes et al., 1994b).

Soy protein concentrates have variable amounts of isoflavones (Table 1). In those protein concentrates derived by water washing of soy flour, the isoflavones are largely

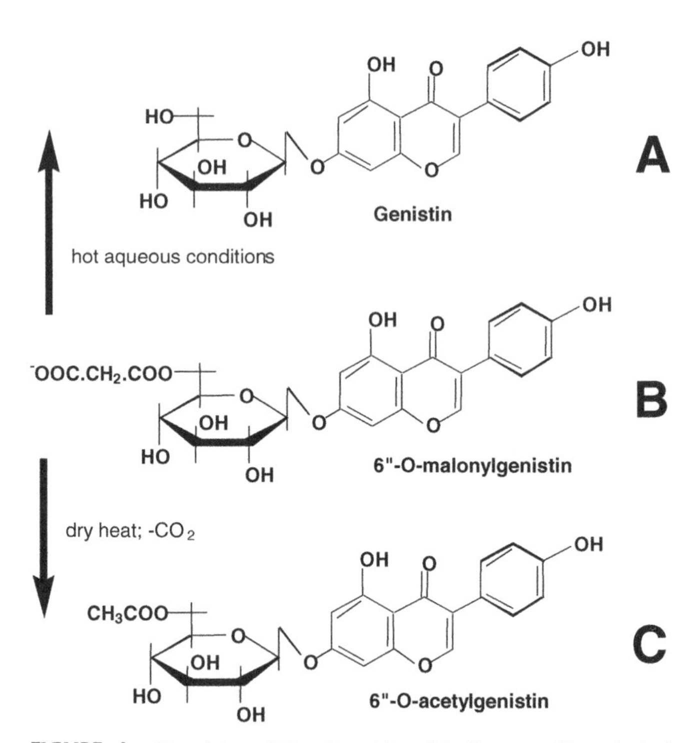

FIGURE 4 **Chemistry of the glycosides of isoflavones.** The principal form of isoflavones *O*-glycosides in the soy and other plants is the 6′-*O*-malonyl ester of the sugar moiety (B). The ester rapidly undergoes hydrolysis to form β-glycoside when heated in aqueous solvents, but also slowly even at room temperature. In the absence of water, the malonate loses CO_2 to form a 6′-*O*-acetyl ester (C). It is also hydrolyzed in aqueous solvents.

retained (Coward et al., 1998). There is some loss of the more hydrophilic isoflavone forms, daidzein > glycitein > genistein and of the conjugates, malonyl esters of β-glycosides > β-glycosides > acetyl esters of β-glycosides > aglycons (Ji Guo-Ping and S. Barnes, unpublished observations). Again, the drying process can lead to more decarboxylation of residual malonyl esters of β-glycosides.

Soy protein isolates have the highest protein content (>91% by weight) of soy food products. They have a lower concentration of the isoflavones than soy flour and water-extracted soy protein concentrate (Table 1). However, high isoflavone-containing soy protein isolates have been prepared for investigational research. The first step in their preparation, treatment with mild alkali, would be expected to dissociate the isoflavones from the now soluble proteins. Isoflavones undergo an interesting reaction with alkalis wherein the heterocyclic ring is opened and then closed to form a five-member ring system (A. Franke and S. Barnes, unpublished observations). The precipitation of the solubilized proteins with a weak acid leads to a further loss of isoflavones, as described for water washing of soy flour. This may account for the larger proportion of isoflavone aglycons in the soy protein isolates (Barnes et al., 1994b).

Uptake and Metabolism of Isoflavones

Unconjugated isoflavones are readily absorbed passively by the cells of the intestine; in this respect, they behave like many other organic compounds used for therapeutic treatment of disease and minor ailments. The more common forms in soy, the *O*-glycosides, have poor passive absorption because of their lower hydrophobicity than the aglycons. Isoflavone β-glucosides may also undergo intestinal transport via the sodium-dependent glucose transporter (SGLT). Phlorizin, a β-glucoside of the 5-hydroxyflavonoid, has long been used as an inhibitor of glucose transport (Dimitrakoudis et al., 1992). However, no *O*-glucosides of isoflavones are found in the blood (Barnes et al., 2001). In contrast, when puerarin, the 8-*C*-glucoside of daidzein, is administered to rats by gavage, it is the only isoflavone that is detected in the blood and urine for the first 24 hours (Prasain et al., 2004). This suggests that puerarin is transported by SGLT.

The lack of isoflavone *O*-glucosides in blood is due to an enzyme, lactose phlorizin hydrolase (LPH), embedded in the apical membrane of the small intestinal mucosal cells that carries out hydrolysis of the β-glycoside conjugates of isoflavones and thereby allows the isoflavone aglycons so formed to be readily absorbed (Day et al., 2000). In the intestinal cells, the isoflavone aglycons are largely converted to β-glucuronide conjugates by uridine diphosphate glucuronosyl transferase (UDPGT) (Sfakianos et al., 1997). This enzyme activity also is present in the liver so that much of the circulating forms of isoflavones in the blood are β-glucuronide conjugates. Only at high-dose levels are unconjugated isoflavones a significant part of the circulating forms of isoflavones (Sfakianos et al., 1997). A second conjugating reaction, *O*-sulfation, is catalyzed by phenol sulfotransferases. The isoflavone sulfates are minor metabolites in female rats but are more common in male rats (Bayer et al., 2001) and in humans (Shelnutt et al., 2002) and by some human breast cancer cell lines (Peterson et al., 1996, 1998).

Enterohepatic Recycling of Isoflavones

If 4-^{14}C–labeled genistein is introduced into the duodenum of female rats with an indwelling cannula in the common bile duct, ~80% of the dose appears in the bile within 3 hours (Sfakianos et al., 1997). If it is introduced into the portal vein, then ~100% of the dose is transported into the collected bile. Furthermore, if the radioactive form in the bile (shown to be the 7-*O*-β-glucuronide) is reinfused into the small intestine, radioactivity quickly reappears in the bile (Sfakianos et al., 1997). If genistein 7-*O*-β-glucuronide is introduced into the duodenum, 25% of the administered dose is recovered in the bile in a 4-hour period; however, if reinfusion occurs in the mid-jejunum, then the recovered dose in the bile rises to 70–80% (Sfakianos et al., 1997). These observations are consistent with genistein undergoing a substantial *enterohepatic circulation* (Figure 5), with formation

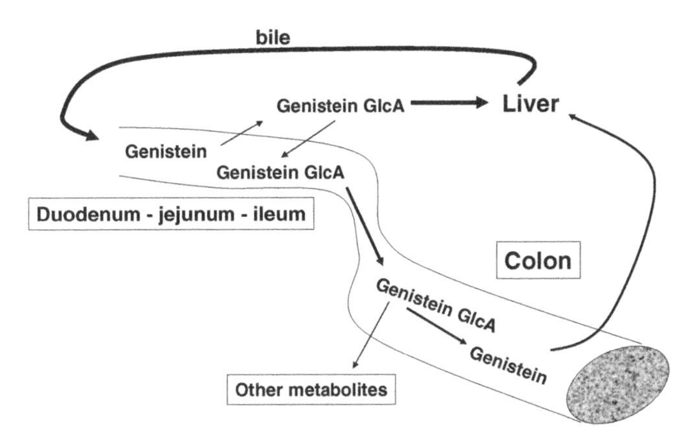

FIGURE 5 **Cartoon of the enterohepatic circulation and pathways of genistein transport and metabolism.** Genistein is readily absorbed from the upper small intestine. Its β-glucoside, genistein, undergoes hydrolysis either due to luminal bacterial β-glucosidases or small intestine apical membrane lactase phlorizin hydrolase. Genistein is absorbed into the enterocytes and there most is converted to its β-glucuronide. Although much of this metabolite enters the bloodstream, some of it refluxes back into the intestinal lumen. Genistein and its β-glucuronide that enter the blood circulation are mostly taken up by the liver and excreted into the bile and thereby reenter the small intestine, completing an enterohepatic circuit. Genistein β-glucuronide undergoes hydrolysis by β-glucuronidases in the mid small intestine, releasing genistein that is taken up into the intestine once again. Some of the genistein β-glucuronide enters the large intestine where hydrolysis is completed and genistein is also reabsorbed. However, in this anaerobic environment degradation of genistein to other metabolites can occur.

of genistein from its β-glucuronide by the action of intestinal β-glucuronidases. Indeed, we have observed genistein β-glucuronide in the bile of rats 1 week after being taken off a diet containing soy and its isoflavones (J. Sfakianos and S. Barnes, unpublished observations).

Bacterial Metabolism of Isoflavones

Isoflavones undergo additional metabolism when they come into contact with intestinal bacteria in the colon. Several metabolites of daidzein (dihydrodaidzein, *O*-desmethylangolensin and equol) (Figure 6) are commonly observed in blood and urine from most species, including humans. These, as for the *primary* isoflavones (daidzein, glycitein, and genistein), undergo β-glucuronidation and sulfation. Very few intact isoflavones are found in feces; the major route of excretion is via the kidney. Up to 60% of orally administered doses of both daidzein and glycitein appears in the urine (Kelly et al., 1995). In contrast, only 15–20% of genistein is excreted in urine. This led some to state that daidzein was more bioavailable than genistein (Xu et al., 1994); however, this statement is misleading because both isoflavones are well absorbed. Instead, daidzein has a higher renal clearance than genistein and therefore actually spends less time in the body. Metabolites of genistein have been less commonly found. These include dihydrogenistein, 6′-hydroxy-*O*-desmethylangolensin, 2-(4-hydroxyphenyl)-propionic acid, and 4-ethyl phenol (Setchell, 1998; Coldham et al., 1999) (Figure 7). The latter accumulates in the prostate of male rats, whereas genistein does not. Interestingly, in elderly Seventh Day Adventists on soy-containing diets, daidzein and its metabolites, but not genistein, accumulate in prostatic fluid to levels up to 50 times their blood concentrations (Hedlund et al., 2005).

Equol, 7,4′-dihydroxyisoflavan, is a major daidzein metabolite in almost all species except in humans. Only one-third of humans have a blood concentration of equol that exceeds 10 nM (the amounts less than this may come from dietary sources such as cow's milk) (Urban et al., 2001). In rats fed soy, the blood equol levels are five to seven times higher than daidzein or genistein (Kim et al., 2004) and are in the 1–3 μM range. Pharmacokinetic analysis suggests that the accumulation of equol in the blood is due not only to its rate of formation from daidzein, but also to it having a lower renal clearance than the other isoflavones (Kim et al., 2004). This marked difference in isoflavone metabolism between experimental animals (rats, mice, monkeys) and humans is a concern because administration of a soy product produces a very different array of isoflavones and their metabolites to tissues of each species. Even in the one third of humans who can consistently generate equol, the blood equol concentra-

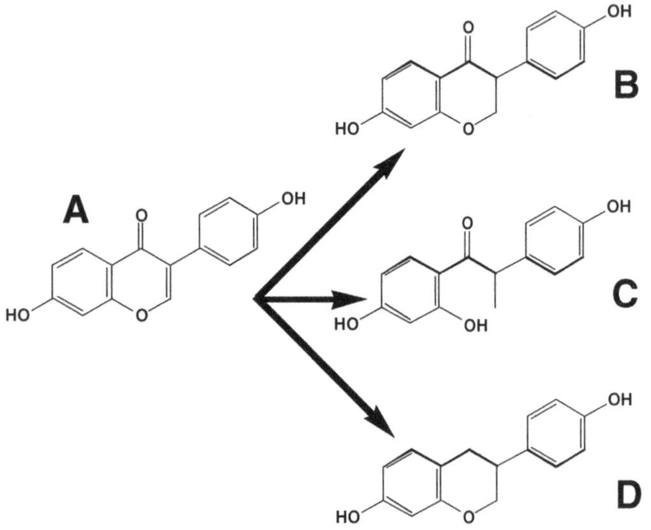

FIGURE 6 **Major bacterial metabolites of daidzein.** Daidzein is either (A) mostly reduced to dihydrodaidzein or (B) undergoes ring opening to form (C) *O*-desmethylangolensin. In most animals, but only in one third of human subjects, daidzein undergoes a more complex reduction to form the isoflavone (D) equol.

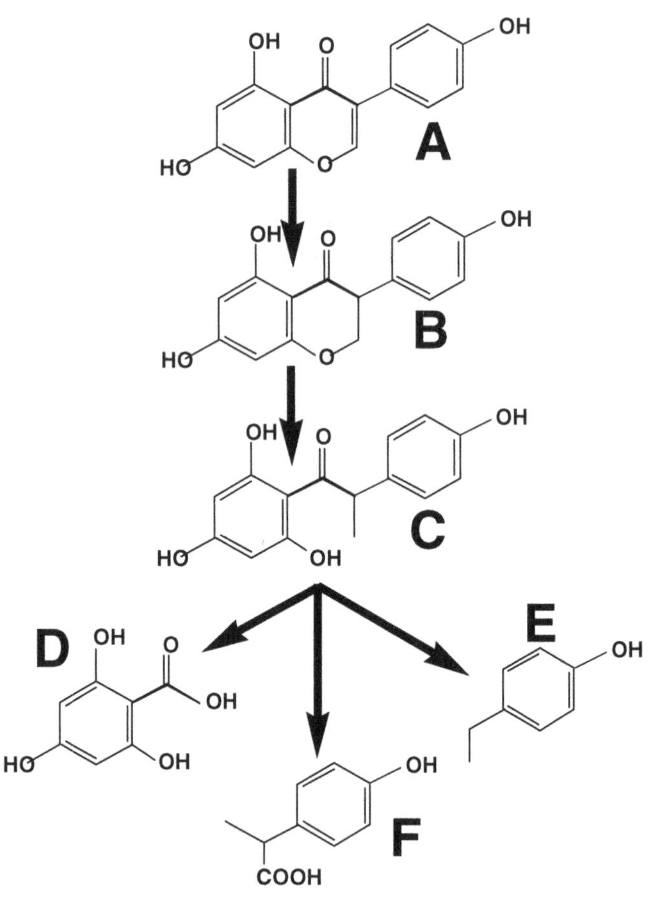

FIGURE 7 **Metabolism of genistein.** Genistein (A) undergoes reduction to form dihydrogenistein (B) or ring opening to form 6′-hydroxy-*O*-desmethylangolensin (C). Although the pathways are not well defined, genistein is also converted to 2,4,6-trihydroxybenzoic acid (D), *p*-ethylphenol (E), and 2-(4-hydroxyphenyl)-propionic acid (F).

tions are substantially lower than in animals (Urban et al., 2001).

Isoflavones and Cytochrome P450

Another relatively unexplored area of metabolism is the hydroxylation of isoflavones by the cytochrome P450 (CYP) system. In experiments *in vitro* with isolated rat and human microsomes (Kulling et al., 2000; Kulling and Lehmann, 2002), hydroxylation can occur slowly in the 6, 8, and 3′ positions. 6- and 8-hydroxydaidzein and genistein have been detected in miso prepared by fermentation (Esaki et al., 1999). These isoflavones are much stronger antioxidants than their parent isoflavones because they are catechols. This property may have prevented their detection in clinical and preclinical animal experiments, unless the blood and urine specimens are treated with an excess of antioxidants (e.g., vitamin C or a metal chelator) before storage, the 6- and 8-hydroxyisoflavones may undergo degradation. We have observed that both 6- and 8-hydroxydaidzein when dissolved in 80% aqueous methanol are unstable and completely disappear when stored for 1 month at 4°C (K. Jones, D.R. Moore, II, and S. Barnes, unpublished observations).

Metabolism of Isoflavones in Inflammatory Cells

The inflammatory response consists of the formation of powerful oxidant species such as superoxide anion, O_2^-, hydrogen peroxide (H_2O_2), hydroxyl radical (OH), hypochlorous acid (HOCl), and peroxynitrite (ONO_2^-), as well as cytokines and hydrolytic enzymes (Schwartsburd, 2004). HOCl and ONO_2^- react with tyrosine residues in proteins to form 3-chloro- and 3-nitrotyrosine (Ischiropoulos et al., 1992; Hazen and Heinecke, 1997). Analogous reactions occur for isoflavones. Genistein and daidzein are nitrated in the B-ring to form 3′-nitro derivatives. Chlorination occurs in both the A- and B-rings to form 6-, 8- and 3′-mono and dichloro derivatives (Boersma et al., 1999). The chloro isoflavones are formed both by differentiated HL-60 cells (Boersma et al., 2003) and by freshly isolated human polymorphonuclear cells (D'Alessandro et al., 2003) following activation with a phorbol ester. The further metabolism of these compounds is not yet defined, but it does not include reaction with glutathione (D'Alessandro et al., 2005).

SOY AND HUMAN HEALTH

As noted earlier, the medical value of the soybean was first appreciated several millennia ago. The modern discovery of the effects of soybeans on human health occurred as medical research in the 1960s and 1970s looked beyond surgical and pharmacological treatments of the major chronic diseases such as atherosclerosis and cancer. It became clear from animal studies that the diet was a variable in models of atherosclerosis and that plant proteins were superior to animal proteins in this context (Hamilton and Carroll, 1976). As a result, a soy protein fraction was used to treat patients with hypercholesterolemia (Sirtori et al., 1977). Over the next 20 years various reports appeared in the literature and led to an important meta-analysis of the effects of soy protein on serum lipids (Anderson et al., 1995). This in turn enabled the establishment in 1999 of a health claim for the use of soy protein to prevent cardiovascular disease (http://vm.cfsan.fda.gov/~lrd/fr991026.html).

Suggestions that soy might also have an important role in lowering the risk of cancer came from several angles. First, Doll and Peto (1981) observed that the worldwide variation in the incidence and death from cancer could not be explained solely by ethnic or genetic origins. They concluded that diet was a major factor (35–70% of the risk). Initially, the much higher fat content of the U.S. and Western European diets was seen as the driving force for the higher risk of breast and prostate cancer in these countries as opposed to Asia. Indeed, international comparisons of fat intake and breast cancer risk were supportive of this hypothesis. However, in Americans there was no correlation between fat content in the diet and breast cancer risk (Willett et al., 1987). A plausible alternative explanation was that the Asian diet contained cancer-preventing substances (Barnes et al., 1990). A hint came from an unintended change in 1986 in the design of chemoprevention experiments in rodent models of breast cancer. The National Cancer Institute decided to switch from a laboratory chow diet to a semi-defined AIN76A diet. It was intended that the change would lead to a more reproducible model to test chemopreventive agents. A chow diet is an unregulated mixture of soymeal, wheat, and fishmeal, the composition of which was dependent on market prices of its components, whereas the AIN76A diet contained casein as the only protein. Surprisingly, the number of mammary tumors induced by the carcinogen N-methyl-N-nitrosourea (NMU) on the AIN76A diet rose sharply, resulting in both a higher incidence and a substantial loss of animals during the observation period to their tumor burden (Grubbs et al., 1985). In 1980, Troll et al. had shown that adding soybeans in the diet of rats reduced the number of mammary tumors in an X-ray model of mammary carcinogenesis. However, it was not clear which soybean component was responsible.

PRECLINICAL EXPERIMENTS EXPLORING THE SOY–CANCER PREVENTION HYPOTHESIS

The introduction of experimental designs where the dietary intake was carefully controlled for caloric and protein content has demonstrated that diets containing soy prevent experimentally induced cancer in most cases. Barnes et al. (1990, 1994a) and Hawrylewicz et al. (1995) showed that various soy fractions lowered the number of tumors in carcinogen-induced mammary carcinogenesis. The rationale for soy's effect was proposed at that time as being due to its isoflavone content, although there are other theories. One of these, a small peptide, the Bowman-Birk inhibitor, was studied in detail by Kennedy (1998). An analogous peptide, lunasin, has been identified by a group of investigators at UC-Davis (Galvez et al., 2001). Phytosterols (Awad et al., 2000; Ju et al., 2004) and inositol phosphates (Shamsuddin et al., 1997) have also had their advocates.

GENISTEIN AND BREAST CANCER MODELS

A test of the role of a dietary substance in disease prevention is to examine it in isolation (i.e., to add it to a standard semisynthetic diet and to ensure that the animal's diet consumption, rate of growth, and final adult weight are unaffected). This is a pharmacological approach to a dietary problem and not necessarily an ideal model to test the effect of a dietary constituent (Barnes and Prasain, 2005). It was fortunate that the initial rodent experiments on the soy isoflavone genistein were carried out in Coral Lamartiniere's laboratory. Dr. Lamartiniere is a toxicologist with an interest in the effects of synthetic estrogen exposure during the perinatal and prepubertal periods of development. Although at that time genistein was a very expensive phytochemical, nonetheless, he demonstrated that rat pups treated i.p. with genistein (in DMSO as the solvent) on postnatal days 2, 4, and 6 had 50% less mammary tumors induced by the carcinogen DMBA than pups treated with DMSO alone (Lamartiniere et al., 1995a). A study where genistein was administered on postnatal days 14, 16, and 18 produced similar data (Lamartiniere et al., 1995b). Because genistein was administered i.p. in these experiments, the question remained as to whether this was relevant to dietary exposure. Subsequently, Fritz et al. (1998) discovered that delivering genistein to the dam's diet (and hence to the pups via her milk) also reduced the number of mammary tumors in a dose-dependent manner. However, a study from our laboratory sowed confusion by showing that administering genistein to adult animals in their diet was not chemopreventive (Kim et al., 2004). Lamartiniere et al. (2002) reported a similar negative finding. However, they went on to show that when prepubertal delivery of genistein (as described earlier) is combined with adding it to the adult diet, there is a significant increase in the level of inhibition of mammary tumors (Table 2). Ironically, in the late 1990s, the National Cancer Institute switched back from the AIN76A diet to a laboratory chow diet. When genistein was administered to adult female Sprague–Dawley rats in the laboratory chow background, it had a strong chemopreventive effect (Figure 8). These data strongly suggest that early life exposure to genistein sets the stage for a beneficial sensitivity to genistein in adult life.

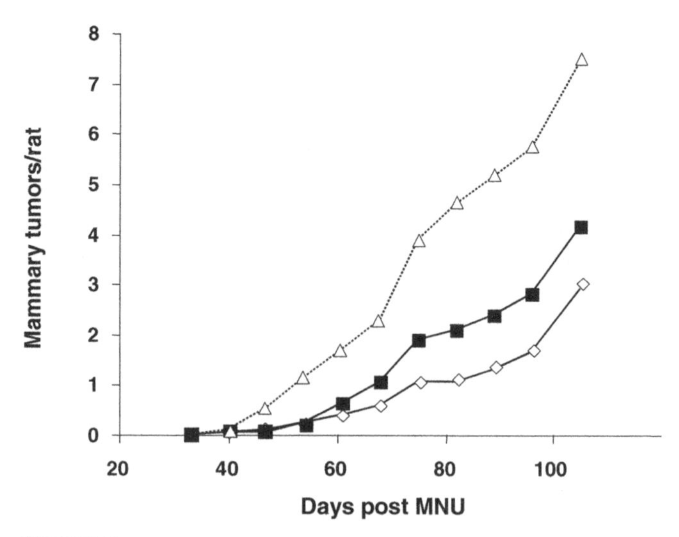

FIGURE 8 **Effect of dietary genistein on mammary rumors in adult female rats treated with the carcinogen, *N*-methyl-*N*-nitrosourea.** The control animals (open triangles) were fed a laboratory chow diet. Genistein was added to this diet at two doses (200 mg/kg diet, closed squares; 2000 mg/kg diet, open diamonds).

TABLE 2 The Effect of Dietary Genistein on the Average Tumor Number per Rat in a Carcinogen-Induced[a] Model of Breast Cancer

Experimental group	Exposure to genistein	Mean no. of mammary tumors per rat
Control	None	8.9
Prepubertal	1–21 days	4.3
Adult	After tumors appear (100 days)	8.2
Prepubertal + adult	From birth to end of study	2.8

Note: The control AIN76A diet contained no phytoestrogen. The other AIN76A diets contained 250 mg of genistein per kilogram of body weight.

[a]All rats were treated with 80 mg of dimethylbenz[a]anthracene per kilogram of body weight at day 50 postpartum.

Source: The data were adapted from Lamartiniere et al. (2002).

Hilakivi et al. (1999) showed that exposure to genistein prenatally by its administration to the dams increased the number of mammary tumors induced by DMBA in rats. However, genistein was administered i.v. and thereby bypassed the enzymes responsible for its metabolism (see previous sections on metabolism). In a subsequent experiment when genistein was administered neonatally, Hilakivi et al. (2001) found that it caused a decrease in the number of mammary tumors, confirming the previous results of Lamartiniere et al. (1995a).

TIMING OF EXPOSURE TO SOY IN HUMANS

Analogous results to the preclinical experiments noted earlier have been observed in epidemiological studies. In a study on breast cancer in Shanghai, China, there was a dose-dependent–negative association between eating soy in adolescence and breast cancer (Shu et al., 2001) (Table 3). However, there was no correlation with other fresh legumes in the diet. In a second study in Asian-Americans in California, it was found that women who ate tofu more than once a week in adolescence, but little in adult life, were less likely to have breast cancer (adjusted odds ratio [OR] = 0.77) than those who ate tofu less than once a month at any stage during life. Those who ate tofu more than once a week only in adult life (adjusted OR = 0.93) were at a similar risk to low tofu eaters (Wu et al., 2002). In contrast, those who ate tofu at least once a week throughout life had the lowest risk of breast cancer (adjusted OR = 0.53, p trend = 0.001). A report on identical twins found that they do not start menstruation (a measure of estrogen sensitivity) at the same time; typically in 50% of the twins, the difference was at least 1 year (Hamilton and Mack, 2003). Importantly, the twin who had two of the first signs of puberty was 5.4 times more likely to have breast cancer than their sibling.

SOY, ISOFLAVONES, AND PREEXISTING BREAST CANCER

There are two quite different views regarding the roles of soy and isoflavones on existing mammary tumors. Hawrylewicz et al. (1995) showed that when female rats treated with DMBA on an AIN76A diet were subjected to resection of the first mammary tumor and then randomly placed on AIN76A diet or AIN76A diet where the casein was replaced by soy protein isolate (containing isoflavones), the soy-free animals had statistically more mammary tumors than those on a soy diet (Figure 9). These data suggest a chemopreventive effect of soy protein in this model.

In contrast, a number of authors (Hsieh et al., 1998; Allred et al., 2001a,b; Ju et al., 2001, 2002) have used an athymic nude mouse model to implant human breast cancer cells into this animal to create a model of recurrent mammary cancer. For this model to work, the mice must be ovariectomized. This maneuver removes the physiological source of estrogens. Under these conditions human MCF-7 cells do not grow. However, adding soy or soy isoflavones to the diet leads to slow but steady growth of the cancer cells (Figure 10). One interpretation of these experimental results is that genistein or soy containing genistein will promote the growth of cancers and therefore should be avoided in women with preexisting breast cancer or at high risk of breast cancer. However, it should be noted that in this animal model, the thymus and hence the source of T cells have been removed. This is the way that the human breast cancer cells can be implanted without rejection by the mouse immune system. Detection of foreign antigens is carried out by the innate immune system (Figure 11). Natural killer (NK) cells respond to *foreignness* by producing interferon-γ (IFN-γ). This in turn causes recruitment of T cells producing antibodies to nonself antigens and clonal expansion of the T cells. It is this aspect of the immune system that is absent in the nude mouse.

It is, therefore, of some interest that a theory of immune tolerance and onset of cancer is emerging (Cheng et al., 2004). There are mouse strains where the onset of breast cancer is age dependent. In a search for a rationale for this, it was noted that the breast cancer cells when grown in culture produce an extracellular fraction that when incubated with natural killer cells or T cells causes an inhibition of

TABLE 3 Epidemiological Data Linking Adolescent Soy Intake and Breast Cancer Risk

Group interviewed	Food	Lowest quintile[a]	Third quintile[a]	Fifth quintile[a]	Trend, p
Premenopausal[b]	Soy	1.00	0.72 (0.54–96)	0.53 (0.39–0.72)	0.0001
	Fresh legumes	1.00	1.04 (0.82–1.33)	0.96 (0.72–1.29)	0.51
Postmenopausal[c]	Soy	1.00	0.65 (0.44–0.97)	0.49 (0.33–0.74)	0.006
	Fresh legumes	1.00	0.92 (0.65–1.30	0.96 (0.67–1.39)	0.82
Mothers[d]	Soy	1.00	0.59 (0.32–1.07)	0.35 (0.21–0.60)	<0.01
	Fresh legumes	1.00	0.88 (0.57–1.38)	0.67 (0.40–1.12)	0.55

[a]Odds ratios were compared with the lowest quintile of intake and adjusted for intake level of rice and wheat products, age, education, family history of breast cancer, history of breast fibroadenoma, WHR, age at menarche, physical activity, ever had livebirth, menopausal status, and age at menopause. The cases came from the Shanghai Cancer Registry and matched controls from the Shanghai Resident Registry.

[b]Number of cases = 952, controls = 990.

[c]Number of cases = 501, controls = 562.

[d]Number of cases = 296, controls = 365; in this set, dietary data during adolescence were provided by the subjects' mothers.

Source: Adapted from Shu et al., 2001.

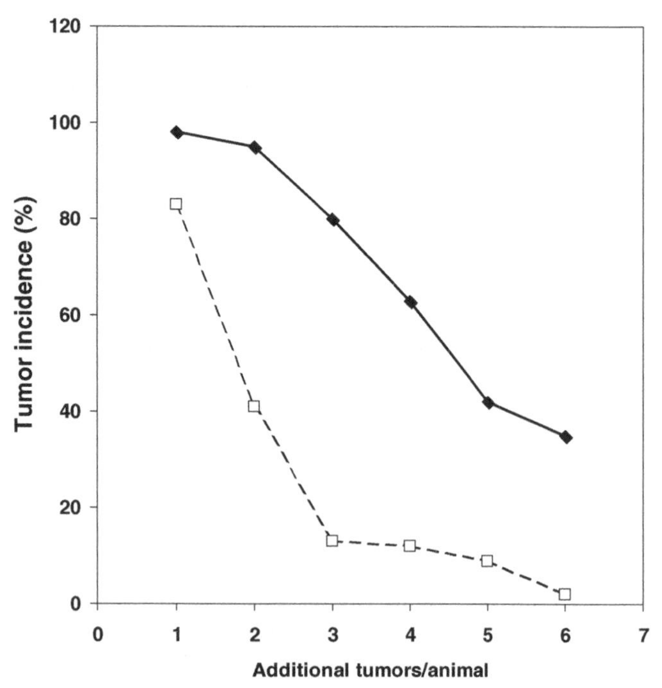

FIGURE 9 **Soy protein isolate (SPI) reduces the number of mammary tumors induced by *N*-methyl-*N*-nitrosourea (NMU).** Female Sprague–Dawley rats were placed on the AIN76A diet with casein (20% w/w) as the source of protein. At 7 weeks of age, they were intravenously injected with NMU. After the first mammary tumor appeared, the tumor was resected and the animals placed either on the same AIN76A diet or on an AIN76A diet in which the casein was replaced by soy protein isolate. The data represent the incidence (%) of additional mammary tumors observed over a 15-week period for each of the diets. The incidences on the SPI diet for the appearance of 2, 3, 4, 5, or more tumors were significantly different from the casein-based diet. (Redrawn from Hawrylewicz et al., 1995.)

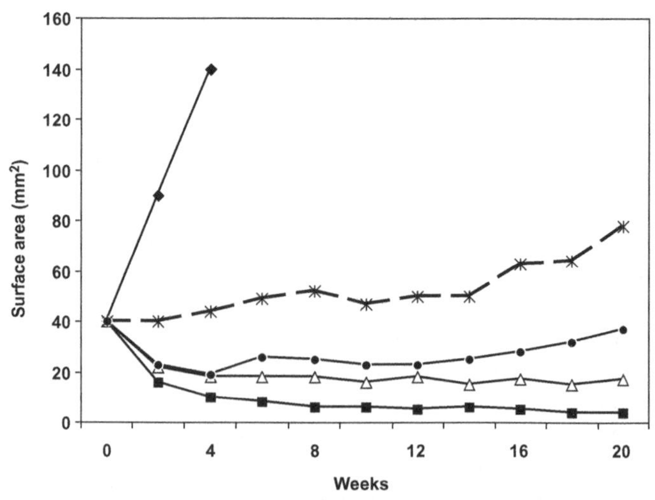

FIGURE 10 **Effect of dietary genistein on growth of human breast cancer MCF-7 cells implanted into ovariectomized athymic nude mice.** After placing estradiol pellets under the skin, tumor cells (1×10^5 cells/site) were injected at four sites. The 17β-estradiol pellets were removed once the surface area of the tumors had grown to 38 mm^2. Animals were fed AIN93 diets with differing levels of genistein (■, 0 ppm; △, 125 ppm; •, 250 ppm; ⋇, 1000 ppm) and tumor surface areas monitored over a 20-week period. In one group of mice, the 17β-estradiol pellets were left under the skin. (Redrawn from Ju et al., 2001.)

the DNA synthesis and production of IFN-γ in response to the cytokine IL-2 (Liu et al., 2005). This fraction contains *exosomes*, multilamellar vesicles from the cancer cells. In the presence of polyphenols in the nanomolar range, these inhibitory effects on the immune response are reversed (Barnes et al., 2005). This implies that one of the functions of isoflavones is to prevent tumor exosome–induced immune tolerance, thereby causing tumors to remain recognized by the immune system. In the intact rat model, mammary tumor growth is inhibited by soy and its isoflavones (Hawrylewicz et al., 1995), whereas in athymic ovariectomized mice, the immune response is ablated by the lack of the thymus, allowing the weak estrogen-like effect of genistein to be observed. Interestingly, in the animal models of breast cancer, the main effect of genistein is to increase the latent period before tumors begin to appear rather than slowing the rate of tumor growth once they are established (Figure 8). Though not proven, this is consistent with genistein extending the period where immune system can still detect the tumor and preventing immune tolerance.

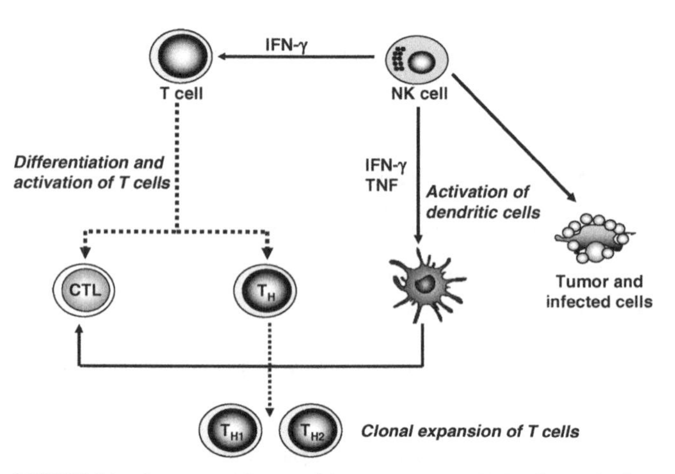

FIGURE 11 **Innate and humoral immune system.** NK cells are the first line of defense in the innate part of the immune system. In conjunction with interferon-γ, activation of NK cells leads to selection of specific T cells that recognize the *foreign tumor* antigens and then their clonal expansion. The latter represent the humoral response. Athymic mice lack T cells and thus the cellular response to tumor antigens.

CONCLUSION

The scientific studies on soy reviewed in this chapter reveal that isoflavones and other polyphenols have several mechanisms of action (Table 4), ranging at the nanomolar level from estrogen-like effects dependent on estrogen receptors (Shao et al., 2000), the synthesis and excretion of

TABLE 4 Mechanisms of Action Attributed to Isoflavones in Cancer Cells

Concentration range	Mechanism	Reference(s)
<10 nM	Estrogen receptor β expression	Kuiper et al., 1998
>10 nM >100 nM	Estrogen receptor α proliferation	Wang and Kurzer, 1997; Zava and Duwe, 1998
	Restores interferon-γ production by T cells	Barnes et al., 2005
>100 nM >1 μM	Blocks production of tumor exosomes	Barnes et al., 2005
>1 μM >10 μM	Inhibition of TNFα/NFκB activation	Davis et al., 1999
	Inhibition of 17β-hydroxysteroid dehydrogenase	Makela et al., 1995
	Inhibition of steroid and phenol sulfotransferases	Kirk et al., 2001
	Alters transforming growth factor β signaling	Kim et al., 1998
	Free radical scavenging	Wei et al., 1993
>10 μM	Protein tyrosine kinase inhibition	Akiyama et al., 1987
	DNA topoisomerase II	Markovits et al., 1989
	Inhibition of metalloproteinase-9	Shao et al., 1998
	Cell cycle progression	Pagliacci et al., 1994

IFN-γ in the immune system (Barnes et al., 2005; Liu et al., 2005), and production of exosomes by tumor cells (Barnes et al., 2005), to effects at the low micromolar level via inhibition of activation of tumor necrosis factor-α (Davis et al., 2001), antioxidant events (Surh, 2003), and tyrosine kinase inhibition (Akiyama and Ogawara, 1991). They are molecules with complex pharmacological effects, and the investigator must be very careful in developing suitable experimental designs that model aspects of human disease. With this in mind, the role of isoflavones, indeed of any preventive or therapeutic agent, on the growth of tumor cells in culture must be viewed very cautiously so as to not draw grandiose conclusions concerning human health and disease from a grossly simplified system.

Acknowledgments

Federal support for research on isoflavones has been in the form of grants-in-aid from the National Center for Complementary and Alternative Medicine for the Purdue University-University of Alabama at Birmingham Botanicals Center for Age-related Disease (P50 AT00477; C. Weaver, PI) and from the National Cancer Institute to the University of Alabama at Birmingham Center for Nutrient–Gene Interaction (U54 CA100949; S. Barnes, PI). Funds for the mass spectrometers used in research at UAB were provided by a Shared Instrumentation Award from the National Center for Research Resources (S10 RR06487).

References

Akiyama, T., Ishida, J., Nakagawa, S., Ogawara, H., Watanabe, S., Itoh, N., Shibuya, M., and Fukami, Y. 1987. Genistein, a specific inhibitor of tyrosine-specific protein kinases. *J Biol Chem* **262**: 5592–5595.

Akiyama, T., and Ogawara, H. 1991. Use and specificity of genistein as inhibitor of protein-tyrosine kinases. *Meth Enzymol* **201**: 362–370.

Allred, C.D., Allred, K.F., Ju, Y.H., Virant, S.M., and Helferich, W.G. 2001a. Soy diets containing varying amounts of genistein stimulate growth of oestrogen-dependent (MCF-7) tumors in a dose-dependent manner. *Cancer Res* **61**: 5045–5050.

Allred, C.D., Ju, Y.H., Allred, K.F., Chang, J., and Helferich, W.G. 2001b. Dietary genistein stimulates growth of oestrogen-dependent breast cancer tumors similar to that observed with genistein. *Carcinogenesis* **22**: 1667–1673.

Anderson, J.W., Johnstone, B.M., and Cook-Newell, M.E. 1995. Meta-analysis of the effects of soy protein intake on serum lipids. *N Engl J Med* **333**: 276–282.

Awad, A.B., Downie, A., Fink, C.S., and Kim, U. 2000. Dietary phytosterol inhibits the growth and metastasis of MDA-MB-231 human breast cancer cells grown in SCID mice. *Anticancer Res* **20**: 821–824.

Barnes, S., Grubbs, C., Setchell, K.D.R., and Carlson, J. 1990. Soybeans inhibit mammary tumors in models of breast cancer. *Prog Clin Biol Res* **347**: 239–253.

Barnes, S., Peterson, T.G., Grubbs, C., and Setchell K.D.R. 1994a. Potential role of dietary isoflavones in the prevention of cancer. *Adv Exp Med Biol* **354**: 135–147.

Barnes, S., Kirk, M., and Coward, L. 1994b. Isoflavones and their conjugates in soy foods: extraction conditions and analysis by HPLC-mass spectrometry. *J Agric Food Chem* **42**: 2466–2474.

Barnes, S., Xu, J., Smith. M., and Kirk, M. 2001. Lack of evidence for the intestinal absorption of isoflavone β-glucosides in the intact rat. Paper presented at the 221st National Meeting of the American Chemical Society, San Diego, CA.

Barnes, S., Wang, C-C., Kirk, M., Smith-Johnson, M., Coward, L., Barnes, N.C., Vance, G., and Boersma B. 2002. HPLC-mass spectrometry of isoflavonoids in soy and the American groundnut, *Apios americana*. *Adv Exp Med Biol* **505**: 77–88.

Barnes, S., Zhang, H.G., Liu, C.R., Liu, P., Yu, S.H., and Prasain, J.K. 2005. Polyphenols inhibit breast cancer cell exosome regulation of T cell and natural killer cell response. *FASEB J* **19**: A1461.

Barnes, S., and Prasain, J.K. 2005. Current progress in the use of traditional medicines and nutraceuticals. *Current Opin Plant Biol* **8**: 324–328.

Bayer, T., Colnot, T., and Dekant, W. 2001. Disposition and biotransformation of the estrogenic isoflavone daidzein in rats. *Toxicol Sci* **62**: 205–211.

Boersma, B.J., Patel, R.P., Kirk, M., Darley-Usmar, V.M., and Barnes, S. 1999. Chlorination and nitration of soy isoflavones. *Arch Biochem Biophys* **368**: 265–275.

Boersma, B.J., D'Alessandro, T., Benton, M.R., Kirk, M., Wilson, L.S., Prasain, J., Botting, N.P., Barnes, S., Darley-Usmar, V.M., and Patel, R.P. 2003. Neutrophil myeloperoxidase chlorinates soy isoflavones and enhances their antioxidant properties. *Free Radic Biol Med* **35**: 1417–1430.

Cheng, F., Gabrilovich, D., and Sotomayor, E.M. 2004. Immune tolerance in breast cancer. *Breast Dis* **20**: 93–103.

Coldham, N.G., Howells, L.C., Santi, A., Montesissa, C., Langlais, C., King, L.J., Macpherson, D.D., and Sauer, M.J. 1999. Biotransformation of genistein in the rat: elucidation of metabolite structure by product ion mass fragmentology. *J Steroid Biochem Mol Biol* **70**: 169–184.

Coward, L., Barnes, N.C., Setchell, K.D.R., and Barnes, S. 1993. The antitumor isoflavones, genistein and daidzein, in soybean foods of American and Asian diets. *J Agric Food Chem* **41**: 1961–1967.

D'Alessandro, T., Prasain, J., Botting, N.P, Moore, R., Darley-Usmar, V.M., Patel, R.P., and Barnes, S. 2003. Polyphenols, inflammatory response, and cancer prevention: chlorination of isoflavones by human neutrophils. *J Nutr* **133**: 3773S–3777S.

D'Alessandro, T.L., Moore, R., Botting, N., and Barnes, S. 2005. *In vivo* glucuronidation of daidzein and its chlorinated isomers. *FASEB J* **19**: A449.

Davis, J.N., Kucuk, O., and Sarkar, F.H. 1999. Genistein inhibits NF-kappa B activation in prostate cancer cells. *Nutr Cancer* **35**: 167–174.

Davis, J.N., Kucuk, O., Djuric, Z., and Sarkar, F.H. 2001. Soy isoflavone supplementation in healthy men prevents NF-kappa B activation by TNF-alpha in blood lymphocytes. *Free Radic Biol Med* **30**: 1293–1302.

Day, A.J., Canada, F.J., Diaz, J.C., Kroon, P.A., Mclauchlan, R., Faulds, C.B., Plumb, G.W., Morgan, M.R., and Williamson, G. 2000. Dietary flavonoid and isoflavone glycosides are hydrolyzed by the lactase site of lactase phlorizin hydrolase. *FEBS Lett* **468**: 166–170.

Dimitrakoudis, D., Vranic, M., and Klip, A. 1992. Effects of hyperglycemia on glucose transporters of the muscle: use of the renal glucose reabsorption inhibitor phlorizin to control glycemia. *J Am Soc Nephrol* **3**: 1078–1091.

Doll, R., and Peto, R. 1981. The causes of cancer: quantitative estimates of avoidable risks of cancer in the United States today. *J Natl Cancer Inst* **66**: 1291–1308.

Esaki, H., Kawakishi, S., Morimitsu, Y., and Osawa, T. 1999. New potent antioxidative o-dihydroxyisoflavones in fermented Japanese soybean products. *Biosci Biotechnol Biochem* **63**: 1637–1639.

Foster, S. 1994. Kudzu root monograph. *Q Rev Nat Med* **Winter**: 303–308.

Fritz, W.A., Coward, L., Wang, J., and Lamartiniere, C.A. 1998. Dietary genistein: perinatal mammary cancer prevention, bioavailability and toxicity testing in the rat. *Carcinogenesis* **19**: 2151–2158.

Galvez, A.F., Chen, N., Macasieb, J., and de Lumen, B.O. 2001. Chemopreventive property of a soybean peptide (lunasin) that binds to deacetylated histones and inhibits acetylation. *Cancer Res* **61**: 7473–7478.

Grubbs, C.J., Farnell, D.R., Hill, D.L., and McDonough, K.C. 1985. Chemoprevention of N-nitroso-N-methylurea-induced mammary cancers by pretreatment with 17β-estradiol and progesterone. *J Natl Cancer Inst* **74**: 927–931.

Hamilton, R.M., and Carroll, K.K. 1976. Plasma cholesterol levels in rabbits fed low fat, low cholesterol diets: effects of dietary proteins, carbohydrates and fibre from different sources. *Atherosclerosis* **24**: 47–62.

Hamilton, A.S., and Mack, T.M. 2003. Puberty and genetic susceptibility to breast cancer in a case–control study in twins. *N Engl J Med* **348**: 2313–2322.

Hawrylewicz, E.J., Zapata, J., and Blair, W.H. 1995. Soy and experimental cancer: animal studies. *J Nutr* **125**(3 Suppl): 698S–708S.

Hazen, S.L., and Heinecke, J.W. 1997. 3-Chlorotyrosine, a specific marker of myeloperoxidase-catalyzed oxidation, is markedly elevated in low-density lipoprotein isolated from human atherosclerotic intima. *J Clin Invest* **99**: 2075–2081.

Hedlund, T.E., Maroni, P.D., Ferucci, P.G., Dayton, R., Barnes, S., Jones, R., Moore, D.R., Ogden, L.G., Wähälä, K., Sackett, H.M., and Gray, K.J. 2005. Long-term dietary habits influence soy isoflavone metabolism in Caucasian men: selective accumulation of isoflavonoids within prostatic fluid. *J Nutr* **135**: 1400–1406.

Hilakivi-Clarke, L., Cho, E., Onojafe, I., Raygada, M., and Clarke, R. 1999. Maternal exposure to genistein during pregnancy increases carcinogen-induced mammary tumorigenesis in female rat offspring. *Oncol Rep* **6**: 1089–1095.

Hilakivi-Clarke, L., Cho, E., deAssis, S., Olivo, S., Ealley, E., Bouker, K.B., Welch, J.N., Khan, G., Clarke, R., and Cabanes, A. 2001. Maternal and prepubertal diet, mammary development and breast cancer risk. *J Nutr* **131**: 154S–157S.

Horn-Ross, P.L., Barnes, S., Kirk, M., Coward, L., Parsonnet, J., and Hiatt, R.A. 1997. Urinary phytoestrogen levels in young women from a multiethnic population. *Cancer Epidemiol Biomark Prev* **6**: 339–345.

Horn-Ross, P.L., Barnes, S., Lee, M., Coward, L., Mandel, E., Koo, J., John, E.M., and Smith, M. 2000. Assessing phytoestrogen exposure in epidemiologic studies: development of a database (United States). *Cancer Causes Control* **11**: 289–298.

Hsieh, C.Y., Santell, R.C., Haslam, S.Z., and Helferich, W.G. 1998. Oestrogenic effects of genistein on the growth of oestrogen receptor–positive human breast cancer (MCF-7) cells *in vitro* and *in vivo*. *Cancer Res* **58**: 3833–3838.

Hymowitz, T. 1990. Soybeans: The success story. *In* "Advances in New Crops" (J. Janick and J.E. Simon, eds.), pp. 159–163. Timber Press, Portland, OR.

Ischiropoulos, H., Zhu, L., Chen, J., Tsai, M., Martin, J.C., Smith, C.D., and Beckman, J.S. 1992. Peroxynitrite-mediated tyrosine nitration catalyzed by superoxide dismutase. *Arch Biochem Biophys* **298**: 431–437.

Ju, Y.H., Allred, C.D., Allred, K.F., Karko, K.L., Doerge, D.R., and Helferich, W.G. 2001. Physiological concentrations of dietary genistein dose-dependently stimulate growth of oestrogen-dependent human breast cancer (MCF-7) tumors implanted in athymic nude mice. *J Nutr* **131**: 2957–2962.

Ju, Y.H., Doerge, D.R., Allred, K.F., Allred, C.D., and Helferich, W.G. 2002. Dietary genistein negates the inhibitory effect of tamoxifen on the growth of estrogen-dependent human breast cancer (MCF-7) cells implanted in athymic mice. *Cancer Res* **62**: 2474–2477.

Ju, Y.H., Clausen, L.M., Allred, K.F., Almada, A.L., and Helferich, W.G. 2004. Beta-sitosterol, beta-sitosterol glucoside, and a mixture of beta-sitosterol and beta-sitosterol glucoside modulate the growth of estrogen-responsive breast cancer cells *in vitro* and in ovariectomized athymic mice. *J Nutr* **134**: 1145–1151.

Kelly, G.E., Joannou, G.E., Reeder, A.Y., Nelson, C., and Waring, M.A. 1995. The variable metabolic response to dietary isoflavones in humans. *Proc Soc Exp Biol Med* **208**: 40–43.

Kennedy, A.R. 1998. The Bowman-Birk inhibitor from soybeans as an anticarcinogenic agent. *Am J Clin Nutr* **68**(6 Suppl): 1406S–1412S.

Kim, H., Peterson, T.G., and Barnes, S. 1998. Mechanisms of action of the soy isoflavone genistein: emerging role of its effects through transforming growth factor beta signaling pathways. *Am J Clin Nutr* **68**: 1418S–1425S.

Kim, H., Hall, P., Smith, M., Kirk, M., Prasain, J.K., Barnes, S., and Grubbs, C. 2004. Chemoprevention by grape seed extract and genistein in carcinogen-induced mammary cancer in rats is diet-dependent. *J Nutr* **134**: 3445S–3552S.

Kirk, C.J., Harris, R.M., Wood, D.M., Waring, R.H., and Hughes, P.J. 2001. Do dietary phytoestrogens influence susceptibility to hormone-dependent cancer by disrupting the metabolism of endogenous oestrogens? *Biochem Soc Trans* **29**: 209–216.

Kudou, S., Fleury, Y., Welti, D., Magnolato, D., Uchida, T., Kitamura, K., and Okubo, K. 1991. Malonyl isoflavone glycosides in soybean seeds (Glycine max Merrill). *Agric Biol Chem* **55**: 2227–2233.

Kulling, S.E., Honig, D.M., Simat, T.J., and Metzler, M. 2000. Oxidative *in vitro* metabolism of the soy phytoestrogens daidzein and genistein. *J Agric Food Chem* **48**: 4963–4972.

Kulling, S.E., and Lehmann, L. 2002. Metzler M. Oxidative metabolism and genotoxic potential of major isoflavone phytoestrogens. *J Chromatogr B Anal Technol Biomed Life Sci* **777**: 211–218.

Lamartiniere, C.A., Moore, J., Holland, M., and Barnes, S. 1995a. Genistein and chemoprevention of breast cancer. *Proc Soc Exp Biol Med* **208**: 120–123.

Lamartiniere, C.A., Moore, J.B., Brown, N.A., Thompson, R., Hardin, M.J., and Barnes, S. 1995b. Genistein suppresses mammary cancer in rats. *Carcinogenesis* **16**: 2833–2840.

Lamartiniere, C.A., Cotroneo, M.S., Fritz, W.A., Wang, J., Mentor-Marcel, R., and Elgavish, A. 2002. Genistein chemoprevention: timing and mechanisms of action in murine mammary and prostate. *J Nutr* **132**: 552S–558S.

Liu, C.R., Yu, S.H., Grizzle, W.E., Kimberly, R.P., Wang, J.H., Liu, P., Zhang, L.M., Hsu, H.C., Barnes, S., Mountz, J.D., and Zhang, H.G. 2005. Breast tumor exosomes promote tumor growth by immune suppression of NK cells. *FASEB J* **19**: A39–A40.

Makela, S., Poutanen, M., Lehtimaki, J., Kostian, M.L., Santti, R., and Vihko, R. 1995. Estrogen-specific 17 beta-hydroxysteroid oxidoreductase type 1 (E.C. 1.1.1.62) as a possible target for the action of phytoestrogens. *Proc Soc Exp Biol Med* **208**: 51–59.

Markovits, J., Linassier, C., Fosse, P., Couprie, J., Pierre, J., Jacquemin-Sablon, A., Saucier, J.M., Le Pecq, J.B., and Larsen, A.K. 1989. Inhibitory effects of the tyrosine kinase inhibitor genistein on mammalian DNA topoisomerase II. *Cancer Res* **49**: 5111–5117.

Pagliacci, M.C., Smacchia, M., Migliorati, G., Grignani, F., Riccardi, C., and Nicoletti, I. 1994. Growth-inhibitory effects of the natural phyto-oestrogen genistein in MCF-7 human breast cancer cells. *Eur J Cancer* **30A**: 1675–1682.

Peterson, T.G., Coward, L., Kirk, M., Falany, C.N., and Barnes, S. 1996. Isoflavones and breast epithelial cell growth: the importance of genistein and biochanin A metabolism in the breast. *Carcinogenesis* **17**: 1861–1869.

Peterson, T.G., Ji, G-P., Kirk, M., Coward, L., Falany, C.N., and Barnes, S. 1998. Metabolism of the isoflavones genistein and biochanin A in human breast cancer cell lines. *Am J Clin Nutr* **68**: 1505–1511.

Prasain, J.K., Jones, K., Kirk, M., Wilson, L., Smith-Johnson, M., Weaver, C.M., and Barnes, S. 2003. Identification and quantitation of isoflavonoids in Kudzu dietary supplements by HPLC and electrospray ionization tandem mass spectrometry. *J Agric Food Chem* **51**: 4213–4218.

Prasain, J.K., Jones, K., Brissie, N., Moore, D.R. II, Wyss, J.M., and Barnes, S. 2004. Identification of puerarin and its metabolites in rats by liquid chromatography-tandem mass spectrometry. *J Agric Food Chem* **52**: 3708–3712.

Schultz, G. 1965. Isoflavone glucoside formononetin-7-glucoside and biochanin A-7-glucoside in *Trifolium pratense* L. *Naturwissenschaften* **52**: 517.

Schwartsburd, P.M. 2004. Age-promoted creation of a pro-cancer microenvironment by inflammation: pathogenesis of dyscoordinated feedback control. *Mech Age Develop* **125**: 581–590.

Sfakianos, J., Coward, L, Kirk, M., and Barnes, S. 1997. Intestinal uptake and biliary excretion of the isoflavone genistein in the rat. *J Nutr* **127**: 1260–1268.

Shamsuddin, A.M., Vucenik, I., and Cole, K.E. 1997. IP6: a novel anti-cancer agent. *Life Sci* **61**: 343–354.

Shao, Z.M., Wu, J., Shen, Z.Z., and Barsky, S.H. 1998. Genistein exerts multiple suppressive effects on human breast carcinoma cells. *Cancer Res* **58**: 4851–4857.

Shao, Z.M., Shen, Z.Z., Fontana, J.A., and Barsky, S.H. 2000. Genistein's "ER-dependent and independent" actions are mediated through ER pathways in ER-positive breast carcinoma cell lines. *Anticancer Res* **20**: 2409–2416.

Shelnutt, S.R., Cimino, C.O., Wiggins, P.A., Ronis, M.J., and Badger, T.M. 2002. Pharmacokinetics of the glucuronide and sulfate conjugates of genistein and daidzein in men and women after consumption of a soy beverage. *Am J Clin Nutr* **76**: 588–594.

Shu, X.O., Jin, F., Dai, Q., Wen, W., Potter, J.D., Kushi, L.H., Ruan, Z., Gao, Y.T., and Zheng, W. 2001. Soyfood intake during adolescence and subsequent risk of breast cancer among Chinese women. *Cancer Epidemiol Biomark Prev* **10**: 483–488.

Simoons, F.J. 1978. The geographic hypothesis and lactose malabsorption: a weighing of the evidence. *Am J Dig Dis* **23**: 963–980.

Sirtori, C.R., Agradi, E., Conti, F., Mantero, O., and Gatti E. 1977. Soybean-protein diet in the treatment of type-II hyperlipoproteinaemia. *Lancet* **1**(8006): 275–277.

Surh, Y.J. 2003. Cancer chemoprevention with dietary phytochemicals. *Nature Rev Cancer* **3**: 768–780.

Troll, W., Wiesner, R., Shellabarger, C.J., Holtzman, S., and Stone, J.P. 1980. Soybean diet lowers breast tumor incidence in irradiated rats. *Carcinogenesis* **1**: 469–472.

U.S. Department of Agriculture, Agricultural Research Service. 2002. USDA-Iowa State University Database on the Isoflavone Content of Foods, Release 1.3—2002. Available at the Nutrient Data Laboratory web site: http://www.nal.usda.gov/fnic/foodcomp/Data/isoflav/isoflav.html.

Urban, D., Irwin, W., Kirk, M., Markiewicz, M.A., Myers, R., Smith, M., Weiss, H., Grizzle, W.E., and Barnes, S. 2001. The effect of isolated soy protein on plasma biomarkers in elderly men with elevated serum prostate specific antigen. *J Urol* **165**: 294–300.

Wei, H., Wei, L., Frankel, K., Bowen, R., and Barnes, S. 1993. Inhibition of tumor promoter induced hydrogen peroxide formation *in vitro* and *in vivo* by genistein. *Nutr Cancer* **20**: 1–12.

Willett, W.C., Stampfer, M.J., Colditz, G.A., Rosner, B.A., Hennekens, C.H., and Speizer, F.E. 1987. Dietary fat and the risk of breast cancer. *N Engl J Med* **316**: 22–28.

Wu, A.H., Wan, P., Hankin, J., Tseng, C-C., Yu, M.C., and Pike, M.C. 2002. Adolescent and adult soy intake and risk of breast cancer in Asian-Americans. *Carcinogenesis* **23**: 1491–1496.

Xu, X., Wang, H.J., Murphy, P.A., Cook, L., and Hendrich, S. 1994. Daidzein is a more bioavailable soymilk isoflavone than is genistein in adult women. *J Nutr* **124**: 825–832.

Zava, D.T., and Duwe, G. 1997. Estrogenic and antiproliferative properties of genistein and other flavonoids in human breast cancer cells *in vitro*. *Nutr Cancer* **27**: 31–40.

CHAPTER

33

Selenium and Cancer Prevention

CLEMENT IP, JAMES MARSHALL, YOUNG-MEE PARK, HAITAO ZHANG, YAN DONG, YUE WU, AND ALLEN C. GAO

INTRODUCTION

Research over the past 35 years has demonstrated a role for selenium (Se) in cancer prevention. Low blood Se levels were found to be associated with an increased incidence and mortality from various types of cancers. The role of selenium in the prevention of a number of degenerative conditions including cancer, inflammatory diseases, cardiovascular disease, neurological diseases, aging, infertility, and infections has been established by laboratory experiments, clinical trials, and epidemiological data. Most of the effects in these conditions are related to the function of selenium in antioxidant enzyme systems. Replenishing selenium in deficiency conditions appears to have immune-stimulating effects, particularly in patients undergoing chemotherapy. However, increasing the levels of selenoprotein antioxidant enzymes (glutathione peroxidase, thioredoxin reductase, etc.) appears to be only one of many ways in which selenium-based metabolites contribute to normal cellular growth and function. Animal data, epidemiological data, and intervention trials have shown a clear role for selenium compounds in both prevention of specific cancers and antitumorigenic effects in post-initiation phases of cancer.

Redox regulation of protein thiols is a fundamental aspect of protein chemistry that is known to have a significant impact on cell biology. Because of its strong nucleophilic nature, methylselenol (an active selenium metabolite) can react avidly with protein thiols and result in either a gain or a loss of these thiol groups. Using a display thiol-proteomics approach, studies have demonstrated that methylselenol is able to cause global thiol modification of proteins. These changes are manifested in distinct quantifiable patterns as a function of time. There is increasing recognition that many cellular processes are sensitive to the integration of redox-sensitive signals. Each reactive thiol-containing protein may act as a unique cellular sensor to monitor the redox status of the microenvironment. Based on this paradigm, selenium may activate or inactivate a circuitry of switches in controlling the fate of cell proliferation, differentiation, or apoptosis. In summary, genomics and proteomics technologies have provided evidence that selenium affects not just a few key targets, but a multitude of targets. A challenge is to validate these discoveries in innovative human intervention trials. This chapter reviews the evidence supporting an association of selenium with common forms of cancer. In some detail, the evidence for the SELECT trial of selenium and vitamin E in prostate cancer is also considered as an illustration of the types of controlled trials necessary to establish the effectiveness of selenium in cancer prevention.

BREAST CANCER

Selenium is effective in the reduction of cancer incidence when provided to animals at nontoxic doses only 5- to 10-fold above the nutritional requirement (Ip, 1986; El-Bayoumy, 1991). Numerous studies have indicated the efficacy of selenium in the significant reduction of mammary tumor incidence after exposure to carcinogens, including 2-acetylaminofluorene, methylnitrosourea, and 7,12-dimethylbenz(*a*)anthracene, and selenium has also been shown to be effective against the development of spontaneous mammary tumors in the C3H mouse model (El-Bayoumy, 1991). The relationship between selenium status and the incidence of breast cancer remains somewhat controversial, with one

Copyright © 2006, Elsevier Inc.
All rights of reproduction in any form reserved.

study indicating a protective role (McConnell et al., 1980) and other studies not (Hunter et al., 1990; Garland et al., 1993, 1995; Ghadirian et al., 2000).

COLON CANCER

Progress in chemoprevention research has brought about innovative approaches to the prevention and control of colon cancer (Reddy, 1986; Wattenberg, 1992; Giovannucci and Willett, 1994; Kelloff, 2000). Epidemiological studies have pointed to an inverse association between dietary intake of selenium and colorectal cancer risk in humans (Clark, 1986; El-Bayoumy, 1991). A clinical trial by Clark et al. (1996) demonstrated that administration of selenium-enriched yeast significantly inhibited colon cancer incidence in humans. A series of experiments in laboratory animals also showed that supplementation of sodium selenite inhibits carcinogenesis in the colon (El Bayoumy, 1995). Generally, humans ingest organic forms of selenium, such as SM and SC; however, cancer prevention studies in preclinical models have not revealed any significant differences between the inorganic forms of selenium and those naturally occurring forms of selenium (Nayini et al., 1991; El Bayoumy et al., 1995). A preclinical study indicated that dietary SM, one of the major forms of selenium in the selenium-enriched yeast, lacked chemopreventive efficacy against AOM-induced colon carcinogenesis in F344 rats (Nayini et al., 1991). There are also studies to indicate that chronic feeding of inorganic and certain organic forms of selenium at >5 ppm induces toxic effects (Wilber, 1980; Fan and Kizer, 1990). Therefore, substantial efforts have been made to develop organoselenium compounds with maximal chemopreventive efficacy but low toxicity. Organoselenium compounds hold great promise as chemopreventive agents (Fan and Kizer, 1990; Nayini, 1991) against cancers of the colon, at least, in preclinical models (Reddy et al., 1992, 1997; Rao et al., 2000).

SELENIUM AND PROSTATE CANCER

Selenium supplementation showed great promise in lowering prostate cancer risk in a previous controlled intervention trial. The complete 13 years' worth of results of the Nutritional Prevention of Cancer Trial (Clark et al., 1996; Duffield-Lillico et al., 2003) have been analyzed, confirming that Se supplementation was associated with marked reductions in risks to total (all-site except skin) carcinomas and to cancers of the prostate and colon-rectum. Of the treatment effects, the most robust was for prostate cancer, which was more frequent and was confirmed by serum prostate-specific antigen (PSA) level. Therefore, the role of selenium supplementation is considered in some detail in the following with regard to prostate cancer.

Androgen signaling plays an important role in the development of prostate cancer. Laboratory findings indicate that exposure of androgen-responsive human prostate cancer cells to an active monomethylated selenium metabolite decreases the expression of androgen receptor (AR) and its trans-activating activity. PSA is a gene known to be positively regulated by AR and is a well-accepted biomarker for the diagnosis and prognosis of prostate cancer. As expected, selenium also depresses PSA transcript and protein in a dose response and time schedule similar to that for AR. In addition to PSA, microarray data mining analysis suggests that the expression of many androgen-responsive genes can also be reversed by selenium. This information supports a mechanism-driven role of selenium in prostate cancer chemoprevention.

The Nutritional Prevention of Cancer Trial Results

A number of case–control studies have demonstrated an inverse relationship between selenium status and prostate cancer risk (Yoshizawa et al., 1998; Helzlsouer et al., 2000; Nomura et al., 2000; Brooks et al., 2001; Li et al., 2004). The litmus test of the efficacy of a chemopreventive agent is a randomized intervention design involving an appropriate cohort of subjects. One of the more important studies of selenium as a chemopreventive agent is the Nutritional Prevention of Cancer (NPC) study initiated by Larry Clark. Clark et al. (1996) and Duffield-Lillico et al. (2003) reported that supplementation of people with selenized yeast is capable of reducing the overall cancer morbidity by nearly 50%. The study was a randomized, double-blind, placebo-controlled trial involving 1312 patients (mostly men) who were recruited initially because of a history of basal cell or squamous cell carcinoma of the skin. Individuals in the treatment arm were given Se at 200 μg/day (average daily intake in the United States is ~100 μg) for a mean of 4.5 years. After a total follow-up of 8271 person-years, selenium treatment did not decrease the incidence of these nonmelanoma skin cancers. However, patients receiving the supplement showed a much lower prevalence of developing lung (relative risk [RR] = 0.54), colon (RR = 0.42), or prostate cancer (RR = 0.37).

Larry Clark passed away in 2000; his colleague James Marshall (then at the Arizona Cancer Center but since relocated to Roswell Park) assumed responsibility for completing the trial. The original report by Clark et al. (1996) was based on an interim analysis of the data collected from 1983 to 1993, even though the follow-up of all participants actually continued until 1996. There were justifiable reasons behind this rather unusual decision. Although the trial was still blinded, a decrease in overall cancer morbidity and mortality in the selenium-supplemented cohort became apparent. In 1994, the Safety Monitoring and Advisory

Committee recommended that the trial be unblinded and the results published. After the completion of an audit of the study by the National Cancer Institute (NCI) in 1995, the blinded phase of the trial was terminated early the following year. At this time, all participants were informed of their treatment status, given the opportunity to take selenium supplement, and reconsented to enroll in the open-label phase of the trial. Extending the analysis for an additional 3 years to the end of the blinded phase in 1996, an update by Duffield-Lillico et al. (2002) reaffirmed the significant reduction in prostate cancer incidence by selenium (RR = 0.48, 95% confidence interval [CI] = 0.28–0.80).

Because of the randomized and double-blinded nature of the trial design, the NPC results command a high degree of credibility. The one caveat about the NPC trial is that the observed preventive effects of selenium are secondary endpoints that were not hypothesized at the start of the study. They were instead proposed after the investigators had noticed a trend for differential cancer incidence and mortality between the placebo and treatment groups.

The SELECT Trial

The fact that the hypothesis for selenium protection of prostate cancer in the NPC was not stated *a priori* raised suspicion that the findings might represent a statistical artifact. Nonetheless, the NPC prostate cancer data were instrumental in leading to the development of the current Selenium and Vitamin E Chemoprevention Trial (SELECT), which is aimed specifically to determine the efficacy of these two agents, either alone or in combination, in reducing prostate cancer incidence among average-risk men (Klein et al., 2001). In spite of the value of SELECT, it will not be possible to use this trial to gain insight into the mechanism of action of selenium in prostate cancer prevention. The selenium chemoprevention research team at Roswell Park is working on a translational model to address this gap of knowledge.

An intriguing piece of information from the NPC prostate cancer results is that baseline plasma selenium is highly correlated with the impact of selenium treatment (Duffield-Lillico et al., 2003). For those in the lowest and middle tertile of baseline selenium, treatment decreased the risk of prostate cancer by fivefold and threefold, respectively. However, for those in the highest tertile of baseline selenium, treatment failed to produce any significant protective effect. It is not yet understood whether this suggests that selenium is protective only within a narrow range, that differences in baseline selenium reflect variations in metabolic capacity, or that exposure to other environmental agents might modify the impact of selenium. This issue is revisited in the section "Future Directions."

An analysis of the blood PSA data also turned out to be quite illuminating. PSA is a well-accepted marker for the diagnosis and prognosis of prostate cancer. In brief, the PSA trajectory over time in placebo- and selenium-treated patients who did not develop prostate cancer is not statistically different from each other. However, among those who developed prostate cancer, the PSA trajectory of the selenium-treated patients is significantly less steep than that of the placebo-treated patients. This divergence suggests that PSA might be a reliable biomarker to monitor the responsiveness to selenium. Statistical analysis of this result is under way. Laboratory studies to elucidate the mechanism underlying the effect of selenium on PSA production are discussed in the section "MSA Interference of Androgen Receptor Signaling in Human Prostate Cancer Cells."

Methylseleninic Acid

In a previous review, Ip et al. (2002) pointed out the need to use a direct- and fast-acting selenium compound to investigate the mechanism of action of selenium. Selenomethionine, the supplement used in SELECT and presumably the major form of selenium in selenized yeast, was studied extensively in the early 1990s. It was originally proposed (Ip and Ganther, 1990; Ip et al., 1991; Ip, 1998) that the metabolism of selenomethionine to methylselenol (CH_3SeH) would be important for the expression of chemopreventive efficacy. In the whole animal, liver and kidney are the major organs for selenium metabolism; the conversion of selenomethionine to methylselenol requires five enzymatic steps (Ip, 1998) (Figure 1). Tissues such as breast and prostate have a low capacity to produce the monomethylated selenium metabolite from selenomethionine. For this reason, cultured breast or prostate cells generally are growth inhibited by selenomethionine only when it is present at levels of 100–400 μM in the medium. These concentrations of selenium are much higher than the plasma concentrations of 2–4 μM attainable by supplementation. The dose of 200 μg/day in the NPC study increased blood concentrations of selenium-treated subjects from a baseline of 1.4 μM to ~2.5 μM (Clark et al., 1996).

Methylselenol is highly reactive, difficult to prepare, and cannot be tested as is. To obviate this problem, Ip et al. (2000) developed a stable metabolite called methylseleninic acid (CH_3SeO_2H, abbreviated to *MSA*) for cell culture studies. Once taken up by cells, MSA is readily reduced to CH_3SeH through nonenzymatic reactions involving glutathione or NADPH. Therefore, biochemically, MSA serves as a ready-made reagent to generate CH_3SeH endogenously as soon as it enters into cells. We found that mouse and human cancer cells are sensitive to MSA at a concentration as low as 2.5 μM (Ip et al., 2000; Dong et al., 2002). Thus, both selenomethionine and MSA produce the same active metabolite. The notable difference is that whereas selenomethionine has to be added to the culture medium at exceedingly high levels, a physiological concentration of MSA is sufficient to elicit biological responses. As expected, MSA

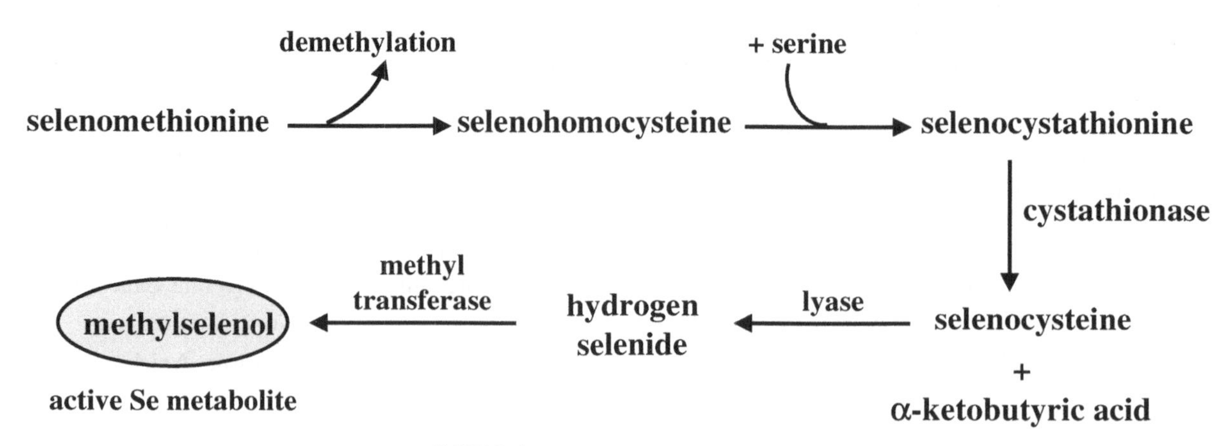

FIGURE 1 Selenium metabolic pathway.

has excellent anticancer activity *in vivo*; its efficacy is similar to that of selenoamino acids (Ip et al., 2000).

MSA Interference of Androgen Receptor Signaling in Human Prostate Cancer Cells

In vitro studies with human prostate cancer cells showed that exposure to MSA results in cell cycle arrest and induction of apoptosis (Jiang et al., 2001, 2002; Wang et al., 2002; Dong et al., 2003, 2004; Zu and Ip, 2003). These events are accompanied by changes in the expression of many key cell cycle– and apoptosis-regulatory molecules, as well as by changes in the activities of a number of survival and death signaling pathways. The clonal expansion of prostate cancer at the early stage is mostly dependent on androgen stimulation. Androgen response is mediated by binding to the AR, which subsequently translocates into the nucleus and interacts with specific androgen-responsive elements (AREs) in the promoters of target genes. The interaction leads to the activation or repression of genes involved in the proliferation and differentiation of the prostate cells (Jenster, 1999).

Almost all patients with advanced prostate cancer respond initially to treatments that interfere with the AR signaling process. However, these treatments fail after prolonged use and the growth of the cancer recurs (Koivisto et al., 1998). Recurrent prostate cancer is generally androgen independent, although the expression of AR is maintained regardless of the clinical stage of the disease (Sadi et al., 1991; Hobisch et al., 1996). The fact that PSA continues to be produced by the pathologically advanced cancer suggests that the AR signal transduction pathway is still intact. Several hypotheses have been proposed to explain this phenomenon. Mutations of the AR may enable the cells to be sensitized by very low levels of androgens, perhaps even by non-androgen steroids (Zhao et al., 2000). Alternatively, the receptor may become promiscuous and can be activated by nonsteroidal growth factors and cytokines (Culig et al., 1998). Prostate cancer may also adapt to androgen deprivation by increasing the expression of AR through gene amplification (Visakorpi et al., 1995; Koivisto et al., 1997; Ford et al., 2003). Therefore, an intervention strategy aimed at dampening the intensity of AR signaling would be helpful not only for controlling prostate cancer in high-risk men but also for preventing relapses after endocrine therapy.

We reported that MSA is able to markedly depress AR transcript and protein levels in a dose-dependent manner within hours in the androgen-responsive human LNCaP prostate cancer cells (Dong et al., 2004). PSA is a gene known to be positively regulated by AR. As expected, decreases in PSA transcript and protein follow a dose response and time schedule similar to that for AR upon exposure to MSA. The reduction of AR and PSA expression by MSA occurs well before any detectable change in cell number. With the use of a luciferase reporter construct linked to either the PSA promoter or the ARE, we found that MSA inhibits the transactivating activity of AR in cells transfected with the wild-type AR expression vector. MSA also suppresses the binding of AR to the ARE site, as evidenced by electrophoretic mobility shift assay of the AR–ARE complex. However, we cannot distinguish whether this is due to a block in nuclear translocation of the activated AR or to physical interference of AR association with the ARE through modulation of other co-regulators. These various possibilities will be investigated systematically.

Incidentally, cellular PSA is inhibited to a greater magnitude by MSA compared with secretory PSA (Cho et al., 2004), suggesting that the turnover of PSA might also be affected by MSA. The half-life of PSA is about 3.6 hours in control untreated cells but is reduced to 1.5 hr in MSA-treated cells, thus confirming that PSA degradation is indeed enhanced by MSA. The decrease in the half-life of PSA is reversed by lysosomal inhibitor, but not by proteasomal inhibitor. This finding is consistent with our preliminary data that MSA greatly enhances the transcript level of lysosomal cathepsin B and cathepsin L. There could be two mechanisms by which MSA decreases cellular PSA expression. The first is at the gene transcription level and the second at the level of protein degradation. For this reason, cellular, rather than secretory, PSA may provide a better handle to study mechanisms of selenium intervention. The NPC finding of a decreased PSA trajectory by selenium in prostate cancer patients might reflect an important biological response that is happening in the prostate tissue.

MICROARRAY METHODS SEARCHING FOR POTENTIAL Se TARGETS

It has been widely recognized that microarray gene expression analysis offers great promise in unraveling the mechanisms of anticancer agents. Bioinformatics holds the key to unlocking the treasure of data from these array studies. We described a data mining approach to gain further insight into selenium biology utilizing published microarray datasets (Zhang et al., 2004). The paradigm combines laboratory- and bioinformatics-based research to identify molecular targets of prostate cancer intervention by selenium. Previously we had profiled gene expression changes in PC-3 and LNCaP prostate cancer cells treated with MSA, using either the Affymetrix oligonucleotide U95A chip or a custom cDNA array. Zhao et al. (2004) had also performed microarray analysis in MSA-treated LNCaP cells using a high-density cDNA array. Our goal was to use these three selenium datasets and develop a systematic data mining strategy to earmark putative prostate cancer genes that are sensitive to selenium intervention; these genes are derived from three newly published microarray datasets generated by using human surgical prostate tumor specimen. The first is an Affymetrix oligonucleotide array study in 50 normal and 52 prostate cancers reported by Singh et al. (2002). The second, described by Welsh et al. (2001), is similar to the first with the exception that a fewer number of samples were examined (9 normal and 25 prostate cancers). The third is an analysis of 41 normal and 62 prostate cancers by Lapointe et al. (2004), using a 26K-gene cDNA microarray. These three prostate cancer datasets proffer a fountain of information of dysregulated genes implicated in prostate carcinogenesis.

First, we devised a method to merge and methodically analyze the three selenium microarray datasets according to standardized criteria. Second, we subjected the prostate cancer datasets to permutation *t*-test analysis to identify a list of genes consistently dysregulated in prostate carcinogenesis. Then we matched the first analysis with the second analysis to cull a subset of dysregulated prostate cancer genes of which expression could be reversed or restored to normal by selenium intervention. With the above procedure, we pared down to 42 genes, which are reciprocally regulated; many of them are involved in controlling cell cycle progression and/or cell death. Selenium modulates their expression in a way that is consistent with cell growth inhibition, cell cycle block, and apoptosis induction. Our bioinformatics exercise also revealed four genes with tumor-suppressing activities (SERPINA5, gelsolin, CYLD, and SSBP2), which can be upregulated by selenium.

The finding that selenium decreases the expression and transactivation of AR fueled our interest in applying a similar microarray analysis approach to investigate whether the transcription of AR-regulated genes, in addition to PSA, might be counteracted by selenium. Recent events have made this query possible. In separate studies by DePrimo et al. (2002) and Nelson et al. (2002), LNCaP cells were treated with synthetic androgen and microarray analyses were then performed to identify genes responsive to androgen stimulation. These two androgen datasets are well suited to serve as a tool to mine the selenium datasets for fresh clues. Altogether, 92 genes are commonly modulated by both selenium and androgen, and slightly less than half of them (38 out of 92) are altered in opposite directions. A plausible explanation for this is that genes have multiple regulatory elements, both positive and negative, in their promoter regions. Selenium is known to alter the expression of many transcription factors, co-activators, and co-repressors (Dong et al., 2003). The ARE is but one of many regulatory elements controlling the transcription of androgen-responsive genes. Thus, it is not surprising that selenium could counteract the expression of some, but not all, androgen-regulated genes. Collectively, the above information has provided us with a trove of exciting clues to investigate the mechanism of selenium chemoprevention of prostate cancer. Moreover, these selenium target genes could also serve as biomarkers in clinical trials to gauge the efficacy of selenium intervention.

REDOX MODIFICATION OF PROTEINS BY MSA

Redox regulation of protein cysteines is a fundamental aspect of protein chemistry that is known to have a significant impact on cell biology. As discussed earlier, the generation of a monomethylated selenium metabolite is critical for the anticancer activity of selenium. At physiological pH, methylselenol is present in an ionic form (i.e., CH_3Se^-). Because of its strong nucleophilic nature, methylselenol is expected to react avidly with protein thiols. However, because most protein thiols exhibit a pK_a value of 8.0–8.5, few cellular protein thiols would react with micromolar concentrations of methylselenol at physiological pH, even under conditions of oxidative stress. But some protein cysteine residues exist as thiolate anion at neutral pH, because their pK_a values are lowered as a result of the influence of neighboring nucleophilic groups. More often than not, the thiolate is stabilized by salt bridges to positively charged residues (Polgar and Halasz, 1978; Page and West, 1986). Those thiols with lower pKa values may thus exhibit enhanced reactivity because of the nature of the thiolate, and they are called "reactive thiols." The interaction of proteins with a methyl selenium metabolite could potentially result in a gain or loss of reactive thiols, depending on the reduction potential. These modifications have never been examined systematically before because of the lack of a reliable methodology to quantify reactive protein thiols globally in cells.

We completed a study to investigate the extent of protein thiol modification by MSA in human prostate cancer cells using a biotinylated iodoacetamide (BIAM)–based display proteomics approach (Park et al., 2004). The labeling of reactive thiols with BIAM was adapted from a previously published method (Kim et al., 2000) with minor modifications. PC-3 cells were treated with MSA for different times ranging from 0.5 to 24 hours (no cell growth inhibition was evident during this period), and the protein extract was labeled with BIAM. After two-dimensional (2D) gel electrophoresis, the samples were processed for the detection of reactive thiol-containing proteins by reaction with HRP-conjugated streptavidin. The image data were analyzed by the Self Organizing Maps (SOMs) clustering algorithm. Out of 194 reactive thiol-containing protein spots on the 2D gel display, 100 of them (cluster 1) were not sensitive to MSA modulation. The remaining 94 were categorized into three distinct patterns of change. Cluster 2 showed an immediate but sustained loss of reactive thiols for at least 24 hours; cluster 3 showed a transient loss of reactive thiols followed by rapid rebound; and cluster 4 showed a transient gain followed by a rapid return to normal. Because of limitations in the methodology, the present approach is likely to underestimate the number of redox-sensitive proteins amenable to modification by selenium.

Our attention is focused on the idea that global protein redox changes induced by selenium represent a form of cellular stress because these changes are likely to lead to protein misfolding, unfolding, or aggregation. The concept of quality control monitoring of newly synthesized proteins in the endoplasmic reticulum (ER) is well described (Kaufman, 2002; Rao et al., 2004). An accumulation of misfolded or unfolded proteins in the ER triggers a defined set of sensor and modulator signals to stop protein synthesis and to refold or degrade the aberrant proteins so that the cells may continue to survive. Our preliminary data showed that exposure of PC-3 cells to MSA induces a number of signature ER stress molecular markers, including phospho-PERK, phospho-eIF2α, and GRP-78, within a few hours. GRP-78 belongs to the family of chaperones; it is a key protein charged with promoting folding and preventing aggregation of proteins in the ER (Kaufman, 2002). MSA also greatly increases GADD153 and caspase 12 activation. The latter two markers are usually associated with cell cycle exit and/or apoptosis when ER stress due to protein unfolding is too severe and beyond repair. These same cellular changes have been demonstrated by numerous studies to occur in cancer cells (but not necessarily normal untransformed cells) treated with selenium. Based on this information, we are proposing a novel hypothesis that typical ER stress signaling responses governing the balance between survival and death may also be initiated by selenium as a result of damage to mature and newly synthesized proteins. Because metabolic oxidative stress is greater in cancer cells than in normal cells, cancer cells may be more susceptible to redox stress than normal cells (Spitz et al., 2000). This might be one reason that normal untransformed cells are not nearly as sensitive as cancer cells to selenium inhibition of growth (Ip and Medina, 1987; Menter et al., 2000).

It has been well documented that the redox status of proteins has a profound effect on their functions/activities. Two examples are cited to illustrate how selenium causes defined redox changes, which are accompanied by either a gain or a loss of function/activity of the protein. First, using a 20-kDa carboxyl-terminal fragment of p53 with two cysteines at codons 275 and 277, Seo et al. (2002) reported that a reduction of these two thiols by selenium significantly increases sequence specific DNA binding and transactivation of p53. MSA and selenite are more potent than selenomethionine in inducing p53 redox changes (Smith et al., 2004). The finding is congruent with the interpretation that MSA and selenite are converted to the reactive monomethylated metabolite much more efficiently than selenomethionine. A second example is provided by the work of Gopalakrishna et al. (1997) regarding the redox modification of protein kinase C by selenite. There are two cysteine-rich regions in protein kinase C: The regulatory domain contains 12 cysteine residues, and the catalytic domain contains 6 or 7 cysteine residues. At low concentrations, selenite converts four cysteine residues to two disulfides; and at high concentrations, it converts eight cysteine residues to four disulfides. The former modification is associated with a loss of affinity to ATP, whereas the latter with a lower V_{max} of the enzyme. Thus, in addition to causing ER stress, these studies raise the provocative suggestion that selenium might act as a chemical switch to turn a protein on or off without affecting the expression level of the protein.

FUTURE DIRECTIONS

Thiol methyltransferase (TMT) is a key enzyme involved in generating the active metabolite, methylselenol, from selenomethionine. TMT is a membrane-bound enzyme and is extremely labile once separated from the membrane. Therefore, this enzyme is very difficult to purify, and efforts to clone and sequence the TMT gene have failed mainly for this reason. As a result, molecular pharmacogenetic studies on the polymorphism of this gene could not be conducted. However, TMT is expressed on the membrane of human red blood cells, which are easily accessible, and a radiochemical assay has been developed to study its enzymatic activity (Weinshilboum et al., 1979). Using this assay, Price et al. (1989) observed a fivefold variation in TMT activity in a large random sample. Ninety-eight percent of this variation was attributed to heredity. This study suggests the presence of polymorphisms in this genetic locus; at least one allele encoding high TMT activity may be responsible.

TMT plays a critical role in selenium metabolism by catalyzing the reaction from hydrogen selenide to methylselenol, the active selenium metabolite (Figure 1). Variations in the enzymatic activity of TMT could conceivably affect an individual's ability to metabolize selenium and lead to differences in responsiveness to selenium supplementation. As described earlier, the NPC trial showed that among individuals with low and medium levels of baseline plasma selenium, selenium treatment decreased prostate cancer incidence by threefold or more, whereas no protective effect by selenium was observed among those with high levels of baseline selenium. The differences in baseline selenium could be explained by the differences in the enzymatic activity of TMT. In individuals with high TMT activity, selenium can be efficiently metabolized and excreted, resulting in low baseline selenium levels. Therefore, we hypothesize that individuals with higher TMT activity are likely to benefit more from selenium supplementation.

The level of methylselenol would be a direct measurement of the ability to generate the active selenium metabolite. However, methylselenol is very difficult to speciate. To the best of our knowledge, no methodology has been developed for quantifying the level of methylselenol in biological fluids. On the other hand, a simple assay for determining TMT activity in red blood cells is available. We plan to examine the activity of TMT in the cohort of pre-brachytherapy patients and assess the value of using TMT activity to predict the responsiveness to selenium supplementation. The outcome could have significant clinical implications, as it could provide important information in designing custom-tailored intervention strategy for prostate cancer.

CONCLUSION

There is a great deal of evidence from epidemiological studies and basic science that has informed our understanding of the anticancer effects of selenium. The application of genomics and proteomics technologies will open new avenues of research into uncharted frontiers of selenium action. Based on the microarray data, we have shown that selenium affects not just a few key targets, but a multitude of targets. In doing so, the impact of selenium is amplified. The diversity of the molecular targets also makes it difficult for cancer cells to escape the inhibitory effects of selenium. Through the methodology of display thiol-proteomics, we have, for the first time, provided convincing evidence that selenium is capable of inducing global redox modification of proteins. This finding has significant implications in terms of cellular stress response and activation/inactivation of protein function. A challenge is to design innovative intervention trials that will allow us to validate these discoveries from the laboratory.

References

American Cancer Society. 2004. Cancer Facts and Figures Pamphlet. American Cancer Society.

Brooks, J.D., Jeffrey, M.E., Chan, D.W., Sokoll, L.J., Landis, P., Nelson, W.G., Muller, D., Andres, R., and Carter, H.B. 2001. Plasma selenium level before diagnosis and the risk of prostate cancer development. *J Urol* **166**: 2034–2038.

Cho, S.D., Jiang, C., Malewicz, B., Dong, Y., Young, C.Y.F., Kang, K.-S., Lee, Y.-S., Ip, C., and Lu, J. 2004. Methyl selenium metabolites decrease prostate-specific antigen expression by inducing protein degradation and suppressing androgen-stimulated transcription. *Mol Cancer Ther* **3**: 605–611.

Clark, L.C. 1986. The epidemiology of selenium and cancer. *Fed Proc* **44**: 2584–2589.

Clark, L.C., Combs, G.F., Turnbull, B.W., Slate, E.H., Chalker, D.K., Chow, J., Davis, L.S., Glover, R.A., Graham, G.F., Gross, E.G., Krongrad, A., Lesher, J.L., Park, K., Sanders, B.B., Smith, C.L., and Taylor, R. 1996. Effects of selenium supplementation for cancer prevention in patients with carcinoma of the skin: A randomized controlled trial. *JAMA* **276**: 1957–1985.

Culig, Z., Hobisch, A., Hittmair, A., Peterziel, H., Cato, A.C.B., Bartsch, G., and Klocker, H. 1998. Expression, structure, and function of androgen receptor in advanced prostatic carcinoma. *Prostate* **35**: 63–70.

DePrimo, S.E., Diehn, M., Nelson, J.B., Reiter, R.E., Matese, J., Fero, M., Tibshirani, R., Brown, P.O., and Brooks, J.D. 2002. Transcriptional programs activated by exposure of human prostate cancer cells to androgen. *Genome Biol* **3**: research0032.

Dong, Y., Ganther, H.E., Stewart, C., and Ip, C. 2002. Identification of molecular targets associated with selenium-induced growth inhibition in human breast cells using cDNA microarrays. *Cancer Res* **62**: 708–714.

Dong, Y., Zhang, H., Hawthorn, L., Ganther, H.E., and Ip, C. 2003. Delineation of the molecular basis for selenium-induced growth arrest in human prostate cancer cells by oligonucleotide array. *Cancer Res* **63**: 52–59.

Dong, Y., Lee, S.O., Zhang, H., Marshall, J., Gao, A.C., and Ip, C. 2004. Prostate specific antigen (PSA) expression is down-regulated by selenium through disruption of androgen receptor signaling. *Cancer Res* **64**: 19–22.

Duffield-Lillico, A.J., Reid, M.E., Turnbull, B.W., Combs, G.F. Jr., Slate, E.H., Fischbach, L.A., Marshall, J.R., and Clark, L.C. 2002. Baseline characteristics and the effect of selenium supplementation on cancer incidence in a randomized clinical trial: a summary report of the nutritional prevention of cancer trial. *Cancer Epidemiol Biomarkers Prev* **11**: 630–639.

Duffield-Lillico, A.J., Dalkin, B.L., Reid, M.E., Turnbull, B.W., Slate, E.H., Jacobs, E.T., Marshall, J.R., and Clark, L.C. 2003. Selenium supplementation, baseline plasma selenium and incidence of prostate cancer: an analysis of the complete treatment period of the Nutritional Prevention of Cancer Trial. *Br J Urol Int* **91**: 608–612.

El-Bayoumy, K. 1991. The role of selenium in cancer prevention. *In* "Cancer Prevention" (V.T. DeVita, Jr., S. Hellman, and S.A. Rosenberg, eds.), pp. 1–15. J.B. Lippincott Co., Philadelphia.

El-Bayoumy, K., Upadhyaya, P., Chae, Y-H., Sohn, O.S., Rao, C.V., Fiala, E.S., and Reddy, B.S. 1995. Chemoprevention of cancer by organoselenium compounds. *J Cell Biochem* **22S**: 92–100.

Fan, A.M., and Kizer, K.W. 1990. Selenium: nutritional toxicological, and clinical aspects. *West J Med* **153**: 160–167.

Ford, O.H., III, Gregory, C.W., Kim, D., Smitherman, A.B., and Mohler, J.L. 2003. Androgen receptor gene amplification and protein expression in recurrent prostate cancer. *J Urol* **170**: 1817–1821.

Garland, M., Morris, J.S., Stampfer, M.J., Colditz, G.A., Spate, V.L., Baskett, C.K., Rosner, B., Speizer, F.E., Willett, W.C., and Hunter, D.J. 1995. Prospective study of toenail selenium levels and cancer among women. *J Natl Cancer Inst Bethesda* **87**: 497–505.

Garland, M., Willett, W.C., Manson, J.E., and Hunter, D.J. 1993. Antioxidant micronutrients and breast cancer. *J Am Coll Nutr* **12**: 400–411.

Ghadirian, P., Maisonneuve, P., Perret, C., Kennedy, G., Boyle, P., Krewski, D., and Lacroix, A. 2000. A case–control study of toenail selenium and cancer of the breast, colon, and prostate. *Cancer Detect Prev* **24**: 305–313.

Giovannucci, E., and Willett, W.C. 1994. Dietary factors and risk of colon cancer. *Ann Med* **26**: 443–452.

Gopalakrishna, R., Gunimeda, U., and Chen, Z.-H. 1997. Cancer-preventive selenocompounds induce a specific redox modification of cysteine-rich regions in Ca^{2+}-dependent isoenzymes of protein kinase C. *Arch Biochem Biophys* **348**: 25–36.

Helzlsouer, K.J., Huang, H.Y., Alberg, A.J., Hoffman, S., Burke, A., Norkus, E.P., Morris, J.S., and Comstock, G.W. 2000. Association between α-tocopherol, γ-tocopherol, selenium, and subsequent prostate cancer. *J Natl Cancer Inst* **92**: 2018–2023.

Hobisch, A., Culig, Z., Radmayr, C., Bartsch, G., Klocker, H., and Hittmair, A. 1996. Androgen receptor status of lymph node metastases from prostate cancer. *Prostate* **28**: 129–135.

Hunter, D.J., Morris, J.S., Stampfer, M.J., Colditz, G.A., Speizer, F.E., and Willett, W.C. 1990. A prospective study of selenium status and breast cancer risk. *JAMA* **264**: 1128–1131.

Ip, C. 1986. Selenium and experimental cancer. *Ann Clin Res* **18**: 22–22.

Ip, C. 1998. Lessons from basic research in selenium and cancer prevention. *J Nutr* **128**: 1845–1854.

Ip, C., Dong, Y., and Ganther, H.E. 2002. New concepts in selenium chemoprevention. *Cancer Metastasis Rev* **21**: 281–289.

Ip, C., and Ganther, H.E. 1990. Activity of methylated forms of selenium in cancer prevention. *Cancer Res* **50**: 1206–1211.

Ip, C., Hayes, C., Budnick, R.M., and Ganther, H.E. 1991. Chemical form of selenium, critical metabolites, and cancer prevention. *Cancer Res* **51**: 595–600.

Ip, C., and Medina, D. 1987. Current concepts of selenium and mammary tumorigenesis. *In* "Cellular and Molecular Biology of Breast Cancer" (D. Medina, W. Kidwell, G. Heppner, and E.P. Anderson, eds), pp. 479–494. Plenum Press, New York.

Ip, C., Thompson, H.J., Zhu, Z., and Ganther, H.E. 2000. *In vitro* and *in vivo* studies of methylseleninic acid: evidence that a monomethylated selenium metabolite is critical for cancer chemoprevention. *Cancer Res* **60**: 2882–2886.

Jenster, G. 1999. The role of androgen receptor in the development and progression of prostate cancer. *Semin Oncol* **26**: 407–421.

Jiang, C., Wang, Z., Ganther, H., and Lu, J. 2001. Caspases as key executors of methyl selenium-induced apoptosis (anoikis) of DU-145 prostate cancer cells. *Cancer Res* **61**: 3062–3070.

Jiang, C., Wang, Z., Ganther, H., and Lu, J. 2002. Distinct effects of methylseleninic acid versus selenite on apoptosis, cell cycle, and protein kinase pathways in DU145 human prostate cancer cells. *Mol Cancer Ther* **1**: 1059–1066.

Kaufman, R.J. 2002. Orchestrating the unfolded protein response in health and disease. *J Clin Invest* **110**: 1389–1398.

Kelloff, G.J., Sigman, C.C., Johnson, K.M., Boone, C.W., Greenwald, P., Crowell, J.A., Hawk, E.T., and Doody, L.A. 2000. Perspectives on surrogate end points in the development of drugs that reduce the risk of cancer. *Cancer Epidemiol Biomarkers Prev* **9**: 127–137.

Kelloff, G.J. Perspectives on cancer chemoprevention research and drug development. *Adv Cancer Res* **78**: 199–334.

Kim, J.R., Yoon, H.W., Kwon, K.S., Lee, S.R., and Rhee, S.G. 2000. Identification of proteins containing cysteine residues that are sensitive to oxidation by hydrogen peroxide at neutral pH. *Anal Biochem* **283**: 214–221.

Klein, E.A., Thompson, I.M., Lippman, S.M., Goodman, P.J., Albanes, D., Taylor, P.R., and Coltman, C. 2001. SELECT: the next prostate cancer prevention trial. *J Urol* **166**: 1311–1315.

Koivisto, P., Kononen, J., Palmberg, C., Tammela, T., Hyytinen, E., Isola, J., Trapman, J., Cleutjens, K., Noordzij, A., Visakorpi, T., and Kallioniemi, O.P. 1997. Androgen receptor gene amplification: a possible molecular mechanism for androgen deprivation therapy failure in prostate cancer. *Cancer Res* **57**: 314–319.

Koivisto, P., Kolmer, M., Visakorpi, T., and Kallioniemi, O.P. 1998. Androgen receptor gene and hormonal therapy failure of prostate cancer. *Am J Pathol* **152**: 1–9.

Kristal, A.R., and Lampe, J.W. 2002. Brassica vegetables and prostate cancer risk: A review of the epidemiological evidence. *Nutr Cancer* **42**: 1–9.

Lapointe, J., Li, C., Higgins, J.P., van de, R.M., Bair, E., Montgomery, K., Ferrari, M., Egevad, L., Rayford, W., Bergerheim, U., Ekman, P., DeMarzo, A.M., Tibshirani, R., Botstein, D., Brown, P.O., Brooks, J.D., and Pollack, J.R. 2004. Gene expression profiling identifies clinically relevant subtypes of prostate cancer. *Proc Natl Acad Sci USA* **101**: 811–816.

Li, H., Stampfer, M.J., Giovannucci, E.L., Morris, J.S., Willett, W.C., Gaziano, J.M., and Ma, J. 2004. A prospective study of plasma selenium levels and prostate cancer risk. *J Natl Cancer Inst* **96**: 696–703.

McConnell, K.P., Jager, R.M., Bland, K.I., and Blotcky, A.J. 1980. The relationship of dietary selenium and breast cancer. *J Surg Oncol* **15**: 67–70.

Menter, D.G., Sabichi, A.L., and Lippman, S.M. 2000. Selenium effects on prostate cell growth. *Cancer Epidemiol Biomarkers Prev* **9**: 1171–1182.

Nayini, J.R., Sugie, S., El-Bayoumy, K., Rao, C.V., Rigotty, J., Sohn, O.-S., Fiala, E., and Reddy, B.S. 1991. Effect of dietary benzylselenocyanate on azoxymethane-induced colon carcinogenesis in male F344 rats. *Nutr Cancer* **15**: 129–139.

Nelson, P.S., Clegg, N., Arnold, H., Ferguson, C., Bonham, M., White, J., Hood, L., and Lin, B. 2002. The program of androgen-responsive genes in neoplastic prostate epithelium. *Proc Natl Acad Sci USA* **99**: 11890–11895.

Nomura, A.M.Y., Lee, J., Stemmermann, G.N., and Combs, G.F. 2000. Serum selenium and subsequent risk of prostate cancer. *Cancer Epidemiol Biomarkers Prev* **9**: 883–887.

Page, M.G., and West, I.C. 1986. Characterization *in vivo* of the reactive thiol groups of the lactose permease from *Escherichia coli* and a mutant; exposure, reactivity and the effects of substrate binding. *Biochim Biophys Acta* **858**: 67–82.

Park, E.-M., Ip, C., Choi, K.-S., Park, S.-Y., Kong, E.-S., Zhang, H., and Park, Y.-M. 2004. A display thiol-proteomics approach to identify molecular targets sensitive to redox regulation by selenium. Frontiers in Cancer Prevention Research, Third Annual AACR International Conference, Seattle, WA.

Polgar, L., and Halasz, P. 1978. Evidence for multiple reactive forms of papain. *Eur J Biochem* **88**: 513–521.

Price, R.A., Keith, R.A., Spielman, R.S., and Weinshilboum, R.M. 1989. Major gene polymorphism for human erythrocyte (RBC) thiol methyltransferase (TMT). *Genet Epidemiol* **6**: 651–662.

Reddy, B.S. 1986. Diet and colon cancer: evidence from human and animal model studies. *In* "Diet, Nutrition and Cancer: A Critical Evaluation" (B.S. Reddy and L.A. Cohen, eds), pp. 47–65. CRC Press, Inc., Boca Raton, FL.

Reddy, B.S., Rivenson, A., Kulkarni, N., Upadhyaya, P., and El-Bayoumy, K. 1992. Chemoprevention of colon carcinogenesis by the synthetic organoselenium compound 1,4-phenylenebis(methylene) selenocyanate. *Cancer Res* **52**: 5635–5640.

Reddy, B.S., Upadhyaya, P., Simi, B., and Rao, C.V. 1994. Evaluation of organoselenium compounds for potential chemopreventive properties in colon carcinogenesis. *Anticancer Res* **14**: 2509–2514.

Reddy, B.S., Rivenson, A., El-Bayoumy, K., Upadhyaya, P., Pittman, B., and Rao, C.V. 1997. Chemoprevention of colon cancer by organoselenium compounds and impact of high- or low-fat diets. *J Natl Cancer Inst* **89**: 506–512.

Reddy, B.S., Hirose, Y., Lubet, R.A., Steele, V.E., Kelloff, G.J., and Rao, C.V. 2000. Lack of chemopreventive efficacy of DL-selenomethionine in colon carcinogenesis. *Int J Mol Med* **5**: 327–330.

Rao, R.V., Ellerby, H.M., and Bredesen, D.E. 2004. Coupling endoplasmic reticulum stress to the cell death program. *Cell Death Differ* **11**: 372–380.

Rao, C.V., Cooma, I., Rosa, J.G., Simi, B., El-Bayoumy, K., and Reddy, B.S. 2000. Chemoprevention of familial adenomatous polyposis development in the APC^{min} mouse model by 1,4-phenylene*bis*(methylene) selenocyanate. *Carcinogenesis London* **21**: 617–621.

Sadi, M.V., Walsh, P.C., and Barrack, E.R. 1991. Immunohistochemical study of androgen receptors in metastatic prostate cancer—comparison of receptor content and response to hormonal therapy. *Cancer* **67**: 3057–3064.

Seo, Y.R., Kelley, M.R., and Smith, M.L. 2002. Selenomethionine regulation of p53 by a Ref1-dependent redox mechanism. *Proc Natl Acad Sci USA* **99**: 14548–14553.

Singh, D., Febbo, P.G., Ross, K., Jackson, D.G., Manola, J., Ladd, C., Tamayo, P., Renshaw, A.A., D'Amico, A.V., Richie, J.P., Lander, E.S., Loda, M., Kantoff, P.W., Golub, T.R., and Sellers, W.R. 2002. Gene expression correlates of clinical prostate cancer behavior. *Cancer Cell* **1**: 203–209.

Smith, M.L., Lancia, J.K., Mercer, T.I., Kelley, M.R., and Ip, C. 2004. Selenium compounds regulate p53 by common and distinctive mechanisms. *Anticancer Res* **24**: 1401–1408.

Spitz, D.R., Sim, J.E., Ridnour, L.A., Galoforo, S.S., and Lee, Y.J. 2000. Glucose deprivation-induced oxidative stress in human tumor cells. A fundamental defect in metabolism? *Ann NY Acad Sci* **899**: 349–362.

Visakorpi, T., Hyytinen, E., Koivisto, P., Tanner, M., Keinanen, R., Palmberg, C., Palotie, A., Tammela, T., Isola, J., and Kallioniemi, O.P. 1995. *In vivo* amplification of the androgen receptor gene and progression of human prostate cancer. *Nature Genet* **9**: 401–406.

Wang, Z., Jiang, C., and Lu, J. 2002. Induction of caspase-mediated apoptosis and cell-cycle G_1 arrest by selenium metabolite methylselenol. *Mol Carcinogen* **34**: 113–120.

Wattenberg, L.W. 1992. Chemoprevention of cancer by naturally occurring and synthetic compounds. *In* "Cancer Chemoprevention" (L. Wattenberg, M. Lipkin, C.W. Boone, and G.J. Kelloff, eds.), pp. 19–39. CRC Press, Inc., Boca Raton, FL.

Weinshilboum, R.M., Sladek, S., and Klumpp, S. 1979. Human erythrocyte thiol methyltransferase: radiochemical microassay and biochemical properties. *Clin Chim Acta* **97**: 59–71.

Welsh, J.B., Sapinoso, L.M., Su, A.I., Kern, S.G., Wang-Rodriguez, J., Moskaluk, C.A., Frierson, H.F., Jr., and Hampton, G.M. 2001. Analysis of gene expression identifies candidate markers and pharmacological targets in prostate cancer. *Cancer Res* **61**: 5974–5978.

Wilber, C.G. 1980. Toxicology of selenium: a review. *Clin Toxicol* **17**: 171–230.

Yoshizawa, K., Willett, W.C., Stampfer, M.J., Spiegelman, D., Rimm, E.B., and Giovannucci, E. 1998. Study of prediagnostic selenium level in toenails and the risk of advanced prostate cancer. *J Natl Cancer Inst* **90**: 1219–1224.

Zhang, H., Dong, Y., Zhao, H., Brooks, J.D., Hawthorn, L., Nowak, N., Marshall, J.R., Gao, A.C., and Ip, C. 2004. Microarray data mining for potential selenium targets in chemoprevention of prostate cancer. *Cancer Genom Proteom* **2**: 97–114.

Zhao, H., Whitfield, M.L., Xu, T., Botstein, D., and Brooks, J.D. 2004. Diverse effects of methylseleninic acid on the transcriptional program of human prostate cancer cells. *Mol Biol Cell* **15**: 506–519.

Zhao, X.Y., Malloy, P.J., Krishnan, A.V., Swami, S., Navone, N.M., Peehl, D.M., and Feldman, D. 2000. Glucocorticoids can promote androgen-independent growth of prostate cancer cells through a mutated androgen receptor. *Nat Med* **6**: 703–706.

Zu, K., and Ip, C. 2003. Synergy between selenium and vitamin E in apoptosis induction is associated with activation of distinctive initiator caspases in human prostate cancer cells. *Cancer Res* **63**: 6988–6995.

CHAPTER

34

Glucosinolates

RADHA M. BHEEMREDDY AND ELIZABETH H. JEFFERY

INTRODUCTION

Epidemiological studies have associated diets rich in cruciferous vegetables and other glucosinolate-containing plants with reduced risk for a number of cancers. Animal studies have identified several glucosinolate derivatives from cruciferous vegetables that exhibit these chemopreventive properties. A large body of literature shows that glucosinolate derivatives modify many mammalian detoxification enzymes that make up part of our host defense against foreign chemicals, by inhibiting carcinogen activation and increasing carcinogen detoxification, resulting in clearance of carcinogens from the body. For more than 3 decades, these effects have been considered responsible for the reduced cancer initiation or decreased promotion and progression of tumors seen in animal and human studies. These same glucosinolate derivatives have been shown to arrest the cell cycle, slow or stop proliferation, and enhance apoptosis in cancer cell lines. Some of these compounds, in purified form, have either already shown encouraging results or are poised ready for testing in clinical trials of cancer prevention in high-risk groups. In this chapter, we summarize some epidemiological, clinical, animal, and cell culture studies on cancer prevention by dietary crucifers and glucosinolate derivatives and highlight the areas that need further research.

OCCURRENCE AND DISTRIBUTION OF GLUCOSINOLATES IN EDIBLE PLANTS

Glucosinolates have been a topic of agricultural research for more than a century, although frequently focused on adverse effects in animals fed concentrated crucifer-based feeds (Price et al., 1993). There has been renewed interest in these compounds because of the bioactivity of their aglucon metabolites that may be responsible for lowered cancer risk in persons eating cruciferous vegetables. Glucosinolates are the thioglucosides of modified amino acids, which are formed as secondary metabolites in a limited number of plant families. There are >120 glucosinolates identified, belonging to 16 families of angiosperms. The Brassicaceae, which include the cruciferous vegetables, are an economically important family because of their role in the human diet (Fahey et al., 2001) (Table 1). Most plant species contain more than one glucosinolate, and whereas concentrations vary considerably across varieties, the same spectrum or profile of glucosinolates usually occurs across all varieties of any given subspecies. Although some plants contain many glucosinolates, typically relatively few (one to four) predominate (Rosa et al., 1997). Interestingly, the distribution of glucosinolates frequently differs both qualitatively and quantitatively among plant parts (roots, leaves, seeds, etc.) of a single plant. Seeds, some of which are used as condiments, contain higher concentrations of glucosinolates than other edible parts (Carlson et al., 1987) (Table 2). Furthermore, the glucosinolate content depends not only on the genetic makeup, but also on the growing environment (Brown et al., 2002). Storage and processing may lead to either enhancement or loss of bioactivity depending on the specific conditions. For these reasons, it is often difficult to estimate intake of bioactive components in a population. For a more detailed discussion of the occurrence, distribution, and concentrations of glucosinolates, the reader is directed to several extensive review articles (Fenwick et al., 1983; Rosa et al., 1997; Fahey et al., 2001; Jeffery and Jarrell, 2001).

Copyright © 2006, Elsevier Inc.
All rights of reproduction in any form reserved.

TABLE 1 List of Widely Consumed Edible Plants and Their Prominent Glucosinolates

Common name	Scientific name	Average Glucosinolate (mg/100 g)	Prominent glucosinolates
Arugula	*Eruca sativa*	—	Glucoerucin, Glucoraphanin
Broccoli	*Brassica oleracea* var. *italica*	62	Glucoraphanin, Sinigrin, Gluconapin, Glucobrassicin
Brussels sprouts	*Brassica olerace* var. *gemmifera*	237	Sinigrin, Gluconapin, Progoitrin, Glucoraphanin, Glucoiberin, Glucobrassicin
Cabbage	*Brassica oleracea* var. *capitata*	59	Sinigrin, Glucoiberin, Progoitrin, Glucobrassicin
Chinese cabbage	*Brassica oleracea* var. *pekinensis*	21	Sinigrin, Progoitrin, Glucobrassicin, Gluconasturtiin
Cauliflower	*Brassica oleracea* var. *botrytis*	43	Sinigrin, Glucoraphanin, Glucoiberin, Glucobrassicin
Collard greens	*Brassica oleracea* var. *acephala*	201	Sinigrin, Glucoiberin, Glucobrassicin
Drumstick	*Moringa oleifera*	20,200	Glucoconringiin (rhamnopyranosyloxy), benzyl glucosinolate
Garden cress	*Lepidium sativum*	390	Glucotropaeolin
Horseradish	*Armoracia lapathifolia*	160	Sinigrin, Gluconapin, Glucoputranjivin, Gluconasturtiin
Kohlrabi	*Brassica oleracea* var. *gongylodes*	73	Gluconapin, Glucoerucin, Glucoraphanin, Gluconasturtiin, Glucobrassicin
Mustard Black	*Brassica nigra*	4,630	Sinigrin, Gluconapin, Gluconasturtiin, 1-Methylpropyl Glucosinolate
Brown	*Brassica juncea*	4,660	Sinigrin, Progoitrin, Gluconapin, Glucobrassicanapin
White	*Sinapis alba*	6,410	Glucosinalbin, Glucoputranjivin
Water cress	*Nasturtium officinale*	95	Gluconasturtiin, Glucobrassicin, Glucosiberin, Glucohirsutin
Rutabaga	*Brassica oleracea* var. *napobrassica*	92	Sinigrin, Gluconapin, Progoitrin, Glucoerucin, Glucoraphanin, Gluconasturtiin
Radish	*Raphunus sativa*	93	Sinigrin, Glucoerucin, Glucotropaeolin, Gluconasturtiin, Glucobrassicin
Turnip	*Brassica campestris*	93	Gluconapin, Glucobrassicanapin

Source: Fenwick et al., 1983; Rosa et al., 1997; Kiddle et al., 2001; Bennett et al., 2003; McNaughton and Marks, 2003.

TABLE 2 Glucosinolate Content of Seed and Vegetative Tissue

Cruciferous vegetable	Seed (μmol/g)	Fresh tissue (μmol/g)
Broccoli	151.6	1.9
Brussels sprouts	135.8	5.5
Cauliflower	140.2	1.0
Collard greens	176.0	4.4
Kale	186.6	3.2
Mustard greens	185.0	11.9
Kohlrabi	193.9	0.9

Source: Carlson et al., 1987.

Glucosinolate Structure and Diversity

Glucosinolate structure consists of a β-D-thioglucose group linked to a sulfonated aldoxime moiety and a side chain (R group) derived from one of several amino acids (Figure 1A). Based on the amino acid precursors, glucosinolates are grouped as aliphatic, aromatic, or indolyl glucosinolates when derived from methionine, phenylalanine, or tryptophan, respectively (Mithen et al., 2000). Extensive research has identified enzymes that elongate the aliphatic side chain (three to six carbons in length are commonly

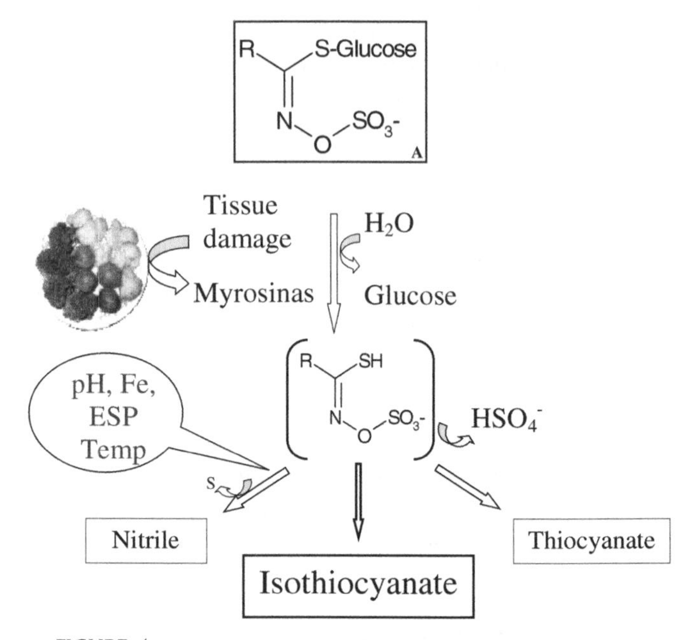

FIGURE 1 Schematic representation of glucosinolates hydrolysis.

found in dietary crucifers). Other enzymes support desaturation, oxidation, or reduction, steps that follow side-chain elongation and that produce, for example, sulfinyl, sulfonyl, sulfide, and de-sulfo products (Wittstock and Halkier, 2002). Further, in the Moringaceae family (producing the Indian fruit drumstick), there may be an additional sugar moiety (rhamnose or arabinose) glycosylated to the benzene ring of the phenylalanine-derived side chain (Fahey et al., 2001). The abundance and the type of glucosinolate present in each species is dependent on the presence of the enzymes involved in these synthetic pathways and therefore may be genetically modified to breed for vegetables with the desired glucosinolate profile. Broccoli is one vegetable that has already been genetically modified to provide about 80 times the efficacy, when compared with the standard broccoli (Mithen et al., 2003).

Glucosinolate Hydrolysis to Bioactive Derivatives

Glucosinolates are not bioactive but must undergo hydrolysis to an aglucon, followed by rearrangement, to form the bioactive glucosinolates derivatives. This hydrolysis may occur either within the plant tissue, catalyzed by the plant enzyme myrosinase, or following ingestion, catalyzed by the gut microflora (Mithen et al., 2000). Mammalian cells do not possess an active thioglucosidase. In intact plants, glucosinolates are physically separated from myrosinase, so glucosinolates remain chemically stable until the plant tissue is disrupted due to food preparation or chewing. When glucosinolates come into contact with myrosinase, the glucose is lost, and an unstable aglucon intermediate remains, which rapidly rearranges nonenzymatically to form an isothiocyanate, nitrile, or thiocyanate (Figure 1). These different products that are formed vary in their potency as anticancer agents. Some isothiocyanates with a hydroxyl group in the 2 position spontaneously cyclize to form oxazolidine-2-thiones; aglucons with terminal double bonds form epithionitriles in the presence of a myrosinase cofactor, the epithiospecifier protein (Wittstock and Halkier, 2002; Matusheski et al., 2004). Under acid conditions, in the presence of millimolar concentrations of iron or in the presence of the epithiospecifier protein and micromolar concentrations of iron, a nitrile can be formed from any aglucon (Matusheski, personal communications). The importance of this is that of all the hydrolysis products, isothiocyanates appear to be the most bioactive. Table 3 lists several bioactive compounds, their parent glucosinolates, and the vegetables in which they are abundant.

Dietary Intake of Glucosinolates

Detailed information on dietary glucosinolate or isothiocyanate intake is difficult to obtain. However, rough estimates can be made from available data on consumption of cruciferous vegetables. Estimated *per capita* consumption of fresh and frozen broccoli, cabbage, and cauliflower within the United States (USDA-NASS Agriculture Statistics, 2003) is presented in Table 4. The total *per capita* consumption of crucifers for year 2001 was reported at 19.7 lbs: roughly 1/3 cup or 24 g/person/day, based on total commercial production divided by total population. Glucosinolate content of commonly consumed vegetables varies from 500 to 2000 μg/g (Table 1), giving an average daily consumption in the range of ~13 mg glucosinolates per day per person within the United States. Intake is substantially greater in a number of Asian countries. For example, in a study of 1724 Shanghai women, average cruciferous vegetable consumption was 98 g/day, four times higher than in the United States (Fowke et al., 2003b). Also, different cruciferous vegetables are popular in different parts of the world. The Japanese

TABLE 3 Bioactive Glucosinolates Derivatives

Glucosinolate	Bioactive compound
Sinigrin	Allyl isothiocyanate (AITC)
Glucotropaeolin	Benzyl isothiocyanate (BITC)
Gluconaturtiin	Phenylethyl isothiocyanate (PEITC)
Glucoraphanin	Sulforaphane (SF)
Glucobrassicin	Indole-3-carbinol (I3C)
Progoitrin	Crambene (CHB)

TABLE 4 Consumption of Glucosinolate-Containing Vegetables in the United States (2001)

Vegetable	Fresh (g/yr)	GS content (mg/g)	Frozen (g/yr)	GS content (mg/g)	TVC (g/yr)	Total GS consumption (mg/yr)
Cabbage	4044	0.59			4044	2382
Broccoli	2578	0.62	978	0.51	3556	1698
Cauliflower	889	0.43	267	0.41	1156	492
Total	7511		1244		8755	4573

Source: USDA-NASS Agricultural Statistics (2003).
GS, glucosinolates; TVC, total vegetable consumption.

consume substantial amounts of wasabi, a Japanese horseradish, as a condiment with sushi, and the Koreans consume kimchi, a fermented cabbage or cabbage/radish product with almost every meal, whereas Americans consume mostly cabbage and broccoli (Fenwick et al., 1983). A database of glucosinolate content of common vegetables may soon be available, greatly simplifying calculation of glucosinolates consumption (McNaughton and Marks, 2003).

EPIDEMIOLOGICAL INVESTIGATIONS RELATING GLUCOSINOLATES AND CANCER PREVENTION

Individuals with a high intake of fruits and vegetables appear to be at lower risk for developing a number of cancers (Table 5). A cohort study of survivors of ovarian cancer reported a statistically significant survival advantage for women in the highest quartile of intake for all vegetables in general (adjusted hazard ratio [HR] = 0.75, $p < .01$) and for those in the highest quartile of intake for cruciferous vegetables in particular (HR = 0.75, $p < .03$) (Nagle et al., 2003). A case-control study investigating the association between renal cell carcinoma incidence and diet identified a strong inverse relationship between renal cell carcinoma and intake of both dark green vegetables ($p < .001$) and cruciferous vegetables ($p < .001$); the protective effect of crucifers persisted even when data were adjusted for known nutrients in the crucifers, such as vitamin C and carotenoids (Yuan et al., 1998). The authors concluded that nonnutrients such as glucosinolate derivatives may play a role in protecting against renal cell carcinoma (Yuan et al., 1998).

The results of many studies support the possibility that consumption of cruciferous vegetables has a stronger inverse association to cancer risk than the consumption of all vegetables (Jain et al., 1999; Cohen et al., 2000; Kolonel et al., 2000). For example, the Health Professionals' Follow-up Study monitored 47,909 men over 10 years and reported 252 cases of bladder cancer. Analysis of food frequency questionnaires collected three times during that 10-year period revealed a significant reduction in risk (relative risk [RR], 0.49; $p = .008$) for bladder cancer in individuals ingesting five or more servings of cruciferous vegetables a week, compared wtih those ingesting one or fewer servings per week (Michaud et al., 1999). A similar calculation for consumption of green leafy vegetables or for total fruits and vegetables did not show a significant risk reduction.

Data are accumulating to suggest that, as one might expect, the protective response varies with the amount of cruciferous vegetables consumed: Risk is typically decreased most in the highest quartile of intake. For example, one study reported a significant 40% reduction in prostate cancer risk in individuals who consumed three to five servings or more of cruciferous vegetables per week, compared with those consuming only one serving or fewer (Cohen et al., 2000; Kolonel et al., 2000). Similarly, a meta-analysis of 20 studies, controlling for total vegetable intake, found an 8% decrease in risk for colon cancer with every 10-g increase in cruciferous vegetables consumed per day (Kohlmeier and Su, 1997). In the Nurses' Health Study, a significant reduction in risk (RR, 0.67; $p = .03$) for non-Hodgkin's lymphoma was seen among women who consumed five or more servings per week in comparison with women who consumed fewer than two servings per week (Zhang et al., 2000).

Whereas the number of studies showing an inverse relation between cruciferous vegetable intake and a decrease in risk for cancer is growing, there are a substantial number of well-controlled studies that do not show this effect. A review of 94 studies concluded that consumption of cruciferous vegetables is associated with reduced risk of cancer at several sites (Verhoeven et al., 1996). However, in that review, only 58 of the 87 case-control studies evaluated showed an inverse association between consumption of cruciferous vegetables and cancer risk, and findings were only statistically significant in 39 of these studies. Cohort studies showed the same trend as case-control studies, with five of seven studies showing an inverse effect. Studies continue to

TABLE 5 Epidemiological Studies Showing the Effect of Dietary Cruciferous Vegetables on Risk of Cancer

Cancer site	Study type	Intake	Risk	*p* value	Reference
Bladder	Prospective	>5 ser/wk	RR 0.49	0.008	Michaud et al., 1999
Lung	Case-control	0.5 ser/day	OR 0.31	CI (0.1–0.92)	Zhao et al., 2001
Lymphoma	Prospective	>5 ser/wk	RR 0.67	0.03	Zhang et al., 2000
Prostrate	Case-control	>3 ser/wk	OR 0.59	0.02	Cohen et al., 2000
Prostrate	Case-control	5 ser/wk	OR 0.61	0.006	Kolonel et al., 2000
Breast	Case-control	Quartile 4	OR 0.50	0.01	Fowke et al., 2003a
Kidney	Case-control	Quartile 4	OR 0.53	0.001	Yuan et al., 1998
Ovarian	Case-control	>0.83 ser/day	HR 0.75	0.03	Nagle et al., 2003

CI, confidence interval; HR, hazard ratio; OR, odds ratio; RR, relative risk; ser, serving.

show protection in a preponderance of studies, but not in all studies (Kristal and Lampe, 2002).

One possible cause for these inconsistent findings may be the genetic variability in the makeup of the individuals. Cancer protective effects of cruciferous vegetables are mostly attributed to their ability to modulate the xenobiotic metabolizing enzymes. A number of studies have uncovered the fact that human genetic polymorphisms in xenobiotic metabolizing enzymes can change both an individual's risk for cancer and the extent to which cruciferous vegetables can protect that individual (Spitz et al., 2000; Lin et al. 2002). In a study of the relationship between incidence of colon cancer and ingestion of cruciferous vegetables, sensitivity to protection by cruciferous vegetables was found to vary substantially with polymorphism in the family of glutathione *S*-transferase (GST) enzymes. Thus, a greater protective effect of broccoli specifically, and cruciferous vegetables in general, was seen in individuals who were missing the GSTM1 isoenzyme (GSTM1-null genotype) than in the general study population (Lin et al., 2002). A similar study conducted among lung cancer patients showed that a protective effect of cruciferous vegetables was significant in current smokers who were both GSTM1- and GSTT1-null genotype (Spitz et al., 2000). Whereas Spitz et al. (2000) found no significant protective effect of cruciferous vegetables against lung cancer incidence in former smokers, Zhao et al. (2001) showed a protective effect in nonsmoking Singapore Chinese women who were GSTM1 null. The different results from these two studies may reflect a difference in the range of cruciferous vegetable intake in the United States and Singapore: The latter study reported a mean intake very similar to that reported for the United States (~50 μmol isothiocyanates/wk), but the range of intake was up to 10-fold greater (Zhao et al., 2001).

Most of the cited epidemiological studies calculate dietary intake of cruciferous vegetables using food frequency questionnaires. That method of data collection might, however, cause some inaccuracy because of multiple causes including poor recall, recall bias, errors in identification of cruciferous vegetables, variation in glucosinolate levels due to variety, growing, and storage conditions, as well as difficulty in estimation of serving size. Several studies have used urinary isothiocyanate excretion as a measure of dietary exposure to cruciferous vegetables (Spitz et al., 2000; Zhao et al., 2001; Fowke et al., 2003a). This can give a precise measure of excretion and therefore a relative measure of intake. However, it is limited by the fact that much of a dose is excreted during the first 12 hours, and therefore, it is difficult to interpret period urine samples if intake varies substantially day to day (Shapiro et al., 1998). Albeit, when viewed together, the epidemiological studies strongly support a role for cruciferous vegetables in dietary prevention of cancer.

CHEMOPREVENTION STUDIES IN ANIMAL MODELS

The capacity for cruciferous vegetables to modulate metabolism of carcinogens and prevent mutagenic and carcinogenic outcomes has been demonstrated in numerous animal models (Verhoeven et al., 1997; Hecht, 2000; Jeffery and Jarrell, 2001; Murillo and Mehta, 2001; Conaway et al., 2002). In addition, studies using animal models of cancer have found that in addition to the whole vegetable, purified dietary isothiocyanates and indoles, bioactive metabolites of glucosinolates, are also effective chemopreventive agents (Table 6). Animal feeding studies that evaluate changes in detoxification enzymes as an endpoint of efficacy have employed a broad range of cruciferous vegetables including broccoli and watercress. In contrast, feeding studies evaluating tumor incidence or tumor size as an endpoint have mostly utilized Brussels sprouts or cabbage. For example, in a study by Kassie et al. (2003), male F344 rats were given the liver and colon carcinogen 2-amino-3-methylimidazoquinoline (IQ) by gavage. In addition, some of these rats received either Brussels sprouts or red cabbage juice (5% v/v) in their drinking water. Dietary Brussels sprouts and red cabbage juice both significantly decreased IQ-induced glutathione-*S*-transferase-P-positive foci ($GST\text{-}P^{+}$) number (a measure of initiation) and size (a measure of promotion/progression) in the livers of these rats. The Brussels sprouts diet effectively decreased initiation, but not progression in colon, and the red cabbage juice was without effect on initiation or progression in the colon. In this study, cooking did not diminish the cancer protective effects of this vegetable diet. These studies included the feeding of juices from two varieties of each vegetable. Although the glucosinolate content varied substantially among varieties, there appeared little difference in efficacy. The authors speculated that the interactive effect of all glucosinolate derivatives might have more impact than the content of any single glucosinolate. Another possibility is that the percentage yield of bioactive isothiocyanates, relative to the less active nitriles or thiocyanates, was greater from the variety with lower glucosinolate levels, equalizing the bioactive isothiocyanate yield (Keck et al., 2003).

The majority of whole animal studies evaluating cancer prevention by cruciferous vegetables or glucosinolate derivatives have focused on prevention of initiation. However, several studies report efficacy of isothiocyanates given either before or after exposure to carcinogens, demonstrating that at least in some cancer models, cruciferous vegetables, glucosinolates, or isothiocyanates may be protective during both initiation and promotion/progression. For example, when rats were given the purified glucosinolate sinigrin, starting 22 hours after administration of the carcinogen 1,2-dimethylhydrazine (DMH), a significant

TABLE 6 Effect of Glucosinolate Derivatives on Chemical-Induced Cancers

Anticarcinogen[a]	Carcinogen[b]	Test system	Type of cancer	Effect
2-Phenethyl isothiocyanate (PEITC)[e]				
Before	NNK	Mouse	Lung	Inhibition
Before	BaP	Mouse	Forestomach	Inhibition
Before	BaP	Mouse	Lung	No effect
Before	BOP	Hamster	Lung	Inhibition
Before	DMBA	Rat	Mammary	Inhibition
During	DMBA	Mouse	Lung and forestomach	Inhibition
Before and during	NNK	Rat	Lung	Inhibition
Before, during, and after	NMBA	Rat	Esophageal	Inhibition
Before and after	DEN	Mouse	Liver	Inhibition
Before and after	DMBA	Rat	Mammary	No effect
After	NNK	Mouse	Lung	No effect
PEITC-NAC conjugates[g]				
Before or after	AOM	Rat	Colon	Inhibition
Benzyl isothiocyanate (BITC)[e]				
Before	NNK	Mouse	Lung	No effect
Before	DEN	Mouse	Forestomach	Inhibition
Before	DEN	Mouse	Lung	No effect
Before	BaP	Mouse	Lung and forestomach	Inhibition
Before	BaP	Mouse	Skin and forestomach	No effect
During	DMBA/BaP	Mouse	Lung and forestomach	Inhibition
Before and after	NMBA	Rat	Esophageal	No effect
Before and after	DMBA	Rat	Mammary	Inhibition
Before and after	DEN	Rat	Lung	Inhibition
After	DMBA	Rat	Mammary	Inhibition
After	DMH	Mouse	Colon	Inhibition
After	NNK	Mouse	Lung	Inhibition
Sulforaphane (SF)[g,c,d]				
Before and after	DMBA	Rat	Stomach	Inhibition
Before, during, and after	BaP	Mice	Stomach	Inhibition
Before or after	AOM	Rat	Colon (ACF)	Inhibition
Indole-3-carbinol (I3C)[e]				
Before	AFB1	Rainbow trout	Liver	Inhibition
After	AFB1	Rainbow trout	Liver	Enhanced
Before, during, and after	DMH	Rat	Colon	Enhanced
Before and after	MNU/ DMBA	Rat	Mammary	Inhibition
After	DEN and MNU and DBN	Rat	Liver and lung	Inhibition
I3C, DIM, I3A[e]				
Before	DMBA/BaP	Rat/Mouse	Mammary/forestomach	Inhibition
I3C, Sinigrin[e]				
Before, during, and after	DEN/4NQO	Rat	Liver/tongue	Inhibition
Singirin[j]				
After	DMH	Rat	Colon	Inhibition
Cabbage[e]				
Before	MNU	Rat	Mammary	Inhibition
During	AFB1/DMH	Rat/Mouse	Liver	Inhibition
Brussels sprouts[e,f]				
Before or after	AOM	Rat	Colon (ACF)	Inhibition
During or after	DMBA	Rat	Mammary	Inhibition
Cabbage Cauliflower Broccoli[e]				
After	DMBA	Rat	Mammary	Inhibition
Gardencress juice[i]				
Before	IQ	Rat	Colon (ACF)	Inhibition
Broccoli sprouts[h]				
Before and after	DMBA	Rat	Mammary	Inhibition

[a]Dosing schedule of potential anticarcinogen, relative to dosing of carcinogen.

[b]Carcinogen abbreviations: AFB1 Aflatoxin B1; AOM, azoxymethane; BaP, benz(*a*)pyrene; BOP, *N*-nitrosobis(2-oxopropyl)amine; DBN, *N,N*-dibutyl nitrosamine; DEN, diethylnitrosamine; DMBA, 9,10-dimethyl-1,2-benzanthracene; DMH, 1,2-dimethylhydrazine dihydrochloride; IQ, 2-amino-3-methylimidazoquinoline; MNU, *N*-methyl-*n*-nitrosourea; 4NQO, 4-nitroquinoline1-oxide; NMBA, *N*-nitrosomethylbenzylamine; NNK, 4-(*N*-nitrosomethylamino)-1-(3-pyfldyl)-1-butanone; ACF, aberrant crypt foci; DIM, 3,3′-diindolylmethane; I3A, indole-3-acetonitrile (Zhang et al., 1994; Fahey et al., 1997, 2002; Verhoeven et al., 1997; Rijken et al., 1999; Chung et al., 2000; Kassie et al., 2002; Smith et al., 2003).

inhibition of appearance of colonic aberrant crypt foci was seen (Smith et al., 1998). Also, the purified glucosinolate derivatives sulforaphane (SF) and phenethyl isothiocyanate (PEITC) have been shown to significantly decrease ($p < .01$) azoxymethane-induced colonic aberrant crypt foci in F344 rats, when given in the diet before or after the carcinogen, suggesting protection against both initiation and promotion/progression (Chung et al., 2000). It is possible that the preponderance of anti-initiation studies in the literature may not reflect a lack of inhibition of proliferation, but that until recently the effect of isothiocyanates on carcinogenesis was frequently limited to anti-initiation studies (Table 6). Two reasons may have been responsible. Because inhibition of proliferation requires feeding of the test substance for a prolonged period, often months, it may have been technically difficult to produce sufficient test substance, when purification and/or synthetic systems were first under development. More significant, hypothesis-driven research demanded that initiation be the target of experiments, since the accepted hypothesis for the mechanism of action of glucosinolate derivatives was improved metabolism and clearance of chemical carcinogens. Studies using cultured cells have identified that isothiocyanates also arrest the cell cycle and cause apoptosis (see later discussion). This has led to a strong rationale for evaluating the effect of isothiocyanates on progression/proliferation. For example, Smith et al. (2003) focused on effects of Brussels sprouts on apoptosis and mitosis in the colonic mucosa of male Wistar rats given DMH. Oral Brussels sprouts juice or dietary freeze-dried uncooked Brussels sprouts increased apoptosis and decreased mitosis in colonic mucosa of DMH-treated rats. Importantly, in rats not receiving the carcinogen, neither juice nor freeze-dried Brussels sprouts had any inhibitory effect on normal mitosis. In contrast to the study described earlier, where cooking Brussels sprouts or red cabbage juice had no effect on efficacy (Kassie et al., 2003), when the Brussels sprouts were blanched before freeze-drying for addition to the diet, the protective effect was lost. Further studies are necessary to determine the cause of the lack of consistency in results from studies evaluating the effect of cooked cruciferous vegetables on cancer prevention.

Effects of cruciferous vegetables on cancer prevention are not limited to any one vegetable type, carcinogen, or species of animal tested. The studies compiled in Table 6 are taken from several review articles and research papers to give an overall perspective on the breadth of the cancer-preventive action of glucosinolate derivatives that has been reported in studies using animal models of cancer. Efficacy has been reported for juice, raw and cooked cruciferous vegetables, purified glucosinolates, isothiocyanates, and even the *N*-acetylcysteine conjugate metabolites of isothiocyanates. Efficacy appears to cross species, type of cancer, carcinogen, treatment protocol, initiation, and promotion/progression, although the extent of protection appears to depend on a number of factors, including the frequency and amount ingested, the stage of carcinogenesis, and the type of cancer (Xu et al., 2001). Even though one cannot extrapolate these findings from animal studies directly to human efficacy, these data do strongly implicate glucosinolate derivatives from cruciferous vegetables in chemoprevention.

MECHANISMS OF CANCER PREVENTION BY GLUCOSINOLATE DERIVATIVES

Our understanding of mechanisms involved in cancer prevention by cruciferous vegetables has evolved concurrently with the fields of xenobiotic metabolism and cancer biology. Cruciferous vegetables were first shown to modify the enzymes that metabolize drugs and other xenobiotics in the 1970s, as our knowledge of these enzymes first began to unfold (Pantuck et al., 1979). With this knowledge arose the hypothesis that induction of detoxification enzymes might decrease the activity of carcinogens. In support of this, cancer prevention, decreased formation of DNA adducts, and an increase in elimination of carcinogens were found to occur in parallel with the increase in detoxification enzymes (Verhoeven et al., 1997). Glucosinolate derivatives have been found to trigger signal transduction events leading to cell cycle arrest and apoptosis. It remains to be determined whether these effects are secondary to changes in detoxification enzymes or changes in the antioxidant/redox status of the cell, whether they are primary mechanisms for anticarcinogenesis, or whether these mechanisms work in conjunction with enzyme induction to provide anticarcinogenesis. In addition, glucosinolate metabolites may also have epigenetic effects; by inhibiting histone, deacetylase be able to slow or even reverse tumor formation (Myzak et al., 2004).

Detoxification Enzymes

The rate of metabolism and clearance of many environmental procarcinogens and carcinogens is enhanced by a diet rich in cruciferous vegetables or glucosinolate derivatives. Phase I detoxification enzymes, also called *bioactivation enzymes*, are primarily made up from the family of cytochrome P450 (CYP) isoenzymes. Phase I reactions support oxidation, reduction, and hydrolysis of carcinogens and other xenobiotics, and the products may be more reactive (bioactivated) or less reactive (detoxified). The products of bioactivation, reactive carcinogenic or toxic products, may cause adverse effects on the body such as DNA damage leading to initiation of carcinogenesis, or they may immediately undergo further phase II metabolism to form detoxified conjugation products. Conjugation enhances hydrophilicity of the metabolites, thus facilitating elimination of the carcinogen from the body. The compounds that are detoxified, rather than bioactivated, by phase I metabolism may be excreted directly or undergo further metabolism by phase II conjugation enzymes. Glucosinolate derivatives have been found to induce a few CYP enzymes, inhibit a few more CYP enzymes, and induce several phase II conjugation enzymes. Therefore, if CYP-dependent bioactivation of a carcinogen could be inhibited and detoxification and clearance enhanced, this could slow or prevent the initiation of carcinogenesis by chemical carcinogens, leading to lowered risk of developing cancer.

One example of glucosinolates altering metabolism is seen with 4-methylnitrosamino-1-(3-pyridyl)-1-butanone (NNK), a carcinogen present in tobacco smoke. NNK undergoes CYP-dependent bioactivation (carbonyl reduction) to form 4-(methylnitrosamino)-1-(3-pyridyl)-1-butanol (NNAL), a direct-acting carcinogen that can methylate DNA (Hecht, 1999) (Figure 2). In humans, metabolism of NNAL by phase II conjugation results in detoxification and excretion of NNAL as a glucuronide. Another metabolic route for NNK is through CYP-dependent carbon hydroxylation to form the mutagenic metabolite diazohydroxide, which can cause DNA point mutations (Hecht, 1999). A third route is via CYP-dependent *N*-oxidation to pyridine *N*-oxide, which has no carcinogenic effect and can be excreted without further metabolism. The glucosinolate derivative PEITC prevents NNK lung cancer in rats and mice and enhances NNAL and NNAL glucuronide excretion in rats and humans, supporting the theory that PEITC has diverted metabolism away from formation of the carcinogenic diazohydroxide. In humans, bioactivation appears to involve several CYP enzymes, including CYP 1A2, 2A6, and 3A4, whereas detoxification through *N*-oxidation is supported by CYP 2B1, and possibly CYP 3A4. Thus, induction of glucuronidation and inhibition of the specific CYP enzymes that bioactivate NNK could be responsible for the decreased carcinogenic potential of NNK. The shared role of CYP enzymes in bioactivation and detoxification has led some scientists to suggest that induction of phase II conjugating enzymes and/or inhibition of phase I CYP enzymes may be more reliably anticarcinogenic than induction of phase I enzymes (Talalay and Fahey, 2001). Yet whole vegetables protect against cancer in epidemiological studies even though they contain indolyl derivatives like indole-3-carbinol, known to cause induction of some CYP enzymes.

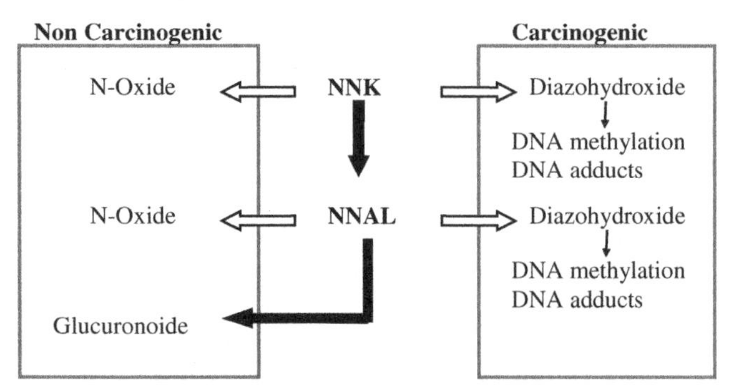

FIGURE 2 NNK metabolism.

A broad range of glucosinolate derivatives have been studied for the ability to affect both phase I and phase II detoxification enzymes in whole animals and in cell culture systems. Table 7 lists some of the enzymes that have been studied in this context. The mechanism of enzyme induction by these derivatives has been reviewed (Lampe and Peterson, 2002; Thornalley, 2002). In brief, promoter regions of the genes of upregulated enzymes contain one or both of two regulatory regions that respond to glucosinolate derivatives, the xenobiotic response element (XRE) and the antioxidant response element (ARE) (Figure 3). Indolyl isothiocyanate derivatives, such as indole-3-carbinol and its metabolite diindolylmethane, trigger the XRE through binding to a

TABLE 7 Partial List of Enzymes Modulated by Glucosinolate Derivatives

Aflatoxin aldehyde reductase
Cytochrome P450 1A and 2E
Epoxide hydrolases
Ferritin
Glutathione reductase
Glutathione peroxidase
Glutathione *S*-transferases
γ-Glutamylcysteine synthetase
Heptoglobin
Multidrug resistance protein (MRP-1)
NAD(P)H: quinone oxidoreductase
P-glycoprotein
Thioredoxin reductase
UDP-glucuronosyltransferases

Source: Thimmulappa et al., 2002; Hintze et al., 2003.

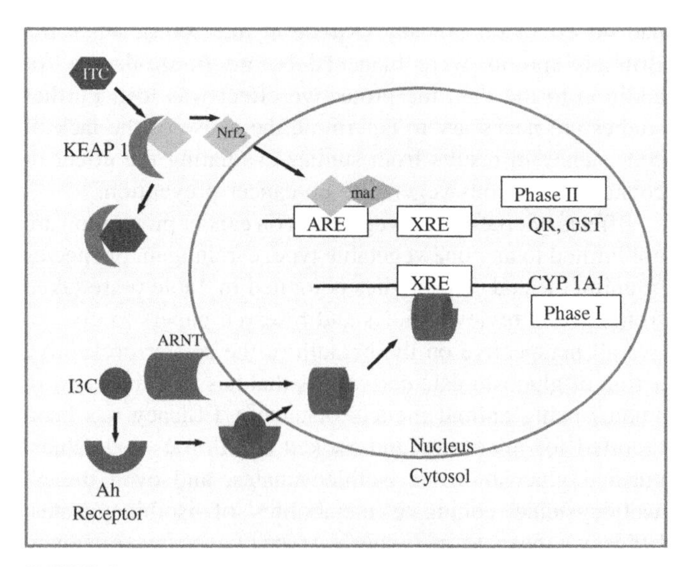

FIGURE 3 Transcriptional regulation of detoxification enzymes by glucosinolate derivatives.

cytosolic receptor. This complex of the metabolite and the Ah receptor then translocates to the nucleus, where the complex binds and activates the XRE, leading to the induction of a battery of enzymes, including both phase I (CYP 1A) and phase II enzymes. Other glucosinolate derivatives, such as the isothiocyanates allyl isothiocyanate (AITC) and SF, cause the endogenous cytosolic transcription factor Nrf2 to translocate to the nucleus and activate the ARE, but the isothiocyanates themselves are not bound to the Nrf2 transcription factor. Comparing the potency with which different isothiocyanates upregulate phase II enzymes in cell culture, SF appears very much more potent than other isothiocyanates (Talalay and Fahey, 2001). One possible reason for this is that SF accumulates rapidly in cultured cells, increasing the intracellular concentration by several orders of magnitude over the concentration of SF added to the medium (Zhang and Callaway, 2002). Whether this occurs within the body or only in cell culture remains to be determined because SF does not appear to maintain this potency advantage in animal feeding experiments (Keck et al., 2002; Munday and Munday, 2004)

Modulation of Signal Transduction, Cell Cycle Arrest, and Apoptosis

Studies have established the ability of glucosinolate derivatives to induce cell cycle arrest and apoptosis in cancer cells in culture while having little or no cytotoxic effect on normal noncancerous cells (Xiao et al., 2003). The mechanisms involved in triggering these events are under investigation Chen and Kong, 2004). One study evaluated the effect of four common isothiocyanate derivatives of glucosinolates—benzyl isothiocyanate (BITC), AITC, PEITC, and SF—on cultured cancer cell lines from several major organ sites: liver (HepG2 cells), breast (MCF-7 cells), colon (HT-29 cells), skin (HaCaT cells), and blood (HL60/S and 8226/S cells) (Zhang et al., 2003). Interestingly, both BITC and AITC were more potent in arresting cell growth than either PEITC or SF, even though SF had earlier been shown to be the most potent in induction of phase II enzymes in cultured cells (Zhang and Callaway, 2002). These results suggest that there may be distinct mechanisms involved in the induction of phase II enzymes and the arrest of the cell cycle by these compounds. Because both mechanisms may play a role in prevention of cancer, vegetables that contain a mixture of glucosinolate derivatives acting through different mechanisms may prove synergistic in their action.

Studies employing xenografts of tumor cells grown under the dorsal skin of immune-deficient mice show that glucosinolate derivatives can induce apoptosis in this model also. In a mouse xenograft model implanted with PC-3 human prostate cells, 10 μmol AITC given i.p. three times a week significantly inhibited tumor growth ($p = .05$). Prostate cancer cell xenografts excised from mice receiving AITC exhibited a significant increase in apoptosis, together with a decrease in mitotic cell number compared with xenografts from mice with no AITC (Srivastava et al. 2003). These findings using the immune-compromised mouse xenograft model are in agreement with the chemical carcinogenesis model in immune-sufficient rats, in which rats given the carcinogen DMH to induce colon carcinogenesis, dietary sinigrin caused enhanced apoptosis of the aberrant crypt cells (Smith et al., 1998).

The pathways leading to cell cycle arrest and apoptosis are still under investigation. Phenethyl isothiocyanate has been reported to induce apoptosis through a p53-dependent pathway, in studies using the JB6 cell line (Huang et al., 1998). In another study, activation of ERK, but not JNK, was implicated in PEITC-induced apoptosis of PC-3 cells (Xiao and Singh, 2002). In HeLa, Jurkat, and 293 cells, it was found that PEITC-dependent JNK activation was associated with apoptosis (Xiao and Singh, 2002; Hu et al., 2003). Taken together, these studies suggest that there are multiple pathways by which isothiocyanates trigger apoptosis, and that involvement of any one pathway may be specific to the cell line under study.

CLINICAL STUDIES WITH GLUCOSINOLATE DERIVATIVES

Absorption and Metabolic Effects of Glucosinolate Derivatives

Metabolism studies using rodents have shown that ingested isothiocyanates are conjugated to glutathione, further metabolized, and excreted in urine as *N*-acetylcysteine conjugates. These conjugates can be individually identified and quantified by high-performance liquid chromatography (HPLC)/UV (Duncan et al., 1997). Several clinical studies have used urinary excretion of individual conjugates as biomarkers and a relative measure of absorption of various cruciferous vegetables (Shapiro et al., 1998; Conaway et al., 2000; Fowke et al., 2003a,b). Total urinary isothiocyanates, measured as compounds that react with 1,2-benzenedithiol to form cyclic condensation products, have also been used as a measure of dietary intake (Ye et al., 2002). The cyclic condensation assay has the advantage that a single analysis can be used regardless of the particular vegetable in the diet. However, the measure of specific isothiocyanates is less easily confounded and can be used to evaluate intake of specific crucifers more accurately.

Clinical studies have also used urinary products to estimate modification of carcinogen metabolism by diets rich in cruciferous vegetables. A broccoli/Brussels sprouts diet significantly decreased urinary excretion of 2-amino-3,8-dimethylimidazo(4,5-f) quinoxaline (MeIQx) and 1-amino-1methyl-6-phenylimidazo(4,5-b)pyridine (PhIP), carcinogenic heterocyclic aromatic amine metabolites from cooked meats (Murray et al., 2001). These data were interpreted to mean that phase I bioactivation to carcinogens had been inhibited. Similarly, a group of individuals given cruciferous vegetables together with fried meat over the 6-week study period excreted approximately twofold more conjugates than a group receiving noncruciferous vegetables with the fried meat (DeMarini et al., 1997). This was interpreted to mean that carcinogenic products formed were twice as likely to be metabolized by phase II enzymes and excreted.

Based on rodent studies that show that PEITC enhances detoxification and excretion of the tobacco carcinogen NNK, a clinical trial evaluated the effect of watercress, a rich source of PEITC, on urinary tobacco metabolites in smokers (Hecht, 1995). Similar to results from the rodent studies, an increased excretion of NNAL and its glucuronide was observed in smokers following ingestion of watercress. Because in the rodent studies this change in metabolism correlated with PEITC protection from lung cancer, it has been proposed that PEITC should be developed as prophylactic therapy for addicted smokers (Hecht et al., 1995). Furthermore, a second tobacco carcinogen, benzo(a)pyrene, shows a shift in metabolic products and decreased carcinogenicity in rodents fed BITC (Lin et al., 1993). Therefore, PEITC and BITC may best function together to prevent lung cancer from the mixture of carcinogens present in cigarette smoke (Hecht, 1995).

Clinical studies also support the hypothesis that cruciferous vegetables modulate estrogen metabolism in a manner consistent with reduced risk for estrogen-dependent cancers such as breast or endometrial cancers (Kall et al., 1996; Fowke et al., 2000) (Figure 4). Indole-3-carbinol is present in most cruciferous vegetables as its parent compound glucobrassicin and has been identified as the main contributor to the shift in estrogen urinary metabolites seen following ingestion of cruciferous vegetables. The change in urinary metabolites is from production of 16α-hydroxyestrone to the less estrogenic metabolite 2-hydroxyestrone (Figure 4). Women given 250 g of broccoli twice daily for 12 days exhibited this shift, with a 29.5% ($p > .05$) increase in the ratio of urinary 2 : 16α-hydroxyestrone metabolites (Kall et al., 1996). Similarly, a dietary intervention trial in healthy postmenopausal women found that for each 10-g incremental increase in cruciferous vegetable consumption per day, there was an 0.08% (CI 95%, 0.02–0.15) increase in the urinary 2 : 16α-hydroxyestrone ratio (Fowke et al., 2000). Enzymes associated with formation of 2-hydroxy metabolites are CYP 1A1 and 1B1 in extrahepatic tissue and CYP 3A4/5 and 1A2 in hepatic tissue; CYP 1A and possibly 1B are upregulated by indole 3-carbinol and its metabolites (Sanderson et al., 2001). These promising results have prompted phase I trials with indole-3-carbinol. The collection of urine samples is both minimally invasive and safer than handling blood samples. This methodology will no doubt be expanded to include measurement of additional metabolites for determination of efficacy of glucosinolate derivatives in slowing or preventing many cancers.

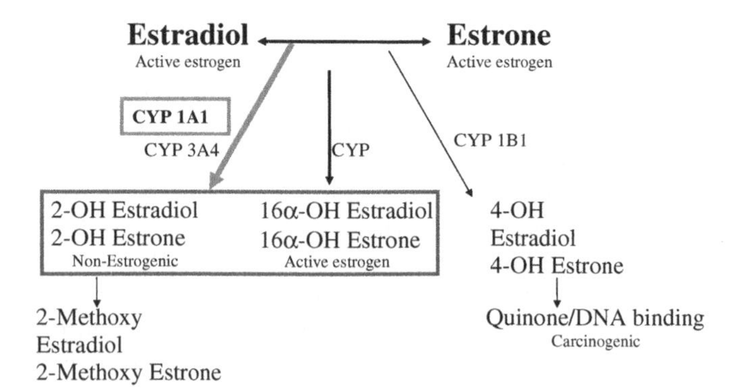

FIGURE 4 Effect of indole-3-carbinol and its metabolites on estrogen metabolism. Alteration of estrogen metabolism results in an increased 2-OH/16-OH estrogen ratio (box in figure), which has been found to correlate with reduced risk of female cancers.

Cancer Prevention

Clinical trials of cancer prevention and treatment are still very few and are typically, as a result of clearcut prevention studies in rodents, linked to urinary biomarkers of altered metabolism. As described earlier, indole-3-carbinol and its more potent metabolite diindolylmethane protect against estrogen-dependent breast cancer in rats (Wattenberg and Loub, 1978; Chen et al., 1998), this protection is linked to an increase in the urinary 2 : 16α-hydroxyestrone ratio (Jellinck et al., 1993), and this change in metabolite ratio can be seen in women ingesting cruciferous vegetables. Epidemiological studies have shown clearly that a low urinary 2 : 16α-hydroxyestrone ratio is a risk factor for breast cancer and that a high crucifer diet, indole-3-carbinol, or diindolylmethane can each elevate the ratio (Bradlow and Sepkovic, 2002). Furthermore, tamoxifen and diindolylmethane appear to work by independent means, possibly suggesting a role for indolyl products in addition to tamoxifen in women at high risk for breast cancer (Cover et al., 1999).

Patients with laryngeal papillomas require periodic surgery. When patients were given daily indole-3-carbinol for 8 months, there was a cessation in the growth of papillomas in six patients and these patients did not require surgery. Six patients showed reduced papilloma growth, and the other six did not respond to the treatment (Rosen et al., 1998). Another small trial evaluated the effect of indole-3-carbinol on women with cervical epithelial neoplasia (CIN). Thirty individuals in stage II or III CIN were randomized to placebo, 200 or 400 mg/day of oral indole-3-carbinol. After 12 weeks of treatments, 50% of those taking 200 mg and

45% of those taking 400 mg exhibited complete regression and did not need surgery (Bell et al., 2000). Although a key stumbling block has been the purification of sufficient quantities to perform clinical trials, there is a move toward developing isothiocyanates as prophylactic treatment for individuals at high risk for recurrent adenoma or papilloma. Phase I pharmacokinetic studies have been initiated using PEITC (Conaway et al., 2002), and methods are being developed for the estimation of urinary products of other isothiocyanates. The next few years should see considerable development in the evaluation of glucosinolate derivatives as chemopreventive tools in medicine.

Safety of Glucosinolate Derivatives

Before glucosinolate derivatives can be used in supernutritional amounts, they must be evaluated for adverse effects. Early studies on feeding rapeseed meal to livestock can act as pointers to suggest which adverse effects might occur at higher than usual intake levels. Rapeseed meal is a rich source of the nitrile crambene (cyanohydroxybutene), which may be present at 10- or even 50-fold the amount typically found in cruciferous vegetables. Hepatic, renal, and pancreatic lesions, as well as thyroid enlargement, have been associated with these high doses (Papas et al., 1979; Wallig et al., 1992). Feeding a rapeseed meal diet to both poultry and laboratory animals has been reported to cause growth retardation, weight loss, and liver necrosis (Tookey et al., 1980). Such adverse effects have not been reported in individuals consuming a crucifer-rich diet because the content of glucosinolates in a serving of cruciferous vegetables, 500 mg or less, is a fraction of that present in a 40% rapeseed meal diet, 3–5 g/00 g feed (Kloss et al., 1994). Cruciferous vegetables are a rich source of vitamin K, often providing the entire daily requirement in a single serving, causing physicians to advise patients taking coumadin or related anticoagulant drugs to exclude crucifers from their diets, because coumadin functions by inhibiting the recycling of vitamin K. Another concern has been raised that consumption of a diet rich in cruciferous vegetables might cause goiter. The oxzaolidine-2-thione derivatives of glucosinolates have been shown to inhibit incorporation of iodine into precursors of thyroxine and thus to interfere with secretion of thyroxine hormone (Tookey et al., 1980). Even if glucosinolate-containing foods are not the primary cause of goiter, it is possible that they might aggravate goiter formation in individuals with very low iodine intake. However, even taking this into consideration, based on serving size, several studies have concluded that eating cruciferous vegetables is not a public health concern (Tookey et al., 1980). Nevertheless, there may be a need to examine the antinutritional effects of glucosinolate derivatives, because over the past decade, with the growing interest in glucosinolate derivatives for their anticarcinogenic properties, intake has increased in some sectors of society (Mithen et al., 2000). For example, encapsulated broccoli concentrates are available over the counter as dietary supplements. Manufacturers of dietary supplements are not required to carry out extensive preclinical or clinical safety evaluations on their products. Whereas a small randomized trial evaluating the use of a broccoli supplement reported no adverse effects, no beneficial effects were reported either, suggesting that larger doses may soon be evaluated (Clapper et al., 1997). With the use of extracts or concentrates, the daily intake of glucosinolates has the potential to be increased many fold, highlighting the need for safety studies. In one study, purified PEITC (0.1% of the diet) was fed to rats for 32 weeks and caused weight loss and bladder carcinoma in >50% of the rats over the following 16-week period (Sugiura et al., 2003). Thus, administration of glucosinolate derivatives in supplements and purified powders may cause harm at the elevated doses possible with supplements. Another possibility is that ingestion of purified glucosinolates or derivatives may have very different effects to the whole food, even if taken in similar amounts to those found in the diet. For these reasons, there is a growing need for research to determine the safe upper levels for intake of glucosinolate derivatives, both purified and within cruciferous vegetables. However, it is also necessary to maintain a perspective on the need for concern due to adverse effects that are only reported for extremely high intake levels.

CONCLUSION

There is an abundant literature on epidemiological, animal, and mechanistic studies strongly supporting a role for cruciferous vegetables in prevention of cancers. These have led to promising results in a few small clinical trials. They have also encouraged plant breeders and food manufacturers to take up projects to improve the content of glucosinolates and their bioactive derivatives in crucifers and crucifer-containing food products. There are ongoing research efforts to create both vegetable varieties with enhanced glucosinolate levels and a database quantifying glucosinolates in many commonly consumed cruciferous vegetables. Dietary supplements containing glucosinolates or their bioactive derivatives are also commonly available. However, there are still areas that need further research if the full health benefits of dietary crucifers are to be recognized. Further details on absorption, metabolism, and mechanism of action are necessary if we are to determine an effective dietary portion/quota/allocation. Most importantly, safety studies are needed that evaluate both safe upper limits and potential interactions between these bioactive compounds and cancer chemotherapeutics. With the advances that are occurring in the field, the goal of using cruciferous vegetables for dietary cancer prevention may soon become a reality.

References

Bell, M.C., Crowley-Nowick, P., Bradlow, H.L., Sepkovic, D.W., Schmidt-Grimminger, D., Howell, P., Mayeaux, E.J., Tucker, A., Turbat-Herrera, E.A., and Mathis, J.M. 2000. Placebo-controlled trial of indole-3-carbinol in the treatment of CIN. *Gynecol Oncol* **78**(2): 123–129.

Bennett, R.N., Mellon, F.A., Foidl, N., Pratt, J.H., Dupont, M.S., Perkins, L., and Kroon, P.A. 2003. Profiling glucosinolates and phenolics in vegetative and reproductive tissues of the multi-purpose trees *Moringa oleifera* L. (horseradish tree) and *Moringa stenopetala* L. *J Agric Food Chem* **51**(12): 3546–3553.

Bradlow, H.L., and Sepkovic, D.W. 2002. Diet and breast cancer. *Ann N Y Acad Sci* **963**: 247–267.

Brown, A.F., Yousef, G.G., Jeffery, E.H., Klein, B.P., Wallig, M.A., Kushad, M.M., and Juvik, J.A. 2002. Glucosinolates profiles in broccoli: variation in levels and implications in breeding for cancer chemoprotection. *J Am Soc Hortic Sci* **127**(5): 807–813.

Carlson, D.G., Daxenbichler, M.E., and VanEtten, C.H. 1987. Glucosinolates in cruciferous vegetables: broccoli, Brussels sprouts, cauliflower, collards, kale, mustard greens and kohlrabi. *J Am Soc Hortic Sci* **112**(1): 173–178.

Chen, C., and Kong, A.N. 2004. Dietary chemopreventive compounds and ARE/EpRE signaling. *Free Radic Biol Med* **36**(12): 1505–1516.

Chen, I., McDougal, A., Wang, F., and Safe, S. 1998. Aryl hydrocarbon receptor-mediated antiestrogenic and antitumorigenic activity of diindolylmethane. *Carcinogenesis* **19**(9): 1631–1639.

Chung, F.L., Conaway, C.C., Rao, C.V., and Reddy, B.S. 2000. Chemoprevention of colonic aberrant crypt foci in Fischer rats by sulforaphane and phenethyl isothiocyanate. *Carcinogenesis* **21**(12): 2287–2291.

Clapper, M.L., Szarka, C.E., Pfeiffer, G.R., Graham, T.A., Balshem, A.M., Litwin, S., Goosenberg, E.B., Frucht, H., and Engstrom, P.F. 1997. Preclinical and clinical evaluation of broccoli supplements as inducers of glutathione S-transferase activity. *Clin Cancer Res* **3**(1): 25–30.

Cohen, J.H., Kristal, A.R., and Stanford, J.L. 2000. Fruit and vegetable intakes and prostate cancer risk. *J Natl Cancer Inst* **92**(1): 61–68.

Conaway, C.C., Getahun, S.M., Liebes, L.L., Pusateri, D.J., Topham, D.K., Botero-Omary, M., and Chung, F.L. 2000. Disposition of glucosinolates and sulforaphane in humans after ingestion of steamed and fresh broccoli. *Nutr Cancer* **38**(2): 168–178.

Conaway, C.C., Yang, Y.M., and Chung, F.L. 2002. Isothiocyanates as cancer chemopreventive agents: their biological activities and metabolism in rodents and humans. *Curr Drug Metab* **3**(3): 233–255.

Cover, C.M., Hsieh, S.J., Cram, E.J., Hong, C., Riby, J.E., Bjeldanes, L.F., and Firestone, G.L. 1999. Indole-3-carbinol and tamoxifen cooperate to arrest the cell cycle of MCF-7 human breast cancer cells. *Cancer Res* **59**(6): 1244–1251.

DeMarini, D.M., Hastings, S.B., Brooks, L.R., Eischen, B.T., Bell, D.A., Watson, M.A., Felton, J.S., Sandler, R., and Kohlmeier, L. 1997. Pilot study of free and conjugated urinary mutagenicity during consumption of pan-fried meats: possible modulation by cruciferous vegetables, glutathione S-transferase-M1, and N-acetyltransferase-2. *Mutat Res* **381**(1): 83–96.

Duncan, A.J., Rabot, S., and Nugon-Baudon. 1997. Urinary mercapturic acids as markers for the determination of isothiocyanate release from glucosinolates in rats fed a cauliflower diet. *J Sci Food Agric* **73**: 214–220.

Fahey, J.W., Zhang, Y., and Talalay, P. 1997. Broccoli sprouts: an exceptionally rich source of inducers of enzymes that protect against chemical carcinogens. *Proc Natl Acad Sci USA* **94**(19): 10367–10372.

Fahey, J.W., Zalcmann, A.T., and Talalay, P. 2001. The chemical diversity and distribution of glucosinolates and isothiocyanates among plants. *Phytochemistry* **56**(1): 5–51.

Fahey, J.W., Haristoy, X., Dolan, P.M., Kensler, T.W., Scholtus, I., Stephenson, K.K., Talalay, P., and Lozniewski, A. 2002. Sulforaphane inhibits extracellular, intracellular, and antibiotic-resistant strains of *Helicobacter pylori* and prevents benzo[a]pyrene-induced stomach tumors. *Proc Natl Acad Sci USA* **99**(11): 7610–7615.

Fenwick, G.R., Heaney, R.K., and Mullin, W.J. 1983. Glucosinolates and their breakdown products in food and food plants. *Crit Rev Food Sci Nutr* **18**(2): 123–201.

Fowke, J.H., Longcope, C., and Hebert, J.R. 2000. Brassica vegetable consumption shifts estrogen metabolism in healthy postmenopausal women. *Cancer Epidemiol Biomarkers Prev* **9**(8): 773–779.

Fowke, J.H., Chung, F.L., Jin, F., Qi, D., Cai, Q., Conaway, C., Cheng, J.R., Shu, X.O., Gao, Y.T., and Zheng, W. 2003a. Urinary isothiocyanate levels, Brassica, and human breast cancer. *Cancer Res* **63**(14): 3980–3986.

Fowke, J.H., Shu, X.O., Dai, Q., Shintani, A., Conaway, C.C., Chung, F.L., Cai, Q., Gao, Y.T., and Zheng, W. 2003b. Urinary isothiocyanate excretion, Brassica consumption, and gene polymorphisms among women living in Shanghai, China. *Cancer Epidemiol Biomarkers Prev* **12**(12): 1536–1539.

Hecht, S.S. 1995. Chemoprevention by isothiocyanates. *J Cell Biochem Suppl* **22**: 195–209.

Hecht, S.S. 1999. Chemoprevention of cancer by isothiocyanates, modifiers of carcinogen metabolism. *J Nutr* **129**(3): 768S–774S.

Hecht, S.S. 2000. Inhibition of carcinogenesis by isothiocyanates. *Drug Metab Rev* **32**(3-4): 395–411.

Hecht, S.S., Chung, F.L., Richie, J.P., Jr., Akerkar, S.A., Borukhova, A., Skowronski, L., and Carmella, S.G. 1995. Effects of watercress consumption on metabolism of a tobacco-specific lung carcinogen in smokers. *Cancer Epidemiol Biomarkers Prev* **4**(8): 877–884.

Hintze, K.J., Keck, A.S., Finley, J.W., and Jeffery, E.H. 2003. Induction of hepatic thioredoxin reductase activity by sulforaphane, both in Hepa1c1c7 cells and in male Fisher 344 rats. *J Nutr Biochem* **14**(3): 173–179.

Hu, R., Kim, B.R., Chen, C., Hebbar, V., and Kong, A.N. 2003. The roles of JNK and apoptotic signaling pathways in PEITC-mediated responses in human HT-29 colon adenocarcinoma cells. *Carcinogenesis* **24**(8): 1361–1367.

Huang, C., Ma, W.Y., Li, J., Hecht, S.S., and Dong, Z. 1998. Essential role of p53 in phenethyl isothiocyanate-induced apoptosis. *Cancer Res* **58**(18): 4102–4106.

Jain, M.G., Hislop, G.T., Howe, G.R., and Ghadirian, P. 1999. Plant foods, antioxidants, and prostate cancer risk: findings from case–control studies in Canada. *Nutr Cancer* **34**(2): 173–184.

Jeffery, E.H., and Jarrell, V. 2001. Cruciferous vegetables and cancer prevention. *In* "Handbook of Nutraceuticals and Functional Foods" (W.R.E.C.), pp. 169–191. CRC Press, Boca Raton, FL.

Jellinck, P.H., Forkert, P.G., Riddick, D.S., Okey, A.B., Michnovicz, J.J., and Bradlow, H.L. 1993. Ah receptor binding properties of indole carbinols and induction of hepatic estradiol hydroxylation. *Biochem Pharmacol* **45**(5): 1129–1136.

Kall, M.A., Vang, O., and Clausen, J. 1996. Effects of dietary broccoli on human *in vivo* drug metabolizing enzymes: evaluation of caffeine, oestrone and chlorzoxazone metabolism. *Carcinogenesis* **17**(4): 793–799.

Kassie, F., Rabot, S., Uhl, M., Huber, W., Qin, H.M., Helma, C., Schulte-Hermann, R., and Knasmuller, S. 2002. Chemoprotective effects of garden cress (*Lepidium sativum*) and its constituents towards 2-amino-3-methyl-imidazo[4,5-f]quinoline (IQ)–induced genotoxic effects and colonic preneoplastic lesions. *Carcinogenesis* **23**(7): 1155–1161.

Kassie, F., Uhl, M., Rabot, S., Grasl-Kraupp, B., Verkerk, R., Kundi, M., Chabicovsky, M., Schulte-Hermann, R., and Knasmuller, S. 2003. Chemoprevention of 2-amino-3-methylimidazo[4,5-f]quinoline (IQ)–induced colonic and hepatic preneoplastic lesions in the F344 rat by cruciferous vegetables administered simultaneously with the carcinogen. *Carcinogenesis* **24**(2): 255–261.

Keck, A.S., Staack, R., and Jeffery, E.H. 2002. The cruciferous nitrile crambene has bioactivity similar to sulforaphane when administered to

Fischer 344 rats but is far less potent in cell culture. *Nutr Cancer Int J* **42**(2): 233–240.

Keck, A.S., Qiao, Q., and Jeffery, E.H. 2003. Food matrix effects on bioactivity of broccoli-derived sulforaphane in liver and colon of F344 rats. *J Agric Food Chem* **51**(11): 3320–3327.

Kiddle, G., Bennett, R.N., Botting, N.P., Davidson, N.E., Robertson, A.A., and Wallsgrove, R.M. 2001. High-performance liquid chromatographic separation of natural and synthetic desulphoglucosinolates and their chemical validation by UV, NMR and chemical ionisation-MS methods. *Phytochem Anal* **12**(4): 226–242.

Kloss, P., Jeffrey, E., Wallig, M., Tumbleson, M., Parsons, C., Johnson, L., and Reuber, M. 1994. Efficacy of feeding glucosinolate-extracted crambe meal to broiler chicks. *Poult Sci* **73**(10): 1542–1551.

Kohlmeier, L., and Su, L. 1997. Cruciferous vegetables consumption and colorectal cancer risk: meta-analysis of the epidemiological evidence. *FASEB J* **11**(A369).

Kolonel, L.N., Hankin, J.H., Whittemore, A.S., Wu, A.H., Gallagher, R.P., Wilkens, L.R., John, E.M., Howe, G.R., Dreon, D.M., West, D.W., and Paffenbarger, R.S., Jr. 2000. Vegetables, fruits, legumes and prostate cancer: a multiethnic case–control study. *Cancer Epidemiol Biomarkers Prev* **9**(8): 795–804.

Kristal, A.R., and Lampe, J.W. 2002. Brassica vegetables and prostate cancer risk: a review of the epidemiological evidence. *Nutr Cancer* **42**(1): 1–9.

Kushad, M.M., Brown, A.F., Kurilich, A.C., Juvik, J.A., Klein, B.P., Wallig, M.A., and Jeffery, E.H. 1999. Variation of glucosinolates in vegetable crops of *Brassica oleracea*. *J Agric Food Chem* **47**(4): 1541–1548.

Lampe, J.W., and Peterson, S. 2002. Brassica, biotransformation and cancer risk: genetic polymorphisms alter the preventive effects of cruciferous vegetables. *J Nutr* **132**(10): 2991–2994.

Lin, H.J., Zhou, H., Dai, A., Huang, H.F., Lin, J.H., Frankl, H.D., Lee, E.R., and Haile, R.W. 2002. Glutathione transferase GSTT1, broccoli, and prevalence of colorectal adenomas. *Pharmacogenetics* **12**(2): 175–179.

Lin, J.M., Amin, S., Trushin, N., and Hecht, S.S. 1993. Effects of isothiocyanates on tumorigenesis by benzo[a]pyrene in murine tumor models. *Cancer Lett* **74**(3): 151–159.

Matusheski, N.V., Juvik, J.A., and Jeffery, E.H. 2004. Heating decreases epithiospecifier protein activity and increases sulforaphane formation in broccoli. *Phytochemistry* **65**(9): 1273–1281.

McNaughton, S.A., and Marks, G.C. 2003. Development of a food composition database for the estimation of dietary intakes of glucosinolates, the biologically active constituents of cruciferous vegetables. *Br J Nutr* **90**(3): 687–697.

Michaud, D.S., Spiegelman, D., Clinton, S.K., Rimm, E.B., Willett, W.C., and Giovannucci, E.L. 1999. Fruit and vegetable intake and incidence of bladder cancer in a male prospective cohort. *J Natl Cancer Inst* **91**(7): 605–613.

Mithen, R., Faulkner, K., Magrath, R., Rose, P., Williamson, G., and Marquez, J. 2003. Development of isothiocyanate-enriched broccoli, and its enhanced ability to induce phase 2 detoxification enzymes in mammalian cells. *Theor Appl Genet* **106**(4): 727–734.

Mithen, R.F., Dekker, M., Verkerk, R., Rabot, S., and Johnson, I.T. 2000. The nutritional significance, biosynthesis and bioavailability of glucosinolates in human foods. *J Sci Food Agric* **80**(7): 967–984.

Munday, R., and Munday, C.M. 2004. Induction of phase II detoxification enzymes in rats by plant-derived isothiocyanates: comparison of allyl isothiocyanate with sulforaphane and related compounds. *J Agric Food Chem* **52**(7): 1867–1871.

Murillo, G., and Mehta, R.G. 2001. Cruciferous vegetables and cancer prevention. *Nutr Cancer* **41**(1-2): 17–28.

Murray, S., Lake, B.G., Gray, S., Edwards, A.J., Springall, C., Bowey, E.A., Williamson, G., Boobis, A.R., and Gooderham, N.J. 2001. Effect of cruciferous vegetable consumption on heterocyclic aromatic amine metabolism in man. *Carcinogenesis* **22**(9): 1413–1420.

Myzak, M.C., Karplus, P.A., Chung, F.L., and Dashwood, R.H. 2004. A novel mechanism of chemoprotection by sulforaphane: inhibition of histone deacetylase. *Cancer Res* **64**(16): 5767–5774.

Nagle, C.M., Purdie, D.M., Webb, P.M., Green, A., Harvey, P.W., and Bain, C.J. 2003. Dietary influences on survival after ovarian cancer. *Int J Cancer* **106**: 264–269.

Pantuck, E.J., Pantuck, C.B., Garland, W.A., Min, B.H., Wattenberg, L.W., Anderson, K.E., Kappas, A., and Conney, A.H. 1979. Stimulatory effect of Brussels sprouts and cabbage on human drug metabolism. *Clin Pharmacol Ther* **25**(1): 88–95.

Papas, A., Ingalls, J.R., and Campbell, L.D. 1979. Studies on the effects of rapeseed meal on thyroid status of cattle, glucosinolate and iodine content of milk and other parameters. *J Nutr* **109**(7): 1129–1139.

Price, W.D., Lovell, R.A., and McChesney, D.G. 1993. Naturally occurring toxins in feedstuffs: Center for Veterinary Medicine Perspective. *J Anim Sci* **71**(9): 2556–2562.

Rijken, P.J., Timmer, W.G., van de Kooij, A.J., van Benschop, I.M., Wiseman, S.A., Meijers, M., and Tijburg, L.B. 1999. Effect of vegetable and carotenoid consumption on aberrant crypt multiplicity, a surrogate end-point marker for colorectal cancer in azoxymethane-induced rats. *Carcinogenesis* **20**(12): 2267–2272.

Rosa, E.A.S., Heaney, R.K., Fenwick, G.R., and Portas, C.A.M. 1997. Glucosinolates in crop plants. *In* "Horticultural Reviews" (J. Janick, ed.), Vol. 19, pp. 99–215. John Wiley & Sons, Indianapolis, IN.

Rosen, C.A., Woodson, G.E., Thompson, J.W., Hengesteg, A.P., and Bradlow, H.L. 1998. Preliminary results of the use of indole-3-carbinol for recurrent respiratory papillomatosis. *Otolaryngol Head Neck Surg* **118**(6): 810–815.

Sanderson, J.T., Slobbe, L., Lansbergen, G.W., Safe, S., and van den Berg, M. 2001. 2,3,7,8-Tetrachlorodibenzo-p-dioxin and diindolylmethanes differentially induce cytochrome P450 1A1, 1B1, and 19 in H295R human adrenocortical carcinoma cells. *Toxicol Sci* **61**(1): 40–48.

Shapiro, T.A., Fahey, J.W., Wade, K.L., Stephenson, K.K., and Talalay, P. 1998. Human metabolism and excretion of cancer chemoprotective glucosinolates and isothiocyanates of cruciferous vegetables. *Cancer Epidemiol Biomarkers Prev* **7**(12): 1091–1100.

Smith, T.K., Lund, E.K., and Johnson, I.T. 1998. Inhibition of dimethylhydrazine-induced aberrant crypt foci and induction of apoptosis in rat colon following oral administration of the glucosinolate sinigrin. *Carcinogenesis* **19**(2): 267–273.

Smith, T.K., Mithen, R., and Johnson, I.T. 2003. Effects of Brassica vegetable juice on the induction of apoptosis and aberrant crypt foci in rat colonic mucosal crypts *in vivo*. *Carcinogenesis* **24**(3): 491–495.

Spitz, M.R., Duphorne, C.M., Detry, M.A., Pillow, P.C., Amos, C.I., Lei, L., de Andrade, M., Gu, X., Hong, W.K., and Wu, X. 2000. Dietary intake of isothiocyanates: evidence of a joint effect with glutathione *S*-transferase polymorphisms in lung cancer risk. *Cancer Epidemiol Biomarkers Prev* **9**(10): 1017–1020.

Srivastava, S.K., Xiao, D., Lew, K.L., Hershberger, P., Kokkinakis, D.M., Johnson, C.S., Trump, D.L., and Singh, S.V. 2003. Allyl isothiocyanate, a constituent of cruciferous vegetables, inhibits growth of PC-3 human prostate cancer xenografts *in vivo*. *Carcinogenesis* **24**(10): 1665–1670.

Sugiura, S., Ogawa, K., Hirose, M., Takeshita, F., Asamoto, M., and Shirai, T. 2003. Reversibility of proliferative lesions and induction of non-papillary tumors in rat urinary bladder treated with phenylethyl isothiocyanate. *Carcinogenesis* **24**(3): 547–553.

Talalay, P., and Fahey, J.W. 2001. Phytochemicals from cruciferous plants protect against cancer by modulating carcinogen metabolism. *J Nutr* **131**(11 Suppl): 3027S–3033S.

Thimmulappa, R.K., Mai, K.H., Srisuma, S., Kensler, T.W., Yamamoto, M., and Biswal, S. 2002. Identification of Nrf2-regulated genes induced by the chemopreventive agent sulforaphane by oligonucleotide microarray. *Cancer Res* **62**(18): 5196–5203.

Thornalley, P.J. 2002. Isothiocyanates: mechanism of cancer chemopreventive action. *Anticancer Drugs* **13**(4): 331–338.

Tookey, H.L., VanEtten, C.H., and Daxenbichler, M.E. 1980. Glucosinolates. *In* "Toxic Constituents of Plant Foodstuffs" (I.E. Liener, ed.), pp. 103–141. Academic Press, New York.

USDA-NASS Agricultural Statistics: Vegetables and melons (2003). Available at: http://www.usda.gov/nass/pubs/agr03/03_ch4.pdf, IV-31 and IV-35.

Verhoeven, D.T., Goldbohm, R.A., van Poppel, G., Verhagen, H., and van den Brandt, P.A. 1996. Epidemiological studies on Brassica vegetables and cancer risk. *Cancer Epidemiol Biomarkers Prev* **5**(9): 733–748.

Verhoeven, D.T., Verhagen, H., Goldbohm, R.A., van den Brandt, P.A., and van Poppel, G. 1997. A review of mechanisms underlying anticarcinogenicity by Brassica vegetables. *Chem Biol Interact* **103**(2): 79–129.

Wallig, M.A., Kore, A.M., Crawshaw, J., and Jeffery, E.H. 1992. Separation of the toxic and glutathione-enhancing effects of the naturally occurring nitrile, cyanohydroxybutene. *Fundam Appl Toxicol* **19**(4): 598–606.

Wattenberg, L.W., and Loub, W.D. 1978. Inhibition of polycyclic aromatic hydrocarbon-induced neoplasia by naturally occurring indoles. *Cancer Res* **38**(5): 1410–1413.

Wittstock, U., and Halkier, B.A. 2002. Glucosinolate research in the Arabidopsis era. *Trends Plant Sci* **7**(6): 263–270.

Xiao, D., and Singh, S.V. 2002. Phenethyl isothiocyanate-induced apoptosis in p53-deficient PC-3 human prostate cancer cell line is mediated by extracellular signal-regulated kinases. *Cancer Res* **62**(13): 3615–3619.

Xiao, D., Srivastava, S.K., Lew, K.L., Zeng, Y., Hershberger, P., Johnson, C.S., Trump, D.L., and Singh, S.V. 2003. Allyl isothiocyanate, a constituent of cruciferous vegetables, inhibits proliferation of human prostate cancer cells by causing G2/M arrest and inducing apoptosis. *Carcinogenesis* **24**(5): 891–897.

Xu, M., Orner, G.A., Bailey, G.S., Stoner, G.D., Horio, D.T., and Dashwood, R.H. 2001. Post-initiation effects of chlorophyllin and indole-3-carbinol in rats given 1,2-dimethylhydrazine or 2-amino-3-methyl-imidazo. *Carcinogenesis* **22**(2): 309–314.

Ye, L., Dinkova-Kostova, A.T., Wade, K.L., Zhang, Y., Shapiro, T.A., and Talalay, P. 2002. Quantitative determination of dithiocarbamates in human plasma, serum, erythrocytes and urine: pharmacokinetics of broccoli sprout isothiocyanates in humans. *Clin Chim Acta* **316**(1-2): 43–53.

Yuan, J.M., Gago-Dominguez, M., Castelao, J.E., Hankin, J.H., Ross, R.K., and Yu, M.C. 1998. Cruciferous vegetables in relation to renal cell carcinoma. *Int J Cancer* **77**(2): 211–216.

Zhang, S.M., Hunter, D.J., Rosner, B.A., Giovannucci, E.L., Colditz, G.A., Speizer, F.E., and Willett, W.C. 2000. Intakes of fruits, vegetables, and related nutrients and the risk of non-Hodgkin's lymphoma among women. *Cancer Epidemiol Biomarkers Prev* **9**(5): 477–485.

Zhang, Y., Kensler, T.W., Cho, C.G., Posner, G.H., and Talalay, P. 1994. Anticarcinogenic activities of sulforaphane and structurally related synthetic norbornyl isothiocyanates. *Proc Natl Acad Sci USA* **91**(8): 3147–3150.

Zhang, Y., and Callaway, E.C. 2002. High cellular accumulation of sulphoraphane, a dietary anticarcinogen, is followed by rapid transporter-mediated export as a glutathione conjugate. *Biochem J* **364**(Pt 1): 301–307.

Zhang, Y., Tang, L., and Gonzalez, V. 2003. Selected isothiocyanates rapidly induce growth inhibition of cancer cells. *Mol Cancer Ther* **2**(10): 1045–1052.

Zhao, B., Seow, A., Lee, E.J., Poh, W.T., Teh, M., Eng, P., Wang, Y.T., Tan, W.C., Yu, M.C., and Lee, H.P. 2001. Dietary isothiocyanates, glutathione S-transferase -M1, -T1 polymorphisms and lung cancer risk among Chinese women in Singapore. *Cancer Epidemiol Biomarkers Prev* **10**(10): 1063–1067.

C H A P T E R

35

Green Tea

JANELLE M. LANDAU, JOSHUA D. LAMBERT, AND CHUNG S. YANG

INTRODUCTION

Many studies suggest that green tea consumption may promote good health and prevent cancer. Scientific investigation in cell culture and animal studies continues to show promise in this regard. Ambiguous results from epidemiological studies, however, prevent forming a declarative statement for the cancer preventive effects of tea in humans. Possible explanations for the varied results from human studies could be related to the organ site investigated, the type and amount of tea consumed, or lifestyle confounding factors. In this chapter, we discuss the chemistry, oxidative-reduction properties, metabolism, and bioavailability of green tea polyphenols, as well as their possible cancer prevention activities and mechanisms in animals and humans.

More than 12 centuries ago, tea became a popular drink in China. When sailors began to bring tea to England from Asia around 1644, tea began to replace ale as the national drink of England. Tea shrubs were introduced in the United States in 1799, and in 1901, Thomas Sullivan developed the first tea bag. Tea is now second only to water as the world's most consumed beverage.

All tea comes from *Camellia sinensis*, a warm-weather evergreen. Tea is grown in thousands of tea gardens around the world, resulting in thousands of flavorful variations. Leaves of the *C. sinensis* plant are dried for stability and shelf life. Various processing techniques and the extent of oxygen exposure determine the type of tea that is produced from the fresh tea leaves. In the manufacturing of green tea, the leaves are steamed, rolled, and dried with minimum oxidation of the constituents. In black tea production, the leaves are crushed to allow enzyme-catalyzed oxidation of polyphenolic compounds, leading to polymerization and other chemical reactions that produce the distinctive color and taste of black tea. Oolong tea falls somewhere between green and black teas, in that the polyphenols in leaves are only partially oxidized. Tea is also divided by grades, determined by the leaf size. Herbal teas are not from the *C. sinensis* plant and, therefore, require completely different categorizing. For the purposes of this chapter, we discuss green tea, whose composition is similar to that of fresh tea leaves.

The notion that tea may aid in the prevention of certain diseases and may promote good health is quite popular. Indeed, many animal studies and *in vitro* experiments have shown beneficial health effects of green tea, including the prevention of cardiovascular disease and cancer. Strong evidence for such beneficial health effects in humans, however, is scarce. This chapter discusses the chemistry, oxidative properties, and bioavailability of green tea polyphenols, as well as their possible cancer prevention activities and mechanisms in animals and humans.

TEA CHEMISTRY AND OXIDATION-REDUCTION PROPERTIES

The dried green tea leaves preserve the original constituents in the tea leaves. The characteristic polyphenolic compounds in tea are known as *catechins*, which include (−)-epigallocatechin-3-gallate (EGCG), (−)-epigallocatechin (EGC), (−)-epicatechin-3-gallate (ECG), and (−)-epicatechin (EC), with EGCG being the major catechin in tea (Figure 1) (Balentine et al., 1997). Polyphenolic structures are characterized by several hydroxyl groups on aromatic rings. These catechins (or flavonols) are made in plants for the purpose of defense against ultraviolet (UV) radiation, herbivores, and

Copyright © 2006, Elsevier Inc.
All rights of reproduction in any form reserved.

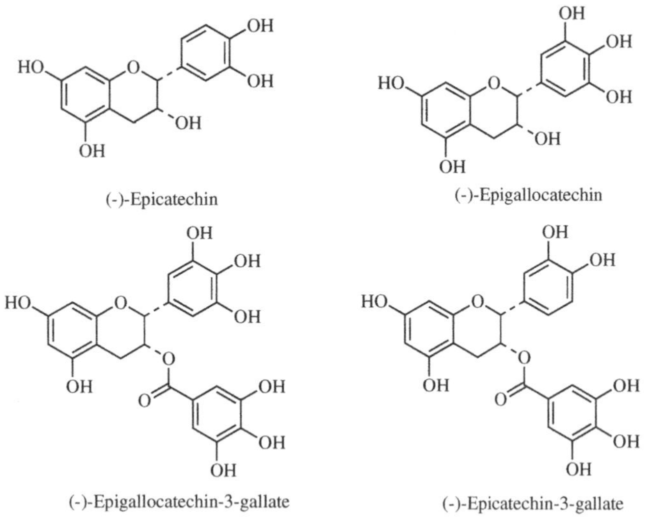

(-)-Epicatechin

(-)-Epigallocatechin

(-)-Epigallocatechin-3-gallate

(-)-Epicatechin-3-gallate

FIGURE 1 Catechin structures.

pathogens. Tea leaves also contain other polyphenols in small quantities such as quercetin, kaempferol, and myricetin, as well as the alkaloids caffeine and theobromine. A typical brewed green tea beverage (e.g., 2.5 g tea leaves in 250 ml of hot water) contains 240–320 mg of catechins and 20–50 mg of caffeine (Balentine et al., 1997).

Tea catechins and other tea polyphenols are efficient scavengers of free radicals. Several functional groups in their structures appear to be important in conferring their low reduction potentials. All catechins have two hydroxyl groups in *ortho* position in the B-ring (Figure 1), which participate in electron delocalization. Both EGC and EGCG have three hydroxyl groups in the B-ring. In ECG and EGCG, the hydroxyl group at the 3 position in the C-ring is esterified with gallic acid, thus providing three more hydroxyl groups. The tri-hydroxyl group in both the B-ring and the gallate moiety have been associated with increased antioxidant activity. There is also some evidence that the A-ring of EGC and EGCG may provide an antioxidant site (Zhu et al., 2000).

Whereas tea polyphenols have been shown to have strong antioxidant activity *in vitro*, such activity has been demonstrated only in some *in vivo* experiments (reviewed by Higdon and Frei, 2003). An intervention trial among smokers found that green tea consumption decreased oxidative DNA damage (Hakim et al., 2003). Urinary 8-hydroxydeoxyguanosine (8-OHdG) levels were 31% lower after 4 months of decaffeinated green tea (4 cups/day) consumption. The relevance of this biomarker and the importance of this antioxidative mechanism in the inhibition of carcinogenesis require further investigation. On the other hand, studies have suggested that the cell-killing activity of tea polyphenols, at least *in vitro*, may be related to their pro-oxidant activity. For example, we have shown that EGCG-induced apoptosis in H661 human lung cancer cells and Ras-transformed human bronchial cells is completely or partially blocked by the inclusion in the medium of catalase, which catalyzes the decomposition of H_2O_2 (Yang et al., 1998, 2000). When EGCG was added to cell culture medium, H_2O_2 was produced (Hong et al., 2002). Preincubation of cells with EGCG has been shown to block signaling systems induced by the epidermal growth factor (EGF) and platelet-derived growth factor (PDGF). Our results with esophageal squamous cells indicated that this blockage of EGF signaling was associated with the inactivation or degradation of the EGF receptor, and the effect could be abolished by the inclusion of superoxide dismutase, which converts oxygen radicals to H_2O_2, in the preincubation system (unpublished results). The addition of superoxide dismutase also stabilized EGCG and increased its growth inhibition effect. Both of these observations suggest the involvement of EGCG pro-oxidation in some of the reported activities of EGCG *in vitro*. It is not known whether such reactions occur in tissues where antioxidative capacity is much higher and oxygen partial pressure is much lower than that in cell culture medium.

INHIBITION OF CARCINOGENESIS IN ANIMAL MODELS

Green tea has been shown to inhibit carcinogenesis induced by UV light and chemical carcinogens in rodents, as well as spontaneous tumorigenesis in wild-type and genetically modified mice. The organs for which tea has demonstrated a protective effect include the lung, skin, oral cavity, esophagus, stomach, liver, pancreas, bladder, small intestine, colon, and prostate (Yang and Wang, 1993; Yang et al., 2002; Chung et al., 2003).

The lung tumorigenesis model, which exposes A/J mice to 4-(methylnitrosamino)-1-(3-pyridyl)-1-butanone (NNK), has demonstrated that green tea can inhibit tumor formation at several stages. In this model, treatment of female A/J mice with a single dose of NNK results in the formation of pulmonary tumors in nearly every mouse with an average of 9.3 tumors/mouse after 16 weeks. Decaffeinated green tea given as the sole source of drinking fluid during the initiation stage, during the post-initiation stage, or after lung adenoma formation inhibited the number of tumors that were formed (Yang et al., 1998). These results suggest that tea can inhibit lung tumorigenesis at the initiation and promotion stages. Inhibition of tumor invasion and metastasis in transplanted and spontaneous metastatic tumor models by intragastric infusion of green tea or EGCG has also been reported (Sazuka et al., 1995; Taniguchi et al., 1992). Tea has also been shown to inhibit spontaneous lung tumorigenesis (e.g., administration of 1% freshly brewed green tea inhibited the spontaneous development of lung adenoma and rhabdomyosarcoma in A/J mice [Landau et al., 1997]). In this study, the body weights and retroperitoneal fat-pad weights of mice drinking 1% green tea were 14% and 35% lower, respectively, than those of the control mice. Likewise, the inhibition of skin tumorigenesis by caffeine or tea was shown to be closely correlated to the reduction of body fat (Conney et al., 2002). The relationship between tea consumption, lower body fat, and carcinogenesis requires further investigation. Inhibition of lung tumorigenesis by tea preparations has not, however, been unequivocally demonstrated. For example, Witschi et al. (1998) reported that green tea extract did not reduce lung tumor multiplicity in male A/J mice treated with one dose of NNK or in a cigarette smoke–induced lung tumorigenesis model.

Whereas the NNK experiments already described in this chapter used decaffeinated green tea and the cancer preventive activity of EGCG has been demonstrated (Yang et al., 1998), the caffeine in tea is also important in the inhibition of carcinogenesis in some animal models. In the UVB-induced skin carcinogenesis mouse model, caffeine plays a significant role. Orally administered green tea and black tea were effective in reducing the incidence and multiplicity of UVB-induced skin tumors, whereas orally administered decaffeinated teas were much less or not effective (Huang et al., 1997). The addition of caffeine restored the protective activity to the decaffeinated teas. Topical application of caffeine or EGCG to hairless mice that had been pretreated twice weekly for 20 weeks with UVB decreased the multiplicity of skin tumors by 44–72% or 55–66%, respectively (Lu et al., 2002). In addition, both compounds were shown to increase the apoptotic index of the tumors by 56–92%.

The bioavailability of tea constituents is apparently a key factor in determining the effectiveness of tea in inhibiting tumor formation. The oral cavity and digestive tract, which have direct contact with orally administered tea, may receive the most benefit from tea consumption. For example, in the 7, 12-dimethylbenz[a]anthracene (DMBA)–induced hamster model of oral carcinogenesis, treatment with 0.6% green tea, as the sole source of drinking fluid, reduced the number of visible tumors by 35% and tumor volume by 57% (Li et al., 2002). Immunohistochemical assays showed that tea increased the apoptotic index (the percent of cells undergoing programmed cell death) of the tumors while it decreased the proliferation index and microvessel density. Tea preparations have been shown to inhibit esophageal, forestomach, and intestinal cancer. Tea preparations have also been shown to inhibit colon carcinogenesis in several studies, although such an effect was not observed in others (reviewed by Yang et al., 2002).

The transgenic adenocarcinoma of the mouse prostate (TRAMP) model emulates the progressive forms of human prostate cancer without the need for induction with chemicals or hormones. When these mice were given 0.1% green tea extract (which contains the polyphenol levels equivalent to 6 cups of green tea per day) as the source of drinking fluid for 24 weeks, prostate cancer development was inhibited and no metastasis was seen (Gupta et al., 2001). In addition, green tea infusion to TRAMP mice caused inhibition of insulin-like growth factor-1 (IGF-1), restoration of IGF-binding protein-3, and elevation of apoptosis. In a breast cancer model in SCID female mice, IGF-1 was also inhibited by green tea in combination with soy phytochemical concentrate (Zhou et al., 2004). Green tea (1.5%) as the sole source of drinking fluid reduced the mammary tumor weight significantly. A second transplanted tumor model in mice also showed reductions in tumor size with green tea extract consumption (Sartippour et al., 2001). In two other breast cancer models, green tea extract significantly increased the latency period to first tumor formation (Kavanagh et al., 2001; Yanaga et al., 2002). Studies using DMBA to induce mammary tumors in rats, however, showed little or no effect of green tea polyphenols on inhibiting post-initiation, promotion, or progression of mammary carcinogenesis (Hirose et al., 1997; Tanaka et al., 1997).

MECHANISMS OF CANCER PREVENTION

Alterations in Intracellular Signaling Cascades

Activation of the transcription factors activator protein 1 (AP-1) and nuclear factor-κB (NFκB) is commonly seen in carcinogenesis. These transcription factors promote the uncontrolled growth of cells. EGCG and other tea polyphenols have been shown to inhibit the activation of AP-1 and NFκB. Although the antioxidative mechanisms have been implicated in this activity, the results can be better explained by the direct inhibition of specific protein kinases by these tea polyphenols. Several studies using different cell lines have shown that EGCG inhibits the activity of various kinases (Ahmad et al., 2000; Chung et al., 2001; Yang et al., 2001). These include direct inhibition of MAP kinases, and the results are consistent with previous observations that EGCG (5–20 μM) inhibited the phosphorylation of *jun* N-terminal kinase, activation of AP-1, and the transformation of mouse epidermal cells, as well as the suppression of AP-1 activity by topical application of EGCG to B6D2 transgenic mice. Downregulation of AP-1 by tea polyphenols may contribute to the p53 increase and the stress-induced elevation of apoptosis seen in tea-treated cells (Chung et al., 2001).

EGCG has been shown to inhibit the activity of IκB kinase in tumor necrosis factor-α (TNF-α)–stimulated intestinal epithelial cells and lipopolysaccharide (LPS)-stimulated murine macrophages (Yang et al., 2001). In both cases, there was diminished IκB degradation and NFκB activity in response to stimulation. Likewise, Ahmad et al. (2000) demonstrated that EGCG inhibited the activity of NFκB in TNF-α– and LPS-stimulated human epidermoid carcinoma cells. This effect could also be mediated by inhibition of IκB phosphorylation and degradation. The transcription factor NFκB plays important roles in inflammation and in suppressing apoptosis in cancer cells.

Regulation of Cell Cycle

The development of tumors has been associated with the dysfunction of the cell cycle checkpoints and overexpression of growth-promoting cell cycle factors such as cyclin D1 and cyclin-dependent kinases (CDKs) (Diehl, 2002; Semczuk and Jakowicki, 2004). EGCG has been reported to inhibit CDK-2 and -4 (Liang et al., 1999), leading to the inhibition of hyperphosphorylation of the retinoblastoma (Rb) protein and causing G_0/G_1-phase arrest. This type of cell cycle arrest by EGCG has been demonstrated in several human tumor cell lines, including breast, epidermal, prostate, and head and neck squamous cell cancers. The direct inhibition of CDK by EGCG may be a primary event (Liang et al., 1999).

Induction of Apoptosis

Apoptosis is the process by which a damaged cell degrades itself to prevent the proliferation of the genetic damage. Typically, in cancer cells, this cell death is inhibited. EGCG has been reported to induce apoptosis in many cell lines, including leukemia, skin, lung, stomach, and prostate cancer cells (Ahmad et al., 1997; Mukhtar et al., 1999; Yang and Chung, 1999). The H_2O_2 generated in the cell culture system due to autoxidation of EGCG could account for some of the reported apoptotic activity. It appears that EGCG can induce apoptosis by H_2O_2-dependent and H_2O_2-independent pathways. A study by Leone et al. (2003) suggested that certain green tea polyphenols bind to the antiapoptotic proteins Bcl-2 and Bcl-xL and, thus, may prevent inhibition of apoptosis. Using a combination of advanced physical measurements and computational docking studies, these investigators determined that tea polyphenols with a gallate moiety inhibit the aforementioned antiapoptotic proteins at nanomolar levels. If this action does indeed take place in the cells, one would expect to observe the induction of apoptosis with nanomolar amounts of EGCG. However, enhanced apoptosis was usually observed with much higher concentrations of EGCG (20–100 μM) (Yang et al., 2002). Caspase 3 activation has been demonstrated to be required for green tea polyphenol-induced apoptosis. Caspase 3 activity was increased in cells that were treated with green tea polyphenols, and caspase 3–deficient tumor cells did not undergo apoptosis when exposed to polyphenols (Hsu et al., 2003).

Inhibition of Angiogenesis, Invasion, and Metastasis

Angiogenesis, the formation of new blood vessels, is important for tumor development. Tumors induce new blood cell growth to provide a pathway for nutrient and waste transport as it grows larger. Cao and Cao (1999) demonstrated the inhibition of endothelial growth and angiogenesis in the chorioallantoic membrane assay by EGCG (20 μM). They also showed that oral administration of 1.25% green tea to mice inhibited new corneal vessel formation stimulated by vascular endothelial growth factor (VEGF). Several investigators have demonstrated the EGCG inhibits the expression of VEGF in head and neck, breast, and colon carcinoma cells (Jung et al., 2001; Masuda et al., 2002; Sartippour et al., 2002). In the TRAMP mouse model using gene array techniques and immunoblot analysis, the expression of VEGF and matrix metalloproteinases (MMP-2 and MMP-9) were shown to be elevated in the transgenic mice, and these gene expressions were inhibited in TRAMP mice consuming green tea extract (Adhami et al., 2003). EGF receptor (EGFR) is frequently overexpressed in neoplastic cells, activating signaling transduction pathways that promote cell proliferation and tumor progression. EGCG inhibited the autophosphorylation of EGFR in head and neck and breast carcinoma cell lines (Masuda et al., 2001, 2002). Overexpression of MMP has been shown to increase the invasive and metastatic potential of tumor cells, whereas the suppression of these zinc-dependent proteases has been shown to inhibit tumor growth and invasion. EGCG inhibited the activity of secreted MMP-2 and MMP-9 with fairly low doses (8–13 μM) (Garbisa et al., 2001).

Inhibition of Aberrant Arachidonic Acid Metabolism

Arachidonic acid is metabolized by cyclooxygenase (COX) to form prostaglandin E_2 and by 5-, 12-, or 15-lipoxygenase (LOX) to form leukotrienes. Overexpression of COX-2, 5-LOX, and other LOX enzymes is observed in several types of cancers. EGCG has been shown to inhibit the induction of COX-2 in both *in vitro* and *in vivo* systems. EGCG at doses of 100–200 μM reduced COX-2 protein expression and activity in human cartilage cells (Ahmed et al., 2002). Whereas these findings are potentially interesting, the concentrations of EGCG used in the study are 10–100 times greater than those observed *in vivo*. The results must, therefore, be confirmed in animal model or in humans. Mice consuming EGCG before 12-tetradecanoyl-phorbol-13-acetate application to the skin had significantly less COX-2 expression in their skin compared to control mice (Kundu et al., 2003). Inhibition of COX-2 with the ingestion of green tea extract was observed in the colons of rats (Metz et al., 2000) and the skin of mice (Katiyar et al., 1992). Within our laboratory, various catechins were shown to inhibit the formation of COX and LOX-dependent metabolites in human normal and tumor colon microsomes (Hong et al., 2001). ECG and EGCG were the most potent inhibitors.

BIOAVAILABILITY AND METABOLISM

Human Data

An understanding of the processes involved in the absorption, distribution, and metabolism of tea polyphenols is essential for determining their potential actions *in vivo* and their overall significance in human disease prevention. Interindividual variation in the plasma and tissue bioavailability of active tea components is substantial and may result, in part, from genetic polymorphisms in the enzymes involved in polyphenol metabolism and individual variation in colonic microflora (Scalbert and Williamson, 2002).

Several studies of the systemic bioavailability of orally administered green tea and catechins in human volunteers have been conducted (Yang et al., 1998; Chow et al., 2001; Van Amelsvoort et al., 2001; Lee et al., 2002). Most recently, we have shown that oral administration of 20 mg green tea solids/kg body weight resulted in the maximum concentration (C_{max}) of 223, 124, and 77.9 ng/ml in the plasma for EGC, EC, and EGCG, respectively (Lee et al., 2002). Time to reach a maximum concentration (T_{max}) was found to range from 1.3 to 1.6 hours with half-lives ($t_{1/2}$ of 3.4, 1.7, and 2 hours for EGCG, EGC, and EC, respectively). The T_{max} increased with greater dose of catechins (Chow et al., 2001). When the catechins (EGCG, EGC, or ECG) were given individually in a single 1.5-mmol dose with breakfast, the plasma kinetics showed a difference in appearance among the catechins (Van Amelsvoort et al., 2001). The peak value of EGCG, EGC, and ECG occurred at 2.9, 1.4, and 4 hours, respectively; the half-lives were 4, 1.7, and 7, respectively. Plasma EC and EGC were present mainly in the conjugated form, whereas 77% of the EGCG was in the free form (Lee et al., 2002). The data support earlier findings that plasma EGC was present as glucuronide (57–71%) and sulfate (23–36%) with only a small fraction of free EGC (Yang et al., 1998; Chow et al., 2001). Likewise, plasma EC was largely in the sulfated form (66%) with less glucuronide (33%). EGC was also methylated (4′-*O*-methyl-EGC) in humans, and its plasma and urine levels were higher than those of EGC (Lee et al., 2002). Pharmacokinetics and toxicity of EGCG at a dose of 800 mg in pure form or in Polyphenon E (a mixture of the main green tea polyphenols) have been investigated (Chow et al., 2003). These doses were found to be safe and acceptable to humans. However, in a Phase II trial investigating the effect of green tea on patients with prostate carcinomas, a daily dose of 6 g green tea (given in six 1-g doses/day) led to adverse effects in 69% of the subjects, which included nausea, vomiting, insomnia, fatigue, diarrhea, abdominal pain, and confusion (Jatoi et al., 2003). In contrast to previous studies in rodents employing multiple-dose regimens, Chow et al. (2003) have shown that daily dosing with 800 mg EGCG to human volunteers for 4 weeks resulted in a 60% increase in the systemic exposure to free EGCG. This increased availability may be due to alterations in drug-metabolizing enzymes or the accumulation of EGCG in a nonplasma compartment.

Comparison of Human to Rat and Mouse

The pharmacokinetics of EGCG and the other catechins have been investigated in rats, mice, and humans (Yang et al., 2002). Studies of [^{3}H]-EGCG in both rats and mice showed that following a single intragastric (i.g.) dose, radioactivity was distributed throughout the body (Suganuma et al., 1998; Kohri et al., 2001). After 24 hours, 10% of the initial dose of radioactivity was found in the blood with ~1% in the prostate, heart, lungs, liver, kidneys, and other tissues of rats and mice. The major route of elimination was through the feces in both species. In the rat, 77% of an intravenous (IV) dose of [^{3}H]-EGCG was eliminated in the bile, whereas only 2% was eliminated through the urine. Treatment of rats with a green tea polyphenol preparation (0.6% w/v in distilled water) resulted in increased plasma levels of polyphenols over a 14-day period, with levels of EGC and EC being higher than those of EGCG (Kim et al., 2000). Plasma levels then decreased over the subsequent 14 days, suggesting an adaptive effect. EGCG levels were found to be the highest in the rat esophagus, intestine, and colon, which have direct contact with tea catechins, whereas EGCG levels were lower in the bladder, kidneys, liver, lungs, and prostate, which depend on systemic bioavailability. When the same polyphenol preparation was given to mice, the EGCG levels in the plasma, lungs, and liver were much higher than in rats (Kim et al., 2000). On the basis of the numerous biotransformation studies that have been conducted, it appears that mice are more similar to humans than rats in terms of enzymatic ability to conjugate tea catechins.

Metabolites Formed in the Body

Tea polyphenols are extensively metabolized by intestinal and hepatic enzymes and by the intestinal microflora. Knowledge of their bioavailability and metabolism is necessary to evaluate their biological activity within target tissues. The metabolites that are found in blood and target organs may differ from the native substances in terms of biological activity. Our laboratory has proposed a schematic describing the possible factors governing the bioavailability of catechins (Figure 2). This model includes several biotransformations including methylation, glucuronidation,

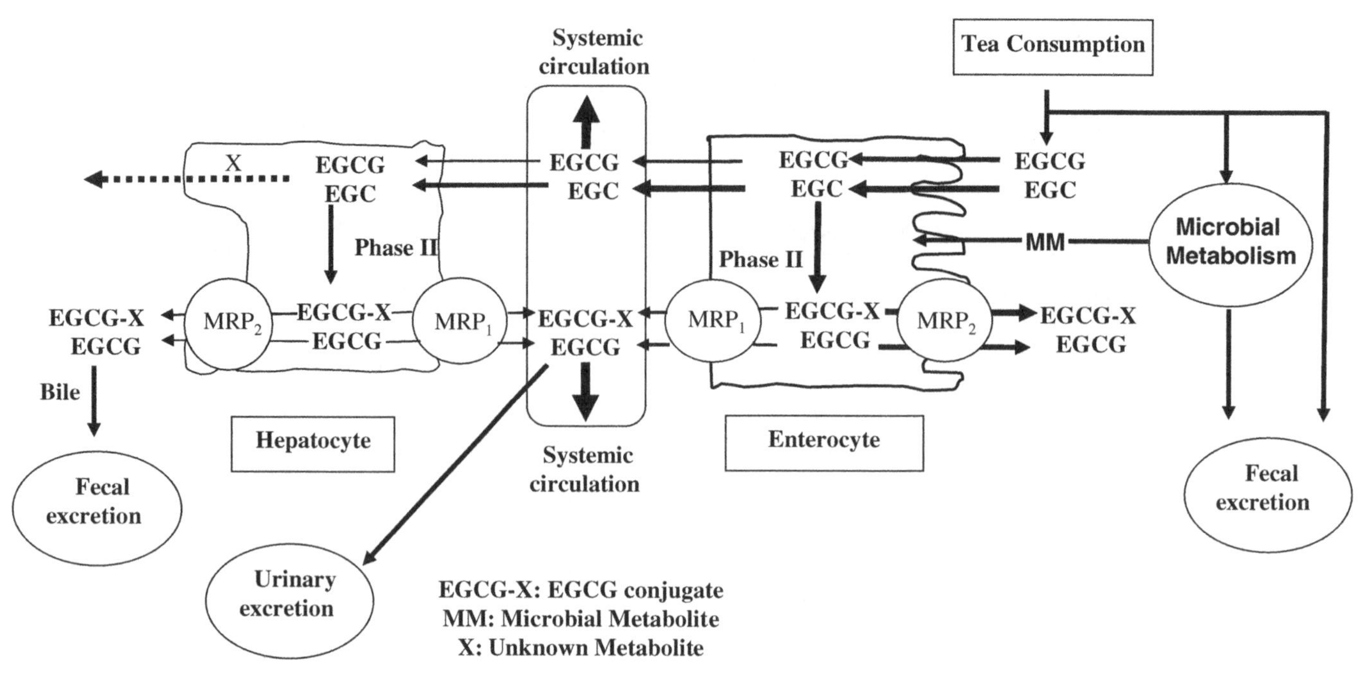

FIGURE 2 **Factors governing bioavailability.** Proposed model illustrating the possible factors governing the bioavailability of tea catechins. Multidrug resistance–associated proteins (MRPs) include MRP1, which is expressed on the basolateral membrane of most cell types, and MRP2, which is expressed on the apical side of cells of the liver, kidney, and intestine.

sulfation, and ring-fission metabolism. For example, anaerobic fermentation of EGC, EC, and ECG with human fecal microflora has been shown to result in the production of the ring fission products, 5-(3′,4′,5′-trihydroxyphenyl)-γ-valerolactone (M4), 5-(3′,4′-dihydroxyphenyl)-γ-valerolactone (M6), and 5-(3′,5′-dihydroxyphenyl)-γ-valerolactone (M6′) (Figure 3), and these are detectable in urine (Meselhy et al., 1997; Meng et al., 2002). These compounds contain a valerolactone structure while retaining the polyphenolic character of the parent compound and may, therefore, have biological activities. EGCG has also been shown to undergo methylation, forming 4′,4″-di-*O*-methyl-EGCG (Meng et al., 2002). As another example, EGCG has been observed to rapidly oxidize in intestinal fluid (pH 8.5) with the amount of EGCG decreasing 81.6% in only 5 minutes, whereas a similar incubation in mouse plasma (pH 7.4) resulted in only a 29.3% decrease in EGCG (Yoshino et al., 1999). This oxidation, however, was found to create dimerized products, which had greater superoxide radical scavenging activity than EGCG. Investigation into the biological activities of the metabolites of green tea is an open area of research.

EPIDEMIOLOGICAL STUDIES

The plethora of animal studies demonstrating protective effects of tea against tumorigenesis suggests that one would expect to see such an effect in humans. The effect of tea consumption on human cancer has been studied extensively and reviewed in the literature (Yang and Wang, 1993; Blot et al., 1996; Kohlmeier et al., 1997; Buschman, 1998; Yang et al., 2002; Higdon and Frei, 2003). Many case-control studies have shown that subjects who consume large amounts of tea had lower cancer risk; in particular, risk of gastric and esophageal cancers was lower in green tea consumers in Japan and China. However, many other studies did not observe this protective effect. For example, a systematic review of 21 epidemiological investigations of gastrointestinal cancer or precancerous lesions suggested a protective effect of green tea on adenomatous polyps and chronic atrophic gastritis formation, but no clear support for green tea's preventive role in stomach and intestinal cancer (Borrelli et al., 2004).

A population-based case-control study of breast cancer was conducted among women of Asian descent living in Los Angeles to investigate the effect of green and black tea (Wu et al., 2003a). Green tea drinkers had a significantly reduced risk of breast cancer that was maintained even after adjusting for several potential confounding factors including smoking, alcohol, coffee, and black tea intake, family history of breast cancer, physical activity, and intake of soy and dark green vegetables. Among women who carried at least one low-activity catechol-*O*-methyltransferase (COMT) allele, both green and black tea drinkers showed a significantly reduced risk of breast cancer (Wu et al., 2003b), as opposed to the initial study (Wu et al., 2003a), in which

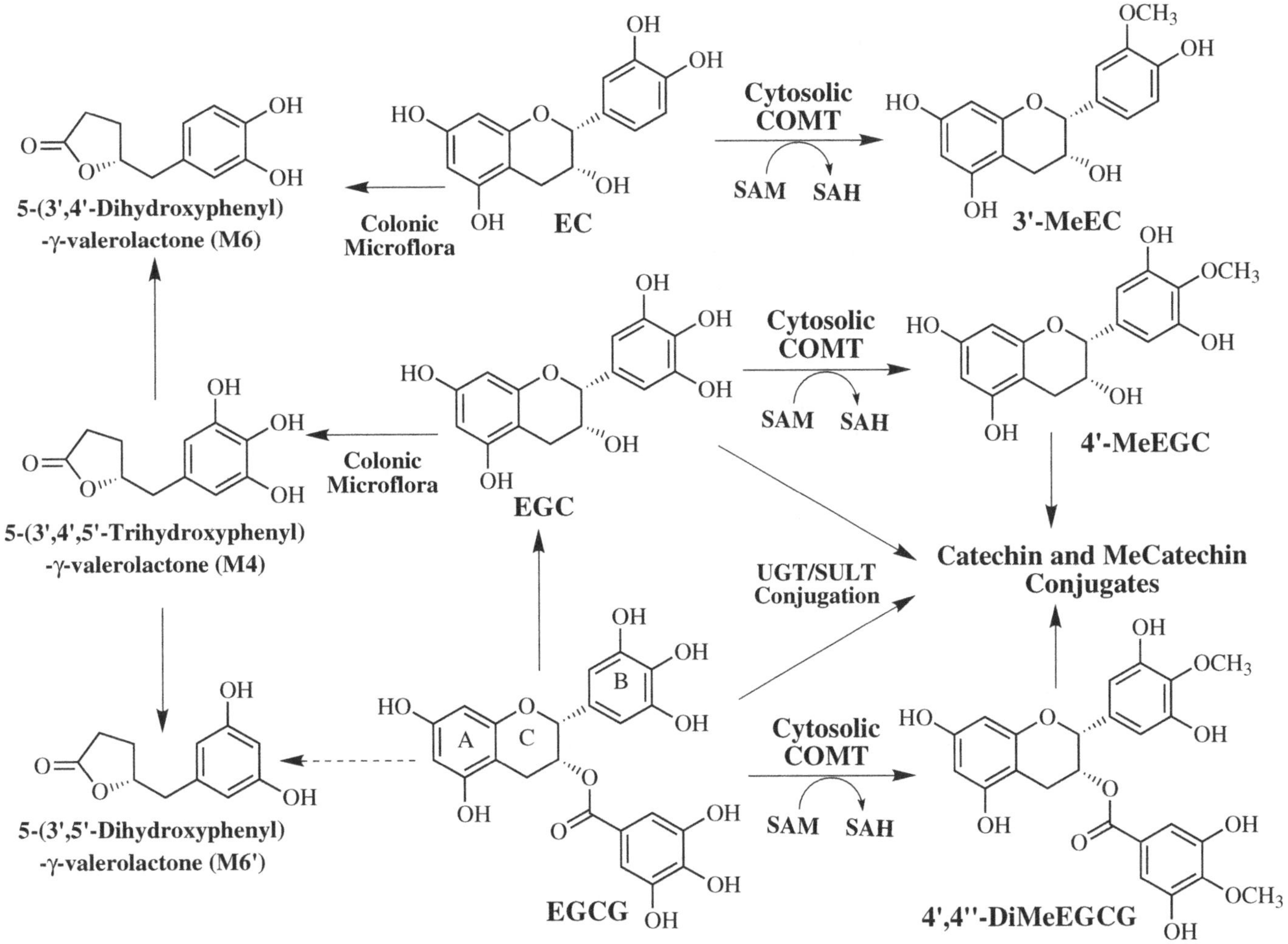

FIGURE 3 **Ring fission products.** Metabolic fate of tea catechins (COMT, catechol-*O*-methyltransferase; SAM, *s*-adenosylmethionine; SAH, homocysteine; SULT, sulfotransferase; UGT, uridine 5′-diphosphoglucuronosyltransferase).

no effect of black tea was seen. The authors concluded that individuals with a low-activity COMT allele have a reduced risk of breast cancer because they metabolize tea polyphenols less efficiently and, therefore, had prolonged exposure to these compounds. In two prospective studies in Japan, green tea was not, however, associated with decreased breast cancer risk when women drinking five or more cups of tea per day were compared with women drinking less than one cup (Suzuki et al., 2004). A case-control study of prostate cancer in southeast China found that prostate cancer risk declined with increasing frequency, duration, and quantity of green tea consumed (Jian et al., 2003). One Japanese cohort study found that total cancer risk was significantly lower in women who drank >10 cups of green tea per day, but not men (Imai et al., 1997).

One explanation for the difficulty in interpreting epidemiological results is that "tea" is a diverse beverage. The polyphenolic content depends on how the leaves are processed before drying, the geographic location, and growing conditions. Within a particular tea beverage, the polyphenol concentration varies among the type of tea (e.g., blended, instant, or decaffeinated) and preparation (e.g., amount used, brew time, and temperature). The highest amounts of polyphenols are found in brewed hot tea (541–692 μg/ml), less in instant preparations (90–100 μg/ml), and lower amounts in iced and ready-to-drink tea (Hakim et al., 2000). Despite some early controversy, it is now widely accepted that the addition of milk to tea does not interfere with polyphenol absorption (Hollman et al., 2001). Yet other issues such as tea drinking alone or with meals remain to be investigated further.

INTERVENTION STUDIES

Several intervention trials have investigated the effect of tea consumption on various biomarkers in smokers. In one intervention trial, 143 heavy smokers were randomized to drink 4 cups/day of green tea, black tea, or water (Hakim et al., 2003). After 4 months of intervention, the green tea group had significantly lower urinary 8-OHdG levels after adjusting for baseline measurement and other potential confounding factors. A double-blind intervention trial in which 64 smokers with oral leukoplakia were given daily capsules containing a mixture of tea polyphenols and topical applied tea mixture was conducted (Li et al., 1999). Oral lesions were significantly reduced in 38% of the experimental patients as compared with 10% of the placebo control patients. The incidence of micronucleated exfoliated oral mucosal cells was significantly lower in the tea-treated group.

Patients with androgen-independent prostate carcinoma were given 1 g of green tea six times per day and monitored monthly for changes in prostate-specific antigen (PSA) levels (Jatoi et al., 2003). After 1 month of treatment, no beneficial effects were seen on the PSA levels of these patients, and many patients complained about side effects. Certainly, intervention trials with other high-risk groups are warranted.

CONCLUSIONS

Because of the wide consumption of tea beverages worldwide, the biological activity of tea constituents continues to be an important topic for scientific investigation. The biological mechanisms discussed in this chapter suggest that tea possesses cancer-preventive activities. Nevertheless, these activities have not been convincingly demonstrated in humans, in spite of the many epidemiological studies. Studies using a more quantitative assessment of tea consumption (Sun et al., 2002) and analyzing subgroups of the population (Wu et al., 2003b) have begun to demonstrate the expected protective effect. More positive results are expected when methodology in epidemiological studies is further refined. Another consideration is that at the levels of human tea consumption, which are usually lower than those used in animal cancer chemoprevention studies, the amount of the tea polyphenols that reaches the target tissues is a limiting factor. For cancer prevention, one possible approach is to increase the amount of tea intake, but this may be limited by the taste and possible undesirable side effects. At moderate levels of tea consumption, the organ sites that are more accessible to tea polyphenols, such as the oral cavity and intestinal tract, are likely to be protected by tea. This concept could be tested in future epidemiological and intervention human studies.

References

Adhami, V.M., Ahmad, N., and Mukhtar, H. 2003. Molecular targets for green tea in prostate cancer prevention. *J Nutr* **133**: 2417S–2424S.

Ahmad, N., Feyes, D.K., Nieminen, A.L., Agarwal, R., and Mukhtar, H. 1997. Green tea constituent epigallocatechin-3-gallate and induction of apoptosis and cell cycle arrest in human carcinoma cells. *J Natl Cancer Inst* **89**: 1881–1886.

Ahmad, N., Gupta, S., and Mukhtar, H. 2000. Green tea polyphenol epigallocatechin-3-gallate differentially modulates nuclear factor-kappa B in cancer cells versus normal cells. *Arch Biochem Biophys* **376**: 338–346.

Ahmad, S., Rahman, A., Hasnain, A., Lalonde, M., Goldberg, V.M., and Haqqi, T.M. 2002. Green tea polyphenol epigallocatechin-3-gallate inhibits the IL-1 beta-induced activity and expression of cyclooxygenase-2 and nitric oxide synthase-2 in human chondrocytes. *Free Radic Biol Med* **33**: 1097–1105.

Balentine, D.A., Wiseman, S.A., and Bouwens, L.C. 1997. The chemistry of tea flavonoids. *Crit Rev Food Sci Nutr* **37**: 693–704.

Blot, W.J., Chow, W.H., and McLaughlin, J.K. 1996. Tea and cancer: a review of the epidemiological evidence. *Eur J Cancer Prev* **5**: 425–438.

Borrelli, F., Capasso, R., Russo, A., and Ernst, E. 2004. Systematic review: green tea and gastrointestinal cancer risk. *Aliment Pharmacol Ther* **19**: 497–510.

Buschman, J.L. 1998. Green tea and cancer in humans: a review of the literature. *Nutr Cancer* **31**: 151–159.

Cao, Y., and Cao, R. 1999. Angiogenesis inhibited by drinking tea. *Nature* **398**: 381.

Chow, H.H., Cai, Y., Alberts, D.S., Hakim, I., Dorr, R., Shahi, F., Crowell, J.A., Yang, C.S., and Hara, Y. 2001. Phase I pharmacokinetic study of tea polyphenols following single-dose administration of epigallocatechin gallate and polyphenon E. *Cancer Epidemiol Biomarkers Prev* **10**: 53–58.

Chow, H.H., Cai, Y., Hakim, I.A., Crowell, J.A., Shahi, F., Brooks, C.A., Dorr, R.T., Hara, Y., and Alberts, D.S. 2003. The pharmacokinetics and safety of green tea polyphenols after multiple-dose administration of epigallocatechin gallate and polyphenon E in healthy individuals was studied. *Clin Cancer Res* **9**: 3312–3319.

Chung, F.L., Schwartz, J., Herzog, C.R., and Yang, Y.M. 2003. Tea and cancer prevention: studies in animals and humans. *J Nutr* **133**: 3268S–3274S.

Chung, J.Y., Park, J.O., Phyu, H.P., Dong, Z., and Yang, C.S. 2001. Mechanisms of inhibition of the ras-MAP kinase signaling pathway in 30.7b ras 12 cells by tea polyphenols (–)-epigallocatechin-3-gallate and theaflavin-3,3′-digallate. *FASEB* J **15**: 2022–2024.

Conney, A.H., Lu, Y.P., Lou, Y.R., and Huang, M.T. 2002. Inhibitory effects of tea and caffeine on UV-induced carcinogenesis: relationship to enhanced apoptosis and decreased tissue fat. *Eur J Cancer Prev* **11**: S28–S36.

Diehl, J.A. 2002. Cycling to cancer with cyclin D1. *Cancer Biol Ther* **1**: 226–231.

Garbisa, S., Sartor, L., Biggin, S., Salvato, B., Benelli, R., and Albini, A. 2001. Tumor gelatinases and invasion inhibited by green tea flavonol epigallocatechin-3-gallate. *Cancer* **91**: 822–832.

Gupta S., Hastak K., Ahmad N., Lewin J.S., and Mukhtar H. 2001. Inhibition of prostate carcinogenesis in TRAMP mice by oral infusion of green tea polyphenols. *Proc Natl Acad Sci USA* **28**: 10350–10355.

Hakim, I.A., Harris, R.B., Brown, S., Chow, H.H., Wiseman, S., Agarwal, S., and Talbot, W. 2003. Effect of increased tea consumption on oxidative DNA damage among smokers: a randomized controlled study. *J Nutr* **133**: 3303S–3309S.

Hakim, I.A., Weisburger, U., Harris, R.B., Balentine, D., van-Mierlo, C., and Paetau-Robinson, I. 2000. Preparation, composition and consumption patterns of tea-based beverages in Arizona. *Nutr Res* **20**: 1715–1724.

Higdon, J.V., and Frei, B. 2003. Tea catechins and polyphenols: health effects, metabolism, and antioxidant functions. *Crit Rev Food Sci Nutr* **43**: 89–143.

Hirose, M., Mizoguchi, Y., Yaono, M., Tanaka, H., Yamaguchi, T., and Shirai, T. 1997. Effects of green tea catechins on the progression or late promotion stage of mammary gland carcinogenesis in female

Sprague–Dawley rats pretreated with 7,12-dimethylbenz[a]anthracene. *Cancer Lett* **112**: 141–147.

Hollman, P.C., Van Het Hof, K.H., Tijburg, L.B., and Katan, M.B. 2001. Addition of milk does not affect the absorption of flavonols from tea in man. *Free Radic Res* **34**: 297–300.

Hong, J., Smith, T.J., Ho, C.T., August, D.A., and Yang, C.S. 2001. Effects of purified green and black tea polyphenols on cyclooxygenase- and lipoxygenase-dependent metabolism of arachidonic acid in human colon mucosa and colon tumor tissues. *Biochem Pharmacol* **62**: 1175–1183.

Hong, J-I., Lu, H., Meng, X.F., Ryu, J-H., Hara, Y., and Yang, C.S. 2002. Stability, cellular uptake, biotransformation and efflux of tea polyphenol (–)-epigallocatechin-3-gallate in ht-29 human colon adenocarcinoma cells. *Cancer Res* **62**: 7241–7246.

Hsu, S., Lewis, J., Singh, B., Schoenlein, P., Osaki, T., Athar, M., Porter, A.G., and Schuster, G. 2003. Green tea polyphenol targets the mitochondria in tumor cells inducing caspase 3-dependent apoptosis. *Anticancer Res* **23**: 1533–1539.

Huang, M.T., Xie, J.G., Wang, Z.Y., Ho, C.T., Lou, Y.R., Wang, C.X., Hard, G.C., and Conney, A.H. 1997. Effects of tea, decaffeinated tea, and caffeine on UVB light-induced complete carcinogenesis in SKH-1 mice: demonstration of caffeine as a biologically important constituent of tea. *Cancer Res* **57**: 2623–2629.

Imai, K., Suga, K., and Nakachi, K. 1997. Cancer-preventive effects of drinking green tea among a Japanese population. *Prev Med* **26**: 769–775.

Jatoi, A., Ellison, N., Burch, P.A., Sloan, J.A., Dakhil, S.R., Novotny, P., Tan, W., Fitch, T.R., Rowland, K.M., Young, C.Y., and Flynn, P.J. 2003. A phase II trial of green tea in the treatment of patients with androgen-independent metastatic prostate carcinoma. *Cancer* **97**: 1442–1446.

Jian, L., Xie, L.P., Lee, A.H., and Binns, C.W. 2003. Protective effect of green tea against prostate cancer: a case–control study in southeast China. *Int J Cancer* **108**: 130–135.

Jung, Y.D., Kim, M.S., Shin, B.A., Chay, K.O., Ahn, B.W., Liu, W., Bucana, C.D., Gallick, G.E., and Ellis, L.M. 2001. EGCG, a major component of green tea, inhibits tumour growth by inhibiting VEGF induction in human colon carcinoma cells. *Br J Cancer* **84**: 844–850.

Katiyar, S.K., Agarwal, R., Wood, G.S., and Mukhtar, H. 1992. Inhibition of phorbol ester tumor promoter 12-*O*-tetradecanoylphorbol-13-acetate-caused tumor promotion in 7,12-dimethylbenz[a]-anthracene–initiated SENCAR mouse skin by a polyphenolic fraction isolated from green tea. *Cancer Res* **52**: 6890–6897.

Kavanagh, K.T., Hafer, L.J., Kim, D.W., Mann, K.K., Sherr, D.H., Rogers, A.E., and Sonenshein, G.E. 2001. Green tea extracts decrease carcinogen-induced mammary tumor burden in rats and rate of breast cancer cell proliferation in culture. *J Cell Biochem* **82**: 387–398.

Kim, S., Lee, M.J., Hong, J., Li, C., Smith, T.J., Yang, G.Y., Seril, D.N., and Yang, C.S. 2000. Plasma and tissue levels of tea catechins in rate and mice during chronic consumption of green tea polyphenols. *Nutr Cancer* **37**: 41–48.

Kohlmeier, L., Weterings, K.G., Steck, S., and Kok, F.J. 1997. Tea and cancer prevention: an evaluation of the epidemiologic literature. *Nutr Cancer* **27**: 1–13.

Kohri, T., Nanjo, F., Suzuki, M., Seto, R., Matsumoto, N., Yamakawa, M., Hojo, H., Hara, Y., Desai, D., Amin, S., Conaway, C.C., and Chung, F.L. 2001. Synthesis of (–)-[4-3H] epigallocatechin gallate and its metabolite fate in rats after intravenous administration. *J Agric Food Chem* **49**: 1042–1048.

Kundu, J.K., Na, H.K., Chun, K.S., Kim, Y.K., Lee, S.J., Lee, S.S., Lee, O.S., Sim, Y.C., and Surh, Y.J. 2003. Inhibition of phorbol ester-induced COX-2 expression by epigallocatechin gallate in mouse skin and cultured human mammary epithelial cells. *J Nutr* **133**: 3805S–3810S.

Landau, J.M., Wang, Z.Y., Yang, G.Y., Ding, W., and Yang, C.S. 1997. Inhibition of spontaneous formation of lung tumors and rhabdomyosarcomas in A/J mice by black and green tea. *Carcinogenesis* **19**: 501–507.

Lee, M.J., Maliakal, P., Chen, L., Meng, X., Bondoc, F.Y., Prabhu, S., Lambert, G., Mohr, S., and Yang, C.S. 2002. Pharmacokinetics of tea catechins after ingestion of green tea and (–)-epigallocatechin-3-gallate by humans: formation of different metabolites and individual variability. *Cancer Epidemiol Biomarkers Prev* **11**: 1025–1032.

Leone, M., Zhai, D., Sareth, S., Kitada, S., Reed, J.C., and Pellecchia, M. 2003. Cancer prevention by tea polyphenols is linked to their direct inhibition of antiapoptotic Bcl-2-family proteins. *Cancer Res* **63**: 8118–8121.

Li, N., Sun, Z., Han, C., and Chen, J. 1999. The chemopreventive effects of tea on human oral precancerous mucosa lesions. *Proc Soc Exp Biol Med* **220**: 218–224.

Li, N., Chen, X., Liao, J., Yang, G., Wang, S., Josephson, Y., Han, C., Chen, J., Huang, M.T., and Yang, C.S. 2002. Inhibition of 7, 12-dimethylbenz[a]anthracene (DMBA)-induced oral carcinogenesis in hamsters by tea and curcumin. *Carcinogenesis* **23**: 1307–1313.

Liang, Y.C., Lin-Shiau, S.Y., Chen, C.F., and Lin, J.K. 1999. Inhibition of cyclin-dependent kinases 2 and 4 activities as well as induction of Cdk inhibitors p21 and p27 during growth arrest of human breast carcinoma cells by (–)-epigallocatechin-3-gallate. *J. Cell Biochem.* **75**: 1–12.

Lu, Y.P., Lou, Y.R., Xie, J.G., Peng, Q.Y, Liao, J., Yang, C.S., Huang, M.T., and Conney A.H. 2002. Topical applications of caffeine or (–)-epigallocatechin gallate (EGCG) inhibit carcinogenesis and selectively increase apoptosis in UVB-induced skin tumors in mice. *Proc Natl Acad Sci USA* **99**: 12455–12460.

Masuda, M., Suzui, M., and Weinstein, I.B. 2001. Effects of epigallocatechin-3-gallate on growth, epidermal growth factor receptor signaling pathways, gene expression, and chemosensitivity in human head and neck squamous cell carcinoma cell lines. *Clin Cancer Res* **7**: 4220–4229.

Masuda, M., Suzui, M., Lim, J.T., Deguchi, A., Soh, J.W., and Weinstein, I.B. 2002. Epigallocatechin-3-gallate decreases VEGF production in head and neck and breast carcinoma cells by inhibiting EGFR-related pathways of signal transduction. *J Exp Ther Oncol* **2**: 350–359.

Meng, X., Sang, S., Zhu, N., Lu, H., Sheng, S., Lee, M.J., Ho, C.T., and Yang C.S. 2002. Identification and characterization of methylated and ring-fission metabolites of tea catechins formed in humans, mice, and rats. *Chem Res Toxicol* **15**: 1042–1050.

Meselhy, M.R., Nakamura, N., and Hattori, M. 1997. Biotransformation of (–)-epicatechin 3-O-gallate by human bacteria. *Chem Pharm Bull Tokyo* **45**: 888–893.

Metz, N., Lobstein, A., Schneider, Y., Gosse, F., Schleiffer, R., Anton, R., and Raul, F. 2000. Suppression of azoxymethane-induced preneoplastic lesions and inhibition of cyclooxygenase-2 activity in the colonic mucosa of rats drinking a crude green tea extract. *Nutr Cancer* **38**: 60–64.

Mukhtar, H., and Ahmad, N. 1999. Mechanism of cancer chemopreventive activity of green tea. *Proc Soc Exp Biol Med* **220**: 234–238.

Sartippour, M.R., Heber, D., Ma, J., Lu, Q., Go, V.L., and Nguyen, M. 2001. Green tea and its catechins inhibit breast cancer xenografts. *Nutr Cancer* **40**: 149–156.

Sartippour, M.R., Shao, Z.M., Heber, D., Beatty, P., Zhang, L., Liu, C., Ellis, L., Liu, W., Go, V.L., and Brooks, M.N. 2002. Green tea inhibits vascular endothelial growth factor (VEGF) induction in human breast cancer cells. *J Nutr* **132**: 2307–2311.

Sazuka, M., Maurakami, S., Isemura, M., Satoh, K., and Nukiwa, T. 1995. Inhibitory effects of green tea infusion on *in vitro* invasion and *in vivo* metastasis of mouse lung carcinoma cells. *Cancer Lett* **98**: 27–31.

Scalbert, A., and Williamson, G. 2002. Dietary intake and bioavailability of polyphenols. *J Nutr* **130**: 2073S–2085S.

Semczuk, A., and Jakowicki, J.A. 2004. Alterations of pRb1-cyclin D1-cdk4/6-p16(INK4A) pathway in endometrial carcinogenesis. *Cancer Lett* **203**: 1–12.

Suganuma, M., Okabe, S., Oniyama, M., Tada, Y., Ito, H., and Fujiki, H. 1998. Wide distribution of [^{3}H](−)-epigallocatechin gallate, a cancer preventive tea polyphenol, in mouse tissue. *Carcinogenesis* **19**: 1771–1776.

Sun, C.L., Yuan, J.M., Lee, M.J., Yang, C.S., Gao, Y.T., Ross, R.K., and Yu, M.C. 2002. Urinary tea polyphenols in relation to gastric and esophageal cancers: a prospective study of men in Shanghai, China. *Carcinogenesis* **23**: 1497–1503.

Suzuki, Y., Tsubono, Y., Nakaya, N., Suzuki, Y., Koizumi, Y., and Tsuji, I. 2004. Green tea and the risk of breast cancer: pooled analysis of two prospective studies in Japan. *Br J Cancer* **90**: 1361–1363.

Tanaka, H., Hirose, M., Kawabe, M., Sano, M., Takesada, Y., Hagiwara, A., and Shirai, T. 1997. Post-initiation inhibitory effects of green tea catechins on 7,12-dimethylbenz[a] anthracene-induced mammary gland carcinogenesis in female Sprague-Dawley rats. *Cancer Lett* **116**: 47–52.

Taniguchi, S., Fujiki, H., Kobayashi, H., Go, H., Miyado, K., Sadano, H., and Shimokawa, R. 1992. Effect of (−)-epigallocatechin gallate: the main constituent of green tea: on lung metastasis with mouse B16 melanoma cell lines. *Cancer Lett* **65**: 51–54.

Van Amelsvoort, J.M., Van Hof, K.H., Mathot, J.N., Mulder, T.P., Wiersma, A., and Tijburg, L.B. 2001. Plasma concentrations of individual tea catechins after a single oral dose in humans. *Xenobiotica* **31**: 891–901.

Witschi, H., Espiritu, I., Yu, M., and Willits, N.H. 1998. The effects of phenethyl isothiocyanate, N-acetylcysteine and green tea on tobacco smoke-induced lung tumors in strain A/J mice. *Carcinogenesis* **19**: 1789–1794.

Wu, A.H., Yu, M.C., Tseng, C.C., Hankin, J., and Pike, M.C. 2003a. Green tea and risk of breast cancer in Asian Americans. *Int J Cancer* **106**: 574–579.

Wu, A.H., Tseng, C.C., Van Den Berg, D., and Yu, M.C. 2003b. Tea intake, COMT genotype, and breast cancer in Asian-American women. *Cancer Res* **63**: 7526–7529.

Yanaga, H., Fujii, T., Koga, T., Araki, R., and Shirouzu, K. 2002. Prevention of carcinogenesis of mouse mammary epithelial cells RIII/MG by epigallocatechin gallate. *Int J Mol Med* **10**: 311–315.

Yang, C.S., and Wang, Z.Y. 1993. Tea and cancer: a review. *J Natl Cancer Inst* **58**: 1038–1049.

Yang, C.S., Chen, L., Lee, M.J., Balentine, D., Kuo, M.C., and Schantz, S.P. 1998. Blood and urine levels of tea catechins after ingestion of different amounts of green tea by human volunteers. *Cancer Epidemiol Biomarkers Prev* **7**: 351–354.

Yang, C.S., Yang, G.Y., Landau, J.M., Kim, S., and Liao, J. 1998. Tea and tea polyphenols inhibit cell hyperproliferation, lung tumorigenesis, and tumor progression. *In* "Experimental Lung Research: First International Symposium on Mouse Pulmonary Carcinogenesis" (G. Stoner and A. Malkinson, eds.), Vol. 24, pp. 629–639. Taylor & Francis, Philadelphia.

Yang, C.S., and Chung, J. 1999. Growth inhibition of human cancer cell lines by tea polyphenols. *Curr Pract Med* **2**: 163–166.

Yang, C.S., Maliakal, P., and Meng, X. 2002. Inhibition of carcinogenesis by tea. *Annu Rev Pharmacol Toxicol* **42**: 25–54.

Yang, F., Oz, H.S., Bavre, S., de Villiers, W.J., McClain, C.J., and Varilek, G.W. 2001. The green tea polyphenol (−)-epigallocatechin-3-gallate blocks nuclear factor-kappaB activation by inhibiting Ikappa B kinase activity in the intestinal epithelial cell line IEC-6. *Mol Pharmacol* **60**: 528–533.

Yang, G-Y., Liao, J., Kim, K., Yurkow, E.J., and Yang, C.S. 1998. Inhibition of growth and induction of apoptosis in human cancer cell lines by tea polyphenols. *Carcinogenesis* **19**: 611–616.

Yang, G-Y., Liao, J., Li, C., Chung, J.Y., Yurkow, E.J., Ho, C-T., and Yang, C.S. 2000. Effect of black and green tea polyphenols on c-jun phosphorylation and H_2O_2 production in transformed and non-transformed human bronchial cell lines: Possible mechanisms of cell growth inhibition and apoptosis induction. *Carcinogenesis* **21**: 2035–2039.

Yoshino, K., Suzuki, M., Sasaki, K., Miyase, T., and Sano, M. 1999. Formation of antioxidants from (−)-epigallocatechin gallate in mild alkaline fluids, such as authentic intestinal juice and mouse plasma. *J Nutr Biochem* **10**: 223–229.

Zhou, J.R., Yu, L., Mai, Z., and Blackburn, G.L. 2004. Combined inhibition of estrogen-dependent human breast carcinoma by soy and tea bioactive components in mice. *Int J Cancer* **108**: 8–14.

Zhu, N., Huang, T.C., Yu, Y., LaVoie, E.J., Yang, C.S., and Ho, C.T. 2000. Identification of oxidation products of (−)-epigallocatechin gallate and (−)-epigallocatechin with H(2)O(2). *J Agric Food Chem* **48**: 979–982.

CHAPTER

36

Garlic

JOHN MILNER

INTRODUCTION

Mounting evidence continues to raise the possibility that garlic is a protective factor against cancer. Studies using fresh garlic extracts, aged garlic, garlic oil, and a number of specific organosulfur compounds arising from processed garlic provide support for a reduction in cancer risk and a modification in tumor behavior, although there is considerable variability in response. Regardless, the ability of garlic and related allyl sulfur compounds to block models for colon, lung, breast, and liver suggests general mechanisms of action are a real possibility. The anticancer characteristics appear to arise through both a dose- and a temporal-related change in a number of cellular events involved with the cancer process, including those involving drug metabolism, inflammation, hormonal regulation, immunocompetence, cell cycle regulation, apoptosis, and angiogenesis. When using chemical carcinogens in animal models, there is little difference in the relative efficacy of water- and lipid-soluble allyl sulfur compounds. However, the tumor proliferation/apoptosis response is highly dependent on the species provided. A shift in sulfhydryl groups, alterations in glutathione/oxidized glutathione ratios, and resultant changes in cellular redox status may be involved in some of the phenotypic changes caused by allyl sulfur compounds. Although the anticarcinogenic and antitumorigenic data are intriguing, additional studies are necessary with more reasonable exposures over prolonged periods to verify efficacy in humans. Finally, it is critical that genomic, epigenomic, proteomic, and metabolomic factors are considered so that models can be developed to predict who might benefit most from expanded use of garlic or its allyl sulfur components.

Allium vegetables including garlic, onion, leeks, chives, and scallions are used throughout history for their sensory characteristics and their apparent health benefits (Rivlin, 2001). The ability of these foods to serve as antimicrobial, antithrombotic, antitumor, hypolipidemic, antiarthritic, and hypoglycemic agents has surely been important to the widespread belief in these vegetables as medicinal foods. Although clinical studies provide some important insights into the potential physiological significance of dietary garlic and individual variability, especially for heart disease (Rahman, 2001; Dhawan and Jain, 2004; Franco et al., 2004; Tattelman, 2005), the most compelling evidence linking garlic and related foods with cancer comes from preclinical studies using cultured cells or animal models (Milner, 2001; Thomson and Ali, 2003). Epidemiological support for the anticancer effects of garlic, admittedly sparse, is suggestive that those with higher intakes have increased protection against some cancer (Fleischauer and Arab, 2001; Hsing et al., 2002; Khanum et al., 2004; Sengupta et al., 2004). Cohort studies provide evidence, though not overly compelling, that an inverse association existed between garlic intake and the incidence of colorectal cancer and possibly the incidence at several other cancer sites (Fleischauer and Arab, 2001). Evidence again suggests that increased garlic intake, as well as related allium foods, was associated with a reduction in prostate cancer risk (Hsing et al., 2002). The apparent protection was independent of body size, intake of other foods, and total calories. Although data relating garlic intake to human cancer risk are tantalizing, it is likely that variation in a variety of genetic and environmental factors may influence the response found among individuals. Thus, it should not be surprising that variability occurs in the literature about the importance of garlic and related allium foods and overall cancer risk and/or tumor behavior.

The role of genomics is increasingly being recognized as a key factor in the biological response to foods and their

Copyright © 2006, Elsevier Inc.
All rights of reproduction in any form reserved.

components (Davis and Milner, 2004; Fenech, 2005). Collectively, genetic background (nutrigenetic effects), DNA methylation and histone regulation (nutritional epigenomic effects), ability to induce or repress gene expression patterns (nutritional transcriptomics effects), the occurrence and activity of specific proteins (nutriproteomic effects), and/or the dose and temporal changes in cellular small molecular weight compounds (metabolomics effects) can influence the overall response to any food (Hsing et al., 2002). Knowledge about each of these genomic variables will allow for a preemptive approach to those who will benefit most from the ingestion of garlic or other related allium foods (Figure 1). This "omic" information may also provide valuable clues about specificity in response and will assist in the identification of surrogate fluids/tissues and associated biomarkers that can be used for predicting responders or identify anyone who might be placed at risk because of dietary change (Ommen and Groten, 2004). Unraveling the importance of each of the potential sites of regulation within the "omics" is particularly challenging but holds promise to help explain the mounting inconsistencies in the scientific literature about diet and cancer prevention interrelationships, especially those related to garlic and cancer prevention.

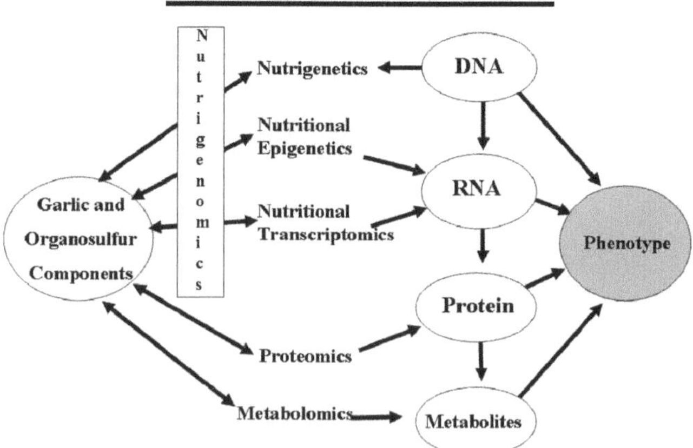

FIGURE 1 **Garlic and the "omics."** Evidence indicates that a number of processes associated with genes and their products are influenced by garlic or one or more of its allyl sulfur components. Thus, genes may influence absorption, metabolism, or the site of action of bioactive components within garlic. Each of these potential gene and gene product modifiers of the action of garlic are briefly discussed in the text.

BIOACTIVE FOOD COMPONENTS AND THEIR METABOLITES

The most important constituent within garlic that accounts for its anticancer properties in a model system remains to be determined. Nevertheless, there is a wealth of evidence suggesting that organosulfur constituents are likely significant contributors. Sulfur in garlic is known to reach concentrations as high as 1% of its dry weight (Amagase et al., 2001). Within the allium family, considerable variability occurs in the content and chemical sulfur species, which can be markedly influenced by the vegetation period examined, as well as plant genetics (Krest et al., 2000; Brandolini et al., 2005). Thus, it is not surprising that considerable variability is observed when food disappearance data for garlic or associated allium foods are correlated with cancer risk and mortality. The complexity of this interrelationship can also be further modified by constituents other than sulfur content and speciation including the rather significant amount of oligosaccharide that occurs. Oligosaccharides have been reported to influence gastrointestinal (GI) flora or GI function, both of which are associated with a cancer risk in some experimental models (VanLoo, 2004). Although garlic has a moderate amount of protein, it is a relatively rich source of the amino acid arginine, which has experimentally been reported to suppress inflammatory processes, which again has been linked to reduced cancer risk (Lind, 2004). The presence of several other factors, including selenium and flavonoids, may also influence several cellular processes that have been linked experimentally to cancer incidence and tumor behavior (Borek, 2001; Dong et al., 2001; Sengupta et al., 2004).

The intracellular metabolite actually accounting for the change in cell signaling due to garlic and thereby leading to a phenotypic change has also yet to be defined. Although considerable information points to the ability of garlic to suppress the incidence and multiplicity of chemically induced tumors, it does not do so by changing the growth of the host. Thus, normal nonneoplastic cells do not appear to be as sensitive to the effects of garlic or its organosulfur constituents as neoplastic cells. In fact, some of the allyl sulfur compounds may be protective to normal functioning cells. Data from Koh et al. (2005) suggest that low concentration of diallyl disulfide (DADS) was neuroprotective possibly by activating PI3K/Akt and by inhibiting GSK-3 activation, cytochrome *c* release, caspase-3 activation, and PARP cleavage. However, when exposures were raised to excess, cytotoxicity occurred. Likewise, normal liver cells appear to be more resistant to the toxic effects of selected allyl sulfur compounds than neoplastic cells (Sundaram and Milner, 1993; Liu and Yeh, 2000). These inconsistencies indicate that biological responses reflect the uptake and/or the formation of the active intermediate and its rate of removal, which is likely variable across cell types. Differences in each of these variables likely explains the variation in sensitivity of various neoplastic cells to the organosulfur compounds, as well as the lower susceptibility of nonneoplastic cells to growth inhibition by these agents (Sundaram and Milner, 1996).

It is certainly possible that the active organosulfur intermediate may be a radical. Koh et al. (2005) have provided some of the strongest evidence that enhanced radical formation is likely involved because growth inhibition was found to correlate with the occurrence of free radicals and membrane lipid peroxidation in neuronal cells (nPC12) treated with DADS. Other cellular events started to change when exposures were increased to ~50 μM DADS, including a block in PI3K/Akt and the activation of GSK-3 and caspase-3, the release of cytochrome *c*, and the cleavage of PARP (Koh et al., 2005). It remains to be determined whether a block in radical formation would prevent these subsequent cellular responses. These observations also raise the possibility that the protective effects of garlic against chemical carcinogenesis might relate to its antioxidant properties (Khanum et al., 2004). However, its ability to alter the growth of an existing tumor may relate to the ability to increase intracellular oxidative damage (Koh et al., 2005). Clearly, additional studies are necessary to resolve this interesting conundrum.

Not all allyl sulfur compounds appear equally toxic to cells. Water-soluble compounds found in deodorized garlic, such as S-allyl cysteine (SAC), are far less toxic than the lipid-soluble compounds such as DADS (Liu and Yeh, 2000; Knowles and Milner, 2001; Elango et al., 2004). Generally, the antiproliferative effects of the allyl sulfur compounds increase as the number of sulfur atoms increases (Sundaram and Milner, 1996; Knowles and Milner, 2001; Elango et al., 2004). Although all cells will ultimately become susceptible to the toxic effects of allyl sulfur compounds when the concentration becomes sufficiently high, there are clear differences in response among various cell types. More attention to how uptake, metabolism, and excretion of specific allyl sulfur compounds vary should help explain why these differences in sensitivity exist and help point to which tissue(s) may be most responsive to dietary fortification with garlic.

FREE RADICALS AND GARLIC

Reactive oxygen species (ROS) are known to arise from endogenous processes and exogenous exposures. These ROS are believed to cause genetic oxidation/damage to DNA and other macromolecules. Unchecked, this oxidative damage may lead to a host of conditions including cancer. Normally, this process is held in check by elaborate endogenous or exogenous antioxidant processes. Garlic is one of several foods with proposed antioxidant properties (Milner, 2001; Riblin, 2001; Thomson and Ali, 2003). Deodorized garlic preparations also appear to be protective against oxidative damage. Studies by Gedik et al. (2005) revealed that long-term administration of aqueous garlic extract (AGE) alleviated liver fibrosis and oxidative damage, as indicated by reduced myeloperoxidase activity in rats with biliary obstruction. Using another model, Sener et al. (2003) reported that peeled crushed garlic extracts reversed the decrease in GSH level and the increase in fatty acid oxidation radicals (malondialdehyde) and MPO activity resulting from thermal stress. Although it remains unclear whether a block in oxidation accounts for the plethora of published manuscripts about the anticarcinogenic and properties associated with garlic and its sulfur constituents, there is evidence to the contrary. Because disulfides and trisulfides arising from garlic can deplete intracellular glutathione, oxidative stress might be involved in the upregulation of carcinogen metabolism, especially those involved with phase II detoxifying enzymes. Adding glutathione and *N*-acetylcysteine to HepG2 cells was discovered to markedly reduce the induction of glutathione *S*-transferase (GST), presumably by blocking antioxidant-responsive element (ARE) activity, presumably because it helped maintain Nrf2 in a complex form in the cytosol, thus preventing its migration to the nucleus (Chen et al., 2004). Diallyl compounds are also known to form volatile epoxide intermediates by way of unsaturated double-bond oxidation and, thus, may contribute to the induction of phase II enzymes. Support for the idea that oxidative intermediates are involved in the response to diallyl trisulfide (DATS) comes from the observation that addition of epoxide hydrolase will decrease, at least partially, the ability of diallyl compounds to increase ARE activity while also slightly attenuating Nrf2 protein induction (Chen et al., 2004).

EPIGENOMICS AND GARLIC

Epigenomics can also influence genetic expression patterns. Several regulatory proteins including DNA methyltransferases, methyl-cytosine guanine dinucleotide binding proteins, histone-modifying enzymes, chromatin remodeling factors, and their multimolecular complexes are involved in controlling epigenomic processes (Ross, 2003; Gallou-Kabani and Junien, 2005). Because several dietary components may influence epigenomic events, these processes represent additional control sites at which bioactive food components in garlic may reduce cancer burden. Although the impact of garlic on DNA methylation has not been adequately investigated, it is known that allyl sulfurs can influence DNA methylation processes indirectly by influencing blocking carcinogen metabolism. Carcinogen bind-ing to DNA is known to influence DNA methylation patterns (Zhang et al., 2005), and this process is recognized to be influenced by dietary fortification with garlic and many of its sulfur constituents (Milner, 2001; Khanum et al., 2004).

There is also evidence that the components of garlic can affect histone homeostasis. Druesne et al. (2004) found that DADS and allyl mercaptan were very effective in increasing histone H3 acetylation in Caco-2 and HT-29 cells in culture. The reason for the histone H4 hyperacetylation occurring preferentially at the lysine residues 12 and 16 remains to be resolved but appears to relate to reduction in histone deacetylase activity (Druesne et al., 2004). The DADS-induced hyperacetylation was accompanied by an increase in p21 (waf1/cip1) expression, at mRNA and protein levels, again demonstrating that epigenomic events can influence subsequent gene expression patterns. Such intracellular changes may account for the ability of DADS and other allyl sulfur compounds to cause the accumulation of cells in the G_2 phase of the cell cycle (Knowles and Milner, 2003). DADS and allyl mercaptan are rather unique in that they join a relatively short list of dietary factors that have been found to alter histone homeostasis (i.e., caloric restriction, butyrate, catechins, and sulforaphane).

Studies by Lea and Randolph (2001) indicate that the ability of allyl sulfurs to affect epigenomic events is not consistent across all cell types. Interestingly, their data suggest that normal liver cells are more responsive to histone regulation than other nonneoplastic cells. More comparative studies are necessary to explain why these differences exist among various types of nonneoplastic and neoplastic cells. Regardless, such changes would typically be associated with differentiation of cells and, therefore, may have profound implications in the role of diet in the regulation of stem cells.

GARLIC AND TRANSCRIPTOMICS

Data from cDNA array studies reveal that the antiproliferative effects of DADS may relate to changes in the expression of a host of genes including those related to alterations in cellular matrix gene expression (Frantz et al., 2000). Specifically, DADS exposure was shown to downregulate the expression of aggrecan 1, tenascin R, vitronectin, and cadherin 5, whereas it upregulated 40S ribosomal protein SA, platelet-derived growth factor–associated protein, and glia-derived neurite-promoting factor levels. These changes in matrix protein expression may influence cellular adhesion, as sometimes observed in studies using allicin and other allyl sulfides (Ledezma et al., 2004; Sela et al., 2004). Frantz et al. (2000) reported that the increase in HT-29 cell detachment by aqueous garlic extracts related to an increase in epidermal growth factor receptor and integrin-α6 mRNA expressions. Additional studies are necessary to characterize more fully which changes in gene expression patterns explain the likely multiple targets involved with the anticancer and antitumorigenic properties associated with increased intake of garlic and its related sulfur constituents.

The GST family of xenobiotic-metabolizing enzymes is involved in the metabolic detoxification of various environmental carcinogens and may influence a number of cellular processes including the clearance of oxidative stress products and the modulation of cell proliferation and apoptosis signaling pathways (Mahajan and Atkins, 2005). Andorfer et al. (2004) compared in a short-term feeding study the effects of DADS, diallylthiosulfinate (allicin), and butylated hydroxyanisole on GST expression in the GI tract and liver of mice. The effects of DADS and allicin on GST expression were especially prominent in stomach and small intestine, where there were major coordinate changes in GST subunit profiles. In particular, the transcripts of the mGSTM1 and mGSTM4 genes, which share large segments of common 5′-flanking sequences, and their corresponding subunits were selectively induced. Although liver and colon GSTs were also increased, but to a lesser extent, there was no effect on heart, brain, and testis, suggesting gene expression patterns are not equally influenced across all tissues. Their data also indicate these organosulfur compounds may operate on GST transcription through a reversible modification of certain protein sulfhydryl groups, shifts in reduced glutathione/oxidized glutathione ratios, and resultant changes in cellular redox status. Additional studies are necessary to clarify the role of thiol switches as a site of action of organosulfur compounds occurring in garlic and other foods.

As mentioned previously, studies by Chen et al. (2004) demonstrate that the ability of DATS to cause ARE gene activation and Nrf2 protein accumulation correlated with phase II gene expression induction. Using transient transfection HepG2 cells, they found that DATS-induced ARE activity was inhibited by dominant-negative Nrf2 Kelch-like ECH-associating protein 1 and constructs. The ability of DATS to influence cellular thiol status may account for this phenomenon. Pretreatment with various upstream protein kinase inhibitors revealed that the protein kinase C pathway was not directly involved in this induction of ARE activity, but that a calcium-dependent signaling pathway was involved (Chen et al., 2004).

GARLIC AND PROTEOMICS

The examination of patterns of changes in protein expression and their modifications, or proteomics, presents a formidable challenge to the scientific community (Barnes and Kim, 2004). Undeniably, considerable evidence points to the ability of essential nutrient deficiencies to alter the rate of protein synthesis and degradation. Today, it is clear that both essential and nonessential nutrients can influence not only protein anabolism and catabolism but markedly influence post-translation processes by influencing the degree of phosphorylation, glycosylation, nitration, and ubiquitination. New information generated by a proteomic approach will undeniably have a major impact on understanding how subtle changes in diet can influence protein signals involved with cancer. Understanding proteomics will require a greater attention to not only which food exposure causes a change but how this response is influenced by the duration of consumption and how compensatory cellular processes influence these changes.

The occurrence and post-translation patterns of specific proteins have been observed to be modified by the ingestion of allium vegetables or their associated sulfur constituents. Although in many cases scientists have focused on the impact of allyl sulfur compounds on enzymatic activity, it is clear that activity may reflect a difference in the protein content and the amount occurring in the active state. For example, diallyl sulfide (DAS) was found to induce the expression of the wild-type p53 and to downregulate the expression of mutant (mut) p53 in cells in culture when Western blot analysis and immunohistochemical protein detection were combined with multivariable flow cytometry (Wen et al., 2004). The increase in the expression of the wild-type tumor suppressor gene protein p53 was accompanied by elevation of the levels of cyclin-dependent kinase inhibitor p21/waf1.

Changes in activity may also be a result of a combination in the quantity and activity of specific cellular proteins. Exposure of synchronized colonic cells to DADS increased p34(cdc2) hyperphosphorylation by 15% (Knowles and Milner, 2000). Consistent with its ability to slightly increase the quantity of hyperphosphorylated p34 (cdc2), DADS also decreased cdc25C protein expression. These findings suggest that the ability of DADS to inhibit p34(cdc2) kinase activation occurs because of decreased p34(cdc2)/cyclin B1 complex formation and a shift in the p34(cdc2) hyperphosphorylation state (Knowles and Milner, 2000). Similar conclusions were reached by Wu et al. (2004) when the effects of DAS, DADS, and DATS were found to modify the cell cycle of human liver tumor cells (J5) in culture.

MULTIPLE TARGETS

There is compelling evidence that several organosulfur compounds in garlic can influence a number of processes involved with cancer. Interestingly, both water-soluble and lipid-soluble allyl sulfurs have been reported to influence these molecular events (Figure 2). Some of the processes modified include the blocking of mutagenesis, blocking carcinogen-DNA adduct formation, serving as a free-radical scavenger, blocking cell proliferation, promoting differentiation, and decreasing angiogenesis. Although there is a large body of evidence supporting each of these plus other mechanisms, there is a need for additional research to determine which change is causally related to a cancer-preventive activity associated with garlic and its allyl sulfur components. The following is a brief account of some of the evidence linking garlic and related sulfur components with some of the processes associated with cancer.

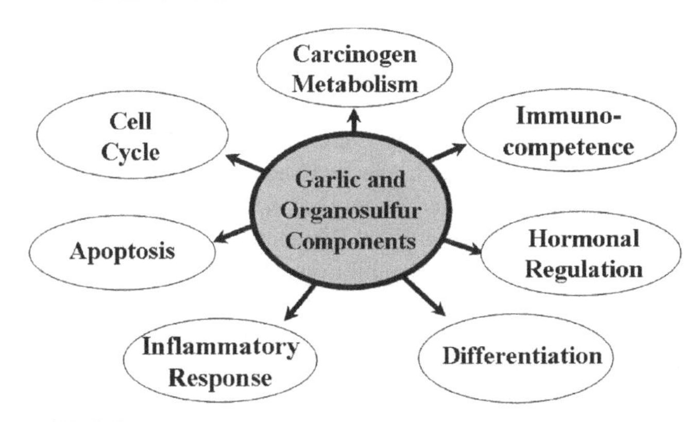

FIGURE 2 **Garlic may influence multiple cancer processes.** Dietary garlic may influence genetic and epigenetic events associated with several diseased states including cancer. Alterations in each of these processes is highly dependent on the form and quantity of allyl sulfur provided and the duration of exposure.

Carcinogen Bioactivation

By far the most compelling evidence about the mechanism by which allyl sulfur compounds can inhibit the cancer process comes from studies demonstrating that they can markedly suppress carcinogen bioactivation and the subsequent formation of DNA adducts. Studies with several chemical carcinogens document the fact that the anticancer properties associated with garlic are not limited to a specific animal model or to a particular tissue. Moreover, these studies demonstrate that both water- and lipid-soluble allyl sulfur compounds are effective in retarding chemical carcinogenesis. Because several types of allyl sulfur compounds offer protection against chemical carcinogenesis, multiple mechanisms are possible (Borek, 2001; Milner, 2001; Yang et al., 2001; Thomson and Ali, 2003; Andorfer et al., 2004; Khanum et al., 2004; Sengupta et al., 2004). Certainly, it does not appear that a single cytochrome P450 (CYP) enzymatic change could account for the observed protection based on the variety of carcinogens examined. Nevertheless, one class of carcinogens that appear to be particularly sensitive to water- and lipid-soluble allyl sulfurs is the nitrosamines (Yang et al., 2001). Much of the evidence in the literature suggests that garlic may promote the formation of nitrosothiols, thereby reducing their ability to form carcinogenic nitrosamines (Dion et al., 1997). The decrease in carcinogenicity observed may also arise from a block in the formation and/or bioactivation of nitrosamines (Gao et al., 2002). A competitive block or autocatalysis of CYP 2E1 may account for part of this inhibition, at least for lipid-soluble organosulfur agents (Gao et al., 2002). DAS is sequentially converted to diallyl sulfoxide (DASO) and diallyl sulfone ($DASO_2$) by CYP 2E1. Studies by Davenport and Wargovich (2005) found that although DADS and AMS decreased CYP 2E1, adding dipropyl sulfide, dipropyl disulfide, propyl methyl sulfide, or SAC did not influence the expression of hepatic protein or influence CYP 2E1 mRNA levels. Although polymorphisms in CYP 2E1 might be logically assumed to influence the response to garlic, no such relationship has been observed, at least with the risk of esophageal and stomach cancer (Gao et al., 2002). Nevertheless, several studies have shown that different garlic compounds can reduce CYP 2E1 activity, presumably by serving as competitive inhibitors. Because allyl sulfurs inhibit the actions of several carcinogens not requiring CYP 2E1 activity, it is logical to assume that alterations in other phase I, or also II (Andorfer et al., 2004; Chen et al., 2004), enzymatic targets are involved.

Hormonal Regulation

The association between estrogen exposure, either with or without progestin, and breast cancer risk continues to be a topic of immense interest and debate (Creasman, 2005). Although no significant effect of garlic or its constituents on estradiol have been reported, a change in the biological response to diethylstilbestrol (DES), a synthetic estrogen known to increase mammary cancer in animal models, has been observed (Green et al., 2003). Part of the effects of DAS may arise from its ability to block DES metabolism and the subsequent formation of DNA adducts by blocking lipid hydroperoxides in mammary tissue (Green et al., 2003).

The androgen dependence of the growth of some tumor types including prostate cancer is well recognized. Adding several allyl sulfur compounds, in particular S-allylmercaptocysteine (SAMC), was found to enhance the rate of testosterone disappearance from cells in culture and may have accounted in part for the antitumorigenic properties observed (Pinto et al., 2000). Adding SAMC created a situation similar to androgen deprivation. Although the mechanism responsible for this effect remains to be determined, it is conceivable that it involves the conversion of testosterone to metabolites that have less affinity for androgen receptors (Pinto et al., 2000). Other hormones may also be involved, including luteinizing hormone, as demonstrated in research by Oi et al. (2001).

Inflammation and Immunocompetence

The anticancer properties linked with garlic may also arise from suppression of inflammation and promotion of immunocompetence. Garlic oil derivatives have been found to differentially suppress the production of nitric oxide and prostaglandin E_2 (PGE_2) in activated macrophages (Chang and Chen, 2005). These studies found that DAS decreased stimulated nitric oxide and PGE_2 production by inhibiting inducible synthase and cyclooxygenase-2 expressions. DADS inhibited activated nitric oxide production by decreasing inducible synthase expression and by directly clearing nitric oxide (Chang and Chen, 2005). Cytokine production has also been reported to be reduced significantly in the presence of garlic extract (Hodge et al., 2002).

Studies by Lang et al. (2004) suggest that another organosulfur compound, allicin, exerts its immunomodulatory effect on intestinal epithelial cells by attenuating intestinal inflammation. Allicin was found to markedly inhibit the spontaneous and tumor necrosis factor-α (TNF-α)–induced secretion of IL-1β, IL-8, IP-10, and MIG from the two cell lines in a dose-dependent manner and suppressed the expression of IL-8 and IL-1β mRNA levels. Allicin was also found to suppress the degradation of IκB, which may have mediated these effects. However, the effects are complex because garlic derivatives appear to have both stimulatory and inhibitory properties in lymphocyte proliferation and lipopolysaccharide (LPS)-induced TNF-α generation (Romano et al., 1997; Salman et al., 1999). Whether these variations in response relate to the type of sulfur compound tested, the duration of exposure, or some other modifier remains to be determined.

Evidence exists that a nonsteroidal anti-inflammatory drug (NSAID)–activated gene (NAG-1) possesses both proapoptotic and antitumorigenic activities. Data in the literature reveal that this gene is upregulated by anticancer agents such as DADS and NSAIDs (Bottone et al., 2002). Adding DADS *in vitro* produced a dose-dependent increase in NAG-1. Induction of p53 was found to precede that of NAG-1. DADS did not induce NAG-1 or p53 in a p53 mutant cell line (Bottone et al., 2002).

Antiproliferation and Apoptosis

A variety of allyl sulfur compounds have been reported to reduce the growth of neoplastic cells in culture and *in vivo* (Sundaram and Milner, 1993, 1996; Knowles and Milner, 2001; Wen et al., 2004; Wu et al., 2004). At least part of this reduced growth relates to a blockage in the cell cycle, most frequently in the G_2/M phase (Wen et al., 2004; Wu et al., 2004). The transitory nature of this inhibition suggests that the rates of clearance of allyl sulfur are likely an important determinant of the magnitude of the response. Certainly, all cells are not equally susceptible to the antiproliferative effects of these sulfur compounds, and in particular nonneoplastic cells tend to be less responsive. Generally, as the concentration of the allyl sulfur compound increases, there is also a shift from a depression in cell proliferation to a greater involvement of apoptosis. However, insufficient attention has been given to which process is actually influenced first. Considerable evidence points to the dependence of the allyl component and the number of sulfur atoms as determinants of the degree of antiproliferative and apoptotic response. DATS has been reported to be >10 times as effective as DADS in retarding some tumors. As reviewed previously, alterations in several molecular targets may explain the antiproliferative and apoptotic effects of allyl sulfur compounds.

As additional information about the molecular targets for the various organosulfur compounds arises, it will be possible to develop better predictive models for determining which individuals will benefit most from dietary change with allium foods. The use of this "nutritional preemption" approach should allow for the use of specific foods, such as garlic, at critical points that allow for a block in the initiation and progression of a pathway that leads to an unhealthy or lethal phenotype.

INTERACTION WITH OTHER FOOD COMPONENTS

It is certainly conceivable that a variety of food components might influence the ability of garlic to suppress the cancer process. It is somewhat logical that variation in the sulfur content of the diet might be one variable (Amagase et al., 1996). Although the amount of evidence is not overwhelming, it appears that variation in dietary sulfur amino acids, unsaturated fats, and selenium can influence the response to allyl sulfur compounds (Amagase et al., 1996). When carcinogen-DNA adducts were used as the biomarker, there was a beneficial effect of combining garlic, selenite, and retinyl acetate beyond that caused by each ingredient alone. The effects of combining garlic with tomatoes were examined for their ability to synergistically inhibit hamster buccal pouch cancer (Bhuvaneswari et al., 2005). Combining garlic and tomatoes suppressed the incidence and mean tumor burden of hamster buccal pouch carcinomas possibly by decreasing phase I enzyme activities and by increasing phase II enzyme activities. The effect of combining bioactive food components on the antitumorigenic properties of allyl sulfur compounds has not been adequately examined.

As the era of molecular nutrition unfolds, we will gain a greater understanding about which of the many processes modified by garlic is critical to induce a phenotypic change. This information will be fundamental to the development of tailored strategies for reducing cancer burden. The identification of biomarkers that can be used to predict who will respond is essential for effective intervention to occur.

References

Amagase, H., Schaffer, E.M., and Milner, J.A. 1996. Dietary components modify the ability of garlic to suppress 7,12-dimethylbenz(a) anthracene-induced mammary DNA adducts. *J Nutr* **126**: 817–824.

Amagase, H., Petesch, B.L., Matsuura, H., Kasuga, S., and Itakura, Y. 2001. Intake of garlic and its bioactive components. *J Nutr* **131**: 955S–962S.

Andorfer, J.H., Tchaikovskaya, T., and Listowsky, I. 2004. Selective expression of glutathione S-transferase genes in the murine gastrointestinal tract in response to dietary organosulfur compounds. *Carcinogenesis* **25**: 359–367.

Barnes, S., and Kim, H. 2004. Nutriproteomics: identifying the molecular targets of nutritive and non-nutritive components of the diet. *J Biochem Mol Biol* **37**: 59–74.

Bhuvaneswari, V., Abraham, S.K., and Nagini, S. 2005. Combinatorial antigenotoxic and anticarcinogenic effects of tomato and garlic through modulation of xenobiotic-metabolizing enzymes during hamster buccal pouch carcinogenesis. *Nutrition* **21**: 726–31.

Borek, C. 2001. Antioxidant health effects of aged garlic extract. *J Nutr* **131**: 1010S–1015S.

Bottone, F.G., Jr., Baek, S.J., Nixon, J.B., and Eling, T.E. 2002. Diallyl disulfide (DADS) induces the antitumorigenic NSAID-activated gene (NAG-1) by a p53-dependent mechanism in human colorectal HCT 116 cells. *J Nutr* **132**: 773–778.

Brandolini, V., Tedeschi, P., Cereti, E., Maietti, A., Barile, D., Coisson, J.D., Mazzotta, D., Arlorio, M., and Martelli, A. 2005. Chemical and genomic combined approach applied to the characterization and identification of Italian Allium sativum L. *J Agric Food Chem* **53**: 678–683.

Chang, H.P., and Chen, Y.H. 2005. Differential effects of organosulfur compounds from garlic oil on nitric oxide and prostaglandin E2 in stimulated macrophages. *Nutrition* **21**: 530–536.

Chang, H.S., Yamato, O., Yamasaki, M., Ko, M., and Maede, Y. 2005. Growth inhibitory effect of alk(en)yl thiosulfates derived from onion and garlic in human immortalized and tumor cell lines. *Cancer Lett* **223**: 47–55.

Chen, C., Pung, D., Leong, V., Hebbar, V., Shen, G., Nair, S., Li, W., and Kong, A.N. 2004. Induction of detoxifying enzymes by garlic organosulfur compounds through transcription factor Nrf2: effect of chemical structure and stress signals. *Free Radic Biol Med* **37**: 1578–1590.

Creasman, W.T. 2005. Breast cancer: the role of hormone therapy. *Semin Reprod Med* **23**: 167–171.

Davenport, D.M., and Wargovich, M.J. 2005. Modulation of cytochrome P450 enzymes by organosulfur compounds from garlic. *Food Chem Toxicol* Jul 4 [Epub ahead of print].

Davis, C.D., and Milner, J. 2004. Frontiers in nutrigenomics, proteomics, metabolomics and cancer prevention. *Mutat Res* **551**: 51–64.

Dhawan, V., and Jain, S. 2004. Effect of garlic supplementation on oxidized low density lipoproteins and lipid peroxidation in patients of essential hypertension. *Mol Cell Biochem* **266**: 109–115.

Dion, M.E., Agler, M., and Milner, J.A. 1997. S-allyl cysteine inhibits nitrosomorpholine formation and bioactivation. *Nutr Cancer* **28**: 1–6.

Dong, Y., Lisk, D., Block, E., and Ip, C. 2001. Characterization of the biological activity of gamma-glutamyl-Se-methylselenocysteine: a novel, naturally occurring anticancer agent from garlic. *Cancer Res* **61**: 2923–2928.

Druesne, N., Pagniez, A., Mayeur, C., Thomas, M., Cherbuy, C., Duee, P.H., Martel, P., and Chaumontet, C. 2004. Diallyl disulfide (DADS) increases histone acetylation and p21(waf1/cip1) expression in human colon tumor cell lines. *Carcinogenesis* **25**: 1227–1236.

Elango, E.M., Asita, H., Nidhi, G., Seema, P., Banerji, A., and Kuriakose, M.A. 2004. Inhibition of cyclooxygenase-2 by diallyl sulfides (DAS) in HEK 293T cells. *J Appl Genet* **45**: 469–471.

Fenech, M. 2005. The Genome Health Clinic and Genome Health Nutrigenomics concepts: diagnosis and nutritional treatment of genome and epigenome damage on an individual basis. *Mutagenesis* **20**: 255–269.

Fleischauer, A.T., and Arab, L. 2001. Garlic and cancer: a critical review of the epidemiologic literature. *J Nutr* **131**: 1032S–1040S.

Franco, O.H., Bonneux, L., de Laet, C., Peeters, A., Steyerberg, E.W., and Mackenbach, J.P. 2004. The Polymeal: a more natural, safer, and probably tastier (than the Polypill) strategy to reduce cardiovascular disease by more than 75%. *BMJ* **329**: 1447–1450.

Frantz, D.J., Hughes, B.G., Nelson, D.R., Murray, B.K., and Christensen, M.J. 2000. Cell cycle arrest and differential gene expression in HT-29 cells exposed to an aqueous garlic extract. *Nutr Cancer* **38**: 255–264.

Gallou-Kabani, C., and Junien, C. 2005. Nutritional epigenomics of metabolic syndrome: new perspective against the epidemic. *Diabetes* **54**: 1899–1906.

Gao, C., Takezaki, T., Wu, J., Li, Z., Wang, J., Ding, J., Liu, Y., Hu, X., Xu, T., Tajima, K., and Sugimura, H. 2002. Interaction between cytochrome P-450 2E1 polymorphisms and environmental factors with risk of esophageal and stomach cancers in Chinese. *Cancer Epidemiol Biomarkers Prev* **11**: 29–34.

Gedik, N., Kabasakal, L., Sehirli, O., Ercan, F., Sirvanci, S., Keyer-Uysal, M., and Sener, G. 2005. Long-term administration of aqueous garlic extract (AGE) alleviates liver fibrosis and oxidative damage induced by biliary obstruction in rats. *Life Sci* **76**: 2593–2606.

Green, M., Thomas, R., Gued, L., and Sadrud-Din, S. 2003. Inhibition of DES-induced DNA adducts by diallyl sulfide: implications in liver cancer prevention. *Oncol Rep* **10**: 767–771.

Hodge, G., Hodge, S., and Han, P. 2002. Allium sativum (garlic) suppresses leukocyte inflammatory cytokine production *in vitro*: potential therapeutic use in the treatment of inflammatory bowel disease. *Cytometry* **48**: 209–215.

Hsing, A.W., Chokkalingam, A.P., Gao, Y.T., Madigan, M.P., Deng, J., Gridley, G., and Fraumeni, J.F., Jr. 2002. Allium vegetables and risk of prostate cancer: a population-based study. *J Natl Cancer Inst* **94**: 1648–1651.

Khanum, F., Anilakumar, K.R., and Viswanathan, K.R. 2004. Anticarcinogenic properties of garlic: a review. *Crit Rev Food Sci Nutr* **44**: 479–488.

Knowles, L.M., and Milner, J.A. 2000. Diallyl disulfide inhibits p34(cdc2) kinase activity through changes in complex formation and phosphorylation. *Carcinogenesis* **21**: 1129–1134.

Knowles, L.M., and Milner, J.A. 2001. Possible mechanism by which allyl sulfides suppress neoplastic cell proliferation. *J Nutr* **131**: 1061S–1066S.

Knowles, L.M., and Milner, J.A. 2003. Diallyl disulfide induces ERK phosphorylation and alters gene expression profiles in human colon tumor cells. *J Nutr* **133**: 2901–2906.

Koh, S.H., Kwon, H., Park, K.H., Ko, J.K., Kim, J.H., Hwang, M.S., Yum, Y.N., Kim, O.H., Kim, J., Kim, H.T., Do, B.R., Kim, K.S., Kim, H., Roh, H., Yu, H.J., Jung, H.K., and Kim, S.H. 2005. Protective effect of diallyl disulfide on oxidative stress-injured neuronally differentiated PC12 cells. *Brain Res Mol Brain Res* **133**: 176–186.

Krest, I., Glodek, J., and Keusgen, M. 2000. Cysteine sulfoxides and allinase activity of some Allium species. *J Agric Food Chem* **48**: 3753–3760.

Lang, A., Lahav, M., Sakhnini, E., Barshack, I., Fidder, H.H., Avidan, B., Bardan, E., Hershkoviz, R., Bar-Meir, S., and Chowers, Y. 2004. Allicin inhibits spontaneous and TNF-alpha induced secretion of proinflammatory cytokines and chemokines from intestinal epithelial cells. *Clin Nutr* **23**: 1199–1208.

Lea, M.A., and Randolph, V.M. 2001. Induction of histone acetylation in rat liver and hepatoma by organosulfur compounds including diallyl disulfide. *Anticancer Res* **21**: 2841–2845.

Ledezma, E., Apitz-Castro, R., and Cardier, J. 2004. Apoptotic and anti-adhesion effect of ajoene, a garlic derived compound, on the murine melanoma B16F10 cells: possible role of caspase-3 and the alpha(4)beta(1) integrin. *Cancer Lett* **206**: 35–41.

Lind, D.S. 2004. Arginine and cancer. *J Nutr* **134**: 2837S–2841S.

Liu, L., and Yeh, Y.Y. 2000. Inhibition of cholesterol biosynthesis by organosulfur compounds derived from garlic. *Lipids* **35**: 197–203.

Mahajan, S., and Atkins, W.M. 2005. The chemistry and biology of inhibitors and pro-drugs targeted to glutathione S-transferases. *Cell Mol Life Sci* **62**: 1221–1233.

Milner, J.A. 2001. Mechanisms by which garlic and allyl sulfur compounds suppress carcinogen bioactivation. Garlic and carcinogenesis. *Adv Exp Med Biol* **492**: 69–81.

Oi, Y., Imafuku, M., Shishido, C., Kominato, Y., Nishimura, S., and Iwai, K. 2001. Garlic supplementation increases testicular testosterone and decreases plasma corticosterone in rats fed a high protein diet. *J Nutr* **131**: 2150–2156.

Ommen, B., and Groten, J.P. 2004. Nutrigenomics in efficacy and safety evaluation of food components. *World Rev Nutr Diet* **93**: 134–152.

Pinto, J.T., Qiao, C., Xing, J., Suffoletto, B.P., Schubert, K.B., Rivlin, R.S., Huryk, R.F., Bacich, D.J., and Heston, W.D. 2000. Alterations of prostate biomarker expression and testosterone utilization in human LNCaP prostatic carcinoma cells by garlic-derived S-allylmercaptocysteine. *Prostate* **45**: 304–314.

Rahman, K. 2001. Historical perspective on garlic and cardiovascular disease. *J Nutr* **131**(3s): 977S–979S.

Rivlin, R.S. 2001. Historical perspective on the use of garlic. *J Nutr* **131**(3s): 951S–954S.

Romano, E.L., Montano, R.F., Brito, B., Apitz, R., Alonso, J., Romano, M., Gebran, S., and Soyano, A. (1997). Effects of Ajoene on lymphocyte and macrophage membrane-dependent functions. *Immunopharmacol Immunotoxicol* **19**: 15–36.

Ross, S.A. 2003. Diet and DNA methylation interactions in cancer prevention. *Ann NY Acad Sci* **983**: 197–207.

Salman, H., Bergman, M., Bessler, H., Punsky, I., and Djaldetti, M. 1999. Effect of a garlic derivative (alliin) on peripheral blood cell immune responses. *Int J Immunopharmacol* **21**: 589–597.

Saravanan, G., and Prakash, J. 2004. Effect of garlic (Allium sativum) on lipid peroxidation in experimental myocardial infarction in rats. *J Ethnopharmacol* **94**: 155–158.

Sela, U., Ganor, S., Hecht, I., Brill, A., Miron, T., Rabinkov, A., Wilchek, M., Mirelman, D., Lider, O., and Hershkoviz, R. 2004. Allicin inhibits SDF-1alpha–induced T cell interactions with fibronectin and endothelial cells by down-regulating cytoskeleton rearrangement, Pyk-2 phosphorylation and VLA-4 expression. *Immunology* **111**: 391–399.

Sener, G., Satyroglu, H., Ozer Sehirli, A., and Kacmaz, A. 2003. Protective effect of aqueous garlic extract against oxidative organ damage in a rat model of thermal injury. *Life Sci* **73**: 81–91.

Sengupta, A., Ghosh, S., and Bhattacharjee, S. 2004. Allium vegetables in cancer prevention: an overview. *Asian Pac J Cancer Prev* **5**: 237–245.

Sundaram, S.G., and Milner, J.A. 1993. Impact of organosulfur compounds in garlic on canine mammary tumor cells in culture. *Cancer Lett* **74**: 85–90.

Sundaram, S.G., and Milner, J.A. 1996. Diallyl disulfide inhibits the proliferation of human tumor cells in culture. *Biochim Biophys Acta* **1315**: 15–20.

Tattelman, E. 2005. Health effects of garlic. *Am Fam Physician* **72**(1): 103–106.

Thomson, M., and Ali, M. 2003. Garlic [*Allium sativum*]: a review of its potential use as an anti-cancer agent. *Curr Cancer Drug Targets* **3**: 67–81.

Van Loo, J.A. 2004. Prebiotics promote good health: the basis, the potential, and the emerging evidence. *J Clin Gastroenterol* **38**: S70–75.

Wen, J., Zhang, Y., Chen, X., Shen, L., Li, G.C., and Xu, M. 2004. Enhancement of diallyl disulfide-induced apoptosis by inhibitors of MAPKs in human HepG2 hepatoma cells. *Biochem Pharmacol* **68**: 323–331.

Wu, C.C., Chung, J.G., Tsai, S.J., Yang, J.H., and Sheen, L.Y. 2004. Differential effects of allyl sulfides from garlic essential oil on cell cycle regulation in human liver tumor cells. *Food Chem Toxicol* **42**: 1937–1947.

Yang, C.S., Chhabra, S.K., Hong, J.Y., and Smith, T.J. 2001. Mechanisms of inhibition of chemical toxicity and carcinogenesis by diallyl sulfide (DAS) and related compounds from garlic. *J Nutr* **131**: 1041S–1045S.

Zhang, Y.J., Chen, Y., Ahsan, H., Lunn, R.M., Chen, S.Y., Lee, P.H., Chen, C.J., and Santella, R.M. 2005. Silencing of glutathione S-transferase P1 by promoter hypermethylation and its relationship to environmental chemical carcinogens in hepatocellular carcinoma. *Cancer Lett* **221**: 135–143.

C H A P T E R

37

Berries

NAVINDRA P. SEERAM

INTRODUCTION

Studies suggest that consumption of a phytochemical-rich diet, which includes fruits and vegetables, contributes toward reducing the risk of certain types of human cancers. Among fruits, berries such as blackberries, black raspberries, blueberries, cranberries, raspberries, and strawberries are popularly consumed in our diet in fresh and in processed forms such as beverages, yogurts, jellies, and jams. In addition, berry extracts are widely consumed in dietary supplement forms for their potential human health benefits. A wide number of laboratory and animal studies have shown that berries have anticancer properties that are attributed to their high content of a diverse range of bioactive phytochemicals. These compounds include flavonoids (anthocyanins, flavonols, and flavanols), condensed tannins (proanthocyanidins [PAs]), hydrolyzable tannins (ellagitannins [ETs] and gallotannins [GTs]), stilbenoids (e.g., resveratrol), phenolic acids (hydroxybenzoic and hydroxycinnamic acids), and lignans. Berry bioactives may impart anticancer effects through various complementary and overlapping mechanisms of action. These include antioxidant effects as free radical scavengers, as well as acting indirectly through antioxidant actions that protect DNA from damage, the regulation of enzymes important in metabolizing xenobiotics and carcinogens, the modulation of nuclear receptors, gene expression, and subcellular signaling pathways of proliferation, angiogenesis, and apoptosis. This chapter reviews the research progress, advances, future challenges, and impact of berry consumption on cancer prevention.

STRUCTURAL TYPES OF BERRY BIOACTIVES

Over the past few decades, knowledge of the composition of berry fruits in fresh, freeze-dried, and extract forms has rapidly expanded with the advent of highly sensitive analytical methods, allowing researchers to establish phytochemical profiles or "chemical fingerprints" of these fruits. These bioactive phytochemicals have been identified as flavonoids (anthocyanins, flavonols, and flavanols), condensed tannins (PAs), hydrolyzable tannins (ETs and GTs), stilbenoids, phenolic acids (hydroxybenzoic and hydroxycinnamic acids), and lignans (Seeram and Nair, 2002; Manach et al., 2004). The considerable diversity in the skeletal structures of these compounds imparts unique biological properties to each class that affects their absorption, distribution, metabolism, and excretion in humans (Beecher, 2003; Manach et al., 2004, 2005; Williamson and Manach, 2005). The structural diversity of berry bioactives can be observed by the varying types and oxidation levels of their heterocycle ring, their substitution patterns of hydroxylation (bearing an -OH group), the existence of stereoisomers, their glycosylation by various sugars, and/or acylation by organic and phenolic acids, and by conjugation with themselves to form polymers, etc. The main structural classes of berry bioactives are shown in Figure 1 and are discussed in the following subsections.

Anthocyanins and Anthocyanidins

Of the numerous phytochemicals found in berries, the anthocyanins are probably the best known. Anthocyanins are

Copyright © 2006, Elsevier Inc.
All rights of reproduction in any form reserved.

R1 = R2 = H; Pelargonidin
R1 = OH; R2 = H; Cyanidin
R1 = R2 = OH; Delphinidin

Anthocyanidins

R1 = R2 = OH; R3 = H; Quercetin
R1 = R3 = H; R2 = OH; Kaempferol
R1 = R2 = R3 = OH; Myricetin

Flavonols

R1 = R2 = R3 = OH; Catechin
R1 = R2 = OH; R3 = gallate; Gallocatechin

Flavanols

$R_1 = R_2 = H$, Propelargonidins
$R_1 = H$, $R_2 = OH$, Procyanidins
R_1, $R_2 = OH$, Prodelphinidins

Proanthocyanidins

R1 = R2 = R3 = OH; Gallic acid

Hydroxybenzoic acid

R1 = R2 = OH; Caffeic acid
R1 = OH; Coumaric acid

Hydroxycinnamic acid

Resveratrol

Stilbenoids

Secoisolariciresinol

Lignans

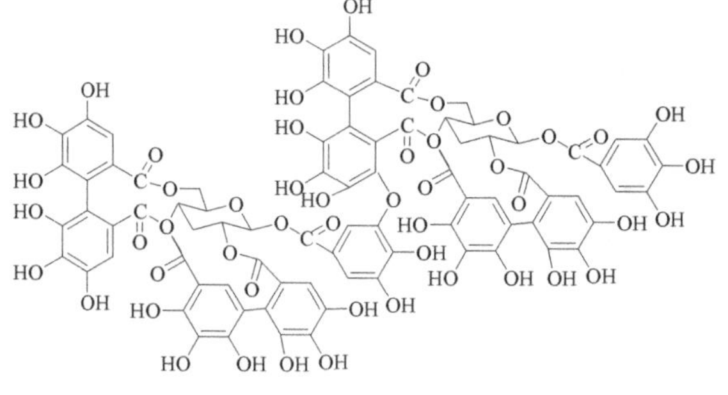

Sanguiin H-6

Ellagitannin

FIGURE 1 Structural classes of bioactives found in berries: anthocyanins, flavonol, flavanols, proanthocyanidins, ellagitannins, hydroxycinnamic and hydroxybenzoic acids, stilbenoids, and lignans.

the pigments that impart the attractive red, blue, purple, violet, and intermediate red-purple to berries and many other fruits, vegetables, and grains (Mazza and Miniati, 1993; Seeram et al., 2001a,b; Wu and Prior, 2005). Similar to most other flavonoids, anthocyanins occur naturally in fruits and vegetables as glycosides. The de-glycosylated or aglycone forms of anthocyanins are known as *anthocyanidins*, which exist as different chemical structures, both colored and uncolored, according to variations in pH (Seeram et al., 2001b). Several hundred anthocyanins are known varying in the basic anthocyanidin skeleton, with the six most common being cyanidin (the most ubiquitous), delphinidin, pelargonidin, malvidin, petunidin, and peonidin (Seeram and Nair, 2002; Seeram et al., 2003) (Figure 1). Apart from variations in the anthocyanidin core, structural diversification is further achieved by the identity and extent and position at which glycosides and/or acyl groups are attached to the skeleton. The most common glycosides encountered on anthocyanins are glucose, galactose, rhamnose, and arabinose usually as 3-glycosides or as 3,5-diglycosides. However, rutinosides (6-*O*-L-rhamnosyl-D-glucosides), sophorosides (2-*O*-D-glucosyl-D-glucosides), and sambubiosides (2-*O*-D-xylosyl-D-glucosides) are also common, as are some 3,7-diglycosides and 3-triosides (Clifford, 2000). Common acylating agents include phenolic acids (caffeic, *p*-coumaric, ferulic, and sinapic), which may themselves bear glycosidic sugars, and a range of aliphatic acids (e.g., acetic, malic, malonic, oxalic, and succinic).

Flavonols

Flavonols are the most ubiquitous flavonoids found in foods and, similar to anthocyanins, also occur naturally in glycosylated forms where the associated sugar moiety is often glucose or rhamnose, although other substituents such as galactose, arabinose, xylose, and glucuronic acid may also be involved. The most common flavonol aglycons are quercetin (the most ubiquitous), kaempferol, and myricetin (Figure 1). Because their biosynthesis is stimulated by light, flavonols accumulate in the outer and aerial tissues of plants (in leaves) and fruits (in skin). However, in berries, they are commonly found in the flesh and achenes of the fruits such as in strawberries (Seeram et al., 2006) and in raspberries (Kaehkoenen et al., 2001).

Flavanols

Flavanols are the only class of flavonoids that do not occur naturally as glycosides. Flavanols exist in both monomeric (catechins) and polymeric (PAs; see later discussion) forms (Figure 1). Catechins and epicatechin are the main flavanols found in berry fruits, whereas gallocatechin, epigallocatechin, and epigallocatechin gallate are found in certain seeds of leguminous plants, in grapes, and in tea (Manach et al., 2004).

Condensed Tannins (Proanthocyanidins)

Condensed tannins, or PAs, are dimers, oligomers, and polymers of catechins that are bound together by links between C4 and C8 (or C6) (Buelga-Santos and Scalbert, 2000) (Figure 1). However, in addition to C–C linkages, PAs can also have ether linkages between C2–O5 or C2–O7, referred to as *A-type linkages*. PAs can also be classified based on their constituent units that are produced on acid hydrolysis. In this case, they are referred to by the nomenclature system established for anthocyanidins. The most ubiquitous PAs are procyanidins, consisting of individual (epi)catechin units. Others include the less common propelargonidins, consisting of (epi)afzelechin units, and prodelphinidins, consisting of (epi)gallocatechin units. It is difficult to estimate the PA content of berries and other foods because they have a wide range of structures and molecular weights and their mean degree of polymerization in foods has rarely been determined (Manach et al., 2004; Gu et al., 2004). Among common edible berries, blueberries and cranberries contain high levels of PAs (Gu et al., 2004).

Hydrolyzable Tannins (Ellagitannins and Gallotannins)

Hydrolyzable tannins are categorized into GTs and ETs. GTs are esters of gallic acid, whereas ETs are composed of esters of hexahydroxydiphenic acid (HHDP: 6,6′-dicarbonyl-2,2′,3,3′,4,4′-hexahydroxybiphenyl moiety). On hydrolysis of ETs, the HHDP moiety spontaneously rearranges to release ellagic acid, hence, their name (Clifford and Scalbert, 2000). The hydrolysis reaction to form ellagic acid is usually employed for the detection and quantification or ETs in berry fruits (Amakura et al., 2000). ET monomers can be further oxidized in plants and form dimers, trimers, and tetramers with molecular weights up to 4000 Da. Among common edible berries, strawberries, raspberries, blackberries, and black raspberries contain high levels of ETs (Maeaettae-Riihinen et al., 2004a,b).

Phenolic Acids

Berries contain a wide variety of phenolic acids (Zadernowski et al., 2005), which occur as derivatives of hydroxybenzoic acid (e.g., gallic acid) and hydroxycinnamic acid (e.g., caffeic acid) (Figure 1). The hydroxycinnamic acids are more common than the hydroxybenzoic acids and consist chiefly of *p*-coumaric, caffeic, ferulic, and sinapic acids. Hydroxycinnamic acids are found in all parts of fruits, although the highest concentrations are seen in the outer parts of ripe fruits. Concentrations generally decrease during the course of ripening, but total quantities increase as the fruit increases in size (Clifford, 2004). Although phenolic acids are found in berries in free forms, they can be considered components of complex polymers such as hydrolyzable tannins (GTs or ETs) or PAs. Hence, they can be released from their "parent" compounds *in vivo* by changes in physiological pH, enzymatic, or gut bacterial action, or *in vitro* by storage, processing conditions, and so on (see the section "Bioavailability and Metabolism of Berry Bioactives").

Stilbenoids

Stilbenes are phenolic-based compounds, of which the most widely recognized is resveratrol (3,4′,5-trihydroxystilbene) (Figure 1). Resveratrol has attracted immense attention because of its biological properties including its anticancer effects (reviewed in Aggarwal et al., 2004). Resveratrol has a number of closely related analogs (e.g., pterostilbene and piceatannol), and it plays an important role as the parent molecule of oligomers known as the *viniferins* (Aggarwal et al., 2004). Among edible berries, resveratrol and its analogs have been reported in members of the *Vaccinum* genus, for example, blueberry, bilberry, lingonberry, and cranberry (Rimando et al., 2004).

Lignans

Lignans are formed from two phenylpropane units. Although the richest dietary sources of lignans are flaxseed and linseed, which contain secoisolariciresinol (Figure 1) and low quantities of matairesinol (Scalbert and Williamson, 2000; Clifford, 2004), some cereals, grains, fruits, and certain vegetables also contain traces of lignans. Lignans have been reported in berries such as strawberry, blackberry, raspberry, cloudberry, cranberry, lingonberry, and blueberry (Mazur et al., 2000).

Triterpenes and Sterols

Although the predominant bioactive phytochemicals in berries are phenolic compounds (see previous subsections), there have been reports of nonpolar compounds such as ursolic acid, triterpene hydroxycinnamates, and β-sitosterol in members of the *Vaccinum* species, for example, cranberries (Murphy et al., 2003; Schmandke, 2004).

DISTRIBUTION OF BERRY BIOACTIVES

Berries contain a wide range of phytochemicals, the most predominant of which are phenolic (aromatic ring bearing hydroxyl, -OH, group) in nature. Phenolic contents have been reported to vary considerably among different berry genera. For example, in the *Vaccinum* genus, anthocyanins are reported as the main phenolics in bilberry, bog-whortleberry, and cranberry, but in cowberries, flavanols and procyanidins predominate (Kaehkoenen et al., 2001). In the genus *Rubus* (e.g., cloudberry and raspberry), the main phenolics are ETs, and in the genus *Fragaria* (e.g., strawberry), ETs are the second largest group after anthocyanins (Kaehkoenen et al., 2001). Flavonols based on quercetin and kaempferol aglycons are also reported to be present in substantial quantities in strawberries (Seeram et al., 2006). Phenolic acids are found in high levels in rowanberries (genus *Sorbus*) and anthocyanins in chokeberries (genus *Aronia*). In the genus *Ribes* (currants and gooseberries), anthocyanins predominate, as well as in crowberries (genus *Empetrum*) (Kaehkoenen et al., 2001).

Maeaettae-Riihinen (2004) identified and quantified soluble and insoluble phenolics in 18 species of berries belonging to the families Grossulariaceae, Ericaceae, Rosaceae, Empetraceae, Elaeagnaceae, and Caprifoliaceae. The berry phenolics were identified as conjugated hydroxycinnamic acids, flavonol glycosides, and anthocyanins. The study showed similarities in the distribution of conjugated forms of phenolics among berry species of the same family and differences in the profiles and compositions of anthocyanins among individual types of berries.

Mechanisms of Chemoprevention by Berry Bioactives

Epidemiological evidence has shown that the consumption of a phytochemical-rich diet contributes toward reducing the risk of certain types of human cancers (Steinmetz and Potter, 1991; Meyskens and Zabo, 2005). Although the predominant phytochemicals in berry fruits are phenolic compounds such as anthocyanins, its other phytochemicals may also contribute synergistically and/or additively to its anticancer activities (Camire, 2002; Seeram et al., 2004). Hence, berries contain a wide range of phytochemicals that may impart anticancer effects through various complementary and overlapping mechanisms of action (Liu, 2003; Heber, 2004). The individual constituents of berries, as well as total berry extracts, have been shown in *in vitro* and *in vivo* studies to exert anticancer properties through different mechanisms. For example, berry bioactives may exert anticancer effects through their antioxidant properties as free radical scavengers while acting indirectly through antioxidant actions that protect DNA from damage, the regulation of enzymes important in metabolizing xenobiotics and carcinogens, the modulation of nuclear receptors, gene expression, and subcellular signaling pathways of proliferation, angiogenesis, and apoptosis.

Although an effort has been made to categorize the actions of berry bioactives in the following discussion, the reader will notice overlap between sections, which is due to the multimechanistic and complementary pathways through which berry phytochemicals exert their anticancer effects.

Modulation of Signaling Pathways of Proliferation, Apoptosis, and Cell Cycle Arrest

Studies have investigated the subcellular signaling and molecular mechanisms through which berry phytochemicals may exert their anticancer properties. These include the ability of berry extracts and their purified bioactives to inhibit cell proliferation and modulate cell cycle arrest, induce DNA repair and signal transduction, and apoptosis in cancer cells while having little or no cytotoxic effect on normal noncancerous cells. Although many of these studies have focused on evaluating whole berry extracts, a significant number of bioassay-guided fractionations, aimed at isolating and identifying the active constituents present in the berry extracts, have been done. Some of the *in vitro* anticancer studies conducted on berries are discussed in the following paragraphs.

Blueberry, black chokeberry, lingonberry, and raspberry extracts were shown to decrease the proliferation of human colon HT-29 and breast MCF-7 cancer cells in a dose-dependent manner (Olsson et al., 2004). Similarly, whole cranberry fruit extracts were assayed for tumor growth inhibition using seven tumor cell lines and selective inhibition of K562 leukemia, and HT-29 colon cells were observed from a methanolic extract in the range of 16–125 μg/ml (Yan et al., 2002). Bilberry extract was shown to inhibit the growth of human HL60 leukemia cells and HCT116 colon carcinoma cells and induce apoptotic cell bodies and nucleosomal DNA fragmentation in the HL60 leukemia cells (Katsube et al., 2003). Juranic (2005) compared the antiproliferative action of red raspberries to malignant human colon carcinoma LS174 cells and to normal immune competent cells, with the action of ellagic acid (a bioactive constituent of berries) alone. Results from this study showed that raspberry extracts possess the potential for antiproliferative action against human colon carcinoma cells, which was correlated with its content of ellagic acid. In this study, the cytotoxic activity of the extracts was not pronounced on normal human PBMC colon cells (Juranic, 2005).

A bioactivity-guided fractionation of cranberries identified triterpenoid esters that inhibited the growth of MCF-7 breast, ME180 cervical, and PC3 prostate tumor cell lines (Murphy et al., 2003). The major bioactives were identified as the *cis*- and *trans*- isomers of 3-*O*-*p*-hydroxycinnamoyl ursolic acid. The authors reported that the *cis*- isomer showed superior antiproliferative activity when compared with its *trans* counterpart and to quercetin and cyanidin-3-galactoside. Phenylboronic acid was also isolated from the cranberry extract, but it did not exhibit significant antitumor activity (Murphy et al., 2003).

Ramos (2005) investigated the effects of individual purified berry bioactives, quercetin, chlorogenic acid, and epicatechin, as well as whole strawberry fruit extract on the viability and apoptosis of human hepatoma HepG2 cells. Quercetin and the strawberry fruit extract inhibited cell viability in a dose-dependent manner, whereas chlorogenic acid and epicatechin had no prominent effects on the cell death rate. Similarly, quercetin and the strawberry extract, but not chlorogenic acid and epicatechin, induced apoptosis in hepatoma HepG2 cells. In cell cycle progression experiments, quercetin and the strawberry extract were observed to arrest the G_1 phase in the cell cycle before apoptosis (Ramos et al., 2005).

In a study to identify the chemopreventive phytochemicals in black raspberries, Han et al. (2005) identified two of its bioactives as ferulic acid and β-sitosterol. In the bioassay-guided fractionation experiment, Han (2005) also demonstrated that a purified fraction eluted with ethanol during chromatography of the organic extract of freeze-dried black raspberries inhibited the growth of premalignant and malignant but not normal human oral epithelial cell lines. However, purified ellagic acid alone was found to inhibit the growth of normal, premalignant, and malignant human oral cell lines. Using flow cytometry and Western blotting of cell cycle–regulatory proteins, these workers also investigated molecular mechanisms by which ferulic acid, β-sitosterol, and the berry ethanol fraction could selectively inhibit the growth of premalignant and malignant oral cells. They observed no discernible change in the cell cycle distribution following treatment of cells with the berry ethanol fraction. Premalignant and malignant cells redistributed to the G_2/M phase of the cell cycle following incubation with ferulic acid, whereas β-sitosterol–treated premalignant and malignant cells accumulated in the G_0/G_1 and G_2/M phases. The berry ethanol fraction reduced the levels of cyclin A and cell division cycle gene 2 (cdc2) in premalignant cells and cyclin B1, cyclin D1, and cdc2 in the malignant cell lines. The berry ethanol fraction also elevated the levels of p21waf1/cip1 in the malignant cell line. Ferulic acid treatment led to increased levels of cyclin B1 and cdc2 in both cell lines, and p21waf1/cip1 was induced in the malignant cell line; on the other hand, β-sitosterol reduced the levels of cyclin B1 and cdc2 while increasing p21waf1/cip1 in both the premalignant and the malignant cell lines. The authors concluded that the growth-inhibitory effects of black raspberries on premalignant and malignant human oral cells may reside in specific components that target aberrant signaling pathways regulating cell cycle progression (Han et al., 2005).

Cell lines of differing origins have been shown to respond with varying degrees of sensitivity in growth toward berry extracts. For example, a cranberry presscake (the material remaining after squeezing the juice from berries) extract inhibited proliferation of eight human tumor cell lines of multiple origins (Ferguson et al., 2004). The androgen-dependent prostate cell line, LNCaP, was the most sensitive of those tested, whereas the estrogen-independent breast line, MDA-MB-435, and the androgen-independent prostate line, DU145, were the least sensitive. Other human tumor lines originating from breast (MCF-7), skin (SK-MEL-5), colon (HT-29), lung (DMS114), and brain (U87) had intermediate sensitivities to the cranberry extract. Using flow cytometric analyses of DNA distribution (for cell cycle) and annexin V positivity (for apoptosis), the authors showed that a purified fraction blocked cell cycle progression and induced cells to undergo apoptosis in a dose-dependent manner in MDA-MB-435 breast cells (Ferguson et al., 2004). In another study, human oral, prostate, and colon cancer cells responded with differing sensitivities to cranberry bioactives (Seeram et al., 2004). In this study, Seeram et al. (2004) showed that although the individual cranberry phytochemicals, such as its flavonols, organic acids, PAs, and anthocyanins, inhibited the growth of the tumor cells, when they were combined, as found in a total cranberry extract, antiproliferative activities were significantly enhanced.

The effects of berry extracts on signal transduction pathways have also been reported. For example, Huang (2002) reported on the effects of a black raspberry methanol extract and its purified fractions on transactivation of activated protein-1 (AP-1) and nuclear factor-κB (NFκB) induced by the carcinogen BaP diol-epoxide (BPDE) in mouse epidermal cells. AP-1 and NFκB are transcription factors associated with carcinogenesis (Bode and Dong, 2000). Inhibition of AP-1 activity has been shown to lead to the suppression of cell transformation (Dong et al., 1997). NFκB is also an important regulator in deciding cell fate, such as programmed cell death and proliferation control, and is critical in tumorigenesis (Baldwin, 1996). The inhibitory effects of a purified black raspberry fraction on AP-1 and NFκB were mediated via inhibition of mitogen-activated protein kinase (MAPK) activation and inhibitory subunit κB phosphorylation, respectively. Pretreatment of cells with purified berry fractions did not result in an inhibition of BPDE binding to DNA, which suggested that this was not a mechanism of reduced AP-1 and NFκB activities. In addition, none of the purified fractions were found to affect p53-dependent transcription activity. In view of the important roles of AP-1 and NFκB in tumor promotion and progression, the authors concluded that the ability of black raspberries to inhibit tumor development may be mediated by impairing signal transduction pathways, leading to activation of AP-1 and NFκB (Huang et al., 2002).

The inhibitory effects of strawberry on tetradecanoylphorbol-13-acetate (TPA)—or ultraviolet B (UVB)–induced AP-1 and NFκB were recently demonstrated by Wang (2005). TPA and UVB are well-known tumor promoters and can produce reactive oxygen species (ROS) and stimulate AP-1 and NFκB activities by activating MAPK signaling pathways such as the extracellular signal–regulated kinases 1/2 (ERK1/2), c-Jun amino-terminal kinases (JNKs), and the p38 MAPK (Schulze-Osthoff et al., 1997; Hou et al., 2004). These workers also evaluated strawberry extracts for inhibition of proliferation and transformation of human and mouse cancer cells. The strawberry extracts inhibited the proliferation of human lung epithelial cancer cell line A549 and decreased TPA-induced neoplastic transformation of mouse epidermal cells. In addition, pretreatment of the mouse epidermal cells with strawberry extracts resulted in the inhibition of both UVB- and TPA-induced AP-1 and NFκB transactivation. Furthermore, the strawberry extracts also blocked TPA-induced phosphorylation of ERKs and UVB-induced phosphorylation of ERKs and JNK kinase in the mouse epidermal cell culture. These results suggest that the ability of strawberries to block UVB- and TPA-induced AP-1 and NFκB activation might be due to their antioxidant properties and their ability to reduce oxidative stress. The authors concluded that the oxidative events that regulate AP-1 and NFκB transactivation could be important molecular targets for cancer prevention. Therefore, strawberries may be highly effective as chemopreventive agents that act by targeting the downregulation of AP-1 and NFκB activities, blocking MAPK signaling, and suppressing cancer cell proliferation and transformation (Wang et al., 2005).

In another study, freeze-dried strawberries and freeze-dried black raspberries were extracted with methanol, partitioned, and chromatographed into several fractions (Xue et al., 2001). The extracts, along with ellagic acid, were analyzed for anti-transformation activity in a Syrian hamster embryo (SHE) cell transformation model. None of the extracts or ellagic acid alone produced an increase in morphological transformation. For assessment of chemopreventive activity, SHE cells were treated with test samples and benzopyrene for 7 days. Ellagic acid and two of the purified fractions produced a dose-dependent decrease in transformation compared with the benzopyrene treatment only. Ellagic acid and the two purified fractions were further examined using a 24-hour co-treatment with benzopyrene or a 6-day treatment following 24 hours with benzopyrene. Ellagic acid showed inhibitory ability in both protocols. The two purified fractions significantly reduced benzopyrene-induced transformation when co-treated with benzopyrene for 24 hours. The authors concluded that the possible mechanism by which the purified fractions inhibited cell transformation appear to involve interference of uptake, activation, detoxification of benzopyrene, and/or intervention of DNA binding and DNA repair (Xue et al., 2001).

Angiogenesis

Antiangiogenic (the ability to reduce unwanted growth of blood vessels) approaches to treat cancer represent a priority area in vascular tumor biology. Angiogenesis-inhibiting agents have the potential for inhibiting tumor growth and limiting the dissemination of metastasis, thus keeping cancers in a static growth state for prolonged periods.

Extracts of blueberry, bilberry, cranberry, elderberry, raspberry, and strawberry were studied for antioxidant efficacy, cytotoxic potential, cellular uptake, and antiangiogenic properties (Roy et al., 2002; Bagchi et al., 2004). The authors evaluated various combinations of the extracts and showed that a "synergistic extract" significantly inhibited both hydrogen peroxide (H_2O_2) and tumor necrosis factor-α (TNF-α)–induced vascular endothelial growth factor (VEGF, a key regulator of tumor angiogenesis) expression by human keratinocytes (Roy et al., 2002; Bagchi et al., 2004). The same research group also studied the synergistic extract in an *in vivo* mice model of angiogenesis and observed that it significantly inhibited basal monocyte chemotactic protein-1 (MCP-1), a protein responsible for facilitating angiogenesis (Atalay et al., 2003). In addition, the synergistic extract significantly inhibited inducible NFκB transcription. Endothelioma cells pretreated with the synergistic berry extract showed a diminished ability to form hemangioma and markedly decreased tumor growth by >50% (Atalay et al., 2003).

Liu (2005) reported that black raspberry extract showed antiangiogenic properties in a human tissue–based *in vitro* fibrin clot angiogenesis assay. Bioassay-guided fractionation of the berry extract resulted in a highly potent antiangiogenic fraction that completely inhibited angiogenic initiation and vessel growth. Further subfractionation of this active fraction revealed the coexistence of multiple antiangiogenic compounds, one of which has been identified as gallic acid (a bioactive constituent of berries). However, the authors concluded that the whole fraction was superior to its subfractions and that the active ingredients may be additive and/or synergistic in their antiangiogenic effects (Liu et al., 2005).

Antimutagenicity

The initial step in the formation of cancer is damage to the genome of a somatic cell producing a mutation in an oncogene or a tumor suppressor gene. Strawberry, blueberry, and raspberry juices and extracts were evaluated for their ability to inhibit the production of mutations by the direct-acting mutagen methyl methanesulfonate and the metabolically activated carcinogen benzopyrene (Hope et al., 2004). The berry juices significantly inhibited mutagenesis caused by both carcinogens. Ethanol extracts from freeze-dried fruits of strawberry and blueberry cultivars were also evaluated, and hydrolyzable tannin-containing fractions from strawberries were found to be most effective at inhibiting mutations.

Induction of Antioxidant Enzymes

ROS are formed during the normal endogenous metabolic process and from exogenous factors such as ionizing radiation, diet, and xenobiotics (Davis, 1987; Halliwell and Gutteridge, 1989). Oxidative stress arises either from the overproduction of ROS or from the deficiency of antioxidant defense or repair mechanisms, resulting in reversible or irreversible damage to critical cellular macromolecules such as lipids, proteins, and DNA (Davis, 1987). Oxidative stress has been implicated in initiation, promotion, and progression phases of carcinogenesis (Cerutti, 1985), and the resulting unrepaired oxidative damage has been suggested to play a role in other chronic diseases, including cancer (Ames et al., 1993). Aerobic organisms constantly battle the adverse effects of ROS by increasing the production of biochemical antioxidants (such as glutathione and ascorbate) or by inducing endogenous antioxidant enzymes including superoxide dismutase (SOD), catalase, glutathione peroxidase (G-POD), and glutathione reductase (GR). These scavenging antioxidant molecules and the endogenous antioxidant enzymes attenuate the ROS concentration to maintain an intracellular reduction and oxidation (redox) balance.

Strawberries have been shown to have antioxidant capacity against ROS such as ROO, O_2^-, H_2O_2, OH, and $^1O_2$ (Wang and Lin, 2000; Wang and Zheng, 2001). These workers also demonstrated the activities of antioxidant enzymes including SOD, G-POD, and GR in strawberries (Wang et al., 2005). The activities of antioxidant enzymes in blackberries have also been shown (Jiao and Wang, 2000). The activities of antioxidant enzymes in both berries were shown to be positively correlated with their antioxidant capacity (Jiao and Wang, 2000; Wang et al., 2005).

Studies have been designed to investigate correlations between antioxidative potential and antiproliferative activities of berries. For example, Meyers (2003) investigated eight strawberry cultivars to find out if their antioxidant capacities, by the total oxyradical scavenging capacity (TOSC) assay, can be correlated with their antiproliferative activities. Overall, although the proliferation of HepG2 human liver cancer cells was significantly inhibited in a dose-dependent manner after exposure to all strawberry cultivar extracts, these workers found no relationship between antiproliferative activity and antioxidant content. In another study, similar results were observed when extracts of four raspberry cultivars were evaluated for total antioxidant capacity and cancer cell antiproliferative activity (Weber and Liu, 2002). In this study, the antioxidant activity of each cultivar was directly related to the total amount of phenolics, but no significant relationship was found between antiproliferative activity and the total amount of phenolics (Weber and Liu, 2002).

Berry extracts and their purified bioactives have been investigated for effects on the production of cytokines such as TNF-α, which mediates a variety of cell functions including stimulation of nitric oxide (NO) production. TNF-α has been related to oxidative stress and diseases such as chronic inflammation (Park et al., 2000). Wang (2002) investigated common purified berry phenolics and anthocyanin-enriched blueberry, blackberry, Saskatoon berries, and black currant extracts for their effects on the production of TNF-α in RAW 264.7 macrophages. Gallic acid and catechin showed small but significant effects, whereas chlorogenic acid had no effect on TNF-α production. The flavonol quercetin inhibited TNF-α production, whereas kaempferol and myricetin induced the secretion of TNF-α. The individual anthocyanidins (pelargonidin, cyanidin, delphinidin, peonidin, and malvidin), anthocyanins (malvidin 3-glucoside and malvidin 3,5-diglucosides), and anthocyanin-enriched blueberry extracts induced TNF-α production and acted as modulators of the immune response in the activated macrophages (Wang and Mazza, 2002).

Inhibitors of Detoxification Enzymes

Phase I and phase II metabolizing enzymes play an important role in the biotransformation of carcinogens and xenobiotics in the human body. In phase I reactions, these chemicals undergo bioactivation catalyzed by cytochrome, P450 (CYP) isozymes to produce strong electrophiles which are capable of interacting with cellular nucleophiles such as DNA to form adducts eventually culminating in mutagenesis and neoplastic transformation. In normal cells, the reactive intermediates formed by phase I reactions are then conjugated via phase II enzymes with glucuronides, sulfate, or glutathione, facilitating their excretion. Phase II xenobiotic detoxification enzymes include glutathione *S*-transferase, sulfotran ferases, UDP-glucuronyl transferases, and quinone reductase (QR). Conjugation enhances hydrophilicity of the metabolites, thus facilitating elimination of the carcinogen from the body. Although phase I enzymes increase the carcinogenic potency of a chemical, phase II enzymes serve to detoxify the electrophilic metabolites. An imbalance in phase I and phase II carcinogen-metabolizing enzymes has been documented in a wide range of malignant tumors including breast cancer (Williams and Phillips, 2000).

Kansanen et al. (1996) investigated the *in vitro* effects of some flavonoids and phenolic acids common to berries, as well as extracts of strawberry and black currant, on CYP 1A1 isozyme. These workers found that the flavonoid aglycons and berry extracts were effective inhibitors of CYP 1A1, whereas the flavonoid glycosides and phenolic acids were not (Kansanen et al., 1996). Other studies have shown that flavonoid-rich fractions from *Vaccinium* species, such as cranberries, induce QR *in vitro* (Bomser et al., 1996). This study also showed that a cranberry extract inhibited expression of ornithine decarboxylase (ODC), a key enzyme responsible for polyamine biosynthesis (Bomser et al., 1996).

Inhibitors of Metalloproteinase Enzymes

Matrix metalloproteinases (MMPs) are enzymes essential for development, and remodeling of tissues and aberrant overexpression of these enzymes contributes to several pathological conditions. In particular, MMP overexpression in cancer plays a significant role in metastasis by providing a mechanism for invasion and progression. MMPs are involved in proteolysis of the extracellular matrix, which can lead to the progression of tumors (Pupa et al., 2002). Raspberries and blackberries have been shown to inhibit the activities of MMP-2 and MMP-9 (Tate et al., 2004). Quercetin, a typical berry flavonol, has been shown to have a chemoprotective role through complex effects on signal transduction involved in cell proliferation, including increased expression of endogenous tissue inhibitors of MMPs (Morrow et al., 2001). Ursolic acid, which has been reported in berries such as cranberries (Murphy et al., 2003), reduced the expression of MMP-9 in HT-1080 fibrosarcoma cells and consequently inhibited tumor invasion (Cha et al., 1996, 1998).

As part of a study to determine the effects of cranberry extracts on prostate tumor proliferation, evaluation of the effects of whole cranberry extract and purified fractions on MMP expression in DU145 prostate cells was conducted (Kondo et al., 2004; Neto et al., 2006). The whole cranberry extract inhibited expression of MMP-2 and MMP-9 in the cells at 100 μg/ml concentrations. A purified PA fraction, at 500 μg/ml, inhibited MMP-2 expression completely and resulted in ~75% inhibition of MMP-9 activity (Kondo et al., 2004; Neto et al., 2006).

CHEMOPREVENTION STUDIES WITH BERRY BIOACTIVES

Animal Studies

The chemopreventive potential of freeze-dried berries against aerodigestive tract cancers, such as oral cavity and esophageal cancers, has been demonstrated in a number of animal studies (Stoner et al., 1999; Kresty et al., 2001; Aziz et al., 2002; Casto et al., 2002). Studies have suggested that berries, which contain high amounts of ETs and ellagic acid (e.g., strawberries and black raspberries), show better effects against these cancers than those that contain PAs as their predominant tannins (e.g., blueberries) (Aziz et al., 2002). However, although ellagic acid, an abundant component in berries, has been shown to inhibit carcinogenesis both *in vitro* and *in vivo*, several studies have reported that other compounds in berries may also contribute to the observed anticancer effects (Stoner et al., 1999).

Studies have been designed to investigate the chemopreventive effects of berries during initiation and progression phases of cancer. Lyophilized black raspberries (LBRs) were evaluated against N-nitrosomethylbenzylamine (NMBA)–induced esophageal tumorigenesis in the F344 rat during initiation and post-initiation phases of carcinogenesis

(Kresty et al., 2001). Anti-initiation studies included a 30-week tumorigenicity period, quantification of DNA adducts, and NMBA metabolism study. Feeding 5 and 10% LBRs, for 2 weeks prior to NMBA treatment and throughout a 30-week period significantly reduced tumor multiplicity (39 and 49%, respectively). The post-initiation inhibitory potential of berries was evaluated in a second experiment with administration of LBRs after NMBA treatment. In this experiment, animals were sacrificed at 15, 25, and 35 weeks. The LBRs were found to inhibit tumor progression as evidenced by significant reductions in the formation of preneoplastic esophageal lesions, decreased tumor incidence and multiplicity, and reduced cellular proliferation. At 25 weeks, both 5 and 10% LBRs significantly reduced tumor incidence, tumor multiplicity, proliferation rates, and preneoplastic lesion development. At 35 weeks, only the 5% LBRs significantly reduced tumor incidence and multiplicity, proliferation indices, and preneoplastic lesion formation. The authors concluded that dietary administration of LBRs inhibited events associated with the initiation, promotion, and progression stages of carcinogenesis.

In another study with LBRs, the hamster cheek pouch (HCP) assay was used to evaluate the ability of the berries to inhibit oral cavity tumors (Casto et al., 2002). Hamsters were fed 5 and 10% LBRs in the diet for 2 weeks prior to treatment with dimethylbenzanthracene (DMBA) and for 10 weeks thereafter. HCPs were painted with the DMBA to induce tumor formation. The animals were sacrificed 12–13 weeks after the beginning of DMBA treatment and the number and volume of tumors were determined. The authors observed a significant difference in tumor number between the LBR-treated and control groups (Casto et al., 2002).

Blueberries were evaluated for their ability to inhibit NMBA tumorigenesis in the rat esophagus (Aziz et al., 2002). As previously mentioned, blueberries differ in phytochemical content from strawberries and black raspberries in that their predominant tannins are PAs and not ETs. Two weeks prior to NMBA treatment, animals were placed on a control diet or diets containing 5 and 10% freeze-dried blueberries. At 25 weeks, animals on 5 and 10% blueberries produced no significant differences in tumor incidence, multiplicity, or size when compared with NMBA-treated controls. In addition, blueberries did not reduce the formation of NMBA-induced O6-methylguanine adducts in esophageal DNA when fed at 10% of the diet. The authors concluded that blueberries appear to lack components that inhibit the initiation and progression of NMBA-induced tumori-genesis in the rat esophagus (Aziz et al., 2002). It should be noted that although blueberries did not show anticancer properties in these studies, its consumption has been correlated with other health benefits such as anti-neurodegenerative properties and so on (Joseph et al., 1998, 2003).

Human Studies

A survey of the literature revealed no published human clinical studies examining the anticancer effects of berries. However, data are available on the absorption, distribution, metabolism, and excretion of berry bioactives in humans obtained from foods, beverages, extracts, and as singly purified compounds (see the section "Bioavailability and Metabolism of Berry Bioactives," later in this chapter).

A phase I study sought to examine tolerance for high dietary levels of freeze-dried berries that would be necessary for chemoprevention studies (The James 2002/2003 Annual Report, Comprehensive Cancer Center, Arthur G. James Cancer Hospital and Richard J. Solove Research Institute, Ohio State University). Because the berries were well tolerated, studies are being designed to test the anticancer effects of these berries among individuals with precancerous lesions and at high risk for esophageal, colon, and oral cancers (www.jamesline.com/patientsandpublic/research/index.cfm).

A human study (Moller et al., 2004) investigated the effects of black currant anthocyanins on the steady state level of oxidative DNA damage in mononuclear blood cells of 57 healthy human subjects, determined as strand breaks, as well as endonuclease III and formamidopyrimidine DNA glycosylase (Fpg). The baseline level of oxidative DNA damage was low, and Fpg-sensitive sites increased during the intervention within the black currant anthocyanin group, whereas there were no differences between treatments in any of the DNA damage markers. The authors concluded that even large amounts of berry antioxidants did not decrease the already low steady state levels of oxidative DNA damage in healthy, adequately nourished humans (Moller et al., 2004).

DIETARY INTAKE OF BERRY BIOACTIVES

As previously discussed, phenolics are the predominant phytochemicals present in berry fruits. Unfortunately, because of the considerable number of factors that can modify their concentrations, reference food composition tables are not available. Their estimation in foods is also extremely challenging because of their wide structural diversity existing as different conjugated forms and complex polymeric nature, ill-defined structures, and unavailability of commercial standards. As a result, data on their dietary intake, as well as data on their bioavailability and pharmacokinetics in humans, are limited. Only partial data for certain phenolics, such as flavonols, have been published on the basis of direct food analysis or bibliographic compilations (Manach et al., 2004). In the United States, agencies such as the U.S. Department of Agriculture (USDA) have established databases in which the flavonoid contents of selected foods, compiled from varying bibliographic sources, are available (USDA web site).

Studies have shown a high variability in polyphenol intake based on variations in individual food preferences. A diet consisting of several servings of fruit and vegetables per day can provide up to 1 g of phenolics consisting of the following: 16% flavonols, flavones, and flavanones; 17% anthocyanins; 20% catechins; and 45% PAs, ETs, and other "bioflavonoids" (Kuhnau, 1976). Among the berry bioactives, research has targeted individual data for specific classes of compounds. For example, consumption of flavonols has been estimated at 20–25 mg/day in the United States, Denmark, and Holland (Hertog et al., 1993; Justesen et al., 1997; Sampson et al., 2002). In Italy, consumption ranged from 5 to 125 mg/day, and the mean value was 35 mg/day (Pietta et al., 1996). In Finland, where high amounts of berries are eaten, anthocyanin consumption was found to be 82 mg/day on average, although some intakes exceeded 200 mg/day (Heinonen, 2001). Intake of phenolic acids ranged from 6 to 987 mg/day in Germany (Radtke et al., 1998).

Dietary burden, nature, and occurrence of specific classes of berry bioactives have been previously reviewed. These include anthocyanins (Clifford, 2000a); ETs (Clifford and Scalbert, 2000); PAs (Santos-Buelga and Scalbert, 2000); sterols (Piironen, 2000); hydroxybenzoic acid derivatives (Tomás-Barberán and Clifford, 2000); chlorogenic acid and other cinnamates (Clifford, 2000b); lignans and stilbenes (Cassidy et al., 2000); and flavonols, flavones, and flavanols (Hollman and Art, 2000).

BIOAVAILABILITY AND METABOLISM OF BERRY BIOACTIVES

Several review articles have been published on the bioavailability and metabolism of phenolics (Scalbert and Williamson, 2000; Rechner et al., 2002; Manach et al., 2004, 2005a; Walle, 2004; Williamson and Manach, 2005). A wide body of studies has shown that although phenolics are the predominant phytochemicals in human diet, they are not necessarily the most active *in vivo*, either because they are poorly absorbed from the gut, highly metabolized, or rapidly eliminated. In addition, because of digestive and hepatic activities, the bioactivities of phenolic metabolites that are bioavailable in blood and target organs may differ significantly from their native forms. Hence, extensive knowledge of the bioavailability of phenolics is essential if their health effects are to be understood.

Because most phenolics are present in food in the form of esters, glycosides, or polymers that cannot be absorbed in their native form, they must be hydrolyzed by intestinal enzymes or by the colonic microflora before they can be absorbed, for example, into aglycons, which can then be absorbed from the small intestine. When the gut microflora is involved, the efficiency of absorption is often reduced because the flora also degrades the aglycons that it releases and produces various simple phenolic and aromatic acids in the process. During the course of absorption, phenolics are conjugated (usually methylated, sulfated, and glucuronidated) in the small intestine and later in the liver, a metabolic detoxification process that facilitates biliary and urinary elimination. Because the conjugation mechanisms are highly efficient, aglycons are either absent in blood or present in very low concentrations after consumption of nutritional doses. Circulating phenolics are conjugated derivatives that are extensively bound to albumin (Scalbert and Williamson, 2000). Phenolics are able to penetrate tissues, particularly those in which they are metabolized, but reports on their ability to accumulate within specific target tissues are scarce (Manach et al., 2004). Phenolics are secreted via the biliary route into the duodenum, where they are subjected to the action of bacterial enzymes, especially β-glucuronidase, in the distal segments of the intestine, after which they may be reabsorbed. This enterohepatic recycling may lead to a longer presence of phenolics within the body.

The metabolism of the major classes of berry bioactives is discussed in the following subsections.

Metabolism of Anthocyanins

Among berry bioactives, the metabolism and bioavailability of anthocyanins in both human and animal models have been well studied (Prior, 2002). Human studies with anthocyanins have shown that albeit at low concentrations, they are detectable intact in human plasma (Cao and Prior, 1999; Cao et al., 2001; Milbury et al., 2002; Mazza et al., 2002; Bitsch, 2004). The elimination of plasma anthocyanins appears to follow first-order kinetics, and most anthocyanins were excreted in the urine within 4 hours of feeding (Milbury et al., 2002). Other studies have shown that anthocyanins and their metabolites are detectable in human urine after consumption of boysenberries (Cooney et al., 2004), strawberries (Felgines et al., 2003), and elderberries (Murkovic et al., 2001). The bioavailability of 15 structurally different anthocyanins from blueberry, boysenberry, black raspberry, and black currant in both humans and rats was investigated (McGhie et al., 2003). This study showed that intact and unmetabolized anthocyanins were detected in urine, although the relative concentrations of dosing varied, indicating that differences in bioavailability were due to variations in chemical structure. Anthocyanin metabolites and tissue distribution in digestive organs (stomach, jejunum, liver), kidney, and brain were studied in male Wistar rats fed with blackberry anthocyanins for 15 days (Talavera et al., 2005). Intact blackberry anthocyanins were detected in the stomach, while other organs (jejunum, liver, kidney) contained the anthocyanins in their intact and in their methylated and monoglucuronidated forms. Jejunum and blood plasma also contained anthocyanins in their aglycon forms. In the brain, the total anthocyanin content reached 0.25 nmol/g tissue (Talavera et al., 2005). Milbury et al. (2005) also demonstrated that berry anthocyanins cross the blood–brain barrier.

Metabolism of Flavonols

Among berry flavonols, quercetin, the most ubiquitous flavonol in plant foods, is probably the most investigated. Hollman (1995, 1996) showed that quercetin is bioavailable in human plasma and demonstrated that glucosides of quercetin were more efficiently absorbed than quercetin itself, whereas the rhamnoglucoside (rutin) was less efficiently and less rapidly absorbed. The bioavailability of quercetin differs among food sources, depending on the type of glycosides they contain. For example, onions, which contain glucosides, are better sources of bioavailable quercetin than apples and tea, which contain rutin and other glycosides.

The presence of intact glycosides of quercetin in plasma had been debated, but it is now accepted that such compounds are absent from plasma after nutritional doses (Manach et al., 2005). On metabolism, phenolic acids can also be produced from flavonols by the gut microflora. Quercetin degradation produces mainly 3,4-dihydroxyphenylacetic, 3-methoxy-4-hydroxyphenylacetic (homovanillic acid), and 3-hydroxyphenylacetic acids (Manach et al., 2005).

Metabolism of Tannins (Proanthocyanidins and Ellagitannins)

Assessment of the bioavailability and metabolism of tannins (PAs, ETs, and GTs) remains a challenge because of their ill-defined structures, lack of authentic standards, and lack of accurate data on their compositions in foods. Because of these challenges, there are few human studies reporting bioavailability of PAs and ETs (Seeram et al., 2004; Manach et al., 2005). Although the detection of PA dimers B1 and B2 in human plasma has been reported (Holt et al., 2002), studies done both *in vitro* and in animals have shown that polymerization greatly impairs intestinal absorption (Déprez et al., 2001; Donovan et al., 2002). An ET, punicalagin (MW 1084), was detected intact in rat plasma and was reported as the largest polyphenol observed *in vivo* (Cerda et al., 2003). Given the poor absorption of these molecules in their intact forms, it is possible that their biological effects may be attributable not only to direct actions of tannins themselves, but to the actions of some of their metabolites that can be more readily absorbed. PAs and ETs may be degraded into various phenolic and aromatic acids and other metabolites by the microflora (Cerda et al., 2005a,b; Manach et al., 2005). ETs have been shown to release ellagic acid in human plasma (Seeram et al., 2004). Whereas the microbial metabolism of PAs has never been studied in humans after consumption of purified PA polymers (Manach et al., 2005), that of ETs has been reported (Cerda et al., 2004, 2005a,b). Therefore, further investigations into the degradation of PAs into microbial metabolites must be further evaluated in humans.

CONCLUSIONS AND FUTURE DIRECTIONS

In conclusion, an overwhelming number of cell culture and animal studies suggest that berries may have immense potential for the prevention and treatment of cancer. Berry bioactives may act individually, additively, and synergistically to exert their chemopreventive properties. Because extrapolations cannot be made between *in vitro* and animal studies to humans, future clinical trials should be designed to investigate the potential of berries for the prevention and treatment of human cancers. In addition, further details on absorption, distribution, metabolism, and mechanisms of action of berry bioactives in humans are necessary to determine effective dietary portions of berries. Whether bioactivities of berries are made stronger by the interactions of the many substances within a particular fruit, as well as in combination with phytochemicals from other fruits and vegetables, should be investigated. In addition, interactions of berries with prescription drugs and other herbal medicines, through their ability to modulate enzymes or cell receptors, should be investigated in carefully planned and controlled human clinical studies.

References

Aggarwal, B.B., Bhardwaj, A., Aggarwal, R.S., Seeram, N.P., Shishodia, S., and Takada, Y. 2004. Role of resveratrol in prevention and therapy of cancer: preclinical and clinical studies. *Anticancer Res* **24**: 2783–2840.

Amakura, Y., Okada, M., Tsuji, A., and Tonogai, Y. 2000. High-performance liquid chromatography determination with photodiode array detection of ellagic acid in fresh and processed fruits. *J Chromatogr B* **896**: 87–93.

Ames, B.N., Shigena, M.K., and Hagen, T.M. 1993. Oxidants, antioxidants and the degenerative diseases of aging. *Proc Natl Acad Sci USA* **90**: 7915–7922.

Atalay, M., Gordillo, G., Roy, S., Rovin, B., Bagchi, D., Bagchi, M., and Sen, C.K. 2003. Antiangiogenic property of edible berry in a model of hemangioma. *FEBS Lett* **544**: 252–257.

Aziz, R.M., Nines, R., Rodrigo, K., Harris, K., Hudson, T., Gupta, A., Morse, M., Carlton, P., and Stoner, G.D. 2002. The effect of freeze-dried blueberries on N-nitrosomethylbenzylamine tumorigenesis in the rat esophagus. *Pharm Bio* **40**: 43–49.

Bagchi, D., Sen, C.K., Bagchi, M., and Atalay, M. 2004. Anti-angiogenic, antioxidant, and anticarcinogenic properties of a novel anthocyanin-rich berry extract formula. *Biochem Trans Biokhimiya* **69**: 75–80.

Baldwin, A.S. 1996. The NF-kappa B and I kappa B proteins: new discoveries and insights. *Annu Rev Immunol* **14**: 649–683.

Beecher, G.R. 2003. Overview of dietary flavonoids: nomenclature, occurrence, and intake. *J Nutr* **133**: 3248S–3254S.

Bitsch, I., Janssen, M., Netzel, M., Strass, G., and Frank, T. 2004. Bioavailability of anthocyanidin-3 glycosides following consumption of elderberry extract and blackcurrant juice. *Int J Clin Pharm Ther* **42**: 293–300.

Bode, A.M., and Dong, Z. 2000. Signal transduction pathways: targets for chemoprevention of skin cancer. *Lancet Oncol* **1**: 181–188.

Bomser, J., Madhavi, D.L., Singletary, K., and Smith, M.A.L. (1996). *In vitro* anticancer activity of fruit extracts from *Vaccinium* species. *Planta Med* **62**: 212–216.

Buelga-Santos, C., and Scalbert, A. 2000. Proanthocyanidins and tannin-like compounds-nature, occurrence, dietary intake and effects on nutrition and health. *J Sci Food Agric* **80**: 1094–1117.

Cao, G., and Prior, R.L. 1999. Anthocyanins are detected in human plasma after oral administration of an elderberry extract. *Clin Chem* **45**: 574–576.

Cao, G., Muccitelli, H.U., Sanchez-Moreno, C., and Prior, R.L. 2001. Anthocyanins are absorbed in glycated forms in elderly women: a pharmacokinetic study. *Am J Clin Nutr* **73**: 920–926.

Camire, M.E. 2002. Phytochemicals in the *Vaccinium* family: bilberries, blueberries, and cranberries. *In* "Phytochemicals: Their Role in Nutrition and Health" (M.S. Meskin, W.R. Bidlack, A.J. Davies, and S.T. Omaye, eds), pp. 19–40. CRC Press, Boca Raton, FL.

Cassidy, A., Hanley, B., and Lamuela-Raventos, R.M. 2000. Isoflavones, lignans and stilbenes—origins, metabolism and potential importance to human health. *J Sci Food Agric* **80**: 1044–1062.

Casto, B.C., Kresty, L.A., Kraly, C.L., Pearl, D.K., Knobloch, T.J., Schut, H.A., Stoner, G.D., Mallery, S.R., and Weghorst, C.M. 2002. Chemoprevention of oral cancer by black raspberries. *Anticancer Res* **22**: 4005–4015.

Cerda, B., Llorach, R., Ceron, J.J., Espin, J.C., and Tomas-Barberan, F.A. 2003. Evaluation of the bioavailability and metabolism in the rat of punicalagin, an antioxidant polyphenol from pomegranate juice. *Eur J Nutr* **42**: 18–28.

Cerda, B., Espin, J.C., Parra, S., Martinez, P., and Tomas-Barberan, F.A. 2004. The potent *in vitro* antioxidant ellagitannins from pomegranate juice are metabolised into bioavailable but poor antioxidant hydroxy-6H-dibenzopyran-6-one derivatives by the colonic microflora of healthy humans. *Eur J Nutr* **43**: 205–220.

Cerda, B., Periago, P., Espin, J.C., and Tomas-Barberan, F.A. 2005a. Identification of urolithin A as a metabolite produced by human colon microflora from ellagic acid and related compounds. *J Agric Food Chem* **53**: 5571–5576.

Cerda, B., Tomas-Barberan, F.A., and Espin, J.C. 2005b. Metabolism of antioxidant and chemopreventive ellagitannins from strawberries, raspberries, walnuts, and oak-aged wine in humans: identification of biomarkers and individual variability. *J Agric Food Chem* **53**: 227–235.

Cerutti, P.A. 1985. Pro-oxidant states and tumor promotion. *Science* **227**: 375–381.

Cha, H.J., Bae, S.K., Lee, H.Y., Lee, O.H., Sato, H., Seiki, M., Park, B.C., and Kim, K.W. 1996. Anti-invasive activity of ursolic acid correlates with the reduced expression of matrix metalloproteinase-9 (MMP-9) in HT1080 fibrosarcoma cells, *Cancer Res* **56**: 2281–2284.

Cha, H.J., Park, M.T., Chung, H.Y., Kim, N.D., Sato, H., Seiki, M., and Kim, K.W. 1998. Ursolic acid–induced down-regulation of MMP-9 gene is mediated through the nuclear translocation of glucocorticoid receptor in HT1080 fibrosarcoma cells. *Oncogene* **16**: 771–778.

Clifford, M.N. 2000a. Anthocyanins—nature, occurrence and dietary burden. *J Sci Food Agric* **80**: 1063–1072.

Clifford, M.N. 2000b. Chlorogenic acids and other cinnamates—nature, occurrence, dietary burden, absorption and metabolism. *J Sci Food Agric* **80**: 1033–1043.

Clifford, M.N., and Scalbert, A. 2000. Ellagitannins—nature, occurrence and dietary burden. *J Sci Food Agric* **80**: 1118–1125.

Cooney, J.M., Jensen, D.J., and McGhie, T.K. 2004. LC-MS identification of anthocyanins in boysenberry extract and anthocyanin metabolites in human urine following dosing. *J Sci Food Agric* **84**: 237–245.

Davies, K.J. 1987. Protein damage and degradation by oxygen radicals. I. General aspects. *J Biol Chem* **62**: 9895–9901.

Déprez, S., Mila, I., Huneau, J-F., Tomé, D., and Scalbert, A. 2001. Transport of proanthocyanidin dimer, trimer and polymer across monolayers of human intestinal epithelial Caco-2 cells. *Antiox Redox Signal* **3**: 957–967.

Dong, Z., Huang, C., Brown, R.E., and Ma, W.Y. 1997. Inhibition of activator protein 1 activity and neoplastic transformation by aspirin. *J Biol Chem* **272**: 9962–9970.

Donovan, J.L., Manach, C., Rios, L., Morand, C., Scalbert, A., and Remesy, C. 2002. Procyanidins are not bioavailable in rats fed a single meal containing a grapeseed extract or the procyanidin dimer B3. *Br J Nutr* **87**: 299–306.

Felgines, C., Talavera, S., Gonthier, M-P., Texier, O., Scalbert, A., Lamaison, J-L., and Remesy, C. 2003. Strawberry anthocyanins are recovered in urine as glucuro- and sulfoconjugates in humans. *J Nutr* **133**: 1296–1301.

Ferguson, P.J., Kurowska, E., Freeman, D.J., Chambers, A.F., and Koropatnick, D.J. 2004. A flavonoid fraction from cranberry extract inhibits proliferation of human tumor cell lines. *J Nutr* **134**: 1529–1535.

Gu, L., Kelm, M.A., Hammerstone, J.F., Beecher, G., Holden, J., Haytowitz, D., Gebhardt, S., and Prior, R.L. 2004. Concentrations of proanthocyanidins in common foods and estimations of normal consumption. *J Nutr* **134**: 613–617.

Halliwell, B., and Gutteridge, J.M.C. 1989. "Free Radicals in Biology and Medicine," 2nd ed. Clarendon Press, Oxford, U.K.

Han, C.H., Ding, H., Casto, B., Stoner, G.D., and D'Ambrosio, S.M. 2005. Inhibition of the growth of premalignant and malignant human oral cell lines by extracts and components of black raspberries. *Nutr Cancer* **51**: 207–217.

Hertog, M.G.L., Hollman, P.C.H., Katan, M.B., and Kromhout, D. 1993. Intake of potentially anticarcinogenic flavonoids and their determinants in adults in the Netherlands. *Nutr Cancer* **20**: 21–29.

Heber, D. 2004. Phytochemicals beyond antioxidation. *J Nutr* **134**: 3175S–3176S.

Heinonen, M. 2001. Anthocyanins as dietary antioxidants. *In* "Third International Conference on Natural Ontioxidants and Anticarcinogens in Food, Health, and Disease" (S. Voutilainen and J.T. Salonen, eds), Vol. 25, June 6–9, 2001. Helsinki: Kuopion Yliopisto, Finland.

Hollman, P.C.H., Devries, J.H.M., Vanleeuwen, S.D., Mengelers, M.J.B., and Katan, M.B. 1995. Absorption of dietary quercetin glycosides and quercetin in healthy ileostomy volunteers. *Am J Clin Nutr* **62**: 1276–1282.

Hollman, P.C.H., Vandergaag, M., Mengelers, M.J.B., Vantrijp, J.M.P., Devries, J.H., and Katan, M.B. 1996. Absorption and disposition kinetics of the dietary antioxidant quercetin in man. *Free Radic Biol Med* **21**: 703–707.

Hollman, P.C.H., and Ilja, C.W.A. 2000. Flavonols, flavones and flavanols—nature, occurrence and dietary burden. *J Sci Food Agric* **80**: 1081–1093.

Hou, D.X., Kai, K., Li, J.J., Lin, S., Terahara, N., Wakamatsu, M., Fujii, M., Young, M.R., and Colburn, N. 2004. Anthocyanidins inhibit activator protein 1 activity and cell transformation: structure-activity relationship and molecular mechanisms. *Carcinogenesis* **25**: 29–36.

Hope, S.S., Tate, P.L., Huang, G., Magee, J.B., Meepagala, K.M., Wedge, D.E., and Larcom, L.L. 2004. Antimutagenic activity of berry extracts. *J Med Food* **7**: 450–455.

Huang, C., Huang, Y., Li, J., Hu, W., Aziz, R., Tang, M-S., Sun, N., Cassady, J., and Stoner, G.D. 2002. Inhibition of benzo(a)pyrene diol-epoxide–induced transactivation of activated protein 1 and nuclear factor κB by black raspberry extracts. *Cancer Res* **62**: 6857–6863.

Jiao, H., and Wang, S.Y. 2000. Correlation of antioxidant capacities to oxygen radical scavenging enzyme activities in blackberry. *J Agric Food Chem* **48**: 5672–5676.

Joseph, J.A., Shukitt-Hale, B., Denisova, N.A., Prior, R.L., Cao, G., Martin, A., Taglialatela, G., and Bickford, P.C. 1998. Long-term dietary strawberry, spinach, or vitamin E supplementation retards the onset of age-related neuronal signal-transduction and cognitive behavioral deficits. *J Neurosci* **18**: 8047–8055.

Joseph, J.A., Denisova, N.A., Arendash, G., Gordon, M., Diamond, D., Shukitt-Hale, B., and Morgan, D. 2003. Blueberry supplementation enhances signaling and prevents behavioral deficits in an Alzheimer disease model. *Nutr Neurosci* **6**: 153–162.

Juranic, Z., Zizak, Z., Tasic, S., Petrovic, S., Nidzovic, S., Leposavic, A., and Stanojkovic, T. 2005. Antiproliferative action of water extracts of seeds or pulp of five different raspberry cultivars. *Food Chem* **93**: 39–45.

Justesen, U., Knuthsen, P., and Leth, T. 1997. Determination of plant polyphenols in Danish foodstuffs by HPLC-UV and LC-MS detection. *Cancer Lett* **114**: 165–167.

Kaehkoenen, M.P., Hopia, A.I., and Heinonen, M. 2001. Berry phenolics and their antioxidant activity. *J Agric Food Chem* **49**: 4076–4082.

Kansanen, L., Mykkanen, H., and Torronen, R. 1996. Flavonoids and extracts of strawberry and black currant are inhibitors of the carcinogen-activating enzyme CYP1A1 *in vitro*. *Natural Antioxidants Food Quality Atheroscl Cancer Prev* **181**: 386–388.

Katsube, N., Iwashita, K., Tsushida, T., Yamaki, K., and Kobori, M. 2003. Induction of apoptosis in cancer cells by bilberry (*Vaccinium myrtillus*) and the anthocyanins. *J Agric Food Chem* **51**: 68–75.

Kondo, M., Lamoureaux, T.L., Neto, C.C., Hurta, R.A.R., Curtis, S., Matchett, M.D., Yeung, H., Sweeney-Nixon, M.I., and Vaisberg, A.J. 2004. Proanthocyanidins, anthocyanins and triterpenoids from cranberry fruits: antitumor activity and effects on matrix metalloproteinase expression. *J Nutr* **134**: 3521S–3547S.

Kresty, L.A., Morse, M.A., Morgan, C., Carlton, P.S., Lu, J., Gupta, A., Blackwood, M., and Stoner, G.D. 2001. Chemoprevention of esophageal tumorigenesis by dietary administration of lyophilized black raspberries. *Cancer Res* **61**: 6112–6119.

Kuhnau, J. 1976. The flavonoids. A class of semi-essential food components: their role in human nutrition. *World Rev Nutr Diet* **24**: 117–191.

Liu, R.H. 2003. Health benefits of fruits and vegetables are from additive and synergistic combination of phytochemicals. *Am J Clin Nutr* **78**: 517S–520S.

Liu, Z., Schwimer, J., Liu, D., Greenway, F.L., Anthony, C.T., and Woltering, E.A. 2005. Black raspberry extract and fractions contain angiogenesis inhibitors. *J Agric Food Chem* **53**: 3909–3915.

Maeaettae-Riihinen, K.R., Kamal-Eldin, A., Mattila, P.H., Gonzalez-Paramas, A.M., and Toerroenen, A.R. 2004a. Distribution and contents of phenolic compounds in eighteen Scandinavian berry species. *J Agric Food Chem* **52**: 4477–4486.

Maeaettae-Riihinen, K.R., Kamal-Eldin, A., and Toerroenen, A.R. 2004b. Identification and quantification of phenolic compounds in berries of *Fragaria* and *Rubus* species (family Rosacea). *J Agric Food Chem* **52**: 6178–6187.

Manach, C., Scalbert, A., Morand, C., Rémésy, C., and Jimenez, L. 2004. Polyphenols: food sources and bioavailability. *Am J Clin Nutr* **79**: 727–747.

Manach, C., Williamson, G., Morand, C., Scalbert, A., and Rémésy, C. 2005. Bioavailability and bioefficacy of polyphenols in humans. I. Review of 97 bioavailability studies. *Am J Clin Nutr* **81**: 230S–242S.

Mazur, W.M., Uehara, M., Wahala, K., and Adlercreutz, H. 2000. Phytooestrogen content of berries, and plasma concentrations and urinary excretion of enterolactone after a single strawberry-meal in human subjects. *Br J Nutr* **83**: 381–387.

Mazza, G., and Miniati, E. 1993. "Anthocyanins in Fruits, Vegetables and Grains." CRC Press, Boca Raton, FL.

Mazza, G., Kay, C.D., Cottrell, T., and Holub, B.J. 2002. Absorption of anthocyanins from blueberries and serum antioxidant status in human subjects. *J Agric Food Chem* **50**: 7731–7737.

McCord, J.M. 1979. Superoxide dismutases: occurrence, structure, function and evolution. *In* "Isozyme: Current Topics in Biological and Medical Research" (M. Rattazzi, J. Scandalios, and G.S. Whitt, eds), Vol. 3, pp. 1–21. Alan R. Liss, Inc., New York.

McGhie, T.K., Ainge, G.D., Barnett, L.E., Cooney, J.M., and Jensen, D.J. 2003. Anthocyanin glycosides from berry fruit are absorbed and excreted unmetabolized by both humans and rats. *J Agric Food Chem* **51**: 4539–4548.

Meyers, K.J., Watkins, C.B., Pritts, M.P., and Liu, R.H. 2003. Antioxidant and antiproliferative activities of strawberries. *J Agric Food Chem* **51**: 6887–6892.

Meyskens, F.L., and Szabo, E. 2005. Diet and cancer: the disconnect between epidemiology and randomized clinical trials. *Cancer Epidemiol Biomarkers Prev* **14**: 1366–1369.

Milbury, P.E., Cao, G., Prior, R.L., and Blumberg, J. 2002. Bioavailability of elderberry anthocyanins. *Mech Ageing Dev* **123**: 997–1006.

Milbury, P.E., Graf, B.A., Blumberg, J.B., Curran-Celentano, J.M., McDonald, J., Doncaster, K.L., Vinqvist, M., and Kalt, W. 2005. Anthocyanins cross the blood brain barrier: effects on oxidative stress-induced apoptosis [Abstract]. Paper presented at: 229th ACS National Meeting, AGFD-171, San Diego, California, United States.

Moller, P., Loft, S., Alfthan, G., and Freese, R. 2004. Oxidative DNA damage in circulating mononuclear blood cells after ingestion of black currant juice or anthocyanin-rich drink. *Mutat Res* **551**: 119–126.

Morrow, D.M.P., Fitzsimmons, P.E.E., Chopra, M., and McGlynn, H. 2001. Dietary supplementation with the antitumor promoter quercetin: its effects on matrix metalloproteinase gene regulation. *Mutat Res* **480–481**: 269–276.

Murkovic, M., Mülleder, U., Adam, U., and Pfannhauser, W. 2001. Detection of anthocyanins from elderberry juice in human urine. *J Sci Food Agric* **81**: 934–937.

Murphy, B.T., MacKinnon, S.L., Yan, X., Hammond, G.B., Vaisberg, A.J., and Neto, C.C. 2003. Identification of triterpene hydroxycinnamates with *in vitro* antitumor activity from whole cranberry fruit (*Vaccinium macrocarpon*). *J Agric Food Chem* **51**: 3541–3545.

Neto, C.C., Krueger, C.G., Lamoureaux, T.L., Kondo, M., Vaisberg, A.J., Hurta, R.A.R., Curtis, S., Matchett, M.D., Yeung, H., Sweeney-Nixon, M.I., and Reed, J.D. 2005. MALDI-TOF MS characterization of proanthocyanidins from cranberry fruit (*Vaccinium macrocarpon*) that inhibit tumor cell growth and matrix metalloproteinase expression *in vitro*. *J Sci Food Agric* **86**: 18–25.

Olsson, M.E., Gustavsson, K.E., Andersson, S., Nilsson, A., and Duan, R-D. 2004. Inhibition of cancer cell proliferation *in vitro* by fruit and berry extracts and correlations with antioxidant levels. *J Agric Food Chem* **52**: 7264–7271.

Park, Y.C., Rimbach, G., Saliou, C., Valacchi, G., and Packer, L. 2000. Activity of monomeric, dimeric, and trimeric flavonoids on NO production, TNF-α secretion, and NF-κB–dependent gene expression in RAW 264.7 macrophages. *FEBS Lett* **464**: 93–97.

Pietta, P., Simonetti, P., and Roggi, C. 1996. Dietary flavonoids and oxidative stress. *In* "Natural Antioxidants and Food Quality in Atherosclerosis and Cancer Prevention" (J.T. Kumpulainen and J.T. Salonen, eds), pp. 249–255. Royal Society of Chemistry, London.

Piironen, V., Lindsay, D.G., Miettinen, T.A., Toivo, J., and Lampi, A-M. 2000. Plant sterols: biosynthesis, biological function and their importance to human nutrition. *J Sci Food Agric* **80**: 939–966.

Prior, R.L. 2004. Absorption and metabolism of anthocyanins: potential health effects. *In* "Phytochemicals: Mechanisms of Action," pp. 1–19. 4th International Phytochemical Conference, Pomona, California, United States.

Pupa, S.M., Menard, S., Forti, S., and Tagliabue, E. 2002. New insights into the role of extracellular matrix during tumor onset and progression. *J Cell Physiol* **192**: 259–267.

Radtke, J., Linseisen, J., and Wolfram, G. 1998. Phenolic acid intake of adults in a Bavarian subgroup of the national food composition survey. *Z Ernahrungswiss* **37**: 190–197.

Ramos, S., Alia, M., Bravo, L., and Goya, L. 2005. Comparative effects of food-derived polyphenols on the viability and apoptosis of a human hepatoma cell line (HepG2). *J Agric Food Chem* **53**: 1271–1280.

Rechner, A.R., Kuhnle, G., Bremner, P., Hubbard, G.P., Moore, K.P., and Rice-Evans, C.A. 2002. The metabolic fate of dietary polyphenols in humans. *Free Radic Biol Med* **33**: 220–235.

Rimando, A.M., Kalt, W., Magee, J.B., Dewey, J., and Ballington, J.R. 2004. Resveratrol, pterostilbene, and piceatannol in *Vaccinium* berries. *J Agric Food Chem* **52**: 4713–4719.

Roy, S., Khanna, S., Alessio, H.M., Vider, J., Bagchi, D., Bagchi, M., and Sen, C.K. 2002. Antiangiogenic property of edible berries. *Free Radic Res* **36**: 1023–1031.

Sampson, L., Rimm, E., Hollman, P.C., de Vries, J.H., and Katan, M.B. 2002. Flavonol and flavone intakes in US health professionals. *J Am Diet Assoc* **102**: 1414–1420.

Schmandke, H. 2004. Ursolic acid and its derivatives with antitumor activity in berries of *Vaccinium* species. *Ernaehrungs-Umschau* **51**: 235–237.

Schulze-Osthoff, K., Ferrari, D., Riehemann, K., and Wesselborg, S. 1997. Regulation of NF-kappa β activation by MAP kinase cascades. *Immunobiology* **198**: 35–49.

Seeram, N.P., Momin, R.A., Bourquin, L.D., and Nair, M.G. 2001a. Cyclooxygenase inhibitory and antioxidant cyanidin glycosides from cherries and berries. *Phytomedicine* **8**: 362–369.

Seeram, N.P., Bourquin, L.D., and Nair, M.G. 2001b. Degradation products of cyanidin glycosides from tart cherries and their bioactivities. *J Agric Food Chem* **49**: 4924–4929.

Seeram, N.P., and Nair, M.G. 2002. Inhibition of lipid peroxidation and structure-activity–related studies of the dietary constituents, anthocyanins, anthocyanidins and catechins. *J Agric Food Chem* **50**: 5308–5312.

Seeram, N.P., Zhang, Y., and Nair, M.G. 2003. Inhibition of proliferation of human cancer cell lines and cyclooxygenase enzymes by anthocyanidins and catechins. *Nutr Cancer* **46**: 101–106.

Seeram, N.P., Adams, L.S., Hardy, M.L., and Heber, D. 2004a. Total cranberry extract versus its phytochemical constituents: antiproliferative and synergistic effects against human tumor cell lines. *J Agric Food Chem* **52**: 2512–2517.

Seeram, N.P., Lee, R., and Heber, D. 2004b. Bioavailability of ellagic acid in human plasma after consumption of ellagitannins from pomegranate (*Punica granatum* L.) juice. *Clin Chim Acta* **348**: 63–68.

Seeram, N.P., Lee, R., Scheuller, H.S., and Heber, D. 2005. Identification of phenolics in strawberries by liquid chromatography electrospray ionization mass spectroscopy. *Food Chem* **97**: 1–11.

Steinmetz, K.A., and Potter, J.D. 1991. Vegetable, fruit and cancer. I. Epidemiology. *Cancer Causes Control* **2**: 325–357.

Stoner, G.D., Kresty, L.A., Carlton, P.S., Siglin, J.C., and Morse, M.A. 1999. Isothiocyanates and freeze-dried strawberries as inhibitors of esophageal cancer. *Toxicol Sci* **52**: 95–100.

Tate, P., God, J., Bibb, R., Lu, Q., and Larcom, L.L. 2004. Inhibition of metalloproteinase activity by fruit extracts. *Cancer Lett* **212**: 153–158.

Talavera, S., Felgines, C., Texier, O., Besson, C., Gil-Izquierdo, A., Lamaison, J-L., and Remesy, C. 2005. Anthocyanin metabolism in rats and their distribution to digestive area, kidney, and brain. *J Agric Food Chem* **53**: 3902–3908.

Tomás-Barberán, F.A., and Clifford, M.N. 2000. Dietary hydroxybenzoic acid derivatives—nature, occurrence and dietary burden. *J Sci Food Agric* **80**: 1024–1032.

US Department of Agriculture. 2003. USDA database for the flavonoid content of selected foods. Available at: www.nal.usda.gov/fnic/foodcomp/. Accessed July 2005.

Walle, T. 2004. Absorption and metabolism of flavonoids. *Free Radic Biol Med* **36**: 829–837.

Wang, J., and Mazza, G. 2002. Effects of anthocyanins and other phenolic compounds on the production of tumor necrosis factor α in LPS/IFN-γ-activated RAW 264.7 macrophages. *J Agric Food Chem* **50**: 4183–4189.

Wang, S.Y., and Lin, H.S. 2000. Antioxidant activity in fruit and leaves of blackberry, raspberry, and strawberry is affected by cultivar and maturity. *J Agric Food Chem* **48**: 140–146.

Wang, S.Y., and Zheng, W. 2001. Effect of plant growth temperature on antioxidant capacity in strawberry. *J Agric Food Chem* **49**: 4977–4982.

Wang, S.Y., Feng, R., Lu, Y., Bowman, L., and Ding, M. 2005. Inhibitory effect on activator protein-1, nuclear factor-kappa B, and cell transformation by extracts of strawberries (*Fragaria* × *ananassa* Duch). *J Agric Food Chem* **53**: 4187–4193.

Weber, C., and Liu, R.H. 2002. Antioxidant capacity and anticancer properties of red raspberry. *Acta Hort* **585**: 451–457.

Williams, J.A., and Phillips, D.H. 2000. Mammary expression of xenobiotic metabolizing enzymes and their potential role in breast cancer. *Cancer Res* **60**: 4667–4677.

Williamson, G., and Manach, C. 2005. Bioavailability and bioefficacy of polyphenols in humans. II. Review of 93 intervention studies. *Am J Clin Nutr* **81**: 243S–255S.

Wu, X., and Prior, R.L. 2005. Systematic identification and characterization of anthocyanins by HPLC-ESI-MS/MS in common foods in the United States: fruits and berries. *J Agric Food Chem* **53**: 2589–2599.

Xue, H., Aziz, R.M., Sun, N., Cassady, J.M., Kamendulis, L.M., Xu, Y., Stoner, G.D., and Klaunig, J.E. 2001. Inhibition of cellular transformation by berry extracts. *Carcinogenesis* **22**: 351–356.

Yan, X., Murphy, B.T., Hammond, G.B., Vinson, J.A., and Neto, C.C. 2002. Antioxidant activities and antitumor screening of extracts from cranberry fruit (*Vaccinium macrocarpon*). *J Agric Food Chem* **50**: 5844–5849.

Zadernowski, R., Naczk, M., and Nesterowicz, J. 2005. Phenolic acid profiles in some small berries. *J Agric Food Chem* **53**: 2118–2124.

C H A P T E R

38

Isoprenoids and Novel Inhibitors of Mevalonate Pathway Activities

HUANBIAO MO AND CHARLES E. ELSON

INTRODUCTION

The mevalonate pathway supports pools of farnesyl diphosphate, geranylgeranyl diphosphate, and dolichol phosphate, products essential for cell survival and proliferation (Figure 1). Chemotherapeutic agents in clinical evaluation inhibit either the activities providing mevalonate-derived intermediates (statins, phenylacetate, and phenylbutyrate) or the activity transferring the farnesyl moiety to small G proteins (farnesyl protein transferase inhibitors). The inhibitory actions attributed to the cyclic isoprenoids, perillyl alcohol and *d*-limonene, include inhibition of farnesyl protein transferase and activation of allyl diphosphate diphosphatase with a concomitant increase in the signaling molecule farnesol, triggering 3-hydroxy-3-methylglutaryl coenzyme A (HMG-CoA) reductase degradation and inhibiting translation of HMG-CoA reductase mRNA. An overexpressed and sterol-feedback resistant HMG-CoA reductase activity in tumors, coupled with post-transcriptional down-regulation of reductase activity triggered by isoprenoids, may afford isoprenoids tumor-targeted growth-suppressive potential.

ISOPRENOIDS: PURE AND MIXED

Members of a broad class of plant products collectively termed *isoprenoids*, differing in size, complexity, and function derived from diverse mevalonate pathway activities operative in plants, suppress the growth of cultured cells, with selectivity for tumor cells and in preclinical studies suppress tumor growth with no evidence of host toxicity (Adany et al., 1994; Yazlovitskaya and Melnykovych, 1995; Stayrook et al., 1997; Ura et al., 1998; Yaguchi et al., 1998; Ariazi et al., 1999; Elson et al., 1999; Mo and Elson, 1999; Mo et al., 1999; Sahin et al., 1999; McIntyre et al., 2000; Rioja et al., 2000; Crowell and Elson, 2001; Smalley and Eisen, 2002; Beaupre et al., 2003; Clark et al., 2003). Reviews record the characterization of 23,000 isoprenoids. Some of the mevalonate-derived secondary products are "pure" isoprenoids of varying structural complexity (Sacchettini and Poulter, 1997) but consisting only of multiples of the five-carbon isoprene unit (×), for example, monoterpenes (2×), sesquiterpenes (3×), diterpenes (4×), triterpenes (6×), tetraterpenes (8×), and polyterpenes (n×) (Bach, 1995). Prominent among the monocyclic monoterpenes reported to suppress tumor growth are a hydrocarbon (*d*-limonene), several alcohols (carvacrol, cresol, eugenol, perillyl alcohol, thymol), aldehydes (menthal, perillaldehyde), and a ketone (menthone). Bicyclic monoterpenes of interest include an alcohol (myrentol) and a ketone (verbenone). Acyclic monoterpenes include alcohols (geraniol, linalool) and an aldehyde (geranial). Corresponding acyclic monoterpenes containing a *cis* bond (nerol, neral) have lower tumor-suppressive potency (Tatman and Mo, 2002). The acyclic sesquiterpenoid alcohol, *trans*, *trans* farnesol is reportedly the most potent of the simple (volatile) isoprenoids (Tatman and Mo, 2002).

Others are "mixed" isoprenoids: the prenylated coumarins, flavones, flavanols, isoflavones, chalcones, quinones, and chromanols, each with only a part of the molecule geraniol or farnesol being derived via the mevalonate pathway (Barron and Ibrahim, 1996). Among the mixed isoprenoids widely distributed in nature, the farnesylated chromanols δ-*d*- and γ-*d*-tocotrienol (He et al., 1997) and the farnesylated quinone menaquinone-3 (Yaguchi et al., 1997,

Copyright © 2006, Elsevier Inc.
All rights of reproduction in any form reserved.

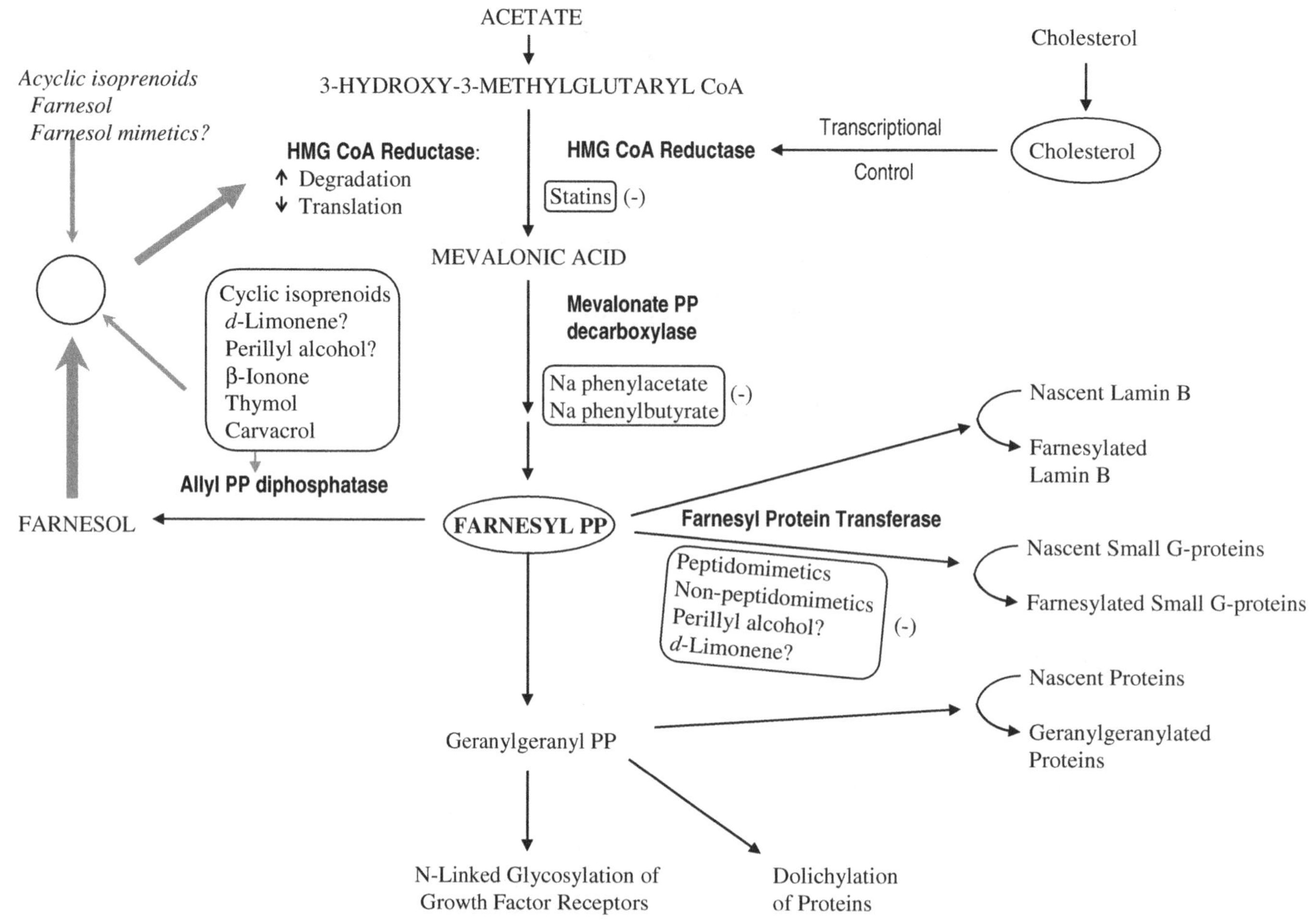

FIGURE 1 The mevalonate pathway supports pools of farnesyl diphosphate, geranylgeranyl diphosphate, and dolichol phosphate, products essential for cell survival and proliferation. Chemotherapeutic agents in clinical evaluation inhibit either the activities providing mevalonate-derived intermediates (statins, phenylacetate, and phenylbutyrate) or the activity transferring the farnesyl moiety to small G proteins (farnesyl protein transferase inhibitors). The inhibitory actions attributed to the cyclic isoprenoids, perillyl alcohol and *d*-limonene, include inhibition of farnesyl protein transferase, activation of allyl diphosphate diphosphatase with a concomitant increase in the signaling molecule, farnesol, triggering HMG-CoA reductase degradation and inhibiting translation of HMG-CoA reductase mRNA. An overexpressed and sterol-feedback–resistant HMG-CoA reductase activity in tumors, coupled with post-transcriptional downregulation of reductase activity triggered by isoprenoids, may afford isoprenoids tumor-targeted growth suppressive potential.

1998; Miyazawa et al., 2001) are reported to have very significant tumor-suppressive activity.

Pure and mixed isoprenoids play regulatory roles in germination, growth, differentiation, flowering, senescence, abscission, and dormancy; provide antioxidant activity; attract pollinating insects; and provide a defense against predatory insects and fungi (Hemming, 1983; Dahiya et al., 1984; Janssen et al., 1987; De Rosa et al., 1994; Tahara et al., 1994; Gagnon et al., 1995; Rahalison et al., 1995; Klepzig et al., 1996; Saito et al., 1996; Pare and Tumlinson, 1997; Sadof and Grant, 1997). Consumers continue to enjoy the nutritional, antimicrobial, and sensory properties a number of diverse isoprenoids contribute to the food supply. Sadly missing are the databanks required for estimating the quantities of pure and mixed isoprenoids presented in a typical diet (Tatman and Mo, 2002).

Isoprenoids Suppress Growth of Tumor Cells

As a consequence of the structural diversity encompassing differences in number of isoprene residues, double bonds, bond configuration, cyclization, and head group polarity, isoprenoids differ substantially in tumor-suppressive potency (Elson, 1995, 1996; Elson et al., 1999; Mo et al., 1999, 2000; Tatman and Mo, 2002) and diverse tumor cell lines differ substantially in sensitivity to an individual isoprenoid (Mo and Elson, 1999; Mo et al., 1999). Although the differential impact of isoprenoids on the growth of tumor and normal cells has been broadly demonstrated, there remains uncertainty regarding the initiating event triggered by isoprenoids (Crowell and Elson, 2001). The growth of tumor cells reflects a "positive" balance between two factors, cell division and cell death. Definitive studies employing cell cycle analysis demonstrate that isoprenoids have an impact on both sides of the "balance" equation (Crowell and Elson, 2001).

Isoprenoids Arrest Tumor Cells at the G_1/S Interface of the Cell Cycle

Farnesol (Chakrabarti et al., 1991; Voziyan et al., 1993; Burke et al., 1997), farnesol derivatives (Mo et al., 2000; McAnally et al., 2003), geraniol (Shoff et al., 1991; Carnesecchi et al., 2004), geraniol derivatives (McAnally et al., 2004), β-ionone (Mo and Elson, 1999; Liu et al., 2004a, 2004b), perillyl alcohol (Bardon et al., 1998; Ferri et al., 2001; Shi and Gould, 2002; Elegbede et al., 2003), perillaldehyde (Elegbede et al., 2003), perillic acid (Beaupre et al., 2003), γ-tocotrienol (Mo and Elson, 1999), and menaquinone-3 (Miyazawa et al., 2001) slow the progress of diverse lines of tumor cells through the cell cycle with a resultant buildup of cells in the G_1 phase.

The G_1 phase of the cell cycle represents the interval (gap) between mitosis (M phase) and DNA replication (S phase) in proliferating cells. Passage from G_1 to S is regulated by a family of cyclins that act as regulatory subunits for cyclin-dependent kinases (cdks). Myc, a mitogen-activated transcription factor with downstream target genes encoding cyclins D2, D1, and E, modulates the cyclin/cdk complex that regulates the G_1-to-S progression of cells. The cyclin/cdk complex is activated by the sequential phosphorylation and dephosphorylation of key residues located primarily in the cdk subunits. The cyclin/cdk complex of early G_1 consists either of cdk2, cdk4, or cdk6 bound to a cyclin D isoform. When stabilized as a consequence of DNA damage, p53 upregulates expression of the cdk inhibitor, $p21^{Waf1/Cip1}$, thereby holding cells in G_1. Activation of transforming growth factor-β (TGF-β) receptors also leads to the inhibition of cyclin D/cdk activity preventing the phosphorylation of the retinoblastoma protein (Rb). Transition to the S phase is triggered by the phosphorylation of Rb following activation of the cyclin D/cdk complex. Phosphorylated Rb dissociates from transcription factor E2F, which is then free to initiate myc expression and DNA replication. Cyclin E/cdk2 accumulates during late G_1 phase and triggers passage into S phase. An indirect action of myc is the sequestration of the cyclin E/cdk2 inhibitor, $p27^{kip1}$, into cyclin D/cdk4 complexes (Harbour and Dean, 2000; Bartek and Lukas, 2001).

Cells exposed to the cyclic monoterpenes, *d*-limonene or perillyl alcohol, geraniol, and β-ionone are arrested in G_1 with concomitant decreased expression of c-myc (Giri et al., 1999), cyclin D1 (Bardon et al., 1998, 2002; Park et al., 2001; Shi and Gould, 2002), cyclin E (Ariazi *et al.*, 1999), cdk2 (Bardon et al., 1998, 2002; Ariazi et al., 1999; Shi and Gould, 2002), and cdk4 (Bardon et al., 2002). Also reported as a consequence of exposure to cyclic monoterpenes (Ariazi et al., 1999; Bardon et al., 2002; Shi and Gould, 2002) and tocotrienols (Agarwal et al., 2004) is the increased expression of a cdk inhibitor, $p21^{Waf1/Cip1}$; the resulting inhibition of cyclin D/cdk–mediated phosphorylation of Rb (Bardon et al., 2002; Shi and Gould, 2002) blocks the dissociation of the inactive Rb/E2F complex. Geraniol and β-ionone downregulate the expression of cyclins D1, E, and A1 and cdk2 (Duncan et al., 2004). Tocotrienols also downregulate the expression of c-myc (Nesaretnam et al., 2000). Acyclic isoprenoid derivatives suppress E2F activity (Ura et al., 1998) and induce $p27^{kip1}$ expression (Miyazawa et al., 2001; Reuveni et al., 2003) with a concomitant suppression of cyclin E/cdk2 activity (Reuveni et al., 2003). The tocotrienol (Shun et al., 2004) and perillyl alcohol–stimulated upregulation of TGF-β2 and insulin-like growth factor-2 (IGF-2) receptors (Jirtle et al., 1993; Mills et al., 1995; Ariazi and Gould, 1996; Ariazi et al., 1999) may facilitate the trafficking of mitogens into lysosomes for degradation (Ariazi and Gould, 1996). All of the aforementioned reported responses to cyclic monoterpenes presage the arrest of cells in G_1.

Isoprenoids Initiate Apoptotic Cell Death

On the other side of the equation, farnesol (Adany et al., 1994; Haug et al., 1994; Voziyan et al., 1995; Miquel et al., 1996, 1998; Stayrook et al., 1997; Rioja et al., 2000), farnesyl derivatives (Perez-Sala et al., 1998; Ura et al., 1998; Mo et al., 2000; Smalley and Eisen, 2002; McAnally et al., 2004), geraniol (Shoff et al., 1991; Duncan et al., 2004), carotenoids (Yaguchi et al., 1998; Zhang et al., 1999; Briviba et al., 2001; Kotake-Nara et al., 2002; McAnally et al., 2004; Li et al., 2002; Palozza et al., 2002a, 2002b), β-ionone (Mo and Elson, 1999; Duncan et al., 2004; Liu et al., 2004a), limonene (Jirtle et al., 1993), perillyl alcohol (Mills et al., 1995; Reddy et al., 1997; Ariazi et al., 1999; Elegbede et al., 2003), perillic acid (Beaupre et al., 2003), and γ-tocotrienol (Mo and Elson, 1999; Sylvester and Shah, 2005; Birringer et al., 2003; Shah et al., 2003; Agarwal et al., 2004; Sakai et al., 2004; Takahashi and Loo, 2004) initiate apoptotic cell death.

The relative abundance of proapoptotic (Bad, Bak, Bax, Bid, Bim) and antiapoptotic (Bcl-2, Bcl-XL) proteins determines the susceptibility of cells to programmed death. The proapoptotic proteins trigger caspase activation. Cyclic and acyclic carotenoids (Li et al., 2002; Palozza et al., 2002a,

2002b), cyclic monoterpene, perillyl alcohol (Broitman et al., 1996; Burke et al., 2002), the acyclic sesquiterpene, farnesol (Broitman et al., 1996; Burke et al., 2002), and tocotrienols (Agarwal et al., 2004) suppress the expression of antiapoptotic Bcl-2; β-carotene (Palozza et al., 2002b), perillyl alcohol (Broitman et al., 1996; Burke et al., 2002), and farnesol (Broitman et al., 1996; Burke et al., 2002) suppress Bcl-XL expression. Tocotrienols (Agarwal et al., 2004), a finding requiring additional work (Takahashi and Loo, 2004), and perillyl alcohol induce expression of proapoptotic Bad, Bak, and Bax (Stayrook et al., 1997; Ariazi et al., 1999; Burke et al., 2002). Caspase activity is activated in cells incubated with perillyl alcohol (Beaupre et al., 2003), farnesol (Flach et al., 2000), tocotrienols (Sylvester and Shah, 2005; Shah et al., 2003; Sakai et al., 2004), and a farnesol mimetic vitamin K2 (Miyazawa et al., 2001). Expression of c-jun and c-fos, signal-transducing transcription factors of the AP-1 family, which appear to play roles in both cell proliferation and cell death (Ameyar et al., 2003; Eferl and Wagner 2003), are induced transiently in cells following exposure to perillyl alcohol (Ariazi et al., 1999; Satomi et al., 1999). Tocotrienols (Shun et al., 2004) and farnesylamine, an acyclic sesquiterpene derivative (Ura et al., 1998), similarly induce c-jun. The dynamic balance between fos- and jun-related proteins might play a decisive role in whether a cell survives or undergoes apoptosis (Bossy-Wetzel et al., 1997). The mechanism of the Rb-regulated p53-dependent apoptotic pathway requires study (Harbour and Dean, 2000); as delineated earlier, the cyclin D/cdk–mediated phosphorylation of Rb and its subsequent dissociation from E2F is suppressed in cells incubated with perillyl alcohol. The isoprenoid-mediated initiation of apoptosis may be independent of a p53 function. β-Ionone and γ-tocotrienol initiate apoptosis in B16 and MCF-7 cells (Mo and Elson, 1999) that express wild-type p53 (Parker et al., 1994; David-Pfeuty et al., 1996; Gudas et al., 1996), in Caco-2 cells that express mutated p53 (Gartel et al., 1996), and in p53-null HL-60 cells (Koeffler et al., 1986; Parker et al., 1994). The suppressed post-translational processing of lamin B in nuclei of promyelocytic leukemia cells exposed to β-ionone interferes with the assembly of daughter nuclei and renders DNA available to p53-independent apoptotic endonuclease activities (Mo and Elson, 1999). Annexin I is upregulated in cells exposed to perillyl alcohol (Ariazi et al., 1999); upregulation of annexin I and facilitation of the recognition phosphatidylserine by the phosphatidylserine receptor (Fadok and Henson, 2003) might explain the redistribution of phosphatidylserine in cellular membranes (Clark et al., 2002) and changes in MAPK (Clark et al., 2003; Shun et al., 2004), as well as caspase-3 (Flach et al., 2000; Miyazawa et al., 2001; Shah et al., 2003; Agarwal et al., 2004; Sakai et al., 2004) activities in cells following exposure to isoprenoids. All of these reported responses to isoprenoids are proapoptotic.

PART A: POSTULATED ISOPRENOID-MEDIATED ACTION: SUPPRESSION OF FARNESYL PROTEIN TRANSFERASE ACTIVITY

The diverse responses described earlier tend to be those that occur at midpoint or late in signal transduction pathways; this suggests that isoprenoids modulate an initiating event that has downstream impact on signal transduction. Interest has focused on the inhibition of farnesyl protein transferase (Figure 1), the activity catalyzing the transfer of a farnesyl moiety to the cysteine residue in the conserved carboxyl-terminus sequence (generally CAAX) of the small G proteins that are early components of interlocking signaling cascades (Coleman et al., 1997). Reviews of the effects of various farnesyl protein transferase inhibitors cited changes in the cell cycle with cells accumulating in G_1 in some cell lines and G_2 in others and the induction of apoptosis (Vitale et al., 1999; Tamanoi et al., 2001). The early investigations of the mechanism underlying the tumor-suppressive action of perillyl alcohol recorded a lower incorporation of C^{14}- mevalonate into $p21^{ras}$ and other 21–26 kDA proteins in cells incubated with lovastatin and perillyl alcohol when compared with that in cells incubated with lovastatin (Crowell et al., 1991). These findings reflected either the inhibition of farnesyl protein transferase or the inhibition of the synthesis of farnesyl diphosphate and geranylgeranyl diphosphate. These mevalonate-derived substrates and a third, dolichyl phosphate, are required for the post-translational modification, membrane anchoring, and biological activity of small G proteins (Zhang and Casey, 1996), nuclear lamins (Hutchison et al., 1994), and growth factor receptors (Girnita et al., 2000), activities prominent in rapidly proliferating cells (Figure 1). Subsequent findings that perillyl alcohol suppressed C^{14}-mevalonate incorporation into Rap1 and Rab6 but not into Ras suggest that perillyl alcohol inhibits type I and type II geranylgeranyl protein transferases but not farnesyl protein transferase (Ren et al., 1997). At physiologically attainable levels perillic acid methyl ester, a minor metabolite of perillyl alcohol, proved to be a potent inhibitor of the incorporation of farnesyl diphosphate and geranylgeranyl diphosphate into Ras and G25K proteins by mammalian farnesyl protein transferase and geranylgeranyl protein transferase (Gelb et al., 1995). The potency of diverse monoterpenes in suppressing protein isoprenylation parallels their potency in suppressing tumor cell proliferation (Crowell et al., 1994), albeit the latter action requires substantially lower concentrations of the metabolites. Monoterpenes suppress the prenylation of other proteins that may be oncogenic, for example, ras-related TC21/R-Ras2 (Graham et al., 1994) and the PRL-1/PTPCAAX tyrosine phosphatases (Cates et al., 1996). In one study, perillyl alcohol arrested the growth and initiated apoptosis in Bcr/Abl-transformed hematopoietic cells in the absence of an inhibitory impact on ras prenylation and ras activity (Clark et al., 2003).

Acyclic isoprenoid derivatives suppress farnesyl protein transferase activity. Farnesylamine (Ura et al., 1998), but not the sesquiterpene, *trans, trans*-farnesol (Miquel et al., 1998), has an impact on the prenylation of small G proteins. Cellular kinases may provide substrate for the farnesylation of the small G proteins by activating farnesol (Westfall et al., 1997; Bentinger et al., 1998). Another derivatized form of farnesol farnesylthiosalicyclic acid is variously reported to inhibit *in vitro* methyltransferase activity, the final step in the post-translational processing of ras (Marciano et al., 1995), to prevent the membrane attachment of mature ras (Haklai et al., 1998) or dislodge membrane-bound ras (Egozi et al., 1999; Gana-Weisz et al., 2002), therein facilitating its degradation. Another farnesol derivative, farnesylpyridinium, appears to have detergent-like properties (Hamada et al., 2002).

Clinical Evaluations of Farnesyl Protein Transferase Inhibitors

Phase I studies of *d*-limonene (Vigushin et al., 1998; Chow et al., 2002) and phase I (Ripple et al., 1998, 2000; Hudes et al., 2000; Murren et al., 2002; Azzoli et al., 2003) and II (Bailey et al., 2002; Liu et al., 2003; Meadows et al., 2002) studies of perillyl alcohol revealed dose-limiting toxicities: nausea, vomiting, anorexia, unpleasant taste, and eructation. Hypokalemia due to decreased absorption of dietary potassium was reversed with modest oral potassium supplementation (Hudes et al., 2000). Stable disease and/or modest clinical responses were attained in trials with doses ranging from 1.2 to 8.4 g/m^2/day administered in three (Ripple et al., 1998; Hudes et al., 2000; Murren et al., 2002) or four (Ripple et al., 2000; Azzoli et al., 2002; Bailey et al., 2002; Morgan-Meadows et al., 2003) doses in some, but not all, trials (Liu et al., 2003). The maximum tolerated dose determined for perillyl alcohol was determined to be ~15–16 g (~8.4–9.0 g/m^2) per day delivered orally in four doses (Azzoli et al., 2003; Morgan-Meadows et al., 2003). Although the gastrointestinal toxicity associated with the maximum dose, 16.2 g/day, was not dose limiting, a dose of 8.1 g/day (4 × 2.025 g) was recommended for Phase II trials, as no pharmacological advantage was achieved with higher doses (Morgan-Meadows et al., 2003).

Four non-peptidomimetic farnesyl protein transferase inhibitors, R115777 (Zujewski et al., 2000; Karp et al., 2001; Punt et al., 2001; Crul et al., 2002; Johnston et al., 2003; Adjei et al., 2003; Cohen et al., 2003), SCH66336 (Adjei et al., 2000; Eskens et al., 2001; Awada et al., 2002; Sharma et al., 2002), BMS-214662 (Haluska et al., 2002; Caponigro et al., 2003), and tipifarnib (Patnaik et al., 2003), are undergoing clinical trials with each achieving significant clinically relevant responses. Shared dose-limiting toxicities include nausea, vomiting, and diarrhea. Agent-specific toxicities include myelosuppression, neurological complications, and skin sensitivity (R115777); myelosuppression and renal and neurological complications (SCH66336); abdominal cramping, anorexia, fatigue, fever, and gastrointestinal and liver toxicity (BMS-214662); and myelosuppression (tipifarnib). Clinical investigations of a peptidomimetic FT inhibitor (L-778,123) were discontinued because of evidence of drug-related cardiac conduction abnormalities (Britten et al., 2001; Hahn et al., 2002; Haluska et al., 2002).

Alternative to the Suppression of Farnesyl Protein Transferase: Suppression of Mevalonic Acid–Pyrophosphate Decarboxylase Activity

An alternative to the inhibition of farnesyl protein transferase is to suppress the synthesis of isopentenyl diphosphate (Figure 1), the precursor of farnesyl diphosphate and geranylgeranyl diphosphate; the substrates required for the post-translational modification of small G proteins and nuclear lamins; and dolichyl phosphate, the substrate required for the dolichylation of proteins and glycosylation of growth factor receptors. Cells incubated with an inhibitor of mevalonic acid–pyrophosphate decarboxylase, sodium phenylacetate, or sodium phenylbutyrate (Samid et al., 1994) accumulate in the G_1 phase of the cell cycle or undergo apoptotic cell death (Harrison et al., 1998; DiGiuseppe et al., 1999; Finzer et al., 2003).

Clinical Evaluations of Mevalonic Acid–Pyrophosphate Decarboxylase Inhibitors

Preclinical evaluations demonstrated the significant chemotherapeutic potential of high-dose sodium phenylacetate (550 mg/kg of body weight) (Samid et al., 1994, Harrison et al., 1998); the results of clinical trials have shown less promise. These inhibitors of mevalonic acid–pyrophosphate decarboxylase activity have been evaluated in Phase I (Thibault et al., 1994, 1995; Piscitelli et al., 1995; Carducci et al., 1996) and Phase II (Buckner et al., 1999; Chang et al., 1999) studies. Although modest responses were recorded with circa 300–400 mg/kg/day infusions, toxicities including emesis, central nervous system depression, transient somnolence, confusion, and fatigue were dose limiting.

Alternative to the Suppression of Farnesyl Protein Transferase: Suppression of 3-Hydroxy-3-Methylglutaryl Coenzyme A Reductase Activity

A second approach employs the inhibition of HMG-CoA reductase activity (Figure 1), the rate-limiting activity in the pathway (Brown and Goldstein, 1980; Goldstein and Brown, 1990). As a consequence of mevalonate starvation, cells incubated with diverse inhibitors of HMG-CoA reductase, the statins, accumulate in the G_1 phase of the cell cycle or undergo apoptotic death (reviewed by Elson et al., 1999; Mo and Elson, 1999; Mo et al., 1999). Findings that supplemental mevalonate reverses the geraniol-mediated arrest of cells grown in suspension culture support the concept offered herein (Shoff et al., 1991), whereas findings that cells grown on monolayers (Shoff et al., 1991; Duncan et al., 2004) may point to an isoprenoid-mediated impact at a later site in the mevalonate pathway, allyl diphosphate diphosphatase (Case et al., 1995) (Figure 1).

Statins Arrest Cells at the G_1/S Interface of the Cell Cycle

Cells exposed to statins are arrested in G_1 with concomitant decreased expression of c-myc (Dricu et al., 1997; Park et al., 2001; Denoyelle et al., 2003), cyclin D1 (Oda et al., 1999; Park et al., 2001; Wachtershauser et al., 2001; Denoyelle et al., 2003), cyclin E (Oda et al., 1999; Park et al., 1999; Garcia-Roman et al., 2001; Ukomadu et al., 2003a), cdk2 (Gray-Bablin et al., 1997; Rao et al., 1998; Park et al., 1999), and cdk4 (Rao et al., 1998; Park et al., 1999; Wachtershauser et al., 2001), and increased expression of a cdk inhibitor, $p21^{Waf1/Cip1}$ (Gray-Bablin et al., 1997; Lee et al., 1998; Ghosh et al., 1999; Fenig et al., 2002; Denoyelle et al., 2003; Ukomadu and Dutta, 2003b; Wang and Macaulay, 2003). Inhibition of the cyclin/cdk–mediated phosphorylation of Rb (Lee et al., 1998; Lukas et al., 1996; Ghosh et al., 1999; Ukomadu and Dutta, 2003a; Ukomadu and Dutta, 2003b) blocks the dissociation of the inactive Rb/E2F complex. Statins suppress E2F activity (Park et al., 2001) and induce $p27^{kip1}$ expression (Gray-Bablin et al., 1997; Ghosh et al., 1999; Oda et al., 1999; Park et al., 1999, 2001; Garcia-Roman et al., 2001; Wang and Macaulay, 2003) with a concomitant suppression of cyclin E/cdk2 activity (Ghosh et al., 1999).

Statins Initiate Apoptotic Cell Death

Statins suppress the expression of antiapoptotic Bcl-2 (Agarwal et al., 1999; Park et al., 1999; Dimitroulakos et al., 2000; Garcia-Roman et al., 2001; Blanco-Colio et al., 2002) and Bcl-XL (Blanco-Colio et al., 2003) and induce proapoptotic Bax expression (Agarwal et al., 1999) and caspase-7 activity (Marcelli et al., 1998). On one hand, statins induce the expression of c-fos (Martinez-Gonzalez et al., 1997) and, on the other, suppress AP-1 binding activity (Vrtovsnik et al., 1997; Wang et al., 2000).

Proposed Mechanism Underlying Statin-Mediated Suppression of Cell Growth

As a consequence of the reduced pools of farnesyl diphosphate, geranylgeranyl diphosphate, and dolichyl phosphate imposed by the inhibition of HMG-CoA reductase activity by statins, activities early in the signal transducing pathways requiring the prenylation of small G proteins (Hohl and Lewis, 1995; Coleman et al., 1997; Holstein et al., 2002a, 2002b; Wang et al., 2000; Blanco-Colio et al., 2002) and N-linked glycosylation of growth factor receptors (Engstrom and Larsson, 1988; Larsson, 1993, 1994; Dricu et al., 1997; McCarty, 2001) are attenuated as are mitotic activities requiring the prenylation of the nuclear lamins (Beck et al., 1988; Hancock et al., 1989; Schafer et al., 1989).

Clinical Evaluations of 3-Hydroxy-3-Methylglutaryl Coenzyme A Reductase Inhibitors

Although preclinical evaluations demonstrated the significant chemotherapeutic potential of high-dose statins (15–70 mg/kg of body weight), the results of clinical trials have shown only modest promise and significant dose-limiting toxicity (Thibault et al., 1996; Larner et al., 1998; Kawata et al., 2001; Kim et al., 2001; Minden et al., 2001). Toxicities associated with high-dose lovastatin include gastrointestinal dysfunction, myalgia, muscle weakness, elevated creatine phosphokinase, anorexia, and ulcerative lesions. Doses approaching levels normally prescribed for cholesterol control (20–80 mg/day) may have limited efficacy (Anonymous, 1993, Blais et al., 2000).

PART B: POSTULATED ISOPRENOID-MEDIATED ACTION: SUPPRESSION OF HMG CoA REDUCTASE ACTIVITY

The isoprenoid-mediated impact on signal transduction pathway, cell division, and apoptosis might be explained, like that of the statins, by mevalonate starvation. Farnesol (Correll and Edwards, 1994; Meigs et al., 1996; Meigs and Simoni, 1997), farnesol derivatives (farnesyl acetate (Bradfute and Simoni, 1994), ethyl farnesyl ether (Bradfute and Simoni, 1994), farnesol homologs (tocotrienols) (Parker et al., 1993), and geranylated tocol analogs (Pearce et al., 1994) accelerate the degradation of HMG-CoA reductase by a nonlysosomal cysteine protease. Tocotrienols (Parker et al., 1993) and farnesol (Peffley and Gayen, 1997) decrease the efficiency of HMG-CoA reductase mRNA translation. Geraniol suppresses HMG-CoA reductase activity by suppressing both HMG-CoA reductase transcription and mRNA translation (Peffley and Gayen, 2003). Limonene (Clegg et al., 1982; Peffley and Gayen, 2003) and perillyl alcohol (Peffley and Gayen, 2003) decrease reductase mass by decreasing the efficiency of HMG-CoA reductase mRNA translation (Peffley and Gayen, 2003). Geranyl geraniol stimulates the Insig-dependent ubiquitination and degradation of HMG-CoA reductase (Sever et al., 2003); β-carotene also decreases HMG-CoA reductase mass via a post-translational action (Moreno et al., 1995).

Parallel Responses to Statins and Isoprenoids

The statins and isoprenoids suppress HMG-CoA reductase activity and concomitantly the post-translational processing of small G proteins, nuclear lamins, and growth factor receptors required for their biological activities. A brief recap of responses triggered by statins and by pure and mixed isoprenoids underlying the arrest of cells in G_1 includes the suppression of various activities including the N-linked glycosylation of growth factor receptors, cyclin D1 and E expression, cdk expression, cyclin D1/cdk and cyclin E/cdk activity, c-myc expression, and Rb phosphorylation, and the induction of $p21^{CiP1/WAF1}$, $p27^{Kip1}$, and c-fos expression. A recap of responses triggered by statins and by pure and mixed isoprenoids underlying the initiation of apoptosis includes the suppression of the expression of anti-apoptotic Bcl-2 and Bcl-xL expression and induction of proapoptotic bax expression and caspase activity.

Opposing Responses to Statins and Isoprenoids; Attenuation of Lovastatin-Mediated Responses by Isoprenoids

The statins and isoprenoids suppress HMG-CoA reductase activity, the former by inhibition (Goldstein and Brown, 1990), the latter by post-transcriptional downregulation (Clegg et al., 1982; Parker et al., 1993; Bradfute and Simoni, 1994; Correll and Edwards, 1994; Pearce et al., 1994; Meigs and Simoni, 1997; Chao et al., 2002; Peffley and Gayen, 2003) of the enzyme. As a consequence of the depletion of cellular cholesterol by lovastatin, HMG-CoA reductase synthesis is upregulated and reductase stability increased (Brown and Goldstein, 1980). The post-transcriptional actions triggered by isoprenoids attenuate the statin-mediated upregulation of HMG-CoA reductase (Parker et al., 1993; Bradfute and Simoni, 1994; Correll and Edwards, 1994; Yu et al., 1994; Meigs et al., 1996; Meigs and Simoni, 1997; Peffley and Gayen, 2003).

Depletion of the farnesyl diphosphate pool secondary to statin-mediated mevalonate deprivation attenuates ras farnesylation (Wang et al., 2000; Blanco-Colia et al., 2002). In response to the indiscriminant inhibition of HMG-CoA reductase imposed by lovastatin, the depleted pools of cellular prenyl diphosphate upregulate the synthesis of small G proteins with a resultant accumulation of nascent small G proteins (Holstein et al., 2002b). Co-incubation with an isoprenoid (perillyl alcohol) suppresses this upregulation (Holstein et al., 2002a; Holstein and Hohl, 2003). As previously delineated, findings that the incorporation of labeled farnesyl diphosphate into small G proteins in cells incubated with perillyl alcohol and lovastatin is less than that recorded in cells incubated with lovastatin have been widely interpreted as being a consequence of perillyl alcohol–mediated inhibition of farnesyl protein transferase activity; findings now demonstrate that it is the limiting pool of small G proteins rather than the inhibition of farnesyl protein transferase activity that is responsible (Holstein et al., 2002a; Holstein and Hohl, 2003).

Tumor-Specific Action of the Isoprenoids

The differential impact on the growth of malignant cells compared with normal cells, noted with isoprenoids (Adany et al., 1994; Yazlovitskaya and Melnykovych, 1995; Stayrook et al., 1997; Ura et al., 1998; Yaguchi et al., 1998; Ariazi et al., 1999; Elson et al., 1999; Mo and Elson, 1999; Mo et al., 1999; Rioja et al., 2000; Sahin et al., 1999; Crowell and Elson, 2001; McIntyre et al., 2000; Smalley and Eisen, 2002; Clark et al., 2003; Beaupre et al., 2003; Duncan et al., 2004; Sakai et al., 2004) but not with the indiscriminant inhibitors of HMG-CoA reductase activity, the statins (Brown and Goldstein, 1980) traces, we propose, to a fundamental lesion of malignant cells, the uncoupling of HMG-CoA reductase activity from sterol-mediated feedback regulation, thereby permitting the synthesis of the nonsterol products of the mevalonate pathway essential for cell survival in a sterol-rich environment (reviewed by Elson and Yu, 1994; Elson, 1995; Elson, 1996; Elson et al., 1999; Mo et al., 1999).

The dysregulation of reductase activity in tumors (Siperstein and Fagan, 1964; Chen et al., 1978; George and Goldfarb, 1980; Gregg et al., 1982; Yachnin et al., 1984; Bruscalalupi et al., 1985; Engstrom and Schofield, 1987; Erickson et al., 1988; Azrolan and Coleman, 1989; Kawata et al., 1990; Bennis et al., 1993) is confirmed by our findings of several-fold higher copies of HMG-CoA reductase mRNA in human colon tumor (Caco2) and leukemic (CEM) cells compared with levels present in normal colon cells (CCD18) and normal human lymphocytes (Hentosh et al., 2001). Findings that HMG-CoA reductase promoter activity was threefold higher in Caco2 tumor cells than in CCD18 normal cells suggest that the differential binding of transcription factor(s) on the reductase promoter is responsible for the attenuation of the normal sterol-mediated regulation of reductase activity (Hentosh et al., 2001). Observations of the inverse correlation between DNA methylation and gene expression levels (Laird and Jaenisch, 1994), the hypomethylation of protooncogenes, Ha-ras, Ki-ras, c-fos, c-myc, Erb-A1, and bcl-2 in human leukemias and liver tumors (Laird and Jaenisch, 1994) and of the hypomethylation of Ha-ras, c-fos, c-myc, and HMG-CoA reductase in nodules in livers of rats exposed to diverse carcinogens (Coni et al., 1992; Rossiello et al., 1994) led us to examine the methylation status of the promoter regions of HMG-CoA reductase genes from solid tumor, leukemic, and normal cells. On finding that the reductase promoter sequences in both normal and malignant cells were hypomethylated, we concluded that an aberrant methylation pattern does not alter the binding of transcription factors to the promoter region of the HMG-CoA reductase gene (Hentosh et al., 2001). We, therefore, propose alternate hypotheses to explain the overexpression of HMG-CoA reductase gene in tumor cells, cells with membranes enriched in cholesterol (Coleman et al., 1997). A perturbation, either in the precursors of the sterol regulatory element-binding proteins (SREBPs) or of the SREBP cleavage activation protein (SCAP), might support the overexpression of HMG-CoA reductase (Brown and Goldstein, 1997; Osborne, 2000; Horton et al., 2002). Cholesterol depletion in cultured cells initiates the proteolytic cascade leading to the elevation of transcription factors SREBP-1a and SREBP-2, increased HMG-CoA reductase mRNA transcription and translation with the resultant increase in HMG-CoA reductase mass (Shimano et al., 1996). The addition of sterols suppresses the processing of SREBP-2 but not of SREBP-1a (Hannah et al., 2001). Contrary to the relative abundance of SREBP-1c, a transcription factor targeting lipogenic genes, to SREBP-1a in liver tissue (Shimano et al., 1997; Shimomura et al., 1997), in embryonic and hepatoma cells, the expression of SREBP-1a is reported to exceed that of SREBP-1c (Brown and Goldstein, 1997; Shimomura et al., 1997; Osborne, 2000; Hannah et al., 2001). SREBP-1a, expressed in tumors (Hannah et al., 2001), does not respond to sterol-mediated downregulation. Alternatively, a mutation in SCAP, a G → A transition at codon 443 of SCAP, changing aspartic acid to asparagine, enhances its cleavage-stimulating activity, thereby rendering HMG-CoA reductase resistant to sterol regulation (Hua et al., 1996).

The overexpression of members of the type 1 receptor tyrosine kinase family, especially ErbB-2 (HER-2, Neu) has been implicated in multiple forms of cancer (Hainsworth et al., 2000; Hellstrom et al., 2001; Yarden, 2001; Hempstock et al., 1998). Incubation of ErbB-2–expressing cells with tyrosine kinase inhibitors induces concentration- and time-dependent reductions in HMG-CoA reductase activity (Asslan et al., 1998; Sindermann et al., 2001). Both HMG-CoA reductase mRNA levels and the rate of HMG-CoA reductase synthesis are significantly lower (Asslan et al., 1998). In normal cells treated with lovastatin, there is a compensatory increase in HMG-CoA reductase mRNA and reductase mass (Brown and Goldstein, 1980); the overexpression is tentatively associated with an increase in phosphotyrosine levels (Sindermann et al., 2001) and tyrosine kinase activity (Mutoh et al., 1999).

The metabolic error underlying the widely reported upregulation of HMG-CoA reductase activity in tumors (reviewed by Elson and Yu, 1994; Elson, 1995, 1996; Elson et al., 1999; Mo et al., 1999) remains to be delineated. Although the basis of the dysregulated activity remains to be resolved, the activity retains high sensitivity to isoprenoid-mediated post-transcriptional downregulation (Parker et al., 1993, 1994; Peffley and Gayen, 2003).

Preclinical and Clinical Evaluation of Isoprenoids

Preclinical evaluations of farnesyl protein transferase, mevalonic acid–pyrophosphate decarboxylase, and HMG-CoA reductase inhibitors yield dramatic responses. When administered at maximum tolerated levels in clinical trials, the responses are not encouraging. The dose-limiting toxicity noted with perillyl alcohol, gastrointestinal discomfort, differs from those toxicities recorded for the other mevalonate pathway–targeted agents. With revised formulations and dosing schedules, the severity of the dose-limiting toxicities elicited by perillyl alcohol might be eased, thereby permitting the administration of chemotherapeutically effective doses. The application of more potent isoprenoids might prove clinically effective absent the gastrointestinal discomfort accompanying high-dose perillyl alcohol. Another approach envisions the potentiation of the statin action with the co-administration of a tumor-targeted isoprenoid.

CANCER PREVENTION

Efficacy and follow-up studies provide evidence that cancer incidence is modestly lower in hypercholesterolemic populations undergoing lovastatin therapy (Anonymous, 1993). A search for volatile isoprenoid constituents of fruits, vegetables, and herbs spanning seven plant families identified 179 monoterpenes and sesquiterpenes. Of these, 41 were screened for tumor-suppressive potency. Volatile isoprenoids differed substantially in potency as determined with a melanoma B16 screen; IC_{50} values fell generally within the range 200–400 μmol/liter. Sixteen of the isoprenoids evaluated proved to have greater potency than perillyl alcohol and 33 had greater potency than *d*-limonene, the two isoprenoids advanced to clinical evaluation. The finding that blends of isoprenoids suppressed tumor cell proliferation with efficacy greater than that of the sum of individual agents demonstrates the cumulative impact of diverse volatile isoprenoid constituents of the diet (Tatman and Mo, 2002).

The modest protection from breast cancer associated with dietary vitamin E may be due to the effects of the associated tocotrienols. Laboratory studies show that α-tocopherol alone has little effect on mammary tumors, whereas the tocotrienols have potent antiproliferative and proapoptotic effects (Guthrie et al., 1997; Netsaretnam et al., 1998; Mo and Elson, 1999; McIntyre et al., 2000), which would be expected to reduce risk of breast cancer (Schwenke, 2002).

Isoprenoids complement the tumor-suppressive activity of other dietary agents. Incubation of tumor cells with tyrosine kinase inhibitors induces concentration- and time-dependent reductions in HMG-CoA reductase activity (Asslan et al., 1998; Sindermann et al., 2001). Incubation of prostate tumor cells with isoprenoids or genistein, a tyrosine kinase inhibitor in soy products, yielded a concentration-dependent suppression of growth. When applied in combination, the resulting suppression of growth was significantly greater than that predicted by the sum of the activities of the two classes of agents (Mo, unreported observations).

SUMMARY

Contrary to the promise shown in preclinical studies, dose-limiting toxicities diminish the prospects for the development of chemotherapeutic agents targeting the mevalonate pathway. An aberrant pathway activity, an overexpressed sterol feedback-resistant HMG-CoA reductase activity broadly present in tumors, offers a novel target for chemopreventive and nutritional intervention. Isoprenoids impacting only on the post transcriptional regulatory actions controlling reductase activity effectively starve tumor cells of the mevalonate-derived products required for the maturation and biological activity of proteins having essential roles in maintaining cell proliferation and blocking apoptosis.

Acknowledgments

This work was supported by the Texas Woman's University (TWU) Research Enhancement Program, TWU Chancellor's Research Fellow Program, Human Nutrition Research Fund, Texas Food and Fiber Commission, American Cancer Society–University of North Texas Institutional Grant, and the Wisconsin Alumni Research Foundation.

References

Adany, I., Yazlovitskaya, E.M., Haug, J.S., Voziyan, P.A., and Melnykovych, G. 1994. Differences in sensitivity to farnesol toxicity between neoplastically- and non-neoplastically-derived cells in culture. *Cancer Lett* **79**: 175–179.

Adjei, A.A., Erlichman, C., Davis, J.N., Cutler, D.L., Sloan, J.A., Marks, R.S., Hanson, L.J., Svingen, P.A., Atherton, P., Bishop, W.R., Kirschmeier, P., and Kaufmann, S.H. 2000. A Phase I trial of the farnesyl transferase inhibitor SCH66336: evidence for biological and clinical activity. *Cancer Res* **60**: 1871–1877.

Adjei, A.A., Maue, A., Bruzek, L., Marks, R.S., Hillman, S., Geyer, S., Hanson, L.J., Wright, J.J., Erlichman, C., Kaufmann, S.H., and Vokes, E.E. 2003. Phase II study of the farnesyl transferase inhibitor R115777 in patients with advanced non–small-cell lung cancer. *J Clin Oncol* **21**: 1760–1766.

Agarwal, M.K., Agarwal, M.L., Athar, M., and Gupta, S. 2004. Tocotrienol-rich fraction of palm oil activates p53, modulates Bax/Bcl2 ratio and induces apoptosis independent of cell cycle association. *Cell Cycle* **3**: 205–211.

Agarwal, B., Bhendwal, S, Halmos, B., Moss, S.F., Ramey, W.G., and Holt, P.R. 1999. Lovastatin augments apoptosis induced by chemotherapeutic agents in colon cancer cells. *Clin Cancer Res* **5**: 2223–2229.

Ameyar, M., Wisniewska, M., and Weitzman, J.B. 2003. A role for AP-1 in apoptosis: the case for and against. *Biochimie* **85**: 747–752.

Anonymous. 1993. Lovastatin 5-year safety and efficacy study. Lovastatin Study Groups I through IV. *Arch Intern Med* **153**: 1079–1087.

Ariazi, E.A., and Gould, M.N. 1996. Identifying differential gene expression in monoterpene-treated mammary carcinomas using subtractive display. *J Biol Chem* **271**: 29286–29294.

Ariazi, E.A., Satomi, Y., Ellis, M.J., Haag, J.D., Shi, W., Sattler, C.A., and Gould, M.N. 1999. Activation of the transforming growth factor beta signaling pathway and induction of cytostasis and apoptosis in mammary carcinomas treated with the anticancer agent perillyl alcohol. *Cancer Res* **59**: 1917–1928.

Asslan, R., Pradines, A., Favre, G., and Le Gaillard, F. 1998. Tyrosine kinase-dependent modulation of 3-hydroxy-3-methylglutaryl-CoA reductase in human breast adenocarcinoma SKBR-3 cells. *Biochem J* **330**: 241–246.

Awada, A., Eskens, F.A., Piccart, M., Cutler, D.L., van der Gaast, A., Bleiberg, H., Wanders, J., Faber, M.N., Statkevich, P., Fumoleau, P., and Verweij, J. 2002. Phase I and pharmacological study of the oral farnesyltransferase inhibitor SCH 66336 given once daily to patients with advanced solid tumours. *Eur J Cancer* **38**: 2272–2278.

Azrolan, N.I., and Coleman, P.S. 1989. A discoordinant increase in the cellular amount of 3-hydroxy-3-methylglutaryl-CoA reductase results in the loss of rate-limiting control over cholesterogenesis in a tumor cell-free system. *Biochem J* **258**: 421–425.

Azzoli, C.G., Miller, V.A., Ng, K.K., Krug, L.M., Spriggs, D.R., Tong, W.P., Riedel, E.R., and Kris, M.G. 2003. A phase I trial of perillyl alcohol in patients with advanced solid tumors. *Cancer Chemother Pharmacol* **51**: 493–498.

Bach, T.J. 1995. Some new aspects of isoprenoid biosynthesis in plants—a review. *Lipids* **30**: 191–202.

Bailey, H.H., Levy, D., Harris, L.S., Schink, J.C., Foss, F., Beatty, P., and Wadler, S. 2002. A phase II trial of daily perillyl alcohol in patients with advanced ovarian cancer: Eastern Cooperative Oncology Group Study E2E96. *Gynecol Oncol* **85**: 464–468.

Bardon, S., Foussard, V., Fournel, S., and Loubat, A. 2002. Monoterpenes inhibit proliferation of human colon cancer cells by modulating cell cycle–related protein expression. *Cancer Lett* **181**: 187–194.

Bardon, S., Picard, K., and Martel, P. 1998. Monoterpenes inhibit cell growth, cell cycle progression, and cyclin D1 gene expression in human breast cancer cell lines. *Nutr Cancer* **32**: 1–7.

Barron, D., and Ibrahim, R.A. 1996. Isoprenylated flavonoids—a survey. *Phytochem* **43**: 921–982.

Bartek, J., and Lukas, J. 2001. Pathways governing G1/S transition and their response to DNA damage. *FEBS Lett* **490**: 117–122.

Beaupre, D.M., McCafferty-Grad, J., Bahlis, N.J., Boise, L.H., and Lichtenfield, M.G. 2003. Farnesyl transferase inhibitors enhance death receptor signals and induce apoptosis in multiple myeloma cells. *Leuk Lymp* **44**: 2123–2134.

Beck, L., Hosick, T.J., and Sinensky, M. 1988. Incorporation of a product of mevalonic acid metabolism into proteins of Chinese hamster ovary cell nuclei. *J Cell Biol* **107**: 1307–1316.

Bennis, F., Favre, G., Le Gaillard, F., and Soula, G. 1993. Importance of mevalonate-derived products in the control of HMG-CoA reductase activity and growth of human lung adenocarcinoma cell line A549. *Int J Cancer* **55**: 640–645.

Bentinger, M., Grunler, J., Peterson, E., Swiezewska, E., and Dallner, G. 1998. Phosphorylation of farnesol in rat liver microsomes: properties of farnesol kinase and farnesyl phosphate kinase. *Arch Biochem Biophys* **353**: 191–198.

Birringer, M., EyTina, J.H., Salvatore, B.A., and Neuzil, J. 2003. Vitamin E anologues as inducers of apoptosis: structure-function relation. *Br J Cancer* **88**: 1948–1955.

Blais, L., Desgagne, A., and LeLorier, J. 2000. 3-Hydroxy-3-methylglutaryl coenzyme A reductase inhibitors and the risk of cancer: a nested case–control study. *Arch Intern Med* **160**: 2363–2368.

Blanco-Colio, L.M., Justo, P., Daehn, I., Lorz, C., Ortiz, A., and Egido, J. 2003. Bcl-xL overexpression protects from apoptosis induced by HMG-CoA reductase inhibitors in murine tubular cells. *Kidney Int* **64**: 181–191.

Blanco-Colio, L.M., Villa, A., Ortego, M., Hernandez-Presa, M.A., Pascual, A., Plaza, J.J., and Egido, J. 2002. 3-Hydroxy-3-methyl-glutaryl coenzyme A reductase inhibitors, atorvastatin and simvastatin, induce apoptosis of vascular smooth muscle cells by downregulation of Bcl-2 expression and Rho A prenylation. *Atherosclerosis* **161**: 17–26.

Bossy-Wetzel, E., Bakiri, L., and Yaniv, M. 1997. Induction of apoptosis by the transcription factor c-jun. *EMBO J* **16**: 1695–1709.

Bradfute, D.L., and Simoni, R.D. 1994. Non-sterol compounds that regulate cholesterogenesis. Analogues of farnesyl pyrophosphate reduce 3-hydroxy-3-methylglutaryl-coenzyme A reductase levels. *J Biol Chem* **269**: 6645–6650.

Britten, C.D., Rowinsky, E.K., Soignet, S., Patnaik, A., Yao, S.L., Deutsch, P., Lee, Y., Lobell, R.B., Mazina, K.E., McCreery, H., Pezzuli, S., and Spriggs, D. 2001. A phase I and pharmacological study of the farnesyl protein transferase inhibitor L-778,123 in patients with solid malignancies. *Clin Cancer Res* **7**: 3894–3903.

Briviba, K., Schnaebele, K., Schwertle, E., Blockhaus, M., and Rechkemmer, G. 2001. beta-Carotene inhibits growth of human colon carcinoma cells *in vitro* by induction of apoptosis. *Biol Chem* **382**: 1663–1668.

Broitman, S.A., Wilkinson, J., Cerda, S., and Branch, S.K. 1996. Effects of monoterpenes and mevinolin on murine colon tumor CT-26 *in vitro* and its hepatic "metastases" *in vivo*. *Adv Exp Med Biol* **401**: 111–130.

Brown, M.S., and Goldstein, J.L. 1980. Multivalent feedback regulation of HMG CoA reductase, a control mechanism coordinating isoprenoid synthesis and cell growth. *J Lipid Res* **21**: 505–517.

Brown, M.S., and Goldstein, J.L. 1997. The SREBP pathway: regulation of cholesterol metabolism by proteolysis of a membrane-bound transcription factor. *Cell* **89**: 331–340.

Bruscalalupi, G., Leoni, S., Mangiantini, M.T., Minieri, M., Spagnuolo, S., and Trentlanc, A. 1985. True uncoupling between cholesterol synthesis and 3-hydroxy-3-methylglutaryl coenzyme A reductase in an early stage of liver generation. *Cell Mol Biol* **31**: 365–368.

Buckner, J.C., Malkin, M.G., Reed, E., Cascino, T.L., Reid, J.M., Ames, M.M., Tong, W.P., Lim, S., and Figg, W.D. 1999. Phase II study of antineoplastons A10 (NSC 648539) and AS2-1 (NSC 620261) in patients with recurrent glioma. *Mayo Clin Proc* **74**: 137–145.

Burke, Y.D., Stark, M.J., Roach, S.L., Sen, S.E., and Crowell, P.L. 1997. Inhibition of pancreatic cancer growth by the dietary isoprenoids farnesol and geraniol. *Lipids* **32**: 151–156.

Burke, Y.D., Ayoubi, A.S., Werner, S.R., McFarland, B.C., Heilman, D.K., Ruggeri, B.A., and Crowell, P.L. 2002. Effects of the isoprenoids perillyl alcohol and farnesol on apoptosis biomarkers in pancreatic cancer chemoprevention. *Anticancer Res* **22**: 3127–3134.

Caponigro, F., Casale, M., and Bryce, J. 2003. Farnesyl transferase inhibitors in clinical development. *Expert Opin Investig Drugs* **12**: 943–954.

Carducci, M.A., Bowling, M.K., Eisenberger, M.A., Sinibaldi, V., Simons, J.W., Chen, T.L., Noe, D., Grochow, L.B., and Donehower, R.C. 1996. Phenylbutyrate (PB) for refractory solid tumors: a phase I clinical and pharmacologic evaluation. *Proc Am Soc Clin Oncol* **15**: A1542.

Carnesecchi, S., Bras-Goncalves, R., Bradaia, A., Zeisel, M., Gosse, F., Poupan, M-F., and Raul, F. 2004. Geraniol, a component of plant essential oils, modulates DNA synthesis and potentiates 5-fluorouracil efficacy on human tumor xenografts. *Cancer Lett* **215**: 53–59.

Case, G.L., He, L., Mo, H., and Elson, C.E. 1995. Induction of geranylpyrophosphate pyrophosphatase activity by cholesterol-suppressive isoprenoids. *Lipids* **30**: 357–359.

Cates, C.A., Michael, R.L., Stayrook, K.R., Harvey, K.A., Burke, Y.D., Randall, S.K., Crowell, P.L., and Crowell, D.N. 1996. Prenylation of oncogenic human PTP (CAAX) protein tyrosine phosphatases. *Cancer Lett* **110**: 49–55.

Chakrabarti, R., and Engleman, E.G. 1991. Interrelationships between mevalonate metabolism and the mitogenic signaling pathway in T lymphocyte proliferation. *J Biol Chem* **266**: 12216–12222.

Chang, S.M., Kuhn, J.G., Robins, H.I., Schold, S.C., Spence, A.M., Berger, M.S., Mehta, M.P., Bozik, M.E., Pollack, I., Schiff, D., Gilbert, M., Rankin, C., and Prados, M.D. 1999. Phase II study of phenylacetate in patients with recurrent malignant glioma: a North American Brain Tumor Consortium report. *J Clin Oncol* **17**: 984–990.

Chao, J.T., Gapor, A., and Theriault, A. 2002. Inhibitory effect of delta-tocotrienol. A HMG-CoA reductase inhibitor, on monocyte-endothelial cell adhesion. *J Nutr Sci Vitaminol Tokyo* **48**: 332–337.

Chen, H.W., Kandutsch, A.A., and Heineiger, H.J. 1978. The role of cholesterol in malignancy. *Prog Exp Tumour Res* **22**: 275–316.

Chow, H.H., Salazar, D., and Hakim, I.A. 2002. Pharmacokinetics of perillic acid in humans after a single dose administration of a citrus preparation rich in d-limonene content. *Cancer Epidemiol Biomarkers Prev* **11**: 1472–1476.

Clark, S.S., Perman, S.M., Sahin, M.B., Jenkins, G.J., and Elegbede, J.A. 2002. Antileukemic activity of perillyl alcohol (POH): uncoupling apoptosis from G0/G1 arrests suggests that the primary effect of POH on Bcr/Abl-transformed cells is to induce growth arrest. *Leukemia* **16**: 213–222.

Clark, S.S., Zhong, L., Filiault, D., Perman, S., Ren, Z., Gould, M., and Yang, X. 2003. Anti-leukemia effect of perillyl alcohol in Bcr/Abl-transformed cells indirectly inhibits signaling through Mek in a Ras- and Raf-independent fashion. *Clin Cancer Res* **9**: 4494–4504.

Clegg, R.J., Middleton, B., Bell, G.D., and White, D.A. 1982. The mechanism of cyclic monoterpene inhibition of 3-hydroxy-3-methylglutaryl coenzyme A reductase *in vivo* in the rat. *J Biol Chem* **257**: 2294–2299.

Cohen, S.J., Ho, L., Ranganathan, S., Abbruzzese, J.L., Alpaugh, R.K., Beard, M., Lewis, N.L., McLaughlin, S., Rogatko, A., Perez-Ruixo, J.J., Thistle, A.M., Verhaeghe, T., Wang, H., Weiner, L.M., Wright, J.J., Hudes, G.R., Neal, J., and Meropol, N.J. 2003. Meropol Phase II and pharmacodynamic study of the farnesyltransferase inhibitor R115777 as initial therapy in patients with metastatic pancreatic adenocarcinoma. *J Clin Oncol* **21**: 1301–1306.

Coleman, P.S., Chen, L.C., and Sepp-Lorenzino, L. 1997. Cholesterol metabolism and tumor cell proliferation. *Subcellular Biochem* **28**: 363–435.

Coni, P., Pang, J., Pichiri-Coni, G., Hsu, S., Rao, P.M., Rajalakshmi, S., and Sarma, D.S. 1992. Hypomethylation of beta-hydroxy-beta-methylglutaryl coenzyme A reductase gene and its expression during hepatocarcinogenesis in the rat. *Carcinogenesis* **13**: 497–499.

Correll, G.C., and Edwards, P.A. 1994. Mevalonic acid-dependent degradation of 3-hydroxy-3-methylglutaryl-coenzyme A reductase *in vivo* and *in vitro*. *J Biol Chem* **269**: 633–638.

Crowell, P.L., Chang, R.R., Ren, Z., Elson, C.E., and Gould, M.N. 1991. Selective inhibition of isoprenylation of 21–26-kDa proteins by the anticarcinogen d-limonene and its metabolites. *J Biol Chem* **266**: 17679–17685.

Crowell, P.L., and Elson, C.E. 2001. Isoprenoids, health and disease. *In* "Nutraceuticals and Functional Foods" (R.E.C. Wildman, ed.), pp. 31–53. CRC Press, New York.

Crowell, P.L., Ren, Z., Lin, S., Vedejs, E., and Gould, M.N. 1994. Structure–activity relationships among monoterpene inhibitors of protein isoprenylation and cell proliferation. *Biochem Pharmacol* **47**: 1405–1415

Crul, M., de Klerk, G.J., Swart, M., van't Veer, L.J., de Jong, D., Boerrigter, L., Palmer, P.A., Bol, C.J., Tan, H., de Gast, G.C., Beijnen, J.H., and Schellens, J.H. 2002. Phase I clinical and pharmacologic study of chronic oral administration of the farnesyl protein transferase inhibitor R115777 in advanced cancer. *J Clin Oncol* **20**: 2726–2735.

Dahiya, J.S., Strange, R.N., Bilyard, K.G., Cooksey, C.J., and Garratt, P.J. 1984. Two isoprenylated isoflavone phytoalexins from *Cajanus cajan. Phytochemistry* **23**: 871–874.

David-Pfeuty, T., Chakrani, F., Ory, K., and Nouvian-Dooghe, Y. 1996. Cell cycle–dependent regulation of nuclear p53 traffic occurs in one subclass of human tumor cells and in untransformed cells. *Cell Growth Differ* **7**: 1211–1225.

Denoyelle, C., Albanese, P., Uzan, G., Hong, L., Vannier, J.P., Soria, J., and Soria, C. 2003. Molecular mechanism of the anti-cancer activity of cerivastatin, an inhibitor of HMG-CoA reductase, on aggressive human breast cancer cells. *Cellular Signaling* **15**: 327–338.

De Rosa, S., De Giulio, A., and Iodice, C. 1994. Biological effects of prenylated hydroquinones: Structure–activity relationship studies in antimicrobial, brine shrimp, and fish lethality assays. *J Nat Prod* **57**: 1711–1716.

DiGiuseppe, J.A., Weng, L.J., Yu, K.H., Fu, S., Kastan, M.B., Samid, D., and Gore, S.D. 1999. Phenylbutyrate-induced G1 arrest and apoptosis in myeloid leukemia cells: structure–function analysis. *Leukemia* **13**: 1243–1253.

Dimitroulakos, J., Thai, S., Wasfy, G.H., Hedley, D.W., Minden, M.D., and Penn, L.Z. 2000. Lovastatin induces a pronounced differentiation response in acute myeloid leukemias. *Leuk Lymphoma* **40**: 167–178.

Dricu, A., Wang, M., Hjertman, M., Malec, M., Blegen, H., Wejde, J., Carlberg, M., and Larsson, O. 1997. Mevalonate-regulated mechanisms in cell growth control: role of dolichyl phosphate in expression of the insulin-like growth factor-eceptor (IGF-1R) in comparison to Ras prenylation and expression of c-myc. *Glycobiology* **7**: 625–633.

Duncan, R.E., Lau, D., El-Sohemy, A., and Archer, M.C. 2004. Geraniol and b-ionone inhibit proliferation, cell cycle progression, and cyclin-dependent kinase 2 activity in MCF-7 breast cancer cells independent of effects on HMG-CoA reductase activity. *Biochem Pharmacol* **68**: 1739–1747.

Eferl, R., and Wagner, E.F. 2003. AP-1: a double-edged sword in tumorigenesis *Nature Reviews Cancer* **3**: 859–868.

Egozi, Y., Weisz, B., Gana-Weisz, M., Ben-Baruch, G., and Kloog, Y. 1999. Growth inhibition of ras-dependent tumors in nude mice by a potent ras-dislodging antagonist. *Int J Cancer* **80**: 911–918.

Elegbede, J.A., Flores, R., and Wang, R.C. 2003. Perillyl alcohol and perillaldehyde induced cell cycle arrest and cell death in BroTo and A549 cells cultured *in vitro*. *Life Sci* **73**: 2831–2840.

Elson, C.E. 1995. Suppression of mevalonate pathway activities by dietary isoprenoids: Protective roles in cancer and cardiovascular disease. *J Nutr* **125**: 1666s–1672s.

Elson, C.E. 1996. Novel lipids and cancer: Isoprenoids and other phytochemicals. *In* "Dietary Fats, Lipids, Hormones, and Tumorigenesis" (D. Heber and D. Kritchevsky, eds.), pp. 71–86. Plenum Publishing Corporation, New York.

Elson, C.E., Peffley, D.M., Hentosh, P., and Mo, H. 1999. Isoprenoid-mediated inhibition of mevalonate synthesis: potential application to cancer. *Proc Soc Exp Biol Med* **221**: 294–311.

Elson, C.E., and Yu, S.G. 1994. The chemoprevention of cancer by mevalonate-derived constituents of fruits and vegetables. *J Nutr* **124**: 607–614.

Engstrom, W., and Schofield, P.N. 1987. Expression of 3-hydroxy-3-methylglutaryl coenzyme A- reductase and LDL-receptor genes in human embryonic tumors and in normal fetal tissues. *Anticancer Res* **7**: 337–342.

Engstrom, W., and Larsson, O. 1988. The effects of glycosylation inhibitors on the proliferation of a spontaneously transformed cell line (3T6) *in vitro. Cell Sci* **90**: 447–456.

Erickson, S.K., Cooper, A.D., Barnard, G.F., Havel, C.M., Watson, J.A., Feingold, K.R., Moser, A.H., Hughes-Fulford, M., and Siperstein, M.D. 1988. Regulation of cholesterol metabolism in a slow-growing hepatoma *in vivo*. *Biochim Biophys Acta* **960**: 131–138.

Eskens, F.A., Awada, A., Cutler, D.L., de Jonge, M.J., Luyten, G.P., Faber, M.N., Statkevich, P., Sparreboom, A., Verweij, J., Hanauske, A.R., and Piccart, M. 2001. Phase I and pharmacokinetic study of the oral farnesyl transferase inhibitor SCH 66336 given twice daily to patients with advanced solid tumors. *J Clin Oncol* **19**: 1167–1175.

Fadok, V.A., and Hanson, P.M. 2003. Apoptosis: Giving phosphatidylserine recognition an assist—with a twist. *Current Biol* **13**: R655–R657.

Fenig, E., Szyper-Kravitz, M., Yerushalmi, R., Lahav, M., Beery, M., Wasserman, L., Gutman, H., and Nordenberg, J. 2002. Basic fibroblast growth factor mediated growth inhibition in breast cancer cells is independent of ras signaling pathway. *Oncology Rep* **9**: 875–877.

Ferri, N., Arnaboldi, L., Orlandi, A., Yokoyama, K., Gree, R., Granata, A., Hachem, A., Paoletti, R., Gelb, M.H., and Corsini, A. 2001. Effect of S(−) perillic acid on protein prenylation and arterial smooth muscle cell proliferation. *Biochem Pharmacol* **62**: 1637–1645.

Finzer, P., Stohr, M., Seibert, N., and Rosl, F. 2003. Phenylbutyrate inhibits growth of cervical carcinoma cells independent of HPV type and copy number. *J Cancer Res Clin Oncol* **129**: 107–113.

Flach, J., Antoni, I., Villemin, P., Bentzen, C.L., and Niesor, E.J. 2000. The mevalonate/isoprenoid oathway inhibitor apomine (SR-45023A) is antiproliferative and induces apoptosis similar to farnesol. *Biochem Biophys Res Commun* **270**: 240–246.

Gagnon, H., Grandmaison, J., and Ibrahim, R. 1995. Phytochemical and immunocytochemical evidence for the accumulation of 2′-hydroxylupalbigenin in lupin nodules and bacteroids. *Mol Plant Microbe Interact* **8**: 131–137.

Gana-Weisz, M., Halaschek-Wiener, J., Jansen, B., Elad, G., Haklai, R., and Kloog, Y. 2002. The Ras inhibitor S trans, trans-farnesylthiosalicylic acid chemosensitizes human tumor cells without causing resistance. *Clin Cancer Res* **8**: 555–565.

Garcia-Roman, N., Alvarez, A.M., Toro, M.J., Montes, A., and Lorenzo, M.J. 2001. Lovastatin induces apoptosis of spontaneously immortalized rat brain neuroblasts: involvement of nonsterol isoprenoid biosynthesis inhibition. *Mol Cell Neurosci* **17**: 329–341.

Gartel, A.L., Serfas, M.S., Gartel, M., Goufman, E., Wu, G.S., El-Deiry, W.S., and Tyner, A.L. 1996. P21 (WAF1/CIP1) expression is induced in newly nondividing cells in diverse epithelia and during differentiation of the Caco-2 intestinal cell line. *Exper Cell Res* **227**: 171–181.

Gelb, M.H., Tamanoi, F., Yokoyama, K., Ghomashchi, F., Esson, K., and Gould, M.N. 1995. The inhibition of protein prenyltransferases by oxygenated metabolites of limonene and perillyl alcohol. *Cancer Lett* **91**: 169–175.

George, R., and Goldfarb, S. 1980. Inhibition of 3-hydroxy-3-methylglutaryl coenzyme A reductase activity in Morris hepatoma 7800 after intravenous injection of mevalonic acid. *Cancer Res* **40**: 4717–4721.

Ghosh, P.M., Moyer, M.L., Mott, G.E., and Kreisberg, J.I. 1999. Effect of cyclin E overexpression on lovastatin induced G1 arrest and RhoA inactivation in NIH3T3 cells. *J Cell Biochem* **74**: 532–543.

Giri, R.K., Parija, T., and Das, B.R. 1999. d-Limonene chemoprevention of hepatocarcinogenesis in AKR mice: inhibition of c-jun and c-myc. *Oncol Rep* **6**: 1123–1127.

Girnita, L., Wang, M., Xie, Y., Nilsson, G., Dricu, A., Wejde, J., and Larsson, O. 2000. Inhibition of N-linked glycosylation down-regulates insulin-like growth factor-1 receptor at the cell surface and kills

Ewing's sarcoma cells: Therapeutic implications. *Anti-Cancer Drug Design* **15**: 67–72.

Goldstein, J.L., and Brown, M.S. 1990. Regulation of the mevalonate pathway. *Nature (Lond)* **343**: 425–430.

Graham, S.M., Cox, A.D., Drivas, G., Rush, M.G., D'Eustachio, P., and Der, C.J. 1994. Aberrant function of the Ras related protein TC21/R-Ras2 triggers malignant transformation. *Mol Cell Biol* **14**: 4108–4115.

Gray-Bablin, J., Rao, S., and Keyomarsi, K. 1997. Lovastatin induction of cyclin-dependent kinase inhibitors in human breast cells occurs in a cell cycle–independent fashion. *Cancer Res* **57**: 604–609.

Gregg, R.G., Sabine, J.R., and Wilce, P.A. 1982. Regulation of 3-hydroxy-3-methylglutaryl coenzyme A reductase in rat liver and Morris hepatomas 5123C, 9618A and 5123tc. *Biochem J* **204**: 457–462.

Gudas, J.M., Nguyen, H., Li, T., Sadzewicz, L., Robey, R., Wosikowksi, K., and Cowan, K.H. 1996. Drug-resistant breast cancer cells frequently retain expression of a functional wild-type p53 protein. *Carcinogenesis* **17**: 1417–1427.

Guthrie, N., Gapor, A., Chambers, A.F., and Carroll, K.K. 1997. Inhibition of proliferation of estrogen receptor-negative MDA-MB-435 and -positive MCF-7 human breast cancer cells by palm oil tocotrienols and tamoxifen, alone and in combination. *J Nutr* **127**: S544–S548.

Hahn, S.M., Bernhard, E.J., Regine, W., Mohiuddin, M., Haller, D.G., Stevenson, J.P., Smith, D., Pramanik, B., Tepper, J., DeLaney, T.F., Kiel, K.D., Morrison, B., Deutsch, P., Muschel, R.J., and McKenna, W.G. 2002. A Phase I trial of the farnesyltransferase inhibitor L-778,123 and radiotherapy for locally advanced lung and head and neck cancer. *Clin Cancer Res* **8**: 1065–1072.

Hainsworth, J.D., Lennington, W.J., and Greco, F.A. 2000. Overexpression of Her-2 in patients with poorly differentiated carcinoma or poorly differentiated adenocarcinoma of unknown primary site *J Clin Oncol* **18**: 632–635.

Haklai, R., Weisz, MG., Elad, G., Paz, A., Marciano, D., Egozi, Y., Ben-Baruch, G., and Kloog, Y. 1998. Dislodgment and accelerated degradation of Ras. *Biochemistry* **37**: 1306–1314.

Haluska, P., Dy, G., and Adjei, A. 2002. Farnesyl transferase inhibitors as anticancer agents. *Eur J Cancer* **38**: 1685–1700.

Hamada, M., Nishio, K., Doe, M., Usuki, Y., and Tanaka, T. 2002. Farnesylpyridinium, an analog of isoprenoid farnesol, induces apoptosis but suppresses apoptotic body formation in human promyelocytic leukemia cells. *FEBS Lett* **514**: 250–254.

Hancock, J.F., Magee, A.I., Childs, J.E., and Marshall, C.J. 1989. All ras proteins are polyisoprenylated but only some are palmitoylated. *Cell* **57**: 1167–1177.

Hannah, V.C., Ou, J., Luong, A., Goldstein, J.L., and Brown, M.S. 2001. Unsaturated fatty acids down-regulate srebp isoforms 1a and 1c by two mechanisms in HEK-293 cells. *J Biol Chem* **276**: 4365–4372.

Harbour, J.W., and Dean, D.C. 2000. Rb function in cell-cycle regulation and apoptosis. *Nature Cell Biol* **2**: E65–E67.

Harrison, L.E., Wojciechowicz, D.C., Brennan, M.F., and Paty, P.B. 1998. Phenylacetate inhibits isoprenoid biosynthesis and suppresses growth of human pancreatic carcinoma. *Surgery* **124**: 541–550.

Haug, J.S., Goldner, C.M., Yazlovitskaya, E.M., Voziyan, P.A., and Melnykovych, G. 1994. Directed cell killing (apoptosis) in human lymphoblastoid cells incubated in the presence of farnesol: Effect of phosphatidylcholine. *Biochim Biophys Acta* **1223**: 133–140.

He, L., Mo, H., Hadisusilo, S., and Elson, C.E. 1997. Isoprenoids suppress the growth of murine B16 melanomas *in vitro* and *in vivo*. *J Nutr* **127**: 668–674.

Hellstrom, I., Goodman, G., Pullman, J., Yang, Y., and Hellstrom, K.E. 2001. Overexpression of HER-2 in ovarian carcinomas. *Cancer Res* **61**: 2420–2423.

Hemming, F. 1983. The biosynthesis of polyisoprenoid chains. *Biochem Soc Trans* **11**: 497–503.

Hempstock, J., Kavanagh, J.P., and George, N.J. 1998. Growth inhibition of prostate cell lines *in vitro* by phyto-oestrogen. *Br J Urol* **82**: 560–563.

Hentosh, P., Yuh, S.H., Elson, C.E., and Peffley, D.M. 2001. Sterol-independent regulation of 3-hydroxy-3-methylglutaryl coenzyme A reductase in tumor cells. *Mol Carcinog* **32**: 154–166.

Hohl, R.J., and Lewis, K. 1995. Differential effects of monoterpenes and lovastatin on RAS processing. *J Biol Chem* **270**: 17508–17512.

Holstein, S.A., and Hohl, R.J. 2003. Monoterpene regulation of Ras and Ras-related protein expression. *J Lipid Res* **44**: 1209–1215.

Holstein, S.A., Wohlford-Lenane, C.L., and Hohl, R.J. 2002a. Isoprenoids influence expression of Ras and Ras-related proteins. *Biochemistry* **41**: 13698–13704.

Holstein, S.A., Wohlford-Lenane, C.L., and Hohl, R.J. 2002b. Consequences of mevalonate depletion. Differential transcriptional, translational, and post-translational up-regulation of Ras, Rap1a, RhoA, and RhoB. *J Biol Chem* **277**: 10678–10682.

Horton, J.D., Goldstein, J.L., and Brown, M.S. 2002. SREBPs: activators of the complete program of cholesterol and fatty acid synthesis in the liver *J Clin Invest* **109**: 1125–1131.

Hua, X., Nohturfft, A., Goldstein, J.L., and Brown, M.S. 1996. Sterol resistance in CHO cells traced to point mutation in SREBP cleavage-activating protein. *Cell* **87**: 415–426.

Hudes, G.R., Szarka, C.E., Adams, A., Ranganathan, S., McCauley, R.A., Weiner, L.M., Langer, C.J., Litwin, S., Yeslow, G., Halberr, T., Qian, M., and Gallo, J.M. 2000. Phase I pharmacokinetic trial of perillyl alcohol (NSC 641066) in patients with refractory solid malignancies. *Clin Cancer Res* **6**: 3071–3080.

Hutchison, C.J., Bridger, J.M., Cox, L.S., and Kill, I.R. 1994. Weaving a pattern from disparate threads: lamin function in nuclear assembly and DNA replication. *J Cell Sci* **107**: 3259–3269.

Janssen, A.M., Scheffer, J.J.C., and Baerheim-Svendsen, A. 1987. Antimicrobial activities of essential oils. A 1976–1986 literature review of possible applications *Pharm Weekbl., Sci Ed* **7**: 193–197.

Jirtle, R.L., Haag, J.D., Ariazi, E.A., and Gould, M.N. 1993. Increased mannose 6-phosphate/insulin-like growth factor II receptor and transforming growth factor β1 levels during monoterpene-induced regression of mammary tumors. *Cancer Res* **53**: 3849–3852.

Johnston, S.R., Hickish, T., Ellis, P., Houston, S., Kelland, L., Dowsett, M., Salter, J., Michiels, B., Perez-Ruixo, J.J., Palmer, P., and Howes, A. 2003. Phase II study of the efficacy and tolerability of two dosing regimens of the farnesyl transferase inhibitor, R115777, in advanced breast cancer. *J Clin Oncol* **21**: 2492–2499.

Karp, J.E., Lancet, J.E., Kaufmann, S.H., End, D.W., Wright, J.J., Bol, K., Horak, I., Tidwell, M.L., Liesveld, J., Kottke, T.J., Ange, D., Buddharaju, L., Gojo, I., Highsmith, W.E., Belly, R.T., Hohl, R.J., Rybak, M.E., Thibault, A., and Rosenblatt, J. 2001. Clinical and biologic activity of the farnesyltransferase inhibitor R115777 in adults with refractory and relapsed acute leukemias: a phase 1 clinical-laboratory correlative trial. *Blood* **97**: 3361–3369.

Kawata, S., Takaishi, N., Nagase, T., Ito, N., Matsuda, Y., and Tamura, S. 1990. Increase in the active form of 3-hydroxy-3-methylglutaryl coenzyme A reductase in human hepatocellular carcinoma: possible mechanism for alteration of cholesterol bio synthesis. *Cancer Res* **50**: 3270–3273.

Kawata, S., Yamasaki, E., Nagase, T., Inui, Y., Ito, N., Matsuda, Y., Inada, M., Tamura, S., Noda, S., Imai, Y., and Matsuzawa, Y. 2001. Effect of pravastatin on survival in patients with advanced hepatocellular carcinoma. A randomized controlled trial. *Br J Cancer* **84**: 886–891.

Kim, W.S., Kim, M.M., Choi, H.J., Yoon, S.S., Lee, M.H., Park, K., Park, C.H., and Kang, W.K. 2001. Phase II study of high-dose lovastatin in patients with advanced gastric adenocarcinoma. *Invest New Drugs* **19**: 81–83.

Klepzig, K.D., Smalley, E.B., and Raffa, K.F. 1996. Combined chemical defenses against an insect-fungal complex. *J Chem Ecol* **22**: 1367–1388.

Koeffler, H.P., Miller, C., Nicolson, M.A., Ranyard, J., and Bosselman, R.A. 1986. Increased expression of p53 protein in human leukemia cells. *Proc Natl Acad Sci USA* **83**: 4035–4039.

Kotake-Nara, N.E., Kim, S.J., Kobori, M., Miyashita, K., and Nagao, A. 2002. Acyclo-retinoic acid induces apoptosis in human prostate cancer cells. *Anticancer Res* **22**: 689–696.

Laird, P.W., and Jaenisch, R. 1994. DNA methylation and cancer. *Hum Mol Genet* **3**: 1487–1495.

Larner, J., Jane, J., Laws, E., Packer, R., Myers, C., and Shaffrey, M. 1998. A phase I–II trial of lovastatin for anaplastic astrocytoma and glioblastoma multiforme. *Am J Clin Oncol* **21**: 579–583.

Larsson, O. 1993. Cell cycle–specific growth inhibition of human breast cancer cells induced by metabolic inhibitors. *Glycobiology* **3**: 475–479.

Larsson, O. 1994. Effects of isoprenoids on growth of normal human mammary epithelial cells and breast cancer cells *in vitro*. *Anticancer Res* **14**: 123–128.

Lee, S.J., Ha, M.J., Lee, J., Nguyen, P., Choi, Y.H., Pirnia, F., Kang, W.K., Wang, X.F., Kim, S.J., and Trepel, J.B. 1998. Inhibition of the 3-hydroxy-3-methylglutaryl-coenzyme A reductase pathway induces p53-independent transcriptional regulation of p21(WAF1/CIP1) in human prostate carcinoma cells. *J Biol Chem* **273**: 10618–10623.

Li, Z., Wang, Y., and Mo, B. 2002. The effects of carotenoids on the proliferation of human breast cancer cell and gene expression of bcl-2. *Zhonghua Yufang Yixue Zazhi* **36**: 254–257.

Liu, G., Oettel, K., Bailey, H., Van Ummersen, L., Tutsch, K., Staab, M.J., Horvath, D., Alberti, D., Arzoomanian, R., Rezazadeh, H., McGovern, J., Robinson, E., DeMets, D., and Wilding, G. 2003. Phase II trial of perillyl alcohol (NSC 641066) administered daily in patients with metastatic androgen independent prostate cancer. *Invest New Drugs* **21**: 367–372.

Liu, J-R., Chen, B-Q., Yang, B-F., Dong, H-W., Sun, C-H., Wang, Q., Song, G., and Song, Y-Q. 2004a. Apoptosis of human gastric adenocarcinoma cells induced by β-ionone. *World J Gastroenterol* **10**: 348–351.

Liu, J-R., Yang, B-F., Chen, B-Q., Yang, Y-M., Dong, H-W., and Song, Y-Q. 2004b. Inhibition of β-ionone on SGC-7901 cell proliferation and upregulation of metalloproteinases-1 and -2 expression. *World J Gastroenterol* **10**: 167–171.

Lukas, J., Bartkova, J., and Bartek, J. 1996. Convergence of mitogenic signalling cascades from diverse classes of receptors at the cyclin D-cyclin–dependent kinase-pRb–controlled G1 checkpoint. *Mol Cell Biol* **16**: 6917–6925.

Marcelli, M., Cunningham, G.R., Haidacher, S.J., Padayatty, S.J., Sturgis, L., Kagan, C., and Denner, L. 1998. Caspase-7 is activated during lovastatin-induced apoptosis of the prostate cancer cell line LNCaP. *Cancer Res* **58**: 76–83.

Marciano, D., Ben-Baruch, G., Marom, M., Egozi, Y., Haklai, R., and Kloog, Y. 1995. Farnesyl derivatives of rigid carboxylic acids-inhibitors of ras-dependent cell growth. *J Med Chem* **38**: 1267–1272.

Martinez-Gonzalez, J., Vinals, M., Vidal, F., Llorente-Cortes, V., and Badimon, L. 1997. Mevalonate deprivation impairs IGF-I/insulin signaling in human vascular smooth muscle cells. *Atherosclerosis* **135**: 213–223.

McAnally, J.A., Jung, M., and Mo, H. 2003. Farnesyl-O-acetylhydroquinone and geranyl-O-acetylhydroquinone suppress the proliferation of murine B16 melanoma cells, human prostate and colon adenocarcinoma cells, human lung carcinoma cells, and human leukemia cells. *Cancer Lett* **202**: 181–192.

McCarty, M.F. 2001. Suppression of dolichol synthesis with isoprenoids and statins may potentiate the cancer-retardant efficacy of IGF-I down-regulation. *Med Hypotheses* **56**: 12–16.

McIntyre, B.S., Briski, K.P., Gapor, A., and Sylvester, P.W. 2000. Antiproliferative and apoptotic effects of tocopherols and tocotrienols on preneoplastic and neoplastic mouse mammary epithelial cells. *Proc Soc Exp Biol Med* **224**: 292–301.

Meadows, S.M., Mulkerin, D., Berlin, J., Bailey, H., Kolesar, J., Warren, D., and Thomas, J.P. 2002. Phase II trial of perillyl alcohol in patients with metastatic colorectal cancer *Int J Gastrointest Cancer* **32**: 125–128.

Meigs, T.E., Roseman, D.S., and Simoni, R.D. 1996. Regulation of 3-hydroxy-3-methylglutaryl-coenzyme A reductase degradation by the nonsterol mevalonate metabolite farnesol *in vivo*. *J Biol Chem* **271**: 7916–7922.

Meigs, T.E., and Simoni, R.D. 1997. Farnesol as a regulator of HMG-CoA reductase degradation: characterization and role of farnesyl pyrophosphatase. *Arch Biochem Biophys* **345**: 1–9.

Mills, J.J., Chari, R.S., Boyer, I.J., Gould, M.N., and Jirtle, R.L. 1995. Induction of apoptosis in liver tumors by the monoterpene perillyl alcohol. *Cancer Res* **55**: 979–983.

Minden, M.D., Dimitroulakos, J., Nohynek, D., and Penn, L.Z. 2001. Lovastatin induced control of blast cell growth in an elderly patient with acute myeloblastic leukemia. *Leuk Lymphoma* **40**: 659–662.

Miquel, K., Pradines, A., and Favre, G. 1996. Farnesol and geranylgeraniol induce actin cytoskeleton disorganization and apoptosis in A549 lung adenocarcinoma cells. *Biochem Biophys Res Commun* **225**: 869–876.

Miquel, K., Pradines, A., Terce, F., Selmi, S., and Favre, G. 1998. Competitive inhibition of choline phosphotransferase by geranylgeraniol and farnesol inhibits phosphatidylcholine synthesis and induces apoptosis in human lung adenocarcinoma A549 cells. *J Biol Chem* **273**: 26179–26186.

Miyazawa, K., Yaguchi, M., Funato, K., Gotoh, A., Kawanishi, Y., Nishizawa, Y., You, A., and Ohyashiki, K. 2001. Apoptosis/differentiation-inducing effects of vitamin K2 on HL-60 cells: dichomotous nature of vitamin K2 in leukemia cells. *Leukemia* **15**: 1111–1117.

Mo, H., and Elson, C.E. 1999. Apoptosis and cell-cycle arrest in human and murine tumor cells are initiated by isoprenoids. *J Nutr* **129**: 804–813.

Mo, H., Peffley, D.M., and Elson, C.E. 1999. Targeting the action of isoprenoids and related phytochemicals to tumors. *In* "Nutritional Oncology" (D. Heber, G.L. Blackburn, and V.L.W. Go, eds.), pp. 379–391. Academic Press, New York.

Mo, H., Tatman, D., Jung, M., and Elson, C.E. 2000. Farnesyl anthranilate suppresses the growth, *in vitro* and *in vivo*, of murine B16 melanomas. *Cancer Lett* **157**: 145–153.

Moreno, F.S., Rossiello, M.R., Manjeshwar, S., Nath, R., Rao, P.M., Rajalakshmi, S., and Sarma-Dittakavi, S.R. 1995. Effect of beta-carotene on the expression of 3-hydroxy-3-methylglutaryl coenzyme A reductase in rat liver. *Cancer Lett* **96**: 201–208.

Morgan-Meadows, S., Dubey, S., Gould, M., Tutsch, K., Marnocha, R., Arzoomanin, R., Alberti, D., Binger, K., Feierabend, C., Volkman, J., Ellingen, S., Black, S., Pomplun, M., Wilding, G., and Bailey, H. 2003. Phase I trial of perillyl alcohol administered four times daily continuously. *Cancer Chemother Pharmacol* **52**: 361–366.

Murren, J.R., Pizzorno, G., DiStasio, S.A., McKeon, A., Peccerillo, K., Gollerkari, A., McMurray, W., Burtness, B.A., Rutherford, T., Li, X., Ho, P.T., and Sartorelli, A. 2002. Phase I study of perillyl alcohol in patients with refractory malignancies. *Cancer Biol Ther* **1**: 130–135.

Mutoh, T., Kumano, T., Nakagawa, H., and Kuriyama, M. 1999. Involvement of tyrosine phosphorylation in HMG-CoA reductase inhibitor-induced cell death in L6 myoblasts, *FEBS Lett* **444**: 85–89.

Nesaretnam, K., Dorasamy, S., and Darbre, P.D. 2000. Tocotrienols inhibit growth of ZR-75-1 breast cancer cells. *Internat J Food Sci Nutr* **51**: S95–S103.

Nesaretnam, K., Stephen, R., Dils, R., and Darbre, P. 1998. Tocotrienols inhibit the growth of human breast cancer cells irrespective of estrogen receptor status. *Lipids* **33**: 879–892.

Oda, H., Kasiske, B.L., O'Donnell, M.P., and Keane, W.F. 1999. Effects of lovastatin on expression of cell cycle regulatory proteins in vascular smooth muscle cells. *Kidney Int* **71**: S202–S205.

Osborne, T.F. 2000. Sterol regulatory element-binding proteins (SREBPs): key regulators of nutritional homeostasis and insulin action. *J Biol Chem* **275**: 32379–32382.

Palozza, P., Serini, S., Torsello, A., Maggiano, N., Angelini, M., Boninsegna, A., Di-Nicuolo, F., Ranelletti, F.O., and Calviello, G. 2002b. Induction of cell cycle arrest and apoptosis in human colon adenocarcinoma cell lines by beta-carotene through down-regulation of cyclin A and Bcl-2 family proteins. *Oxford* **23**: 11–18.

Palozza, P., Serini, S., Torsello, A., Boninsegna, A., Covacci, V., Maggiano, N., Ranelletti, F.O., Wolf, F.I., and Calviello, G. 2002a. Regulation of cell cycle progression and apoptosis by beta-carotene in undifferentiated and differentiated HL-60 leukemia cells: Possible involvement of a redox mechanism. *Internat J Cancer* **97**: 593–600.

Pare, P.W., and Tumlinson, J.H. 1997. De novo biosynthesis of volatiles induced by insect herbivory in cotton plants. *Plant Physiol* **114**: 1161–1167.

Park, C., Lee, I., and Kang, W.K. 2001. Lovastatin-induced E2F-1 modulation and its effect on prostate cancer cell death. *Carcinogenesis* **22**: 1727–1731.

Park, W.H., Lee, Y.Y., Kim, E.S., Seol, J.G., Jung, C.W., Lee, C.C., and Kim, B.K. 1999. Lovastatin-induced inhibition of HL-60 cell proliferation via cell cycle arrest and apoptosis. *Anticancer Res* **19**: 3133–3140.

Parker, C., Whittaker, P.A., Usmani, B.A., Lakshmi, M.S., and Sherbet, G.V. 1994. Induction of 18A2/mts1 gene expression and its effects on metastasis and cell cycle control. *DNA Cell Biol* **13**: 1021–1028.

Parker, R.A., Pearce, B.C., Clark, R.W., Gordan, D.A., and Wright, J.J.K. 1993. Tocotrienols regulate cholesterol production in mammalian cells by post-transcriptional suppression of 3-hydroxy-3-methylglutaryl-coenzyme A reductase. *J Biol Chem* **268**: 11230–11238.

Patnaik, A., Eckhardt, S.G., Izbicka, E., Tolcher, A.A., Hammond, L.A., Takimoto, C.H., Schwartz, G., McCreery, H., Goetz, A., Mori, M., Terada, K., Gentner, L., Rybak, M.E., Richards, H., Zhang, S., and Rowinsky, E.K. 2003. A phase I, pharmacokinetic, and biological study of the farnesyltransferase inhibitor tipifarnib in combination with gemcitabine in patients with advanced malignancies. *Clin Cancer Res* **9**: 4761–4771.

Pearce, B.C., Parker, R.A., Deason, M.E., Dischino, D.D., Gillespie, E., Qureshi, A.A., Volk, K., and Wright, J.J. 1994. Inhibitors of cholesterol biosynthesis. 2. Hypocholesterolemic and antioxidant activities of benzopyran and tetrahydronaphthalene analogues of the tocotrienols. *J Med Chem* **37**: 526–541.

Peffley, D.M., and Gayen, A.K. 1997. Inhibition of squalene synthase but not squalene cyclase prevents mevalonate-mediated suppression of 3-hydroxy-3-methylglutaryl coenzyme A reductase synthesis at a post-transcriptional level. *Arch Biochem Biophys* **337**: 251–260.

Peffley, D.M., and Gayen, A.K. 2003. Plant-derived monoterpenes suppress hamster kidney cell 3-hydroxy-3-methylglutaryl coenzyme a reductase synthesis at the post-transcriptional level. *J Nutr* **133**: 38–44.

Perez-Sala, D., Gilbert, B.A., Rando, R.R., and Canada, F.J. 1998. Analogs of farnesylcysteine induce apoptosis in HL-60 cells. *FEBS Lett* **426**: 319–324.

Piscitelli, S.C., Thibault, A., Figg, W.D., Tompkins, A., Headlee, D., Lieberman, R., Samid, D., and Myers, C.E. 1995. Disposition of phenylbutyrate and its metabolites, phenylacetate and phenylacetylglutamine. *J Clin Pharmacol* **35**: 368–373.

Punt, C.J., van Maanen, L., Bol, C.J., Seifert, W.F., and Wagener, D.J. 2001. Phase I and pharmacokinetic study of the orally administered farnesyl transferase inhibitor R115777 in patients with advanced solid tumors. *Anticancer Drugs* **12**: 193–197.

Rahalison, L., Benathan, M., Monod, M., Frenk, E., Gupta, M.P., Solis, P.N., Fuzzati, N., and Hostettmann, K. 1995. Antifungal principles of Baccharis pedunculata. *Planta Med* **61**: 360–362.

Rao, S., Lowe, M., Herliczek, T.W., and Keyomarsi, K. 1998. Lovastatin mediated G1 arrest in normal and tumor breast cells is through inhibition of CDK2 activity and redistribution of p21 and p27, independent of p53. *Oncogene* **17**: 2393–2402.

Reddy, B.S., Wang, C.X., Samaha, H., Lubet, R., Steele, V.E., Kelloff, G.J., and Rao, C.V. 1997. Chemoprevention of colon carcinogenesis by dietary perillyl alcohol. *Cancer Res* **57**: 420–425.

Ren, Z., Elson, C.E., and Gould, M.N. 1997. Inhibition of type I and type II geranylgeranyl-protein transferases by the monoterpene perillyl alcohol in NIH3T3 cells. *Biochem Pharmacol* **54**: 113–120.

Reuveni, H., Klein, S., and Levizki, A. 2003. The inhibition of ras farnesylation leads to an increase in p27Kip1 and G1 cell cycle arrest. *Eur J Biochem* **270**: 2759–2772.

Rioja, A., Pizzey, A.R., Marson, C.M., and Thomas, N.S. 2000. Preferential induction of apoptosis of leukaemic cells by farnesol. *FEBS Lett* **467**: 291–295.

Ripple, G.H., Gould, M.N., Arzoomanian, R.Z., Alberti, D., Feierabend, C., Simon, K., Binger, K., Tutsch, K.D., Pomplun, M., Wahamaki, A., Marnocha, R., Wilding, G., and Bailey, H.H. 2000. Phase I clinical and pharmacokinetic study of perillyl alcohol administered four times a day. *Clin Cancer Res* **6**: 390–396.

Ripple, G.H., Gould, M.N., Stewart, J.A., Tutsch, K.D., Arzoomanian, R.Z., Alberti, D., Feierabend, C., Pomplun, M., Wilding, G., and Bailey, H.H. 1998. Phase I clinical trial of perillyl alcohol administered daily. *Clin Cancer Res* **4**: 1159–1164.

Rossiello, M.R., Rao, P.M., Rajalakshmi, S., and Sarma, D.S. 1994. Similar patterns of hypomethylation in the beta-hydroxy-beta-methylglutaryl coenzyme A reductase gene in hepatic nodules induced by different carcinogens. *Mol Carcinog* **10**: 237–245.

Sacchettini, J.C., and Poulter, C.D. 1997. Creating isoprenoid diversity. *Science* **277**: 1788–1789.

Sadof, C.S., and Grant, G.G. 1997. Monoterpene composition of *Pinus sylvestris* varieties resistant and susceptible to *Dioryctria zimmermani*. *J Chem Ecol* **23**: 1917–1927.

Sahin, M.B., Perman, S.M., Jenkins, G., and Clark, S.S. 1999. Perillyl alcohol selectively induces G0/G1 arrest and apoptosis in Bcr/Abl-transformed myeloid cell lines. *Leukemia* **13**: 1581–1591.

Saito, K., Okabe, T., Inamori, Y., Tsujibo, H., Miyake, Y., Hiraoka, K., and Ishida, N. 1996. The biological properties of monoterpenes. Hypotensive effects on rats and antifungal activities on plant pathogenic fungi of monoterpenes. *Mokuzai Gakkaishi* **42**: 677–680.

Sakai, M., Okabe, M., Yamasaki, M., Tachibana, H., and Yamada, K. 2004. Induction of apoptosis by tocotrienol in rat hepatoma dRLh-84 cells. *Anticancer Res* **24**: 1683–1688.

Samid, D., Ram, Z., Hudgins, W.R., Shack, S., Liu, L., Walbridge, S., Oldfield, E.H., and Myers, C.E. 1994. Selective activity of phenylacetate against malignant gliomas: resemblance to fetal brain damage in phenylketonuria. *Cancer Res* **54**: 891–895.

Satomi, Y., Miyamoto, S., and Gould, M.N. 1999. Induction of AP-1 activity by perillyl alcohol in breast cancer cells. *Carcinogenesis* **20**: 1957–1961.

Schafer, W.R., Kim, R., Sterne, R., Thorner, J., Kim, S.H., and Rine, J. 1989. Genetic and pharmacological suppression of oncogenic mutations in ras genes of yeast and humans. *Science* **245**: 379–385.

Schwenke, D.C. 2002. Does lack of tocopherols and tocotrienols put women at increased risk of breast cancer? *J Nutr Biochem* **13**: 2–20.

Sever, N., Song, B-L., Yabe, D., Goldstein, J.L., Brown, M.S., and DeBose-Boyd, R.A. 2003. Insig-dependent ubiquitination and degradation of mammalian 3-hydroxy-3-methylglutaryl-CoA reductase stimulated by sterols and geranylgeraniol. *J Biol Chem* **278**: 52479–52490.

Sharma, S., Kemeny, N., Kelsen, D.P., Ilson, D., O'Reilly, E., Zaknoen, S., Baum, C., Statkevich, P., Hollywood, E., Zhu, Y., and Saltz, L.B. 2002. A phase II trial of farnesyl protein transferase inhibitor SCH 66336, given by twice-daily oral administration, in patients with metastatic colorectal cancer refractory to 5-fluorouracil and irinotecan. *Ann Oncol* **13**: 1067–1071.

Shah, S., Gapor, A., and Sylvester, P.W. 2003. Role of caspase-8 activation in mediating vitamin E-induced apoptosis in murine mammary cancer cells. *Nutr Cancer* **45**: 236–246.

Shi, W., and Gould, M.N. 2002. Induction of cytostasis in mammary carcinoma cells treated with the anticancer agent perillyl alcohol. *Carcinogenesis* **23**: 131–142.

Shimano, H., Horton, J.D., Hammer, R.E., Shimomura, I., Brown, M.S., and Goldstein, J.L. 1996. Overproduction of cholesterol and fatty acids causes massive liver enlargement in transgenic mice expressing truncated SREBP-1a. *J Clin Invest* **98**: 1575–1584.

Shimano, H., Horton, J.D., Shimomura, I, Hammer, R.E., Brown, M.S., and Goldstein, J.L. 1997. Isoform 1c of sterol regulatory element binding protein is less active than isoform 1a in livers of transgenic mice and in cultured cells. *J Clin Invest* **99**: 846–854.

Shimomura, I., Shimano, H., Horton, J.D., Goldstein, J.L., and Brown, M.S. 1997. Differential expression of exons 1a and 1c in mRNAs for sterol regulatory element binding protein-1 in human and mouse organs and cultured cells. *J Clin Invest* **99**: 838–845.

Shoff, S.M., Grummer, M., Yatvin, M.B., and Elson, C.E. 1991. Concentration-dependent increase in murine P388 and B16 population doubling time by the acyclic monoterpene geraniol. *Cancer Res* **51**: 37–42.

Shun, M-C., Yu, W., Gapor, A., Parsons, R., Atkinson, J., Sanders, B.G., and Kline, K. 2004. Pro-apototic mechanisms of action of a novel vitamin E analog (α-TEA) and a naturally occurring form of vitamin E (δ-tocotrienol) in MDA-MB-435 human breast cancer cells. *Nutr Cancer* **48**: 95–105.

Sindermann, J.R., Schmidt, A., Breithardt, G., and Buddecke, E. 2001. Lovastatin controls signal transduction in vascular smooth muscle cells by modulating phosphorylation levels of mevalonate-independent pathways, *Basic Res Cardiol* **96**: 283–289.

Siperstein, M.D., and Fagan, V.M. 1964. Deletion of the cholesterol-negative feedback system in liver tumors. *Cancer Res* **24**: 1108–1115.

Smalley, K.S., and Eisen, T.G. 2002. Farnesyl thiosalicylic acid inhibits the growth of melanoma cells through a combination of cytostatic and pro-apoptotic effects. *Int J Cancer* **98**: 514–522.

Stayrook, K.R., Mckinzie, J.H., Burke, Y.D., Burke, Y.A., and Crowell, P.L. 1997. Induction of the apoptosis-promoting protein BAK by perillyl alcohol in pancreatic ductal adenocarcinoma relative to untransformed ductal epithelial cells. *Carcinogenesis* **18**: 1655–1658.

Swinnen, J.V., Heemers, H., Deboel, L., Foufelle, F., Heyns, W., and Verhoeven, G. 2000. Stimulation of tumor-associated fatty acid synthase expression by growth factor activation of the sterol regulatory element-binding protein pathway. *Oncogene* **19**: 5173–5181.

Sylvester, P.W., and Shah, S.J. 2005. Mechanisms mediating the antiproliferative and apoptotic effects of vitamin E in mammary cancer. *Front Biosci* **10**: 699–709.

Tahara, S., Katagiri, Y., Ingham, J.L., and Mizutani, J. 1994. Prenylated flavonoids in the roots of yellow lupin. *Phytochemistry* **36**: 1261–1271.

Takahashi, K., and Loo, G. 2004. Disruption of mitochondria during tocotrienol-induced apoptosis in MDA-MB-231 human breast cancer cells. *Biochem Pharmacol* **67**: 315–324.

Tamanoi, F, Gau, C.L., Jiang, C., Edamatsu, H., Kato-Stankiewicz, J. 2001. Protein farnesylation in mammalian cells: effects of farnesyltransferase inhibitors on cancer cells. Cell Mol Life Sci **58**: 1636–1649.

Tatman, D., and Mo, H. 2002. Volatile isoprenoid constituents of fruits, vegetables and herbs cumulatively suppress the proliferation of murine B16 melanoma and human HL-60 leukemia cells. *Cancer Lett* **175**: 129–139.

Thibault, A., Cooper, M.R., Figg, W.D., Venzon, D.J., Sartor, A.O., Tompkins, A.C., Weinberger, M.S., Headlee, D.J., McCall, N.A., Samid, D., and Meyers, C.E. 1994. A phase I and pharmacokinetic study of intravenous phenylacetate in patients with cancer. *Cancer Res* **54**: 1690–1694.

Thibault, A., Samid, D., Cooper, M.R., Figg, W.D., Tompkins, A.C., Patronas, N., Headlee, D.J., Kohler, D.R., Venzon, D.J., and Myers, C.E. 1995. Phase I study of phenylacetate administered twice daily to patients with cancer. *Cancer* **75**: 2932–2938.

Thibault, A., Samid, D., Tompkins, A.C., Figg, W.D., Cooper, M.R., Hohl, R.J., Trepel, J., Liang, B., Patronas, N., Venzon, D.J., Reed, E., and Myers, C.E. 1996. Phase I study of lovastatin, an inhibitor of the mevalonate pathway, in patients with cancer. *Clin Cancer Res* **2**: 483–491.

Ukomadu, C., and Dutta, A. 2003a. Inhibition of cdk2 activating phosphorylation by mevastatin. *J Biol Chem* **278**: 4840–4846.

Ukomadu, C., and Dutta, A. 2003b. p21-dependent inhibition of colon cancer cell growth by mevastatin is independent of inhibition of G1 cyclin-dependent kinase. *J Biol Chem* **278**: 43586–43504.

Ura, H., Obara, T., Shudo, R., Itoh, A., Tanno, S., Fujii, T., Nishino, N., and Kohgo, Y. 1998. Selective cytotoxicity of farnesylamine to pancreatic carcinoma cells and Ki-ras–transformed fibroblasts. *Mol Carcinog* **21**: 93–99.

Vigushin, D.M., Poon, G.K., Boddy, A., English, J., Halbert, G.W., Pagonis, C., Jarman, M., and Coombes, R.C. 1998. Phase I and pharmacokinetic study of *d*-limonene in patients with advanced cancer. Cancer Research Campaign Phase I/II Clinical Trials Committee. *Cancer Chemother Pharmacol* **42**: 111–117.

Vitale, M., DiMatola, T., Rossi, G., Laezza, C., Fenzl, G., and Bifulco, M. 1999. Prenyltransferase inhibitors induce apoptosis in proliferating thyroid cells through a p53-independent, CrmA-sensitive, and caspase-3–like protease-dependent mechanism. *Endocrinol* **14**: 698–704.

Voziyan, P.A., Goldner, C.M., and Melnykovych, G. 1993. Farnesol inhibits phosphatidylcholine biosynthesis in cultured cells by decreasing cholinephosphotransferase activity. *Biochem J* **295**: 757–762.

Voziyan, P.A., Haug, J.S., and Melnykovych, G. 1995. Mechanism of farnesol cytotoxicity: further evidence for the role of PKC-dependent signal transduction in farnesol-induced apoptotic cell death. *Biochem Biophys Res Commun* **212**: 479–486.

Vrtovsnik, F., Couette, S., Prie, D., Lallemand, D., and Friedlander, G. 1997. Lovastatin-induced inhibition of renal epithelial tubular cell proliferation involves a p21ras activated, AP-1–dependent pathway. *Kidney Int* **52**: 1016–1027.

Wachtershauser, A., Akoglu, B., and Stein, J. 2001. HMG-CoA reductase inhibitor mevastatin enhances the growth inhibitory effect of butyrate in the colorectal carcinoma cell line Caco-2. *Carcinogenesis* **22**: 1061–1067.

Wang, I.K., Lin-Shiau, S.Y., and Lin, J.K. 2000. Suppression of invasion and MMP-9 expression in NIH 3T3 and v-H-Ras 3T3 fibroblasts by lovastatin through inhibition of ras isoprenylation. *Oncology* **59**: 245–254.

Wang, W., and Macaulay, R.J.B. 2003. Cell-cycle gene expression in lovastatin-induced medulloblastoma apoptosis. *Can J Neurolog Sci* **30**: 349–357.

Wang, X, Sato, R., Brown, M.S., Hua, X., and Goldstein, J.L. 1994. SREBP-1, a membrane-bound transcription factor released by sterol-regulated proteolysis. *Cell* **77**: 53–62.

Westfall, D., Aboushadi, N., Shackelford, J.E., and Krisans, S.K. 1997. Metabolism of farnesol: phosphorylation of farnesol by rat liver microsomal and peroxisomal fractions. *Biochem Biophys Res Commun* **230**: 562–568.

Wolf, D., and Rotter, V. 1985. Major deletions in the gene encoding the p53 tumor antigen cause lack of p53 expression in HL-60 cells. *Proc Natl Acad Sci USA* **82**: 790–794.

Yachnin, S., Toub, D., and Mannickarottu, V. 1984. Divergence in cholesterol biosynthetic rates and 3-hydroxy-3-methylglutaryl-CoA reductase activity as a consequence of granulocyte versus monocyte-macrophage differentiation in HL-60 cells. *Proc Natl Acad Sci USA* **81**: 894–897.

Yaguchi, M., Miyazawa, K., Katagiri, T., Nishimaki, J., Kizaki, M., Tohyama, K., and Toyama, K. 1997. Vitamin K2 and its derivatives induce apoptosis in leukemic cells and enhance the effect of all-trans-retinoic acid. *Leukemia (Basingstoke)* **11**: 779–787.

Yaguchi, M., Miyazawa, K., Otawa, M., Katagiri, T., Nishimaki, J., Uchida, Y., Iwase, O., Gotoh, A., Kawanishi, Y., and Toyama, K. 1998. Vitamin K2 selectively induces apoptosis of blastic cells in myelodysplastic syndrome: Flow cytometric detection of apoptotic cells using APO2.7 monoclonal antibody. *Leukemia (Basingstoke)* **12**: 1392–1397.

Yang, Y.A., Han, W.F., Morin, P.J., Chrest, F.J., and Pizer, E.S. 2002. Activation of fatty acid synthesis during neoplastic transformation: role of mitogen-activated protein kinase and phosphatidylinositol 3-kinase. *Exp Cell Res* **279**: 80–90.

Yang, Y.A., Morin, P.J., Han, W.F., Chen, T., Bornman, D.M., Gabrielson, E.W., and Pizer, E.S. 2003. Regulation of fatty acid synthase expression in breast cancer by sterol regulatory element binding protein-1c. *Exp Cell Res* **282**: 132–137.

Yarden, Y. 2001. Biology of HER2 and its importance in breast cancer *Oncology* **61**: 1–13.

Yazlovitskaya, E.M., and Melnykovych, G. 1995. Selective farnesol toxicity and translocation of protein kinase C in neoplastic HeLa-S3K and non-neoplastic CF-3 cells. *Cancer Lett* **88**: 179–183.

Yu, S.G., Abuirmeileh, N.M., Qureshi, A.A., and Elson, C.E. 1994. Dietary β-ionone suppresses hepatic 3-hydroxy-3-methylglutaryl coenzyme A reductase activity. *J Agric Food Chem* **42**: 1493–1496.

Zhang, F.L., and Casey, P.J. 1996. Protein prenylation: molecular mechanisms and functional consequences. *Annu Rev Biochem* **65**: 241–269.

Zhang, J., Zhang, J., Zhao, Y., Shi, H., Zhu, S., and Cai, M. 1999. Effects of beta-carotene on apoptosis and cell cycle of leukemic cell line HL-60. *Acta Nutrimenta Sinica* **21**: 401–404.

Zujewski, J., Horak, I.D., Bol, C.J., Woestenborghs, R., Bowden, C., End, D.W., Piotrovsky, V.K., Chiao, J., Belly, R.T., Todd, A., Kopp, W.C., Kohler, D.R., Chow, C., Noone, M., Hakim, F.T., Larkin, G., Gress, R.E., Nussenblatt, R.B., Kremer, A.B., and Cowan, K.H. 2000. Phase I and pharmacokinetic study of farnesyl protein transferase inhibitor R115777 in advanced cancer. *J Clin Oncol* **18**: 927–941.

CHAPTER

39

Cancer Anorexia and Cachexia

DAVID HEBER AND N. SIMON TCHEKMEDYIAN

INTRODUCTION

As a result of advances in our understanding of the metabolic and nutritional effects of many common forms of cancer, therapeutic options have been developed to reverse or reduce the effects of cancer anorexia and cachexia. Such options are becoming recognized as an integral part of the care of cancer patients to improve both their quality of life and the outcome of cancer therapies. The development of early and appropriate nutritional interventions holds the promise of improving the cancer patient's ability to undergo and tolerate definitive oncological therapies, including surgery, irradiation, chemotherapy, and the increasing variety of newer treatments, including biological response modifiers, angiogenesis inhibitors, monoclonal antibodies, and other targeted therapies. Implementation of nutritional management can provide a constructive and empowering experience for the patient and family during cancer therapy.

In contrast to uncomplicated starvation, cachexia is an advanced state of wasting marked by excess loss of skeletal muscle mass relative to total body weight loss. Because humans are well adapted to starvation, weight loss occurring gradually because of decreased calorie intake occurs with relative maintenance of lean body mass at the expense of body fat as an energy source. Because of metabolic and nutritional effects accompanying advanced cancer, these adaptations are inhibited or impaired, ultimately leading to advanced malnutrition and life-threatening cachexia. Certain common forms of cancer are more frequently associated with marked weight loss at the time of diagnosis than others, but weight loss is typically present in up to half of all untreated cancer patients.

The metabolic, hormonal, and inflammatory abnormalities associated with cancer anorexia and cachexia can overlap with the effects of chronic infections and surgery and result in marked effects on protein, carbohydrate, and lipid metabolism. Cytokines released by tumor cells, immune cells, and stromal cells mediate many of the observed changes in metabolism leading to anorexia and cachexia. Pharmacological agents that improve appetite, interfere with cytokine production, and inhibit inflammation have been combined with advanced nutritional technologies in attempts to produce weight gain, increase lean tissue, and improve the quality of life. Although pharmacological and adjunctive nutritional therapy of the malnourished cancer patient can ameliorate the impact of malnutrition on the quality of life, the search continues for additional therapeutic targets for reversing, delaying, or preventing cancer anorexia and cachexia.

MALNUTRITION AND CACHEXIA IN CANCER

Malnutrition and cachexia are frequently associated with cancers of the pancreas, lung, head and neck, stomach, and prostate. The overall incidence of malnutrition in cancer patients varies widely, occurring in between 30 and 87% of different populations studied (Shils, 1977; Nixon et al., 1980). For example, in patients with pancreatic and stomach cancers, up to 85% are cachectic, whereas among breast cancer and sarcoma patients, only 40% are cachectic (Monitto et al., 2001).

In our experience with 644 mostly ambulatory cancer patients, we observed weight loss of >5% of baseline body

Copyright © 2006, Elsevier Inc.
All rights of reproduction in any form reserved.

weight in 59% of the cases (Tchekmedyian, 1995). Fifty-nine percent of patients had decreased appetite, 67% had decreased food intake, and 54% were underweight when their weight was compared with the calculated ideal body weight. The advanced starvation state resulting from decreased food intake and hormonal/metabolic abnormalities characteristic of the interaction between tumor and host has been called *cancer cachexia* (Brennan, 1977). A retrospective analysis of patient body weight in early cooperative group chemotherapy trials determined that the presence of >6% weight loss from usual body weight was a significant prognostic factor predictive of a poorer survival (De Wys et al., 1980). In this study, the apparent effect of weight loss at the time of diagnosis in this study on median survival for certain cancers was greater than the impact of chemotherapy. Cachexia is directly associated with poorer survival in patients with many types of cancer, including advanced pancreatic and lung cancer (Persson et al., 2002). Poor quality of life, fatigue, weakness, and poorer responses to cancer therapies are all associated with cachexia.

RELATIVE ROLES OF ANOREXIA AND METABOLIC ABNORMALITIES

Anorexia clearly plays a major role in weight loss in the cancer patient but cannot explain all of the weight loss noted. Anorexia complicates cancer in 15–40% of patients at the time of diagnosis (De Wys, 1972; Evans et al., 1985). However, malnourished patients with localized cancers under metabolic ward conditions fail to gain weight even when given apparently adequate calories for anabolism, suggesting that these patients are hypermetabolic. Moreover, treatment with megestrol acetate, while improving appetite and leading to weight gain, fails to increase lean body mass (LoPrinzi et al., 1993). Decreased caloric intake is a marker of poorer survival in patients with pancreatic cancer (Okusaka et al., 1998), but it is not clear whether this is simply secondary to advanced disease status and an inability to eat. By contrast, the metabolic and body composition changes seen with cachexia are profound with marked reductions in skeletal muscle and adipose tissue resembling those found with surgical trauma, burns, infections, acquired immunodeficiency syndrome (AIDS), and injury rather than those seen with uncomplicated starvation.

Despite the development of advanced technology and delivery systems for total parenteral nutrition and continuous enteral nutrition, nutrition therapy alone does not reverse the weight loss and metabolic abnormalities of cancer malnutrition. Although nutritional rehabilitation can be demonstrated in selected patients who respond to antineoplastic therapy, the application of parenteral or enteral nutrition as adjuncts to chemotherapy in cancer patients has not resulted in increased survival or predictable weight gain (Brennan, 1981; Shike et al., 1984). Although a decrease in caloric intake is characteristically observed in malnourished cancer patients, clinical evidence suggests that decreased food intake alone cannot account for all the weight loss noted in cancer patients. Means of reversing the relentless catabolic progression due to metabolic abnormalities reviewed later in this chapter could potentially have meaningful effects on nutrition and survival time.

Increased whole body protein breakdown, increased lipolysis, and increased gluconeogenesis have been repeatedly demonstrated in malnourished cancer patients. A number of observations made with regard to fat metabolism in cachectic cancer patients may help explain the disproportionate decrease in fat tissue mass including increased lipolysis, decreased lipogenesis, hypertriglyceridemia, increased hepatic secretion of very low density lipoprotein (VLDL), increased *de novo* fatty acid synthesis, and a futile cycle of fatty acids between liver and adipose tissue. High turnover rates of both glycerol and free fatty acids (FFAs) have been observed combined with elevated fatty acid release into the circulation (Shaw and Wolfe, 1987). Fasting plasma FFAs are elevated in weight-losing cancer patients by comparison with weight-stable individuals, and there is increased sensitivity to the lipolytic effects of adrenaline (Yam et al., 1994). In malnourished cancer patients, basal fatty acid turnover was found to be 25% higher than in non-cancer controls and was found to be similar to the rate observed in patients with severe burns (Legaspi et al., 1987). Overall, lipolysis was increased by 40%, and there was a 20% increase in fatty acid oxidation in cancer patients with fat loss. A disproportionate loss of muscle mass, as is the case with fat cell mass, is also seen in malnourished cancer patients. A 75% decrease in skeletal muscle mass has been observed with a 30% loss of weight from preillness weight.

Attempts to Reverse Metabolic Abnormalities

Because predictable renutrition of the cancer patient has not been possible, a great deal of research has been conducted concerning specific hormonal and metabolic abnormalities that could interfere with renutrition. Over the past 15 years, research on the basic pathophysiology of cancer cachexia has resulted in the definition of several metabolic and hormonal abnormalities in malnourished cancer patients. These abnormalities include hypogonadism in male cancer patients (Chlebowski and Heber, 1982), increased glucose production (Holroyde et al., 1975; Chlebowski and Heber, 1986), increased protein catabolism (Heber et al., 1982; Burt et al., 1984), increased lipolysis and fatty acid oxidation (Jeevanandam et al., 1986; Shaw and Wolfe, 1987), and insulin resistance (Bennegard et al., 1986; Byerley et al., 1991).

Based on the metabolic abnormalities observed, a number of strategies using hormonal and metabolic agents were tested to reverse these abnormalities. Hydrazine sulfate has been tested based on its ability to inhibit gluconeogenesis (Chlebowski et al., 1984), and insulin infusion has been attempted to counteract apparent insulin resistance (Moley et al., 1985). Neither of these treatments resulted in weight gain.

Host–Tumor Interactions and the Development of Cachexia

Based on autopsy studies performed in the 1920s (Warren, 1932; Terepka and Waterhouse, 1956) and animal studies done in the 1950s (Fenninger and Mider, 1954), it was postulated that tumors acted to siphon off needed energy and protein from the host. In the 1970s and 1980s, specific abnormalities of intermediary metabolism were identified in cancer patients that could account for the common observation that such patients lost weight even in the face of apparently adequate nutrition. Studies conducted in a number of laboratories, including our own, have demonstrated that maladaptive metabolic abnormalities occur frequently in patients with cancer. In 1983, we demonstrated that adequate calories and protein administered to six patients with active localized head and neck cancer via forced continuous enteral alimentation under metabolic ward conditions for 29 days failed to lead to significant weight gain (Heber et al., 1986). The observed failure of these patients to gain weight despite adequate caloric intake under metabolic ward conditions supports the concept that malnourished cancer patients are hypermetabolic, which may be due in turn to futile cycling with resulting energy inefficiency.

Energy Balance in the Cancer Patient

If metabolic abnormalities promote the development of malnutrition or interfere with renutrition, then there should be some evidence of abnormally increased energy expenditure. A number of investigators have used indirect calorimetry and the abbreviated Weir formula to calculate energy expenditure at rest and then compared this with the basal energy expenditure (BEE) determined using the Harris–Benedict formulas. Long et al. (1981) demonstrated a mean difference of 2% when this comparison was performed in 20 normal controls. In 1980, Bozetti et al. (1980) found that 60% of a group of patients with advanced cancer had basal metabolic rates increased 20% above predicted. Dempsey et al. (1984) studied energy expenditure in a group of 173 malnourished gastrointestinal cancer patients. Fifty-eight percent had abnormal resting energy expenditure (REE) by indirect calorimetry compared with BEE, but a greater percentage were hypometabolic rather than hypermetabolic (36 vs 22%). Knox et al. (1983) studied 200 patients with a variety of cancers and found abnormal energy metabolism in 59% but found more hypometabolic than hypermetabolic individuals (33% vs 26%).

Lean body mass rather than fat mass correlates with the individual variations observed in measured REE. The hypothesis that the malnourished cancer patient may be hypermetabolic relative to the amount of lean body mass remaining has been examined. Peacock et al. (1987) studied REE in noncachectic patients with sarcomas. These patients had no prior treatment, had large localized sarcomas, and no weight loss or history of decreased food intake. REE corrected for body cell mass (BCM) determined by total body potassium counting or body surface area was significantly greater in male sarcoma patients compared with controls. This difference was due to both a decrease in BCM and an increase in REE in these patients before the onset of weight loss.

Glucose and Protein Metabolism in Cancer Patients

Tumors have been demonstrated to increase the rate of glucose utilization in a number of tissues (Heber, 1989). Because there are only ~1200 kcal stored in the body as liver and muscle glycogen, blood glucose levels would be expected to fall. This does not occur, because there is also an increase in hepatic glucose production in cachectic and anorectic tumor-bearing animals and humans. The regulation of protein metabolism is tightly linked to carbohydrate metabolism because these processes are critical to the normal adaptation to starvation or underfeeding. During starvation, there is a decrease in glucose production, protein synthesis, and protein catabolism. The decrease in glucose production occurs because fat-derived fuels, primarily ketones, are used for energy production. Although there are, on average, ~54,000 kcal of protein stored in the BCM, only about half of this is available for energy production. In fact, depletion below 50% of body protein stores is incompatible with life. Whole body protein breakdown is increased in lung cancer patients and has been shown to correlate with the degree of malnutrition such that more malnourished patients have greater elevations of their whole body protein breakdown rates expressed per kilogram of body weight (Heber et al., 1982). Hydrazine sulfate is a noncompetitive inhibitor of gluconeogenesis. When this drug was administered to lung cancer patients in one study, not only did whole body glucose production decrease as expected, but there was also a decrease in the whole body protein breakdown rate (Tayek et al., 1987). Hydrazine sulfate has not been found to improve nutritional parameters, quality of life parameters, or survival in randomized trials in cancer patients, despite these seemingly promising effects (Kosty et al., 1994; Loprinzi et al., 1994).

Glucoregulatory Hormones

The normal adaptation to malnutrition involves changes in the secretion of a number of glucoregulatory hormones, including insulin, growth hormone, cortisol, and thyroid hormones. Because the changes observed in malnourished cancer patients are in the opposite direction of the adaptations observed in uncomplicated starvation, we have studied the secretion of these hormones under standardized conditions in a metabolic ward. In all cases, cancer patients received enteral nutrition calculated to maintain body weight for at least 3 days before study.

Growth hormone levels were measured in the fasting state in 27 patients with lung cancer or colorectal cancer. The mean fasting level was 55.7 ± 10.6 (SEM) pg/ml with a wide range from 30 to 232 pg/ml. In other studies, Tayek and Brasel (1995) have reported that more severely malnourished colorectal cancer patients have more elevated levels of growth hormone. Plasma insulin and growth hormone were also measured following an infusion of 0.5 g/kg of arginine for 30 minutes. There was a rise in growth hormone to normal levels observed 60 minutes after the end of the infusion. Therefore, growth hormone appears to respond normally to fasting and arginine infusion. A standard oral glucose load of 40 g/m^2 was also administered to a group of colon and lung cancer patients. Plasma glucose levels were elevated above the normal range into a range consistent with impaired glucose tolerance, but not diabetes. Plasma growth hormone levels were suppressed in the early part of the test, when insulin and glucose levels were elevated, but rose at 5 hours after the oral glucose load. Plasma cortisol levels were in the normal range. Thus, there was a generally normal response to an oral glucose load except for an elevation of insulin and glucose levels in the first 2 hours of the test. These data are consistent with an insulin-resistant state.

Insulin resistance has been observed in malnourished cancer patients using the euglycemic insulin clamp technique (Bennegard et al., 1986). The infusion of tumor necrosis factor-α (TNF-α) for 12 hours in rats results in both increased uptake of glucose and insulin resistance (Lang et al., 1992). These observations suggest that cytokines, including tumor TNF-α, may play a role in the pathogenesis of the metabolic abnormalities noted in the malnourished cancer patient.

Thyroid Hormones

The production of triiodothyronine (T_3) from thyroxine (T_4) is reduced significantly in uncomplicated starvation, short-term fasting, or malnutrition (Danforth et al., 1978). It has been proposed that the failure to adequately reduce T_3 production during starvation in cancer patients could lead to a hypermetabolic state (Danforth et al., 1978). We examined thyroid function tests in 27 cancer patients and 18 controls after at least 3 days of adequate nutrition under metabolic ward conditions. There were no differences in any of the measured thyroid hormone levels including T_4, T_3, or reverse T_3 between cancer patients and control subjects observed under conditions of adequate nutrition. Therefore, there was no evidence in these studies of increased thyroid hormone levels during refeeding that could impair renutrition. Other studies conducted in outpatient settings have found decreased levels of thyroid hormone as expected in undernourished patients (Persson et al., 1985). However, these changes secondary to malnutrition are apparently reversible in cancer patients with renutrition.

Lipid Metabolism in Cancer Cachexia

Net synthesis of adipose tissue triglyceride normally occurs when there is a net surplus of energy intake over expenditure. This can occur, however, also in the absence of increased food intake, as demonstrated in animals given progesterone under conditions of constant food intake (Hervey and Hervey, 1967). Under these circumstances, increased body fat deposition may result from a decrease in energy expenditure via modulation of the metabolism of fat away from fatty acid oxidation toward more energy efficient storage. In obese subjects, it has been proposed that increased fat mass results from the failure of increased fatty acid oxidation to keep pace with increased fat intake (Schutz et al., 1992). In the cancer patient who cannot maintain or gain weight, the opposite situation of excess fatty acid oxidation, which cannot be eclipsed by fat and calorie intake, may impair renutrition.

Under normal conditions of feeding and fasting, the uptake and breakdown of fat from adipose tissue is controlled by two adipose tissue enzymes: hormone-sensitive lipase (HSL) (Holm et al., 1988) and lipoprotein lipase (LPL) (Eckel, 1987). During early fasting, decreased insulin levels and increased glucagon and epinephrine result in cyclic adenosine monophosphate (cAMP) activation of a protein kinase, which phosphorylates and activates HSL. When activated, HSL hydrolyzes the triglyceride in the lipid droplet of the adipocyte into FFAs to be released into the circulation. Conversely, activated LPL hydrolyzes the core of circulating triglyceride-rich lipoproteins into FFAs and monoacylglycerol (Tayek et al., 1987). These fatty acids are the major source of substrate for adipocyte triglyceride synthesis, because adipocytes synthesize very small amounts of fatty acids *de novo* (Knittle et al., 1977).

Studies using stable isotopes have found that weight-losing cancer patients have increased rates of glycerol and FFA turnover when compared with normal patients and cancer patients without weight loss (Shaw and Wolfe, 1987). A glucose infusion failed to suppress lipolysis in the weight-losing cancer patients, as it did in normal subjects.

Hypertriglyceridemia, depletion of carcass fat stores, and decreased LPL levels have been observed in tumor-bearing animals and malnourished cancer patients (Axelrod and Costa, 1980; Cohn et al., 1981; Devereaux et al., 1984; Thompson et al., 1984). In animals bearing a mammary adenocarcinoma (AC33) for 18 days, decreased adipose tissue LPL activity was observed, together with a decrease in fat cell size but not number, and a decrease in serum insulin levels compared wtih non–tumor-bearing control animals consuming similar amounts of food (Lanza-Jacoby et al., 1984). Increased serum-FFAs, cholesterol, and triglycerides were observed consistent with the decrease in LPL activity.

Tumor and Host Factors Mediating Malnutrition and Cachexia

While studying cachexia in chronic infection, Beutler and Cerami (1986, 1988) and Oliff (1988) found that rabbits infected with trypanosomes lost weight and developed hypertriglyceridemia. They traced this to an inhibition of LPL and found that the serum of animals treated with lipopolysaccharide (LPS) contained the same inhibitor of LPL, suggesting it resulted from immune activation. In view of its potential role in wasting, it was called "cachectin." In earlier studies, it had been reported that the serum of mice treated with BCG and endotoxin had antitumor activity. The factor responsible for this effect was isolated from macrophages and called "tumor necrosis factor" (Norton et al., 1985). The amino acid and genetic sequences of TNF and cachectin were found to be identical, and the protein was called *TNF/cachectin*. Using recombinant DNA methodology, it was possible to produce large amounts of TNF for evaluation of its biological properties. Intravenous administration of TNF caused all the manifestations of toxic shock (Socher et al., 1988). Sublethal doses produced many of the metabolic abnormalities seen with cancer cachexia in a dose-related fashion (Stovroff et al., 1988; Tracey et al., 1988). Oliff et al. (1987) transfected a tumor with the gene for human TNF and implanted the tumor with or without the transfection leading to continuous production of TNF. The mice bearing the TNF-α–secreting tumor developed progressive anorexia, weight loss, fat depletion, and earlier death compared with the animals bearing the nonsecreting tumor. In human studies where TNF was given to cancer patients intermittently, it did not cause weight loss (Blick et al., 1987). This failure may have been due to the failure to consistently elevate TNF levels. However, anorexia was noted consistent with the idea that anorexia secondary to cytokines precedes malnutrition.

As the immune system attempts to clear the body of tumor cells, inflammation is seen in many forms of cancer in various tissues. Both tumor and host factors are released locally and into the circulation during this process. These factors can promote profound metabolic abnormalities that lead to anorexia, malnutrition, and cachexia. These factors are cytokines and include TNF-α interleukin (IL)-1, IL-2, and IL-6, interferon-γ (IFN-γ), and proteolysis-inducing factor (PIF). These cytokines are produced by tumor, immune, and stromal cells and in many cases provide one means of intercellular communication between tumor cells and the cells of the microenvironment in which they grow. A number of hormones regulate lipolysis, including insulin, adrenocorticotrophic hormone (ACTH), epinephrine, growth hormone, insulin-like growth factors (IGFs), and others (Nilsson-Ehle et al., 1980). Cytokines are produced, though not exclusively, by host macrophages and lymphocytes in response to the tumor (Moertel, 1986). These substances usually act in a paracrine fashion in the local environment of the tumor. With disease progression, it is possible that cytokines may circulate to other tissues and act as endocrine factors. Several cytokines have also been shown to increase lipolysis, including TNF-α, IL-1β, and IL-2, IL-6, IFN-γ, lipid-mobilizing factor (LMF), and PIF. For example, LMF and PIF were originally thought to be produced only by tumor cells, but LMF has been shown to be produced by both white and brown adipose tissue in addition to tumor cells (Bing et al., 2004). Other cytokines find their way into the circulation where they can ultimately cross the blood–brain barrier, including TNF-α, IL-1α, IL-2β, and IL-6.

IL-1 is an inflammatory cytokine produced by macrophages in response to endotoxin, but it has also been implicated in the pathogenesis of cancer cachexia. Hellerstein et al. (1989) demonstrated that IL-1 can reduce food intake in meal-fed rats. Moldawer et al. (1988a) showed that doses of IL-1 one-tenth of those that cause fever can reduce food intake in mice. IL-1 can also cause a change in hepatic protein synthesis similar to that seen in tumor-bearing animals. Moldawer et al. (1988b) found IL-1 activity in the plasma of only 1 of 23 cancer patients, but in 5 of 6 patients with septic shock. Jensen et al. (1990) demonstrated increased IL-1 gene expression in the livers of cachectic tumor-bearing rats despite undetectable circulating levels of IL-1.

Evidence for IL-6 playing a role in cancer cachexia comes from the observation that sarcoma-bearing mice have elevated levels of IL-6 (Jablons et al., 1989). In addition, under certain circumstances IL-6 levels are elevated following TNF infusion, so IL-6 may act to mediate in part the effects of TNF (Broukaert et al., 1989).

IFN-γ is produced by activated T cells and is a potent stimulator of macrophages. IFN enhances the effects of TNF and increases the mRNA expression triggered by TNF in macrophages exposed to endotoxin (Koerner et al., 1987). Sarcoma-bearing rats treated with antibody against IFN have reduced degree of weight loss and improved survival compared with control tumor-bearing rats (Langstein et al., 1989).

LMF (Hirai et al., 1998) and PIF (Todorov et al., 1996) appear to have direct effects on fat cells in the periphery and can produce weight loss via lipolysis in the absence of anorexia. Increased production of cytokines may also account for the increased production of acute-phase proteins and increased oxidation products in the circulation of cancer patients. In general, increases in serum levels of cytokines including TNF-α, IL-1, IL-6, and IFN-γ, though detected, are not correlated with the degree of weight loss in patients with advanced cancer (Maltoni et al., 1997). TNF has been detected in the circulation in some, but not all, cancer patients (Flick and Gifford, 1984). However, in a study of pancreatic cancer patients, PIF was detected in the urine of 80% of patients, and those patients with detectable PIF in their urine were more malnourished by comparison with those with no PIF detected (Wigmore et al., 2000). PIF has also been found in urine from patients with breast, ovarian, lung, colon, and rectal cancer who have progressive weight loss of ≥1 kg/mo (Caruik et al., 1997). In one study of breast cancer patients, serum levels of TNF-α were found to correlate with stage of disease rather than weight loss (Karayainnakis et al., 2001). In another study (Sheen-Chen et al., 1997), TNF-α serum levels were measurable in 36.5% of a group of patients with pancreatic cancer and higher levels were found in patients with metastatic disease by comparison with localized disease. In a study of gastric and colorectal cancer patients, the serum levels of soluble IL-2 receptor were most markedly elevated in patients with cachexia (Shibata and Takekawa, 1997).

Effects of Cytokines on Protein Metabolism

We have previously demonstrated increased whole body protein turnover in lung cancer patients (Heber et al., 1982), and it is likely that protein wasting is mediated by cytokines (Melville et al., 1990). Ubiquitin is a 76 amino acid protein with multiple functions, among which is the attachment to proteins that are to be degraded in proteasomes. The ubiquitin–proteasome proteolytic pathway is considered to play the major role in intracellular protein degradation in muscles. In this process, ubiquitin becomes activated and attached to the protein substrate and the polyubiquitinated protein is recognized for degradation by the 26S proteasome complex.

TNF-α (Garcia-Martinez et al., 1993) and PIF (Lorite et al., 1997) inhibit protein synthesis and increase protein degradation in skeletal muscle. PIF (Lorite et al., 2001), TNF-α, or IFN-γ (Llovera et al., 1998), when infused intravenously, cause an increased expression of ubiquitin, while leukemia-inhibitory factor (LIF) and IL-6 do not change ubiquitin expression. IL-6 has also been implicated in the loss of lean body mass seen in cachectic mice bearing tumors such as the colon-26 adenocarcinoma.

Administration of an anti-IL-6 receptor antibody reduced loss of muscle weight and suppressed enzymatic activity of cathepsins B and L (Fujita et al., 1996). On the other hand, some studies suggest that IL-6 does not cause skeletal muscle protein degradation when studied *in vitro* (Garcia-Martinez et al., 1994). Goodman (1994) has shown that rats given IL-6 acutely activated both total and myofibrillar protein degradation in muscle, while mice receiving murine IL-6 over a 7-day period at a dose of 250 μg/kg of body weight per day showed no depression of body weight or food intake (Espat et al., 1996).

IL-1 isolated from adherent human monocytes was shown to stimulate muscle protein degradation in intact muscles by a mechanism sensitive to inhibition of lysosomal thiol proteases (Baracos et al., 1983). However, recombinant human IL-1β was not able to reproduce this effect, which suggests that it was due to another cytokine that was not TNF-α or IFN-α, IFN-β, or IFN-γ (Goldberg et al., 1988). Infusion of IL-1β, together with TNF-α, to rats with Yoshida sarcoma reduced the synthesis rate of tumor fractional protein but had no effect on muscle protein metabolism (Ling et al., 1991).

Pale muscle fibers are affected more than red fibers, and fiber loss is predominantly from myofibrillar protein, determined by the release of 3-methylhistidine (Mitch and Goldberg, 1996). Studies demonstrate specific targeting of myosin heavy chain in muscle (Acharyya et al., 2004). In addition, cancer patients have reduced serum albumin levels and increased levels of acute-phase proteins, such as C-reactive protein (CRP) (Fearon et al., 1998). Elevated levels of CRP are associated with a shorter survival time (Falconer et al., 1995). Both depression of protein synthesis and increased protein degradation contribute to the muscle atrophy. Protein synthesis may be impaired due to an imbalance of amino acids caused by increased utilization of specific amino acids, as well as depression of branched-chain amino acids such as leucine (Yoshizawa, 2004), which not only are substrates for protein synthesis but have the unique ability to initiate signal transduction pathways that modulate the initiation of translation.

The ubiquitin–proteasome proteolytic pathway has been shown to play a significant role in muscle protein degradation in cachexia (Bossola et al., 2003). Ubiquitin also has a role in DNA repair (Jentsch et al., 1987) and mitosis (Glotzer et al., 1991). In addition, the lysosomal pathway has been shown to play a role in lung cancer patients referred for curative resection with average weight losses of 29%. In these patients, an increased expression of the lysosomal protease cathepsin B was observed in skeletal muscle biopsies (Jagoe et al., 2002). In the ubiquitin–proteasome pathway, proteins are marked for degradation by the addition of a polyubiquitin tag and are cleaved within a 26S proteasome structure, which is a cylinder with proteolytic enzymes on the inner surface to prevent their mixing with the cellular cytoplasm. The protein is transferred to the inside of the cylinder by a specific 19S particle. Specific ubiquitin ligases (E3) are also important in the breakdown of myofibrillar proteins in cachexia (Bodine et al., 2001). Tumor or host factors that mediate malnutrition and cachexia are believed to upregulate the ubiquitin–proteasome pathway in skeletal muscle. *In vitro* studies with TNF-α showed that it stimulated ubiquitin conjugation of muscle proteins (Li et al., 1998) and directly induced protein degradation, as determined by the release of tyrosine or 3-methylhistidine (Llovera et al., 1997) and a decrease in myosin, but there was no change in expression of proteasome subunits. Both PIF (Whitehouse and Tisdale, 2003) and TNF-α (Li and Reid, 2000) are thought to stimulate protein degradation through increased nuclear binding of the transcription factor nuclear factor-κB (NFκB), which has a central role in inflammation as well.

Effects of Cytokines on Lipid Metabolism

Cytokines can induce loss of adipose tissue and increases in serum triglycerides and fatty acid oxidation. The enzyme LPL extracts fatty acids from plasma lipoproteins for storage in fat cells so that its inhibition would lead to elevated levels of triglycerides in the circulation. On the other hand, HSL releases FFAs back into the circulation by hydrolyzing stored triglycerides and these fatty acids can be oxidized or taken up by the liver for synthesis into triglycerides. The activities of both LPL and HSL are affected by numerous hormones and cytokines. Hypertriglyceridemia is commonly observed in cancer patients, and stimulation of hepatic lipogenesis has been clearly demonstrated (Grunfeld and Feingold, 1991). Studies have examined the adipose cells of cancer patients to investigate the relative regulation of LPL and HSL. The mRNA for LPL and the total LPL enzyme activity have not been found to be significantly different between cancer patients and healthy controls, and serum TNF-α levels were also normal (Thompson et al., 1993). On the other hand, there was a doubling of mRNA levels for HSL in adipose tissue of cancer patients. The cancer patients also exhibited a twofold elevation of serum triglyceride and fatty acid levels. There was a significant correlation of the serum fatty acid level with the expression of HSL mRNA in adipose tissue, consistent with increased mobilization of stored triacylglycerides and an increased release of FFAs into the circulation. Nonetheless, all of the cytokines demonstrate the ability to inhibit LPL (Strassman and Kambayashi, 1995). Short-term administration of TNF in animals and in some human experiments causes hypertriglyceridemia in addition to increased oxygen consumption, temperature, and whole body protein breakdown (Michie et al., 1988). Thus, there is no single mechanism accounting for fat mobilization. Because fat mobilization is so essential to surviving starvation, it is not surprising that many mechanisms regulating this process are dysregulated in cancer malnutrition and cachexia.

Fatty acid mobilization may be partly due to increased activation of β-adrenergic receptors in the fat cells of cancer patients (Drott et al., 1989). LMF causes lipolysis in adipocytes independent of a direct effect on LPL or HSL (Hirai et al., 1998). Instead, LMF stimulates a β-adrenergic receptor, which increases lipolysis in white adipose tissue and thermogenesis in brown adipose tissue (Russell et al., 2002). In fact, LMF has been shown to be identical to a plasma protein identified as zinc α_2-glycoprotein (ZAG) by Todorov et al. (1996). The levels of ZAG mRNA are elevated 10-fold in the adipose tissue of cachectic mice implanted with MAC16 tumor cells (Bing et al., 2004). In studies of fat cells obtained from cachectic cancer patients, ZAG has not been detected. However, both ZAG mRNA and immunoreactivity have been detected in human omental and subcutaneous white adipose tissue in cancer-free healthy individuals. TNF-α acts through a membrane-bound receptor, which activates mitogen-activated protein kinase (MEK) and extracellular signal-related kinase (ERK) to stimulate lipolysis rather than acting through the adrenergic receptor (Zhang et al., 2002).

CANCER ANOREXIA

Anorexia is simply defined as reduced appetite for food resulting in reduced food intake. It is a common condition among cancer patients with malnutrition and in many cases precedes the development of malnutrition (Moley et al., 1988). Parabiosis experiments, in which a nonmetastasizing tumor is implanted in one animal and its circulation is connected surgically to another non–tumor-bearing animal, demonstrate that the same anorexia, metabolic changes, weight loss, and cachexia occur in the non–tumor-bearing animal, despite no evidence of metastatic tumor at necropsy (Norton et al., 1985). The tumor-bearing and non–tumor-bearing animal only share 1.5% of their total circulation, strongly suggesting a humoral factor such as a cytokine. In humans, anorexia is often multifactorial and may result primarily from effects of cytokines; tumor-related mechanical gastric and bowel compression, such as is seen with hepatomegaly and peritoneal metastases; disorders in hunger satiety regulatory systems; taste disorders often caused by drugs (such as metallic taste or oral mucosal disruption also known as *mucositis*); nausea and vomiting; or psychological problems, including depression (Padilla, 1986).

Although there are no established approaches to reversing cytokine actions on anorexia, there are a number of approaches to treating anorexia, and its early identification in the cancer patient is central to the prevention, or at least amelioration, of the malnutrition associated with cancer. Even in cancer patients where food intake appears to be normal, there is a failure to adapt to metabolic needs if there is coexistent weight loss. Metabolic abnormalities in cancer often lead to an increase in REE, and this occurs in the absence of any increase in food intake. For example, in the latter half of the menstrual cycle (called the *luteal phase*), there is an increase in progesterone production, which leads to an increase in body temperature, appetite, and calorie intake, often associated with increased sweet and fat cravings, resulting in an increase in food intake. This increased food intake can be viewed as adaptive in response to the increased metabolic rate resulting from the increase in body temperature. The failure to adapt to increased metabolic demands in the cancer patient has been identified as relative hypophagia even when food intake measured using current instruments, including food records and food frequency questionnaires, is normal. These instruments are relatively inaccurate and may lead to underestimates of total energy intake as great as 25% when compared with total energy expenditure measured directly with doubly labeled water (Thomson et al., 1990). An additional problem in assessing anorexia is that food intake is rarely measured before the development of cancer (Peacock et al., 1987).

Central Nervous System Mechanisms

Food intake in humans is carefully regulated in the ventromedial nucleus of the hypothalamus. Several neuropeptides including leptin, neuropeptide Y, insulin, galanin, endorphins, and cholecystokinin have been shown to affect both food intake and energy expenditure (Rosenbaum et al., 1997). It is clear from findings on the actions of leptin that there is careful regulation of body fat because circulating blood levels of leptin are proportional to body fat percentage over a significant physiological range (Considine et al., 1996). Leptin is produced by adipocytes in response to the net energy balance at the fat cell (Klein et al., 1996). In fact, glucose or citrate incubated with fat cells has been shown to be the direct signal for leptin secretion rather than insulin, which had been proposed to be the signal. In a number of studies of short-term calorie restriction and refeeding, leptin levels and insulin levels both decrease together with restriction and then increase again with refeeding. The balance of neurotransmitters in the hypothalamus can also affect food intake. Agents that affect serotonin and norepinephrine levels in the neuronal synapse affect appetite. Amphetamines, amphetamine analogs including phentermine, phenylpropanolamine, and norepinephrine reuptake inhibitors reduce appetite and have modest effects on energy expenditure. A number of common selective serotonin reuptake inhibitors (SSRIs) including fluoxetine (Prozac) and sertraline (Zoloft) reduce food intake and body weight at least transiently in obese subjects, especially when weight gain is a symptom of depression. Sibutramine (Meridia) is a combined norepinephrine and serotonin reuptake inhibitor and reduces food intake. On the other hand, other agents used to treat depression including monoamine oxidase (MAO) inhibitors such as amitriptyline (Elavil) and lithium result in an increase in body weight and food intake in some individuals. As discussed earlier, progesterone increases food intake in women in the latter part of the menstrual cycle and has been associated with mild depression, and the glucocorticoids affect food intake by a separate mechanism in the hypothalamus where the type II glucocorticoid receptor has been identified. Appetite, physical activity, and food intake are regulated as carefully as body temperature by a combination of neurotransmitters, neuropeptides, and steroid hormones in the central nervous system. It may be possible to alter these mechanisms in a desired fashion as specific agents are explored in cachexia and obesity research to modulate food intake.

Nausea and Acquired Taste Aversions

Nausea and acquired taste aversions are common problems in the malnourished cancer patient. De Wys and Walters (1975) specifically identified an inability to taste sugar and a heightened sensitivity to bitterness in cancer patients and associated these with observed red-meat aversion and elevated threshold to sweet taste that had been observed clinically. Such taste abnormalities have been associated with reductions in the levels of circulating trace metals, including zinc and nickel. In our own studies, we examined >100 cancer patients and were able to identify increased sweet threshold and red-meat aversion with heightened sensitivity to bitter tastes. However, by using age-matched controls without cancer, all differences in taste observed in our studies could be accounted for by age, sex, and smoking status (Larsen et al., 1983). Nonetheless, patients continue to report taste abnormalities, including metallic tastes secondary to chemotherapy and general losses of taste following head and neck irradiation. Some of these changes are clearly due to direct damage to the papilla in the tongue where the taste receptors are located (Mattes et al., 1992).

In addition to these global taste changes, it is possible for patients to develop specific taste aversions. In experiments by Bernstein (1978), children were exposed to nut-flavored ice cream during chemotherapy, which is a type of ice cream not usually eaten by children. Following the appropriately controlled study designs, Bernstein (1978) was able to demonstrate that children developed a specific acquired taste aversion to nut-flavored ice creams, but not to strawberry, chocolate, or vanilla. As a result of these studies, it is recommended that patients avoid their favorite foods on the days they receive chemotherapy, particularly if they have nausea. This food intake then has to be made up through supplementation as they recover from the effects of chemotherapy. Fortunately, there are newer agents to deal with nausea specifically, including serotonin antagonists such as ondansetron and centrally acting drugs (metoclopramide, dexamethasone), which minimize nausea, acquired taste aversion, and the malnutrition associated with chemotherapy (Rolla et al., 1992). Physicians should consider the effects of frequent tests, procedures, and treatments on a patient's ability to maintain adequate intake over time.

Psychological Causes Including Depression

Stress and depression can lead to reduced food intake in some patients. One physiological basis for this is the increased levels of corticotropin-releasing factor (CRF) found in the cerebrospinal fluid of depressed patients who decrease their food intake by comparison with depressed patients who increase their food intake (Nemeroff et al., 1984). Infusion of CRF into the third ventricle of rats or mice leads to reduced food intake. Similar studies of cerebrospinal fluid have not been performed in cancer patients, but there are a number of surveys documenting the importance of depression in the cancer patient. This depression leads to a reduced quality of life and can lead to anorexia and reduced food intake. Careful attention to the psychological and social aspects of the patient and the family can often be helpful in ameliorating the effects of depression on food intake. However, in some cases pharmacological treatment of depression is required (Haig, 1992). In these cases, careful attention to the effects of the antidepressant therapy on food intake should be maintained.

APPROACHES TO THE TREATMENT OF ANOREXIA AND CACHEXIA

In the 1920s, prior to the era of modern cancer treatment, it was believed that malnutrition was the means by which tumors killed patients (Warren, 1932). Therefore, great effort was expended in force-feeding patients with terminal cancer (Terepka and Waterhouse, 1956). In the 1970s following the introduction of total parenteral nutrition, force-feeding by the parenteral route was utilized in cancer patients with malnutrition. As reviewed by Klein et al. (1986), the net effect of total parenteral nutrition was negative with an increased incidence of hyperglycemia and infection. These two complications are likely related because it is known that hyperglycemia impairs white cell function. In the 1980s, the mechanisms by which cytokines could alter metabolism were demonstrated, as outlined in previous sections. However, no major breakthrough has been made that can reverse the effects of the cytokines released by the immune system in response to cancer. The successful treatment of cancer leads to a regain of lost weight and a reversal of the metabolic abnormalities associated with cancer cachexia. Therefore, the emphasis has now shifted to early diagnosis and recognition of malnutrition, adjunctive treatment of the malnourished patient with antiemetics, appetite enhancement, and enteral nutrition when possible.

Pharmacological agents developed to combat anorexia were selected for study on the basis that they result in weight gain as a side effect in other conditions. Testosterone can be given in injectable form, particularly in patients with hypogonadism associated with cachexia. Anabolic androgens were tested based on their ability to build muscle and to counteract the metabolic effects of hypogonadism observed in male cancer patients (Chlebowski et al., 1986). Oxandrolone, an oral anabolic steroid, has been used to promote weight gain in patients who have had extensive surgery, chronic infection, or severe trauma (Berger et al., 1996). Appetite improvement and a trend toward weight gain were seen in a trial of oxandrolone in patients with AIDS (Berger et al., 1996). Danazol is a synthetic steroid known to cause weight gain. It was assessed in combination with tamoxifen in a randomized double-blind, placebo-controlled trial in patients with advanced cancer (Bishop et al., 1993). It was found that the combination stabilized body weight in patients that did not demonstrate weight gain in response to tamoxifen alone.

In the 1980s, it was serendipitously noted (Tchekmedyian et al., 1986, 1987) that a high dose of megestrol acetate, a progestational steroid, increased appetite and led to weight gain in 30 of 33 patients with advanced breast cancer. Preliminary observations also demonstrated weight gain in 13 of 15 AIDS patients (von Roenn et al., 1988). Two subsequent randomized placebo-controlled trials demonstrated significant improvements in weight, appetite, well-being, and quality of life parameters in patients with AIDS (Oster et al., 1994; von Roenn et al., 1994). Based on these studies, the Food and Drug Administration (FDA) approved the use of megestrol acetate oral suspension in patients with AIDS anorexia. Additional randomized placebo-controlled trials showed appetite improvement in cancer patients given megestrol acetate (Berenstein et al., 2005).

Although it appears that the primary effect of megestrol acetate is to enhance food intake, there may be important effects of megestrol acetate specific to adipocyte lipid metabolism. In animals, an increase in fat mass has been observed in the absence of a change in food intake following progesterone administration (Hervey and Hervey, 1967), and in cell culture studies megestrol acetate induces adipocyte development of lipogenic enzymes (Hamburger et al., 1988).

A traditional medical maneuver of family physicians to increase appetite has been the administration of prednisone, a glucocorticoid. However, randomized trials of prednisone have revealed short-term (4 weeks) improvements in appetite, without weight gain (Moertel et al., 1974). Dronabinol, a marijuana derivative, has been found to improve appetite and mood in patients with AIDS and anorexia, without significant weight gain. FDA approval of this compound for use in AIDS anorexia was based on a placebo-controlled trial (Beal et al., 1995). Treatment with the serotonin antagonist cyproheptadine has been reported to have a weight-enhancing effect, but in a randomized, placebo-controlled, double-blind trial, it had no effect on progressive weight loss in cachectic cancer patients (Kardinal et al., 1990).

Another line of investigation has examined the effects of drugs with anti-inflammatory effects. The nonsteroidal anti-inflammatory drug (NSAID) indomethacin acts by inhibiting cyclooxygenase activity and has been shown to prolong survival of patients with solid tumors and improve some parameters of malnutrition such as hand-grip strength without an increase in body weight (Lundholm et al., 1994). Another NSAID, ibuprofen, has been shown to reduce REE and CRP levels in patients with pancreatic cancer (Wigmore et al., 1995). When combined with megestrol acetate and administered to patients with advanced gastrointestinal cancer, ibuprofen produced an increase in body weight (2.3 kg), compared with megestrol acetate alone, which in this study demonstrated a decrease in body weight (2.8 kg) (McMillan et al., 1999).

Agents that interfere with TNF-α production such as pentoxifylline have been reported to decrease TNF-α mRNA levels in cancer patients. However, pentoxifylline did not affect either anorexia or cachexia in a study of 35 cancer patients (Goldberg et al., 1995). Thalidomide can also reduce production of TNF-α by increasing its degradation rate and has been shown to promote weight gain in human immunodeficiency virus (HIV)–infected patients who are receiving treatment for tuberculosis. No results for its use in cancer cachexia have been reported. A single study reported that the pineal hormone melatonin reduced the mean serum levels of TNF-α in patients with solid tumors and significantly reduced the incidence of high weight loss (>10%) compared with supportive care alone (Lissoni et al., 1996). However, there have been no randomized trials of melatonin.

Eicosapentaenoic acid (EPA), an omega-3 polyunsaturated fatty acid, has been shown to antagonize the action of PIF. In cachectic mice bearing the MAC16 tumor, EPA attenuated protein degradation by downregulation of the increased expression of the proteasome subunits and ubiquitin-conjugating enzyme without any effect on protein synthesis (Whitehouse et al., 2001). EPA acts by interfering with intracellular signalling events, eventually preventing nuclear accumulation of NFκB (Whitehouse et al., 2003). EPA has been investigated as an anticachectic agent, both as a triglyceride (Wigmore et al., 1996) and as the free acid (Wigmore et al., 2000), in patients with pancreatic cancer and was found to produce weight stabilization in patients losing weight at the rate of 2.0–2.9 kg/mo. Combined with nutritional supplementation, EPA produced significant weight gain at 3 weeks (1 kg) and 7 weeks (2 kg) (Barber et al., 1999). Both performance status and appetite were significantly improved, and there was a fall in REE normalized to lean body mass with a weight gain primarily as lean body mass. After 3 weeks of consuming a fish-oil–enriched nutritional supplement formula, a significant fall in IL-6 production, a rise in serum insulin with a fall in the cortisol-to-insulin ratio, and a fall in the proportion of patients that excreted PIF in the urine were observed (Barber et al., 2001). A randomized trial confirmed that there was a net gain of weight and lean tissue and improved quality of life (Fearon et al., 2003).

CLINICAL RECOMMENDATIONS FOR ANOREXIA AND CACHEXIA PREVENTION AND TREATMENT

Early recognition of malnutrition is essential. Improved biomarkers are needed for the detection of early anorexia and metabolic changes associated with the host response to the tumor. Many of the available tools are so insensitive that global assessment of malnutrition clinically is often as discerning as obtaining biochemical measures of malnutrition. For clinical purposes, one should bear in mind that a 5% unintended weight loss is very significant and indicates a late manifestation of this process.

Up to two-thirds of patients with advanced cancer have some degree of weight loss, and more than half are underweight, have loss of appetite, or complain of a decrease in food intake. More than 1.3 million new invasive cancer cases are diagnosed yearly in the United States alone, with an estimated 560,000 yearly cancer deaths. These statistics emphasize the enormous frequency of anorexia and cachexia (Cancer Statistics, 2004). The need for nutritional support depends on the clinical context, patient preferences, and economic considerations. The first step in management is nutritional evaluation, dietary counseling, and follow-up. Severe, persistent anorexia that does not respond to dietary counseling can be reversed with pharmacological treatment such as megestrol acetate. Nutritional support is available in the form of homemade or commercial food supplements, enteral nutrition, and parenteral nutrition. Conservative cost estimates for these interventions range from <$100/mo for homemade food supplements to >$8000/mo for home parenteral nutrition. Clinicians must be familiar with the benefits, risks, and costs of these therapies to suggest appropriate options. Table 1 summarizes the most common interventions utilized and presents benefits, risks, included services and products, and costs. One should note that with regard to androgen replacement, injectable testosterone is rather inexpensive ($2 for a 200-mg dose) compared with oral anabolic steroids. Transdermal testosterone patches have an intermediate cost (Tchekmedyian, 1998).

As research progresses in the field of obesity for the development of various agonists and antagonists that affect

TABLE 1 Benefits, Risks, and Costs of Nutrition Interventions

Intervention	Benefits	Risks	Included services and products	Average monthly charges or costs ($) (range)
Counseling	Patient satisfaction Patient education Nutrition maintenance Adherence to protocols	None	One initial and one follow-up visit by registered dietitian	190 (140–210)[a]
Food supplements:				
Homemade	Nutrition maintenance Avoid or delay need for more expensive therapy	Limited risks: diarrhea (lactose intolerance), nausea	Three 8-oz servings = 750 kcal/day Example: Carnation Instant Breakfast + milk	64 (49–80)[b]
Commercial	Same	Patients may not like taste	Three 8-oz servings = 750–1080 kcal/day	168 (120–240)[b]
Appetite stimulants:				
Megestrol acetate oral suspension	Improved appetite, weight, well being	Male impotence, vaginal bleeding, deep-vein thrombosis	200 mg/day, 1-mo supply 400 mg/day, 1-mo supply 800 mg/day, 1-mo supply	92 (88–109)[c] 184 (177–219) 368 (354–438)
Dronabinol	Improved appetite, no significant weight change	Euphoria, somnolence, dizziness, confusion	2.5 mg/day, 1-mo supply 5 mg/day, 1-mo supply	161 (130–180)[c] 305 (220–354)
Prednisone	Short-term (4-wk) appetite stimulation	Hypokalemia, muscle weakness, cushingoid features, hyperglycemia, immune suppression, others	40 mg/day, 1-mo supply	15 (4–21)[c]
Oxandrolone	Increased appetite at 15-mg/day dose; no significant weight change	Liver toxicity; contraindicated in prostate cancer	5 mg/day, 1-mo supply 15 mg/day, 1-mo supply	344 (327–370)[c] 912 (817–1134)
Enteral nutrition	Maintenance of nutrition via enteral route when oral route is not available	Requires nasogastric, gastrostomy, or jejunostomy tube placement; aspiration, diarrhea, nausea, bloating, infection, bleeding	Feeding supply kit	469[e,f]
Home parenteral	Maintenance of nutrition when no other alternative is appropriate; no evidence of improved survival in end-stage cancer	Catheter-related pneumothorax, sepsis, thrombosis, bleeding; hepatic dysfunction, fluid and electrolyte imbalance	Costs of indwelling venous devices and their placement, as well as care of complications not included	6517[g]

[a]Charges calculated based on prevailing hospital- and office-based dietitian compensation; overhead not included.
[b]Average retail prices in five grocery stores in Long Beach, California (2005).
[c]Average retail prices in five pharmacies in Long Beach, California (2005).
[d]Medicare-allowable charges (Durable Medical Equipment Regional Center, Region D. Supplier Manual. Nashville, TN, Cigna, February 2005).
[e]Based on intake of 2000 kcal/day. (Patient receiving 500-ml bolus four times a day using a 1 kcal/ml feeding.) Basic formula; specialized formulas for specific comorbidities can increase costs substantially.
[f]Feedings are administered through a syringe as bolus feedings.
[g]Estimated needs based on a 70-kg person receiving 25 kcal/kg and 0.8–1.0 g of protein/kg/day.
Source: Modified and updated with permission from Tchekmedyian (2005).

appetite and energy expenditure, the field of cancer cachexia research may benefit by the development of newer pharmacological agents based on this knowledge. In addition to the compounds presented in Table 1, research on the inflammatory response has progressed considerably as well, and it is now clear that the central nervous system senses inflammation via the direct actions of cytokines on brain centers. It has not been possible to separate the peripheral and central aspects of the inflammatory response, but this area deserves further research.

Further research with anticytokine drugs such as thalidomide and anabolic compounds such as growth hormone are ongoing. Research efforts are also focused on the nutritional modulation of the process of tumor progression following initial treatment. This work includes the use of low-fat, high-fiber diets, micronutrients, and some phytochemicals found to have antitumor effects in experimental model systems. Ongoing clinical trials should provide new information on the use of nutritional interventions for the prevention of cancer recurrence and/or progression. In addition, it may be possible to separate the beneficial aspects of the immune response directed against the tumor and the undesirable spillover effects on host metabolism.

Acknowledgment

This research was supported by the UCLA Clinical Nutrition Research Unit, National Institutes of Health grant no. CA 47210.

References

Acharyya, S., Ladner, K.J., Nelsen, L.L., Damrauer, J., Reiser, P.J., Swoap, S., and Guttridge, D.C. 2004. Cancer cachexia is regulated by selective targeting of skeletal muscle gene products. J Clin Invest **114**: 370–378.

Axelrod, L., and Costa, G. 1980. Contribution of fat loss to weight loss in cancer. *Nutr Cancer* **2**: 81–83.

Barber, M.D., Ross, J.A., Voss, A.C., Tisdale, M.J., and Fearon, K.C.H. 1999. The effect of an oral nutritional supplement enriched with fish oil on weight-loss in patients with pancreatic cancer. *Br J Cancer* **81**: 80–86.

Baracos, V., Rodeman, H.P., Dinarello, C.A., and Goldberg, A.L. 1983. Stimulation of muscle protein degradation and prostaglandin E_2 release by leukocyte pyrogen (interleukin-1). *N Engl J Med* **308**: 553–555.

Barber, M.D., Fearon, K.C.H., Tisdale, M.J., McMillan, D.C., and Ross, J.A. 2001. Effect of a fish oil-enriched nutritional supplement on metabolic mediators in patients with pancreatic cancer cachexia. *Nutr Cancer* **40**: 118–124.

Beal, J.E., Olson, R., Laubenstein, L., *et al.* 1995. Dronabinol as a treatment for anorexia associated with weight loss in patients with AIDS. *J Pain Symptom Manage* **10**: 89–97.

Bennegard, K., Lundgren, F., and Lundholm, K. 1986. Mechanisms of insulin resistance in cancer associated malnutrition. *Clin Physiol* **6**: 539–547.

Berger, J.R., Pall, L., Hall, C., *et al.* 1996. Oxandrolone in AIDS-wasting myopathy. *AIDS* **10**: 1657–1662.

Bernstein, I.L. 1978. Learned taste aversions in children receiving chemotherapy. *Science* **200**: 1302–1303.

Berenstein, E., and Ortiz, Z. 2005. Megestrol acetate for the treatment of anorexia-cachexia syndrome. *Cochrane Database Syst Rev* **18**: CD004310.

Beutler, B., and Cerami, A. 1986. Cachectin and tumor necrosis factor as two sides of the same biological coin. *Nature (London)* **320**: 584–588.

Beutler, B., and Cerami, A. 1988. The common mediator of shock, cachexia, and tumor necrosis. *Adv Immunol* **42**: 213–231.

Bing, C., Bao, Y., Jenkins, J., Sanders, P., Manieri, M., Cinti, S., Tisdale, M.J., and Trayhum, P. 2004. Zinc-(2-glycoprotein, a lipid mobilizing factor, is expressed in adipocytes and is up-regulated in mice with cancer cachexia. *Proc Natl Acad Sci USA* **101**: 2500–2505.

Bishop, J.F., Smith, J.G., Jeal, P.N., Murray, R., Drummond, R.M., Pitt, P., Olver, I.N., and Bhowal, A.K. 1993. The effect of danazol on tumour control and weight loss in patients on tamoxifen for advanced breast cancer: a randomised double-blind placebo controlled trial. *Eur J Cancer* **29A**: 814–818.

Blick, M., Sherwin, S.A., and Rosenblum, M. 1987. Phase I study of recombinant tumor necrosis factor in cancer patients. *Cancer Res* **47**: 2986–2989.

Bodine, S.C., Latres, E., Baumheuter, S., *et al.* 2001. Identification of ubiquitin ligases required for skeletal muscle atrophy. *Science* **294**: 1704–1708.

Bossola, M., Muscaritoli, M., Costelli, P., Grieco, G., Bonelli, G., Pacelli, F., Fanelli, F.R., Doglietto, G.B., and Baccino, F.M. 2003. Increased muscle proteasome activity correlates with disease severity in gastric cancer patients. *Ann Surg* **237**: 384–389.

Bozzetti, F., Pagnoni, A.M., and Del Vecchio, M. 1980. Excessive caloric expenditure as a cause of malnutrition in patients with cancer. *Surg Gynecol Obstet* **150**: 229–234.

Brennan, M.F. 1977. Uncomplicated starvation vs. cancer cachexia. *Cancer Res* **58**: 1867–1873.

Brennan, M.F. 1981. Total parenteral nutrition in the cancer patient. *N Engl J Med* **305**: 375–382.

Broukaert, P., Spriggs, D.R., and Demetri, G. 1989. Circulating interleukin 6 during a continuous infusion of tumor necrosis factor and interferon-gamma. *J Exp Med* **169**: 2257.

Bruera, E., Roca, E., Cedaro, L., *et al.* 1985. Action of oral methylprednisolone in terminal cancer patients: a prospective randomized double-blind study. *Cancer Treat Rep* **69**: 751–754.

Burt, M.E., Stein, P.T., Schwade, J.B., and Brennan, M. 1984. Whole body protein metabolism in cancer-bearing man: effect of total parenteral nutrition and associated insulin response. *Cancer (Philadelphia)* **53**: 1246–1252.

Byerley, L.O., Heber, D., Bergman, R.N., Dubria, M., and Chi, J. 1991. Insulin action and metabolism in head and neck cancer patients. *Cancer (Philadelphia)* **67**: 2900–2906.

Cancer Statistics. 2004. *CAJ Cancer J Clin* **54**: 8–29.

Caruik, P., Lorite, M.J., Todorov, P.T., Field, W.N., Wigmore, S.J., and Tisdale, M.J. 1997. Induction of cachexia in mice by a product isolated from the urine of cachectic cancer patients. *Br J Cancer* **76**: 606–613.

Chlebowski, R.T., and Heber, D. 1982. Hypogonadism in male patients with metastatic cancer prior to chemotherapy. *Cancer Res* **42**: 2495–2497.

Chlebowski, R.T., and Heber, D. 1986. Metabolic abnormalities in cancer patients: Carbohydrate metabolism. *Surg Clin North Am* **66**: 957–969.

Chlebowski, R.T., Heber, D., Richardson, B., and Block, J.B. 1984. Influence of hydrazine sulfate on abnormal carbohydrate metabolism in cancer patients with weight loss. *Cancer Res* **44**: 857–861.

Chlebowski, R.T., Herrold, J., Oktay, E., Chlebowski, J., Ponce, A., and Heber, D. 1986. Influence of nandrolone decanoate on weight loss in cancer patients. *Cancer (Philadelphia)* **58**: 183–186.

Cohn, S.H., Bartenhaus, W., Vartsky, D., Sawitsky, A., Zanzi, I., Vaswani, A., Yasumura, S., Rai, K., Cortes, E., and Ellis, K.J. 1981. Body composition and dietary intake in neoplastic disease. *Am J Clin Nutr* **34**: 1997–2004.

Considine, R.V., Sinha, M.D., Heiman, L., *et al.* 1996. Serum immunoreactive leptin concentrations in normal weight and obese humans. *N Engl J Med* **334**: 292–295.

Danforth, E.A., Jr., Burger, A.G., and Wimpfheimer, C. 1978. Nutritionally-induced alterations in thyroid hormone metabolism and thermogenesis. *Experientia Suppl* **32**: 213–217.

Dempsey, D.T., Feurer, I.D., Knox, L.S., Crosby, L.O., Buzby, G.P., and Mullen, J.L. 1984. Energy expenditure in malnourished gastrointestinal cancer patients. *Cancer (Philadelphia)* **53**: 1265–1273.

Devereaux, D.R., Redgrave, T.G., Tilton, M., *et al.* 1984. Intolerance to administered lipids in tumor-bearing animals. *Surgery (St. Louis)* **96**: 414–419.

De Wys, W.D. 1972. Anorexia as a general effect of cancer. *Cancer* **45**: 2013–2019.

De Wys, W.D., and Walters, K. 1975. Abnormalities of taste sensation in cancer patients. *Cancer (Philadelphia)* **36**: 1888–1896.

De Wys, W.D., Begg, C., Lavin, P.T., *et al.* 1980. Prognostic effect of weight loss prior to chemotherapy in cancer patients. *Am J Med* **69**: 491–497.

Drott, C., Perrson, H., and Lundholm, K. 1989. Cardiovascular and metabolic response to adrenaline infusion in weight-losing cancer patients with and without cancer. *Clin Physiol* **9**: 427–439.

Eckel, R.H. 1987. Adipose tissue lipoprotein lipase. *In* "Lipoprotein Lipase" (J. Borenstajn, ed.), pp. 79–132. Evener Publishers, Chicago.

Espat, N.J., Auffenberg, T., Rosenberg, J.J., Martin, R.D., Fang, C.H., Hasselgren, P-O., Copeland, E.M., and Moldawer, L.L. 1996. Ciliary neurotrophic factor is catabolic and shares with IL-6 the capacity to induce an acute phase response. *Am J Physiol* **271**: R185–R190.

Evans, W.K., Makuch, R., and Clamon, G.H., 1985. Limited impact of total parenteral nutrition on nutritional status during treatment for small cell lung cancer. *Cancer Res* **45**: 3347–3353.

Falconer, J.S., Fearon, K.C., Ross, J.A., Elton, R., Wigmore, S.J., Garden, O.J., *et al.* 1995. Acute-phase protein response and survival duration of patients with pancreatic cancer. *Cancer* **75**: 2077–2082.

Fearon, K.C.H. 1992. The mechanism and treatment of weight loss in cancer. *Proc Nutr Soc* **51**: 251–265.

Fearon, K.C.H., Falconer, J.S., Slater, C., McMillan, D.C., Ross, J.A., and Preston, T. 1998. Albumin synthesis rates are not decreased in hypoalbuminemic cachectic cancer patients with an ongoing acute-phase protein response. *Ann Surg* **227**: 249–254.

Fearon, K.C.H., von Megenfeldt, M.F., Moses, A.G.W., *et al.* 2003. Effect of a protein and energy dense n-3 fatty acid enriched oral supplement on loss of weight and lean tissue in cancer cachexia: a randomised double blind trial. *Gut* **52**: 1479–1486.

Fenninger, L.D., and Mider, G.B. 1954. Energy and nitrogen metabolism in cancer. *Adv Cancer Res* **2**: 229–253.

Flick, D.A., and Gifford, G.E. 1984. Cachectin/tumor necrosis factor: Production, distribution and metabolic fate *in vivo*. *J Immunol* **135**: 3972–3977.

Fujita, J., Tsujinaka, T., Yano, M., *et al.* 1996 Anti-interleukin-6 receptor antibody prevents muscle atrophy in colon-26 adenocarcinoma-bearing mice with modulation of lysosomal and ATP-ubiquitin–dependent proteolytic pathways. *Int J Cancer* **68**: 637–643.

Garcia-Martinez, C., Lopez-Soriano, F.J., and Argiles, J.M. 1993. Acute treatment with tumour necrosis factor-α induces changes in protein metabolism in rat skeletal muscle. *Mol Cell Biochem* **125**: 11–18.

Garcia-Martinez, C., Lopez-Soriano, F.J., and Argiles, J.M. 1994. Interleukin-6 does not activate protein breakdown in rat skeletal muscle. *Cancer Lett* **76**: 1–4.

Glotzer, M., Murray, A.W., and Kirschner, M.N. 1991. Cyclin is degraded by the ubiquitin pathway. *Nature* **349**: 132–138.

Goldberg, A.L., Kettlehut, I.C., Foruno, K., Fagan, J.M., and Baracos, V. 1988. Activation of protein breakdown and prostaglandin E_2 production in rat skeletal muscle in fever is signaled by a microphage product distinct from interleukin-1 or other known monokines. *J Clin Invest* **81**: 1378–1383.

Goldberg, R.M., Loprinzi, C.L., Malliard, J.A., *et al.* 1995. Pentoxifylline for treatment of cancer anorexia and cachexia? A randomized, double-blind, placebo-controlled trial. *J Clin Oncol* **13**: 2856–2859.

Gomes-Marcondes, M.C.C., Smith, H.J., Cooper, J.C., and Tisdale, M.J. 2002. Development of an *in vitro* model system to investigate the mechanism of muscle protein catabolism induced by proteolysis-inducing factor. *Br J Cancer* **86**: 1628–1633.

Goodman, M.N. 1994. Interleukin-6 induces skeletal muscle protein breakdown in rats. *Proc Soc Exp Biol Med* **205**: 182–185.

Grunfeld, C., and Feingold, K.R. 1991. Tumor necrosis factor, cytokines and hyperlipidemia of infection. *Trends Endocrinol Metab* **2**: 213–219.

Haig, C. 1992. Management of depression in patients with advanced cancer. *Med J Aust* **156**: 499–503.

Hamburger, A.W., Parnes, H.F., Gordon, G.B., Shantz, L.M., O'Donnell, K.A., and Aisner, J. 1988. Megestrol acetate induced differentiation of 3T3LI adipocytes *in vitro*. *Semin Oncol* **15**: 76–78.

Heber, D. 1989. Metabolic pathology of cancer malnutrition. *Nutrition* **5**: 135–137.

Heber, D., Chlebowski, R.T., Ishibashi, D.E., Herrold, J.N., and Block, J.B. 1982. Abnormalities in glucose and protein metabolism in noncachectic lung cancer patients. *Cancer Res.* **42**: 4815–4819.

Heber, D., Byerley, L.O., Chi, J., Grosvenor, M., Bergman, R.N., Coleman, M., and Chlebowski, R.T. 1986. Pathophysiology of malnutrition in the adult cancer patient. *Cancer (Philadelphia)* **58**: 1867–1873.

Hellerstein, M.D., Meydani, S.N., Meydani, M., Wu, K., and Dinarello, C.K. 1989. Interleukin-1–induced anorexia in the rat. *J Clin Invest* **84**: 228–235.

Hervey, E., and Hervey, G.R. 1967. Energy storage in female rats treated with progesterone in the absence of increased food intake. *Physiol (London)* **200**: 118–119.

Hirai, K., Hussey, H.J., Barber, M.D., Price, S.A., and Tisdale, M.J. 1998. Biological evaluation of a lipid-mobilizing factor isolated from the urine of cancer patients. *Cancer Res* **58**: 2359–2365.

Holm, C., Kirchgessner, T.G., Svenson, K.L., Fredrikson, F., Nielsson, S., *et al.* 1988. Hormone sensitive lipase: Sequence, expression, and chromosonal localization to 19 cent-p 13.3. *Science* **241**: 1503–1506.

Holroyde, C.P., Gabuzda, T., Putnam, R., Paul, P., and Reichard, G. 1975. Carbohydrate metabolism in cancer cachexia. *Cancer Res* **35**: 3710–3714.

Jablons, D.M., McIntosh, K., and Mule, J.J. 1989. Induction of interferon-2/interleukin-6(IL-6) by cytokine administration and detection of circulating interleukin-5 in the tumor-bearing state. *Ann NY Acad Sci* **557**: 157.

Jagoe, R.T., Redfern, C.P.F., Roberts, R.G., Gibson, G.J., and Goodship, T.H.J. 2002. Skeletal muscle mRNA levels for cathepsins B, but not components of the ubiquitin–proteasome pathway, are increased in patients with lung cancer referred for thoracotomy. *Clin Sci* **102**: 353–361.

Jeevanandam, M., Horowitz, G.D., Lowry, S.F., and Brennan, M.F. 1986. Cancer cachexia and the rate of whole body lipolysis in man. *Metab Clin Exp* **35**: 304–310.

Jensen, J.C., Buresh, C.M., and Fraker, D.L. 1990. Enhanced hepatic cytokine gene expression in cachectic tumor bearing rats. *Surg Forum* **41**: 469.

Jentsch, S., McGrath, I.P., and Varshavsky, A. 1987. The yeast DNA repair gene RAD6 encodes a ubiquitin-conjugating enzyme. *Nature* **329**: 131–134.

Karayiannakis, A.J., Syrigos, K.N., Polychronidis, A., Pitiakoudis, M., Bounovas, A., and Simppoulos, K. 2001. Serum levels of tumor necrosis factor-α and nutritional status in pancreatic cancer patients. *Anticancer Res* **21**: 1355–1358.

Kardinal, C.G., Loprinzi, C.L., Schaid, D.J., Hass, A.C., *et al.* 1990. A controlled trial of cyproheptadine in cancer patients with anorexia and/or cachexia. *Cancer* **65**: 2657–2662.

Klein, S., Simes, J., and Blackburn, G.L. 1986. Total parenteral nutrition and cancer clinical trials. *Cancer (Philadelphia)* **58**: 1378–1386.

Klein, S., Coppack, S.W., Mohamed-Ali, V., and Landt, M. 1996. Adipose tissue leptin production and plasma leptin kinetics in humans. *Diabetes* **45**: 984–987.

Knittle, J.L., Ginsberg-Fellner, F., and Brown, R.E. 1997. Adipose tissue development in man. *Am J Clin Nutr* **30**: 762–766.

Knox, L.S., Crosby, L.O., Feurer, I.D., Buzby, G.P., Miller, C.L., and Mullen, J.L. 1983. Energy expenditure in malnourished cancer patients. *Ann Surg* **197**: 152–162.

Koerner, T.J., Adams, D.O., and Hamilton, T.A. 1987. Regulation of tumor necrosis factor (TNF) expression: Interferon enhances the accumulation of mRNA for TNF induced by lipopolysaccharide in murine peritoneal macrophages. *Cell Immunol* **109**: 437–443.

Kosty, M., Fleishman, S., Herndon, J., *et al.* 1994. Cisplatin, vinblastine and hydrazine sulfate in advanced non-small lung cancer: A randomized, placebo-controlled, double-blind phase III study of the Cancer and Leukemia Group. *Br J Clin Oncol* **12**: 1113–1120.

Lang, C.H., Dobrescu, C., and Bagby, G.J. 1992. Tumor necrosis factor impairs insulin action on peripheral glucose disposal and hepatic glucose output. *Endocrinology (Baltimore)* **130**: 43–52.

Langstein, H.W., Fraker, D.L., and Norton, J.A. 1989. Reversal of cachexia by antibodies to interferon gamma but not tumor necrosis factor. *Surg Forum* **15**: 408.

Larsen, C., Byerley, L., Heber, D., and Chlebowski, R. 1983. Factors contributing to altered taste sensations in cancer patients. *Am Soc Parenter Enteral Nutr Clin Congr* 7th, Washington, DC.

Lanza-Jacoby, S., Lansky, S.C., Miller, E.E., and Cleary, M.P. 1984. Sequential changes in the activities of lipoprotein lipase and lipogenic enzymes during tumor growth in rats. *Cancer Res* **44**: 5062–5067.

Legaspi, A., Jeevanandam, M., Starnes, H.F., and Brennan, M.F. 1987. Whole-body lipid and energy metabolism in the cancer patient. *Metabolism* **36**: 958–963.

Li, Y-P., Schwartz, R.J., Waddell, I.D., Holloway, B.R., and Reid, M.B. 1998. Skeletal muscle myocytes undergo protein loss and reactive oxygen-mediated NF-κB activation in response to tumor necrosis factor α. *FASEB J* **12**: 871–880.

Li, Y-P., and Reid, M.B. 2000. NF-κB mediates the protein loss induced by TNF-α in differentiated skeletal muscle myotubes. *Am J Physiol* **279**: R1165–R1170.

Ling, P.K., Istfan, N., Blackburn, G.L., and Bistrian, B.R. 1991. Effects of interleukin 1-β (IL-1) and combination of IL-1 and tumor necrosis factor on tumor growth and protein metabolism. *J Nutr Biochem* **2**: 553–559.

Lissoni, P., Paolorossi, F., Tancini, G., Barni, S., Ardizzoia, A., Brivio, F., Zubelewicz, B., and Chatikhine, V. 1996. Is there a role for melatonin in the treatment of neoplastic cachexia? *Eur J Cancer* **32A**: 1340–1343.

Llovera, M., Carbo, N., Lopez-Soriano, J., Garcia-Martinez, C., Busquets, S., Alvarez, B., *et al.* 1998. Different cytokines modulate ubiquitin gene expression in rat skeletal muscle. *Cancer Lett* **13**: 83–87.

Llovera, M., Garcia-Martinez, C., Agell, N., Lopez-Soriano, F.J., and Argiles, J.M. 1997. TNF can directly induce the expression of the ubiquitin-dependent proteolytic system in rat soleus muscles. *Biochem Biophys Res Commun* **230**: 238–244.

Long, C.L., Schaffel, N., Geiger, J.W., *et al.* 1981. Metabolic response to injury and illness: Estimation of energy and protein needs from indirect calorimetry and nitrogen balance. *J Parenter Enteral Nutr* **5**: 366.

Loprinzi, C.L., Schaid, D.J., Dose, A.M., Burnham, N.L., and Jensen, M.D. 1993. Body-composition changes in patients who gain weight while receiving megestrol acetate. *J Clin Oncol* **11**: 152–154.

Loprinzi, C.L., Goldberg, R.G., Su, J.Q., *et al.* 1994. Placebo-controlled trial of hydrazine sulfate patients with newly diagnosed non–small lung cancer. *J Clin Oncol* **12**: 1126–1129.

Lorite, M.J., Cariuk, P., and Tisdale, M.J. 1997. Induction of muscle protein degradation by a tumour factor. *Br J Cancer* **76**: 1035–1040.

Lorite, M.J., Smith, H.J., Arnold, J.A., Morris, A., Thompson, M.G., and Tisdale, M.J. 2001. Activation of ATP-ubiquitin–dependent proteolysis in skeletal muscle *in vivo* and murine myoblasts *in vitro* by a proteolysis-inducing factor (PIF). *Br J Cancer* **85**: 297–302.

Lundholm, K., Gelin, J., Hyltander, A., *et al.* 1994. Anti-inflammatory treatment may prolong survival in undernourished patients with metastatic solid tumours. *Cancer Res* **54**: 5602–5606.

Maltoni, M., Fabbri, L., Nani, O., Scarpi, E., Pezzi, L., Flamini, E., Riccobon, A., Derni, S., Pallotti, G., and Amadori, D. 1997. Serum levels of tumour necrosis factor and other cytokines do not correlate with weight loss and anorexia in cancer patients. *Support Care Cancer* **5**: 130–135.

Mattes, R.D., Curran, W.J., Alavi, I., Powlis, W., and Whittington, R. 1992. Clinical implications of learned food aversions in cancer patients treated with chemotherapy or radiation therapy. *Cancer (Philadelphia)* **70**: 192–200.

McMillan, D.C., Wigmore, S.J., Fearon, K.C.H., O'Gorman, P., Wright, C.E., and McArdle, C.S. 1999. A prospective randomized study of megestrol acetate and ibuprofen in gastrointestinal cancer patients with weight loss. *Br J Cancer* **79**: 495–500.

Michie, H.R., Spriggs, D.R., Manogue, K.R., Sherman, M.I., Rerhaug, A., *et al.* 1988. Tumor necrosis factor and endotoxin induce similar metabolic responses in human beings. *Surgery (St. Louis)* **104**: 280–286.

Mitch, W.E., and Goldberg, A.L. 1996. Mechanisms of muscle wasting. The role of the ubiquitin–proteasome pathway. *N Engl J Med* **335**: 1897–1905.

Melville, S., McNurlan, M.A., Calder, A.G., and Garlick, P.J. 1990. Increased protein turnover despite normal energy metabolism and responses to feeding in patients with lung cancer. *Cancer Res* **50**: 1125–1131.

Moertel, C.G. 1986. On lymphokines, cytokines, and breakthroughs. *JAMA* **256**: 3141–3143.

Moertel, C.G., Schutt, A.J., Reitemeier, R.J., *et al.* 1974. Corticosteroid therapy of preterminal gastrointestinal cancer. *Cancer (Philadelphia)* **33**: 1607–1609.

Moldawer, L.L., Anderson, C., and Gelin, J. 1988a. Regulation of food intake and hepatic protein synthesis by recombinant derived cytokines. *Am J Physiol* **254**: G450–G456.

Moldawer, L.L., Droft, C., and Lundholm, K. 1988b. Monocytic production and plasma bioactivities of interleukin-1 and tumor necrosis factor in human cancer. *Eur J Clin Invest* **18**: 486–492.

Moley, J.F., Morrison, S.D., and Norton, J.A. 1985. Insulin reversal of cancer cachexia in rats. *Cancer Res* **45**: 4925–4931.

Moley, J.F., Morrison, S.D., Gorschboth, C.M., and Norton, J.A. 1988. Body composition changes in rats with experimental cancer cachexia: Improvement with exogenous insulin. *Cancer Res* **48**: 2784–2787.

Monitto, C.L., Berkowitz, D., Lee, K.M., Pin, S., Li, D., and Breslow, M. 2001. Differential gene expression in a murine model of cancer cachexia. *Am J Physiol* **281**: E289–E297.

Nemeroff, C.B., Widerlov, E., Bissette, G., Walleus, H., Karlsson, I., *et al.* 1984. Elevated concentration of CSF corticotropin releasing factor–like immunoreactivity in depressed patients. *Science* **226**: 1342–1344.

Nilsson-Ehle, P., Garfinkel, A.S., and Schotz, M.C. 1980. Lipolytic enzymes and plasma lipoprotein metabolism. *Annu Rev Biochem* **49**: 667–673.

Nixon, D.W., Heymsfield, S.B., Cohen, A., Kutner, M.H., Ansley, J., *et al.* 1980. Protein–calorie undernutrition in hospitalized cancer patients. *Am J Med* **68**: 683–690.

Norton, J.A., Moley, J.F., and Green, M.V. 1985. Parabiotic transfer of cancer anorexia/cachexia in male rats. *Cancer Res* **45**: 5547–5552.

Okusaka, T., Okada, S., Ishii, H., Ikeda, M., Kosakomoto, H., and Yoshimori, M. 1998. Prognosis of advanced pancreatic cancer patients with reference to calorie intake. *Nutr Cancer* **32**: 55–58.

Oliff, A. 1988. The role of tumor necrosis factor (cachectin) in cachexia. *Cell (Cambridge, Mass)* **54**: 141–142.

Oliff, A., Defeo-Jones, D., and Boyer, M. 1987. Tumors secreting human TNF/cachectin induce cachexia in mice. *Cell (Cambridge, Mass)* **50**: 555–563.

Oster, M.H., Enders, S.R., and Samuels, S. 1994. Megestrol acetate in patients with AIDS and cachexia. *Ann Intern Med* **121**: 400–408.

Padilla, G.V. 1986. Psychological aspects of nutrition and cancer. *Surg Clin North Am* **60**: 1121–1135.

Peacock, J.L., Inculet, R.I., Corsey, R., Ford, D.B., Rumble, W.F., *et al.* 1987. Resting energy expenditure and body cell mass alterations in noncachetic patients with sarcoma. *Surgery (St. Louis)* **102**: 465–472.

Persson, C., and Glimeluis, B. 2002. The relevance of weight loss for survival and quality of life in patients with advanced gastrointestinal cancer treated with palliative chemotherapy. *Anticancer Res* **22**: 3661–3668.

Persson, H., Bennegard, K., Lundberg, P.A., Svaninger, G., and Lundholm, K. 1985. Thyroid hormones in conditions of chronic malnutrition. A study with special reference to cancer cachexia. *Ann Surg* **201**: 45–52.

Popiela, T., Lucchi, R., and Giongo, F. 1989. Methylprednisolone as palliative therapy for female terminal cancer patients. *Eur J Cancer Clin Oncol* **25**: 1823–1829.

Reyo-Teran, G., Sierra-Madero, J.G., Martinez del Cerro, V., *et al.* 1996. Effects of thalidomide on HIV-associated wasting syndrome: a randomized, double-blind, placebo-controlled trial. *AIDS* **10**: 1501–1507.

Roila, F., Tonato, M., and Favall, G. 1992. A multicenter double-blind study comparing the antiemetic efficacy and safety of ondansetron plus dexamethasone vs. metoclopramide plus dexamethasone and diphenhydramine in cisplatin treated cancer patients. *Proc Am Soc Clin Oncol* **11**: 1375A.

Rosenbaum, M., Leibel, R.L., and Hirsch, J. 1997. Obesity. *N Engl J Med* **337**: 397–407.

Russell, S.T., Hirai, K., and Tisdale, M.J. 2002. Role of β3-adrenergic receptors in the action of a tumour lipid mobilizing factor. *Br J Cancer* **86**: 424–428.

Schutz, Y., Tremblay, A., Weinsier, R.L., and Nelson, K.M. 1992. Role of fat oxidation in the long-term stabilization of body weight in obese women. *Am J Clin Nutr* **55**: 670–674.

Shaw, J.H.F., and Wolfe, R.R. 1987. Fatty acid and glycerol kinetics in septic patients and in patients with gastrointestinal cancer. The response to glucose infusion and parenteral feeding. *Ann Surg* **205**: 368–376.

Sheen-Chen, S-M., Chen, W-J., Eng, H-L., and Chou, F-F. 1997. Serum concentrations of tumor necrosis factor in patients with breast cancer. *Breast Cancer Res Treat* **43**: 211–215.

Shibata, M., and Takekawa, M. 1997. Increased serum concentrations of circulatory soluble receptors for interleukin-2 and its effect as a prognostic indicator in cachectic patients with gastric and colorectal cancer. *Oncology* **56**: 54–58.

Shike, M., Russell, D.M., Detsky, A.S., Harrison, J.E., McNeill, K.G., *et al.* 1984. Changes in body composition in patients with non–small cell lung cancer. *Ann Intern Med* **101**: 303–309.

Shils, M.E. 1977. Nutritional problems associated with gastrointestinal and genitourinary cancer. *Cancer Res* **37**: 2366–2372.

Socher, S.H., Friedman, A., and Martinez, D. 1988. Recombinant human tumor necrosis factor induces acute reductions in food intake and body weight in mice. *J Exp Med* **167**: 1957–1962.

Stovroff, M.C., Fraker, D.L., Swedenborg, J.A., and Norton, J.A. 1988. Cachectin/Tumor Necrosis Factor—a possible mediator of cancer anorexia in the rat. *Cancer Res* **48**: 4567–4572.

Strassman, G., and Kambayashi, T. 1995. Inhibition of experimental cancer cachexia by anti-cytokine and anti-cytokine receptor therapy. *Cytokines Mol Ther* **1**: 107–113.

Tayek, J.A., Heber, D., and Chlebowski, R.T. 1987. Effect of hydrazine sulphate on whole body protein breakdown measured by 14-Clysine metabolism in lung cancer patients. *Lancet* **2**: 241–244.

Tayek, J.A., and Brasel, J.A. 1995. Failure of ananbolism in malnourished cancer patients receiving growth hormone. *J Clin Endocrinol Metab* **80**: 2082–2087.

Tchekmedyian, N.S. 1995. Costs and benefits of nutrition support in cancer. *Oncology* **9**: 79–84.

Tchekmedyian, N.S. 1998. Pharmacoeconomics of nutritional support in cancer. *Semin Oncol* **25**(Suppl 6): 62–69.

Tchekmedyian, N.S., Tait, N., Moody, M., and Aisner, J. 1987. High-dose megestrol acetate: a possible treatment for cancer cachexia. *JAMA* **257**: 1105–1108.

Terepka, A.R., and Waterhouse, C. 1956. Metabolic observations during force feeding of patients with cancer. *Am J Med* **20**: 225–238.

Thompson, M.P., Cooper, S.T., Parry, B.R., and Tuckey, J.A. 1993. Increased expression of the mRNA for hormone-sensitive lipase in adipose tissue of cancer patients. *Biochem Biophys Acta* **1180**: 236–242.

Thompson, M.P., Koons, J.E., Tan, E.T.H., *et al.* 1984. Modified lipoprotein lipase activities, rates of lipogenesis, and lipolysis as factors leading to lipid depletion in C57BL mice bearing preputial gland tumor, ESR-586. *Ann Surg* **204**: 637–642.

Thomson, S.R., Hirshberg, A., and Haffejee, A. 1990. Resting metabolic rate of esophageal carcinoma patients. A model for energy expenditure measurement in a homogeneous cancer patient population. *J Parenter Enteral Nutr* **14**: 119–121.

Todorov, P.T., Caruik, P., McDevitt, T., Coles, B., Fearon, K., and Tisdale, M. 1996. Characterization of a cancer cachectic factor. *Nature* **379**: 739–742.

Tracey, K.J., Wei, H., and Manogue, K.R. 1988. Cachectin/tumor necrosis factor induces cachexia. anemia, and inflammation. *J Exp Med* **167**: 1211–1227.

von Roenn, J.H., Murphy, R.L., Weber, K.M., William, L.M., and Weitzman, S.A. 1988. Megestrol acetate for treatment of cancer cachexia associated with human immunodeficiency virus (HIV) infection. *Ann Intern Med* **109**: 840–841.

von Roenn, J.H., Armstrong, D., Kotler, D.P., *et al.* 1994. Megestrol acetate in patients with AIDS-related cachexia. *Ann Intern Med* **12**: 393–399.

Watchorn, T.M., Waddell, I.D., Dowidar, N., and Ross, J.A. 2001. Proteolysis-inducing factor regulates hepatic gene expression via the transcription factors NF-κB and STAT3. *FASEB J* **15**: 562–564.

Whitehouse, A.S., and Tisdale, M.J. 2003. Increased expression of the ubiquitin–proteasome pathway in murine myotubes by proteolysis-inducing factor (PIF) is associated with activation of the transcription factor NF-κB. *Br J Cancer* **89**: 1116–1122.

Whitehouse, A.S., Smith, H.J., Drake, J.L., and Tisdale, M.J. 2001. Mechanism of attenuation of skeletal muscle protein catabolism in cancer cachexia by eicosapentaenoic acid. *Cancer Res* **61**: 3604–3609.

Warren, S. 1932. The immediate causes of death in cancer. *Am J Med Sci* **184**: 610–615.

Wigmore, S.J., Todorov, P.T., Barber, M.D., Ross, J.A., Tisdale, M.J., and Fearon, K.C.H. 2000. Characteristics of patients with pancreatic cancer expressing a novel cancer cachectic factor. *Br J Surg* **87**: 53–58.

Wigmore, S.J., Falconer, J.S., Plester, C.E., Ross, J.A., Maingay, J.P., *et al.* 1995. Ibuprofen reduces energy expenditure and acute-phase protein production compared with placebo in pancreatic cancer patients. *Br J Cancer* **72**: 185–188.

Wigmore, S.J., Ross, J.A., Falconer, J.S., Plester, C.E., Tisdale, M.J., *et al.* 1996. The effect of polyunsaturated fatty acids on the progress of cachexia in patients with pancreatic cancer. *Nutrition* **12**: S27–S30.

Wigmore, S.J., Barber, M.D., Ross, J.A., Tisdale, M.J., and Fearon, K.C.H. 2000. Effect of oral eicosapentaenoic acid on weight loss in patients with pancreatic cancer. *Nutr Cancer* **36**: 177–184.

Wilcox, J., Corr, J., Shaw, J., *et al.* 1984. Prednisone as an appetite stimulant in patients with cancer. *Br Med J Clin Res Edu* **288**: 27.

Yam, D., Ben-Hur, H., Fink, A., Dgani, R., Shani, A., *et al.* 1994. Insulin and glucose status, tissue and plasma lipids in patients with tumours of the ovary or endometrium: possible dietary implications. *Br J Cancer* **70**: 1186–1187.

Yoshizawa, F. 2004. Regulation of protein synthesis by branched-chain amino acids *in vivo*. *Biochem Biophys Res Commun* **313**: 417–422.

Zhang, H.H., Halbleib, M., Ahmad, R., *et al.* 2002. Tumor necrosis factor-α stimulates lipolysis in differentiated human adipocytes through activation of extracellular signal-related kinase and evaluation of intracellular cyclic AMP. *Diabetes* **51**: 2929–2935.

CHAPTER

40

Weight Management in the Breast Cancer Survivor

ANNE MCTIERNAN

INTRODUCTION

Overweight and obesity increase risk for breast cancer development in postmenopausal women (i.e., the age-group at greatest risk for developing the disease). Once they develop breast cancer, women of any age are at increased risk of recurrence and poorer survival if they are overweight or obese. These effects of obesity on cancer outcome are substantial and of potentially great clinical importance. The prevalence of overweight and obesity is higher in women with breast cancer, compared with women from the general population (International Agency for Research on Cancer [IARC], 2002a). Compounding this is that weight gain after diagnosis is common in some breast cancer patients, especially among those receiving systemic adjuvant therapy (Chlebowski et al., 2002; Brown et al., 2003). Weight gain during the post–breast cancer diagnosis period has also been associated with an adverse effect on recurrence risk and survival (Chlebowski et al., 2002). In addition to adversely affecting prognosis, overweight and obesity also increase the risk of several complications from breast cancer treatment and increase the risk of several co-morbidities. There are several potential mechanisms that might explain the link between increased adiposity and reduced prognosis, including hormonal, inflammatory, and immune system effects. Although definitive clinical trials testing weight loss effects on prognosis in breast cancer patients have not been conducted, strategies for weight control may be helpful for breast cancer patients and survivors.

There are several ways to measure body composition and adiposity. Simple, inexpensive, and noninvasive measures include height, weight, body mass index (BMI, kg/m^2), waist and hip circumferences, bioelectric impedance (estimates percent body fat), fat calipers (can be used to estimate overall and regional body fat) (Roche et al., 1996). Other body composition measures give more reliable and valid measures of body composition but are more invasive and expensive. These latter include underwater weighing (considered the "gold standard" for body composition), DEXA scan (measures lean mass, bone mass, and fat mass), computed tomography (CT) and magnetic resonance imaging (MRI) scans (used to estimate intra-abdominal and subcutaneous abdominal fat, typically measured with one cross-sectional slice to reduce radiation exposure and costs).

BMI is the most common measure of adiposity used in studies of obesity and breast cancer and, for comparison purposes, is the one used throughout this chapter. Obesity experts have developed the following categories of adiposity based on BMI (Flegal et al., 1998): underweight (<18.5 kg/m^2), normal weight (18.5–24.9 kg/m^2), overweight (25.0–29.9 kg/m^2), and obese (≥ 30.0 kg/m^2) (Table 1). Obesity is further subclassified; the most important subclassification is ≥ 40.0, or extreme obesity, as individuals often have serious metabolic complications at this level of obesity.

OBESITY AND BREAST CANCER MORTALITY: NONPATIENT POPULATIONS

In the American Cancer Society (ACS) Prevention Study II, a prospective cohort study in 900,000 American adults including 495,477 women, 57,145 cancer deaths were identified during 16 years of follow-up (Calle et al., 2003). Cancer mortality was determined through personal inquiries and linkage with the National Death Index. The relative risks

Copyright © 2006, Elsevier Inc.
All rights of reproduction in any form reserved.

TABLE 1 Classification of Overweight and Obesity by Body Mass Index (BMI)

	BMI (kg/m^2)
Underweight	<18.5
Normal weight	18.5–24.9
Overweight	25.0–29.9
Obese	≥30.0–39.9
Extreme obesity	≥40.0

(RRs) for increasing category of BMI, compared with women with BMI <25.0 kg/m^2, were 1.34 (BMI 25.0–29.9 kg/m^2), 1.63 (BMI 30.0–34.9 kg/m^2), 1.70 (BMI 35.0–39.9 kg/m^2), and 2.12 (BMI ≥ 40.0 kg/m^2). The test for trend was highly significant ($p < .001$). In the Iowa Women's Health study, a cohort of 21,707 women, a positive association of waist/hip ratio with breast cancer mortality was also observed after follow-up of up to 7 years (Folsom et al., 1993).

Because these studies did not focus on a patient population, but risk in an originally cancer-free population, it is not clear how much of the effect of BMI on mortality was due to increased breast cancer incidence with obesity and how much was due to decreased survival among obese breast cancer patients. Indeed, increased adiposity has been found to be adversely associated with incidence of breast cancer (van den Brandt et al., 2000; IARC, 2002a; Morimoto et al., 2002), survival among breast cancer patients (Chlebowski et al., 2002), and stage at diagnosis (Reeves et al., 1996; Wee et al., 2000; Baumgartner et al., 2004).

OVERWEIGHT, OBESITY, AND BREAST CANCER PROGNOSIS

Almost 40 studies have examined the association of obesity with breast cancer outcomes in patient populations (Chlebowski et al., 2002; Brown et al., 2003). A statistically significant association between overweight or obesity and recurrence or survival was seen in 26 reports that included 29,460 women with breast cancer (Table 2), while 8 studies including 3727 women did not see such associations. Negative effects of body weight on breast cancer recurrence and survival have been observed in both premenopausal and postmenopausal women (Holmberg et al., 1994; Lethaby et al., 1996).

Goodwin et al. (1995) published a meta-analysis of studies published before 1992 and estimated that overweight or obesity was associated with a statistically significantly 78–91% increased risk of recurrence and a 36–56% increased risk of death (Goodwin et al., 1995). In another study, obesity was strongly and statistically significantly associated ($p = .005$) with disease-free survival and overall survival in a cohort of 535 women (median age 50 years) with newly diagnosed breast cancer. In addition, obesity at diagnosis was related (hazard rate [HR] = 1.86, 95% confidence interval [CI] = 1.02–3.40) to a significant decrease in survival in postmenopausal women with inflammatory breast cancer (Chang et al., 2001). These associations of obesity and adverse breast cancer outcome are substantial, with differences comparable in magnitude to those associated with adjuvant hormonal and chemotherapy use and of potentially great clinical importance.

A review of published prospective studies of adiposity and breast cancer prognosis (Chlebowski et al., 2002) concluded that most studies identified a significant adverse association of obesity with either recurrence or death. Despite these numerous studies, it is still not clear whether there are interactions with adjuvant therapy. An NSABP analysis of 3385 clinical trial patients from a randomized, placebo-controlled trial evaluating tamoxifen for lymph node–negative, estrogen receptor (ER)–positive breast cancer found that obese women benefited as much as lighter-weight women from tamoxifen therapy (Dignam et al., 2003). Furthermore, in that population, BMI was not adversely associated with breast cancer mortality. Compared with normal-weight women, obese women had greater all-cause mortality (HR = 1.31, 95% CI = 1.12–1.54) and greater risk of deaths due to causes unrelated to breast cancer (HR = 1.49, 95% CI = 1.15–1.92).

Goodwin et al. (2002) reported a prospective cohort study that was designed to examine the prognostic effect of obesity in early-stage breast cancer. Height and weight were measured in a fasting state prior to initiation of adjuvant treatment in 535 women with T1–3, N0–1, M0 breast cancer. After a median 50 months of follow-up, obesity predicted distant disease-free and overall survival ($p < .001$). Women with BMI 20–25 kg/m^2 had the lowest risk of recurrence and death; those with BMI < 20 or BMI > 25 kg/m^2 had an increased risk of recurrence (RR 1.18 and 1.72, respectively) and death (RR 1.21 and 1.78, respectively). The adverse effect of obesity persisted after adjustment for tumor stage, nodal stage, tumor grade, ER and progesterone receptor status, and adjuvant treatment (chemotherapy and/or hormone therapy). All but two of the deaths were due to breast cancer.

Body fat distribution may be relevant to breast cancer prognosis. Researchers in British Columbia, Canada, identified 603 patients with incident breast cancer and collected self-reported anthropometric data before treatment (Borugian et al., 2003). After up to 10 years of follow-up, the RR for breast cancer mortality for highest versus lowest quartile of waist/hip ratio in postmenopausal cases was 3.3 (95% CI 1.1–10.4). The increased mortality risk was limited to those with ER-positive tumors. A small study found that increased truncal obesity significantly predicted breast

TABLE 2 Breast Cancer Studies Showing Statistically Significant Associations among Obesity and Survival or Recurrence

Study	Geographic location	Type of study	N	Stage	Ages	Systemic therapy use (N if given)	Obesity measurements	Results	Notes
Donegan et al. (1978a)	Columbia, MO	Hospital record based	962	A, B, C, D	58.4 years (≤130 lbs); 61.2 years (>130 lbs)	None (962)	Premastectomy body weight	RR for recurrence in women >130 lbs = 1.44**; RR for recurrence in women >130 lbs with negative axillary nodes = 2.65**	Only included women with a standard radical mastectomy without radiation or other adjuvant therapy
Donegan et al. (1978b)	Milwaukee, WA	Hospital based	83	—	22–38; mean: 56.4	—	Weight; OI	Rate of recurrence = 41%** for obese and 8%** for nonobese; 40%** for women ≥160 lbs and 11%** for women <160 lbs; 5-year survival rates were not significantly lower for obese women	OI = (weight [lbs]/height [in.]); obese categorized as >2.45 in OI; included only patients treated by mastectomy
Boyd et al. (1981)	Toronto, Ontario, Canada	Population based	749	I, II, III	35–70	Ovarian ablation (71); ovarian ablation + prednisone (72); none (62)	Weight; BSA; QI	Disease-free survival associated with weight ($\chi^2 = 4.67$*); BSA ($\chi^2 = 3.86$*); QI ($\chi^2 = 5.05$*); among premenopausal women >45 years, recurrence-free survival was significantly longer for those who received adjuvant ovarian ablation ($\chi^2 = 5.75$*)	When association between weight and disease-free survival was adjusted simultaneously for clinical stage, lymph node status, and tumor grade, $\chi^2 = 3.58$, $p = .06$
Tartter et al. (1981)	New York, NY	Hospital based	274	I, II, III	—	—	Weight; QI	Cumulative 5-year disease-free survival = 49%* for women ≥150 lbs and 67%* for <150 lbs; 56% (NS) for QI ≥ 3.5 and 72% (NS) for QI < 3.5	Differences in survival rates among women ≥ and <150 lbs remained significant after stratifying by stage
Greenburg et al. (1985)	London	Multihospital based	582	I, II, III, IV	24–50	—	Weight; QI	Estimated 5-year survival probability = 55% for women >154 lbs; 80% for women <113 lbs; RR for dying for women >154 lbs (baseline <113 lbs) = 1.7* (adjusted for clinical stage, age at diagnosis, other confounders)	Restricted to premenopausal women; other confounders: age at first birth, age at menarche, social class, miscarriage history, family history, oral contraceptive use, smoking, and hospital of diagnosis
Newman et al. (1986)	Canada	Population based	300	—	35–74	—	Weight; QI; dietary intake of calories, total fat, saturated fat	OR of dying from breast cancer associated with weight >63 kg = 1.68*; no other obesity measurements were significantly associated with survival	300 = the number of cases in this case–control study; control/case ratio was 3:1
Mohle-Boetani et al. (1988)	Bay Area, CA	Population based	838	I, II, IIIA, IIIB, IV	22–74 (median: 56)	—	Weight at diagnosis; BMI at diagnosis and age 20; change in BMI from age 20 years	RR of death among premenopausal women = 1.7* for weight >140 lbs (baseline ≤140 lbs); no difference was seen among postmenopausal women. RR of death for all obese women = 1.4* (baseline BMI ≤30.4)	BMI = (1000 * weight [lbs]/height [in.^{2}]); BMI ≥ 34.7 = obese; death rates were adjusted for age at diagnosis, stage at diagnosis, and period of follow-up
Lees et al. (1989)	Northern Alberta, Canada	Population based	1121	I, II, III, IV	<35–80+	Radiation therapy; chemotherapy	Weight	Survival was 71%** for women <66 kg and 61%** for women >66 kg; type of treatment was not shown to influence survival	Percent survival was adjusted for stage, nodal status, age at menarche, and age at first birth
Coates et al. (1990)	Georgia	Hospital based	1960	1, 2, 3, 4	—	Radiation (222); hormonal therapy (35); chemo (111)	Weight; BMI	For all stages, 5-year survival rates were associated with BMI ($\chi^2 = 15.02$, $p < .001$); blacks had a lower probability of survival for 5 years (57%) than whites (76%), and a higher average BMI	Examined only black and white women; BMI = (weight [kg]/height [m]^2)

(continues)

TABLE 2 (*Continued*)

Study	Geographic location	Type of study	N	Stage	Ages	Systemic therapy use (N if given)	Obesity measurements	Results	Notes
Kimura (1990)	Japan	Hospital based	593	I, II, III	—	—	BMI	10-year survival rates for premenopausal women = 80.8% (NS) (lean), 70.4%* (ordinary), and 75.1%* (obese); for postmenopausal women = 87.5%* (lean), 80.2%* (ordinary), and 68.8%* (obese)	Subjects were categorized by BMI: lean <21.0, ordinary 21.1–23.0, obese >23.1; 5-year survival rates were not significant
Kyogoku et al. (1990)	Japan	Multihospital based	213	I, II, III	—	Radiation therapy (16); chemotherapy (87); endocrine therapy (130)	Weight; BSA; RW; OI; QI	RR for death = 3.20* for body weight >60 kg (baseline <45 kg); 3.84* for BSA >1.5 (baseline <1.4); 3.86** for RW >1.2 (baseline <1.0); 4.42** for OI >8.0 (baseline <6.0); 2.51** for QI >25 (baseline <20); 5- and 10-year survival probabilities decreased significantly with increasing BSA and QI; endocrine therapy and chemotherapy were not significantly related to survival	RW = (weight [kg]/height [cm] – 100 * 0.9); OI = (weight [kg]/height $[cm]^{1.7499}$) * 1000; RR adjusted for stage, ages at menarche and first birth, menstrual status, benign breast disease and abortion history, smoking, radiation therapy, chemotherapy, hormonal therapy, and operative procedure
Tretli et al. (1990)	Norway	Population based	8427	I, II, III, IV	30–69	—	QI	RR of dying (95% CI) for the fifth quintile of QI (baseline first quintile) for stage I = 1.70 (1.29, 2.25); for stage II = 1.42 (1.17, 1.73); little or favorable risk was observed among stage III and IV patients	Analyses stratified by menopausal status were not significantly different from nonstratified analyses
Vatten et al. (1991)	Norway	Population based	242	I, II, III, IV	50 ± 5.3	—	BMI	HR (95% CI) for dying among the fourth BMI quartile (baseline first quartile) = 2.1 (1.3, 6.7); χ^2 for survival associated with fourth BMI quartile = 16.52**	BMI quartiles (kg/m^2) = <22; 22–24; 24–27; ≥27; HR adjusted for age at diagnosis, stage at diagnosis, and total serum cholesterol
Ewertz et al. (1991)	Denmark	Population based	1744	I, II, III	<70	Hormone replacement therapy (HRT) (570)	Weight (current, at age 20, 10 and 20 years before diagnosis, changes); BMI; fat consumption	RR of dying for women: currently <50 kg = 1.48*; >70 kg at age 20 = 1.69*; with weight losses ≥5 kg = 1.59*; with advanced disease and weight <50 kg = 1.67*; fat consumption, BMI, and use of menopausal HRT were not associated with survival	Early disease defined as having a tumor size <4 cm, no skin invasion, no positive lymph nodes, and grade I; stratification by early and late disease did not alter association between BMI and survival
Senie et al. (1992)	New York, NY	Hospital based	923	—	24–95, mean: 55.5 ± 11.7	Chemotherapy	Percentage of ideal weight (measured/ideal weight)	HR for recurrence = 1.29* for obese women; HR for recurrence for obese women with negative nodes = 1.59*; for positive nodes = 1.07 (NS)	Ideal weight = midpoint of weight range based on height; obese ≥125% of ideal weight; HR adjusted for tumor size, lymph node status, age at diagnosis, and adjuvant chemotherapy
Törnberg and Carstensen (1993)	Sweden	Population based	1170	I, II, III, IV	62.4 ± 12.0	—	QI	RR of dying for QI ≥28 (baseline ≤22): for all women = 1.7**; for ages 50–59 years = 2.1**; for ≤49 years = 2.4 ($p = .10$)	RR adjusted for current age, while age ranges refer to age at diagnosis
Bastarrachea et al. (1994)	Houston, TX	Hospital record based	735	II, III	—	Chemotherapy (735)	Percentage over ideal weight; QI	RR for recurrence in obese = 1.33*; 10-year disease-free survival rate = 43%** for >30% over ideal weight; 41%** for >29.7 in QI	Ideal weight = upper limit of weight range for a medium body frame given the woman's height; obese ≥20% ideal weight

Holmberg et al. (1994)	Sweden and Norway	Population based	422	—	<45	—	BMI	Relative hazard of death for BMI ≥29 (baseline <19) = 5.93*; risk of death was 8%* higher for every one unit increase in BMI	Association between BMI and survival adjusted for age and country
Jain and Miller (1994)	Canada	Population based	1033	—	40–66	—	Weight; BMI; triceps skinfold (mm); weight/height ratio	RR of dying associated with triceps skinfold >25.7 (baseline <14.9) = 1.21* after adjusting for weight; BMI and weight/height were not associated with the risk of dying after stratification by menopausal status, nodal status, tumor size, and hormone receptor status	Some levels were close to statistical significance but were not detected after stratification (smaller sample sizes); 5-year survival probabilities were not significantly associated with obesity
Mæhle et al. (1996)	Norway	Population based	1238	—	28–91, median: 63	Tamoxifen (33% of ER-positive women)	QI; prediagnosis weight	RR of dying for women in fifth quintile of QI versus first quintile: ER-positive women = 2.18 (p = .06); ER-negative women = 0.36*; ER-positive and PgR-positive women = 3.16 (p = .06); ER-negative and PgR-negative women = 0.17*	RR adjusted for lymph node status, tumor size, and mean nuclear area; ~one-third of ER-positive patients took tamoxifen
Haybittle et al. (1997)	Cambridge, UK	Population based	2455	I, II	<70	Radiotherapy	Weight	RR of death for women >60 kg was only significant in postmenopausal patients (1.27**), even after stratification by stage; RR of death in 5 years for postmenopausal women >60 kg = 1.68 (p = .0001)	Only included women with a simple mastectomy; weight had little effect on deaths from causes other than breast cancer (RR for women >60 kg = 1.03)
Newman et al. (1997)	Northern Alberta, Canada	Population based	1169	I, II, III	25–98 (median: 56.1)	Chemotherapy radiotherapy; hormonal therapy	BMI	HR (endpoint = death from breast cancer) for BMI >28.9 = 2.47*; for BMI 22.8–28.9 = 2.13*; among women with no positive nodes: HR for BMI >28.9 = 2.5*; for BMI 22.8–28.9 = 2.1*; hormonal therapy was not associated with survival	BMI results were only significant when adjusted for size of tumor, number of positive nodes, estrogen receptor level, age, and an interaction between BMI and number of positive nodes
Hebert et al. (1998)	New York, NY	Hospital based	472	I, II, IIIa	52.2 ± 11.9	—	Weight; BMI; 34-question FFQ; total energy intake	RR for BMI and recurrence = 1.09** in premenopausal women; risk of death increased by 6%* in postmenopausal women and by 12%** in premenopausal women for every 1 unit increase in BMI (kg/m^2)	Fitting total energy intake in models in place of BMI led to a higher predictive capability, but no increase in significance
Goodwin et al. (2000)	Toronto, Canada	Hospital based	535	—	50.4 ± 9.7	Tamoxifen (151); Chemotherapy (147); Both (46); None (168)	BMI	Obesity was related to both distant disease-free survival (p = .0005) and overall survival (p = .007)	Obese BMI values not given; women were newly diagnosed, receiving standard adjuvant therapy
Kumar et al. (2000)	Tampa, FL	Hospital based	166	I, II, III, IV	—	—	Weight; skinfold and circumference measurements	HR for survival for weight gain at age 30 = 1.15*; higher suprailiac/thigh ratio = 2.61**; higher Quetelet index = 0.92**	Suprailiac: thigh skinfold ratio used as proxy for upper/lower body skinfold ratio; Quetelet index = (weight [kg]/height [m^2])
Hryniuk et al. (2001)	Detroit, MI	Hospital based	1054	I, II, III	Median: 58	Tamoxifen (540)	Not specified	HR for disease-free survival = 1.5* for obese women ≥50 years; when limited to women on tamoxifen, adjusting for diabetes, HR = 1.2 (NS) for obese women	Significant interaction was detected for tamoxifen and diabetes, leading to an HR for women with diabetes on tamoxifen of 2.4** for mortality from breast cancer

—, Not reported. *P < 0.05. **P < 0.01. NS, Not significant at α = 0.05 level.
RR, relative risk; OR, odds ratio; HR, hazard ratio; QI, Quetelet index; BSA, body surface area; BMI, body mass index; FFQ, food frequency questionnaire; RW, relative weight.

cancer survival (Kumar et al., 2000). In that study, 83 (50%) of 166 breast carcinoma patients with up to 10 years of follow-up died of their breast cancer. Android body fat distribution, as indicated by a higher suprailiac/thigh ratio, was a statistically significant ($p < .0001$) prognostic indicator for survival after controlling for stage of disease, with an HR of 2.6 (95% CI, 1.63–4.17).

Risk of future second primary breast cancer may also be increased with increased adiposity. Results from a population-based cohort of 1285 breast cancer survivors suggest an increased risk for contralateral breast cancer among overweight or obese breast cancer survivors (Li et al., 2003). In the NSABP analysis of 3385 tamoxifen trial patients, contralateral breast cancer hazard was higher in obese women than in underweight/normal-weight women, (HR = 1.58, 95% CI = 1.10–2.25), as was the risk of additional primary breast cancers (HR = 1.62, 95% CI = 1.16–2.24).

WEIGHT GAIN AFTER DIAGNOSIS AND BREAST CANCER OUTCOMES

Weight gain after diagnosis has been frequently reported for breast cancer patients, especially among women receiving systemic adjuvant chemotherapy (Dixon et al., 1978; Donegan et al., 1978a,b; Foltz, 1985; Heasman et al., 1985; Huntington, 1985; Chlebowski et al., 1986; Faber-Langendoen, 1996; Goodwin et al., 1998).

In a prospective cohort of 535 newly diagnosed breast cancer patients, use of adjuvant chemotherapy and onset of menopause were the strongest predictors of weight gain (Goodwin et al., 1999). The causes of this weight gain have not been identified but could be from a mixture of reduced physical activity after diagnosis (Irwin et al., 2003a), changes in dietary intake (Goodwin et al., 1999; Rock et al., 2000), and reduced rates of metabolism (Demark-Wahnefried et al., 1997, 2001).

In the Health, Eating, Activity, Lifestyle (HEAL) Study, a population-based cohort of 1185 women with stage 0–3a breast cancer, levels of recreational physical activity significantly decreased between diagnosis and 1 year after diagnosis regardless of age at diagnosis (Irwin et al., 2003a) (Figure 1). This decrease was seen in women at all stages but was most pronounced in those at the higher stages (Figure 2). Women who had been treated with chemotherapy were more likely to decrease their activity levels, although women with any treatment were likely to have reduced activity levels (Figure 3). Obese women reduced their activity levels more than lighter weight women (Figure 4). The amount of decrease in physical activity could explain the degree of weight gain in those who gained weight after diagnosis, even without changes in dietary composition.

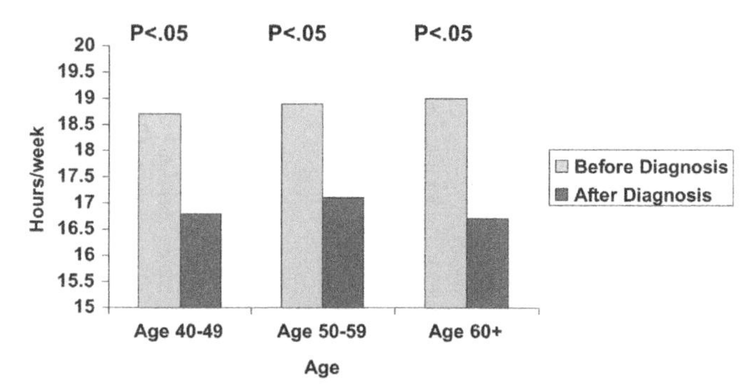

FIGURE 1 Total physical activity before and after diagnosis by age: the HEAL population-based cohort of stage 0–3a breast cancer patients (N = 1185).

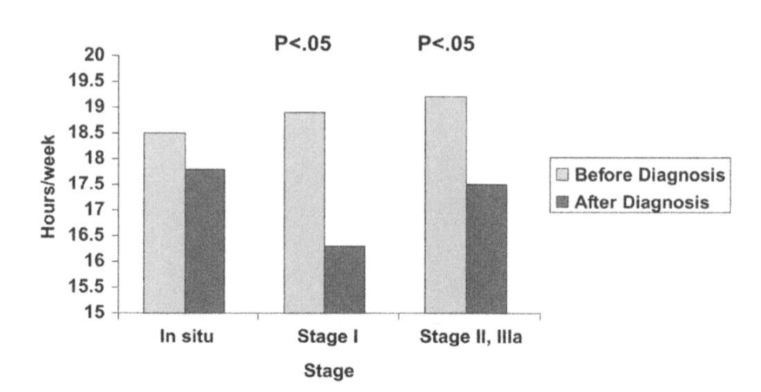

FIGURE 2 Total physical activity before and after diagnosis by stage at diagnosis: the HEAL population-based cohort of stage 0–3a breast cancer patients (N = 1185).

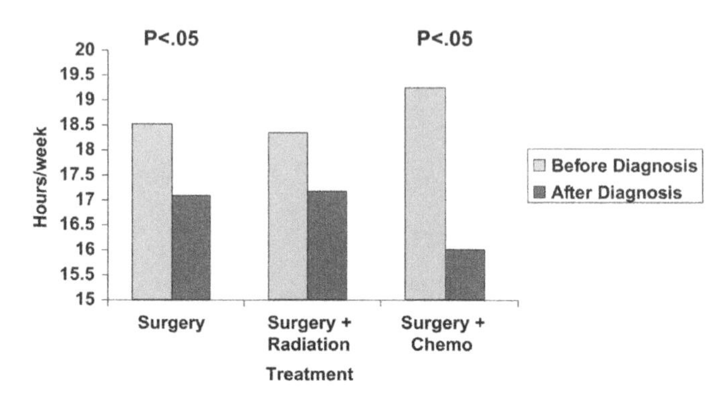

FIGURE 3 Total physical activity before and after diagnosis by primary treatment: the HEAL population-based cohort of stage 0–3a breast cancer patients (N = 1185).

One report suggested associations among obesity, depressive symptomatology, and abnormal eating attitudes in women at risk for breast cancer recurrence, which could compound patients' attempts to maintain or lose excess weight (Rock et al., 2000).

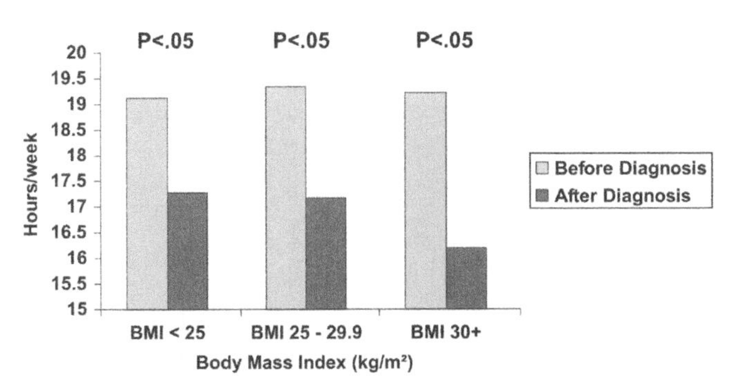

FIGURE 4 Total physical activity before and after diagnosis by adiposity: the HEAL population-based cohort of stage 0–3a breast cancer patients (N = 1185).

Tamoxifen treatment does not appear to influence body weight (Fisher et al., 1998; Goodwin et al., 1999). Although anthracycline chemotherapy may have less effect on weight than other chemotherapy regimens, weight gains between 2 and 4 kg following some chemotherapy regimens such as cyclophosphamide, methotrexate, and 5-fluorouracil (CMF) have been commonly reported (Demark-Wahnefried et al., 1993, 1997, 2001). This weight gain consists primarily of body fat (Cheney et al., 1997; Aslani et al., 1999). In a report of the National Cancer Institute of Canada Clinical Trials Group, adjuvant CMF and CEF (with epirubicin) was associated with average weight increases of 4.36 and 2.93 kg, respectively ($p < .001$ compared with baseline) (Shepard et al., 2001). In breast cancer survivors, return to prediagnosis weight is rare (Camoriano et al., 1990; Faber-Langendoen, 1996).

Four studies have investigated the relationship between weight gain after diagnosis and prognosis (Chlebowski et al., 2002) (Table 3). Three of these studies in early-stage resected breast cancer found that weight gain after diagnosis increased recurrence risk or decreased survival. In a North Central Oncology Group study of 545 early-stage breast cancer patients, women with weight gain greater than the median of 5.9 kg were 1.5 times more likely to relapse and 1.6 times more likely to die (Camoriano et al., 1990). Chlebowski et al. (1986) found that women who gained >10 kg after diagnosis had significantly reduced survival. Prospective studies specifically addressing the effect of weight gain after diagnosis on breast cancer recurrence risk are necessary (Chlebowski et al., 2002).

OBESITY AND DEVELOPMENT OF COMORBIDITIES IN BREAST CANCER PATIENTS

Obese breast cancer patients are at increased risk of developing problems after surgery including wound complication and lymphedema (Barber et al., 1995; Forouhi et al., 1995). Obesity also is a risk factor for endometrial cancer development and may place women on tamoxifen at further increased risk of this disease (Bernstein et al., 1999). Severe obesity strongly predicted ($p = .016$) development of congestive heart failure in women who had received doxorubicin chemotherapy in one report (Kallab et al., 2000).

In a study of 1800 postmenopausal breast cancer patients identified through the National Cancer Institute Surveillance, Epidemiology, and End Results (SEER) and followed for 30 months after diagnosis, only 51% of deaths were attributed to breast cancer (Yancik et al., 2001a,b), and the percentage of deaths ascribed to breast cancer decreased with age. Especially in older, postmenopausal populations, attention to obesity as a risk factor for potentially fatal comorbid conditions such as cardiovascular disease, venous thromboembolic disease, and stroke is of potential major importance in optimizing breast cancer patient outcome. Furthermore, obesity increases the risk of several other cancers, including endometrium, kidney, esophageal, and colon (IARC, 2002b). Women who have had a diagnosis of breast cancer are at increased risk for some of these cancers, and obese women have a further increased risk.

OBESITY AND QUALITY OF LIFE IN BREAST CANCER PATIENTS

Quality of life in some breast cancer patients and survivors may be adversely affected (Ganz et al., 1998, 1996, 2002, 2003; Gelber et al., 1998; Michael et al., 2000). Knobf et al. (1983) reported a correlation between weight gain and anxiety over appearance. In women with advanced breast cancer, therapy-associated weight gain reduced quality of life (Kornblith et al., 1993). Interventions that may reduce weight, conversely, such as physical activity interventions, have been shown to improve quality of life in breast cancer survivors (Courneya, 2003). One randomized clinical trial of three dietary interventions versus control in 48 obese breast cancer patients found that women with a psychiatric diagnosis had less weight loss in a weight reduction program compared with women without such diagnoses (Jenkins et al., 2003). After 30 months of follow-up, subjects with any psychiatric disorder had a mean weight loss of 1.2% of baseline weight compared with 7.8% weight loss in subjects with no diagnosis.

POTENTIAL MECHANISMS FOR AN ADVERSE PROGNOSTIC EFFECT OF OBESITY

Several mechanisms have been proposed for an adverse prognostic effect of obesity in cancer. These mechanisms

TABLE 3 Breast Cancer Studies Showing Nonsignificant Results for the Associations among Survival or Recurrence and Obesity

Study	Geographic location	Type of study	N	Stage	Ages	Systemic therapy use (N if given)	Obesity measurements	Results	Notes
Sohrabi et al. (1981)	Louisville, KY	Hospital based	106	—	—	—	Quetelet score	No significant association was found between obesity and recurrence	Quetelet score = (weight/height); obese defined as having Quetelet score >2.45
Williams et al. (1988)	Manchester, UK	Hospital based	227	—	—	Tamoxifen (200); Ovarian ablation (27)	Weight	Among patients with operable disease, no significant associations were found between weight and overall survival, recurrence-free survival, or survival from the start of endocrine therapy	All patients had advanced breast cancer and were treated with tamoxifen (88%) or by ovarian ablation (12%) subsequent to their first relapse; menopausal status did not affect the results
Kamby et al. (1989)	Denmark	Population based	863	I, II	—	Chemo (138); tamoxifen (155)	BSA (m^2); QI; weight	Recurrence and percent survival after recurrence (stratified by menopausal status) were not associated with weight, BSA, or QI	Calculations of BSA and QI were based on 536 patients for whom both weight and height were available
Katoh et al. (1994)	Pittsburgh, PA	Hospital based	301	I, II, III, IV	Median: 72	Chemo or radiotherapy (112); none (181)	QI; weight	Obesity was not significantly associated with survival or recurrence of breast cancer after both univariate and multivariate analysis	Examined only postmenopausal women; obese >27 in QI; adjusted for age, stage, tumor size, nodal status, hormone receptor status, and level of treatment
den Tonkenlaar et al. (1995)	Utrecht, The Netherlands	Population based	241	A, B, C, D	—	None (241)	Weight; QI at screening and diagnosis; fat distribution	Measures of obesity were not associated with differences in survival; OR for advanced breast cancer (stages B, C, D) = 2.93* for weight ≥75.0 kg (baseline <61.5); 3.09* for QI ≥ 28.0 (baseline <23.0)	Restricted study to women with natural menopause; measured triceps and subscapular skinfolds to determine fat distribution
Obermair et al. (1995)	Vienna, Austria	Hospital based	473	—	—	Tamoxifen (283); chemotherapy (300); irradiation (133)	Percentage over ideal weight	5-year disease-free survival rate = 87.0% for obese and 89.3% for nonobese (NS); adjusted RR for disease-free survival = 0.83 (NS) for obese women; tamoxifen use was not significantly associated with being obese	Obese >25% over ideal weight defined by Broca's index ([height (cm) − 100] − 10%); RR adjusted for tumor size, lymph node involvement, estrogen and progesterone receptor status, menopausal status, and histological grading
Lethaby et al. (1996)	Auckland, New Zealand	Population based	1138	—	—	Various forms of adjuvant treatment (92)	BMI	10-year survival rates for women >50 years = 67% (obese) and 77% (nonobese) (NS); for women <50 years = 67% (obese) and 74% (nonobese) (NS); survival rates did not vary when stratified by adjuvant treatment	BMI was calculated for 73% of study participants; obese categorized as >28 BMI
Galanis et al. (1998)	Hawaii	Population based	378	—	20–72	—	BMI	RR of death among women with BMI 22.7–25.7 (baseline <22.6) = 1.7 (NS); BMI > 25.8 = 2.2 (NS)	Median of BMI distribution = 22.7 kg/m^2; 378 incident cases developed out of a cohort of 17,628 women over an average of 15 years

—, Not reported. *$p < .05$. **$p < .01$. NS, Not significant at $\alpha = 0.05$ level.
RR, relative risk; OR, odds ratio; HR, hazard ratio; QI, Quetelet index; BSA, body surface area; BMI, body mass index; FFQ, food frequency questionnaire; RW, relative weight; OI, obesity index.

include increased levels of circulating hormones such as estrogen and androgens, reduced levels of sex hormone–binding globulin (SHBG), which thereby increases the levels of free estradiol and free testosterone, increased levels of insulin and insulin-like growth factors (IGFs), reduced levels of IGF-binding globulin, increased levels of cortisol and leptin, increased levels of cytokines, effects of diet, reduced immune functioning, and chemotherapy underdosing in obese patients. Although some biological evidence exists to support many of these potential mechanisms, there is little direct evidence of their role.

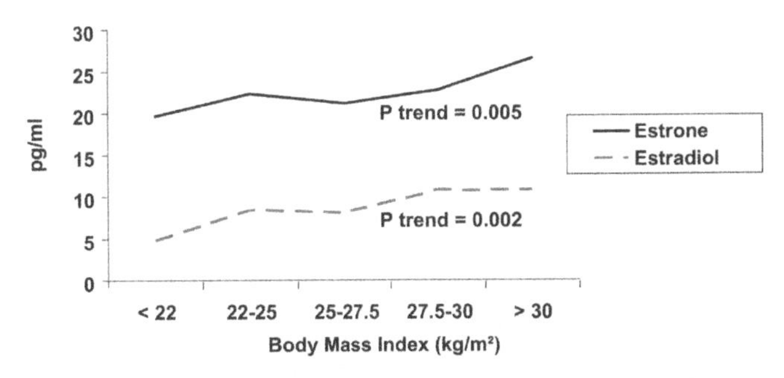

FIGURE 5 Estrone and estradiol concentrations according to body mass index: the HEAL population-based cohort of stage 0–3a breast cancer patients (N = 505 postmenopausal cases).

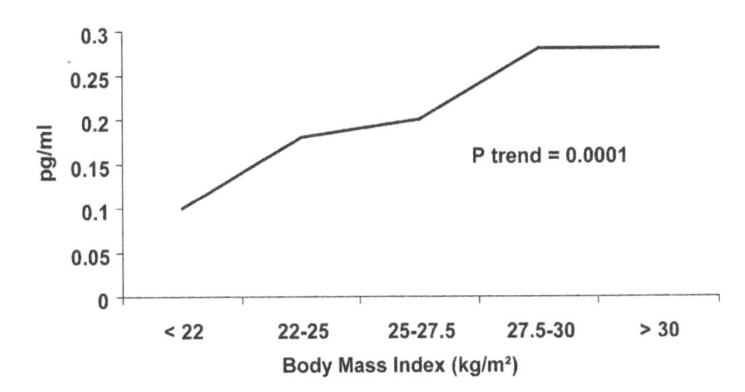

FIGURE 6 Free estradiol concentrations according to body mass index: the HEAL population-based cohort of stage 0–3a breast cancer patients (N = 505 postmenopausal cases).

Estrogens

Postmenopausal women produce estrogens in fat and other tissue through the aromatization of androgens to estrogens (Siiteri, 1987). The enzyme aromatase is abundantly present in adipose tissue, especially subcutaneous fat. Estrogens are tumor promoters *in vitro* and *in vivo*, and women with high circulating levels of estrogens are at increased risk of developing breast cancer (Endogenous Hormones and Breast Cancer Collaborative Group, 2002; Key et al., 2003).

Postmenopausal women who are overweight or obese have elevated levels of estrogens compared with lighter weight women (Cauley et al., 1989; Verkasalo et al., 2001). In a population-based cohort of 505 postmenopausal women with stage 0–3a breast cancer (the HEAL Study), adiposity was positively and statistically significantly associated with circulating levels of estrone, estradiol, and free estradiol (McTiernan et al., 2003) (Figures 5 and 6). Women were identified to this study through the SEER cancer registries of western Washington and New Mexico and were primarily non-Hispanic and Hispanic Whites. Between 4 and 12 months after diagnosis, anthropometric measures and blood draws were obtained on all women and DEXA scans were obtained on 415 women. Obese women (BMI $\geq$ 30 kg/m^2) had 35% higher concentrations of estrone and 130% higher concentrations of estradiol, compared with lighter women (BMI < 22.0 kg/m^2) (p trend, .005 and .002, respectively). Similar associations were observed for DEXA-derived body fat mass and percent body fat and waist circumference. Concentrations of free estradiol were doubled to tripled in overweight and obese women compared with lighter weight women (p trend = .0001).

Androgens

Overweight, obese, and sedentary postmenopausal women have elevated concentrations of circulating total and free androgens (Cauley et al., 1989; Newcomb et al., 1995), and one report suggests that this association may be due to increased amounts of 17β-hydroxysteroid dehydrogenase in subcutaneous and intra-abdominal fat (Corbould et al., 1998). A combined analysis of nested case–control studies within nine cohort studies, which included data from 663 breast cancer cases and 1765 women without breast cancer, found that postmenopausal women with serum hormone concentrations in the top quintile for testosterone, androstenedione, dehydroepiandrosterone (DHEA), and DHEA-sulfate (DHEA-S) were approximately twice as likely to develop breast cancer compared with women with serum hormones in the bottom quintile (Endogenous Hormones and Breast Cancer Collaborative Group, 2002). In the same analysis, a doubling of androgen concentration resulted in a 20–40% increase in risk for breast cancer. When estradiol and testosterone were included in the same model, the effect of doubling of testosterone on breast cancer risk was greater than that of estradiol (RR 1.32 and 1.18, respectively), and similar results were observed for androstenedione when combined in a model with estradiol. These androgens may increase cell proliferation by being converted to estradiol and estrone in the circulation or target tissue (Siiteri, 1987). In addition, androgens may affect breast cancer risk by directly stimulating the growth and division of breast cells (Endogenous Hormones and Breast Cancer Collaborative Group, 2002).

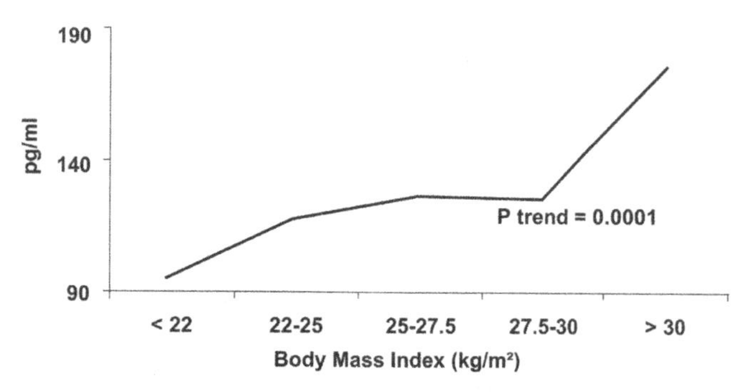

FIGURE 7 Testosterone concentrations according to body mass index: the HEAL population-based cohort of stage 0–3a breast cancer patients (N = 505 postmenopausal cases).

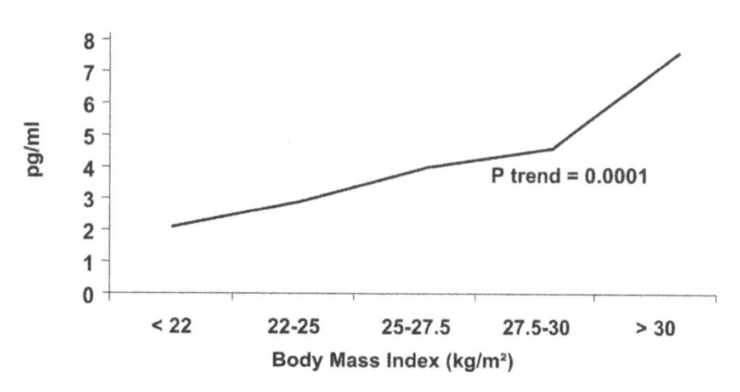

FIGURE 8 Free testosterone concentrations according to body mass index: the HEAL population-based cohort of stage 0–3a breast cancer patients (N = 505 postmenopausal cases).

In the HEAL cohort of breast cancer patients, overweight and obese women had statistically significantly elevated levels of testosterone, free testosterone, and DHEA-S (McTiernan et al., 2003) (Figures 7 and 8). Levels of DHEA-S and free testosterone were higher in women in the top quartiles for body fat mass compared with the leanest women, although the trend was only statistically significant for free testosterone.

Insulin and Insulin-Like Growth Factors

High levels of insulin and C peptide have been associated with increased risk for some common cancers (Kaaks et al., 200), and insulin has mitogenic effects on breast cells (Belfiore et al., 1996; Papa and Belfiore, 1996). In a study of 535 women with early-stage breast cancer, Goodwin et al. (2002) investigated several of these potential mediators. Fasting insulin levels were significantly associated with both distant recurrence and death. Women in the highest quartile of insulin levels had a 2.1 times increased risk of distant recurrence compared with those in the lowest quartile (95% CI 1.2–3.6, $p = .01$) and a 3.3 times greater risk of death (95% CI 1.5–7.0, $p = .002$) (adjusted for age, nodal stage, tumor stage, tumor grade, hormone receptor status, adjuvant chemotherapy, adjuvant tamoxifen). The effect of insulin on survival was independent of BMI. Circulating IGF-1, IGF-2, IGF-binding protein (IGFBP)-1 and IGFBP-3, and estradiol did not exert independent effects on distant recurrence or death.

Hyperinsulinemia could affect breast cancer prognosis in several ways. Insulin has been found to stimulate ER-α in breast cancer cells *in vitro* (Yee and Lee, 2000). Insulin also stimulates the production of estrogens and androgens, increasing production of these by adipose tissue, and down-regulates sex hormone–binding protein, the major carrier molecule for estradiol and testosterone (Plymate et al., 1990).

Abdominal Fat

The body fat that is stored in the intra-abdominal area is thought to have special physiological properties and is more associated than other body fat with risk factors for diabetes and cardiovascular disease. Increased intra-abdominal fat is associated with increased levels of insulin and total and low-density lipoprotein (LDL) cholesterol (Irwin et al., 2003b).

The role of visceral fat on breast cancer prognosis has not been established. Increased intra-abdominal fat, however, is associated with increased circulating levels of serum insulin and glucose (Irwin et al., 2003b), and as described earlier, insulin may be a tumor growth promoter. Therefore, interventions that decrease intra-abdominal fat levels may be hypothesized to improve cancer prognosis. In a small study, a 2-month low-fat diet and structured exercise intervention in women with a history of breast cancer resulted in a significant decrease in waist circumference (McTiernan et al., 1998). In a clinical trial in 173 postmenopausal overweight/obese sedentary women without breast cancer, exercise preferentially and significantly decreased intra-abdominal fat (Irwin et al., 2003b).

Cytokines, Inflammation, and Immune Function

Obesity is also associated with inflammatory markers including C-reactive protein (CRP), serum amyloid A (SAA), interleukin (IL)-6, IL-1, and tumor necrosis factor-α (TNF-α), some of which have been shown to be higher in women with metastatic breast cancer compared with normal controls and with women with early breast cancer (Blann et al., 2002; Mahmoud and Rivera, 2002; O'Hanlan et al., 2002). Despite a paucity of data, it seems plausible that women with depressed immune function might be at increased risk of breast tumor progression. Studies suggest decreased immune function in obese women (Nieman et al., 1999), in women who participate in "yo-yo" dieting (Shad et al., 2004), and increased immune function with exercise in breast cancer survivors (Nieman et al., 1995).

TABLE 4 Breast Cancer Studies of Weight Gain after Diagnosis and Clinical Outcome

Study	Geographic location	Type of study	N	Stage	Ages	Mean weight gain observation (range)	Results	Notes
Bonomi et al. (1984)	Chicago, IL	Hospital based	67	II	—	18 lbs	62/67 women gained at least 5 lbs; weight gain analyzed as % of ideal weight was negatively associated to disease-free survival (χ^2 = 12.34*)	Out of 67 women receiving adjuvant chemotherapy, 47 of these women also received tamoxifen
Chlebowski et al. (1986)	Western, US	Multicenter	62	—	—	3.7 kg for CMF group; 2.0 kg for 5-FU group	In 1 year, 91% of women in CMF group gained weight, 3% lost weight; 74% of women in 5-FU group gained weight, 26% lost weight; none of the five women who gained >10 kg survived*	Overall survival rates were 31% in CMF group and 51% in 5-FU group
Camoriano et al. (1990)	Minnesota and Illinois	Hospital based	545	—	20–75	Median: 5.9 kg** (premenopausal; 3.6 kg** (treated postmenopausal); 1.8 kg** (observed postmenopausal)	For premenopausal women: RR of recurrence = 1.5 (NS) for women who gained more weight than the median after 60 weeks; RR of death = 1.6* for women who gained more weight than the median	RR adjusted for nodal status, age, estrogen receptor status, tumor size, baseline Quetelet index, and nuclear grade
Levine et al. (1991)	Birmingham, AL	Hospital based	32	—	26–68	1.8 kg** (–3.6–10.35)	69% of total sample gained weight. RR of recurrence within 2 years for women who gained weight (baseline = no weight gain) = 1.36 (NS)	No differences were observed among type of chemotherapy, operation, or menopausal status

—, Not reported; *$P < .05$; **$p < .01$; NS, not significant.
CMF, cyclophosphamide, methotrexate, and 5-fluorouracil; CMFVP, CMF, vincristine, prednisone; 5-FU, 5-fluorouracil.

METHODS FOR WEIGHT LOSS AND MAINTENANCE FOR BREAST CANCER PATIENTS

Several methods for weight loss or control have been tested in the general population (Obesity Education Initiative, 1998) or in persons with other obesity-related conditions such as diabetes and cardiovascular disease (Tuomilehto et al., 2001; Knowler et al., 2002). Detailed guidelines for the identification, diagnosis, and treatment of overweight and obesity have been published by several institutes of the National Institutes of Health (Obesity Education Initiative, 1998) and from the U.S. Preventive Task Force (McTigue et al., 2003). There are no specific guidelines for weight loss or maintenance methods in breast cancer patients or survivors, however.

The first step for clinicians should be the assessment of body composition including BMI (McTigue et al., 2003). For overweight (BMI 25.0–29.9 kg/m^2) or obese (BMI $\geq$ 30 kg/m^2) women, physicians can then apply a weight loss strategy as outlined by the National Heart, Lung, and Blood Institute (NHLBI) Obesity Education Initiative Expert Panel (1998). This panel recommends a weight loss treatment algorithm that combines dietary therapy, physical activity, and behavioral treatment, provided on an ongoing basis to promote weight loss and maintenance.

Behavioral Weight Loss Therapy

Reviews of randomized trials in healthy obese individuals and in those at high risk for other diseases (prediabetics, hypertensives) (Perri and Fuller, 1995; Perri, 1998; Wadden and Sarwer, 2000) show that the combination of diet and behavioral treatment typically delivered in 15–24 weekly group sessions produces an average weight loss of ~8.5 kg (mean body weight reduction = 9%). This degree of weight loss is associated with significant improvements in blood pressure, blood glucose, and psychological well-being (Blackburn, 1992, 1999). In the year following behavioral treatment, participants regain typically 30–40% of their lost weight. However, relatively few studies have provided behavioral treatment lasting more than 6 months, and follow-up studies conducted 2–5 years after behavioral treatment have documented a gradual but reliable return to baseline weights (Clark et al., 1991, 1996; Perri and Fuller, 1995; Perri, 1998; Kumanyika et al., 2000). Long-term success is more likely when participants are provided with extended treatment programs. Support for the efficacy of extended lifestyle treatment has been well documented (Graham et al., 1983; Clark et al., 1991, 1996; Perri and Fuller, 1995; Perri, 1998; Wadden and Sarwer, 2000). Compared with behavior therapy without additional therapist contacts, extended treatment in the form of weekly or biweekly group therapy sessions improves the maintenance of treatment effects for as long as 1 year following initial therapy. Similarly, multicomponent approaches that combine ongoing client–therapist contacts (whether in person or by telephone and mail) with relapse prevention training or social support programs have shown improved maintenance compared with behavioral treatment without such programs (Clark et al., 1991, 1996; Perri and Fuller, 1995; Perri, 1998). Continued adherence appears to be the mechanism responsible for the better outcomes observed in extended treatments.

Weight Loss Diets

The success of most dietary weight loss therapies has rested on reducing caloric intake below that required for current weight maintenance (e.g., creating a negative energy balance). A low-fat, reduced-calorie diet has been shown to produce significant weight loss when combined with behavioral change counseling (NHLBI Obesity Education Initiative, 1998). Reduced calorie diets can be achieved through meal replacements, dietary pattern change, or a combination (NHLBI Obesity Education Initiative, 1998). The first step in most weight loss diets is self-monitoring, where the individual records all food eaten each day. Then, the daily intake of calories, fat, fiber, carbohydrates, or all of these can be tallied by the individual or weight loss counselor. Another key step is frequent and regular weighing by a health professional or weight loss counselor. A major key to sustained weight loss is to achieve lifelong dietary pattern changes, rather than short-term "crash" diets (NHLBI Obesity Education Initiative, 1998).

There is preliminary evidence that very low carbohydrate diets may work through additional mechanisms beyond simple calorie restriction and produce greater weight loss compared with low-calorie diets (Foster et al., 2003; Samaha et al., 2003), although over a year, low-carbohydrate diets may not be more efficacious than reduced calorie diets (Foster et al., 2003). All diets have similar issues, in that most patients regain weight within a year after initial weight loss (McTigue et al., 2003).

Weight Loss Pharmacotherapy

For obese patients, or for those with BMI $\geq$ 27 with serious co-morbidities, weight loss medications may be a useful adjunct to diet and exercise therapy (Arterburn and Noel, 2001; McTigue et al., 2003). Two medications are approved for weight loss, and both are efficacious in the short term, although long-term efficacy data are not available. The first is sibutramine, a dopamine, norepinephrine, and serotonin reuptake inhibitor that inhibits appetite through a central mechanism. In a review of seven randomized clinical trials, sibutramine combined with lifestyle change promoted weight loss of 2.8–4.2 kg over 8–52 weeks in healthy adults and those with controlled hypertension

(Arterburn and Noel, 2001). However, patients regained weight after cessation of treatment. The second, orlistat, a gastrointestinal lipase inhibitor, prevents fat absorption. In 10 randomized trials, it has produced an average 3.5 kg weight loss over 1–2 years, in excess of control (lifestyle alone) weight loss. Another review with updated trial data (McTigue et al., 2003) concluded that therapy with sibutramine or orlistat combined with lifestyle change produced weight loss of 3–5 kg over that of control (lifestyle alone), and that prolonged use continued this weight loss past 2 years. Two other medications, phentermine and mazindol, produced similar weight loss in the short term but are not Food and Drug Administration (FDA) approved for long-term use. This same review concluded that three additional medications showed mixed results: metformin, diethylpropion, and fluoxetine. None of these medications has been specifically tested in breast cancer patients or survivors, so their effects on prognosis or other aspects of the breast cancer experience are unknown.

Bariatric Surgery

For severely obese persons (BMI $\geq$ 40.0) or for patients with serious co-morbidities for whom obesity poses an extreme risk, more invasive methods of weight loss can be considered such as bariatric surgery (Brolin, 2002). The effect of weight loss surgery, however, has not been tested in persons who have had cancer.

Exercise and Weight Loss and Maintenance

Physical activity may provide a low-risk method of preventing weight gain and promoting maintenance of weight loss in overweight and obese men and women (Pronk and Wing, 1994). Several studies have shown losses in total body weight from exercise training without dieting (Keim et al., 1990; Katoh et al., 1994; Irwin et al., 2003a). In a review of several hundred studies of exercise training and weight loss, Wilmore (1996) concluded that the average weight loss over 12 months of exercise training would amount to only 3.2 kg. Unlike weight loss dietary interventions, physical activity also increases or maintains muscle mass (Andreoli et al., 2001) and increases cardiorespiratory fitness levels (Hardman et al., 1992).

Weight Loss Studies in Cancer Patients and Survivors

Studies of weight loss reduction have been limited to breast cancer patients and survivors and have been few and with mixed results. The Mayo Clinic randomized 107 breast cancer patients to monthly nonintensive dietitian counseling. Median weight increase at 6 months was 2 kg in the counseling group versus 3.5 kg in the control group, a nonsignificant difference (Loprinzi et al., 1996). Goodwin et al. (1995) evaluated a multidisciplinary approach combining group dietary sessions, psychological support groups, and exercise programs in 61 breast cancer patients. For women with BMI > 25 kg/m^2, weight loss was 1.63 ± 4.22 kg, and aerobic exercise increase was a strong predictor of successful weight loss (Goodwin et al., 1995). In a study of 34 obese breast cancer survivors, a combination of individualized counseling and Weight Watchers program produced greater weight loss than either alone or control (Djuric et al., 2002). Weight change after 12 months of intervention was 0.85 kg in the control group, −2.6 kg in the Weight Watchers program group, −8.0 kg in the individualized counseling group, and −9.4 kg in the comprehensive group that used both individualized counseling and the Weight Watchers program. Weight loss relative to control was statistically significant in the comprehensive group 3, 6, and 12 months after randomization, whereas weight loss in the individualized group was significant only at 12 months. The study resulted in weight loss of 10% or more of initial body weight in 6 of 10 women in the comprehensive group after 12 months. These same researchers found that the comprehensive group experienced significant declines in leptin and improvements in lipids (Jen et al., 2004). Finally, de Waard et al. (1993) randomized 102 postmenopausal women (median BMI 27 kg/m^2) with a recent breast cancer diagnosis to a weight loss program involving stepwise reduction in caloric intake versus a control group. After 1 year, median weight loss was 6.0 kg with the intervention ($p < .05$).

Most studies targeting weight loss in breast cancer patients have not focused on metabolic and hormonal consequences of weight loss. Furthermore, most of the small number of weight loss studies in breast cancer patients have been in newly diagnosed patients undergoing treatment (i.e., during times when attention to diet and exercise are difficult). The emerging science of weight loss combining dietary change, exercise, behavioral intervention, and ongoing contact (Blackburn, 1999; Kiernan and Winkleby, 2000) suggests weight loss programs can now be successfully implemented in breast cancer patients.

Dietary Interventions in Breast Cancer Patients and Survivors

Dietary fat intake represents one possible mediating mechanism for the poor outcome associated with obesity in breast cancer, assuming a greater dietary fat intake in obese than in nonobese persons (Zhang et al., 1995; Herbert et al., 1998; Saxe et al., 1999). Though not without controversy (Holmes et al., 1999), the current evidence (Schatzkin, 1997) on dietary fat intake and breast cancer recurrence supports two ongoing full-scale outcome studies in breast cancer survivors (Chlebowski et al., 1993; Pierce et al., 1997). Feasibility of maintaining dietary fat intake reduction in breast cancer patients and survivors has been established

(Chlebowski et al., 1993, 2000). In women without breast cancer, reduction in estrogen levels in postmenopausal women and decreased mammographic density (a marker of breast cancer risk) (Boyd et al., 1997; Knight et al., 1999) have been associated with fat reduction. The two ongoing clinical trials of dietary fat intake reduction in breast cancer survivors have not targeted weight loss, reduction in BMI, or prevention of weight gain as intervention targets, however. Indeed, these interventions are associated with modest or no weight loss (e.g., ~4-lb difference between intervention and control throughout 3 years in the Women's Intervention Nutrition Study [Chlebowski et al., 2000] and no difference between intervention and control participants in the WHEL Study [Thomson et al., 2004]). Thus, existing studies of dietary fat intake reduction in breast cancer populations are not addressing the question of weight loss in breast cancer patients and survivors.

Exercise Interventions in Breast Cancer Patients and Survivors

In one clinical trial, 121 stage I-II breast cancer patients were randomized to control or self-directed or supervised exercise (Segal et al., 2001). Physical functioning was favorably ($p < .01$) impacted by exercise. Weight loss was not an intervention target, however, and only in the subset "supervised exercise in women not receiving chemotherapy" was reduced body weight (−3.8 kg) seen. Several other randomized trials of exercise in breast cancer patients and survivors have been reported, and all involved much smaller study populations (Courneya, 2003). Typically the intervention lasted only ~12 weeks, with a goal of change in fitness. Thus, existing studies of exercise in cancer populations have not targeted or achieved substantial weight reduction. There may be several quality of life and other beneficial effects of exercise in breast cancer survivors beyond weight loss and maintenance, so it is important to include exercise as part of the weight loss intervention. Furthermore, in women without breast cancer, exercise has been shown to promote weight maintenance after a weight loss intervention (NHLBI Obesity Education Initiative, 1998).

SUMMARY

Overweight and obesity are associated with poor prognosis in breast cancer patients. There have been no randomized clinical trials testing the effect of weight loss on recurrence or survival in overweight or obese breast cancer patients, however. In the absence of clinical trial data, most individual patients should be advised to avoid weight gain through the cancer treatment process. In addition, weight loss is probably safe, and perhaps helpful, for overweight and obese breast cancer survivors who are otherwise healthy.

References

Andreoli, A., Monteleone, M., Van Loan, M., Promenzio, L., Tarantino, U., and De Lorenzo, A. 2001. Effects of different sports on bone density and muscle mass in highly trained athletes. *Med Sci Sports Exerc* **33**(4): 507–511.

Arterburn, D., DeLaet, D., and Flum, D. 2005. Obesity. *Clin Evid* **13**: 707–725.

Aslani, A., Smith, R., and Allen, B. 1999. Changes in body composition during breast cancer chemotherapy with the CMF-regimen. *Breast Cancer Res Treat* **57**(3): 285–290.

Barber, G.R., Miransky, J., Brown, A.E., Coit, D.G., Lewis, F.M., Thaler, H.T., Kiehn, T.E., and Armstrong, D. 1995. Direct observations of surgical wound infections at a comprehensive cancer center. *Arch Surg* **130**(10): 1042–1047.

Bastarrachea, J., Hortobagyi, G.N., Smith, T.L., Kau, S.W., and Buzdar, A.U. 1994. Obesity as an adverse prognostic factor for patients receiving adjuvant chemotherapy for breast cancer. *Ann Intern Med* **120**(1): 18–25.

Baumgartner, K., Baumgartner, R., Hunt, W., Crumley, D., Gilliland, F., McTiernan, A., Bernstein, L., and Ballard-Barbash, R. 2004. Association of body composition and weight history with breast cancer prognostic markers: a divergent pattern between Hispanic and non-Hispanic white women. *Am J Epidemiol* **160**(11): 1087–1097.

Belfiore, A., Frittitta, L., and Costantino, A. 1996. Insulin receptors in breast cancer. *Ann NY Acad Sci* **784**: 173–188.

Bernstein, L., Deapen, D., Cerhan, J.R., Schwartz, S.M., Liff, J., McGann-Maloney, E., Perlman, J.A., and Ford, L. 1999. Tamoxifen therapy for breast cancer and endometrial cancer risk. *J Natl Cancer Inst* **91**(19): 1654–1662.

Blackburn, G.L. 1999. Benefits of weight loss in the treatment of obesity. *Am J Clin Nutr* **69**(3): 347–349.

Blackburn, H. 1992. The three beauties: bench, clinical, and population research. *Circulation* **86**(4): 1323–1331.

Blann, A., Byrne, G., and Baildam, A. 2002. Increased soluble intercellular adhesion molecule-1, breast cancer and the acute phase response. *Blood Coagul Fibrinolysis* 2002; **13**: 165–168.

Bonomi, P., Bunting, N., Fishman, D., Wolter, J., et al. 1984. Weight gain during adjuvant chemotherapy or hormono-chemotherapy for stage II breast cancer evaluated in relation to disease free survival (DFS) [abstract]. *Breast Cancer Res Treat* **4**: 339.

Borugian, M., Sheps, S., Kim-Sing, C., Olivotto, I., Van Patten, C., Dunn, B., Coldman, A., Potter, J., Gallagher, R., and Hislop, T. 2003. Waist-to-hip ratio and breast cancer mortality. *Am J Epidemiol* **158**(10): 963–968.

Boyd, N., Campbell, J., and Germanson, T. 1981. Body weight and prognosis in breast cancer. *J Natl Cancer Inst* **67**(4): 785–789.

Boyd, N.F., Greenberg, C., Lockwood, G., Little, L., Martin, L., Byng, J., Yaffe, M., and Tritchler, D. 1997. Effects at two years of a low-fat, high-carbohydrate diet on radiologic features of the breast: results from a randomized trial. Canadian Diet and Breast Cancer Prevention Study Group. *J Natl Cancer Inst* **89**(7): 488–496.

Brolin, R.E. 2002. Bariatric surgery and long-term control of morbid obesity. *JAMA* **288**(22): 2793–2796.

Brown, J.K., Byers, T., Doyle, C., Coumeya, K.S., Demark-Wahnefried, W., Kushi, L.H., McTieman, A., Rock, C.L., Aziz, N., Bloch, A.S., Eldridge, B., Hamilton, K., Katzin, C., Koonce, A., Main, J., Mobley, C., Morra, M.E., Pierce, M.S., and Sawyer, K.A. 2003. Nutrition and physical activity during and after cancer treatment: an American Cancer Society guide for informed choices. *CA Cancer J Clin* **53**(5): 268–291.

Calle, E.E., Rodriguez, C., Walker-Thurmond, K., and Thun, M.J. 2003. Overweight, obesity, and mortality from cancer in a prospectively studied cohort of U.S. adults. *N Engl J Med* **348**(17): 1625–1638.

Camoriano, J.K., Loprinzi, C.L., Ingle, J.N., Therneau, T.M., Krook, J.E., and Veeder, M.H. 1990. Weight change in women treated with adjuvant therapy or observed following mastectomy for node-positive breast cancer. *J Clin Oncol* **8**(8): 1327–1334.

Cauley, J.A., Gutai, J.P., Kuller, L.H., LeDonne, D., and Powell, J.G. 1989. The epidemiology of serum sex hormones in postmenopausal women. *Am J Epidemiol* **129**(6): 1120–1131.

Chang, S., Alderfer, J., Asmar, L., and Buzdar, A. Inflammatory breast cancer survival: the role of obesity and menopausal status at diagnosis. *Breast Cancer Res Treat* **64**(2): 157–163.

Cheney, C.L., Mahloch, J., and Freeny, P. 1997. Computerized tomography assessment of women with weight changes associated with adjuvant treatment for breast cancer. *Am J Clin Nutr* **66**(1): 141–146.

Chlebowski, R.T., Aiello, E., and McTiernan, A. 2002. Weight loss in breast cancer patient management. *J Clin Oncol* **20**(4): 1128–1143.

Chlebowski, R.T., Blackburn, G., Winters, B., Goodman, M., et al. 2000. Long term adherence to dietary fat reduction in the Women's Intervention Nutrition Study. *Proc Am Soc Clin Oncol* **19**: 207.

Chlebowski, R.T., Blackburn, G.L., Buzzard, I.M., Rose, D.P., Martino, S., Khandekar, J.D., York, R.M., Jeffery, R.W., Elashoff, R.M., and Wynder, E.L. 1993. Adherence to a dietary fat intake reduction program in postmenopausal women receiving therapy for early breast cancer. The Women's Intervention Nutrition Study. *J Clin Oncol* **11**(11): 2072–2080.

Chlebowski, R.T., Weiner, J.M., Reynolds, R., Luce, J., Bulcavage, L., and Bateman, J.R. 1986. Long-term survival following relapse after 5-FU but not CMF adjuvant breast cancer therapy. *Breast Cancer Res Treat* **7**(1): 23–30.

Clark, M.M., Abrams, D.B., Niaura, R.S., Eaton, C.A., and Rossi, J.S. 1991. Self-efficacy in weight management. *J Consult Clin Psychol* **59**(5): 739–744.

Clark, M.M., Cargill, B.R., Medeiros, M.L., and Pera, V. 1996. Changes in self-efficacy following obesity treatment. *Obes Res* **4**(2): 179–181.

Coates, R., Clark, W., and Greenburg, R. 1990. Race, nutritional status, and survival from breast cancer. *J Natl Cancer Inst* **82**: 1684–1692.

Corbould, A.M., Judd, S.J., and Rodgers, R.J. 1998. Expression of types 1, 2, and 3 17 beta-hydroxysteroid dehydrogenase in subcutaneous abdominal and intra-abdominal adipose tissue of women. *J Clin Endocrinol Metab* **83**(1): 187–194.

Courneya, K.S. 2003. Exercise in cancer survivors: an overview of research. *Med Sci Sports Exerc* **35**(11): 1846–1852.

de Waard, F., Ramlau, R., Mulders, Y., de Vries, T., and van Waveren. S. 1993. A feasibility study on weight reduction in obese postmenopausal breast cancer patients. *Eur J Cancer Prev* **2**(3): 233–238.

Demark-Wahnefried, W., Hars, V., and Conaway, M. 1997. Reduced rates of metabolism and decreased physical activity in breast cancer patients receiving adjuvant chemotherapy. *Am J Clin Nutr* **65**(5): 1495–1501.

Demark-Wahnefried, W., Peterson, B., and Winer, E. 2001. Changes in weight, body composition, and factors influencing energy balance among premenopausal breast cancer patients receiving adjuvant chemotherapy. *J Clin Oncol* **19**: 2381–2389.

Demark-Wahnefried, W., Rimer, B.K., and Winer, E.P. 1997. Weight gain in women diagnosed with breast cancer. *J Am Diet Assoc* **97**(5): 519–526, 529; quiz 527–528.

Demark-Wahnefried, W., Winer, E., and Rimer, B. 1993. Why women gain weight with adjuvant chemotherapy for breast cancer. (review). *J Clin Oncol* **11**(7): 1418–1429.

den Tonkelaar, I., de Waard, F., Seidell, J., and Fracheboud, J. 1995. Obesity and subcutaneous fat patterning in relation to survival of postmenopausal breast cancer patients participating in the DOM-project. *Breast Cancer Res Treat* **34**(2): 129–137.

Dignam, J., Wieand, K., Johnson, K., Fisher, B., Xu, L., and Mamounas, E. 2003. Obesity, tamoxifen use, and outcomes in women with estrogen receptor-positive early-stage breast cancer. *J Natl Cancer Inst* **95**(19): 1467–1476.

Dixon, J., Moritz, D., and Baker, F. 1978. Breast cancer and weight gain: an unexpected finding. *Oncol Nurs Forum* **5**(3): 5–7.

Djuric, Z., DiLaura, N.M., Jenkins, I., Darga, L., Jen, C.K., Mood, D., Bradley, E., and Hryniuk, W.M. 2002. Combining weight-loss counseling with the Weight Watchers plan for obese breast cancer survivors. *Obes Res* **10**(7): 657–665.

Donegan, W.L., Hartz, A.J., and Rimm, A.A. 1978a. The association of body weight with recurrent cancer of the breast. *Cancer* **41**(4): 1590–1594.

Donegan, W.L., Jayich, S., Koehler, M.R., et al. 1978b. The prognostic implications of obesity for the surgical cure of breast cancer. *Breast Dis Breast* **4**: 14–17.

Endogenous Hormones and Breast Cancer Collaborative Group. 2002. Endogenous sex hormones and breast cancer in postmenopausal women: reanalysis of nine prospective studies. *J Natl Cancer Inst* **94**(8): 606–616.

Ewertz, M., Gillanders, S., Meyer, L., and Zedeler, K. 1991. Survival of breast cancer patients in relation to factors which affect the risk of developing breast cancer. *Int J Cancer* **49**(4): 526–530.

Faber-Langendoen, K. 1996. Weight gain in women receiving adjuvant chemotherapy for breast cancer. *JAMA* **276**(11): 855–856.

Fisher, B., Costantino, J.P., Wickerham, D.L., Redmond, C.K., Kavanah, M., Cronin, W.M., Vogel, V., Robidoux, A., Dimitrov, N., Atkins, J., Daly, M., Wieand, S., Tan-Chiu, E., Ford, L., and Wolmark, N. 1998. Tamoxifen for prevention of breast cancer: report of the National Surgical Adjuvant Breast and Bowel Project P-1 Study. *J Natl Cancer Inst* **90**(18): 1371–1388.

Flegal, K.M., Carroll, M.D., Kuczmarski, R.J., and Johnson, C.L. 1998. Overweight and obesity in the United States: prevalence and trends, 1960–1994. *Int J Obes Relat Metab Disord* **22**(1): 39–47.

Folsom, A.R., Kaye, S.A., Sellers, T.A., Hong, C-P., Cerhan, J.R., Potter, J.D., and Prineas, R.J. 1993. Body fat distribution and 5-year risk of death in older women. *JAMA* **269**(4): 483–487.

Foltz, A.T. 1985. Weight gain among stage II breast cancer patients: a study of five factors. *Oncol Nurs Forum* **12**(3): 21–26.

Forouhi, P., Dixon, J.M., Leonard, R.C., and Chetty, U. 1995. Prospective randomized study of surgical morbidity following primary systemic therapy for breast cancer. *Br J Surg* **82**(1): 79–82.

Foster, G.D., Wyatt, H.R., Hill, J.O., McGuckin, B.G., Brill, C., Mohammed, B.S., Szapary, P.O., Rader, D.J., Edman, J.S., and Klein, S. 2003. A randomized trial of a low-carbohydrate diet for obesity. *N Engl J Med* **348**(21): 2082–2090.

Galanis, D.J., Kolonel, L.N., Lee, J., and Le Marchand, L. 1998. Anthropometric predictors of breast cancer incidence and survival in a multiethnic cohort of female residents of Hawaii, United States. *Cancer Causes Control* **9**(2): 217–224.

Ganz, P.A., Coscarelli, A., Fred, C., Kahn, B., Polinsky, M.L., and Petersen, L. 1996. Breast cancer survivors: psychosocial concerns and quality of life. *Breast Cancer Res Treat* **38**(2): 183–199.

Ganz, P.A., Desmond, K.A., Leedham, B., Rowland, J.H., Meyerowitz, B.E., and Belin, TR. 2002. Quality of life in long-term, disease-free survivors of breast cancer: a follow-up study. *J Natl Cancer Inst* **94**(1): 39–49.

Ganz, P.A., Greendale, G.A., Petersen, L., Kahn, B., and Bower, J.E. 2003. Breast Cancer in Younger Women: Reproductive and Late Health Effects of Treatment. *J Clin Oncol* **21**(22): 4184–4193.

Ganz, P.A., Rowland, J.H., Meyerowitz, B.E., and Desmond, K.A. 1998. Impact of different adjuvant therapy strategies on quality of life in breast cancer survivors. *Recent Results Cancer Res* **152**: 396–411.

Gelber, R.D., Bonetti, M., Cole, B.F., Gelber, S., and Goldhirsch, A. 1998. Quality of life assessment in the adjuvant setting: is it relevant? International Breast Cancer Study Group. *Recent Results Cancer Res* **152**: 373–389.

Goodwin, P., Esplen, M.J., Butler, K., Winocur, J., Pritchard, K., Brazel, S., Gao, J., and Miller, A. 1998. Multidisciplinary weight management in locoregional breast cancer: results of a phase II study. *Breast Cancer Res Treat* **48**(1): 53–64.

Goodwin, P.J., Ennis, M., and Pritchard, K.I., et al. 2000. Fasting insulin presicts distant disease free survival and overall survival in women with operable breast cancer. *Proc Am Soc Clin Oncol* **19**: 272.

Goodwin, P.J., Ennis, M., Pritchard, K.I., McCready, D., Koo, J., Sidlofsky, S., Trudeau, M., Hood, N., and Redwood, S. 1999. Adjuvant treatment and onset of menopause predict weight gain after breast cancer diagnosis. *J Clin Oncol* **17**(1): 120–129.

Goodwin, P.J., Ennis, M., Pritchard, K.I., Trudeau, M.E., Koo, J., Madarnas, Y., Hartwick, W., Hoffman, B., and Hood, N. 2002. Fasting insulin and outcome in early-stage breast cancer: results of a prospective cohort study. *J Clin Oncol* **20**(1): 42–51.

Goodwin, P.J., Esplen, M.J., Winocur, J., Butler, K., and Pritchard, K.I. 1995. Development of a weight management program in women with newly diagnosed locoregional breast cancer. *In* "Psychosomatic Obstetrics and Gynecology" (J. Bitzer and M. Stauber, Eds), pp. 491–496. Monduzzi Editore, International Proceedings Division, Bologna (Italy).

Graham, L.E., 2nd, Taylor, C.B., Hovell, M.F., and Siegel, W. 1983. Five-year follow-up to a behavioral weight-loss program. *J Consult Clin Psychol* **51**(2): 322–323.

Greenburg, E., Vessey, M., and McPherson, K. 1985. Body size and survival in premenopausal breast cancer. *Br J Cancer* **51**: 691–697.

Hardman, A.E., Jones, P.R., Norgan, N.G., and Hudson, A. 1992. Brisk walking improves endurance fitness without changing body fatness in previously sedentary women. *Eur J Appl Physiol Occup Physiol* **65**(4): 354–359.

Haybittle, J., Houghton, J., and Baum, M. 1997. Social class and weight as prognostic factors in early breast cancer. *Br J Cancer* **75**(5): 729–733.

Heasman, K.Z., Sutherland, H.J., Campbell, J.A., et al. 1985. Dietary fat consumption and survival among women with breast cancer. *J Natl Cancer Inst* **75**: 37–41.

Hebert, J.R., Hurley, T.G., and Ma, Y. 1998. The effect of dietary exposures on recurrence and mortality in early stage breast cancer. *Breast Cancer Res Treat* **51**(1): 17–28.

Holmberg, L., Lund, E., Bergstrom, R., Adami, H.O., and Meirik, O. 1994. Oral contraceptives and prognosis in breast cancer: effects of duration, latency, recency, age at first use and relation to parity and body mass index in young women with breast cancer. *Eur J Cancer* **30A**(3): 351–354.

Holmes, M.D., Stampfer, M.J., Colditz, G.A., Rosner, B., Hunter, D.J., and Willett, W.C. 1999. Dietary factors and the survival of women with breast carcinoma. *Cancer* **86**(5): 826–835.

Hryniuk, W., Banerjee, M., and Du, W. 2001. Adjuvant tamoxifen may be relatively ineffective in women with diabetes and breast cancer. *Proc Am Soc Clin Oncol* **20**: 36a.

Huntington, M.O. 1985. Weight gain in patients receiving adjuvant chemotherapy for carcinoma of the breast. *Cancer* **56**(3): 472–474.

International Agency for Research on Cancer. 2002a. "IARC Handbooks of Cancer Prevention," Vol. 6, "Weight Control and Physical Activity." IARC Press, Lyon.

International Agency for Research on Cancer. 2002b. "Weight Control and Physical Activity." IARC Press, Lyon.

Irwin, M.L., Crumley, D., McTiernan, A., Bernstein, L., Baumgartner, R., Gilliland, F.D., Kriska, A., and Ballard-Barbash, R. 2003a. Physical activity levels before and after a diagnosis of breast carcinoma: the Health, Eating, Activity, and Lifestyle (HEAL) study. *Cancer* **97**(7): 1746–1757.

Irwin, M.L., Yasui, Y., Ulrich, C.M., Bowen, D., Rudolph, R.E., Schwartz, R.S., Yukawa, M., Aiello, E., Potter, J.D., and McTiernan, A. 2003b. Effect of exercise on total and intra-abdominal body fat in postmenopausal women: a randomized controlled trial. *JAMA* **289**(3): 323–330.

Jain, M., and Miller, A.B. 1994. Pre-morbid body size and the prognosis of women with breast cancer. *Int J Cancer* **59**(3): 363–368.

Jen, K., Djuric, Z., DiLaura, N., Buison, A., Redd, J., Maranci, V., and Hryniuk, W. 2004. Improvement of metabolism among obese breast cancer survivors in differing weight loss regimens. *Obes Res* **12**(2): 306–312.

Jenkins, I., Djuric, Z., Darga, L., DiLaura, N., Magnan, M., and Hryniuk, W. 2003. Relationship of psychiatric diagnosis and weight loss maintenance in obese breast cancer survivors. *Obes Res* **11**(11): 1369–1375.

Kaaks, R., Toniolo, P., Akhmedkhanov, A., Lukanova, A., Biessy, C., Dechaud, H., Rinaldi, S., Zeleniuch-Jacquotte, A., Shore, R.E., and Riboli, E. 2000. Serum C-peptide, insulin-like growth factor (IGF)-I, IGF-binding proteins, and colorectal cancer risk in women. *J Natl Cancer Inst* **92**: 1592–1600.

Kallab, A.M., Taturn, P., Dipiro, C., Litaher, M., and Jillella, A. 2000. Severe obesity as a risk factor for congestive heart failure (CHF) in women receiving doxorubicin for breast cancer. *Proc Am Soc Clin Oncol* **19**: 366.

Kamby, C., Ejlertsen, B., Andersen, J., Birkler, N.E., Ryitter, L., Zedeler, K., and Rose, C. 1989. Body size and menopausal status in relation to the pattern of spread in recurrent breast cancer. *Acta Oncol* **28**(6): 795–799.

Katoh, A., Watzlaf, V., and D'Amico, F. 1994. An examination of obesity and breast cancer survival in post-menopausal women. *Br J Cancer* **70**: 928–933.

Katoh, J., Hara, Y., and Narutaki, K. 1994. Cardiorespiratory effects of weight reduction by exercise in middle-aged women with obesity. *J Int Med Res* **22**(3): 160–164.

Keim, N.L., Barbieri, T.F., Van Loan, M.D., and Anderson, B.L. 1990. Energy expenditure and physical performance in overweight women: response to training with and without caloric restriction. *Metabolism* **39**(6): 651–658.

Key, T., Appleby, P., Reeves, G., Roddam, A., Dorgan, J., Longcope, C., Stanczyk, F., Stephenson, H., Jr., Falk, R., Miller, R., Schatzkin, A., Allen, D., Fentiman, I., Key, T., Wang, D., Dowsett, M., Thomas, H., Hankinson, S., Toniolo, P., Akhmedkhanov, A., Koenig, K., Shore, R., Zeleniuch-Jacquotte, A., Berrino, F., Muti, P., Micheli, A., Krogh, V., Sieri, S., Pala, V., Venturelli, E., Secreto, G., Barrett-Connor, E., Laughlin, G., Kabuto, M., Akiba, S., Stevens, R., Neriishi, K., Land, C., Cauley, J., Kuller, L., Cummings, S., Helzlsouer, K., Alberg, A., Bush, T., Comstock, G., Gordon, G., Miller, S., Longcope C., and the Endogenous Hormones Breast Cancer Collaborative Group. 2003. Body mass index, serum sex hormones, and breast cancer risk in postmenopausal women. *J Natl Cancer Inst* **95**(16): 1218–1226.

Kiernan, M., and Winkleby, M. 2000. Identifying patients for weight-loss treatment: an empirical evaluation of the NHLBI obesity education initiative expert panel treatment recommendations. *Arch Intern Med* **160**(14): 2169–2176.

Kimura, M. 1990. Obesity as prognostic factors in breast cancer. *Diabetes Res Clin Pract* **10**(Suppl 1): S247–S251.

Knight, J.A., Martin, L.J., Greenberg, C.V., Lockwood, G.A., Byng, J.W., Yaffe, M.J., Tritchler, D.L., and Boyd, N.F. 1999. Macronutrient intake and change in mammographic density at menopause: results from a randomized trial. *Cancer Epidemiol Biomarkers Prev* **8**(2): 123–128.

Knobf, M.K., Mullen, J.C., Xistris, D., and Moritz, D.A. 1983. Weight gain in women with breast cancer receiving adjuvant chemotherapy. *Oncol Nurs Forum* **10**(2): 28–33.

Knowler, W.C., Barrett-Connor, E., Fowler, S.E., Hamman, R.F., Lachin, J.M., Walker, E.A., and Nathan, D.M. 2002. Reduction in the incidence of type 2 diabetes with lifestyle intervention or metformin. *N Engl J Med* **346**(6): 393–403.

Kornblith, A.B., Hollis, D.R., Zuckerman, E., Lyss, A.P., Canellos, G.P., Cooper, M.R., Herndon, J.E., 2nd, Phillips, C.A., Abrams, J., Aisner, J., et al. 1993. Effect of megestrol acetate on quality of life in a dose-response trial in women with advanced breast cancer. The Cancer and Leukemia Group B. *J Clin Oncol* **11**(11): 2081–2089.

Kumanyika, S.K., Van Horn, L., Bowen, D., Perri, M.G., Rolls, B.J., Czajkowski, S.M., and Schron, E. 2000. Maintenance of dietary behavior change. *Health Psychol* **19**(1 Suppl): 42–56.

Kumar, N., Cantor, A., Allen, K., and Cox, C. 2000. Android obesity at diagnosis and breast carcinoma survival: Evaluation of the effects of anthropometric variables at diagnosis, including body composition and body fat distribution and weight gain during life span, and survival from breast carcinoma. *Cancer* **88**(12): 2751–2757.

Kyogoku, S., Hirohata, T., Takeshita, S., Nomura, Y., and Shigematsu, T., 1990. Horie A. Survival of breast-cancer patients and body size indicators. *Int J Cancer* **46**(5): 824–831.

Lees, A., Jenkins, H., and May, C. 1989. Risk factors and 10-year breast cancer survival in northern Alberta. *Breast Cancer Res Treat* **13**: 143–151.

Lethaby, A.E., Mason, B.H., Harvey, V.J., and Holdaway, I.M. 1996. Survival of women with node negative breast cancer in the Auckland region. *N Z Med J* **109**(1029): 330–333.

Levine, E.G., Raczynski, J.M., and Carpenter, J.T. 1991. Weight gain with breast cancer adjuvant treatment. *Cancer* **67**(7): 1954–1959.

Li, C.I., Malone, K.E., Porter, P.L., and Daling, J.R. 2003. Epidemiologic and molecular risk factors for contralateral breast cancer among young women. *Br J Cancer* **89**(3): 513–518.

Loprinzi, C.L., Athmann, L.M., Kardinal, C.G., O'Fallon, J.R., See, J.A., Bruce, B.K., Dose, A.M., Miser, A.W., Kern, P.S., Tschetter, L.K., and Rayson, S. 1996. Randomized trial of dietician counseling to try to prevent weight gain associated with breast cancer adjuvant chemotherapy. *Oncology* **53**(3): 228–232.

Maehle, B., and Tretli, S. 1996. Pre-morbid body-mass-index in breast cancer: reversed effect on survival in hormone receptor negative patients. *Breast Cancer Res Treat* **41**: 123–130.

Mahmoud, F., and Rivera, N. 2002. The role of C-reactive protein as a prognostic indicator in advanced cancer. *Curr Oncol Rep* **4**: 250–255.

McTiernan, A., Rajan, K.B., Tworoger, S.S., Irwin, M., Bernstein, L., Baumgartner, R., Gilliland, F., Stanczyk, F.Z., Yasui, Y., and Ballard-Barbash, R. 2003. Adiposity and sex hormones in postmenopausal breast cancer survivors. *J Clin Oncol* **21**(10): 1961–1966.

McTiernan, A., Ulrich, C., Kumai, C., Bean, D., Schwartz, R., Mahloch, J., Hastings, R., Gralow, J., and Potter, J.D. 1998. Anthropometric and hormone effects of an eight-week exercise-diet intervention in breast cancer patients: results of a pilot study. *Cancer Epidemiol Biomarkers Prev* **7**(6): 477–481.

McTigue, K.M., Harris, R., Hemphill, B., Lux, L., Sutton, S., Bunton, A.J., and Lohr, K.N. 2003. Screening and interventions for obesity in adults: summary of the evidence for the U.S. Preventive Services Task Force. *Ann Intern Med* **139**(11): 933–949.

Michael, Y.L., Kawachi, I., Berkman, L.F., Holmes, M.D., and Colditz, G.A. 2000. The persistent impact of breast carcinoma on functional health status: prospective evidence from the Nurses' Health Study. *Cancer* **89**(11): 2176–2186.

Mohle-Boetani, J.C., Grosser, S., Whittemore, A.S., Malec, M., Kampert, J.B., and Paffenbarger, R.S., Jr. 1988. Body size, reproductive factors, and breast cancer survival. *Prev Med* **17**(5): 634–642.

Morimoto, L.M., White, E., Chen, Z., Chlebowski, R.T., Hays, J., Kuller, L., Lopez, A.M., Manson, J., Margolis, K.L., Muti, P.C., Stefanick, M.L., and McTiernan, A. 2002. Obesity, body size, and risk of postmenopausal breast cancer: the Women's Health Initiative (United States). *Cancer Causes Control* **13**(8): 741–751.

National Heart, Lung, and Blood Institute Obesity Education Initiative. 1998. "Clinical Guidelines on the Identification, Evaluation, and Treatment of Overweight and Obesity in Adults: The Evidence Report, Executive Summary." National Heart, Lung, and Blood Institute, Bethesda, MD.

Newcomb, P., Klein, R., Klein, B., Haffner, S., Mares-Perlman, J., Cruickshanks, K., and Marcus, P. 1995. Association of dietary and life-style factors with sex hormones in postmenopausal women. *Epidemiology* **6**: 318–321.

Newman, S.C., Lees, A.W., and Jenkins, H.J. 1997. The effect of body mass index and oestrogen receptor level on survival of breast cancer patients. *Int J Epidemiol* **26**(3): 484–490.

Newman, S.C., Miller, A.B., and Howe, G.R. 1986. A study of the effect of weight and dietary fat on breast cancer survival time. *Am J Epidemiol* **123**(5): 767–774.

Nieman, D., Henson, D., Nehlsen-Cannarella, S., Ekkens, M., Utter, A., Butterworth, D., and Fagoaga, O. 1999. Influence of obesity on immune function. *J Am Diet Assoc* **99**(3): 294–299.

Nieman, D.C., Cook, V.D., Henson, D.A., Suttles, J., Rejeski, W.J., Ribisl, P.M., Fagoaga, O.R., and Nehlsen-Cannarella, S.L. 1995. Moderate exercise training and natural killer cell cytotoxic activity in breast cancer patients. *Int J Sports Med* **16**(5): 334–337.

Obermair, A., Kurz, C., and Hanzal, E. 1995. The influence of obesity on the disease-free survival in primary breast cancer. *Anticancer Res* **15**(5B): 2265–2269.

O'Hanlan, D., Lynch, J., Cormican, M., and Given, H. 2002. The acute phase response in breast cancer. *Anticancer Res* **22**: 1289–1293.

Papa, V., and Belfiore, A. 1996. Insulin receptors in breast cancer: biological and clinical role. *J Endocrinol Invest* **19**(5): 324–333.

Perri, M.G. 1998. Maintenance of treatment effects in the long-term management of obesity. *Clin Psychol* **5**: 526–543.

Perri, M.G., and Fuller, P.R. 1995. Success and failure in the treatment of obesity: where do we go from here? *Med Exerc Nutr Health* **4**: 255–272.

Pierce, J., Faerber, S., Wright, F., Newman, V., Flatt, S., Kealey, S., Rock, C., Hryniuk, W., and Greenberg, E.R. 1997. Feasibility of a randomized trial of a high-vegetable diet to prevent breast cancer recurrence. *Nutr Cancer* **28**(3): 282–288.

Plymate, S., Hoop, R., and Jones, R. 1990. Regulation of sex hormone-binding globulin production by growth factors. *Metabolism* **39**: 967–970.

Pronk, N.P., and Wing, R.R. 1994. Physical activity and long-term maintenance of weight loss. *Obes Res* **2**: 587–599.

Reeves, M., Newcomb, P., Remington, P., Marcus, P., and MacKenzie, W. 1996. Body mass and breast cancer. Relationship between method of detection and stage of disease. *Cancer* **77**(2): 301–307.

Roche, A., Lohman, T., and Heymsfield, S. 1996. "Human Body Composition." Human Kinetics Publishers, Portland, OR.

Rock, C., McEligot, A., and Flatt, S. 2000. Eating pathology and obesity in women at risk for breast cancer recurrence. *Int J Eat Disord* **27**(2): 172–179.

Samaha, F.F., Iqbal, N., Seshadri, P., Chicano, K.L., Daily, D.A., McGrory, J., Williams, T., Williams, M., Gracely, E.J., and Stern, L. 2003. A low-carbohydrate as compared with a low-fat diet in severe obesity. *N Engl J Med* **348**(21): 2074–2081.

Saxe, G.A., Rock, C.L., Wicha, M.S., and Schottenfeld, D. 1999. Diet and risk for breast cancer recurrence and survival. *Breast Cancer Res Treat* **53**(3): 241–253.

Schatzkin, A. 1997. Dietary change as a strategy for preventing cancer. *Cancer Metastasis Rev* **16**(3–4): 377–392.

Segal, R., Evans, W., Johnson, D., Smith, J., Colletta, S., Gayton, J., Woodard, S., Wells, G., and Reid, R. 2001. Structured exercise improves physical functioning in women with stages I and II breast cancer: results of a randomized controlled trial. *J Clin Oncol* **19**(3): 657–665.

Senie, R.T., Rosen, P.P., Rhodes, P., Lesser, M.L., and Kinne, D.W. 1992. Obesity at diagnosis of breast carcinoma influences duration of disease-free survival. *Ann Intern Med* **116**(1): 26–32.

Shade, E., Ulrich, C., Wener, M., Wood, B., Yasui, Y., Lacroix, K., Potter, J., and McTiernan, A. 2004. Frequent intentional weight loss is associated with lower natural killer cell cytotoxicity in postmenopausal women: possible long-term immune effects. *J Am Diet Assoc* **104**(6): 903–912.

Shepherd, L., Parulekar, W., and Day, A. 2001. Weight gain during adjuvant therapy in high risk pre/perimenopausal breast cancer patients:

analysis of a National Cancer Institute of Canada Clinical Trials Group (NCIC CTG) Phase III Study. *Proc Am Soc Clin Oncol* **20**: 36a.

Siiteri, P.K. 1987. Adipose tissue as a source of hormones. *Am J Clin Nutr* **45**(1 Suppl): 277–282.

Sohrabi, A., Sandoz, J., Spratt, J.S., et al. 1981. Body weight and prognosis in breast cancer. *J Natl Cancer Inst* **67**: 785–789.

Tartter, P.I., Papatestas, A.E., Ioannovich, J., Mulvihill, M.N., Lesnick, G., and Aufses, A.H., Jr. 1981. Cholesterol and obesity as prognostic factors in breast cancer. *Cancer* **47**(9): 2222–2227.

Thomson, C., Rock, C., Giuliano, A., Newton, T., Cui, H., Reid, P., Green, T., and Alberts, D. 2004. Longitudinal changes in body weight and body composition among women previously treated for breast cancer consuming a high-vegetable, fruit and fiber, low-fat diet. *Eur J Nutr* **5**(1–8).

Tornberg, S., and Carstensen, J. 1993. Serum beta-lipoprotein, serum cholesterol and Quetelet's index as predictors for survival of breast cancer patients. *Eur J Cancer* **29A**(14): 2025–2030.

Tretli, S., and Ottestad, L. 1990. The effect of pre-morbid height and weight on the survival of breast cancer patients. *Br J Cancer* **62**: 299–303.

Tuomilehto, J., Lindstrom, J., Eriksson, J.G., Valle, T.T., Hamalainen, H., Ilanne-Parikka, P., Keinanen-Kiukaanniemi, S., Laakso, M., Louheranta, A., Rastas, M., Salminen, V., and Uusitupa, M. 2001. Prevention of type 2 diabetes mellitus by changes in lifestyle among subjects with impaired glucose tolerance. *N Engl J Med* **344**(18): 1343–1350.

van den Brandt, P.A., Spiegelman, D., Yaun, S-S., Adami, H-O., Beeson, L., Folsom, A.R., Fraser, G., Goldbohm, R.A., Graham, S., Kushi, L., Marshall, J.R., Miller, A.B., Rohan, T., Smith-Warner, S.A., Speizer, F.E., Willett, W.C., Wolk, A., and Hunter, D.J. 2000. Pooled analysis of prospective cohort studies on height, weight, and breast cancer risk. *Am J Epidemiol* **152**(6): 514–527.

Vatten, L., Foss, O., and Kvinnsland, S. 1991. Overall survival of breast cancer patients in relation to preclinically determined total serum cholesterol, body mass index, height and cigarette smoking: a population-based study. *Eur J Cancer Prev* **27**(5): 641–646.

Verkasalo, P.K., Thomas, H.V., Appleby, P.N., Davey, G.K., and Key, T.J. 2001. Circulating levels of sex hormones and their relation to risk factors for breast cancer: a cross-sectional study in 1092 pre- and postmenopausal women (United Kingdom). *Cancer Causes Control* **12**(1): 47–59.

Wadden, T.A., and Sarwer, D.B. 2000. Behavioral treatment of obesity. New approaches to an old disorder. *In* "The Management of Eating Disorders" (D. Goldstein, ed.). Humana Press, Totowa, NJ.

Wee, C., McCarthy, E., Davis, R., and Phillips, R. 2000. Screening for cervical and breast cancer: is obesity an unrecognized barrier to preventive care? *Ann Intern Med* **132**(9): 697–704.

Williams, G., Howell, A., and Jones, M. 1988. The relationship of body weight to response to endocrine therapy, steroid hormone receptors and survival of patients with advance cancer of the breast. *Br J Cancer* **58**: 631–634.

Wilmorem, J.H. 1996. Increasing physical activity: alterations in body mass and composition. *Am J Clin Nutr* **63**(3 Suppl): 456S–460S.

Yancik, R., Ganz, P.A., Varricchio, C.G., and Conley, B. 2001a. Perspectives on comorbidity and cancer in older patients: approaches to expand the knowledge base. *J Clin Oncol* **19**(4): 1147–1151.

Yancik, R., Wesley, M.N., Ries, L.A., Havlik, R.J., Edwards, B.K., and Yates, J.W. 2001b. Effect of age and comorbidity in postmenopausal breast cancer patients aged 55 years and older. *JAMA* **285**(7): 885–892.

Yee, D., and Lee, A. 2000. Crosstalk between the insulin-like growth factors and estrogens in breast cancer. *J Mammary Gland Biol Neoplasia* **5**(107–15).

Zhang, S., Folsom, A.R., Sellers, T.A., Kushi, L.H., and Potter, J.D. 1995. Better breast cancer survival for postmenopausal women who are less overweight and eat less fat. The Iowa Women's Health Study. *Cancer* **76**(2): 275–283.

CHAPTER

41

Nutrition Support of the Adult Cancer Patient

HEIDI J. SILVER, EVE CALLAHAN, AND GORDON L. JENSEN

INTRODUCTION

Twenty-five years ago, Bistrian et al. (1976) recognized that among hospitalized patients, those with cancer had the highest prevalence of undernutrition. Presently, more than half of all cancer patients and ~80% of those with gastrointestinal (GI) malignancies lose weight during the course of their disease (National Cancer Institute [NCI], 2004). More than two-thirds of these patients are adults 65 years or older with coexisting diseases. Weight loss and undernutrition contribute to morbidity and mortality. For example, Conti et al. (1977) found that weight loss in esophageal cancer patients with resectable tumors increased surgical risk. Additionally, Gianotti et al. (1995) showed in multiple regression analysis that preadmission weight loss of ≥10% of usual body weight was a strong predictor of postoperative infection (p = .02). Further, DeWys et al. (1980) observed 31–87% of 3047 patients enrolled in 12 chemotherapy protocols had weight loss before treatment and weight loss was related to decreased median survival. More recent estimates suggest that up to 40% of cancer-related deaths are secondary to impaired nutritional status and mortality is highest in older patients (Zeman, 1991).

The syndrome of cancer cachexia is characterized not only by weight loss but also anorexia and resultant decreased food intake, early meal satiety, alterations in taste and smell, weakness and fatigue, anemia, and edema (Heber et al., 1992). Within the options for medical nutrition therapy (MNT) interventions, nutrition support allows provision of nutrients (protein, carbohydrates, fat, water, vitamins, and trace elements) either through a tube into the stomach or small bowel (enteral nutrition support [EN]) or through a catheter into a peripheral or central vein (parenteral nutrition support [PN]). The primary goal of nutrition support in the cancer patient is to reverse undernutrition in a safe and cost-effective manner (American Society for Parenteral and Enteral Nutrition [ASPEN] Board of Directors and the Clinical Guidelines Task Force, 2002). Despite aggressive attempts to provide nutrition support in patients with cancer cachexia, most patients fail to gain weight consistently (Heber et al., 1992). Secondary goals of nutrition support focus on minimizing antineoplastic treatment side effects and enhancing quality of life.

ENTERAL NUTRITION SUPPORT

Indications

EN is typically provided to head, neck, and upper GI tract cancer patients in acute, community, and long-term care settings when patients are unable to chew, swallow, digest, and/or absorb adequately to meet nutrient requirements. One key reason EN is preferred to PN is that EN is more physiological; EN maintains gut mucosal barrier function and prevents endogenous gut bacterial translocation. For example, Jiang et al. (2003) randomized 40 patients with stomach or colon cancer into an EN or a PN group after tumor resection. Patients received isocaloric and isonitrogenous formulas initiated 3 days postoperatively. Intestinal permeability was measured by urinary excretion of lactulose and mannitol after administration on postoperative days 1, 7, and 12. Lactulose/mannitol ratio was significantly lower in the EN group on days 7 and 12, indicating increased gut mucosal integrity.

Copyright © 2006, Elsevier Inc.
All rights of reproduction in any form reserved.

In a study conducted by Bozzetti et al. (2001), 317 GI cancer patients from 10 institutions in Italy were randomly assigned to isocaloric and isonitrogenous EN or PN solutions for 1 week after surgery. EN patients had significantly fewer total and infectious complications. Additionally, the mean length of hospital stay for the EN group was almost half as long as that of the PN group (5.7 ± 2.9 vs 10.4 ± 4.5 hospital days, respectively).

In contrast, Fish et al. (1997) compared EN to PN of the same energy, nitrogen, and glutamine composition by randomly assigning 17 patients with gastric or pancreatic malignancies who were matched by age and body mass index (BMI) to receive either solution for 5 days postoperatively. No significant differences were observed for plasma amino acid profiles or nitrogen balance. Moreover, Braga et al. (2001) randomized 257 patients with upper GI tract cancer after surgery to early EN or PN solutions that were isocaloric and isonitrogenous for an average of 13 days. These authors observed no significant differences in nutritional variables (albumin, prealbumin, and retinol-binding protein) or immune function variables (delayed hypersensitivity response, polymorphonuclear phagocytosis, T lymphocytes, interleukin [IL]-2 receptors, IL-6, and C-reactive protein [CRP]) in a subgroup of these patients. Additionally, overall complication rate was similar (36% for EN vs 40% for PN). As in most studies comparing EN with PN, the EN group did not achieve their caloric goal as quickly as the PN group (4 days vs 1 day). However, a significant recovery of intestinal oxygen tension was observed earlier in EN patients and occurred from postoperative day 4 to study completion ($p < .01$).

The potential benefits of administering EN have also been investigated in comparison with oral intake and with intravenous fluid without PN or oral intake. Bozzetti et al. (1998) compared EN with a standard oral diet in 50 undernourished patients receiving two cycles (32 days) of concomitant chemotherapy and radiation therapy for esophageal cancer. During the course of treatment, the EN group maintained body weight and visceral proteins, whereas the oral diet group had a significant decrease in body weight and visceral proteins ($p = .01$). Notably, the findings from this study may underestimate the benefits of EN, as the EN group was more undernourished with a greater pretreatment weight loss than the oral diet group (15.5% vs 12.3% of usual body weight, $p < .02$).

In evaluating the provision of early EN (i.e., EN initiated within 24 hours postoperatively), Hochwald et al. (1997) demonstrated that early EN resulted in improved protein metabolism in 29 patients undergoing curative resection for an upper GI tract malignancy. In this study, patients were randomized to standard intravenous fluids (n = 17) or early EN (n = 12). The early EN patients had significantly decreased protein catabolism, as measured by continuous leucine infusion, and improved net whole body protein balance. Similar results in achieving positive nitrogen balance with provision of EN were observed in studies conducted in the late 1980s in nonsurgical cancer patients (Daly et al., 1987).

It is also generally agreed that EN is more cost effective than PN (ASPEN, 2002). However, only a few studies have compared the costs of EN with PN and the only one conducted with cancer patients exclusively was the aforementioned study by Braga et al. (2001). Like other studies, the main focus of these investigators was to compare EN and PN solution costs. Braga et al. (2001) estimated that using EN instead of PN would save $65 daily. In a retrospective comparison of the costs associated with home EN (HEN) to home PN (HPN) based on Medicare charges in 1996, Reddy and Malone (1998) found that the average annual cost per patient for EN solutions ($9535 ± 13,980) was about one-fifth the cost of PN solutions ($55,193 ± 30,596). Yet, the entire cost of both EN and PN may be greater than what has been reported, as it would encompass other costs such as placement of the feeding tube or catheter, infusion pump loan, administration set and dressing kit, and costs of follow-up care including emergency room, physician office or clinic visits, home nursing and other professional therapeutic care, medication therapy, laboratory charges, and hospital readmissions.

Enteral Access

Short-term and long-term techniques of enteral access are available for cancer patients who need EN. Short-time techniques such as nasogastric and nasojejunal feeding tube placement are considered easier to insert and lower in cost. However, these techniques are usually not used longer than 4–6 weeks because of the potential for patient discomfort (e.g., nasal irritation), technical failure (e.g., tube displacement), and/or long-term complications. Nasoenteric tubes are inserted through the nose, into the pharynx, down the esophagus, and into the stomach (nasogastric); or through the stomach into the duodenum (nasoduodenal); or through the duodenum into the jejunum (nasojejunal). Nasogastric feeding may be contraindicated for patients at risk of aspiration or those with delayed gastric emptying.

For long-term EN, access techniques are typically through the abdominal wall (enterostomy) into the stomach (gastrostomy) or the jejunum (jejunostomy). A gastrostomy or jejunostomy can be performed by endoscopy, interventional radiology, or surgically. The percutaneous endoscopic gastrostomy (PEG) technique is the most common method for placing a gastrostomy tube. PEG tubes are usually placed in an endoscopy suite using intravenous conscious sedation and local anesthesia. Three methods have been described for PEG placement commonly referred to as "pull," "push," and "poke" (Sacks et al., 1983; Russell et al., 1984; Ponsky, 1989). Contraindications to PEG tubes for EN are nonfunctioning gut, high risk for aspiration pneumonia, gastroesophageal reflux, ascites, or obstructions of the pharynx or esophagus that prevent passage of the endoscope (Vanek, 2002a). Percutaneous tubes can also be placed by interventional radiology.

Two procedures are most commonly used for surgical placement of gastrostomy tubes in the operating room. The Stamm gastrostomy (1894) is an open surgical procedure that requires an incision through the abdominal wall, suturing the stomach to the abdominal wall, and inserting a catheter through that is sutured in place. The Witzel technique (1891) is more frequently used for jejunal feeding. In comparing the "push" PEG technique with surgical gastrostomy using the Stamm procedure, Steigmann et al. (1990) observed no significant differences in tube function, complication rates, mortality, or costs. Still, the PEG is used most frequently in the adult oncology population, as it can be performed as an ambulatory procedure. Gastric buttons, which are skin-level devices, are often preferable for children and more active ambulatory adult patients because they offer a low-profile tube with a shorter catheter length (Gauderer et al., 1980).

For patients who require small-bowel feeding, such as those at high risk for aspiration or those who have had esophagectomy, small-bore percutaneous endoscopic jejunostomy or surgical jejunostomy tubes have been used with similar outcomes as PEG tubes (Bergstrom et al., 1995). Jejunostomy tubes are often anchored in place with an external suture to prevent migration or removal. Combination gastrojejunal tubes are placed endoscopically to allow simultaneous gastric decompression with jejunal feeding. Both gastrostomy and jejunostomy tubes can be replaced in an established tract.

Enteral Formula Selection

A wide variety of liquid formulas are commercially available for enteral support of cancer patients. Some are also designed to be used as oral supplements depending on the palatability of the formulation. The choice of an enteral formula is typically patient specific. In addition to meeting energy, protein, and volume requirements, formula selection is influenced by the type of feeding access and the potential benefit from formulas enhanced by specialty nutrients. All formulas are supplemented with vitamins, minerals, and trace elements to meet recommended daily allowances (RDA) (Food and Nutrition Board [FNB], 1989). Formulas are typically categorized as polymeric, chemically defined, disease-specific, or specialty formulas.

Polymeric (standard) formulas are usually lactose free and provide 1 kcal/ml. They are composed of intact nutrients (whole proteins, disaccharides, and triglycerides) and formulated so that 12–20% of the total calories are protein, 45–60% are carbohydrate, and 30–40% are fat. Some intact formulas are concentrated to provide more calories in less volume such as 1.5 or 2.0 kcal/ml or a higher nitrogen load per nonprotein calorie for patients with increased protein requirements. Most standard formulas were designed to be low in fiber and residue. Fiber-supplemented formulas are usually enriched with insoluble (soy polysaccharide) fiber and are often used in long-term EN because diarrhea is the most frequently occurring GI complication (Ciocon et al., 1992). Although the etiology of diarrhea is multifactorial and medications are a major factor (Edes et al., 1990), fiber-supplemented formulas may contribute to resolving diarrhea, as fiber fermentation by anaerobic bacteria in the colon produces short-chain fatty acids, which increase sodium and water absorption (Zarling et al., 1994).

Chemically defined formulas are often referred to as *predigested* or *elemental formulas* because the protein source is partially hydrolyzed by digestive enzymes. These formulas are primarily used for patients with reduced absorptive capacity or those with a jejunal feeding access and intolerant of polymeric formulas. The protein content of these formulas is provided as elemental amino acids, dipeptides, and/or tripeptides that can be directly absorbed by enterocytes via active transport. Because the sites on the small-bowel brush–border membrane for absorption of amino acids and small peptides are separate and separate carrier systems exist for transport, it is thought that enteral formulas containing both amino acids and peptides appear in the portal blood faster and allow greater amounts of total nitrogen absorption than formulas composed of amino acids alone (Johnson, 1997). One study conducted by Borlase et al. (1992) showed no significant difference in tolerance to either type of chemically defined formula.

In disease-specific formulas, the nutrient composition has been modified to meet macronutrient or micronutrient needs in a specific disease state. For example, formulas that have increased amounts of the branched-chain amino acids (leucine, isoleucine, and valine) and reduced amounts of the aromatic amino acids (tryptophan, tyrosine, and phenylalanine) have been used in patients with hepatic encephalopathy. Likewise, formulations containing lower amounts of phosphorus, potassium, and sodium have been used in patients with kidney failure and medium-chain triglycerides have been used in lieu of long-chain triglycerides in patients with pancreatitis.

Specialty formulas are designed to enhance immune function with specific nutrient substrates such as conditionally essential amino acids like glutamine and arginine or omega-3 fatty acids or ribonucleic acids (RNA). In 1988, Daly et al. found that supplementing EN with arginine in postoperative cancer patients significantly increased mean

T-lymphocyte response and CD4 count within 1 week of surgery. Similar benefits have been observed for pancreatic, gastric, and colorectal cancer patients who have undergone surgery (Di Carlo et al., 1999; Gianotti et al., 1999; Wu et al., 2001). In 1999, Heys et al. reported findings from a meta-analysis of 11 prospective randomized controlled trials comparing EN using a formula supplemented with "immune-enhancing" nutrients versus a standard enteral formula. Six of these eleven trials involved patients with GI malignancies who were treated postoperatively with early EN. The formula provided to patients in the experimental group in these six studies was enhanced with L-arginine, omega-3 fatty acids, and RNA (Impact). These 243 experimental patients experienced a 47% reduced incidence of postoperative infectious complications (i.e., major wound infections, intra-abdominal abscesses, and/or septicemia). However, the enhanced formula did not have significant effects on the incidence of nosocomial pneumonia or mortality. Yet these patients had significantly shorter hospital stays—by 2.4 hospital days. It is possible the decreased hospital stays provided economic benefits.

In another study by Daly et al. (1995), the effect of immune-enhanced EN was evaluated on prostaglandin E_2 (PGE_2) synthesis, infectious complications, and hospital stay in 60 adults with upper GI tract malignancies who had jejunal tubes placed intraoperatively. Patients were stratified by disease and usual body weight and randomized to either standard enteral feedings or enteral feedings supplemented with L-arginine, omega-3 fatty acids, and RNA beginning 1 day postoperatively. Mean PGE_2 production decreased significantly at day 7 only in the enhanced group. Infectious complications occurred in significantly fewer patients of the enhanced group (10%) compared with the standard group (43%). The enhanced group also had an average hospital stay that was significantly shorter (16 vs 22 hospital days).

Although many cancer patients may benefit from administration of immune-enhanced EN, a meta-analysis conducted by Heyland et al. (1994) raises concerns that the potential benefit of reduced infections and complications may not extend to those patients who are critically ill. A number of studies suggest that provision of arginine, through increasing cytokine release and/or nitric oxide production, increases mortality in critically ill patients who have sepsis (Heyland and Samis, 2003).

De Luis et al. (2003) investigated the effect of arginine-supplemented early EN on ILs in oral and laryngeal cancer patients. Thirty-six patients who had a 5–10% weight loss before surgery were randomized to either standard EN or an isocaloric isonitrogenous arginine-enhanced EN for an average of 9 days. These investigators observed no significant differences in IL-6 and tumor necrosis factor-α (TNF-α) levels of patients in the standard group compared with those receiving arginine supplementation.

Enteral Infusion Regimen

Selecting a method for the EN infusion is based on the type of feeding tube, the enteral formula, the feeding route, and volume of the infusion. Continuous infusions are administered at a steady rate usually over a period of 16–24 hours in the acute-care setting and 8–16 hours in the home environment. Continuous feedings are beneficial for patients with delayed gastric emptying, risk for aspiration pneumonia, reduced absorptive capacity, or dumping syndrome. They are most frequently used for feeding into the duodenum or jejunum to prevent malabsorptive or osmotic diarrhea.

Bolus or intermittent feedings allow infusing enteral formula at specific intervals throughout the day. Typically the total 24-hour volume of formula is divided into three to six feedings daily. Bolus feedings, for gastric access, are usually delivered by syringe or feeding reservoir into the tube with a maximum of 500 ml/feeding. Intermittent feedings are infused by gravity drip over a slower time period such as 30–120 minutes.

After verification of feeding tube placement, EN is usually initiated full strength at a rate of 25–50 ml/h for standard formulas and 15–25 ml/h for hypertonic formulations or small-bowel feeding. The rate of feeding is advanced to the desired volume on the basis of patient tolerance, typically increased by 25 ml in 4–12 hour increments. As most cancer patients receiving EN are undernourished before tube placement, caution should be used in advancing enteral formula rate to prevent refeeding syndrome (i.e., aggressive feeding resulting in increased extracellular fluid volume, hypophosphatemia, hypokalemia, and hypomagnesemia). Gonzalez et al. (1996) observed hypophosphatemia of <2.5 mmol/liter in 25% of 106 undernourished cancer patients 72 hours after initiation of nutrition support. In this study, patients who were older (60 years and older) had twice the risk for refeeding syndrome as compared with younger (38–59 years) patients.

Complications of Enteral Nutrition

Although EN is considered a safer form of nutrition support than PN, there is potential for physical, metabolic, and mechanical complications. GI symptoms are the most commonly reported physical complications of EN. Patients may report diarrhea, constipation, nausea, vomiting, gastroesophageal reflux, abdominal cramping and pain, abdominal distention, and flatus. Other frequent physical complaints derive from oozing, redness, soreness, and pain at the ostomy site. Metabolic complications include dehydration, refeeding syndrome, hyperglycemia, and weight loss. Mechanical complications are those problems that are directly related to the placement and maintenance of the

TABLE 1 Frequency of Complications Related to Enteral Nutrition Support in Adult Patients: Review of Published Literature[a]

Type of complication	Rates	References
Physical		
Diarrhea	8–63%	Rains, 1981; Bruning et al., 1988; Sami, 1990; Silver et al., 2004
Nausea	18–40%	Rains, 1981; Bruning et al., 1988; Roberge et al., 2000; Silver et al., 2004
Vomiting	10–16%	Rains, 1981; Bourdel-Marchasson, 1997; Silver et al., 2004
Reflux	4–33%	Bourdel-Marchasson, 1997; Roberge et al., 2000
Constipation	2–50%	Rains, 1981; Bruning et al., 1988; Silver et al., 2004
Abdominal pain/cramps	15–53%	Bruning et al., 1988; Silver et al., 2004
Abdominal distention	50%	Silver et al., 2004
Flatus	53%	Silver et al., 2004
Peristomal skin problems	6–80%	Larson, 1986; Shike, 1989; Bourdel-Marchasson, 1997; Silver et al., 2004
Sleep interruption	13–42%	Sami, 1990; Roberge, 2000
Metabolic		
Dehydration/thirst	50–77%	Bruning et al., 1988; Roberge, 2000; Silver et al., 2004
Infection	5%	Page, 2002
Weight loss	38–75%	Rains, 1981; Silver et al., 2004
Mechanical		
Pulmonary aspiration	3–14%	Shike, 1989; Rabeneck, 1996; Bourdel-Marchasson 1997; Silver et al., 2004
Tube obstruction	8–33%	Campos et al., 1990; Sami, 1990; Silver et al., 2004
Tube leaking	28–33%	Bourdel-Marchasson 1997; Silver et al., 2004
Tube displacement	2–35%	Larson, 1986; Campos et al., 1990; Bourdel-Marchasson 1997; Page, 2002; Silver et al., 2004
Pump malfunction	31%	Silver et al., 2004

[a]Review included studies of enteral nutrition that included ≥10 subjects with cancer. Only Rains (1981), Bruning (1988), Campos et al. (1990), and Roberge (2000) reported complications in cancer subjects exclusively. Studies investigating enteral immunonutrition were not included.

feeding tube such as pulmonary aspiration, tube clogging, tube leaking, tube displacement, and infusion pump malfunction. Table 1 presents reported rates of the common complications of EN. Though less frequent, electrolyte abnormalities such as hypernatremia, hyponatremia, hyperkalemia, hypokalemia, hyperphosphatemia, hypophosphatemia, and hypomagnesemia can occur. Electrolyte abnormalities in EN are usually related to hydration status, excessive losses, or inappropriate enteral regimen.

PARENTERAL NUTRITION SUPPORT

The contraindications for EN are few; they include intractable vomiting or diarrhea, prolonged postoperative ileus, severe bowel obstruction, mesenteric ischemia, or diffuse peritonitis (ASPEN, 2002). Thus, in most cases PN should be reserved for true intestinal failure. Nevertheless, PN is frequently ordered in acute-care settings for cancer patients. However, only a few studies have shown beneficial outcomes. Three meta-analyses were conducted in the late 1980s and early 1990s evaluating outcomes of PN in cancer patients. In an analysis of 28 randomized controlled trials by Klein et al. (1994), patients with GI cancers receiving PN preoperatively had significantly fewer surgical complications and intraoperative mortality, but those receiving chemotherapy or radiation treatment showed no improvements in tolerance of treatment, response to treatment, or survival. Chemotherapy patients had significantly increased risk of developing infections. Similarly, a meta-analysis published in 1990 by McGeer et al. demonstrated that patients on PN who were undergoing chemotherapy had significantly greater incidence of infectious complications. Because many of these studies used PN formulations now considered excessive, especially in dextrose administration, and did not provide intensive insulin therapy to maintain euglycemia, the potential risks versus benefits of PN need reconsideration. For example, Van der Berghe et al. (2001) compared intensive insulin infusion adjusted to maintain blood glucose between 80 and 110 mg/dl with conventional insulin treatment with insulin infusion initiated when blood glucose reached 215 mg/dl in a randomized trial involving 1548 patients in surgical intensive care. Van der Berghe et al. (2001) observed significantly lower incidence of bloodborne infections ($p < .003$), acute renal failure ($p < .04$), and mortality ($p < .04$) in patients provided with intensive insulin treatment. The greatest mortality was seen with patients who developed multiple organ failure from sepsis.

Most importantly, a study conducted by the Veterans Affairs Total Parenteral Nutrition Cooperative Study Group (1991) elucidated which PN patients would most likely benefit from PN. In the Veterans Affairs study, 395 undernourished patients who required laparotomy or noncardiac thoracotomy were randomized to receive either PN for 7–15 days preoperatively and 3 days postoperatively or only postoperative PN. Only those patients in the preoperative PN group who were severely undernourished (determined by Subjective Global Assessment) benefited from PN, as they had significantly fewer noninfectious complications ($p = .03$).

Parenteral Access

Overall, 150 million vascular access devices are used annually in the United States with an estimated cost in 2003 approximating $1.4 billion (Ryder, 1999). Central venous and pulmonary artery catheters for PN account for 5 million of these 150 million devices (Ryder, 1999; Vanek, 2002b). The expected duration of PN therapy, the condition of the patient's veins, and the osmolality of the parenteral solution determine the site of venous access.

Peripheral access is obtained by standard venipuncture into a peripheral vein. Peripheral parenteral nutrition (PPN) is most often used for short-term therapy up to 14 days until central venous or enteral access is obtained or as a supplement to oral intake. The limited tolerance of peripheral veins to high osmolar solutions dictates the contents of the PPN admixture. Gazitua et al. (1979) evaluated peripheral vein tolerance to amino acid infusions and observed that phlebitis occurred more frequently when amino acids were added to the admixture, and all patients (n = 67) developed phlebitis when osmolarity of the admixture exceeded 600 mOsm/liter. In a prospective randomized trial with 30 gastric cancer patients after resection, Matsusue et al. (1995) compared the simultaneous infusion of lipid emulsion with a parenteral amino acid–dextrose–electrolyte solution for reduction of thrombophlebitis. Patients received equiosmolar amino acid–dextrose solutions with the addition of either 10% lipid or 5% dextrose. The 10% lipid group had significantly less edema on postoperative days 2 and 4, and these inves-

TABLE 2 Types of Central Venous Catheters Available for Use in Cancer Patients[a]

Type of catheter	Description	Indications for use	Advantages	Disadvantages	Length of therapy
Nontunneled CVC	Single or multilumen catheter placed percutaneously into jugular subclavian, or femoral vessel; subclavian is preferred	Acute-care setting for short-term therapy	Economical, easily removed, easy to change over guidewire	Routine care required: heparin flushing, sterile dressing, patient self-care; catheters secured by sutures at exit site, can detach and dislodge catheter	Weeks
Tunneled CVC	Single and multilumen catheters, placed percutaneously in jugular or subclavian veins or via cut down in cephalic vein; Dacron cuff used and tunneled in subcutaneously	Extended IV therapy; utilized in the inpatient and outpatient settings	Can be used for extended periods, minimal dressing needs; patient can easily assume self-care; catheter is secured with subcutaneous	Placement in the operating room; routine heparin flushes are required; may be difficult to remove	Months to years
PICC	Single or double-lumen catheters placed percutaneously into the antecubital vessels	Utilized in the acute-care and outpatient settings	Placement at bedside by trained RN; eliminates risks associated with thoracic CVC placement; removal easy	Requires routine flushing and site care; patient self-care difficult; external catheter breakage is possible	Months
Port-a-cath	Catheter and self-sealing silicone septum placed into anterior chest wall	Long-term intermittent IV access	Site care only when port is accessed, monthly heparin flushes if port not in use; no external components for breakage	Needle access required; needle displacement is possible; surgically placement and removal required	Months to years

Source: From American Society for Parenteral and Enteral Nutrition (ASPEN) practice manual 1998.

tigators concluded that the simultaneous infusion of a lipid emulsion helped decrease the risk for thrombophlebitis.

Central venous catheters (CVCs) commonly used to administer total parenteral nutrition (TPN) are nontunneled CVCs, tunneled CVCs, Port-a-caths, and peripherally inserted central catheters (PICCs). Table 2 compares different types of CVCs. Catheter type for TPN is determined by patient condition, expected duration of TPN, care setting, venous anatomy, coagulation status, and patient and/or health care provider preference (ASPEN, 2002). Many cancer patients have a preexisting CVC (i.e., before TPN initiation) for chemotherapy, medication administration, hemodynamic monitoring, hematopoietic infusions, and/or hydration.

Few studies have been designed to determine the optimal type of access for TPN in cancer patients. Santarpia et al. (2002) compared the prevalence of CVC-related infections according to the type of implanted CVC in a retrospective study of 221 patients that included 159 cancer patients. For the 159 implanted Port-a-caths in 153 patients and 71 tunneled catheters in 68 patients, Port-a-caths were associated with higher rates of infection as compared with tunneled catheters (23% vs 10%, respectively, $p = .03$). Notably, the Port-a-caths had been previously used for chemotherapy in several subjects, while the tunneled catheters had been placed for TPN only and, thus, had less frequent manipulation. Likewise, Bozzetti et al. (2002) compared complications including infections of Port-a-caths versus tunneled catheters in a retrospective study of 447 patients that included 314 cancer patients. Using Cox regression analysis, Port-a-caths had a hazard ratio of 3.0 compared with 2.8 for tunneled catheters.

On the contrary, Bow et al. (1999) were able to demonstrate safe use of Port-a-caths in 120 chemotherapy patients with solid tissue malignancies. Comparing central venous–placed Port-a-caths to standard peripheral intravenous access, Bow et al. (1999) observed a low rate of infectious complications (0.23 per 1000 port-used days) as compared to prior reports of 0.23–0.46 per 1000. These investigators concluded that low infection rates were likely related to a low frequency of prolonged myelosuppression and restricted manipulation of Port-a-caths by a limited number of skilled nurses. In this study, Port-a-cath use was also associated with reduced patient anxiety, pain, and discomfort.

PICCs are being used for TPN. Only a few randomized prospective studies have described usage of PICCs in cancer patients. However, PICCs have been associated with increased rates of thrombophlebitis. For example, Cowl et al. (2000) compared tunneled CVCs inserted into the superior vena cava via the subclavian or internal jugular vein versus PICCs inserted using the cephalic or basilic venous approach in 102 hospitalized patients. Sixty-seven percent of the CVCs were placed without complication (i.e., thrombophlebitis, malposition of insertion, pneumothorax, line occlusion, catheter infection, dislodged catheter, and catheter failure or leak) as compared to only 46% of the PICCs ($p < .05$). Furthermore, Smith et al. (1998) conducted a retrospective review of 283 tunneled CVCs compared to 555 PICCs. In this study, PICCs were associated with a significant increase in catheter malfunction ($p < .001$), arm vein phlebitis ($p < .001$), and total number of complications ($p < .001$). In contrast, Biffi et al. (2001) observed no significant

TABLE 3 Rates of Common Complications of Parenteral Nutrition Support in the Adult Cancer Patient: Review of the Published Research

Type of complication	Rates	References
Mechanical		
Catheter thrombosis	0.2–3%	Smith et al., 1998; Duerksen, 1998; Bozzetti et al., 2002
Catheter occlusion	4–13%	Smith et al., 1998; Cowl et al., 2000; Bozzetti et al., 2002
Pneumothorax	0.2–5%	Duerksen, 1998; Cowl et al., 2000
Phlebitis	2–12%	Smith et al., 1998; Duerksen, 1998
Infectious		
Catheter-related sepsis	4–21%	Smith et al., 1998; Cowl et al., 2000; Santarpia, 2001; Bozzetti et al., 2002
Metabolic		
Altered electrolytes	14%	Braga et al., 2001
Hyperglycemia	9%	Braga et al., 2001
Cholestasis	15%	Chan, 1999
Overhydration/edema	12–30%	Lough et al., 1990; Bozzetti et al., 2002

[a]Review included studies of parenteral nutrition in cancer patients only. Other common complications of parenteral nutrition include infusion pump malfunction, metabolic bone disease, hypoglycemia, altered acid–base balance, and deficiencies or excesses of macronutrients, vitamins, minerals, and trace elements.

differences among adult cancer patients randomly assigned to receive either a Groshong PICC or a Port-a-cath for chemotherapy.

Complications from PN are of four types: mechanical (i.e., those related to infusion apparatus), infectious, metabolic (e.g., imbalances of electrolytes or acid–base balance), and nutritional (i.e., nutrient inadequacies or excesses) (ASPEN, 2002). Table 3 presents complications frequently associated with usage of PN. Overall, the literature suggests from 2 to 43% of patients will experience a catheter-related infection (Verso and Agnelli, 2003). In response to the high rate of infections associated with CVCs, the use of CVCs impregnated with antimicrobials such as chlorhexidine and silver sulfadiazine (silver coated) or with minocycline and rifampin have been investigated for risk of infection when compared with untreated CVCs. Harter et al. (2002) compared silver-coated to untreated catheters by randomizing 233 cancer patients undergoing chemotherapy, including 84 patients receiving autologous hematopoietic stem cell transplantation (HSCT). The incidence of catheter-related infections was significantly less in the silver-coated group (n = 120) compared with the control group (n = 113), 10.2% versus 21.2%, respectively ($p = .01$). A concern remaining for investigation is whether impregnated CVCs will increase the incidence of thrombophlebitis.

Hematopoietic Stem Cell Transplantation

HSCT involves ablative therapy combining chemotherapy with or without total body irradiation to eradicate tumor cells (ASPEN, 2002). During the transplantation process, the phases of cytoreduction, neutropenia, and engraftment challenge patients in maintaining adequate nutritional status secondary to therapy-related toxicity. Toxicity that commonly affects HSCT patients can include mucositis, esophagitis, odynophagia, dysgeusia, cachexia, nausea, emesis, and diarrhea.

The use of TPN in HSCT patients is well documented and has improved long-term survival in some patients. However, because earlier studies involved both allogeneic, autologous, and syngeneic transplanted subjects, it has been suggested that the benefits of TPN use may be most optimal for allogeneic patients only (ASPEN, 2002). Weisdorf et al. (1987) compared TPN versus intravenous hydration in well-nourished HSCT patients in a randomized controlled trial of 104 allogeneic, 32 autologous, and 1 syngeneic hematological cancer patients. Patients were observed from day −7 to day +28 of the transplantation process. Overall, the greatest survival rate was observed in the TPN group (50%) compared with the hydration group (35%), $p = .015$. Furthermore, 41% of TPN group versus 22% of the hydration group had disease free-survival ($p = .026$), and the hydration group had a significantly increased risk of relapse ($p = .008$). No survival advantage was observed for the autologous patients.

Lough et al. (1990) also investigated the effects of TPN compared with intravenous hydration from days 1 to 21 of HSCT in 17 allogeneic and 12 autologous hematological cancer patients. They observed that the TPN group had higher bilirubin and γ-glutamyltransferase levels than the hydration group and more line cultures positive for bacteremia ($p < .05$). However, the hydration group had significantly greater weight loss.

Roberts et al. (2003) compared outcomes in 55 well-nourished breast cancer patients undergoing autologous HSCT in a prospective randomized study comparing the use of TPN (n = 27) versus oral diet (n = 28). Both groups had significant decreases in anthropometric measures (i.e., body weight, $p < .001$; triceps skinfold, $p < .001$; and mid-arm muscle circumference, $p = .017$). The oral diet group had significantly higher weight loss (6.5% subjects vs 2% TPN subjects), and mid-arm muscle circumference decreased more in the oral diet group (7% subjects vs 2% TPN subjects). Thus, it is suggested that TPN in the acute setting of autologous HSCT be reserved for patients with pre-transplantation impaired nutritional status, complications after transplant that interfere with nutrient intake, or prolonged inadequate oral intake.

Charuhas et al. (1997) compared the effect of continuation of TPN versus intravenous hydration fluids in the ambulatory setting on resumption of oral intake after HSCT in a double-blind randomized trial of 200 allogeneic, 53 autologous, and 5 syngeneic patients. Although there was a trend for median time to resumption of 85% of calculated energy need by oral intake to be less (by 6 days) in the hydration group compared with the TPN group ($p = .049$), the hydration group had increased weight loss ($p = .04$). Notably, no significant differences were observed in hospital readmissions and relapse or death at 150 days after transplantation.

Although a number of studies have been designed to examine benefits of glutamine-enriched TPN infusions or oral glutamine in the acute-care setting of HSCT, results have been conflicting. Ziegler et al. (1992) compared standard TPN with glutamine-enriched TPN (0.57 g/kg/day) initiated 1 day after transplantation in 45 allogeneic patients with hematological malignancies in a randomized control trial. The glutamine-enriched TPN group had better nitrogen balance ($p = .002$), decreased number of infections ($p = .04$), and decreased length of hospital stay ($p = .017$). In a later study with a subset of 20 patients, Ziegler et al. (1998) evaluated the effects of glutamine-enriched TPN on circulating lymphocytes and lymphocyte subsets. Patients who received glutamine-enriched PN had an increased total lymphocyte count (332 ± 50 vs 590 ± 71 cells/μl, $p = .01$), greater number of total T lymphocytes (54 ± 19 vs 229 ± 70 cells/μl, $p = .03$), and significantly higher CD4 and CD8 T-lymphocyte counts in peripheral blood. Moreover, Schloerb and Amare (1993) conducted a randomized controlled trial to compare standard TPN with glutamine-enriched TPN (2830 mg of glutamine/100 ml of TPN) in 13 allogeneic and 16 autologous transplant patients who had 26 hematological malignancies and 3 solid tumors. The allogeneic patients in the glutamine-enriched TPN group had no positive blood cultures ($p < .05$) and decreased length of hospital stay of 5.8 days compared with the standard TPN group ($p < .05$).

In another study, Schloerb and Skikne (1999) randomized 43 patients with hematological malignancies and 23 with solid tumor malignancies (18 received allogeneic HSCT and 48 received autologous HSCT) to receive either an oral glutamine dose of 10 g three times daily (n = 35) or oral glycine (n = 31). When TPN became necessary for meeting nutrient needs, patients in the oral glutamine group received glutamine-supplemented TPN at 0.57 g/kg. No significant differences were observed between the glutamine and glycine groups in length of hospital stay, number of days on TPN, time to neutrophil recovery, incidence of positive blood cultures, sepsis, mucositis, diarrhea severity, or incidence of acute graft-vs-host disease. There was a trend toward reduced need for TPN and increased long-term survival ($p = .05$) with glutamine supplementation.

Few clinical trials have investigated the use of EN in adult HSCT patients. Roberts and Miller (1998) reported successful use of EN via PEG tubes for an average of 5 months after HSCT in a retrospective study of 11 allogeneic and 5 autologous patients with 10 hematological malignancies and 6 solid tumors. They observed no significant bleeding or metabolic abnormalities associated with PEG use. Additionally, EN was not interrupted by nausea, vomiting, diarrhea, or gastric residual volume. Weight maintenance was achieved and survival was 81% at 30 days and 62% at 1 year after transplantation. Thus, EN, especially via a PEG tube, is potentially useful in the HSCT population. However, concerns have been raised that using nasoenteric tubes in pancytopenic patients may lead to postnasal hemorrhage and sinusitis (Sefcick et al., 2001).

MEETING NUTRIENT GOALS

Energy and Macronutrients

Meeting nutritional requirements through the provision of nutrition support necessitates attention to patients' macronutrient (carbohydrate, fat, protein, and fiber), micronutrient (vitamins, minerals and trace elements), and water needs. The Harris–Benedict equation is most often used to estimate basal energy expenditure in cancer patients on the basis of sex, age, and body weight. Although little empirical evidence is available, it is usually suggested that cancer patients' energy requirements are ~1.5 times their resting energy expenditure (REE). In contrast, when Bruning et al. (1988) provided cancer patients who were well-nourished orally with EN at this dose postoperatively, they observed significant weight and body fat mass loss after 1 and 3 weeks of nutrition support. Consequently, the next group of patients they treated with postoperative EN received 50% more energy than 1.5 times REE. The second group had no significant changes in body weight or body fat mass. In using indirect calorimetry to measure energy expenditure, Knox et al. (1983) showed that cancer patients can be hypometabolic, normometabolic, or hypermetabolic and, thus, have varying energy needs. The studies of Fredrix et al. (1991a) suggest that metabolic alterations are related to tumor type. For example, these investigators observed no significant increase in REE when comparing gastric and colorectal cancer patients with healthy controls or nonmalignant GI patients (1991b). However, increased REE was observed in patients with non–small-cell lung cancer (1991c).

Unlike the metabolic alterations that are observed in a typical starvation state, cancer-related cachexia mediated by increased levels of circulating cytokines can cause patients to have increased whole body protein turnover and skeletal muscle catabolism. Depletion of muscle mass and nitrogen loss produces a state of negative nitrogen balance. Even with adequate calories from carbohydrate and fat to spare protein for synthesis, reversing protein-energy undernutrition in cancer patients is often unsuccessful. In older cancer patients, inadequate energy intake and resultant weight loss is especially concerning, as it exacerbates age-related sarcopenia (i.e., loss of lean body mass with aging). Sarcopenia predisposes older cancer patients to frailty, disability, and functional dependence (Morley, 2001). Although it is commonly recommended that daily protein need is ~1.5 g/kg for patients with protein-energy undernutrition, the optimal amount of protein in the enteral or parenteral prescription has not been defined by empirical evidence. Thus, the primary goal is to maximize nitrogen retention and preserve or increase lean body mass and muscle function. To meet that aim, undernourished cancer patients may require up to 2 g/kg with adequate nonprotein calories for protein sparing (Hoffer, 2003).

Micronutrients

Vitamins, minerals, and trace elements (i.e., iron, zinc, manganese, selenium, copper, chromium, cobalt, and iodine) are essential to maintenance of health. Detecting deficiencies is difficult because serum values may not reflect intakes. Individuals may respond to micronutrient deficiencies by increasing absorption, mobilizing body stores, increasing efficient utilization, or decreasing losses. The Dietary Reference Intakes (FNB, 2000) are the recommendations for nutrient requirements devised by the FNB of the National Academies of Science National Research Council. Intended as guidelines for assessing and planning intakes of healthy people, each nutrient has four values: an Estimated

Average Requirement (EAR), an RDA, an Adequate Intake (AI) value, and a Tolerable Upper Intake Level (UL).

As enteral formulas are designed to meet the RDAs, micronutrient deficiencies are rare with EN support. Berner et al. (1989) assessed blood and plasma levels of vitamin A, thiamine, riboflavin, niacin, folic acid, pyridoxine, biotin, pantothenic acid, vitamin B12, and vitamin C in eight older cancer patients who received EN for an average of 10 months. The intakes of all vitamins met or exceeded the RDA except for vitamin A, which averaged 93% of the RDA. Likewise, mean blood and plasma levels were within the normal range for all vitamins except mean plasma carotene, which was significantly below normal.

Parenteral requirements for vitamins, minerals, and trace elements are less certain. Typical parenteral multivitamin formulations include vitamins A, C, D, E, niacin, riboflavin, thiamine, pyridoxine, pantothenic acid, folic acid, and vitamins B12 and K. Multiple trace element preparations or single entity products are added to parenteral admixtures. Zinc, copper, chromium, manganese, and in some conditions selenium are considered essential in PN infusions to prevent deficiency states. The electrolyte composition (i.e., amounts of sodium, potassium, magnesium, calcium, chloride, and phosphate) of the PN admixture is altered to meet individual needs and correct imbalances.

Fluid

Three formulas for estimating fluid requirements are most commonly used to calculate the daily water component of the enteral or parenteral prescription. Recognizing the need to balance insensible losses and maintain a tolerable renal solute load, the National Academy of Sciences FNB published the formula of 1 ml/kcal in the 1989 RDAs as a recommendation for adults (FNB, 1989). Chidester and Spangler (1997) have suggested 1500–2000 ml for institutionalized adults. Another recommendation based on body weight is 30 ml/kg with a minimum of 1500 ml/day (Chernoff, 1999). Though not specific to nutrition support, the latest recommendation by the FNB (2004) for adult total fluid intake is 2.7–3.7 liters/day. To achieve euhydration, all sources of fluid intakes and outputs should be assessed. Conditions such as congestive heart failure, renal failure, and ascites require careful monitoring of fluid status.

Although the American Medical Association has stated that dehydration is the most common electrolyte abnormality in older adults, there is no accepted definition of dehydration (Weinberg and Minaker, 1995). Moreover, little empirical evidence is available to determine specific fluid requirements. Older cancer patients are less tolerant of inadequate hydration and more likely to develop dehydration. In a prospective descriptive study with older laryngeal and esophageal cancer patients on HEN, Silver et al. (2004a) observed total water intakes averaging 53% of water need, estimated at 30 ml/kg, which was significantly correlated with decreased urination ($p = .001$).

Most importantly, it should be noted that water comprises ~84% of the fluid in a standard (1-kcal/ml) enteral formula and only ~57% of a condensed (2-kcal/ml) formula. Thus, additional water either being flushed through the feeding tube or consumed orally is necessary to meet requirements. Additional water is also necessary in enteral or parenteral support to compensate for excessive losses in chronic diarrhea or vomiting, draining wounds or fistulas, ostomy output, high urine output, or elevated body temperature.

HOME NUTRITION SUPPORT

Demographics

Although cancer is the greatest indicator for HEN and HPN worldwide, the current incidence and prevalence of HEN and HPN in cancer patients is unknown, as there are no mandatory reporting requirements. The North American Home Parenteral and Enteral Nutrition Patient Registry (The Oley Foundation 1994) showed that 3931 cancer patients received HEN and 5357 cancer patients received HPN for the first time between 1985 and 1992. Combining the registry data with Medicare data, Howard et al. (1995) projected a 25% annual growth rate in U.S. patients on home nutrition support and a shift toward greater usage of nutrition support in cancer patients. Compiling the total numbers of patients on HEN and HPN with Medicare payments, they estimated $1.14 billion paid in 1992 that was 80% of Medicare Part B allowable charges.

Clinical Outcomes

In examining clinical outcomes of the cancer patients on HEN and HPN in the registry, Howard (1993) found that those on HEN were older than those on HPN (mean of 60 vs 43 years) but had a slightly higher 1-year survival rate (32% vs 28%). Comparing complications that led to hospital readmissions in 1 year, Howard (1993) reported that HEN readmissions occurred one-third as frequently as HPN with an average of approximately one readmission per year for the HPN patient. In contrast, the study by Campos et al. (1990) with head, neck, and upper GI tract cancer patients on HEN in the late 1980s reported 52 readmissions for 29 of 39 patients during a period of 176 days. Similarly, the study by Silver et al. (2004a) with older laryngeal and esophageal cancer patients who underwent surgery in 2000/2001 reported one to six hospital visits per patient in the first 3 months after discharge on HEN.

Although about half of patients receiving HEN report consuming food orally in conjunction with their tube feeding, only 10–30% of cancer patients resume a full oral diet (Campos et al., 1990; Howard, 1993; Schneider et al., 2001). In current clinical practice, it is supposed that poor resumption of oral intake may be related to tube feeding schedule. Consequently, it has become standard practice for EN discharge prescriptions to be written as a continuous 8–12 hour nocturnal infusion with the notion that freeing the patient from diurnal or 24-hour infusion would improve appetite and promote oral intake. However, in a within-subject randomized crossover design conducted with healthy men, Stratton et al. (2003) observed similar effects on appetite sensations and no significant differences in oral energy intake among the 3 tube feeding schedules (i.e., nocturnal, diurnal, or 24 hour). Noticeably, this study was only 3 days in duration and earlier work from the same investigators suggested that tube feeding of longer duration may influence appetite and food intake (Stratton et al., 2000). Yet the findings of Stratton et al. indicate that disease or other nutrition-related factors may influence the poor oral intake of HEN patients.

Quality of Life Outcomes

Although not clearly defined, it is generally agreed that assessment of quality of life (QOL) should include physical, cognitive, emotional, social, and functional factors. Some QOL assessments also include patient life satisfaction, spirituality, and finances or availability of resources. Few studies have empirically or prospectively measured QOL in cancer patients on HEN or HPN. In comparison with the general population, QOL is rated poorer by cancer patients on HEN (Schneider et al., 2000). Fatigue, sleep disturbance, body image, subjective rating of health, and impaired social, cognitive, and physical functionality contribute to poor QOL (Callahan et al., 2000; Roberge et al., 2000). Loeser et al. (2003) observed that 13% of the variance in QOL rating was related to nutritional status in a prospective cross-sectional study that included head, neck, and upper GI tract cancer patients. In a randomized trial of a standard EN formula postoperatively, a standard EN formula administered preoperatively and postoperatively and an arginine-supplemented EN formula administered preoperatively and postoperatively in 30 undernourished head and neck cancer patients, Van Bokhorst-de Van der Schuer et al. (2000) found significantly higher rated QOL only for preoperatively treated patients.

Smith (1994) has modernized QOL measurement in home care technologies such as HPN by recognizing the role of informal caregivers (i.e., unpaid family members, relatives, or friends who provide direct care) in daily management of the technology and identifying caregiving factors that affect QOL outcomes. Although primarily developed and tested with nonmalignant patients on HPN, Smith's Caregiving Effectiveness Model incorporates the caregiving context (caregiver characteristics, caregiver–care-recipient interactions, and patient education appraisal), adaptive context (family economic stability, caregiver health status, family adaptation, and reactions to caregiving), and caregiving effectiveness (patient QOL, caregiver QOL, patient condition, and technological side effects). In applying Smith's model to older adults on HEN, Silver et al. (2004b) identified 34 tasks performed daily by informal caregivers in managing HEN for older adults and developed a Home Enteral Nutrition Caregiver Tasks Checklist (Figure 1). In assessing informal caregivers' preparedness for caregiving and self-rated caregiver effectiveness, Silver et al. (2004b) found unmet training needs for an average of 18 of 33 of the tasks delineated on the checklist.

Current Medicare policy restricts the frequency and/or duration of in-home nursing visits and limits professional nutrition services in home and community settings to patients with diabetes mellitus and nondialysis renal disease. Thus, patients on HEN and HPN are forced to rely on informal caregivers for assistance with daily health care. The adequate training and preparation of caregivers along with prudent use of HEN and HPN and multidisciplinary intervention that includes frequent monitoring and reassessment are more likely to result in efficacious care that can lower unnecessary formal health care use, reduce hospital readmissions, reverse malnutrition, and save health care dollars.

In conclusion, nutrition support of the cancer patient requires careful identification of patients already undernourished, those at risk for undernutrition, and/or those who will benefit from aggressive nutrition intervention. Nutrition therapy options, that is, EN vs PN, type of access, and composition of the nutrition infusion should be considered in the context of patient condition, nutritional needs, potential complications or side effects, and potential benefits in nutritional status, functionality, and QOL. Despite relatively little empirical evidence, both EN and PN have appropriate uses in carefully selected patients. Yet the role of PN in mildly or moderately undernourished cancer patients does not seem an appropriate choice. The most promising outcomes of PN seem to be in severely undernourished patients undergoing major abdominal surgery for gastric malignancies and in bone marrow transplant recipients undergoing chemotherapy. Thus, EN continues to be the preferable option for many cancer patients. With either route of nutrition support, a key factor for efficacy of support is the role of a highly skilled multidisciplinary team in early assessment and intervention, routine monitoring, and frequent follow-up in conjunction with adequate preparation and training of the informal caregivers who provide daily home health care. For those patients receiving palliative care, the options of withdrawal or withholding of nutrition support should be discussed so that patients and families can make informed decisions (American Dietetic Association, 2002).

Home Enteral Nutrition Caregiver Tasks Checklist

Instructions: I am going to read a list of tasks that you may or may not be responsible for in taking care of your relative. I want you to tell me if (1) yes, you perform this task or (2) no, you do not perform this task. Next, I want you to tell me if (1) you have had formal teaching and do not need more; (2) you have had formal teaching but feel a need for more; (3) you have not had formal teaching but feel a need for some; or (4) you have not had formal teaching and do not need any. There is no right answer; please give me your best response.

TASKS	(1) Yes I do this	(2) No I do not do this	(1) I have received teaching. I do not need more.	(2) I have received teaching. But I need more.	(3) I have not received teaching. But I need teaching.	(4) I have not received teaching. I do not need any.
1. Bathing and personal hygiene of care recipient						
2. Lifting and positioning care recipient						
3. Helping care recipient walk						
4. Washing hands using aseptic / sterile technique						
5. Preparing, measuring, and mixing tube feeding formula						
6. Storing the tube feed formula						
7. Hooking up / connecting the feeding set and tubing						
8. Turning the feeding pump on and off						
9. Flushing the feeding tube						
10. Changing and/or cleaning the tubing						
11. Monitoring how long the bag of formula hangs						
12. Caring for skin at the tube site						
13. Administering other medications						
14. Organizing home care services						
15. Organizing blood work and/or lab services						
16. Setting-up clinic and doctor appointments						
17. Managing inventory of feeding equipment and supplies						
18. Communicating with the insurance agency						
19. Providing transportation						
20. Doing shopping						
21. Doing household chores						
22. Managing finances						
23. Responding to emergencies						
24. Managing nausea and/or vomiting						
25. Managing stomach cramps and/or gas						
26. Managing diarrhea and/or constipation						
27. Managing a feeding tube leak						
28. Checking formula residuals						
29. Checking the position of the tube						
30. Managing a clogged feeding tube						
31. Monitoring for infection						
32. Monitoring for weight loss or gain						
33. Monitoring for dehydration						
34. Monitoring for nutrient-drug interactions						

FIGURE 1 Home Enteral Nutrition Caregiver Tasks Checklist.

References

American Dietetic Association. 2002. Position of the American Dietetic Association: ethical and legal issues in nutrition, hydration, and feeding. *J Am Diet Assoc* **102**: 716–725.

American Society for Parenteral and Enteral Nutrition [ASPEN] Board of Directors and the Clinical Guidelines Task Force. 2002. Guidelines for the Use of Parenteral and Enteral Nutrition in Adult and Pediatric patients. *J Parenter Enter Nutr* **26**.

Bergstrom, L.R., Larson, D., Zinsmeister, A.R., Sarr, M.G., and Silverstein, M.D. 1995. Utilization and outcomes of surgical gastrostomies and jejunostomies in an era of percutaneous endoscopic gastrostomy: a population-based study. *Mayo Clin Proc* **70**: 829–836.

Berner, Y., Morse, R., Frank, O., Baker, H., and Shike, M. 1989. Vitamin plasma levels in long-term enteral feeding patients. *JPEN J Parenter Enteral Nutr* **13**: 525–528.

Biffi, R., De Braud, F., Orsi, F., Pozzi, S., Arnaldi, P., Goldhirsch, A., Rotmensz, N., Robertson, C., Bellomi, M., and Andreoni, B. 2001. A randomized, prospective trial of central venous ports connected to standard open-ended or Groshong catheters in adult oncology patients. *Cancer* **92**: 1204–1212.

Bistrian, B.R., Blackburn, G.L., Vitale, J., Cochran, D., and Naylor, J. 1976. Prevalence of malnutrition in general medical patients. *JAMA* **235**: 1567–1570.

Borlase, B.C., Bell, S.J., Lewis, E.J., Swails, W., Bistrian, B.R., Forse, R.A., and Blackburn, G.L. 1992. Tolerance to enteral tube feeding diets in hypoalbuminemic critically ill, geriatric patients. *Surg Gynecol Obstet* **174**: 181–188.

Bow, E.J., Kilpatrick, M.G., and Clinch, J.J. 1999. Totally implantable venous access ports systems for patients receiving chemotherapy for solid tissue malignancies: A randomized controlled clinical trial examining the safety, efficacy, costs, and impact on quality of life. *J Clin Oncol* **17**: 1267.

Bozzetti, F., Cozzaglio, L., Gavazzi, C., Bidoli, P., Bonfanti, G., Montalto, F., Soto Parra, H., Valente, M., and Zucali, R. 1998. Nutritional support in patients with cancer of the esophagus: impact on nutritional status, patient compliance to therapy, and survival. *Tumori* **84**: 681–686.

Bozzetti, F., Braga, M., Gianotti, L., Gavazzi, C., and Mariani, L. 2001. Postoperative enteral versus parenteral nutrition in malnourished patients with gastrointestinal cancer: a randomised multicentre trial. *Lancet* **358**: 1487–1492.

Bozzetti, F., Mariani, L., Bertinet, D.B., Chiavenna, G., Crose, N., De Cicco, M., Gigli, G., Micklewright, A., Moreno Villares, J.M., Orban, A., Pertkiewicz, M., Pironi, L., Vilas, M.P., Prins, F., and Thul, P. 2002. Central venous catheter complications in 447 patients on home parenteral nutrition: an analysis of over 100.000 catheter days. *Clin Nutr* **21**: 475–485.

Braga, M., Gianotti, L., Gentilini, O., Parisi, V., Salis, C., and Di Carlo, V. 2001. Early postoperative enteral nutrition improves gut oxygenation and reduces costs compared with total parenteral nutrition. *Crit Care Med* **29**: 242–248.

Bruning, P.F., Halling, A., Hilgers, F.J., Kappner, G., Poelhuis, E.K., Kobashi-Schoot, A.M., and Schouwenburg, P.F. 1988. Postoperative nasogastric tube feeding in patients with head and neck cancer: a prospective assessment of nutritional status and well-being. *Eur J Cancer Clin Oncol* **24**: 181–188.

Callahan, C.M., Haag, K.M., Weinberger, M., Tierney, W.M., Buchanan, N.N., Stump, T.E., and Nisi, R. 2000. Outcomes of percutaneous endoscopic gastrostomy among older adults in a community setting. *J Am Geriatr Soc* **48**: 1048–1054.

Campos, A.C., Butters, M., and Meguid, M.M. 1990. Home enteral nutrition via gastrostomy in advanced head and neck cancer patients. *Head Neck* **12**: 137–142.

Charuhas, P.M., Fosberg, K.L., Bruemmer, B., Aker, S.N., Leisenring, W., Seidel, K., and Sullivan, K.M. 1997. A double-blind randomized trial comparing outpatient parenteral nutrition with intravenous hydration: effect on resumption of oral intake after marrow transplantation. *JPEN J Parenter Enteral Nutr* **21**: 157–161.

Chernoff, R., ed. 1999. "Geriatric Nutrition." ASPEN Publishers, Gaithersburg, MD.

Chidester, J.C., and Spangler, A.A. 1997. Fluid intake in the institutionalized elderly. *J Am Diet Assoc* **97**: 23–28; quiz 29–30.

Ciocon, J.O., Galindo-Ciocon, D.J., Tiessen, C., and Galindo, D. 1992. Continuous compared with intermittent tube feeding in the elderly. *JPEN J Parenter Enteral Nutr* **16**: 525–528.

Conti, S., West, J.P., and Fitzpatrick, H.F. 1977. Mortality and morbidity after esophagogastrectomy for cancer of the esophagus and cardia. *Am Surg* **43**: 92–96.

Cowl, C.T., Weinstock, J.V., Al-Jurf, A., Ephgrave, K., Murray, J.A., and Dillon, K. 2000. Complications and cost associated with parenteral nutrition delivered to hospitalized patients through either subclavian or peripherally-inserted central catheters. *Clin Nutr* **19**: 237–243.

Daly, J.M., Bonau, R., Stofberg, P., Bloch, A., Jeevanandam, M., and Morse, M. 1987. Immediate postoperative jejunostomy feeding. Clinical and metabolic results in a prospective trial. *Am J Surg* **153**: 198–206.

Daly, J.M., Reynolds, J., Thom, A., Kinsley, L., Dietrick-Gallagher, M., Shou, J., and Ruggieri, B. 1988. Immune and metabolic effects of arginine in the surgical patient. *Ann Surg* **208**: 512–523.

Daly, J.M., Weintraub, F.N., Shou, J., Rosato, E.F., and Lucia, M. 1995. Enteral nutrition during multimodality therapy in upper gastrointestinal cancer patients. *Ann Surg* **221**: 327–338.

de Luis, D.A., Izaola, O., Cuellar, L., Terroba, M.C., Arranz, M., Fernandez, N., and Aller, R. 2003. Effect of C-reactive protein and interleukins blood levels in postsurgery arginine-enhanced enteral nutrition in head and neck cancer patients. *Eur J Clin Nutr* **57**: 96–99.

Dewys, W.D., Begg, C., Lavin, P.T., Band, P.R., Bennett, J.M., Bertino, J.R., Cohen, M.H., Douglass, H.O., Jr., Engstrom, P.F., Ezdinli, E.Z., Horton, J., Johnson, G.J., Moertel, C.G., Oken, M.M., Perlia, C., Rosenbaum, C., Silverstein, M.N., Skeel, R.T., Sponzo, R.W., and Tormey, D.C. 1980. Prognostic effect of weight loss prior to chemotherapy in cancer patients. Eastern Cooperative Oncology Group. *Am J Med* **69**: 491–497.

Di Carlo, V., Gianotti, L., Balzano, G., Zerbi, A., and Braga, M. 1999. Complications of pancreatic surgery and the role of perioperative nutrition. *Dig Surg* **16**: 320–326.

Edes, T.E., Walk, B.E., and Austin, J.L. 1990. Diarrhea in tube-fed patients: feeding formula not necessarily the cause. *Am J Med* **88**: 91–93.

Fish, J., Sporay, G., Beyer, K., Jones, J., Kihara, T., Kennedy, A., Apovian, C., and Jensen, G.L. 1997. A prospective randomized study of glutamine-enriched parenteral compared with enteral feeding in postoperative patients. *Am J Clin Nutr* **65**: 977–983.

Food and Nutrition Board. 1989. "Recommended Dietary Allowances," 10th edition. National Academy Press, Washington, DC.

Food and Nutrition Board. 2000. "Dietary Reference Intakes. Applications in Dietary Assessment." National Academy Press, Washington, DC.

Food and Nutrition Board. 2004. "Dietary Reference Intakes for Water, Potassium, Sodium, Chloride, and Sulfate." National Academy Press, Washington, DC.

Fredrix, E.W., Soeters, P.B., Rouflart, M.J., von Meyenfeldt, M.F., and Saris, W.H. 1991b. Resting energy expenditure in patients with newly detected gastric and colorectal cancers. *Am J Clin Nutr* **53**: 1318–1322.

Fredrix, E.W., Soeters, P.B., Wouters, E.F., Deerenberg, I.M., von Meyenfeldt, M.F., and Saris, W.H. 1991a. Effect of different tumor types on resting energy expenditure. *Cancer Res* **51**: 6138–6141.

Fredrix, E.W., Wouters, E.F., Soeters, P.B., van der Aalst, A.C., Kester, A.D., von Meyenfeldt, M.F., and Saris, W.H. 1991c. Resting energy expenditure in patients with non–small cell lung cancer. *Cancer* **68**: 1616–1621.

Gauderer, M.W., Ponsky, J.L., and Izant, R.J., Jr. 1980. Gastrostomy without laparotomy: a percutaneous endoscopic technique. *J Pediatr Surg* **15**: 872–875.

Gazitua, R., Wilson, K., Bistrian, B.R., and Blackburn, G.L. 1979. Factors determining peripheral vein tolerance to amino acid infusions. *Arch Surg* **114**: 897–900.

Gianotti, L., Braga, M., Radaelli, G., Mariani, L., Vignali, A., and Di Carlo, V. 1995. Lack of improvement of prognostic performance of weight loss when combined with other parameters. *Nutrition* **11**: 12–16.

Gianotti, L., Braga, M., Fortis, C., Soldini, L., Vignali, A., Colombo, S., Radaelli, G., and Di Carlo, V. 1999. A prospective, randomized clinical trial on perioperative feeding with an arginine-, omega-3 fatty acid-, and RNA-enriched enteral diet: effect on host response and nutritional status. *JPEN J Parenter Enteral Nutr* **23**: 314–320.

Gonzalez, G., Fajardo Rodriguez, A., and Gonzalez, E. 1996. The incidence of the refeeding syndrome in cancer patients who receive artificial nutritional treatment. *Nutr Hosp* **11**: 98–101.

Harter, C., Salwender, H.J., Bach, A., Egerer, G., Goldschmidt, H., and Ho, A.D. 2002. Catheter-related infection and thrombosis of the internal jugular vein in hematologic-oncologic patients undergoing chemotherapy: a prospective comparison of silver-coated and uncoated catheters. *Cancer* **94**: 245–251.

Heber, D., Byerley, L.O., and Tchekmedyian, N.S. 1992. Hormonal and metabolic abnormalities in the malnourished cancer patient: effects on host–tumor interaction. *JPEN J Parenter Enteral Nutr* **16**: 60S–64S.

Heyland, D.K., Cook, D.J., and Guyatt, G.H. 1994. Does the formulation of enteral feeding products influence infectious morbidity and mortality rates in the critically ill patients? A critical review of the evidence. *Crit Care Med* **22**: 1192–1202.

Heyland, D.K. and Samis, A. 2003. Does immunonutrition in patients with sepsis do more harm than good? *Intensive Care Med* **29**: 669–671.

Heys, S.D., Walker, L.G., Smith, I., and Eremin, O. 1999. Enteral nutritional supplementation with key nutrients in patients with critical illness and cancer: a meta-analysis of randomized controlled clinical trials. *Ann Surg* **229**: 467–477.

Hochwald, S.N., Harrison, L.E., Heslin, M.J., Burt, M.E., and Brennan, M.F. 1997. Early postoperative enteral feeding improves whole body protein kinetics in upper gastrointestinal cancer patients. *Am J Surg* **174**: 325–330.

Hoffer, L.J. 2003. Protein and energy provision in critical illness. *Am J Clin Nutr* **78**: 906–911.

Howard, L. 1993. Home parenteral and enteral nutrition in cancer patients. *Cancer* **72**: 3531–3541.

Howard, L., Ament, M., Fleming, C.R., Shike, M., and Steiger, E. 1995. Current use and clinical outcome of home parenteral and enteral nutrition therapies in the United States. *Gastroenterology* **109**: 355–365.

Jiang, X.H., Li, N., and Li, J.S. 2003. Intestinal permeability in patients after surgical trauma and effect of enteral nutrition versus parenteral nutrition. *World J Gastroenterol* **9**: 1878–1880.

Johnson, L. 1997. Digestion and absorption. "Gastrointestinal Physiology," 5th ed. L. Johnson, ed. St. Louis, MO., Mosby-Year Book, Inc.: 113–134.

Klein, S., and Koretz, R.L. 1994. Nutrition support in patients with cancer: what do the data really show? *Nutr Clin Pract* **9**: 91–100.

Knox, L.S., Crosby, L.O., Feurer, I.D., Buzby, G.P., Miller, C.L., and Mullen, J.L. 1983. Energy expenditure in malnourished cancer patients. *Ann Surg* **197**: 152–162.

Loeser, C., von Herz, U., Kuchler, T., Rzehak, P., and Muller, M.J. 2003. Quality of life and nutritional state in patients on home enteral tube feeding. *Nutrition* **19**: 605–611.

Lough, M., Watkins, R., Campbell, M., Carr, K., Burnett, A., and Shenkin, A. 1990. Parenteral nutrition in bone marrow transplantation. *Clin Nutr* **9**: 97–101.

Matsusue, S., Nishimura, S., Koizumi, S., Nakamura, T., and Takeda, H. 1995. Preventive effect of simultaneously infused lipid emulsion against thrombophlebitis during postoperative peripheral parenteral nutrition. *Surg Today* **25**: 667–671.

McGeer, A.J., Detsky, A.S., and O'Rourke, K. 1990. Parenteral nutrition in cancer patients undergoing chemotherapy: a meta-analysis. *Nutrition* **6**: 233–240.

Morley, J.E. 2001. Anorexia, sarcopenia, and aging. *Nutrition* **17**: 660–663.

National Cancer Institute. Nutrition in Cancer Care: Available at: www.nci.nih.gov/cancerinfo/pdq/supportivecare/nutrition/healthprofessional.

The Oley Foundation. 1994. North America home parenteral and enteral nutrition patient registry 1985–1992. Albany, New York.

Ponsky, J.L. 1989. Percutaneous endoscopic stomas. *Surg Clin North Am* **69**: 1227–1236.

Reddy, P., and Malone, M. 1998. Cost and outcome analysis of home parenteral and enteral nutrition. *JPEN J Parenter Enteral Nutr* **22**: 302–310.

Roberge, C., Tran, M., Massoud, C., Poiree, B., Duval, N., Damecour, E., Frout, D., Malvy, D., Joly, F., Lebailly, P., and Henry-Amar, M. 2000. Quality of life and home enteral tube feeding: a French prospective study in patients with head and neck or oesophageal cancer. *Br J Cancer* **82**: 263–269.

Roberts, S., and Miller, J. 1998. Success using PEG tubes in marrow transplant recipients. *Nutr clin pract* **13**: 74–78.

Roberts, S., Miller, J., Pineiro, L., and Jennings, L. 2003. Total parenteral nutrition vs oral diet in autologous hematopoietic cell transplant recipients. *Bone Marrow Transplant* **32**: 715–721.

Russell, T.R., Brotman, M., and Norris, F. 1984. Percutaneous gastrostomy. A new simplified and cost-effective technique. *Am J Surg* **148**: 132–137.

Ryder, M. 1999. The future of vascular access: Will the benefits be worth the risk? *Nutr Clin Pract* 165–169.

Sacks, B.A., Vine, H.S., Palestrant, A.M., Ellison, H.P., Shropshire, D., and Lowe, R. 1983. A nonoperative technique for establishment of a gastrostomy in the dog. *Invest Radiol* **18**: 485–487.

Santarpia, L., Pasanisi, F., Alfonsi, L., Violante, G., Tiseo, D., De Simone, G., and Contaldo, F. 2002. Prevention and treatment of implanted central venous catheter (CVC)–related sepsis: a report after six years of home parenteral nutrition (HPN). *Clin Nutr* **21**: 207–211.

Schloerb, P.R., and Amare, M. 1993. Total parenteral nutrition with glutamine in bone marrow transplantation and other clinical applications (a randomized, double-blind study). *JPEN J Parenter Enteral Nutr* **17**: 407–413.

Schloerb, P., Skikne, B. 1999. Oral and parenteral glutamine in bone marrow transplantation: a randomized, double-blind study. *J Parenter Enter Nutr* **23**: 117–122.

Schneider, S.M., Pouget, I., Staccini, P., Rampal, P., and Hebuterne, X. 2000. Quality of life in long-term home enteral nutrition patients. *Clin Nutr* **19**: 23–28.

Schneider, S.M., Raina, C., Pugliese, P., Pouget, I., Rampal, P., and Hebuterne, X. 2001. Outcome of patients treated with home enteral nutrition. *JPEN J Parenter Enteral Nutr* **25**: 203–209.

Sefcick, A., Anderton, D., Byrne, J.L., Teahon, K., and Russell, N.H. 2001. Naso-jejunal feeding in allogeneic bone marrow transplant recipients: results of a pilot study. *Bone Marrow Transpl* **28**: 1135–1139.

Silver, H.J., Wellman, N.S., Arnold, D.J., Livingstone, A.S., and Byers, P.M. 2004a. Older adults on home enteral nutrition: Enteral regimen, provider involvement, and health care outcomes. *JPEN J Parenter Enteral Nutr* **28**: 92–98.

Silver, H.J., Wellman, N.S., Galindo-Ciocon, D., and Johnson, P. 2004b. Family caregivers of older adults on home enteral nutrition have multiple unmet task-related training needs and low overall preparedness for caregiving. *J Am Diet Assoc* **104**: 43–50.

Smith, C.E. 1994. A model of caregiving effectiveness for technologically dependent adults residing at home. *ANS Adv Nurs Sci* **17**: 27–40.

Smith, J.R., Friedell, M.L., Cheatham, M.L., Martin, S.P., Cohen, M.J., and Horowitz, J.D. 1998. Peripherally inserted central catheters revisited. *Am J Surg* **176**: 208–211.

Stamm, M. 1894. Gastrostomy: a new method. *Med News* 324–326.

Stiegmann, G.V., Goff, J.S., Silas, D., Pearlman, N., Sun, J., and Norton, L. 1990. Endoscopic versus operative gastrostomy: final results of a prospective randomized trial. *Gastrointest Endosc* **36**: 1–5.

Stratton, R.J., Stubbs, R.J., and Elia, M. 2000. Impact of nasogastric feeding duration on appetite and food intake. *Clin Nutr* **19**(suppl): 54.

Stratton, R.J., Stubbs, R.J., and Elia, M. 2003. Short-term continuous enteral tube feeding schedules did not suppress appetite and food intake in healthy men in a placebo-controlled trial. *J Nutr* **133**: 2570–2576.

The Veterans Affairs Total Parenteral Nutrition Cooperative Study Group. 1991. Perioperative total parenteral nutrition in surgical patients. *New Engl J Med* **325**: 525–532.

Van Bokhorst-de Van der Schuer, M.A., Langendoen, S.I., Vondeling, H., Kuik, D.J., Quak, J.J., and Van Leeuwen, P.A. 2000. Perioperative enteral nutrition and quality of life of severely malnourished head and neck cancer patients: a randomized clinical trial. *Clin Nutr* **19**: 437–444.

Van den Berghe, G., Wouters, P., Weekers, F., Verwaest, C., Bruyninckx, F., Schetz, M., Vlasselaers, D., Ferdinande, P., Lauwers, P., Bouillon, R. Intensive insulin therapy in critically ill patients. 2001. *N Engl J Med* **345**: 1359–1367.

Vanek, V. 2002a. Ins and outs of enteral access: part 2, long-term access—esophagostomy and gastrostomy. *Nutr Clin Pract* 50–74.

Vanek, V. 2002b. The ins and outs of venous access: part I. *Nutr Clin Pract* 85–98.

Verso, M., and Agnelli, G. 2003. Venous thromboembolism associated with long-term use of central venous catheters in cancer patients. *J Clin Oncol* **21**: 3665–3675.

Weinberg, A.D., and Minaker, K.L. 1995. Dehydration. Evaluation and management in older adults. Council on Scientific Affairs, American Medical Association. *JAMA* **274**: 1552–1556.

Weisdorf, S.A., Lysne, J., Wind, D., Haake, R.J., Sharp, H.L., Goldman, A., Schissel, K., McGlave, P.B., Ramsay, N.K., and Kersey, J.H. 1987. Positive effect of prophylactic total parenteral nutrition on long-term outcome of bone marrow transplantation. *Transplantation* **43**: 833–838.

Witzel, O. 1891. Zur technik der magenfistelanlagen. *Centralbl chir*: 601–604.

Wu, G.H., Zhang, Y.W., and Wu, Z.H. 2001. Modulation of postoperative immune and inflammatory response by immune-enhancing enteral diet in gastrointestinal cancer patients. *World J Gastroenterol* **7**: 357–362.

Zarling, E.J., Edison, T., Berger, S., Leya, J., and DeMeo, M. 1994. Effect of dietary oat and soy fiber on bowel function and clinical tolerance in a tube feeding dependent population. *J Am Coll Nutr* **13**: 565–568.

Zeman, F.J. 1991. Nutrition and cancer. *In* "Clinical Nutrition and Dietetics" (F.J. Zeman, ed.), 2nd edition, pp. 571–598. Macmillan Publishing Company, New York.

Ziegler, T.R., Young, L.S., Benfell, K., Scheltinga, M., Hortos, K., Bye, R., Morrow, F.D., Jacobs, D.O., Smith, R.J., and Antin, J.H., et al. 1992. Clinical and metabolic efficacy of glutamine-supplemented parenteral nutrition after bone marrow transplantation. A randomized, double-blind, controlled study. *Ann Intern Med* **116**: 821–828.

Ziegler, T.R., Bye, R.L., Persinger, R.L., Young, L.S., Antin, J.H., and Wilmore, D.W. 1998. Effects of glutamine supplementation on circulating lymphocytes after bone marrow transplantation: a pilot study. *Am J Med Sci* **315**: 4–10.

C H A P T E R

42

Assessing Endocrine Effects of Cancer and Ectopic Hormone Syndromes

DAVID HEBER

Many common forms of cancer originate in tissues having the capacity to produce peptides, steroids, and other bioactive molecules in the microenvironment of tumors, where they can act in a paracrine or autocrine fashion (Odell and Wolfsen, 1982). The paraneoplastic endocrine syndromes ("ectopic" or "inappropriate" hormone production) comprise a wide array of symptom complexes associated with malignant or less commonly benign neoplasms. Most of the syndromes are associated with the production of peptide hormones, which, in some instances, have autocrine stimulatory effects. Hypercalcemia, the most common paraneoplastic endocrine syndrome, may be due to the systemic release of parathyroid hormone–related protein (PTHrP), factors that may be produced locally (cytokines) or by a combination of these mechanisms. A spectrum of other syndromes may be related to the production of specific hormones or growth factors, including insulin-like growth factor (IGF) and fibroblast growth factor 23. Molecular mechanisms responsible for the development of these syndromes are poorly understood. Mutational events not only may initiate neoplastic transformation but may also lead to the activation (reexpression) of genes responsible for hormone production. Additionally, epigenetic events such as methylation may also be responsible for the development of these syndromes. It is likely that a multiplicity of genetic and epigenetic events may contribute to the development of paraneoplastic endocrine syndromes.

Some proteins that are secreted are not active as ligand effector molecules, but even these products sometimes have structural homologies to known hormones. In some cases, these hormones travel through the bloodstream to act in an endocrine fashion (Odell, 1989). These observations support the notion that the abnormalities of gene regulation common to all cancer cells can result in aberrant gene expression evidenced by the production of peptide and steroid hormones. This chapter examines two separate aspects of the endocrinology of cancer. First, there is the problem of endocrine assessment of the patient and diagnosed cancer. Many normal hormones are part of the general tumor–host interaction leading to malnutrition. In some cases, there is an acquired dysregulation of hormone synthesis and secretion secondary to the presence of the tumor. Studies reviewed here show that cytokines involved in the immune response of the host to the tumor may cause insulin resistance and muscle catabolism. Second, there are less common ectopic hormone syndromes. In these cases, peptides such as adrenocorticotropic hormone (ACTH) or corticotrophin-releasing factor are produced ectopically and produce unusual, but clearly identifiable, metabolic syndromes that are diagnostic of an underlying carcinoma that may not have been discovered. Among the most striking and clinically obvious effects of tumors on host metabolism are ectopic hormone syndromes such as severe hypoglycemia, hypercalcemia, and electrolyte abnormalities.

ENDOCRINE ABNORMALITIES IN THE CANCER PATIENT

Patients with cancer often present with endocrine and metabolic abnormalities. These problems can be due to either ectopic hormone syndromes or endocrine dysfunction unrelated to these specific paraneoplastic syndromes.

First, abnormalities of glucose metabolism are common in patients with diagnosed cancer. In fact, hyperglycemia can be the first presentation of an occult carcinoma. This is

Copyright © 2006, Elsevier Inc.
All rights of reproduction in any form reserved.

usually due to the effects of cytokines on host glucose metabolism discussed extensively in Chapter 39. Cancer patients presenting with hyperglycemia likely demonstrate the common genetic predisposition to diabetes mellitus in the general population, which may or may not have been otherwise expressed. In fact, the decrease in muscle mass occurring in the cancer patient with malnutrition has a metabolic consequence for insulin action and glucose metabolism similar to the age-related decrease in muscle mass, which contributes to the increased incidence of diabetes noted in the elderly. Insulin and oral agents can correct this insulin resistance but do not lead to a reversal of cachexia in the human (Byerley et al., 1991). Nonetheless, glycemic control is indicated in cancer patients, considering the known increased incidence of infectious complications observed whenever blood sugar levels exceed 200 mg/dl. This is presumably due to a defect in white blood cell chemotaxis and other poorly defined abnormalities in cellular immune function associated with malnutrition, as well as hyperglycemia (Heber et al., 1986).

Hypercalcemia frequently occurs in patients with cancer (Rodman and Sherwood, 1978). This can be due to either metastatic disease in the bones causing calcium mobilization due to local resorption of bone, which contains 85% of the body's calcium stores, or it can be due to one of a number of paraneoplastic syndromes discussed in this chapter. It is important to remember that immobilization can lead to hypercalcemia (Sherwood, 1980). Adequate hydration, avoidance of urinary tract obstruction and infection, and physical therapy leading to rapid rehabilitation after any period of forced bedrest should minimize problems with hypercalcemia when these are not due to paraneoplastic syndromes. Primary hyperparathyroidism occurs in ~1 per 1000 individuals in the general population and can be unmasked by bedrest (Heath et al., 1980). This possibility should be considered, as well as ectopic hormone syndromes. Second, hypercalcemia is one of the most common paraneoplastic syndromes and usually occurs at the advanced or terminal stage of the illness (Mundy et al., 1984). Hypercalcemia progressively causes diverse clinical symptoms, such as nausea, unconsciousness, and coma, which profoundly affect the morbidity and eventual mortality of patients with cancer (Mundy et al., 1982, 1984). Evidence has accumulated that PTHrP, which is a potent stimulator of bone resorption, is responsible for inducing hypercalcemia (Guise and Mundy, 1998). Clinical studies have reported that ~80% of hypercalcemic patients with solid tumors exhibit increased blood levels of PTHrP (Burtis et al., 1990). Consistent with these clinical studies, it was demonstrated that several human tumors that produce substantial amounts of PTH-rP caused hypercalcemia when implanted into nude mice and that the neutralizing antibodies to PTHrP reversed hypercalcemia in these tumor-bearing animals (Kukreja et al., 1988; Sato et al., 1993).

Third, abnormalities of thyroid function can occur in the cancer patient. Hyperthyroidism can lead to weight loss and muscle catabolism. A distinguishing clinical feature is that hyperthyroidism is associated with weight loss and preserved or increased appetite, while anorexia is usually associated with cachexia not due to hyperthyroidism. When thyroid function was examined systematically, there was no evidence of consistent hyperthyroidism in a series of patients carefully studied by our group (Heber et al., 1986). In fact, with advanced cachexia there is a decrease in triiodothyronine (T_3) and a rise in reverse T_3 consistent with the so-called *euthyroid sick syndrome* (Chopra et al., 1975). This is usually seen only in very advanced cancer cachexia but frequently in malnourished patients hospitalized in intensive care units.

Fourth, hypogonadism can be seen in cancer patients. In one series studied by our group, ~50% of a group of male patients with a variety of types of cancer were hypogonadal (Chlebowski and Heber, 1982). Among these, half had hypothalamic-pituitary hypogonadism, as can be seen with malnutrition, and the other half had primary gonadal disease leading to reduced testosterone synthesis and secretion.

Finally, it is possible for cancer patients to have abnormalities of adrenal gland function, especially when they have received glucocorticoid therapy. Prednisone and other steroids used at pharmacological doses for >1 month led to suppression of the hypothalamic–pituitary–adrenal axis (Cook and Meikle, 1985). Such secondary hypoadrenalism can be detected by measuring a morning cortisol level. A level of <25 μg/dl suggests secondary or primary adrenal insufficiency. When cancer spreads to the adrenal glands causing adrenal insufficiency, both the medulla and the cortex are usually involved, resulting in reduced ability to respond to a hypoglycemic stress with adequate catecholamines to defend against further hypoglycemia (Hasan et al., 1991). Patients with this abnormality will fail to have a racing pulse or diaphoresis when suffering a hypoglycemic episode. Adrenal insufficiency can be life threatening, and patients being given pharmacological doses of adrenal steroids chronically should wear an identifying bracelet so that they can be given supplemental glucocorticoids under any stressful situation such as surgery, trauma, or infection.

The above discussion of routine endocrine evaluation of cancer patients highlights the fact that although ectopic hormone syndromes specifically result from certain forms of cancer, the patient with cancer can suffer from metabolic and endocrine disorders.

PARANEOPLASTIC SYNDROMES

A number of paraneoplastic syndromes have not been proven to result from the actions of a specific hormone. These include weight loss and related metabolic abnormalities, abnormal immune function and connective tissue disorders, neurological disorders, vascular disorders, dermatological disorders, and renal disorders. The role of cytokines in fever, anorexia, and weight loss is discussed further in Chapter 39. Abnormal immune function has been documented in cancer patients. Glasgow et al. (1974) found that 41 of 53 patients with cancer had skin anergy and, of these, 66% had a circulating substance that impaired immune function. Preliminary studies suggested that the factor was a peptide with a molecular weight of <10kD. Cancer patients frequently have peripheral neuropathy, causalgia, degeneration of the dorsal roots, myelopathic disorders, and myasthenia gravis–like disorders. In one study of 250 men with lung cancer and 250 women with breast cancer, 16% of the men and 4.4% of the women had neurological or muscular signs (Croft and Wilkinson, 1965). It is not clear that in all cases the malignancy was responsible for the disorders, but there is clearly an association. A number of vascular disorders including migratory thrombophlebitis, hemorrhage, and nonbacterial endocarditis can be associated with malignancy (Slichter and Harker, 1974).

Dermatological disorders can also be associated with malignancy. For example, acanthosis nigricans, which is associated with insulin resistance, has been shown to be significantly associated with visceral malignancies, especially adenocarcinomas (Curth, 1971). A specific action of a tumor product can cause a skin lesion such as the flushing associated with carcinoid. There can be a genetic relationship between a skin manifestation and cancer, as with Gardner's syndrome or Peutz–Jeghers syndrome. Autoimmune disorders associated with cancer can cause dermatomyositis or bullous pemphigoid.

Renal disorders such as nephrotic syndrome, bilateral venous thrombosis, and amyloidosis can be complications of malignancy or myeloma-like syndromes. Lee et al. (1966) reported that in 101 patients presenting with nephrotic syndrome, an underlying malignancy was diagnosed in 11%. Eight patients had membranous glomerulonephritis, and one had minimal abnormalities. These patients had a variety of types of cancer including lung, cervical, ovarian, kidney, breast, colon, gastrointestinal, and oropharyngeal cancers.

For all of the aforementioned manifestations, there is a clear association. In some cases, potential humoral substances have been identified (cytokines, tumor antigens, thromboplastic factors), but precise characterization of the pathogenesis of these disorders is not yet established.

ECTOPIC HORMONE SYNDROMES

Odell (1989) has proposed that peptide production by tumor is a nearly universal property of tumors. Odell used radioimmunoassay to detect ACTH and related peptides, calcitonin, vasopressin, and chorionic gonadotropin and proved that elevated serum levels were extremely common in cancer patients by comparison with healthy controls. On the other hand, actual clinical syndromes as opposed to radioimmunoassay abnormalities are much less common.

Pearse (1966) originated the concept of the APUD (amine precursor uptake and degradation) cell. On electron microscopy, these cells display a prominent rough endoplasmic reticulum and Golgi complex and are rich in ribosomes. They also contain round secretory granules of 100–250 nm size. These cells originate in the neural crest and migrate through the mesoderm to the primitive intestine. From there, they migrate to many locations, forming what has been proposed to be a complex endocrine system of scattered neuroectodermal tissue in the GI tract and related viscera. The cytochemical commonality of the APUD cells could be used to support the concept that many of the ectopic hormone syndromes are only ectopic in the prominence of the differentiated function of the particular APUD cells, but these cells in reduced numbers are normally scattered throughout these tissues. Moreover, the APUD concept may help explain certain aspects of ectopic hormone syndromes including the production of more than one hormone by a single tumor, the multiple endocrine neoplasia syndrome, and the association of certain neuroendocrine neoplasms with abnormalities of the neural crest such as Hirschsprung's or von Recklinghausen's diseases.

Ectopic ACTH Syndrome

The ectopic ACTH syndrome has been associated primarily with tumors of the lung, thymus, and pancreas (Gewirtz and Yalow, 1974; Odell et al., 1979; Wolfsen and Odell, 1979). Oat cell carcinoma of the lung accounts for 60% of cases. Thymic tumors account for 15%, and pancreatic cancer (usually islet cell) accounts for 10% of cases. Bronchial adenoma of the carcinoid type accounts for 4%, and the remaining 11% are due to a variety of tumors. ACTH is synthesized from a higher molecular weight precursor known as *proopiomelanocortin* (Orth et al., 1978). This protein is glycosylated and contains the sequences of ACTH and β- and γ-lipotropin, β-endorphin, and the enkephalins.

Tumors producing the ectopic ACTH syndrome may also produce corticotropin-releasing hormone (CRH) or CRH-like peptides (Belsky et al., 1985). These CRH peptides then act on the pituitary gland to release ACTH. These tumors can be differentiated from ACTH producers in the fact that dexamethasone, a long-acting steroid, can ameliorate the syndrome by reducing pituitary responsiveness to CRH in some cases.

Wolfsen and Odell (1979) examined both plasma and extracts of lung cancer tissue for pro-ACTH identified by column chromatography. In 100 patients admitted with abnormal chest x-ray films, 53 of 74 with lung cancer had increased plasma ACTH. In 101 patients with chronic obstructive lung disease, 5 of 20 with increased ACTH and only 2 of 81 with normal ACTH developed lung cancer within 2 years. The mean level of ACTH in cancer patients was 131.8 pg/ml, whereas in the healthy subjects it was 52.5 pg/ml.

Most patients with ectopic ACTH syndrome did not have the classic clinical features of Cushing's syndrome. The acute consequences of ACTH and excess of both mineralocorticoid and glucocorticoid predominate. There is generalized muscle weakness due to hypocalcemic alkalosis due to mineralocorticoid effects. There is hyperpigmentation due to the melanotropic peptides produced. There is also polyuria and polydipsia due to glucose intolerance, hypertension, and edema due to the excess mineralocorticoid effect.

Imaging studies are critical in localizing the tumor source in patients with Cushing's syndrome caused by ectopic ACTH secretion (Doppman, 1989). Anatomical imaging with computed tomography and magnetic resonance imaging is used most commonly to localize the source of ACTH. However, in 30–50% of patients with ectopic production, the source of ACTH secretion cannot be found despite repeated studies over time (Doppman, 1989). Up to half of these patients do not respond to medical therapy of hypercortisolism and must undergo bilateral adrenalectomy with lifelong replacement therapy. Functional imaging with nuclear medicine techniques enables *in vivo* imaging of physiological and pathophysiological processes. Among these techniques, positron emission tomography (PET) studies are increasingly used in oncology (Jones, 1996). [^{18}F]Fluorodeoxyglucose (FDG) whole-body scanning is by far the most widely used and recognized application of PET for tumor identification (Anderson and Price, 2000), and although it often fails to visualize the more common differentiated tumors (Adams et al., 1998a), poorly differentiated tumors with high proliferative activity may take up FDG (Eriksson et al., 2000; Nakamoto et al., 2000). Because these tumors express somatostatin receptors, scintigraphy with the somatostatin analog [^{111}In]-diethylenetriaminepentaacetate-D-Phe-pentetreotide (OctreoScan) has been used to detect tumors. Detectability of lesions in scintigraphic studies depends on multiple factors, including lesion size, location, type, or degree of somatostatin receptor expression (Kwekkeboom et al., 1993; Hammond et al., 1994; Adams et al., 1998a; Papotti et al., 2001) and on the amount of radioactivity in the lesion. Increased tumoral metabolic rate and glucose transport through the cell membrane are necessary for increased uptake of FDG (Seregni et al., 1998). FDG-PET is most likely to identify those tumors with high proliferative activity.

Therapy of patients with ectopic ACTH syndrome depends primarily on the nature of the underlying tumor. Because oat cell is the frequent cause, the prognosis depends of the effectiveness of the antineoplastic therapy. Agents such as aminoglutethimide, metyrapone, and the adrenal cytolytic agent (o,p9-DDD) (Cooper and Shucart, 1979; Bertagna et al., 1989) act to inhibit adrenal function.

ECTOPIC PITUITARY, HYPOTHALAMIC, AND PLACENTAL HORMONES

Ectopic production of growth hormone (hGH) is one of the most frequently documented hormonal syndromes (Steiner et al., 1968). It has been suggested that the possibility of an extrapituitary tumor be considered in every patient presenting with acromegaly. The initial identification of hGH ectopic production was in a lung tumor. Following surgical resection, blood levels of hGH fell from 38 ng/ml to 3 ng/ml, but no study of the tumor tissue was conducted (Cameron et al., 1969). Since 1959, approximately 50 cases of ectopic growth hormone-releasing hormone (GHRH) production from extrapituitary tumors have been described to cause this syndrome (Rivier et al., 1982; Osella et al., 2003). Osella et al. (2003) described the case of a 47-year-old Caucasian woman with ectopic GHRH syndrome sustained by a bronchial carcinoid. The criteria for the diagnosis of acromegaly due to ectopic GHRH secretion were satisfied including confirmation of active GH hypersecretion, unequivocal demonstration of GHRH production and secretion from an extrapituitary tumor, and cure of acromegaly after removal of the tumor. The tumor was an atypical carcinoid and there was a familial history of lung and colorectal cancer. Acromegaly was slightly active (mean GH value: 7.4 ng/ml; IGF-1: 436 ng/ml), and after tumor removal, there was a progressive decline of GH levels, consistent with remission of pituitary somatotroph hyperplasia. Pituitary radiology showed an empty sella, demonstrating for the first time its association with ectopic GHRH syndrome. Somatostatin and long-acting somatostatin analogs have been shown to be useful in treating patients with this syndrome.

Ectopic production of human chorionic gonadotropin (hCG) has been demonstrated by Braunstein et al. (1981), who found that 11.6% of patients with nontrophoblastic tumors compared with only 1.5% of patients with benign disorders had elevated β-hCG levels in the blood between 1 and 5 ng/ml. No patient with a benign disorder had levels above 10, whereas 13% of patients with tumors had above this level.

A major problem is that normal tissues produce hCG. Although the finding of hCG is not diagnostic of cancer, it may be a useful biomarker for following the course of individual cancer patients. The production of hCG leads to no symptoms except for the production of gynecomastia in some men. In these cases, it is not clear whether production or conversion of estrogenic substances by the tumor or gonadal response to the hCG has led to the observed gynecomastia.

The ectopic production of free β-hCG is a common phenomenon in epithelial tumors, a phenomenon originally believed to have no biological significance. However, it is now apparent that β-hCG may significantly affect tumor development by increasing cell populations through inhibition of apoptosis (Butler and Iles, 2004). The β,β-hCG homodimer, with topological similarities to growth factors, has been suggested to be the responsible mediator of these novel tumorigenic responses. Isolated β-hCG monomer from β,β-hCG homodimer and the homodimer both demonstrated growth effects on the β-hCG–responding bladder cancer cell line T24. Maximal increases in cell number corresponded to the elution peak of dimeric and monomeric β-hCG. The β,β-hCG homodimer is no more bioactive than its monomeric counterpart in stimulating bladder cancer cell growth. This strengthens the proposition that β-hCG may exert its antiapoptotic effects by antagonistic inhibition of other growth factor receptors and not by a specific receptor-mediated homodimeric interaction, as seen for its topological counterparts transforming growth factor (TGF), platelet-derived growth factor-B (PDGF-B), and NGF.

Ectopic production of antidiuretic hormone (ADH) is well described but must be differentiated from the very common syndrome of inappropriate ADH production (SIADH) (Robertson, 1976; Comis et al., 1980). Hypovolemia, invasion of the vagus nerve, metastases to the hypothalamus, drug administration, carcinomatous neuropathy, and ectopic production of a vasopressin-releasing factor can all lead to increased ADH levels. Stretch receptors in the right atrium can lead to increased ADH when stimulated by intrathoracic lesions. It is important to distinguish ectopic tumor production of ADH from the aforementioned causes. Patients with bronchogenic carcinomas and mesotheliomas frequently have elevated ADH, but it is not always clear to what extent ectopic production versus stimulation of vagal nerves or baroreceptors accounts for the elevated ADH levels found. Clinical findings in this syndrome include water intoxication with complications of anorexia, nausea, vomiting, headache, confusion, and ultimately coma if the serum sodium is low enough. Treatment by fluid restriction is usually successful, although hypertonic saline infusion is sometimes useful as well.

Hypoglycemic Substances

Although tumors have been associated with hypoglycemia, the pathogenesis in many cases is still not established (Olefsky et al., 1962; Unger et al., 1964; Shames et al., 1968; Saeed et al., 1969; Honicky and de Papp, 1973; Lyall et al., 1975; Shetty et al., 1982; Smith et al., 1982). There are two major causes of hypoglycemia associated with tumors: (1) insulin production by islet cell tumors and (2) production of hypoglycemia from extrapancreatic tumors by other mechanisms. For example, cytokines may be able to affect glucose metabolism via effects on the liver directly independent of any effects of insulin. Mice bearing interleukin-1β (IL-1β)–secreting tumor have been used to study the chronic effect of IL-1β on glucose metabolism (Metzger et al., 2004). Mice were injected with syngeneic tumor cells transduced with the human IL-1β gene. Serum IL-1β levels increased exponentially with time. Secretion of IL-1β from the developed tumors was associated with decreased food consumption, reduced body weight, and reduced blood glucose levels. Body composition analysis revealed that IL-1β caused a significant loss in fat tissue without affecting lean body mass and water content. Hepatic phosphoenolpyruvate carboxykinase (PEPCK) and glucose-6-phosphatase (G6Pase) activities and mRNAs levels of these enzymes were reduced, and 2-deoxyglucose (2DG) uptake by peripheral tissues was enhanced. mRNA levels of glucose transporters in the liver were determined by real-time polymerase chain reaction (RT-PCR) analysis. Glut-3 mRNA levels were upregulated by IL-1β. Glut-1 and Glut-4 mRNA levels in IL-1β mice were similar to mRNA levels in pair-fed mice bearing nonsecreting tumor. mRNA level of Glut-2, the major glucose transporter of the liver, was downregulated by IL-1β. Both decreased glucose production by the liver and enhanced glucose disposal resulted in the development of hypoglycemia in mice bearing IL-1β–secreting tumors. The observed changes in expression of hepatic glucose transporters that are not dependent on insulin may have contributed to the increased glucose uptake.

Fasting hypoglycemia from extrapancreatic tumors can also be caused by production of IGF (especially IGF-2), production of substances that stimulate insulin secretion, production of insulin receptors by the tumor, or excessive glucose consumption due to the size of the tumor (usually sarcomas). Fasting hypoglycemia can also be caused by severe liver disease, hypopituitarism, hypothyroidism, and pancreatic disease with reduced glucagon reserves. Production of cytokines, which enhance glucose utilization, preexisting malnutrition, and chemotherapy can also cause hypoglycemia. Several hundred such patients have been reported to date (Marks et al., 1974). In 42%, there are large mesenchymal or mesodermal tumors including fibrosarcomas, mesotheliomas, neurofibromas, and leiomyosarcomas ranging in weight from 800g to 10kg. They are frequently benign, and symptoms abate after tumor resection. Hepatocellular carcinomas and hepatomas account for 22%. Adrenal cortical carcinoma accounts for 9%. Pancreatic, bile duct, and other GI tumors account for 10%. Another 17% are accounted for by miscellaneous tumor types including lung, cervix, ovary, and kidney. In only rare cases are there elevations in serum insulin levels. The prognosis is related to tumor type, and fortunately many of these patients have benign tumors.

Hypercalcemic Substances

Hypercalcemia can be a sign of serious disease. Hyperparathyroidism is the most common cause of hypercalcemia, followed by malignancy (Knecht et al., 1996); up to 58% of hospitalized patients with hypercalcemia have an associated cancer (Crespo et al., 1999).

Malignancy-associated hypercalcemia can be caused by two entities, separately or in combination, based on the mechanisms of hypercalcemia. Humoral hypercalcemia of malignancy (HHM) is due to tumor hormone secretion into the systemic circulation distant to the skeleton with subsequent bone resorption. Local osteolytic hypercalcemia is caused by osteoclastic bone resorption from the release of factors produced by direct skeletal tumor involvement (Wysolmerski and Broadus, 1994).

Squamous cell carcinomas account for ~50% of cases of HHM (Knecht et al., 1996; Crespo et al., 1999). Most cases involve the lung, but carcinomas of the head and neck, oropharynx, and urogenital region have been described. Squamous cell carcinoma of the skin with HHM is unusual, with 13 case reports in the literature associating both (Sparks et al., 1985; Picascia and Caro, 1987; Mori et al., 1996; Reynaud-Mendel et al., 1997; Crespo et al., 1999). The remaining cases of HHM have been seen in renal cortical carcinoma, adult T-cell leukemia, and breast, colorectal, and esophageal adenocarcinoma (Mundy, 1988; Martin and Grill, 1992; Rikimaru et al., 1995; Crespo et al., 1999; Lortholary et al., 1999).

Hypercalcemia in the absence of hyperparathyroidism was described in the 1930s (Knecht et al., 1996), but Albright (1941) was the first to postulate the production of a substance with parathyroid-like properties in a patient with renal cell carcinoma, hypercalcemia, and hypophosphatemia.

As already discussed, the direct invasion of bone by tumor can lead to hypercalcemia. The administration of estrogen or androgen to a patient with breast cancer metastatic to bone can lead to hypercalcemia. Ectopic production of parathyroid hormone (PTH) or PTH-like substances (Sherwood, 1980), production of bone-mobilizing substances such as PGEs, osteoclast-activating factor (OAF), or transforming growth factors, as well as ectopic production of vitamin D, can also lead to hypercalcemia.

Sherwood et al. (1967) using a radioimmunoassay for PTH were able to demonstrate ectopic production in lung carcinoma, an undifferentiated parotid tumor, an adrenal carcinoma, and a histiocytic lymphoma. A PTHrP has also been identified in tumors. The PTH gene is located on chromosome 11, while the PTHrP gene is located on the short arm of chromosome 12. This protein is normally produced in keratinocytes and has been found in mammalian milk and in the sheep fetus, suggesting some role in fetal–maternal calcium homeostasis. The availability of a radioimmunoassay for PTHrP has facilitated differential diagnosis and therapy in a large number of patients. In one study of PTHrP in breast cancer patients with bone metastases, 88% of tumors in patients who eventually developed hypercalcemia contained PTHrP (Bundred et al., 1991).

PGEs may also be involved in ectopic causes of hypercalcemia, but the evidence in humans is variable. It may be that PGEs are important local mediators in bone under the influence of other hypercalcemia hormones. In addition to these hormones, OAF is an important cause of hypercalcemia in patients with multiple myeloma and some lymphomas (Mundy et al., 1977).

Extensive studies showed that some cancers had the ability to produce a substance similar to PTH that caused bone resorption *in vitro* and *in vivo*. It was further shown that this substance was capable of producing many of the characteristics of primary hyperparathyroidism with hypercalcemia produced by bone and renal tubular calcium resorption, reduced renal phosphorus threshold, phosphaturia, and increased urinary excretion of cyclic adenosine monophosphate (cAMP). With this condition, unlike hyperparathyroidism, the PTH level is usually low or undetectable, and levels of 1,25-dihydroxyvitamin D are also decreased (Martin, 1988; Strewler, 2000). Moseley et al. (1987) called this hormone-like substance PTHrP. Animal models of PTHrP-producing tumors with reversal of the hypercalcemic state by anti-PTHrP antibodies confirmed its role in HHM (Martin, 1988; Strewler, 2000). PTHrP has been detected in bone metastasis and may have a role in local osteolytic hypercalcemia (Wysolmerski and Broadus, 1994). It has also been described in a benign tumor of the ovary by Knecht et al. (1996), who called this condition the "humoral hypercalcemia of benignancy."

The human PTH gene is found in the short arm of chromosome 11, and the PTHrP gene is in the short arm of chromosome 12, which is believed to have arisen from a duplication of chromosome 11 (Ng and Martin, 1990; Wysolmerski and Broadus, 1994). The similarities between PTH and PTHrP are maintained in the 13 amino acids of the N-terminal of the molecules; actually, 8 are identical. This similitude in the N-terminal permits PTH and PTHrP to use the same receptors (Martin, 1988; Wysolmerski and Broadus, 1994; Knecht et al., 1996) and probably accounts for their similar biological characteristics (Wysolmerski and Broadus, 1994; Knecht et al., 1996; Strewler, 2000). The remainder of both molecules differs substantially (Martin, 1988), so PTH antisera will not inhibit PTHrP, and current commercial tests to detect PTH will not detect PTHrP (Martin, 1988; Ng and Martin, 1990).

PTHrP is found in healthy epithelia, mesenchymal tissues, endocrine glands, and the central nervous system, where it functions as a local messenger within tissues in an autocrine or paracrine fashion (Wysolmerski and Broadus, 1994; Strewler, 2000). Its presence is necessary for the adequate formation of cartilage and bone, in the development of mammary tissue and possibly milk production by the glandular epithelial cells, for tooth development, as a neuronal cell protector, and in maintaining adequate fetal concentrations of fetal calcium by acting on the placental calcium pump, and it participates in smooth muscle dilatation (Ng and Martin, 1990; Wysolmerski and Broadus, 1994; Strewler, 2000). Its function in skin is unknown. An excellent review on the physiology of PTHrP was done by Strewler (2000).

High levels of cAMP excretion and increased PTHrP have been reported in patients with bronchogenic carcinoma (Ng and Martin, 1990) and other cancers, especially breast cancer (Wysolmerski and Broadus, 1994), without the presence of hypercalcemia, raising the possibility that tumors produce PTHrP and hypercalcemia develops only when calcium homeostasis mechanisms become overwhelmed or tumor burden is increased (Rikimaru et al., 1995).

Other factors may need to be present to actually produce an HHM syndrome. Animal studies have shown IL-6 to be the sole producer of hypercalcemia by promoting osteoclastic activity (Yoneda et al., 1993), and cell line cultures from squamous carcinomas and normal foreskin keratinocytes ceased to cause bone resorption when antibody to IL-1a was added (Nowak, 1990). It is possible that these and other factors, such as tumor growth factor-α and TNF, act synergistically with PTHrP to produce bone resorption and hypercalcemia (Goldman, 2000).

Patients with HHM usually have abrupt onset of symptoms, and serum calcium levels are considerably elevated (Sparks et al., 1985; Picascia and Caro, 1987; Mori et al., 1996; Reynaud-Mendel et al., 1997; Crespo et al., 1999). Prognosis is usually poor despite aggressive therapy, with a median survival of ~6 weeks. Therapy targeted at the malignancy, either by excision or chemotherapy, has caused resolution of the hypercalcemia (Sparks et al., 1985; Picascia and Caro, 1987). General therapy is as with hypercalcemia of any cause. Mobilization to reduce bone resorption and hydration to enhance calcium excretion are the mainstays of treatment. Calcitonin, bisphosphonates (etidronate, pamidronate), plicamycin (mithramycin), and gallium nitrate inhibit osteoclast function and reduce bone resorption. Glucocorticoids are helpful in treating vitamin D–related hypercalcemia (Goldman, 2000).

Therapy of these hypercalcemic syndromes with mithramycin, bisphosphonates, phosphate, glucocorticoids, indomethacin, and calcitonin has been examined (Mundy et al., 1983). Many patients respond to these therapies, but there is no systematic therapy of this condition.

Calcitonin

Ectopic production of calcitonin (CT) has been demonstrated in many patients without medullary carcinoma of the thyroid. As in these patients, there are few symptoms of the overproduction of calcitonin. Schwartz et al. (1979) studied the utility of this hormone as a biomarker and found elevated CT in common forms of cancer including lung (38%), colon, (24%), breast (38%), pancreas (42%), and stomach (30%).

The CALC-1 gene encoding human CT is located on the tip of the short arm of chromosome 11 (11p15.3-15.5). Although the parafollicular C cells of the thyroid gland are the dominant source of circulating mature CT, several other categories of neuroendocrine cells besides the thyroid normally contain and secrete CT.

Mature CT is a 32-amino acid polypeptide with a disulfide bridge and a carboxy-terminal proline amide that play functionally important roles in mature CT (Hofstra et al., 1994). Mature CT results from the post-translational modification of a larger 141-amino acid precursor (preprocalcitonin) within the parafollicular C cells. Preprocalcitonin first undergoes cleavage of a signal peptide to form procalcitonin (proCT), a prohormone consisting of 116 amino acid residues. At the proCT amino-terminus, there is a 57-amino acid peptide, called *aminoproCT* (or *PAS-57*), and at the carboxyl-terminus, there is a 21-amino acid peptide called CT carboxy-terminal peptide-1 (CCP-1 or Katacalcin). The immature CT peptide consisting of 33 amino acids is located centrally within the proCT molecule. The mature, active 32-amino acid CT (which includes an amidated proline at its carboxy-terminus) is produced from immature CT by the enzyme peptidylglycine-amidating monooxidase (PAM).

Erythropoietin

The kidney is the principal source of erythropoietin (EPO), and a number of benign and malignant conditions of the kidney are associated with an increased production of erythropoietin (Sherwood and Goldwasser, 1976). Nonneoplastic lesions such as benign cysts result in increased erythropoietin, suggesting that dysplastic cells can result in increased EPO production (Ghio et al., 1981). Ectopic production of EPO has been associated with cerebellar hemangioblastoma (21%), uterine fibroma (6%), adrenal cortical tumors (3%), ovarian neoplasms (3%), hepatomas (2%), and pheochromocytoma (1%). More than 50% of patients with elevated EPO have malignant renal tumors or benign renal conditions. Increased red blood cell count occurs in 2–5% of patients with renal neoplasms and 9–20% of patients with cerebellar hemangioblastoma (Ghio et al., 1981; Montag et al., 1984).

CONCLUSION

Ectopic peptide hormone production is a common occurrence with many tumors. Ectopic hormone syndromes are relatively uncommon but can be highly significant clinically. Common endocrine disorders also occur in the cancer patient and can contribute to malnutrition, hyperglycemia, hypercalcemia, and other metabolic problems. The endocrine function of tumor tissues can provide new opportunities for developing intermediate markers and therapeutic strategies for cancer prevention and treatment.

Acknowledgment

This research was supported by the UCLA Clinical Nutrition Research Unit NIH Grant no. CA 47210.

References

Adams, S., Baum, R., Rink, T., Schumm-Drager, P.M., Usadel, K.H., and Hor, G. 1998a. Limited value of fluorine-18 fluorodeoxyglucose positron emission tomography for the imaging of neuroendocrine tumours. *Eur J Nucl Med* **25**: 79–83.

Adams, S., Baum, R.P., Hertel, A., Schumm-Draeger, P.M., Usadel, K.H., and Hor, G. 1998b. Comparison of metabolic and receptor imaging in recurrent medullary thyroid carcinoma with histopathological findings. *Eur J Nucl Med* **25**: 1277–1283.

Albright, F. 1941. Case records of the Massachusetts General Hospital. *N Engl J Med* **225**: 789–791.

Anderson, H., and Price, P. 2000. What does positron emission tomography offer oncology? *Eur J Cancer* **36**: 2028–2035.

Belsky, J.L., Cuello, B., Swanson, L.W., et al. 1985. Cushing's syndrome due to ectopic production of corticotropin-releasing factor. *J Clin Endocrinol Metab* **60**: 496–500.

Bertagna, X., Fevrod-Coune, C., Escourolle, H., et al. 1989. Suppression of ectopic adrenocorticotropin secretion by the long-acting somatostatin analogue octreotiols. *J Clin Endocrinol Metab* **68**: 988–991.

Bundred, N.J., Ratcliffe, W.A., Walker, R.A., et al. 1991. Parathyroid hormone–related protein and hypercalcemia in breast cancer. *Br Med J* **303**: 1506–1509.

Burtis, W.J., Brady, T.G., Orloff, J.J., et al. 1990. Immunochemical characterization of circulating parathyroid hormone–related protein in patients with humoral hypercalcemia of cancer. *N Engl J Med* **322**: 1106–1112.

Butler, S.A., and Iles, R.K. 2004. The free monomeric beta subunit of human chorionic gonadotrophin (hCG beta) and the recently identified homodimeric beta-beta subunit (hCG beta beta) both have autocrine growth effects. *Tumour Biol* **25**: 18–23.

Byerley, L.O., Heber, D., Bergman, R.N., Dubria, M., and Chi, J. 1991. Insulin action and metabolism in head and neck cancer patients. *Cancer (Philadelphia)* **67**: 2900–2906.

Cameron, D.P., Burger, H.G., DeKretzer, M.D., et al. 1969. On the presence of immunoreactive growth hormone in a bronchogenic carcinoma. *Australas Ann Med* **18**: 143–146.

Chlebowski, R.T., and Heber, D. 1982. Hypogonadism in male patients with metastatic cancer prior to chemotherapy. *Cancer Res* **42**: 2495–2497.

Chopra, I.J., Chopra, U., Smith, S.R., et al. 1975. Reciprocal changes in serum concentration of 3,39,59-triiodothyronine (reverse T3) and 3,39,5-triiodothyronine (T3) in systemic illnesses. *J Clin Endocrinol Metab* **41**: 1043–1049.

Comis, R.L., Miller, M., and Ginsberg, S.J. 1980. Abnormalities in water homeostasis in small cell anaplastic lung cancer. *Cancer (Philadelphia)* **45**: 2414–2421.

Cook, L.J., and Meikle, A.W. 1985. Factitious Cushing's syndrome. *J Clin Endocrinol Metab* **61**: 385–387.

Cooper, P.R., and Shucart, W.A. 1979. Treatment of Cushing's disease with o,p9-DD [letter]. *N Engl J Med* **301**: 48–49.

Crespo, M., Sopena, B., Orloff, J.J., et al. 1999. Immunohistochemical detection of parathyroid hormone-related protein in a cutaneous squamous cell carcinoma causing humoral hypercalcemia of malignancy. *Arch Pathol Lab Med* **123**: 725–730.

Croft, P.B., and Wilkinson, M. 1965. The incidence of carcinomatous neuromyopathy in patients with various types of carcinoma. *Brain* **88**: 427–434.

Curth, H.O. 1971. Cutaneous manifestations associated with malignant internal disease. *In* "Dermatology in General Medicine" (C.B. Fitzpatrick, K.A. Arndt, W.H. Claude, Jr., et al., eds.). McGraw-Hill, New York.

Doppman, J.L., Nieman, L., Miller, D.L., et al. 1989. Ectopic adrenocorticotropic hormone syndrome: localization studies in 28 patients. *Radiology* **172**: 115–124.

Eriksson, B., Bergstrom, M., Orlefors, H., et al. 2000. Use of PET in neuroendocrine tumors. *In vivo* applications and *in vitro* studies. *Q J Nucl Med* **44**: 68–76.

Expert Committee on the Diagnosis and Classification of Diabetes Mellitus. 1997. *Diabetes Care* **20**: 1183–1197.

Gewirtz, G., and Yalow, R.S. 1974. Ectopic ACTH production in carcinoma of the lung. *J Clin Invest* **53**: 1022–1032.

Ghio, R., Haupt, E., Ratti, M., and Boccaccio, P. 1981. Erythrocytosis associated with a dermoid cyst of the ovary and erythropoietic activity of the tumor fluid. *Scand J Haemotal* **27**: 70–74.

Glasgow, A.H., Nimberg, R.B., Menzoian, H.O., et al. 1974. Association of anergy with an immunosuppressive peptide fraction in the serum of patients with cancer. *N Engl J Med* **291**: 1263–1267.

Goldman, L., and Bennett, J.C., eds. 2000. The parathyroid glands, hypercalcemia, and hypocalcemia. *In* "Cecil Textbook of Medicine" (L. Goldman and J.C. Bennett, eds.), pp. 13998–14004. WB Saunders Co, Philadelphia.

Guise, T.A., and Mundy, G.R. 1998. Cancer and bone. *Endocr Rev* **19**: 18–54.

Hammond, P.J., Jackson, J.A., and Bloom, S.R. 1994. Localization of pancreatic endocrine tumours. *Clin Endocrinol (Oxf)* **40**: 3–14.

Hasan, R.I., Yonan, N.A., and Lawson, R.A. 1991. Adrenal insufficiency due to bilateral metastases from oat cell carcinoma of the esophagus. *Eur J Cardiothorac Surg* **5**: 336–337.

Heath, H., III, Hodgson, S.F., and Kennedy, M.A. 1980. Primary hyperparathyroidism: Incidence, morbidity, and potential economic impact in a community. *N Engl J Med* **302**: 189–193.

Heber, D., Byerley, L.O., Chi, J., et al. 1986. Pathophysiology of malnutrition in the adult cancer patient. *Cancer (Philadelphia)* **58**: 1867–1874.

Hofstra, R.M., Landvaster, R.M., Ceccherini, I., et al. 1994. A mutation in the RET proto-oncogene associated with multiple endocrine neoplasia type 2B and sporadic medullary thyroid carcinoma. *Nature* **367**: 375–376.

Honicky, R.E., and dePapp, E.W. 1973. Mediastinal teratoma with endocrine function. *Am J Dis Child* **126**: 650.

Jones, T. 1996. The imaging science of positron emission tomography. *Eur J Nucl Med* **23**: 807–813.

Knecht, T.P., Behling, C.A., Burton, D.W., et al. 1996. The humoral hypercalcemia of benignancy. *Clin Chem* **105**: 487–492.

Kukreja, S.C., Shevrin, D.H., Wimbiscus, S.A., et al. 1988. Antibodies to parathyroid hormone-related protein lower serum calcium in athymic mouse models of malignancy associated hypercalcemia due to human tumors. *J Clin Invest* **82**: 1798–1802.

Kwekkeboom, D.J., Krenning, E.P., Bakker, W.H., et al. 1993. Somatostatin analogue scintigraphy in carcinoid tumours. *Eur J Nucl Med* **20**: 283–292.

Lee, J.C., Yamaguchi, H., and Hopper, J., Jr. 1966. The association of cancer and the nephrotic syndrome. *Ann Intern Med* **64**: 41–51.

Lortholary, A.H., Cadeau, S.D., Bertrand, G.M., et al. 1999. Humoral hypercalcemia in patients with colorectal carcinoma. *Cancer* **86**: 2217–2221.

Lyall, S.S., Marieb, N.J., Wise, J.K., et al. 1975. Hyperinsulinemic hypoglycemia associated with a neurofibrosarcoma. *Arch Intern Med* **135**: 865–867.

Marks, L.J., Steinke, J., Podolsk, S., and Egdahl, R.H. 1974. Hypoglycemia associated with neoplasia. *Ann NY Acad Sci* **230**: 147–160.

Martin, T.J. 1988. Humoral hypercalcemia of malignancy. *Bone Miner* **4**: 83–89.

Martin, T.J., and Grill, V. 1992. Hypercalcemia in cancer. *J Steroid Biochem Mol Biol* **43**: 123–129.

Metzger, S., Nusair, S., Planer, D., et al. 2004. Inhibition of hepatic gluconeogenesis and enhanced glucose uptake contribute to the development of hypoglycemia in mice bearing IL-1β–secreting tumor. *Endocrinology* **145**: 5150–5156.

Montag, T.W., Murphy, R.E., and Belinson, J.L. 1984. Virilizing malignant lipid cell tumor producing erythropoietin. *Gynecol Oncol* **19**: 98–103.

Mori, H., Aoki, K., Katayama, I., et al. 1996. Humoral hypercalcemia of malignancy with elevated plasma PTHrP, TNFa and IL-6 in cutaneous squamous cell carcinoma. *Dermatology* **23**: 460–462.

Moseley, J.M., Kubota, M., Diefenbach-Jagger, H., et al. 1987. Parathyroid hormone–related protein purified from a human lung cancer cell line. *Proc Natl Acad Sci USA* **84**: 5048–5052.

Mundy, G.R., Rais, L.G., Shapiro, J.L., et al. 1977. Big and little forms of esteoclast-activating factor. *J Clin Invest* **60**: 122–128.

Mundy, G.R., and Martin, T.J. 1982. The hypercalcemia of malignancy: pathogenesis and management. *Metabolism* **31**: 1247–1277.

Mundy, G.R., Wilkinson, R., and Heath, D.A. 1983. Comparative study of available medical therapy for hypercalcemia of malignancy. *Am J Med* **74**: 421–432.

Mundy, G.R., Ibbotson, K.J., D'Souza, S.M., et al. 1984. The hypercalcemia of cancer. Clinical implications and pathogenic mechanisms. *N Engl J Med* **310**: 1718–1727.

Mundy, G.R. 1988. Hypercalcemia of malignancy revisited. *J Clin Invest* **82**: 1–6.

Nakamoto, Y., Higashi, T., Sakahara, H., et al. 2000. Evaluation of pancreatic islet cell tumors by fluorine-18 fluorodeoxyglucose positron emission tomography: comparison with other modalities. *Clin Nucl Med* **25**: 115–119.

Ng, K.W., and Martin, T.J. 1990. Humoral hypercalcemia of malignancy. *Clin Biochem* **23**: 11–16.

Nowak, R.A., Morrison, N.E., Goad, D.L., et al. 1990. Squamous cell carcinomas often produce more than a single bone resorption-stimulating factor: role of interleukin-1a. *Endocrinology* **127**: 3061–3069.

Odell, W.D. 1989. Paraendocrine syndromes of cancer. *Adv Intern Med* **34**: 325–351.

Odell, W.D., and Wolfsen, A.R. 1982. Humoral syndromes associated with cancer: ectopic hormone production. *Prog Clin Cancer* **8**: 57–74.

Odell, W.D., Wolfsen, A.R., Bachelot, I., and Hirose, F.M. 1979. Ectopic production of lipotropin by cancer. *Am J Med* **66**: 631–638.

Olefsky, S., Bailey, I., Samols, E., and Bilkus, D. 1962. A fibrosarcoma with hypoglycemia in a high serum insulin level. *Lancet* **2**: 378–380.

Orth, D.N., Guillemin, R., Ling, N., and Nicholson, W.E. 1978. Immunoreactive endorphins, lipotropins, and corticotropins in human nonpituitary tumor: evidence for a common precursor. *J Clin Endocrinol Metab* **46**: 849–852.

Osella, G., Orlandi, F., and Caraci, P. 2003. Acromegaly due to ectopic secretion of GHRH by bronchial carcinoid in a patient with empty sella. *J Endocrinol Invest* **26**: 163–169.

Papotti, M., Croce, S., Bello, M., et al. 2001. Expression of somatostatin receptor types 2, 3 and 5 in biopsies and surgical specimens of human lung tumours. Correlation with preoperative octreotide scintigraphy. *Virchows Arch* **439**: 787–797.

Pearse, A.G. 1966. Common cytochemical properties of cells producing polypeptide hormones with particular reference to calcitonin and the thyroid C cells. *Vet Rec* **79**: 587–590.

Picascia, D.D., and Caro, W.A. 1987. Cutaneous squamous cell carcinoma and hypercalcemia. *J Am Acad Dermatol* **17**: 347–351.

Reynaud-Mendel, B., Robert, C., Flageul, B., et al. 1997. Malignant hypercalcemia induced by a parathyroid hormone–related protein secreted by a cutaneous squamous cell carcinoma. *Arch Dermatol* **133**: 113.

Rikimaru, K., Matsutomo, F., Hayashi, E., et al. 1995. Evaluation of serum concentration of parathyroid hormone–related protein and its implication in hypercalcemia in squamous cell carcinoma of the head and neck. *Int J Oral Maxillofac Surg* **24**: 365–368.

Rivier, J., Speiss, J., Thorner, M., and Vale, W. 1982. Characterization of a growth hormone–releasing factor from a human pancreatic islet tumor. *Nature (London)* **300**: 276–278.

Robertson, G.L. 1976. The regulation of vasopressin in function in health and disease. *Recent Prog Horm Res* **33**: 333–385.

Rodman, J.S., and Sherwood, L.M. 1978. Disorders of mineral metabolism in malignancy. *In* "Metabolic Bone Disease" (L.V. Avioli and S. Krane, eds.). Academic Press, New York.

Saeed, S.M., Fine, G., and Horn, R.S., Jr. 1969. Hypoglycemia associated with extra-pancreatic tumors: An immunofluorescent study. *Cancer (Philadelphia)* **24**: 158–166.

Saeed uz Zafar, M., Mellinger, R.C., Fine, G., et al. 1979. Acromegaly associated with a bronchial carcinoid tumor: evidence for ectopic production of growth hormone releasing activity. *J Clin Endocrinol Metab* **48**: 66–71.

Sato, K., Yamakawa, Y., Shizume, K., et al. 1993. Passive immunization with anti-parathyroid hormone related protein monoclonal antibody markedly prolongs survival time of hypercalcemic nude mice bearing transplanted human PTHrP-producing tumors. *J Bone Miner Res* **8**: 849–860.

Schwartz, K.E., Wolfsen, A.R., Forster, B., and Odell, W.D. 1979. Calcitonin in non-thyroidal cancer. *J Clin Endocrinol Metab* **49**: 438–444.

Seregni, E., Chiti, A., and Bombardieri, E. 1998. Radionuclide imaging of neuroendocrine tumours: biological basis and diagnostic results. *Eur J Nucl Med* **25**: 639–658.

Shames, J.M., Dhurandhar, N.R., and Blackard, W.G. 1968. Insulin-secreting bronchial carcinoid tumor with widespread metastases. *Am J Med* **44**: 632–637.

Sherwood, J.B., and Goldwasser, E. 1976. Erythropoietin production by human renal carcinoma cells in monolayer culture. *Endocrinology (Baltimore)* **99**: 504–510.

Sherwood, L.M. 1980. The multiple causes of hypercalcemia in malignant disease [editorial]. *N Engl J Med* **303**: 1412–1413.

Sherwood, L.M., O'Riordan, J.L., Aurbach, G.D., and Potts, J.T. 1967. Production of parathyroid hormone by nonparathyroid tumors. *J Clin Endocrinol Metab* **27**: 140.

Shetty, M.R., Boghossian, H.M., Duffell, D., et al. 1982. Tumor-induced hypoglycemia: A result of ectopic insulin production. *Cancer (Philadelphia)* **49**: 1920–1923.

Slichter, S.J., and Harker, L. 1974. Hemostasis in malignancy. *Ann NY Acad Sci* **230**: 252–261.

Smith, N.L., Janelli, D.E., Madariaga, J., and Mishriki, Y. 1982. Hypoglycemia and Hodgkin's disease with hyperinsulinemia. *J Surg Oncol* **19**: 27–30.

Sparks, M.K., Kuhlman, D.S., Prieto, A., et al. 1985. Hypercalcemia in association with cutaneous squamous cell carcinoma. *Arch Dermatol* **121**: 243–246.

Steiner, H., Dahlback, O., and Walenstrom, J. 1968. Ectopic growth-hormone production and osteoarthropathy in carcinoma of the bronchus. *Lancet* **1**: 783–785.

Strewler, G.J. 2000. The physiology of parathyroid hormone–related protein. *N Engl J Med* **342**: 177–185.

Unger, R.H., Lochner, J., and Eisentraut, A.M. 1964. Identification of insulin and glucagon in bronchogenic metastasis. *J Clin Endocrinol Metab* **24**: 823–831.

Wolfsen, A.R., and Odell, W.D. 1979. ProACTH: Use for early detection of lung cancer. *Am J Med* **66**: 765–772.

Wysolmerski, J.J., and Broadus, A.E. 1994. Hypercalcemia of malignancy: the central role of parathyroid hormone–related protein. *Ann Rev Med* **45**: 189–200.

Yoneda, T., Nakai, M., Moriyama, K., et al. 1993. Neutralizing antibodies to human interleukin 6 reverses hypercalcemia associated with a human squamous carcinoma. *Cancer Res* **53**: 737–740.

CHAPTER

43

Counseling the Cancer Survivor

LINDA A. JACOBS AND ELLEN GIARELLI

INTRODUCTION

The concept of "survivorship" after a diagnosis of cancer reflects significant improvements made during the past decade in the quality and quantity of life (Leigh, 2001). Because cancer has been categorized as a chronic disease, patients and families are situated on a continuum of care. The period during which patients are characterized as survivors is lengthened, as many live a long cancer-free life and die of causes other than cancer. Each patient's experience with cancer and, therefore, survivorship is personal, intimate, and unique to the individual and family and is influenced by socioeconomic status, ethnic background, and cultural heritage.

Survivorship issues include surviving the diagnosis and initial treatment, adapting to physical limitations, and managing any late effects. Long-term follow-up will require screening for physiological problems, psychosocial adaptation, and ultimately restoring and maintaining a high quality of life. Many individuals seek nutrition-related information after a diagnosis with cancer, including information regarding diet, supplement use, and nutritional complementary therapies. These issues are covered elsewhere in this text.

The impact of nutrition on the cancer process can be complicated and confusing to patients with cancer. Science-based diet and nutrition information serves as a counterpoint to popular nutrition information that may not always be accurate. Sources of dietary and nutrition information may include friends and family, the popular press, television, the Internet, and self-professed experts promoting nutrition regimens. These sources of information may not always be accurate. The health benefits of recommended treatments, as well as many health promotion and disease prevention activities including dietary recommendations, are based on epidemiological observations and clinical trials. Patients should be provided with adequate information to understand the benefits and risks of complementary and alternative medical (CAM) nutritional therapies. In addition, many CAM therapies are promoted to the general public for wellness and cancer prevention; therefore, cancer survivors have the added burden of assessing the impact of CAM therapies on their type of cancer and cancer treatments. Cancer survivors should be encouraged to be vigilant consumers when considering all nutrition modalities, especially CAM nutritional therapies.

Many aspects of cancer treatment are beyond patient control, and decisions regarding surgery, radiation treatment, and/or the choice of chemotherapy regimens are, for the most part, dictated by the type and extent of the cancer. Patients diagnosed with cancer may think that nutritional deficiencies or excesses may have contributed to the etiology of their diagnosis and to subsequent treatment outcome. Consequently, many factors influence cancer survivors' concerns regarding the nutritional decisions they make after treatment has ended.

Cancer survivors are exposed to information and advice regarding nutrients and dietary changes that claim to alter disease course and outcome. The complexity of cancer treatment decisions can intimidate and confuse patients; some nutritional information that focuses on the impact of nutrients on cancer risk and treatment outcomes can also be complex and create confusion and uncertainty regarding recommended cancer treatment. In contrast, the benefits of alternative nutrition modalities are often presented in simplified, unscientific, and quasi-scientific language more easily understood by the nonmedical community. Confusing

Copyright © 2006, Elsevier Inc.
All rights of reproduction in any form reserved.

and conflicting information, as well as a less personalized medical care system, has contributed to a distrust of conventional medicine for many individuals. In some cases, distrust and confusion regarding the best course of cancer treatment, including nutritional recommendations, can lead patients to more unconventional methods of treatment including the use of certain diets and supplements.

The increased emphasis of research in nutrition and cancer on gene–nutrient interaction and biomarkers derived from research on nutrigenetics and nutrigenomics will result in the need to reevaluate the relationship of health care providers to cancer survivors in terms that were originally developed to deal with patients at risk for heritable cancers in one of two conditions: individuals at risk for cancer not yet diagnosed and those diagnosed and treated but carrying a heightened genetic risk for recurrence.

SURVIVORSHIP

What does it mean to be a survivor? In cancer care, the terms "survivor" and "survivorship" cover a range of states, from mere existence despite disease to total cure. The concept of survivorship applies to many aspects of life after cancer. Quality of life has been called the most common and important measurement of survival (Grant et al., 1996); however, even when quality of life is dismal, one is still surviving. Consequently, conceptual models of survivorship have changed as the options for health care have changed.

The term "survivorship" was historically used to describe family members who survived the loss of a loved one to cancer (Leigh, 1996). When cancer care offered limited treatments, rare cures, and little prospect of hope for patients and their families, the model for survivorship focused on helping family members grieve and accept personal loss. As treatments improved, patients lived longer and survivorship was redefined in terms of disease-free intervals. A newer model of survivorship was constructed with issues faced by the patient who responded to treatment, went into remission, or was cured. A cancer survivor was the individual whose cancer did not recur in the 5, 10, and more years following diagnosis and treatment.

Over the years, the contemporary idea of survivorship after a diagnosis of cancer has evolved along with the scientific advances that improve the quality and quantity of life (Leigh, 2001). Because cancer has been categorized as a chronic disease; patients and families are situated on a continuum of care. The period when patients are characterized as survivors is optimized as they live a longer cancer-free life and die of causes other than cancer. Models of survivorship evolve as cancer treatments improve. Each patient's experiences with illness and therefore survivorship are personal, intimate, and unique to the individual and family's experience with cancer, as well as their socioeconomic status and cultural heritage.

With the advent of increased interest in cancer risk reduction, gene–nutrient interaction, and counseling of patients with hereditary cancers, a new area of genetic cancer care has emerged, which has developed a whole new set of issues to be considered. With the addition of the single word "genetic" to qualify "cancer care," one could assume that there simply has been the inclusion of an additional cause of disease and subsequently another aspect of care. In practice, however, this single qualifier changes the nature of care in disease management, counseling, surveillance, and assessment of the psychosocial impact on patients and family members. Provider and patient discussions expand from individual to generational issues, and surveillance changes from monitoring for recurrence to waiting for expression of the genetic condition. Patients and family members struggle to understand the impact of knowing one's genetic risk of cancer; the fear of losing insurance and employment; and the feelings of grief, fear, relief, and confusion that may be associated with learning genetic test results. Although these shifts in focus may seem merely semantic, underlying them is a scientific revolution that has advanced nursing into the genomic era of medicine and introduced priority areas for nursing research. With the emergence of the genetic theory of disease, there has been a shift in the way we think about cancer, design treatments, and plan lifelong care. What survivorship actually encompasses in genetic cancer care is also expanding.

In June 2003, the Centers for Disease Control and Prevention (CDC) and the Lance Armstrong Foundation conducted a workshop called "Building Partnerships to Advance Cancer Survivorship and Public Health," which focused on developing an action plan that outlined how public health can address critical cancer survivorship issues. This action plan was developed by expert participants who addressed each of the following public health areas in the context of cancer survivorship: surveillance and research; communication, education, and training; programs, policies, and infrastructure; access to quality care and services; and evaluation and quality improvement. In the past year, survivorship has also been identified as a new priority for the National Cancer Institute (NCI), which outlined an action plan for fiscal year 2004 that focuses on survivorship issues as they relate to areas of public health similar to those outlined by the CDC and the Lance Armstrong Foundation. Although the term "cancer survivor" has not been used when describing an individual who has been identified as genetically at risk for developing cancer, the CDC/Lance Armstrong Foundation and National Institutes of Health (NIH) initiatives included a discussion of genetics in the action plans for addressing survivorship issues.

Advances in genetic technology and pharmacotherapeutics have dramatically altered the treatment course and long-term outcomes for many cancer patients and their families. For example, the decoding of the human genome and the identification of genes associated with individual susceptibility to treatment-related late effects affect treatment decisions and are leading to the tailoring of individual cancer treatments (Marshall, 2003; McLeod and Yu, 2003; Watters et al., 2003). In addition, patients with hereditary cancers are surviving longer and reproducing generations of individuals with genetic cancer predisposition. Consequently, the way we apply the concept of survivorship must evolve. For the purpose of discussing survivorship issues, patients are divided into two groups: individuals who have developed cancer and afterward have genetic mutation testing, and those who know they have a genetic alteration (genotype) that predisposes to cancer but have not yet developed a cancer (phenotype).

Cancer Survivor with Genetic Predisposition

A traditional model of survivorship has the prerequisite of a diagnosis of a disease to which one does not succumb. This model of survivorship may be applicable to individuals with cancer who have an inherited genetic predisposition to cancer, insofar as they have been diagnosed with a disease; many of the survivorship issues are similar to the issues of individuals who have had sporadic cancers. These issues include surviving the diagnosis and initial treatment, adapting to physical limitations, and managing the long-term late effects of cancer that will require screening for physiological problems, psychosocial adaptation, and ultimately restoring and maintaining a high quality of life. However, there are survivorship issues encountered by patients with hereditary cancer syndromes that are not relevant for survivors of sporadic cancers. For example, decisions regarding prophylactic surgery and disease-specific surveillance recommendations for the individual diagnosed with a sporadic cancer are very different for an individual with a cancer resulting from an inherited genetic predisposition. The broader family discussion with unaffected siblings, children, and parents regarding their cancer risk, including treatment and long-term surveillance options, are issues that must be considered when managing the care of an individual with a hereditary form of cancer. The broad range of disease-specific survivorship issues that can be identified for every hereditary cancer syndrome are beyond the scope of this chapter. Survival issues for patients and families with *BRCA1* and *MEN2* mutations are used to illustrate many of the complex survivorship issues that may be encountered when dealing with individuals with hereditary cancer syndromes. The intricacies and detail required to dissect the following could be the entire focus of this chapter; however, it is presented with the intent of provoking thought and providing the reader with a general overview of survivorship issues in genetic cancer care.

Case Study 1

A 40-year-old white woman presents with a mass in her left breast noted on mammogram. She reports that her mother was diagnosed with breast cancer at age 46 and died of her disease and her sister was diagnosed at age 38 and is doing well. She has two additional sisters and a brother who are well. The patient is premenopausal, has one daughter and two sons, and is married. A breast biopsy reveals a 2-cm lesion and one to two positive left axillary sentinel lymph nodes. Her tumor is estrogen- and progesterone receptor–positive, and she was treated with a mastectomy, four cycles of doxorubicin and cyclophosphamide, and radiation therapy to her left chest wall, followed by tamoxifen. She tested positive for the *BRCA1* gene. To date, no one else in her family has had genetic testing.

Treatment and Recurrence Issues

Many factors influence treatment decisions for breast cancer patients, whether they have an inherited predisposition to breast cancer or sporadic breast cancer. The effect of genes, hormones, and/or biomarkers on responsiveness to treatment, recurrence risk, and long-term disease-free survival has the potential to alter the course of treatment and ultimately long-term survival for individuals with inherited breast cancer. For example, the clinical significance of *BRCA1* mRNA levels was identified in tumor tissues as possible predictors of response to anthracycline-containing chemotherapy in breast cancer patients (Egawa et al., 2003), and *BRCA*-associated breast cancers have an increased risk of contralateral breast cancer compared with women with sporadic breast cancer (Constant et al., 2002). In addition, the role of radiotherapy and radiation sensitivity of breast tissue in women who are mutation carriers of *BRCA1/2* has been explored, with the ultimate determination that there is no significant difference between toxicity or treatment response between women with heritable breast cancer compared with women with sporadic breast cancers (Sharan et al., 1997; Pierce et al., 2000; Baeyens et al., 2002). By comparison, the role of radiotherapy for patients who are mutation carriers continues to be questioned and associated sequelae evaluated (Pierce et al., 2000). These known germline mutations, with autosomal dominant transmission, explain only part of the familial aggregation of breast cancer. Genetic epidemiology studies have shown evidence of inheritance patterns that are non-Mendelian and familial residual risk caused by the multiplicative effects of several genes that are more common in the population and confer moderate risks for cancer (Bonadona and Lasset, 2003). Consequently, it is evident that ongoing scientific advances influence treatment decisions and, therefore, the nature of the survivorship experience, including surveillance issues and treatment decisions for patients and families with heritable cancers.

Surveillance and Survivorship Issues

During the past few years, numerous studies have explored issues associated with the decision to undergo genetic testing. A number of patients and/or family members continue to choose not to undergo testing, and for many this decision will determine the recommended cancer treatment and surveillance. There are specific recommendations for affected individuals and their close relatives (first- or second-degree relatives) if a germline mutation associated with a particular cancer syndrome has been identified in the affected individual. For example, prophylactic surgery, including prophylactic mastectomy and prophylactic salpingo-oophorectomy, is presented to women who are unaffected *BRCA1* or *BRCA2* mutation carriers as an option to prevent breast and ovarian cancer. For a carrier who has been diagnosed with breast cancer, there is a 20% chance of developing a second primary breast cancer or relapsing within 5 years of their original diagnosis. For these individuals, mastectomy and prophylactic surgery (including prophylactic contralateral mastectomy and prophylactic bilateral salpingo-oophorectomy) may increase survival over surveillance alone and decrease the risk of relapse or a second primary breast cancer (Eeles, 2000; Sakorafas and Tsiotou, 2000). However, though commercially available, genetic testing is not always offered to patients who meet the guidelines for clinical genetic testing nor is it available across care settings, and it is important to understand that standard of care does not mandate that patients and family members who are at increased genetic risk of breast and ovarian cancer be offered genetic testing.

The information gained through genetic testing has the potential to significantly alter the course of treatment and subsequent surveillance recommendations for patients and their families. The survivorship experience may include lifelong uncertainty about recurrence risk, the risk for development of other cancers, as well as worry regarding cancer risk in family members of cancer patients who are identified at risk for a germline mutation and do not undergo testing (Kinnery et al., 2001). Although genetic testing can be beneficial for high-risk individuals, test results can be inconclusive. Consequently, the only time that clinical genetic testing affects the estimation of risk of developing cancer is when a genetic test is a true positive or negative. Women with breast cancer who have a significant family history of breast or ovarian cancer suggestive of an autosomal dominant inheritance pattern related to these cancers should be offered genetic education, counseling, and testing. However, because test results may be uninformative, these individuals should be managed as high-risk patients with appropriate surveillance and management recommendations in the absence of a true-negative test result.

There are general surveillance recommendations for individuals with inherited breast cancer tailored for each individual on the basis of the patient's profile. The American Cancer Society recommendations for breast cancer screening take into account a number of factors including age and family history (Smith et al., 2003). For example, the screening recommendations and survivorship issues for a breast cancer patient with a family history of cancer who is a mutation carrier and was treated with a left mastectomy and chest radiation and did not choose to have bilateral mastectomies or oophorectomies will be different than the recommendations for a similar patient who had prophylactic surgery. Also, if an individual decides to have bilateral mastectomies, he or she can eliminate the need for mammograms and other breast surveillance options such as breast ultrasounds, regular clinical breast examinations, and breast magnetic resonance imaging films. These seemingly complicated options make it critical that cancer patients with hereditary susceptibility to cancer, health care providers, and the general public be informed regarding the risks and benefits of genetic testing, as well as how test results influence treatment options and decisions, and ultimately the course of the survivorship experience, as illustrated in the next example.

The decision-making process regarding *BRCA1/2* testing, as well as testing for all of the inherited cancer mutations, remains potentially complex and difficult despite the benefits to be gained by quantifying individual and familial cancer risk, and the guidance that could be provided for subsequent treatment decisions and long-term surveillance and survivorship issues. Genetic testing decisions affect many psychosocial functions, including health practices, family relationships, reproductive decision-making, insurance issues, and finances. Patients and family members must consider what this information will mean for unaffected family members and have an understanding of the benefits, risks, and limitations of increased surveillance, prophylactic surgery, or other preventive strategies if they are to undergo genetic testing (Meijers-Heijboer et al., 2001).

Survivorship Issues in Individuals at Increased Risk of Cancer

Issues of survivorship arise at the nexus of a patient's health needs and the ability of the health care system to meet them. One may say that survivorship issues are generated from the healing relationship established between a patient and a health care provider. In this relationship, the patient's health care needs are identified and the health care provider offers information, treatment options, and resources to meet these needs. In the case of a patient with known disease, as soon as health care providers inform the patient of the diagnosis, both begin to identify survivorship issues because information and treatment choices must be made that will optimize the quantity and quality of life.

The nature of the healing relationship between the patient and health care provider for at-risk individuals in genetic cancer care is different than for the patient with cancer; therefore, survivorship issues are different. In this case, patients may learn long before a cancer diagnosis that they are at 40–85% risk of developing breast cancer and 20–40% risk of developing ovarian cancer in their lifetime. The individual who tests positive for a gene mutation associated with cancer begins to identify treatment choices that will influence survivorship issues. For example, at-risk individuals who undergo prophylactic surgery consent to removing an otherwise healthy and functioning body part to prevent future disease. The potential side effects of prophylactic surgery should be clearly discussed during education and counseling. Pellegrino (2003) describes three components of the healing relationship in health care: the act of medicine, the fact of illness, and the act of profession. Genetic testing (the act of medicine) generates the diagnosis of heritable risk (the fact of illness) (Giarelli, 2003a). The act of profession generates risk management strategies including lifelong surveillance or watching and waiting for cancer.

Surveillance and Survivorship Issues

When individuals who carry a mutation that predisposes them to developing cancer are identified (e.g., *RET*, *APC*, *BRCA1*, *BRCA2*), they will be asked to think about risk management to improve survival. They will also begin lifelong incidental and planned (Giarelli, 2003b) surveillance for phenotypic expression of the altered genotype. Chemoprevention may also be considered. All of this occurs in the absence of cancer and on a presumption of penetrance or risk of disease. Already the model for understanding survivorship has shifted to include "risk of disease" instead of "actual disease" as the source of survival issues.

In the next scenario, the patient has a positive genetic test and a strong family history that confer an increased risk of cancer. The genetic risk becomes proxy for the diagnosis. Survival issues change from "attempts to improve" to "attempts to guarantee" the quantity and quality of life. This takes the form of watching and waiting for early signs of disease and may also include preventing disease by removing, when possible, the at-risk organs. Survivorship issues in genetic cancer care of someone at risk for cancer are poignantly illustrated by the experiences of a child with an *RET* mutation.

Case Study 2

A single mother, age 35, was found to have nodules on both lobes of her thyroid gland. A biopsy revealed bilateral medullary thyroid carcinoma and c-cell hyperplasia widely dispersed throughout the lobes. A family history and pedigree uncovered significant history of thyroid cancer, Hirschsprung's disease, and adrenal tumors in first- and second-degree relatives in the maternal lineage. Genetic testing was performed on the proband and her 8-year-old daughter. Both had a missense mutation at codon 620 of the *RET* protooncogene on chromosome 10, and both were diagnosed as having multiple endocrine neoplasia type 2a (MEN2a). The mother underwent neck dissection and total thyroidectomy. Her medullary thyroid carcinoma was encapsulated and lymph nodes were negative. The daughter underwent a total prophylactic thyroidectomy. Her thyroid tissue was disease free. After surgery, both mother and daughter began thyroid hormone–replacement therapy and calcium supplementation. Both were advised to adhere to lifelong surveillance guidelines that would include annual 24-hour urine analysis for catecholamines and annual analysis of serum levels of thyroid-stimulating hormone, T_3, T_4, calcium, and calcitonin. Biochemical analyses are used to evaluate the occurrence of adrenal hyperplasia associated with MEN2a, appropriate thyroid hormone activity, hyperparathyroidism, and medullary thyroid carcinoma recurrence or expression, respectively.

In this scenario, the mother's survival can be understood in terms of disease-free intervals. Her survivorship issues will be similar to those of other cancer patients who measure life in 5, 10, and longer years of life after cancer. Her quality of life will be maintained with careful medical management of thyroid hormone replacement therapy and minimization of the complement of adverse physiological effects of thyroidectomy. After this point, the similarities end and survivorship issues unique to genetic cancer care become most apparent. Both mother and daughter have a lifelong variable risk for the development of other tumors associated with MEN2a. They have a 30–50% chance of developing pheochromocytoma and a 10–30% chance of developing parathyroid tumors (Modigliani et al., 1995; Pausova et al., 1996). There are no data to predict the occurrence of medullary thyroid carcinoma from *in situ* thyroid cells after thyroidectomy, and there is a 50% chance that the *RET* mutation will be passed to offspring in the autosomal dominant inheritance pattern characteristic of MEN2a (McKusick, 1997). Because expression is variable, no patient can know when neoplasia will develop. The mother's disease represents the child's risk of disease, and the responsibility for monitoring oneself is extended to monitoring one's offspring.

The child's situation is different. She did not have cancer. She was cancer free. Her survival issues, although not urgent, still focus on quantity and quality of life. They result directly from her genetic predisposition and mutation status, and a critical point is that these issues are not based on the "fact" of disease, but on the probability of disease. The at-risk person will comply with surveillance guidelines on "faith" (or the trust in something without visible proof of its existence) in the accuracy of genetic technology and the state of the science of genetic cancer care. Her daily life may be infused with incidental surveillance events as she attends

TABLE 1 Shifting Concepts Related to "Survivorship"

Cancer care	Genetic cancer care
Individual	Generational
Personal longevity	Family longevity
Absolute risk	Relative risk
Recurrence	Penetrance and expression
Conventional treatment	New models of treatment
Monitoring self	Monitoring self and others
Lifelong surveillance	*Lives*-long surveillance
Nurse–patient relationship	Nurse–extended family relationship
Calculable cost of care	Unknown cost of care
Personal fertility	Reproductive potential

to physical feelings that may (or may not) be associated with *RET* mutation expression or medical management (Giarelli, 2003). Her choice to conceive children will be affected by the probability of passing the genetic mutation to offspring. Thus, the issue of personal fertility becomes an issue of family viability. Personal survival is coexistent with family survival, and cancer prevention is not individual but generational. At this young age, at-risk individuals begin to participate in highly structured, lifelong relationships with health care professionals for the purpose of early detection of a disease from which there may not be a favorable outcome. Her genotype may be further expressed, in which case illness becomes factual. In the event that there is no further expression of MEN2a, she may regret years of worry and question decisions that were made based on her genetic risk.

Although it may not be possible for many, the ideal outcome for cancer-free patients identified at risk for a heritable cancer is that they never develop disease. At-risk individuals may embrace lifelong surveillance as a way to experience a sense of control over an otherwise uncontrollable process. Patients and providers know that genetic technology widens the range of health care options and favorably transforms cancer care and as the nature of the entire survivorship experience. Consequently, previous models of survivorship are of limited value. The paradigm of survivorship is beginning to shift, and in doing so, it will accommodate the constantly advancing fluid science of genomic medicine (Table 1). At this time we have limited terminology to competently describe the survivorship experiences of individuals with heritable cancer syndromes and are only beginning to understand the structure of this fluid model of survivorship in genetic cancer care.

DISCUSSION AND FUTURE DIRECTIONS

Advances in nutritional oncology and the development of biomarkers based on nutrigenetic and nutrigenomic information will necessarily result in a shift to a genomic focus for cancer care, which will require that health care providers reevaluate the assessment, management, and follow-up recommendations for patients and families at risk for and with a diagnosis of a heritable or sporadic cancer. Furthermore, the application of the idea of survivorship in genetic cancer care requires the reconstruction of prior theory and evaluation of the prior fact that, as Kuhn (1962) states, is "an intrinsically revolutionary process." Health care providers cannot take a common body of belief for granted, but they must search for new facts with which to rebuild a field of study, to construct a model that is compatible with the science and suitable for the multifarious survivorship and other issues of a growing cohort of people at genetic risk for cancer.

In conclusion, much more research is necessary in this field and it is time to set aside preconceived models of cancer evaluation, treatment, and survivorship care. Recall the survivorship issues discussed in the scenarios and the components of the healing relationship, and consider the following questions: What are the effects of creating a "fact of illness," as described in this article, on a person's quality of life? How does prophylactic surgery impact quality of life and longevity of families? How can health care providers change lifelong individual surveillance to "lives"-long generational surveillance? And, how can we further individualize treatments according to genotype and gene–environment interactions?

Ultimately, the answers to these and other questions will generate the common language we need to converse with our patients about their genetic cancer survivorship issues and will help to clarify the evolving concepts of cancer survivorship and survivorship in relation to genetic cancer care in an era in which increasing amounts of nutritional biomarker information will arise from the fields of nutrigenetics and nutrigenomics.

References

Baeyens, A., Thierens, H., Claes, K., et al. 2002. Chromosomal radiosensitivity in breast cancer patients with a known or putative genetic predisposition. *Br J Cancer* **87**: 1379–1385.

Bonadona, V., and Lasset, C. 2003. Inherited predisposition to breast cancer: after the BRCA1 and BRCA2 genes, what next? *Bull Cancer* **90**: 587–594.

Constant, M.M.E., Menke-Pluijmers, M.B.E., Seynavet, C., et al. 2002. Clinical experience of prophylactic mastectomy followed by immediate breast reconstruction in women at hereditary risk of breast cancer (HB(O)C) or a proven BRCA1 and BRCA2 germ-line mutation. *Eur J Surg Oncol* **28**: 627–632.

Eeles, R. 2000. Future possibilities in the prevention of breast cancer intervention strategies in BRCA1 and BRCA2 mutation carriers. *Breast Cancer Res* **2**: 283–290.

Egawa, C., Motomura, K., Miyoshi, Y., et al. 2003. Increased expression of BRCA1 mRNA predicts favorable response to anthracycline-containing chemotherapy in breast cancers. *Breast Cancer Res Treat* **78**: 45–50.

Giarelli, E. 2003a. Safeguarding being: a bioethical principle for genetic nursing care. *Nurs Ethics* **10**: 255–268.

Giarelli, E. 2003b. Bringing threat-to-the-fore: participating in life-long surveillance for genetic risk of cancer. *Oncol Nurs Forum* **6**: 945–955.

Grant, M., Padilla, G.V., and Greimel, E.R. 1996. Survivorship and quality of life issues. *In* "Cancer Nursing: A Comprehensive Textbook," (R. McCorkle, M. Grant, M. Frank-Stromborg, and S.B. Baird, eds), 2nd edition, pp. 1313–1321. Saunders, Philadelphia, PA.

Kinney, A., DeVellis, B., Skrzynia, C., and Millikan, R. 2001. Genetic testing for colorectal carcinoma susceptibility. *Cancer* **91**: 57–65.

Kuhn, T.S. 1962. "The Structure of Scientific Revolutions." The University of Chicago Press, Chicago.

Leigh, S. 1996. Defining our destiny. *In* "A Cancer Survivor's Almanac: Charting Your Journey" (B. Hoffman, ed.), pp. 261–271. Chronimed Publishing, Minneapolis.

Leigh, S. 2001. Preface: the culture of survivorship. *Semin Oncol Nurs* **17**: 234–235.

Marshall, E. 2003. Preventing toxicity with a gene test. *Science* **302**: 588–590.

McKusick, F.A. 2003. "Mendelian Inheritance in Man: A Catalog of Human Genes and Genetic Disorders," 12th edition. Johns Hopkins University Press, Baltimore, MD (1997). Available at: www.ncbi.nlm.nih/gov/htbin-post/Omim.htm (accessed October 7, 2003).

McLeod, H.L., and Yu, J. 2003. Cancer pharmacogenomics: SNPS, chips, and the individual patient. *Cancer Invest* **21**: 630–640.

Meijers-Heijboer, E.J., Verhoog, L.C., Brekelmans, C.T.M., et al. 2001. Considerations in genetic testing and prophylactic measures. *Lancet* **5**: 117–120.

Modigliani, E., Vasen, H., Raue, K., et al. Pheochromocytoma in multiple endocrine neoplasia type 2: European study. *J Intern Med* **238**: 363–367.

Pausova, Z., Soliman, E., Amizuka, N., et al. 1996. Role of the RET proto-oncogene in sporadic hyperparathyroidism and in the hyperparathyroidism of MEN type 2a. *J Clin Endocrinol Metab* **81**: 2711–2718.

Pellegrino, E.D. 1979. Toward a reconstruction of medical morality: the primacy of the act of profession and the fact of illness. *J Med Philosophy* **4**: 32–55.

Pierce, L., Strawderman, M., Narod, S., et al. 2000. Effect of radiotherapy after breast-conserving treatment in women with breast cancers and germline BRCA1/2 mutations. *J Clin Oncol* **18**: 3360–3369.

Sakorafas, G.H., and Tsiotou, A.G. 2000. Genetic predisposition to breast cancer: a surgical perspective. *Br J Surg* **87**: 49–162.

Sharan, S.K., Morimatsu, M., Albrecht, U., et al. 1997. Embryonic lethality and radiation hypersensitivity mediated by Rad51 in mice lacking BRCA2. *Nature* **386**: 804–810.

Smith, R., Saslow, D., Sawyer, K.A., et al. 2003. American Cancer Society guidelines for breast cancer screening: update 2003. *CA Cancer J Clin* **53**: 141–169.

Watters, J.W., and McLeod, H.L. 2003. Cancer pharmacogenomics: current and future applications. *Biochim Biophys Acta* **1603**: 99–111.

CHAPTER

44

Nutritional Support and Quality of Life

N. SIMON TCHEKMEDYIAN, DAVID CELLA, AND DAVID HEBER

INTRODUCTION

Few things are more frightening than the diagnosis of cancer. The patient with cancer faces the prospect of difficult treatment choices, debilitating pain, loss of function, and the anxiety associated with risk of mortality. Some of the effects of chemotherapy, such as nausea, profound fatigue, and hair loss, have attained a frightening reputation among patients. In response to these fears, some patients consider delaying or even denying their treatment or elect a nontoxic alternative therapy, which may include nutrition. Many patients who agree to recommended "conventional" therapy also have an interest in adjuvant nutrition therapy. In either case, the practice of nutritional oncology is exemplified by a profound respect for the quality of life (QOL) of the cancer patient. It is only with an understanding of the nature of QOL and how it is assessed and quantified that many of the benefits of nutrition in cancer treatment and prevention can be gauged. It is critical to understand the impact of QOL issues in the cancer patient when determining how to apply nutritional adjuvant therapy as part of the new paradigm of nutritional oncology. This chapter provides an overview of QOL assessment, including how nutrition therapies can be judged on the basis of their impact on QOL.

The past 50 years have seen a shift from the treatment of acute disease to chronic disease and ultimately to primary and secondary prevention. Health care providers concerned with the management of chronic diseases including cancer have begun to strive to improve not only the quantity of life as measured by survival but also the QOL of the cancer patient. Prior to the 1970s, health outcomes in oncology were usually limited to survival and treatment toxicity. However, the concern for documenting a broader concept of patient outcomes has increased dramatically (Fayers and Jones, 1983; Schipper and Levitt, 1985; Aaronson and Beckman, 1987; Cella and Cherin, 1988; Barofsky and Sugarbaker, 1990; Cella and Tulsky, 1990; Osoba, 1991) while not losing sight of the primary goal of reducing mortality (Gill and Feinstein, 1994). For example, QOL is an important consideration in the treatment of patients with advanced lung cancer because treatment is largely palliative. Moreover, QOL predicts survival in non–small-cell lung cancer, and there is increasing acceptance by clinicians and regulatory authorities of symptoms and QOL as primary or co-primary endpoints in clinical trials.

Medicine has a long tradition of concern for the well-being of the people it serves. Every physician is trained to think of an intervention as a potential balance between iatrogenic harm and therapeutic benefit. By and large, people with cancer seek treatments that may extend their lives, but the toll on life quality must be factored in. In some circumstances (e.g., aggressive treatment in advanced disease), QOL has value equal to quantity of life. Recognizing this, the U.S. Food and Drug Administration (FDA) adopted a policy in which QOL is acknowledged as one of two primary criteria for approval of new anticancer agents (Johnson and Temple, 1985). An antitumor drug can be approved if it demonstrates an improvement in QOL, whether or not it shows an advantage over standard therapy in survival. Such thinking is familiar in cancer medicine, as exemplified by developments in breast-sparing surgery, limb and organ prostheses, low toxicity chemotherapy for good prognosis cancers, and palliative care.

This chapter emphasizes QOL in the care of the oncology patient and serves to remind all oncologists of the important role of nutrition in this process.

Copyright © 2006, Elsevier Inc.
All rights of reproduction in any form reserved.

DEFINITION OF QUALITY OF LIFE

There are two fundamental components of the "QOL" concept: subjectivity and multidimensionality. *Subjectivity* refers to the fact that QOL can be understood only from the patient's perspective. Like pain, which is considered to have a subjective component, one can only assess a person's QOL by asking the patient about it directly. Although this consideration may seem obvious, it profoundly affects the types of instruments one uses to measure QOL. It is not possible to estimate QOL by observing patient behaviors because such behaviors do not account for underlying patient perceptions of QOL. These underlying processes include perception of illness, perception of treatment, expectations of self, and appraisal of risk/harm.

When we ask patients how they feel, their response is only partially related to their observable behavior. It is also influenced by their current set of expectations surrounding their actual functional level, as well as their perceptions about the treatment environment. If patients believe we are in a position to help, they may exaggerate their symptom or problem. If they believe we might withhold a treatment option, they may minimize treatment side effects in their response. Patients' assessments of QOL are dynamic over time and in different situations. In general, QOL is best understood as the difference between one's actual functional level and one's ideal standard. Patients who are able to adjust their expectations under duress are also able to adapt better to their illness and treatment. Therefore, given two patients with the same level of functional impairment, the more cognitively flexible of the two will report a higher QOL than the less flexible one. This interplay between expectation, adaptation, and self-report of well-being has been demonstrated with pain (Padilla et al., 1990) and overall QOL (Padilla et al., 1992). Furthermore, it is evident that patients who find themselves in progressively more threatening situations, including deteriorating health status, are inclined to generate more positive evaluations of uncertainty. This results in more positive assessments of QOL than would be expected in the absence of cognitive adjustment (Mishel, 1990). This suggests that patients with more advanced disease are more tolerant of toxic therapies than we would see in "naive" raters, such as healthy reference populations or even expert health providers. In general, people living with cancer prefer more aggressive therapy than therapy based on the projections of proxy raters. The fundamental component of subjectivity must be included in measuring QOL whenever QOL concerns drive treatment decisions.

The second basic aspect of QOL is multidimensionality. This is based on the psychometric tradition of health status measurement. The multidimensionality of QOL refers to the coverage of a broad range of content, including physical, functional, emotional, and social well-being. It is assumed that by aggregating measures of these various aspects of functioning, one can approximate a single index of QOL (Stewart et al., 1981). Little work has been done to determine the relative importance of each of the major determinants of QOL. As a result, measurement devices that aggregate scores do so with little knowledge of what might be distorted by assuming equivalence across dimensions. Rather than make any assumptions about their relative importance, some have opted not to aggregate dimensional scores into a total score or to do so only post hoc (Aaronson et al., 1988; Stewart et al., 1989; Hays and Stewart, 1990; Ware and Sherbourne, 1993). Newer scales under development attempt to measure the importance of each dimension to the patient being questioned.

Subjectivity

Most treatment decisions in oncology are best made with patient input that incorporates their perception of QOL. The decision to undergo radiation treatment versus surgical treatment for prostate cancer involves many dimensions beyond the consideration of survival probability. QOL issues related to sexual and urinary function are equally important. QOL refers to patients' appraisal of and satisfaction with their current level of functioning compared with what they perceive to be possible or ideal (Cella and Cherin, 1988). It is important to consider the appraisal of the extent of dysfunction, as well as the rating of how this appraisal fits with the patient's value system. A rating of dysfunction is valuable because it documents the tangible advantages and disadvantages of various treatments. A value-based rating can be useful because it provides the patient's subjective opinion as to whether that dysfunction is tolerable. For example, cystitis and proctitis following prostatic irradiation are common. Although healthy individuals might not accept such discomfort, it is remarkable to many radiation oncologists how well this dysfunction is tolerated by prostate cancer patients. Many decisions about treatment include this information, at least implicitly. As indicated earlier, many patients' perceptions of their illness are extremely variable. For example, some patients prefer a gastrostomy tube to a nasogastric catheter not because of any medical or physical consideration, but because of the perception of others about the patient's degree of illness with an obvious tube hanging out of the nose compared with a hidden gastrostomy catheter. Similarly, the same degree of nausea and vomiting in two patients can lead to different degrees of disability based not only on the degree of nausea but also on how this interferes with the daily routine of each patient. The degree of dysfunction could also relate to the emotional reaction to the nausea and vomiting. Only a multidimensional assessment of QOL including physical, social, and emotional components would detect this distinction.

Subjectivity should not be confused with lack of validity. The measurement science behind QOL can provide for the collection of reproducible and substantive data.

Multidimensionality

A large number of dimensions have been proposed as part of the global construct of QOL. Activity level, or functional status, has been proposed as a reasonable estimate of overall QOL (Karnofsky and Burchenal, 1949; Zubrod et al., 1960). Single-item estimates of subjective well-being or a personal appraisal of overall QOL have been used to assess QOL (Gough et al., 1983; Bernheim and Buyse, 1984). Such single-item estimates of QOL are not acceptable because they are dimensionless. A one-item measure makes it impossible to determine specific information about the nature of score change. Pain scales, symptom and toxicity ratings, mood scales, scales to measure activities of daily living (Katz et al., 1963), and the classic performance status scales (Karnofsky and Burchenal, 1949; Zubrod et al., 1960) are not QOL measures by this criterion of multidimensionality.

Although there is agreement among experts on the multidimensionality of QOL, there is less agreement on the specific nature of these dimensions. Schipper and Levitt (1985) have stated that there are four dominant contributors to the QOL composite: (1) physical/occupational function, which is the ability to carry on in one's usual role; (2) psychological state, including freedom from depression, anxiety, and other psychological disorders; (3) sociability encompassing the ability to maintain social interactions; and (4) somatic comfort such as freedom from pain and discomfort. Other dimensions included by some investigators are general life satisfaction and the ability to engage in personal leisure pursuits.

Although there are many potential QOL dimensions, most can be grouped into one of four areas: physical, functional, emotional, and social (Cella, 1991). QOL scales vary with regard to the names given to the dimensions measured. Furthermore, there are frequently discrepancies between the dimensions reported to be measured by a scale and the actual item content. Psychometric data that could help determine the underlying dimensionality are rarely reported, presumably because of the small numbers of patients studied in the development and validation of scales, making statistical evaluation difficult. Available factor analyses and scale aggregation have generally supported the validity of the four primary dimensions of health-related QOL described earlier (physical, emotional, functional, and social) (Stewart et al., 1981; Schipper et al., 1984; Aaronson, 1986; Aaronson and Beckman, 1987; DeHaes et al., 1987; Hays and Stewart, 1990; Cella, 1991, 1997).

Physical Well-Being

Physical well-being refers to perceived and observed physical functions and disorders. Common problems encountered in the cancer patient include fatigue, nausea, vomiting, and pain. The distinction between physical dysfunction related to disease status versus treatment is an important distinction for the physician. However, patients usually consider both the disease and the treatment-related dysfunctions as a single entity and may interpret disease symptoms as side effects. Some investigators have specifically separated gastrointestinal (GI) toxicity as a separate measure (Schipper et al., 1984; DeHaes et al., 1987).

Functional Well-Being

Functional status refers to the patient's ability to perform daily activities related to personal needs, ambitions, and social roles. The most basic of these activities include walking, feeding, bathing, and dressing. It also includes the ability to carry out expected responsibilities with family, friends, and colleagues. It is sometimes important to differentiate functional from physical well-being. For example, a patient may be able to continue to work despite significant physical dysfunction.

Emotional Well-Being

Emotional well-being is both correlated with and distinct from physical well-being (Hays and Stewart, 1990). A comprehensive health-related QOL measure assesses both sides of this spectrum. The onset of cancer and its treatment can lead to the blunting of positive emotional experience. Patients with cancer usually demonstrate little evidence of emotional distress by comparison with patients undergoing outpatient psychotherapy treatment (Cella et al., 1989; Guadagnoli and Mor, 1989). However, this observation does not minimize the impact of positive affect (well-being) and negative affect (distress) on the cancer patient.

Social Well-Being

As an aspect of QOL, social well-being is the most difficult to define. The content of this dimension is diverse, ranging from perceived social support, maintenance of leisure activities, and family functioning to intimacy, including sexuality. The diverse nature of social well-being has made it difficult to define. Nonetheless, it is clearly important to patients adapting and coping with illness. This dimension includes maintenance of gratifying relationships with friends and acquaintances, as well as closer relationships with family and significant others. Most QOL questionnaires for cancer patients ask few, if any, questions about this dimension or simply ask about overall level of social or family activity compared with premorbid baseline.

Other Considerations

Some of the aspects of QOL listed in the previous subsections, such as sexuality, cut across several of the four dimensions discussed earlier. Sexuality is mediated by both physical and functional status, which contribute to desire and arousal capability and to physical comfort with sexual activity. However, sexuality is also dependent on emotional well-being and the level of intimacy within the relationship.

A number of other important areas of health-related QOL are not included in the four-domain scheme described earlier. For example, treatment satisfaction and spirituality are important aspects of the cancer treatment experience. However, there have been no convincing factor analysis studies of existing measures to suggest that these are separate dimensions of QOL. This is an area that requires first-hand study, because of the importance of treatment satisfaction and spiritual well-being to the person with cancer. For example, treatment satisfaction is clearly important from the standpoint of perceived well-being and quality of care. Treatment satisfaction is itself a multidimensional concept (Ware et al., 1983). Therefore, though related to QOL, it is often evaluated separately. As a result, data combining both QOL and treatment satisfaction are rarely reported.

Spirituality, though very important to some patients, is of little importance to others. It also means very different things to different people. To some, it is primarily an emotional (i.e., mental) dimension because it involves an inner belief system. To others, its meaning derives from the social contacts created by participating in worship or community activity. And among those patients who regard spirituality highly, some find that the challenges of illness promote spiritual growth, whereas others find difficulty resolving the spiritual crisis they face as a result of their illness. Perhaps because of these complications, the highly personalized realm of spirituality is a poor statistical fit with QOL questions from the four primary domains (Cella, 1997). Therefore, like treatment satisfaction, it tends to be considered separately from QOL (if at all). In fact, however, it may be extremely important. Some have suggested that spirituality be considered a separate QOL domain in its own right (Donovan et al., 1989).

PURPOSE OF QUALITY OF LIFE MEASUREMENT

Investigators may want to measure QOL in cancer patients for at least three reasons: (1) to assess rehabilitation needs, (2) to evaluate treatment outcome, and (3) to predict response to future treatment. All of these aspects clearly have relevance to nutritional support in the cancer patient and to nutrition adjuvant therapy.

Assessing Rehabilitation Needs

In clinical settings, patients are confronted by a host of physical and psychological challenges to their coping ability. Itemizing the likely problems and clustering them into groups can help clinicians attempting to promote optimal patient adaptation. Carefully constructed psychometric scales can help clinicians assess and better treat the rehabilitation needs, including nutritional rehabilitation needs of their patients. Because cancer is likely to cause disruption in a number of areas, a good instrument will be sensitive enough to detect problems in a number of areas. Inventories such as the Cancer Rehabilitation Evaluation System (CARES) (Ware et al., 1983; Schag and Heinrich, 1988; Ganz et al., 1992) or the Sickness Impact Profile (SIP) (Bergner et al., 1976, 1981) make such assessments possible.

Because cancer tends to limit functional ability and role performance, patients' expectations of themselves are likely to change as the disease progresses. Those patients who successfully lower their expectations in parallel to decreased functional ability will better avoid disappointment, thereby maintaining a higher QOL than patients who maintain unrealistically high expectations of themselves. As a result, self-reported QOL is improved by this down-modification of expectation. Psychotherapeutic treatment can be geared toward changing patient expectations when functionality is chronically compromised. Effective palliative care often involves compassionate patient education that addresses patients' needs for understanding and modification of expectations in addition to pure symptom control.

Evaluating Treatment Outcome

The most common reason for measuring QOL is to obtain a broader, more comprehensive measure of health outcome. In this application, the purpose is not to identify problems for the treatment team, but to compare the QOL across alternative treatments. Examples of this approach are found throughout the literature (Baum et al., 1980; Silverfarb and Maurer, 1980; Sugarbaker et al., 1982; Silverfarb et al., 1983; Coates et al., 1987).

Investigators evaluating new cancer treatments are often as concerned with treatment toxicity as they are with efficacy. In fact, this application of QOL measurement is best characterized as a form of extended toxicity rating by which to judge the value of treatment. In this way, QOL becomes an important aspect of the cost/benefit ratio in evaluating treatment recommendations on the basis of clinical trial data.

In the past, when this has been the purpose of QOL measurement, the scales selected have usually been simple, easy-to-administer measures with less sensitivity and specificity than those selected for investigations of clinical rehabilitation. Usually, these methods have placed an emphasis on physical and functional dimensions. This has changed with the advent of more easily administered broad-based scales (Schipper et al., 1984; Aaronson et al., 1988; Stewart et al., 1989; Ware and Sherbourne, 1993; Cella, 1997).

Predicting Response to Future Treatment

Pretreatment activity level or performance status is a significant predictor of survival in certain tumor types (e.g., lung cancer). This has usually been measured using either the Karnofsky or Zubrod single-item rating scales (Karnofsky and Burchenal, 1949; Zubrod et al., 1960). In fact, reports of QOL as a predictor of survival have been published (Ruckdeschel and Plantados; 1989; Ganz et al., 1991). It is likely that a more broad-based questionnaire including other dimensions of QOL would be an even more useful predictor of survival.

The value of multidimensional instruments to evaluate the complexities of QOL, particularly patients' self-evaluation as distinguished from clinicians' observations, has become evident in clinical cancer research (Osoba, 1994). Several widely used scales measure more than one dimension of QOL, often using graded response choices that offer better accuracy and distinctions between people than dichotomous choices that merely reflect the presence or absence of a problem. By definition, QOL instruments query patients directly because the concept of QOL is inherently subjective. Measurement science and application enable reliable and valid summary scores of the patient's subjective experience.

Nutritional QOL Assessment Options: Advanced Lung Cancer as a Model

The EORTC QLQ-C30 with its lung cancer module and the FACT-L with its Lung Cancer Subscale (LCS) and Trial Outcome Index (TOI) are often used in clinical research and occasionally even in clinical practice in patients with lung cancer. They provide valuable information on patient well-being, but they also have inherent limitations in their ability to provide complete information. Only a representative sample of questions can reasonably be asked, and there is always the chance that the selected sample does not reflect the priorities of a given patient being assessed. Even when the questions are well suited to the patient, missing data over time can result in a loss of statistical power to produce clinically relevant and unbiased findings. Because the underlying factors that affect a patient's ability to complete a questionnaire over time are often related to the patient's actual condition, longitudinal data with more than a small amount of missing data can be uninterpretable and challenging to analyze.

The EORTC QLQ-C30 is a 30-item questionnaire that assesses overall function, symptoms, and QOL. This questionnaire, widely cited in clinical trials, requires about 10 minutes for patients to complete (Aaronson , 1993). An additional assessment, the 13-item lung cancer module, consists of items querying side effects of treatment and disease symptoms (Bergman et al., 1994). The QLQ-C30, which measures global QOL, function (physical, role, cognitive, emotional, and social), and symptoms (fatigue, pain, and nausea and vomiting), is designed to measure distinct aspects of well-being and show responsiveness to change in a patient's health status (Aaronson , 1993).

The FACT-L, similar in item content to the EORTC QLQ-C30, is also widely used to assess several aspects of QOL in patients with lung cancer. Several refinements have resulted in the current 36-item survey that assesses four general QOL domains (physical, social/family, emotional, and functional well-being), along with additional patient symptoms and concerns, such as appetite loss, chest tightness, shortness of breath, and hair loss. This LCS of the FACT-L queries patients' disease symptoms using nine questions, to which patients respond "not at all," "a little bit," "somewhat," "quite a bit," or "very much" (Cella et al., 1995; Cella, 2004). A summary higher order physical summary score, the TOI, provides an efficient (21 items), precise, and relevant measurement of the physical dimensions of patient-reported health. It comprises physical well-being, functional well-being, and the LCS and integrates them into an index (Cella et al., 1995; Cella, 2004).

In addition to the usual subscales scored on FACT-L (www.facit.org), a very brief, 14-item, symptom-focused assessment for use in clinical practice and clinical trials has been added (Table 1). All items (except the last item) come from the longer (36-item) FACT-L, so validity data are abundant. Because of its flexibility, the FACT-L and its derivatives (e.g., TOI and FACT-Lung Symptom Index) can offer a highly customizable and informative approach.

Other instruments in current use focus specifically on symptoms. The Lung Cancer Symptom Scale is a 15-item questionnaire that consists of nine patient and six clinician questions. Its measurement focuses on palliation and control of symptoms in patients treated in clinical trials. The Lung Cancer Symptom Scale is highly reliable and feasible for use in clinical trials. Administration requires about 5 minutes.

TABLE 1 FACT-L Symptom Index

1. I have a lack of energy.
2. I have pain.
3. I have nausea.
4. I am short of breath.
5. I am losing hair.
6. My thinking is clear.
7. I have been coughing.
8. I have a good appetite.
9. I feel tightness in my chest.
10. Breathing is easy for me.
11. I am bothered by side effects of treatment.
12. I am content with the quality of my life right now.
13. I have been emotionally distressed.
14. Compared to one week ago, would you say that in the above areas you are overall better, worse, or about the same?

Note: FACT-L, Functional Assessment of Cancer Therapy—Lung.

Its content is narrower in scope than that of the EORTC and FACT questionnaires, but the Lung Cancer Symptom Scale is unique in that it includes both clinician and patient input (Hollen et al., 1994).

The Rotterdam Symptom Checklist, a 34-item questionnaire that summarizes psychological and physical distress in general cancer populations, requires around 10 minutes to complete (de Haes et al., 1990). The Memorial Symptom Assessment Scale is a 32-item survey that assesses physical and psychological symptoms in general cancer populations (Portenoy, 1994). The Symptom Distress Scale has also been used often to evaluate symptoms in patients with advanced lung cancer (McCorkle and Young, 1978).

Each of the QOL instruments has unique strengths and usefulness in various clinical settings of cancer, but the most widely used in lung cancer are the EORTC QLQ-C30 + the 13-item lung cancer module and the FACT-L; both have been extensively validated and translated into >30 languages. Experience has shown that they are valuable in elucidating the effects of lung cancer on QOL.

QUALITY OF LIFE AND NUTRITION

Patients with advanced cancer depend on relief from uncomfortable symptoms to recover a basic sense of physical comfort and well-being. Nausea, vomiting, anorexia, fatigue, weakness, and weight loss are common nutritional problems encountered by the cancer patient.

The nausea associated with chemotherapy is unlike the nausea associated with minor bacterial illnesses, viruses, or mild irritable bowel syndrome. The central stimulation of the emesis centers in the brain can lead to an acquired aversion to associated stimuli including any foods eaten before chemotherapy. Vomiting associated with chemotherapy is also influenced by anxiety and conditioning. Patients undergoing cancer therapy know that it can make them very ill, and this affects their QOL.

Fortunately, much can be done to alleviate symptoms of nausea and even prevent vomiting altogether in patients undergoing chemotherapy using some of the newer drugs that are available. For example, 5-HT_3 receptor antagonists have markedly improved the ability to control GI symptoms associated with chemotherapy.

Anorexia, because of its impact on food intake, can lead to depletion of energy stores and a catabolic state that eventually results in profound weakness. A meal is often a gratifying experience and an opportunity for the family to be together, so anorexia has psychological and social implications.

EXERCISE AND QUALITY OF LIFE

Emerging evidence suggests that exercise may influence QOL outcomes in breast cancer survivors. Kendall et al. (2005) collected information using the short form-36 (sf-36) during telephone interviews with 374 breast cancer patients, diagnosed between 1983 and 1988 at ages 40 years or younger and interviewed, on average 13.2 years after diagnosis. These women previously participated in a case-control study soon after their diagnoses, providing information on breast cancer risk factors including exercise activity. The impact of changes in exercise activity (comparing prediagnosis to postdiagnosis levels) on the sf-36 mental and physical health summary scales was compared using regression analyses. A positive change in exercise activity was associated with a higher score on the sf-36 physical health summary scale at follow-up (p = .005). However, a change in exercise activity was not associated with the sf-36 mental health summary scale score. Patients who increased their activity levels did not differ from those who did not in terms of medical or demographic characteristics. Nonetheless, this study provides one of the longest follow-up periods of breast cancer survivors to date among studies that focus on QOL and is unique in its focus on women diagnosed at a young age. The results demonstrate high levels of functioning and well-being among long-term breast cancer survivors and indicate that women whose exercise activity increased following diagnosis score higher on the sf-36 physical health summary scale. These findings suggest a potential role for exercise activity in maintaining well-being after a cancer diagnosis.

In a systematic review of exercise interventions in oncology, 34 randomized clinical trials and controlled clinical trials were identified and reviewed for substantive results and assessed for methodological quality (Knols et al., 2005). Although a variety of exercise modalities were used, differing in content, frequency, intensity, and duration, positive results were reported for a diverse set of outcomes, including physiological measures, objective performance indicators, self-reported functioning and symptoms, psychological well-being, and overall health-related QOL. It was concluded that although cancer patients may benefit from physical exercise both during and after treatment, the specific beneficial effects of physical exercise may vary as a function of the stage of disease, the nature of the medical treatment, and the current lifestyle of the patient. Further research is warranted to improve study design, including the use of larger sample sizes and appropriate comparison groups, to identify patients who will most benefit from exercise and to assess motivation and adherence to an exercise program.

CONCLUSION

The role of nutritional intervention in cancer at different stages has not been firmly established. In previous chapters, various roles have been examined. When nutrition is being used for secondary prevention in a patient where an early cancer has been treated through surgery or radiation, a preventive approach using a diet rich in fruits, vegetables, cereals, and grains is used to achieve a low-fat and high-fiber dietary goal. Various dietary supplements are also used in this setting. All of these aspects of intervention can contribute to a positive feeling for many patients who can contribute to their care by controlling their food intake. The demonstration of the increase in autonomy that results in these patients remains to be demonstrated. In some patients undergoing active therapy for advanced malignancy, taking on a nutritional regimen may be overwhelming. For these patients, it is often desirable to postpone active involvement of the patient in dietary changes until their therapeutic course nears completion. In the patient with advanced cancer and weight loss, an established goal of nutritional intervention is to stabilize or reverse underlying progressive undernutrition. Early detection of anorexia and undernutrition can also help initiate steps to prevent cancer cachexia. In the setting of treatable malignancies (such as lymphoma and ovarian cancer), nutritional support can be an essential component of an overall aggressive strategy of antitumor therapy. Reversing or entirely preventing cachexia in patients with end-stage malignancies may not be possible, but even in this setting, anorexia can be palliated. A future research direction is the study of diets that may enhance immune function in the advanced cancer patient. There is little or no evidence to suggest that nutritional therapies ever lead to rapid tumor growth or deterioration of the patient. The few case reports in the literature of tumor flares while patients received total parenteral nutrition are rare associations rather than proven cause and effect. Although there is some evidence that vitamin supplementation may palliate conditions such as mucositis without an obvious neutralization of therapeutic effects on head and neck cancer, there is a need for further study on the interaction of nutrition during the course of cancer therapies.

Nutritional intervention offers the advanced cancer patient supportive care and enhanced QOL, in addition to the therapeutic benefits ordinarily attributed to this form of intervention. Cancer patients who are relieved of uncomfortable symptoms can recover a basic sense of well-being and comfort. Meticulous and consistent attention to the assessment and treatment of such common complaints as nausea, vomiting, pain, anorexia, dyspnea, constipation, and a variety of other diseases and treatment-related problems is essential to the patient's QOL. Increased interest in QOL has led to the development of valid means of measurement of health-related QOL, and these instruments should be included in studies of nutrition in the cancer patient whenever possible. A strong and consistent concern for improving the QOL of cancer patients has become as important as the previously all-encompassing concern for extending quantity of life.

Acknowledgment

This research is supported by the UCLA Clinical Nutrition Research Unit and by NIH Grant no. CA 47210.

References

Aaronson, N.K. 1986. Methodological issues in psychosocial oncology with special reference to clinical trials. *In* "Assessment of Quality of Life and Cancer Treatment" (V. Ventafridda, P.S.A.M. van Dam, R. Yancik, and M. Tamburini, eds), pp. 29–42. Elsevier, Amsterdam.

Aaronson, N.K., and Beckman, I. 1987. "The Quality of Life of Cancer Patients," Vol. 17, "Monograph Series of the European Organization for Research and Treatment of Cancer (EORTC)." Raven Press, New York.

Aaronson, N.K., Bullinger, M., and Admedzai, S. 1988. A modular approach to quality-of-life assessment in cancer clinical trials. *Recent Results Cancer Res* **111**: 231–249.

Aaronson, N.K., Ahmedzai, S., and Bergman, B. 1993. The European Organization for Research and Treatment of Cancer QLQ-C30: a quality-of-life instrument for use in international clinical trials of in oncology. *J Natl Cancer Inst* **85**: 365–376.

Barofsky, I., and Sugarbaker, P. 1990. Cancer. *In* "Quality of Life Assessments in Clinical Trials" (B. Spilker, ed.), pp. 419–439. Raven Press, New York.

Baum, M., Priestman, T., West, R.R., and Jones, E.M. 1980. A comparison of subjective responses in a trial comparing endocrine with cytotoxic treatment in advanced carcinoma of the breast. *Eur J Cancer* **16**: 223–226.

Bergman, B., Aaronson, N.K., and Ahmedzai, S. 1994 The EORTC QLQ-LC13: A modular supplement to the EORTC Core Quality of Life Questionnaire (EORTC QLQ-C30) for use in lung cancer clinical trials. *Eur J Cancer* **330A**: 635–642.

Bergner, M., Bobbitt, R.A., Carter, W.B., and Gilson, B.S. 1976. The Sickness Impact Profile: Validation of a health status measure. *Med Care* **14**: 57–61.

Bergner, M., Bobbitt, R.A., Carter, W.B., and Gilson, B.S. 1981. The Sickness Impact Profile: development and final revision of a health status measure. *Med Care* **19**: 787–806.

Bernheim, J.L., and Buyse, M. 1984. The anamnestic comparative self-assessment for measuring the subjective quality of life of cancer patients. *J Psychosoc Oncol* **1**: 25–38.

Cella, D.F. 1991. Functional status and quality of life: current views on measurement and intervention. *In* "Functional Status and Quality of Life in Persons with Cancer", pp. 1–12. American Cancer Society, Atlanta, GA.

Cella, D.F. 1997. "Manual for the Functional Assessment of Clinical Illness Therapy (FACIT) Scales." Evanston Northwestern Healthcare, Evanston, IL.

Cella, D.F., and Cherin, E.A. 1988. Quality of life during and after cancer treatment. *Compr Ther* **14**: 69–75.

Cella, D.J., Tross, S., Orav, E.J., Holland, J.C., Silberfarb, P.M., and Rafla, S. 1989. Mood states of patients after the diagnosis of cancer. *J Psychosoc Oncol* **7**: 45–54.

Cella, D.F., and Tulsky, D.S. 1990. Measuring quality of life today: methodological aspects. *Oncology* **5**: 29–38.

Cella, D.F., Bonomi, A.E., and Lloyd, S.R. 1995. Reliability and validity of the Functional Assessment of Cancer Therapy Lung (FACT-L) quality of life instrument. *Lung Cancer* **12**: 199–220.

Cella, D. 2004. The Functional Assessment of Cancer Therapy-Lung and Lung Cancer Subscale assess quality of life and meaningful symptom improvement in lung cancer. *Semin Oncol* **31**: 11–15.

Coates, A., Gebsky, V., Bishop, J.F., et al. 1987. Improving the quality of life during chemotherapy for advanced breast cancer. *N Engl J Med* **317**: 1490–1495.

DeHaes, J.C.J.M., Raatgever, J.W., van der Bug, M.E.L., Hamersma, E., and Neijt, J.P. 1987. Evaluation of the quality of life of patients with ovarian cancer treated with combination chemotherapy. *In* "The Quality of Life of Cancer Patients" (N.K. Aaronson and J. Beckman, eds.), pp. 215–226. Raven Press, New York.

de Haes, J.C., van Knippenberg, F.C., and Neijt, J.P. 1990. Measuring psychological and physical distress in cancer patients: structure and application of the Rotterdam Symptom Checklist. *Br J Cancer* **62**: 1034–1038.

Donovan, K., Sanson-Fisher, R.W., and Redman, S. 1989. Measuring quality of life in cancer patients. *J Clin Oncol* **7**: 959–968.

Functional Assessment of Chronic Illness Therapy (FACIT) questionnaire page. FACIT web site. Available at: www.facit.org/qview/qlist.aspx. Accessed June 6, 2005.

Fayers, P.M., and Jones, D.R. 1983. Measuring and analyzing quality of life in cancer clinical trials. A review. *Stat Med* **2**: 429–446.

Ganz, P.A., Lee, J.J., and Siau, J. 1991. Quality of life assessment: an independent prognostic variable for survival in lung cancer. *Cancer (Philadelphia)* **67**: 3131–3135.

Ganz, P.A., Schag, A.C., Lee, J.J., and Sim, M.-S. 1992. The CARES. A generic measure of health-related quality of life for patients with cancer. *Qual Life Res* **1**: 19–29.

Gill, T.M., and Feinstein, A.R. 1994. A critical appraisal of the quality of quality of life measurements. *JAMA* **272**: 619–646.

Gough, J.R., Furnival, C.M., Schilder, L., and Grove, W. 1983. Assessment of the quality of life of patients with advanced cancer. *Eur J Cancer Clin Oncol* **19**: 1161–1165.

Guadagnoli, E., and Mor, V. 1989. Measuring cancer patients' affect: Revision and psychometry properties of the Profile of Mood States (POMS) psychological assessment. *Am J Consult Clin Psychol* **1**: 150–154.

Hays, R.D., and Stewart, A.L. 1990. The structure of self-reported health in chronic disease patients. Psychological assessment. *J Consult Clin Psychol* **2**: 22–30.

Hollen, P.J., Gralla, R.J., and Kris, M.G. 1994. Measurement of quality of life in patients with lung cancer in multicenter trials of new therapies: psychometric assessment of the Lung Cancer Symptom Scale. *Cancer* **73**: 2087–2098.

Johnson, J.R., and Temple, R. 1985. Food and Drug Administration requirements for approval of new anticancer drugs. *Cancer Treat Rep* **69**: 1155–1157.

Karnofsky, D.A., and Burchenal, J.H. 1949. The clinical evaluation of chemotherapeutic agents in cancer. *In* "Evaluation of Chemotherapeutic Agents" (C.M. McCleod, ed.), pp. 191–205. Columbia University Press, New York.

Katz, S.T., Ford, A.B., Moskowitz, R.W., Jackson, B.A., and Jaffee, M.W. 1963. Studies of illness in the aged. The Index of ADL. *JAMA* **185**: 914–919.

Kendall, A.R., Mahue-Giangreco, M., Carpenter, C.L., Ganz, P.A., and Bernstein, L. 2005. Influence of exercise activity on quality of life in long-term breast cancer survivors. *Qual Life Res* **14**: 361–371.

Knols, R., Aaronson, N.K., Uebelhart, D., Fransen, J., and Aufdemkampe, G. 2005. Physical exercise in cancer patients during and after medical treatment: a systematic review of randomized and controlled clinical trials. *J Clin Oncol* **23**: 3830–3842.

McCorkelle, R., and Young, K. 1978. Development of a symptom distress scale. *Cancer Nurs* **1**: 373–378.

Mishel, M.H. 1990. Reconceptualization of the uncertainty of illness theory. *Image J Nurs Scholarship* **22**: 256–264.

Osoba, D., ed. 1991. "Effect of Cancer on Quality of Life." CRC Press, Boca Raton, FL.

Osoba, D. 1994. Lessons learned from measuring health-related quality of life in oncology. *J Clin Oncol* **12**: 608–616.

Padilla, G.V., Ferrell, B., Grant, M.M., and Rhiner, M. 1990. Defining the content domain of quality of life for cancer patients with pain. *Cancer Nurs* **13**: 108–115.

Padilla, G.V., Mishel, M.H., and Grant, M.M. 1992. Uncertainty, appraisal, and quality of life. *Qual Life Res* **1**: 155–165.

Portenoy, R.K., Thaler, H.T., and Kornblith, A.B. 1994. The Memorial Symptom Assessment Scale: an instrument for the evaluation of symptom prevalence, characteristics, and distress. *Eur J Cancer* **30A**: 1326–1336.

Ruckdeschel, J.C., and Plantadosi, S. 1989. Assessment of quality of life by the Functional Living Index-Cancer (FLIC) is superior to performance status for prediction of survival in patients with lung cancer. *Proc Am Soc Clin Oncol*: 311. Abstract no. 1209.

Schipper, H., and Levitt, M. 1985. Measuring quality of life: risks and benefits. *Cancer Treat Rep* **69**: 1115–1123.

Schag, A.C., and Heinrich, R.L. 1988. "CARES: Cancer Rehabilitation Evaluation System." CARES Consultants, Los Angeles.

Schipper, H., Clinch, J., McMurray, A., and Levitt, M. 1984. Measuring the quality of life of cancer patients. The Functional Living Index—Cancer. Development and validation. *J Clin Oncol* **2**: 472–483.

Silberfarb, P.M., and Maurer, L.H. 1980. Psychosocial aspects of neoplastic disease. I. Functional status of breast cancer patients during different treatment regimens. *Am J Psychiatry* **137**: 450–455.

Silberfarb, P.M., Holland, J.C.B., Anbar, D., Bahna, G., Maurer, L.H., Chahinian, A.P., and Comis, R. (1983). Psychological responses of patients receiving two drug regimens for lung carcinoma. *Am J Psychiatry* **140**: 110–111.

Stewart, A.L., Ware, J.F., and Brook, R.H. 1981. Advances in the measurement of functional status. Construction of aggregate indexes. *Med Care* **19**: 473–488.

Stewart, A.L., Greenfield, S., Hays, R.D., Wells, K., Rogers, W.H., Berry, S.D., McGlynn, E.A., and Ware, J.E. 1989. Functional status and well-being of patients with chronic conditions. Results from the Medical Outcomes Study. *JAMA* **262**: 907–913.

Sugarbaker, P.H., Barofsky, I., Rosenberg, S.A., et al. 1982. Quality of life assessment of patients in extremity sarcoma trials. *Surgery (St. Louis)* **91**: 17–23.

Ware, J.F., and Sherbourne, C.D. 1992. A 36 item short-form health survey (SF-36) I. Conceptual framework and item selection. *Med Care* **30**: 473–483.

Ware, J.F., Snyder, M.K., Wright, W.R., and Davies, A.R. 1983. Defining and measuring patient satisfaction with medical care. *Eval Program Plan* **6**: 247–263.

Zubrod, C.G., Schneiderman, M., Frei, F., Brindley, C., Gold, G.L., Shnider, B., Orieto, C., Gorman, J., Jones, R., Jonsson, R., Colsky, J., Chalmers, T., Ferguson, B., Dederick, M., Holland, J., Selawry, O., Regelson, W., Lasagna, L., and Owens, A.H. 1960. Appraisal of methods for the study of chemotherapy of cancer in man: comparative therapeutic trial of nitrogen mustard and triethylene thiophosphoramide. *J Chronic Dis* **11**: 7–33.

CHAPTER

45

Modern Statistical Methods in Clinical Nutrition

ROBERT M. ELASHOFF

INTRODUCTION

Modern methods of statistical analysis are required when conducting large clinical trials in nutrition and cancer prevention. As an example of the challenges faced in clinical research in this new interdisciplinary field of nutritional oncology, the statistical analysis of the Women's Intervention Nutrition Study (WINS) is described in some detail. WINS is based on a wealth of epidemiological and experimental evidence as reviewed elsewhere (Cohen et al., 1993; Wynder et al., 1997). The study was designed as a two-arm randomized trial comparing the effectiveness of an intensive dietary intervention, 15% energy from fat, versus a control group. Women who had either a total mastectomy or segmental mastectomy with axillary lymph node dissection were randomized equally into two groups under the stratification of nodal status and clinics. The primary outcome of this study is the time to recurrence of breast cancer.

In these many respects, the WINS trial is not unlike other large clinical intervention trials in nutrition and cancer, which have used dietary interventions with somewhat different endpoints, such as the Colon Polyp Prevention Trial (polyps) and the Women's' Health Initiative (heart disease and cancer). It is critical to determine that we are asking the right questions of these large trials, which hold the promise of providing definitive answers to important questions in nutrition and cancer prevention research.

DESCRIPTION OF THE WINS STUDY

A Case Study of Nutrition and Cancer Prevention Trials

The ultimate endpoints of the WINS study will not be discussed here, as this is an ongoing trial. Therefore, what follows is a description of the study design and a previous trial conducted by the same group examining adherence to the dietary intervention.

The WINS study was designed to compare the effectiveness of an intensive nutrition intervention versus a non-intensive nutrition intervention in the treatment of breast cancer. All subjects received systemic adjuvant therapy, which is a combination of chemotherapy and/or tamoxifen. The goal is to compare the primary endpoint of the study (relapse-free survival) between the two treatment arms. Major aspects of the study include:

1. Comparison of relapse-free survival between the treatment groups
2. Comparison of overall survival between the treatment groups
3. Evaluation of the association between lipid profile and treatment arm
4. Evaluation of the association between lipid profile and dietary fat intake

Copyright © 2006, Elsevier Inc.
All rights of reproduction in any form reserved.

Participants are stratified according to two pre-randomization factors. They are:

1. Systemic therapy: tamoxifen alone, tamoxifen + chemotherapy, chemotherapy alone
2. Nodal status: positive, negative, and undetermined (The undetermined group includes the case of no axillary lymph node dissection [ALND], fewer than six lymph nodes examined at ALND, negative sentinel node. This group is not considered in the sample size calculation.)

The major response variables are as follows in the trial:

A. First, the primary endpoint for statistical analysis is relapse-free survival. The following occurrences are considered events for the relapse-free survival analysis:
   1. Local recurrence
   2. Regional recurrence
   3. Distant recurrence
   4. In-breast local recurrence
   5. Opposite breast cancer events
B. Secondary Outcome: Overall Survival
   1. Overall survival is also analyzed. The endpoint for overall survival analysis is death from any causes.
C. Other Secondary Outcomes: Nutritional and Metabolic Variables
   1. Nutritional and Metabolic variables dealing with adherence and expected changes in body weight (body mass index [BMI]) and dietary intake are used to investigate whether observed changes are associated with treatment group and with observed dietary fat intake. These variables will include:
      a. Plasma fatty acid measurements
      b. Total cholesterol
      c. Triglycerides
      d. Low-density lipoprotein (LDL) and high-density lipoprotein (HDL) cholesterol
      e. BMI
      f. Adherence to diet
      g. Potential adverse effects of the diet intervention

The data analysis of this study involved the following aspects: (1) accrual and retention; (2) recurrence comparisons; (3) compliance with the diet; (4) additional aspects of the nutrient data; (5) brief review of the anthropometrics; (6) brief analysis of quality of life questionnaire, medical events, and alcohol and smoking intakes. Note that the actual data analysis presented here refers to our previous adherence trial and not to the ongoing WINS, because it is inappropriate to report the results of a yet uncompleted trial. The background discussion here is an abbreviated summary of the detailed report on the adherence trial with the purpose of emphasizing the crucial points that led to the design, funding, and implementation of this previous study.

The essential questions that motivated this WINS adherence study are as follows:

1. Will the required number of patients be accrued to this study?
2. Will the patients assigned to the intensive dietary arm adhere to the diet?
3. Will patients who withdraw from the study permit clinical endpoints to be obtained by the study physicians?
4. Is their evidence that the breast cancer recurrence rate is reduced in the intensive dietary intervention arm compared with the nonintensive intervention arm?
5. Are the answers to questions 1–4 in the affirmative so that there exists consistency of results in the important aspects of this study?

DESIGN ISSUES

There are a number of critical design issues that must be considered in planning any cancer and nutrition prevention trial. First, the key to any nutritional cancer prevention trial is the relationship of the physicians and nutritionists to the patients. Thus, to enhance compliance, it is important that there be a strong and direct involvement on the part of the research physician with patients during the trial. The frequency of such physician involvement will depend on the funding levels available to the trial. Second, in recurrence trials, specifically, the precise definition of recurrence must be well defined and agreed upon prior to the initiation of the trial, including significant discussion with the Data Safety Monitoring Board and expert oncologists in the field of interest. Third, it should be recognized that stratification can significantly reduce the statistical power of a study, so there should be considerable evidence presented justifying any proposed stratification variables. Indeed, Peto et al. (1977) have recommended either no stratification factors or an extremely limited number of such factors. Moreover, these should have major prognostic significance. It is possible, after the description of the patient prognostic factors in the study, to plausibly adjust via covariance for imbalances, although there are statisticians who regard this approach as controversial. Fourth, the nutrition trials should be carefully monitored by sending certified nutritionists, data managers, and, in some cases, physicians to the multiple clinical sites. Clearly, in advance of any patient accrual, there must be workshops describing the nutritional intervention to both physicians and nutritionists, the procedures to be followed, the ways in which data are to be collected and the specific forms completed, and the operation of the web-based data management system. Finally, there should be frequent meetings of the Executive Committee of the trial and the site Principal Investigators should be contacted periodically for teleconference meetings.

IMPORTANT STATISTICAL ISSUES

There are a plethora of important statistical issues in any clinical trial. Many of these are identified by carrying out quite detailed and descriptive statistical analyses. Such analyses include not only various tabulations but most importantly figures and graphical studies of the data. Such studies can delineate errors in the data, considerable patient heterogeneity on the primary and secondary endpoints of the study, and possibly unusual relationships not previously recognized. Thus, it is not possible to do an inferential statistical analysis without trying to find concordance between a statistical model that attempts to represent the data and the data itself. In this way, one can make efforts to assess all the assumptions appropriate for the statistical model from which inferences about the nutritional intervention, prognostic factors, and other design issues can be assessed. In this section, we simply focus on a few statistical problems that we addressed in the WINS feasibility study (also called the *WINS adherence study*).

Typical two-arm randomized nutritional intervention studies are longitudinal in nature. That is, study participants are monitored at regularly scheduled milestone visits over the course of the study. Measurements of the study endpoints are taken during these milestone visits and may include (depending on the purpose of the study) weight, BMI, lipid profiles, tumor recurrence, food records, and so on. Statistical analyses of these endpoints (or outcomes) are commonly performed on a milestone-by-milestone (commonly referred to as *time-by-time analysis of variance* [ANOVA]) basis (Chlebowski et al., 1993), which ignores within-subject correlation over time, or by fixed effects repeated-measures ANOVA (Savendahl et al., 1997; Davidson et al., 1998; Lipkin, 1998). Despite their relative simplicity, these methods suffer weaknesses. The time-by-time ANOVA has two weaknesses. First, it cannot address questions regarding treatment effects that relate to the longitudinal development of the mean response profiles, such as changes over time in weight or blood lipid profiles for each group as a whole or for individuals. Second, inferences made within each of the separate analyses are not independent. With weakly correlated data, marginally significant differences at each milestone may be compelling as a whole; however, if the data are strongly correlated over time within subjects, this may not be true (Diggle et al., 1994). Further, time-by-time ANOVA implicitly assumes that the outcome is measured at exactly the same time for each participant after the onset of the nutritional intervention. This assumption is usually not valid. Although the study design may call for the milestone visits to be, say, 3 months apart, many participants do not show up for their scheduled visits and must be rescheduled at a later date.

Consider, for example, a weight loss study. Analysis of the 3-month weight data may have included a significant proportion of participants who actually were weighed at 4 or 5 months. There are two problems with this. First, these participants have had a significantly longer amount of time to lose weight than those who came in on time. Second, those who do not come in as scheduled may be those who are not complying with the study protocol. In either case, results are unreliable and may include significant bias. Furthermore, it is rare to have complete data and it is not uncommon to perform the analysis on a complete case basis. The repeated-measures ANOVA can be considered a first attempt at a single analysis of a longitudinal dataset (Diggle et al., 1994). However, it requires a complete, balanced array of data, with strong assumptions about the correlation structure and normality. These ANOVA methods do not give a viable approach to longitudinal data analysis. Current mainstream statistical modeling of longitudinal data overcomes the shortcomings of these ANOVA models. Using data from the WINS Feasibility study (Chlebowski et al., 1993), it is possible to compare and contrast two methodologies for analyzing longitudinal data that explicitly account for the correlations between successive observations on each unit. These are the linear mixed effects (LME) model approach (Laird and Ware, 1982) and the generalized estimating equations (GEE) approach (Liang and Zeger, 1986; Zeger and Liang, 1986). We discuss the strengths and weaknesses of each of these models and when they should be used.

Parameter estimates and their standard errors are compared with those from a standard linear regression model (which ignores within unit correlation). We also demonstrate a flexible semi-parametric approach (B-spline regression) (Wang and Taylor, 1995; Shi et al., 1996) to modeling the time-trend curves. Lastly, we demonstrate an objective method, developed by Leung and Elashoff (1996) and based on their time-trend curves. These clusters separate the participants into adherers and nonadherers. By an *adherer*, we mean a participant who followed study protocol. These clusters may then be used in conjunction with baseline variables such as those from psychosocial questionnaires to predict who will adhere to the study protocol "Modeling the Drop-Out Mechanism in Repeated-Measures Studies" and who will not.

The WINS Feasibility study was a multicenter study to determine the degree to which women having had early stage breast cancer will adhere to a program involving a significant reduction of dietary fat. WINS is based on a wealth of epidemiological and experimental evidence as reviewed elsewhere (Cohen et al., 1993; Wynder et al., 1997). The study was designed as a two-arm randomized trial comparing the effectiveness of an intensive dietary intervention, 15% energy from fat, versus a control group. Major aspects of the study include:

- Comparison of fat intake between two dietary arms to monitor the adherence to the intervention

- Identifying a set of behavioral and psychosocial variables that can be used as predictors of adherence
- Investigation of the association between fat intake and plasma fatty acid, or fat intake and lipid profile
- Investigation of the association between fat intake and other dietary and behavioral variables
- The effect of tamoxifen on cholesterol, triglycerides, HDL, and LDL

It is, of course, recognized that the key issues of patients leaving the trial early for various reasons, patients agreeing to stay in the study without periodic visits, and other reasons for incomplete data collection are all extremely important to address. There is some quite useful information about the handling of incomplete data in the text by Little and Rubin (2002) and in other review articles, which are outside the scope of this chapter.

CONDUCT OF THE TRIAL

A total of 290 women, who had either a total mastectomy or segmental mastectomy with axillary lymph node dissection, were randomized equally into two groups under the stratification of nodal status and clinics. These participants were accrued from November 1988 to September 1992 from seven clinics: Methodist Hospital, Houston; Emory University School of Medicine, Atlanta; Harbor-UCLA, Los Angeles; Deaconess Hospital, Boston; American Health Foundation, New York; Evanston Hospital, Illinois; and Wayne State University, Detroit. Prior to joining the study, all participants provided written informed consent meeting all federal and institutional requirements including an expressed willingness to accept either group.

The inclusion criteria for the study included women at 50 years of age or older and localized Stage I or 2 breast cancer. The exclusion criteria were as follows:

- The interval between the randomization and the definitive surgery >180 days
- Segmental mastectomy patient with dominant mass within ipsilateral breast remnant
- Segmental mastectomy patient with tumor size >4 cm
- Malignant breast cancer other than carcinoma or distant metastatic disease
- Patients in the category of more advanced disease
- Patients with previous breast malignancy
- Patients consuming <25% calories from fat at baseline

Registered dietitians from the clinical centers were trained centrally at a 4-day training session that included 2 days of dietary intervention training and training in standardized procedures for documenting food records and collecting anthropometric data. As part of the training, dietitians were certified to collect actual study food records after successful collection and documentation of dietary data from subjects similar to the study population. WINS participants were instructed to keep 4-day food records (4DFR) before each clinic visit, which included a prerandomization visit and 3, 6, 12, 18, and 24 months postrandomization visits. The 4DFR consisted of 4 consecutive days, including three weekdays and one weekend day. Participants were given detailed instructions on keeping accurate records of food intake. Food weighing scales, measuring spoons, cups, and rulers were provided to participants to enhance accuracy in reporting amounts. To ensure accurate documentation, the 4DFR were reviewed by the dietitians certified in the WINS dietary assessment techniques. The 4DFR were analyzed for nutrient intake using the database maintained at the University of Minnesota's Nutrition Coordinating Center (version 20, 1991). Mean daily intakes of energy and fat were calculated for the 4DFR using equal weighting for each of the 4 days (three weekdays and one weekend day).

Following randomization, those participants assigned to the treatment arm were given an individualized fat gram goal and received nutrition education sessions every 2 weeks for the first 8 weeks. In December 1990, the WINS Executive Committee met and reviewed preliminary data on adherence. These data showed that it was quite feasible for the participants to achieve the 20% of calories from fat intake goal. In light of these and Japanese data that suggest a favorable prognosis when a population intake is closer to 15% energy from fat, they voted to reduce the fat gram target to 15% as an additional approach to achieve group differences in fat intake.

If a woman had not met her fat gram goal or did not achieve >25% reduction in calories from fat after the biweekly sessions, the sessions were repeated as needed over the next 2 months. After the initial intensive meetings, subsequent nutrition contacts (visits, calls, or mailings) were monthly through 8 months, then bimonthly through 12 months, and then quarterly through 24 months. The nutrition education sessions in the treatment arm were from the WINS low-fat eating plan (LFEP) that had been developed and pilot tested with postmenopausal breast cancer patients and detailed elsewhere (Buzzard et al., 1990). Briefly, the LFEP is a step-by-step individualized counseling approach to reduce total fat intake based on behavioral and social teaming conceptualizations of dietary behavioral change (Bandura, 1969). The LFEP includes education, goal setting, evaluation, and feedback components.

The controls received minimal nutritional counseling except guidance on nutrient adequacy as defined by a nutrient intake that was <67% of the recommended dietary allowances (RDAs), as determined by the analysis of their food records. Counseling for adequacy of RDAs was also provided for women in the treatment arm.

The clinical nutritionists did not counsel either the treatment or the control participants on reductions or any changes in their caloric intake or exercise levels. All subjects were discouraged from initiating use of dietary supplements. Blood samples were collected at baseline and at 6, 12, 18, and 24 months into the study. Participants provided data for demographic, dietary adherence, and quality-of-life questionnaires. Results from the blood analysis and other questionnaires will be reported elsewhere.

STATISTICAL ANALYSIS OF THE TRIAL DATA

The statistical analyses here are from the WINS adherence trial. We have two primary interests herein. First, we investigate the mean structure of the variables of interest (weight, daily fat grams, and percentage of daily calories from fat) for the two groups over time using two modern regression methods. Both of these account for the serial correlation of an individual's measurements over time. The two methods we are interested in comparing are the LME model (Laird and Ware, 1982) and the GEE (Zeger and Liang, 1986; Diggle et al., 1994). We also compare parameter estimates and their standard errors with standard linear regression, which does not take into account the serial correlation over time.

Second, in addition to determining whether it is feasible to keep a group of women on a low-fat diet, we want to be able to determine, with some type of objective criteria, which women adhered with the study protocol and which did not. Given this information, it may be possible to predict, based on baseline covariates and psychosocial questionnaires, who is most likely to adhere and who is not. This information could then be used to target those most likely not to adhere and give them specialized counseling. Within each group (control and treatment), we subclassified participants into adherent and nonadherent participants. A control group participant is nonadherent if she changes her dietary habits in accordance with the treatment group protocol. A participant assigned to the treatment group is nonadherent if she does not meet the dietary goal of daily fat intake reduction to <20% fat calories and maintenance of this goal thereafter. These data have previously been analyzed by Chlebowski et al. (1993). However, their analysis did not account for the longitudinal nature of the study and no attempt was made to cluster the groups into adherent and nonadherent participants.

At each milestone visit, namely at baseline and at 3, 6, 12, 18, and 24 months, they performed a one-way ANOVA on percentage fat calories and on weight. This method of analysis is commonly referred to as *time-by-time ANOVA* (Diggle et al., 1994) and implicitly assumes that outcomes are not correlated over time. We reiterate the two major weaknesses to this approach. First, it cannot address questions regarding treatment effects that relate to the longitudinal development of the mean response profiles, for example, changes in daily fat consumption over time for each group as a whole or for individuals. Second, inferences made within each of the separate analyses are not independent (Diggle et al., 1994). Another drawback of this methodology, as applied to the data presented in this article, is that one tacitly assumes that all participants are monitored at, for instance, 6 months postbaseline or at least within a few-week window around 6 months. However, the data for the 6-month visit were actually collected from 5.3 months postbaseline up to 10 months postbaseline. One could argue that those who do not come in for visits on schedule are those most likely not adhering to the study protocol and that the data at 6 and 10 months are not comparable and should not be included together in the 6-month analysis. Current mainstream statistical modeling of longitudinal data overcomes these shortcomings of the time-by-time ANOVA analysis. To address our first question (i.e., what are the mean response profiles of the two groups and do the mean response profiles of the two groups differ from each another?), we fit LME and GEE models for each of the outcomes of interest. The strengths of these two models are outlined in the next two subsections. Mathematical details of these models can be found in the literature referenced below.

Linear Mixed Effects

For a longitudinal data analysis, the typical scientific interest is either in the pattern of change over time (e.g., growth) of the outcome or in the dependence of the outcome on covariates. An LME model addresses both of these interests simultaneously. An LME model (so named because both fixed and random effects are modeled) is a two-stage model based on explicit identification of population and individual characteristics. During the first stage, population parameters (the fixed effects), individual effects, and within-person variability are modeled. Between-person variation is introduced at Stage 2 (see Laird and Ware, 1982). This model improves on the ANOVA models with regard to several important facets. First, there is no need for balance in the data (i.e., the number and timing of the measurements among individuals need not be equal). Second, serial correlation of an individual's measurements is explicitly modeled during the first stage. The ANOVA analyses completely ignore these two facets of the data. The major drawback of this model is that for continuous outcomes, the error structure is assumed to be multivariate normal.

Generalized Estimating Equations

When the main interest of a longitudinal analysis is in the population mean regression structure (i.e., the dependence of the outcome on the covariates), the time dependence among the repeated measurements for a participant is a nuisance but must be appropriately dealt with, nonetheless. In this case, the GEE (Liang and Zeger, 1986; Zeger and Liang, 1986) approach has several advantages over the LME approach. For continuous outcomes, the likelihood-based LME approach assumes that the outcomes have a multivariate normal distribution (or at least approximately normal or that there exists a transformation to normality). For the GEE approach, we need only to specify that a known function of the marginal expectation of the outcome variable is a linear function of the covariates and assume that the variance is a known function of this mean. In other words, we only need to specify the first two moments (mean and variance) of the distribution and not the entire distribution. Furthermore, we specify a "working" correlation matrix for the observations for each participant. Liang and Zeger (1986) show that this method gives consistent and robust estimators of the regression coefficients and of their variances even when the "working" correlation matrix is mis-specified as long as missing data are missing completely at random in the sense of Rubin (1976). More recent work (Robins et al., 1995) has modified the GEE approach to yield consistent estimates under the weaker condition that the data are missing at random (Rubin, 1976).

There are at least two occasions when the GEE model is not warranted and one should use the LME model. These arise when individual patterns of change over time are the scientific interest or when the correlation structure of the covariates is the primary interest.

Modeling the Mean Structure's Dependence on Time through B-spline Regression

For many longitudinal studies, the expected outcome depends on time. For example, a study that follows a cohort of children over several years, recording their heights at specified intervals, will reveal that their expected height is strongly dependent on time. The expected outcome of interest may simply be a smooth (infinitely differentiable) function of time such as a linear or quadratic function (or higher order polynomial) or a transcendental function of time. In other cases, such as the present one, the expected outcome may only be a continuous, nondifferentiable function of time (consider the height example where children experience a growth spurt or where a patient takes a sudden drastic turn for the worse or better). In such cases, polynomials and transcendental functions may be inappropriate. Fortunately, in these cases, the analyst has another tool at his/her disposal: B-spline longitudinal regression (Wang and Taylor, 1995; Shi et al., 1996).

Suppose we have a sequence of time points (called *knots* in the theory of splines), $t_0 < t_1 < \ldots < t_n$. A *k*th-order spline function is a set of *n* piecewise *k*th-order polynomials, P_i, defined on $[t_i, t_{i+1}$ such that at each knot, t_i, the $(i - 1)$th and *i*th polynomials agree along with their first $k - 1$ derivatives (these conditions ensure continuity and smoothness).

The *k*th-order B-spline functions are a basis consisting of a set of overlapping, continuous ($k = 1$) or smooth ($k > 1$), unimodal, nonnegative, linearly independent functions that sum to one at all time points in the interval $[t_0, t_n]$. A nice feature of B-splines is that any *k*th-order spline function defined on the knot sequence $t_0, t_1, \ldots, t_n$ can be written as a linear combination of the *k*th-order B-spline (B for basis) functions. If only the two boundary knots are supplied, B-spline regression reduces to polynomial regression. The analyst is at liberty to choose a series of knots in the interior of the interval of definition and are typically placed at time points with high curvature and/or where many data points are collected. An algebraic definition of B-splines here would only detract from the main theme of this paper, and the interested reader is referred to Cheney and Kincaid (1994) and DeBoor (1978). Once the knots have been selected, the B-splines are computed. We want to model the time dependence of the outcome with a *k*th-order spline. Because the *k*th-order B-splines are a basis for all *k*th-order splines with the given knot sequence, the B-spline basis can be included in the design matrix of any regression model and we can estimate the B-spline parameters, which are the weights used in the linear combination of the B-splines (which in turn defines the appropriate spline function and hence the time trend of the outcome of interest).

We placed a single knot at $t = 3$ (first follow-up visit at 3 months). The study was designed to get the women in the treatment arm of the trial to reduce fat intake to 20% of their daily energy requirement by their first follow-up visit and then maintain it thereafter. Hence, the study design suggests that two piecewise polynomials, with a single knot at 3 months, would suffice.

Cluster Analysis Using a Finite Support Distributional Model

To address our second question—specifically, are there adherers and nonadherers—we use the methodology developed by Leung and Elashoff (1996). Their model is a generalized LME model. It is more general than the model of Laird and Ware (1982) with regard to several aspects. First, the assumption of normality is replaced with the more general assumption that, conditional on the random effects, $\mathbf{b}_i$, the density of the outcome $\mathbf{y}_i$, is assumed to be a member of the exponential family of distributions (of which the normal distribution is a member). Second, they assume that the independent, unobservable vectors, $\mathbf{b}_i$ are a random sample from some finite-support random-effects distribution, *G*. This distribution is a linear combination of unit atomic distributions consisting of distinct elements over the parameter space of *G*. The support size, *m*, of *G* (i.e., the number of unit atomic distributions) is unknown and is estimated from the data. This, in turn, defines *m* expected, time-dependent, outcome profiles about which the individual outcomes are clustered. Classification of individuals into these clusters is a natural byproduct of their method. Individual classification into clusters is determined by computing the posterior probability that an individual belongs to one of the clusters. Protection from estimating "too many" clusters is provided by estimating the parameters using a maximum-penalized-likelihood method. This classification, or clustering feature, of their method is used to classify participants into protocol adherers and nonadherers. Third, it provides robust variance estimates of the fixed parameter that remain consistent in the presence of mis-specification of the conditional distribution of the outcome given the random effects. We assume that the conditional distribution of the outcome given the random effects is normal.

Handling Incomplete Data

Regression models generally include several variables that enter the model. In the generalized exponential family of regression models with random regression coefficients and random and fixed variables, the problem of how to deal with missing data must be addressed so that trend curves can be estimated and treatment effects can be tested, allowing all parameters and distributions to be properly estimated. Papers by Little (1995) and Robins et al. (1995) dealing with our models and inference approaches when there are missing data show that using GEE on all the data when some of the data are missing at random will produce consistent estimates of the statistical quantities needed in time-trend estimation and significance testing. This consistency is obtained using the techniques of Robins et al. (1995). Little (1995) provides a general formulation to consider nonrandom missing data in repeated-measures studies. Additionally, the work by Leung and Elashoff (1996) rests on likelihood methods, and there, all the data can be used and consistent estimates obtained for all the statistical quantities noted earlier.

RESULTS OF THE STATISTICAL ANALYSIS OF THE TRIAL DATA

Parameter estimates and their standard errors obtained by the LME and GEE methods are compared in Tables 1–3. We cannot directly compare the time-by-time ANOVA method with the LME and GEE because of the additional B-spline parameters included in the longitudinal models. However, we can compare these methods with standard linear regression that does not account for the within-unit serial correlation. We fit a first-order B-spline model with a single interior knot at 3 months.

Recall that a first-order spline function is a set of piecewise linear functions; as such we have fit a piecewise linear longitudinal model. Baseline values and treatment arm were treated as covariates. Covariate interactions with the B-splines were also considered. The expected outcome for an individual is the same for all three of these models and is:

. . . .

$$E(\mathbf{y}_i) = (\alpha + \beta_m I(i \in T) + \beta_b y_{i,0})\mathbf{l} + X(\mathbf{t_i}), \gamma_1 + I(i \in T)X(\mathbf{t_i}), \gamma_2 + y_{i,0}X(\mathbf{t_i}), \gamma_3$$

Here, $\mathbf{y}_i$ is an n_i-dimensional column vector of outcomes, $I(i \in T)$ is an indicator function and is equal to 1 if participant i is in the treatment arm and zero otherwise. **1** is a t_i-dimensional column vector of 1's. $X(\mathbf{t}_i)$ is the $n_i \times 2$ matrix of B-spline bases (each column is one component of the basis) where $\mathbf{t}_i$ is the n_i-vector of times at which $\mathbf{y}_i$ was measured. (The dependence of the outcome on time is mediated through the B-spline basis functions. Hence, we explicitly write the B-spline basis as a function of time.) α is the intercept parameter, β_{trt} is the treatment group effect, β_b is the baseline variable effect parameter, γ_1 is the vector of B-spline effects, and γ_2 and γ_3 are the time by treatment group interaction effects and time by baseline variable interaction effects, respectively. For the LME model, the B-splines were treated as both random and fixed effects.

The first three columns of these tables give the parameter estimates, their standard errors, and p values for the standard linear regression model. The middle three columns correspond to the LME model and the last three to the GEE model. All three outcomes of interest—weight, percentage of daily energy from fat, and daily fat grams—were highly skewed, so a natural log transformation was taken to make the data more normally distributed. Even after this transformation, there are several notable differences in the parameter estimates and/or their standard errors between these methods. In Table 1, the intercept estimate for the GEE method is 67% larger than that from the LNIE method. More striking, however, are the differences in the standard errors for the estimates of the intercept, baseline outcome, and treatment group in Tables 1–3. The standard errors of these estimates from the GEE model are much smaller than those from the LME model. As a result, the intercept and treatment groups are marginally significant under the GEE model, whereas under the LME model and the linear regression model, there is no evidence of a significant intercept or group effect. These differences are a result of the assumption of normality that must be made to apply the LME and linear regression models. Comparing the linear regression model with the LME and GEE models, we note that, with respect to weight (Table 3), the estimate of the second B-spline basis function parameter is about twice as large when linear regression is used than when either the LME or GEE model is applied to the data. The result is a significant value in the former case and insignificant values in the latter two cases. A similar result can be seen with the baseline weight by second B-spline interaction. The reason for these inflated estimates from the linear regression model is that the weight measurements within individuals are highly correlated over time. The linear regression model completely ignores this correlation, whereas the LME and GEE models do not.

Because of the non-normality of the data, we think that the standard errors obtained from the GEE model (recall these standard errors are robust to mis-specification of the correlation structure) more correctly reflect the true underlying variability in these data.

Figures 1–3 display the mean response profiles for the control group and the treatment group from the final fitted GEE models. These response profiles overlay the observed data in the first two frames of each figure. The final model includes the intercept and those parameters that are significantly different from zero (Tables 1–3).

From these tables, one can see that the baseline weight, baseline daily fat grams, and baseline percentage fat calories are highly significant in their respective models. Furthermore, there is a very strong treatment group by time interaction, via the group-spline interactions. For percentage fat calories and fat grams, there is also a significant baseline outcome variable by time interaction. From the third frame

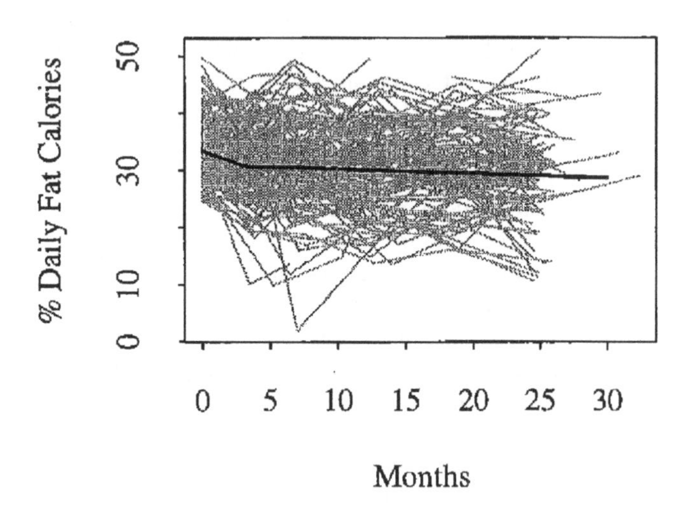

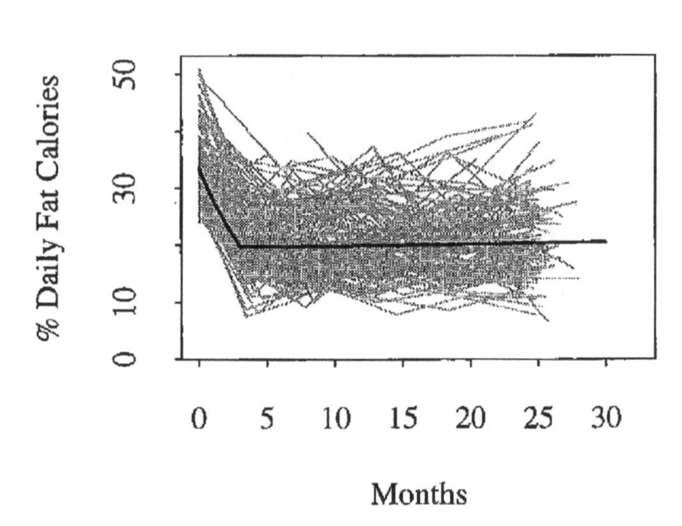

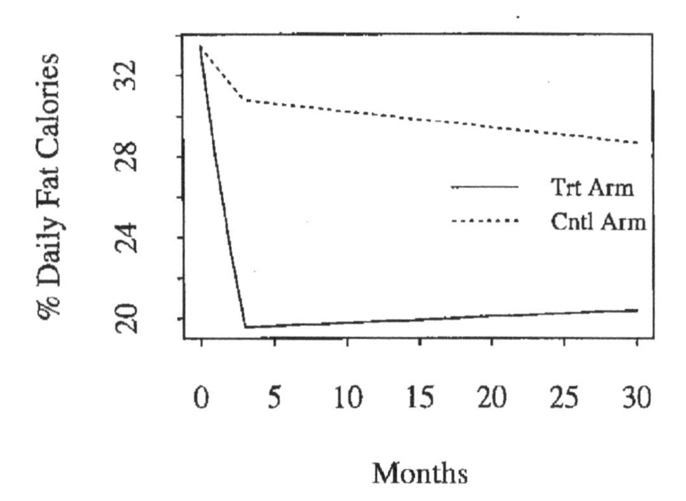

FIGURE 1 Observed data and mean response profiles for the treatment and control arms. Response: Percentage calories from fat. (From first edition of *Nutritional Oncology*.)

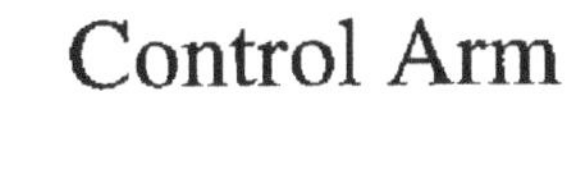

Treatment Arm

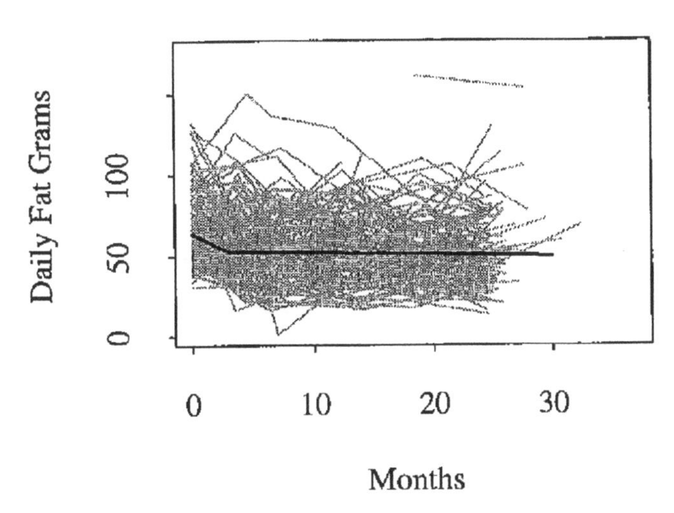

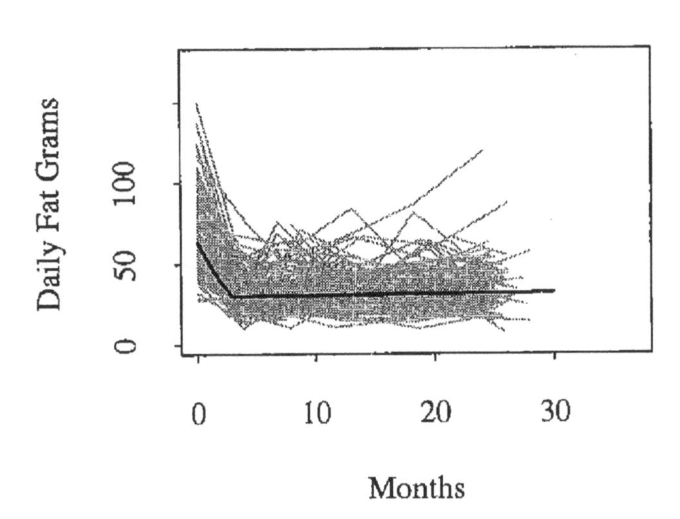

Predicted Response Profile

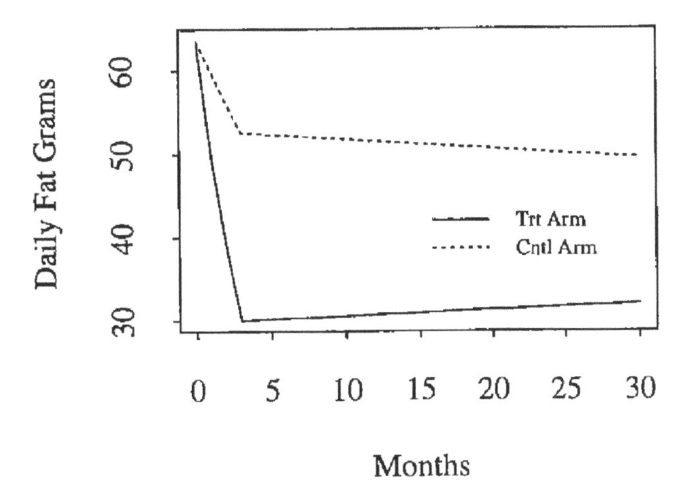

FIGURE 2 Observed data and mean response profiles for the treatment and control arms. Response: Daily Fat grams. (From first edition of *Nutritional Oncology*.)

in Figure 1, one can see that the percentage of fat calories for the treatment arm was reduced to ~20% and that the participants were able to maintain it for >2 years with only a slight increase. Although there is not a significant group effect, there is a significant group by time interaction. During the first 3 months of the trial, the treatment group reduced their daily percentage fat calories from >32 to <20%, while the control group only reduced their percentage fat calories by 1%. Over the subsequent 2 years, there is relatively little change in percentage fat calories in either group. The intervention (treatment) group reduced their fat grams from >60 g/day to just under 30 g/day by the third month. Over the following 21 months, their fat grams per day increased slightly to ~32 g/day. During the first 3 months of the trial, the treatment group lost a small amount of weight; however, by the end of the second year, they had gained it back.

Applying the methodology of Leung and Elashoff (1996), we found that we could subclassify the treatment into two clusters—adherers and nonadherers—with respect to per-

Control Arm

Weight (kg)
60 100 140
0 5 10 15 20 25 30
Months

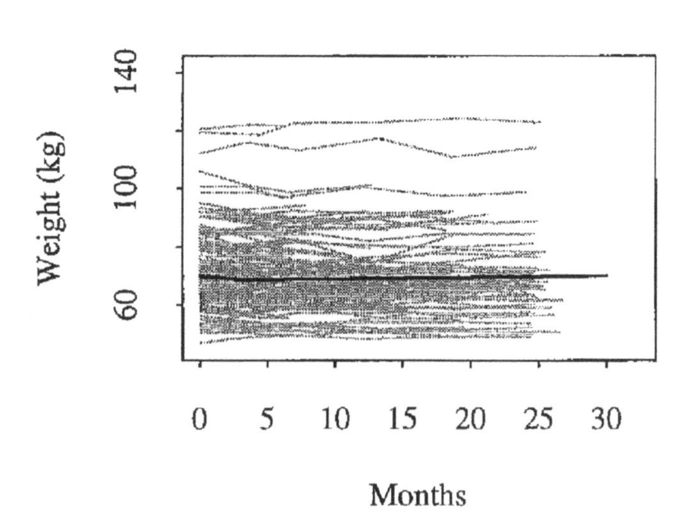

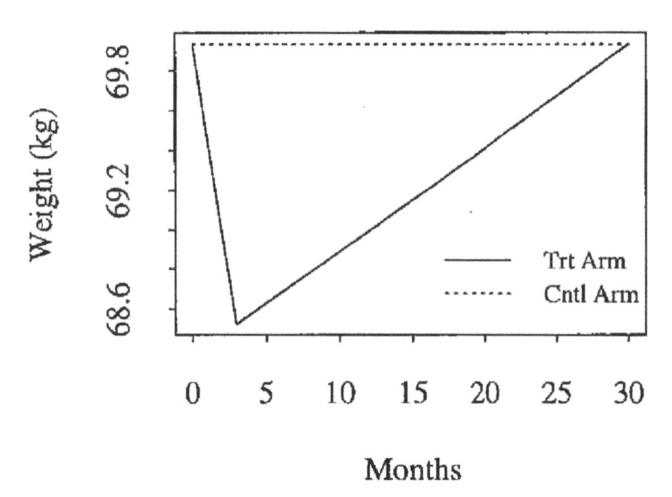

FIGURE 3 Observed data and mean response profiles for the treatment and control arms. Response: Weight. (From first edition of *Nutritional Oncology*.)

centage calories from fat and daily fat grams. The mean response profiles of these two clusters are shown in Figures 4 and 5, respectively. It is interesting to note that after the first 3 months of the trial, the mean profile for the treatment arm was ~20% calories from fat (see Figure 1). This mean is made up of the two clusters: adherers and nonadherers. The adherers, after the third month, have a mean of ~16% fat calories, while the nonadherers are >25%. A total of 44.4% (63/142) of the participants in the treatment group were classified as adherers with respect to percentage of fat calories. Because the cluster classification is based on the expected posterior probability of belonging to a particular cluster, it may turn out that a participant is placed in Cluster 1 with a probability of 0.5–1.0. In this case, we are not very certain whether this participant belongs in this cluster or the other. Sixty-seven out of seventy-nine participants (84.8%) classified as nonadherent had a posterior probability of ≥60% of belonging to the nonadherent cluster. Sixty-two out of sixty-three participants (98.4%) classified as adherent had a posterior probability of ≥60% of belonging to the adherent cluster. This is a very high percentage of participants that were classified into a cluster with >60% probability, so we

TABLE 1 Comparison of Parameter Estimates and Standard Errors for the Different Methodologies; Outcome: Log of % Daily Energy from Fat

	Linear regression			LME			GEE		
Covariate	**Est.**	**S.E.**	***P***	**Est.**	**S.E.**	***p***	**Est.**	**S.E.**	***p***
Intercept	−0.002	0.314	0.994	−0.003	0.207	0.990	−0.005	0.003	0.103
bfat[a]	1.001	0.089	0.000	1.001	0.059	0.000	1.001	0.001	0.000
grp[b]	0.000	0.030	0.992	0.000	0.020	0.986	−0.001	0.000	0.085
BS1[c]	1.340	0.404	0.001	1.327	0.384	0.001	1.318	0.304	0.000
BS2[c]	1.124	0.593	0.058	1.330	0.572	0.020	1.210	0.602	0.045
bfat × BS1	−0.407	0.115	0.000	−0.403	0.109	0.000	−0.402	0.085	0.000
bfat × BS2	−0.370	0.168	0.028	−0.426	0.163	0.009	−0.387	0.170	0.023
grp × BS1	−0.450	0.039	0.000	−0.447	0.037	0.000	−0.440	0.032	0.000
grp × BS2	−0.323	0.058	0.000	−0.325	0.056	0.000	−0.350	0.052	0.000

[a]Log of baseline % daily energy from fat.
[b]Treatment group coded 1 for treatment; 0 for control.
[c]BS1, first B-spline; BS2, second B-spline.

TABLE 2 Comparison of Parameter Estimates and Standard Errors for the Different Methodologies; Outcome: Log of Daily Fat Grams

	Linear regression			LME			GEE		
Covariate	**Est.**	**S.E.**	***p***	**Est.**	**S.E.**	***p***	**Est.**	**S.E.**	***p***
Intercept	−0.003	0.268	0.991	−0.002	0.189	0.993	−0.003	0.005	0.564
bfat[a]	1.001	0.064	0.000	1.000	0.045	0.000	1.001	0.001	0.000
grp[b]	0.000	0.041	0.991	0.000	0.029	0.985	0.001	0.001	0.089
BS1[c]	2.118	0.346	0.000	2.062	0.337	0.000	2.095	0.270	0.000
BS2[c]	1.156	0.515	0.003	1.636	0.488	0.001	1.553	0.527	0.003
bfat × BS1	−0.555	0.083	0.000	−0.541	0.081	0.000	−0.550	0.065	0.000
bfat × BS2	−0.433	0.123	0.000	−0.460	0.117	0.000	−0.434	0.127	0.000
grp × BS1	−0.570	0.053	0.000	−0.566	0.052	0.000	−0.559	0.043	0.000
grp × BS2	−0.379	0.078	0.000	−0.398	0.074	0.000	−0.435	0.069	0.000

[a]Log of baseline daily fat grams.
[b]Treatment group coded 1 for treatment; 0 for control.
[c]BS1, first B-spline; BS2, second B-spline.

TABLE 3 Comparison of Parameter Estimates and Standard Errors for the Different Methodologies; Outcome: Log of Weight

	Linear regression			LME			GEE		
Covariate	**Est.**	**S.E.**	***p***	**Est.**	**S.E.**	***p***	**Est.**	**S.E.**	***p***
Intercept	−0.000	0.066	0.999	0.000	0.028	0.999	0.000	0.000	0.112
bwt[a]	1.000	0.015	0.000	1.000	0.007	0.000	1.000	0.000	0.000
grp[b]	0.000	0.006	0.995	7.956	0.003	0.997	0.000	0.000	0.121
BS1[c]	0.092	0.090	0.310	0.133	0.068	0.054	0.117	0.072	0.106
BS2[c]	0.367	0.125	0.003	0.177	0.183	0.330	0.203	0.145	0.161
bwt × BS1	−0.020	0.021	0.353	−0.029	0.016	0.070	−0.025	0.017	0.125
bwt × BS2	−0.081	0.029	0.006	−0.037	0.043	0.396	−0.041	0.035	0.232
grp × BS1	−0.028	0.008	0.000	−0.027	0.006	0.000	−0.027	0.005	0.000
grp × BS2	−0.038	0.012	0.000	−0.038	0.016	0.017	−0.042	0.015	0.006

[a]Log of baseline weight.
[b]Treatment group coded 1 for treatment; 0 for control.
[c]BS1, first B-spline; BS2, second B-spline.

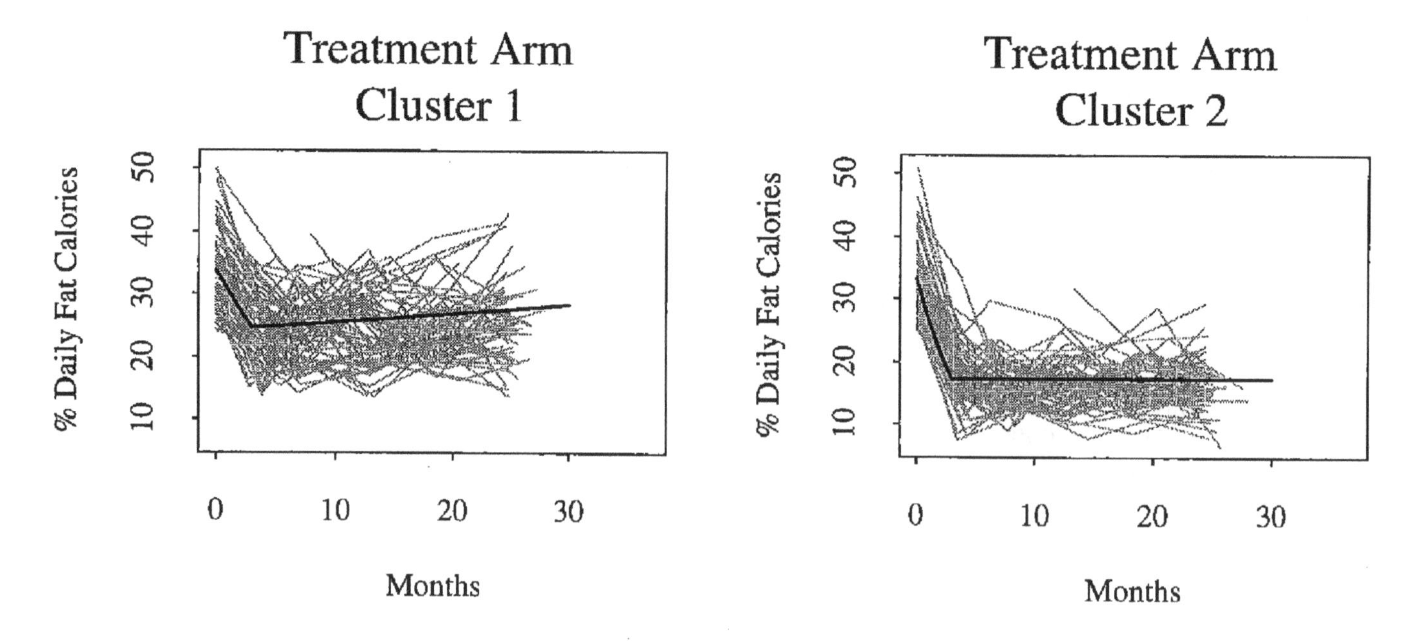

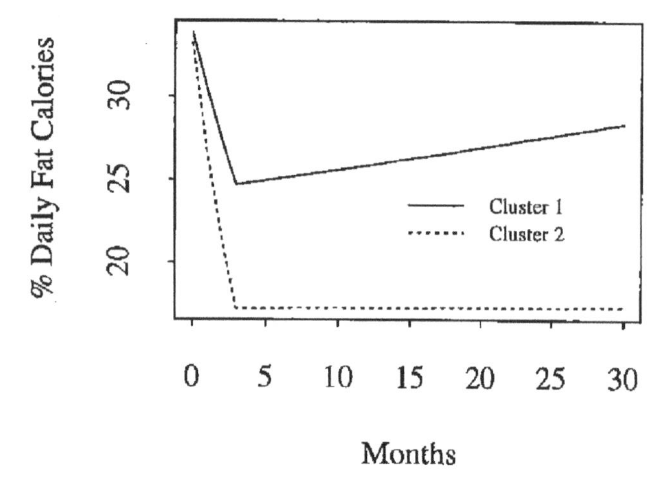

FIGURE 4 Observed data and mean response profiles for the treatment clusters around percentage of calories from fat. (From first edition of *Nutritional Oncology*.)

think that these clusters represent a real finding and not some weak artificial outcome.

With regard to total daily fat grams, 29.6% (42/142) of the participants in the treatment arm were classified into Cluster 2 (Figure 5), which we consider adherers. Of these adherers, 97.6% (41/42) of them were classified into this cluster with posterior probability >60%. Ninety-eight out of one-hundred (98%) of those classified as nonadherers were classified into this cluster with posterior probability >60%.

We also clustered the controls into two groups with respect to percent fat calories and total fat grams. Nonadherence in the control group is a little more difficult to assess. Figure 6 shows the two clusters of participants, with regard to percentage fat calories, with their mean responses. The participants in the first cluster clearly adhere (i.e., do not change their dietary habits). However, the participants in the second cluster changed their dietary habits and consumed a lower percentage of their calories from fat. By 2 years, the mean percentage fat calories in this cluster is <20%—the goal for the treatment group. A total of 121 (99.2%) out of 122 of the controls in Cluster 1 were classified into that cluster with a probability of ≥60%, and 24

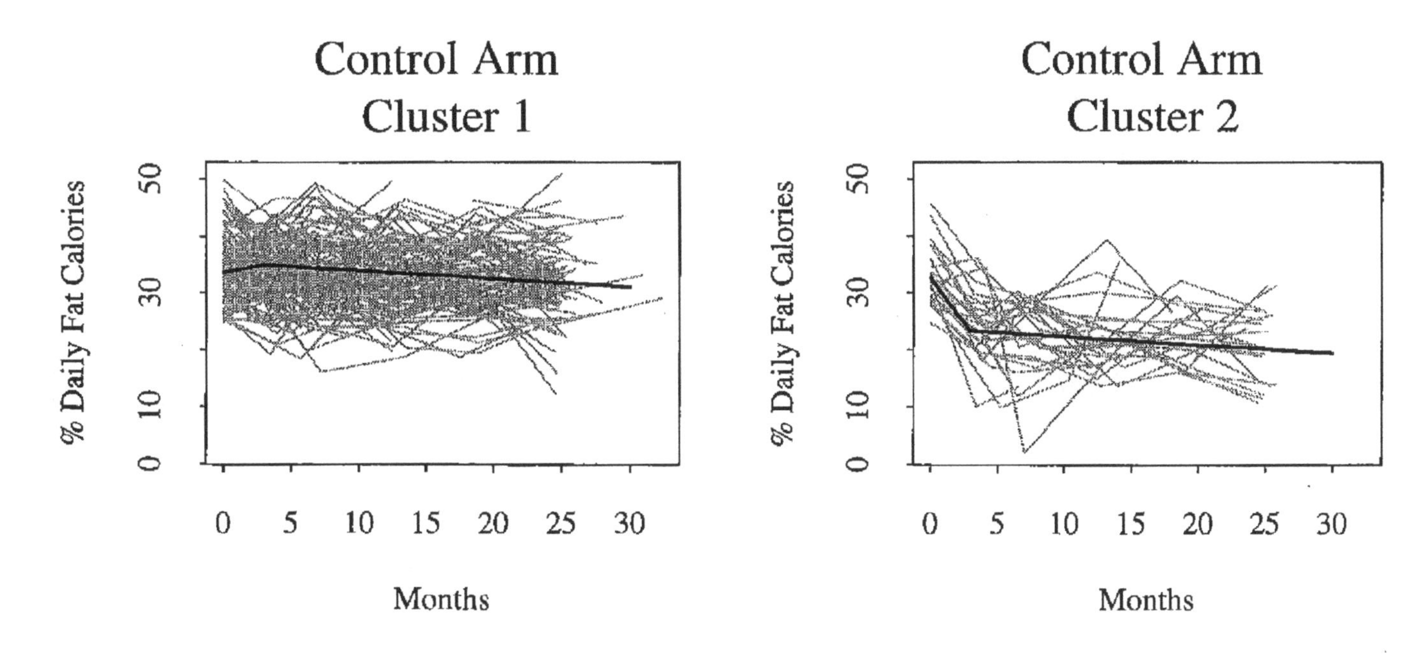

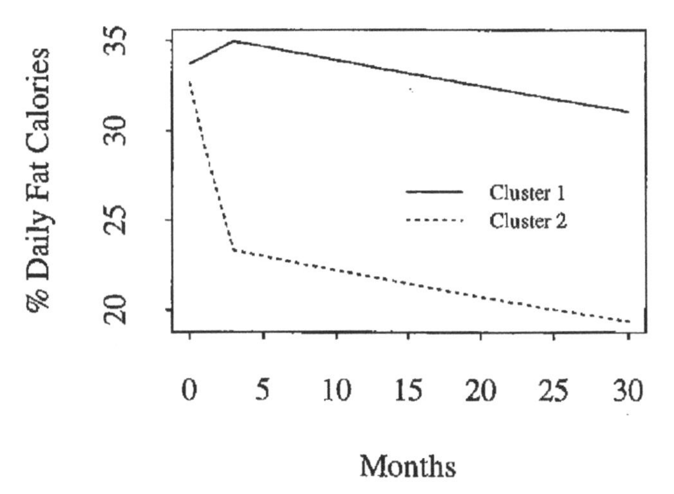

FIGURE 5 Observed data and mean response profiles for the treatment clusters around daily fat grams. (From first edition of *Nutritional Oncology*.)

(92.3%) out of 26 were classified into Cluster 2 with a probability of ≥60%. Furthermore, 82.4% of the controls adhered to the study protocol.

With respect to total fat grams, 74.3% (110/148) of the participants in the control arm adhered to the study protocol (Cluster 1 in Figure 7). The remaining 38 participants reduced their daily fat grams intake from ~60 g/day to just >30 g/day during the first 3 months of the trial (see Figure 7). Classification probabilities again were quite high. A total of 107 (97.3%) out of 110 of the control participants that were classified into Cluster 1 were done so with posterior probability >60%.

It is interesting to look at how many participants in each arm of the trial were classified as adherers with respect to both percent fat calories and daily fat grams. Table 4 displays this cross-tabulation. In the treatment arm, 72.3% of the participants were classified the same with respect to both percentage fat calories and daily fat grams. In the control arm, 87.8% were classified the same. A possible explanation of why only 72.3% of the treatment arm participants were

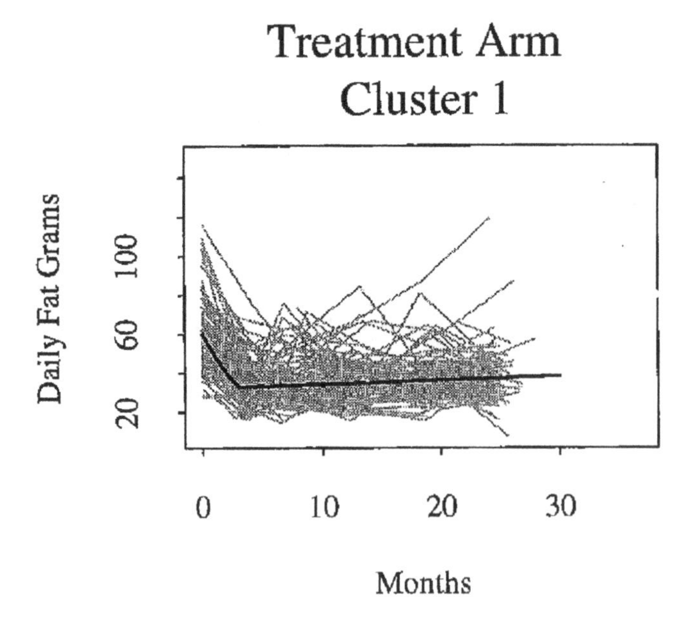

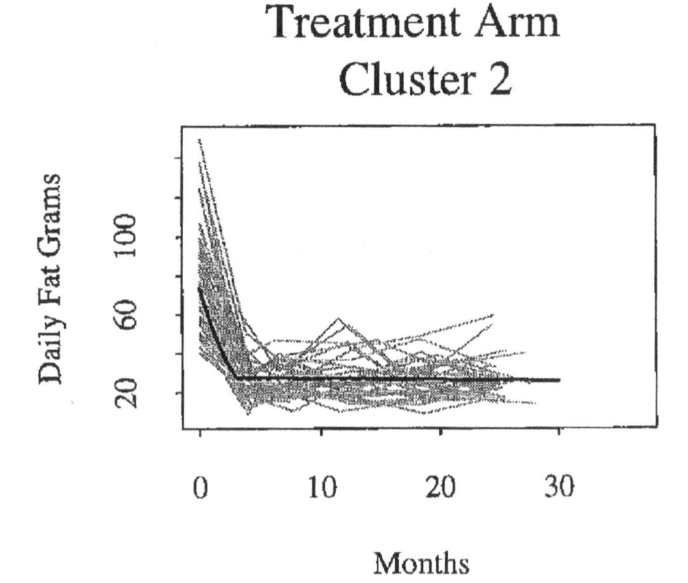

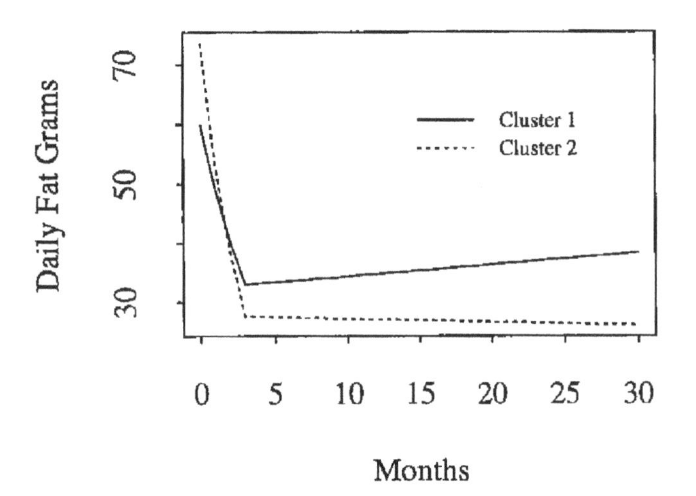

FIGURE 6 Observed data and mean response profiles for the control clusters around daily fat grams. (From first edition of *Nutritional Oncology*.)

classified the same is that a large number, 30, of the participants were adherers with respect to percentage fat calories and nonadherers with respect to total fat grams. This suggests that these women may have achieved their goal with respect to percentage fat calories by keeping their total fat grams relatively constant while eating more.

The strengths, weaknesses, and potential for errors in dietary assessment methods are well known (Beaton, 1994; Buzzard, 1994; Wynder et al., 1997). The possibility for inaccurate measurements exists with most measures because they rely on self-report, as in the case of WINS use of 4DFR. The major strengths in food-record methods include the precision in measuring food intake and the limited reliance on memory in reporting intakes. The major limitation in 4DFR is the tendency for people to eat differently when recording their intake (Witschi, 1990; Schakel et al., 1998). This limitation is of particular concern in dietary intervention studies because of the potential for participants in the low-fat group to better adhere when recording their intake compared with other times. This behavior, generally known

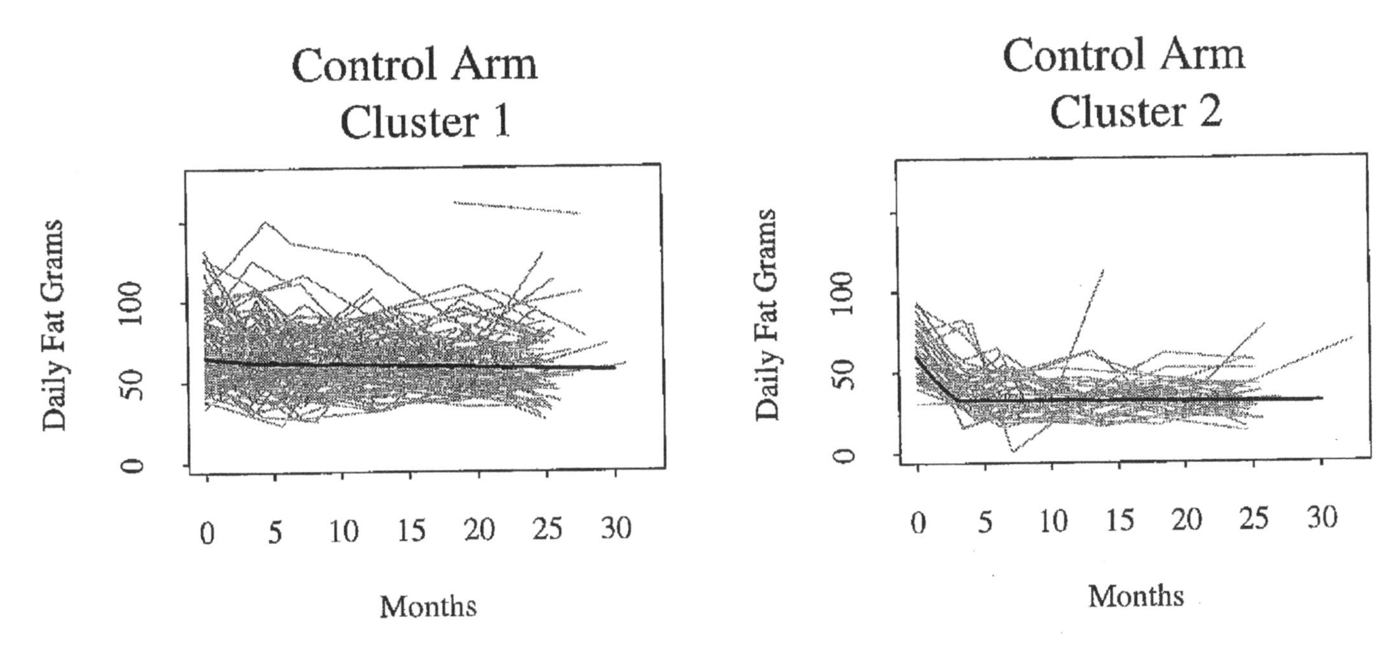

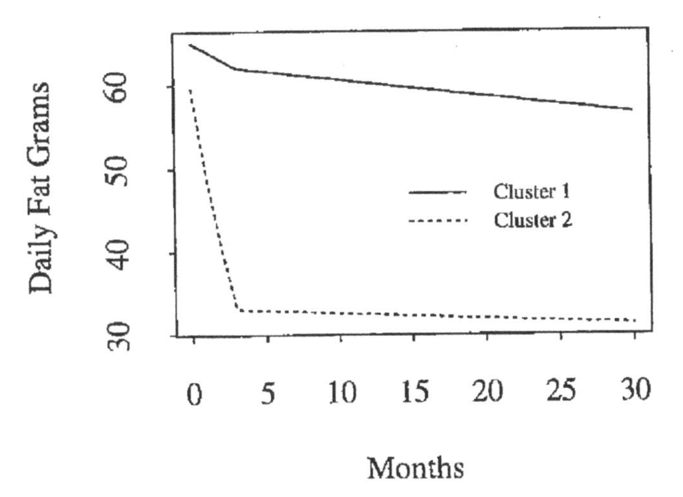

FIGURE 7 Observed data and mean response profiles for the control clusters around daily fat grams. (From first edition of *Nutritional Oncology*.)

TABLE 4 Cross-Tabulation of Adherers and Nonadherers in Both Arms of the Trial (Treatment/Control)

	Percentage fat grams		
	Adherers	Nonadherers	Total
Total fat grams			
Adherers	33/107	9/3	42/110
Nonadherers	30/15	70/23	100/38
Total	63/122	79/26	142/148

as "response-set bias" (Kristal et al., 1998) cannot be controlled for and must be considered in the interpretation of the results herein.

The WINS Feasibility Study was designed to investigate the viability of permanently changing the dietary habits of a randomly selected group of women who met certain inclusion/exclusion criteria (see Chlebowski et al., 1993). For the two responses investigated, weight and percentage of fat calories, the intervention was successful in changing dietary habits as evidenced by the group by time interaction.

However, the specific goal of the study was to effect change that would result in a diet that consisted of 20% (or less) of daily calories from fat.

Our cluster analysis shows that 44.4% of the women randomly assigned to the treatment group were successful (16.4% daily calories from fat). The remaining 55.6% reduced their percentage of calories from fat and achieved a mean of ~25% fat calories. This suggests that a more intensive intervention would be useful, followed by an aggressive maintenance program. It could be speculated that those women whose percentage fat calories were higher at baseline were those who could not adhere to the study protocol. However, we adjusted for baseline percentage of calories from fat in our model. This, in effect, removes any bias due to the baseline value. The mean baseline percentage of calories from fat for the adherers in the treatment group was 33.6% and that for the nonadherers was 34.4%. These are not significantly different from one another ($p = 0.45$, using the Wilcoxon Rank Sum Test) (Lehmann, 1975).

SUMMARY

The usefulness of approaches to longitudinal analyses has been clearly shown. The newer methodologies initiated by Laird and Ware (1982), Jennrich and Schluchter (1986), and Liang and Zeger (1986) and further developed by almost a generation of statisticians have produced methods to importantly enhance our ability to obtain much more information from the longitudinal design. This work does not require the analyst to "fudge factor" the data; it makes minimal use of normal distributions (including some methodologies in which normal distribution assumptions are nowhere required); it does not require us to assume correlation structures of questionable accuracy; it enables us to make inferences with missing data; and it provides us with valid significance tests.

Sample Size Considerations

Sample size computations for this study are based on relapse-free survival as the primary outcome. Additionally, all subjects who are randomized, except the strata of undetermined lymph node group, will be included in the primary analysis within their randomized treatment assignments (i.e., an intent-to-treat analysis). Sample size calculations are not exact computations but are approximations based on an assumed model. We utilized published information from NSABP trials involving tamoxifen treatment in postmenopausal breast cancer populations to estimate the required survival probabilities that we expect to observe in the current study. The undetermined lymph node strata patients were not considered in sample size calculation because the survival or relapse-free survival information about the undetermined lymph node strata patient was not available.

The power calculations were carried out non-parametrically using a flexible program that obtains power estimates for survival analyses via simulation. Options in the program include: up to 10 strata; general subject accrual proportions; two treatment groups; a variety of disease-free survival or survival distributions; drop-in or drop-out rates; loss to follow-up and withdrawal distributions; years of accrual and follow-up; and three methods of interim testing to maintain the overall significance level of the test (including Pocock, Tsiatis, and Fleming). The survival, loss-to-follow-up, withdrawal, and accrual distributions may be either empirical, Rayleigh, exponential, gamma, Weibull, or uniform.

The power calculations for the WINS are based on a comparison of disease-free survival time between the two treatment groups (IIG and NIG) and the following assumptions:

A. Stratification factor (only one stratification factor is used because the surgical consultant of SCU indicates that the three groups of systemic therapy do not have different disease-free survival rates.)

Nodal status: Several accrual proportions by nodal status were considered.

Nodal status		–	+
Proportion of patients accrued	Option 1	10%	90%
	Option 2	25%	75%
	Option 3	55%	45%
	Option 4	60%	40%

B. Accrual and follow-up time: 417 subjects accrued per year for 6 years, with 3 years of additional follow-up.

C. Drop-in rate from NIG to IIG and drop-out rate from IIG to NIG:

Drop-in rate	**Drop-out rate**
0.10	0.30

D. Uniform accrual distributions

E. Random censoring model

F. No qualitative interaction

G. Five interim analyses using the Fleming–Harrington method

H. Two-sided significance level of .05

I. Withdrawals folded into the drop-out rate

J. Upward adjustment of sample size to handle noncancer death rate without recurrence

K. All centers follow the same survival distribution (i.e., there is no interaction of treatment by center)

L. The final power was computed by carrying out 1000 simulations of the study design

TABLE 5 Assumed Cumulative Disease-Free Survival Rates

Nodal status	ER level	Time (years)	Group I	Group II
–	+	0.0	1.000	1.000
		1.0	0.990	0.995
		2.0	0.920	0.970
		3.0	0.870	0.940
		4.0	0.800	0.870
		10.0	0.700	0.800
		100.0	0.000	0.000
–	–	0.0	1.000	1.000
		1.0	0.920a	0.950
		2.0	0.900	0.940
		3.0	0.880	0.930
		4.0	0.850	0.900
		10.0	0.750	0.850
		100.0	0.000	0.000
+	+	0.0	1.000	1.000
		1.0	0.950	0.970
		2.0	0.850	0.920
		3.0	0.750	0.820
		4.0	0.700	0.780
		5.0	0.650	0.730
		10.0	0.500	0.600
		100.0	0.000	0.000
+	–	0.0	1.000	1.000
		1.0	0.900	0.950
		2.0	0.750	0.820
		3.0	0.650	0.720
		4.0	0.600	0.680
		5.0	0.550	0.630
		10.0	0.400	0.500
		100.0	0.000	0.000

TABLE 6 Results of Power Calculations

Accrual time	6 years
Follow-up time	3 years
No. of accrual patients per year	417
Nodal status –:+ %	60%:40%
ER status –:+	20%:80%
Drop in:out rate	10%:30%
Power	84.4%

M. The disease-free survival probabilities assumed within each stratum are summarized in Table 5; these values were based on published data from NSABP breast cancer trials involving tamoxifen.

Table 6 summarizes the result of final power calculations.

In summary, if 2500 subjects are accrued over a 6-year period and subsequently followed for 3 additional years, there would be 84% power to detect the assumed differences in disease-free survival at 9 years, using the assumed models. Based on these computations, our goal is to accrue at least 2502 subjects over a 6-year period.

CONCLUSIONS

The statistical design is that of a randomized, two-arm study with two stratification factors: systemic therapy and nodal status. The primary endpoint of the study is disease-free survival. A secondary endpoint includes overall survival defined as death from any cause. Both of these endpoints may be right-censored because of subjects who are lost to follow-up or who have not yet reached the study endpoint. Other secondary endpoints include the lipid profile measurements. These outcomes, as well as other measured covariates, may be binary, polychotomous, or continuous and may consist of repeated measurements over time.

References

Bandura, A. 1969. "Principles of Behavior Modification." Holt, Rinehart & Winston, New York.

Beaton, G.H. 1994. Approaches to analysis of dietary data: relationship between planned analyses and choice of methodology. *Am J Clin Nutr* **59**: 253s–261s.

Buzzard, I.M., Asp, E.H., Chlebowski, R.T., Boyer, A.P., Jeffery, R.W., Nixon, D.W., Blackburn, G.L., Joehimsen, P.R., Scanlon, E.F., Insull, W.J., Elashoff, R.M., Butrum, R., and Wynder, E.L. 1990. Diet intervention methods to reduce fat intake: Nutrient and food group composition of self-selected low-fat diets. *J Am Diet Assoc* **90**: 42–50.

Buzzard, I.M. 1994. Rationale for an international conference series on dietary assessment methods. *Am J Clin Nutr* **59**(Suppl): 143s–145s.

Cheney, W., and Kincaid, D. 1994. "Numerical Mathematics and Computing." Brooks/Cole, Pacific Grove, CA.

Chlebowski, R.T., Blackburn, G.L., Buzzard, I.M., Rose, D.P., Martino, S., Khandokar, J.D., York, R.M., Jeffery, R.W., Elashoff, M.E., and Wynder, E.L. 1993. Adherence to a dietary fat intake reduction program in postmenopausal women receiving therapy for early breast cancer. *J Clin Oncol* **11**: 2072–2080.

Cohen, L.A., Rose, D.P., and Wynder, E.L. 1993. A rationale for dietary intervention in postmenopausal breast cancer patients: an update. *Nutr Cancer* **90**: 1–10.

Davidson, M.H., Maki, K.C., Kong, J.C., Dugan, L.D., Torri, S.A., Hall, H.A., Drennan, K.B., Anderson, S.M., Fulgoni, V.Z., Saldanha, L.G., and Olson, B.H. 1998. Long term effects of consuming foods containing psyllium seed husks on serum lipids in patients with hypercholesterolemia. *Am J Clin Nutr* **67**: 367–376.

DeBoor, C. 1978. "A Practical Guide to Splines." Springer-Verlag, New York.

Diggle, P.J., Liang, K., and Zeger, S.L. 1994. "Analysis of Longitudinal Data." Oxford University Press, New York.

Jennrich, R.J., and Schluchter, M.D. 1986. Unbalanced repeated measures models with structured covariance matrices. *Biometries* **42**: 805–820.

Kristal, A.F., Andrilla, H.A., Koepsell, T.D., Diehr, P.H., and Cheadle, A. 1998. Dietary assessment instruments are susceptible to intervention-associated response set bias. *J Am Diet Assoc* **98**: 40–43.

Laird, N.M., and Ware, J.H. 1982. Random-effects models for longitudinal data. *Biometrics* **38**: 963–974.

Lehmann, E.L. 1975. "Nonparametries: Statistical Methods Based on Ranks." Holden-Day, San Francisco.

Leung, M.K., and Elashoff, M.E. 1996. Generalized linear mixed-effects models with a finite-support random-effects distribution: a maximum-penalized likelihood approach. *Biometr J* **38**: 135–151.

Liang, K., and Zeger, S.L. 1986. Longitudinal data analysis using generalized linear models. *Biometrika* **73**: 13–22.

Lipkin, E.W. 1998. A longitudinal study of calcium regulation in a non-human primate model of parenteral nutrition. *Am J Clin Nutr* **67**: 246–254.

Little, R.J.A. 1995. Modeling the drop-out mechanism in repeated-measures studies. *JASA J Am Stat Assoc* **90**: 1112–1121.

Little, R., and Rubin, D. 2002. "Statistical Analysis with Missing Data," 2nd edition. Wiley InterScience, Hoboken, NJ.

Peto, R., Pike, M.C., Armitage, P., Breslow, N.E., Cox, D.R., Howard, S.V., Mantel, N., McPherson, K., Peto, J., and Smith, P.G. 1977. Design and analysis of randomized clinical trials requiring prolonged observation of each patient. II. analysis and examples. *Br J Cancer* **35**: 1–39.

Robins, J.M., Rotnitzky, A., and P, Z.L. 1995. Analysis of semiparametric regression models for repeated outcomes in the presence of missing data. *JASA J Am Stat Assoc* **90**: 106–121.

Rubin, D.B. 1976. Inference and missing data. *Biometrika* **63**: 81–92.

Savendahl, L., Mars, M.H., Underwood, L.E., and Zeisel, S.H. 1997. Prolonged fasting in humans results in diminished plasma choline concentrations but does not cause liver dysfunction. *Am J Clin Nutr* **66**: 622–625.

Schakel, S., Sievert, Y.A., and Buzzard, I.M. 1998. Sources of data for developing and maintaining a nutrient database. *J Am Diet Assoc* **88**: 1268–1271.

Shi, M., Weiss, R.E., and Taylor, J.M.G. 1996. An analysis of paediatric CD4 counts for acquired immune deficiency syndrome using flexible random curves. *Appl Stat* **45**: 151–163.

Wang, Y., and Taylor, J.M.G. 1995. Flexible methods for analysing longitudinal data using piecewise cubic polynomials. *J Stat Comput Simul* **52**: 133–150.

Witschi, J.C. 1990. Short-term dietary recall and recording methods. *In* "Nutrition Epidemiology" (W. Willett, ed.), pp. 42–50. Oxford University Press, New York.

Wynder, E.L., Cohen, L.A., Muscat, J.E., Winters, B., Dwyer, J.T., and Blackburn, G. 1997. Breast cancer: weighing the evidence for a promoting role of dietary fat. *J Natl Cancer Inst* **89**: 766–775.

Zeger, S.L., and Liang, K. 1986. Longitudinal data analysis for discrete and continuous outcomes. *Biometries* **42**: 121–130.

CHAPTER

46

Evidence-based Practice Management in Cancer Prevention and Treatment

GEORGE L. BLACKBURN

INTRODUCTION

Methodologies for summarizing, assessing, and judging the strength of scientific evidence on diet, nutrition, and the causation and prevention of cancer have evolved from Sir Austin Bradford Hill's inference of etiology in a broad biological context (e.g., criteria for establishing scientific causation) (Bradford Hill, 1965) to evidence-based medicine's (EBM) focus on efficacy of treatment.

The evidence-based approach is considered state of the art in efforts to synthesize research findings as a basis for practice, guidelines, and recommendations (U.S. Preventive Services Task Force, 1996; Heggie et al., 2003; Morris and Carson, 2003; American Diabetes Association, 2005a) (Tables 1 and 2). The aim of EBM (Evidence-based Medicine Working Group, 1992) is to promote clinical decision-making based on the best available scientific evidence (Bero and Rennie, 1995; Blackburn et al., 2005). The standards against which evidence is judged are designed to be overt and predefined, with studies classified according to grades of evidence based on research design. The result is a hierarchy of evidence that puts the highest weighting on randomized controlled trials (RCTs) rather than on observational studies (Heggie et al., 2003) (Table 3).

Considerable evolution has occurred in the evaluation of scientific evidence. Advances in study design methodology, along with data showing parity of outcomes between RCTs and observational interventions (Benson and Hartz, 2000; Concato et al., 2000), have challenged assumptions that underlie the hierarchy of evidence. In part, they have also served as an impetus for the development of new methods to assess the quality of research findings.

These new approaches include modification of traditional levels of evidence to accommodate outcomes from well-conducted observational studies (Blackburn et al., 2005) and evaluation of evidence beyond that of efficacy alone. The U.S. Preventive Services Task Force has acknowledged these changes by citing the need to consider evidence as a whole, including trade-offs among benefits, harms, costs, and net benefits relative to optimal allocation of resources (Harris et al., 2001; Blackburn et al., 2005).

CANCER RATES AND CAUSATION

Background

Cancer is a major cause of mortality throughout the world. It accounts for 7.1 million deaths annually (12.5%) of the global total. Approximately 20 million people suffer from cancer—a figure projected to rise to 30 million within 20 years (World Health Organization, 2005a). The latest data from the American Cancer Society (ACS) (2006b) indicate that cancer is the leading cause of death among all Americans younger than 85 years. This year in the United States, the ACS estimates that 1,372,910 new cases of cancer will be diagnosed and that 570,260 people will die from the disease. Lung cancer, which is largely preventable, is the leading cause of cancer death, accounting for one in three deaths in men and one in four in women.

Trends

In many countries, >25% of deaths are attributable to cancer. In 2000, 5.3 million men and 4.7 million women

Copyright © 2006, Elsevier Inc.
All rights of reproduction in any form reserved.

TABLE 1 U.S. Preventive Services Task Force Hierarchy of Research Design

I	Evidence obtained from at least one properly randomized controlled trial
II-1	Evidence obtained from well-designed controlled trials without randomization
II-2	Evidence obtained from well-designed cohort or case-control analytical studies, preferably from more than one center or research group
II-3	Evidence from multiple time series with or without the intervention; dramatic results in uncontrolled experiments (such as results of the introduction of penicillin treatment in the 1940s)
III	Opinions of respected authorities, based on clinical experience, descriptive studies and case reports, or reports of expert committees

Note: The Third U.S. Preventive Services Task Force added a three-category rating (good, fair, poor) of internal validity to its standard hierarchy of research design. A well-performed randomized controlled trial, for example, would be rated 1-good; a fair cohort study would be rated II-2-fair (Agency for Healthcare Research and Quality, 2001; Harris et al., 2001).

TABLE 2 American Diabetes Association Grading System for Clinical Practice Recommendations

Level of Evidence Description
A
Clear evidence from well-conducted, generalizable, randomized controlled trials that are adequately powered, including:
• Evidence from a well-conducted multicenter trial
• Evidence from a meta-analysis that incorporated quality ratings in the analysis
• Compelling nonexperimental evidence, i.e., "all or none" rule developed by the Center for Evidence-Based Medicine at Oxford[a]
Supportive evidence from well-conducted randomized controlled trials that are adequately powered, including:
• Evidence from a well-conducted trial at one or more institutions
• Evidence from a meta-analysis that incorporated quality ratings in the analysis
B
Supportive evidence from well-conducted cohort studies, including:
• Evidence from a well-conducted prospective cohort study or registry
• Evidence from a well-conducted meta-analysis of cohort studies
Supportive evidence from a well-conducted case-control study
C
Supportive evidence from poorly controlled or uncontrolled studies, including:
• Evidence from randomized clinical trials with one or more major or three or more minor methodological flaws that could invalidate the results
• Evidence from observational studies with high potential for bias (such as case series with comparison with historical controls)
• Evidence from case series or case reports
Conflicting evidence with the weight of evidence supporting the recommendation
E
Expert consensus or clinical experience

Note: The latest American Diabetes Association grading system assigns ratings of A, B, or C depending on the quality of evidence. Expert Opinion (E) is a separate category for recommendations that do not yet have clinical trial evidence, clinical trials might be impractical, or there is conflicting evidence.

Source: From the American Diabetes Association, 2006.

[a]Either all patients died before therapy and at least some survived with therapy, or some patients died without therapy and none died with therapy; for example, use of insulin in the treatment of diabetic ketoacidosis.

developed a malignant tumor, and 6.2 million of them died from the disease. Cancer has emerged as a major public health problem in developing countries, with an impact equal to that in industrialized nations (International Agency for Research on Cancer[IARC], 2004); it is becoming an increasingly important factor in the global burden of disease.

The number of new cancer cases annually is expected to increase an estimated 50%, rising from 10 million in 2000 to 15 million by 2020 (Stewart and Kleihues, 2003). This predicted rise will be due mainly to steadily aging populations in both developed and developing countries, as well as growing adoption of unhealthy lifestyles. Approximately 60% of new cancer cases will occur in the less developed parts of the world (WHO). Cancer is strongly associated with social and economic status, with risk factors highest in groups with the least education (WHO, 2005a).

In most developed countries, cancer is the second leading cause of death after cardiovascular disease (CVD), and epidemiological evidence points to this trend emerging in the less developed world. This is particularly true of countries in "transition," or middle income countries such as South America and Asia. Already more than half of all cancer cases occur in developing countries. The incidence of lung cancer and cancers of the colon, rectum, breast, and prostate generally increases in parallel with economic development, while stomach cancer declines.

Environmental Causes

From a global perspective, the three main cancer-causing agents are tobacco, diet and exercise, and infections (IARC/WHO, 2006). Dietary modification and regular physical activity are significant elements in cancer prevention and control. Overweight and obesity are both serious risk factors for cancer. After tobacco, overweight and obesity appear to be the most important avoidable causes of cancer (WHO, 2005a).

Dietary factors account for up to 30% of cancers in Western countries (Doll and Peto, 1996). The proportion is thought to be ~20% in developing countries and is expected to grow (IARC, 2006). As developing nations become urbanized, patterns of cancer, particularly those most strongly associated with diet and physical activity, tend to shift toward those of economically developed countries. Cancer rates also change as populations move between countries and adopt different dietary patterns.

TABLE 3 Evidence-based Medicine Conventional Hierarchy of Study Design

Experimental studies
Meta-analysis of randomized controlled trials
Randomized controlled trials
Quasi-experimental
Observational studies
Cohort study
Case-control study
Cross-sectional study
Before and after study
Case series

Note: Evidence-based medicine's traditional hierarchy of evidence puts the highest weighting on randomized controlled trials rather than on observational studies.

Source: From NHS Centre for Reviews and Dissemination, 2001.

Migrants from regions with low rates of colon cancer to those with high rates of colon carcinogenesis (or vice versa) show rapid changes in their risk of colon cancer. In the United States, colon and rectal cancers are increasing, with ~1 million new cases every year. These tumors are most prevalent in the economically developed world, but their incidence is rising in developing countries as well (Bingham et al., 2003; IARC, 2006). Dietary effects are presumed to underlie many of the large international differences in incidence seen for most cancers (McCullough and Giovannucci, 2004).

Dietary Factors and Cancer

Alcohol consumption is an established cause of cancers of the oral cavity, pharynx, larynx, esophagus, liver, and breast. For each of these cancers, risk increases substantially with intake of more than two drinks per day (ACS, 2005a). Prolonged high consumption of red and processed meat is also thought to increase the risk of cancer in the distal portion of the large intestine (Chao et al., 2005).

Data show an association between intake of dietary fiber and risk of colon and rectal cancers. Bingham et al. (2003) report that an approximate doubling of total fiber from foods could reduce the risk of colorectal cancer by 40%. Similarly, Peters et al. (2003) suggest that dietary fiber, particularly from grains, cereals, and fruits, is associated with decreased risk of distal colon adenoma.

Findings from the Women's Health Initiative (WHI) Dietary Modification Trial suggest that the risk of brest cancer may be modified by reducing the intake of total fat to 20% of total energy and increasing the daily consumption of vegetables and fruit and grain (Buzdar, 2006; Prentice et al., 2006). These data are complemented by initial results from another prospective dietary study, the Women's Intervention Nutrition Study (WINS), which show that a lifestyle intervention resulting in dietary fat intake reduction can improve the relapse-free survival of postmenopausal breast cancer patients (Chlebowski et al., 2005).

Studies indicate that consumption of fruits and vegetables may protect against cancers of the mouth, pharynx, larynx, stomach, colorectum, and lung (IARC/WHO, 2005). However, van Giles et al. (2005) suggest that the intake of fruits and vegetables, once thought to protect against breast cancer, provides no significant risk reduction. These data run counter to those of the EPIC study (Miller et al., 2004).

Obesity, insulin resistance, and low physical activity may mask or negate biologically consequential benefits from consumption of fruits and vegetables. Using the cumulative average of repeated dietary assessments could introduce systematic measurement error and further distort diet–cancer relations (Schatzkin and Kipnis, 2004). As originally reported in *Food, Nutrition and the Prevention of Cancer: A Global Perspective* (World Cancer Research Fund, 1997), confounding can interfere with the interaction of dietary factors and cancer in nutritional intervention studies, leading to misinterpretation of data, misleading results, and missed opportunities to prevent and/or control cancer. Further investigation is necessary to assess whether adjustment for these variables can lead to protection against cancer, earlier detection of existing cancers, or improved prognosis.

A priority exists to prevent and treat obesity, insulin resistance, and physical inactivity so that patients can gain the health benefits contained within the *2005 Dietary Guidelines for Americans* (Department of Health and Human Services [HHS] and the U.S. Department of Agriculture [USDA], 2005). Dietary patterns, physical activity, and weight control can substantially affect the risk of developing cancer and modify cancer risk at all stages of its development (ACS, 2006a).

The Obesity-Cancer Connection

In the United States, current patterns of overweight and obesity are thought to account for 14% of all deaths from cancer in men and 20% of those in women. Calle et al. (2003) report a relation between increased body weight and higher death rates for all cancers combined and for cancers at multiple specific sites. Obesity has been linked to significantly higher death rates from cancers of the esophagus, colon, rectum, liver, gallbladder, pancreas, and kidney. It has also been implicated in higher death rates from non-Hodgkin's lymphoma and multiple myeloma (Calle et al., 2003; ACS, 2006a).

Significant trends of increasing risk with higher body mass index (BMI) have also been seen in death rates from stomach and prostate cancers in men, and cancers of the breast (in women), uterus, cervix, and ovaries (Calle et al., 2003; ACS, 2006a). A study indicates that obesity may be associated with more advanced-stage prostate cancer and lower overall survival rates (Baillargeon et al., 2005).

A substantial body of evidence (Chlebowski et al., 2004) suggests that biological mechanisms for these associations and trends include increased levels of endogenous hormones (sex steroids, insulin, and insulin-like growth factor-1 [IGF-1]) associated with overweight and obesity. Longer exposure of breast tissue to circulating estrogen has been linked to increased risk of breast cancer (ACS, 2006a). Components of the metabolic syndrome—for example, hyperinsulinemia (Lawlor et al., 2004), insulin resistance (Muti et al., 2002), low high-density lipoprotein cholesterol (HDL-C) (Furberg et al., 2005)—are known to be associated with cancers of the breast, colon, and other sites (ACS, 2005a).

Malin et al. (2004) report that insulin resistance and IGFs may synergistically increase breast cancer risk. These data are consistent with those from other studies (Chlebowski et al., 2004, 2005; Winters et al., 2004). As mechanisms underlying human carcinogenesis are better understood, dietary research will increasingly focus on intermediate markers, such as the IGFs and potential carcinogenic metabolites (McCullough and Giovannucci, 2004).

Prevalence of Obesity

The prevalence of obesity worldwide has risen sharply during the past four decades. Substantial evidence shows a relation among overweight, obesity, and many types of cancer, such as those of the esophagus, colorectum, breast, endometrium, and kidney (WHO). In the United States, the number of obese adults doubled to ~63 million between 1976–1980 and 2001–2002. The ranks of those with severe obesity, with >100 lbs of excess weight, grew to nearly 11 million people in 2001/2002 (Lehman Center Weight Loss Surgery Expert Panel, 2005).

The WHO estimates that of the more than one billion people who are overweight (BMI $\geq$ 30 kg/m^2) worldwide, 300 million are obese (BMI $\geq$ 40 kg/m^2) (Sanchez-Castillo et al., 2004). The *2005 Dietary Guidelines for Americans* (Bero and Rennie, 1995) underscores the health risks associated with overweight, obesity, and a sedentary lifestyle by highlighting the need for physical activity and calorie control as well as a healthy balance of nutritious foods.

Physical Activity

The nature of the associations among physical activity, obesity, nutrition, and cancer remains unclear. However, regular activity is thought to improve metabolic syndrome and reduce risk of colon, breast, endometrial, and prostate cancers (Calle et al., 2003; Chlebowski et al., 2004, 2005; Winters et al., 2004; WHO, 2004). Regular physical activity can contribute to the maintenance of a healthy body weight by balancing caloric intake and energy expenditure (ACS, 2006a).

Data from the IARC and the WHO (IARC, 2006) indicate that limiting weight gain reduces the risk of cancer at several sites, including breast (in postmenopausal women), endometrium, kidney (renal cell), and esophagus. Modern chronic diseases, including type 2 diabetes, coronary heart disease, and cancer are the leading killers in Westernized society and are increasing at a rampant pace in developing nations. Overwhelming evidence from a variety of sources—including epidemiological, prospective cohort, and intervention studies—links most chronic diseases seen in the world today to physical inactivity and inappropriate dietary consumption (Roberts and Barnard, 2005).

GRADING OF SCIENTIFIC EVIDENCE

Overview of Causation Science

Reliance on medical statistics and clinical applications of epidemiology are developments of the twentieth century, especially the latter half of the period. Through the 1940s, medical research was carried out by physician–investigators guided by observation of patients, pathophysiological reasoning, and small-scale experimentation at the bedside (Lewis, 1945; Bernard, 1966). The nature of clinical research changed in conjunction with, and in response to, advances in cellular analysis and molecular biology; development of quantification in therapeutic evaluation; the emergence of probabilistic thinking; and the application of statistical methods and theory (Chalmers, 2001).

Bradford Hill's influence on medical statistics and clinical research has been considerable. He authored an influential textbook on medical statistics, which was published in 1937 (Hill, 1937). He also played a pivotal role in the evaluation of streptomycin in the treatment of tuberculosis. The results of that trial, published in 1948 (Medical Research Council Streptomycin in Tuberculosis Trials Committee, 1948), marked the start of the modern era of clinical research. Bradford Hill and his colleague, Sir Richard Doll, also played key roles in the development of observational epidemiological research. Major case-control studies conducted in 1950 by Hill and Doll in the United Kingdom (Doll and Hill, 1950) and Wynder and Graham (1950) in the United States showed that smoking was a cause of most cancer deaths. In 1951, Hill and Doll (1954) also initiated the first major cohort study of British doctors, their smoking habits, and lung cancer.

In 1965, Bradford Hill (1965) established criteria for scientific causation, broad guidelines that have served as a model for standards since developed to assess the quality of research evidence. Originally developed for use in occupational medicine, the criteria have been widely applied in a variety of fields (Rom, 1992). They include nine points of consideration, not all of which must be fulfilled to establish scientific causation. Key criteria, those with the highest priority in judging a causal relationship, are (1) consistency of the association across studies, (2) strength of the association, (3) and temporal relationship.

In the case of dietary fat intake and prostate cancer risk, for example, a series of *in vitro* laboratory, animal, and clinical studies were required to meet criteria for substantial scientific evidence. Though epidemiological investigations suggested an association of dietary fat intake with prostate cancer risk, there was limited supporting evidence from animal studies (Zhou and Blackburn, 1997). The failure of the Alpha-Tocopherol and Beta Carotene (ATBC) Cancer Prevention Study (Alpha-Tocopherol and Beta Carotene Cancer Prevention Study Group, 1994) underscores the need to develop strong supporting data in animal models (De Luca and Ross, 1996). Although conceived on the basis of epidemiological and mechanistic evidence, the trial went forward without published evidence that B-carotene prevented lung cancer in animal models (Wynder et al., 1997).

The Causes of Cancer (Doll and Peto, 1981), a landmark review by British epidemiologists Richard Doll and Richard Peto, included estimates of the extent to which cancer in general, and specific cancers, could be avoided by changes in diet. Published 16 years after Hill defined causality, *The Causes of Cancer* concluded that environmental carcinogens, other than those in tobacco and diet, were relatively unimportant causes of cancer. Doll and Peto's review, which is still frequently cited, set the agenda for current thinking on nutritional oncology.

HISTORY OF EVIDENCE-BASED MEDICINE

The traditional paradigm of medical education and practice considers understanding of basic pathophysiological mechanisms of disease, coupled with clinical experience (Haynes, 2002), sufficient grounds for clinical decision-making. In contrast, EBM promotes the centrality of scientific evidence as the basis for treatment and policy decisions. The underlying philosophy of EBM suggests that a formal set of rules must complement medical training and common sense for clinicians to effectively interpret the results of clinical research (Guyatt et al., 2000).

However, challenges in applying new knowledge (e.g., abundance of literature, the tiny fraction of adequately tested and clinically valid reports, and limitations of time and resources) are considerable (Haynes, 2002). To help clinicians, health systems, and policy makers overcome these obstacles, advocates of EBM have created procedures to objectively summarize and assess the quality of scientific evidence, and make recommendations based on those assessments (Table 3).

Charged with developing recommendations for clinical preventive services, the Canadian Task Force on the Periodic Health Examination published its first report in 1979, a seminal work using systematic rules of evidence to support the strength of recommendations for a wide variety of preventive services (Table 4). The report applied a hierarchy of evidence to rank recommendations according to the available type and amount of evidence. The same approach, which was used to derive a grading of recommendations, appears to have been the first practical application of such levels of evidence (Centre for Evidence-based Medicine. Oxford-Centre for Evidence-based Medicine, 2001; Kroke et al., 2004) (Table 5).

TABLE 4 Canadian Task Force on Preventive Health Care Levels of Evidence

Levels of evidence	
I	Evidence from at least one well-designed randomized controlled trial
II-1	Evidence from well-designed controlled trials without randomization
II-2	Evidence from well-designed cohort or case-control analytical studies, preferably from more than one center or research group
II-3	Evidence from comparisons between times or places with or without the intervention; dramatic results from uncontrolled studies could be included here
III	Opinions of respected authorities, based on clinical experience; descriptive studies or reports of expert committees

Note: The 1979 report of the Canadian Task Force on the Periodic Health Examination was the first to use systematic rules of evidence to support the strength of recommendations for a wide variety of preventive services. The report applied a hierarchy of evidence to rank recommendations according to the available type and amount of evidence (Canadian Task Force on the Periodic Health Examination, 1979).
Source: From Levine et al., 2001.

The U.S. Preventive Services Task Force (Task Force/USPSTF) (Table 1) was established in 1984 to extend the approach of the Canadian Task Force by systematically reviewing the scientific evidence for individual clinical preventive services, and making recommendations for practitioners about what services should be routinely offered. Its controversial *Guide to Clinical Preventive Services*, released in 1989, downplayed expert opinion as a basis for making recommendations and took a neutral position when evidence was lacking (USPSTF, 1989). It also accelerated a growing movement to replace traditional "expert consensus" methods for developing clinical recommendations with a systematic and explicit process for reviewing evidence and linking clinical practice guidelines directly to the quality of the science (Woolf, 1990).

Within health care, the evidence-based paradigm has become all-pervasive. At both basic and continuing education levels, skills in finding and appraising evidence are now central to many curricula. Databases, journals, and Internet sites, often free at the point of delivery, provide an accessible infrastructure to support the adoption of evidence-based

TABLE 5 Oxford Centre for Evidence-based Medicine Levels of Evidence (May 2001)

Level	Therapy/prevention: etiology/harm	Prognosis	Diagnosis	Differential diagnosis/symptom prevalence study	Economic and decision analyses
1a	SR (with homogeneity[a]) of RCTs	SR (with homogeneity[a]) of inception cohort studies; CDR[b] validated in different populations	SR (with homogeneity[a]) of Level 1 diagnostic studies; CDR[b] with 1b studies from different clinical centres	SR (with homogeneity[a]) of prospective cohort studies	SR (with homogeneity[a]) of Level 1 economic studies
1b	Individual RCT (with narrow confidence interval[c])	Individual inception cohort study with ≥80% follow-up; CDR[b] validated in a single population	Validating[k] cohort study with good[i] reference standards; or CDR[b] tested within one clinical center	Prospective cohort study with good follow-up[m]	Analysis based on clinically sensible costs or alternatives; systematic review(s) of the evidence; and including multiway sensitivity analyses
1c	All or none[d]	All or none case series	Absolute SpPins and SnNouts[g]	All or none case series	Absolute better-value or worse-value analyses[j]
2a	SR (with homogeneity[a]) of cohort studies	SR (with homogeneity[a]) of either retrospective cohort studies or untreated control groups in RCTs	SR (with homogeneity[a]) of Level >2 diagnostic studies	SR (with homogeneity[a]) of 2b and better studies	SR (with homogeneity[a]) of Level >2 economic studies
2b	Individual cohort study (including low-quality RCT; e.g., <80% follow-up)	Retrospective cohort study or follow-up of untreated control patients in an RCT; derivation of CDR[b] or validated on split-sample[f] only	Exploratory[k] cohort study with good[i] reference standards; CDR[b] after derivation, or validated only on split-sample[f] or databases	Retrospective cohort study, or poor follow-up	Analysis based on clinically sensible costs or alternatives; limited review(s) of the evidence or single studies; and including multiway sensitivity analyses
2c	"Outcomes" research; ecological studies	"Outcomes" research[h]		Ecological studies	Audit or outcomes research
3a	SR (with homogeneity[a]) of case-control studies		SR (with homogeneity[a]) of 3b and better studies	SR (with homogeneity[a]) of 3b and better studies	SR (with homogeneity[a]) of 3b and better studies
3b	Individual case-control study		Nonconsecutive study or without consistently applied reference standards	Nonconsecutive cohort study or very limited population	Analysis based on limited alternatives or costs, poor quality estimates of data, but including sensitivity analyses incorporating clinically sensible variations
4	Case series (and poor quality cohort and case-control studies[e])	Case series (and poor quality prognostic cohort studies[l])	Case-control study, poor or nonindependent reference standard	Case series or superseded reference standards	Analysis with no sensitivity analysis
5	Expert opinion without explicit critical appraisal, or based on physiology, bench research or "first principles"	Expert opinion without explicit critical appraisal, or based on physiology, bench research or "first principles"	Expert opinion without explicit critical appraisal, or based on physiology, bench research or "first principles"	Expert opinion without explicit critical appraisal, or based on physiology, bench research or "first principles"	Expert opinion without explicit critical appraisal, or based on economic theory or "first principles"

Note: The Oxford Centre for Evidence-Based Medicine has adopted five categories related to diagnosis, prognosis, and harm, with 10 separate levels of evidence for each category (Oxford Centre for Evidence-based Medicine, 2001; Atkins et al., 2004a). Available at www.cebm.net/levels_of_evidence.asp.

Users can add a minus sign (–) to denote the level that fails to provide a conclusive answer because of

TABLE 5 *(Continued)*

- EITHER a single result with a wide confidence interval (such that, for example, an ARR in an RCT is not statistically significant but its confidence intervals fail to exclude clinically important benefit or harm)
- OR a systematic review with troublesome (and statistically significant) heterogeneity.

Such evidence is inconclusive and, therefore, can only generate Grade D recommendations, which include the following:

A consistent level 1 studies
B consistent level 2 or 3 studies *or* extrapolations from level 1 studies
C level 4 studies *or* extrapolations from level 2 or 3 studies
D level 5 evidence *or* troublingly inconsistent or inconclusive studies of any level

[a] By *homogeneity*, we mean a systematic review that is free of worrisome variations (heterogeneity) in the directions and degrees of results between individual studies. Not all systematic reviews with statistically significant heterogeneity need be worrisome, and not all worrisome heterogeneity need be statistically significant. As noted earlier, studies displaying worrisome heterogeneity should be tagged with a minus sign (–) at the end of their designated level.

[b] Clinical decision rule. (These are algorithms or scoring systems that lead to a prognostic estimation or a diagnostic category.)

[c] See note no. 2 for advice on how to understand, rate, and use trials or other studies with wide confidence intervals.

[d] Met when *all* patients died before the Rx became available, but some now survive on it; or when some patients died before the Rx became available, but *none* now die on it.

[e] By *poor-quality cohort study*, we mean one that failed to clearly define comparison groups and/or failed to measure exposures and outcomes in the same (preferably blinded) objective way in both exposed and nonexposed individuals and/or failed to identify or appropriately control known confounders and/or failed to carry out a sufficiently long and complete follow-up of patients. By *poor-quality case-control study*, we mean one that failed to clearly define comparison groups and/or failed to measure exposures and outcomes in the same (preferably blinded), objective way in both cases and controls and/or failed to identify or appropriately control known confounders.

[f] Split-sample validation is achieved by collecting all the information in a single tranche, then artificially dividing this into "derivation" and "validation" samples.

[g] An "Absolute SpPin" is a diagnostic finding whose *S*pecificity is so high that a *P*ositive result rules-*in* the diagnosis. An "Absolute SnNout" is a diagnostic finding whose *S*e*n*sitivity is so high that a *N*egative result rules-*out* the diagnosis.

[h] *Good, better, bad,* and *worse* refer to the comparisons between treatments in terms of their clinical risks and benefits.

[i] *Good* reference standards are independent of the test, and are applied blindly or objectively to all patients. *Poor* reference standards are haphazardly applied but still independent of the test. Use of a nonindependent reference standard (where the "test" is included in the "reference," or where the "testing" affects the "reference") implies a Level 4 study.

[j] Better-value treatments are clearly as good but cheaper or better at the same or reduced cost. Worse-value treatments are as good and more expensive or worse and equally or more expensive.

[k] Validating studies test the quality of a specific diagnostic test, based on prior evidence. An exploratory study collects information and trawls the data (e.g., using a regression analysis) to find which factors are "significant."

[l] By *poor-quality prognostic cohort study*, we mean one in which sampling was biased in favor of patients who already had the target outcome, or the measurement of outcomes was accomplished in <80% of study patients, or outcomes were determined in an unblinded, nonobjective way, or there was no correction for confounding factors.

[m] Good follow-up in a differential diagnosis study is >80%, with adequate time for alternative diagnoses to emerge (e.g., 1–6 months acute, 1–5 years chronic).

practice (The University of Sheffield). Other indications of widespread acceptance include new research institutions devoted to the subject of EBM; recurring editorials discussing its importance; innovations in methodologies and criteria for gathering and evaluating data; and a surge of RCTs in medical research (Timmermans and Mauck, 2005).

Over the past 20 years, an explicit methodology (Mulrow et al., 1997) for systematic reviews and meta-analyses has been popularized by the Cochrane Collaboration's *Cochrane Library* (Bero and Rennie, 1995; Cochrane Library). The reviews summarize the current status of medical scientific research and are used to resolve clinical questions, develop practice guidelines, determine research agendas, and establish health care policy.

The *Cochrane Library* (Cochrane Library) is the leading source of information on the efficacy of health care interventions. The Library contains the full text of Cochrane reviews, which bring together information on controlled studies (mostly RCTs) in a standard format (Mallett and Clarke, 2003). The Cochrane Central Register of controlled trials (CENTRAL) (Dickersin et al., 2002, 2003) is the main source used by Cochrane reviewers to locate studies. It contains citations to >300,000 reports of studies. Other evidence-based databases and resources include the Agency for Health Care Research and Quality: Evidence-based Practice, the National Guidelines Clearinghouse (*AHRQ. National Guidelines Clearinghouse*), and various practice guidelines developed by professional and academic medical societies (*AHRQ. National Guidelines Clearinghouse*).

HIERARCHIES OF EVIDENCE

Current levels of evidence have been developed mainly to address clinical research questions and, therefore, place major emphasis on RCTs as the primary and most convincing evidence in the evaluation process (Kroke et al., 2004). However, problems (Claxton and Thompson, 2001) and limitations associated with this approach (Claxton and Thompson, 2001; Kroke et al., 2004) have prompted numerous initiatives to broaden concepts of evidence away from the rigor of research design alone. Many groups, including the USPSTF (Harris et al., 2001), have developed guidelines based on grading hierarchies and other approaches for classifying and using disparate sources of evidence (Agency for Healthcare Research and Quality, 2004; Lehman Center Weight Loss Surgery Expert Panel, 2005).

The Executive Report from the Betsy Lehman Center for Patient Safety and Medical Error Reduction Expert Panel on

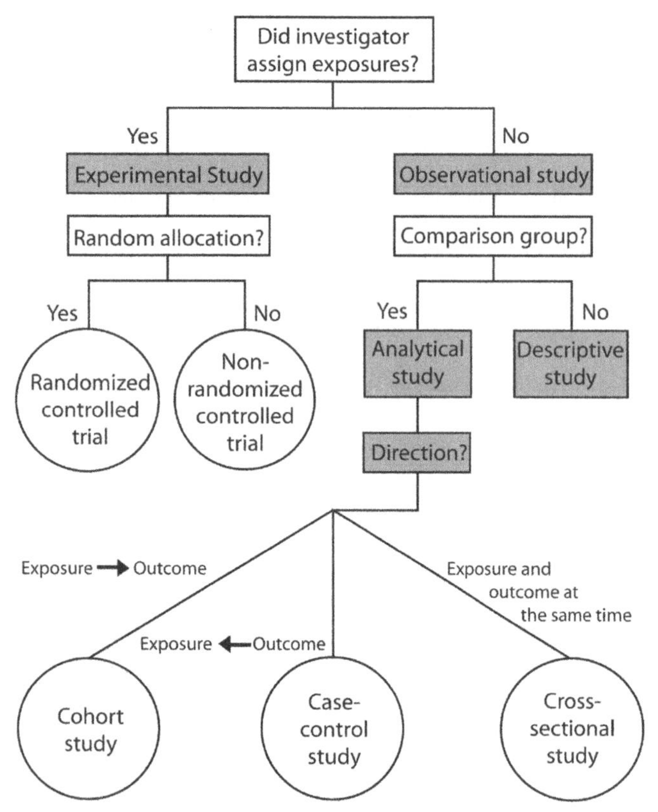

FIGURE 1 Algorithm for classifying types of clinical research. Each type of study design has particular strengths and weaknesses; all, however, are vital to a comprehensive understanding of the links between diet and cancer. The strongest evidence indicating that food and nutrition modify the risk of cancer comes from a combination of different types of epidemiological studies, supported by experimental findings and by identification of plausible biological pathways (World Cancer Research Fund and American Institute for Cancer Research, 1997). (Used with permission from Grimes and Schulz, 2002.)

BOX 1 Types of Clinical Research

Overview

Two types of studies—experimental and observational—are most relevant to hierarchies of evidence. The former includes controlled trials, either randomized or nonrandomized; and the latter, cohort, case-control, and cross-sectional studies. These are also known as *analytical studies*. Like controlled trials, they have comparison or control groups. The major difference between experimental and observational studies lies in whether investigators assign exposures (e.g., treatments) (Feinstein, 1985; Rothman, 1986; Hennekens and Buring, 1987; Hulley et al., 2001; Kelsey et al., 1996) or track them over time. Only comparative studies (both analytical and experimental) enable assessment of possible causal associations (Grimes and Schulz, 2002) (Figure 1).

Of these study designs, clinical trials and cohort studies usually require large sample sizes and lengthy follow-up periods to provide adequate statistical power to measure differences in outcome (U.S. Preventive Services Task Force, 1996). As a result, they can be slow to yield results and very expensive. The following descriptions summarize the general strengths and weaknesses of the most frequently used experimental and observational study designs.

Randomized Controlled Trials

Randomized controlled trials (RCTs) assign subjects by chance to either a study group (intervention) or a control (which receives standard treatment, e.g., no intervention or a placebo). Blinded trials conceal upcoming assignments from either investigators or subjects; double blind, from both. In nonrandomized controlled trials, assignments are made by some other allocation scheme, such as alternate assignment (Schulz et al., 1994).

The design of RCTs eliminates confounding biases, both known and unknown, enhancing comparability between groups and providing a more valid basis for inferring that the intervention caused the observed outcome. Properly designed and implemented RCTs are likely to have internal validity (i.e., measure what they set out to measure and be free of all biases; e.g., selection, information, and outcome). External validity, the extent to which results can be generalized to the broader community, is a potential problem with RCTs; people who volunteer to participate in clinical trials may differ in important ways from those who do not (Lilienfeld and Lilienfeld, 1980). Ethical issues are another limiting factor: RCTs cannot be used if subjects would be harmed by withdrawal or denial of effective treatment or intentionally exposed to noxious substances (e.g., toxins or bacteria).

Nonrandomized Controlled Trials

Nonrandomized controlled trials follow exposed and unexposed subjects forward in time to measure frequency of outcomes. Advantages of this study design include use of a concurrent control group and uniform measurement of outcomes for both groups. Selection bias, however, is a potential disadvantage.

The U.S. Preventive Services Task Force (Agency for Healthcare Research and Quality, 2001) and the Canadian Task Force on Preventive Health Care (Canadian Task Force on the Periodic Health Examination, 1994) have designated the nonrandomized controlled trial design as class II-1, indicating less scientific rigor than RCTs, but more than analytical studies.

Cohort, Case–Control, and Cross-Sectional Studies

Cohort studies follow already-exposed individuals (e.g., smokers) forward over time (longitudinally) to measure outcomes (e.g., cancer). In contrast, case-control studies start with an outcome and then look back in time for exposures that might have caused the outcome. In case-control studies of cancer screening, for example, prior exposure to a cancer-screening test is compared between patients with cancer (cases) and those without (controls). Cross-sectional studies are sometimes called *frequency surveys* or *prevalence studies* (Last, 1988). They examine the presence or absence of disease and the presence or absence of exposure at one point in time (e.g., obesity in women with arthritis vs women without arthritis) (U.S. Preventive Services Task Force, 1996).

All of these study designs are subject to potential systematic bias in that choice of treatments, risk factors, or other covariables might be made on the basis of important (or unrecognized) factors that could affect outcome. There is the potential for bias in the measurement and interpretation of data; the recall of medical histories or prior exposures; and the selection of patients who might differ from the general population in important ways. Confounding is a key concern with observational study designs. Unlike RCTs, which automatically adjust for known and unknown confounding variables, cohort and case-control study designs can only account for known confounders; the onus is, therefore, on investigators to make sure that such studies are free of bias.

BOX 2 Quantification of Risk

Cohort studies allow for calculation of true incident rates, relative risks, and attributable risks (i.e., the rate of a disease or other outcome in exposed individuals that can be attributed to the exposure). Relative risk compares the risk of disease among people with a particular exposure to that among people without that exposure. Relative risk above 1.0 indicates higher risk among exposed than unexposed persons; below 1.0 indicates an inverse association between a risk factor and the disease, or a protective effect. The higher the relative risk, the stronger the evidence of a causal relationship. A relative risk of 2.0 for high meat consumption implies a doubling of risk; a relative risk of 12.0 for certain levels of smoking and drinking implies a twelvefold increase in risk, as well as strong evidence of causation. Odds ratios, which provide a good proxy for relative risk, are used as the outcome measure in case-control studies.

Absolute risk, the observed or calculated probability of an event in a population under study, is also important. A large relative risk of a rare cancer amounts to a small absolute risk. In contrast, a small relative risk may amount to a large absolute risk for common cancers. For example, a relative risk of 1.10 (or a 10% increased risk) translates into many extra cases of colon and breast cancer cases in Europe and North America, where those cancers are very common.

Weight Loss Surgery (WLS), for example, brought together multidisciplinary task groups to develop best practices in WLS. Each task group conducted a systematic review of the literature and prepared an evidence-based report. Most of evidence came from observational or experimental data.

Traditional evidence-based analysis was used to critically assess all selected studies for internal validity; the studies were then ranked according to similar levels of evidence on the basis of study design. Expert opinion—including clinical experience, the opinions of respected authorities, reports from expert committees, and consensus of the Expert Panel—was used in conjunction with RCTs or observational studies to develop recommendations (Lehman Center Weight Loss Surgery Expert Panel, 2005).

A 15-member Task Force (*Guide to Community Preventive Services*, 2005; Pappaioanou and Evans, 1998) charged with developing *The Guide to Community Preventive Services: Systematic Reviews and Evidence-based Recommendations (the Guide)* (Guide to Community Preventive Services, 2004) is using a similar approach to synthesize evidence derived primarily from observational or experimental data (Briss et al., 2000). The methodology allows for a broad range of public health interventions to be evaluated in ways that incorporate scientific rigor, as well as the feasibility and appropriateness of the evaluation (Atkins et al., 2004b).

THE ROLES OF RCTs AND OBSERVATIONAL STUDIES

For some years, the standard approach to evaluating the quality of individual studies has been based on the hierarchical grading system of research design in which RCTs receive the highest score (Table 3) (i.e., a stratification scheme that implies a trade-off between vulnerability to bias and external validity) (Hadorn et al., 1996). However, as critical appraisal techniques have matured, attention has been drawn to the limitations of this approach (Lohr and Carey, 1999), especially its focus on internal validity.

Susceptibility to bias is an important indicator of the internal validity of a study, but lack of bias does not inform about the appropriateness of a study design, its external validity, or its relevance to the research question at hand (Kroke et al., 2004). In certain instances (e.g., studies of diseases that take many years to develop or lifestyle interventions), well-designed cohort studies may provide more compelling evidence than an inadequately powered or poorly conducted RCT.

RCTs are also rarely available for lifestyle-related factors (Kroke et al., 2004) and might be inappropriate, unfeasible, or unethical to obtain. Observational studies dominate the literature (Funai et al., 2001) of preventive medicine and nutritional oncology and are primarily used to identify risk factors and prognostic indicators (Naylor and Guyatt, 1996). They have several advantages over RCTs—including lower cost, greater timeliness, and a broader range of patients (Feinstein, 1989)—but concern about inherent bias has limited their use in comparing treatments (Moses, 1995; Kunz and Oxman, 1998).

METHODOLOGY ADVANCES IN OBSERVATIONAL STUDIES

The ascendancy of RCTs was hastened by a landmark article (Sacks et al., 1982) comparing published RCTs with those that used observational designs. That review of the literature concluded that biases in patient selection may irretrievably weight the outcome of historical controlled trials in favor of new therapies (Sacks et al., 1982). Other comparative studies (Chalmers et al., 1977, 1983; Sacks et al., 1982; Colditz et al., 1989; Miller et al., 1989) drew similar conclusions about cohort studies with concurrent selection of control subjects, as well as case-control designs. On the basis of these findings, many leading experts declared that observational studies were inappropriate for use in defining evidence-based medical care.

Historical milestones developed between 1662 and 1948 (Chalmers, 2001) challenge the fundamental criticism of observational studies (i.e., that unrecognized confounding factors may lead to distorted, and therefore, misleading results) (Benson and Hartz, 2000; Chalmers, 2001; Concato, 2004; Concato and Horwitz, 2004; Sacks et al., 1982). So do more recent data. In a comparison of observational studies and RCTs in certain clinical situations, Concato et al. (2000) concluded that data from well-conducted observational studies did not appear to produce results that were biased compared with randomized trials. Benson and Hartz (2000) reported similar findings from a comparison of observational studies and RCTs.

Rigorous methodologies that mimic those used in the design of randomized clinical trials have much to do with those outcomes. A specific method to strengthen observational studies (the "restricted cohort" design) (Horwitz et al., 1990) adapts principles of RCT design for use in observational studies. It identifies a "zero time" for determining a patient's eligibility and baseline features; uses inclusion and exclusion criteria similar to those of clinical trials; adjusts for differences in baseline susceptibility to the outcome; and uses statistical methods (e.g., intention-to-treat analysis) similar to those used in RCTs (Mannucci et al., 2004).

FACTORS PROMOTING EVOLUTION IN HIERARCHIES OF EVIDENCE

The influence of dietary and nutritional exposures on the development of cancer has underscored the need to reassess criteria used to evaluate the quality of research. Cancer develops slowly, over years or decades. Consequently, single clinical trials, which rarely last >5 years, cannot address the whole span of cancer development. This does not mean that they are not an important component of the evidence base, only that they should not be seen as offering overriding evidence (Heggie et al., 2003).

During the past decade, rapid expansion in a number of pertinent scientific fields and, in particular, the amount of population-based epidemiological evidence has helped clarify the role of diet in preventing and controlling morbidity and premature mortality resulting from cancer and other noncommunicable diseases (NCDs). Some of the specific dietary components that increase the probability of occurrence of these diseases in individuals, and interventions to modify their impact, have also been identified (Report of a Joint WHO/FAO Expert Consultation, 2003).

Growing insight into the impact of diet and exercise on the risk of developing cancer has put preventive medicine at the center of efforts to reduce incidence rates. The most promising role for prevention in current medical practice may lie in changing the personal health behaviors of patients long before clinical disease develops. The importance of this aspect of clinical practice is evident from a growing literature linking some of the leading causes of death to a handful of personal health behaviors (Manson et al., 2004).

Following recommended diets, together with maintenance of physical activity and appropriate body mass, can reduce global incidence of cancer by 30–40% (World Cancer Research Fund, 1997). In the United States, excess weight and inactivity alone play such an important role in disease burden that *Healthy People 2010*, a nationwide health promotion and disease prevention agenda, lists physical inactivity and obesity as the top two health indicators, followed by tobacco use (U.S. Department of Health and Human Services, 2000).

It is surprisingly rare for the evidence to show clearly and unambiguously what course of action should be recommended for any given question (Scottish Intercollegiate Guidelines Network, 2002). Nevertheless, organizations using evidence-based methodologies to develop guidelines on clinical preventive services are finding broad agreement on a core set of services of proven effectiveness that can be recommended to primary care providers and their patients (World Cancer Research Fund, 1997; National Institutes of Health, 1998; Report of a WHO Consultation, 2000; Report of a Joint WHO/FAO Expert Consultation, 2003). Basing preventive health care decisions on the evidence for their effectiveness is an important step in the progress of disease prevention and health promotion (U.S. Preventive Services Task Force, 1996).

EVOLUTIONS IN EVIDENCE-BASED ASSESSMENTS OF RESEARCH QUALITY

Shifting clinical priorities, methodology advances that reduce potential bias in observational studies, and rapid growth in the epidemiological database are validating the credibility of hierarchies that differ from conventional models and prompting reassessments of how scientific literature is categorized and judged. Trends include reordered hierarchies of evidence and growing awareness of the need to base appraisals of quality on a wider range of study designs. Levels of evidence have been updated to incorporate the understanding that different medical areas require different sets of levels of evidence.

The developers of *The Guide to Community Preventive Services: Systematic Reviews and Evidence-based Recommendations* (*the Guide*) (Pappaioanou and Evans, 1998) are assessing the quality of study execution in detail and considering it along with study design. This approach allows a well-conducted case-control or prospective cohort study, for example, to receive greater weight than a poorly conducted RCT (Briss et al., 2000).

The Canadian Task Force on Preventive Health Care has differentiated four research categories (i.e., therapy, prevention, etiology, and harm; prognosis; diagnosis; and economic analysis) with separate levels of evidence for each of these categories (Canadian Task Force on Periodic Health Examination, 1999). The Oxford Centre for Evidence-Based Medicine has adopted five categories related to diagnosis, prognosis, and harm, with 10 separate levels of evidence for each category (Atkins et al., 2004a; Oxford Centre for Evidence-based Medicine, 2001) (Table 5).

Evolutions in the USPSTF hierarchy of evidence have led to revisions in some aspects of methodology (Atkins et al., 2001; Harris et al., 2001; Woolf and Atkins, 2001); consideration of elements of evidence beyond study design (Atkins et al., 2004a); and the use of outcomes tables to help categorize magnitude of benefits, harms, and net benefits from implementation of a preventive service (Harris et al., 2001).

SIGN's revised grading system (Table 6), introduced in 2000 (Scottish Intercollegiate Guidelines Network. Methodology Review Group, 1999; Harbour and Miller, 2001), combines study type and quality rating in the evidence level (Harbour and Miller, 2001) and allows more weight to be given to recommendations supported by good-quality observational studies where RCTs are not available for practical or ethical reasons. It also incorporates a considered judg-

TABLE 6 Revised SIGN Grading System (Harbour and Miller, 2001)

Levels of evidence	
1++	High-quality meta-analyses, systematic reviews of RCTs, or RCTs with a very low risk of bias
1+	Well-conducted meta-analyses, systematic reviews of RCTs, or RCTs with a low risk of bias
1–	Meta-analyses, systematic reviews of RCTs, or RCTs with a high risk of bias
2++	High-quality systematic reviews of case-control or cohort studies High-quality case-control or cohort studies with a very low risk of confounding, bias, or chance and a high probability that the relationship is causal
2+	Well-conducted case-control or cohort studies with a low risk of confounding, bias, or chance and a moderate probability that the relationship is causal
2–	Case-control or cohort studies with a high risk of confounding, bias, or chance and a significant risk that the relationship is not causal
3	Nonanalytical studies, e.g., case reports, case series
4	Expert opinion

Note: SIGN's revised grading system, introduced in 2000 (Scottish Intercollegiate Guidelines Network. Methodology Review Group, 1999; Harbour and Miller, 2001), combines study type and quality rating in the evidence level and allows more weight to be given to recommendations supported by good-quality observational studies when RCTs are not available (Scottish Intercollegiate Guidelines Network, 2002).

ment process that allows guideline developers to downgrade a recommendation when they perceive that the evidence is weaker than a simple evaluation of the methodology would suggest (Scottish Intercollegiate Guidelines Network, 2002).

ADAPTING TO UNCERTAINTY

Ideally, the definition of increased or decreased risk should be based on a relationship that has been established by multiple RCTs of interventions on populations that are representative of the target of a recommendation. In the absence of such evidence (Report of a Joint WHO/FAO Expert Consultation, 2003), the WHO/FAO has modified criteria used by the World Cancer Research Fund (World Cancer Research Fund, 1997) to include the results of controlled trials where relevant and available.

In addition, consistent evidence on community and environmental variables that lead to behavior changes, and thereby modify risks, has been taken into account in categorizing risks. This applies in particular to the complex interaction among environmental factors that affect excess weight gain, a risk factor recognized as contributing to many chronic diseases and cancers. The WHO/FAO uses four categories to describe strength of evidence: convincing, probable, possible, and insufficient (Table 7).

The first two categories rely on epidemiological data showing consistent associations between exposure and disease, with little or no evidence to the contrary. Available evidence is based on substantial numbers of studies, including prospective observational studies, and where relevant, RCTs of sufficient size, duration, and quality that show consistent effects. Possible evidence is based mainly on findings from case-control and cross-sectional studies, while insufficient evidence is based on the findings of a few studies that are suggestive, but insufficient to establish an association between exposure and disease.

AN EMERGING STATE OF THE ART

It has been recognized for some time that inferring causation of chronic disease requires a comprehensive view of the evidence base in a broad biological context; indeed, Bradford Hill described the need to adapt existing models to the peculiarities of observational studies in 1965. In that evidence underpinning an inference of causation is inherently more diverse than that required to demonstrate clinical efficacy, an approach identical to EBM's conventional hierarchy of study design (NHS Centre for Reviews and Dissemination, 2001) is inadequate to address the challenge of questions related to the influence of dietary and nutritional exposures on the development of cancer.

Since the 1970s, a growing number of organizations have employed various systems to grade the quality (level) of evidence and the strength of recommendations. Methods for assessing quality differ in the characteristics considered (e.g., measures of internal, external, statistical, and construct validity) and in the way these characteristics are measured (Atkins et al., 2004a). The impact of various approaches on the quality of reported study evidence (Moher et al., 1998) and on the results of meta-analyses is an area of considerable research interest (Atkins et al., 2004b; Briss et al., 2000).

In 2006, a rigorous assessment of thousands of published studies on the subject of diet and cancer is scheduled for publication by the American Institute for Cancer Research and the World Cancer Research Fund International (WCRF/AICR) (Heggie et al., 2003). That evidence-based

TABLE 7 WHO/FAO Strength of Evidence

Convincing evidence: Evidence based on epidemiological studies showing consistent associations between exposure and disease, with little or no evidence to the contrary; a substantial number of studies, including prospective observational studies, and where relevant, randomized controlled trials of sufficient size, duration, and quality showing consistent effects; and biologically plausible associations.

Probable evidence: Evidence based on epidemiological studies showing consistent associations between exposure and disease, with perceived shortcomings in the available evidence, or some evidence to the contrary that precludes a more definite judgment; usually supportive laboratory evidence; and biologically plausible associations. Shortcomings in the evidence may include insufficient duration of trials (or studies); insufficient trials (or studies) available; inadequate sample sizes; or incomplete follow-up.

Possible evidence: Evidence based mainly on findings from case-control and cross-sectional studies, with insufficient randomized controlled trials, observational studies, or nonrandomized controlled trials available; supportive evidence from nonepidemiological studies, such as clinical and laboratory investigations; and biologically plausible associations. Additional trials are required to support tentative associations.

Insufficient evidence: Evidence based on findings of a few studies that are suggestive but insufficient to establish an association between exposure and disease. Limited or no evidence is available from randomized controlled trials. More well-designed research is required to support tentative associations.

Criteria used by the World Health Organization/UN Food and Agriculture Organization (WHO/FAO) include results from controlled trials, where relevant and available. They also take into account environmental factors that effect excess weight gain, a risk factor for many cancers (Report of a Joint WHO/FAO Expert Consultation, 2003).

report will admit data from all study designs (e.g., ecological, prospective cohort, case-control, and laboratory studies); human and animal mechanistic data (*in vivo* only) will be analyzed separately, giving more weight to the human mechanistic data (Wynder et al., 1997; Zhou and Blackburn, 1997; Heggie et al., 2003).

Other leading-edge systems are also being developed for judging the quality of evidence. The latest American Diabetes Association (ADA) grading system assigns ratings of A, B, or C, depending on the quality of evidence (Table 2). Expert Opinion (E) is a separate category for recommendations when evidence from clinical trials is not yet available, clinical trials might be impractical, or there is conflicting evidence (ADA, 2006).

The system used by the Grades of Recommendation Assessment, Development and Evaluation (GRADE) Working Group (Table 8) (Atkins et al., 2004b) takes into account study design, study quality, consistency, and directness of evidence for each important outcome. For randomized trials, for example, reviewers might use criteria such as the adequacy of allocation concealment, blinding, and follow-up. Overall quality of evidence is explicitly judged across outcomes on the basis of the lowest quality of evidence for any of the critical outcomes (Atkins et al., 2004a).

Over the past 30 years, research on carcinogenesis has yielded a tremendous knowledge base (Go et al., 2004). The link between diet and cancer is now fully appreciated. Many lines of evidence show that nutrients and nonnutrients in dietary patterns (Blackburn, 2001) ("Dietary Patterns for Weight Management and Health. Proceedings of a symposium. Dallas, Texas, USA. April 27–29, 2001," 2001) have the potential to influence cancer development, but much work remains to identify the roles of diet, obesity, and physical activity in the prevention, progression, and treatment of cancer.

TABLE 8 The GRADE Working Group System for Grading the Quality of Evidence

Criteria for assigning grade of evidence

Type of evidence

Randomized trial = high

Observational study = low

Any other evidence = very low

Decrease grade if:

- Serious (−1) or very serious (−2) limitation to study quality
- Important inconsistency (−1)
- Some (−1) or major (−2) uncertainty about directness
- Imprecise or sparse data (−1)
- High probability of reporting bias (−1)

Increase grade if:

- Strong evidence of association—significant relative risk of >2 (<0.5) based on consistent evidence from two or more observational studies with no plausible confounders (+1)
- Very strong evidence of association—significant relative risk of >5 (<0.2) based on direct evidence with no major threats to validity (+2)
- Evidence of a dose–response gradient (+1)
- All plausible confounders would have reduced the effect (+1)

A leading-edge system being developed by the Grades of Recommendation Assessment, Development and Evaluation (GRADE) Working Group assesses study design, study quality, consistency, and directness of evidence for each important outcome when judging quality of evidence. For randomized trials, for example, reviewers might use criteria such as the adequacy of allocation concealment, blinding, and follow-up (Atkins et al., 2004a, 2004b).

References

Agency for Healthcare Research and Quality. 2001. Current methods of the U.S. Preventive Services Task Force: a review of the process. Available at www.ahrq.gov/clinic/ajpmsuppl/harris1.htm. Accessed February 13, 2006.

Agency for Healthcare Research and Quality. 2004. Evidence-based Practice Centers Overview. Available at www.ahrq.gov/clinic/epc/. Accessed February 16, 2006.

AHRQ. National Guidelines Clearinghouse. Available at www.guideline.gov/resources/guideline_index.aspx. Accessed February 13, 2006.

Alpha-Tocopherol and Beta Carotene Cancer Prevention Study Group. 1994. The effect of vitamin E and beta carotene on the incidence of lung cancer and other cancers in male smokers. *N Engl J Med* **330**: 1029–1035.

American Cancer Society. 2006a. "Cancer Facts & Figures 2006." Available at www.cancer.org/downloads/STT/CAFF2006PWSecured.pdf. Accessed February 13, 2006.

American Cancer Society. 2006b. "Statistics for 2006." Available at www.cancer.org/docroot/STT/stt_0.asp. Accessed February 13, 2006.

American Diabetes Association. 2005. Clinical practice recommendations 2005. *Diabetes Care* **28**(Suppl 1): S1–79.

American Diabetes Association. 2006. Standard of medical care in diabetes. Diabetes Care 29: S4–S42. Available at http://care.diabetesjournals.org/cgi/content/full/29/suppl_1/s4/T1. Accessed February 13, 2006.

Atkins, D., Best, D., Briss, P.A., Eccles, M., Falck-Ytter, Y., Flottorp, S., et al. 2004a. GRADE Working Group. Grading quality of evidence and strength of recommendations. *BMJ* **328**: 1490.

Atkins, D., Best, D., and Shapiro, E.N. 2001. The Third U.S. Preventive Services Task Force: background, methods and first recommendations. *Am J Prev Med* **20**(3 Suppl): 1–108.

Atkins, D., Eccles, M.S.F., Guyatt, G.H., Henry, D., Hill, S., et al. 2004b. The GRADE Working Group. Systems for grading the quality of evidence and the strength of recommendations I: Critical appraisal of existing approaches. The GRADE Working Group. *BMC Health Serv Res* **4**: 38.

Baillargeon, J., Pollock, B.H., Kristal, A.R., Bradshaw, P., Hernandez, J., Basler, J., Higgins, B., Lynch, S., Rozanski, T., Troyer, D., Thompson, I. 2005. The association of body mass index and prostate-specific antigen in a population-based study. *Cancer* **203**(5): 1092–1095.

Benson, K., and Hartz, A.J. 2000. A comparison of observational studies and randomized, controlled trials. *N Engl J Med* **342**: 1878–1886.

Bernard, C.I. 1966. "Introduction a la Medecine Experimentale." Garnier-Flammarion, Paris.

Bero, L., and Rennie, D. 1995. The Cochrane Collaboration: preparing, maintaining, and disseminating systematic reviews of the effects of health care. *JAMA* **24**: 1935–1938.

Bingham, S.A., Day, N.E., Luben, R., Ferrari, P., Slimani, N., Norat, T., et al. 2003. Dietary fibre in food and protection against colorectal cancer in the European Prospective Investigation into Cancer and Nutrition (EPIC): an observational study. *Lancet* **1**: 1496–1501.

Blackburn, G.L. 2001. Treatment approaches: food first for weight management and health. *Obes Res* **9**(Suppl 4): 223S–227S.

Blackburn, G.L., Hu, F.B., and Harvey, A.M. 2005. Evidence-based recommendations for best practices in weight loss surgery. *Obes Res* **13**: 203–204.

Blue Cross Blue Shield Association. Technology Evaluation Center. Special Report: The Relationship between Weight Loss and Changes in Morbidity Following Bariatric Surgery for Morbid Obesity. Assessment Program, Vol. 18. 2003. Available at www.bcbs.com/tec/vol18/18_09.html. Accessed February 13, 2006.

Bradford Hill, A. 1965. The environment and disease: association or causation? *Proc R Soc Med* **58**: 295–300.

Briss, P.A., Zaza, S., Pappaioanou, M., Fielding, J., Wright-De Aguero, L., Truman, B.I., et al. 2000. Developing an evidence-based Guide to Community Preventive Services—methods. The Task Force on Community Preventive Services. *Am J Prev Med* **18**(1 Suppl): 35–43.

Buzdar, A.U. 2006. Dietary modification and risk of breast cancer. *JAMA* **295**: 691–692.

Calle, E.E., Rodriguez, C., Walker-Thurmond, K., and Thun, M.J. 2003. Overweight, obesity, and mortality from cancer in a prospectively studied cohort of U.S. adults. *N Engl J Med* **348**: 1625–1638.

Canadian Task Force on Periodic Health Examination. 1999. Levels of evidence and grades of recommendations: Canadian Task Force on Periodic Health Examination.

Canadian Task Force on the Periodic Health Examination. 1979. The periodic health examination. *Can Med Assoc J* **121**: 1193–1254.

Canadian Task Force on the Periodic Health Examination. 1994. "The Canadian Guide to Clinical Preventive Care." Minister of Supply and Services Canada, Ottowa.

Centre for Evidence-based Medicine. Oxford-Centre for Evidence-based Medicine. 2001. Levels of evidence and grades of recommendation. Available at www.cebm.net/levels_of_evidence.asp. Accessed February 13, 2006.

Chalmers, I. 2001. Comparing like with like: some historical milestones in the evolution of methods to create unbiased comparison groups in therapeutic experiments. *Int J Epidemiol* **30**: 1156–1164.

Chalmers, T.C., Celano, P., Sacks, H.S., and Smith, H.J. 1983. Bias in treatment assignment in controlled clinical trials. *N Engl J Med* **309**: 1358–1361.

Chalmers, T.C., Matta, R.J., Smith, H.J., and Kunzler, A.M. 1977. Evidence favoring the use of anticoagulants in the hospital phase of acute myocardial infarction. *N Engl J Med* **297**: 1091–1096.

Chao, A., Thun, M.J., Connell, C.J., McCullough, M.L., Jacobs, E.J., Flanders, W.D., et al. (2005). Meat consumption and risk of colorectal cancer. *JAMA* **293**: 172–182.

Chlebowski, R.T., Blackburn, G.L., Elashoff, R.E., Thomsom, C., and Goodman, M.T. 2005. Dietary fat reduction in postmenopausal women with primary breast cancer: Phase III Women's Intervention Nutrition Study (WINS) [abstract]. *Proc Am Soc Clin Oncol* **23**(16S): 3S Abstract 10.

Chlebowski, R.T., Pettinger, M., Stefanick, M.L., Howard, B.V., Mossavar-Rahmani, Y., and McTiernan, A. 2004. Insulin, physical activity, and caloric intake in postmenopausal women: breast cancer implications. *J Clin Oncol* **22**: 4507–4513.

Claxton, K., and Thompson, K.M. 2001. A dynamic programming approach to the efficient design of clinical trials. *J Health Econ* **20**: 797–882.

Cochrane Library. Available at www.cochrane.org/index0.htm. Accessed February 13, 2006.

Colditz, G.A., Miller, J.N., and Mosteller, F. 1989. How study design affects outcomes in comparisons of therapy. I: Medical. *Stat Med* **8**: 441–454.

Concato, J. 2004. Observational versus experimental studies: what's the evidence for a hierarchy? *NeuroRx* **1**: 341–347.

Concato, J., and Horwitz, R.I. 2004. Beyond randomised versus observational studies. *Lancet* **363**: 1660–1661.

Concato, J., Shah, N., and Horwitz, R.I. 2000. Randomized, controlled trials, observational studies, and the hierarchy of research designs. *N Engl J Med* **342**: 1887–1892.

De Luca, L.M., and Ross, S.A. 1996. Beta-carotene increases lung cancer incidence in cigarette smokers. *Nutr Rev* **54**: 178–180.

Department of Health and Human Services (HHS) and the Department of Agriculture (USDA). 2005. Dietary Guidelines for Americans 2005. Available at www.healthierus.gov/dietaryguidelines/. Accessed February 12, 2006.

Dickersin, K., Manheimer, E., Wieland, S., Robinson, K.A., Lefebvre, C., and McDonald, S. 2002. Development of the Cochrane Collaboration's CENTRAL Register of controlled clinical trials. *Eval Health Prof* **25**: 38–64.

Dietary Patterns for Weight Management and Health. Proceedings of a symposium. Dallas, Texas, USA. April 27–29, 2001. 2001. *Obes Res* **9**(Suppl 4): 217S–358S.

Doll, R., and Hill, A.B. 1950. Smoking and carcinoma of the lung. Preliminary report. *Br Med J* **2**: 739–748.

Doll, R., and Hill, A.B. 1954. The mortality of doctors in relation to their smoking habits. *Br Med J* **1**: 1451–1455.

Doll, R., and Peto, R. 1981. The causes of cancer: quantitative estimates of avoidable risks of cancer in the United States today. *J Natl Cancer Inst* **66**: 1191–1308.

Doll, R., and Peto, R. 1996. Epidemiology of cancer. *In* "Oxford Textbook of Medicine" (D.J. Weatherall, J.G.G. Ledingham, and D.A. Warrell, eds), pp. 197–221. Oxford University Press, Oxford.

Evidence-based Practice Centers Overview. 2004. Available at www.ahrq.gov/clinic/epc. Accessed February 13, 2006.

Feinstein, A.R. 1985. "Clinical Epidemiology: The Architecture of Clinical Research." WB Saunders Co, Philadelphia.

Feinstein, A.R. 1989. Epidemiologic analyses of causation: the unlearned scientific lessons of randomized trials. *J Clin Epidemiol* **42**: 481–489.

Funai, E.F., Rosenbush, E.J., Lee, M.J., and Del Priore, G. 2001. Distribution of study designs in four major US journals of obstetrics and gynecology. *Gynecol Obstet Invest* **51**: 8–11.

Furberg, A.S., Jasienska, G., Bjurstam, N., Torjesen, P.A., Emaus, A., Lipson, S.F., et al. 2005. Metabolic and hormonal profiles: HDL cholesterol as a plausible biomarker of breast cancer risk. The Norwegian EBBA Study. *Cancer Epidemiol Biomarkers Prev* **14**: 33–40.

Go, V.L., Wong, D.A., Wang, Y., Butrum, R.R., Norman, H.A., and Wilkerson, L. 2004. Diet and cancer prevention: evidence-based medicine to genomic medicine. *J Nutr* **134**(12 Suppl): 3513S–3516S.

Grimes, D.A., and Schulz, K.F. 2002. An overview of clinical research: the lay of the land. *Lancet* **359**: 57–61.

Guide to Community Preventive Services. 2004. Available at www.thecommunityguide.org/. Accessed February 13, 2006.

Guide to Community Preventive Services. About Us. July 2005. Available at www.thecommunityguide.org/about/default.htm. Accessed February 13, 2006.

Guyatt, G.H., Haynes, R.B., Jaeschke, R.Z., Cook, D.J., Green, L., Naylor, C.D., et al. 2000. Users' Guides to the Medical Literature: XXV. Evidence-based medicine: principles for applying the Users' Guides to patient care. Evidence-Based Medicine Working Group. *JAMA* **284**: 1290–1296.

Hadorn, D.C., Baker, D., Hodges, J.S., and Hicks, N. 1996. Rating the quality of evidence for clinical practice guidelines. *J Clin Epidemiol* **49**: 749–754.

Harbour, R., and Miller, J.N. 2001. A new system for grading recommendations in evidence-based guidelines. *BMJ* **323**: 334–336.

Harris, R.P., Helfand, M., Woolf, S.H., Lohr, K.N., Mulrow, C.D., Teutsch, S.M., et al. 2001. Methods Work Group, Third U.S. Preventive Services Task Force. Current methods of the U.S. Preventive Services Task Force: a review of the process. *Am J Prev Med* **20**: 21–35.

Haynes, R.B. 2002. What kind of evidence is it that Evidence-Based Medicine advocates want health care providers and consumers to pay attention to? *BMC Health Services Res* **2**: 3.

Heggie, S.J., Wiseman, M.J., Cannon, G.J., Miles, L.M., Thompson, R.L., Stone, E.M., et al. 2003. Defining the state of knowledge with respect to food, nutrition, physical activity, and the prevention of cancer. *J Nutr* **133**: 3837S–3842S.

Hennekens, C.H., and Buring, J.E. 1987. "Epidemiology in Medicine." Little, Brown and Company, Boston.

Hill, A.B. 1937. "Principles of Medical Statistics," Vol. 3. The Lancet, London.

Horwitz, R.I., Viscoli, C.M., Clemens, J.D., and Sadock, R.T. 1990. Developing improved observational methods for evaluating therapeutic effectiveness. *Am J Med* **89**: 630–638.

Hulley, S.B., Cummings, S.R., Browner, W.S., Grady, D., Hearst, N., and Newman, R.D., eds. 2001. "Designing Clinical Research: An Epidemiologic Approach," 2nd edition. Lippincott Williams & Wilkins, Baltimore.

International Agency for Research on Cancer. 2006. Available at www.iarc.fr/. Accessed February 13, 2006.

International Agency for Research on Cancer/World Health Organization. 2005. Vegetables and fruits do not protect against breast cancer. Available at www.iarc.fr/ENG/Press_Releases/pr157a.html. Accessed February 13, 2006.

Kelsey, J.L., Whittemore, A.S., Evans, A.S., and Thompson, W.D. 1996. "Methods in Observational Epidemiology," 2nd edition. Oxford University Press, New York.

Kroke, A., Boeing, H., Rossnagel, K., and Willich, S.N. 2004. History of the concept of "levels of evidence" and their current status in relation to primary prevention through lifestyle interventions. *Public Health Nutr* **7**: 279–284.

Kunz, R., and Oxman, A.D. 1998. The unpredictability paradox: review of empirical comparisons of randomised and non-randomised clinical trials. *BMJ* **317**(7167): 1185–1190.

Last, J.M., ed. 1988. "A Dictionary of Epidemiology," 2nd edition. Oxford University Press, New York.

Lawlor, D.A., Smith, G.D., and Ebrahim, S. 2004. Hyperinsulinaemia and increased risk of breast cancer: findings from the British Women's Heart and Health Study. *Cancer Causes Control* **15**: 267–275.

Lehman Center Weight Loss Surgery Expert Panel. 2005. Commonwealth of Massachusetts. Betsy Lehman Center for Patient Safety and Medical Error Reduction. Expert Panel on Weight Loss Surgery: executive report. *Obes Res* **13**(2): 205–226.

Levine, M., Moutquin, J., Walton, R., and Feightner, J. 2001. Chemoprevention of breast cancer. A joint guideline from the Canadian Task Force on Preventive Health Care and the Canadian Breast Cancer Initiative's Steering Committee on Clinical Practice Guidelines for the Treatment of Breast Cancer. *CMAJ* **164**(12): 1681–1690.

Lewis, T. 1945. "Research in Medicine and Other Addresses," 2nd edition. Lewis and Co, London.

Lilienfeld, A.M., and Lilienfeld, D.E. 1980. "Foundations of Epidemiology," 2nd edition. Oxford University Press, New York.

Lohr, K.N., and Carey, T.S. 1999. Assessing "best evidence": issues in grading the quality of studies for systematic reviews. *Jt Comm J Qual Improv* **25**(9): 470–479.

Malin, A., Dai, Q., Yu, H., Shu, X.O., Jin, F., Gao, Y.T., et al. 2004. Evaluation of the synergistic effect of insulin resistance and insulin-like growth factors on the risk of breast carcinoma. *Cancer Causes Control* **100**: 694–700.

Mallett, S., and Clarke, M. 2003. EBM notebook. *EBM* **8**: 100–101.

Mannucci, E., Monami, M., Masotti, G., and Marchionni, N. 2004. All-cause mortality in diabetic patients treated with combinations of sulfonylureas and biguanides. *Diabetes Metab Res Rev* **20**: 44–47.

Manson, J.E., Skerrett, P.J., Greenland, P., and VanItallie, T.B. 2004. The escalating pandemics of obesity and sedentary lifestyle: a call to action for clinicians. *Arch Intern Med* **164**: 249–258.

McCullough, M.L., and Giovannucci, E.L. 2004. Diet and cancer prevention. *Oncogene* **23**: 6349–6364.

Medical Research Council Streptomycin in Tuberculosis Trials Committee. 1948. Streptomycin treatment for pulmonary tuberculosis. *BMJ* **ii**: 769–782.

Miller, A.B., Altenburg, H.P., Bueno-de-Mesquita, B., Boshuizen, H.C., Agudo, A., Berrino, F., et al. 2004. Fruits and vegetables and lung cancer: Findings from the European Prospective Investigation into Cancer and Nutrition. *Int J Cancer* **108**: 269–276.

Miller, J.N., Colditz, G.A., and Mosteller, F. 1989. How study design affects outcomes in comparisons of therapy. II: Surgical. *Stat Med* **8**: 455–466.

Moher, D., Pham, B., Jones, A., Cook, D.J., Jadad, A.R., Moher, M., et al. 1998. Does quality of reports of randomised trials affect estimates of intervention efficacy reported in meta-analyses? *Lancet* **352**: 609–613.

Morris, C.D., and Carson, S. 2003. Routine vitamin supplementation to prevent cardiovascular disease: a summary of the evidence for the U.S. Preventive Services Task Force. *Ann Intern Med* **139**: 56–70.

Moses, L.E. 1995. Measuring effects without randomized trials? Options, problems, challenges. *Med Care* **33**: AS8–14.

Mulrow, C.D., Cook, D.J., and Davidoff, F. 1997. Systematic reviews: critical links in the great chain of evidence. *Ann Intern Med* **126**: 389–391.

Muti, P., Quattrin, T., Grant, B.J., Krogh, V., Micheli, A., Schunemann, H.J., et al. 2002. Fasting glucose is a risk factor for breast cancer: a prospective study. *Cancer Epidemiol Biomarkers Prev* **11**: 1361–1368.

National Institutes of Health. 1998. "Clinical Guidelines on the Identification, Evaluation, and Treatment of Overweight and Obesity in Adults. The Evidence Report (No. 98-4083)." Washington, DC: National Institutes of Health. National Heart, Lung, and Blood Institute.

Naylor, C.D., and Guyatt, G.H. 1996. Users' guides to the medical literature. X. How to use an article reporting variations in the outcomes of health services. The Evidence-Based Medicine Working Group. *JAMA* **275**: 554–558.

NHS Centre for Reviews and Dissemination. 2001. "CRD Report Number 4: Undertaking Systematic Reviews of Research on Effectiveness. CRD's Guidance for Those Carrying Out or Commissioning Reviews," 2nd edition. University of York, United Kingdom.

Oxford Centre for Evidence-based Medicine. 2001. Oxford Centre for Evidence-based Medicine Levels of Evidence. Available from www.musckids.com/~annibald/ebm/oxford_levels_of_evidence.pdf. Accessed February 13, 2006.

Pappaioanou, M., and Evans, C.J. 1998. Development of the Guide to Community Preventive Services: a U.S. Public Health Service initiative. *J Public Health Manag Pract* **4**: 48–54.

Peters, U., Sinha, R., Chatterjee, N., Subar, A.F., Ziegler, R.G., Kulldorff, M., et al. 2003. Dietary fibre and colorectal adenoma in a colorectal cancer early detection programm. *Lancet* **361**: 1491–1495.

Prentice R.L., Caan B., Chlebowski R.T., Patterson R., Kuller L.H., Ockene J.K., et al. 2006. Low-fat dietary pattern and risk of invasive breast cancer: the Women's Health Initiative randomized controlled Dietary Modification. *JAMA* **295**: 629–642.

Report of a Joint WHO/FAO Expert Consultation. 2003. Diet, Nutrition and the Prevention of Chronic Diseases. WHO Technical Report Series No. 916. World Health Organization, Geneva.

Report of a WHO Consultation. 2000. Obesity: Preventing and Managing the Global Epidemic. WHO Technical Report Series 894. World Health Organization, Geneva.

Roberts, C.K., and Barnard, R.J. 2005. Effects of exercise and diet on chronic disease. *J Appl Physiol* **98**: 3–30.

Rom, W.N. 1992. "Environmental and Occupational Medicine," 2nd edition. Little, Brown and Company, Boston.

Rothman, K.J. 1986. "Modern epidemiology." Little, Brown and Company, Boston.

Sacks, H., Chalmers, T.C., and Smith, H.J. 1982. Randomized versus historical controls for clinical trials. *Am J Med* **72**: 233–240.

Sanchez-Castillo, C.P., Pichardo-Ontiveros, E., and Lopez-R, P. 2004. The epidemiology of obesity. *Gac Med Mex* **140**(Suppl 2): S3–S20.

Schatzkin, A., and Kipnis, V. 2004. Could exposure assessment problems give us wrong answers to nutrition and cancer questions? *J Natl Cancer Inst* **96**: 1564–1565.

Schulz, K.F., Chalmers, I., Grimes, D.A., and Altman, D.G. 1994. Assessing the quality of randomization from reports of controlled trials published in obstetrics and gynecology journals. *JAMA* **272**: 125–128.

Scottish Intercollegiate Guidelines Network. 2002, April. SIGN 50: A guideline developer's handbook. Section 6. Available at www.sign.ac.uk/guidelines/fulltext/50/index.html. Accessed February 13, 2006.

Scottish Intercollegiate Guidelines Network. Methodology Review Group. 1999. "Report on the Review of the Method of Grading Guideline Recommendations." SIGN, Edinburgh.

Steinmetz, K.A., and Potter, J.D. 1996. Vegetables, fruit, and cancer prevention: a review. *J Am Diet Assoc* **96**(10): 1027–1039.

Stewart, B.W., and Kleihues, P. 2003. World Cancer Report. Available at www.iarc.fr/WCR/index.html. Accessed February 13, 2006.

The Cochrane Central Register of Controlled Trials (CENTRAL). 2003. "The Cochrane Library," Issue 2, Vol. 2005. Update Software Ltd, Oxford.

The University of Sheffield. An appraisal of Evidence Based Health Care. The impact of Evidence Based Health Care. Available at www.shef.ac.uk/scharr/ir/mschi/unit12/4impact.htm. Accessed February 13, 2006.

Timmermans, S., and Mauck, A. 2005. The promises and pitfalls of evidence-based medicine. *Health Aff (Millwood)* **24**: 18–28.

U.S. Department of Health and Human Services. 2000. "Healthy People 2010: Understanding and Improving Health," 2nd edition. US Government Printing Office, Washington, DC.

U.S. Preventive Services Task Force. 1989. "Guide to Clinical Preventive Services: An Assessment of the Effectiveness of 169 Interventions." Williams and Wilkins, Baltimore.

U.S. Preventive Services Task Force. 1996. "Guide to Clinical Preventive Services," 2nd edition. Williams & Wilkins, Baltimore.

van Gils, C.H., Peeters, P.H., Bueno-de-Mesquita, H.B., Boshuizen, H.C., Lahmann, P.H., Clavel-Chapelon, F., et al. 2005. Consumption of vegetables and fruits and risk of breast cancer. *JAMA* **293**: 183–193.

Winters, B.L., Mitchell, D.C., Smiciklas-Wright, H., Grosvenor, M.B., Liu, W., and Blackburn, G.L. 2004. Dietary patterns in women treated for breast cancer who successfully reduce fat intake: the Women's Intervention Nutrition Study (WINS). *J Am Diet Assoc* **104**: 551–559.

Woolf, S.H. 1990. Practice guidelines: a new reality in medicine. I. Recent developments. *Arch Intern Med* **150**: 1811–1818.

Woolf, S.H., and Atkins, D. 2001. The evolving role of prevention in health care: contributions of the U.S. Preventive Services Task Force. *Am J Prev Med* **20**(3 Suppl): 13–20.

World Cancer Research Fund. 1997. "Food, Nutrition and the Prevention of Cancer: A Global Perspective." American Institute for Cancer Research, Washington, DC.

World Cancer Research Fund and American Institute for Cancer Research. 1997. "Expert Panel Report Summary—Food Nutrition and the Prevention of Cancer: A Global Perspective." American Institute for Cancer Research, Washington, DC.

World Health Organization. Global strategy on diet, physical activity and health. Cancer: diet and physical activity's impact. Available at www.who.int/dietphysical_activity/publications/facts/cancer/en/. Accessed February 13, 2006.

World Health Organization. 2004. Fifty-seventh World Health Assembly. Global strategy on diet, physical activity and health. Available at http://www.who.int/gb/ebwha/pdf_files/WHA57/A57_R17-en.pdf. Accessed February 13, 2006.

Wynder, E.L., Cohen, L.A., Muscat, J.E., Winters, B., Dwyer, J.T., and Blackburn, G.L. 1997. Breast cancer: weighing the evidence for a promoting role of dietary fat. *J Natl Cancer Inst* **89**: 766–775.

Wynder, E.L., and Graham, E.A. 1950. Tobacco smoking as a possible etiological factor in bronchiogenic carcinoma. A study of six hundred and eighty-four proved cases. *JAMA* **143**: 855–874.

Zhou, J.R., and Blackburn, G.L. 1997. Bridging animal and human studies: what are the missing segments in dietary fat and prostate cancer? *Am J Clin Nutr* **66**: 1572S–1580S.

APPENDIX

Glossary of Terms in Evidence-based Medicine (The University of Sheffield)

Absolute risk reduction (ARR) is the difference in the event rate between control group (CER) and treated group (EER): ARR = CER – EER.

Case-Control Study involves identifying patients who have the outcome of interest (cases) and control patients without the same outcome, and looking back to see whether they had the exposure of interest.

Case series is a report on a series of patients with an outcome of interest. No control group is involved.

Control event rate (CER): see *Event Rate*.

Clinical practice guideline is a systematically developed statement designed to assist practitioner and patient to make decisions about appropriate health care for specific clinical circumstances.

Cohort study involves identification of two groups (cohorts) of patients: one that did receive the exposure of interest and one that did not, and following these cohorts forward for the outcome of interest.

Cost-benefit analysis converts effects into the same monetary terms as the costs and compares them.

Cost-effectiveness analysis converts effects into health terms and describes the costs for some additional health gain (e.g., cost per additional MI prevented).

Cost-utility analysis converts effects into personal preferences (or utilities) and describes how much it costs for some additional quality gain (e.g., cost per additional quality-adjusted life-year, or QALY).

Crossover study design is the administration of two or more experimental therapies one after the other in a specified or random order to the same group of patients.

Cross-sectional study is the observation of a defined population at a single point in time or time interval. Exposure and outcome are determined simultaneously. See also glossary of study designs.

Decision analysis is the application of explicit, quantitative methods to analyze decisions under conditions of uncertainty.

Ecological survey: based on aggregated data for some population as it exists at some point or points in time; to investigate the relationship of an exposure to a known or presumed risk factor for a specified outcome.

Experimental event rate (EER): see *Event Rate*.

Event rate is the proportion of patients in a group in whom the event is observed. Thus, if out of 100 patients, the event is observed in 27, the event rate is 0.27. CER and EER are used to refer to this in control and experimental groups of patients, respectively.

Evidence-based health care extends the application of the principles of evidence-based medicine (see below) to all professions associated with health care, including purchasing and management.

Evidence-based medicine is the conscientious, explicit, and judicious use of current best evidence in making decisions about the care of individual patients. The practice of evidence-based medicine means integrating individual clinical expertise with the best available external clinical evidence from systematic research.

Likelihood ratio is the likelihood of a given test result in a patient with the target disorder compared with the likelihood of the same result in a patient without that disorder.

Meta-analysis is an overview that uses quantitative methods to summarize the results.

N-of-1 trials The patient undergoes pairs of treatment periods organized so that one period involves the use of the experimental treatment and one period involves the use of an alternative or placebo therapy. The patients and physician are blinded, if possible, and outcomes are monitored. Treatment periods are replicated until the clinician and patient are convinced that the treatments are definitely different or definitely not different.

Negative predictive value (–PV) is the proportion of people with a negative test result who are free of disease. See also *SpPins and SnNouts*.

Number needed to treat (NNT) is the number of patients who need to be treated to prevent one bad outcome. It is the inverse of the ARR:

$$NNT = 1/ARR$$

Odds are a ratio of events to nonevents, for example, if the event rate for a disease is 0.2 (20%), its nonevent rate is 0.8 (80%), and its odds are 0.2/0.8 = 0.25 (see also *Odds Ratio*).

Odds ratio is the odds of an experimental patient suffering an event relative to the odds of a control patient.

Overview is a systematic review and summary of the medical literature.

Positive predictive value (+PV) is the proportion of people with a positive test result who have disease. Also called the post-test probability of disease after a positive test. See also *SpPins and SnNouts*.

Randomized controlled clinical trial is when a group of patients are randomized into an experimental group and a control group. These groups are followed up for the variables/outcomes of interest.

Relative risk reduction (RRR) is the percent reduction in events in the treated group event rate (EER) compared with the control group event rate (CER):

$$RRR = (CER - EER)/CER \times 100$$

Risk ratio is the ratio of risk in the treated group (EER) to the risk in the control group (CER): RR = EER/CER. RR is used in randomized trials and cohort studies.

Sensitivity is the proportion of people with disease who have a positive test. See also *SpPins and SnNouts*.

SnNout: when a sign/test has a high sensitivity, a negative result rules out the diagnosis; for example, the sensitivity of a history of ankle swelling for diagnosing ascites is 92%; therefore, if a person does not have a history of ankle swelling, it is highly unlikely that the person has ascites.

Specificity is the proportion of people free of a disease who have a negative test result. See also *SpPins and SnNouts*.

SpPin: when a sign/test has a high specificity, a positive result rules in the diagnosis; for example, the specificity of fluid wave for diagnosing ascites is 92%. Therefore, if a person has a fluid wave, it is highly likely that the person has ascites.

CHAPTER

47

Dietary Guidelines in Cancer Prevention

JOHANNA DWYER

INTRODUCTION: HISTORY OF NUTRITION GUIDELINES IN PUBLIC HEALTH

Nutritional recommendations consisting of guidelines, eating plans, and icons have been issued by public health authorities in the United States for more than a hundred years. The recommendations have been driven largely by nutrition-related concerns. However, broader problems in society and the state of the science are also influential. Early dietary guidance issued in the first part of the twentieth century by the federal government emphasized avoiding deficiency, a foundation or "core" diet, and getting enough to eat and enough of the essential nutrients. It gradually shifted and by mid-century paid more attention to balance, variety and moderation, and avoidance of excess, especially caloric excess. By the dawn of the twenty-first century, these notions pervaded most official federal guidance for energy, as well as all of the micronutrients and macronutrients. The highlights of each era are described in the following subsections.

1900–World War I: Emphasis on Sufficiency and Food Costs

In the United States, national dietary goals and recommendations began with advice issued by the President's Home Commission in the Theodore Roosevelt administration (Haughton et al., 1987; Hogbin et al., 2003). The early nutritional recommendations were guides to healthful eating for those on various food budgets. They were qualitative rather than quantitative and stressed what to eat, rather than why or how much of various foods to eat. During World War I, the "Basic 5" eating guide was developed. It focused on conserving food for the war effort, getting enough to eat, and variety. The Basic 5 included fish (which conserved more grain than beef and other animal flesh foods), starchy foods, "watery" fruits, vegetables, and sweets.

Incorporating Newer Knowledge of Nutrition: 1920s

During the 1920s, the number of nutrients known to be essential expanded to include many new vitamins and minerals. The concept of a "foundation diet" of basic or staple foods needed to ensure nutrient adequacy became popular. Dietary guidelines included admonitions to eat more of the "healthy" or "protective" foods high in specific nutrients (often called *protective factors* because their chemical structure was frequently still unknown) and in nutrient density, such as meats, milk and other animal protein foods, leafy green vegetables, and citrus fruits.

1930s Great Depression and Getting Enough

The Great Depression of the 1930s brought poverty and hunger to many and the need for economy to all. Dietary recommendations stressed economy and conservation of food. Federal nutritionists published menus that met all minimal nutritional needs as they were then known. Several versions of menus were developed for consumers on different food budgets. Since some nutrients had not yet been discovered and for other nutrients the levels needed for health were unknown, the adequacy of the recommendations for all nutrients was difficult to determine.

Copyright © 2006, Elsevier Inc.
All rights of reproduction in any form reserved.

World War II: Recommended Allowances, the Basic 7 Graphic, and Conserving Food for the War Effort

In 1941, just prior to America's entry into World War II, the first edition of the Recommended Dietary Allowances (RDAs) was issued under the auspices of the National Academy of Sciences. The goal was to ensure the health of the population. The concept of adequacy of "protective" nutrients such as protein, vitamins, and mineral elements could now be more fully operationalized in recommendations for choices from food groups that were rich in them because most of the essential nutrients were known. The RDAs were accompanied by menus illustrating how the nutrient recommendations could be put to use. Also, to aid in communication, the "Basic 7" food guide icon was developed and named for the seven groups it recommended (citrus and other fruits, green leafy, deep green vegetables, dark yellow vegetables, milk and milk products, meat and meat substitutes, cereals and grains, and butter and margarine). It was widely popularized.

World War II also brought increased attention to conservation of the food supply and to keeping the population healthy for the war effort during the period of food rationing. Nutritional guidance incorporated information on choices among available foods that would meet nutrient needs in a responsible manner from the standpoint of the war effort.

1950 Cold War, Abundance, the Baby Boom, and the Basic 4

In the postwar period, food supplies became more abundant and dietary guidance was altered to encourage liberal food consumption. In an effort to simplify food guidance and to focus only on the foundation diet needed to ensure adequacy of nutrients other than calories, the fruits and vegetables were combined into a single group and the butter-margarine group was omitted because it was not needed in a guide that focused only on the "basics" or groups that were essential for obtaining required nutrients. Sufficiency in calories could be achieved by simply eating whatever other foods were desired.

From the 1950s until 1977, the Basic 4 food groups constituted the major federal guidance about eating patterns. The Basic 4 foundation diet consisted of grains, vegetables and fruit, milk and milk products, and meat and meat substitutes. The Basic 4 targeted only nutrient adequacy, stressed choices from all of the food groups, emphasizing micronutrient dense foods in amounts up to ~1200 kcal, and provided at least 80% of eight key nutrients (Davis and Saltos, 1995).

1970s Growing Concerns about Overconsumption and the "Basic 5"

During the mid-1970s public health concerns about overconsumption and obesity increased, and a fifth "optional" food group was added to the U.S. Department of Agriculture's (USDA) Basic 4 food guide. The new Basic 5 guide was designed to call attention to the need for moderation and avoidance of obesity. The addition of an "extraneous" or low nutrient density/high calorie group was viewed as realistic by some and unfortunate by others.

1970s: Dietary Goals for the United States and Dietary Guidelines for Americans: Emphasis on Balance and Moderation

In the 1960s and 1970s the associations between diet and coronary artery disease and other chronic degenerative diseases such as alcoholic liver disease became clearer. In 1977, the role of diet in chronic degenerative disease was examined in a series of oversight hearings by the U.S. Senate Select Committee on Nutrition and Human Needs. The committee issued a staff report entitled "Dietary Goals for the United States" that provided national and individual targets for consumption. There was much dissent and discussion in Congress and in the nutrition science community about the dietary goals document and its recommendations (Dwyer, 1983). In order to evaluate the evidence for the diet–disease links, an expert group was assembled by the American Society for Clinical Nutrition (ASCN). It issued a set of recommendations that supported many but not all of those proposed in the Senate Select Committee report (Report of the Task Force, 1979). At the same time, the Surgeon General of the United States commissioned the National Academy of Sciences to develop recommendations for expanding national plans for preventive services that included nutrition. These had been formulated in a document called "Promoting Health, Preventing Disease: Objectives for the Nation" in the Ford administration. The report, entitled "Healthy People," was published in 1977 by the then Department of Health Education and Welfare (now the Department of Health and Human Services) (Surgeon General, 1977). In 1980, the USDA and the U.S. Department of Health, Education and Welfare issued the first edition of the *Dietary Guidelines for Americans*, which reflected the recommendations provided by ASCN (U.S. Department of Health and Human Services/USDA, 1980). The ASCN recommendations provided qualitative goals, rather than the quantitative Dietary Goals recommendations of the Senate Select Committee because experts believed the evidence was not yet sufficient for quantitative guidelines. Similar qualitative guidelines were incorporated into the first edition of "Healthy People," which were recommendations from the National Academy of Sciences to the Department of Health,

TABLE 1 Changes in the Dietary Guidelines for Americans 1980–2000

Guideline	Changes
Variety	"Eat a variety of foods" remained until 2000 when it was changed to "Let the pyramid guide your food choices"
Weight	"Maintain a desirable weight" in 1980 changed to "Maintain a healthy weight" in 1990, and in 1995 to "Balance the food you eat with physical activity to maintain and improve your weight." In 2000 it was changed to "Aim for a healthy weight."
Physical activity	Added as "Be physically active each day," in 2000
Fat	The 1980 and 1985, "Avoid too much fat, saturated fat and cholesterol," guides changed to, "Choose a diet low in fat, saturated fat and cholesterol," for 1990 and 1995. By 2000 it had changed to, "Choose a diet low in saturated fat and cholesterol and moderate in fat."
Starch and fiber	In 1980 and 1985 the guideline was "Eat foods with adequate starch and fiber."
Sugars	The 1980 and 1985 guideline, "Avoid too much sugar," changed in 1990 to "Use sugar only in moderation." In 1995 this changed again to "Choose a diet moderate in sugar," and in 2000 it became "Choose beverages and foods to moderate your intake of sugars."
Vegetables, fruits, and grains	No guideline was included until 1990, when "Choose a diet with plenty of vegetables, fruits, and grain products" was introduced. In 1995 it changed to "Choose a diet with plenty of grains, vegetables, and fruits," and in 2000 it became "Choose a variety of fruits and vegetables daily."
Grains	None until 2000, "Choose a variety of grains, including whole grains."
Sodium	The 1980 and 1985 guideline was "Avoid too much sodium." In 1990 it became "Use salt and sodium only in moderation." In 1995 it changed to "Choose a diet moderate in salt and sodium," and in 2000 to "Choose and prepare foods with less salt."
Alcohol	"If you drink alcohol, do so in moderation" has remained the same from 1980 to 2000.
Food safety	Only in 2000 was the guideline "Keep foods safe to eat" added.

Education and Welfare on dietary and other objectives for promoting health and preventing disease in the United States (Surgeon General, 1977). The recommendations emphasized not only achieving nutritional adequacy but balance, variety and moderation, and directions rather than absolute amounts for macronutrients like fat, saturated fat, sugar, sodium, and cholesterol where data were less secure.

The *Dietary Guidelines for Americans* reports appeared first in 1980 and have been issued approximately every 5 years since 1980 (U.S. Department of Health and Human Services/USDA, 1980, 1985, 1990, 1995, 2000, and 2005). Table 1 summarizes them from 1980 to 2000.

1980s: Growing Acceptance of the New Diet–Chronic Disease Risk Paradigm

Following the publication of the *Dietary Guidelines*, many other groups issued guidelines. During the 1970s and 1980s, there was a good deal of contention about the proliferation and validity of various dietary recommendations to reduce each chronic degenerative disease risk. However, over time, the utility of dietary guidelines that were appropriate for the reduction in risk of many different chronic degenerative diseases at the same time gained support. This culminated in publication of the *National Academy of Sciences on Diet and Health* in 1989 (Committee on Diet and Health, 1989). It strongly endorsed the concepts of balance, variety and moderation, and physical activity. This report, issued by the Committee on Diet and Health of the National Research Council, National Academy of Sciences, was a comprehensive study on diet, health, and chronic disease risk that reified the importance of addressing the diet–disease relationships already discussed in the *Dietary Guidelines*. It provided its own dietary recommendations that were similar to the *Dietary Guidelines* but more quantitative (Committee on Diet and Health, 1989). An accompanying report summarized recommendations for implementing the guidelines (Committee on Dietary Guidelines Implementation, 1990).

Since the 1990s, professional, voluntary groups, and the government have been broadly supportive of the principles embodied in the *Dietary Guidelines* and the process of formulating them has been marked with less bitterness. Also, the notion of a single set of guidelines that decreased risks of many chronic degenerative diseases has continued to be popular.

1990s: Coordination of Dietary Guidance Tools

During the 1990s, new nutrition education tools were developed and existing guidance was refined (Davis and Saltos, 1995). These included the *USDA Food Guide Pyramid* and the first *Healthy Eating Index*, the tool for evaluating adherence to some of the guidelines was also published during the 1990s (Kennedy et al., 1994).

Graphics or icons for healthy eating have been used for many years in this country and abroad. They have increasingly been incorporated into food guidance systems to provide a graphic representation of the basic concepts they embody: adequacy, balance, variety, moderation, and proportionality among others. The graphic was only one element of nutrition education, with a focus only on major messages rather than all of the subtleties of healthy eating. Nevertheless, it provided a pictorial representation of key points in a healthy eating pattern for those who want one.

During the early 1990s, nutrition scientists in the USDA crafted this visual graphic or icon to depict ideal consumption patterns that conformed to the 1990 *Dietary Guidelines* and met the most current RDAs. This followed earlier and somewhat less successful efforts that date to the early 1980s, which involved a "food wheel" that included the total diet concept and energy balance. The 1992 food guide graphic's food group categories were based on both the distribution of nutrients in various food groups and existing food consumption patterns. Extensive argument ensued about whether a bowl, a pyramid, or some other graphic was most appropriate to convey concepts of balance, variety, moderation, and proportionality, and which foods should be placed in each food group—an argument that continues until today. Market research was done to examine the various shapes and settle the argument. The Pyramid was adopted as the best graphic for conveying these concepts on the advice of the expert consultants, and in 1992, the USDA Food Group Pyramid was released (Kennedy, 1994). It quickly became popular. Similar pyramids and other graphics followed in the United States and abroad (Dwyer et al., 2002).

Age-specific pyramid icons developed in the later 1990s, and the USDA issued a child pyramid on dietary guidance for children younger than 5 years, who have different needs than older individuals. The Jean Mayer USDA Human Nutrition Research Center on Aging at Tufts University produced a Tufts "Elder Pyramid" for individuals older than 70 years because elders' needs are slightly different than younger adults for vitamins B 12, D, calcium, nutrient dense foods, calories, and water. These pyramids involved very few changes from the 1992 Pyramid and were also likely to provide a diet that was adequate in nutrients.

During the 1990s, many other nongovernmentally based pyramids proliferated, including those for various ethnic eating patterns such as the Mediterranean Diet, the Asian Diet, special eating patterns (e.g., vegetarian), and for special age-groups. They varied in their nutrient adequacy; some were carefully tested to make sure that they made nutrient targets, while others were not.

1995 Dietary Guidelines: Foods instead of Nutrients

The 1995 edition of the *Dietary Guidelines for Americans* mentioned the USDA Pyramid's utility in the guideline on "Eat a Variety of Foods" (US Department of Health and Human Services/USDA, 1995). Until 1995 only seven dietary guidelines were included. The focus of the guidelines continued to be either on constituents (such as sugar, fat, cholesterol, sodium, starch, fiber, and alcohol rather than emphasizing foods to eat) or on total diet. Also the tone emphasized limiting and avoiding rather than adding or substituting foods. The major change in 1995 was a greater emphasis on a total diet concept in the dietary guidance.

Year 2000 Dietary Guidelines: The Pyramid and Weight in the Spotlight

In the year 2000, ten dietary guidelines were issued. These were categorized in three groups: Aim for fitness, Build a healthy diet, and Choose wisely (ABC). Greater emphasis was placed on achieving or maintaining a healthy weight and a healthy physical activity level than in prior guidelines. Also, a guideline on keeping food safe to eat and one on consuming a variety of grains, especially whole grains, was added for the first time (USDA/U.S. Department of Health and Human Services, 2000).

In the year 2000 *Dietary Guidelines*, after much debate over whether the USDA's food group pyramid should be mentioned, the pyramid concept was given a guideline of its own. The "Eat a variety of foods" guideline of 1995 was changed to "Let the pyramid guide your food choices" to provide more specificity as to meaning and to stress the guidelines goal of achieving variety among food groups. The year 2000 *Dietary Guidelines* also emphasized variety within food groups in the grains and fruit and vegetables guideline, endorsed the notion that plant foods were the foundation of the diet, and stressed the necessity of proportionality in dietary choice, and added a food safety guideline (Murphy, 2001; Read, 2004).

CURRENT NUTRITION GUIDELINES

Since the year 2000, the trend has been toward a fusion of the dietary guidelines with the newly reformulated dietary reference intakes for nutrients and the USDA's food guide pyramid, which was just issued in revised form.

Year 2005 Dietary Guidelines: Fusion and Harmonization of Guidance

A comparison of the 2005 and 2000 dietary guidelines is provided in Table 2. The 2005 Dietary Guidelines Committee revised the guidelines because dietary standards for all essential nutrients had been updated by the Food and Nutrition Board, Institute of Medicine, and National Academy of Sciences since the year 2000 guidelines were issued and now included recommendations not only for adequate amounts of many nutrients but also for acceptable ranges and upper safe levels for nutrient intakes (Barr et al., 2002; Dwyer, 2004). Also, many aspects of the food label had been

TABLE 2 The 2005 Dietary Guidelines for Americans Highlighting Changes Since the Year 2000 Dietary Guidelines

- Increased recommendation for fruits and vegetables (5–13 servings)
- Increase fat-free, low-fat dairy recommendations (to 3 cups/day)
- Increase whole grains to ≥3-oz equivalents/day
- Popularize the concept of discretionary calories (breakout solid fats from soft margarines and liquid oils, added sugars)
- Specify physical activity at 30 minutes moderate intensity to reduce chronic disease risk, and 90 minutes moderated to help maintain body weight and prevent body gain, and 60–90 min/day moderate intensity to sustain weight loss
- Trans fat singled out for keeping them as low as possible
- Decreasing sodium to <2300 mg/day (Pyramid recommendations could not meet that goal but did reduce it)
- Increase potassium to 4700 mg/day
- Keep alcohol if consumed at all at 1 drink/day for women, and 2 for men.

TABLE 3 The Recommended Revised Dietary Guidelines for Americans

1. Consume a variety of foods within and among the basic food groups while staying within energy needs
2. Control calorie intake to manage body weight
3. Be physically active every day
4. Increase daily intake of fruits and vegetables, whole grains, and nonfat or low-fat milk and milk products
5. Choose fats wisely for good health
6. Choose carbohydrates wisely for good health
7. Choose and prepare foods with little salt
8. If you drink alcoholic beverages, do so in moderation
9. Keep foods safe to eat

altered by the Food and Drug Administration (FDA), the effects of fortification of grains with folic acid were becoming apparent, and much new science had been published on clinical trials involving various nutrients, making an update of the dietary guidelines imperative.

The 2005 Dietary Guidelines Advisory Committee (DGAC) explored evidence in nine areas of focus; adequate nutrients within calorie needs; weight management; physical activity; food groups to encourage consumption of fats, carbohydrates, sodium and potassium, and alcoholic beverages; and food safety. The committee examined the best of the recent science, using an evidence-based system that involved a systematic evaluation of the strength of the evidence linking cause and effect in a statement. Most federal statements on diet–disease relationships, including the health claims approved by the FDA, now rely on such evidence-based reviews so the data used conform to the Data Quality Act enacted by Congress in 2000 to ensure policy making based on sound science. The process involves defining the questions or statements to be examined, collecting all relevant studies, and evaluating each study independently for its type (since this determines in part the strength of the causal inference that can be made) and the quality of the study. The strength of the science is reported in some of the recommendations. The major advantage of the systematic review process is reliability; different but knowledgeable scientists should come to the same conclusions after review of the evidence. It is also more objective. The process uses predetermined search strategies, and this lessens the chances that literature reviews might be limited by selective searches of the evidence to support preconceived conclusions.

For the evidence-based reviews, the Dietary Guidelines Committee selected associations that involved key nutrients and important health outcomes. The questions asked were the strength of the association or relationship between nutrient intakes and decreased risks of disease. Although the 2005 guidelines were qualitative in nature, the committee referred to quantitative targets provided by the Food and Nutrition Board's *Dietary Reference Intakes*. These included the RDAs, the tolerable upper intake levels (ULs) for several micronutrients, and ranges of Acceptable Macronutrient Distribution Ranges for Healthy Adults (AMDR), as well as guidance on targets for energy needs and energy output (Barr et al., 2004; Dwyer, 2004).

The scientific report of the 2005 *Dietary Guidelines* is a comprehensive document that reviews the new scientific evidence. It provides 23 specific technical recommendations for the general public and 18 additional recommendations for specific population groups, along with the rationales for each. It is available on the web at www.health.gov/dietaryguidelines and is discussed in depth elsewhere (McMurray et al., 2003; Dwyer, 2005).

In the 2005 version of the *Dietary Guidelines*, there are nine guidelines, although the final wording for communications to lay persons is summarized in only three major statements for consumers (Table 3). The two major themes in the 2005 guidelines are consuming a variety of foods from the basic food groups and controlling calorie intakes that are intertwined and interdependent. Table 2 summarizes the major differences between the year 2000 and the 2005 guidelines. Until the year 2000, the guidelines started with an emphasis on variety; after the year 2000 the first guideline emphasized aiming for fitness (Aim for a healthy weight and Be physically active each day), and the concept was given even more emphasis in the 2005 guidelines. The emphasis on avoidance of overweight and sedentary lifestyles was maintained in the 2005 committee report. The major difference between the 2005 and 2000 and previous guidelines was that sugars were not explicitly mentioned, although the committee did provide a recommendation for limiting intake of added sugars under the topic listed as "choosing carbohydrates wisely" and, where calorie intake levels were stressed, limitations in added sugars were mentioned.

In early 2005, the two cabinet-level departments issued the official executive summary of the 2005 *Dietary Guidelines*. Based on the scientific report and developed by a committee of federal employees, it provided recommendations for eating patterns to fulfill the dietary guidelines (Dietary Guidelines Advisory Committee, 2004). It was aimed at policy makers, health care providers, and nutrition educators. It is available on the web at www.healthierus.gov/dietaryguidelines.

The vast majority of changes involved simplification and not distortion or change in the scientific committee's document. For example, the goal for saturated fat was fixed at <10% and dietary cholesterol at <300 mg rather than by low-density lipoprotein (LDL)–cholesterol levels as recommended by the committee, largely for practical reasons. Also, the recommended levels of N-6, N-3 fatty acids and recommendations about consuming two servings of fish high in EPA/DHA were not included. A goal of keeping trans fat as low as possible was adopted. When changes in the 2005 *Dietary Guidelines* were applied to foods, this meant more emphasis on consuming unsaturated fats and oils, whole grains, legumes, and dark green vegetables in eating patterns.

In mid 2005, a consumer brochure called "Finding Your Way to a Healthier You" was developed for consumers (U.S. Department of Health and Human Services/USDA, 2005). Three key messages for a healthier lifestyle were highlighted:

- Making smart choices from every food group: The emphasis here was on fruits, vegetables, whole grains, and fat-free or low-fat milk and milk products, as well as lean meats, poultry, fish, beans, eggs, and nuts; such a pattern is low in saturated fats, trans fats, cholesterol, salt, and added sugars.
- Finding your balance between food and physical activity
- Getting the most nutrition from your calories

2005 MyPyramid: New USDA Food Group "Radiant" Pyramid Debuts

The latest revision of the USDA Food Pyramid, *MyPyramid* or the Food Guidance System, as it is sometimes called, is based on standards for nutrient intakes provided in the Dietary Reference Intakes (DRIs). More general dietary guidance such as that provided in the *Dietary Guidelines for Americans* is also incorporated. In an effort to make the Pyramid a realistic eating guide, the USDA spent considerable time analyzing recent dietary data and planning the Pyramid recommendations to build on existing habits while filling in gaps by making minimal recommendations necessary to achieve nutrient adequacy. The Pyramid was designed to also be in line with other federal nutrition guidance, such as *Healthy People 2010* of the U.S. Department of Health and Human Services (2000), the Nutrient Facts label on foods, and the Supplement Facts label on dietary supplements.

The DRIs were completed in late 2003, followed by the 2005 *Dietary Guidelines for Americans* and the *USDA MyPyramid,* its new pyramid and food guidance system, in mid 2005. The Pyramid was revised to take into account changes in the underlying science as reflected in the DRI and the *Dietary Guidelines*, and the results of focus groups and public comment. For the first time, public comment was used extensively to identify the current strengths and weaknesses of the Pyramid. All of these nutrition guidance documents are being revised more or less in tandem. They are now somewhat better integrated than they were in the past, and this may make them easier for consumers to use. The Nutrient Facts panel on food labels is also being examined. Unfortunately it continues to lag behind the other federal food guidance tools, perhaps in part because of the difficulty in changing the standards used without changing regulations, which is an onerous, time-consuming, and politically charged process.

The reasons that the 1992 Pyramid needed revision in 2005 included the fact that it was based on now outdated standards, calorie levels and portion sizes were not clearly understood by consumers, and food consumption had changed considerably over the 10 years since the Pyramid was first developed.

Since the *USDA Food Group Pyramid* is so closely associated with the *Dietary Guidelines for Americans*, it was fortunate that its revision proceeded in parallel with the revision of the 2005 Guidelines. Public comment was used extensively. The issues that were identified in public comment as specifically needing attention in revising the Pyramid included provision of recommendations on calorie intakes and finding ways to highlight achieving adequacy, but not excess, in energy intakes. It quickly became apparent that there was a need to emphasize nutrient density, especially since so many Americans have very low levels of energy output because of their sedentary lifestyles. Also, Pyramid revisions needed to focus attention on fostering consumption of foods that currently did not meet recommendations (e.g., consumption of whole grains, dark green and yellow-orange vegetables, and legumes). It was also important to make dietary guidance, especially with respect to serving size, more understandable, which it was not to most consumers.

Meeting Altered and New Nutrient Standards (DRI and 2005 Dietary Guidelines)

Nutritional standards and goals had changed a good deal since 1992, when the Pyramid was first established. All of the former recommended dietary allowances for vitamins, elements, protein, and fatty acids had been reexamined, and new DRI standards were issued, the last being published in 2004. In addition, the new DRIs also include the AMDR for certain macronutrients; protein, carbohydrate and added sugars, total fiber, total fat, linoleic acid, and α-linoleic acid are also included. Food Group Pyramid recommendations needed updating with these up-to-date scientific standards.

For adequacy, the primary sources of information for the new 2005 Pyramid were the many reports on DRIs of nutrients issued by the Food and Nutrition Board, Institute of Medicine, National Academy of Sciences and Health Canada over the past decade. The nutrients most likely to be consumed by the general public in amounts low enough to be of concern were given special attention, including, for adults, vitamins A, C, E, calcium, magnesium, potassium, and fiber. For children vitamin E, calcium, magnesium, potassium, and fiber were found to be low in national survey data.

For moderation, the upper levels of the DRI and the year 2005 *Dietary Guidelines for Americans* were employed to generate first approximations of intakes to use in the Pyramid. The nutrients judged to be in excess by the Dietary Guidelines Committee were fat, especially saturated and trans fat, salt, and "added sugar." The Pyramid plan met most of these concerns. It was not possible to meet the sodium goal of 2300 mg in the DRI without extensive changes in food patterns. For some nutrients, like sodium, levels were not low enough to meet the RDAs, but they were substantially lower than the prior RDA was, and so the trend was in the appropriate direction. The new Pyramid came closer than prior versions to reaching the sodium goal and the 4700-mg potassium goal. Thus, the Pyramid was revised to keep the nutrient targets in line with the new *Dietary Guideline* recommendations while preserving the concept of gradual changes and small steps.

Specifying Energy Levels

Although the calorie levels for the Pyramid were always provided in the nutrition guidance material that accompanied the Pyramid, the information about calorie levels and that consumers could not eat as much as they desired were not clearly understood by many consumers. Unfortunately, few people read the nutrition education material accompanying the Pyramid on how to use it, and so they met the Pyramid recommendations by eating more food of all sorts. A major advance in the 2005 revisions of the Pyramid was the inclusion of personalized pyramids at 12 different calorie levels. Now, calorie levels are more numerous and are explicitly specified so that individuals can choose what fits them the best. The exact calorie levels are not shown in the summary graphic, but an interactive web site is available that tailors a pyramid to each individual on the basis of his or her age, sex, and physical activity level. Information is provided so that consumers can choose the appropriate Pyramid for their needs. Current debate includes whether a graphic and web site should include a pyramid for elders that includes the lower energy and high micronutrient needs of older persons.

Coping with Low Energy Intakes and the Nutrient Density Problem

The basic rule is that the more physically active people are, the more food they can eat. Because most Americans are sedentary, for most people dietary recommendations must be based on the energy needs of *sedentary* persons (e.g., the energy needs of those who take <3000 steps or the equivalent in other physical activity per day). This amounts to ~1500 kcal for women and 2000 kcal for men. At low energy outputs, since nutrient adequacy must be achieved in a relatively small number of calories, the USDA focused particular attention on foods within each group that had a high nutrient density for the key nutrients of concern to ensure that those who followed the Pyramid would obtain the nutrients they needed for health. Nutrient density is the percent of nutrients to calories of foods within each of the food groups. Of greatest concern in considering nutrient density are nutrients of public health significance because these are the ones that are likely to be low or lacking in existing diets. Thus, particular consideration needs to be paid to vitamins A, C, E, calcium, magnesium, potassium, and fiber in adults, and vitamins E, calcium, magnesium, potassium, and fiber in children, since these nutrients were found to be low in population-based surveys such as the National Health and Nutrition Evaluation Survey (NHANES). Whether these same nutrients remain problematic when intakes of dietary supplements and fortified foods are included remains to be determined as data become more adequate on these sources of nutrients in the years to come.

When and if people become more physically active than the sedentary pattern, as is certainly highly desirable, they can add more foods and/or lower nutrient density foods to the recommended eating pattern. For example, low-activity individuals (who take at least 3000–6000 steps/day) could have more food and greater choice and still meet the DRI/Dietary Guideline targets, if they expended more energy. Moderately active persons (≥6000 steps/day) could include even greater amounts and types of food while still meeting their nutrient needs.

Coping with Different Calorie Levels

In order to construct pyramids for different calorie levels, the amounts of each food group that meet nutrient adequacy goals at each level of energy needs were assessed, and 12 age and energy intake groups were considered. Additional constraints were considered and built in, and the results were compared with goals and readjusted. The final results were given to communications experts to put them into language that consumers could understand. The challenge that remains is conveying the concept of nutrient density both to health professionals and to consumers.

The "radiant" *MyPyramid* attempts to convey these notions, with the food groups arranged vertically within the pyramid, and the size of each colored band representing the relative proportion of each food group within the overall diet. The eater is urged to choose foods within each group from the "leanest" selections that are lowest in calories (especially fat and added sugars) and highest in micronutrients.

Assigning Nutritional Goals to Each Specific Food Intake Pattern and Nutrient Content to Each Food Group and Subgroup

In addition to using up-to-date scientific standards, recent information on food consumption was also considered to make the Pyramid guide practical and actionable for those who have typical food consumption patterns using commonly eaten foods. The USDA used the most current food consumption and food choice data to update the nutrient profiles for the Pyramid food groups so that they reflected current food choice realities within each of these categories. The updating process then involved taking account of changes in food consumption within different food groups over the 10 years since the first Pyramid was developed and updating the nutrient content of each food group and subgroup to reflect these changes. The food groups were constructed as composites on the basis of the types and amounts of foods currently consumed by Americans. However, in constructing the food groups and their nutrient profiles, the "leanest" lowest calorie versions of recipes were chosen. Additional fats, oils, soft margarines, and added sugars were considered separately in the "discretionary calories" category, to be added as individuals wished after micronutrient needs were met from food sources. Finally, the amounts of each new food group were determined for individuals at each caloric level. For example, while an individual with a calorie allowance of 1200 kcal would be recommended 4 ounces of bread a day, a person with an allowance of 3200 might need more.

Translating Nutrient Goals into Realistic Food Selection Recommendations for Each Food Group and Subgroup in the Food Guide Pyramid for Those at Each Energy Level

The USDA examined the current food consumption and nutrient profiles and identified gaps in nutrient levels for overall diets. Particular attention was paid to nutrients that are considered to be problems of public health significance, either because they were lacking in the food supply or because they were viewed by federal and other experts as being of special public health concern for many groups, such as vitamins A, C, calcium, and iron. Additional nutrients such as folic acid need special attention in some specific groups, such as women of childbearing age because of links between deficiency of it during the preconception period and birth defects. These nutrients of public health significance are all on the Nutrient Facts labels on processed foods. Vitamin E is a nutrient that is not viewed as a public health problem in the United States, because no deficiency of it has been identified, although it is lower in the food supply and it is difficult to meet current vitamin E recommendations from food sources alone.

Changes in the Pyramid Food Patterns

The major changes in food patterns in the 2005 Food Pyramid were in providing 12 servings at many calorie levels and increasing the amounts of vegetables recommended for some calorie levels. Also, there were changes in the relative amounts of some of the vegetable subgroups. The amounts of dark green vegetables and legumes were increased. The remaining vegetable subgroups were held constant or decreased. Also, the amount of whole grains was increased to at least one-half of the total amount in every pattern. Enriched grains were decreased proportionally. These alterations have led some individuals to advocate for fortification of whole grains with folic acid, since whole grains are not now fortified, and a shift toward whole grains might lead to decreased intakes of folacin.

Incorporating Less Nutritious Foods into Patterns: Discretionary Calories

Once the fundamental diet–disease relationships were established by the DRI process and the Dietary Guidelines Committee, nutritious food patterns could be established. Then these patterns could be incorporated into a food guidance pattern that also allowed for less highly nutritious foods and encouraged cultural diversity. The discretionary fats category was divided into solid fats and oils and soft margarines, and a shift in the proportions recommended was made in the 2005 revision of the Pyramid to 40% solid fats and 40% oils.

Clearing up Existing Confusion

There were also some changes in the Pyramid that were attempts to clear up confusion. For example, legumes are classified as vegetables and as members of the meat group as beans. They could theoretically be placed as legumes or nuts and seeds in a separate group or as a subgroup of the meat group.

Making Portions and Servings Understandable

Another criticism of the 1992 Pyramid was that the servings or portions it recommended were confusing to consumers. Such confusion often led to overeating because the portions specified were very small in food guidance materials compared with what was actually being served in restaurants and many homes. The amount of food offered influences consumption to some extent; the larger the portion offered, the more that is eaten. American consumers are confused about portions because they are not accustomed to noting or using food weights; they prefer household measures, and household measures are not always clear. Also, the standard portions used on other government guidance, such as servings on food labels, are not always the same as the size of servings used in the Pyramid and the specified calorie levels (2000 calories is the standard on the food label's Nutrient Facts panel) are not necessarily similar. Finally, recommended servings and serving sizes as actually served or eaten in restaurants, as well as at home, are often widely different. USDA adopted the use of household measures such as cups and ounces in providing guidance. However, more needs to be done to lessen confusion and ensure that consumers understand these changes because ounces, which can be both weight and volume measurements, are difficult to understand and inherently confusing.

Finishing Touches on the Pyramid

Before the newly refurbished *MyPyramid* could be released, the USDA did a series of modeling studies to verify that nutrient adequacy and moderation were in fact achieved, excess was avoided, and recommended patterns were likely to be acceptable to consumers. It used the nutrient goals of the DRI report and food consumption data from the 1999/2000 cycle of the NHANES to do this and found that for the key nutrients the pyramid was satisfactory. The revised version of the USDA Pyramid released in 2005 incorporated the newly revised DRI, the 2005 *Dietary Guidelines for Americans*, and other recent federal guidance, such as the report on nutrient labeling emphasizing the importance of energy that was recently released by the FDA.

INDIVIDUALIZING THE RADIANT PYRAMID

The new USDA Pyramid, "*MyPyramid*," included an accompanying web site (www.mypyramid.gov). The web site permits the viewer to individualize the pyramid to his or her own special needs. There are 12 pyramids that are keyed to different caloric needs and further customization is of course possible by altering choices within and among the food groups. This individualization goes a long way to quelling some of the former criticisms of the Food Group Pyramid; consumers often failed to adopt the prior graphic and personalize it to their own needs. The person can enter age, sex, and physical activity level and get personalized recommendations based on an appropriate energy intake. Then the nutrient recommendations can be converted into food-based recommendations. The individual can find general food guidance and suggestions for making wise choices from each food group that meet DRI recommendations for almost all nutrients. This step forward is laudable. However, there is little material available for low-income, low-literacy, or noncomputer users who often need such food guides. Nutrition educators must develop materials tailored to these audiences.

The *MyPyramid* presents educational challenges. A major difference with the new MyPyramid approach compared with prior tools is that more than five food groups are necessary to meet the DRI and AMDR for nutrient intakes. Particular emphasis is needed on increasing consumption of deep green and leafy vegetables, lesser amounts of starchy vegetables, and other changes. Also, the individual needs to have a way of keeping track of the fat contained in milk products and meats, fats, and added sugars and calories from added sugars that are not included in the guide, because the pyramid servings assume the leanest lower calorie options. In fact, many people eat higher calorie options, and if they fail to account for that, they are likely to consume excessive numbers of calories. Unfortunately the mechanisms regulating food intakes are not precise enough to assume that automatic self-regulation will occur.

The MyPyramid.gov web site provides a number of tools for helping consumers help themselves. The MyPyramid Plan provides a quick estimate of what and how much food an individual of a given age, gender, and activity level should eat. The MyPyramid Tracker provides detailed information on the individual's dietary quality and physical activity status by allowing the person to compare a day's worth of foods eaten with current nutrition guidance. Also, it provides advice depending on a person's desires to lose weight or maintain their current weight. On the web site, MyPyramid provides in-depth information for every food group, including servings in commonly used measures, recommendations for choosing healthy oils, physical activity, and "discretionary" calories. Finally the Start Today area of the web site provides downloadable tips and resources for all the food groups and for physical activity, and a worksheet to track intake. When the web site is fully operational and can meet consumer capacity, it will be a valuable tool.

A second innovation in the 2005 version of the pyramid is the new symbol: the "radiant" MyPyramid to introduce the concept of nutrient density. The radiant pyramid is called by this name because the food groups are arrayed across the base of the pyramid and then radiate down from the top. There are six colored bands to symbolize the five food groups and oils. The MyPyramid symbol represents the recommended proportion of foods from each food group and focuses on the importance of making smart food choices in every food group, every day. The concept of proportionality is shown by the different widths of the food group bands. The widths suggest how much food a person should choose from each group. The widths are general guides rather than exact proportions. The concept of variety is that foods from each food group should be included each day. This new format also depicts balance across groups at the bottom of the pyramid. Moderation is another important concept. It is represented by the narrowing of each food group from bottom to top of the pyramid. The wide base includes foods with little or no solid fats, added sugars, or caloric sweeteners; these should be selected more often to get the most nutrition from calories consumed. The importance of moderating intakes with wise food choices is also emphasized; as one eats more and goes up the pyramid, the amounts that are eaten need to be less if energy intakes are not to be exceeded. The guiding principle for choices within each food group is nutrient density:nutrients per calorie. This concept is helpful in that it is an aid for maximizing nutrient intakes without caloric excess. MyPyramid is part of an overall food guidance system that emphasizes the need for a more individualized approach to improving diet and lifestyle. The web site MyPyramid.gov includes additional information for helping consumers to incorporate their choices into their own lifestyles.

The third innovation is that there is now a stick figure on the side of the radiant MyPyramid and a staircase on the side of the pyramid. This is to integrate physical activity, which is a new element on the icon, into food guidance. Fourth, the food groups are color-coded and these colors are coordinated with those used in the 2005 *Dietary Guidelines* to refer to the same food groups.

MyPyramid places emphasis on gradual improvement of dietary habits by again using the steps analogy: "steps to a healthier you"; the notion is that individuals can benefit from taking small steps to improve their diets and lifestyles each day. Even small steps can be helpful. A child-friendly version of MyPyramid for children 6–11 years old is being developed by USDA.

The new dietary guidance materials are among the best ever developed by the federal government. However, some of the concepts that have been introduced have not been fully elucidated. These concepts include the notion of "discretionary calories" and that of "nutrient density"—two concepts that until recently had even eluded clear understanding by many nutrition scientists.

Discretionary calories refers to the calories left over after one has chosen enough of each of the food groups to meet one's appropriate RDA for each nutrient, while not exceeding energy needs or consuming excessive amounts of each nutrient and while moderating intakes appropriately. For sedentary individuals who have relatively low energy intakes, the number of discretionary calories is extremely limited. For example, at 1400 kcal, only 172 calories, or ~12%, are discretionary and remain after the food pattern has been fulfilled; this would amount to 5 tsp of sugar and a few pats of butter. Many elderly people have such low calorie intakes. As people become more physically active, the situation improves; at 3200 kcal, 334 calories are discretionary, also ~12%, but with almost twice the leeway in terms of choices. To make more discretionary calories available, the easiest solution is to become more physically active because needs for most micronutrients do not rise with increasing levels of energy output and so less nutrient dense, higher calorie items are acceptable choices. To increase the amount of discretionary calories available, the consumption of nutrient-rich foods that are relatively low in energy density is also an important strategy—one that is built into MyPyramid already. The use of fortified foods and dietary supplements to provide additional nutrients would provide somewhat more leeway, although not everyone is likely to do this.

The second unfamiliar concept in the new "radiant pyramid" is *nutrient density*; that is, the ratio of the amount of a nutrient in foods to the energy provided by these same foods, for example, nutrients per calorie. This is difficult for most consumers to grasp as well. The basic ideas are well described in an article by Kennedy and Zelman (2005). Both naturally nutrient dense foods (e.g., those that naturally provide appropriate nutrient/calorie ratios) and fortified foods that have nutrients added to them are nutrient dense. However, only the naturally nutrient dense foods and those fortified by federal regulations (such as vitamins D in milk products) are used in calculating the nutrient contributions of food groups in the USDA pyramid. Those who use highly fortified cereals or calcium-fortified orange juice on a regular basis, for example, might be able to meet their micronutrient needs with fewer of certain food groups. Similarly, the contribution of dietary supplements is not included even though approximately half of the U.S. population uses dietary supplements, most of which contain nutrients, on a regular basis. However, the use of fortified foods would not necessarily make it any easier to achieve balance or moderation, particularly as it relates to macronutrients or fiber. Another problem is that the individualized radiant pyramids have been constructed using the leanest choices (e.g., low-fat milk and skinless chicken) and the least amounts of added sugars.

The major shortcoming with MyPyramid is that for those who are not sophisticated at using computers and web sites, it is still relatively difficult to get print copies of the pyramid and the *Dietary Guidelines*. Also, the pyramid has never been assessed in a human study to ascertain whether biomarkers of risk or of nutritional status are altered for the better.

CANCER-SPECIFIC GUIDELINES

Dietary recommendations, which are designed to alter the types and amounts of substrates provided to the body, are essentially a chemoprevention strategy with the bioactive substances of interest provided in foods rather than in the more isolated constituents in dietary supplements. It may be possible to design diets of foods that provide some of the benefits with fewer of the risks involved in drug therapies such as tamoxifen for the prevention of certain cancers. Three important concepts in understanding how and why diet might work as a chemoprevention strategy are first to recognize that many common diet-related cancers are epithelial in nature and appear to be affected by alterations in nutrient intakes (Tsao et al., 2004). The development of the cancers involves multiple steps to encompass a multifocal field in the carcinogenesis process. The multistep nature of cancer development is important because it implies that action at one or several of the steps may impede or delay cancer development. The classic stages of carcinogenesis include initiation (DNA binding and damage of a rapid and irreversible nature to the cell), promotion (which involves epigenetic mechanisms that lead to a series of irreversible defects and lead to premalignancy), and progression, which is also irreversible. *Multifocal field carcinogenesis* refers to the fact that rather than a single cell being affected, a whole area of epithelial cells is affected and the various genetic changes, which are such that they increase the likelihood of premalignant or malignant lesions developing in other cells as well. These later types of cancers are called *second primary tumors*. The process of carcinogenesis may result in the formation of second primary tumors. Most dietary strategies appear to operate in retarding or impeding promotion, but all are thought to work by altering the carcinogenesis process at various points.

Prevention strategies are also multiple. Primary prevention prevents malignancies from ever appearing. Secondary prevention decreases risks among those who have premalignant lesions. Tertiary prevention focuses on prevention of second primary tumors among those in recovered individuals.

Why Have Cancer-Specific Guidelines?

There is a place for cancer-specific nutritional recommendations that work with general dietary recommendations for the population as a whole. One reason for such guidelines is that there is an enormous amount of evidence to be covered on many dietary constituents and food. Some of this information is of interest chiefly to those at very high risk or who are already afflicted with cancer and searching for all means to lower their risks of recurrence. Therefore, cancer-specific evidence-based guidelines are best formulated by experts in cancer. Cancer-specific guidelines can cover issues of interest to the general public in primary prevention, as well as issues of greater concern to those who are at high risk of specific cancers, who have already fallen ill, who are recovering, and who have ongoing disease. Nutritional measures that are appropriate for one cancer stage may not be so for other stages. Also, site-specific and general dietary recommendations can sometimes be made and cancer-specific guidelines are necessary for them. Cancer-specific guidelines permit the dietary recommendations to be put into an overall context of other preventive and curative measures, which are highly relevant, such as cancer screening, not smoking, physical activity, and other measures. Cancer-specific guidelines can also address concerns of those whose cancers are in remission or who are actively undergoing therapy. As time goes on, more needs to be learned about the role of diet in secondary prevention or as adjuvant therapy in cancer treatment and of changes in nutrient needs during cancer therapy. Cancer-specific nutrition guidelines also permit discussion of such issues as phytochemicals or food additives, which are of great interest or concern to many individuals because of their purported links to cancer development but of lesser concern to more general audiences. They also interest many people because they provide hope that they can lessen their chances from suffering from a disease that most people greatly fear. Cancer-specific guidelines are also useful public relations and fundraising tools for professional and disease-related organizations.

The evidence on the links between diet and cancer is considerable. It ranges from epidemiological to *in vitro* studies on cancer prevention and diet, so the sheer mass of material to be covered is large. Thus, it is helpful to have systematic reviews done by experts and to have guidelines constructed by experts; there are few generalists who can comprehend, much less master, the subtleties of all of these different types of evidence for the 100 or more different conditions that are called *cancers*.

There are also arguments against cancer-specific dietary recommendations. Some experts assert that general dietary guidelines are better, because no individual actually knows the diseases from which they are likely to suffer from later in life. Another argument is that very little is known for certain about the links between diet and cancer that would give rise to different dietary advice than that for the general public; so, for the most part, the guidelines are fairly similar for all chronic degenerative diseases and little differences are present. Some argue that to keep the message simple, it may be better to have general guidelines.

Misconceptions about Diet and Cancer

Table 4 summarizes some misconceptions about diet and cancer that are common among lay persons and even health professionals. It is important for all those who use dietary

TABLE 4 Myths and Realities about Dietary Recommendations for Cancer

Myth	Reality
Cancer will never develop among those who follow diet-cancer guidelines.	There is no assurance that those who follow cancer dietary guidelines will not develop cancer; however, risks may be reduced for some of the diet-related cancers. There is no diet that absolutely protects people against all forms of cancer. At this stage in our knowledge, it is inappropriate to say that if the patient had eaten differently, the cancer would never have developed.
Cancer patients are the best source of nutritional advice about cancer.	More specific, objective, and evidence-based advice is available from health care professionals and authoritative expert groups. Fellow patients lack access to the specialized training, experience, and the medical records that inform health professionals. Fellow patients may be enthusiastic about unproven or even harmful cancer therapies.
The same dietary recommendations that reduce risk of cancer are also helpful in treating cancer.	This depends on the specific stage and site of the cancer, and theory often may be quite different.
Dietary recommendations are a substitute for dietitians, and for nutrition counseling and education by the doctor and nurse.	Both general guidelines and specific advice by the physician, others on the nutrition care team, and the dietitian are necessary. The dietitian is the most knowledgeable about adopting recommendations to individual patient needs.
Each health professional should give dietary advice to patients on the basis of his or her own best judgments.	Every patient deserves an evidence-based, agreed-upon nutrition care plan that the entire health care team implements.
Cancer patients can get their own dietary recommendations over the Internet.	Information over the Internet on diet and cancer is not necessarily evidence based and may be not only inefficacious but harmful to health and financially costly. Dietary recommendations provided should be from authoritative sources (the federal government, American Cancer Society, or American Institute for Cancer Research) that strive for evidence-based recommendations.
Most people understand what nutrition can do in cancer prevention and treatment.	There is much confusion and misconceptions are rife, some overly optimistic and others overly pessimistic. Goals are to bring expectations more in line with realities and to assist patients to use nutrition to support cancer risk reduction, treatment, or therapy if needed.
Dietary recommendations and nutrition education of the family can be ignored.	The general population, high-risk individuals, and cancer patients all need help if they are to follow dietary recommendations, especially if they are already ill. Well-informed spouses and families assist in this effort, especially when someone other than the patient does the cooking.
Only hospitalized patients have a need for dietary recommendations and nutrition guidelines.	Everyone needs nutrition guidelines to reduce risk of cancer; special guidelines for the growing number of cancer survivors in the general population and for those who have ongoing disease are also necessary.
People at highest risk of cancer will be those most likely to change their diets.	There is little reason to suggest that this is the case unless health professionals devote particular effort to helping such individuals understand why dietary changes are necessary.

recommendations to use them correctly within a larger context that clearly describes what diet can and cannot do and its place among prevention and treatment measures.

Cancer-Specific Guidelines Available

Several sets of sound cancer-specific dietary recommendations are available. Each is described briefly in the following subsections.

American Institute for Cancer Research Guidelines for Primary Prevention

During the 1990s the World Cancer Research Fund/American Institute for Cancer Research (WCRF/AICR) did a comprehensive global review of the evidence associating diet with cancer. It developed a systematic means for integrating the epidemiological data with that from experimental studies of diet and cancer development and evaluated it in a comprehensive review, entitled "Food, Nutrition and the Prevention of Cancer: A Global Perspective" (WCRF/AICR, 1997). The full report can be viewed at www.aicr.org. The panel summarized and reviewed all of the available evidence by cancer site in the body (breast, lung, colon, etc.), by the various dietary components (vegetables, fruits, etc.) and by a variety of other factors such as obesity, physical activity, and food preparation methods that might also be relevant and affect results. Each potential association was graded as either "convincing," "probable," "possible," or "insufficient." From the standpoint of recommendations, the "convincing" links are the ones that deserve the most attention because they suggest actions that those interested in reducing their risk might take. The associations were graded as convincing if a substantial number of epidemiological studies were strongly consistent and laboratory studies also showed a clear plausible mechanism that could explain why that particular dietary component or other factor might affect cancer risk.

Among the evidence that was judged to be *convincing* were the following observations:

- Diets high in vegetables and fruits decrease the risk of cancer of the colon, rectum, stomach, lung, esophagus, mouth, and pharynx.
- Regular physical activity decreases the risk of colon cancer.
- Obesity increases the risk of endometrial cancer.
- Alcohol increases the risk of cancers of the liver, esophagus, larynx, mouth, and pharynx.

Other evidence was considered consistent but not convincing and, therefore, was judged "probable" in its causal association with cancer. The total number of epidemiological studies was smaller, but laboratory studies showed a clear plausible mechanism. Diets high in vegetables and fruits decreased the risk of breast, bladder, and laryngeal cancers. Obesity increases the risk of breast and kidney cancer. Alcohol increases risk of cancers of the breast, colon, and rectum. Meat increases risk of colorectal cancer.

When epidemiological studies were generally supportive but small in number and the laboratory studies did not necessarily show clear mechanisms, the rating of "possible" was given. For example, the contention that diets high in vegetables and fruits decrease risk of cancers of the liver, ovaries, endometrium, cervix, prostate, thyroid, and kidney was judged as possible.

After several years of work, the panel concluded the chief causes of cancer were tobacco and inappropriate diets, and that between 30 and 40% of all cancers could be prevented by feasible and appropriate diets and related actions. On the basis of the work of the panel, the AICR developed a set of guidelines for cancer prevention (Table 5). In addition, a set of public health goals and advice to individuals that applied globally was also issued, based on the findings of the systematic evidence review. These are presented in Table 6 (AICR, 2005).

In a related effort, the AICR developed a campaign to change eating habits toward patterns that were more in line with the WCRF-AICR guidelines and that encouraged attaining and maintaining a healthy weight. This campaign was entitled the "New American Plate."

TABLE 5 American Institute for Cancer Research Diet and Health Guidelines for Cancer Prevention

1. Choose a diet rich in a variety of plant-based foods
2. Eat plenty of vegetables and fruits
3. Maintain a healthy weight and be physically active
4. Drink alcohol only in moderation, if at all
5. Select foods low in fat and salt
6. Prepare and store food safely
And always remember: do not use tobacco in any form.

In 2005, the AICR produced a cookbook with recipes and advice on the basis of the WCRF-AICR's report (AICR, 2005). The AICR newsletter (available from the web site www.aicr.org) also provides tips and hints for eating in line with the recommendations.

It is anticipated that in 2006 another WCRF-AICR evidence review will be completed and dietary recommendations will be updated accordingly.

American Cancer Society Guidelines for Cancer

For many years, the ACS has issued guidelines on nutrition and cancer prevention; the focus is on reducing the risk of cancer with healthy food choices and physical activity. Statements made in 1999 (Byers) have updated the guidelines. The ACS and the National Cancer Institute (NCI) have also supported guidelines addressing not only the cancers but also other chronic degenerative diseases (Prentice et al., 2004; Eyre et al., 2005). The latest ACS guidelines are provided in Table 7.

Guidelines for Cancer Treatment

Cancer treatment is highly individualized, and for that reason, public health guidelines may be inappropriate to guide diets during active treatment. Health care professionals should provide such advice. Adjuvant nutritional therapy as a cancer treatment should only be undertaken under the direction of a physician who is providing the other oncological therapy.

Complementary and alternative medicine therapies, special dietary therapies not prescribed by the oncologist, and special foods or supplements should not be used without discussion with the physician and examination of evidence-based reviews of the pros and cons of such therapies. Means of addressing these issues, current controversies, and reviews of specific complementary therapies are available (Holland, 1982; Ades et al., 2001; Ades and Rosenthal, 2001; Harpham, 2001; Vickers, 2004). Dietary counseling by a registered dietitian or other knowledgeable health professional can be helpful in developing sensible steps that improve health and equality of life (Rock, 2005).

Guidelines for Cancer Survivors Living in Recovery

Diets that may be helpful in cancer risk reduction and/or prevention may also not be helpful when individuals are in the midst of therapy or already have been treated for cancer, or when they are afflicted with advanced cancer. However, individuals who have survived cancer often want to and do

TABLE 6 Public Health Goals and Advice to Individuals Older Than Age 2 Years Worldwide: American Institute for Cancer Research Recommendations 1997

Public health goal	Individual advice
Food supply, eating and related factors	
Nutritionally adequate and varied diets based on foods of plant origin	Choose a predominantly plant-based diet rich in a variety of vegetables and fruits, legumes, and minimally processed starchy staple foods
Maintain populations body weight within ranges body mass index (BMI) 21 and 23 so that individual BMI is between 18.5 and 25.0	Avoid underweight or overweight and limit weight gain during adulthood to <11 pounds
Maintain physical activity in population with a physical activity level (PAL) of at least 1.75, with opportunities for vigorous physical activity	If occupational activity is low or moderate, take an hour's brisk walk or similar exercise daily and exercise vigorously for at least 1 hour in a week
Foods and drinks	
Vegetables and fruits: promote year-round consumption of a variety of vegetables and fruits, providing ≥7% of total energy	Eat 400–800 g (15–30 oz) or five or more servings a day of a variety of vegetables and fruits, all year round
Other plant foods: a variety of starchy or protein rich foods of plant origin, preferably minimally processed should provide 45–60% total energy	Eat 600–800 g (20–30 oz), or more than seven servings a day of a variety of cereals and grains, legumes, roots, tubers, and plantains; prefer minimally processed foods; limit consumption of refined sugar
Alcoholic drinks: Consumption of alcohol is not recommended and excessive consumption is discouraged, restricted to <5% total energy for men and <2.55 total energy for women	Alcohol consumption is not recommended; if consumed at all, limit alcoholic drinks to fewer than two drinks a day for men and one for women
Meat: If eaten at all, red meat should provide <10% total energy	If eaten at all, limit intake of red meat to <80 g (3 oz) daily; it is preferable to choose fish, poultry, or meat from nondomesticated animals in place of red meat
Total fats and oils: Total fats and oils should provide 15% and no more than 30% total energy	Limit consumption of fatty foods, particularly those of animal origin; choose modest amounts of appropriate vegetable oils
Food processing	
Salt and salting: salt from all sources should amount to <6 g/day (0.25 oz) for adults	Limit consumption of salted foods and use of cooking and table salt; use herbs and spices to season foods
Storage: Store perishable food in ways that minimize fungal contamination	Do not eat food that as a result of prolonged storage at ambient temperatures is liable to contamination with aflatoxins
Preservation: Perishable food, if not consumed promptly, should be kept frozen or chilled	Use refrigeration and other appropriate methods to preserve perishable food as purchased and at home
Additives and residue: Establish and monitor the enforcement of safety limits for food additives, pesticides and their residues, and other chemical contaminants in the food supply	When levels of additives, contaminants, and other residue are properly regulated, their presence in food and drink is not known to be harmful; however, unregulated or improper use can be a health hazard, and this applies particularly in economically developing countries
Preparation: When meat and fish are eaten, encourage relatively low-temperature cooking	Do not eat charred food; for meat and fish eaters, avoid burning of meat juices; consume the following only occasionally: meat and fish grilled (broiled) in direct flame, cured, and smoked meats
Dietary supplements	
Community dietary patterns should be consistent with reduction of cancer risk without the use of dietary supplements	For those who follow the recommendations presented here, dietary supplements are probably unnecessary and possibly unhealthful for reducing cancer risk
Tobacco	
Discourage production, promotion, and use of tobacco in any form	Do not smoke or chew tobacco

make radical changes in their diets (Thomson et al., 2002). It is important to ensure that their nutrition is adequate for supporting recovery and other therapy and for avoiding secondary malnutrition. It is also important to answer the many questions those who are living in recovery have about nutrition. Moreover, because cancer survivors often have diet-related risk factors not only for cancers but also for other chronic degenerative diseases that may need attention, these need to be dealt with as well. Indeed, in some cases these other dietary risk factors may confer considerable risk and may be more likely to cause illness if they are not attended to than risks related to cancer occurrence or recurrence. Examples include obesity, cardiovascular disease, type 2 diabetes, and sedentary lifestyles, for example. The ACS and AICR have begun to provide more specific information to such individuals (Brown et al., 2003).

TABLE 7 American Cancer Society Guidelines on Nutrition and Physical Activity for Cancer Prevention 2003

Guideline	Specific recommendations
Eat a variety of healthful foods, with an emphasis on plant sources	Eat 5 or more servings of a variety of vegetables and fruits each day Choose whole grains in preference to processed (refined) grains and sugars Limit consumption of red meats, especially those high in fat and processed Choose foods that help you maintain a healthful weight
Adopt a physically active lifestyle	Adults: engage in at least moderate activity for 30 minutes or more on five or more days for the week; 45 minutes or more of moderate to vigorous activity on 5 or more days per week may further enhance reductions in the risk of breast and colon cancer Children and adolescence: engage in at least 60 min/day of moderate to vigorous physical activity for at least 5 days per week
Maintain a healthful weight throughout life	Balance calorie intake with physical activity Lose weight if currently overweight or obese
If you drink alcoholic beverages, limit consumption	

It is likely but not proven that guidelines for reducing risk for the occurrence of cancer to begin with may also be helpful in reducing risks of second cancers, although there is much less certainty about this because there are so few studies of survivors. Actions deserving special emphasis are to get weight in line if it is not at a healthy level, to keep up physical activity, and to ensure that food is safe to eat, particularly if the individual is immunosuppressed. If dietary supplements are used, they should be used in levels approximating the daily value (DV) or RDA and not exceed the upper levels (ULs) for intakes of nutrients. During treatment, a multivitamin mineral supplement at 100% DV may be helpful for those who have trouble eating.

As evidence accumulates and new clinical trials of adjuvant dietary therapy are completed, even more specific advice may be possible. Site-specific advice is probably particularly relevant (Denmark-Wahnefried and Rock, 2002). The ACS now presents the evidence for the likelihood of various dietary measures to benefit cancer survivors by specific sites of the cancer. This is useful data and should be consulted by clinicians (Brown et al., 2003).

Nutrition Guidelines for Advanced Cancers

Advanced cancer presents formidable nutritional challenges to the clinician, but this is no reason to ignore the problem. At present, general guidelines are not available. Counseling along with adequate supportive care of other types is necessary on an individual basis.

Why Do Cancer-Specific Nutrition Recommendations Disagree?

Among the common dietary and nutritional recommendations, there is a fair degree of agreement, but they differ on particulars. At first glance, it is puzzling that since evidence-based reviews are touted as being reliable, if different scientists review the same evidence, they should come to the same conclusions. Some of the causes of these differences between various sets of guidelines are straightforward. Some of the guidelines were developed more recently than others and had access to more up-to-date data. The focus or audiences differ; some, such as the WCRF-AICR guidelines, were designed for the entire world, while others, such as the ACS guidelines, were designed for the English-speaking countries of North America, with different realities in terms of physical activity, means of food preparation, traditional diets, and the like. In some cases recommendations were geared to answer only a specific question rather than to be all-encompassing recommendations for the total diet. For example, one specific question might be "do high doses of certain vitamins prevent cancer?" Also, although all of the guidelines tend to be evidence based, the processes for evaluating the evidence and the relative weighting systems used by different groups varied. For example, in certain studies of these links by the Office of Medical Applications of Research and the Agency for Health Care Research on Quality (OMAR-AHRQ) of the U.S. Department of Health and Human Services, randomized clinical trials were given the heaviest weight and in some cases nonrandomized studies or observational studies were given very much less weight or totally excluded, and animal and laboratory studies were also excluded. Such procedures leave very little evidence to evaluate because very few randomized studies of diet and cancer prevention have been done. Therefore, by its very nature, this sort of a rating process is likely to be more conservative than the procedures followed by the WCRF-AICR, or those used by ACS, where the prevailing philosophy is to include epidemiological studies of many different types, as well as other forms of evidence in examining associations.

Systematic reviews also differ in the credence they place on the relevance of animal tests for forecasting human cancer risks and the assumptions that are used to make such conclusions. At present a realistic prediction of risk of cancer in humans from animal studies is sometimes difficult. Whether it is, therefore, reasonable to adopt the Lalonde doctrine (e.g., that action is necessary even if all the scientific evidence is not yet in) or the precautionary principle is a matter on which judgments are likely to vary widely.

Another possible cause of differences between evidence reviews is that many rely on the volunteer effort and goodwill of individuals who have other responsibilities. They may vary in the thoroughness with which they search the literature and in how complete their reviews are. The expert panels that make the final judgment call may still have conflicts of commitment and disposition, even if they are free of financial bias or conflicts of interest, and these may color their deliberations and cause differences.

NUTRITION GUIDELINES AND THE FUTURE

What kinds of nutritional recommendations are likely to emerge? Several trends deserve consideration in this regard, which are also discussed elsewhere (Dwyer, 2001).

Improving Documentation: Systemic Evidence-Based Reviews as the Basis of Guidelines

It is unsettling to professionals and consumers alike to find that some so-called *systematic evidence reviews* come to different conclusions and for reasons that are not easily discernible by users of the final product. For systematic reviews to develop better diet-related recommendations, there is a need to agree on standard protocols to be used and to apply them. Current evidence-based systematic review methods leave much to be desired. There is no commonly agreed upon framework and set of standards for investigating dietary recommendations in a systematic manner; each expert group uses its own criteria, which often differ in ways that are important enough to result in different advice. A commonly agreed upon standard and format for systematic reviews would be helpful.

There is a need for further development of systematic, evidence-based review methods for developing diet-related recommendations. Dietary recommendations involve many different dietary components and interactions among them. Relevant randomized double-blinded clinical trials of sufficient length to yield definitive data on health outcomes are rarely available. Therefore, other less definitive types of evidence must be used. At the same time, there is often a great deal of material not only from human studies but also from animal experiments and *in vitro* studies that may be informative. All experts agree that the criteria for inferring causality in the diet–disease interrelationship includes the strength of the association or magnitude of the effect, consistency of the association, temporality of the association, dose–response relationships, specificity of the association, and biological plausibility. However, the relative weights given to these different types of evidence, and particularly non-clinical trials, epidemiological, and animal studies remains under dispute. Evidence reviews may differ in that some include the use of surrogate or intermediate markers of disease development, whereas others include only health outcomes with respect to actual disease or death. Risks and safety issues and benefits must also be considered. Finally, the level of certainty about the evidence needs to be indicated in systematic reviews and kept in mind when making recommendations.

Bioactives

A particularly nettlesome set of problems is what to do about providing advice on intakes of various bioactives, and what kinds of data are necessary to do this. At the very least, the unique functions of the various phytochemicals and zoochemicals and other bioactive substances in foods that are not the classic nutrients need to be elucidated, the amounts of these substances in foods determined, animal testing results evaluated, bioavailability in humans assessed, and both short- and long-term feeding trials completed in order to determine their potency for health enhancement. Quantitative recommendations and whether such bioactives should be used for food fortification and dietary supplements await the development of such information.

More Realistic Recommendations

Systematic reviews represent the beginning, and not the end, of generating useful dietary recommendations to the public on diet and cancer. Because dietary advice involves total diet and applies to one of the major activities of daily living, additional considerations, such as cost, ease of preparation, and palatability, must also be taken into account. These are issues not needing attention in most studies of drug therapies. The degree to which recommendations vary from current diets and the alterations in supply and demand that might be called for in the food supply if the recommendations are followed also need to be examined. The use of mathematical modeling may be helpful in these regards; it was used by the 2005 Dietary Guidelines Committee with good results. The Dietary Guidelines Committee used a series of food patterns with a range of intakes; food groups were established and assigned nutrients values based on the actualities of what people really ate, not on what foods in the group might be optimal. Then successive approximations were made to develop estimates of the types and amounts of each of the traditional food groups, or subgroups, were necessary to meet the DRI. Finally, because most dietary issues involve public policy, consultation and discussion within the broad scientific community about the recommendations is important, especially in areas where emerging science seems to be particularly promising, but results are not yet definitive.

Greater Complexity of Nutrition Guidelines

Over the past century, dietary advice has become increasingly well documented, complex, and quantitative. Recommendations now include not only quantitative goals for achieving nutrient adequacy but also goals that are increasingly quantitative relating to variety, moderation, balance, proportionality, and avoidance of excess. And the cancer-specific systematic reviews include the possible effects of diet at particular sites and stages, as well as overall. Some preliminary recommendations have been made on secondary prevention. The guidelines are likely to become even more complex and specific and more prescriptive. Health professionals will need to help consumers interpret and apply them.

Encouraging Greater Adherence

In spite of the proliferation of dietary guidelines and the widespread availability of tasty and reasonably priced foods, there is little evidence that consumers today find it easier to make healthful choices than they did with simpler advice given in the past. Population dietary intakes may have improved, but most of that increase is probably due to the greater affluence of the population, food availability, and distributive justice with respect to income. Nutrition educators and communicators recognize that even when consumer motivation is high, consumers find it is very difficult for such advice to be incorporated into healthful choices. The advice is simply too complicated to apply in daily living without additional help. More tailoring of advice to individuals can help to remedy these problems (Dwyer, 1993).

Striking the Appropriate Balance between Simplicity and Complexity in Providing Dietary Guidelines

Striking the appropriate balance between simple actionable messages and more complex and complete ones remains a challenge for all of those giving nutritional advice.

Strategies Other than Dietary Recommendations for Changing the American Diet in More Healthful Directions

Dietary change is not easy and requires more than simply the promulgation of guidelines; alterations in the food supply, the food acquisition environment, and additional nutrition education efforts are also necessary. "Blaming the cook" for failing to provide appropriate food choices is inappropriate; cooks and eaters need assistance to make, serve, and choose more healthful foods and to make what the recommendations say what is served and eaten (Dwyer, 1993). What is important is to have a rationally thought through set of options that can be acted upon, regardless of the method chosen to bring about the dietary change.

Dietary recommendations are a path to improving diets in healthful directions that are based on a demand-driven strategy. Two other options are to make the most healthful foods more readily available by a variety of mechanisms that alter supply rather than demand and marketing foods or dietary supplements high in one or more of the healthful constituents. The most effective way to alter dietary intake depends on what the target group is intended to benefit, the narrowness of the therapeutic versus the toxic threshold for the dietary constituent, and many other issues that vary from one dietary component to another. There is no one strategy that is correct.

Individualization of Dietary Guidance

Various eating patterns are evident that differ in use of the food groups, nutrient adequacy, and health outcomes. However, each of the dietary patterns have some positive nutritional points, and each provides a start for building healthier diets and a way to meet preferences and give joy to eating while promoting the individual's personal ownership in health. Thus, it is vital to tailor nutritional guidance on the basis of eating realities. One step to make nutrition recommendations more accessible and more easily implemented is the individualization movement. Individualization aims at trying to find ways that help people to tailor their eating in actionable and practical ways that do not require detailed advice by a personal dietary counselor or coach. Originally dietary guidelines were conceived of as broad population-based advice that could be used by all adults as guides for planning sensible eating. In fact, consumer research revealed that most people do not want general guidance; they want guidance that is very specific to their particular condition, likes, and dislikes (Borra et al., 2001). No matter what nutritionists say, people eat as they wish. Consumers demand nutritional advice tailored to them as eaters.

Until recently individualization implied "going it alone" to customize these tools for one's own specific purposes by oneself. In the past few years, federal dietary guidance has begun to recognize the need to individualize and to tailor guidance to individuals' particular needs and wants. It also provides some of the help people need to apply dietary guidance to their own lifestyles in actionable ways. Government web sites now include interactive programs to assist consumers in the process. For example, the Healthy Eating Index is now available on the web, in an interactive form that allows people to self assess their own intakes. (See www.nal.usda.gov/fnic/HEI/HEI.html, accessed May 2005.) In addition, the USDA food group pyramid (see www.mypyramid.gov) can now be customized, individualized, and fine-tuned to a greater extent than ever before; and other nutrition education tools have also been individualized (Hoolihan, 2003).

No perfect diet exists that is desired by everyone and ideal for everyone from the health standpoint. Individualization trends are likely to continue and expand in the next few years to help consumers achieve the additional flexibility they want and need in eating. This can be done by careful planning that considers the relative nutrient content of different foods, especially foods within each group, and makes appropriate substitutions. Food availability and cost must also be considered because it is impractical and makes little sense to provide a pattern that specifies foods that are unavailable or cost too much for consumers to afford.

It may be helpful to develop special sets of dietary guidelines and pyramids for certain groups. For example, adolescent girls and women of childbearing age need extra iron and folic acid. The elderly need a readily available source of vitamin B12 and a dietary source of vitamin D, especially if they have dark skin and are not exposed to sufficient ultraviolet light. Individualized eating plans can incorporate these considerations.

It is also possible and desirable to tailor individualized eating by demographics, lifestyles, preferences, and other goals. There is a need to do this and to customize diets for different consumer segments by age, sex, energy level, social factors, and health status.

In the meantime, people still need advice to help them choose wisely, to eat well, and to enjoy their food. They also need ways to individualize their eating in healthful directions that fit their lifestyles and preferences. The most recent ACS guidelines provide somewhat more individualization than prior versions; they focus on foods and dietary patterns rather than specific nutrients and on physical activity and obesity prevention. They permit more personal ownership of healthy lifestyles and incorporate the individual's likes and dislikes, increasing the pleasure that comes from eating and minimizing nonadherence. The ACS guidelines have also done a good job of identifying key consumer segments with similar health concerns, such as those at different stages in cancer prevention or recovery or those with different cancers if they are already ill or in recovery. The ACS guidelines provide the evidence for individualizing and customizing or tailoring on the basis of what is known about the biology and responses to various dietary strategies of the different cancers.

Much remains to be done in tailoring and customizing dietary advice by social and psychological factors. Eating habits and patterns are quite disparate; starting with existing patterns, it is possible to make all of them more healthful with some relatively straightforward dietary advice. The stage of readiness for change is thought to be important and associated with outcomes. Additional tailoring for large consumer groups with common needs, wants, and demographics will be important in the future. Data are now at hand to do this by age, stage in cancer, site of the cancer, and various lifestyle factors using a market segmentation model. Thus, the goal of developing advice for similar groups from the biological standpoint and similar lifestyles and preferences is within reach.

To make individualization a reality, four factors that may be helpful are (1) to use an individualized template or graphic (such as the USDA pyramid); (2) concerns must be prioritized; (3) the focus should be on liked foods; and (4) the time segments for eating foods and meals should be individualized and make sense to users.

Individuals and patients will get information from some source even if health professionals do not provide it. The alternative sources (the Internet, friends, family, and the mass media) are less likely to be soundly based in the evidence than are health professionals. Therefore, health professionals owe it to consumers to provide them with assistance on how to interpret information.

Do Gene-Specific Dietary Guidelines Make Sense Today?

Consumers are interested but also frightened about the implications of genetic information. One concern is genetic determinism—that genes predict everything about the individual's future. Such forebodings of inevitability are overblown, and for most of the common diseases including cancer, it is impossible to predict when, how severely, or even whether a person with a genetic predisposition will ultimately develop the disease.

Genetic influences in monogenic diseases are already well understood. In contrast, for many of the most common chronic degenerative diseases such as for the cancers, the specific molecular mechanisms, and the relevant genes are only beginning to be completed. Thus, for many of these diseases genetic information is not yet available or identified in sufficient detail. For others, the information is very expensive to obtain and may not be sufficiently reliable to be definitive.

Even when information is available and reliable, a second quandary is whether the genetic information will be used, especially for preventive or therapeutic measures. Some individuals might in fact use such information; others are unlikely to, because they often fail to act on other health-related information.

There are also practical concerns about genetic testing, such as who requests genetic testing, who decides whether a genetic test is done, who pays for it, and who decides how to disseminate the results of such a test. Others are concerned about the use of genetic information and how it might be misused to restrict access to health insurance (Clayton, 2003). Indeed, these concerns are serious enough that Congress has taken action to ensure that much genetic information on individuals is kept private and that discrimination on the basis of it is not permitted.

What about including the genetic profile in tailoring? Can diets be personalized by recourse to genetics? Nutrigenetics, or exploring genetic variations among individuals in their nutritional responses, is done today for phenylketonuria (PKU) and with respect to the LDL heterogeneity that occurs on low-fat diets, and polymorphisms to MTHFR and folic acid metabolism. The idea of nutrigenomic diets is to use food to prevent disease by identifying genetic predispositions for chronic conditions that can be mitigated by proper diet. The promise of being able to provide gene-specific dietary guidelines that factor in the genetic variability that accounts for a good deal of our individual responses to diet is alluring and has great appeal to consumers and health professionals alike (Young, 2001; DeBusk et al., 2005). Indeed, in certain respects gene-specific dietary tailoring is already upon us. Some examples include dietary therapy for monogenic defects such as PKU, dietary advice to avoid foods that alter the cytochrome P450 system and some of the drug metabolizing enzymes, and the natural aversion many people have to saccharin because they are genetically bitter tasters, whereas others are not.

However, the soundness of nutrigenomic diet plans for chronic disease risk reduction remains to be determined. Unfortunately, although systems biology is moving forward rapidly, scientists are still far from identifying the common polymorphisms involved in the major diseases including the cancers that are genetically relevant and that can be altered by dietary counseling. Seamless mechanisms from the "omics" to eating that include not only genetics but epigenetic changes and lifetime experience, as well as one's current diet, in diet planning are not yet in place. That is, nutrigenomic diets for chronic diseases such as cancer are not yet ready for "prime time." All that exists is proof of concept. There is questionable reduction in risk with nutritional advice provided by those advocating such measures. Even seemingly similar diseases, including such diseases as breast cancer, may be quite disparate genetically. Nevertheless, it is apparent that a wide range of genes and related single nucleotide polymorphisms are modifiable by nutrients, and once identified, it should be possible to devise diet strategies. However, the major chronic diseases are extremely heterogeneous genetically. Although a number of kits are available on the market that purport to provide dietary advice on the basis of genetic information, in fact their utility or veracity of dietary advice based on them remains dubious and their cost prohibitive, and beneficial health outcomes from their use have not been reported. Therefore, the benefits are clearly unproven. Individualized nutritional recommendations based on genetic information will be possible when we have identified most of the genetically relevant polymorphisms and genetic variability in these diseases. Also, inexpensive complete and available genetic or metabolic profiles of risk factors for complex chronic diseases also will be necessary. Additional needed information includes metabolite measures, databases on phenotypes, a clearer understanding of causal pathways, and effects of diet changes on biochemical and metabolic events. In addition to knowing and measuring the risks, the appropriate dietary interventions must be identified. Personalized disease is a reality today. As we learn more about the genome, personalized nutritional therapy may become a reality, but today it remains a goal for the future.

What Will Government Programs Do to Implement the Guidelines?

What individuals do about adhering to the dietary guidelines is up to them. However, government also has a role in disseminating information about what constitutes healthful eating, to educate people about food choice, and to ensure a food supply that accurately reflects its own dietary advice. Government has produced excellent evidence-based information on what constitutes healthful eating. The problem is that it is accessible largely over the Internet and World Wide Web; this means a sizable proportion of the population will be unaware of it. A few excellent fledgling federal and state efforts have begun on nutrition education, although these are largely web-based, and this again limits their reach. However, what government has so far failed to do is to indicate how federal food policy and federal food programs will change as a result of these documents. The *Dietary Guidelines* are supposed to underpin government nutritional policy and federal food programs including school meals. As yet there has been little movement among political authorities in charge of these programs to alter them in ways that bring them more in line with the guidelines.

Restoring Energy Balance and Healthy Weights

The greatest challenge the *Dietary Guidelines* and MyPyramid face is finding ways to restore energy balance at a healthy weight in a sedentary population that is surrounded by tasty foods everywhere. The 2005 guidelines make it clear that the healthiest way to reduce calories is to avoid added sugars, certain fats, and alcohol, all of which are high in calories and low in essential nutrients. The concept of discretionary calories hammers the point home about how little discretion is available for persons with very sedentary lifestyles. However, energy output must be increased, and this is another considerable challenge.

Policy on Foods to Avoid

It is more palatable from the standpoint of advice to emphasize foods that need to be eaten. Trade associations readily endorse such advice and commodity interests that stand to benefit from such recommendations. The devil is in the details when foods that are to be avoided are mentioned; then there is often great pressure from the affected industries not to make such statements. If the advice is wrong, it can wreak economic havoc. The dietary guidelines have been faulted both for not specifying foods to avoid more precisely and for mentioning other foods prominently.

Testing Health Outcomes of the Guidelines

The literature is far from definitive when it comes to recommending the "best" diet for health. This is because there are very few randomized, long-term, well-controlled clinical trials available to provide data. Instead, observational epidemiology must be employed (Schneider, 2005). The Dietary Approaches to Stop Hypertension (DASH) diet was originally developed in an NIH-sponsored clinical intervention study to reduce blood pressure levels in persons with hypertension. The 2005 MyPyramid recommendations are fairly similar to the DASH diet, although the DASH diet has less discretionary fat and sugar than MyPyramid. DASH has been tested in a controlled feeding situation and found to be effective. However, it remains to be seen what the effects of this diet are on risk reduction in free-living, free-eating community settings.

The most pressing issues remaining are to truly test whether following the *Dietary Guidelines* actually does improve nutrient intakes and metabolic biomarkers of health (e.g., body mass index, lipid metabolism, cardiovascular disease, type 2 diabetes, cancer, osteoporosis). Also of interest is whether teaching children or adults to eat according to the dietary guidelines and MyPyramid pattern or according to cancer-specific guidelines actually carries over into better health during adulthood.

What Health Professionals and Consumers Can Do Now

Experience with the *Dietary Guidelines*, the Pyramid, and cancer-specific guidelines suggests that they have been helpful, but that more attention needs to be paid to them by Americans in their eating choices. Therefore, the advice set forth in the following subsections is appropriate to all consumers.

Look for the Dietary Guidelines and Your Pyramid

Dietary guidelines and pyramids are good for nutrition education because they catch people's attention and turn their thoughts, however fleetingly, toward nutrition. They are popular nutrition education tools and suitable guides for much policy, but they cannot do everything. Additional nutrition information and education are also necessary to bring about eating behavior change.

Do More, Then Eat More

Those who are more physically active can eat more food and eat food that is less nutrient dense and still stay in energy balance while still meeting their nutrient needs.

Make Dietary Choices at the Appropriate Calorie Level, and Do Not Forget Physical Activity

Most Americans and many persons elsewhere in the world are very sedentary. Ultimately, the answer is to increase energy output and to become more physically active. Until they do, they may need only ~1500–2000 kcal/day. They need to find a pyramid that provides an eating plan at their level, and then they must follow the *Dietary Guidelines* quite closely. The lower the energy output, the more constrained are dietary choices if the *Dietary Guidelines* are to be followed.

Eat by the Dietary Guidelines and YourPyramid

There is no question that an eating plan based on current science as embodied in the *Dietary Guidelines* is better than willy-nilly selection of whatever food is available. The differences between the guidelines issued by professional and health organizations are relatively small compared with lack of a pattern altogether.

Choose Nutrient Dense Foods within each Group if you are Sedentary

For those who are sedentary, nutrient density is important in making food choices. They must choose foods within each food group that are high in nutrient density if they are to meet the DRI and the *Dietary Guidelines* without consuming excessive amounts of calories, or undue reliance on fortified foods and supplements to provide micronutrients.

Take Small Steps toward the Dietary Guidelines Today

Behavior change is clearly necessary. The proposed intakes in all of the *Dietary Guidelines* and Pyramids, including the likely revisions in these tools today, are quite different from current eating patterns. Therefore, in order to follow them, people are going to have to change their diets considerably.

Use Additional Tools Such as Cancer-Specific Guidelines if Necessary

On top of these recommendations, some individuals may also choose to use cancer-specific guidelines for planning their eating lives.

CONCLUSIONS

Nutritional guidelines based on systematic reviews of the scientific evidence that are well interpreted can have positive effects on the health of the public and ultimately upon the public health (Schneider, 2005). Nutritional recommendations have changed little from those of the early twentieth century, when a plant-based diet with liberal amounts of fruits and vegetables was first suggested, to today. However, the rationale for such recommendations has changed from an emphasis solely on economy to greater understanding of why such recommendations are healthful. Unfortunately, adherence to dietary recommendations remains relatively low. In order to decrease cancer risks and maximize quality of life, diet must be placed in the context of overall risk reduction strategies. Recommendations for cancer risk reduction and cancer treatment or postrecovery differ and need to be geared to the target population of interest.

References

Ades, T., Gansler, T., Miller, M., and Rosenthal, D.S. 2001. PC-SPES: current evidence and remaining questions. *CA Cancer J Clin* **51**: 199–205.

American Institute for Cancer Research. 2005. "The New American Plate Cookbook; Recipes for a Healthy Weight and a Healthy Life." University of California Press, Berkeley, CA.

American Institute of Cancer Research/World Cancer Research Fund. 1997. "Food, Nutrition, and the Prevention of Cancer: A Global Perspective Summary." Washington, DC.

Barr, S.I., Murphy, S.P., and Poos, M.I. 2002. Interpreting and using the dietary reference intakes in dietary assessment of individuals and groups. *J Am Dietet Assoc* **2**: 780–788.

Borra, S., Kelly, L., Tuttle, M., and Neville, K. 2001. Developing actionable dietary guidance messages: dietary fat as a case study. *J Am Dietet Assoc* **101**: 678–684.

Brown, J.K., Byers, T., Doyle, C., Courneya, K.S., Demark-Wahnefried, W., Kushi, L.H., McTiernann, A., Rock, C.L., Aziz, N., Bloch, A.S., Eldridge, B., Hamilton, K., Katzin, C., Koonce, A., Main, J., Mobley, C., Morra, M.E., Pierce, M.S., and Sawyer, D.A. 2003. Nutrition and physical activity during and after cancer treatment: an American cancer society Guide to Informed Choices. *CA Cancer J Clin* **53**: 268–291.

Byers, T. 1999. The role of epidemiology in developing nutritional recommendations: past, present and future. *Am J Clin Nutr* **69**: 11304S–11305S.

Clayton, E.W. 2003. Ethical, legal and social implications of genomic medicine. *N Engl J Med* **348**: 562–569.

Committee on Diet and Health Diet and Health. 1989. "Implications for Chronic Disease Risk," National Academy Press, Washington, DC.

Committee on Dietary Guidelines Implementation. 1990. "Improving America's Diet and Health: From Recommendations to Action" (Paul R. Thomas, ed.). National Academy Press, Washington, DC.

Davis, C., and Saltos, E. 1995. "Dietary Recommendations and How They Have Changed over Time." US Department of Agriculture and Economic Research Service, Washington, DC.

DeBusk, R.M., Fogarty, C.M., and Ordovas, J. 2005. Nutritional genomics in practice: where do we begin? *J Am Dietet Assoc* **105**: 585–598.

Dietary Guidelines Advisory Committee. 2004. "Report of the Dietary Guidelines for Americans." US Department of Agriculture and Agricultural Research Science, Washington, DC, Lippincott Williams and Wilkins.

Dwyer, J.T. 2005. Dietary guidelines: national perspective. *In* "Modern Nutrition in Health and Disease" (M.E. Shils, M. Shike, A.C. Ross, B. Cabellero, and R.J. Cousins, eds.), 9th edition.

Dwyer, J. 1983. Dietary recommendations and policy implications. *In* "Nutrition Update" (J. Weininger, and G.M. Briggs, eds.), pp. 315–355. John Wiley, New York.

Dwyer, J. 2004. Nutritional requirements and dietary assessment. *In* "Harrison's Principles of Internal Medicine" (Kasper et al., ed.), 16th edition, Chapter 60, pp. 399–403. McGraw-Hill, New York.

Dwyer, J., Bermudez, O.I., Chwang, L.C., Koehn, K., and Chen, C.L. 2002. Dietary guidelines in three regions of the world. *In* "Handbook of Nutrition and Food" (Berdanier, Carlyn D., ed.), pp. 353–371. CRC Press, Boca Raton, FL.

Dwyer, J.T. 1993. Diet and nutritional strategies for cancer risk reduction: focus on the 21st century. *Cancer Res* **72**: 1024–1031.

Dwyer, J.T. 2001. Nutrition guidelines and education of the public. *J Nutr* **131**: 3074S–3077S.

Eyre, H., Kahn, R., Robertson, R.M., Clark, N.G., Doyle, C., Hong, Y., Gaisler, T., Glynn, T., Smith, R.A., Taubert, K., and Thun, M.J. 2005. Preventing cancer, cardiovascular disease and diabetes: a common agenda for American Cancer Society, the American Diabetes Association and the American Heart Association. Submitted to *Stroke*.

Harpham, W.S. 2001. Alternative therapies for curing cancer: what do patients want? What do patients need? *CA Cancer J Clin* **51**: 131–136.

Haughton, B., Gussow, J.D., and Dodds, J.M. 1987. An historical study of underlying assumptions for US food guides from 1917 through the Basic 4 Food Group. *Guide J Nutr* **19**: 169–175.

Hogbin, M., Lyon, J., and Davis, C. 2003. Comparison of dietary recommendations using the dietary guidelines for Americans as a framework. *Nutr Today* **38**: 204–217.

Holland, J.C. 1982. Why patients seek unproven cancer remedies: a psychological perspective. *CA Cancer J Clin* **32**: 10–14.

Hoolihan, L.E. 2003. Individualization of nutrition recommendations and food choices. *Nutr Today* **38**: 225–231.

Kennedy, E. 1994. Dietary guidelines, food guidance and dietary quality. *In* "Handbook of Nutrition and Food" (Berdanier, C.D., ed.), Chapter 11, pp. 339–352. CRC Press, Boca Raton, FL.

Kennedy, E., Ohls, J., Carlson, S., and Fleming, K. 1994. "Healthy Eating Index, Final Report." Food and Nutrition Service, US Department of Agriculture, Alexandria, VA.

McMurray, K.Y. 2003. Setting dietary guidelines: the US process. *J Am Dietet Assoc* **103**(Suppl 2): S10–S16.

Murphy, S.P. 2001. Nutrition guidelines to maintain health. *In* "Nutrition in the Prevention and Treatment of Disease" (A.M. Coulston, C.L. Rock, and E.R. Monsen, eds.), Chapter 48, pp. 753–771. Academic Press, San Diego.

Prentice, R.L., Willett, W.C., Greenwald, P., Alberts, D., Bernstein, L., Boyd, N.F., Byers, T., Clinton, S.K., Fraser, G., Freedman, L., Hunter, D., Kipnis, V., Kolonel, L.N., Kristal, A, Kristal, B.S., Lampe, J.W., McTiernan, A., Milner, J., Patterson, R.E., Potter, J.D., Riboli, E., Schatzkin, A., Yates, A., and Yetley, E. 2004. Nutrition and physical activity and chronic disease prevention: research strategies and recommendations. *J Natl Cancer Inst* **96**: 1276–1287.

Read, M. 2004. The health promoting diet throughout life: adults. *In* "Report of the Dietary Guidelines for Americans Advisory Committee," Chapter 9, pp. 299–316. US Department of Health and Human Services and US Department of Agriculture, Washington, DC.

Report of the Task Force, American Society for Clinical Nutrition. 1979. The evidence relating 6 dietary factors to the nation's health: symposium." *Am J Clin Nutr* **32**(Suppl): 2610–2748S.

Rock, C.L. 2005. Dietary counseling is beneficial for the patient with cancer. *J Clin Oncol* **23**: 1348–1349.

Rock, C.L., and Demark-Wahnefried, W. 2002. Nutrition and survival after the diagnosis of breast cancer: a review of the evidence. *J Clin Oncol* **20**: 3302–3316.

Rosenthal, D., and Ades, T. 2001. Complementary and alternative methods. *CA Cancer J Clin* **51**: 316–320.

Schneider, A. 2005. Food FAQ's. *Nature* **433**: 798–799.

Surgeon General of the United States. 1977. Healthy People: Surgeon General's Report on Health Promotion and Disease Prevention. US Department of Health, Education and Welfare, Public Health Service. PHS Pub. 70: 55011, Washington, DC.

Thomson, C.A., Flatt, S.A., Rock, C.L., Ritenbaugh, C., Newman, V., and Pierce, J.P. 2002. Increased fruit, vegetable, and fiber intake and lower fat intake reported among women previously treated for invasive breast cancer. *J Am Dietet Assoc* **102**: 301–308.

Tsao, A.S, Kim, E.S., and Hong, W.K. 2004. Chemoprevention of cancer. *CA Cancer J Clin* **54**: 150–180.

US Department of Agriculture and US Department of Health and Human Services. 1980. "Nutrition and Your Health: Dietary Guidelines for Americans," 1st edition. Home and Garden Bulletin No. 232, US Government Printing Office, Washington, DC.

US Department of Agriculture and US Department of Health and Human Services. 1985. "Nutrition and Your Health: Dietary Guidelines for Americans," 2nd edition. Home and Garden Bulletin No. 232, US Government Printing Office, Washington, DC.

US Department of Agriculture and US Department of Health and Human Services. 1990. "Nutrition and Your Health: Dietary Guidelines for Americans," 3rd edition. Home and Garden Bulletin No. 232, US Government Printing Office, Washington, DC.

US Department of Agriculture and US Department of Health and Human Services. 1995. "Nutrition and Your Health: Dietary Guidelines for Americans," 4th edition. Home and Garden Bulletin No. 232, US Government Printing Office, Washington, DC.

US Department of Agriculture and US Department of Health and Human Services. 2000. "Nutrition and Your Health: Dietary Guidelines for Americans," 5th edition. Home and Garden Bulletin No. 232, US Government Printing Office, Washington, DC.

US Department of Agriculture and US Department of Health and Human Services. 2005. "Dietary Guidelines for Americans," 6th edition. Home and Garden Bulletin No. 232, US Government Printing Office, Washington, DC.

US Department of Health and Human Services, and US Department of Agriculture. 2005. "Finding Our Way to a Healthier You." US Government Printing Office, Washington, DC.

US Department of Health and Human Services. 2000. Healthy People 2010: Promoting Health, Preventing Disease—Objectives for the Nutritionist. Washington, DC.

Vickers, A. 2004. Alternative cancer cures: unproven or disproven. *CA Cancer J Clin* **54**: 100–118.

World Cancer Research Fund/American Institute for Cancer Research. 1997. Food, Nutrition and the Prevention of Cancer: A Global Perspective. American Institute for Cancer Research, Washington, DC.

Young, V.R. 2002. WO Atwater Award Lecture and 2001 ASNS President's Lecture; Human nutrient requirements: the challenges in a post-genomic era. *J Nutr* **132**: 624–619.

Zelman, K., and Kennedy, E. 2005. Naturally nutrient rich: putting more power on Americans' plates. *Nutrition Today* **40**: 60–70.

C H A P T E R

48

Dietary Interventions

LALITA KHAODHIAR AND GEORGE L. BLACKBURN

Ample evidence suggests that lifestyle and environmental factors can affect cancer risk (World Cancer Research Fund, American Institute for Cancer Research, 1997; Heggie et al., 2003; Blackburn, 2005; Blackburn and Waltman, 2005). In addition to tobacco use, which is associated with cancers of several sites, other modifiable risk factors include alcohol consumption (associated with increased risk of oral, esophageal, breast, and other cancers), physical inactivity (associated with increased risk of colon, breast, and possibly other cancers), and overweight (associated with colon, rectum, and prostate cancer in men, and endometrial, breast, and gallbladder cancer in women) (Vainio and Bianchini, 2002). Data from epidemiological studies have shown that avoiding excessive alcohol consumption, being physically active, and maintaining a healthy body weight may all contribute to reduction in the risk of certain cancers.

In obesity, increased release of free fatty acids, tumor necrosis factor-α (TNF-α), and resistin and reduced release of adiponectin from adipose tissue lead to the development of insulin resistance and compensatory chronic hyperinsulinemia. Increased insulin concentrations result in increased concentrations of bioavailable insulin-like growth factor-1 (IGF-1), which signal through respective receptors to promote cellular proliferation and inhibit apoptosis in a way that might contribute to tumorigenesis (Calle and Kaaks, 2004). Because many cancers do not respond to cancer therapy, it is important to recognize that the risk of developing obesity-associated diseases can be diminished or avoided through dietary and lifestyle interventions.

When compared with tobacco use, however, the effect of dietary intervention can be modest, and the strength of evidence is often weaker. The role of dietary intervention has been compromised by the epidemic of obesity and its correlates: sedentary behavior, poor nutrition, and chronic disease. Because of the major change in the American diet, the homogeneity of the diet, and weak assessment instruments (Bingham et al., 2003), certain cohort studies may distort the evaluation of dietary intervention. This will be particularly true of subjects in these cohorts with the metabolic syndrome. Thus, obesity is a major covariant and must be controlled for accordingly.

The role of nutrition in the etiology and prevention of cancer has also been of intense interest. In the past 25 years, the period in which the obesity epidemic has escalated, hundreds of observational studies have examined the relation between diet and cancers (Blackburn, 2005). Certain international studies have shown that fruit and vegetable consumption reduces risk for a number of cancers (Sauvaget et al., 2003; Miller et al., 2004; Rashidkhani et al., 2005; Shannon et al., 2005), whereas other studies indicate that dietary fat intake may increase risk (Wynder et al., 1997; Bingham et al., 2003; Chlebowski et al., 2005). Results from several prospective studies fail to find evidence of a protective effect from fruits and vegetables or a deleterious effect from dietary fat (Blackburn and Waltman, 2005). For example, published data from two large cohort studies, the Nurses' Health Study (NHS) and the Health Professionals' Follow-up Study (HPFS) (which together include >109,000 participants), found no correlation between fruit and vegetable intake and overall cancer incidence (Hung et al., 2004).

In addition, data from several randomized, placebo-controlled clinical trials on the role of vitamins and/or minerals (alone or in combination) in preventing total or site-specific cancers have not been promising. This may reflect an impaired response due to the increasing prevalence

Copyright © 2006, Elsevier Inc.
All rights of reproduction in any form reserved.

of obesity and the decrease in physical activity. The main micronutrients tested include β-carotene, α-tocopherol, selenium, and retinol. Evidence-based investigation requires results for RCTs, case-control studies, and prospective epidemiology studies with a sufficient range of food intake, macronutrient intake, and vitamin/mineral nutrient intake to investigate the relationship between dietary habits and cancer (Blackburn, 2005). This chapter reviews evidence from epidemiological studies, results from clinical trials on nutrition strategies in the prevention of major cancers, and the mechanisms by which individual constituents of diet may affect the cancer process.

UPPER AERODIGESTIVE TRACT CANCERS (HEAD AND NECK CANCERS)

Oral cancers and those of the pharynx and larynx are usually referred to as *upper aerodigestive tract cancers* or *head and neck cancers*. In the United States, head and neck cancers account for ~3% of all malignancies, with an estimated 37,200 new cases and 11,000 deaths annually (U.S. Department of Health and Human Services, 2004). Oral cancer is more common in men than in women, with the highest incidence in black men. Oral premalignant lesions (i.e., leukoplakia, oral submucous fibrosis, erythroplakia) and dysplasia often precede invasive oral cancers.

Squamous cell carcinoma accounts for >90% of upper aerodigestive tract cancers. Between 40 and 50% of head and neck cancers are diagnosed early, at stages I and II. Treatment given at this stage is relatively successful, and such patients usually have a good prognosis, with a 5-year relative survival rate of 60–90%. However, many of the patients develop local recurrence or secondary primary cancers in other sites within the head and neck. Secondary primary tumors are estimated to occur at an annual rate of 3–10% and are significant threats to long-term survival (Cooper et al., 1989; Rhee et al., 2004).

Dietary Risk Factors

It is well known that tobacco use is a major cause of cancers of the head and neck and is responsible for 90% of oral cancer deaths in men (Cinciripini and McClure, 1998). The combination of alcohol consumption and tobacco use substantially and synergistically increases the risk compared with the risk of either alone. Both tobacco and alcohol use are associated with development of oral premalignant lesions (Hashibe et al., 2000; Thomas et al., 2003).

Epidemiological studies worldwide have suggested that dietary and nutritional factors are involved in the development of upper aerodigestive tract cancers (Winn et al., 1984; McLaughlin et al., 1988; Gridley et al., 1990; Negri et al., 1991; Zheng et al., 1992; Kune et al., 1993; Levi et al., 1998; De Stefani et al., 1999a,b; Franceschi et al., 1999; Bosetti et al., 2000; Tavani et al., 2001; Rajkumar et al., 2003; Sanchez et al., 2003; Rodriguez et al., 2004). Dietary information in these case-control studies was collected using food frequency questionnaires. These case-control studies have consistently reported that high fruit intake decreases the risk of oropharyngeal and laryngeal cancers, particularly in those who use tobacco and/or drink alcohol. It is estimated that high intake of fruits may decrease the risk of oral and pharyngeal cancers by 20–80% (Winn, 1995; Levi et al., 1998). Most but not all of these studies have also shown a protective effect from fiber in the form of vegetable intake. Some studies have also reported an inverse association among whole grain foods, legumes, fish, milk, cereal, monounsaturated fat, β-carotene, vitamin C–containing foods, and risk of cancer.

One study, performed in African Americans, reported that the relation of fruits and vegetables and cancer was stronger in men than in women, and that consumption of vitamin C and fiber was protective only in men. Conversely, high meat intake, particularly red and processed meat, has been shown to increase cancer risk. One study from Switzerland reported that high meat intake accounted for ~50% of oral and pharyngeal cancer in that population (Levi et al., 1998). Another study found that risk also increased with certain indigenous dietary practices, including high intake of chili powder and wood stove cooking (Notani and Jayant, 1987). To date, the most consistent dietary findings across multiple cultural backgrounds are the carcinogenic effect of high alcohol consumption and the protective effect of high fruit intake.

Nutrition Interventions

Several chemoprevention studies of head and neck squamous cell carcinomas have been conducted. Chemoprevention is defined as the use of specific natural or synthetic chemical agents to reverse, suppress, or prevent carcinogenesis. Primary prevention studies entail the treatment of oral premalignant lesions with chemopreventive agents to prevent malignant conversion. Secondary prevention is the use of chemopreventive agents to reduce the rate of secondary primary cancers. The agents most often studied include retinoids, β-carotene, α-tocopherol, and ascorbic acid.

Most early intervention trials for head and neck cancer have shown good overall response with these substances, particularly in primary prevention. However, high relapse rates and serious side effects have been reported, most related to the retinoid compounds (Benner et al., 1993; Sankaranarayanan and Mathew, 1996; Sankaranarayanan et al., 1997). In addition, large prospective randomized chemoprevention trials showed no benefit for supplementation with α-tocopherol, β-carotene, or retinyl palmitate (Gridley et al., 1992; Mayne et al., 2001a; Omenn et al., 1996a). The optimal dose and duration of treatment with these agents are yet to be resolved. Chemoprevention for head and neck cancer (and other cancers) remains investigational.

Vitamin A

Low levels of vitamin A (retinyl palmitate) are frequently seen in patients with stage III and IV head and neck cancers, as well as those with secondary primaries, suggesting a possible role of vitamin A deficiency as a cause of head and neck cancers (Murr et al., 1988). In animal studies, natural and synthetic vitamin A metabolites and analogs (retinoids) were found to suppress head and neck and lung carcinogenesis (Lotan, 1997a). The precise mechanism of vitamin A and its derivatives in the prevention of head and neck cancers is not fully understood. It is thought that these agents restore the expression of genes that regulate cell growth and differentiation. Most of these effects are mediated by nuclear retinoic acid receptors (RARα, β, and γ) and retinoid X receptors (RXRα, β, and γ), which function as retinoid-activated transcription factors (Lotan, 1996, 1997a,b; Lotan et al., 1995; Youssef et al., 2004).

An early randomized controlled study of tobacco chewers with oral leukoplakias showed that administration of vitamin A (60 mg/wk) for 6 months led to full remission in 57% of patients and complete suppression of new lesions in 100% of them. β-carotene (2.2 mmol/wk) induced remission of leukoplakias in 14.8% of patients and suppressed formation of new lesions in 50%. However, oral leukoplakias reappeared after vitamin A or β-carotene treatment was discontinued (Stich et al., 1988, 1991). Several other studies have also reported significant chemoprotective efficacy of retinoids, although none have examined their benefit in regard to mortality.

The European Study on Chemoprevention with Vitamin A and *N*-Acetylcysteine (EUROSCAN) was a large randomized study in >2500 patients with head and neck cancer or lung cancer; 93.5% were previous or current smokers. Participants were randomly assigned to receive retinyl palmitate (300,000 IU/day for 1 year followed by 150,000 IU/day for the second year), *N*-acetylcysteine (600 mg daily for 2 years), both compounds, or no intervention. After a median follow-up of 49 months, supplementation of retinyl palmitate and/or *N*-acetylcysteine resulted in no benefit in survival, event-free survival, or secondary primary tumors in patients with cancers of the head and neck and lungs (de Vries et al., 1999; van Zandwijk et al., 2000).

The potential roles of other retinoid compounds in chemoprevention of head and neck cancer have also been of interest. A landmark study published in 1986 showed that high doses of isotretinoin (13-cis-retinoic acids) (1–2 mg/kg/day for 3 months) were effective in treating for oral leukoplakias (Hong et al., 1986). There were major decreases in the size of the lesions in 67% of those given the drug and in 10% of those given placebo. Dysplasia was reversed in 54% of the drug group compared with 10% of the placebo group. However, >50% of patients who responded to treatment relapsed within 3 months after treatment. In addition, side effects were common, including cheilitis, facial erythema, and dryness and peeling of the skin. These side effects precluded widespread clinical use.

To overcome high rates of relapse and toxic reactions, the same group of investigators conducted further studies using lower doses of isotretinoin (Lippman et al., 1993). In one study, patients with leukoplakia were initially treated with high-dose isotretinoin (1.5 mg/kg/day) for 3 months. Those who had stable or improved lesions were then randomized to receive either 30 mg of β-carotene or low-dose isotretinoin (0.5 mg/kg/day) for 9 months. More than 90% of patients who received isotretinoin and 45% of those who received β-carotene responded to maintenance therapy with minimal toxicity.

A randomized trial of isotretinoin for the prevention of secondary primary cancers in patients previously curatively treated for head and neck cancer has been published (Perry et al., 2005). One hundred fifty-one patients were randomized to high-dose isotretinoin (1 mg/kg/day for 1 year followed by 0.5 mg/kg/day for 2 years), moderate-dose isotretinoin (0.5 mg/kg/day for 3 years), or placebo. The endpoint was the diagnosis of secondary primary cancer of the head and neck, lung, or bladder. After 3 years of treatment, isotretinion provided no advantages over placebo in the occurrence of secondary primary disease, recurrence of primary disease, or disease-free time.

β-Carotene

Epidemiological studies suggest that low dietary intake and low plasma concentration of antioxidant vitamins and minerals are associated with increased risk of cancer (Peto et al., 1981; Hong et al., 1986; Hennekens, 1994). Antioxidant vitamins, which include β-carotene (pro-vitamin A), vitamin E, and vitamin C, are hypothesized to decrease cancer risk, preventing tissue damage by trapping organic free radicals and/or deactivating excited oxygen molecules, a byproduct of many metabolic functions. In animal studies, β-carotene has been shown to inhibit oral carcinogenesis.

Earlier human studies have reported the response rate of oral leukoplakia to β-carotene to be as high as 44–71%, without significant toxicities (Garewal et al., 1990; Toma et al., 1992). One study used a combination of 30 mg of β-carotene, 1000 mg of ascorbic acid, and 800 IU of α-tocopherol per day for 9 months; clinical improvement was seen in 56% of the patients (Kaugars et al., 1994, 1996). The authors also noted that patients who reduced their use of alcohol or tobacco were more likely to respond to the treatment.

In a randomized, double-blinded, placebo-controlled clinical trial, 264 patients who had been curatively treated for early-stage head and neck cancer were randomized to receive 50 mg of β-carotene/day or placebo. After a median follow-up of 51 months, there were no differences between the two groups in overall mortality, local recurrence, and/or secondary primary tumors (Mayne et al., 2001a). Findings from two large randomized controlled trials reported an increase in lung cancer incidence and overall mortality with the combination of β-carotene and vitamin A (Omenn et al., 1996a) or β-carotene alone (Albanes et al., 1996). These outcomes prompted the discontinuation of β-carotene from many chemoprevention studies.

Vitamin E

α-Tocopherol (the most prevalent chemical form of vitamin E found in vegetable oils, seeds, grains, nuts, and other foods) has been used alone or in combination with other antioxidants in chemoprevention studies. In a single arm phase II study, 43 patients with symptomatic leukoplakia or dysplasia were treated orally with α-tocopherol (400 IU) twice daily for 24 weeks; 20 (46%) had clinical responses and 9 (21%) had histological responses (Benner et al., 1993).

In contrast, a randomized placebo-controlled trial in 540 patients with stage I or II head and neck cancer found unexpected adverse effects (Bairati et al., 2005). In the study, patients received supplementation with α-tocopherol, β-carotene, or placebo beginning on the first day of radiation therapy and for 3 years after radiation therapy. In the course of the trial, β-carotene was discontinued after 156 patients were enrolled. During the supplementation period, patients who received α-tocopherol had a higher rate of secondary primary cancers (hazard ratio [HR] 2.88) than patients who received placebo. However, after supplementation was discontinued (with a median follow-up of 52 months), prior users of α-tocopherol had a lower rate of primary cancers (HR = 0.41). After 8 years of follow-up, the incidence of secondary primary cancers was similar in both arms.

ESOPHAGEAL CANCER

In the year 2005, it is estimated that 14,520 Americans will be diagnosed with esophageal cancer and 13,570 will die of this cancer annually (American Cancer Society, 2005).

Two histological types account for the majority of esophageal cancers: adenocarcinoma and squamous cell carcinoma. In the 1960s, >90% of these cancers were squamous cell carcinomas, but in the United States and Western Europe, the incidence of esophageal adenocarcinoma has been steadily increasing. By the early 1990s, adenocarcinoma had become the most common cell type of esophageal cancer among white patients, although squamous cell cancers are still prevalent among black patients (Blot and McLaughlin, 1999). The prognosis for both types of cancer is poor, with a 5-year survival rate of <10%.

Dietary Risk Factors

Squamous Cell Carcinoma

In the United States and Western Europe, squamous cell carcinoma of the esophagus is strongly associated with tobacco and alcohol use. In China, where there are both high- and low-risk areas, esophageal cancer is associated with deficiencies of micronutrients and with exposure to specific carcinogens (e.g., *N*-nitroso compounds) (World Cancer Research Fund, 1997). These compounds are known to be animal carcinogens and can cause various alkyl DNA damages (Wang et al., 1997). Certain types of pickled vegetables and other food products consumed in high-risk areas are rich in *N*-nitroso compounds (Siddiqi et al., 1992). In other endemic regions, such as Iran, Russia, and South Africa, ingestion of very hot foods and beverages has been associated with this type of cancer (Ghadirian, 1987; Ghadirian et al., 1992).

Certain dietary factors may be protective. In a meta-analysis of 1 cohort study and 12 case-control studies, high intake of fruits and vegetables conferred significant protection against esophageal cancer (Riboli and Norat, 2003). Studies from Linxian, north-central China, where the incidence rate of esophageal and gastric cancer is among the world's highest, reported a 20% risk reduction with high consumption of eggs and fresh vegetables (Guo et al., 1994). Vitamins and minerals in these foods are believed to contribute to the reduced cancer risk. Low levels of serum selenium, retinol, and α-tocopherol have been linked to the development of squamous cell cancer of the esophagus and gastric cardia (Mark et al., 2000; Abnet et al., 2003; Taylor et al., 2003).

Adenocarcinoma

Adenocarcinoma of the esophagus is strongly associated with gastroesophageal reflux disease (GERD) and obesity (Lagergren et al., 1999; Mayne and Navarro, 2002). The risk increases with more frequent, more severe, and longer-lasting symptoms of reflux. Long-standing GERD is associated with Barrett's esophagus, a condition in which abnormal intestinal epithelium replaces the normal esophageal squamous epithelium (intestinal metaplasia). There are few dietary studies of adenocarcinoma of the esophagus. A series of case-control studies conducted in Sweden found that high fruit and vegetable intake contributed to a 50% lower risk of adenocarcinoma and a 40% lower risk of squamous cell carcinoma. Consuming fewer than three servings of fruits and vegetables per day accounted for ~20% of both types of cancer (Terry et al., 2001b).

Subjects with a high parallel intake of vitamin C, β-carotene, and α-tocopherol had a 40–50% decreased risk of both histological types of esophageal cancer compared with subjects with a low parallel intake (Terry et al., 2000). The risk reduction of esophageal cancers was more pronounced with vitamin C and β-carotene than with α-tocopherol. In addition, there was an inverse relation between total dietary cereal fiber intake in gastric cardia and esophageal adenocarcinoma, but not in squamous cell carcinoma (Terry et al., 2001c). Highest intake was defined as >14.7 g/day of cereal fiber from whole grain bread, crisp bread, oats, muesli, and other cold and hot breakfast cereals, pasta, and rice.

The authors hypothesized that the protective effects may be due to the ability of wheat fiber to neutralize mutagen formation from the conversion of salivary nitrites to nitrosamines. Another study from the United States found that diets high in total fat, saturated fat, and cholesterol were associated with an increased risk of adenocarcinoma of the esophagus and gastric cardia, while diets high in fiber, vitamin C, β-carotene, and folate were associated with reduced risk (Mayne and Navarro, 2002).

Nutrition Interventions

More than 20% of the population in Linxian (a rural county in Henan Province in north-central China) die from a combination of esophageal squamous cell carcinoma and gastric cardia cancer; both occur at the highest rates in the world. Persons with esophageal basal cell hyperplasia or dysplasia, a premalignant lesion affecting >20% of adults in this area, are at high risk of cancers of the esophagus and/or gastric cardia (Li, 1982). Chronically low intake of several nutrients and certain foods have been implicated in the pathogenesis of the cancers. Nutrition Intervention Trials (NITs), two separate randomized trials, were conducted in this region (Blot et al., 1993, 1995; Dawsey et al., 1993, 1994; Li et al., 1993; Guo et al., 1994; Taylor et al., 1994).

The first trial (NIT General Population Trial) assessed the effect of daily supplementation with four nutrient combinations: retinol and zinc; riboflavin and niacin; vitamin C and molybdenum; and β-carotene, α-tocopherol, and selenium. The sample included nearly 30,000 adults 40–69 years of age. Doses ranged from one to two times the U.S. Recommended Daily Allowances (RDAs) and were designed to supplement low levels rather than provide pharmacological doses. In the second trial (NIT Dysplasia Trial), 3318 people 40–69 years of age with biopsy-proven esophageal dysplasia received daily multiple vitamin-mineral supplementation (14 vitamins and 12 minerals) or placebo for 6 years. Doses two to three times the U.S. RDA were designed to normalize serum levels.

In the first trial, after 5.25 years of supplementation, small but significant reductions in mortality from total dysplasia (9%), total cancer (13%), and gastric cancer (cardia and noncardia combined) (21%) were seen in subjects receiving β-carotene, α-tocopherol, and selenium (but not the other nutrients). None of the four supplementation regimens affected the incidence of esophageal squamous cell and gastric cardia cancers.

There were no significant adverse effects on cause-specific mortality or cancer incidence for any of the four regimens. In the dysplasia trial, after 6 years of multiple vitamin and mineral supplementation, there were small but not significant reductions in mortality rates for total dysplasia (7%), total cancer (4%), and esophageal squamous cell cancer (16%). These studies suggested that restoring adequate intake of certain nutrients might lower the risk of cancer in high-risk populations.

To determine whether dietary supplementation affected precancerous esophageal lesions, 400 subjects with esophageal lesions (basal cell hyperplasia or dysplasia) in a high-risk area in China were randomly divided into two groups for intervention studies with calcium or decaffeinated green tea (Wang et al., 1993, 2002). In the calcium study, subjects were randomized to receive either 1200 mg/day of calcium carbonate or placebo for 11 months, while subjects in the green tea study were randomly assigned to receive either 5 mg of green tea or placebo for 12 months. Esophageal biopsies were performed at the beginning and end of the studies. At the end of the interventions, neither calcium supplementation nor decaffeinated green tea resulted in an improvement in precancerous lesions or abnormal cell proliferation patterns.

After 11 years of follow-up in the calcium study, 10 subjects (10%) in the calcium group developed esophageal cancer, compared with 8 (8%) in the placebo group. Thus, calcium supplementation showed no short- or long-term effects on esophageal cancer. In contrast, a study using multiple vitamin and mineral supplementation for 30 months suggested a modest benefit in squamous cell proliferation of the esophagus in high-risk populations (Rao et al., 1994).

GASTRIC CANCER

Gastric cancer is the fourth most common cancer and the second leading cause of cancer deaths worldwide (Parkin et al., 1999, 2005; Pisani et al., 1999; Plummer et al., 2004). Almost two-thirds of the cases occur in developing countries, 42% in China alone. In the United States, it is estimated that 21,860 Americans will be diagnosed with gastric cancer and 11,550 will die from the disease in 2005. There has been a steady decline in gastric cancer incidence and mortality in most countries. Most cancers in the United States are advanced at diagnosis, with an overall 5-year survival rate of 22.5%.

Dietary Risk Factors

Data from epidemiological studies show that high intake of salt and salted foods is a risk factor for gastric cancer (Tsugane, 2005). Salt intake is associated with *Helicobacter pylori* infection, a major risk factor for the disease. Together, salt and salted foods can act synergistically to promote the development of gastric cancer. A decline in the daily intake of salt in most developed countries may be partly responsible for a decline in gastric cancer rates.

Several case-control and cohort studies report protective effects of fruits and vegetables on gastric cancer (Riboli and Norat, 2003). Low levels of serum selenium, retinol, and α-tocopherol are associated with squamous cell cancer of the gastric cardia (Mark et al., 2000; Abnet et al., 2003; Taylor et al., 2003). Low levels of vitamin C and high lutein/zeaxanthin concentrations are associated with gastric noncardia cancer (Mark et al., 2000; Mayne et al., 2001b; Abnet et al., 2003). Serum levels of vitamin C and vitamin E have been found to be inversely associated with the severity of gastritis, gastric dysplasia, and gastric precancerous lesions (Su et al., 2000).

Nutrition Interventions

Results from NIT General Population Trials showed that supplementation with retinol and zinc resulted in a 41% reduction in mortality from gastric noncardia cancer, while supplementation with β-carotene, selenium, and α-tocopherol produced a 21% reduction in mortality from gastric cardia and noncardia cancer combined. In the NIT Dysplasia Trial, there was a small but not significant benefit from multiple vitamin and mineral supplementation on combined gastric and esophageal cancer mortality. However, total stomach cancer mortality was slightly increased in the supplemented group (18% higher than placebo, $p > .05$), an outcome attributable to differences in gastric noncardia cancer. There was also a significant increase in gastric noncardia incidence (14 cases in the supplement group and 4 in placebo).

A secondary analysis of the Alpha-Tocopherol, Beta-Carotene Cancer Prevention (ATBC) Study conducted among middle-aged male smokers in Finland evaluated the effect of supplementation on gastric cancer incidence (Malila et al., 2002). Neither α-tocopherol (50 mg/day) or β-carotene (20 mg/day) supplementation had a protective effect against gastric cancer after 6 years of follow-up. Moreover, the data suggested an increased risk of intestinal-type stomach cancer for β-carotene.

There was a randomized controlled trial of anti–*H. pylori* triple therapy and/or dietary supplementation with ascorbic acid and β-carotene for the treatment of gastric precancerous lesions (Correa et al., 2000). Subjects with confirmed histological diagnoses of multifocal nonmetaplastic atrophy and/or intestinal metaplasia were included. All three interventions resulted in significantly increased rates of regression of the cancer precursor lesions. Combinations of the treatments did not improve the regression rates. Thus, these data suggested that anti–*H. pylori* treatment and dietary supplementation with antioxidants may be an effective strategy to prevent gastric cancer.

COLORECTAL CANCER

Colorectal cancer is the third most common cancer worldwide. It accounted for ~1 million new cases in 2002 (Parkin et al., 2005). In the United States, it is estimated that there will be 145,290 new cases diagnosed and 56,290 deaths from the disease in 2005 (American Cancer Society, 2005). The 5-year survival rate (in men) is 65% in North America. The incidence of the disease varies worldwide. The highest incidence rates are in North America, Australia/New Zealand, Western Europe, and Japan.

Dietary Risk Factors and Nutrition Interventions

Studies show that colorectal cancer results from complex interactions between genetic susceptibility and environmental factors. It has been suggested that several nutritional factors may play a significant role in cancer development. There are strong correlations between risk of colorectal cancer and per capita consumption patterns of meat, fat (specifically animal fat), and fiber (Rose et al., 1986; Prentice and Sheppard, 1990; McKeown-Eyssen, 1987, 1994). Epidemiological evidence consistently shows that obesity (particularly central obesity) and physical inactivity are major risk factors for colon cancer (Giovannucci, 2003).

Dietary Fat and Meat Intake

Colon cancer occurs more frequently in populations with high fat and meat intake (National Cancer Institute [NCI], 2005a). In animal studies, exposure to high-fat diets leads to an increased rate of colon cancer (Nauss et al., 1983, 1987). The mechanisms by which dietary fat or meat promote colon carcinogenesis are poorly understood, and human data are scarce. In animal model studies, type of fat affects carcinogenesis. Omega-6 polyunsaturated fatty acids have been shown to upregulate cyclooxygenase-2 (COX-2) expression, alter prostaglandin biosynthesis, enhance enzyme protein kinase C (PKC), inhibit tumor suppressor gene p53-mediated mitochondria-dependent apoptosis, and increase Ras-p21 gene expression (Cheah, 1990; Singh et al., 1997a,b; Reddy, 2004; Wu et al., 2004).

In contrast, omega-3 fatty acids have been found to exhibit antitumor activity by inhibiting COX-2 expression, suppressing PKC activity, and interfering with post-translational modification and membrane localization of Ras-p21. In regard to red meat, it has been hypothesized that heterocyclic amines formed when fish or meat are cooked at high temperature may contribute to increased risk of colon cancer (Hirayama, 1992). In humans, several case-control studies showed positive associations between meat or fat intake and colon cancer, but the results have not always been statistically significant.

In addition, results from prospective cohort studies are inconsistent. One study in the Netherlands, conducted among 120,852 men and women aged 55–69 years, found an increased risk only with processed meat (Slattery et al., 1997). Similarly, a prospective study from Norway found no evidence of association between intake of meat and fat and risk of colon cancer; there was, however, increased risk in women who consumed sausages frequently (Gaard et al., 1996).

In a cohort of 47,949 U.S. male health professionals, intakes of total fat, saturated fat, and animal fat were not related to risk of colon cancer (Giovannucci et al., 1994). However, an elevated risk of colon cancer was associated with red meat intake. Men who ate beef, pork, or lamb as a main dish five or more times per week were 3.5 times more likely to develop cancer than men who ate these foods less than once per month.

In the NHS, a cohort of 88,764 U.S. female nurses aged 34–59 years showed that both red meat and animal fat, but not vegetable fat, were positively associated with the risk of colon cancer. Women who ate beef, pork, or lamb as a main dish every day were 2.5 times more likely to develop colon cancer than those who ate those meats less than once a month. Processed meats and liver were also significantly associated with increased risk (Willett et al., 1990). In contrast, there was no association between meat or fat consumption and colon cancer in two other large prospective studies: the American Cancer Society's Cancer Prevention Study II and the Iowa Women's Health Study (Thun et al., 1992; Bostick et al., 1994). However, follow-up data from the Cancer Prevention Study II cohort found that risk of colorectal cancer increased with prolonged high consumption of red and processed meat (Chao et al., 2005).

Some explanations for the conflicting results on dietary fat intake and colon cancer risk include: (1) validity of the dietary questionnaire used, (2) differences in age, gender, and race of the population studied, (3) variations in methods of meat preparation, and (4) variability in consumption of other foods, such as fiber, fruits, and vegetables.

A meta-analysis of case-control and prospective studies that compared the highest category of meat consumption with the lowest estimated mean relative risk (RR) for colorectal cancer to be 1.35 for red meat and 1.31 for processed meat (Norat et al., 2002). It was also estimated that colorectal cancer risk would decrease 7–24% if average red meat intake was reduced to 70 g/wk. Another meta-analysis of 13 prospective studies showed that a daily increase of 100 g of total meat or red meat consumption was associated with a 12–17% increased risk of colorectal cancer. A daily increase of 25 g of processed meat was associated with a 49% increased risk (Sandhu et al., 2001). An update from the European Prospective Investigation into Cancer and Nutrition (EPIC) study indicates a positive association between colorectal cancer risk and high intake of red and processed meats (Norat et al., 2005).

Six case-control studies and two cohort studies have examined the association of dietary factors with the incidence of colorectal adenomatous polyps, precursors of most colorectal malignancies (Neugut et al., 1993; Kampman et al., 1994; Voskuil et al., 2002; Tiemersma et al., 2004; NCI, 2005a). Three of the eight studies found that high fat intake was a risk factor. The Polyp Prevention Trial (PPT) was a multicenter randomized controlled trial of 2079 men and women 35 years or older with one or more histologically confirmed colorectal adenomas. It found that a diet low in fat (20% of total energy intake), high in fiber (18 g/1000 kcal), and high in vegetables and fruits (five to eight daily servings) did not reduce the risk of recurrence of colorectal adenomas (Schatzkin et al., 1996, 2000).

Dietary Fiber, Vegetables, and Fruit

Evidence of the association between dietary fiber and colorectal cancer is inconclusive. Most animal and epidemiological studies report a protective effect of dietary fiber on the large bowel cancer. Fiber has been thought to affect colon carcinogenesis by binding to bile acids, increasing fecal weight and water (possibly diluting carcinogenesis), and decreasing colonic transit time, which reduces the length of time waste is in contact with intestinal cells (Steinmetz and Potter, 1991a,b; Cummings et al., 1992; Lampe et al., 1992; Macrae, 1999; Muir et al., 2004; NCI, 2005a). Bile acids have been implicated in the etiology of colon cancer, although the exact mechanism is not known (Cheah, 1990). In addition, fiber may act as a substrate for bacterial fermentation, which results in short-chain fatty acid (i.e., butyrate) generation in the colon (Ferguson et al., 2000).

Butyrate acid inhibits the preneoplastic proliferation and growth of colon cancer cells *in vitro* and regulates the substance involved in colon cell growth and adhesion (Macrae, 1999). Review of 37 observational epidemiological studies and meta-analyses of data from 16 of 23 case-control trials showed that most studies found evidence of a protective effect of fiber-rich diets; comparison of the highest and lowest quintiles of intake produced an estimated odds ratio (OR) of 0.57 (Trock et al., 1990a,b).

Similarly, a meta-analysis of 13 case-control studies from nine countries found an inverse relation between dietary fiber intake and risk of colon and rectal cancers. The association was seen in 12 of the 13 studies and was similar in magnitude for left- and right-sided colon and rectal cancers, for men and women, and for different age-groups. It has been suggested that the inverse association with fiber may result from some other closely associated dietary components, such as phenolic compounds, sulfur-containing compounds, or flavones found in fruits, vegetables, nuts, legumes, and grain (NCI, 2005a). In contrast to earlier case-control studies, results from the NHS found no association between the intake of dietary fiber and the risk of colorectal cancer, after adjustment for age, established risk factors, and total energy intake (Fuchs et al., 1999). It should be noted that women in this cohort generally consumed low amounts of dietary fiber.

The protective effects of fruits and vegetables on colorectal cancer risk have been inconsistent. To date, the NHS (88,764 women) and the HPFS (47,325 men) (Michels et al., 2000) have been the largest cohort studies to examine the association between fruit and vegetable consumption and incidence of colon and rectal cancers (Michels et al., 2000). The two studies together included 1,743,645 person-years of follow-up with 937 cases of colon cancer and 244 cases of rectal cancers. Based on analysis adjusted for multiple covariates, no association was found between colon cancer incidence and overall fruit and vegetable intake in women and men. The covariate-adjusted RR of both colon and rectal cancer for a difference in fruit and vegetable intake of one additional serving per day was 1.02 in women and men combined.

In a population-based prospective cohort study of 61,463 women in Sweden, total fruit and vegetable consumption was inversely associated with colorectal cancer risk (Terry et al., 2001a). This association was due largely to fruit consumption and was strongest for risk of rectal cancer. For total colorectal cancer risk, the inverse association was stronger and the dose–response effect more evident among individuals who consumed very low amounts of fruits and vegetables (<2.5 servings of fruits and vegetables/day). This study had several limitations, including no dietary reassessment during the follow-up period, no data on physical activity, and possible reporting errors (data collected from food frequency questionnaires [FFQs]).

A meta-analysis of 17 case-control studies, 10 cohort studies on vegetables, 10 case-control studies, and 9 cohort studies on fruits found that high intake of fruits and vegetables moderately but significantly decreased risk of colorectal cancer (Riboli and Norat, 2003). For vegetables, the protective effect was significantly stronger in case-control than in cohort studies, while there was no significant difference for fruits. In general, the cohort studies found statistically significant protective effects of vegetable intake on risk of colon cancer but not rectal cancer. Fruit had a stronger protective effect against rectal rather than colon cancer.

Six case-control and three cohort studies have examined the relation between dietary risk factors and colorectal cancer; four of the nine found an association between dietary fiber, carbohydrates, and/or vegetables and reduced risk (NCI, 2005a). The result from the NHS found no protective effect of dietary fiber against colorectal adenoma (Fuchs et al., 1999).

Several randomized controlled trials have examined the effect of dietary interventions on the development of adenomatous polyps (Macrae, 1999). In a familial adenomatous polyposis trial, 58 patients were enrolled in the study after total colectomy and ileorectal anastomosis at least 1 year before the study (DeCosse et al., 1989). They were randomly assigned to one of three treatment groups. The control group received placebo plus 2.2 g/day of low-fiber supplement; the vitamin group received 4 g of ascorbic acid plus 400 mg of α-tocopherol and a low-fiber supplement; and the high-fiber group received the two vitamins plus a high-fiber supplement (22.5 g/day) over a 4-year period. Wheat bran was the fiber used in this study. On an actual intake basis, the combined intervention inhibited the development of rectal polyps.

In the Toronto Polyp Prevention Trial, patients were included if they had undergone polypectomy for adenomatous polyps (McKeown-Eyssen et al., 1994). There were no significant differences in polyp recurrence rates between patients who received nutrition counseling to follow a low-fat, high-fiber diet (20% calories from fat, at least 50 g fiber/day) and patients who consumed a typical Western diet with placebo fiber. After 12 months, average fat and fiber intake in the treatment group was 25% and 35 g, while the corresponding numbers for the control group were 33% and 16 g, respectively. Only 86% of patients in the treatment group attended at least two-thirds of their plan counseling.

In the Phase III Colorectal Adenomatous Polyp Prevention trial, 1429 men and women, 40–80 years of age, with one or more histologically confirmed colorectal adenomas resected within 3 months before recruitment were randomized to receive either a high-fiber supplement (13.5 g/day) or a low-fiber supplement (2 g/day) of wheat-bran cereal (Alberts et al., 2000). After 3 years, data showed that wheat-bran fiber had no protective effect against recurrent colorectal adenomas. The Australian Polyp Prevention Project reported that the combination of fat reduction and a supplement of wheat bran reduced the incidence of large colorectal adenomas. The authors concluded that a low-fat diet plus wheat bran supplementation may reduce the transition from smaller to larger adenomas, which may be a critical step in determining which adenomas progress to malignancy (MacLennan et al., 1995).

Calcium

It has been hypothesized that dietary calcium reduces risk of colon cancer by binding secondary bile acids and ionized fatty acids in the lumen of the colon, thus reducing the proliferative stimulation of these compounds on mucosal cells (Wargovich et al., 1983; Newmark et al., 1984; Wargovich et al., 1984; Alberts et al., 2000; Boyapati et al., 2003). In addition, calcium may directly regulate the proliferative activity of colonic epithelium (Wargovich et al., 1992).

A review of >20 published case–control and cohort studies suggests that calcium intake is not associated with a substantially lower risk of colorectal cancer. Findings from large prospective cohort studies have consistently shown weak and inverse associations that were not significant (Martinez and Willett, 1998). Data from two prospective cohorts, the NHS and the HPFS (which included 88,764 women and 47,344 men, respectively), found the protective effects of calcium on distal but not proximal colon cancer (Wu et al., 2002).

There were no associations between calcium or milk intake and colorectal adenomas (Kampman et al., 1994). Interestingly, the benefit was seen mostly in people with calcium intake of 700–800 mg/day from either diet or supplement. Higher calcium intake beyond these amounts did not provide any additional benefit. A pooled analysis of primary data from 10 cohort studies in five countries found an inverse relation between calcium and milk intake and colorectal cancer (Cho et al., 2004b). The effect of milk was limited to cancers of the distal colon and rectum.

A randomized controlled trial among 930 participants investigated the effect of calcium supplementation (calcium carbonate 3 g daily; 1200 mg elemental calcium) on colorectal adenoma recurrence. The primary endpoint was new adenoma found at 1 and/or 4 year follow-up colonoscopies (Baron et al., 1999a,b). Calcium supplementation moderately decreased risk of recurrence for one or more adenomas and the total number of them. The adjusted RR for any adenoma recurrence with calcium compared with placebo was 0.85. Similar reductions were found in the European Cancer Prevention trial (Bonithon-Kopp et al., 2000), which also showed an adverse effect of fiber supplementation in participants with high dietary calcium intake.

Vitamins

Several epidemiological studies indicate that high folate intake from dietary sources or supplements may lower the risk of colorectal adenoma and cancer. Dietary folate influences DNA methylation, synthesis, and repair. Abnormalities in these DNA processes may enhance carcinogenesis, particularly in rapidly proliferative tissues, such as the colorectal mucosa (Giovannucci, 2002a). Inadequate folate may cause incorporation of uracil into DNA and increase frequency of chromosome breaks (Giovannucci, 2003). Findings from the NHS showed a lower risk of colon cancer with high folate intake and prolonged use (>15 years) of multivitamins containing folic acid (Giovannucci et al., 1998).

In the Swedish women cohorts, there was an inverse association between dietary folate intake and risk of colon cancer, but not rectal cancer. This association was most pronounced in smokers (Larsson et al., 2005). A meta-analysis of seven cohort and nine case-control studies reported the stronger association between folate consumption and colorectal cancer risk for dietary folate (folate from foods alone) than for total folate (folate from foods and supplements) (Sanjoaquin et al., 2005).

The role of antioxidant micronutrients in colorectal cancer prevention has also been investigated. In a prospective cohort study of 35,215 Iowa women, total vitamin E intake was inversely associated with the risk of colon cancer (Bostick et al., 1993). The benefit was seen only in women younger than 65 years. There were no benefits of high total intakes of vitamin A, vitamin C, β-carotene, or selenium. In a meta-analysis of 14 randomized trials involving 170,525 participants, supplementation with β-carotene, vitamins A, C, and E, and selenium (alone or in combination) did not prevent colorectal adenomas or cancers or other gastrointestinal cancers (esophageal, gastric, pancreatic, and liver) (Bjelakovic et al., 2004).

Alcohol Consumption

Many case-control and prospective cohort studies have found an association between high alcohol consumption and colorectal cancer (Giovannucci, 2003). Pooled analysis of data from eight cohort studies in five countries in North America and Europe found an increased risk of colorectal cancer limited to persons with an alcohol intake of ≥30 g/day (approximately ≥2 drinks/day) (Cho et al., 2004a). Compared with nondrinkers, the pooled multivariate RRs were 1.16 for persons who consumed 30 to <44 g/day and 1.41 for those who consumed ≥45 g/day.

It should be noted that the study included only one measure of alcohol consumption at baseline and did not investigate lifetime alcohol consumption, alcohol consumption at younger ages, or changes in alcohol consumption during follow-up. Another review of 52 studies found an association between alcohol and colorectal cancer in both females and males. Statistically significant elevations of risk for rectal cancer were often seen in male beer drinkers. Alcohol consumption was also associated with colorectal adenoma (Baron et al., 1998).

Alcohol has been hypothesized to interfere with folate metabolism, stimulate mucosal cell proliferation, activate intestinal procarcinogens, and possibly provide a source of unabsorbed carcinogens (Giovannucci, 2003). Compared with alcohol alone, the risk for colorectal cancer increases substantially with combined intakes of high alcohol and low folate.

Ongoing studies of dietary and other interventions in the chemoprevention of colorectal cancers are listed in Table 1.

Obesity and Physical Activity

Obesity and physical inactivity have been shown to increase risk of colorectal cancer and adenoma (Giovannucci et al., 1995a, 1996; Davidow et al., 1996; Hill, 1999; Giovannucci, 2003). Findings from epidemiological studies have consistently shown excessive weight as a predictor of colon cancer in men (Giovannucci, 2002b; Wei et al., 2004).

TABLE 1 Phase III Clinical Trials in Colorectal Cancer

Phase III trials			
Investigator/institution	**Patient population**	**Interventions**	**Status of patient accrual**
D. Alberts/University of Arizona	Prior sporadic adenoma	Ursodeoxycholic acid vs placebo	Closed
M. Bertagnolli/Multicenter	Prior sporadic adenoma	Celecoxib vs placebo	Closed
Women's Health Initiative/National Institutes of Health	Postmenopausal women	Low-fat diet vs calcium + vitamin D vs HRT vs placebo	Closed
J. Burn/CAPP-1, University of Newcastle	Prephenotypic FAP	Aspirin vs resistant starch vs both vs placebo	Closed
uk-CAP/Cancer Research U.K.	Prior sporadic adenoma	Aspirin vs folate vs both vs placebo	Closed
P. Lance/University of Arizona	Prior sporadic adenoma	Celecoxib vs selenium vs both vs placebo	Open
J. Baron /Dartmouth University	Prior sporadic adenoma	Aspirin ± folate vs placebo; also, folate arm is ongoing	Aspirin arm completed
H. Berkel/Hipple Cancer Research Center	Prior sporadic adenoma	Piroxicam vs calcium carbonate vs both vs placebo	Open
E. Giovannucci/Harvard	Prior sporadic adenoma	Folate vs placebo	Open
J. Burn/CAPP-2, University of Newcastle	HNPCC patients or mutation carriers	Aspirin vs resistant starch vs both vs placebo	Open

Note: ACF, aberrant crypt foci; CAPP, Concerted Action Polyposis Prevention Study; FAP, familial adenomatous polyposis; HNPCC, hereditary nonpolyposis colorectal cancer; HRT, hormone replacement therapy; uk-CAP, U.K. Colorectal Adenoma Prevention Study.

Source: From National Cancer Institute. U.S. National Institutes of Health. Available at www.cancer.gov.

In women, data have been less consistent, although abdominal obesity in women has been associated with colon cancer (Bruce et al., 2000). In a cohort of 89,835 Canadian women, obesity (BMI > 30 mg/m^2) was associated with a twofold increase in the risk of colorectal cancer in premenopausal women (Terry et al., 2002).

Obesity, particularly visceral obesity, is associated with hyperinsulinemia and insulin resistance (Freeman, 2004). Chronic exposure to high insulin levels may increase risk of colon cancer (Giovannucci, 1995, 2001; Bruce et al., 2000). Insulin is an important growth factor of colonic epithelial cells and is a mitogen of tumor cell growth *in vitro*. Several studies show that dietary patterns that stimulate insulin secretion, such as those with high intake of sucrose, high glycemic index, and saturated fat, are associated with a higher risk of colon cancer.

Several epidemiological studies have investigated the relation between physical activity and colon cancer risk (Friedenreich, 2001a,b; Friedenreich and Orenstein, 2002). Of the 46 colon, colorectal cancer, and physical activity studies, 38 have found a large reduction in risk of colon cancer in the most physically active male and female participants (Friedenreich, 2001a). The average RR reduction was 40–50%. The effect was particularly strong for the left colon. In contrast, most studies found no association between physical inactivity and rectal cancer. It should be noted that there are several limitations with epidemiological studies, including crude and incomplete physical activity assessment, lack of adequate control for confounding and effect modification, and a lack of consideration of underlying operative biological mechanisms.

BREAST CANCER

The lifetime risk of breast cancer in women is 1 in 8, with an increasing incidence in each decade of life after age 40 years (Lindley, 2002). In the United States, it was estimated that approximately 211,240 U.S. women would be diagnosed with breast cancer, and 40,410 would die from the disease in 2005 (American Cancer Society, 2005). Only lung cancer accounts for more deaths in women. Breast cancer also occurs in men; an estimated 1690 new cases will be diagnosed per year. Risk of recurrence for the >2 million breast cancer survivors persists at a relatively constant rate for 10–15 years after diagnosis (Early Breast Cancer Trialists' Collaborative Group, 1998). The incidence of breast cancer has gradually increased. However, data from the Centers for Disease Control and Prevention (CDC) have shown that from 1990 to 2000, the female breast cancer mortality rate decreased by 2.3%/year (Stewart et al., 2004).

Dietary Risk Factors and Nutrition Interventions

Evidence suggests that a low-fat diet may influence breast cancer risk through hormonal mechanisms. Ecological comparisons show a positive association between international age-adjusted breast cancer mortality rates and estimated per capita consumption of dietary fat (Rose et al., 1986; Hursting et al., 1990; Yu et al., 1991; Hebert and Rosen, 1996). Although results from case-control studies support this hypothesis, data from prospective cohort studies do not corroborate the association.

A pooled analysis of the results from seven prospective cohort studies in four countries (involving 4980 incident cases in 337,819 women) found no evidence of an association between total dietary fat intake and the risk of breast cancer. There was no reduction in risk even among women whose energy intake from fat was <20% of total energy intake (Hunter et al., 1996). When total data in the NHS were analyzed, there were no relations between dietary fat intake and breast cancer risk (Holmes et al., 1999). However, among premenopausal women, high intake of animal fat, mainly from red meat and high-fat dairy foods (but not vegetable fat), was associated with an increased risk of breast cancer (Cho et al., 2003).

High intakes of fruits and vegetables have been shown to reduce risk of breast cancer in some epidemiological studies. When all studies were considered together, a meta-analysis of 15 case-control and 10 cohort studies found a significant protective effect of vegetables (Riboli and Norat, 2003). When case-control and cohort studies were analyzed separately, the protective effect was found only in case-control studies. Neither type of study showed that fruit had a protective effect against breast cancer. Similar findings were reported in a pooled analysis of eight cohort studies involving 7377 incidents of invasive breast cancer in 351,825 women (Smith-Warner et al., 2001).

A comparison of the highest to lowest quartiles of intake showed multivariate RRs for breast cancer of 0.93 for total fruits, 0.96 for total vegetables, and 0.93 for total fruits and vegetables. No associations were observed for any specific fruits and vegetables tested. Likewise, published results from the European Prospective Investigation into Cancer and Nutrition (EPIC) study (which involved 285,526 women between the ages of 25 and 70 years from eight European countries) showed no association between total or specific vegetable and fruit intake and the risk of breast cancer (van Gils et al., 2005).

The role of micronutrient intake and breast cancer risk has also been examined. Low levels of serum β-carotene, plasma folate, and vitamin B6 have been associated with increased risk of breast cancer (Toniolo et al., 2001; Zhang et al., 2003). In an NHS cohort, intakes of β-carotene from food and supplements, lutein/zeaxanthin, and vitamin A from foods were inversely associated with breast cancer risk in premenopausal women. This association was particularly strong in premenopausal women with a family history of breast cancer or those who consumed ≥15 g of alcohol per day (Zhang et al., 1999). The Women's Health Study, a controlled trial in which ~40,000 women were randomized to receive β-carotene or placebo, found that supplementation had no effect on overall cancer or breast cancer rates (Lee et al., 1999).

Fenretinide, a vitamin A analog, has been shown to inhibit breast carcinogenesis in preclinical studies. A phase III randomized trial compared the effects of 5 years of treatment with fenretinide (orally 200 mg/day) or no treatment. The cohort included 2972 Italian women, 30–70 years of age, with surgically removed stage I breast cancer or ductal carcinoma *in situ*. At a median observation of 97 months, fenretinide had no effect on the incidence of contralateral breast cancer, ipsilateral breast cancer, tumors in other organs, distant metastasis, and all-cause mortality. The results, however, suggested a possible benefit in preventing second breast malignancies in premenopausal women (De Palo et al., 1997; Veronesi et al., 1999).

Several large-scale nutrition intervention trials for the prevention/recurrence of breast cancer are being conducted. These include the Women's Healthy Living and Eating (WHEL) study, the Women's Health Initiative (WHI), and the Women's Intervention Nutritional Study (WINS). Results, when available, are expected to resolve many conflicting findings from epidemiological studies.

Alcohol Consumption

Epidemiological studies have shown a positive association between alcohol consumption and breast cancer risk. A meta-analyses of 53 case-control and cohort studies included 58,515 women with invasive breast cancer and 95,067 controls. Compared with women who reported drinking no alcohol, the RR of breast cancer was 1.32 for an alcohol intake of 35–44 g/day and 1.46 for ≥45 g/day (Hamajima et al., 2002). The RR of breast cancer increased by 7.1% for each additional 10 g (1 drink) intake of alcohol per day. This increase was the same whether women had ever been smokers.

Obesity and Physical Activity

Obesity is associated with hormonal profiles thought to favor growth of breast cancer (Chlebowski et al., 2002). As a potential mediator, obesity is associated with higher concentrations of estrogens, androgens, insulin, IGFs, and lower concentrations of sex hormone binding globulin, and IGF-binding protein (IGF-BP). These hormones may stimulate tumor growth and increase risk of breast cancer recurrence.

Obesity is associated with an increased risk of postmenopausal breast cancer, particularly in women who do not use hormone replacement therapy. Data from 95,256 U.S. female nurses have confirmed this finding. Postmenopausal women with BMI > 31 kg/m^2, who never used hormone replacement, had RR of breast cancer of 1.59 when compared with those with BMI = 20 kg/m^2 (Huang et al., 1997). In women who never used postmenopausal hormones, weight gain after age 18 years was also important; the RR for women who gained >20 kg compared with those who had no weight change was 1.99. Abdominal obesity determined by waist circumference was also a predictor for postmenopausal breast cancer (Huang et al., 1999).

Epidemiological evidence suggests an association between physical activity and breast cancer. The Shanghai Breast Cancer Study (Malin et al., 2005), a population-based study of 1459 incident breast cancer cases and 1556 age frequency–matched controls, found that lack of exercise/sport activity, low occupational activity, and high BMI were all individually associated with increased risk of breast cancer (OR ranged from 1.49 to 1.86). In general, women with lower exercise/sport activity level and higher BMI, or those with higher energy intake, were at an increased risk compared with women who reported more exercise/sport activities, had lower BMIs, or reported less energy intake.

There was a significant multiplicative interaction (p = .02) between adult exercise/sport activity and BMI, with inactive women in the upper quartile being at increased risk (OR 2.16; 95% confidence interval [CI], 1.25–3.74) compared with their active and lean counterparts. This association was stronger in postmenopausal than in premenopausal women, and nonexercising postmenopausal women with higher BMIs were at substantially increased risk (OR 4.74; 95% CI, 2.05–12.20).

The data are consistent with those found in a review of 36 cohort and case-control studies. Of those studies, 24 found a reduction in breast cancer risk in women who were most active in their occupational and/or recreational activity (Friedenreich, 2001a). The average reduction in RR was 30–40%. However, there were several limitations in these studies, such as inadequate measurement of physical activity, incomplete control for confounding, and lack of assessment of effect modifications.

In addition, very few studies have examined the relation between breast cancer and menopausal status. In the Women's Health Study, physical activity among 39,322 women, 45 years or older, was assessed; higher levels of physical activity were found to decrease the risk of breast cancer only in postmenopausal women (Lee et al., 2001). In a Japanese cohort, a strong protective effect of physical activity was observed in premenopausal women with BMI = 25 kg/m^2 (multivariable-adjusted OR = 0.57); risk reduction was also found (OR = 0.71) in postmenopausal women with BMI of 22 to –25 kg/m^2 (Hirose et al., 2003).

Risk Factors Associated with Dietary Fat

Evidence linking breast cancer and dietary fat, particularly saturated and unsaturated fatty acids, has been strong enough to warrant investigation in three major epidemiological studies (WINS, WHI, and WHEL). Results from WINS—which involved 2437 postmenopausal U.S. women aged 48–79 years with early-stage resected primary breast cancer—showed that lifestyle interventions resulting in dietary fat intake reduction might improve the relapse-free survival of postmenopausal breast cancer patients.

Participants, who had already received currently recommended treatment with tamoxifen or chemotherapy, were randomized to either a diet in which 15% of caloric intake was from fat or a nonintervention group (control diet) in which ~30% of caloric intake was from fat (Chlebowski et al., 1993, 2005). After 12 months, the reduction in dietary fat gram intake per day was greater in the intervention group than in control: 33.3 ± 16.7 versus 51.3 ± 24.4 (p < .001), respectively. After 60 months of median follow-up, relapse rate events were significantly lower in the intervention arm compared with control (Chlebowski et al., 2005). A substudy of the WINS trial has randomly selected women from the low-fat diet arm of WINS to examine their successful dietary strategies (Chlebowski et al., 1993, 2005; Buzzard et al.; 1996; Winters et al., 2004).

LUNG CANCER

Lung cancer is the most common cancer worldwide, in both incidence and mortality (Parkin et al., 2005). It is by far the most common cancer of men, with the highest rates observed in North America and Europe. In the United States, lung cancer now accounts for 13% of new cancer cases and 29% of all cancer deaths each year. In 2005, an estimated 172,570 new cases were diagnosed and 163,510 deaths occurred (American Cancer Society, 2005). Lung cancer is now the leading cause of cancer death in both men and women (NCI, 2005b).

Dietary Risk Factors

Cigarette smoking is undoubtedly the primary risk factor for lung cancer. High intakes of fruits and vegetables have been associated with a lower risk of lung cancer in many epidemiological studies, but the effect is not enough to counteract the risk from tobacco. Data from two large cohorts—77,283 women in the NHS and 47,778 men in the HPFS—reported an inverse association between high fruit and vegetable intake and the risk of lung cancer in women but not men (Feskanich et al., 2000). In the EPIC cohort, high intake of fruit significantly reduced the risk of lung cancer, after adjustment for age, smoking status, height, weight, and gender. The association at baseline was strongest in the Northern European centers and among current smokers. There was no association between vegetable intake and lung cancer risk (Miller et al., 2004).

A meta-analysis of case-control and cohort studies found a significant protective effect from fruit in men, but not women (Riboli and Norat, 2003). The protective effects of vegetables were found only in case-control but not cohort studies. A pooled analysis of eight cohort studies involving 3206 incidents of lung cancer in 430,281 women and men found a modest reduction in lung cancer risk with high fruit and vegetable consumption. The result was mostly attributable to fruit, not vegetable, intake. After controlling for smoking habits and other lung cancer risk factors, a 16–23% reduction in lung cancer risk was observed for quintiles 2 through 5 compared with the lowest quintile of consumption for total fruits and for total fruits and vegetables (Smith-Warner et al., 2003).

Nutrition Interventions

Studies have investigated roles of chemopreventive agents in the prevention of lung cancer. There are three chemoprevention settings: primary (healthy), secondary (premalignant lesions), and tertiary (prevention of second primary tumors in previously treated patients) (Lippman and Spitz, 2001). In most studies, attention has been on α-tocopherol, β-carotene, and other vitamin A compounds because of their antioxidant properties and the effect of vitamin A on cell differentiation.

Primary Chemoprevention

Two primary chemoprevention studies in lung cancer have been conducted in healthy individuals at high risk for the development of lung cancer due to smoking or asbestos exposure.

The Alpha-Tocopherol, Beta-Carotene (ATBC) trial was conducted in Finland, where male lung cancer rates were the highest in the world, a finding attributed primarily to smoking. The trial included 29,133 Finnish male smokers 50–69 years of age in a 2 × 2 factorial design of α-tocopherol (50 mg/day) and β-carotene (20 mg/day). Participants were randomly assigned to one of four daily supplement regimens: α-tocopherol alone, β-carotene alone, both α-tocopherol and β-carotene, or placebo for 5–8 years (median 6.1 years) (Albanes et al., 1996).

Eight hundred ninety-four new cases of lung cancer were diagnosed. Supplementation with α-tocopherol produced no overall effect on lung cancer (RR = 0.99) or total mortality, although deaths from hemorrhagic stroke were significantly increased by 50%. Supplementation with β-carotene, however, was associated with increased lung cancer risk (RR = 1.16), as well as total mortality (RR = 1.08). The effect of β-carotene was more pronounced in men who were heavy smokers (at least 1 pack/day) with high alcohol intake (at least one drink per day). Four years after the end of the intervention, the RR of lung cancer among participants who received β-carotene returned to 1 (Virtamo et al., 2003).

The Beta-carotene and Retinol Efficacy Trial (CARET) was initiated to address the large burden of lung cancer in the United States. The study compared the combination of 30 mg of β-carotene and 25,000 IU of retinyl palmitate (retinol) with placebo. Subjects included 18,314 men and women, 50–69 years of age, with at least a 20-pack/year history of smoking (current or recent ex-smokers), and men older than 45 years with occupational asbestos exposure (Omenn et al., 1994).

The study was terminated early after a mean follow-up of 4 years because participants in the active intervention group were found to have a 28% increase in incidence of lung cancer, a 46% increase in lung cancer mortality, a 17% increase in total mortality, and a 26% higher rate of cardiovascular disease mortality compared with participants in the placebo group (Omenn et al., 1996a,b). An increased risk attributed to β-carotene supplementation appeared to be stronger in current smokers (as opposed to former smokers) and in those with high alcohol intake (Omenn et al., 1996a).

CARET participants were followed for ~6 more years after β-carotene and retinol supplementation were stopped. Increased risks of lung cancer (12%) and all-cause mortality (8%) with the active intervention persisted but were no longer statistically significant. Subgroup analyses suggested that the persistent excess risks of lung cancer were restricted primarily to females and cardiovascular disease mortality to females and former smokers (Goodman et al., 2004).

The Physicians' Health Study was a randomized controlled trial designed to test the effect of aspirin and β-carotene in the primary prevention of cardiovascular disease and cancer (Hennekens et al., 1996). The study included 22,071 U.S. male physicians aged 40–84 years; 11% were current smokers and 39% were former smokers. Participants were randomly assigned to one of four groups: aspirin (325 mg on alternate day), β-carotene (50 mg on alternate days), both aspirin and β-carotene, or placebo. After an average of 12 years of treatment and follow-up, there was no significant effect of β-carotene on overall risk of cancer (RR = 0.98), of lung cancer among current (RR = 0.9) or former (RR = 1) smokers, or of overall mortality.

The overall findings from the ATBC and CARET studies suggest that pharmacological doses of β-carotene increase lung cancer risk in relatively heavy smokers. Lung cancer risk was not increased in ATBC participants who smoked less than 1 pack/day or in CARET participants who had already stopped smoking. In addition, other studies, including the Physicians' Health Study, did not show that β-carotene supplementation increased risk of lung cancer in nonsmokers. The mechanism of this adverse effect is not known. It has been postulated that β-carotene supplementation may affect the growth of preclinical tumors rather than *de novo* tumors because of the rapid increase in lung cancer incidence within a year or two of intervention in both studies.

In animal studies, high doses of β-carotene have increased conversion of carcinogen-metabolizing enzymes and caused overgeneration of oxidative stress (Paolini et al., 1999, 2001, 2003; Perocco et al., 1999). It has also been suggested that the oxidative stress induced by cigarette smoke in the lungs may result in a change in β-carotene metabolism, resulting in increased mutagenicity of tobacco carcinogens (Salgo et al., 1999). Studies conducted in the ferret found that high-dose β-carotene in smoke-exposed animals led to squamous metaplasia, a precancerous lesion in the lung.

These animals were found to have an increased number of transient oxidative metabolites, including P450 enzymes that resulted in the destruction of retinoic acid, diminished retinoid signaling, and enhanced cell proliferation. In addition, eccentric cleavage β-carotene metabolites facilitated the binding of smoke derived carcinogens to DNA. In other ferret studies, low-dose β-carotene combined with smoke exposure provided mild protection against squamous metaplasia. Thus, it appears that the effect of β-carotene on lung cancer may be related to dose (Liu et al., 2003, 2004; Russell, 2004).

Secondary Chemoprevention

In head and neck cancer, the role of vitamin A and its derivative for the reversal of premalignant lung lesions has been investigated. In a randomized trial of 86 smokers with bronchoscopic biopsy–proven squamous dysplasia and/or a metaplasia, subjects were randomly assigned to either isotretinoin 1 mg/kg/day or placebo for 6 months (Lee et al., 1994). Both isotretinoin and placebo groups had a similar reduction in the extent of squamous metaplasia (54.3% vs 58.8%, respectively). In both groups, 20% of the subjects had a complete reversal of lesions. These results suggested that isotretinoin had no effect on reversal of squamous metaplasia.

A similar finding was reported in a randomized study of synthetic retinoid etretinate. One hundred and fifty smokers with sputum atypia were treated daily for 6 months with either 25 mg etretinate or placebo. There was no difference in the degree of atypia between the two treatment arms. Toxicity of etretinate was mild.

Another study investigated the effect of retinol in current and former smokers on bronchial dysplasia, nuclear morphometry, and retinoic acid receptor-β (RARβ) mRNA expression (marker of specific retinoid effect) (Lam et al., 2003). Eighty-one current or former smokers with a history of ≤30 pack-years smoking were randomized to receive placebo or retinol (50,000 IU/day) for 6 months. There was no significant difference in the regression rate between the retinol and placebo groups in histopathology and nuclear morphometry.

The likelihood of regression was lower in those who continued to smoke during the study compared with ex-smokers. Retinol was not effective in the upregulation of RARβ in lesions with bronchial dysplasia. The authors hypothesized that the lack of effect of retinol on RARβ expression among current smokers may be due to a suppressive effect of tobacco smoke components on RARβ expression and/or altered cellular metabolism of retinol to retinoic acid and its isomers.

A randomized controlled clinical trial of β-carotene and retinol was conducted with 755 former asbestos workers. At a median treatment of 58 months, supplementation with 50 mg β-carotene/day and 25,000 IU retinol/day on alternate days resulted in no significant reduction in the incidence and prevalence of sputum atypia (McLarty et al., 1995).

Tertiary Chemoprevention

The lifetime risk of second primary tumors in patients with early stage lung cancer is 20–30%. This high rate allows second primary chemoprevention trials for smaller sample sizes than primary prevention trials (NCI, 2005b). The European Study on Chemoprevention with Vitamin A and *N*-Acetylcysteine (EUROSCAN) was a randomized study in patients with head and neck cancer or lung cancer. Supplementation of retinyl palmitate (300,000 IU/day for 1 year followed by 150,000 IU/day for the second year) provided no benefit in survival, event-free survival, or second primary tumors for patients with lung cancer (de Vries et al., 1999; van Zandwijk et al., 2000).

An NCI Intergroup phase III trial involved 1166 patients with pathological stage I non–small-cell lung cancer (NSCLC) 6 weeks to 3 years from definitive resection, with no prior radiotherapy or chemotherapy (Lippman et al., 2001). Patients were randomly assigned to receive placebo or retinoid isotretinoin (30 mg/day) for 3 years. After a median follow-up of 3.5 years, there were no statistically significant differences between the two treatment arms in the time to second primary tumors (unadjusted hazard ratio [HR] = 1.08), recurrences (HR = 0.99), or mortality (HR = 1.07).

Secondary multivariate and subset analyses found an increase in mortality and recurrence in current smokers but decreased mortality and recurrence in never smokers in the isotretinoin arm, suggesting a harmful effect of isotretinoin in current smokers and a beneficial effect in never smokers. Statistically significant treatment-related toxic effects included cheilitis, skin dryness, conjunctivitis, and arthralgia.

PROSTATE CANCER

Prostate cancer is the most common cancer and the second leading cause of cancer-related death in U.S. men. It is estimated that 232,090 new cases will be diagnosed and 30,350 individuals will die from the disease in 2005 (American Cancer Society, 2005). The cost of treating prostate cancer is more than 5 billion dollars annually (Saigal and Litwin, 2002).

Analyses of the database of the SEER Program of the NCI, which included 180,605 men diagnosed with prostate cancer in the United States between 1990 and 2000, showed that median age at diagnosis was 70 years and about one-third of patients were 75 years or older (Brenner and Arndt, 2005). More than 80% of the patients were white. Two-thirds of patients were diagnosed with localized/regional prostate cancer, whereas 6.5% of patients already had distant tumor spread at the time of diagnosis. Absolute survival rates 5 and 10 years after diagnosis were estimated to be 79% and 54%, respectively. Overall, 5- and 10-year relative survival rates were 99% and 95%. Compared with the general population, these outcomes indicated excess mortality of 1% and 5% within 5 and 10 years following diagnosis. Prognosis remained very poor among patients with distant tumor spread, and moderate excess mortality was observed among patients with poorly differentiated or undifferentiated localized/regional prostate cancer.

Dietary Risk Factors

Dietary Fat

Despite significant advances in the early detection and treatment of prostate cancer, little is known about environmental and genetic factors that cause the disease. The major issue in prostate cancer carcinogenesis is not the initiation of disease, but its promotion and progression (Fleshner et al., 2004). Findings from autopsies showed that ~80% of men had microscopic foci of prostate cancer by age 80 years (Sakr et al., 1996). Although the incidence of these foci of latent cancer is similar throughout the world, it can vary from country to country by as much as 20-fold (Wynder et al., 1971). These foci also appear to be more extensive, multifocal, and of higher grade in men from Western countries (Breslow et al., 1977).

Evidence—that men who migrate tend to obtain the incident rate of the host country (Haenszel and Kurihara, 1968) and that prostate cancer rates vary drastically in the same ethnic populations living in different geographic locations (Kolonel et al., 1999)—strongly suggests that environmental factors may influence the progression of latent cancer into a more aggressive state (Haenszel and Kurihara, 1968; Kolonel et al., 1999). Ecological studies show a direct relation between the international prostate cancer mortality rate and the estimated per capita consumption of dietary fat (Rose et al., 1986). In the animal model of prostate cancer, a low-fat diet decreased rates of tumor growth (Wang et al., 1995).

In a review of 33 published case-control and cohort studies on the relation between prostate cancer and dietary fat or specific fatty food types, 8 studies found a significant association. Furthermore, many studies have suggested associations for specific types of fatty foods (Fleshner et al., 2004). Among case-control studies, about half found an increased risk with high intake of dietary fat, animal fat, and saturated and monounsaturated fat (Zhou and Blackburn, 1997; Fleshner et al., 2004). Among seven cohort studies, only the HPFS found an association between total fat consumption and the risk of advanced prostate cancer (RR = 1.79, highest vs lowest quintile of intake) (Giovannucci et al., 1993).

In that study, the association rested primarily with animal fat, especially fat from red meat (but not vegetable fat). Fat from dairy products (with the exception of butter) or fish was unrelated to risk. Two other cohort studies reported positive associations with either saturated fat or food containing fat (such as milk, cheese, butter, meat, and eggs). In a cohort of men of Japanese ancestry living in Hawaii, milk, eggs, and cheese were associated with the risk of prostate cancer, although total fat, saturated, and unsaturated fat were not (Severson et al., 1989). Similarly, a cohort of Seventh Day Adventist adults showed positive associations between fatal prostate cancer and the consumption of milk, cheese, and eggs (Snowdon et al., 1984; Snowdon, 1988).

Mechanisms responsible for the possible association between dietary fat and prostate cancer are not known. Several hypotheses have been proposed, including the following:

1. Dietary fat may increase serum androgen levels. Androgen is likely to play a role in the etiology of prostate cancer (Kolonel et al., 1999). Androgens control cell growth in the prostate (Ford et al., 1994), and a reduction in androgen production is a mainstay in the treatment of prostate cancer. In addition, men castrated at a young age do not develop prostate carcinoma (Sakr et al., 1996). Observational studies found that changes in dietary fat intake affect serum and urinary levels of androgens in men (Hill et al., 1979; Howie and Shultz, 1985). In a twin study, the twin who consumed more fat had higher testosterone levels (Bishop et al., 1988). In a randomized crossover study of a low-fat, high-fiber and high-fat, low-fiber dietary intervention, men on the high-fat, low-fiber diet had 13–15% higher plasma concentrations of total and sex hormone–binding globulin (SHBG)–bound testosterone and urinary testosterone than men on the low-fat, high-fiber diet (Dorgan et al., 1996).
2. Specific types of fatty acids or their metabolites may initiate or promote prostate cancer. Although data are limited, *in vitro* studies have shown that linoleic acid, an omega-6 polyunsaturated fatty acid, can stimulate growth of human prostate cancer, while docosahexaenoic acid (DHA) and eicosapentaenoic acid (EPA), two omega-3 fatty acids present in fish oils, inhibit it (Rose and Connolly, 1991; Connolly et al., 1997). Another *in vitro* study reported that low concentrations of linolenic acid (also an omega-3 fatty acid) and EPA promoted prostate cell

growth (Pandalai et al., 1996). A human case-control study in Uruguay reported a positive association between α-linolenic acid and prostate cancer (De Stefani et al., 2000). Similarly, data from the HPFS found α-linolenic acid, but not linoleic acid, to be associated with advanced prostate cancer risk (Giovannucci et al., 1993). The main sources of linolenic acid in these studies included red meat, dairy foods, mayonnaise, margarine, and butter.

3. Dietary fat is a prooxidant and can increase markers of oxidative stress (Fleshner and Klotz, 1998). The polyunsaturated fatty acids offer a susceptible target for many of these oxidizing species, forming lipid radicals and hydroperoxides that can generate additional oxygen radicals and/or DNA damage (Kolonel et al., 1999).

Fruit, Vegetables

The evidence for a protective effect from vegetables, fruits, and legumes against prostate cancer is neither strong nor consistent. In a multicenter case-control study of African-American, white, Japanese, and Chinese men in the United States and Canada, intakes of legumes and yellow-orange and cruciferous vegetables were associated with lower risk of prostate cancer (Kolonel et al., 2000). In contrast, data analyzed from the cohort of 130,544 men in seven countries recruited into EPIC between 1993 and 1999 found no associations between consumption of total fruits, total vegetables, cruciferous vegetables, or combined total fruits and vegetables and prostate cancer risk (Key et al., 2004).

In the HPFS, an association between cruciferous vegetables and risk for prostate cancer was examined (Giovannucci et al., 2003). Overall there was no association between cruciferous vegetables and prostate cancer risk. However, an inverse relation was observed for younger men (age younger than 65 years at diagnosis) and for organ-confined cancers. The findings suggested that cruciferous vegetables might be important in early stages of prostate cancer. Cruciferous vegetables contain high levels of the isothiocyanate sulforaphane, which is a very potent phase II detoxication enzyme–inducing agent (Zhang et al., 1992, 1994; Talalay et al., 1995; Fahey et al., 1997). Induction of phase 2 enzymes (e.g., glutathione transferases, epoxide hydrolase, NAD(P)H: quinone reductase, and glucuronosyltransferases) plays an important role in the body's protection against carcinogenesis, mutagenesis, and reactive forms of oxygen.

Nutritional Interventions

Dietary Prevention with Fruit, Vegetables, and a Low-Fat Diet

A randomized study of 1350 men examined the effect of a diet low in fat and high in fruits, vegetables, and fiber on serial levels of serum prostate-specific antigen (PSA) (Shike et al., 2002). The intervention group received intensive nutrition counseling, while the control group received a standard brochure on a healthy diet. High consumption of fruits, vegetables, and fiber over a 4-year period had no impact on serum PSA levels. The incidence of prostate cancer during the 4 years was also similar in the two groups.

Chemoprevention

Several compounds such as vitamin E, selenium, lycopene, vitamin D, and phytoestrogens have demonstrated potential for chemoprevention of prostate cancer in clinical or laboratory studies (NCI, 2005c). Currently, there are several ongoing randomized controlled trials in the United States designed to investigate the efficacy of dietary supplements for the prevention of prostate cancer (Barqawi et al., 2004).

Vitamin E

Interest in the role of vitamin E in prevention of prostate cancer is primarily due to its antiproliferative and antioxidant properties. Vitamin E has been shown to enhance the growth inhibitory effects of adriamycin on prostate cancer cells *in vitro* and in animal experiments (Ripoll et al., 1986; Nesbitt et al., 1988). In a cohort of 2974 men from Basel, Switzerland, followed for 17 years, low vitamin E levels in smokers were related to an increased risk for prostate cancer (Eichholzer et al., 1996, 1999).

A nested case-control study examined serum obtained in 1974 from 25,802 persons in Washington County, Maryland. Serum levels of vitamins in 103 men who developed prostate cancer during the subsequent 13 years were compared with levels in 103 men with no cancer matched for age and race. There were no significant associations among β-carotene, lycopene, or tocopherol and prostate cancer (Hsing et al., 1990).

The largest evaluation of the impact of α-tocopherol on prostate cancer risk came from the ATBC study. The prostate cancer incidence was one of many secondary cancer endpoints. Supplementation with α-tocopherol resulted in a 32% reduction in prostate cancer incidence (number of cases 99 compared with 151) (Albanes et al., 1995). The beneficial effect persisted during post-intervention follow-up (12% risk reduction 6 years after supplement was discontinued) (Virtamo et al., 2003).

Baseline serum concentrations of vitamin E fractions, α-tocopherol, and γ-tocopherol were also examined in 100 randomly selected incident prostate cancer case patients and 200 matched controls from the ATBC study (Weinstein et al., 2005). Inverse associations between prostate cancer risk and circulating concentrations of α-tocopherol and γ-tocopherol were observed. Odds ratios for the highest vs the lowest tertiles were 0.49 for α-tocopherol and 0.57 for γ-tocopherol. The association was particularly strong in men supplemented with the α-tocopherol.

Selenium

Selenium is an essential trace element occurring in organic and inorganic forms (Klein, 2004). The organic form is found predominantly in grains, meat, poultry, fish, dairy products, and eggs. It enters the food chain via plant consumption. Marked geographic variability of selenium in food exists because of its local soil content. Studies of geographical areas with different levels of dietary selenium have demonstrated an inverse relation between selenium intake and cancer mortality rate (Shamberger et al., 1976; Schrauzer et al., 1977). However, results from several epidemiological studies have been inconsistent (NCI, 2005c).

After a mean of 7 years of follow-up, men in the HPFS with higher toenail selenium levels had a reduced risk of advanced prostate cancer. After controlling for family history of prostate cancer, BMI, calcium intake, lycopene intake, saturated fat intake, vasectomy, and geographical region, the OR was 0.35 (highest vs lowest quintile) (Yoshizawa et al., 1998). In the Honolulu Heart Program, a nested case-control study was conducted in a cohort of 9345 Japanese-American men. Serum selenium levels at study entry of 249 incident cases diagnosed during 12.4 years of follow-up were compared with those of 249 matched controls. The multivariate OR for the highest quartile of serum selenium was 0.5. This association was more notable for those with advanced disease, diagnosed in 5–15 years, and in current or past smokers (Nomura et al., 2000).

A Nutrition Prevention of Cancer (NPC) study was a randomized control trial designed to determine whether supplementation with selenium would prevent skin cancer. A total of 1312 patients from seven dermatology clinics in the United States with a history of nonmelanoma (basal cell carcinoma and squamous cell carcinoma) skin cancer were randomized to either oral administration of 200 μg of selenium/day or placebo. After an average treatment of 4.5 years and follow-up of 6.4 years, the initial report showed that selenium did not affect the incidence of nonmelanoma skin cancer. However, there were significant reductions in total cancer mortality (50%), total cancer incidence (46%), prostate cancer incidence (63%), lung cancer incidence (46%), and colorectal cancer incidence (58%) in the selenium group (Clark et al., 1996, 1998; Combs et al., 1997a,b).

Subsequent reports of analyses from the entire study period and 2 more years of intervention showed less favorable results than those from the initial reports. Selenium significantly increased risk of squamous cell carcinoma of the skin (25%). In the selenium group, there remained significant reductions in total cancer mortality (41%), total cancer incidence (25%), and prostate cancer incidence (52%), but not in lung cancer or colorectal cancer incidence. The protective effect of selenium on prostate cancer risk appeared to be confined to those with lower baseline PSA levels (≤ 4 tng/ml) and lower baseline plasma selenium concentrations (<123.2 ng/ml) (Duffield-Lillico et al., 2002, 2003a,b; Reid et al., 2004). No patients experienced toxicity due to selenosis.

Selenium reduced incidence of prostate cancer in several animal models and inhibited the growth of prostate cancer cell lines. The exact mechanism of action is not clear, but several hypotheses exist. These include antioxidant effects, enhancement of immune function, induction of apoptosis, inhibition of cell proliferation and protein synthesis, alteration of the metabolism of carcinogens, production of cytotoxicity selenium metabolites, and influence of testosterone production (NCI, 2005c; Klein, 2004).

Vitamin A, Retinoids, and Carotenoids

Findings from observational studies and randomized controlled clinical trials do not support an association between dietary or supplement vitamin A and prostate cancer risk (Kristal and Cohen, 2000; Kristal, 2004). Case-control and cohort studies have reported inconsistent results, and positive studies appear to be confounded by other dietary factors. Only one clinical trial, the CARET, has reported a prostate cancer endpoint (Omenn et al., 1996b). There were no differences in incidence of prostate cancer between the β-carotene, retinyl palmitate, and the placebo groups.

The synthetic retinoid that has been studied most in relation to prostate cancer is fenretinide. Although *in vitro* and animal studies show antiproliferative and apoptotic effects in the prostate tissue (Webber et al., 1999; Sharp et al., 2001), human prostate has a low uptake for fenretinide. This makes it unlikely to be effective for prostate cancer prevention or treatment (Thaller et al., 2000). Several synthetic retinoids are now being developed and tested for chemoprevention.

Most case-control and cohort studies also reported no association between dietary β-carotene, total carotenoids, or supplementation and prostate cancer risk (Kristal, 2004). Results from the ATBC study showed a 23% increased risk for prostate cancer with β-carotene supplementation (Albanes et al., 1995). In contrast, findings from the Physicians' Health Study suggested that β-carotene supplementation may benefit prostate carcinoma risk in a subgroup of men with a low baseline level (Cook et al., 1999).

The association between lycopene and prostate cancer risk is also of interest. In 1995, the Physicians' Health Study reported the protective effect of lycopene on prostate cancer risk. Primary sources of lycopene in that study were tomato sauce, tomatoes, and pizza (Giovannucci et al., 1995b). However, subsequent findings from several case-control studies were mixed (Key et al., 1997; Jain et al., 1999; Norrish et al., 2000). A phase II randomized trial of 26 men with newly diagnosed, clinically localized prostate cancer examined the effect of preoperative lycopene supplementation. Men assigned to the lycopene group had clinical characteristics that were more favorable at prostatectomy, including less involvement of surgical margins and/or extraprostatic tissues, smaller tumor size, and less involvement of the prostate by high-grade prostatic intraepithelial neoplasia; these suggested that lycopene may decrease growth of prostate cancer (Kucuk et al., 2001, 2002).

Two U.S. National Institutes of Health (NIH)–funded studies are under way investigating the effects of lycopene supplement on human prostate cancer. One study is examining lycopene for the prevention of prostate cancer in healthy men. The other is comparing the effect of isoflavones versus lycopene (prior to radical prostatectomy) on intermediate biomarkers (e.g., indices of cell proliferation and apoptosis) and surrogate markers of disease progression in patients with localized prostate cancer.

Phytoestrogen

Phytoestrogens, which are derived from plants, are a broad group of nonsteroidal compounds of diverse structure that have been shown to bind to estrogen receptors (ERs) in animals and humans. They consist of a number of classes, including isoflavones, flavonoids, lignans, and coumestans (Ganry, 2005). Isoflavones such as genistein, daidzein, and glycitein are the most frequently studied phytoestrogens. Genistein and daidzein are found in rich supply in soybeans and soy products, as well as red clover.

In animal models, soy, isoflavones, and rye bran inhibited prostate cancer growth (Landstrom et al., 1998; Zhou et al., 1999, 2002; Bylund et al., 2000). Genistein, the predominant isoflavone found in soy, has been extensively studied and seems to be a promising cancer protective agent. It has been shown to inhibit carcinogenesis through the modulation of genes related to the control of cell cycles, apoptosis, and the inhibition of the activation of nuclear factor-κB (NFκB) and Akt signaling pathways, both of which are known to maintain a homeostatic balance between cell survival and apoptosis (Davis et al., 1999, 2000, 2001; Li and Sarkar, 2002; Sarkar and Li, 2002; Hussain et al., 2003; Sarkar and Li, 2003).

To date, there are few human studies examining the direct relation between individual dietary intake of soy products and other phytoestrogens and the risk of prostate cancer. A review of epidemiological studies found no significant protective effects of phytoestrogens on prostate cancer risk (Ganry, 2005). Currently, there are ongoing NIH-sponsored studies investigating the role of phytoestrogens—such as genistein for the treatment of patients with localized prostate cancer, and soy protein supplement for preventing prostate cancer in patients with elevated PSA levels—in prostate cancer treatment and prevention.

CONCLUSIONS

Compliance with "prudent" dietary patterns based on current national guidelines is associated with decreased risk of chronic diseases (Krauss et al., 2000; Byers et al., 2002; McCullough and Giovannucci, 2004) and is a crucial step in the prevention of cardiovascular disease, diabetes, stroke, and cancer (Eyre et al., 2004). It is estimated that 30–40% of cancers worldwide may be preventable through dietary and lifestyle changes (Eyre et al., 2004).

The 2005 *Dietary Guidelines for Americans* (U.S. Department of Health and Human Services, 2004) features Institute of Medicine reference intakes for macronutrients (Institute of Medicine. Food and Nutrition Board. Dietary Reference Intakes for Energy) and nine, easy-to-understand key messages for good health. The thrust of the 2005 *Dietary Guidelines for Americans* is away from the Western diet, which is higher in saturated fats, red meat, and refined flours, and toward a diet rich in fruits, vegetables, whole grains, and lean meats. The latter is classified as a prudent dietary pattern (Fung et al., 2001; Hu, 2002).

Diets low in saturated fats and high in fruits, vegetables, and high-fiber carbohydrates appear to be safe and effective for maintaining weight and health (Harnack et al., 2002) and may directly benefit some cancers (Eyre et al., 2004). The Shanghai Breast Cancer Study (Malin et al., 2005) has found strong evidence that more exercise together with less weight gain have a considerable effect on the risk of contracting breast cancer.

All large studies have focused on the diets of adults. However, it is possible that diets during childhood and adolescence may play a role in carcinogenesis. Research on diet and cancer prevention is a complex, dynamic, and fast-changing area, one in which many new theories and findings continue to emerge. Although much is known, far more remains to be learned.

References

Abnet, C.C., Qiao, Y.L., Dawsey, S.M., Buckman, D.W., Yang, C.S., Blot, W.J., Dong, Z.W., Taylor, P.R., and Mark, S.D. 2003. Prospective study of serum retinol, beta-carotene, beta-cryptoxanthin, and lutein/zeaxanthin and esophageal and gastric cancers in China. *Cancer Causes Control* **14**(7): 645–655.

Albanes, D., Heinonen, O.P., Huttunen, J.K., Taylor, P.R., Virtamo, J., Edwards, B.K., Haapakoski, J., Rautalahti, M., Hartman, A.M., Palmgren, J., et al. 1995. Effects of alpha-tocopherol and beta-carotene supplements on cancer incidence in the Alpha-Tocopherol Beta-Carotene Cancer Prevention Study. *Am J Clin Nutr* **62**(6 Suppl): 1427S–1430S.

Albanes, D., Heinonen, O.P., Taylor, P.R., Virtamo, J., Edwards, B.K., Rautalahti, M., Hartman, A.M., Palmgren, J., Freedman, L.S., Haapakoski, J., et al. 1996. Alpha-Tocopherol and beta-carotene supplements and lung cancer incidence in the alpha-tocopherol, beta-carotene cancer prevention study: effects of base-line characteristics and study compliance. *J Natl Cancer Inst* **88**(21): 1560–1570.

Alberts, D.S., Martinez, M.E., Roe, D.J., Guillen-Rodriguez, J.M., Marshall, J.R., van Leeuwen, J.B., Reid, M.E., Ritenbaugh, C., Vargas, P.A., Bhattacharyya, A.B., et al. 2000. Lack of effect of a high-fiber cereal supplement on the recurrence of colorectal adenomas. Phoenix Colon Cancer Prevention Physicians' Network. *N Engl J Med* **342**(16): 1156–1162.

American Cancer Society. 2005. "Cancer Facts and Figures." American Cancer Society, New York.

Bairati, I., Meyer, F., Gelinas, M., Fortin, A., Nabid, A., Brochet, F., Mercier, J.P., Tetu, B., Harel, F., Masse, B., et al. 2005. A randomized trial of antioxidant vitamins to prevent second primary cancers in head and neck cancer patients. *J Natl Cancer Inst* **97**(7): 481–488.

Baron, J.A., Beach, M., Mandel, J.S., van Stolk, R.U., Haile, R.W., Sandler, R.S., Rothstein, R., Summers, R.W., Snover, D.C., Beck, G.J., et al. 1999a. Calcium supplements for the prevention of colorectal adenomas. Calcium Polyp Prevention Study Group. *N Engl J Med* **340**(2): 101–107.

Baron, J.A., Beach, M., Mandel, J.S., van Stolk, R.U., Haile, R.W., Sandler, R.S., Rothstein, R., Summers, R.W., Snover, D.C., Beck, G.J., et al. 1999b. Calcium supplements and colorectal adenomas. Polyp Prevention Study Group. *Ann N Y Acad Sci* **889**: 138–145.

Baron, J.A., Sandler, R.S., Haile, R.W., Mandel, J.S., Mott, L.A., and Greenberg, E.R. 1998. Folate intake, alcohol consumption, cigarette smoking, and risk of colorectal adenomas. *J Natl Cancer Inst* **90**(1): 57–62.

Barqawi, A., Thompson, I.M., and Crawford, E.D. 2004. Prostate cancer chemoprevention: an overview of United States trials. *J Urol* **171**(2 Pt 2): S5–S8; discussion S9.

Benner, S.E., Winn, R.J., Lippman, S.M., Poland, J., Hansen, K.S., Luna, M.A., and Hong, W.K. 1993. Regression of oral leukoplakia with alpha-tocopherol: a community clinical oncology program chemoprevention study. *J Natl Cancer Inst* **85**(1): 44–47.

Bingham, S.A., Luben, R., Welch, A., Wareham, N., Khaw, K.T., and Day, N. 2003. Are imprecise methods obscuring a relation between fat and breast cancer? *Lancet* **362**: 182–183.

Bishop, D.T., Meikle, A.W., Slattery, M.L., Stringham, J.D., Ford, M.H., and West, D.W. 1988. The effect of nutritional factors on sex hormone levels in male twins. *Genet Epidemiol* **5**(1): 43–59.

Bjelakovic, G., Nikolova, D., Simonetti, R.G., and Gluud, C. 2004. Antioxidant supplements for prevention of gastrointestinal cancers: a systematic review and meta-analysis. *Lancet* **364**(9441): 1219–1228.

Blackburn, G.L., and Waltman, B.A. 2005. Obesity and insulin resistance. *In* "Cancer Prevention and Management thgrouh Exercise and Weight Control" (A. McTiernan, ed). Marcel Dekker, Inc, New York.

Blot, W.J., Li, J.Y., Taylor, P.R., Guo, W., Dawsey, S., Wang, G.Q., Yang, C.S., Zheng, S.F., Gail, M., Li, G.Y., et al. 1993. Nutrition intervention trials in Linxian, China: supplementation with specific vitamin/mineral combinations, cancer incidence, and disease-specific mortality in the general population. *J Natl Cancer Inst* **85**(18): 1483–1492.

Blot, W.J., Li, J.Y., Taylor, P.R., Guo, W., Dawsey, S.M., and Li, B. 1995. The Linxian trials: mortality rates by vitamin-mineral intervention group. *Am J Clin Nutr* **62**(6 Suppl): 1424S–1426S.

Blot, W.J., and McLaughlin, J.K. 1999. The changing epidemiology of esophageal cancer. *Semin Oncol* **26**(5 Suppl 15): 2–8.

Bonithon-Kopp, C., Kronborg, O., Giacosa, A., Rath, U., and Faivre, J. 2000. Calcium and fibre supplementation in prevention of colorectal adenoma recurrence: a randomised intervention trial. European Cancer Prevention Organisation Study Group. *Lancet* **356**(9238): 1300–1306.

Bosetti, C., Negri, E., Franceschi, S., Conti, E., Levi, F., Tomei, F., and La Vecchia, C. 2000. Risk factors for oral and pharyngeal cancer in women: a study from Italy and Switzerland. *Br J Cancer* **82**(1): 204–207.

Bostick, R.M., Potter, J.D., Kushi, L.H., Sellers, T.A., Steinmetz, K.A., McKenzie, D.R., Gapstur, S.M., and Folsom, A.R. 1994. Sugar, meat, and fat intake, and non-dietary risk factors for colon cancer incidence in Iowa women (United States). *Cancer Causes Control* **5**(1): 38–52.

Bostick, R.M., Potter, J.D., McKenzie, D.R., Sellers, T.A., Kushi, L.H., Steinmetz, K.A., and Folsom, A.R. 1993. Reduced risk of colon cancer with high intake of vitamin E: the Iowa Women's Health Study. *Cancer Res* **53**(18): 4230–4237.

Boyapati, S.M., Bostick, R.M., McGlynn, K.A., Fina, M.F., Roufail, W.M., Geisinger, K.R., Wargovich, M., Coker, A., and Hebert, J.R. 2003. Calcium, vitamin D, and risk for colorectal adenoma: dependency on vitamin D receptor BsmI polymorphism and nonsteroidal anti-inflammatory drug use? *Cancer Epidemiol Biomarkers Prev* **12**(7): 631–637.

Brenner, H., and Arndt, V. 2005. Long-term survival rates of patients with prostate cancer in the prostate-specific antigen screening era: population-based estimates for the year 2000 by period analysis. *J Clin Oncol* **23**(3): 441–447.

Breslow, N., Chan, C.W., Dhom, G., Drury, R.A., Franks, L.M., Gellei, B., Lee, Y.S., Lundberg, S., Sparke, B., Sternby, N.H., et al. 1977. Latent carcinoma of prostate at autopsy in seven areas. The International Agency for Research on Cancer, Lyons, France. *Int J Cancer* **20**(5): 680–688.

Bruce, W.R., Wolever, T.M., and Giacca, A. 2000. Mechanisms linking diet and colorectal cancer: the possible role of insulin resistance. *Nutr Cancer* **37**(1): 19–26.

Buzzard, I.M., Faucett, C.L., Jeffery, R.W., McBane, L., McGovern, P., Baxter, J.S., Shapiro, A.C., Blackburn, G.L., Chlebowski, R.T., Elashoff R.M., et al. 1996. Monitoring dietary change in a low-fat diet intervention study: advantages of using 24-hour dietary recalls vs food records. *J Am Diet Assoc* **96**: 574–579.

Byers, T., Nestle, M., McTiernan, A., Doyle, C., Currie-Williams, A., Gansler, T., and Thun, M. 2002. American Cancer Society 2001 Nutrition and Physical Activity Guidelines Advisory Committee. American Cancer Society guidelines on nutrition and physical activity for cancer prevention: reducing the risk of cancer with healthy food choices and physical activity. *CA Cancer J Clin* **52**: 92–119.

Bylund, A., Zhang, J.X., Bergh, A., Damber, J.E., Widmark, A., Johansson, A., Adlercreutz, H., Aman, P., Shepherd, M.J., and Hallmans, G. 2000. Rye bran and soy protein delay growth and increase apoptosis of human LNCaP prostate adenocarcinoma in nude mice. *Prostate* **42**(4): 304–314.

Calle, E.E., and Kaaks, R. 2004. Overweight, obesity and cancer: epidemiological evidence and proposed mechanisms. *Nat Rev Cancer* **4**: 579–591.

Chao, A., Thun, M.J., Connell, C.J., McCullough, M.L., Jacobs, E.J., Flanders, W.D., Rodriguez, C., Sinha, R., and Calle, E.E. 2005. Meat consumption and risk of colorectal cancer. *JAMA* **293**(2): 172–182.

Cheah, P.Y. 1990. Hypotheses for the etiology of colorectal cancer—an overview. *Nutr Cancer* **14**(1): 5–13.

Chlebowski, R.T., Aiello, E., and McTiernan, A. 2002. Weight loss in breast cancer patient management. *J Clin Oncol* **20**(4): 1128–1143.

Chlebowski, R.T., Blackburn, G.L., Buzzard, I.M., et al. 1993. Adherence to a dietary fat intake reduction program in postmenopausal women receiving therapy for early stage breast cancer. *J Clin Oncol* **11**: 2072–2080.

Chlebowski, R.T., Blackburn, G.L., and Elashoff, R.E. 2005. Dietary fat reduction in postmenopausal women with primary breast cancer: Phase III Women's Intervention Nutrition Study (WINS). *Proc Am Soc Clin Oncol* **24**(10).

Cho, E., Smith-Warner, S.A., Ritz, J., van den Brandt, P.A., Colditz, G.A., Folsom, A.R., Freudenheim, J.L., Giovannucci, E., Goldbohm, R.A., Graham, S., 2004a. Alcohol intake and colorectal cancer: a pooled analysis of 8 cohort studies. *Ann Intern Med* **140**(8): 603–613.

Cho, E., Smith-Warner, S.A., Spiegelman, D., Beeson, W.L., van den Brandt, P.A., Colditz, G.A., Folsom, A.R., Fraser, G.E., Freudenheim, J.L., Giovannucci, E., et al. 2004b. Dairy foods, calcium, and colorectal cancer: a pooled analysis of 10 cohort studies. *J Natl Cancer Inst* **96**(13): 1015–1022.

Cho, E., Spiegelman, D., Hunter, D.J., Chen, W.Y., Stampfer, M.J., Colditz, G.A., and Willett, W.C. 2003. Premenopausal fat intake and risk of breast cancer. *J Natl Cancer Inst* **95**(14): 1079–1085.

Cinciripini, P.M., and McClure, J.B. 1998. Smoking cessation: recent developments in behavioral and pharmacologic interventions. *Oncology (Huntingt)* **12**(2): 249–256, 259; discussion 260, 265, 2.

Clark, L.C., Combs, G.F., Jr., Turnbull, B.W., Slate, E.H., Chalker, D.K., Chow, J., Davis, L.S., Glover, R.A., Graham, G.F., Gross, E.G., et al. 1996. Effects of selenium supplementation for cancer prevention in patients with carcinoma of the skin. A randomized controlled trial. Nutritional Prevention of Cancer Study Group. *JAMA* **276**(24): 1957–1963.

Clark, L.C., Dalkin, B., Krongrad, A., Combs, G.F., Jr., Turnbull, B.W., Slate, E.H., Witherington, R., Herlong, J.H., Janosko, E., Carpenter, D., et al. 1998. Decreased incidence of prostate cancer with selenium supplementation: results of a double-blind cancer prevention trial. *Br J Urol* **81**(5): 730–734.

Combs, G.F., Jr., Clark, L.C., and Turnbull, B.W. 1997a. Reduction of cancer mortality and incidence by selenium supplementation. *Med Klin (Munich)* **92**(Suppl 3): 42–45.

Combs, G.F., Jr., Clark, L.C., and Turnbull, B.W. 1997b. Reduction of cancer risk with an oral supplement of selenium. *Biomed Environ Sci* **10**(2–3): 227–234.

Connolly, J.M., Coleman, M., and Rose, D.P. 1997. Effects of dietary fatty acids on DU145 human prostate cancer cell growth in athymic nude mice. *Nutr Cancer* **29**(2): 114–119.

Cook, N.R., Stampfer, M.J., Ma, J., Manson, J.E., Sacks, F.M., Buring, J.E., and Hennekens, C.H. 1999. Beta-carotene supplementation for patients with low baseline levels and decreased risks of total and prostate carcinoma. *Cancer* **86**(9): 1783–1792.

Cooper, J.S., Pajak, T.F., Rubin, P., Tupchong, L., Brady, L.W., Leibel, S.A., Laramore, G.E., Marcial, V.A., Davis, L.W., Cox, J.D., et al. 1989. Second malignancies in patients who have head and neck cancer: incidence, effect on survival and implications based on the RTOG experience. *Int J Radiat Oncol Biol Phys* **17**(3): 449–456.

Correa, P., Fontham, E.T., Bravo, J.C., Bravo, L.E., Ruiz, B., Zarama, G., Realpe, J.L., Malcom, G.T., Li, D., Johnson, W.D., et al. 2000. Chemoprevention of gastric dysplasia: randomized trial of antioxidant supplements and anti-helicobacter pylori therapy. *J Natl Cancer Inst* **92**(23): 1881–1888.

Cummings, J.H., Bingham, S.A., Heaton, K.W., and Eastwood, M.A. 1992. Fecal weight, colon cancer risk, and dietary intake of nonstarch polysaccharides (dietary fiber). *Gastroenterology* **103**(6): 1783–1789.

Davidow, A.L., Neugut, A.I., Jacobson, J.S., Ahsan, H., Garbowski, G.C., Forde, K.A., Treat, M.R., and Waye, J.D. 1996. Recurrent adenomatous polyps and body mass index. *Cancer Epidemiol Biomarkers Prev* **5**(4): 313–315.

Davis, J.N., Kucuk, O., Djuric, Z., and Sarkar, F.H. 2001. Soy isoflavone supplementation in healthy men prevents NF-kappa B activation by TNF-alpha in blood lymphocytes. *Free Radic Biol Med* **30**(11): 1293–1302.

Davis, J.N., Kucuk, O., and Sarkar, F.H. 1999. Genistein inhibits NF-kappa B activation in prostate cancer cells. *Nutr Cancer* **35**(2): 167–174.

Davis, J.N., Muqim, N., Bhuiyan, M., Kucuk, O., Pienta, K.J., and Sarkar, F.H. 2000. Inhibition of prostate specific antigen expression by genistein in prostate cancer cells. *Int J Oncol* **16**(6): 1091–1097.

Dawsey, S.M., Wang, G.Q., Taylor, P.R., Li, J.Y., Blot, W.J., Li, B., Lewin, K.J., Liu, F.S., Weinstein, W.M., Wiggett, S., et al. 1994. Effects of vitamin/mineral supplementation on the prevalence of histological dysplasia and early cancer of the esophagus and stomach: results from the Dysplasia Trial in Linxian, China. *Cancer Epidemiol Biomarkers Prev* **3**(2): 167–172.

Dawsey, S.M., Wang, G.Q., Weinstein, W.M., Lewin, K.J., Liu, F.S., Wiggett, S., Nieberg, R.K., Li, J.Y., and Taylor, P.R. 1993. Squamous dysplasia and early esophageal cancer in the Linxian region of China: distinctive endoscopic lesions. *Gastroenterology* **105**(5): 1333–1340.

De Palo, G., Camerini, T., Marubini, E., Costa, A., Formelli, F., Del Vecchio, M., Mariani, L., Miceli, R., Mascotti, G., Magni, A., et al. 1997. Chemoprevention trial of contralateral breast cancer with fenretinide. Rationale, design, methodology, organization, data management, statistics and accrual. *Tumori* **83**(6): 884–894.

De Stefani, E., Deneo-Pellegrini, H., Boffetta, P., Ronco, A., and Mendilaharsu, M. 2000. Alpha-linolenic acid and risk of prostate cancer: a case–control study in Uruguay. *Cancer Epidemiol Biomarkers Prev* **9**(3): 335–338.

De Stefani, E., Deneo-Pellegrini, H., Mendilaharsu, M., and Ronco, A. 1999a. Diet and risk of cancer of the upper aerodigestive tract—I. Foods. *Oral Oncol* **35**(1): 17–21.

De Stefani, E., Ronco, A., Mendilaharsu, M., and Deneo-Pellegrini, H. 1999b. Diet and risk of cancer of the upper aerodigestive tract—II. Nutrients. *Oral Oncol* **35**(1): 22–26.

de Vries, N., van Zandwijk, N., and Pastorino, U. 1999. Chemoprevention of head and neck and lung (pre)cancer. *Recent Results Cancer Res* **151**: 13–25.

DeCosse, J.J., Miller, H.H., and Lesser, M.L. 1989. Effect of wheat fiber and vitamins C and E on rectal polyps in patients with familial adenomatous polyposis. *J Natl Cancer Inst* **81**(17): 1290–1297.

Dorgan, J.F., Judd, J.T., Longcope, C., Brown, C., Schatzkin, A., Clevidence, B.A., Campbell, W.S., Nair, P.P., Franz, C., Kahle, L., et al. 1996. Effects of dietary fat and fiber on plasma and urine androgens and estrogens in men: a controlled feeding study. *Am J Clin Nutr* **64**(6): 850–855.

Duffield-Lillico, A.J., Dalkin, B.L., Reid, M.E., Turnbull, B.W., Slate, E.H., Jacobs, E.T., Marshall, J.R., and Clark, L.C. 2003a. Selenium supplementation, baseline plasma selenium status and incidence of prostate cancer: an analysis of the complete treatment period of the Nutritional Prevention of Cancer Trial. *BJU Int* **91**(7): 608–612.

Duffield-Lillico, A.J., Reid, M.E., Turnbull, B.W., Combs, G.F., Jr., Slate, E.H., Fischbach, L.A., Marshall, J.R., and Clark, L.C. 2002. Baseline characteristics and the effect of selenium supplementation on cancer incidence in a randomized clinical trial: a summary report of the Nutritional Prevention of Cancer Trial. *Cancer Epidemiol Biomarkers Prev* **11**(7): 630–639.

Duffield-Lillico, A.J., Slate, E.H., Reid, M.E., Turnbull, B.W., Wilkins, P.A., Combs, G.F., Jr., Park, H.K., Gross, E.G., Graham, G.F., Stratton, M.S., et al. 2003b. Selenium supplementation and secondary prevention of nonmelanoma skin cancer in a randomized trial. *J Natl Cancer Inst* **95**(19): 1477–1481.

Early Breast Cancer Trialists' Collaborative Group. 1998. Tamoxifen for early breast cancer: an overview of the randomised trials. *Lancet* **351**(9114): 1451–1467.

Eichholzer, M., Stahelin, H.B., Gey, K.F., Ludin, E., and Bernasconi, F. 1996. Prediction of male cancer mortality by plasma levels of interacting vitamins: 17-year follow-up of the prospective Basel study. *Int J Cancer* **66**(2): 145–150.

Eichholzer, M., Stahelin, H.B., Ludin, E., and Bernasconi, F. 1999. Smoking, plasma vitamins C, E, retinol, and carotene, and fatal prostate cancer: seventeen-year follow-up of the prospective Basel study. *Prostate* **38**(3): 189–198.

Eyre, H., Kahn, R., Robertson, R.M., Clark, N.G., Doyle, C., Hong, Y., Gansler, T., Glynn, T., Smith, R.A., Taubert, K., et al. 2004. Preventing cancer, cardiovascular disease, and diabetes: a common agenda for the American Cancer Society, the American Diabetes Association, and the American Heart Association. *Stroke* **35**: 1999–2010.

Fahey, J.W., Zhang, Y., and Talalay, P. 1997. Broccoli sprouts: an exceptionally rich source of inducers of enzymes that protect against chemical carcinogens. *Proc Natl Acad Sci USA* **94**(19): 10367–10372.

Ferguson, L.R., Tasman-Jones, C., Englyst, H., and Harris, P.J. 2000. Comparative effects of three resistant starch preparations on transit time and short-chain fatty acid production in rats. *Nutr Cancer* **36**(2): 230–237.

Feskanich, D., Ziegler, R.G., Michaud, D.S., Giovannucci, E.L., Speizer, F.E., Willett, W.C., and Colditz, G.A. 2000. Prospective study of fruit and vegetable consumption and risk of lung cancer among men and women. *J Natl Cancer Inst* **92**(22): 1812–1823.

Fleshner, N., Bagnell, P.S., Klotz, L., and Venkateswaran, V. 2004. Dietary fat and prostate cancer. *J Urol* **171**(2 Pt 2): S19–S24.

Fleshner, N.E., and Klotz, L.H. 1998. Diet, androgens, oxidative stress and prostate cancer susceptibility. *Cancer Metastasis Rev* **17**(4): 325–330.

Ford, L.G., Brawley, O.W., Perlman, J.A., Nayfield, S.G., Johnson, K.A., and Kramer, B.S. 1994. The potential for hormonal prevention trials. *Cancer* **74**(9 Suppl): 2726–2733.

Franceschi, S., Favero, A., Conti, E., Talamini, R., Volpe, R., Negri, E., Barzan, L., La Vecchia, C. 1999. Food groups, oils and butter, and cancer of the oral cavity and pharynx. *Br J Cancer* **80**(3–4): 614–620.

Freeman, H.J. 2004. Risk of gastrointestinal malignancies and mechanisms of cancer development with obesity and its treatment. *Best Pract Res Clin Gastroenterol* **18**(6): 1167–1175.

Friedenreich, C.M. 2001a. Physical activity and cancer prevention: from observational to intervention research. *Cancer Epidemiol Biomarkers Prev* **10**(4): 287–301.

Friedenreich, C.M. 2001b. Physical activity and cancer: lessons learned from nutritional epidemiology. *Nutr Rev* **59**(11): 349–357.

Friedenreich, C.M., and Orenstein, M.R. 2002. Physical activity and cancer prevention: etiologic evidence and biological mechanisms. *J Nutr* **132**(11 Suppl): 3456S–3464S.

Fuchs, C.S., Giovannucci, E.L., Colditz, G.A., Hunter, D.J., Stampfer, M.J., Rosner, B., Speizer, F.E., and Willett, W.C. 1999. Dietary fiber and the risk of colorectal cancer and adenoma in women. *N Engl J Med* **340**(3): 169–176.

Fung, T.T., Rimm, E.B., Spiegelman, D., Rifai, N., Tofler, G.H., Willett, W.C., and Hu, F.B. 2001. Association between dietary patterns and plasma biomarkers of obesity and cardiovascular disease risk. *Am J Clin Nutr* **73**: 61–67.

Gaard, M., Tretli, S., and Loken, E.B. 1996. Dietary factors and risk of colon cancer: a prospective study of 50,535 young Norwegian men and women. *Eur J Cancer Prev* **5**(6): 445–454.

Ganry, O. 2005. Phytoestrogens and prostate cancer risk. *Prev Med* **41**(1): 1–6.

Garewal, H.S., Meyskens, F.L., Jr., Killen, D., Reeves, D., Kiersch, T.A., Elletson, H., Strosberg, A., King, D., and Steinbronn, K. 1990. Response of oral leukoplakia to beta-carotene. *J Clin Oncol* **8**(10): 1715–1720.

Ghadirian, P. 1987. Thermal irritation and esophageal cancer in northern Iran. *Cancer* **60**(8): 1909–1914.

Ghadirian, P., Ekoe, J.M., and Thouez, J.P. 1992. Food habits and esophageal cancer: an overview. *Cancer Detect Prev* **16**(3): 163–168.

Giovannucci, E. 1995. Insulin and colon cancer. *Cancer Causes Control* **6**(2): 164–179.

Giovannucci, E. 2001. Insulin, insulin-like growth factors and colon cancer: a review of the evidence. *J Nutr* **131**(11 Suppl): 3109S–3120S.

Giovannucci, E. 2002a. Epidemiologic studies of folate and colorectal neoplasia: a review. *J Nutr* **132**(8 Suppl): 2350S–2355S.

Giovannucci, E. 2002b. Obesity, gender, and colon cancer. *Gut* **51**(2): 147.

Giovannucci, E. 2003. Diet, body weight, and colorectal cancer: a summary of the epidemiologic evidence. *J Womens Health (Larchmt)* **12**(2): 173–182.

Giovannucci, E., Ascherio, A., Rimm, E.B., Colditz, G.A., Stampfer, M.J., and Willett, W.C. 1995a. Physical activity, obesity, and risk for colon cancer and adenoma in men. *Ann Intern Med* **122**(5): 327–334.

Giovannucci, E., Ascherio, A., Rimm, E.B., Stampfer, M.J., Colditz, G.A., and Willett, W.C. 1995b. Intake of carotenoids and retinol in relation to risk of prostate cancer. *J Natl Cancer Inst* **87**(23): 1767–1776.

Giovannucci, E., Colditz, G.A., Stampfer, M.J., and Willett, W.C. 1996. Physical activity, obesity, and risk of colorectal adenoma in women (United States). *Cancer Causes Control* **7**(2): 253–263.

Giovannucci, E., Rimm, E.B., Colditz, G.A., Stampfer, M.J., Ascherio, A., Chute, C.C., and Willett, W.C. 1993. A prospective study of dietary fat and risk of prostate cancer. *J Natl Cancer Inst* **85**(19): 1571–1579.

Giovannucci, E., Rimm, E.B., Liu, Y., Stampfer, M.J., and Willett, W.C. 2003. A prospective study of cruciferous vegetables and prostate cancer. *Cancer Epidemiol Biomarkers Prev* **12**(12): 1403–1409.

Giovannucci, E., Rimm, E.B., Stampfer, M.J., Colditz, G.A., Ascherio, A., and Willett, W.C. 1994. Intake of fat, meat, and fiber in relation to risk of colon cancer in men. *Cancer Res* **54**(9): 2390–2397.

Giovannucci, E., Stampfer, M.J., Colditz, G.A., Hunter, D.J., Fuchs, C., Rosner, B.A., Speizer, F.E., and Willett, W.C. 1998. Multivitamin use, folate, and colon cancer in women in the Nurses' Health Study. *Ann Intern Med* **129**(7): 517–524.

Goodman, G.E., Thornquist, M.D., Balmes, J., Cullen, M.R., Meyskens, F.L., Jr., Omenn, G.S., Valanis, B., and Williams, J.H., Jr. 2004. The Beta-Carotene and Retinol Efficacy Trial: incidence of lung cancer and cardiovascular disease mortality during 6-year follow-up after stopping beta-carotene and retinol supplements. *J Natl Cancer Inst* **96**(23): 1743–1750.

Gridley, G., McLaughlin, J.K., Block, G., Blot, W.J., Gluch, M., and Fraumeni, J.F., Jr. 1992. Vitamin supplement use and reduced risk of oral and pharyngeal cancer. *Am J Epidemiol* **135**(10): 1083–1092.

Gridley, G., McLaughlin, J.K., Block, G., Blot, W.J., Winn, D.M., Greenberg, R.S., Schoenberg, J.B., Preston-Martin, S., Austin, D.F., and Fraumeni, J.F., Jr. 1990. Diet and oral and pharyngeal cancer among blacks. *Nutr Cancer* **14**(3–4): 219–225.

Guo, W., Blot, W.J., Li, J.Y., Taylor, P.R., Liu, B.Q., Wang, W., Wu, Y.P., Zheng, W., Dawsey, S.M., Li, B., et al. 1994. A nested case–control study of oesophageal and stomach cancers in the Linxian nutrition intervention trial. *Int J Epidemiol* **23**(3): 444–450.

Haenszel, W., and Kurihara, M. 1968. Studies of Japanese migrants. I. Mortality from cancer and other diseases among Japanese in the United States. *J Natl Cancer Inst* **40**(1): 43–68.

Hamajima, N., Hirose, K., Tajima, K., Rohan, T., Calle, E.E., Heath, C.W., Jr., Coates, R.J., Liff, J.M., Talamini, R., Chantarakul, N., et al. 2002. Alcohol, tobacco and breast cancer—collaborative reanalysis of individual data from 53 epidemiological studies, including 58,515 women with breast cancer and 95,067 women without the disease. *Br J Cancer* **87**(11): 1234–1245.

Harnack, L., Nicodemus, K., and Jacobs, D.R., Jr. 2002. An evaluation of the Dietary Guidelines for Americans in relation to cancer occurrence. *Am J Clin Nutr* **76**: 889–896.

Hashibe, M., Sankaranarayanan, R., Thomas, G., Kuruvilla, B., Mathew, B., Somanathan, T., Parkin, D.M., and Zhang, Z.F. 2000. Alcohol drinking, body mass index and the risk of oral leukoplakia in an Indian population. *Int J Cancer* **88**(1): 129–134.

Hebert, J.R., and Rosen, A. 1996. Nutritional, socioeconomic, and reproductive factors in relation to female breast cancer mortality: findings from a cross-national study. *Cancer Detect Prev* **20**(3): 234–244.

Heggie, S.J., Wiseman, M.J., Cannon, G.J., Miles, L.M., Thompson, R.L., Stone, E.M., Butrum, R.R., and Kroke, A. 2003. Defining the state of knowledge with respect to food, nutrition, physical activity, and the prevention of cancer. *J Nutr* **133**(Suppl 1): 3837S–3842S.

Hennekens, C.H. 1994. Antioxidant vitamins and cancer. *Am J Med* **97**(3A): 2S–4S; discussion 22S–28S.

Hennekens, C.H., Buring, J.E., Manson, J.E., Stampfer, M., Rosner, B., Cook, N.R., Belanger, C., LaMotte, F., Gaziano, J.M., Ridker, P.M., et al. 1996. Lack of effect of long-term supplementation with beta carotene on the incidence of malignant neoplasms and cardiovascular disease. *N Engl J Med* **334**(18): 1145–1149.

Hill, M.J. 1999. Mechanisms of diet and colon carcinogenesis. *Eur J Cancer Prev* **8**(Suppl 1): S95–S98.

Hill, P., Wynder, E.L., Garbaczewski, L., Garnes, H., and Walker, A.R. 1979. Diet and urinary steroids in black and white North American men and black South African men. *Cancer Res* **39**(12): 5101–5105.

Hirayama, T. 1992. Life-style and cancer: from epidemiological evidence to public behavior change to mortality reduction of target cancers. *J Natl Cancer Inst Monogr* **12**: 65–74.

Hirose, K., Hamajima, N., Takezaki, T., Miura, S., and Tajima, K. 2003. Physical exercise reduces risk of breast cancer in Japanese women. *Cancer Sci* **94**(2): 193–199.

Holmes, M.D., Hunter, D.J., Colditz, G.A., Stampfer, M.J., Hankinson, S.E., Speizer, F.E., Rosner, B., and Willett, W.C. 1999. Association of dietary intake of fat and fatty acids with risk of breast cancer. *JAMA* **281**(10): 914–920.

Hong, W.K., Endicott, J., Itri, L.M., Doos, W., Batsakis, J.G., Bell, R., Fofonoff, S., Byers, R., Atkinson, E.N., Vaughan, C., et al. 1986. 13-cis-retinoic acid in the treatment of oral leukoplakia. *N Engl J Med* **315**(24): 1501–1505.

Howie, B.J., and Shultz, T.D. 1985. Dietary and hormonal interrelationships among vegetarian Seventh-Day Adventists and nonvegetarian men. *Am J Clin Nutr* **42**(1): 127–134.

Hsing, A.W., Comstock, G.W., Abbey, H., and Polk, B.F. 1990. Serologic precursors of cancer. Retinol, carotenoids, and tocopherol and risk of prostate cancer. *J Natl Cancer Inst* **82**(11): 941–946.

Hu, F.B. 2002. Dietary pattern analysis: a new direction in nutritional epidemiology. *Curr Opin Lipidol* **13**: 3–9.

Huang, Z., Hankinson, S.E., Colditz, G.A., Stampfer, M.J., Hunter, D.J., Manson, J.E., Hennekens, C.H., Rosner, B., Speizer, F.E., and Willett, W.C. 1997. Dual effects of weight and weight gain on breast cancer risk. *JAMA* **278**(17): 1407–1411.

Huang, Z., Willett, W.C., Colditz, G.A., Hunter, D.J., Manson, J.E., Rosner, B., Speizer, F.E., and Hankinson, S.E. 1999. Waist circumference, waist: hip ratio, and risk of breast cancer in the Nurses' Health Study. *Am J Epidemiol* **150**(12): 1316–1324.

Hung, H.C., Joshipura, K.J., Jiang, R., Hu, F.B., Hunter, D., Smith-Warner, S.A., Colditz, G.A., Rosner, B., Spiegelman, D., and Willett, W.C. 2004. Fruit and vegetable intake and risk of major chronic disease. *J Natl Cancer Inst* **96**(21): 1577–1584.

Hunter, D.J., Spiegelman, D., Adami, H.O., Beeson, L., van den Brandt, P.A., Folsom, A.R., Fraser, G.E., Goldbohm, R.A., Graham, S., Howe, G.R., et al. 1996. Cohort studies of fat intake and the risk of breast cancer—a pooled analysis. *N Engl J Med* **334**(6): 356–361.

Hursting, S.D., Thornquist, M., and Henderson, M.M. 1990. Types of dietary fat and the incidence of cancer at five sites. *Prev Med* **19**(3): 242–253.

Hussain, M., Banerjee, M., Sarkar, F.H., Djuric, Z., Pollak, M.N., Doerge, D., Fontana, J., Chinni, S., Davis, J., Forman, J., et al. 2003. Soy isoflavones in the treatment of prostate cancer. *Nutr Cancer* **47**(2): 111–117.

Institute of Medicine. Food and Nutrition Board. 2004. "Dietary Reference Intakes for Energy C, Fiber, Fat, Fatty Acids, Cholesterol, Protein, and Amino Acids (Macronutrients)." The National Academies of Science.

Jain, M.G., Hislop, G.T., Howe, G.R., and Ghadirian, P. 1999. Plant foods, antioxidants, and prostate cancer risk: findings from case–control studies in Canada. *Nutr Cancer* **34**(2): 173–184.

Kampman, E., Giovannucci, E., van 't Veer, P., Rimm, E., Stampfer, M.J., Colditz, G.A., Kok, F.J., and Willett, W.C. 1994. Calcium, vitamin D, dairy foods, and the occurrence of colorectal adenomas among men and women in two prospective studies. *Am J Epidemiol* **139**(1): 16–29.

Kaugars, G.E., Silverman, S., Jr., Lovas, J.G., Brandt, R.B., Riley, W.T., Dao, Q., Singh, V.N., and Gallo, J. 1994. A clinical trial of antioxidant supplements in the treatment of oral leukoplakia. *Oral Surg Oral Med Oral Pathol* **78**(4): 462–468.

Kaugars, G.E., Silverman, S., Jr., Lovas, J.G., Thompson, J.S., Brandt, R.B., and Singh, V.N. 1996. Use of antioxidant supplements in the treatment of human oral leukoplakia. *Oral Surg Oral Med Oral Pathol Oral Radiol Endod* **81**(1): 5–14.

Key, T.J., Allen, N., Appleby, P., Overvad, K., Tjonneland, A., Miller, A., Boeing, H., Karalis, D., Psaltopoulou, T., Berrino, F., et al. 2004. Fruits and vegetables and prostate cancer: no association among 1104 cases in a prospective study of 130544 men in the European Prospective Investigation into Cancer and Nutrition (EPIC). *Int J Cancer* **109**(1): 119–124.

Key, T.J., Silcocks, P.B., Davey, G.K., Appleby, P.N., Bishop, D.T. 1997. A case–control study of diet and prostate cancer. *Br J Cancer* **76**(5): 678–687.

Klein, E.A. 2004. Selenium: epidemiology and basic science. *J Urol* **171**(2 Pt 2): S50–S53; discussion S53.

Kolonel, L.N., Hankin, J.H., Whittemore, A.S., Wu, A.H., Gallagher, R.P., Wilkens, L.R., John, E.M., Howe, G.R., Dreon, D.M., West, D.W., et al. 2000. Vegetables, fruits, legumes and prostate cancer: a multiethnic case–control study. *Cancer Epidemiol Biomarkers Prev* **9**(8): 795–804.

Kolonel, L.N., Nomura, A.M., and Cooney, R.V. 1999. Dietary fat and prostate cancer: current status. *J Natl Cancer Inst* **91**(5): 414–428.

Krauss, R.M., Eckel, R.H., Howard, B., Appel, L.J., Daniels, S.R., Deckelbaum, R.J., Erdman, J.J., Kris-Etherton, P., Goldberg, I.J., Kotchen, T.A., et al. 2000. AHA Dietary Guidelines: revision 2000: A statement for healthcare professionals from the Nutrition Committee of the American Heart Association. *Stroke* **31**: 2751–2766.

Kristal, A.R. 2004. Vitamin A, retinoids and carotenoids as chemopreventive agents for prostate cancer. *J Urol* **171**(2 Pt 2): S54–S58; discussion S58.

Kristal, A.R., and Cohen, J.H. 2000. Invited commentary: tomatoes, lycopene, and prostate cancer. How strong is the evidence? *Am J Epidemiol* **151**(2): 124–127; discussion 128–130.

Kucuk, O., Sarkar, F.H., Djuric, Z., Sakr, W., Pollak, M.N., Khachik, F., Banerjee, M., Bertram, J.S., and Wood, D.P., Jr. 2002. Effects of lycopene supplementation in patients with localized prostate cancer. *Exp Biol Med (Maywood)* **227**(10): 881–885.

Kucuk, O., Sarkar, F.H., Sakr, W., Djuric, Z., Pollak, M.N., Khachik, F., Li, Y.W., Banerjee, M., Grignon, D., Bertram, J.S., et al. 2001. Phase II randomized clinical trial of lycopene supplementation before radical prostatectomy. *Cancer Epidemiol Biomarkers Prev* **10**(8): 861–868.

Kune, G.A., Kune, S., Field, B., Watson, L.F., Cleland, H., Merenstein, D., and Vitetta, L. 1993. Oral and pharyngeal cancer, diet, smoking, alcohol, and serum vitamin A and beta-carotene levels: a case–control study in men. *Nutr Cancer* **20**(1): 61–70.

Lagergren, J., Bergstrom, R., Lindgren, A., and Nyren O. 1999. Symptomatic gastroesophageal reflux as a risk factor for esophageal adenocarcinoma. *N Engl J Med* **340**(11): 825–831.

Lam, S., Xu, X., Parker-Klein, H., Le Riche, J.C., Macaulay, C., Guillaud, M., Coldman, A., Gazdar, A., and Lotan, R. 2003. Surrogate end-point biomarker analysis in a retinol chemoprevention trial in current and former smokers with bronchial dysplasia. *Int J Oncol* **23**(6): 1607–1613.

Lampe, J.W., Slavin, J.L., Melcher, E.A., and Potter, J.D. 1992. Effects of cereal and vegetable fiber feeding on potential risk factors for colon cancer. *Cancer Epidemiol Biomarkers Prev* **1**(3): 207–211.

Landstrom, M., Zhang, J.X., Hallmans, G., Aman, P., Bergh, A., Damber, J.E., Mazur, W., Wahala, K., and Adlercreutz, H. 1998. Inhibitory effects of soy and rye diets on the development of Dunning R3327 prostate adenocarcinoma in rats. *Prostate* **36**(3): 151–161.

Larsson, S.C., Giovannucci, E., and Wolk, A. 2005. A prospective study of dietary folate intake and risk of colorectal cancer: modification by caffeine intake and cigarette smoking. *Cancer Epidemiol Biomarkers Prev* **14**(3): 740–743.

Lee, I.M., Cook, N.R., Manson, J.E., Buring, J.E., and Hennekens, C.H. 1999. Beta-carotene supplementation and incidence of cancer and cardiovascular disease: the Women's Health Study. *J Natl Cancer Inst* **91**(24): 2102–2106.

Lee, I.M., Rexrode, K.M., Cook, N.R., Hennekens, C.H., and Burin, J.E. 2001. Physical activity and breast cancer risk: the Women's Health Study (United States). *Cancer Causes Control* **12**(2): 137–145.

Lee, J.S., Lippman, S.M., Benner, S.E., Lee, J.J., Ro, J.Y., Lukeman, J.M., Morice, R.C., Peters, E.J., Pang, A.C., Fritsche, H.A., Jr., et al. 1994. Randomized placebo-controlled trial of isotretinoin in chemoprevention of bronchial squamous metaplasia. *J Clin Oncol* **12**(5): 937–945.

Levi, F., Pasche, C., La Vecchia, C., Lucchini, F., Franceschi, S., and Monnier, P. 1998. Food groups and risk of oral and pharyngeal cancer. *Int J Cancer* **77**(5): 705–709.

Li, J.Y. 1982. Epidemiology of esophageal cancer in China. *Natl Cancer Inst Monogr* **62**: 113–120.

Li, J.Y., Taylor, P.R., Li, B., Dawsey, S., Wang, G.Q., Ershow, A.G., Guo, W., Liu, S.F., Yang, C.S., Shen, Q., et al. 1993. Nutrition intervention trials in Linxian, China: multiple vitamin/mineral supplementation, cancer incidence, and disease-specific mortality among adults with esophageal dysplasia. *J Natl Cancer Inst* **85**(18): 1492–1498.

Li, Y., and Sarkar, F.H. 2002. Inhibition of nuclear factor kappaB activation in PC3 cells by genistein is mediated via Akt signaling pathway. *Clin Cancer Res* **8**(7): 2369–2377.

Lindley, C. 2002. Developments in breast cancer therapy. *J Am Pharm Assoc (Wash)* **42**(5 Suppl 1): S30–S31.

Lippman, S.M., Batsakis, J.G., Toth, B.B., Weber, R.S., Lee, J.J., Martin, J.W., Hays, G.L., Goepfert, H., and Hong, W.K. 1993. Comparison of low-dose isotretinoin with beta carotene to prevent oral carcinogenesis. *N Engl J Med* **328**(1): 15–20.

Lippman, S.M., Lee, J.J., Karp, D.D., Vokes, E.E., Benner, S.E., Goodman, G.E., Khuri, F.R., Marks, R., Winn, R.J., Fry, W., et al. 2001. Randomized phase III intergroup trial of isotretinoin to prevent second primary tumors in stage I non–small-cell lung cancer. *J Natl Cancer Inst* **93**(8): 605–618.

Lippman, S.M., and Spitz, M.R. 2001. Lung cancer chemoprevention: an integrated approach. *J Clin Oncol* **19**(18 Suppl): 74S–82S.

Liu, C., Russell, R.M., and Wang, X.D. 2003. Exposing ferrets to cigarette smoke and a pharmacological dose of beta-carotene supplementation enhance in vitro retinoic acid catabolism in lungs via induction of cytochrome P450 enzymes. *J Nutr* **133**(1): 173–179.

Liu, C., Russell, R.M., and Wang, X.D. 2004. Low dose beta-carotene supplementation of ferrets attenuates smoke-induced lung phosphorylation of JNK, p38 MAPK, and p53 proteins. *J Nutr* **134**(10): 2705–2710.

Lotan, R. 1996. Retinoids and their receptors in modulation of differentiation, development, and prevention of head and neck cancers. *Anticancer Res* **16**(4C): 2415–2419.

Lotan, R. 1997a. Retinoids and chemoprevention of aerodigestive tract cancers. *Cancer Metastasis Rev* **16**(3–4): 349–356.

Lotan, R. 1997b. Roles of retinoids and their nuclear receptors in the development and prevention of upper aerodigestive tract cancers. *Environ Health Perspect* **105** Suppl 4: 985–988.

Lotan, R., Xu, X.C., Lippman, S.M., Ro, J.Y., Lee, J.S., Lee, J.J., and Hong, W.K. 1995. Suppression of retinoic acid receptor-beta in premalignant oral lesions and its up-regulation by isotretinoin. *N Engl J Med* **332**(21): 1405–1410.

MacLennan, R., Macrae, F., Bain, C., Battistutta, D., Chapuis, P., Gratten, H., Lambert, J., Newland, R.C., Ngu, M., Russell, A., et al. 1995. Randomized trial of intake of fat, fiber, and beta carotene to prevent colorectal adenomas. *J Natl Cancer Inst* **87**(23): 1760–1766.

Macrae, F. 1999. Wheat bran fiber and development of adenomatous polyps: evidence from randomized, controlled clinical trials. *Am J Med 106*(1A): 38S–42S.

Malila, N., Taylor, P.R., Virtanen, M.J., Korhonen, P., Huttunen, J.K., Albanes, D., and Virtamo, J. 2002. Effects of alpha-tocopherol and beta-carotene supplementation on gastric cancer incidence in male smokers (ATBC Study, Finland). *Cancer Causes Control* **13**(7): 617–623.

Malin, A., Matthews, C.E., Shu, X.O., Cai, H., Dai, Q., Jin, F., Gao, Y.T., and Zheng, W. 2005. Energy balance and breast cancer risk. *Cancer Epidemiol Biomarkers Prev* **14**: 1496–1501.

Mark, S.D., Qiao, Y.L., Dawsey, S.M., Wu, Y.P., Katki, H., Gunter, E.W., Fraumeni, J.F., Jr., Blot, W.J., Dong, Z.W., and Taylor, P.R. 2000. Prospective study of serum selenium levels and incident esophageal and gastric cancers. *J Natl Cancer Inst* **92**(21): 1753–1763.

Martinez, M.E., and Willett, W.C. 1998. Calcium, vitamin D, and colorectal cancer: a review of the epidemiologic evidence. *Cancer Epidemiol Biomarkers Prev* **7**(2): 163–168.

Mayne, S.T., Cartmel, B., Baum, M., Shor-Posner, G., Fallon, B.G., Briskin, K., Bean, J., Zheng, T., Cooper, D., Friedman, C., et al. 2001a. Randomized trial of supplemental beta-carotene to prevent second head and neck cancer. *Cancer Res* **61**(4): 1457–1463.

Mayne, S.T., and Navarro, S.A. 2002. Diet, obesity and reflux in the etiology of adenocarcinomas of the esophagus and gastric cardia in humans. *J Nutr* **132**(11 Suppl): 3467S–3470S.

Mayne, S.T., Risch, H.A., Dubrow, R., Chow, W.H., Gammon, M.D., Vaughan, T.L., Farrow, D.C., Schoenberg, J.B., Stanford, J.L., Ahsan, H., et al. 2001b. Nutrient intake and risk of subtypes of esophageal and gastric cancer. *Cancer Epidemiol Biomarkers Prev* **10**(10): 1055–1062.

McCullough, M.L., and Giovannucci, E.L. 2004. Diet and cancer prevention. *Oncogene* **23**: 6349–6364.

McKeown-Eyssen, G. 1994. Epidemiology of colorectal cancer revisited: are serum triglycerides and/or plasma glucose associated with risk? *Cancer Epidemiol Biomarkers Prev* **3**(8): 687–695.

McKeown-Eyssen, GE. 1987. Fiber intake in different populations and colon cancer risk. *Prev Med* **16**(4): 532–539.

McKeown-Eyssen, G.E., Bright-See, E., Bruce, W.R., Jazmaji, V., Cohen, L.B., Pappas, S.C., and Saibil, F.G. 1994. A randomized trial of a low fat high fibre diet in the recurrence of colorectal polyps. Toronto Polyp Prevention Group. *J Clin Epidemiol* **47**(5): 525–536.

McLarty, J.W., Holiday, D.B., Girard, W.M., Yanagihara, R.H., Kummet, T.D., and Greenberg, S.D. 1995. Beta-Carotene, vitamin A, and lung cancer chemoprevention: results of an intermediate endpoint study. *Am J Clin Nutr* **62**(6 Suppl): 1431S–1438S.

McLaughlin, J.K., Gridley, G., Block, G., Winn, D.M., Preston-Martin, S., Schoenberg, J.B., Greenberg, R.S., Stemhagen, A., Austin, D.F., Ershow, A.G., et al. 1988. Dietary factors in oral and pharyngeal cancer. *J Natl Cancer Inst* **80**(15): 1237–1243.

Michels, K.B., Edward, G., Joshipura, K.J., Rosner, B.A., Stampfer, M.J., Fuchs, C.S., Colditz, G.A., Speizer, F.E., and Willett, W.C. 2000. Prospective study of fruit and vegetable consumption and incidence of colon and rectal cancers. *J Natl Cancer Inst* **92**(21): 1740–1752.

Miller, A.B., Altenburg, H.P., Bueno-de-Mesquita, B., Boshuizen, H.C., Agudo, A., Berrino, F., Gram, I.T., Janson, L., Linseisen, J., Overvad, K., et al. 2004. Fruits and vegetables and lung cancer: Findings from the European Prospective Investigation into Cancer and Nutrition. *Int J Cancer* **108**(2): 269–276.

Muir, J.G., Yeow, E.G., Keogh, J., Pizzey, C., Bird, A.R., Sharpe, K., O'Dea, K., and Macrae, F.A. 2004. Combining wheat bran with resistant starch has more beneficial effects on fecal indexes than does wheat bran alone. *Am J Clin Nutr* **79**(6): 1020–1028.

Murr, G., Kostelic, F., Donkic-Pavicic, I., Grdinic, B., and Subic, N. 1988. Comparison of the vitamin A blood serum level in patients with head-neck cancer and healthy persons. *Hno* **36**(9): 359–362.

National Cancer Institute. U.S. National Institutes of Health. 2005a. Colorectal Cancer (PDQ): Prevention. Available at www.cancer.gov.

National Cancer Institute. U.S. National Institutes of Health. 2005b. Lung Cancer (PDQ): Prevention. Available at www.cancer.gov.

National Cancer Institute. U.S. National Institutes of Health. 2005c. Prostate Cancer (PDR) Prevention. Available at www.cancer.gov.

Nauss, K.M., Bueche, D., and Newberne, P.M. 1987. Effect of beef fat on DMH-induced colon tumorigenesis: influence of rat strain and nutrient composition. *J Nutr* **117**(4): 739–747.

Nauss, K.M., Locniskar, M., and Newberne, P.M. 1983. Effect of alterations in the quality and quantity of dietary fat on 1,2-dimethylhydrazine-induced colon tumorigenesis in rats. *Cancer Res* **43**(9): 4083–4090.

Negri, E., La Vecchia, C., Franceschi, S., D'Avanzo, B., and Parazzini, F. 1991. Vegetable and fruit consumption and cancer risk. *Int J Cancer* **48**(3): 350–354.

Nesbitt, J.A., Smith, J., McDowell, G., and Drago, J.R. 1988. Adriamycin-vitamin E combination therapy for treatment of prostate adenocarcinoma in the Nb rat model. *J Surg Oncol* **38**(4): 283–284.

Neugut, A.I., Garbowski, G.C., Lee, W.C., Murray, T., Nieves, J.W., Forde, K.A., Treat, M.R., Waye, J.D., and Fenoglio-Preiser, C. 1993. Dietary risk factors for the incidence and recurrence of colorectal adenomatous polyps. A case–control study. *Ann Intern Med* **118**(2): 91–95.

Newmark, H.L., Wargovich, M.J., and Bruce, W.R. 1984. Colon cancer and dietary fat, phosphate, and calcium: a hypothesis. *J Natl Cancer Inst* **72**(6): 1323–1325.

Nomura, A.M., Lee, J., Stemmermann, G.N., and Combs, G.F., Jr. 2000. Serum selenium and subsequent risk of prostate cancer. *Cancer Epidemiol Biomarkers Prev* **9**(9): 883–887.

Norat, T., Bingham, S., Ferrari, P., Slimani, N., Jenab, M., Mazuir, M., Overvad, K., Olsen, A., Tjonneland, A., Clavel, F., et al. 2005. Meat, fish, and colorectal cancer risk: the European Prospective Investigation into cancer and nutrition. *J Natl Cancer Inst* **97**: 906–916.

Norat, T., Lukanova, A., Ferrari, P., and Riboli, E. 2002. Meat consumption and colorectal cancer risk: dose–response meta-analysis of epidemiological studies. *Int J Cancer* **98**(2): 241–256.

Norrish, A.E., Jackson, R.T., Sharpe, S.J., and Skeaff, C.M. 2000. Prostate cancer and dietary carotenoids. *Am J Epidemiol* **151**(2): 119–123.

Notani, P.N., and Jayant, K. 1987. Role of diet in upper aerodigestive tract cancers. *Nutr Cancer* **10**(1–2): 103–113.

Omenn, G.S., Goodman, G., Thornquist, M., Grizzle, J., Rosenstock, L., Barnhart, S., Balmes, J., Cherniack, M.G., Cullen, M.R., Glass, A., et al. 1994. The beta-carotene and retinol efficacy trial (CARET) for chemoprevention of lung cancer in high risk populations: smokers and asbestos-exposed workers. *Cancer Res* **54**(7 Suppl): 2038s–2043s.

Omenn, G.S., Goodman, G.E., Thornquist, M.D., Balmes, J., Cullen, M.R., Glass, A., Keogh, J.P., Meyskens, F.L., Jr., Valanis, B., Williams, J.H., Jr., et al. 1996a. Risk factors for lung cancer and for intervention effects in CARET, the Beta-Carotene and Retinol Efficacy Trial. *J Natl Cancer Inst* **88**(21): 1550–1559.

Omenn, G.S., Goodman, G.E., Thornquist, M.D., Balmes, J., Cullen, M.R., Glass, A., Keogh, J.P., Meyskens, F.L., Valanis, B., Williams, J.H., et al. 1996b. Effects of a combination of beta carotene and vitamin A on lung cancer and cardiovascular disease. *N Engl J Med* **334**(18): 1150–1155.

Pandalai, P.K., Pilat, M.J., Yamazaki, K., Naik, H., and Pienta, K.J. 1996. The effects of omega-3 and omega-6 fatty acids on in vitro prostate cancer growth. *Anticancer Res* **16**(2): 815–820.

Paolini, M., Abdel-Rahman, S.Z., Sapone, A., Pedulli, G.F., Perocco, P., Cantelli-Forti, G., Legator, M.S. 2003. Beta-carotene: a cancer chemopreventive agent or a co-carcinogen? *Mutat Res* **543**(3): 195–200.

Paolini, M., Antelli, A., Pozzetti, L., Spetlova, D., Perocco, P., Valgimigli, L., Pedulli, G.F., and Cantelli-Forti, G. 2001. Induction of cytochrome P450 enzymes and over-generation of oxygen radicals in beta-carotene supplemented rats. *Carcinogenesis* **22**(9): 1483–1495.

Paolini, M., Cantelli-Forti, G., Perocco, P., Pedulli, G.F., Abdel-Rahman, S.Z., and Legator, M.S. 1999. Co-carcinogenic effect of beta-carotene. *Nature* **398**(6730): 760–761.

Parkin, D.M., Bray, F., Ferlay, J., and Pisani, P. 2005. Global cancer statistics, 2002. CA *Cancer J Clin* **55**(2): 74–108.

Parkin, D.M., Pisani, P., and Ferlay, J. 1999. Global cancer statistics. *CA Cancer J Clin* **49**(1): 33–64.

Perocco, P., Paolini, M., Mazzullo, M., Biagi, G.L., and Cantelli-Forti, G. 1999. Beta-carotene as enhancer of cell transforming activity of powerful carcinogens and cigarette-smoke condensate on BALB/c 3T3 cells in vitro. *Mutat Res* **440**(1): 83–90.

Perry, C.F., Stevens, M., Rabie, I., Yarker, M.E., Cochrane, J., Perry, E., Traficante, R., and Coman, W. 2005. Chemoprevention of head and neck cancer with retinoids: a negative result. *Arch Otolaryngol Head Neck Surg* **131**(3): 198–203.

Peto, R., Doll, R., Buckley, J.D., and Sporn, M.B. 1981. Can dietary beta-carotene materially reduce human cancer rates? *Nature* **290**(5803): 201–208.

Pisani, P., Parkin, D.M., Bray, F., and Ferlay, J. 1999. Estimates of the worldwide mortality from 25 cancers in 1990. *Int J Cancer* **83**(1): 18–29.

Plummer, M., Franceschi, S., and Munoz, N. 2004. Epidemiology of gastric cancer. *IARC Sci Publ*(157): 311–326.

Prentice, R.L., and Sheppard, L. 1990. Dietary fat and cancer: consistency of the epidemiologic data, and disease prevention that may follow from a practical reduction in fat consumption. *Cancer Causes Control* **1**(1): 81–97; discussion 99–109.

Rajkumar, T., Sridhar, H., Balaram, P., Vaccarella, S., Gajalakshmi, V., Nandakumar, A., Ramdas, K., Jayshree, R., Munoz, N., Herrero, R., et al. 2003. Oral cancer in Southern India: the influence of body size, diet, infections and sexual practices. *Eur J Cancer Prev* **12**(2): 135–143.

Rao, M., Liu, F.S., Dawsey, S.M., Yang, K., Lipkin, M., Li, J.Y., Taylor, P.R., Li, B., Blot, W.J., Wang, G.Q., et al. 1994. Effects of vitamin/mineral supplementation on the proliferation of esophageal squamous epithelium in Linxian, China. *Cancer Epidemiol Biomarkers Prev* **3**(3): 277–279.

Rashidkhani, B., Lindblad, P., and Wolk, A. 2005. Fruits, vegetables and risk of renal cell carcinoma: a prospective study of Swedish women. *Int J Cancer* **113**: 451–455.

Reddy, B.S. 2004. Omega-3 fatty acids in colorectal cancer prevention. *Int J Cancer* **112**(1): 1–7.

Reid, M.E., Stratton, M.S., Lillico, A.J., Fakih, M., Natarajan, R., Clark, L.C., and Marshall, J.R. 2004. A report of high-dose selenium supplementation: response and toxicities. *J Trace Elem Med Biol* **18**(1): 69–74.

Rhee, J.C., Khuri, F.R., and Shin, D.M. 2004. Advances in chemoprevention of head and neck cancer. *Oncologist* **9**(3): 302–311.

Riboli, E., and Norat, T. 2003. Epidemiologic evidence of the protective effect of fruit and vegetables on cancer risk. *Am J Clin Nutr* **78**(3 Suppl): 559S–569S.

Ripoll, E.A., Rama, B.N., and Webber, M.M. 1986. Vitamin E enhances the chemotherapeutic effects of adriamycin on human prostatic carcinoma cells in vitro. *J Urol* **136**(2): 529–531.

Rodriguez, T., Altieri, A., Chatenoud, L., Gallus, S., Bosetti, C., Negri, E., Franceschi, S., Levi, F., Talamini, R., and La Vecchia, C. 2004. Risk factors for oral and pharyngeal cancer in young adults. *Oral Oncol* **40**(2): 207–213.

Rose, D.P., Boyar, A.P., and Wynder, E.L. 1986. International comparisons of mortality rates for cancer of the breast, ovary, prostate, and colon, and per capita food consumption. *Cancer* **58**(11): 2363–2371.

Rose, D.P., and Connolly, J.M. 1991. Effects of fatty acids and eicosanoid synthesis inhibitors on the growth of two human prostate cancer cell lines. *Prostate* **18**(3): 243–254.

Russell, R.M. 2004. The enigma of beta-carotene in carcinogenesis: what can be learned from animal studies. *J Nutr* **134**(1): 262S–268S.

Saigal, C.S., and Litwin, M.S. 2002. The economic costs of early stage prostate cancer. *Pharmacoeconomics* **20**(13): 869–878.

Sakr, W.A., Grignon, D.J., Haas, G.P., Heilbrun, L.K., Pontes, J.E., and Crissman, J.D. 1996. Age and racial distribution of prostatic intraepithelial neoplasia. *Eur Urol* **30**(2): 138–144.

Salgo, M.G., Cueto, R., Winston, G.W., and Pryor, W.A. 1999. Beta carotene and its oxidation products have different effects on microsome mediated binding of benzo[a]pyrene to DNA. *Free Radic Biol Med* **26**(1–2): 162–173.

Sanchez, M.J., Martinez, C., Nieto, A., Castellsague, X., Quintana, M.J., Bosch, F.X., Munoz, N., Herrero, R., and Franceschi, S. 2003. Oral and oropharyngeal cancer in Spain: influence of dietary patterns. *Eur J Cancer Prev* **12**(1): 49–56.

Sandhu, M.S., White, I.R., and McPherson, K. 2001. Systematic review of the prospective cohort studies on meat consumption and colorectal cancer risk: a meta-analytical approach. *Cancer Epidemiol Biomarkers Prev* **10**(5): 439–446.

Sanjoaquin, M.A., Allen, N., Couto, E., Roddam, A.W., and Key, T.J. 2005. Folate intake and colorectal cancer risk: a meta-analytical approach. *Int J Cancer* **113**(5): 825–828.

Sankaranarayanan, R., and Mathew, B. 1996. Retinoids as cancer-preventive agents. *IARC Sci Publ* (139): 47–59.

Sankaranarayanan, R., Mathew, B., Varghese, C., Sudhakaran, P.R., Menon, V., Jayadeep, A., Nair, M.K., Mathews, C., Mahalingam, T.R., Balaram, P., et al. 1997. Chemoprevention of oral leukoplakia with vitamin A and beta carotene: an assessment. *Oral Oncol* **33**(4): 231–236.

Sarkar, F.H., and Li, Y. 2002. Mechanisms of cancer chemoprevention by soy isoflavone genistein. *Cancer Metastasis Rev* **21**(3–4): 265–280.

Sarkar, F.H., and Li, Y. 2003. Soy isoflavones and cancer prevention. *Cancer Invest* **21**(5): 744–757.

Sauvaget, C., Nagano, J., Hayashi, M., Spencer, E., Shimizu, Y., and Allen, N. 2003. Vegetables and fruit intake and cancer mortality in the Hiroshima/Nagasaki Life Span Study. *Br J Cancer* **88**: 689–694.

Schatzkin, A., Lanza, E., Corle, D., Lance, P., Iber, F., Caan, B., Shike, M., Weissfeld, J., Burt, R., Cooper, M.R., et al. 2000. Lack of effect of a low-fat, high-fiber diet on the recurrence of colorectal adenomas. Polyp Prevention Trial Study Group. *N Engl J Med* **342**(16): 1149–1155.

Schatzkin, A., Lanza, E., Freedman, L.S., Tangrea, J., Cooper, M.R., Marshall, J.R., Murphy, P.A., Selby, J.V., Shike, M., Schade, R.R., et al. 1996. The polyp prevention trial I: rationale, design, recruitment, and baseline participant characteristics. *Cancer Epidemiol Biomarkers Prev* **5**(5): 375–383.

Schrauzer, G.N., White, D.A., and Schneider, C.J. 1977. Cancer mortality correlation studies—III: statistical associations with dietary selenium intakes. *Bioinorg Chem* **7**(1): 23–31.

Severson, R.K., Nomura, A.M., Grove, J.S., and Stemmermann, G.N. 1989. A prospective study of demographics, diet, and prostate cancer among men of Japanese ancestry in Hawaii. *Cancer Res* **49**(7): 1857–1860.

Shamberger, R.J., Tytko, S.A., and Willis, C.E. 1976. Antioxidants and cancer. Part VI. Selenium and age-adjusted human cancer mortality. *Arch Environ Health* **31**(5): 231–235.

Shannon, J., Ray, R., Wu, C., Nelson, Z., Gao, D.L., Li, W., Hu, W., Lampe, J., Horner, N., Satia, J., et al. 2005. Food and botanical groupings and risk of breast cancer: a case–control study in Shanghai, China. *Cancer Epidemiol Biomarkers Prev* **14**: 81–90.

Sharp, R.M., Bello-DeOcampo, D., Quader, S.T., and Webber, M.M. 2001. N-(4-hydroxyphenyl)retinamide (4-HPR) decreases neoplastic properties of human prostate cells: an agent for prevention. *Mutat Res* **496**(1–2): 163–170.

Shike, M., Latkany, L., Riedel, E., Fleisher, M., Schatzkin, A., Lanza, E., Corle, D., and Begg, C.B. 2002. Lack of effect of a low-fat, high-fruit, -vegetable, and -fiber diet on serum prostate-specific antigen of men without prostate cancer: results from a randomized trial. *J Clin Oncol* **20**(17): 3592–3598.

Siddiqi, M., Kumar, R., Fazili, Z., Spiegelhalder, B., and Preussmann, R. 1992. Increased exposure to dietary amines and nitrate in a population at high risk of oesophageal and gastric cancer in Kashmir (India). *Carcinogenesis* **13**(8): 1331–1335.

Singh, J., Hamid, R., and Reddy, B.S. 1997a. Dietary fat and colon cancer: modulating effect of types and amount of dietary fat on ras-p21 function during promotion and progression stages of colon cancer. *Cancer Res* **57**(2): 253–258.

Singh, J., Hamid, R., and Reddy, B.S. 1997b. Dietary fat and colon cancer: modulation of cyclooxygenase-2 by types and amount of dietary fat during the postinitiation stage of colon carcinogenesis. *Cancer Res* **57**(16): 3465–3470.

Slattery, M.L., Potter, J.D., Duncan, D.M., and Berry, T.D. 1997. Dietary fats and colon cancer: assessment of risk associated with specific fatty acids. *Int J Cancer* **73**(5): 670–677.

Smith-Warner, S.A., Spiegelman, D., Yaun, S.S., Adami, H.O., Beeson, W.L., van den Brandt, P.A., Folsom, A.R., Fraser, G.E., Freudenheim, J.L., Goldbohm, R.A., et al. 2001. Intake of fruits and vegetables and risk of breast cancer: a pooled analysis of cohort studies. *JAMA* **285**(6): 769–776.

Smith-Warner, S.A., Spiegelman, D., Yaun, S.S., Albanes, D., Beeson, W.L., van den Brandt, P.A., Feskanich, D., Folsom, A.R., Fraser, G.E., Freudenheim, J.L., et al. 2003. Fruits, vegetables and lung cancer: a pooled analysis of cohort studies. *Int J Cancer* **107**(6): 1001–1011.

Snowdon, D.A. 1988. Animal product consumption and mortality because of all causes combined, coronary heart disease, stroke, diabetes, and cancer in Seventh-day Adventists. *Am J Clin Nutr* **48**(3 Suppl): 739–748.

Snowdon, D.A., Phillips, R.L., and Choi, W. 1984. Diet, obesity, and risk of fatal prostate cancer. *Am J Epidemiol* **120**(2): 244–250.

Steinmetz, K.A., and Potter, J.D. 1991a. Vegetables, fruit, and cancer. I. Epidemiology. *Cancer Causes Control* **2**(5): 325–357.

Steinmetz, K.A., and Potter, J.D. 1991b. Vegetables, fruit, and cancer. II. Mechanisms. *Cancer Causes Control* **2**(6): 427–442.

Stewart, S.L., King, J.B., Thompson, T.D., Friedman, C., and Wingo, P.A. 2004. Cancer mortality surveillance—United States, 1990–2000. *MMWR Surveill Summ* **53**(3): 1–108.

Stich, H.F., Hornby, A.P., Mathew, B., Sankaranarayanan, R., and Nair, M.K. 1988. Response of oral leukoplakias to the administration of vitamin A. *Cancer Lett* **40**(1): 93–101.

Stich, H.F., Mathew, B., Sankaranarayanan, R., and Nair, M.K. 1991. Remission of precancerous lesions in the oral cavity of tobacco chewers and maintenance of the protective effect of beta-carotene or vitamin A. *Am J Clin Nutr* **53**(1 Suppl): 298S–304S.

Su, L., Fontham, E., Ruiz, B., Schmidt, S., Correa, P., and Bravo, L. 2000. Association of dietary antioxidants on the severity of gastritis in a high risk population. *Ann Epidemiol* **10**(7): 468.

Talalay, P., Fahey, J.W., Holtzclaw, W.D., Prestera, T., and Zhang, Y. 1995. Chemoprotection against cancer by phase 2 enzyme induction. *Toxicol Lett* **82–83**: 173–179.

Tavani, A., Gallus, S., La Vecchia, C., Talamini, R., Barbone, F., Herrero, R., and Franceschi, S. 2001. Diet and risk of oral and pharyngeal cancer. An Italian case–control study. *Eur J Cancer Prev* **10**(2): 191–195.

Taylor, P.R., Li, B., Dawsey, S.M., Li, J.Y., Yang, C.S., Guo, W., and Blot, W.J. 1994. Prevention of esophageal cancer: the nutrition intervention trials in Linxian, China. Linxian Nutrition Intervention Trials Study Group. *Cancer Res* **54**(7 Suppl): 2029s–2031s.

Taylor, P.R., Qiao, Y.L., Abnet, C.C., Dawsey, S.M., Yang, C.S., Gunter, E.W., Wang, W., Blot, W.J., Dong, Z.W., and Mark, S.D. 2003. Prospective study of serum vitamin E levels and esophageal and gastric cancers. *J Natl Cancer Inst* **95**(18): 1414–1416.

Terry, P., Giovannucci, E., Bergkvist, L., Holmberg, L., and Wolk, A. 2001a. Body weight and colorectal cancer risk in a cohort of Swedish women: relation varies by age and cancer site. *Br J Cancer* **85**(3): 346–349.

Terry, P., Lagergren, J., Hansen, H., Wolk, A., and Nyren, O. 2001b. Fruit and vegetable consumption in the prevention of oesophageal and cardia cancers. *Eur J Cancer Prev* **10**(4): 365–369.

Terry, P., Lagergren, J., Ye, W., Nyren, O., and Wolk, A. 2000. Antioxidants and cancers of the esophagus and gastric cardia. *Int J Cancer* **87**(5): 750–754.

Terry, P., Lagergren, J., Ye, W., Wolk, A., and Nyren, O. 2001c. Inverse association between intake of cereal fiber and risk of gastric cardia cancer. *Gastroenterology* **120**(2): 387–391.

Terry, P.D., Miller, A.B., and Rohan, T.E. 2002. Obesity and colorectal cancer risk in women. *Gut* **51**(2): 191–194.

Thaller, C., Shalev, M., Frolov, A., Eichele, G., Thompson, T.C., Williams, R.H., Dillioglugil, O., and Kadmon, D. 2000. Fenretinide therapy in prostate cancer: effects on tissue and serum retinoid concentration. *J Clin Oncol* **18**(22): 3804–3808.

Thomas, G., Hashibe, M., Jacob, B.J., Ramadas, K., Mathew, B., Sankaranarayanan, R., Zhang, Z.F. 2003. Risk factors for multiple oral premalignant lesions. *Int J Cancer* **107**(2): 285–291.

Thun, M.J., Calle, E.E., Namboodiri, M.M., Flanders, W.D., Coates, R.J., Byers, T., Boffetta, P., Garfinkel, L., and Heath, C.W., Jr. 1992. Risk factors for fatal colon cancer in a large prospective study. *J Natl Cancer Inst* **84**(19): 1491–1500.

Tiemersma, E.W., Voskuil, D.W., Bunschoten, A., Hogendoorn, E.A., Witteman, B.J., Nagengast, F.M., Glatt, H., Kok, F.J., and Kampman, E. 2004. Risk of colorectal adenomas in relation to meat consumption, meat preparation, and genetic susceptibility in a Dutch population. *Cancer Causes Control* **15**(3): 225–236.

Toma, S., Benso, S., Albanese, E., Palumbo, R., Cantoni, E., Nicolo, G., and Mangiante, P. 1992. Treatment of oral leukoplakia with beta-carotene. *Oncology* **49**(2): 77–81.

Toniolo, P., Van Kappel, A.L., Akhmedkhanov, A., Ferrari, P., Kato, I., Shore, R.E., and Riboli, E. 2001. Serum carotenoids and breast cancer. *Am J Epidemiol* **153**(12): 1142–1147.

Trock, B., Lanza, E., and Greenwald, P. 1990a. Dietary fiber, vegetables, and colon cancer: critical review and meta-analyses of the epidemiologic evidence. *J Natl Cancer Inst* **82**(8): 650–661.

Trock, B.J., Lanza, E., and Greenwald, P. 1990b. High fiber diet and colon cancer: a critical review. *Prog Clin Biol Res* **346**: 145–157.

Tsugane, S. 2005. Salt, salted food intake, and risk of gastric cancer: epidemiologic evidence. *Cancer Sci* **96**(1): 1–6.

U.S. Department of Health and Human Services, Centers for the Disease Control and Prevention, Center for Chronic Disease Prevention and Health Promotion, Office on Smoking and Health. 2004. The Heath Consequences of Smoking. A Report of the Surgeon General. Rockville, MD.

Vainio, H., and Bianchini, F. 2002. Weight control and physical activity. IARC handbooks of cancer prevention. Volume 6. Lyon, France: International Agency for Research on Cancer.

van Gils, C.H., Peeters, P.H., Bueno-de-Mesquita, H.B., Boshuizen, H.C., Lahmann, P.H., Clavel-Chapelon, F., Thiebaut, A., Kesse, E., Sieri, S., Palli, D., et al. 2005. Consumption of vegetables and fruits and risk of breast cancer. *JAMA* **293**(2): 183–193.

van Zandwijk, N., Dalesio, O., Pastorino, U., de Vries, N., and van Tinteren, H. 2000. EUROSCAN, a randomized trial of vitamin A and N-acetylcysteine in patients with head and neck cancer or lung cancer. For the EUropean Organization for Research and Treatment of Cancer Head and Neck and Lung Cancer Cooperative Groups. *J Natl Cancer Inst* **92**(12): 977–986.

Veronesi, U., De Palo, G., Marubini, E., Costa, A., Formelli, F., Mariani, L., Decensi, A., Camerini, T., Del Turco, M.R., Di Mauro, M.G., et al. 1999. Randomized trial of fenretinide to prevent second breast malignancy in women with early breast cancer. *J Natl Cancer Inst* **91**(21): 1847–1856.

Virtamo, J., Pietinen, P., Huttunen, J.K., Korhonen, P., Malila, N., Virtanen, M.J., Albanes, D., Taylor, P.R., and Albert, P. 2003. Incidence of cancer and mortality following alpha-tocopherol and beta-carotene supplementation: a postintervention follow-up. *JAMA* **290**(4): 476–485.

Voskuil, D.W., Kampman, E., Grubben, M.J., Kok, F.J., Nagengast, F.M., Vasen, H.F., van 't Veer, P. 2002. Meat consumption and meat preparation in relation to colorectal adenomas among sporadic and HNPCC family patients in The Netherlands. *Eur J Cancer* **38**(17): 2300–2308.

Wang, L., Zhu, D., Zhang, C., Mao, X., Wang, G., Mitra, S., Li, B.F., Wang, X., and Wu, M. 1997. Mutations of O6-methylguanine-DNA methyltransferase gene in esophageal cancer tissues from Northern China. *Int J Cancer* **71**(5): 719–723.

Wang, L.D., Qiu, S.L., Yang, G.R., Lipkin, M., Newmark, H.L., and Yang, C.S. 1993. A randomized double-blind intervention study on the effect of calcium supplementation on esophageal precancerous lesions in a high-risk population in China. *Cancer Epidemiol Biomarkers Prev* **2**(1): 71–78.

Wang, L.D., Zhou, Q., Feng, C.W., Liu, B., Qi, Y.J., Zhang, Y.R., Gao, S.S., Fan, Z.M., Zhou, Y., Yang, C.S., et al. 2002. Intervention and follow-up on human esophageal precancerous lesions in Henan, northern China, a high-incidence area for esophageal cancer. *Gan To Kagaku Ryoho* **29**(Suppl 1): 159–172.

Wang, Y., Corr, J.G., Thaler, H.T., Tao, Y., Fair, W.R., and Heston, W.D. 1995. Decreased growth of established human prostate LNCaP tumors in nude mice fed a low-fat diet. *J Natl Cancer Inst* **87**(19): 1456–1462.

Wargovich, M.J., Eng, V.W., and Newmark, H.L. 1984. Calcium inhibits the damaging and compensatory proliferative effects of fatty acids on mouse colon epithelium. *Cancer Lett* **23**(3): 253–258.

Wargovich, M.J., Eng, V.W., Newmark, H.L., and Bruce, W.R. 1983. Calcium ameliorates the toxic effect of deoxycholic acid on colonic epithelium. *Carcinogenesis* **4**(9): 1205–1207.

Wargovich, M.J., Isbell, G., Shabot, M., Winn, R., Lanza, F., Hochman, L., Larson, E., Lynch, P., Roubein, L., and Levin, B. 1992. Calcium supplementation decreases rectal epithelial cell proliferation in subjects with sporadic adenoma. *Gastroenterology* **103**(1): 92–97.

Webber, M.M., Bello-DeOcampo, D., Quader, S., Deocampo, N.D., Metcalfe, W.S., and Sharp, R.M. 1999. Modulation of the malignant phenotype of human prostate cancer cells by N-(4-hydroxyphenyl) retinamide (4-HPR). *Clin Exp Metastasis* **17**(3): 255–263.

Wei, E.K., Giovannucci, E., Wu, K., Rosner, B., Fuchs, C.S., Willett, W.C., and Colditz, G.A. 2004. Comparison of risk factors for colon and rectal cancer. *Int J Cancer* **108**(3): 433–442.

Weinstein, S.J., Wright, M.E., Pietinen, P., King, I., Tan, C., Taylor, P.R., Virtamo, J., Albanes, D. 2005. Serum alpha-tocopherol and gamma-tocopherol in relation to prostate cancer risk in a prospective study. *J Natl Cancer Inst* **97**(5): 396–399.

Willett, W.C., Stampfer, M.J., Colditz, G.A., Rosner, B.A., and Speizer, F.E. 1990. Relation of meat, fat, and fiber intake to the risk of colon cancer in a prospective study among women. *N Engl J Med* **323**(24): 1664–1672.

Winn, D.M. 1995. Diet and nutrition in the etiology of oral cancer. *Am J Clin Nutr* **61**(2): 437S–445S.

Winn, D.M., Ziegler, R.G., Pickle, L.W., Gridley, G., Blot, W.J., and Hoover, R.N. 1984. Diet in the etiology of oral and pharyngeal cancer among women from the southern United States. *Cancer Res* **44**(3): 1216–1222.

Winters, B.L., Mitchell, D.C., Smiciklas-Wright, H., Grosvenor, M.B., Liu, W., and Blackburn, G.L. 2004. Dietary patterns in women treated for breast cancer who successfully reduce fat intake: the Women's Intervention Nutrition Study (WINS). *J Am Diet Assoc* **104**: 551–559.

World Cancer Research Fund, American Institute for Cancer Research. 1997. Food, Nutrition, and the Prevention of Cancer: A Global Perspective. Washington, DC: The Institute.

Wu, B., Iwakiri, R., Ootani, A., Tsunada, S., Fujise, T., Sakata, Y., Sakata, H., Toda, S., and Fujimoto, K. 2004. Dietary corn oil promotes colon cancer by inhibiting mitochondria-dependent apoptosis in azoxymethane-treated rats. *Exp Biol Med (Maywood)* **229**(10): 1017–1025.

Wu, K., Willett, W.C., Fuchs, C.S., Colditz, G.A., and Giovannucci, E.L. 2002. Calcium intake and risk of colon cancer in women and men. *J Natl Cancer Inst* **94**(6): 437–446.

Wynder, E.L., Cohen, L.A., Muscat, J.E., Winters, B.L., Dwyer, J.T., and Blackburn, G.L. 1997. Breast Cancer: Weihging the evidence for a promoting role of dietary fat. *J Natl Cancer Inst* **89**: 766–775.

Wynder, E.L., Mabuchi, K., and Whitmore, W.F., Jr. 1971. Epidemiology of cancer of the prostate. *Cancer* **28**(2): 344–360.

Yoshizawa, K., Willett, W.C., Morris, S.J., Stampfer, M.J., Spiegelman, D., Rimm, E.B., and Giovannucci, E. 1998. Study of prediagnostic selenium level in toenails and the risk of advanced prostate cancer. *J Natl Cancer Inst* **90**(16): 1219–1224.

Youssef, E.M., Lotan, D., Issa, J.P., Wakasa, K., Fan, Y.H., Mao, L., Hassan, K., Feng, L., Lee, J.J., Lippman, S.M., et al. 2004. Hypermethylation of the retinoic acid receptor-beta(2) gene in head and neck carcinogenesis. *Clin Cancer Res* **10**(5): 1733–1742.

Yu, H., Harris, R.E., Gao, Y.T., Gao, R., and Wynder, E.L. 1991. Comparative epidemiology of cancers of the colon, rectum, prostate and breast in Shanghai, China versus the United States. *Int J Epidemiol* **20**(1): 76–81.

Zhang, S., Hunter, D.J., Forman, M.R., Rosner, B.A., Speizer, F.E., Colditz, G.A., Manson, J.E., Hankinson, S.E., and Willett, W.C. 1999. Dietary carotenoids and vitamins A, C, and E and risk of breast cancer. *J Natl Cancer Inst* **91**(6): 547–556.

Zhang, S.M., Willett, W.C., Selhub, J., Hunter, D.J., Giovannucci, E.L., Holmes, M.D., Colditz, G.A., and Hankinson, S.E. 2003. Plasma folate, vitamin B6, vitamin B12, homocysteine, and risk of breast cancer. *J Natl Cancer Inst* **95**(5): 373–380.

Zhang, Y., Kensler, T.W., Cho, C.G., Posner, G.H, and Talalay, P. 1994. Anticarcinogenic activities of sulforaphane and structurally related synthetic norbornyl isothiocyanates. *Proc Natl Acad Sci USA* **91**(8): 3147–3150.

Zhang, Y., Talalay, P., Cho, C.G., and Posner, G.H. 1992. A major inducer of anticarcinogenic protective enzymes from broccoli: isolation and elucidation of structure. *Proc Natl Acad Sci USA* **89**(6): 2399–2403.

Zheng, W., Blot, W.J., Shu, X.O., Gao, Y.T., Ji, B.T., Ziegler, R.G., and Fraumeni, J.F., Jr. 1992. Diet and other risk factors for laryngeal cancer in Shanghai, China. *Am J Epidemiol* **136**(2): 178–191.

Zhou, J.R., and Blackburn, G.L. 1997. Bridging animal and human studies: what are the missing segments in dietary fat and prostate cancer? *Am J Clin Nutr* **66**(6 Suppl): 1572S–1580S.

Zhou, J.R., Gugger, E.T., Tanaka, T., Guo, Y., Blackburn, G.L., and Clinton, S.K. 1999. Soybean phytochemicals inhibit the growth of transplantable human prostate carcinoma and tumor angiogenesis in mice. *J Nutr* **129**(9): 1628–1635.

Zhou, J.R., Yu, L., Zhong, Y., Nassr, R.L., Franke, A.A., Gaston, S.M., and Blackburn, G.L. 2002. Inhibition of orthotopic growth and metastasis of androgen-sensitive human prostate tumors in mice by bioactive soybean components. *Prostate* **53**(2): 143–153.

CHAPTER

49

Future Directions in Cancer and Nutrition Research: Gene–Nutrient Interactions, Networks, and the Xenobiotic Hypothesis

DAVID HEBER, JOHN MILNER, GEORGE BLACKBURN, AND VAY LIANG W. GO

INTRODUCTION

Since the publication of the first edition of this text, there has been a period of tremendous growth in the field of nutritional oncology. There has been an explosion in the application of gene expression microarrays and other general molecular profiling technologies to a wide range of biological issues relevant to carcinogenesis including proliferation, apoptosis, DNA repair, antioxidant defenses, intercellular communications, and xenobiotic metabolism.

Significant discoveries relating to the complex network of biochemical processes underlying living systems, gene discovery, and structure determination have resulted from the widespread use of microarrays in cancer research. Microarrays have also helped to identify biomarkers, disease subtypes, and mechanisms of toxicity, and more recently, to elucidate the genetics of gene expression in human populations and reconstruct gene networks via the integration of gene expression and genetic data. Although there have been some signal achievements leading to new approaches to prevention, which are being tested, the use of molecular profiling technologies as a tool to identify genes responsible for common forms of cancer has been less successful. Although the identification of hundreds or even thousands of genes whose expression changes are associated with disease traits is relatively straightforward, determining which of the genes are causative drivers of disease as opposed to responders to the disease state has proven difficult.

Future research in the field of nutritional oncology will have to examine factors affecting causation and treatment through multifactorial mechanisms involving interactions of genes and the environment because these interactions are the etiological basis of common forms of cancer. The example of the expression of the BRCA1 mutation by differences in physical activity is just one of many examples demonstrating the ability of diet and lifestyle to modify genetic expression.

The process of identifying complex interactions that increase cancer susceptibility and are amenable to prevention will ultimately require the application of systems biology. The goal of systems biology is to define all of the elements present in a given system and to create an interaction network between these components so that the behavior of the system, as a whole and in parts, can be explained under specified conditions. The elements constituting the network that influences carcinogenesis could include genes, epigenetic modulation, metabolic pathways, transcript levels, proteins, or physiological traits. At present, the analytical methods do not exist to fully take advantage of the promise of systems biology. The most advanced systems biology scientists can at best describe the network governing the functioning of a single bacterial enzyme system.

Therefore, the next period in nutrition oncology research will require the stepwise identification of metabolic pathways affected by genetic polymorphisms that can be modulated through diet and lifestyle. Necessarily, there will be duplication as the same mechanisms will be operative in many types of cancer. Once these metabolic pathways and their genetics are understood, they can hopefully be assembled into interacting networks that can be analyzed using systems biology. However, there will be a number of types of research necessary for the successful application of this science to cancer prevention.

Copyright © 2006, Elsevier Inc.
All rights of reproduction in any form reserved.

GENE–NUTRIENT INTERACTION AND THE XENOBIOTIC HYPOTHESIS OF CANCER

The Xenobiotic Hypothesis first raised in the 1999 edition of this textbook is still a valid notion worthy of investigation.

Phytochemicals are being investigated aggressively as potential cancer chemopreventive agents. Cellular research has established that phytochemicals inhibit the proliferation of cancer cells. Cancer cells, particularly those that are highly invasive or metastatic, appear to require a certain level of oxidative stress to maintain a balance of proliferation and apoptosis. They constitutively generate large but tolerated amounts of H_2O_2 that apparently function as signaling molecules in the mitogen-activated protein kinase pathway to constantly activate redox-sensitive transcription factors and responsive genes that are involved in the survival of cancer cells as well as in their proliferation. With such a reliance of cancer cells on H_2O_2, it follows that if the excess H_2O_2 can be scavenged by phenolic phytochemicals having antioxidant activity, the oxidative stress-responsive genes can be suppressed and, consequently, cancer cell proliferation inhibited. On the other hand, phytochemicals can also induce the formation of H_2O_2 following the activation of cytochrome P450 enzymes to achieve an intolerable level of high oxidative stress in cancer cells. As an early response, the stress genes are activated. However, when the critical threshold for cancer cells to cope with the induced oxidative stress has been reached, key cellular components such as DNA are damaged irreparably. In conjunction, genes involved in initiating cell cycle arrest and/or apoptosis are activated. Therefore, phytochemicals can either scavenge the constitutive H_2O_2 or paradoxically generate additional amounts of H_2O_2 to inhibit the proliferation of cancer cells.

The effects of reactive oxygen species (ROS) are dose related. Low doses appear to support tumor cells, whereas higher doses either inhibit cell growth or activate apoptosis.

The complexity of the genetics of cancer is evident from the observation that only in 10% of cases is cancer inherited in a familial fashion. The majority of cancers are multifactorial involving complex gene–gene and gene–nutrient interactions. As high-throughput genotyping and gene sequencing technology advances, we will be able to ask new questions related to these interactions. This new frontier for cancer and nutrition research is very promising.

The somatic genetic changes that occur in precancerous cells are potentially modifiable through nutrition. Increased knowledge in the nutritional sciences and an improved understanding of the cellular and molecular basis of cancer now make it possible to approach research on nutrient–gene interactions relevant to cancer prevention and treatment, as proposed by several authors in their respective chapters. In this concluding chapter, we present a new, unifying hypothesis that may provide a framework for future research at the interface of nutrient–gene interactions. We call this the *xenobiotic hypothesis* because it highlights the relationship of genetic polymorphisms of the enzymes metabolizing ligand-effectors to oxidant stress, nutrient and hormone metabolism, and carcinogenesis. The key to exploring this hypothesis will be to study the nutrient–gene interactions discussed earlier in this book, first presented and discussed in a report by the Expert Committee of the American Institute for Cancer Research in 1997.

Many common forms of cancer, as well as other chronic diseases and the process of aging, have been related to the process of oxidative stress. Drug-metabolizing enzymes (DMEs) are enzymes that metabolize drugs, carcinogens, and other environmental pollutants. It has been proposed that DME genes existed on this planet >2 billion years before the presence of plants, animals, or drugs. An early role for these enzymes in prokaryocytes probably included energy substrate utilization, such as splitting a molecule or inserting an oxygen atom into inaccessible carbon or other food sources, making them susceptible to further metabolism. Another early role for DMEs probably related to their metabolic ability to control the steady state levels of the ligands modulating cell division, growth, morphogenesis, and reproduction. It is quite possible that these roles diversified into a very large number of additional complex signal transduction pathways existing in all eukaryocytes today. Moreover, the enzymatic activities coded for by these genes can, under different circumstances, either detoxify substances or activate procarcinogens into carcinogens critical in the process of tumor promotion.

In this book, the general areas of knowledge and research currently active in the field of nutritional oncology have been reviewed, and methodologies used in fields such as genetics, cellular and molecular biology, epidemiology, clinical investigation, and clinical medicine fields such as medical and surgical oncology have been presented. How will this new field grow and provide new directions for the field of cancer prevention and treatment research?

This field will grow through defining and exploiting the science within the various approaches identified by researchers in nutritional oncology so that the discipline will contribute significantly to the prevention and treatment of cancer. Although the contributions of large multicenter trials such as the SELECT trial in prostate cancer will have major impacts on preventive practices, the efforts of individuals and small groups of investigators in pursuing particular metabolic pathways based on technological breakthroughs resulting from the genetics revolution will continue to play an important role in advancing the scientific agenda of cancer prevention research.

Increased recognition of the contributions of nutritional oncology among patients, clinicians, and government officials charged with the oversight of the National Institutes of

Health, the U.S. Department of Agriculture, the Food and Drug Administration, and the Centers for Disease Control and Prevention has been seen over the past 5 years as the result of significant breakthroughs that have changed the basic paradigms of cancer prevention and treatment.

To this point, there has been widespread recognition of the connections between food and health by consumers. Many areas of traditional and complementary medicine have been utilized to explore the connection between nutrition and cancer, but the full potential of nutritional oncology to have an impact on the survival of the cancer patient has not been realized.

This book has emphasized several themes that can be used to set the course for future research:

- Cancer is a multistep process involving the expression of aberrant genes.
- Nutrigenetics will define the differences in how individuals respond to the same nutritional interventions.
- Nutrigenomics will define the pleiotropic effects of bioactive substances on the multistep process of carcinogenesis.
- Carcinogenesis can be influenced by nutrition through hormonal, paracrine, autocrine, immune, and metabolic mechanisms that modulate cellular proliferation, differentiation, and apoptosis.
- Immune function can be modulated by nutrition and genetics and is integral to the understanding of the effects of nutrition on cancer.
- Obesity is understood in terms of energetics, as well as diet and physical activity, and obesity management is an important component of cancer prevention efforts.
- There are significant excesses of fat and calories in the diet. At the same time, there are deficiencies of micronutrients, fiber, and phytochemicals, which are important for cancer prevention in the U.S. diet and in some diets around the world. This is especially problematic in developing countries where undernutrition and the rapid adoption of modern diets can result in the simultaneous occurrence of starvation and obesity in the same country, and an increase in common forms of cancer related to obesity and the suboptimal intake of micronutrients, fiber, and phytochemicals in the modern diet coupled with physical inactivity.
- The development of plant-based diets with reductions in fat and calories and increases in fiber, micronutrients, and phytochemicals, coupled with programs to increase physical activity and exercise, is the public health approach to cancer prevention.
- Physicians, including primary care physicians and oncologists, have a significant role to play in individualizing approaches to cancer patients and in acting as "agents of change" in the teachable moment of cancer management.

CONCLUSION

The existence of nutrient–gene interactions is a proof of principle of the important influence that nutrition can have on the process of carcinogenesis. The stage was set for this realization by epidemiological work that demonstrated that migrating populations assumed the cancer risk profile of their environment, as well as experimental work showing that animals with the same genetic changes have different expressions of carcinogenesis depending on dietary intake. However, it was only through an improved understanding of the cellular and molecular basis of cancer that it is now possible to define the nutritional influences on the development and progression of common forms of cancer.

There are four key areas where the study of nutrient–gene interaction will be helpful: First, gene–nutrient interaction studies provide a more accurate view of cancer causation than either genetic or nutritional studies done separately. Second, nutrient–gene interaction studies improve the ability to conduct cancer surveillance activities to define at-risk populations. Third, nutrient–gene interactions can provide an approach to the development of smaller and more cost-effective nutrition intervention studies by providing an enhanced ability to recruit at-risk populations. Finally, nutrient–gene interaction effects provide critical data helpful in interpreting the results of nutrition intervention studies. This future area of research promises to yield significant new insights into how nutritional strategies can be devised and applied to prevent and treat cancer in the next century.

The molecular role of nutrition in the multistep process of carcinogenesis at the levels of cell, organ, and organism is now a well-accepted concept. The relative importance in the context of the clinical evolution of cancer, especially in regard to the concomitant treatment of cancer patients with chemotherapy, radiation, and surgery, remains to be defined. We have seen that a single micronutrient such as β-carotene, when used in the context of continued smoking, can promote rather than retard the process of carcinogenesis. We still have limited information on nutrients used in the context of treatment rather than in primary or secondary prevention.

Future studies will require the development of improved biomarkers of cancer progression and perhaps a different paradigm than studying single nutrients individually in prospectively randomized controlled trials. There are a number of special populations that offer opportunities for developing new information. These populations include (1) family members of patients with markedly increased genetic susceptibility to cancer, (2) patients with prior cancer, (3) patients with premalignant lesions, and (4) elderly cancer patients with more indolent cancers where expectant therapy or watchful waiting permits the examination of nutritional parameters in the absence of any other treatment.

Human behavior research and improved food science technology will be critical in translating the scientific advances in the laboratory into public health strategies that work. We know that simply telling people to stop smoking can be highly effective, but food messages are more complex and must deal with interrelated sets of psychological, social, and economic factors. The development of functional foods for cancer prevention may make behavior change more feasible than it is today, but these efforts will still require behavioral research. Functional food research will need to include considerations of taste, cost, and convenience, as well as food production, distribution, and marketing. Efforts in marketing are largely behavioral in nature, while the economics of food involve taste and other biological considerations. Partnership of the food industry, agriculture, and medical science could significantly accelerate the development of nutritional oncology.

As clinical care models evolve, oncology networks may play important roles in facilitating research on nutrition and cancer. Carefully designed multicenter protocols for nutritional adjunctive treatment involving medical oncologists but implemented through allied health professional such as nurses and dietitians will answer many important clinical questions. Patient support groups provide one important source for recruitment to such efforts. These types of studies will require advanced statistical analysis methods to model longitudinal changes in multiple relevant variables over time.

Although all of these new directions for the future are of interest, ultimately there are two basic messages that should be derived from this text. First, nutritional oncology must be clearly defined as part of oncology. Historically, metabolism was an integral part of oncology until the era of molecular biology and genetics. Nutritional oncology can serve to hasten the return of metabolism to oncology where it can now be integrated with genetics and molecular biology. The current dogma that cancer is the result of genetic changes and is not influenced by nutrition must be changed by conducting and publishing research while disseminating the established scientific information presented here in the context of nutritional oncology through medical school curricula and continuing medical education programs. Second, if you are a clinical oncologist or primary care physician treating cancer patients, you should incorporate nutrition into your practice. We know enough about nutrition now to allow you to counsel your patients on avoiding unnecessary malnutrition, depression, and weakness as the result of decreased food intake. We know enough now to prescribe a healthy diet for patients with a treated primary cancer. We need more information on adjuvant nutrition during cancer treatment.

This book is only a beginning. This work will need to be carried on by the young researchers and clinicians reading this book. It is our profound hope that this is the beginning of the new, exciting, and promising field of nutritional oncology.

Index

Page numbers followed by b *indicate boxes;* f, *figures;* t, *tables.*

Copyright © 2006, Elsevier Inc.
All rights of reproduction in any form reserved.

C

E

H

I

K

L

M

N

Q

R

S

T

U

V

W

X

Lightning Source UK Ltd.
Milton Keynes UK
UKOW06n0201171114

241674UK00022B/193/P